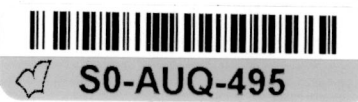

OCCUPATIONAL MEDICINE

Principles and Practical Applications

Second Edition

Occupational Medicine

PRINCIPLES AND PRACTICAL APPLICATIONS

Second Edition

Carl Zenz, M.D., Sc.D.

Consultant in Occupational Medicine
Clinical Professor
University of Wisconsin
Madison, Wisconsin
Medical College of Wisconsin
Milwaukee, Wisconsin
Professor, School of Public Health
University of Illinois
Chicago, Illinois

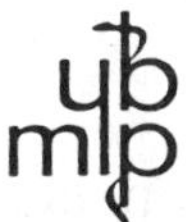

YEAR BOOK MEDICAL PUBLISHERS, INC.
Chicago • London • Boca Raton

2 3 4 5 6 7 8 9 0 KC 92 91 90 89 88

Library of Congress Cataloging-in-Publication Data

Occupational medicine.

Includes bibliographies and index.
1. Medicine, Industrial. I. Zenz, Carl, 1923-
[DNLM: 1. Occupational Diseases. 2. Occupational Health Services. 3. Occupational Medicine.
WA 400 015]
RC963.023 1988 616.9′803 86-24598
ISBN 0-8151-9865-5

Sponsoring Editor: James D. Ryan, Jr./Kevin M. Kelly
Assistant Director, Manuscript Services: Frances M. Perveiler
Production Project Manager: Carol A. Reynolds
Proofroom Supervisor: Shirley E. Taylor

Contributors

ANTERO AITIO, M.D., PH.D.
Professor and Director
Department of Hygiene and Toxicology
Institute of Occupational Health
Helsinki, Finland

ROLF ALEXANDERSSON, M.D.
Associate Professor
Department of Occupational Medicine
Karolinska Hospital
Stockholm, Sweden

OLAV AXELSON, M.D.
Professor, Department of Occupational Medicine and Industrial Ergonomics
University Hospital
Linköping University
Linköping, Sweden

WALTER E. BAKER, PH.D.
Senior VDT Ergonomics Advisor
IBM Corporation
Purchase, New York

MARIO C. BATTIGELLI, M.D., M.P.H.
Director, Rocky Mountain Center for Occupational and Environmental Health
Department of Family and Community Medicine
The University of Utah
Salt Lake City, Utah
Formerly Professor of Medicine and Professor of Public Health
School of Public Health
The University of North Carolina School of Medicine
Chapel Hill, North Carolina

JAMES J. BEAUMONT, PH.D.
Associate Director
Occupational and Environmental Health Unit
University of California
Davis, California

LOUIS S. BELICZKY, M.S., M.P.H.
Director of Industrial Hygiene
United Rubber Workers International
Akron, Ohio

THOMAS BERGGREN, PH.D.
Associate Professor
University of Örebro
Örebro, Sweden

MARCUS B. BOND, M.D.
Consultant in Occupational Medicine
Clinical Professor
Department of Preventive Medicine Biostatistics
University of Colorado Health Sciences Center
Denver, Colorado
Formerly Medical Director
American Telephone & Telegraph Company
Basking Ridge, New Jersey

DUDLEY BRIGGS, M.D.
Consultant in Occupational Medicine
Clinical Assistant Professor
Preventive Medicine
Ohio State University College of Medicine
Physician Advisor for Mount Carmel Hospitals
Columbus, Ohio
Formerly Medical Director
AT&T Network Systems
Columbus, Ohio

DON B. CHAFFIN, PH.D.
Professor, Industrial and Operational Engineering
University of Michigan
Ann Arbor, Michigan

JEFFREY E. COE, M.D.
Liberty Mutual Company
Chicago, Illinois
Formerly Medical Director
Chicago District
LTV Steel
Chicago, Illinois

EDWARD M. CORDASCO, M.D.
Director, Occupational Chest Clinic
Cleveland Clinic Foundation
Cleveland, Ohio

RICHARD J. COSTELLO, P.F., C.I.H.
Industrial Hygienist
Industrywide Studies Branch
Division of Surveillance, Hazard Evaluations and Field Studies
National Institute for Occupational Safety and Health
Cincinnati, Ohio

DAVID L. DAHLSTROM, B.S., M.S.
Associate and Principal-in-Charge of Industrial Hygiene and Occupational Health Programs
Danes and Moore, Ltd.
Atlanta, Georgia
Formerly Corporate Director of Industrial Hygiene
Ecology and Environment, Inc.
Buffalo, New York

JOE A. DELEON, M.D., P.A.
University of Texas Health Science Center at Houston
School of Public Health
Houston, Texas

STEPHEN L. DEMETER, M.D.
Associate Professor of Medicine
Head of the Pulmonary Division
Northeastern Ohio Universities College of Medicine
Akron, Ohio

ROBERT T.P. DETREVILLE, M.D., SC.D.
Colonel, M.C.
United States Air Force (retired)
San Antonio, Texas

O. BRUCE DICKERSON, M.D., M.P.H.
Corporate Director of Health and Safety
IBM Corporation
White Plains, New York

VERNON N. DODSON, M.D.
Professor of Medicine and Preventive Medicine
University of Wisconsin
Madison, Wisconsin

KELLEY J. DONHAM, M.S., D.V.M.
Professor, Institute of Agricultural Medicine and Occupational Health
University of Iowa College of Medicine
Department of Preventive Medicine and Environmental Health
Oakdale, Iowa

ROBERT B. DOUGLAS, PH.D.
Senior Lecturer in Applied Physiology
Department of Occupational Health
London School of Hygiene and Tropical Medicine
London, England

FLORENCE EBERT, R.N., C.O.H.N.
Occupational Health Nurse Consultant
Compliance Consultants, Inc.
Chicago, Illinois

CHRISTER EDLING, M.D.
Department of Occupational Medicine
University of Uppsala
Uppsala, Sweden

DAVID EGILMAN, M.D., M.P.H.
Medical Director
Greater Cincinnati Occupational Health Center
Providence Hospital
Cincinnati, Ohio

KERSTIN EKBERG, PH.D.
Clinical Psychologist
Department of Occupational Medicine
University Hospital
Linköping, Sweden

JOHN M. FAJEN, M.S.
Industrial Hygiene
Industrywide Studies Branch
Division of Surveillance, Hazard Evaluations and Field Studies
National Institute for Occupational Safety and Health
Cincinnati, Ohio

MARILYN A. FINGERHUT, PH.D.
Chief, Epidemiology Section II
Industrywide Studies Branch
Division of Hazard Evaluations and Field Studies
National Institute for Occupational Safety and Health
Cincinnati, Ohio

JORDAN N. FINK, M.D.
Professor of Medicine
Chief of Allergy Division
Medical College of Wisconsin
Milwaukee, Wisconsin

William E. Halperin, M.D., M.P.H.
Chief, Industrywide Studies Branch
Division of Surveillance, Hazard Evaluations and Field Studies
National Institute for Occupational Safety and Health
Cincinnati, Ohio

Monica Hane, Ph.D.
Director, Foundation for Occupational Health Research and Development
Department of Occupational Medicine
Medical Center Hospital
Örebro, Sweden

Jan-Erik Hansson
Ergonomist, Director of Unit of Technical Work Physiology
National Institute of Occupational Health
Solna, Sweden

Raymond D. Harbison, Ph.D.
Professor and Director
Division of Interdisciplinary Toxicology
University of Arkansas for Medical Sciences
Little Rock, Arkansas

Sven Hernberg, M.D., Ph.D.
Director, Department of Epidemiology and Biometry
Scientific Director and Professor
Institute of Occupational Health
Helsinki, Finland

Bruce Hills, M.S.
Industrial Hygienist
Industrywide Studies Branch
Division of Surveillance, Hazard Evaluations and Field Studies
National Institute for Occupational Safety and Health
Cincinnati, Ohio

Christer Hogstedt, M.D.
Professor, Department of Occupational Medicine
Karolinska Hospital
Department of Occupational Medicine
National Institute of Occupational Health
Stockholm, Sweden

Edward P. Horvath, Jr., M.D., M.P.H.
Medical Director
BP America (Formerly The Standard Oil Company)
Cleveland, Ohio
Formerly Section Chief, Occupational Medicine
The Marshfield Clinic
Medical Director
National Farm Medical Center
Marshfield, Wisconsin

Harold R. Imbus, M.D., Sc.D.
Health and Hygiene, Inc.
Greensboro, North Carolina
Formerly Medical Director
Burlington Industries
Greensboro, North Carolina

Jorma Järvisalo, M.D., Ph.D.
Occupational Health Officer
WHO Regional Office for Europe
Copenhagen, Denmark

Julius Kerkay, Ph.D.
Professor of Chemistry and Biology
Cleveland State University
Cleveland, Ohio

A. Johann Kielblock, D.Sc.
Director, Industrial Hygiene Laboratory
Research Organization
Chamber of Mines of South Africa
Johannesburg, Republic of South Africa

D. Jack Kilian, M.D.
Professor of Occupational Medicine
University of Texas
School of Public Health
Houston, Texas

Eric P. Kindwall, M.D.
Director, Department of Hyperbaric Medicine
St. Luke's Hospital
Milwaukee, Wisconsin

Prof. Dr. Peter Knauth
Director, Department of Ergonomics
Institute of Industrial Production
University of Karlsruhe
Karlsruhe, West Germany

Arthur L. Knight, M.D.
Director of Health Services
Ingersoll-Rand Company
Phillipsburg, New Jersey

JON L. KONZEN, M.D.
Medical Director
Owens-Corning Fiberglas Corporation
Toledo, Ohio

JOSEPH LADOU, M.D.
Medical Director
Peninsula Industrial Medical Clinic
Sunnyvale, California
Associate Professor
University of California at San Francisco School of Medicine
San Francisco, California

SANFORD LEFFINGWELL, M.D., M.P.H.
Chief, Research Analysis Section
Priorities and Research Analysis Branch
Division of Standards Development and Technology Transfer
National Institute for Occupational Safety and Health
Cincinnati, Ohio

STUART A. LEVY, M.D.
Chairman, Section of Pulmonary Disease
St. Luke's Hospital
Milwaukee, Wisconsin

LARRY A. LINDESMITH, M.D.
Chief, Pulmonary Medicine
Gunderson Clinic
LaCrosse, Wisconsin

ERNEST MASTROMATTEO, M.D.
E.Mastromatteo Consultants, Inc.
Toronto, Canada
Formerly Director, Occupational Health
INCO Ltd.
Toronto, Canada

C. G. TOBY MATHIAS, M.D.
Chief of Dermatology
Industrywide Studies Branch
Division of Surveillance, Hazard Evaluations and Field Studies
National Institute for Occupational Safety and Health
Cincinnati, Ohio
Formerly Associate Professor
Division of Dermatology
University of California at San Francisco School of Medicine
San Francisco, California

WILLIAM B. MCCLELLAN, M.D.
Clinical Professor
Graduate School of Public Health
University of Pittsburgh
Department of Industrial Environmental Health Services
Pittsburgh, Pennsylvania

GEOFFREY B. MEESE, B.SC., M.SC., PH.D.
Environmental Engineering Division
National Building Research Institute
Council for Scientific and Industrial Research
Pretoria, Republic of South Africa

THEODORE J. MEINHARDT, PH.D.
Epidemiologist, Division of Standards Development and Technology Transfer
National Institute for Occupational Safety and Health
Cincinnati, Ohio

JAMES M. MELIUS, M.D., DR.P.H.
Division of Environmental Health Assessment
New York State Department of Health
Albany, New York

JACQUELINE MESSITE, M.D.
Executive Secretary of the Committee of Public Health
New York Academy of Medicine
Formerly Regional Program Consultant
National Institute for Occupational Safety and Health in Region II
New York, New York

JOHANN T. METS, M.D.
Senior Specialist
Community Health
Senior Lecturer
Occupational Health
University of Cape Town
Republic of South Africa

DANA B. MIRKIN, M.D.
Regional Medical Director
BP of America
Lima, Ohio

PATRICIA L. MOODY, M.D., M.P.H.
Medical Officer
Industrywide Studies Branch
Division of Surveillance, Hazard Evaluations and Field Studies
National Institutes for Occupational Safety and Health
Cincinnati, Ohio

J. Steven Moore, M.D., C.I.H.
Medical-Surgical Clinic of Milwaukee
Assistant Clinical Professor
Medical College of Wisconsin
Milwaukee, Wisconsin

Leela I. Murthy, Ph.D.
Medical Officer
Industrywide Studies Branch
Division of Surveillance, Hazard Evaluations and Field Studies
National Institute for Occupational Safety and Health
Cincinnati, Ohio

Julian B. Olishifski, P.E., C.S.P.
Industrial Hygienist (retired)
Alliance of American Insurers
Chicago, Illinois
Formerly Director, Industrial Hygiene
National Safety Council
Adjunct Assistant Professor of Occupational and Environmental Medicine
University of Illinois
Chicago, Illinois

Karl K. Pearson, Ph.D.
Professor of Analytical Chemistry
Cleveland State University
Cleveland, Ohio

Otto P. Preuss, M.D.
Corporate Medical Director (Retired)
Brush Wellman, Inc.
Cleveland, Ohio

Jennifer M. Ratcliffe, Ph.D., M.Sc.
Epidemiologist, Industrywide Studies Branch
Division of Surveillance, Hazard Evaluations and Field Studies
National Institute for Occupational Safety and Health
Cincinnati, Ohio

Gordon R. Reeve, Ph.D.
Assistant Chief
Epidemiology Section II
Industrywide Studies Branch
Division of Surveillance, Hazard Evaluations and Field Studies
National Institute for Occupational Safety and Health
Cincinnati, Ohio

Vesa Riihimäki, M.D., Ph.D.
Deputy Director
Department of Occupational Hygiene and Toxicology
Institute of Occupational Health
Helsinki, Finland

Donald M. Rowe, M.D.
Director, Medical Services
Kohler Company
Kohler, Wisconsin

Joseph Rutenfranz, M.D., Ph.D.
Professor, Dr. Dr.
Institute für Arbeitsphysiologie an der Universität Dortmund
Dortmund, West Germany

Howard J. Sawyer, M.D.
Director, Occupational, Environment and Preventive Medicine
Henry Ford Hospital
Detroit, Michigan
Adjunct Associate Professor
Occupational and Environmental Health
Wayne State University
Detroit, Michigan
Lecturer, School of Public Health
University of Michigan
Ann Arbor, Michigan

Teresa Schnorr, Ph.D.
Epidemiologist, Industrywide Studies Branch
Division of Surveillance, Hazard Evaluations and Field Studies
National Institute for Occupational Safety and Health
Cincinnati, Ohio

Petrus C. Schutte, M.Sc.
Chief, Physiological Stress Division
Industrial Hygiene Laboratory
Research Organization
Chamber of Mines of South Africa
Johannesburg, Republic of South Africa

Anna Marie Seppäläinen, M.D.
Department of Neurology
University of Helsinki
Helsinki, Finland

Bengt Sjögren, M.D.
Department of Occupational Medicine
National Institute of Occupational Safety and Health
Solna, Sweden

Alexander Blair Smith, M.D., M.S.
Chief, Medical Section
Hazard Evaluations and Technical Assistance Branch
National Institute for Occupational Safety and Health
Cincinnati, Ohio

Thomas H. F. Smith, Ph.D.
Corporate Toxicologist
Corporate Health and Safety
IBM Corporation
Purchase, New York

Joseph A. Solomayer, M.D., Sc.D.
Department of Occupational Medicine
Northeastern Ohio Universities College of Medicine
Rootstown, Ohio
Formerly Medical Director
Terex Division of General Motors Corporation
Hudson, Ohio

Marja Sorsa, Ph.D.
Research Professor
Institute of Occupational Health
Helsinki, Finland

Leslie Stayner, M.S.
Epidemiologist, Industrywide Studies Branch
Division of Surveillance, Hazard Evaluations and Field Studies
National Institute for Occupational Safety and Health
Cincinnati, Ohio

Kyle Steenland, Ph.D.
Epidemiologist, Industrywide Studies Branch
Division of Surveillance, Hazard Evaluations and Field Studies
National Institute of Occupational Safety and Health
Cincinnati, Ohio

Frank B. Stern, M.S.
Epidemiologist, Industrywide Studies Branch
Division of Surveillance, Hazard Evaluations and Field Studies
National Institute for Occupational Safety and Health
Cincinnati, Ohio

Shiro Tanaka, M.D., M.S.
Medical Officer
Industrywide Studies Branch
Division of Surveillance, Hazard Evaluations and Field Studies
National Institute for Occupational Safety and Health
Cincinnati, Ohio

William Taylor, M.D., D.Sc.
Professor (Emeritus)
University of Dundee
Dundee, Scotland

Hans J. van der Merwe, M.B., Ch.B., D.O.H., D.T.M.&H., D.P.H.
Company Medical Officer
AECI Chlor-Alkali and Plastics Limited
Sasolburg, Republic of South Africa

George L. Voelz, M.D.
Medical Advisor for Occupational Medicine
Los Alamos National Laboratory
Los Alamos, New Mexico

Bryant W. Walker, C.S.P.
Director, Safety and Loss Prevention
Automotive Coatings
PPG Industries, Inc.
Cleveland, Ohio

Elizabeth Ward, M.S., Ph.D.
Epidemiologist, Industrywide Studies Branch
Division of Surveillance, Hazard Evaluation and Field Studies
National Institute for Occupational Safety and Health
Cincinnati, Ohio

Donald E. Wasserman, M.S.E.E.
Director, Human Vibration Engineering
Anatrol Corporation
Noise and Vibration Consultants
Cincinnati, Ohio
Formerly Chief of Occupational Noise and Vibration
National Institute of Occupational Safety and Health
Cincinnati, Ohio

Eugene S. Welter, M.D.
Medical Director
The Business and Industrial Health Group
Kansas City, Missouri

Robert H. Wheater, M.S.
Assistant Director
Environmental and Occupational Health Program
American Medical Association
Chicago, Illinois

Ralph P. White, Jr., M.D.
Assistant Clinical Professor of Medicine
Northeastern Ohio University
Rootstown, Ohio

M. Donald Whorton, M.D., M.P.H.
Environmental Health Associates, Inc.
Oakland, California

Carl Zenz, M.D., Sc.D.
Consultant in Occupational Medicine
Clinical Professor
University of Wisconsin
Madison, Wisconsin
Medical College of Wisconsin
Milwaukee, Wisconsin
Professor, School of Public Health
University of Illinois
Chicago, Illinois

R. L. Zielhuis, M.D., Ph.D.
Professor, Medical Faculty (Retired)
Director, Coronel Laboratories
University of Amsterdam
The Netherlands

Foreword to the First Edition

No specialty in medicine is greater than the scientific literature that it creates. No physician is greater than his degree of familiarity with the literature provided by his field of activities.

These statements are strikingly true for occupational medicine, for the pace of that specialty is the pace of industry itself. Occupational medicine did not set that pace. It was forced to conform to it. The creations of this present culture of industry are prodigious. At every sunrise, the occupational physician wakes up to a different world of obligations and opportunities.

Occupational medicine yearly contributes more medical newness than any other specialty. It is within reason to believe that yearly at least 200 medical entities appear, all unknown the year before. All this is akin to the plight of Dukas' "Sorcerer's Apprentice." For every situation solved, ten new ones arise. All is kaleidoscopic—all is bewildering. Whether all this is boon or bane is moot.

It takes a brave physician to be willing to enter occupational medicine. It takes even greater bravery for any group of editors and authors to be willing to attempt to reduce to orderliness the endless medical impositions—all unwillingly and unwittingly created by industry. The boldness of the editor and the contributors to this volume is more than adequate to the staggering tasks assumed, knowing that as they toiled, new newness soon would erase some of their accomplishments. As ever, that is progress.

This book, like every good book, is a miniature garden of greenery and brightness. All that goes on in a garden is a chain reaction. This book, too, is a chain reaction, promising to provide betterment for those who perpetuate this amazing industrial culture.

Carey P. McCord, M.D.
(1886–1979)
Professor Emeritus
University of Michigan
Ann Arbor, Michigan

Preface to the First Edition

Marked progress has occurred in occupational health during the past three decades, and occupational medicine has become a specialty in its own right, occupying a position with aerospace medicine and public health under the American Board of Preventive Medicine since 1955. Based on preventive medicine, the broad purpose of occupational medicine is the promotion and maintenance of the physical and mental health of persons at work. In 1950, the World Health Organization defined occupational health as follows:

> Occupational health should aim at: the promotion and maintenance of the highest degree of physical, mental and social well-being of workers in all occupations; the prevention among workers of departures from health caused by their working conditions; the protection of workers in their employment from risks resulting from factors adverse to health; the placing and maintenance of the worker in an occupational environment adapted to his physiological and psychological equipment; and, to summarize: the adaptation of work to man and of each man to his job.

This is the era of environmental awareness. Environmental influences on the health of workers have encouraged the growth of industrial hygiene and industrial hygiene engineering as specialties concerned with solving industrial health problems by recognizing, evaluating and controlling potential health hazards in the occupational environment.

The enactment of the Williams-Steiger Occupational Safety and Health Act of 1970 (OSHA) has generated tremendous interest in the development of occupational health programs. Covering more than 57 million workers in the United States, the law will involve almost all physicians, medical students, nurses, practicing physicians and management. Therefore, personnel concerned with health and safety must be knowledgeable in new requirements, criteria and standards to meet the need for preventing occupational diseases. The National Institute for Occupational Safety and Health (NIOSH) is charged with the collection of data, review and consultation to formalize development of criteria on which standards can be established to protect the health of workers from exposure to hazards of chemical and physical agents. Relevant data are made available for use "by the Secretary of the Department of Health, Education, and Welfare . . . on the basis of such research, demonstration, and experiments and any other information available to him . . . to effectuate the purposes of this Act . . . by providing medical criteria which will assure insofar as practicable that no employee will suffer diminished health, functional capacity, or life expectancy as a result of his work experience. . . ."

This volume, therefore, is intended to provide basic information to aid in meeting the challenges for new knowledge and requirements for the protection of all workers while still retaining the traditional concepts dealing with occupational disease and trauma. In addition to the occupational environmental factors, occupational health now includes the physiologic and psychologic adaptations of man to work. This shift in emphasis calls for methods devised to improve relationships with workers, labor groups, management and government at all levels.

This book is arranged into major sections consisting of important administrative factors, clinical occupational medicine, the physical occupational environment, the chemical occupational environment and behavioral or psychosocial considerations.

The major goal is to acquaint practicing physicians with the basic operations of various occupational medical departments, including growing employee health services in hospitals with their 1.5 million workers, relationships to the community practice of medicine, an outline of certain administrative functions and some fundamentals of Workmen's Compensation. Teamwork among physicians, nurses, industrial hygienists, psychologists and engineers is highlighted. For the first time, a book on occupational medicine describes the engineering and biomechanics of manual materials handling and low back pain. Biomechanics and ergonomics are assuming greater roles in consideration of placement of workers, assessment of fatigue and repeated low-level physical stresses, which deserve greater awareness among occupational health personnel, and special chapters are devoted to these areas of concern. The sections on work physiology and ergonomics include practical methods to determine physical working capacity and energy expenditure in relationship to certain environmental factors such as effects of prolonged and intermittent heavy work, heat stress, cold, vibration, noise and conditions such as hypobaric and hyperbaric pressures. Occupational exposure to noise presents far-reaching implications requiring physicians and management to become more knowledgeable in the conservation of hearing, both at the work site and in the community, and an in-depth chapter deals with this topic.

With diminishing natural resources from the geographically conventional sources, man will be forced to seek the unexplored reservoirs of oil and mineral wealth in the depths of the oceans under hostile conditions. Therefore, medical aspects of commercial diving and compressed air and work under low temperatures are discussed in considerable detail.

It is not the intent to describe in detail all substances encountered in every work place or occupation. Those ubiquitous and potentially troublesome materials in various work places are comprehensively discussed such as lead, beryllium, cadmium, mercury, certain other important metals and their compounds, toxic substances such as carbon monoxide, other hazardous chemicals and some of the most commonly used solvents.

ACKNOWLEDGMENTS

I wish to thank friends and colleagues throughout the world for their stimulating discussions and for arranging visits to institutes, factories and mines. Appreciation for guidance is given to Jay P. Bartlett, M.D., San Francisco, California; Gerald W. Grawey, M.D., Peoria, Illinois; Robert A. Kehoe, M.D., Cincinnati, Ohio; Mr. Walter M. Tammi, Milwaukee, Wisconsin; Norman Williams, M.D., Philadelphia, Pennsylvania; Peter Wolkonsky, M.D., Chicago, Illinois; C. Craig Wright, M.D., Rochester, New York; and my wife, Lillian S. Nelson, M.D. Special thanks to Mrs. Eleanor Sperry, Librarian, St. Luke's Hospital of Milwaukee, for her valuable assistance.

Especially, I extend my gratitude to the management of Allis-Chalmers Corporation for their enthusiastic support.

Carl Zenz, M.D., Sc.D.

Preface to the Second Edition

Occupational Medicine: Principles and Practical Applications, published in 1975, an internationally recognized reference work, is now combined with *Developments in Occupational Medicine*, published in 1980. The previous, practical organizational format has been followed, consisting of eight major sections: Administrative, Clinical Occupational Medicine, Occupational Pulmonary Diseases, The Physical Occupational Environment, The Chemical Occupational Environment, Selected Work Categories of Concern, Psychosocial Considerations, and Epidemiology: Principles and Practical Examples. Ninety-five authoritative and experienced contributors have meticulously prepared revised and expanded chapters, most completely rewritten; 26 contributors are from other countries, conferring a global perspective to this book. Important new chapters containing new subject matter and latest concepts are included, many for the first time in an occupational medical text: Biologic Monitoring, Occupational Neurotoxicology, Occupational Genotoxicology, Ocular Responses to Chemical and Physical Injury, Effects of Gases and Particles in Welding and Soldering, Hazardous Waste Sites, The Effects of Moderate Thermal Stress on Comfort and Productivity, An Ergonomic Checklist for Industrial Trucks, Investigating Environmental Health Hazards, Firefighters, Agricultural Occupational Medicine, and The Role of the Primary Care Physician in Occupational Medicine.

With expanding uses of new materials found in adhesives, coatings (paints and finishes), a multitude of plastics and other synthetic entities, more workers are potentially exposed, at various levels of risk, often unintentionally. Those concerned with occupational health practices (preventive programs) should and must be aware of the more commonly encountered substances and have some knowledge of what is going on in factories in their communities. The immense quantities of certain hazardous materials used are awesome. Indeed, some chemicals being produced and used for primary and other processes range into and beyond millions to billions of kilograms each year. In the smaller workshops particularly, points of concern may be found in processing and formulating, packaging, storage, shipping, reformulating, applications, maintenance work, laboratory testing, etc. Often overlooked is that these varied activities occur over widely scattered geographic areas and mainly involve small numbers of groups of workers. Despite technological advances, excessive occupational exposures continue to occur. Even today, well-known and heavily used or produced substances, i.e., acids and caustics, benzene, carbon monoxide, ethylene oxide, formaldehyde, hydrogen sulfide, numerous solvents, and other by-products still cause sickness; even radon, long recognized as naturally occurring, has gained prominent concern.

Industrial activities and productivity are steadily increasing in all countries, often accompanied with untold quantities of potentially hazardous and toxic materials present in agriculture, homes, manufacturing, mining, transport, storage, product use and ultimate disposal, at times leading to contamination of workplaces and the surrounding environment.

Although most countries and their jurisdictional areas do not have central registers for occupational exposure data collection, increasingly, news media report industrial accident exposure details and only a few recent events are mentioned for emphasis: "Findings of toxic leakage in Silicon Valley" (California, 1984); "ammonia-line rupture injures 25" (a slaughter house in Texas, 1986); "Fumes sicken 30 workers at landfill" (carbon dioxide and methane, Staten Island, New York, 1986); "100 flee tanker spill of aniline" (Maryland, 1986); "Radioactive gas leaks for 7 days" (uranium hexafluoride, Ohio, 1986); "Chemical accident in uranium processing plant contaminates plant and surrounding community" (Oklahoma, hydrofluoric acid and uranium hexafluoride, 1986); "Chemical plant warehouse fire results in massive spill of pesticides, mercury, solvents, coloring agents, emulsifiers and other chemicals, resulting in severe pollution of the Rhine River and grave damage to the river's ecosystem" (Switzerland, 1986).

These critical but limited examples are overshadowed by other disastrous and deadly accidents in India (massive community contamination by methyl isocyanate, 1984); the Soviet Union (nuclear power plant explosion, 1986), and the natural eruption of heavy amounts of toxic gases in West Africa in 1986, inducing illnesses and deaths of catastrophic scope. To understand and cope with these unfortunate occurrences, knowledge of occupational medicine can be indispensable. This book offers clarification and guidance for those concerned with these and other perplexing aspects of the broad spectrum of occupational medicine.

Terms used to describe "exposure limits" and their applications are carefully discussed in the chapter Industrial Hygiene. The American Conference of Governmental Industrial Hygienists

(ACGIH) publishes annually the threshold limit values for chemical substances and physical agents in the working environment and also prepares and publishes at appropriate intervals documentation of these values, found in Appendix A. Clarification and use of the International System of Measurements (SI) with helpful conversion tables are given in Appendix B.

To further aid the reader, more than 400 illustrations and figures along with numerous tables and references are appropriately placed throughout the book.

CARL ZENZ, M.D., SC.D.

Acknowledgments

My deepest gratitude is given to the contributors for their cooperation and their devotion and for giving valuable time in preparation of this second edition, and chief credit goes to them. For support, advice, and other assistance I offer hearty thanks to Mrs. Thelma Aro, Helsinki, Finland; Harvey V. Davis, Ph.D., Chicago, Illinois; Mr. Bertil Delin, Stockholm, Sweden; Jean S. Felton, M.D., Irvine, California; Gideon Gerhardsson, Ph.D., Stockholm, Sweden; Roy L. Gibson, M.D., Pittsburgh, Pennsylvania; Gerald W. Grawey, M.D., Peoria, Illinois; Mr. William D. Kelley, Cincinnati, Ohio; Marcus M. Key, M.D., Houston, Texas; Mr. Jussi Lehti, Germantown, Wisconsin; Lillian S. Nelson, M.D., Milwaukee, Wisconsin; Mr. Roy Page-Shipp, Pretoria, Republic of South Africa; Yoshimichi Sakai, M.D., Tokyo, Japan; Mrs. Siv Söderlund, Stockholm, Sweden; Lennart Sundell, M.D., Örebro, Sweden; James S. Taylor, M.D., Cleveland, Ohio; Juan Antonio Legaspi Velasco, M.D., Mexico City, Mexico; John T. Wilson, Jr., M.D., Seattle, Washington; and Mrs. Magdalene Wos, medical librarian, and her staff, St. Luke's Hospital, Milwaukee, Wisconsin.

CARL ZENZ, M.D., SC.D.

Contents

PART I

Administrative and Clinical Aspects

1

Occupational Safety in Industry

Bryant W. Walker, C.S.P.

HISTORICAL PERSPECTIVE

Historically, occupational safety as a scientific discipline began to develop at the end of the nineteenth century as the industries in the United States and Europe began their steady climb to the "High-Tech Age" of today. The labor force at this time was subjected to working conditions never before confronted in the small craft shops that had preceded the industrial revolution. Then, the prevailing attitude in industry was "let the worker beware" of the risks that were encountered on the job. Production and output were the primary concerns, not employee safety. It wasn't until 1867 that various factions in society began to notice the losses associated with industrial accidents. Studies were conducted and workers' compensation laws were drafted to provide some measure of protection for workers. Labor unions began to organize in an effort to change industry labor practices and correct job hazards. Industry also began to review the safety and health problems that were causing so much concern. Although there was only a limited amount of safety research available, businesses began providing engineering changes, along with various forms of safety programs that dealt with accident prevention.[20] Safety practitioners were employed to begin a new field of science by studying job environments, defining the causes of accidental injuries, and developing methods to control them.[26]

Safety occupations in the early stages of development were filled by the most available or most qualified individuals who could define the causes and reduce the occurrence of occupational injuries. Many of these individuals had additional responsibilities to occupy their time, which limited their availability for accident prevention activities. Knowledge of accident prevention was also limited, since the field of study was so new to everyone concerned. Most published information came from European practitioners. The American Society of Safety Engineers was founded in 1911 by a group of individuals from New York City insurance associations.[8] The lack of knowledge in the field of safety also gave rise to the First Cooperative Safety Congress, which met in Milwaukee, Wisconsin, in 1912. The Milwaukee Safety Congress began an organized movement to eliminate accidents in the workplace. It later gave birth to the National Safety Council, which continues today to offer assistance to industry and the general public from its headquarters in Chicago, Illinois. Other organizations concerned with worker health and safety, such as the American Occupational Medical Association, chartered in 1916, began to appear between 1900 and 1920.[26] In the 1920s, organized safety programs increased in the larger industries as new technology, such as special respirators contributed by World War I, became available for worker protection.[12]

The newly established National Safety Council began to collect data on the frequency of deaths that occurred in industry, providing an accurate measure of the seriousness of the problem. Frequency rates were developed by comparing the number of deaths to the total population or the population of workers. In 1912, the frequency rate was estimated to be 21 deaths for every 100,000 persons in the United States. In 1933, the frequency rate was 37 deaths for every 100,000 workers and 11.6 deaths per 100,000 population. The latest figures from the 1984 edition of *Accident Facts*, published by the National Safety Council, indicates a frequency of 11 deaths for every 100,000 workers and 4.8 deaths per 100,000 population in 1983. In addition to the deaths in 1983, there were 1.9 million disabling injuries, which caused a loss of 40 million work days. The National Safety Council estimated the cost of the losses in 1983 at $33.4 billion. These figures for the past and the present graphically illustrate the cause for concern and the need for successful safety and health programs in industry.

As interest in safety programs progressed through the years, specialized fields of study emerged to cover the rapidly expanding knowledge devoted to industrial safety and health. The study of occupational safety, having already branched into the two distinct fields of safety engineering and industrial hygiene, was making rapid progress toward addressing the safety concerns of industry and the public. Both fields of study were unique but had the same objective of providing a safe and healthful working environment in industry. The outcome of this split allowed each profession to devote more time to its specialty areas and to introduce new methods to make the workplace safer. Other professions also developed as the fields of study expanded into distinct disciplines in the interest of safety and health: environmental engineers, product safety engineers, fire protection engineers, and various plant engineering specialists. These related professionals working together with occupational health professionals are referred to as the "safety and health team." Since no single profession can resolve all safety and health issues, the team concept is employed to solve problems collectively and meet the challenges of the future.

OCCUPATIONAL SAFETY AND HEALTH TEAM

The safety and health team must be recognized as an integral part of any business organization, requiring financing and staffing proportional to the size of the business or the degree of hazard associated with the specific business operation. A good safety and health program should begin with a minimum staff consisting of a safety specialist and a consulting occupational health professional. As the size of the organization increases, the size of the safety and health team must also increase if successful program results are expected. Although many owners of small businesses may not find it feasible to hire their own professionals, they can consider one or more of the consulting specialists that abound today. Most government agencies offer safety and health consulting services to businesses that need assistance. The Occupational Safety and Health Administration (OSHA), under the Department of Labor, a cabinet of the U.S. government, offers a consultation service to interested businesses. Various professional associations, such as the National Safety Council, American Society of Safety Engineers, Industrial Health Foundation, American Industrial Hygiene Association, and others offer seminars or courses that provide information on safety and health activities.[22] With the availability of information today, every business can have an appropriate program for protecting workers on the job. Even in small businesses, safety and health teams can be organized as management committees to evaluate and control safety and health concerns, and such a committee may consult with professionals to supplement, enhance, or guide their efforts. A physician can be employed, either individually or through a clinic, to provide information on matters pertinent to worker health. The physician can also be a useful consultant on safety and health needs by advising the committee on personal protective equipment requirements and hazard analysis and assist in the elimination of certain health concerns of the workers. Small businesses might develop their programs through other professional groups, such as "employee relations," "personnel," or "human resource specialists," using resources that are available today. Organizations that can employ safety and health teams should create a group similar to that shown on the organizational chart in Figure 1–1. The group can be modified according to the size and needs of the business organization but should maintain the basic reporting structure.

The duties of the various staff members noted may vary according to the different occupations employed or not employed. For example, if an industrial hygienist is not available on staff, the safety engineer may be assigned the role that would normally apply to a hygienist. An occupational health nurse may also be assigned

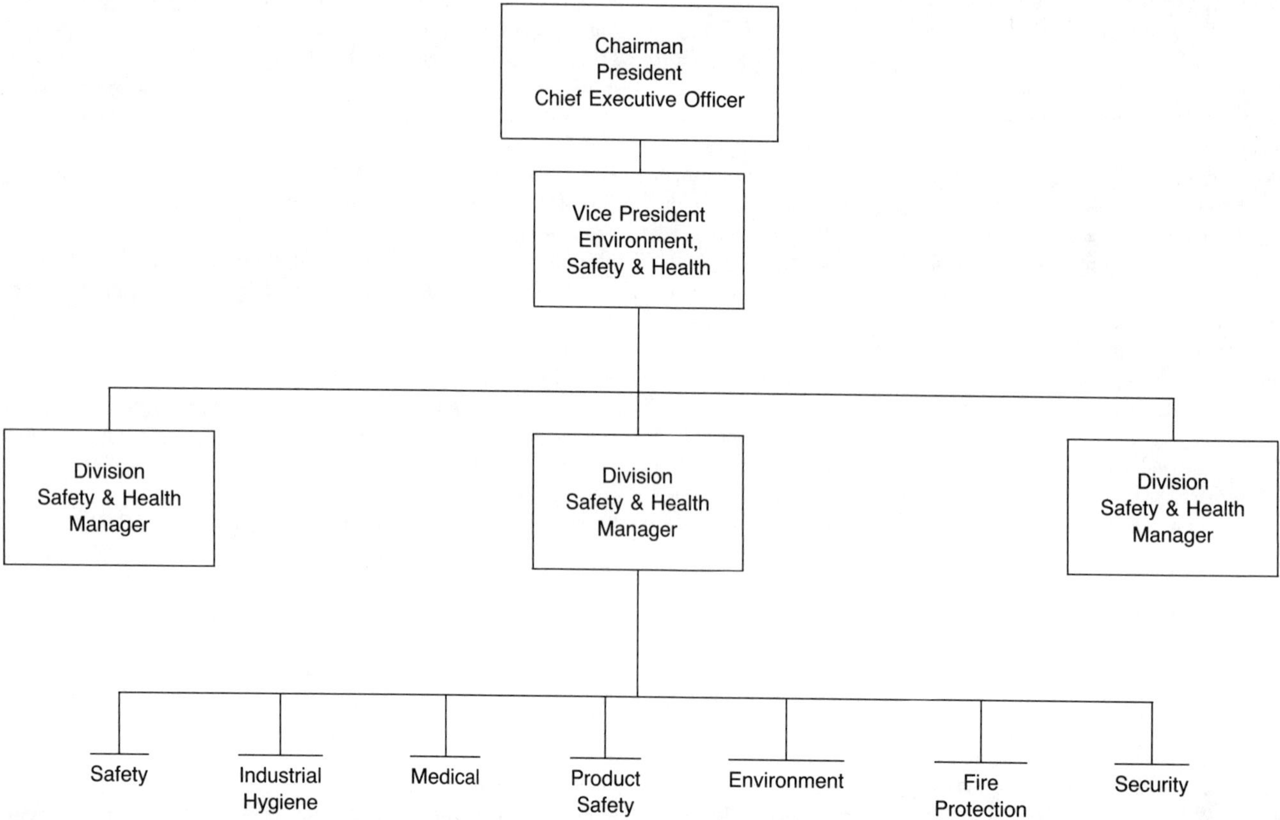

FIG 1–1.
Safety and health organizational chart.

the responsibility of the medical program, with assistance from a consulting physician or local occupational health clinic. In any case, a business will have to concern itself with all areas of occupational safety and health, regardless of the staff employed. The professional group shown in Figure 1–1 represents a well-rounded safety and health team that can eliminate or control most of the safety and health problems that may confront their organization.

In industries that employ professionals, safety engineering is the occupation found most often in individual operating units of a company.[25] This results from the educational development of safety engineers as general practitioners, similar to a general practitioner in the field of medicine. The safety engineer is normally responsible for the total occupational safety and health program at the plant level except in large operations, where industrial hygienists or other safety and health professionals share the responsibilities. The safety engineer will be occupied with various duties, such as fire protection programs, the safe design of equipment and work areas, safety and health training, monitoring environmental hazards, record keeping, and advising other members of management.

An occupational nurse may be the second professional selected for the team after the safety engineer. In some cases, a nurse may be the first team member when resources exclude the employment of a full-time safety engineer. In either case, the occupational nurse is an invaluable member of the team who can lend knowledge to controlling hazards as well as maintaining the health program. The nurse can advise management on health concerns, provide certain physical examination services, act as liaison with a consulting physician, develop information on suspected health problems, maintain accurate health records, and provide health training for employees, including management.

An industrial hygienist is another important member of the team due to a specialized knowledge base that overlaps into both safety engineering and health-related fields (for details, see Chapter 2). The hygienist can help manage environmental control measures, chemical exposure analyses and controls, ergonomics, employee health protection, chemical hazard evaluation, and health-related training.

The occupational physician is also a vital member of any safety and health team. A physician can provide evaluative health services and advise management on methods for maintaining a healthy work force. The physician can screen prospective workers, periodically review the physical condition of workers, evaluate the physiologic requirements of job tasks, and develop health consciousness among managers and the other workers.

As the organization increases in size or needs, it may require additional specialized team members, such as an environmental engineer, fire protection engineer, security specialist, human factors engineer, or others. A close working relationship between team members is essential to a successful organization, since these specialized occupations interface with each other often. The team has to work in unity to achieve the common goal of ensuring a safe and healthful working environment.[9, 2]

MANAGEMENT RESPONSIBILITY

Management must be committed to safety and health if the program is to be successful. This commitment can be confirmed by activity that shows a sincerity equal to that which is devoted toward production, quality, and cost control. When commitment is lacking, it may be more difficult to achieve safety and health goals. The commitment must extend from the top corporate level, beginning with the board of directors, down to line supervisors, to ensure total cooperation on issues relevant to safety and health. Numerous studies have shown that companies with a firm and active management commitment to safety and health have lower accident rates than companies without such a commitment.[3, 4] A policy statement should be issued at all levels of the organization to communicate this commitment effectively. The statement should clearly define management's commitment, the safety and health objectives, the methods of achieving the objectives, and the methods of measuring the success of the objectives.

Management must be committed to the safety and health team by including the team members in all decisions that may have an impact on their areas of responsibility.[28] Such decisions may involve the design or redesign of facilities and changes in production processes, equipment, products, or manpower. Safety and health decisions must begin with every management plan that will affect the workplace and the worker. One of the first steps in defining the scope of a new decision should be to define the risks to employees and available physical assets. The decision tree (Fig 1–2) can be used in the initial evaluation of any projected change that management may be considering. When evaluating the risk factors in a decision, all potential problems must be defined and quantified, since the elimination of such risks must be justified. The safety and health team can often save valuable time and expense in the decision process if they are included at the beginning of the planning stage. They can provide a clear understanding of the safety and health needs before the needs become apparent by way of worker encounters with unexpected hazards. Defining hazards before they become evident is not always an easy task, especially in the case of hazards that have not yet been recognized in the industry. The difficulty lies in the absence of physical or mathematical proof that a hazard may be expected to occur given the conditions of the decision.[24] Analytic tools available for evaluating risks, such as "fault tree analysis" and "systems safety analysis," may offer some assistance, but they are limited to hypothetical proof if no known events are available to establish the probability of expected events. Risk analysis is one area where professionals may have an advantage over nonprofessionals, due to their educational background and field experience. Having safety or health professionals on staff may not be a panacea for all such situations, but they can provide management with a definite edge in early recognition of problems that may be created as a result of business decisions. Eliminating hazards before they affect the environment in an undesirable manner is defined as prevention, and prevention will always be the key to successful safety and health programs.

Accident prevention decisions today cannot be confined to the traditional theory that attributes the cause of most accidents to "unsafe acts." Although many studies have concluded this by statistical analyses, including the Heinrich study,[13] these conclusions are based on the results of limited investigations that have not included a thorough review of the man-environment relationships. The conclusions were developed from an erroneous definition of the cause of accident as the action that created the last event which resulted in the injury. Additional causes, e.g., psychologic factors, inadequate training, inadequate communication of a safe procedure, or actions of other individuals, were not considered in

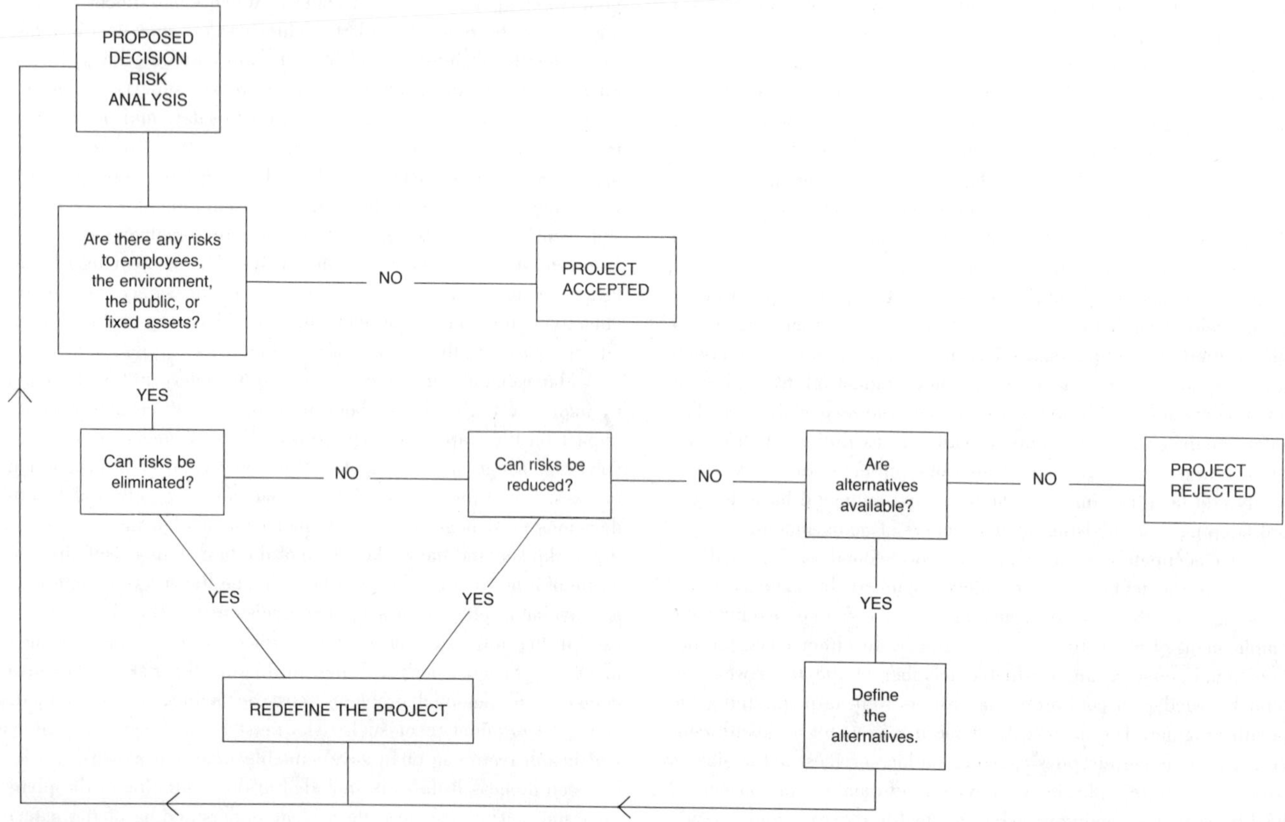

FIG 1–2.
Project risk-analysis decision tree.

the final analysis of the accident. Because of the nearsighted theory that 88% of all accidents are the direct result of an unsafe act committed by the injured person, many critical factors that could lead to a greater reduction in accidents are overlooked.[8] The final act at the time of the accident may be unsafe, but the individual may be predisposed to commit the action as a result of other factors influencing the judgment of the risk associated with the action.

Decisions made concerning accident prevention must consider systems methodology, which will include all influential factors concerning the worker. Risk analysis decisions must encompass the whole process of the worker-environment interface to uncover the potential risks that may surface when the decision becomes a reality.[18] Ergonomists or human factors engineers have long recognized the importance of this concept and have professed that safety practitioners are more effective if they design the environment to fit the worker instead of attempting to fit the worker to the environment. Any changes made to a worker's environment should include a psychophysical analysis of the human characteristics required to perform the job and an analysis of the job mechanics to define the best working relationship between the two. This approach does not exclude training or education to prepare workers for the designed tasks but integrates the worker and the task in such a manner that training becomes less complex.[18] The evaluations should also include a review of psychosocial factors, which play such a significant role in accidents that the World Health Organization convened a special meeting at Geneva in 1982 to discuss their impact.[29]

SAFETY AND HEALTH PROGRAMS

The structure of a safety and health program can vary considerably in industry, but successful programs contain several basic elements that contribute significantly to such successes.[3, 6] The elements are:

1. Management commitment
2. Facility and equipment design
3. Safety and health training and education
4. Safety and health inspection
5. Accident investigation
6. Health hazard evaluations

Management Commitment

Management commitment to safety and health programs has been discussed earlier in this chapter, but it cannot be overemphasized as a key element in any successful safety and health program. A lack of sincere commitment can impede accident prevention programs and delay expected reductions in the frequency of injuries in the workplace. A positive commitment by management is essential to the implementation of other elements in the safety and health program. Once management commitment has been established, the remaining elements of the program can be developed.

Facility and Equipment Design

The design of a manufacturing facility, equipment, process operation or any other part of the job environment should include a safety and health analysis. The expertise of the safety and health team can be employed to assist the design team with the analysis. A thorough analysis in the design stage can uncover hazards that may result from the human interaction with the designed environment. The analysis of the proposal can begin with the use of a decision process such as the one in Figure 1–2. The team performing the analysis can make good use of "Fault Tree" method of defining probable hazards and their causes. This process evaluates each part or subpart of the design in search of probable component failures that could lead to a system failure or accident with potential to cause injury or equipment damage. Progressing beyond the initial discovery of a hazard, the decision process should include a detailed study of the hazard with an objective of removing it from the environment or reducing its impact on the environment or the worker.

Any decision to provide the best method of dealing with a hazard should always include the following three principles of accident prevention, listed in their order of importance.

1. Eliminate the hazard.
2. Isolate the hazard from the worker.
3. Insulate the worker from the hazard.

The first and most important principle, elimination of the hazard, can best be accomplished in the design stage, when the hazard is normally created. If the hazard is already present in the workplace, it may be eliminated by redesigning the source of the hazard so that the exposure is removed. A simple example is the use of an air supply for breathing purposes that is separate from a general utility air supply. The initial cost will increase in proportion to the supply service needed, but the hazard of a worker breathing contaminated or oxygen deficient air will be eliminated. Another example may be the location of manually operated valves or equipment. Valves and equipment should be located for ease of access at the normal level of activity by the average size worker, or else a safe and reasonable means of access to a different level should be provided. In any case, the worker should not be required to devise his own method of access. Other methods of eliminating hazards from the workplace may include changing from the use of a toxic chemical to a nontoxic chemical in a process or formula, using electric vehicles in place of fuel-operated vehicles in a closed or confined area that lacks proper ventilation, or mechanically conveying heavy materials or objects in place of manual methods of conveyance. All hazards should be evaluated to determine if they can be eliminated before proceeding to the use of the next two principles.

Isolating the hazard from the worker is an acceptable method of protection when elimination of the hazard is not feasible. This method is often seen in the design of closed process systems or the use of closures which establish a barrier between the hazard and the worker. An example is the use of permanent connecting piping to transfer a liquid in a closed condition from one point to another rather than using a means of transfer that will expose the worker to the liquid. Barrier guarding such as closures around moving mechanical parts are effective isolating devices. Disconnect switches and pull-out devices, such as those used on power presses, can also be included in this approach. Ventilation systems used to capture and remove contaminants from the workers' breathing zone are excellent methods of isolating a hazard. Robotics or remote operating equipment are also popular methods of isolating the worker from the hazards when elimination is not feasible. This approach is gaining in popularity today due to the ease of removing the worker from jobs with inherent hazards that cannot be eliminated, such as repetitive motion operations or common metal-stamping operations.

The third principle applies to insulating the worker from the hazard by the use of personal protective equipment. Protective clothing or other insulating devices such as hearing protectors are an effective means of protecting workers from certain hazards, but the protection provided is only as good as the programs for selection, training, and enforcement. When used in accordance with recommended practices, which consider the limitations of the equipment and the person wearing the equipment, they can provide suitable protection when methods of elimination and isolation are not feasible. The key factor in the use of this principle is the proper selection of protective devices. The safety and health team or other competent individuals, such as the equipment manufacturer's representative, should select them.

Safety and Health Training and Education

When a hazard is still present in the workplace, the workers must be apprised of the hazard and the methods that will be used to protect them from the hazard. This means that training and education must be considered an integral part of the isolation and insulation principles of accident prevention. There are many commercial programs available today to meet most of the training needs in industry. Some of these programs can be purchased or rented from organizations specializing in safety and health. The following list does not include all organizations but will provide a good base for safety and health information.

National Safety Council
425 N. Michigan Ave.
Chicago, IL 60611

Industrial Health Foundation, Inc.
5231 Centre Ave.
Pittsburgh, PA 15232

American Society of Safety Engineers
850 Busse Hwy.
Park Ridge, IL 60068

American Industrial Hygiene Association
66 S. Miller Rd.
Akron, OH 44313

American Conference of Governmental Industrial Hygienists
P.O. Box 1937
Cincinnati, OH 45201

Occupational Safety and Health Administration (OSHA)
U.S. Department of Labor
Department of Labor Building
Washington, D.C. 20210

National Institute of Occupational Safety and Health (NIOSH)
U.S. Department of Health and Human Services
Centers for Disease Control
Robert A. Taft Laboratories
4676 Columbia Parkway
Cincinnati, OH 45226

There are many more organizations in the United States, serving the public and industry, that readily provide information on safety and health subjects to anyone upon request. Some written publications, training information, or programs may require a fee from the organization. The National Safety Council has compiled an excellent listing of information sources in its *Accident Prevention Manual for Industrial Operations,* dedicating a chapter to the subject.[22] Safety and health training needs should be integrated with job skills training to emphasize the importance of safety and health as a part of the job activities and not as a separate concern. Many of the commercial training programs can be supplemented with specific information related to the individual needs of the user to enhance the effectiveness of the training. Some businesses may want to develop their own program to ensure that a specific subject is addressed or that important procedures are included. Others may want to hire a professional training development company to create a special program. Regardless of the source, training and education is essential in influencing safe job performance where hazards are present in the occupational environment.

Training and education can be accomplished with various media, such as slides, recorded messages, movies, charts, video tapes, computer programs, or other audio-visual aids. The most effective medium will be the one that depicts the subject matter in the best manner while holding the attention of the audience. Selection of a trainer or teacher will be subject to organizational preference, but it should be someone with experience in training and who possesses sound knowledge of the subject. Line supervisors make good trainers, since they are close to the subject and have first-hand experience. The individual assigned to present the information should be familiar with the media being used and how to produce the best results from their use. Proper presentation of training and education programs can produce positive results, but the results may not last unless they are reinforced. Reinforcement can be accomplished in various ways, including repeating the training, providing written procedures or manuals, rewarding good behavior, or applying progressive discipline when undesirable behavior occurs.

Some training subjects are required by government regulations such as the federal Occupational Safety and Health Act and Resources Conservation and Recovery Act. Some of the requirements for hazardous materials standards, such as lead, vinyl chloride, and other specific chemicals, are normally well-defined, to ensure consistency in training all workers affected by the material. Although information about the handling of hazardous material is written in an outline format and not presented as a complete training program, this information can be used effectively in developing the required programs. The most comprehensive information and training requirements are the "employee right-to-know laws" enacted by several states and a similar amendment to the Occupational Safety and Health Act adopted by OSHA in 1984. The basic requirement of the OSHA standard is that industry must educate and train all workers on the hazards of all materials found in their work environment. The standards also provide for reinforcement of the information by requiring that all materials be identified with a label stating the hazards of the chemical and methods of protecting workers while handling the chemical. The standard also requires chemical producers to provide users with hazard information in the form of material safety data sheets on each chemical found in the workplace. Hazardous material labeling is the most difficult part of the standards for industry to comply with, since there are no current industry standards on the style of the label or the information presented on such labels. There are some standardized label formats available from various organizations and private industries, but no universal standard has been adopted for all applications.[10]

An excellent example of a hazardous materials information and training program is one developed by an industrial company that handles thousands of different chemicals in its operations as a coatings and resins manufacturer. The program has been adopted by the National Paint and Coatings Association as an industry standard. It contains the methods of identifying the health, flammability, and reactivity hazards of all chemicals, and a format for a label which defines the chemical, the hazard information, and the minimum personal protective equipment required. This system also includes a training program to inform the workers of the hazards.[16] The company industrial hygienists develop the information for the labels and publish a standard for all company locations to follow. The hygienists define the hazard for each of the three categories of health, flammability, and reactivity with a numerical rating on a scale of zero to four, zero being no significant hazard and four indicating a severe hazard. A label with such defined hazard ratings is shown in Figure 1–3. The personal protective equipment requirements are noted by a letter, shown in Figure 1–4, that can be displayed on a poster in the work areas.

Safety and Health Inspections

Safety and health inspections are control measures used to evaluate the effectiveness of established programs. Inspections can be conducted by one who knows the programs and their objectives. It is important to have an inspector who recognizes the value of the programs and the need for the inspections. Inspections should be designed to provide feedback which will serve as a measure of effectiveness. The inspection results may be recorded on a formal inspection document (safety and health checklist) or may be notes made by the inspector to be transcribed later into a more formal

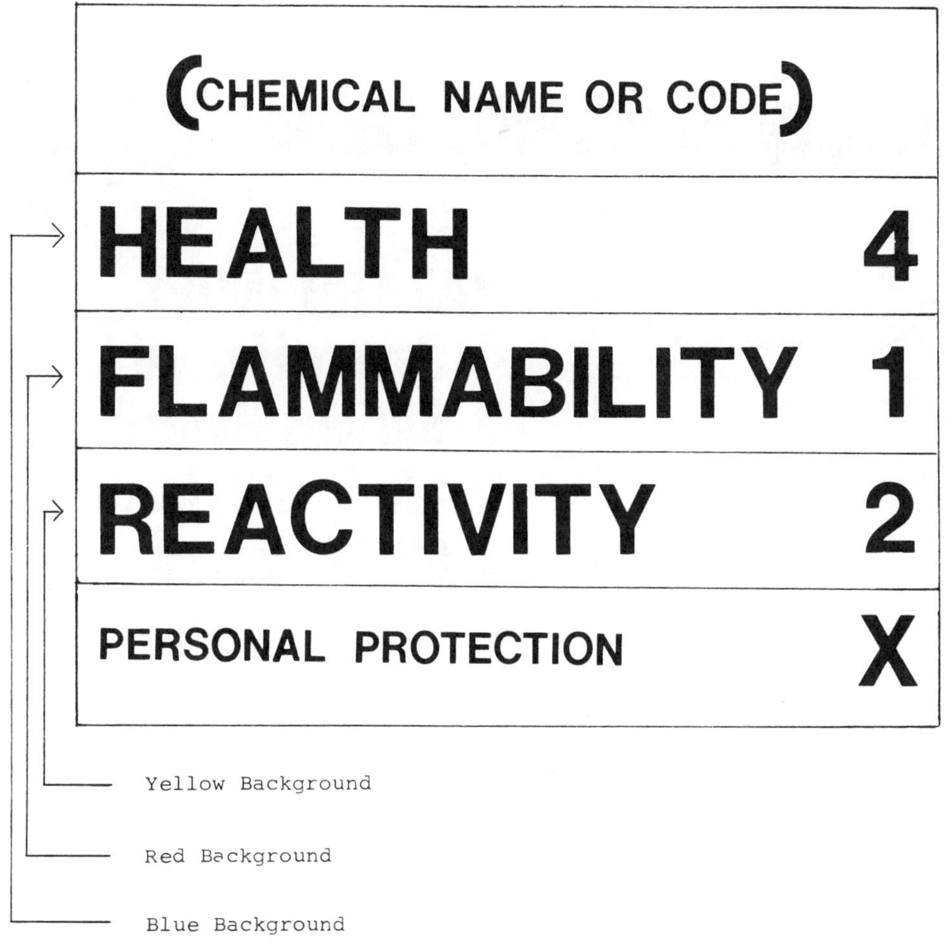

FIG 1–3.
Safety and health warning label for chemicals.

report.[22] The use of formal inspection documents can increase the probability that all areas of concern are inspected with consistency. The document can cue the inspector to look for the key elements of the program and provide the desired feedback for analytical comparison with accumulated data from previous inspections. The need for formal documentation will become more evident as the complexities of the programs increase. Documentation may also serve as legal evidence of safety and health actions, should the initiation or effectiveness of the program be questioned.

Selection of inspectors will depend on the available manpower, but the line supervisor should always be considered as a candidate to conduct the inspections or as a member of the inspection team. The line supervisors have direct contact with the workers and work environment on a daily basis, providing regular control over the application of the safety and health programs. Their intimate knowledge of work activities can provide valuable assistance in defining the successes or failures in the programs. Members of the safety and health team should conduct frequent inspections, collectively or as individuals, to enhance the supervisors' inspections and provide professional feedback to management. Inspectors should be trained to evaluate the work environment for potential hazards as well as known hazards. Suspect situations, such as any man-environment interface, should include an assessment of the risk, for example, evaluation of the (1) probability of an accident-causing event occurring, (2) probability of a worker being involved in the event, and (3) possible consequences of the event.

The National Safety Council developed an "Ergonomics Checklist" in February 1983, which can be used to evaluate specific jobs for potential hazards. The checklist uses specific questions related to problem sources in task design, workspace, manual materials handling, machinery and tools, controls and displays, and hand tools. Unfortunately, some situations can be overlooked without some type of checklist or other structured method of inspection, and this can lead to the recognition of a problem only *after* an accident. The occurrence of these unwanted events can be greatly reduced through competent training and education programs for the inspectors. Prevention, based on a hazard's potential to cause accidents, should always be the impetus for safety and health actions.

The types of inspections conducted will vary in scope from one subject to multiple subjects, depending on the organizational needs or predetermined inspection format. Inspections can also be precipitated by a medical evaluation, a single accident, or an ac-

Safety & Health Label

Coatings & Resins Division

PPG INDUSTRIES

(CHEMICAL NAME OR CODE)	
HEALTH	4
FLAMMABILITY	1
REACTIVITY	2
PERSONAL PROTECTION	X

HAZARD INDEX
4 Severe Hazard
3 Serious Hazard
2 Moderate Hazard
1 Slight Hazard
0 Minimal Hazard

PERSONAL PROTECTION INDEX

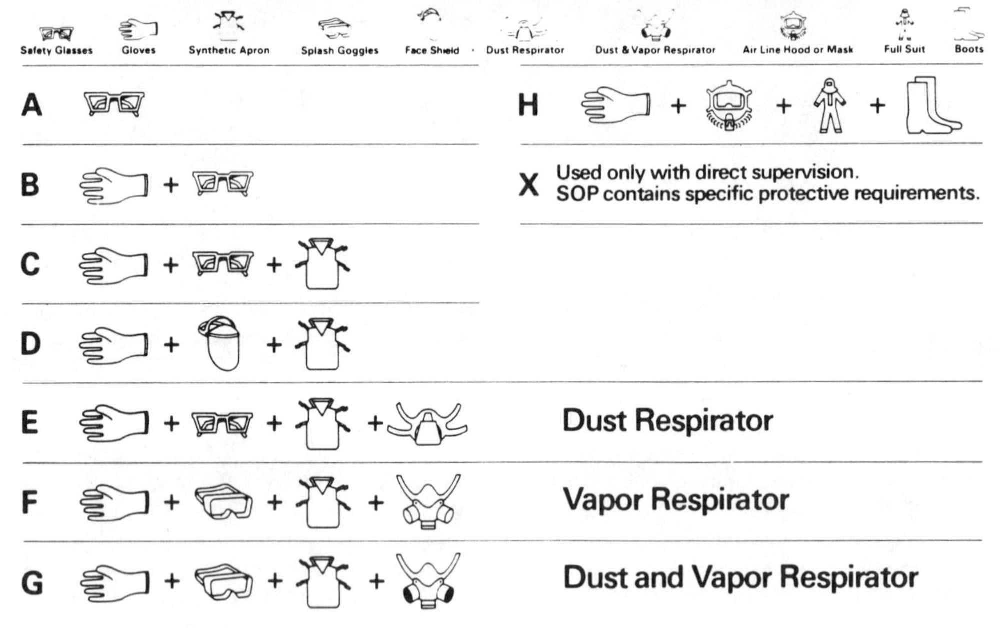

FIG 1–4.
Safety and health label poster.

cident trend, in which case they become corrective in nature rather than preventive. Accident information is invaluable as a source of accident prevention methodology, but the cost of such information is unacceptable. Specific subject inspections, e.g., punch presses, chemical reactors, overhead cranes, and portable electric tools, should be preferable to general inspections, since the inspector can concentrate on specific details. General inspections may become so broad that some important information might be overlooked. Inspections, as with other evaluative programs, should also include an ergonomic review of each work station to determine if the environment is designed to fit the worker's psychophysical characteristics. Inspection programs are not always designed to search for hazards but to be used as a preventive maintenance tool to ensure the integrity of established safety and health programs. Development of inspection programs should include consideration of government regulatory requirements, accident history in the organization, the type of industry hazards, risk information, and organizational safety and health requirements.

Accident Investigation

The most unpleasant part of any safety and health program will undoubtedly be accident investigations. Accidents create the motivation for all safety and health actions, which should be specifically aimed at preventing such events. When an accident occurs, the result of the accident may or may not involve an injury to a worker. Theoretically, the event may not result in any material damage, in which case it is commonly defined as a "near miss" accident. Regardless of the terminology used, an accident is an undesirable event that must be investigated in order to eliminate all equivalent or similar events.

Accident investigations can benefit safety and health programs by providing important information on the causes of accidents. How this information is used is even more important than the results of the investigation. It serves no purpose to investigate accidents without initiating some type of corrective action to prevent future occurrences of similar accidents. All accident investigations should answer several basic questions, such as:

Who was involved in the accident?
What was involved in the accident?
Where did the accident take place?
When did the accident occur?
How did the accident occur?
Why did the accident occur?

Answering the above questions will provide the investigator with enough information to analyze the accident cause or causes properly. Any investigation should begin immediately after the accident is reported. The facts in the case will be fresh in the minds of witnesses, and any physical evidence should remain undisturbed at the site of the accident. The *who, what, where,* and *when* questions are not normally difficult to answer. The *how* question may require additional time and effort to piece the facts together into a clear picture of the events leading to the accident. The *why* question should be answered after all of the information resulting from the previous questions have been recorded.

The investigation should begin with a review of the accident scene as soon as possible after the accident. Photographs may be of value in some cases to preserve elements of the scene which can be reviewed at a later date. All individuals involved, including witnesses who saw the accident or were in the vicinity at the time of the accident, should be interviewed. The interview begins by letting the individuals explain their version of the accident, without interruption. Afterwards, questions are asked on important points where clarification is needed. After obtaining an accurate description of the accident, the analysis should begin with the last event in the sequence of events that resulted in the accident.

In the case of a finger that is cut by contact with a knife, the last event would be the knife-finger contact which results in the laceration. The first question may be, "Why did the knife contact the finger or why did the finger contact the knife?" We can assume that either the finger or the knife was in the wrong position at the time of the event, since it is not likely that the injury was intentional. If one or the other were improperly positioned, was the position dictated by environmental factors or established practice or was it an inadvertent choice of the individual? The answers to such questions will supply clues to the cause of each event that led to the accident. As the investigation regresses through the accident events, additional *why* questions will be created. Sufficient information is then developed which will lead the investigator to reasonable conclusions that can be converted into corrective action.

Health Hazard Evaluations

Health hazard evaluations are used to collect environmental data on the condition of existing hazards and to detect any new hazards in the workplace. The evaluation can be used as a tool to determine the level of risk associated with exposure as well as measure the effectiveness of any hazard control mechanisms. Evaluations should be conducted by an industrial hygienist or an occupational health physician, with other team members lending assistance in collecting field data. The evaluation should include a study of all suspected biologic, chemical, or physical hazards, including ergonomic factors. Quantitative or qualitative methods of measuring the relationship of the hazard with the worker or the results of the relationship should be used when collecting the data. These may include air monitoring to collect and measure air contaminants, noise measurements, radiation measurements, psychophysical examinations, or other methods dictated by a specific hazard encountered in the evaluation.

Health hazard evaluations should be conducted on each job and production process. The evaluations can provide the safety and health team and management with the neccessary data to establish appropriate control measures or eliminate the hazard where control is not feasible. The three principles of accident prevention mentioned previously in this chapter, i.e., elimination, isolation, and insulation, should always be employed in the decision process. If a decision is made to control the hazard, periodic evaluations must be conducted to maintain the integrity of the control measures. A formal review process should be established, based on a specific hazard or as a multiple-hazard review. An industrial hygienist should be consulted to develop specific procedures for local management to use in auditing the controls when a hygienist is not available at the facility. A periodic visit by an industrial hygienist may be necessary to measure accurately the effectiveness of some controls, such as ventilation systems or noise attenuating equipment.

Acknowledgments

I express my appreciation to David C. Swenson for his suggestions and untiring reviews of the drafts prepared for this chapter. I also thank C. D. Johnson and L. W. Keller for their professional critique and support. My greatest appreciation is extended to Carl Zenz, M.D., for providing the opportunity to write this chapter and for his confidence in my ability to do so.

REFERENCES

1. Ahmed MS, Wu D: Chemical safety and health information and decision-making. *Natl Saf News* 1981; 124:3, 44.
2. Chovil A, Alexander GR: Use of industrial hygiene and safety professionals: A survey of South Carolina manufacturing plants. *Am Ind Hyg Assoc J* 1984; 45:365.
3. Cohen A, Smith M, Cohen HH: *Safety Program Practices in High Versus Low Accident Rate Companies—An Interim Report*, NIOSH PB-298332. US Dept of Health, Education, and Welfare, US Government Printing Office, 1975.
4. Cohen HH, Cleveland RJ: Safety program practices in record-holding plants. *Prof Saf* 1983; 28:3, 26.
5. Crutchfield CD: Managing occupational safety and health programs—An overview. *Am Ind Hyg Assoc J* 1981; 42:226.
6. Decker LR: A hierarchy of safety and health program elements. *Prof Saf* 1984; 29:1, 21.
7. Denton DK: A strategy for improving safety problems solving. *Prof Saf* 1983; 28:6, 25.
8. DeReamer R: *Modern Safety and Health Technology*. New York, John Wiley & Sons, 1980.
9. Dionne ED: How to put teamwork in your hazard control program. *Natl Saf News* 1983; 128:4, 57.
10. Fawcett HH, Wood WS: *Safety and Accident Prevention in Chemical Operations*. New York, John Wiley & Sons, 1982.
11. Ferry TS: Safety on the board. *Prof Safety* 1984; 29:6, 27.
12. Forman J: 1920–1929: The Jazz Age—America's joyride ends with a crash. *Occup Hazards* 1975; 37:9, 70.
13. Heinrich HW: *Industrial Accident Prevention*. New York, McGraw-Hill Book Co, 1959.
14. Kalis DB: 1960–1969: The turbulent sixties—Soaring aspirations and deepening disenchantment. *Occup Hazards* 1975; 37:9, 89.
15. Kalis DB: 1776–1850: The Post Revolutionary Period—The first stirrings of industrialism in America. *Occup Hazards* 1975; 37:9, 53.
16. Keller LW, Schaper KL, Johnson CD: A hazardous materials identification system for the coatings and resins industry. *Am Ind Hyg Assoc J* 1980; 41:901.
17. Kinsley GR: Potential accident analysis. *Prof Saf* 1983; 28:7, 25.
18. Kroemer KHE: *Material Handling: Loss Control Through Ergonomics*. Chicago, Alliance of American Insurers, 1979.

18a. LaDou J (ed): *Introduction to Occupational Health and Safety*. Chicago, National Safety Council, 1986.

19. Lucas RE: 1940–1949: War and Peace—America becomes a global superpower. *Occup Hazards* 1975; 37:9, 81.
20. Musacchio C: 1850–1900: The Industrial Revolution—What price progress? *Occup Hazards* 1975; 37:9, 57.
21. Musacchio C: 1930–1939: The Depression Years—An emerging federal presence. *Occup Hazards* 1975; 37:9, 75.
22. National Safety Council: *Accident Prevention Manual for Industrial Operations*. Chicago, National Safety Council, 1974.
23. Olishifski JB, McElroy FE: *Fundamentals of Industrial Hygiene*, ed 3. Chicago, National Safety Council, 1987.
24. Roland HE: Risk and safety value analysis. *Prof Safety* 1983; 28:9, 26.
25. Saltzman BE: Adequacy of current industrial hygiene and occupational professional manpower. *Am Ind Hyg Assoc J* 1982; 43:254.
26. Sheridan PJ: 1900–1916: The Progressive Period—Reform charges the American air. *Occup Hazards* 1975; 37:9, 65.
27. Sheridan PJ: 1970–1976: America in Transition–Which way will the pendulum swing? *Occup Hazards* 1975; 37:9, 95.
28. Walters NK: Safety management accountability process: An effective approach at Du Pont. *Prof Safety* 1983; 28:8, 35.
29. World Health Organization: *Psychosocial Factors in Injury Prevention*. Geneva, World Health Organization, 1982.

2

Industrial Hygiene

Julian B. Olishifski, P.E.

Industrial hygiene may be defined as that science (or art) devoted to the recognition, evaluation, and control of those environmental hazards—chemical, physical, biologic and ergonomic—that may cause sickness, impaired health, or significant discomfort to employees or residents of the community.

Environmental health hazards include conditions that potentially may cause legally compensable occupational illness or they may refer to any condition in the workplace that impairs the health of employees enough to make them lose time from work or to work at less than full efficiency. Both are undesirable. Both are preventable. Their correction is properly a responsibility of management.

The industrial hygienist effectively provides information on the manufacturing operations and other activities of an organization to its medical department. The occupational health physician depends on the skills, techniques, and knowledge of the hygienist to provide insight into the magnitude of environmental factors or stresses as they relate to the health background of an employee's job. In many cases, it is extremely difficult to differentiate between the symptoms of occupational and nonoccupational disease. The industrial hygienist, by pointing out the danger areas, can enable the physician to correlate better the employee's condition and complaints with the potential health hazards arising out of his occupation.

Industrial hygiene is an essential component of occupational health programs. In some companies, the industrial hygiene function may be a part of the medical department, whereas in others it may be a separate, parallel organization, or be part of the research, engineering, or safety department. Regardless of where the industrial hygiene activity is placed, it is an integral part of the company's loss control and accident prevention program.

To run an effective accident prevention program, the services and skills of several professions are needed.

Through engineering, education of the worker, and supervisory techniques, the safety professionals have ably demonstrated their ability to reduce the frequency of accidental injury by control of the many hazards arising out of the industrial environment.

Occupational medicine plays an important role, with physicians being specially trained in occupational and preventive medicine. Application of occupational health principles also ensures that workers are placed in jobs according to their physical capacities, mental abilities, and emotional makeup.

The industrial hygienist, a professional development of this technologic age, serves as the analytic, preventive engineering arm to the safety professional and industrial physician by applying specialized knowledge to the measurement and control of health hazards in the work environment.

Working individually and collectively, the safety professional, industrial physician, and industrial hygienist have helped to improve the industrial health and safety records of many industries. In some companies, the application of these talents is so well organized and effective in the anticipation and correction of hazards that the employees are unquestionably safer and healthier at work than they are at home.

GOALS

The goals of industrial hygiene are reached through competence in a variety of scientific fields—principally chemistry, engineering, physics, biology, and medicine. Trained initially in one of these fields, most industrial hygienists have acquired, by experience and postgraduate study, a knowledge of the other allied disciplines.

Many larger corporations utilize industrial hygiene teams composed of analytical chemists, physicists, engineers, toxicologists, nurses, and physicians, each applying his own specialty to combat occupational health problems. Many smaller companies rely on the comprehensive knowledge of an individual industrial hygienist who is ablest in his specialty and well qualified in related aspects.

The industrial hygienist's aim is to engineer the work area so that hazardous agents or materials are minimized, collected, confined, or otherwise kept away from employees. Specialized knowledge is required to design health protection at lowest cost and maximal effectiveness. The industrial hygienist checks control methods with air analyses or other measurements, including the physician's clinical studies of an employee's health status to verify the adequacy of environmental controls.

Industrial hygiene operates in areas related to those ordinarily covered by medical and safety programs. The industrial hygienist can provide a unique perspective to the company operation and can offer specialized solutions to many problems.

The physician frequently is required to make a decision as to the degree of health hazard arising out of an industrial operation. In emergency situations, in the absence of an industrial hygienist, it becomes the occupational physician's duty to see that proper action toward evaluation and control of health hazards is taken.

The variety of substances and industrial processes that present occupational health hazards steadily increases. Recently developed raw materials and methods of manufacture or new processes may create new environmental stresses. Improved techniques for the prevention and control of existing hazards and stresses are also required.

In some instances, a survey of raw materials, by-products produced intentionally and unintentionally, source and method of dispersion of airborne contaminants, exposure to physical agents, and control measures in use will indicate the effectiveness of the control measures. A more complex problem will require a complete and detailed study by a qualified industrial hygiene engineer.

HAZARD COMMUNICATION AND WORKER RIGHT-TO-KNOW LEGISLATION

There has been a dramatic upsurge in federal and state activity for passage of hazard communication and right-to-know legislation. Approximately 17 states and 9 municipalities have enacted some form of employee or community hazard communication or right-to-know legislation. Hazard communication and the right of workers to be informed of past or current exposures to hazardous or toxic substances intertwine with many other issues involving monitoring and enforcement activities by governmental agencies, trade secrecy protection, legislation dealing with occupational health and safety regulation, product safety and liability aspects, and contamination of the community environment. Few individuals would disagree that workers exposed on the job to substances that are clearly toxic or hazardous have a right to know that such exposures have occurred.

The common features found in most legislative proposals require (1) that the employer furnish information on toxic substances to a governmental agency; (2) that the employer post notices concerning the availability of information on toxic or hazardous materials; (3) that the employer have available material safety data sheets (MSDS) and an alphabetized list of toxic substances in the workplace; (4) that containers be labeled or that signs be posted giving information on toxic or hazardous chemicals found in the workplace; and (5) that training be provided to employees on safe handling procedures.

Since May 27, 1986, employers have been required to label in-plant containers, to inform employees of workplace hazards, to make material safety data sheets or comparable written information available to employees, and to train workers in protective measures when dealing with specific chemical hazards. Employers will have to develop written hazard communication programs outlining their plans to accomplish these objectives.

Intent of Regulation.—The primary intent of the Occupational Safety and Health Administration (OSHA) in promulgating this final hazard communication regulation is to ensure that employees will receive as much information as needed concerning the hazards in their workplaces and that this information will be presented to them in a usable, readily accessible form. The secondary intent of OSHA was to write the regulation in such a way that those companies who have voluntarily instituted effective programs of hazard communication for their employees may continue to use them without substantial modification. The latter goal is accomplished by presenting the provisions of the final regulation in performance language wherever possible.

Labels.—The labels must include the identity of the chemical, hazard warnings, and the name and address of the manufacturer, importer, or responsible party. Chemical distributors also must adhere to the labeling requirements, making sure that material safety data sheets are provided as required. The purpose of labels on hazardous chemicals, or on products containing them, is to warn about potential danger or significant risk. Labels for hazardous materials should be printed on or attached to a container so that they will remain legible and affixed to the container at least as long as the product remains within. They must convey critically important information in a limited space and allow for a limited amount of time and degree of attention from the reader.

Material Safety Data Sheets.—In the final OSHA hazard communication regulation, material safety data sheets serve as the primary vehicle for transmitting detailed hazard information to both downstream employers and employees.

A material safety data sheet is essentially a technical bulletin, generally two or four pages in length, which contains information about a hazardous chemical, such as chemical composition, chemical and physical characteristics, health and safety hazards, and precautions for safe handling and use. Some state right-to-know laws also require the availability of MSDSs, but most of the bulletins have been generated as good business practice, rather than a response to legal requirements.

Employee Information and Training.—The final component of the comprehensive hazard communication regulation promulgated by OSHA is employee information and training. Under the provisions of the final regulation, the employer would be required to provide employees with training about the nature of the hazards they work with and protective measures to be taken at the time of initial assignment and whenever a new hazardous chemical is introduced into the workplace.

Training serves to explain and reinforce the information presented to employees through the media of labels and material safety data sheets. Labels and material safety data sheets will be successful only when employees understand the information presented and are aware of the actions to be taken to avoid or minimize exposure and of the occurrence of adverse effects. Training is critical to effective hazard communication—it is the best way to ensure that workers take protective action and thus decrease the possibility of occupation-related, chemical-source illnesses and injuries.

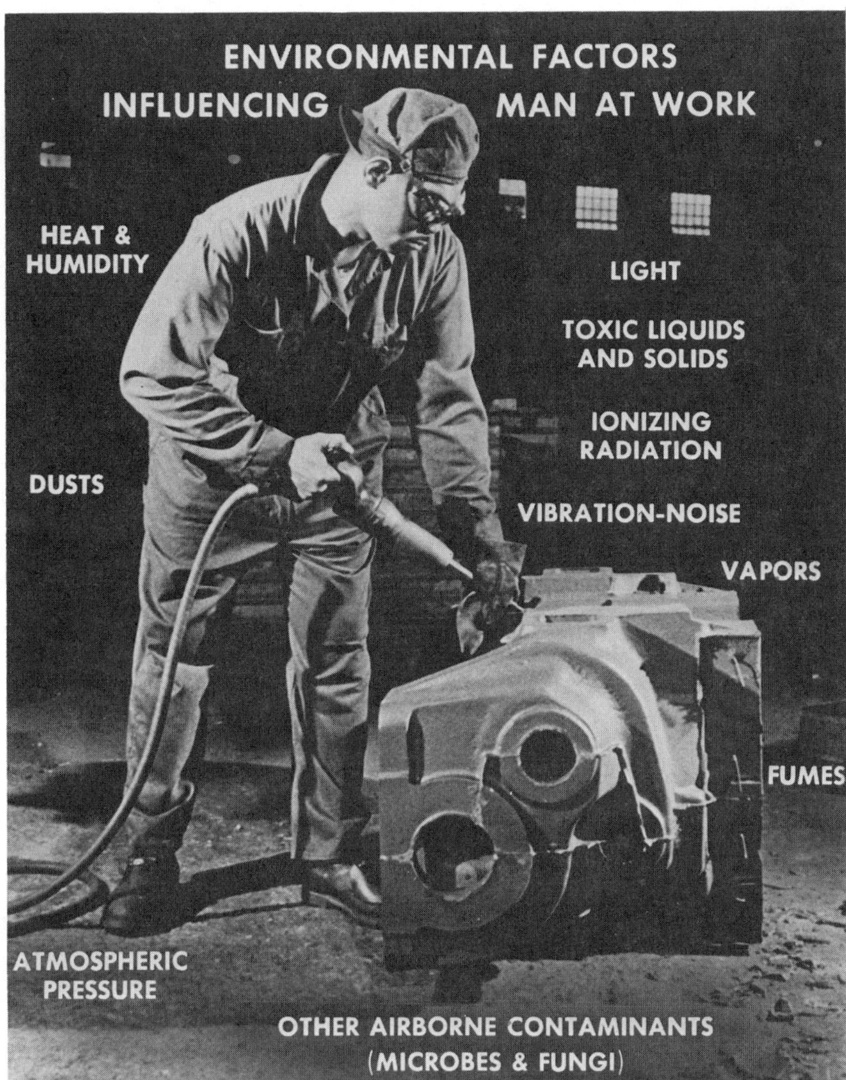
ENVIRONMENTAL FACTORS
INFLUENCING
MAN AT WORK
HEAT &
HUMIDITY
LIGHT
TOXIC LIQUIDS
AND SOLIDS
IONIZING
RADIATION
DUSTS
VIBRATION-NOISE
VAPORS
FUMES
ATMOSPHERIC
PRESSURE
OTHER AIRBORNE CONTAMINANTS
(MICROBES & FUNGI)

FIG 2–1.
Environmental factors influencing man at work.

TYPES OF HAZARDS

The various environmental factors or stresses may be classified as chemical, physical, biologic, or ergonomic (Fig 2–1).

Chemical hazards would be excessive airborne concentrations of mists, vapors, gases, or solids in the form of dusts or fumes. In addition to the hazard of inhalation, some of these materials may act as skin irritants or may be toxic by absorption through the skin.

Physical hazards would include excessive levels of electromagnetic and ionizing radiation, noise, vibration, and extremes of temperature and pressure.

Biologic hazards would include insects, molds, fungi, and bacterial contamination, including defects in sanitation and housekeeping procedures, such as providing potable water, removal of industrial waste and sewage, food handling, and personal cleanliness.

Ergonomic factors would include improperly designed tools or work areas, unusual and unnecessary lifting or reaching, poor visual conditions, or repeated motions in an awkward position that may be responsible for fatigue, stress, and strain and may lead to accidents in the occupational environment. Designing the tools and the job to be done to fit the man should be of prime importance. Intelligent application of engineering and biomechanical principles is required to eliminate hazards of this kind.

Exposure of an employee to any of the harmful stresses or hazards listed may produce an immediate response due to the intensity of the hazard; or the response may result from longer exposure at a lower intensity.

Basically, an effective industrial hygiene program would consist of (1) knowledge and recognition of health hazards arising out of work operations and processes, (2) evaluation and measurement of the magnitude of the hazard, based on past experience and study, and (3) control of the hazard by isolation, substitution, change of process, local exhaust ventilation, general ventilation, and training and education.

DEFINITION OF TERMS

Occupational physicians must be aware of the precise meanings of certain words commonly used in industrial hygiene if they are going to communicate effectively with workers in this area. A fume respirator, for instance, is worthless as protection against gases or vapors. Too frequently, terms such as gases, vapors, fumes, and mists are used interchangeably. Each term has a definite meaning and describes a certain state of matter that can be achieved only by certain physical changes to the substance itself.

Basic to the industrial hygiene vocabulary are states of matter. As defined by the American National Standards Institute, these are as follows.

Dusts.—Solid particles generated by handling, crushing, grinding, rapid impact, detonation, and decrepitation of organic or inorganic materials, such as rock, ore, metal, coal, wood, and grain. Dusts do not tend to flocculate except under electrostatic forces; they do not diffuse in air but settle under the influence of gravity.

Dust is a term used to describe airborne solid particles that range in size from 0.1 to 25μ (1μ = 1/10,000 cm = 1/25,000 in.) (μ is the abbreviation for micron). Dusts above 25μ in size usually will not remain airborne long enough to present an inhalation problem to exposed employees.

Dust may enter the workroom air from various sources. It may be dispersed when a dusty material is handled, such as when lead oxide is dumped into a mixer or a product is dusted with talc. When solid materials are reduced to small sizes in such processes as grinding, crushing, blasting, shaking, and drilling, the mechanical action of the grinding or shaking device supplies a source of energy to disperse the dust formed.

Fumes.—Solid particles generated by condensation from the gaseous state, generally after volatilization from molten materials. This physical change often is accompanied by a chemical reaction, such as oxidation. Fumes flocculate and sometimes coalesce.

A fume is formed when a volatilized solid, such as a metal, condenses in cool air. The solid particles that make up a fume are extremely fine, usually less than 0.1μ. In most cases, the hot material reacts with the air to form an oxide. Examples are lead oxide fume from smelting and iron oxide fume from arc welding. A fume also can be formed when a material such as magnesium metal is burned or when welding or gas cutting is done on galvanized metal (Fig 2–2).

Gases and vapors are not fumes, even if newspaper columnists often (and incorrectly) call them that.

Smoke.—Carbon or soot particles less than 0.1μ in size that result from the incomplete combustion of carbonaceous materials, such as coal or oil. Smoke generally contains droplets as well as dry particles. Tobacco, for instance, produces a wet smoke composed of minute tarry droplets. The size of the particles contained in tobacco smoke is about 0.25μ.

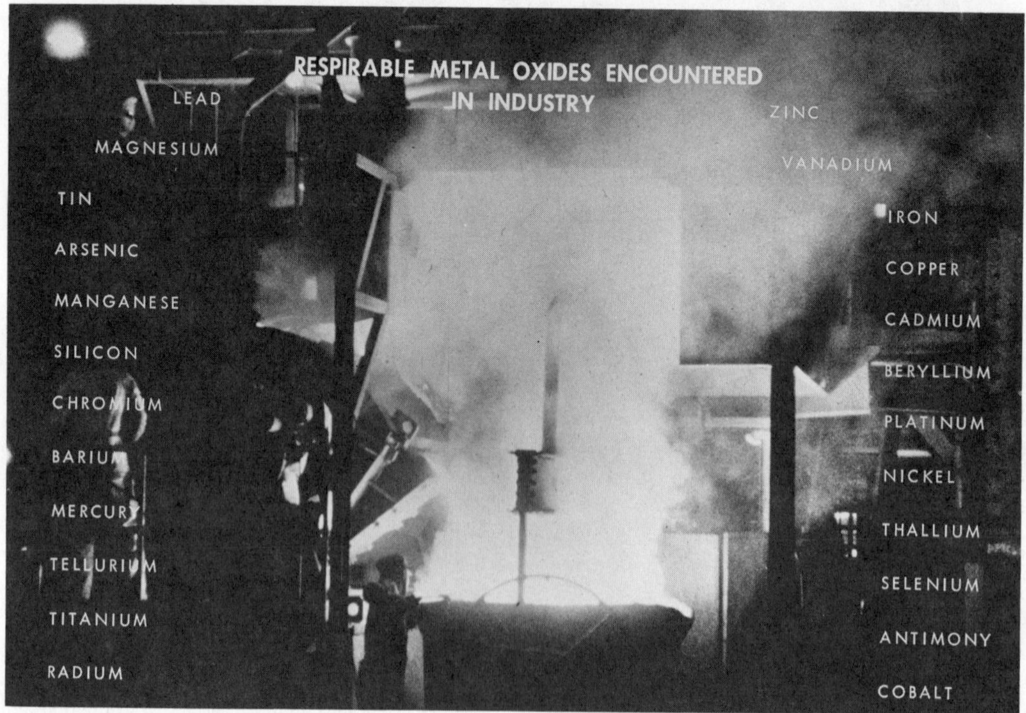

FIG 2–2.
Some respirable metal oxides encountered in industry.

Aerosols.—Liquid droplets or solid particles dispersed in air that are of a fine enough particle size to remain airborne for an extended period.

Mists.—Suspended liquid droplets generated by condensation from the gaseous to the liquid state or by breaking up a liquid into a dispersed state, such as by splashing, foaming, or atomizing. Mist is formed when a finely divided liquid is suspended in the atmosphere. Examples are the oil mist produced during cutting and grinding operations, acid mists from electroplating, acid or alkali mists from pickling operations, paint spray mist from spraying operations, and the condensation of water vapor to form a fog or rain (Fig 2–3).

Gases.—Normally formless fluids that occupy the space or enclosure and can be changed to the liquid or solid state only by the combined effects of increased pressure and decreased temperature. Gases diffuse. Examples are welding gases, internal combustion engine exhaust gases, and air.

Vapors.—The gaseous form of substances that normally are in the solid or liquid state at room temperature and normal pressure. The vapor can be changed back to the solid or liquid state by either increasing the pressure or decreasing the temperature alone. Vapors also diffuse. Evaporation is the process by which a liquid is changed into the vapor state and mixed with the surrounding atmosphere. Solvents with low boiling points will volatilize readily (Fig 2–4).

In addition to the definitions concerning states of matter, which find daily usage in the vocabulary of the industrial hygienist, other terms used to describe degree of exposure are

ppm—Parts of vapor or gas per million parts of contaminated air by volume

mppcf—Millions of particles of a particulate per cubic foot of air

mg/m^3—Milligrams of a substance per cubic meter of air

The occupational health physician will recognize that air contaminants exist as a gas, dust, fume, mist, or vapor in the workroom air. In evaluating the degree of exposure, the measured concentration of the air contaminant is compared to limits that appear in the published standards on levels of exposure. This will be discussed in greater detail later in this chapter.

CHEMICAL AGENTS

The majority of the environmental health hazards to employees arise from exposure to chemical agents in the form of vapors,

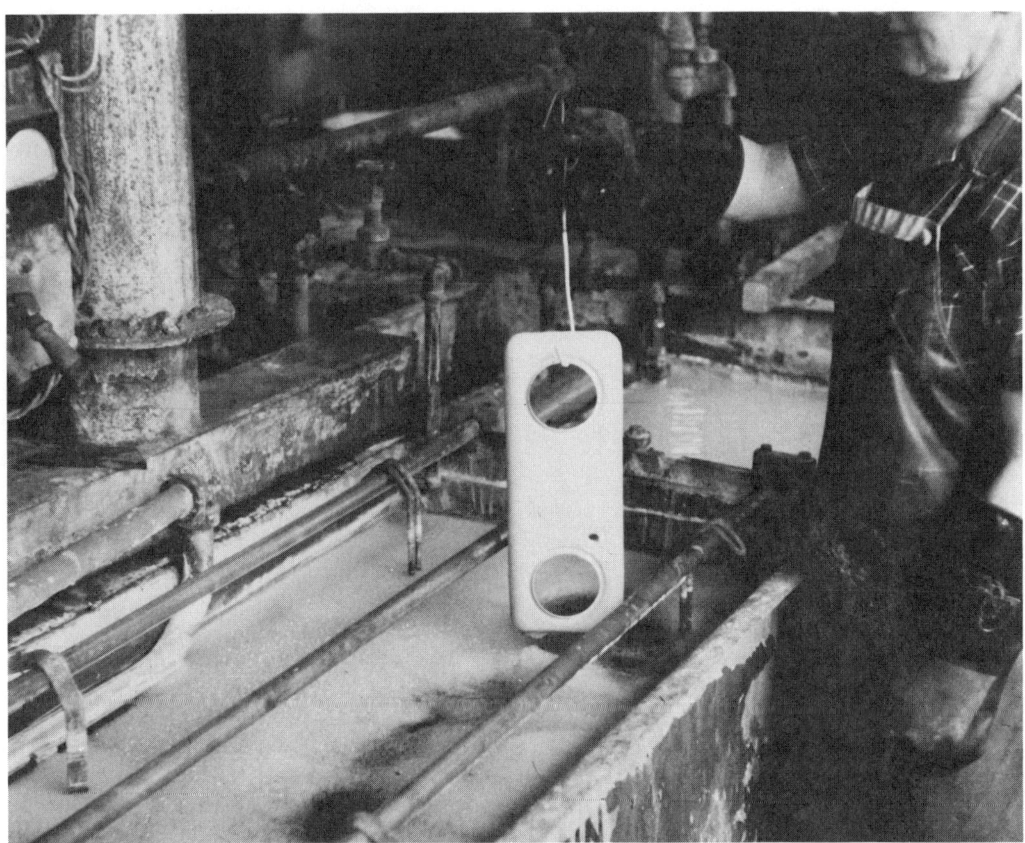

FIG 2–3.
Worker and electroplating tank. Note frothy surface of solution and its corrosiveness, especially seen at the exhaust duct opening. Special clothing, including eye protection, is required, as well as a raised wooden floor to permit washing the area with copious amounts of water.

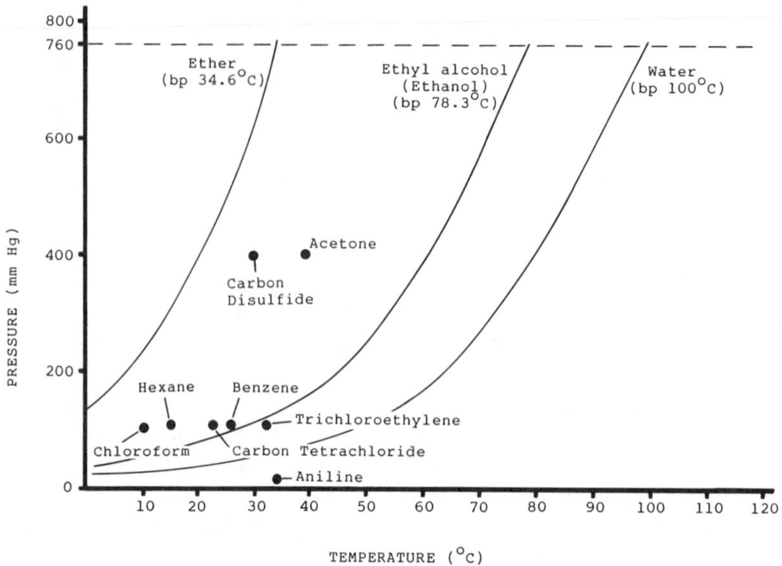

FIG 2–4.

The ability and rate of evaporation of a substance can be exceedingly important when considering all aspects of occupational exposures and potential intake of the substance by the worker. Evaporation involves the transfer of molecules from a liquid phase to a gas phase; the molecules exerting a pressure as any gas ("vapor" referring to the gas state of a substance which is liquid at room temperature, i.e., acetone, ether; and a "gas" as a substance that must be cooled well below room temperature to become a liquid, i.e., oxygen, carbon dioxide, hydrogen sulfide). The pressure of a gas in equilibrium with its liquid phase is called the *vapor pressure,* a measureable point, indicating the capability of a liquid to vaporize, *specific* for each liquid substance at a given temperature (i.e., at room temperature, ether evaporates faster than trichloroethylene). As the temperature of a liquid increases, so does its vapor pressure. The vapor pressure of water at 37° C is 47 mm Hg (the value of PH_2O in alveolar and expired air). When the *boiling point is reached,* the vapor pressure of a liquid equals the atmospheric pressure. The standard normal boiling point is the boiling point at one standard atmosphere, 760 mm Hg. Thus, when observing working conditions, the ambient work room and the process temperatures must be noted. Furthermore, climatic and geographic (altitude) factors can contribute to higher concentrations of vapors and gases on the job. Note the vapor pressures of commonly used solvents, indicating high evaporative capability with small increases of temperature.

gases, dusts, fumes, and mists, or by skin contact with these materials.

In order for the harmful agent to exert its toxic effect on an individual, the chemical must come into contact with a body cell. The routes of entry in work exposures are inhalation, skin absorption, ingestion, and/or any combination of these.

Inhalation Hazards

Inhalation of chemical agents resulting in respiratory hazards may be broken down into two main groups:

1. Oxygen deficiency, in which the oxygen concentration (or partial pressure of oxygen) is below that level considered safe for human exposure.
2. Air containing harmful or toxic contaminants.

Oxygen-Deficient Atmospheres

Each living cell in the body requires a constant supply of oxygen. Some cells are more dependent on a constant oxygen supply than are others. Cells in the brain and nervous system may die after four to six minutes without oxygen. These cells cannot be regenerated or replaced, and permanent changes result from such damage.

Normal air at sea level contains approximately 21% oxygen and 79% nitrogen and other inert gases. At sea level and normal barometric pressure (760 millimeters of mercury), the partial pressure of oxygen would be 21% of 760 mm, or 160 mm. The partial pressure of nitrogen and inert gases would be 600 mm (79% of 760 mm).

At higher altitudes or under conditions of reduced barometric pressure, the relative proportions of oxygen and nitrogen would remain the same, but the partial pressure of each gas would be decreased.

The partial pressure of oxygen at the lung surface is critical, because it determines the rate of diffusion through the moist membranes. Men working at reduced pressure are subject to oxygen starvation, which can have very serious and insidious effects on the senses and judgment.

Reduced pressure is not the only condition under which oxygen starvation may occur. Deficiency of oxygen in the atmosphere of confined spaces is experienced commonly in industry. For this reason, the oxygen content of any tank or other confined space should be checked before entry is made. Instruments such as the oxygen analyzer are commercially available for this purpose.

The first physiologic signs of a deficiency of oxygen (anoxia) are increased rate and depth of breathing. Oxygen concentrations of less than 16% by volume cause dizziness, rapid heartbeat, and headache. A worker should never enter or remain in areas where tests have indicated such concentrations, unless he is wearing some form of supplied air or self-contained respiratory equipment.

Oxygen-deficient atmospheres may cause an inability to move and a semiconscious lack of concern about the imminence of death. In cases of sudden entry into areas containing little or no oxygen, the individual usually has no warning symptoms but immediately loses consciousness and has no recollection of the incident if he is rescued and revived. The senses cannot be relied on to alert or warn an individual of atmospheres deficient in oxygen.

Oxygen-deficient atmospheres may occur in tanks, vats, holds of ships, silos, mines, or in areas where the air may be diluted or displaced by gases or vapors or where the oxygen may be consumed by chemical or biologic reactions.

Airborne Contaminants

Breathing of harmful materials may irritate the upper respiratory tract and lung tissue or the terminal passages of the lungs and the air sacs, depending on the solubility of the material.

Inhalation of biologically inert gases may dilute the atmospheric oxygen below the normal blood saturation value and disturb cellular processes.

Other gases and vapors that have entered the respiratory system may prevent the blood from carrying oxygen to the tissues or interfere with its transfer from the blood to the tissues, producing chemical asphyxia.

Inhaled contaminants that adversely affect the body fall in three general categories:

1. Particulates, which, when deposited in the lungs, may produce either tissue damage, tissue reaction, disease, or physical obstruction.

2. Toxic vapors and gases that produce adverse reaction in the tissue of the lungs themselves.

3. Toxic vapors or gases that do not affect the lung tissue but are passed from the lung into the bloodstream, where they are carried to other body organs or have adverse effects on the oxygen-carrying capacity of the bloodstream itself.

Particulates.—An example of the first type (particulates) is asbestos fiber, which causes fibrotic growth in the alveolar tissue, plugging the ducts or limiting the effective area of the alveolar lining. Other harmful particulates are silica and certain metal fumes.

Vapors and gases.—An example of the second type (toxic gases) is hydrogen fluoride, a gas that directly affects lung tissue. It is a primary irritant of mucous membranes, causing chemical burns. Inhalation of this gas will cause pulmonary edema and direct interference with the gas transfer function of the alveolar lining.

An example of the third type is carbon monoxide, a toxic gas passed into the bloodstream without essentially harming the lung. The carbon monoxide passes through the alveolar walls into the blood, where it ties up the hemoglobin so that it cannot accept oxygen, thus causing oxygen starvation. Cyanide gas has another effect—it prevents utilization of molecular oxygen by cells.

Sometimes several types of lung hazards occur simultaneously. In coal mining operations, for example, explosives release oxides of nitrogen. These impair the bronchial clearance mechanism, so that coal dust associated with the explosions is not efficiently cleansed from the lungs.

The physiologic reactions caused by the inhalation of airborne matter will vary with different types of gases, vapors, and particulate contaminants. The reactions include:

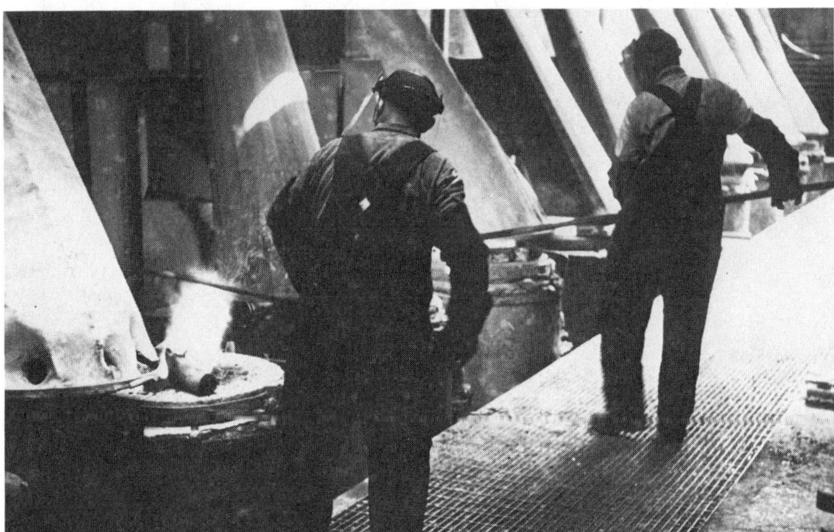

FIG 2–5.
A view of a nonferrous foundry melting room showing exhaust hoods and workers charging melting pots.

1. Cardiopulmonary reactions, which consist of the pneumoconioses, such as silicosis and asbestosis. In certain cases, specific types of lung pathology result, and the heart may be affected (cor pulmonale) when the fibrosis is advanced. In other cases, there is mainly just an accumulation of a relatively inert dust in the lungs.

2. Systemic reactions, which are caused by toxic dusts of such elements as lead, manganese, cadmium and mercury, by their compounds, and by certain organic materials.

3. Metal fume fever, which results from the inhalation of finely divided and freshly generated fumes of zinc or possibly of magnesium or of their oxides (Figs 2–2 through 2–8).

4. Allergic and sensitization reactions, which may be caused by inhalation of, or skin contact with, such materials as organic dusts from flour, grains, and some woods, and dusts of a few organic and inorganic chemicals.

5. Bacterial and fungal infections, which occur from inhalation of dusts containing active organisms, such as wool or fur dust containing anthrax spores or wood bark or grain dust containing parasitic fungi.

6. Irritation of the nose and throat that is caused by acid, alkali, or other irritating dusts or mists. Some dusts, such as soluble chromate dusts, may cause ulceration of the nasal passages or even lung cancer (Figs 2–9, 2–10, and 2–11).

7. Damage to internal tissues that may result from inhaled radioactive materials, such as radium or other isotopes that emit highly ionizing radiation.

Dust Hazards

To evaluate dust exposures properly requires knowledge of the chemical composition, particle size, dust concentration in air, how it is dispersed, and many other factors described here.

In the case of gases, the concentration that reaches the alveolar sacs will be nearly like the concentration in the air breathed. With aerosols or dust particles this is not the case. Large particles, more than 10μ aerodynamic diameter, will be deposited long before they reach the alveolar sacs, through gravity and impaction. Only the smaller particles will reach the alveoli. In the sacs, brownian movement of the particles results in deposition by diffusion.

With the exception of some fibrous materials, dust particles usually must be smaller than 5μ in order to enter the alveoli or inner recesses of the lungs.

Although a few particles, up to 10μ in size, may enter the lungs occasionally, nearly all the larger particles are trapped in the nasal passages, throat, larynx, trachea, and bronchi, from which they are expectorated or swallowed into the digestive tract.

A person with normal eyesight can detect dust particles as small as 50μ in diameter. Smaller airborne particles can be de-

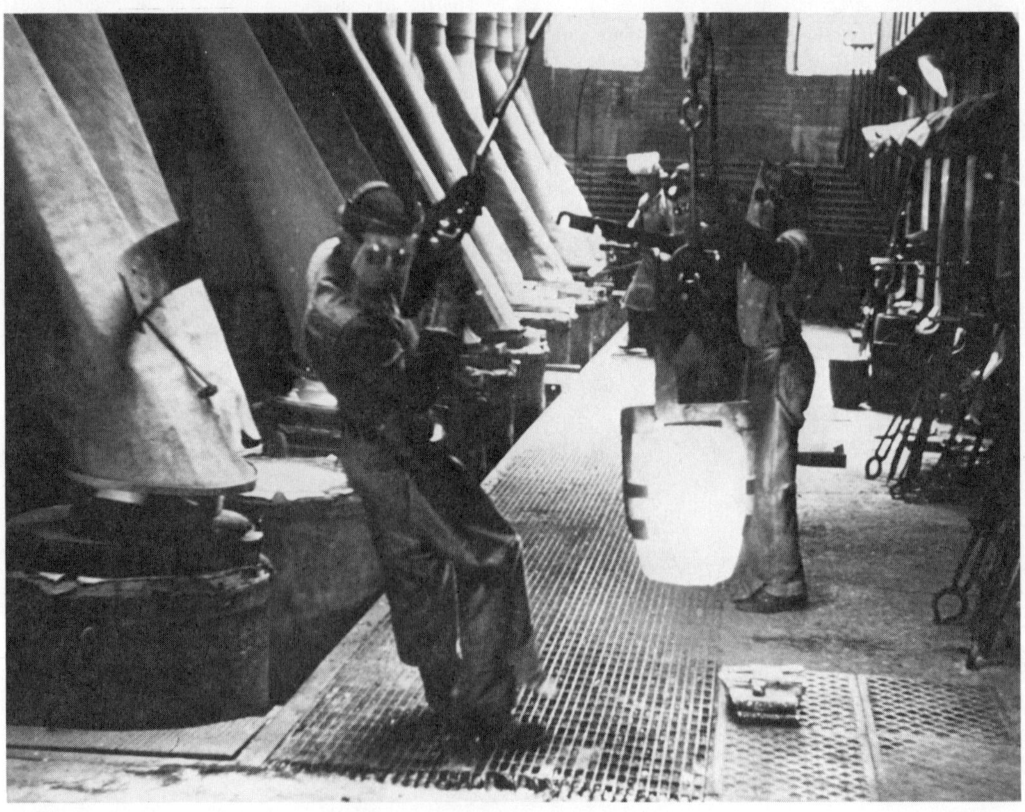

FIG 2–6.
Transporting refractory melting pot from melting room on overhead monorail. Note movable natural gravity hoods over melting stations along left wall.

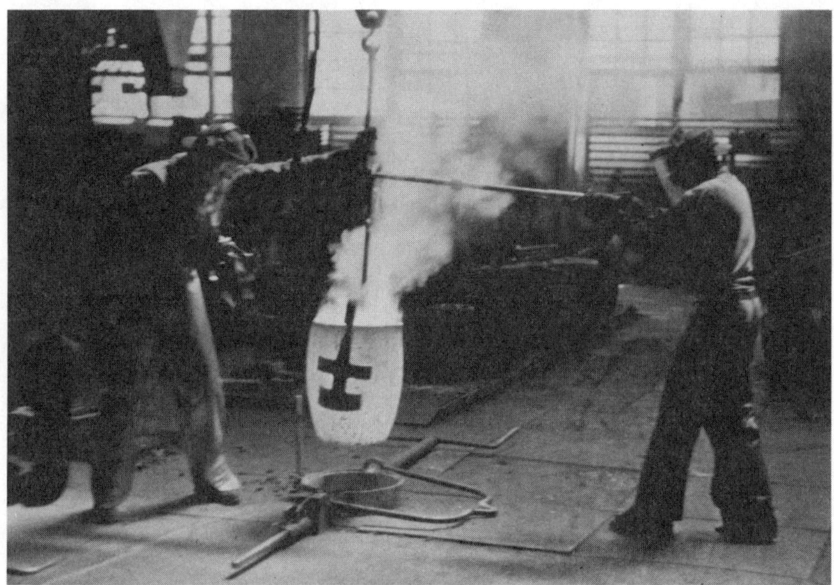

FIG 2–7.
Transferring refractory melting pot from monorail to traveling crane on pouring floor. Note uncontrolled fume from pot spreading throughout foundry.

tected individually by the naked eye only when strong light is reflected from them. Dust of respirable size (less than 10μ) cannot be seen without the aid of a microscope.

Most industrial dusts consist of particles that vary widely in size, with the small particles greatly outnumbering the large ones. Consequently (with few exceptions), when dust is noticeable in the air around an operation, probably more invisible dust particles than visible ones are present.

As a rough approximation, macroscopic particles (those large enough to be visible to the naked eye) are considered to be dispersed by dynamic projection. Microscopic particles (those visible only through a microscope) are considered to have a mass so small that their movement is dependent on the containing air mass. Contaminants, such as the larger dust particles, mists, and sprays, which are dispersed by dynamic projection, can cause external injury (such as acid burns, eye damage, and dermatitis). The microscopic particles may be dangerous to health if inhaled.

Dust in the air may or may not have the same composition as

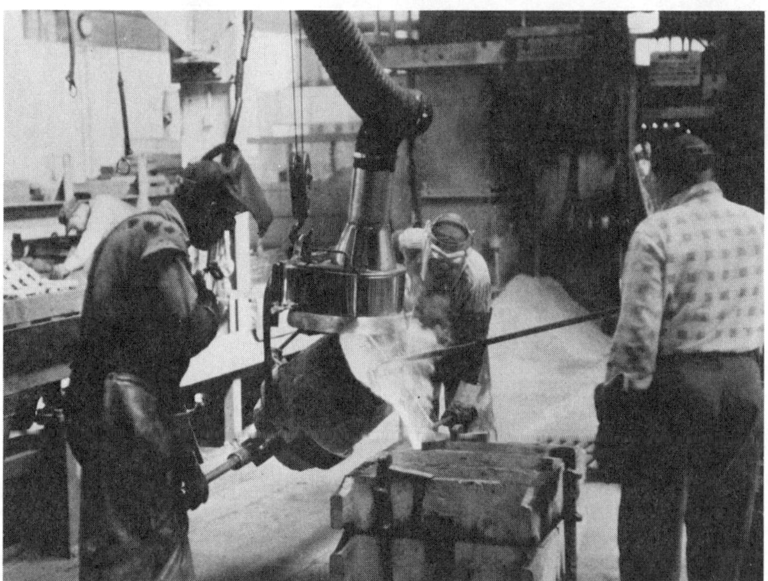

FIG 2–8.
Stainless steel exhaust hood and flexible duct suspended from traveling crane, with complete capture of fumes from pouring operation.

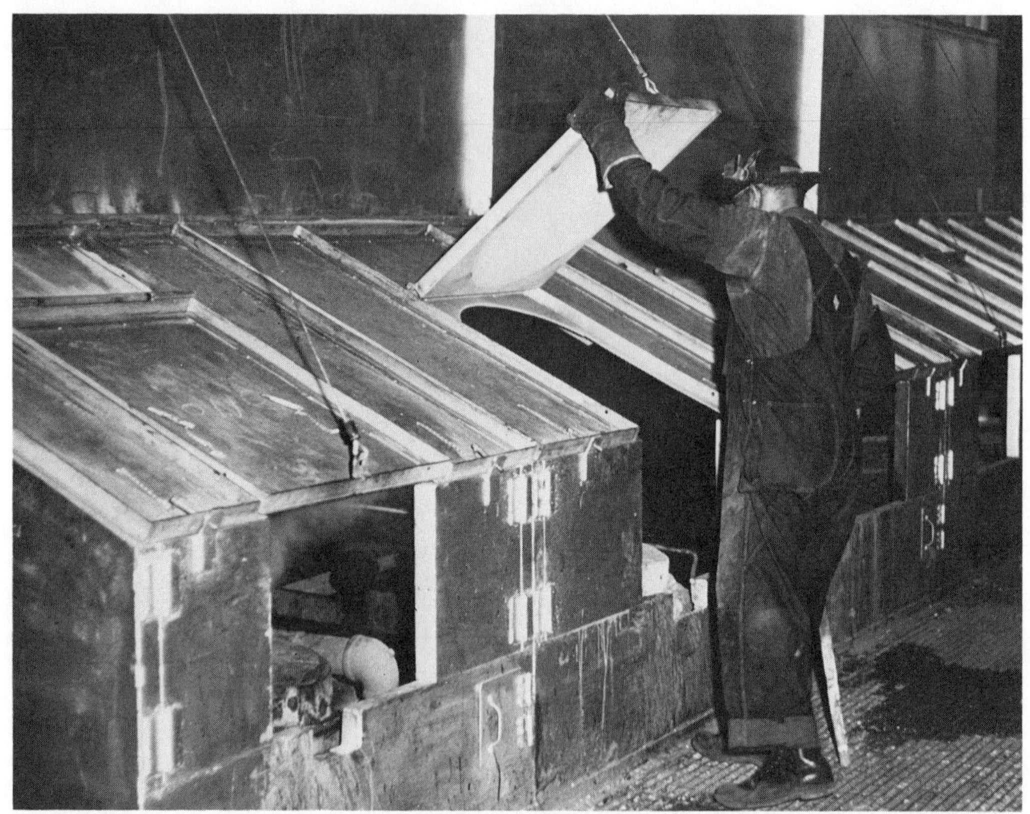

FIG 2–9.
Melting room after installation of enclosure over entire bank of melting stations. Exhaust system maintains constant, inward airflow through ports in front of every station. Counterbalanced door swings back for access to removable refractory melting pot.

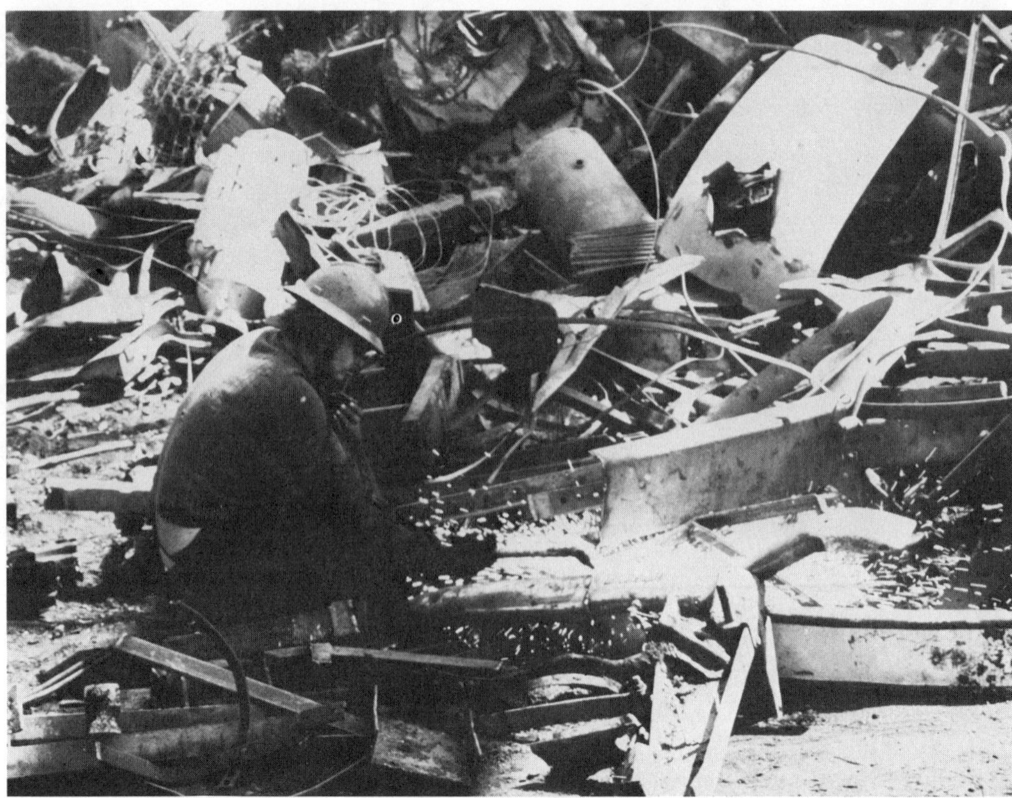

FIG 2–10.
Cutting scrap metal with an oxyacetylene torch. Even when performed outdoors, toxic exposures are possible.

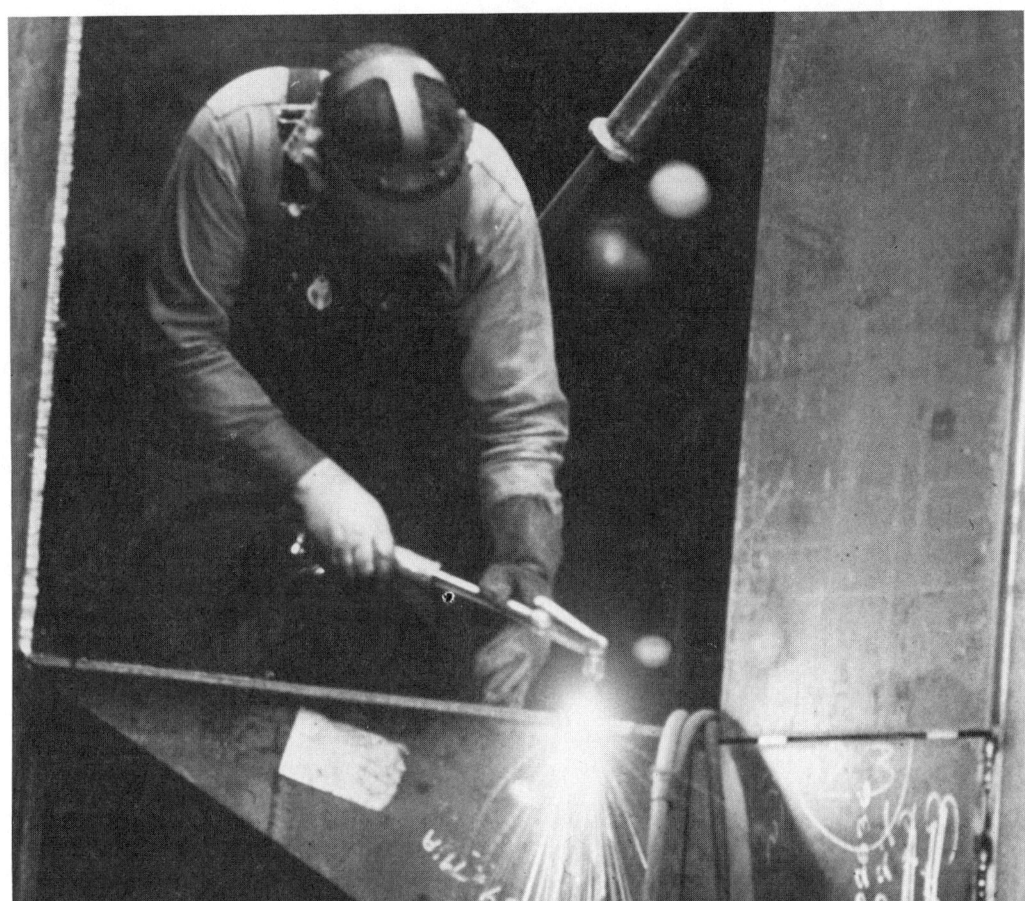

FIG 2–11.
Oxyacetylene torch cutting in a relatively confined space.

its parent material. The determining factors are the particle size and density of each component in the original mixture and the hardness of the material. (Hard materials will resist the pulverizing action of a mechanical device.)

The respiratory system serves as the portal of entry into the body for a great variety of airborne substances, both gaseous and particulate. Many of these atmospheric contaminants are capable of producing injury and disease when they are deposited and accumulate in sufficient amounts in the lungs or, after transfer from the lungs, to sensitive sites deeper within the body. Fine particles that escape upper respiratory removal are deposited from the inhaled air at different depths in the respiratory system and in varying degrees. This depends on a number of factors, including the density, shape, and size of the particles and the pattern of air flow into and out of the lungs.

There is no simple one-to-one relationship between the concentration of an atmospheric contaminant and duration of exposure and the rate of dosage by the hazardous agent to the critical site within the body. For a given magnitude of atmospheric exposure to a potentially toxic particulate contaminant, the resulting hazard can range all the way from an insignificant level to one of great danger, depending on the size of the inhaled particles and other factors that determine their fate in the respiratory system.

In order to quantify the dose-response relationship at the critical site, one must first estimate how much of the inhaled aerosol is deposited initially and at what sites within the respiratory tract and lungs and, finally, what fraction of the retained material reaches the critical site within the lungs or other parts of the body to produce damage.

Ingestion

Toxic and irritant dusts can also be ingested in amounts that may cause trouble. If the toxic dust swallowed with food or saliva is not soluble in body fluids, it is eliminated directly through the intestinal tract. Toxic materials that are readily soluble in body fluids can be absorbed in the digestive system and picked up by the blood.

Skin Absorption

A third way in which toxic and irritant substances may enter the human body is through skin absorption. Many organic compounds, such as TNT, cyanides, and most aromatic amines, amides, and phenols, can produce systemic poisoning by direct contact with the skin. Contact of irritant chemical agents with the skin may result in skin irritation also.

Inhalation as a route of entry is particularly important because of the rapidity with which a toxic material can be absorbed in the lungs, pass into the bloodstream, and reach the brain. This same material, if ingested, would be considerably diluted with the contents of the stomach.

It is important that all routes of entry be studied when an evaluation of the work environment is being made—candy bars or lunches in the work area, solvents being used to clean work clothing and hands, in addition to airborne contaminants in work areas.

Many industrial materials, such as resins and polymers, are relatively inert and nontoxic under normal conditions of use, but when heated or machined, they may decompose to form highly toxic by-products. Information concerning products and by-products can be obtained from the supplier and the chemical and engineering departments within your company.

Solvents

The widespread industrial use of solvents presents a major problem to the industrial hygienist, the industrial physician, and others charged with the responsibility for maintaining a safe, healthful working environment. Getting the job done without hazard to employees or property is dependent on the proper selection, application, handling, and control of solvents and an understanding of their properties.

The term "solvent" commonly refers to those organic liquids used to dissolve other organic materials. It includes materials such as naphtha, mineral spirits, gasoline, turpentine, benzine, alcohol and trichloroethylene (Fig 2–12).

A good working knowledge of the physical properties, nomenclature, and effects of exposure is very helpful in making a proper assessment of an exposure to solvent.

Nomenclature can be misleading. For example, "benzine" sometimes is referred to by the worker as "benzene"—a completely different solvent. Some commercial grades of benzine may contain benzene as a contaminant.

A complete list of all solvents used in the plant should be maintained. Where proprietary solvent mixes are utilized, every effort should be made to determine their composition.

With the extensive publicity given to the severe health hazards of carbon tetrachloride, it would seem that everybody should know that this should not be used as a general solvent. However, the experience has been repeated at times in which a highly toxic solvent has been substituted for one of less toxicity, but at some later date the more toxic solvent, desirable for good solvent properties or low price, has been brought back into the plant without the health and safety personnel being aware of its reintroduction.

Physiologic Effects

Physiologic effects from industrial organic solvent exposures come principally from skin contact and inhalation of the vapors. Ingestion, with resultant absorption into the digestive tract, is not normally considered a major hazard in industry. If the solvent is present in such amounts that skin contact becomes a hazard, there probably always will be an inhalation hazard.

Inhalation of excessive amounts of solvent vapors may produce various physiologic effects.

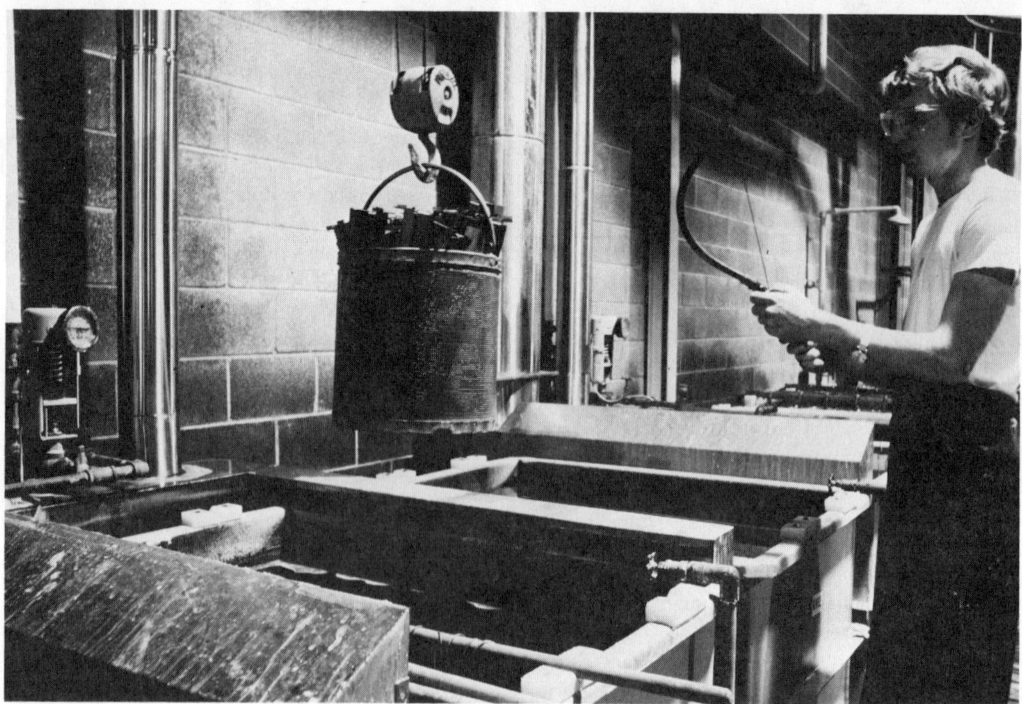

FIG 2–12.
A metal degreasing operation using trichloroethylene as solvent. Note the stainless steel exhaust ventilation system.

Narcosis, irritation of the respiratory tract, and asphyxiation characterize the acute effects produced on high-level exposure to toxic organic vapors. On extended high-level exposures, most organic vapors are capable of producing a gradual, continuous paralysis of the central nervous system. This is expressed in loss of consciousness and may result in respiratory failure.

Many symptoms of narcosis and asphyxiation are quite similar in that the primary effect in each is to impair the functioning of the brain—in narcosis by direct action and in asphyxiation by denying the brain sufficient oxygen. Asphyxiation may also be brought about by oxygen deficiency or the reduction of the partial pressure of oxygen in the inspired air.

Low-level exposures to organic solvents may result in impairments, such as lack of coordination, drowsiness, and similar symptoms, that may lead to increased accident proneness. Other effects may include damage to the blood, lungs, liver, kidney, gastrointestinal system, and other critical organs or tissues.

There is a wide range of hazard potential among the many solvents used in industry. This is governed by the volatility, the concentration, the toxicity, and the duration of exposure to the solvent.

Gases

Carbon Monoxide

In general, potentially hazardous exposure to gases is not obvious in industrial environments. For example, carbon monoxide may occur from the operation of internal combustion engines, such as in forklift trucks, by impingement of a gas flame on a cold surface, with resultant incomplete combustion, or by its use as a reducing gas in a heat-treating department. In addition, the possibility of accidental liberation of high concentrations of carbon monoxide from manufacturing operations that may result in asphyxiation should be kept in mind.

It would seem that due to all the publicity, everybody should be well informed concerning the hazardous nature of carbon monoxide. This gas is responsible for more hazardous exposures and incidents than the sum total of all the other gases. Carbon monoxide is also responsible for the greatest number of cases of fatal asphyxiation.

In areas where excessive levels of carbon monoxide may exist, such as in chemical plants or blast furnace operations, there tends to be an increasing use of automatic, monitoring, carbon monoxide alarm systems.

Fortunately, natural gas is practically in universal use for most fuel gas purposes, and this, of course, contains no carbon monoxide. It is, of course, important always to keep in mind that imperfect combustion of natural or liquefied propane gas in confined areas can produce a sufficient level of carbon monoxide to cause asphyxiation.

Cases of carbon monoxide asphyxiation have occurred over the years where cold systems (such as furnaces) are being heated with natural gas. Here, the impingement of the burning gas on cold surfaces results in incomplete combustion, with markedly greater amounts of carbon monoxide present in the products of combustion.

One part of carbon monoxide gas in 99 parts of air, resulting in a 1% mixture, would be in the safe range in regard to fire hazard, but it would be deadly (10,000 ppm) in terms of a health hazard. The point here is that, in most cases, by protecting against the health hazard, that is, keeping the airborne chemical contaminants within safe limits, the safety professional would eliminate the fire and explosion hazard.

Hydrogen Sulfide

Among the gases that might well be listed with those that may cause sudden death on exposure to relatively moderate concentrations is hydrogen sulfide. Hydrogen sulfide is formed wherever there is decomposition of materials containing sulfur under reducing conditions.

Wherever operations or processes are such that hydrogen sulfide could be generated, all workers should be briefed about the rapidly asphyxiating properties of this gas. It should be emphasized that at the higher concentrations the sense of smell does not provide the warning to which one is accustomed on exposure to the lower concentrations of hydrogen sulfide.

Workers should know ahead of time that if one of them should collapse in some confined area where hydrogen sulfide could be the cause, the fellow workers should not enter the confined area to rescue the victim without adequate respiratory protection.

Dermatitis Hazards

The phase of the survey dealing with dermatitis-producing materials may best start with an inquiry as to the incidence of dermatoses. For example, if no cases from cutting oils and compounds have been reported, this source of dermatoses may require no further investigation, but if a number of minor cases, with an occasional serious case, have occurred, this situation should be investigated thoroughly.

Skin diseases resulting from occupational exposure are reported to account for more than one half of all workmen's compensation claims for occupational diseases. These claims have appeared in all types of industry and sometimes appear where occupational skin diseases may be least expected.

There are two general types of dermatitis: primary irritation and sensitization.

Primary Irritation Dermatitis.—Nearly all persons will suffer primary irritation dermatitis from mechanical agents, such as friction; from physical agents, such as heat or cold; and from chemical agents, such as acids, alkalis, irritant gases and vapors. Brief contact with a high concentration of a primary irritant or prolonged exposure to a low concentration will cause inflammation. Allergy is not a factor in these conditions.

Sensitization Dermatitis.—This is the result of an allergic reaction to a given substance. The sensitivity becomes established during the induction period, which may be a few days to a few months. In most cases, it is ten days to one month. After the sensitivity has become established, exposure to even a small amount of the sensitizing material is likely to produce a severe reaction.

Some substances can produce both primary irritation dermatitis and sensitization dermatitis. Among them are organic solvents, formaldehyde, chromic acid, and epoxy resin systems.

Before new processes are introduced and prior to the adoption of new or different chemicals in an established process, possible dermatitis hazards, including those that may be caused by trace impurities, should be considered carefully. Only a highly skilled and experienced chemist can make analyses for trace impurities, and often this requires highly specialized equipment and techniques. Such analyses are justified, however, by the possibility that considerable benefit may be derived from them. Once the dermatitis hazards have been determined, suitable engineering controls should be devised and built into the processes.

Although general preventive measures can be outlined, it is advisable to solve each exposure problem individually after complete information on the conditions surrounding the job has been obtained.

Attention should be given to washing facilities and the kinds of soaps and cleansers that are used. Personal washing procedures as well as such protective measures as barrier creams, gloves, and other equipment should be checked also.

In addition to solvents, innumerable other primary irritants and sensitizers cause skin affections. Wherever there is skin contact with primary irritants, which may include not only strong acids and alkalis but also many other substances, there may be some incidence of dermatitis.

The type and quantity of skin irritants used in various industrial processes affect the degree of control that can be obtained, but the primary objective in every case should be complete elimination of skin contact. Preventive measures include substituting less-toxic materials, changing the process, wet methods ventilation, protective ointments, and personal protective equipment.

Some processes may require special control. For example, it may be possible to reduce exposure by lowering the temperature of the process and decreasing the air motion around the operation. (Under some conditions, however, decreased air motion may promote rather than reduce exposure. It should be kept well in mind, therefore, that every exposure may require special study.)

PHYSICAL STRESSES

Exposure to extremes of temperature or pressure, as well as radiation and noise, may impose stresses on individuals in the working environment. The industrial hygienist recognizes and evaluates these stresses as having immediate or cumulative effects on the worker's health and well-being. The recognition of these physical stresses, therefore, is as important as are the chemical and ergonomic hazards.

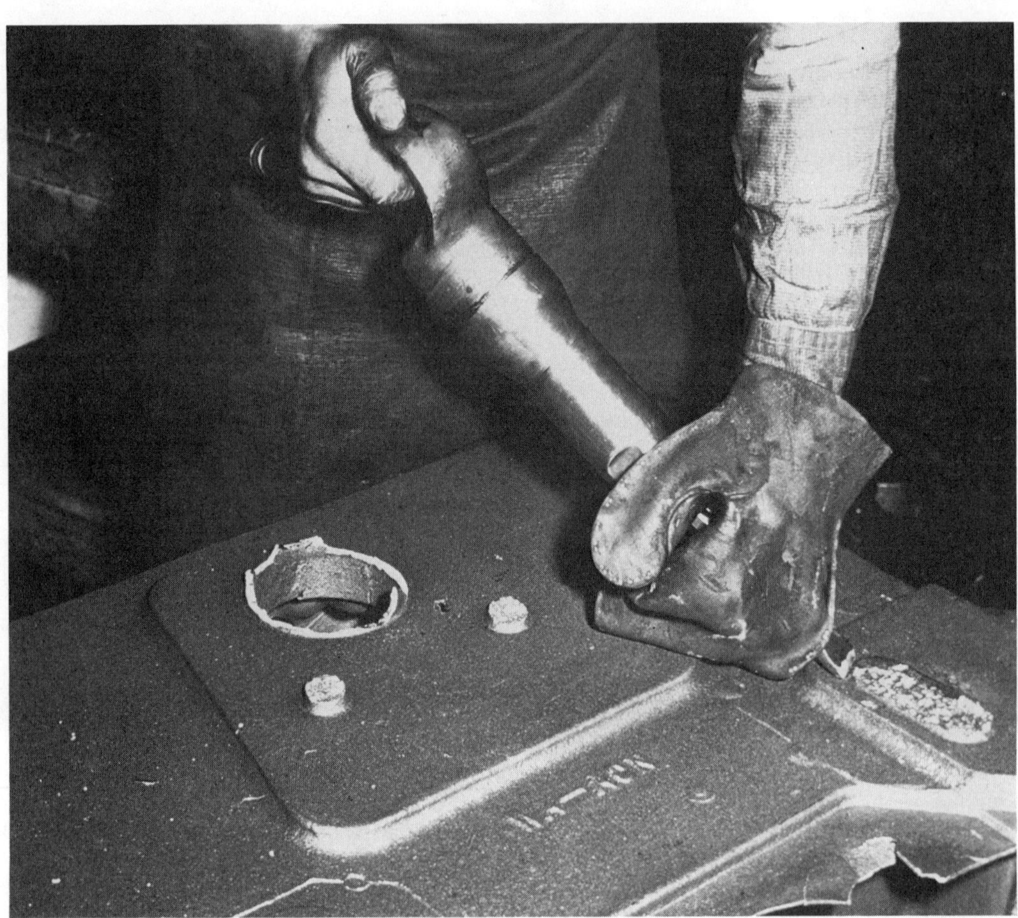

FIG 2–13.
Chipping a large iron casting using an air hammer and hardened chisel, which produces high-level noise along with vibration and at an energy expenditure that could be classified as moderate work load. Proper antinoise devices must be worn by worker.

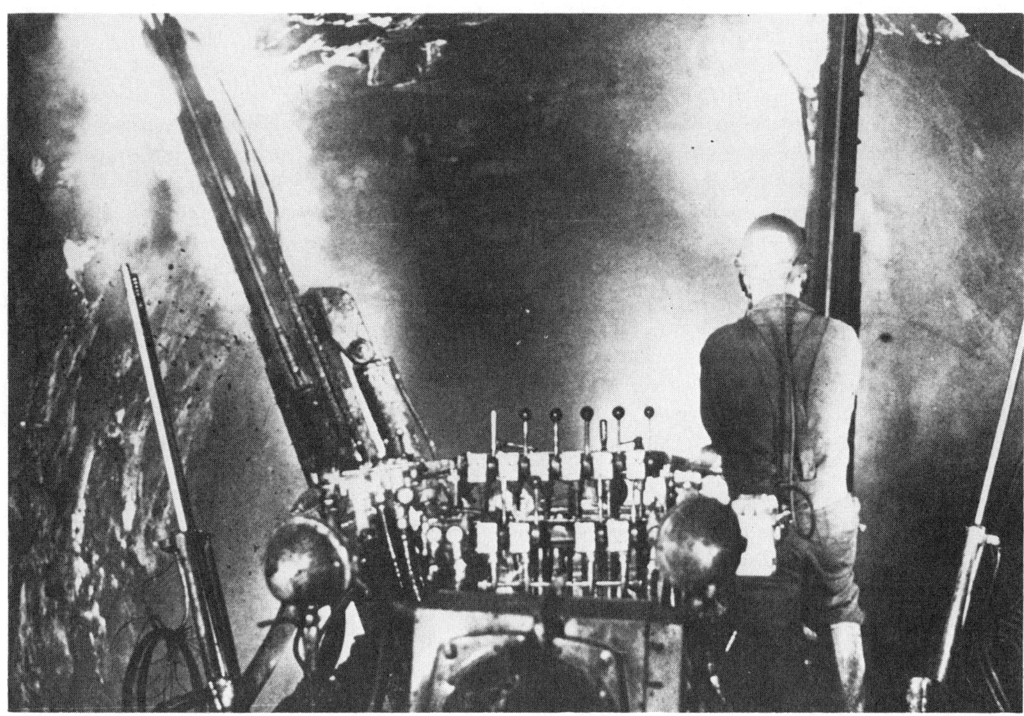

FIG 2–14.
Drilling rig in tunneling work. With hard-rock tunneling and mining, noise is a common physical stress, as are several other hazards, such as dusts, mists, gases, and, often, high temperatures and increased humidity.

Noise

Noise may be defined as "unwanted sound." It is a form of vibration that may be conducted through solids, liquids, or gases.

Noise has psychologic effects; for example, it can startle, annoy, and disrupt concentration, sleep, or relaxation.

Noise can interfere with communication by speech and, as a consequence, interfere with job performance and safety.

Noise has physiologic effects; for example, noise-induced loss of hearing, or aural pain and nausea (when the exposure is severe) (Figs 2–13 and 2–14).

Damage Risk Criteria

If the ear is subjected to high levels of noise for a sufficient period, some loss of hearing may occur. A number of factors can influence the effect of the noise exposure. Among these are

1. Variation in individual susceptibility
2. The total energy of the sound
3. The frequency distribution of the sound
4. Other characteristics of the noise exposure, such as whether it is continuous, intermittent, or made up of a series of impacts
5. The total daily time of exposure
6. The length of employment in the noise environment

Because of the complex relationships of noise and exposure time to threshold shift (reduction in hearing level) and the many possible contributory causes, establishment of criteria for protecting workers against hearing loss presents many difficulties. An added complication is whether such criteria should be designed to protect against any hearing loss or just loss in the speech frequency range, which is the only portion ordinarily considered for compensation purposes.

An effective hearing conservation program should be undertaken where exposure to industrial noise is capable of producing hearing loss. Such a program should include (1) noise exposure analysis, (2) control of noise exposure, and (3) measurement of hearing. (See Chapter 20.)

Ionizing Radiation

A brief description of ionizing radiation hazards is given here; there is an extensive discussion in Chapter 26.

Gamma radiation from radioactive materials and X radiation are highly penetrating and may produce damage in any tissue of the body. What tissue will be damaged depends in part on the energy of the radiation and in part on the relative sensitivity of the tissue.

Alpha and beta radiation are generally also considered with gamma and X radiation, although they are not as penetrating and usually are warded off by the skin. Their danger arises when the materials that produce them have been ingested and fixed in some tissue where the radiations can carry on their destruction at close range.

In the handling of some types of radioactive materials and in the operation of the high-powered particle accelerators now being used, bombardment by high-speed protons and by both high-speed and thermal neutrons must also be considered a possible hazard to health.

These types of radiation all cause injury by ionizing the tissue in which they are absorbed. Such injuries differ widely in location and extent, but the determining factors are the ability of the particular radiation to penetrate through the tissues and the amount of ionization produced by a given physical amount of the radiation. Alpha radiation, for instance, is classed as 20 times as biologically effective as X radiation because the alpha particles are heavy and possess a great ability to disrupt and ionize the tissue molecules with which they come into contact.

X radiation is produced by high-potential electrical discharge in a vacuum and should be anticipated in evacuated electrical apparatus operating at a potential of 10,000 volts or more. Although X radiation is certain to be produced in such apparatus, it is dangerous only if it penetrates the jacket of the apparatus and enters the inhabited part of the workroom.

If one is being overexposed to the radiation of a comparatively low-voltage x-ray tube, an x-ray dermatitis of the hand generally is the first result to be seen. It is characterized by a rough, dry skin, a wart-like growth, and dry, brittle nails. With continuing exposure and somewhat more penetrating X radiation, bone destruction will develop.

Although this discussion is concerned primarily with X radiation and gamma radiation because they are the best known, the same statements apply qualitatively to other types of penetrating radiation. The general method for preventing injuries from any penetrating radiation is separation from them by distance or by shielding with heavy substances in sufficient quantity to reduce the radiation received to below the maximal permissible dose and by limiting the time of exposure.

Nonionizing Radiation

Electromagnetic radiation has varying effects on the body, depending largely on the particular wavelength of the radiation involved. Some hazards associated with different regions of the nonionizing electromagnetic radiation spectrum are described in this section.

The longer wavelengths—including power frequencies, broadcast radio and shortwave radio—can produce general heating of the body. The health hazard from these radiations is very small, however, since it is unlikely that they would be found in intensities great enough to cause significant effect.

Microwaves have wavelengths of 3 m to 3 mm (100–100,000 megahertz [MHz]). They are found in radar, communications, diathermy applications, and food-cooking devices. Microwave intensities may be sufficient to cause significant local heating of tissues.

The effect is related to wavelength, power intensity, and time of exposure. Generally, the longer wavelengths will produce a greater temperature rise in deeper tissues than will the shorter wavelengths. However, for a given power intensity there is less subjective awareness to the heat from longer wavelengths than there is to the heat from shorter wavelengths because of its absorption beneath the body's surface.

An intolerable rise in body temperature, as well as localized damage, can result from an exposure of sufficient intensity and time. In addition, flammable gases and vapors may ignite when they are inside metallic objects located in a microwave beam.

Power intensities for microwaves are given in units of watts per square centimeter. Areas having a power intensity of more than 0.01 watt per sq cm should be avoided. In such areas, dummy loads should be used to absorb the energy output while equipment is being operated or tested. If a dummy load cannot be used, adjacent populated areas should be protected by adequate shielding.

Infrared radiation does not penetrate below the superficial layer of the skin, so its only effect is to heat the skin and the tissues immediately below it. Except for thermal burns, the health hazard on exposure to conventional infrared radiation sources is negligible.

Excessive exposure of the eyes to radiation, mainly visible and infrared radiation, from furnaces and similar hot bodies has been said for many years to produce "glass blower's cataract" or "heat cataract." This condition is an opacity of the rear surface of the lens of the eye.

Visible radiation and ultraviolet radiation also do not penetrate appreciably below the skin; their effect is essentially heating on the surface. The effects of the ultraviolet (UV) waves are much more violent than are those of the visible or infrared—a severe burn can be produced with no warning whatever and significant damage to the lens of the eye can occur from excessive exposure.

Since ultraviolet radiation in industry may be found around electrical arcs, they should be shielded by materials opaque to the ultraviolet. Opacity in the ultraviolet has no relation to opacity in the visible part of the spectrum. Ordinary window glass, for instance, is almost completely opaque to the ultraviolet although transparent to the visible. A piece of plastic dyed a deep red-violet may be almost entirely opaque in the visible part of the spectrum and transparent in the near ultraviolet.

Electric welding arcs (Figs 2–15 and 2–16) and germicidal

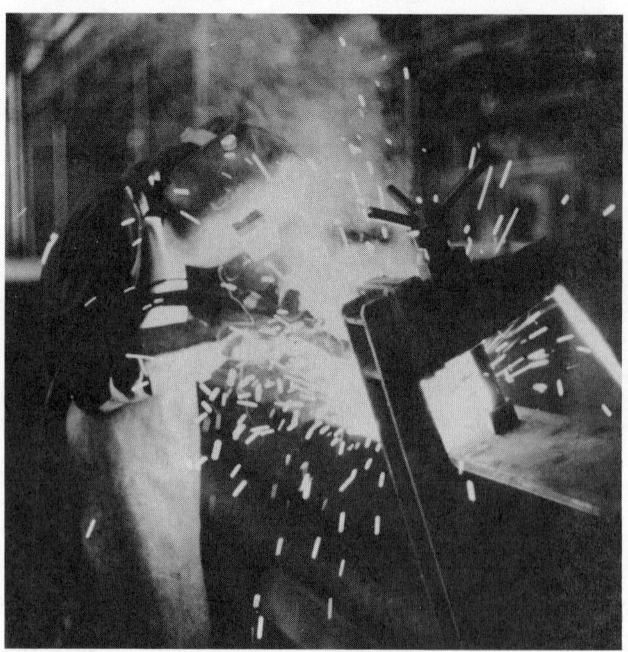

FIG 2–15.
A typical welding scene.

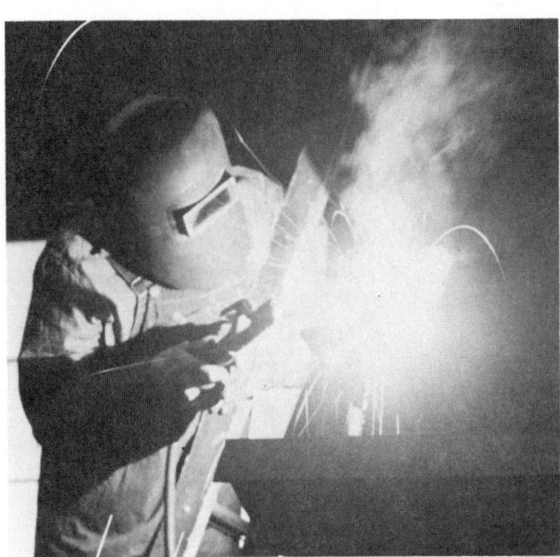

FIG 2–16.
A typical welding scene.

lamps are the most common strong producers of ultraviolet in industry. The ordinary fluorescent lamp generates a good deal of ultraviolet inside the bulb, but it is essentially absorbed in the glass bulb and its fluorescent coating.

The most common exposure to ultraviolet radiation is from direct sunshine. Persons who continually work outdoors in the full light of the sun may develop tumors on exposed areas of the skin, and these tumors occasionally turn malignant.

Ultraviolet radiation from the sun also increases the skin effects of some industrial materials. After exposure to such compounds as cresols, the skin is exceptionally sensitive to the sun. Even a short exposure in the late afternoon when the sun is low is likely to produce a severe sunburn. There are compounds that minimize the effect of UV rays. Some of these are used in certain protective creams. (See Chapter 27 for greater discussion.)

Lasers

Lasers emit beams of coherent light of a single color or wavelength and frequency, in contrast to conventional light sources, which produce random, disordered light wave mixtures of various frequencies. The laser (*l*ight *a*mplification by *s*timulated *e*mission of *r*adiation) is made up of light waves that are nearly parallel to one another, all traveling in the same direction. Light-emitting atoms are "pumped" full of energy and stimulated to fall to a lower energy level, giving off light waves that are directed to produce the coherent laser beam.

The maser, the laser's predecessor, emits microwaves instead of light. Some companies call their lasers "optical masers." Proposed uses for the laser include machining and cutting of metals, and welding of microscopic parts and systems for high-capacity communications.

Since the laser is highly collimated (has a small divergence angle), it can have a large energy density in a narrow beam. Direct viewing of the laser, therefore, should be avoided. The work area should contain no reflective surfaces (such as mirrors or highly polished furniture), for even a reflected laser beam can be hazardous. Suitable shielding to contain the laser beam should be provided.

Biologic Effects

The eye is the organ most vulnerable to injury induced by laser energy. The reason for this is the ability of the cornea and lens to focus the parallel laser beam on a small spot on the retina.

The fact that infrared radiation of certain lasers may not be visible to the naked eye contributes to the potential hazard.

Lasers generating in the ultraviolet range of the electromagnetic spectrum produce corneal burns rather than retinal damage because of the way the eye handles ultraviolet light.

Other factors that have a bearing on the degree of eye injury induced by laser light are (1) the pupil size—the smaller the pupil diameter the less the amount of laser energy permitted to the retina, (2) the power of the cornea and lens to focus the incident light on the retina, (3) the distance from the source of energy to the retina, (4) the energy and wavelength of the laser, (5) the pigmentation of the subject, (6) the place on the retina where the light is focused, (7) the divergence of the laser light, and (8) the presence of scattering media in the light path.

Effects of Temperature Extremes

Probably the most elementary factor of environmental control is control of the thermal environment in which people work. General experience shows that extremes of temperature affect the amount of work that a person can do and the manner in which it is done. The industrial problem more often is that of exposure to high temperatures rather than low temperatures (Figs 2–17 and 2–18).

The body is continually producing heat through its metabolic processes. Since the body processes are so designed that they can operate only within a very narrow limit of temperature, they must dissipate this heat as rapidly as it is produced if the body is to function efficiently and well. A sensitive and rapidly acting set of thermostatic devices in the body must also control the rates of its temperature-regulating processes.

Sweating probably is the most important of the temperature-regulating and heat-dissipating processes. Almost all parts of the skin are provided with sweat glands, which excrete a liquid (mostly water and a little salt) to the surface of the body. This goes on continually, even under conditions of rest.

In an individual who is resting and not under stress, the sweating rate is approximately 1 L per day, which is evaporated as rapidly as it is excreted. Under the stress of heavy work or high temperature, this sweating rate may increase to as much as 4 L (approximately 1 gal) in four hours. As much as 10–12 gm (150–190 grains) of salt per day will be lost with the water. Both the water and salt loss must be made up rather promptly if good health is to continue. In terms of stress, an individual's ability to acclimate is variable, and such stress is dangerous for those with cardiovascular problems.

If the sweat can be evaporated as rapidly as it is formed and if the heat stress is not such as to exceed the maximal sweating rate of which the body is capable, the body can maintain the necessary constant temperature.

The rate of evaporation depends on the moisture content, the

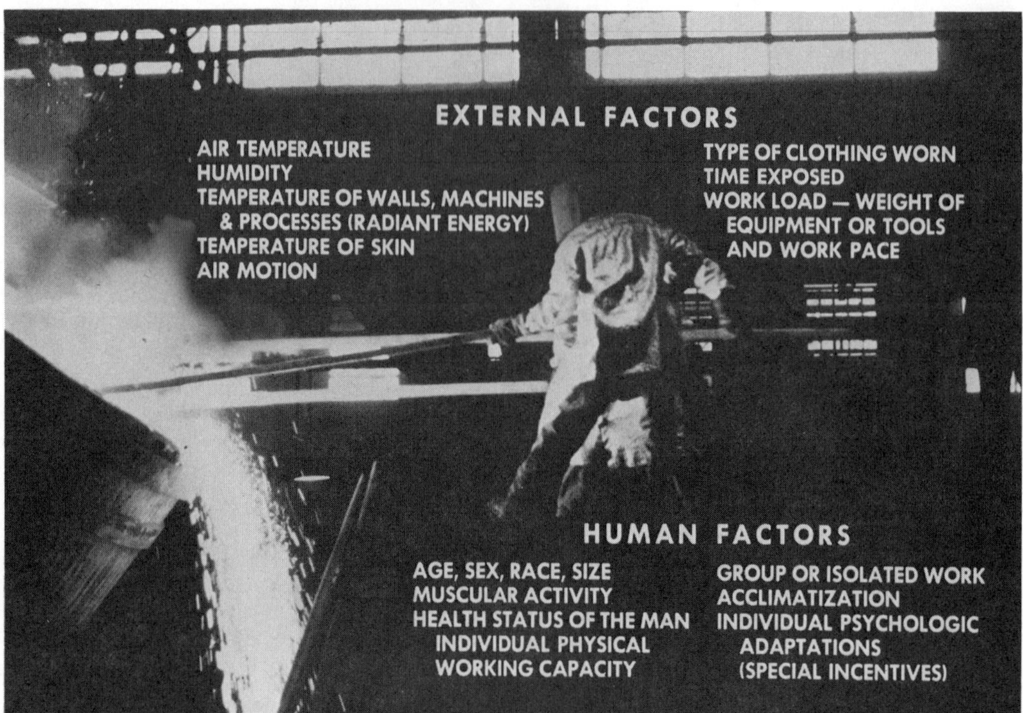

FIG 2–17.
Skimming molten iron—note special protective garment to protect against heat stress.

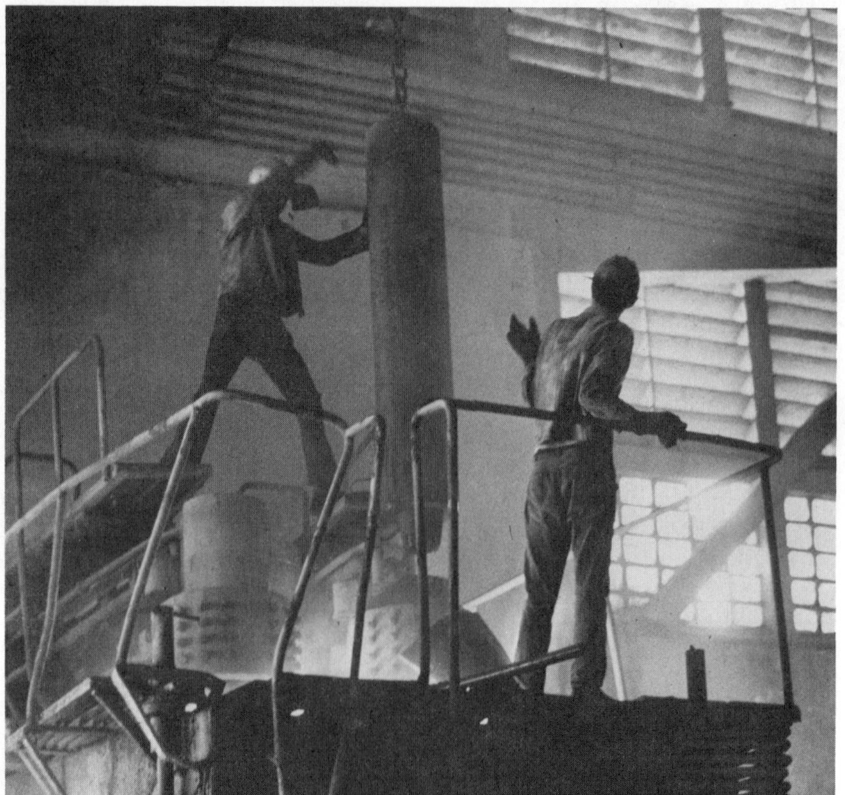

FIG 2–18.
Changing a carbon electrode for an electric furnace in a steel plant. This is an extremely hot job; fortunately, it is of short duration. Improved protective clothing would aid these workers.

rate of air movement, and the temperature of the surrounding air. The industrial hygienist must simultaneously deal with all of these factors in an attempt to determine the effect of the thermal environment on man.

Radiation accounts for some of the body's thermal equilibrium with its surroundings. If an object in the surroundings is far below body temperature, such as a large glass window on a subzero day, a large amount of heat can be radiated and the person may feel chilled even if the air in his immediate environment is fairly warm. If an object in the surroundings, such as a furnace wall, is very much above body temperature, a person may receive a large amount of heat by radiation, and it may be extremely difficult to keep him cool enough by the other available means to maintain a constant body temperature.

Radiant heat is electromagnetic energy that does no heating whatsoever until it strikes some object, such as a person, where it is absorbed. No relief from it whatsoever results from blowing air around. The only protection is to set up an invisible infrared "shadow." This can be done by placing any kind of opaque shield or screen between the person and the radiating surface. If the screen itself, however, does not reflect radiant heat, it will absorb the energy, heat up, and reradiate. Fortunately, commercial aluminum foil, aluminum sheets, and corrugated aluminum siding are all highly reflective in the infrared and are inexpensive. After locating the sources of radiant heat, shields placed between them and the employees will bring welcome relief (Fig 2–19).

Conduction through the clothing and dissipation into the air by conduction is the source of some cooling to the body. This usually is not an important means of cooling, because the conductivity of clothing and the heat capacity of air usually are low.

Conduction and convection become important means of heat loss when the body is in contact with a good cooling agent, such as water. For this reason, when people are exposed to cold water, they become chilled much more rapidly and effectively than when exposed to air at the same temperature.

Air movement cools the body by conduction and convection and also removes the film of saturated air that is formed by evaporation of sweat and replaces it with a fresh layer of air that is capable of accepting more moisture.

The *effects of high temperature* are counteracted by the body's attempt to keep the internal temperature down by increasing the rate of heartbeat. The capillaries in the skin then dilate to bring more blood to the surface so that both the rate of cooling and, gradually, the body temperature are increased.

If the thermal environment is tolerable, these measures rather soon will lead to an equilibrium where the heart rate and the body temperature remain constant. If this equilibrium is not reached until the body temperature is about 102°F (38.9°C), corresponding to a sweating rate of about 2 L per hour, there is imminent danger of heatstroke. Intermittent rest periods for persons necessarily exposed to extreme heat reduce this danger.

Heatstroke (also known as sunstroke) is not necessarily the result of exposure to the sun. It is caused by exposure to an environment in which the body is unable to cool itself sufficiently. As a result, the body temperature rises and reaches a point at which the heat-regulating mechanism breaks down completely. The body temperature then rises rapidly.

The symptoms are hot, dry skin, severe headache, visual disturbances, rapid temperature rise, and loss of consciousness. The condition is recognizable by the flushed face and high temperature. The victim should be removed from the heat immediately and his body cooled as rapidly as possible, most readily by being wrapped in cool, wet sheets. Since the condition may be quickly fatal, medical help should be obtained as soon as possible.

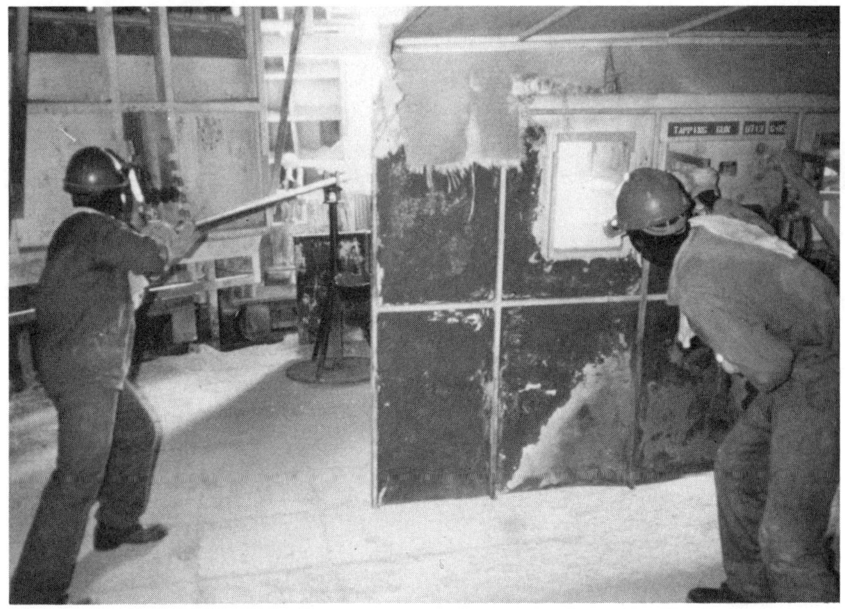

FIG 2–19.
Tapping a carbide producing furnace; intense radiant heat stress present. A practical heat reflective shield constructed mainly of aluminum and counter-balanced. (See Chapter 22 for discussion of physical work and heat stress.)

Heatstroke is a much more serious condition than heat cramps or heat exhaustion. An important predisposing factor is excessive physical exertion.

Heat cramps may result from exposure to high temperature for a relatively long time, particularly if accompanied by heavy exertion, with excessive loss of salt and moisture from the body. Even if the moisture is replaced by drinking water copiously, the excessive loss of salt may provoke heat cramps or heat exhaustion.

Heat cramps are characterized by the cramping of the muscles of either the skeletal system or the intestines. In either case, the condition may be relieved in a few hours under proper treatment, although soreness may persist for several days.

Heat exhaustion may result from physical exertion in a hot environment when vasomotor control and cardiac output are inadequate to meet the increased demand placed on them by peripheral vasodilation. Its signs are a relatively low temperature, pallor, weak pulse, dizziness, profuse sweating, and a cool, moist skin.

Experience has shown that workers do not stand a hot job very well at first but develop tolerance rapidly and acquire full endurance within a week to a month. (A complete discussion of acclimatization and physiologic responses to cold, heat, humidity, and work is to be found in Chapters 22 and 23.)

Effects of Atmospheric Pressure Changes

It has been recognized from the beginning of caisson work, dating back to about 1850, that persons working under greater than normal atmospheric pressures are subject to various ills connected with the job. The main effect (decompression sickness, commonly known as "the bends") results from the release of nitrogen bubbles into the circulation and tissues during decompression. The bubbles lodge at the joints and under muscles, causing severe cramps. To prevent this trouble, decompression is carried out slowly and by stages so that the nitrogen can be eliminated slowly and without the formation of bubbles.

Deep-sea divers are supplied with a mixture of helium and oxygen for breathing. Since helium is an inert diluent and is less soluble in blood and tissue than in nitrogen, it presents a less formidable decompression problem.

The effects of reduced pressure on the worker are much the same as the effects of decompression from a high pressure. If pressure is reduced too rapidly, decompression sickness and ear disturbances similar to, if not identical with, the divers' conditions may result.

Persons working at reduced pressure are also subject to oxygen starvation, which can have very serious and insidious effects on the senses and judgment. There is a considerable amount of evidence that exposure of unacclimatized individuals for three to four hours to an altitude of 9,000 feet above sea level without breathing an atmosphere enriched in oxygen can result in severely impaired judgment. Even if pure oxygen is provided, the altitude should be limited to that giving the same partial pressure of oxygen as air at 8,000 feet. (Hypobaric and hyperbaric conditions are discussed fully in Chapters 25 and 57.)

ERGONOMIC STRESSES

Ergonomic principles involve the interactions between the worker and such traditional environmental elements as atmospheric contaminants, heat, light, sound, and all tools and equipment pertaining to the workplace. The modern concept is that the worker is to be considered the monitoring link of a worker-machine environment system.

The components of a system can cover a wide range, including machines, tools, materials, environmental factors, people, operating instructions, and training manuals or computer programs. As parts of a system, the components usually interact and complement one another, but it is essential to recognize that a failure or malfunction of any component can affect the other components and thus degrade performance.

The environment is an important consideration in a system. Most components (worker, tools) in a system will perform their task properly only under a given set of conditions. A component that works well at normal temperatures may malfunction or fail if placed in a system near another component that generates excessive temperatures.

In any activity, a person receives and processes information and then acts on it. The receptor function occurs largely through the sense organs of the eyes and the ears, but information may also be conveyed through the sense of smell, through touch, or through sensations of heat and cold. This information is conveyed to the central mechanism of the brain and spinal cord, where the information is processed to arrive at a decision. This may involve the integration of the information that already has been stored in the brain, and decisions may vary from responses that are automatic to those that involve a high degree of reasoning or logic.

Having received the information and processed it, the individual then will take action as a result of the decision, and this he or she usually will do through muscular activity based on the skeletal framework of the body. When the activity involves the operation of a piece of equipment, the individual often will form part of a "closed-loop servo system," displaying many of the feedback characteristics of such a system. The human being usually will form the part of the system that makes decisions and he or she has a fundamental part to play in the efficiency of the system.

To achieve maximal efficiency, a worker-machine system must be designed as a whole, with the worker being complementary to the machine and the machine being complementary to the abilities of the worker. Consideration should be given to the general physical and mental demands of the task, so as not to overload the operator. There are many situations that can make excessive demands on operators, and overload can develop, unless information reaches them at a speed with which they can cope and in a form that they can easily understand. The demands should be properly spaced in time, so that they can act on them without undue mental stress. If a study of the demands of the task suggests that overload is possible, steps should be taken to bring the demands within the expected capacity of the operator and so reduce the load.

The human body can endure considerable discomfort and stress and can perform many awkward and unnatural movements—for a limited time. When, however, unnatural conditions or motions are continued for prolonged periods, the physiologic limitations of the worker may be exceeded. To ensure a high level of performance on a continuing basis, work systems must be tailored to human capacities and limitations.

Biomechanics is that phase of engineering devoted to the improvement of the worker-machine-task relationship in an effort to reduce operator discomfort and fatigue.

Biotechnology is a broader term. It encompasses biomechanics, human factors, engineering, and engineering psychology. To arrive at biotechnologic solutions to work-stress problems, the sciences of anatomy, physiology, psychology, anthropometry, and kinesiology need to be brought into play.

Program areas of concern are

1. Strictly biomechanical aspects—the consideration of stress on muscles, bones, nerves, and joints

2. Sensory aspects—the consideration of eye fatigue, color, audio signals, and the like

3. External environment—such as lighting, glare, temperature, humidity, noise, atmospheric contaminants, and vibration

4. The psychologic and social aspects of the working environment

Information obtained from a study of the above-mentioned factors can be translated into tangible changes in work environments. Among the changes that are proving to have positive effects insofar as fatigue and stress reduction are concerned are redesigned hand tools, adjustable chairs and workbenches, improvements in lighting, control of heat and humidity, and noise reduction. For additional details of ergonomic and biomechanic factors, see Chapters 19 and 28.

EVALUATION OF HEALTH HAZARDS

Evaluation may be defined as the decision-making process resulting in an opinion as to the degree of health hazard from chemical or physical agents arising out of industrial operations. The basic approach to controlling occupational disease consists of an evaluation of the potential hazard and control of the specific hazard by suitable industrial hygiene techniques.

Evaluation involves a judgment, based on the individual's past experience, of the magnitude of the environmental factors and qualitative or quantitative (or both) measurement of the chemical, physical, biologic, or ergonomic stresses. The decision as to whether a health hazard exists is based on comparing data collected in the industrial environment with hygienic guides, threshold limit values, maximal acceptable concentrations, or reports in the literature.

Hazard evaluation also requires knowledge of the properties of the air contaminants and a knowledge of their relative toxicity. Evaluation involves a measurement of the quantity that is potentially available for absorption by the user, the amount of time that is available for absorption, the frequency with which the exposure occurs, the physical form of the material or air contaminant and the presence of other toxic or nontoxic additives or contaminants.

Appropriate control measures, such as ventilation, housekeeping, protective clothing, and pertinent training for safe handling procedures, may diminish any hazard that might exist.

Hazard evaluation, therefore, requires individuals such as safety professionals, engineers, chemists, and physicians, who have been trained in the fields of toxicology, industrial hygiene, and occupational health, to recognize, measure, and control these environmental hazards.

Evaluation, in the broad sense, also refers to determining the levels of physical and chemical agents arising out of a process for purposes of studying that process and determining the effectiveness of a given piece of equipment used to control the hazards arising out of that process.

Recognition of industrial health hazards involves knowledge and understanding of the environmental stresses of the workplace and the effect of these stresses on the health of the worker. Control involves the reduction of environmental stress to values that the worker can tolerate without impairment of productivity or his health. Measurement and quantitative evaluation of environmental stress is the essential ingredient that has made modern industrial hygiene a tool for conserving the health and well-being of workers.

Basic Hazard Recognition Procedures

There is a basic, systematic procedure that can be followed in the recognition and evaluation of environmental health hazards:

What is produced?

What raw material is used?

What materials are added in the process?

What by-products are produced?

What equipment is involved?

What is the cycle of operations?

What operational procedures are used?

What health and safety controls are utilized?

What is the level of exposure to harmful chemical or physical agents?

How many employees are exposed and for how long?

Detailed information should be obtained regarding what hazardous materials are used within a plant, type of job operation, how the workers are exposed, work pattern, levels of air contamination, duration of exposure, what control measures are used, and other pertinent information. The hazard potential of the material is determined not only by its inherent toxicity but also by the conditions of use—who uses what, where, and for how long?

To recognize hazardous environmental factors or stresses, a safety professional must first know about the raw materials used and the nature of the products and by-products manufactured. Sometimes this requires considerable effort. If you do not find the information you need, ask your supplier. Use caution in applying the information from one supplier to the product of another supplier. If your supplier simply says, "We don't have any trouble handling it," ask how the supplier handles it so that there is no trouble. Any material can be handled safely if the proper handling procedures are observed.

Any individual who is responsible for the maintenance of a safe, healthful work environment should be thoroughly acquainted with the levels of harmful materials, stress, or other potentially

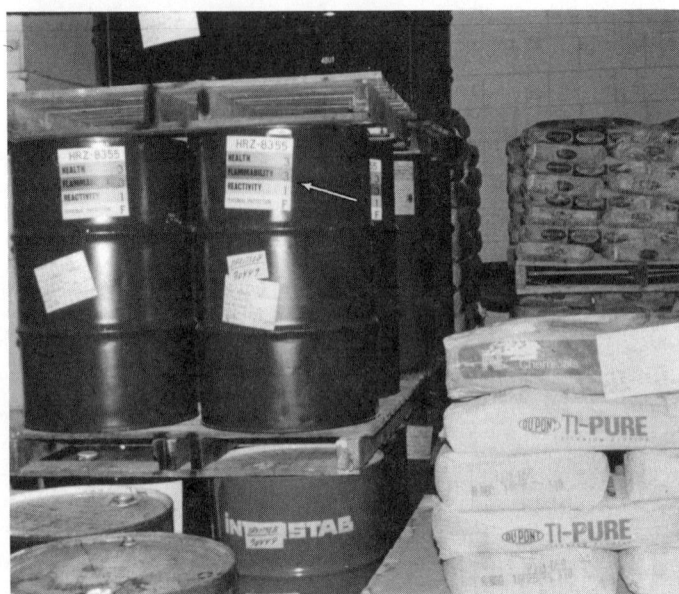

FIG 2–20.
Good housekeeping evident along with clear labels (arrow). (See Chapter 1 for label details.)

hazardous conditions that may be encountered in the industrial environment for which he or she is responsible (Fig 2–20) (see Chapter 1).

If a plant is going to handle a hazardous material, it is necessary for the safety professional to consider all the unexpected events that can occur and what precautions need to be taken to prevent atmospheric release of a toxic material. After these considerations have been studied and proper countermeasures installed during the design of the operation, process, or plant, it is necessary to instruct operating and maintenance personnel on the proper operation of the health and safety control measures. Only in this way can they be made aware of the hazards that could exist and the reasons for the requirements for certain built-in safety features.

The operating and maintenance personnel should set up a routine procedure (at frequent stated intervals) for testing the industrial hygiene and safety provisions that are not used in normal, ordinary plant operations.

A list should be prepared of all raw materials actually in use within the plant, together with those that may be contemplated for early future use. Possibly the best and earliest source of information concerning such materials is the purchasing agent. Accordingly, it is strongly recommended that a close liaison be set up between the purchasing agent and health and safety personnel so that early information will be provided concerning materials in use and those that are to be ordered.

Checklists

A checklist for evaluating environmental hazards arising out of industrial operations is presented here. It should be modified to fit each particular situation.

Overall Process or Operation

1. List all hazardous chemical or physical agents used or formed in the process. For each chemical agent or material:

List the conditions necessary for it to be released to the workroom atmosphere. (Does it normally occur in the process as a dust, mist, fume, or vapor, as a low-volatile liquid, or as a solid? What process conditions could cause material to be sprayed or discharged into the workroom atmosphere as a liquid aerosol or dust cloud?)

List the airborne concentration levels in the workroom atmosphere that normally would be present as a function of time. List the peak airborne concentration levels as a function of event duration.

2. For all raw materials used in the process, consider chemical reactions that could take place to produce other toxic materials (for example, vapors from a degreaser drifting into an arc-welding area).

3. List the levels of those physical agents that normally may be present such as electromagnetic radiations or noise.

Process Equipment

1. List those pieces of equipment containing sufficient hazardous material to produce a hazard if their contents were suddenly released to the environment.

2. List those pieces of equipment that could produce hazardous levels of physical agents during normal or abnormal plant operations.

3. List the machinery and equipment that may produce hazardous concentrations of airborne contaminants.

For each item listed under 1, 2, and 3 indicate the control measures installed to minimize the hazard. Is the health and safety control measure adequate and reliable?

After the list of processes and operations that produce chemical and physical agents to which employees are exposed has been prepared, it is necessary to determine which of the process operations produce conditions that could result in hazardous exposures and need further study.

After the materials and processes are named or determined, material properties, effects and process flows, including pressures, temperatures, and humidity involved, should be reviewed.

A simple process flow sheet could be drawn that will show, stepwise, the introduction of each material and the product of each step. A material and process hazard-and-effects checklist should be established. Some sources of information to assist in preparing this list are data sheets published by the National Safety Council, the American Industrial Hygiene Association, and the Manufacturing Chemists' Association.

In many industrial operations, many different hazards may exist simultaneously. Therefore, it is necessary to examine carefully the overall process in order not to overlook potentially hazardous conditions.

There are many types of industrial operations that should arouse immediate suspicion of a health hazard, unless there is specific information that a process is controlled adequately.

The list of industrial operations shown in Table 2–1 is adapted from the OSHA Compliance Operations Manual and may be of help in alerting the industrial physician to the source and types of possible health hazards.

TABLE 2–1.
Typical Plant Processes That May Produce Health Hazards*

PROCESS OR OPERATION	NATURE AND DESCRIPTION OF HAZARDS
Abrasive blasting	Abrasive blasting equipment may be automatic or manually operated. Either type may use sand, steel shot or artificial abrasives. The dust levels of workroom air should be examined to make certain that the operators are not overexposed
Assembly operations	Improper positioning of equipment and handling of work parts present ergonomic hazards due to repeated awkward motion resulting in excessive stresses
Babbitting	Fumes and dusts of oxides of antimony, lead, tin, and zinc
Bagging and handling of dry materials	Conveying, sifting, sieving, screening, packaging, or bagging of any dry material may present a dust hazard. The transfer of dry, finely divided powder may result in the formation of considerable quantities of airborne dust. Inhalation and skin contact hazards may be present
Ceramic coating	Ceramic coating may present the hazard of airborne dispersion of toxic pigments plus hazards of heat stress from the furnaces and hot ware
Coal handling	Dusts and gases of carbon monoxide, coal, free silica, and sulfur dioxide
Coke handling	Coke and free silica dust
Coking	Contaminants encountered: ammonia, benzene, carbon disulfide, carbon monoxide, cyanamides, hydrogen sulfide, naphthalene and other polycyclics, phenols, pyridine, and sulfur dioxide
Dry grinding	Dry grinding operations should be examined for airborne dust and ergonomic hazards
Dry mixing	Mixing of dry material may present a dust hazard and should take place in completely enclosed mixers whenever air sampling indicates that excessive amounts of airborne dust are present
Electro-tinning (alkaline and halogen)	Mists of caustics, chromates, fluorides, and sulfuric acid
Electron beam welding	Any process involving an electric discharge in a vacuum may be a source of ionizing radiation. Such processes include electron beam equipment and similar devices
Fabric and paper coating	The coating and impregnating of fabric and paper with plastic or rubber solutions may involve evaporation into the workroom air of large quantities of solvents
Ferromanganese handling	Dust and gases of ferromanganese and hydrogen
Forming and forging	Hot bending, forming, or cutting of metals or nonmetals may have the hazards of lubricant mist, decomposition products of the lubricant, skin contact with the lubricant, heat stress (including radiant heat), noise, and dust
Furnace operations	Dusts, fumes, and gases of carbon monoxide, iron oxide, other combustion products and metal oxides, and sulfur dioxide
Galvanizing	Production of fumes, gases and mists of ammonium chloride, chromates, hydrochloric acid, hydrogen chloride, lead oxides, and zinc oxide
Gas furnace or oven heating operations (annealing, baking, drying, etc.)	Any gas- or oil-fired combustion process should be examined to determine the level of by-products of combustion that may be released into the workroom atmosphere. Noise measurements should also be made to determine the level of burner noise
Grinding	Grinding, crushing, or comminuting of any material may present the hazard of contamination of workroom air due to the dust of the material being processed or of the grinding wheel (Figs 2–21 and 2–22)

(continued)

TABLE 2–1. *Continued*

PROCESS OR OPERATION	NATURE AND DESCRIPTION OF HAZARDS
High temperatures from hot castings, unlagged steam pipes, process equipment, etc.	Any process or operation involving high ambient temperatures (dry-bulb temperature), radiant heat load (globe temperature) or excessive humidity (wet-bulb temperature) should be examined to determine the magnitude of the physical stresses that may be present
Leaded steelmaking	Dusts and fumes of iron oxide and lead oxide
Materials handling, warehousing	Work areas should be checked for levels of carbon monoxide and oxides of nitrogen arising from internal combustion engine fork-lift operations
Metalizing	A high-temperature coating of parts ("spraying," Fig 2–23) with molten metals presents hazards of dust and fumes of metals and their oxides, fluxes, carbon monoxide, in addition to heat and nonionizing radiation
Microwave and radiofrequency heating operations	Any process or operation involving microwaves or induction heating should be examined to determine the magnitude of heating effects and, in some cases, noise exposure on the employees
Molten metals	Any process involving the melting and pouring of molten metals should be examined to determine the level of air contaminants of any toxic gas, metal fume or dust produced in the operation (see Fig 2–2). Acrolein often is produced
Ore handling	Dusts of fluorides, free silica, and iron oxide
Paint spraying	Paint spraying operations should be examined for the possibility of hazards from inhalation and skin contact with toxic and irritating solvents and inhalation of toxic pigments (cadmium, chromates and lead). The solvent vapor evaporating from the sprayed surface also may be a source of hazard, because ventilation may be provided only for the paint spray booth (Figs 2–24 and 2–25)
Pickling	Generation of gases and mists of hydrochloric acid, hydrogen chloride, hydrogen fluoride, oxides of nitrogen, and sulfuric acid
Plating	Electroplating processes involve risk of skin contact with strong chemicals and, in addition, may present a respiratory hazard if mist or gases from the plating solutions are dispersed into the workroom air. Most commonly, these can be acids, alkalis, chromic acid mist, etc. (see Fig 2–3)
Punch press, press brake, drawing operations, etc.	Cold bending, forming, or cutting of metals or nonmetals should be examined for hazards of contact with lubricant, inhalation of lubricant mist, and excessive noise
Refractories handling	Free silica dust
Sintering	Dusts and gases of carbon monoxide, fluorides, free silica, iron oxides, and sulfur dioxide
Solvent degreasing	Vapors of perchloroethylene, trichloroethylene, vapor decomposition products (e.g., phosgene), and others
Steelmaking (material handling)	Dusts of fluorspar, graphite, iron oxide, limestone, mill scale, and ore
Tandem rolling mills	Oil mist
Vapor degreasing	The removal of oil and grease from metal products may present hazards. This operation should be examined to determine that excessive amounts of vapor are not being released into the workroom atmosphere
Welding, gas or electric-arc (also "Brazing")	Any process involving the melting and joining of metal parts should be examined for fumes and gases. Oxides of cadmium, chromium, fluorides, iron, manganese, nickel, nitrogen, and vanadium may form, as well as pyrolysis by-products from fluxes and coatings. If there is an arc or spark discharge, the effects of radiation and the products of destruction of the electrodes should be investigated. These operations also commonly involve hazards of high-potential electrical circuits of low internal resistance (see Fig 2–16)
Wet grinding	Wet grinding of any material may produce possibly hazards of mist, dust, and noise
Wet mixing	Mixing of wet materials may present possible hazards of solvent vapors, mists, and possibly dust. The noise levels produced by the associated equipment should be checked

*This material is adapted in part and expanded from the OSHA *Compliance Operations Manual.*

Exposure Levels

To determine exposure levels atmospheric contaminants quantitatively, as well as to measure physical energy stresses, direct-reading instruments or laboratory analytical methods can be used. The particular exposure can be evaluated by chemical analyses of air samples and a detailed step-by-step investigation of the operations conducted to find the areas in which employees are exposed to hazardous amounts of airborne material. The operational analysis should also determine how the material becomes airborne and is dispersed.

The type and extent of controls will depend on the evaluation made of the exposure and the operation that disperses the contaminant.

Industrial hygiene investigations are performed to determine a five-dimensional pattern. The three dimensions of space determine simply where the harmful chemical or physical agent is. By adding a fourth dimension of time, we determine when it is where.

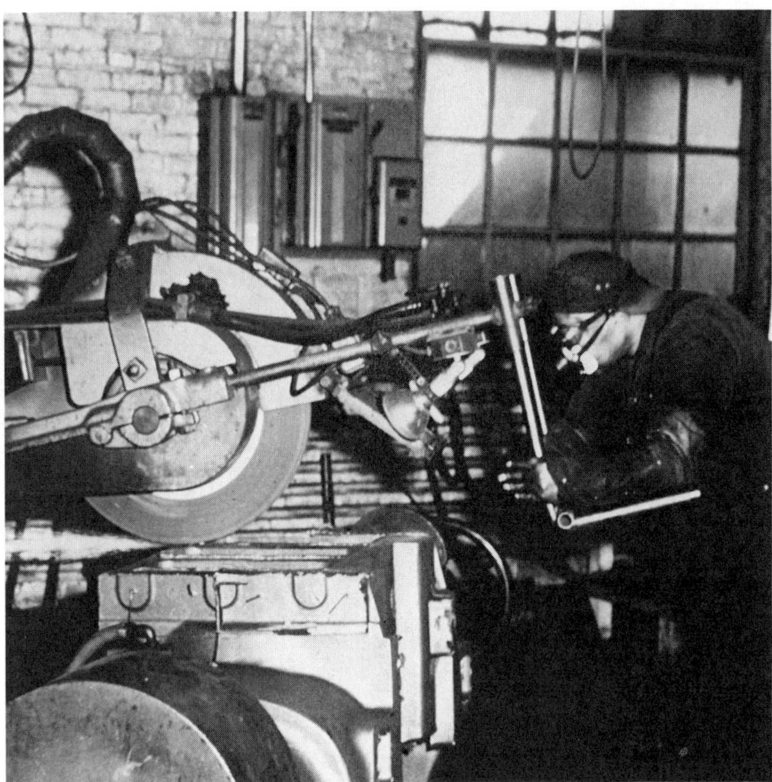

FIG 2–21.
"Swing grinder" grinding a large casting. Note local exhaust ventilation to collecting system. In addition, the worker uses a respirator.

The fifth dimension is man's movement within the space-time envelope, which recognizes that man's exposure depends on where he is when. Although the integration and expression of all this is not a simple matter, it is the best definition of the probability of exposure in a given set of circumstances. This concentration-space-time-man movement pattern is not a constant but a highly variable circumstance.

The harmful effects of deleterious chemical agents are determined by the amount accumulated in the body—by the total dosage. The number of milligrams of harmful material per kilogram of body weight deposited at sensitive sites determines the toxic effect produced. This often is overlooked when expressing individual exposures only in terms of concentration (parts per million) in the air breathed and the length of time of exposure. The amount in the inspired air is not necessarily the amount absorbed.

Differences in particle size or solubility, which, in many cases, are practically impossible to measure accurately, determine the fraction of inhaled impurity that is retained or absorbed. For example, the concentration in the inspired air of Parathion, or solvents, may not be a valid indication of the true exposure of an individual. The absorbed dose also depends on whether or not there is significant skin absorption or ingestion.

There are situations in which analyses of the workroom air alone are not adequate to evaluate precisely the degree of hazard, because the amount absorbed by exposed individuals cannot be predicted from the data obtained by such determinations. In such situations, it is highly desirable to have other means of estimating exposure. With many substances, this can be done by analyzing suitable biologic specimens or excretion products for the toxic agent or a metabolite derived therefrom.

The only biologic fluid finding much application for such exposure tests is blood; limited use has been made of biopsy specimens of lung, skin, and fat, but these are not very practicable for periodic sampling. The excretory products analyzed most frequently are urine and breath; sweat, another major excretion product, is not well adapted for exposure tests.

Special medical examinations, preplacement and periodic, may be required for those employees in occupations involving exposure to some hazardous materials. For example, employees to be placed in occupations involving exposure to a pneumoconiosis-producing dust should be given a chest x-ray and those to be exposed to toxic substances should be given the same clinical tests that will be used later in periodic examinations to provide baseline values in addition to a complete medical examination.

The intervals at which these special procedures are conducted should be determined by the severity of the hazard and modified as the hazard is brought under control.

Representative Air Samples

The importance of the sampling location, the proper time to sample, and the number of samples to be taken during the course

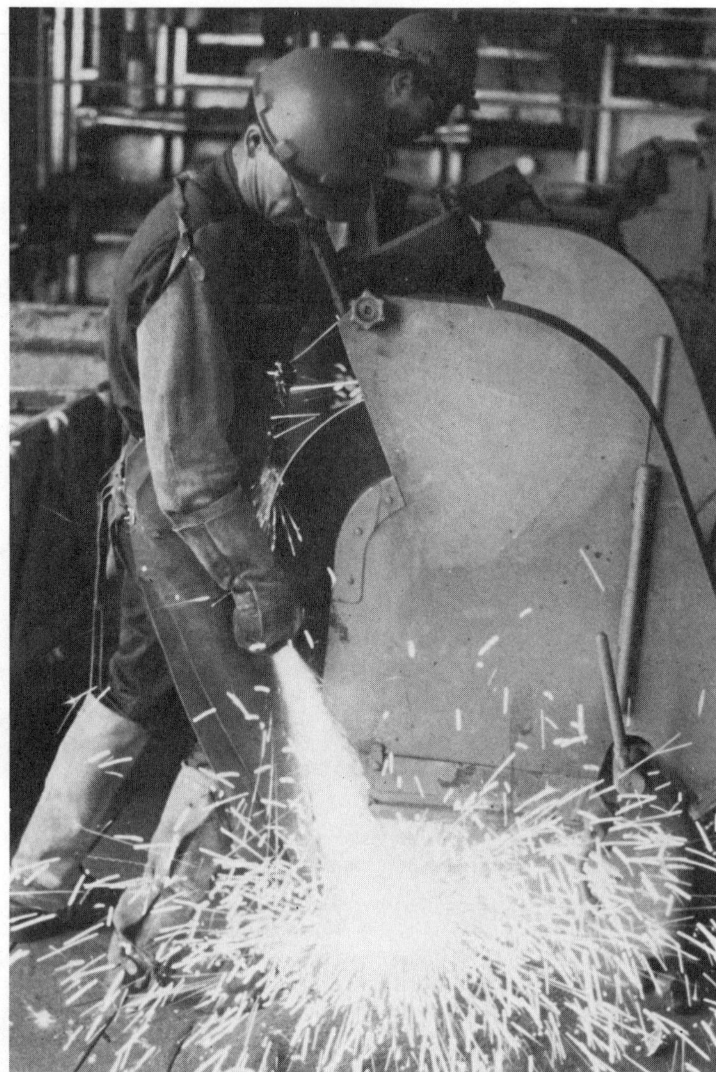

FIG 2–22.
Grinding a steel casting with an inadequate local exhaust system.

of an investigation of the work environment cannot be overstressed.

The selection of an air-sampling method to determine the levels of air contaminants is so dependent on the particular substances and operation involved that no single outline of approach is universally acceptable. Although spot samples, which are also called grab samples, have their useful aspects when used intelligently, they are not sufficient to define every work environment in all cases.

Chemical and physical agents that do not represent too serious a problem may be sampled for and measured periodically in accordance with good industrial hygiene practices. These samples must be so taken as to be truly representative of the concentrations inhaled by workers under actual working conditions. Enough samples should be taken in the breathing zone of workers to define peak concentrations and allow for the calculation of a time-weighted average.

Where there is a potential for serious difficulty, particularly where high-hazard materials are handled in large quantities, continuous monitoring of levels of atmospheric concentration is very desirable. Sampling points should be located at work stations, in areas frequented by workers and in areas where leakage of contaminants to the atmosphere is most likely to occur. The sampling method used should give a valid and reliable measure of the concentration of the air contaminant in space and time.

Number of Tests

An adequate number of tests should be performed to enable one to define the time-weighted average exposure. Air samples must be taken to characterize the peak emissions during various portions of the entire process cycle, in addition to those taken to determine the average level. Air samples collected within an extremely short sampling period may miss the peak concentrations that occur between tests.

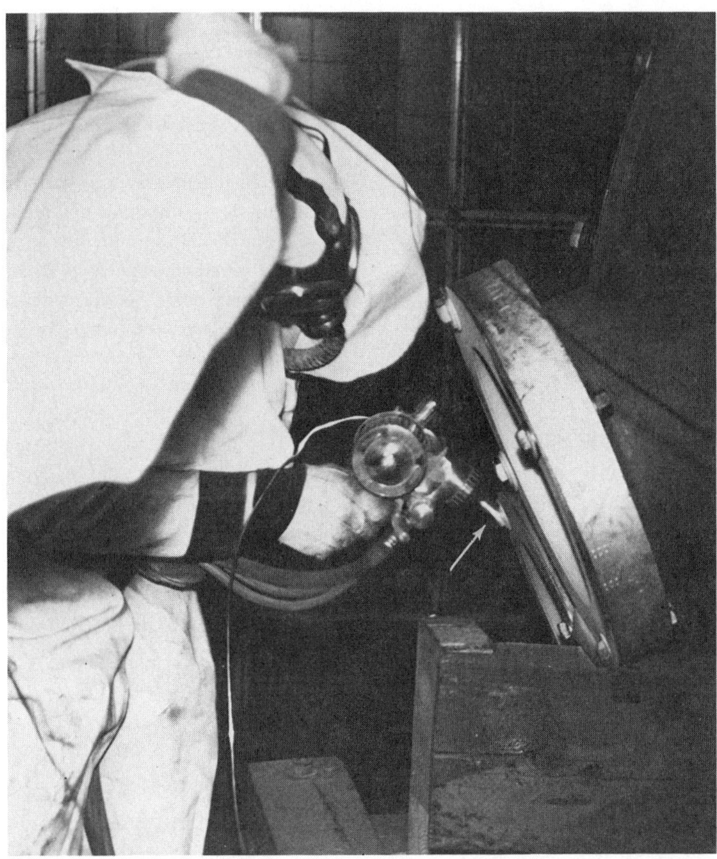

FIG 2–23.
A metalizing operation spraying pure lead *(arrow)*. Although the large object being coated with lead is enclosed in a paint spray booth, the workers are further protected with full-body suits and external air supply.

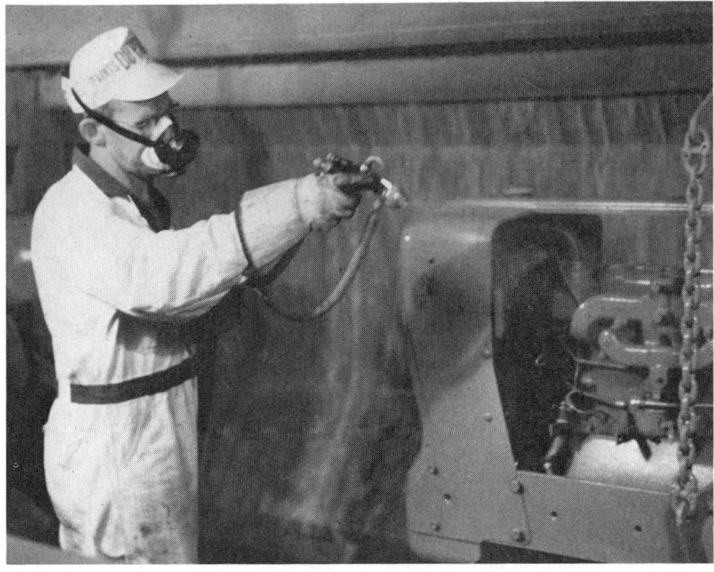

FIG 2–24.
Spray painting in a highly exhausted paint spray booth with water circulating in back of booth to trap particulate matter. Solvent vapors are exhausted away from the worker; in addition, he wears protective clothing.

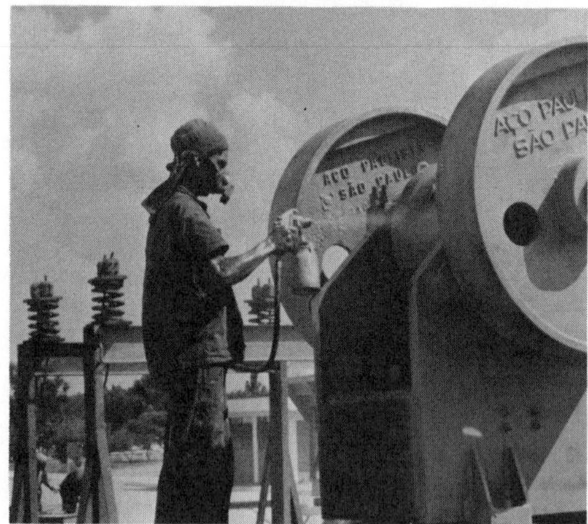

FIG 2–25.
Spray painting outdoors also requires proper protective equipment as is shown here.

In ambient air sampling, a paradox may be encountered. An analysis of a spot or grab sample can be a fairly precise measurement of a small, well-defined sample volume. However, if sampling is continued, using a single sample collector over an extended period, an average value will be obtained, but this does not indicate how the concentration may have varied during the sampling period. It does give information as to the average overall level.

Other Factors

Other factors to be considered in the evaluation of hazards are changes that occur in plant operations during the day or night shifts, contributions to exposure from adjacent operations, and seasonal variations. Another factor to consider is whether the presence of the sampler affects the test result.

Inexperienced personnel, when confronted with an analysis of an isolated air sample of high concentration, conceivably might shut down a relatively safe operation, resulting in considerable embarrassment and financial loss. In other situations, if the limitations of the sampling method and instruments are not understood by the investigator, a serious exposure may be overlooked—it is quite possible to obtain low, seemingly safe average readings but have an extremely hazardous condition. Professional judgment is necessary to reach an intelligent decision, depending on the nature of the hazard.

Sufficient knowledge of the operation or process, particularly its relative magnitude at a given time, is essential for good evaluation of exposure. For example, air samples taken during a production cutback would yield low results, not representative of conditions of exposure under normal operating conditions.

Concentrations of atmospheric contaminants fluctuate as a process cycles, as leaks occur or as misoperation occurs. Do not assume that all manufacturing operations produce air contaminants at the same steady level all day long.

Prior to making any test of the workroom air, the user must have a thorough knowledge of the nature of the contaminant in question and of the other substances likely to be present in the atmosphere in order to make a proper choice of sampling method.

WHERE TO MEASURE

What must be measured and evaluated in industrial hygiene sampling is the duration of exposure and concentration. For the concentration measurement, a test can be made on the air in the worker's breathing zone (Figs 2–26, 2–27, and 2–28).

In some cases, the measuring instrument can be attached directly to the worker, and he can carry it throughout the working day. This is done, for example, with a noise dosimeter for measuring noise exposure or a battery-powered air sampler to collect particulates. This gives an integrated sample.

The other technique is to measure the concentration in the employee's breathing zone over carefully selected intervals, then average the results and weight each measurement according to the length of exposure—the result is a time-weighted average concentration.

Obtaining a satisfactory average exposure measurement during a particular time period is affected by changes from day shift to night shift, from winter to summer, routine changes in process operations, or daily changes in rate and direction of air movement

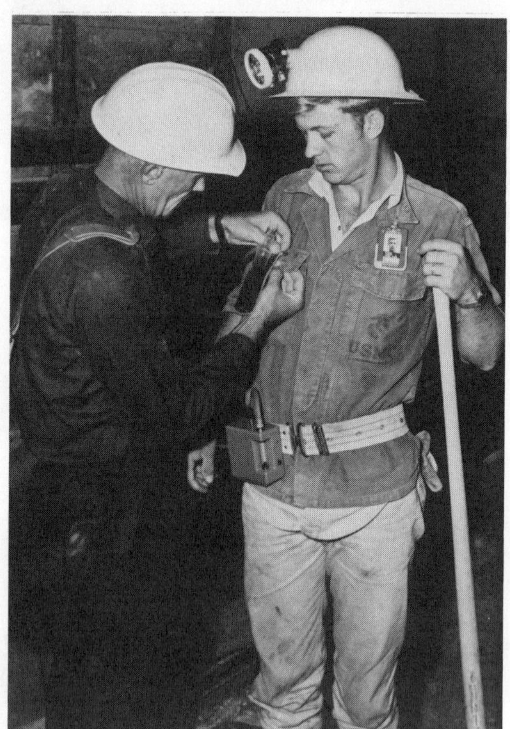

FIG 2–26.
A miner at the Nevada Atomic Test Site is equipped with a midget impinger and Mine-Safety-Appliance Monitaire Sampler. The portable instrument measures toxic and combustible gases and vapors, radioactive dusts, fumes and mists, and air pollutants. The M-S-A Monitaire Sampler is used in tunnels, shafts, emplacement rooms near the bottom of vertical cased holes, open work areas, and shops.

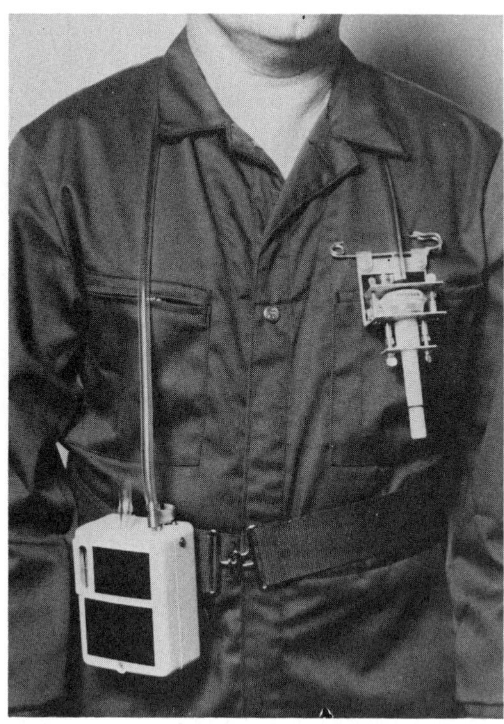

FIG 2–27.
A close-up view of a portable personal sampling pump and miniature filter collecting device attached to the worker's clothing, enabling air samples to be obtained in the worker's immediate area without interfering with freedom of movement.

or temperature. Then, too, one must ask: Will the presence of the sampler alter the routine of the operation in any manner? What is the particle size distribution? What is its chemical nature? (Organic mercury, for example, acts quite differently from mercury vapor, which, in turn, is quite distinct from mercury oxide.) Finally, are there limitations on the peak emission rates as there are for those compounds having a "C" listing in the list of Threshold Limit Values?

If the samples are collected at the right places and combined with a time study of the worker's activity, they can give a measure of the worker's intake of the toxic substance. The results obtained must be compared with a threshold limit value with a full knowledge of its limitation and consideration of other factors in the situation. (The mere history of an exposure does not mean that intoxication or toxic response has occurred.) Breath, blood, or urine assays add to the facts available for making an evaluation of exposure. These, in turn, must be combined with knowledge obtained by the physician directing an adequate medical program. All this serves to emphasize the basic teamwork approach of the industrial health program.

TYPES OF MEASURING INSTRUMENTS

The chemical environmental hazards can be conveniently divided into (1) the particulates and (2) the gases or vapors. Particulates are mixtures or dispersions of solid or liquid particles in air, and they include dust, fume, smoke, mist, and similar materials. Some of these are practically insoluble in body fluids and exert their effect in the lungs, whereas others are soluble and produce systemic poisoning.

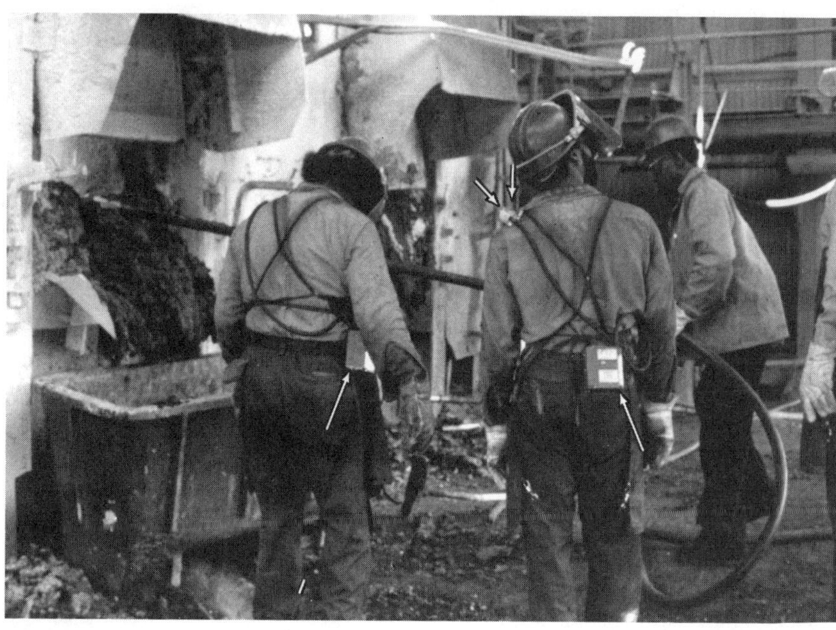

FIG 2–28.
Portable, battery operated pump-monitors *(single arrow)* with collecting filter near breathing zone *(double arrow)* to sample for contaminants in the work area, in this instance for lead in a bronze producing factory. In evaluation of analytic results, the possibility of accidental contamination by the worker must be kept in mind. (See Chapter 36 for further discussion.)

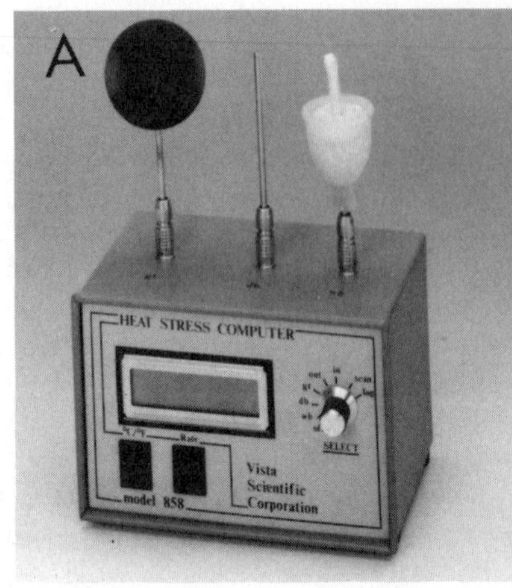

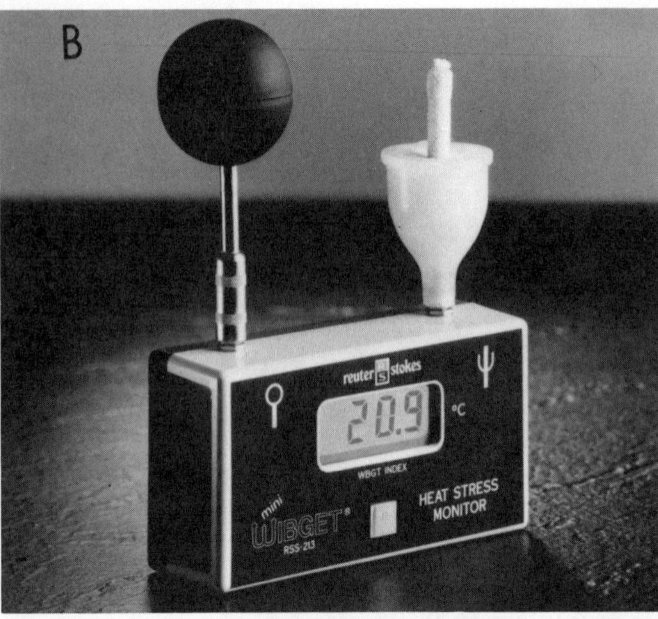

FIG 2–29.
A and **B,** environmental heat stress measuring and analyzing devices have become miniaturized and nearly completely automatic. They utilize the well known and long-used wet bulb, globe temperature index (WBGT). These models determine dry bulb temperature, wet bulb temperature (humidity), air movement, and globe temperature (replacing the conventional 6-inch globe). These instruments are accurate with a fast response (less than 3 minutes), with readout of the individual factors, remote sensors available, connectable to computers or strip chart recorders. (The basis for application to human physiologic responses is described in Chapter 22.) (Courtesy Reuter-Stokes, Cambridge, Ontario, Canada, and Vista Scientific Corp., Ivyland, Pennsylvania.)

Portable direct-reading instruments for the insoluble materials are difficult to make, because such an instrument must count or otherwise determine the number of particles suspended in air. Direct-reading instruments for this purpose do exist, but they are quite bulky. These instruments usually work on the principle of measuring the light scattered at right angles to the beam.

The concentration of gases and vapors in air can be determined more readily by direct-reading instruments, as they form more homogeneous mixtures with air, and separation from the containing air mass often is unnecessary. This group of instruments includes those for measuring concentrations of such common materials as carbon monoxide, mercury vapor, hydrogen cyanide, benzene, carbon tetrachloride, and many others.

The physical hazards—heat and cold, ionizing and nonionizing radiation, noise and atmospheric pressure—usually are measured by direct-reading instruments. In the field of ionizing radiation alone there are literally hundreds of instruments available (Figs 2–29 and 2–30).

Electrical Direct-Reading Instruments

The first general class of instruments comprises those that give a direct reading on a dial. These instruments contain an electrical meter of some sort and electronic circuitry, which requires careful maintenance to function properly.

In one type of electrical direct-reading instrument, the air that is being analyzed is passed over a heated wire. The combustible contaminant in the airstream is ignited, and the resultant rise in wire temperature (which varies with the concentration of the contaminant) is measured by means of an electrical circuit, which usually contains a Wheatstone bridge.

This is related to the gas concentration on the basis of calibration standards. The calibration may be done with any combus-

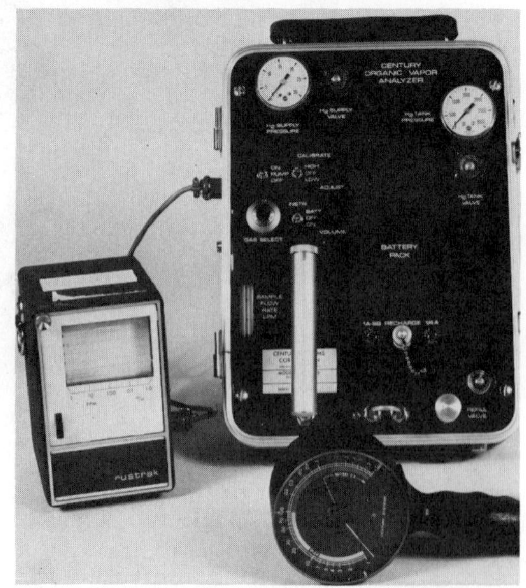

FIG 2–30.
A portable direct reading organic vapor instrument.

tible vapor or gas and the response then is related to its equivalent value for the sample gas. If the sample gas is sufficiently different from the calibration material, the results would be only approximately correct. Therefore, it is advisable to have the units checked on gas composition that is similar to the anticipated sample. Some units are adversely affected by moisture in the incoming sample and a drier is placed in line. When the drying agent becomes saturated, the unit will respond with a different calibration.

It is essential to not only ensure that the batteries and unit are operating as indicated but to be sure that pretreatment equipment is in operating condition. In addition, some materials, such as hydrogen, methane, alcohols, and other oxygenated hydrocarbons, give an unusual response in the combustible gas indicator. Thus, the specific calibration should be performed whenever a special mixture is being evaluated.

Examples of electrical direct-reading instruments that measure the amount of combustible gas or vapor in air are combustible gas indicators, vapor testers, and explosimeters (see Fig 2–30).

Great care must be taken to interpret the instrument reading properly when evaluating contaminants present in concentrations above their upper flammable range. In some instruments, the meter needle rises rapidly to the end of the scale and falls back down to zero and stays down. This may indicate a very rich gas mixture that is above the upper flammable limit. It is important to watch the needle very closely during the test to observe whether it rises and then falls back to zero or a very low reading. If the investigator did not see the needle rise and come back, he or she might erroneously assume the level of gases and vapors in the atmosphere to be safe. Also, electrical direct-reading instruments of this type will not function properly in oxygen-deficient atmospheres.

Portable electrical direct-reading instruments include many other types operating on a variety of principles. Mercury vapor in air can be measured by absorption of ultraviolet light of a specific wavelength. The same technique has also been used for certain chlorinated hydrocarbons. Portable gas chromatographs now are available for on-the-spot sampling and field analysis of gases and vapors. Highly sensitive detection of certain hydrocarbons has been accomplished by measuring their effect on the ionization produced by a hydrogen flame. Oxygen concentration can be measured accurately and quickly by the reduction polarization produced at a sensitive electrode.

Other portable direct-reading instruments contain electrochemical sensors in which a gas-permeable membrane selectively passes a gas of interest, such as oxygen or carbon monoxide, into a cell in which its presence is detected. These devices provide simplified measurement methods for some gases. Some of these devices do not require any external power. In order to prolong the life of the electrochemical sensors, they should be stored in an atmosphere free from the gas to which they normally respond.

The accuracy of the analysis made with electrical direct-reading instruments may be affected by improper maintenance, component unreliability, lack of calibration, poisoning of the catalysts by interfering substances in the atmosphere, changes in airflow rates and volumes, and weak batteries. For this reason, a routine schedule of maintenance and calibration of electrical direct-reading air sampling instruments is necessary.

Color-Change and Stain-Length Instruments

The second class of direct-reading instruments of interest to the safety professional is composed of those that produce a color change in a sensitive chemical through which the air to be tested is drawn. This is a more numerous class and one that has had a great deal of development in recent years.

For the determination of air contaminants, there are three types of direct-reading colorimetric indicators: (1) liquid reagents, (2) chemically treated papers, and (3) glass indicating tubes containing solid chemicals, also known as detector tubes.

Liquid reagents are supplied in sealed ampules or in solid form, which subsequently is diluted or dissolved prior to use. Unstable reagents often are prepared by breaking an ampule containing one component inside a container containing another. The reproducibility of the chemical sampling solution may be difficult. Interference or temperature also can modify the color change, which will be a problem in interpreting the color intensity. The quantity of the air sampled is vital to the proper determination of concentration. If the optical read-out is designed for a fixed volume, and the flow is incorrect because the flow rate is in error or the sampling time is not correct, an incorrect concentration will be indicated. The manufacturer's instructions should be followed carefully and calibration checks performed periodically.

Chemically treated papers hanging unattended in the work area can only give an indication of the contamination level because the volume of air exposed to the paper is not known and the color change in the paper is influenced by air currents and temperature.

Particulate contaminants, such as chromic acid and lead, can also be determined, usually by the addition of liquid reagents to the sample on the filter paper after collection. Evaluation of the stains developed is made visually by comparison with color charts or by photoelectric instruments. Accuracy of the paper detection systems depends on the uniform sensitivity of the paper, the stability of the chemicals employed, and careful calibration.

The third and most popular type of direct-reading colorimetric indicator is the glass indicating tube containing a solid chemical. Presently there are about 100 different types of commercially available detector tubes. Because of their compactness and ready availability, they are convenient for evaluation of exposure to toxic materials in industry (Fig 2–31).

Limitations

The pitfalls and problems in direct-reading colorimetric indicators are basically similar. Each system requires calibration of both the colorimetric reaction and air flow measurement. Since this type of device is destroyed when used, individual units from a lot should be calibrated. The National Institute for Occupational Safety and Health (NIOSH) is developing a detector tube certification program whereby manufacturers will be required to conduct specified calibration tests on each lot of tubes. Although this will minimize the need for calibration in the future, it by no means will obviate the need for calibration checks.

The colorimetric tubes and pumps are deceptively simple to operate. Air usually is drawn through the tube with a pump or squeeze bulb—this means no motor to fail or battery to replace. However, there have been and still are variations from one tube to another due to manufacturing conditions, which are hard to con-

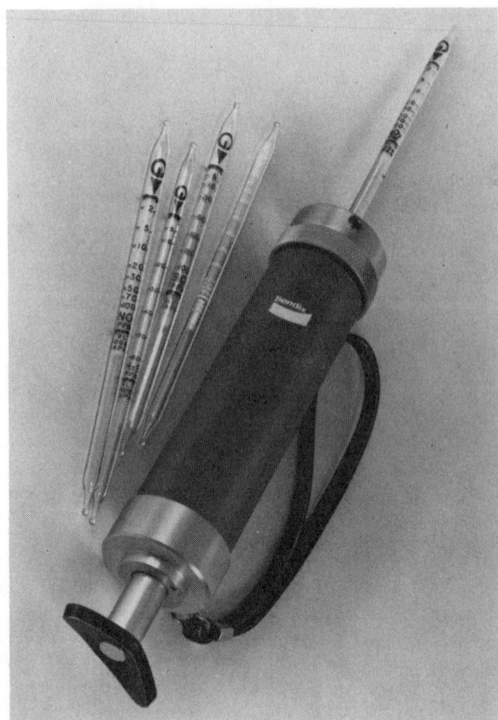

FIG 2–31.
A direct reading colorimetric indicator device.

trol. Practically all colorimetric tubes have been improved as experience has been gained by users and makers.

One form of variability that has been troublesome but is obvious to the user of stain-length tubes is that produced by nonuniformity in the particle size of the medium (usually silica gel) that supports the reacting chemical. The result in some tubes is that, in transportation, the gel fractionates into various sizes by gravity, and the line between stain and no-stain is not sharp but stretches irregularly across the tube, and it may extend much farther up one side than the other, thus making it impossible to obtain an accurate reading of stain-length.

The chemical reactants in the tubes also vary considerably in their degree of chemical stability, although their useful storage life often can be prolonged considerably by storage in a refrigerator.

Rates of chemical reaction are very dependent on temperature; many tubes will give incorrect readings at very high or low ambient temperatures. When colorimetric tubes must be used in cold locations, they should be carried in an inside pocket next to the body, where they can be kept warm and used quickly after removing them from the pocket. Even then, the air drawn through the tube is cold, and the results obtained must be interpreted with caution. Extreme temperatures change the volume of air drawn through the tube, which also affects results.

Perhaps one of the most difficult problems associated with the use of indicator tubes is that of interfering gases and vapors. Other constituents in the workroom air may react with the chemical on the impregnated granules and prevent any color change indication at the concentration of the gas being measured. In other cases, interfering gases may react with the indicating chemical in the tube and produce stains comparable to the test gas being measured. Thus, interferences may result in high, low, or negative readings for the test gas. It is extremely important to interpret properly the results of the tests when interfering gases or vapors are present (Fig 2–32).

It is the responsibility of the manufacturer to point out all the possible substances that produce interferences with a test, at least to the best of his knowledge. However, it is the responsibility of the user to determine the presence or absence of any interfering airborne substances in the workroom environment.

Calibration of these instruments is not difficult but requires facilities not always available in an industrial situation—some method of producing an atmosphere containing a known concentration of the contaminants in a closed chamber. Because a tube once used for calibration is worthless for further use, this method does not give complete reassurance concerning the accuracy of measurement with other successive tubes. The reliability of the color tube method of air analysis, therefore, differs from the electrical devices or the collection of samples for laboratory analysis. The best that can be done is to test a definite number of tubes from each lot produced by the manufacturer.

There is no substitute for experience gained in making tests on known concentrations. By such means, the instrument user learns important factors, such as whether to measure the length up to the beginning or end of the stain front or what portion of an irregularly shaped stain is to be used as the interface or boundary. In some cases, the stains may change with time. Therefore, test results should be recorded immediately.

The problems and pitfalls of using direct-reading indicators are overcome most easily by initially understanding the nature of work operations and the chemicals involved. This requires a preliminary survey to ascertain all the factors involved in the work environment and gives guidance as to the numbers and types of samples needed. Direct-reading indicators are a type of sampling device that can be applied to the assessment of chemical exposures; their limitations are primarily those of calibration and understanding the inherent deficiencies in such devices. Interfering materials as well as variations in temperature and pressure can adversely affect the results. Air sample flow is critical to the maintenance of their calibration. No device is foolproof, and so the

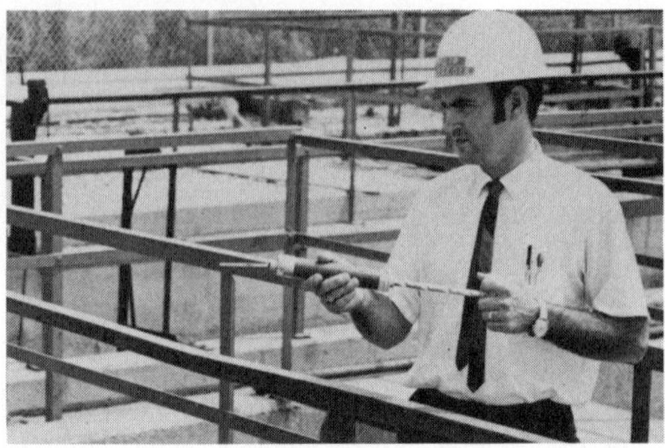

FIG 2–32.
A direct reading device used in the field in a sewage treatment plant, where many organic vapors may be present.

operator of such units must be aware of the limitations in order to understand the results that are obtained. With such knowledge and the operator's ability to apply the sampling results to acceptable concentrations, assessment of workers' occupational exposure can be obtained with reasonable accuracy.

Laboratory Analytic Methods

When it comes to laboratory analytical methods, they are so variable and so dependent on the individual substance and the circumstance that they cannot be discussed in great detail in this general discussion. It should be emphasized, however, that any method that is to be used should be investigated thoroughly by the individual who is to use it. The apparatus should be checked carefully and the method verified, so that it is certain that it is appropriate for the particular operations with which one is concerned. One cannot overemphasize the importance of frequent calibration of the apparatus to be certain that the results will be valid.

Interpretation of Results

The necessity for enough air samples from enough sampling points over a sufficient period of time to give a good estimate of the probable ceiling value during normal operation, the distribution of peaks above the ceiling under exceptional circumstances and a reasonably accurate time-weighted average have been emphasized. Not all operations require such complete information all the time. What is required in any particular operation must be left to the judgment of the people responsible for that operation, and this includes not only the plant superintendent but his or her chief advisors—the safety professional, industrial hygienist, or plant physician. There is no general overall rule of thumb that can be used.

Even when you have a good space-time analysis of the environmental circumstances, you have a very difficult problem of determining the "fifth dimension," which is human movement within space-time. It requires very careful observation to get an accurate picture of human movement within the space-time environment.

Clinical examination of workers, particularly biochemical analysis, can give us some exceedingly valuable clues, but they must be taken in relation to all of the other information obtained.

Problems of skin contact are even more difficult to quantitate than exposure to air dispersion. A "wipe" test may give some clues to surface contamination. Analysis of clothing and biochemical analysis of the worker may give some clues. Here, again, careful and prolonged study of work habits can be helpful.

The industrial physician should have good toxicologic information from the research laboratory, information from good clinical and biochemical studies of workers in known environmental circumstances, and a quantitative and qualitative evaluation of the environmental circumstances in the work area. When put together intelligently, these factors can give a good understanding of whether or not the work environment is healthful.

TOXIC SUBSTANCES LIST

The Occupational Safety and Health Act of 1970 (commonly termed OSHA), Section 20(a) (6), requires that the Secretary of Health, Education, and Welfare (HEW) shall publish a list of all known toxic substances by generic family or other useful grouping and the concentrations at which toxicity is known to occur. The first such list was prepared in 1971. The 1974 edition represents a substantial revision and expansion of the earlier list. Under the Occupational Safety and Health Act, the Secretary of Labor must issue regulations requiring employers to monitor employee exposure to toxic materials and to keep records of any such employee exposure. This requirement is set forth in Section 8(c) (3) of the Act.

The purpose of the toxic substances list published by the National Institute for Occupational Safety and Health (NIOSH) is to identify "all known toxic substances" in accordance with definitions that may be used by all sections of our society to describe toxicity. It should be emphasized to the user that the entry of a substance on the toxic substances list does not automatically mean that this material cannot be used or that contact with it is to be avoided. A listing does mean, however, that the listed substance has the documented potential of being hazardous if misused, and, therefore, proper care must be exercised to prevent harmful or tragic consequences.

The absence of a substance from the toxic substances list does not necessarily indicate that a substance is not toxic. Some hazardous substances may not qualify for the list, because the dose that causes the toxic effect is not known or toxic effects have gone unreported.

Other chemicals associated with skin sensitization and carcinogenicity may be omitted from the list, because these effects have not been reproduced in experimental animals or because the human data are not definitive.

Of necessity, there had to be reliance on the published comments and evaluations of the scientific community; also, there has been no attempt at an evaluation of the degree of hazard that might be expected from substances on the toxic substances list—that being an ultimate goal of the hazard evaluation studies. It is not the purpose of the list to quantitate the hazard by way of the toxic concentration or dose that is presented with each of the substances listed.

AIR QUALITY STANDARDS

In the area of occupational health, standards of environmental quality specifying levels of airborne contaminants are a useful means of expressing and communicating the summation of experimental information and experience.

Many years ago, the American National Standards Institute set up the Z-37 Committee to establish standards of environmental quality for work areas where toxic dusts and gases were of concern. These early standards were expressed as Maximum Allowable Concentrations (commonly expressed as MAC) and later as Acceptable Concentrations, or AC.

More recently, the American Conference of Governmental Industrial Hygienists (ACGIH) established what they called threshold limit values, or TLVs. The TLV not having a "C" listing is a time-weighted average for an eight-hour workday. A time-weighted average is an attempt to summate the daily potential exposure to air contaminants in a variable work environment. Both threshold limit values and acceptable concentrations, where available, have been adopted into the OSHA regulations. (See Appendix A for threshold limit values for chemical substances and physical agents in the work environment.)

Approximately 500 start-up standards for the most common hazardous substances have been published in the various amendments to Part 1910 of Title 29—"Occupational Safety and Health Standards," Federal Register, Volume 36, No. 157, pages 15,101 through 15,104, Aug. 13, 1971.

CRITERIA DOCUMENTS

Development of criteria documents, which are used as a basis for preparing new standards for substances or for recommending more complete standards, is a continuing NIOSH activity under OSHA.

These criteria documents are publications that are prepared from a critical evaluation of all published medical, biologic, engineering, chemical, and trade information and data for the purpose of establishing the concentration of a substance in the occupational environment that has been found to cause no harmful—"toxic"—effects in people working for eight hours per day, five days per week, for a normal work life.

An advocate-adversary approach is utilized by NIOSH in the preparation of these criteria documents. That is, expert critics are called in who have specific experience in handling and controlling the hazards of a substance and who not only represent widely divergent views to the proposed document but also represent organized labor, industry, government, scientific associations, and universities.

The resulting criteria document provides detailed support for the standard recommended by NIOSH. The Secretary of HEW, after review, then submits the criteria document with the recommended standard to the Secretary of the Department of Labor, who has responsibilities for promulgating the final standard.

U.S. Occupational Standard

The U.S. Occupational Standard (USOS) promulgated by the U.S. Department of Labor includes, within the limits of technical feasibility: the concentration of the substance that has been determined to provide a safe, healthful work environment for all persons; the methods for collecting, sampling, and analyzing of the substance; the engineering controls necessary for maintaining a safe environment; appropriate equipment and clothing for the safe handling of the substance; emergency procedures in the event of an accident; medical surveillance procedures necessary for the prevention of illness or injury from inadvertent overexposure; the use of signs and labels to identify the hazardous substances.

In order to ensure that the U.S. Occupational Standards promulgated by the U.S. Department of Labor reflect the best information available at the time of preparation, all individuals with publicly available information should respond to notices published in the Federal Register.

American National Standards Institute (ANSI) Z-37 Standards

In the past, a standard for airborne contaminants was conceived as a single limit, threshold, or boundary between what is healthful and what is not healthful. But there is no such single boundary. The pattern of exposure in space and time may be variable. Therefore, multiple boundaries are needed. As the boundaries are not sharp lines between what is healthful and what is not healthful, we need an explanation of the basis and significance of each of these boundaries that must act as guidelines in maintaining a healthful work environment.

The Z-37 ANSI Committee established several boundaries for a particular substance that they termed "acceptable concentrations," or just AC. They are as follows:

First, an acceptable ceiling concentration of the contaminant in the workroom air for protection of health, assuming an eight-hour workday.

Second, an acceptable time-weighted average value of the air contaminant for protection of health, assuming an eight-hour workday. This is within the limits of a specified ceiling indicated as the first acceptable concentration. This is also limited by defined peaks beyond this ceiling.

Finally, acceptable maximum for peak values of the air contaminant above the acceptable ceiling concentration for an eight-hour workday.

In a particular manufacturing process or operation there occasionally may be an excursion of the air contaminant concentration beyond the acceptable ceiling for a brief period.

There are many substances for which such excursions would be quite acceptable if defined properly. This assumes that the level of exposure is otherwise limited to the acceptable ceiling and acceptable time-weighted average.

Also included in the Z-37 standard is any other level (or levels) considered by experts to be pertinent to a particular substance under consideration.

Under general properties, information is given in the Z-37 standard to indicate the minimal level for sensory detection and to indicate what might or might not be its usefulness as a warning of significant exposure.

The purpose of these multiple boundaries is to give maximal assistance to the safety professional who must determine that a specific design and operation are compatible with a healthful environment. The Z-37 Committee believed that these standards should have the breadth to be informative and, at the same time, a pattern that allows for dynamic growth in concept as well as a change in numbers assigned to acceptable concentrations.

The standard for each substance should contain sufficient information to indicate clearly the basis on which each level was determined, the consequences of overexposure and the relative adequacy of the information. There are instances in which adequate information is not available. If so, this should be clearly stated. Many useful environmental air quality standards in the past have been guesses by experienced people. These are perfectly in order until such time as better information is available, but the fact that they have this limitation should be clearly stated and understood.

Not only must physicians constantly search for a better understanding of the response of human beings to their environment, but they must also realize that the application of any standard as a guideline for control of the work environment will always require the professional judgment of a competent and well-informed individual.

CONTROL OF HEALTH HAZARDS

General methods of controlling environmental factors or stresses that may cause sickness, impaired health, or significant discomfort among workers are given in this section. They include the following:

1. Substitution of a less harmful material for one that is dangerous to health.

2. Change or alteration of a process to minimize worker contact.

3. Isolation or enclosure of a process or work operation to reduce the number of persons exposed.

4. Wet methods to reduce generation of dust in such operations as mining and quarrying.

5. Local exhaust at the point of generation or dispersion of contaminants.

6. General or dilution ventilation with clean air to provide a safe atmosphere.

7. Personal protective devices, such as special clothing or eye and respiratory protection.

8. Good housekeeping, including cleanliness of the workplace, waste disposal, adequate washing, toilet and eating facilities, healthful drinking water, and control of insects and rodents.

9. Special control methods for specific hazards, such as reduction of exposure time, film badges and similar monitoring devices, continuous sampling with preset alarms, and medical programs to detect intake of toxic materials.

10. Medical controls.

11. Training and education to supplement engineering controls.

Substitution

Replacement of a toxic material with a harmless one is a very practical method of eliminating an industrial health hazard. In many cases, a solvent with a lower order of toxicity or flammability may be substituted for a more hazardous one.

In a solvent substitution, it is always advisable to experiment on a small scale before making the new solvent part of the operation or process. For example, carbon tetrachloride can be replaced by such solvents as methyl chloroform, dichloromethane, aliphatic petroleum hydrocarbons, or one of the fluorochlorohydrocarbons. (Precautions listed earlier in this chapter should be reviewed.) Detergent-and-water cleaning solutions can be considered for use in place of organic solvents. Benzene can be replaced by toluene in most lacquers, synthetic-rubber solutions, and paint removers. Natural rubber cements with aliphatic hydrocarbon solvents can perform virtually the same function as benzene cements. The felt hat industry has controlled the hazard of mercurialism by substituting mercury-free carroting materials. Foundries using parting compounds that contain free silica can minimize the silicosis hazard by substituting relatively harmless powders. Silica-containing sandstone grinding wheels have been largely replaced by artificial abrasive wheels usually made of aluminum oxide, considered inert.

Change in Process

A change in process often offers an ideal chance to improve working conditions. Most such changes, of course, are made to improve quality or reduce cost of production—only occasionally to improve the in-plant environment. Yet, we must always keep this possible benefit in mind. This applies to the safety professional more than anyone else.

In some cases, a process can be modified to reduce the exposure to a dust or fume and thus markedly reduce the hazard. In the automobile industry, the amount of lead dust created by grinding solder seams with small, rotary, high-speed sanding disks was greatly reduced by changing to low-speed, oscillating-type sanders. Brush-painting or dipping instead of spray painting will minimize the concentration of airborne contaminants from toxic pigments. Other examples of process changes are arc welding in place of riveting, vapor degreasing with adequate controls to replace hand-washing of parts in open containers, airless spraying techniques and electrostatic devices to minimize overspray as replacements for hand-spraying, and machine application of lead oxide to battery grids, which reduces lead exposure to operators in making storage batteries.

Isolation or Enclosure

Some potentially dangerous operations can be isolated from the people nearby, which solves the exposure problem. The isolation can be by a physical barrier (such as an acoustic box to contain noise from a whining blower or a screaming ripsaw) or by time (such as providing semiautomatic equipment so a person does not have to stay near the noisy machine constantly) or by distance (remote controls).

Isolation is particularly useful for limited operations requiring relatively few workers or where control by any other method is too difficult or too expensive. The job is isolated from the rest of the operation and thus the majority of the workers are not exposed to the hazard. The workers actually concerned with the operation then can be protected by installing a ventilation system that probably would not have been satisfactory if the operation had not been isolated and thus able to be enclosed.

In the chemical industry, the isolation of hazardous processes in closed systems is a widespread practice, which is one reason why the manufacture of toxic substances often is less hazardous than their use under less-well-controlled conditions. In the mechanical industries, complete enclosure frequently is the best solution for control of severe dust or fume hazards, such as those from sandblasting or metal-spraying operations.

Wet Methods

Dust hazards frequently can be minimized or greatly reduced by application of water or other suitable liquid at the source of dust, a method often used for silica and loose dusts. Wetting of floors before sweeping to keep down the dispersion of harmful dust is advisable when better methods, such as vacuum cleaning, cannot be applied.

"Wetting down" is one of the simplest methods of dust control. Its effectiveness, however, depends on proper wetting of the dust. This may require the addition of a wetting agent to the water and proper disposal of the wetted dust before it dries out and is redispersed. Tremendous reductions in dust concentrations have been achieved by the use of water forced through the drill bits used in rock-drilling operations. Many foundries successfully use water under high pressure in place of sandblasting for cleaning castings. Airborne dust concentrations can be kept down if molding sand is kept moist, if castings are wet down before shakeout, and if the floors are wetted intermittently.

Local Exhaust Ventilation

A local exhaust system traps the air contaminant near its source so that a worker standing at the process is not exposed to harmful concentrations. This method usually is preferred to general ventilation but should be used when the contaminant cannot be controlled by substitution, changing the process, isolation, or enclosure. Even though a process has been isolated, it still may require a local exhaust system (Figs 2–33 to 2–39).

After the system is installed and set in operation, its performance should be checked to see that it meets engineering specifications—correct rates of air flow, duct velocities, negative pressures, and the others. Its performance should be checked periodically as a maintenance measure (Fig 2–40).

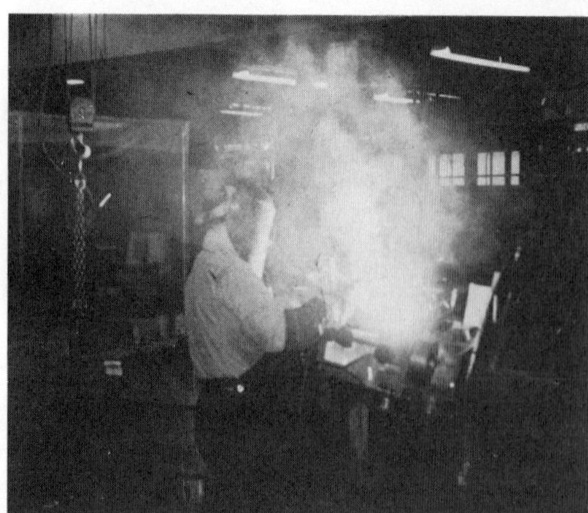

FIG 2–33.
Production welding before exhaust system was installed. Note dense fumes, which are mainly iron oxide.

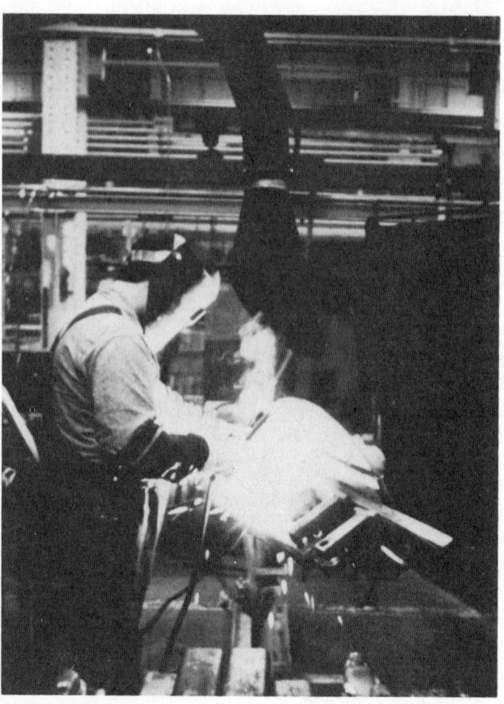

FIG 2–34.
Welding fumes effectively captured by local exhaust. The materials in the air are collected on a special filter, similar to that of a vacuum cleaner.

General or Dilution Ventilation

General or dilution ventilation—adding or removing air to keep the concentration of a contaminant below hazardous levels—uses natural convection through open doors or windows, roof ventilators and chimneys, or artificial air currents produced by fans or blowers. Exhaust fans through roofs, walls, or windows constitute positive all-season dilution ventilation. Consideration must be given to providing make-up air, especially during winter months. Dilution ventilation is practicable only if the degree of air contamination is not excessive and particularly if the contaminant is released at a substantial distance from the worker's breathing zone. Under more adverse conditions, the contaminated air will not be diluted sufficiently before inhalation.

General ventilation should not be used where there are major, localized sources of contamination (especially highly toxic dusts and fumes); local exhaust is more effective and economical in such cases. Where comparatively small amounts of the less-toxic solvents are vaporized, general or dilution ventilation can be a satisfactory method of control.

Personal Protective Equipment

When it is not feasible to render the environment completely safe, it may be necessary to protect the worker from the environ-

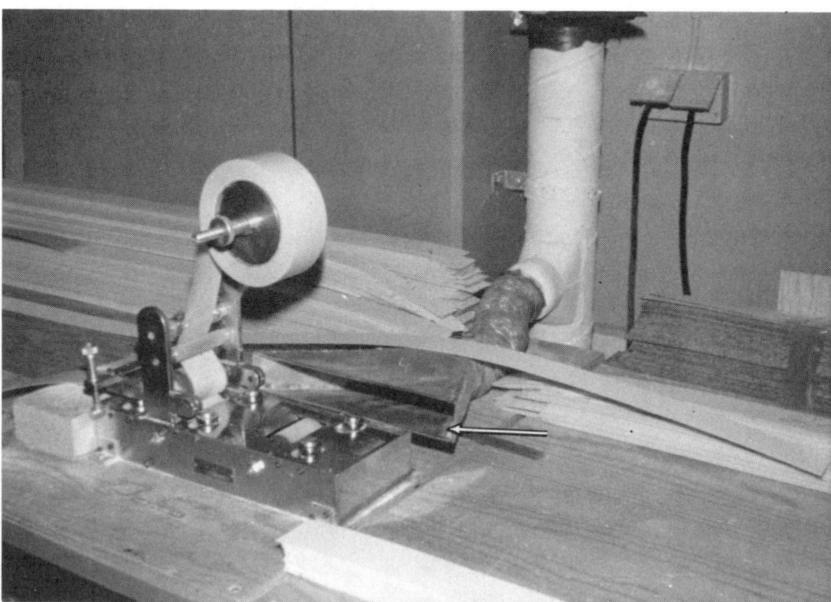

FIG 2–35.
Arrow indicates the local exhaust at the cutting stage in the manufacture of skis with epoxy-fiberglass material for the outer laminations.

ment. Personal protective equipment normally is considered to be secondary to the controls mentioned previously. Where it is not possible to enclose or isolate the process or equipment, provide ventilation or other control measures and where there are short exposures to hazardous concentrations of contaminants—for example, where unavoidable spills may occur—personal protective equipment should be provided and used (see Fig 2–40).

Personal protective devices have one serious drawback—they do nothing to reduce or eliminate the hazard. Their failure means immediate exposure to the hazard, so the fact that a protective device may become ineffective without the knowledge of the wearer is particularly serious. Excellent equipment that meets accepted national standards and specifications is commercially available in great variety. Such equipment, however, is intended for emergency or temporary use only.

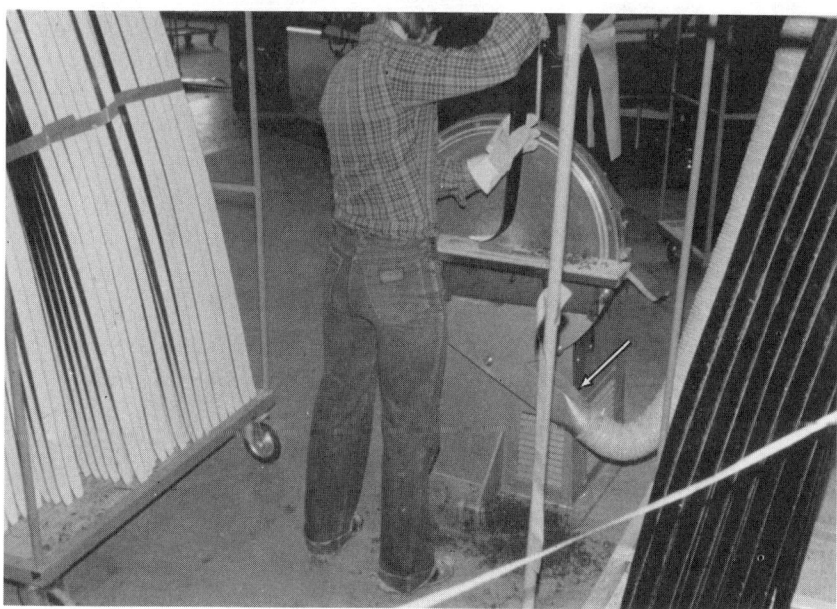

FIG 2–36.
Exhaust system at the grinding stations in the ski manufacturing plant.

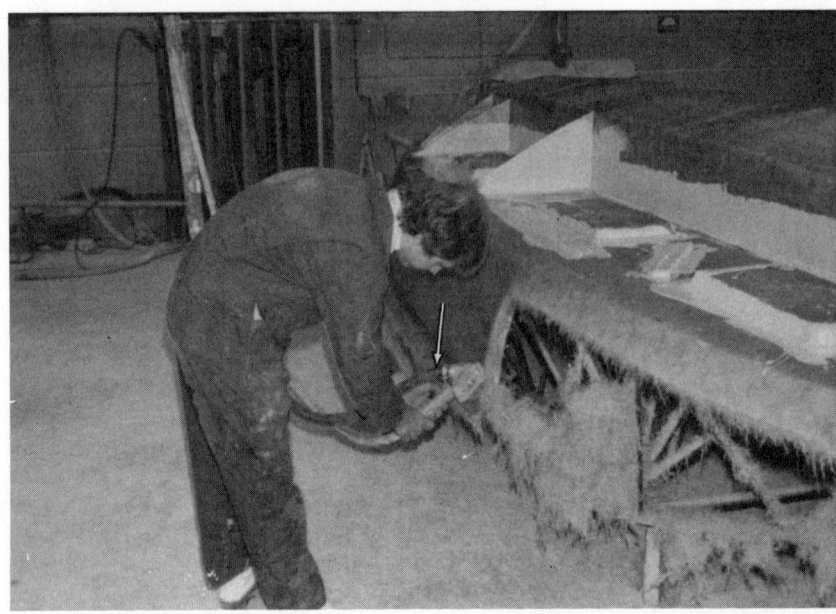

FIG 2–37.
Boat building factory where all tools used to cut, drill, or grind on the fiberglass materials are connected to an exhaust system, thereby eliminating the need for respiratory protective devices such as "face masks."

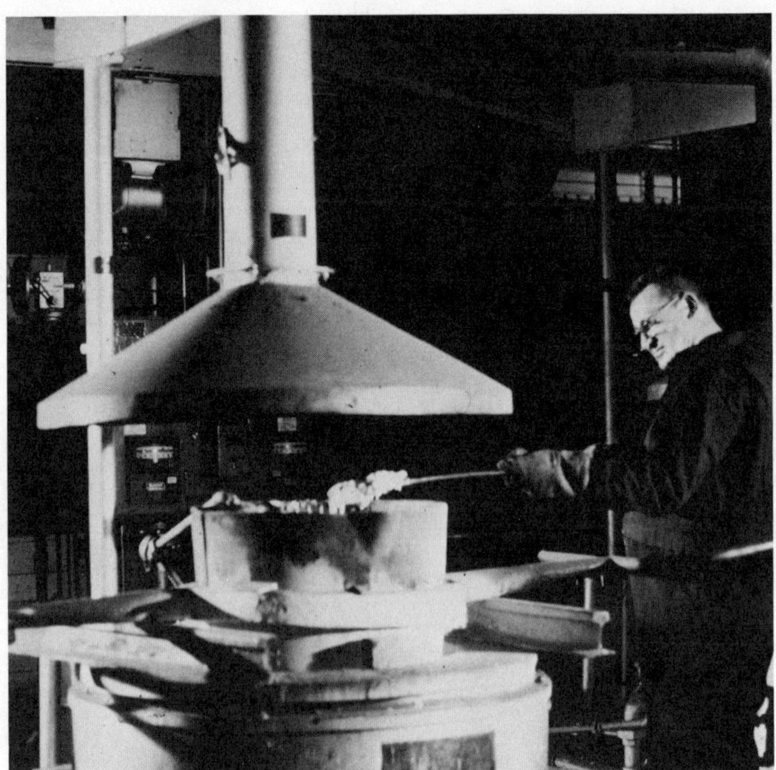

FIG 2–38.
Local exhaust ventilation used in preparing babbitt bearing alloys.

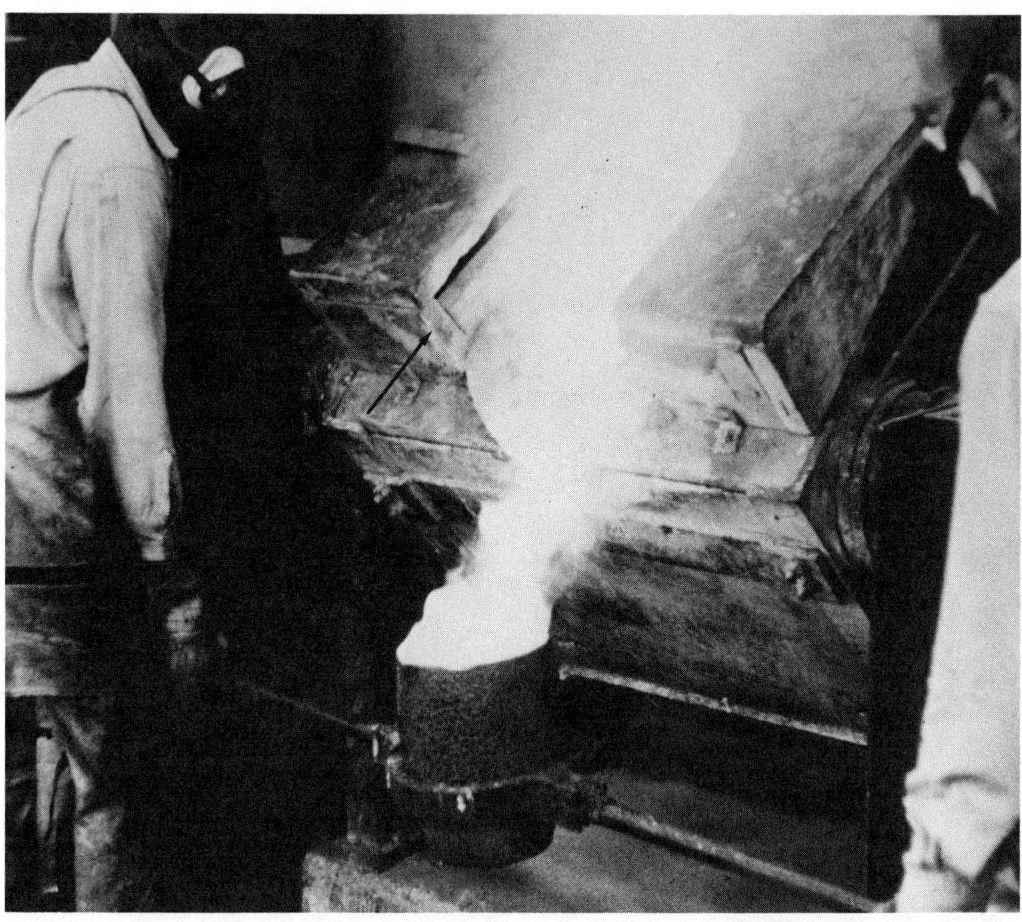

FIG 2–39.
Electric melting furnace used in a centrifugal casting foundry. Considerable fume is seen because the exhaust duct system is badly corroded and nearly clogged. Installation of a new collecting hood eliminated airborne contaminants.

Eye and Face Protection

These include safety goggles, face shields, and similar items used to protect against corrosive solids, liquids, and vapors and foreign bodies. Shaded lenses are used to screen out ultraviolet and infrared radiations. Of the many types of eye and face protection available, there is a correct type for each job and it should be worn at all times on that job.

Hearing Protection

Protection against noise-induced hearing impairment, such as earplugs or earmuffs, often may present special difficulties. First, as with air contaminants, the real answer is to reduce the exposure. But in plants with old machines and processes, and even in new plants, this problem may loom as insoluble. It may be overwhelmingly costly to lower the noise. In such cases, wearing of car protection may be mandatory.

Protective Clothing

Gloves, aprons, boots, coveralls, and other items made of impervious materials should be worn to control or eliminate prolonged or repeated contact with dermatitis-producing solvents or chemicals that may cause systemic poisoning through skin absorption. Again, care must be taken in choosing the correct article for the specific application. For example, some types of rubber that will withstand trichloroethylene will become spongy and disintegrate in lacquer solvent.

For intermittent protection against radiant heat, reflective aluminized clothing can be used. Such garments need special care to preserve their essential shiny surface. Air-cooled jackets and suits are available to make endurable a high convective heat load. Lead-bearing materials are available to protect against ionizing radiation.

Respiratory Protective Devices

Respiratory protective devices normally are restricted to intermittent exposures or those that are impracticable to control by other methods. Respiratory protection should not be substituted for engineering control methods. Exceptions are supplied-air devices for protection in sandblasting (Fig 2–41) or for operations in confined spaces, where an oxygen deficiency may exist.

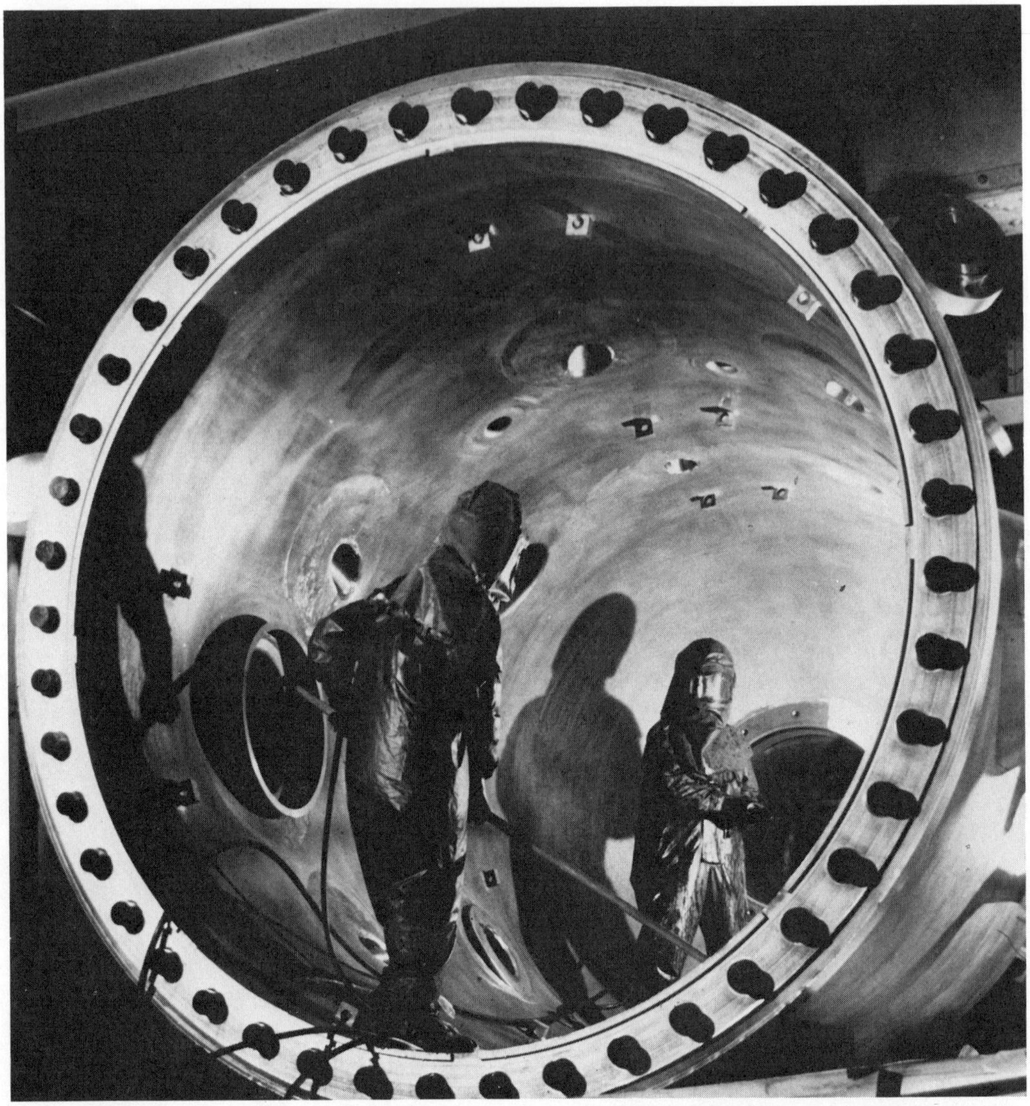

FIG 2–40.
Complete protection for the workers who are etching a large reactor vessel with nitric acid.

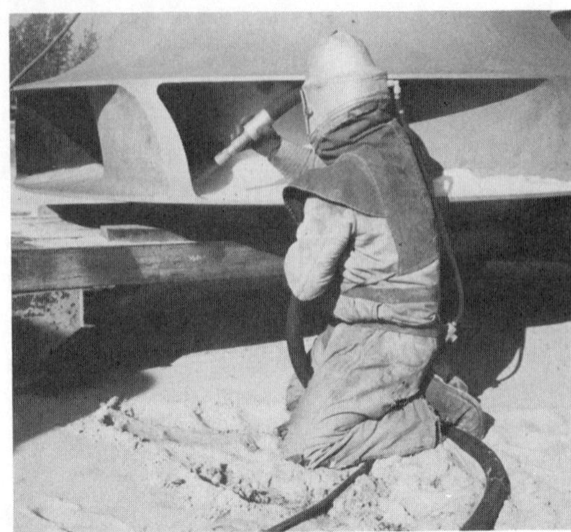

FIG 2–41.
Sandblasting an impeller. Note large amount of silica (sand) used.

Elements of Respiratory Protection

Julian B. Olishifski, P.E.

Carl Zenz, M.D.

Many types of respirators are used for protection against a variety of conditions that may be encountered in different work activities. Each has a particular field of application and limitations from the viewpoint of protection, as well as advantages and disadvantages from the viewpoint of operational procedures and maintenance. Ordinarily, "respirators" are not intended to constitute "first-line defense" against hazardous materials but rather to offer a worker temporary protection. The most effective control measures must be built on engineering principles, described previously and shown in the figures throughout this chapter.

The conditions to be protected against range from those that are mainly a nuisance, such as odor or mild "irritation," to those that are immediately dangerous to life. The hazard may be due to one or more toxic contaminants or to an atmosphere deficient in oxygen. The contaminants may be in the gaseous or particulate state or in combination. Protection may be needed for only minutes, as in rescue operations, or for several hours, i.e., for "sand blasting" (see Fig 2–41) or paint spraying.

Respirators generally fall in these classifications: (1) atmosphere-supplying respirators, (2) air-purifying respirators (gas and vapor [gas mask and chemical cartridge], particulate [dust, fog, fumes, mist, smoke and sprays], and combination gas, vapor, and particulate), and (3) combination atmosphere-supplying and air-purifying respirators (Figs 2–42 to 2–48).

It is the responsibility of the employer to provide a respiratory protection program meeting established requirements. The employer must provide respirators, ensure that employees use the respirators in a proper manner when wearing of respirators is required, and ensure that employees are properly instructed in the use of respirators assigned to their use and to test for leakage, proper fit, and proper operation. The employer must provide a program of cleaning, sanitizing, inspecting, maintaining, repairing, and storing of respirators to ensure that employees are provided with clean respirators in good operating condition.

Requirements for approval of many types of respirators have been established by the Secretary of the Interior and the Secretary of Health, Education, and Welfare and are published as Title 30, Code of Federal Regulations, Part II (30 CFR 11).[27]

An air-purifying respirator for protection against particulates is equipped with a mechanical filter designed to remove particulate matter from the inspired air by capture on the filter, usually a fibrous pad (see Figs 2–24 and 2–25). These respirators consist of a soft, resilient, full, half, or quarter mask facepiece to which is attached one or two filters through which the inspired air is drawn. Check valves, present in most mechanical-filter respirators, pre-

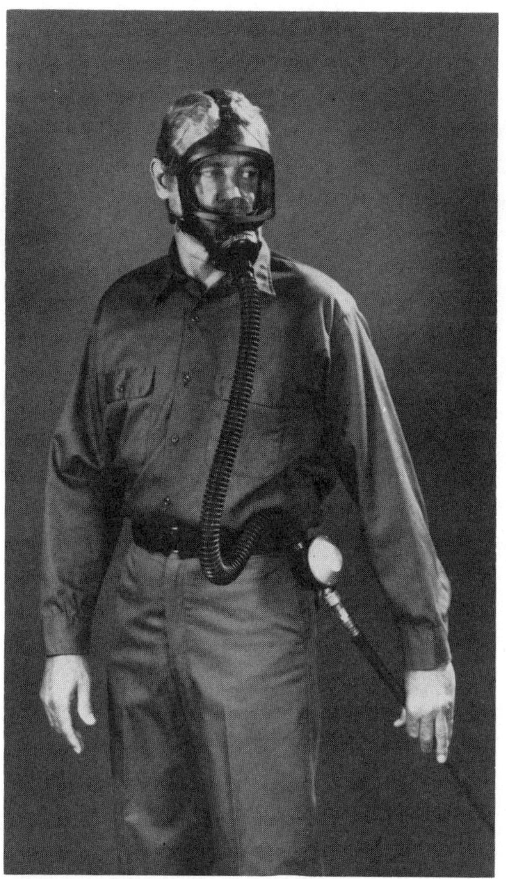

FIG 2–42.
A demand-flow airline respirator with belt-mounted regulator, used with hose to an approved respirable compressed air source, up to 100 meters. (Courtesy of Mine Safety Appliance Co.)

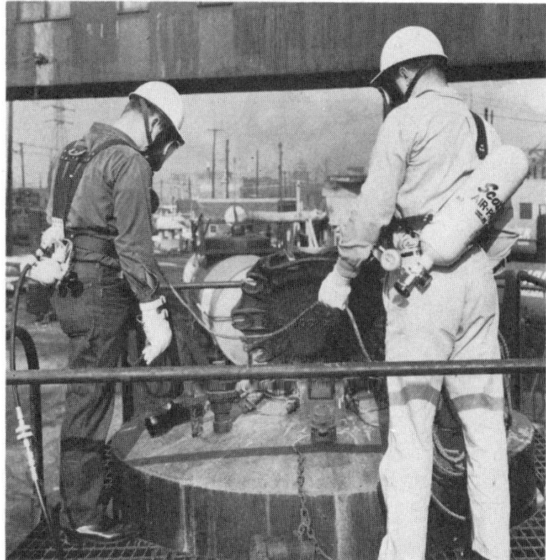

FIG 2–43.
Examples of emergency respirators. The airline respirator has an auxiliary air supply to allow escape in case the line should break.

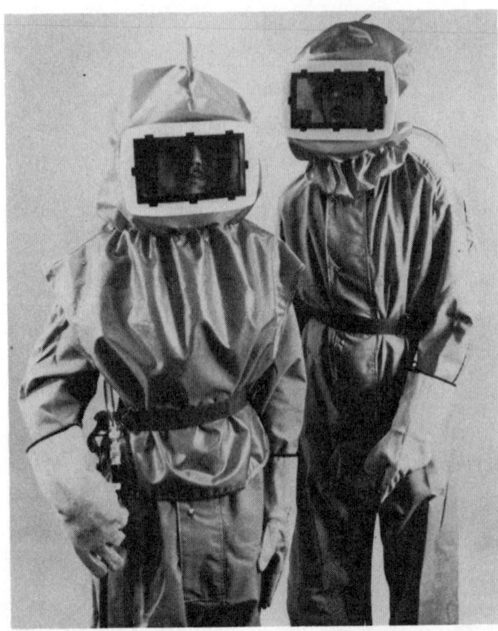

FIG 2–44.
Continuous supplied-air respirators affording full face, head, and neck protection. Useful during paint spraying, chemical handling, bagging, buffing, grinding, sandblasting, pesticide applying, etc. (Courtesy of E.D. Bullard Co.)

vent exhaled breath from passing through the filters, and allow it to be forced out through an exhalation valve in the facepiece to the surrounding atmosphere. The facepiece is held securely to the wearer's face by the head harness or headband.

The useful life of the mechanical filters is limited by the buildup of resistance to inhalation as the contaminant is removed by the filter. The higher the concentration of contaminant in the air drawn into the filter, and the greater the wearer's requirement for ventilation when using a nonpowered respirator, the more rapidly the resistance to inhalation increases. The requirement for ventilation depends on several variables. The most obvious is the amount of energy a worker is expending. This is a function of the task per-

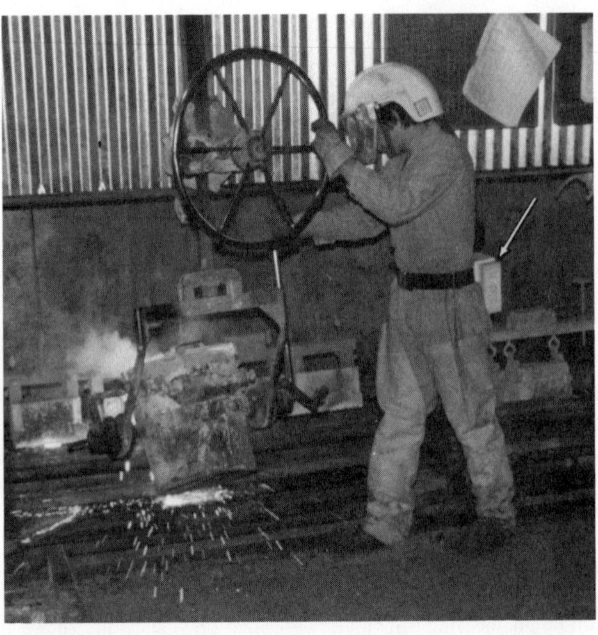

FIG 2–46.
A battery powered air-purifying unit *(arrow)* and helmet (Racal Airstream, Inc.) in use on a pouring line in a brass foundry. These have excellent characteristics—good worker acceptance and ensure that the air breathed by the worker contains no detectable contaminants such as lead dust or fumes. (See Chapter 36 for environmental and clinical details.)

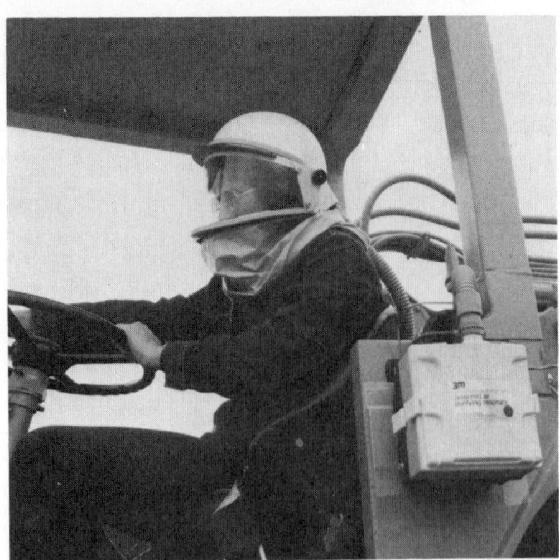

FIG 2–45.
A powered air-purifying helmet, useful in certain jobs, such as pesticide applications in agriculture, forestry, and construction work. (Courtesy of 3M Co.)

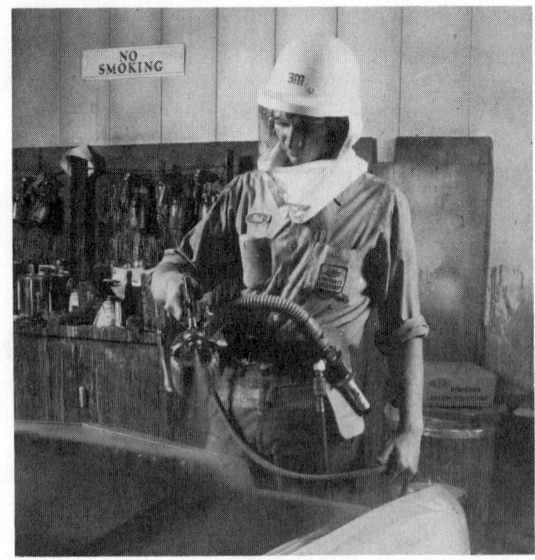

FIG 2–47.
A lightweight air-supplied hood for respiratory protection, useful in many occupations. (Courtesy of 3M Co.)

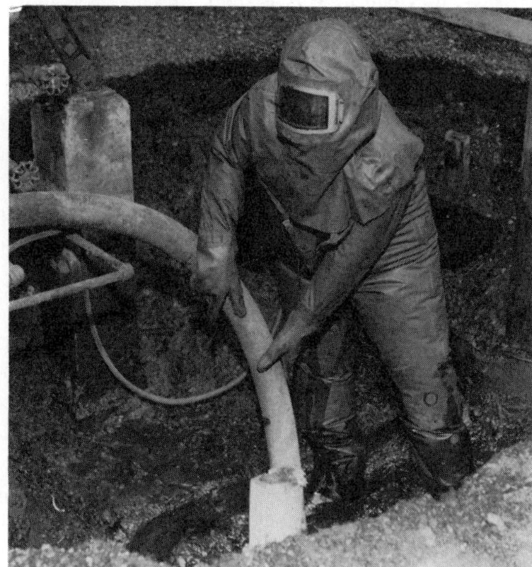

FIG 2–48.
The worker is encased from the neck down in a one-piece suit with integral boots and gloves. His head and shoulders are covered with an airline-fed hood. Fabric is butyl-covered cotton.

formed, the position in which it is performed, and other external stresses, such as heat and humidity, that the worker is subjected to during the performance of the task.[22] The resting respiratory ventilation of a worker depends on body size. It has been thought that women have a lower tidal volume and minute volume ventilation on the basis of sex. This, however, does not seem to be true. Differences in ventilation are related to body size and conditioning rather than to sex. Resting and exercise ventilation studies on normal young women show ventilation to be equivalent to that of males of equal body size. For exposures within threshold limit values, men and women must be considered equally in terms of potential respirable exposures.

A powered air-purifying positive-pressure respirator contains a motor-blower that draws the contaminated air of the workplace through a mechanical filter and discharges pure air into a facepiece, hood, or helmet. The device can be designed to ensure a positive pressure in the facepiece, so that high protection can be achieved. Since leakage through the facepiece seal is reduced and inhalation resistance is eliminated, lower facepiece sealing forces can be used. In addition, the air sweeping through the mask may provide some facial cooling, reducing moisture buildup in the mask. Acceptance of this device by the worker is higher than that of the conventional air-purifying respirators.

The air supply system for the powered air-purifying respirator may be designed to be worn by a worker or separately mounted with an airline connection to the worker, but this additional weight and bulk may be uncomfortable to some workers. As with the nonpowered air-purifying respiratory devices, the filter service life will depend on the concentration of air contaminant(s) (see Figs 2–45 and 2–46).

The positive-pressure-supplied air respirator is an airline respirator consisting of a half mask or full facepiece to which respirable air is supplied through a small-diameter hose. The airline respirator is the most comfortable to wear for prolonged periods, offers little or no resistance to inhalation and the flow of air usually provides a cooling and refreshing effect. The worker supports little weight other than the facepiece and a short connecting hose. A limitation is the necessity for trailing the small-diameter hose connecting the facepiece to the air source, which limits the range of travel (see Fig 2–47).

Problems and Precautions.—Providing adequately fitting respirators is complicated by the wide range of facial sizes and shapes that must be accommodated because of factors such as age, sex and race. Women have need for smaller-sized face-fitted equipment, as pointed out in Chapter 53. Facial hair, such as beards or sideburns, *makes it difficult to achieve an airtight seal* between the facepiece and the face, particularly with the half-mask type of respirator. Hair stubble resulting from failure to shave daily can cause inward leakage of contaminated air. Therefore, workers who must wear respirators with half or full facepiece should be instructed about the need for regular shaving habits. Even in cool environments, there is a buildup of moisture between the skin and the seal, which may compensate for small amounts of hair growth, and the rubber or plastic seal between the mask and face also improves with time because of gradual conformation of the skin to the edge of the mask.

Most respirators affect workers' visual capabilities. The half mask and the attached elements can appreciably restrict normal downward vision. Diminished vision in the full-face mask may be caused not only by the facepiece but also by the design and placement of the eyepieces. Respiratory protection for individuals wearing safety or corrective glasses may pose certain drawbacks, since the device often rests high on the face, making wearing of glasses uncomfortable. For a full-face mask, a proper face seal may not be established if the temple bars of the eyeglasses extend through the sealing edge. Some full-facepiece designs provide for the mounting of special corrective lenses within the facepiece. Although more expensive, these types are preferred for regular use by workers with need for visual correction.

Speech transmission through a respirator is decreased, annoying and fatiguing to workers. Movements of the jaws in speaking may cause leakage between the facepiece and face, especially with the commonly used half-mask respirator. The worker's comfort and acceptance of the distress caused by wearing a respirator are no less important than the device's effectiveness. These factors, such as improperly fitted respirators and uncomfortable resistance to breathing as a result of increased physical effort on the job (the energy requirements of some heavier jobs result in *respiratory air movement up to 50–60 L/min*, which can severely impede air flow), are the major drawbacks to respirator use in the absence of suitable exhaust systems.

Whole-body protective suits (see Fig 2–48) significantly increase respiratory work loads, altering cardiorespiratory and thermoregulatory responses, resulting in early onset of fatigue. When occupational hazards exist, demanding use of such suits or a self-contained breathing apparatus (which can weigh 15 kg or more), submaximal and maximal work performance is greatly reduced and rest pauses are required. Limitations of air supply pose serious risks, especially in firefighters and other emergency or rescue workers who must use self-contained breathing devices. These factors were reported by Levy et al.[15] and by Raven et al.[22, 23]

When making recommendations concerning workers' use of positive-pressure respirators, the clinical entities that may cause problems include severe or uncontrolled asthma, emphysema (bullous or otherwise), and a history of recurrent pneumothorax. Workers with any of these findings may have a higher risk than expected for barotrauma when using positive-pressure respirators.

To reiterate, prevention of occupational respiratory diseases is dependent on recognition of potential hazards in the workplace, minimizing, reducing, and eliminating the hazard(s), protecting the worker by engineering controls and other methods described and illustrated in this and other chapters, medical awareness and assistance in worker selection, education, training, and safe placement. Physical examinations, including chest x-rays and pulmonary function tests, *must not be relied on* to ensure long-term good health of workers but may be used to preselect workers who may be inadvertently exposed to potentially hazardous substances, and who may have existing medical conditions which may be aggravated or exacerbated by work exposures.

To summarize: Selection of the proper type of respiratory protective equipment should be based on the following basic procedures:

1. Identify the substance or substances against which protection is necessary.

2. Know the hazards of each substance and its significant properties.

3. Determine the levels of air contamination, oxygen deficiency, and the conditions of exposure.

4. Determine if any personal capabilities and characteristics are essential to the safe use of the devices or procedures required.

5. Determine what facilities are needed for maintenance.

Since a respirator often becomes uncomfortable after wearing for extended periods, workers must fully realize the need for protection or they will not wear it. To get the workers' cooperation, the following factors are important:

1. Prescribe respiratory protective equipment only after every effort has been made to eliminate the hazard.

2. Explain the situation fully to the worker.

3. Fit the respirator carefully.

4. Provide for maintenance and cleanliness, including sterilization before reissue.

5. Instruct the workers in the proper use of the respirator.

For further discussion of respirators, refer to various NIOSH documents and other reports.[4, 25, 27]

Protective Creams and Lotions

Creams and lotions help minimize skin contact with irritant chemicals. Their effectiveness varies, but, if selected properly and used correctly, they can be very helpful. The cream or lotion must be selected on the basis of competent medical advice. The worker then must be instructed in the value of the protection and its proper application.

Housekeeping

Good housekeeping plays a key role in occupational health protection. Basically, it is another tool in addition to those already listed for preventing dispersion of dangerous contaminants. Dust on overhead ledges and on the floor can readily be dispersed to the in-plant atmosphere by traffic, vibration, and random air currents. Housekeeping is always important; where there are toxic materials, it is paramount.

Immediate cleanup of any spills of toxic material is a very important control measure. A regular cleanup schedule using vacuum cleaners or lines is the only truly effective method of removing dust from the work area. An air hose for blowing away dust should not be used.

Good housekeeping is also essential where solvents are stored, handled, and used. Leaking containers or spigots should be remedied immediately by transferring the solvent to sound containers or by repairing the spigots. Spills should be cleaned up promptly by workers wearing protective equipment. All solvent-soaked rags or absorbents should be disposed of in airtight metal receptacles and removed daily from the plant.

It is impossible to have an effective health program unless maintenance housekeeping is good and the worker has been informed of the need for those measures. For example, if the thermostat on a vapor degreaser fails or is accidentally broken, excessive concentrations of trichloroethylene might quickly build up in the work area unless the equipment is shut down and the necessary repairs are made immediately.

Waste Disposal

Orderly controlled disposition of all hazardous materials should be done by highly trained individuals under strict supervision. Most regulations prohibit the disposal of dangerous substances in any sewer system. Actually, it is not desirable to dispose of any material that gives off objectionable odors in the sewer systems.

Procedures should be established for the disposal of unused dangerous chemicals, toxic residues and contaminated waste, containers of chemicals that no longer are needed, and containers from which labels have been lost or obliterated.

Final disposal of dangerous chemicals should be carried out at a disposal area remote from inhabited areas by controlled burning in a pit with large quantities of fuel—either scrap lumber or flammable liquid—if this is permitted by local regulations.

Each disposal method should be considered individually before emergency disposal is imminent, and prior knowledge and the proper neutralizing materials should be available. If possible, have a remote disposal area, collect the materials in adequately designed containers and have trained personnel dispose of them safely without creating a nuisance or hazardous pollution problem.

Medical Program and Basic Guidelines for Occupational Health and Hygiene

Hans J. Van der Merwe, M.B., Ch.B., D.P.H.

An effective medical control program will help prevent cases of occupational disease. Such a program can also serve as a check on the engineering controls, because symptoms of exposure in a group of workers will indicate a failure that must be corrected. The extent of the medical program will depend on the hazards and seriousness of the exposures. An industrial hygiene program should parallel the medical program. Both are essential to protect the health of employees.

The physical examination for new employees should include a thorough pre-employment history, with the occupational background given in detail (see Chapter 3, Fig 3–5). Chest x-rays should be made of all new employees who will be working in dust exposures that could produce pneumoconiosis. The examining physician should decide what physical capabilities are needed to perform the required work and to screen out those individuals who cannot meet these qualifications.

Occupational hygiene and occupational health have a longstanding interrelationship. Greenburg in 1939[10] and his colleagues presented an epidemiologic study of benzene exposure in the printing industry in terms of monitoring the working environment. Obtaining retrospective information can be difficult because of past working conditions and constraints on availability of relevant information, placing especially severe limitations on epidemiologic studies. It is important to have accurate and pertinent information for case-finding studies of dose response based on time-on-job from work history records and intensity-of-exposure from hygiene measurements, job description, and work history.[9, 13]

Framework on the Basic Concepts

Each stage on the flow diagram in Figure 2–49 is described in terms of activities concerning the technical process. This ought to be presented in an understandable manner to all incumbents involved.

A block diagram (see *column 2,* Fig 2–49) presents each stage in the flow diagram indicating inflow, processed, and outflow materials.

Hazardous Substances, Physical State, and Conditions of Use

Substances: Materials and Products and By-products.—They are numerically indicated in terms of the block diagram. Hazardous substances are also recorded in terms of trade and chemical names.

Physical State of Substances.—Comments on the physical state of substances, e.g., dust, gaseous—vapor, fume, mist, aerosol, solid, or liquid must be recorded.

Other Potentially Hazardous Conditions or Influencing Factors.—Climatic, noise, vibration, radiation, and ergonomic conditions of importance are also indicated.

Exposure Code

Each stage in the flow diagram makes provision for at least three basic exposure codes to workers:

1. (E), enclosed process/nonexposure
2. (M), exposure on maintenance operations only
3. (Ex), exposure during normal working activities

Health Response Groups

The health response groups in Figure 2–50 determine the health effects due to the degree of exposure.

The health response to toxic/hazardous substances on exposure could be outlined as follows (see Fig 2–1):

*Group 1:** Localized skin/surface irritation without systemic effects (potentially nonfatal). Examples: hydrochloric acid, caustic soda, hydrogen fluoride.

*Group 2:** Localized skin/surface irritation with reversible systemic effects (potentially nonfatal).

Group 3: The systemic effects of this group are either potentially nonfatal and irreversible or potentially fatal but reversible. Example: chlorine and carbon tetrachloride.

Group 4: The effects of this group are potentially fatal and irreversible. Example: carginogenic, mutagenic and teratogenic substances.

Exposure Categories

Exposure categories (Figs 2–49 and 2–51) are a useful index to qualify and quantify individual worker exposure in relation to potential environmental chemical substance exposure.

Various categories of exposure are noted in terms of job titles/individual worker exposure by means of physical monitoring of the working environment upon individual exposure (static or personal sampling). The frequency of static-personal sampling could be determined by the exposure category, e.g., higher exposure(s) are sampled more frequently.

Medical Screening/Surveillance

Medical screening or surveillance is the periodic assessment of individual worker(s) in terms of occupational history, medical history, and symptoms and signs related to hazardous substances(s)/condition(s) exposure.

*Chemical substances in both groups 1 and 2 must have adequate warning properties, e.g., smell or sensation upon contact. Example: perchloroethylene.

PROCESS DESCRIPTION	BLOCK DIAGRAM	RAW MATERIALS, INTERMEDIATE END PRODUCTS (COMMON & CHEMICAL NAMES)	PHYSICAL STATE	HAZARDOUS	EXPOSURE	HEALTH RESPONSE GROUPS (SEE FIG 2–2)	EXPOSURE CATEGORIES PHYSICAL SAMPLING-PERSONAL/STATIC: I 1A AND 1B T.L.V-T.W.A 1/10 1A 1B	II T.L.V-T.W.A 1/10 AL	III T.L.V - T.W.A AL PEL	IV T.L.V-T.W.A PEL	PHYSICAL SAMPLING (QUALITATIVE & QUANTITATIVE)	MEDICAL SCREENING/ SURVEILLANCE	BIOLOGICAL SCREENING/ SURVEILLANCE
Reaction takes place between (1–3) at 575° C–595° C to form (1), (4–7)	1–3 (substances) REACTOR	1. Chlorine	Vapour		E,M	3					***	***	***
		2. Propylene	"		"	2							
		3. Ethylene	"		"	2							
		4. Hydrochloric Acid	"		"	1							
		5. Hexachlorobenzene	"		"	4							
	4–7	6. Carbontetrachloride	"		"	3(4)	Shift Foreman						
	(substances)	7. Perchloroethylene	Liquid		"	2	(4)	- - - - -	- - - - - -	- - - - -	Annually Φ	Annually Φ	Annually Φ
Separation takes between (1), (4–7) (7) is boiled off & Hexes filled in 220 liter drums	QUENCH COLUMN HEX SYSTEM						Panel Operators (4) Outside Operators (4) Filters (5) Filters Asst (5)	- - -	- - - - - -	- - - - -	Six Monthly Φ	Six Monthly Φ	Six Monthly Φ
	Hexes dump	HEXES: Hexachlorobenzene Hexachlorobutadine Hexachlorobenzene	) solids) vapour)	Vapour Noise	Ex, " "	4 4 4			Effluent Operator (1)	- - - - -	Monthly Φ	Monthly Φ	Monthly, Φ
	Process continues 7 6 (substances) PCE CTC				E,M				- - -	- - - - -	Continuous/ Weekly Φ (I)	Weekly Φ (II)	Weekly Φ (II)

FIG 2–49.

Flow diagram summary of a perchloroethylene and carbon tetrachloride manufacturing plant. Key: *E* = enclosed process; *M* = maintenance contract; *Ex* = exposed process. ** = Health response to chemical exposure; I-IV = categories of worker exposure for personal/static sampling; *** = Frequency of sampling/screening/surveillance for job titles in terms of "HIGH RISK" substance—Hexachlorobutadine (TLVs - American Conference of Governmental Industrial Hygienists)[6]; ϕ = Guidelines: (i) continuous physical monitoring (personal/static) for health response—groups III and IV on exposure > P.E.L.; (ii) weekly screening/surveillance for health response groups III and IV on exposure > P.L.E.—depending on amount of exposure; † = exposure to complete process; ‡ = exposure to hexes only; # = no workers exposed under normal working conditions; AL = action level—approximately 50% T.L.V. − T.W.A; PEL = permissible exposure limit (T.L.V. − T.W.A − ppm or mg/m^9); Ia = undetected amount(s) of exposure; Ib = trace amount(s) but less than 1/10 T.L.V–T.W.A; ≥ = equal or more; ≤ = equal or less.

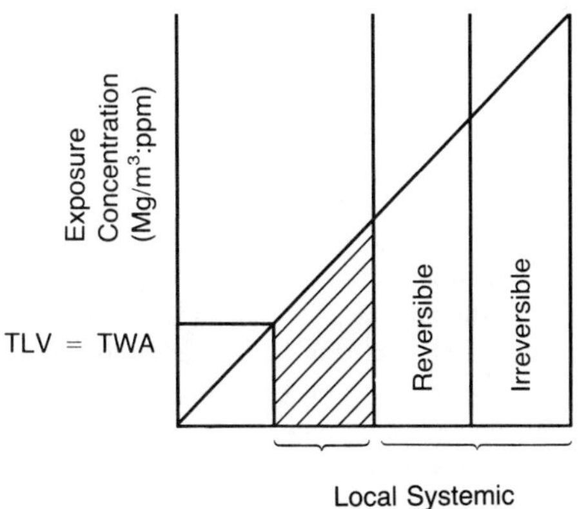

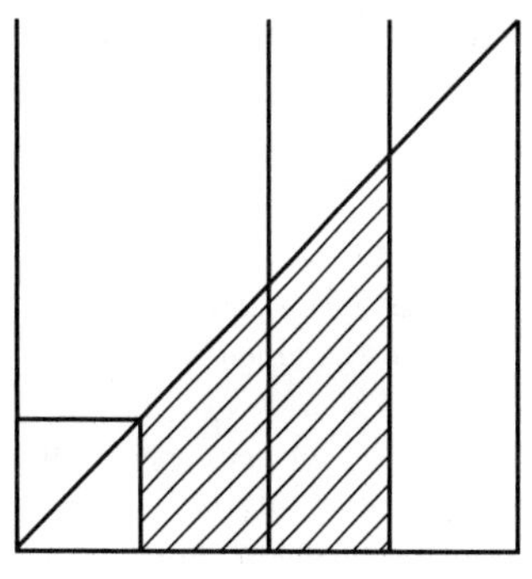

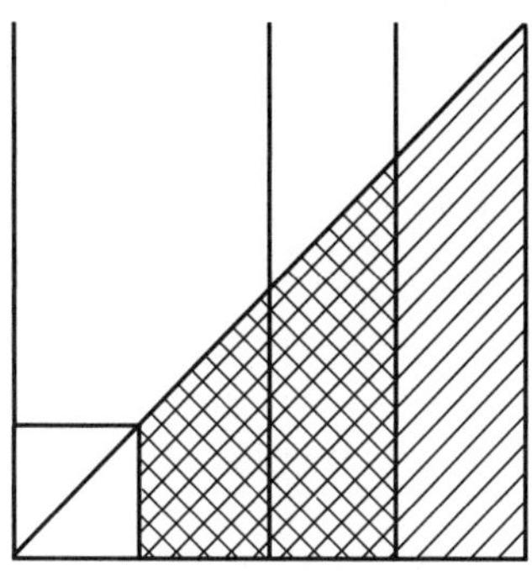

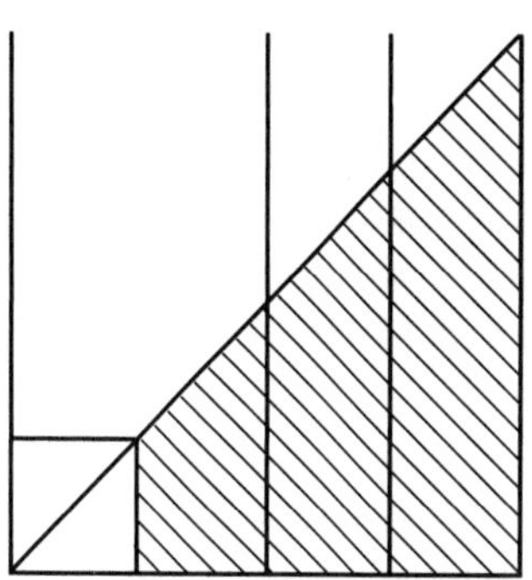

FIG 2–50.
Schematic drawing of health response to toxic/hazardous substances on overexposure. ⧅ = potentially fatal; ⧄ = potentially nonfatal.

Exposure Category Ia	: Undetected amounts of exposure
Exposure Category Ib	: Trace amounts but less than 1/10 T.L.V. = T.W.A.
Exposure Category II	: Equal or more than 1/10 T.L.V. − T.W.A. but less than 1/2 T.L.V. − T.W.A. (A.L = approximately 50% T.L.V. − T.W.A.)
Exposure Category III	: Equal or more than 1/2 T.L.V. − T.W.A. but equal or less than T.L.V. − T.W.A. (P.E.L = permissible exposure limit)
Exposure Category IV	: More than T.L.V − T.W.A. exposure
	: Following engineering prevention, corrective and control measures and worker safety protection such as:
	• Elimination by substitution of chemical substance
	• Enclosure of process
	• Segregation of process
	• Suppression to exposure
	• Local exhaust ventilation
	• General ventilation
	• General cleanliness and personal hygiene
	• Personal protection–safety wear

FIG 2–51.
Employee exposure assessment strategy—exposure categories.

Biologic Screening/Surveillance

Biologic screening is the period assessment of individual worker(s) in terms of special investigations, e.g., blood or urine tests, related to exposure to hazardous substances(s) or condition(s).

It is important to note that the physical monitoring exercise does not always precede medical and biologic screening/surveillance. The latter screening/surveillance programs may take priority, in that individual worker exposure and response are determined, as in lead poisoning. However, TLV (threshold limit value) and TWA (time-weighted average) guidelines establish assurance to both employer and employee in terms of any possible risks concerned. (Refer to Chapters 13 and 29 and Appendix A).

SUMMARY

The most effective method of control is at the source—prevent exposure to harmful physical energy stresses and contamination of workroom air and thus prevent inhalation of harmful chemical agents. The importance of personal hygiene should not be overlooked. The periodic medical examinations provide a good opportunity for instruction of employees in various personal hygiene measures.

Good washing facilities, clean lunchrooms and clean work clothes can help prevent additional, even though minor, exposure to toxic materials. Also, contaminated work clothes should not be taken home, where a toxic dust could contaminate the home or expose other members of the family.

The degree of health hazard to an individual arising from exposure to environmental factors or stresses depends on four factors: (1) the nature of the environmental factor or stress, (2) the intensity of exposure, (3) the duration of exposure, and (4) human variability or individual differences.

It is of the utmost importance to obtain a list of all the chemicals used as raw materials and to determine the nature of the products and by-products arising out of industrial operations.

After the list of chemical and physical conditions to which employees are exposed has been prepared, it is necessary to determine which of the chemical or physical agents result in hazardous exposures and need further evaluation.

Valuable information can be obtained by observing the manner in which health hazards are generated, the number of people involved and the control measure in use.

The kind of provisions that must be made to protect against health hazards will vary from plant to plant, from one toxic material to another, and from process to process. It is not possible to lay down formal rules or standards that would cover every kind of operation in every kind of plant.

The intensity of exposure is determined by direct-reading instruments or by collecting air samples for laboratory analysis at various times and under different operating conditions. Ordinarily, the industrial hygiene engineer collects the contaminant samples in the field; later, these samples are analyzed in the laboratory by the chemist. Nearly all physical agents can be evaluated by means of direct-reading instruments.

To determine the duration of exposure for an individual, a detailed job description must be obtained.

The overall process or operation must be broken down into a series of successive steps. The equipment, materials, and time necessary for each step should be checked with the operator. The potential health hazards for each step should be identified as to time and magnitude.

The final step in evaluating an environmental exposure is the interpretation of results obtained in the field survey.

From the information developed in preparing a job description and the measurements made of the magnitude of the environmental factor or stress, a daily eight-hour and peak exposure can be calculated, and a decision can be made as to the degree of exposure of an individual or a group of individuals.

A SAMPLE INDUSTRIAL HYGIENE STUDY

Reports of industrial hygiene studies must be made available to all concerned, especially to the designated facility physician or physicians, regardless of the physician's specialty, experience, or employment relationships (whether or not the physician is in private practice, practices solo or in a multiphysician group, receives a fee for service or a retainer or consultancy fee, or is a part-time employee of the organization.

An excellent example of an actual factory hygienic survey is presented:

September 19, 1985

Attached is the report of the industrial hygiene survey performed at the San Luis Potosi facility during the week of May 6, 1985. Sampling was performed to evaluate potential employee exposure to butyl mercaptan, xylene, carbon disulfide, and zineb dust.

Carbon disulfide and xylene levels were below both the OSHA permissible exposure limit (PEL) and the American Conference of Governmental Industrial Hygienists (ACGIH) recommended limits. Sampling for both n-butyl mercaptan and zineb dust indicated exposure levels exceeding the ACGIH recommended limits.

A number of recommendations have been included within this report to reduce employee exposure potential.

We recommend that this report (and the attached summary in Spanish) be made available to all employees in accordance with the corporate industrial hygiene survey report notification procedures.

Please contact me if you have any questions regarding the contents of this report.

Sincerely,

Harvey V. Davis, Ph.D.
Director of Environmental Health & Hygiene

Industrial Hygiene Survey Report
San Luis Potosi, Mexico
Summary

The survey was performed to evaluate potential employee exposure to butyl mercaptan, xylene, carbon disulfide, and zineb dust. Both personal breathing zone and area samples were obtained in the merphos unit, the endrin production area and zineb packaging. All carbon disulfide and xylene samples were below the OSHA and ACGIH recommended limits. Area sampling for n-butyl mercaptan indicated levels above the limits recommended by the American Conference of Governmental Industrial Hygienists, yet below the OSHA permissible exposure limit of 10 ppm. The sample results for zineb

TABLE 2–2
Exposure Limits Outlined in Industrial Hygiene Survey Report

SUBSTANCE	AGENCY		
	OSHA PEL	*ACGIH TLV*	*NIOSH*
N-butyl mercaptan	10 ppm	0.5 ppm	*
Carbon disulfide	20 ppm	10 ppm	1 ppm
Xylene	100 ppm	100 ppm	100 ppm
Zineb	*	*	*
Nuisance Particulates	15 mg/m^3	10 mg/m^3	*

*An exposure limit has currently not been established.

dust during the packaging process also indicate a potential for excessive exposure based on the ACGIH limit for nuisance particulates. The installation of engineering controls to reduce dust levels in this area are currently being reviewed. To protect against the current exposure concentrations, respirators must be worn at all times when working in the packaging process area.

The report includes detailed recommendations and summaries of health effects for the substances monitored: "The following health effects are based on animal toxicology studies and/or information from the literature reporting adverse human health effects due to overexposure. The reported health effects are not expected to occur in operations employing sound industrial hygiene practices."

The report includes a brief discussion of exposure limits (Table 2–2).

The manufacturing processes are described and addenda are included giving sample sites, numbers, employee names, sampling duration, volumes, concentrations found, and comments, if needed. The sampling devices and methods of analyses are mentioned and described where pertinent, and the accredited laboratories performing the analyses are listed.

Experience, discussion with others in the field, and a thorough knowledge of the particular chemical or physical agent and manufacturing operations are required to evaluate and control properly the hazards arising out of the industrial environment.

REFERENCES

1. American Conference of Governmental Industrial Hygienists: *Air Sampling Instruments Manual*, ed 5, 1978; Threshold Limit Values, Cincinnati, 1984.
2. American Industrial Hygiene Association: *Respiratory Protective Devices Manual*. Lansing, Michigan, Committee on Respirators, 1963.
3. American Industrial Hygiene Association: *Hygienic Guide Series; Respiratory Protective Devices Manual*. Akron, Ohio, 1984.
4. American National Standards Institute, Inc.: *Acceptable Concentrations*. No ANSIZ-37; *Practices for Respiratory Protection*. No Z88.2, New York, 1969
5. Astleford W: *Engineering Control of Welding Fumes*. U.S.D.H.E.W., NIOSH, September, 1974.
6. Barr HS, Hocutt RH, Smith JB: *Cotton Dust Controls in Yarn Manufacturing*. U.S. Department of Health, Education, and Welfare, Public Health Service, Center for Disease Control, National Institute for Occupational Safety and Health, Division of Laboratories and Criteria Development, Cincinnati, 1974.
7. Bryan H: *Handbook of Occupational Hygiene (Installment 1)*. Hingham, Mass, Kluwer Publishing, 1983.
8. Cralley LV, Cralley LJ, Clayton GH: *Industrial Hygiene Highlights*, Vol 1. Pittsburgh, Industrial Health Foundation of America, 1968.
9. Gamble J, Spirtas R: Job classification and utilization of complete work histories in occupational epidemiology. *J Occup Med* 18:399–404, 1976.
10. Greenburg L, Mayer MR, Goldwater L, et al: Benzene (Benzol) poisoning in the rotogravure printing industry in New York City. *J Ind Hyg Toxicol* 1939; 21:395–420.
11. Hallenbeck WH, Cunningham KM: *Quantitative Risk Assessment for Environmental and Occupational Health*. Chelsea, Mich, Lewis, 1986.
12. Hatch TF, Gross P: *Pulmonary Deposition and Retention of Inhaled Aerosols*. New York, Academic Press, Inc, 1964.
13. Hoyle HR, Langner RR, Scharnweber HC: Linking industrial hygiene and health records. *Am Ind Hyg Assoc J* 1975; 36: 760–766.
14. Langer RR, Norwood SK, Socha GE, et al: Two methods for establishing industrial hygiene priorities. *Am Ind Hyg Assoc J* 1979; 40:1039.
15. Levy SA, Margolis I, Zenz C: Ergonomics study shows effect of full-body suit on energy use. *Occup Health Saf* 1976; 15:12.
16. Linch AL: *Evaluation of Ambient Air Quality by Personnel Monitoring*. Boca Raton, Fla, CRC Press, Inc, 1974.
17. Nelson KW: The place of biological measurements in standard-setting concepts. *JOM* 1973; 15:439–440.
18. NIOSH: *Occupational Exposure Sampling Strategy Manual*, 1977.
19. *Occupational Health Guidelines for Chemical Hazards*. National Institute of Occupational Safety and Health, Cincinnati, Ohio, 1981, publication no 81-123.
20. Olishifski JB: *Fundamentals of Industrial Hygiene*, ed 3. Chicago, National Safety Council, 1987.
21. Patty FA: *Industrial Hygiene and Toxicology*, Vol 2. New York, John Wiley & Sons, Inc, 1981.
22. Raven PB, Dodson A, Davis TO: Stresses involved in wearing PVC-supplied air suits: A review. *Am Ind Hyg Assoc J* 1979; 40:592.
23. Raven PB, et al: Maximal stress test performance while wearing a self-contained breathing apparatus. *J Occup Med* 1977; 19:802.
24. Sanderson JT: *CEFIC Report on Occupational Exposure Limits and Monitoring Strategy*. Brussels, Belgium, European Council of Chemical Manufacturers Federations, 1981.
25. *The Welding Environment* (a research report on fumes and gases generated during welding operations). Miami, American Welding Society, 1974.
26. *Safety and Health*. Morgantown, West Virginia, U.S. Department of Health and Human Services, 1974.
27. U.S. Department of Health, Education, and Welfare: *The Industrial Environment—Its Evaluation & Control*, Public Health Service, Center for Disease Control, National Institute for Occupational Safety and Health, 1973.
28. U.S. Department of Labor: *Compliance Operations Manual*, No OSHA-2006. Washington, D.C., Occupational Safety and Health Administration, January, 1972.

3

The Role of the Primary Care Physician in Occupational Medicine: Principles, Practical Observations, and Recommendations

Eugene S. Welter, M.D.

In this chapter we will examine the role of the primary care physician's practice as it pertains to medicine, patient, and employer. The subjects will be handled on the assumption that the primary care physician is reading about these concepts for the first time and up until now has believed that his only responsibility has been to his patients. The full-time occupational physician is also encouraged to read this section, since I think he or she needs to understand the viewpoint of the private practice sector, in order to ensure better communication between physician, patient, and industry.

ETHICS

The first area the private or personal physician needs to clarify is the ethics of his or her relationship to the patient's employer. Does this relationship occur often enough for the physician to be concerned about it? For many primary care physicians the answer is "yes," since they are engaged in some form of occupational medical care if they perform preplacement examinations, give emergency care of workplace injuries, and perhaps, provide physical examinations for the managerial candidates of local companies. For other physicians, the relationship is not as clear, but nevertheless, is as binding, as when the need arises to fill out the insurance form certifying disability, to write the note that allows the patient to return to work after a sickness or injury that was not work-related, to advise the pregnant worker who is worried about work exposure to her unborn child or the work demands on her already-taxed physical condition, or to consider the ever-present possibility that a patient's condition may be directly or indirectly related to the workplace.

Considering that over half of the population of the United States is at one time or another employed, and that less than 4,000 physicians in the United States belong to an organized occupational medicine group, that leaves a lot of working patients (more than 80% of the work force) cared for by primary care physicians.

The ethics of health care services to the worker has come under particularly close scrutiny lately. The American Occupational Medical Association has responded with a "Code of Ethical Conduct for Physicians" which is applicable to all physicians, not just those who are members of the American Occupational Medical Association. In regard to the ethics of occupational medicine, three major issues must be addressed:

1. Loyalty: to whom does the physician respond and to whom is he or she accountable?

2. Confidentiality: who should have access to what medical information?

3. Reporting: to whom should suspected or known work-related hazards or illnesses be reported?

Loyalty to the Patient

The subject of ethics and liability has been addressed by several authors[15, 13, 6] at various national meetings. The Arizona Center for Occupational Safety and Health has published a project module entitled *Ethical Dilemmas Facing Clinicians Who Provide Health Services To Workers*,[21] which reviews the subject in detail. Tabershaw[23] has answered the question, "Whose agent is the occupational physician?": "The physician works for no other purpose than the benefit of his patients. In occupational medicine, this is the worker. As with other third-party payers, the patient is still primary. The physician is not an 'agent' of industry."

The American Occupational Medical Association Code of Ethics stresses that (1) the highest priority is to be given to the health and safety of the individual (patient); (2) the physician must practice on a scientific basis, with objectivity and integrity, and (3) the physician must give an honest opinion and avoid having his or her medical judgment influenced by any conflict of interest.

It must not be overlooked that a similar or parallel code has not been established for employers, nor is an employer bound by any ethical behavior beyond that set forth by existing legal agreements and specific state or federal laws.

In my role as instructor to medical students and family practice residents, I can always rely on this question being raised: "How do you deny that you are a 'company' man when the company employs you and pays you?" As to pay, I reply, if most industrial-medical associations are traced back far enough, it will be discovered that medical care was established by joint employee-employer agreements and that the employee gave up some monetary reward to get medical coverage, so it is the employee who is indirectly paying the doctor or financing the medical care. As to company pressure on physicians to do anything unethical, there are opportunities for physicians to move on to other jobs. On the other side of the coin, I ask: "Who is under more pressure, the occupational physician or the private health care provider? Who must keep the patient happy so that he can collect his fee, prevent bad publicity, and make sure malpractice suits are not filed?" Usually, after some thought, the residents I teach admit that the pressure on the occupational physician is not so great, when viewed in that light.

Confidentiality

The question of who should have access to what medical information has now been decided by the Occupational Safety and Health Act (OSHA) and other legal opinions. The courts[17, 25, 19] have ruled that, with preplacement examinations, the patient has waived his or her rights to confidentiality and that the information obtained is the property of the employer. Occupational Safety and Health Administration regulations that deal with employers having employees exposed to toxic substances or harmful physical agents are very specific with regard to who has rights to which records: . . . "employees and their designated representatives (have) a right of access to relevant exposure and medical records; and . . . representatives of the Assistant Secretary (for OSHA) (have) a right of access to these records." *Access* means the right and opportunity to examine and copy no later than 15 days after the request is made. *Designated representative* means any individual or organization to whom an employee gives written authorization to exercise a right of access. An employee's *medical record* includes medical and employment questionnaires or histories, the results of medical examinations, laboratory tests, medical opinions, diagnoses, progress notes and recommendations, descriptions of treatments and prescriptions, and employee medical complaints. It does *not* include records concerning voluntary employee assistance programs, if these are maintained separately from the employer's medical program and its records.[24] The OSHA regulations also allow the physician the discretion to determine if direct access to the information would be detrimental to the employee's health, and if so, to provide the information to a designated representative by having specific written consent.

Inappropriate release of medical information can have serious adverse consequences on job security, so the physician should be sure of his position both legally and ethically when he does commit himself. The patient should sign a "release of information form" (Fig 3–1) before any record is disclosed to a third party, and the patient should be made aware of what he is signing. These "release of information" forms are usually incorporated into preplacement examination and insurance forms. When a worker's compensation claim is filed, confidentiality can no longer be protected, since the employer and appropriate agencies are entitled to access to that information. When in doubt as to the legal obligations, the physician should consult a lawyer knowledgeable in medical records law.

Occasionally, the wishes of the patient cannot be honored because withholding information would have adverse overriding personal or public health consequences. A case such as this presents real ethical problems and must be handled on an individual basis. The American Medical Association's Canon of Medical Ethics states, "A physician may not reveal the confidences entrusted to him in the course of medical attendance, or the deficiencies he may observe in the character of patients, unless he is required to do so by law or unless it becomes necessary in order to protect the welfare of the individual or the community."

The rules and regulations about the release of medical information apply to oral communication as well as written. Often a physician is asked by another health care provider for information (as when a private-care physician is called by the employer's nurse or doctor). The private physician should ask why the information is needed and what will be done with it. Again, to protect confidentiality and not jeopardize the patient's work situation, a written permit to release information should be obtained if at all possible, unless the situation appears to dictate that this is not necessary. This release may have already been accomplished as part of an insurance claim. Always be guided by the principle of what is best for the health and welfare of the patient, as long as no overriding public good is involved. However, remember to be honest in all information given; do not take it upon yourself to protect your patients by falsification or deliberate omission in records or information (especially in diagnosis—i.e., "flu" rather than "acute alcoholic intake"), since ultimately truth will prevail and "protectionism" may only delay much needed care as well as reduce or destroy credibility.

Reporting Health Risks

The reporting of job health risks may make the employer liable for damages, cause unfavorable publicity and possibly a plant closedown or production delays, or even result in company retaliation against the patient-employee. However, as stated earlier, the physician's medical responsibility is to ensure the health of his patient as well as the health of the patient's fellow workers. Disclosure of health risks may take the form of patient counseling, communicating findings to companies and government agencies, and publishing pertinent cases and findings in scientific journals.

Disclosures to the patient should be made on the basis of medical fact and not on social and political suppositions. (The methodology of making a diagnosis of work-related condition will be discussed later.) When reporting to employers, every effort should be made to protect the identity of the patient, unless by prior agreement the patient-employee has consented to full disclosure. Remember, however, it does no good to keep as a profound secret something that has come out on an insurance claim form.

State and federal agencies are readily identified in the phone directory under Department of Labor/Occupational Health and Safety listings. Again, remember to discuss your disclosure with

PATIENT INFORMATION

Name____________ Address____________

Soc. Sec. # ____________ ____________

DOB:________ Age:______ Phone: ____________

Allergies:____________

INJURY INFORMATION

Date of Injury: ________ Part of Body Affected:____________

Statement of Accident:____________

COMPANY INFORMATION

Company Name:____________ Contact Person:____________

Address:____________ Phone No.____________

INSURANCE INFORMATION

Company Name:____________ Contact Person:____________

Address:____________ Phone No.____________

CONSENT FOR TREATMENT

This is to certify that I the undersigned consent to the administration of whatever anesthetics and the performance of whatever procedures may be decided to be necessary or advisable in the opinion of the attending physician.

I further consent to having personnel of The Business and Industry Health Group obtain saliva, blood or urine specimen to determine the use of controlled substances or alcohol content if so requested by my employer.

Signed____________
Patient Date

Signed____________
Witness Date

AUTHORIZATION TO RELEASE INFORMATION

I hereby authorize The Business and Industry Health Group to release all or any portion of my records, including x-rays or laboratory results, and to permit any doctors or other employees to be interviewed regarding my diagnosis, care and treatment rendered by The Business and Industry Health Group.

This authorization includes, but is not limited to, my employer, insurance companies, unemployment and worker's compensation carriers.

Signed____________
Patient Date

Signed____________
Witness Date

____________Case

____

C L R D P Y N

BIHG-020

FIG 3–1.
A release-of-information form.

the patient-employee and abide by an agreed-upon decision, unless an overriding public health situation exists.

DETERMINING PATIENT EMPLOYABILITY

Conducting Job Placement Examinations

Routine job placement examinations can be boring. Most company health forms require similar answers, but they are frequently worded in many different ways, which is frustrating, because so much time is spent deciding what is wanted and where. However, if examinations are viewed as "treasure hunts" or "health hazard appraisals," they can be much more meaningful to both the physician and the patient.

The first question I ask a patient is, "What is the reason for this examination?" Specifically, what type of work is the person being considered for? What kind of equipment will the person be using? All too often, patients reply that they don't know what the examination is for. Job dissatisfaction may be anticipated in these individuals, because they are accepting a job without knowing what it entails. But for those workers who do know, use your knowledge, as well as what the patient knows about the job, to tailor the examination so that you can ascertain that the patient has the specific physical capabilities the job requires. For example, a federal Department of Transportation physical examination for interstate truck drivers, which must be done every two years, is intended to protect the public who use the highways from an accident that might be caused by an incapacitated driver. A physician examining a candidate for a truck driver's job would not just listen to his heart and lungs. Good vision and hearing are needed to operate a truck, so the eyes and ears must be thoroughly examined. Upper and lower extremity coordination and muscle power are also needed and the examination of these is vital. Several health risk factors may be connected to truck driving, and the patient should be counseled about these risks, if necessary. For instance, the enforced inactivity of truck driving, the stress of meeting delivery dates, and the high fat content of truckstop meals may pose a threat to the driver's health if he is not advised to control his weight and cholesterol intake, avoid smoking, and exercise during his off hours. This is an ideal chance to practice preventive medicine in a worker who might not otherwise have visited a physician for an examination. (See Chapter 60 for more information on the health hazards of truck driving.)

When conducting preplacement physical examinations, the object of the physician is to help minimize injuries and to make sure the worker can be productive. Should a physician have the full responsibility of determining employability? The U.S. Department of Labor says no. The physician should advise the patient and the patient's employer if physical or mental impairments exist, and if they do, how they would affect job performance. The employer then must decide if the prospective employee can be safely placed at work. The argument that "only hale and healthy bodies" are wanted "because of insurance liability" and "less absenteeism" is not valid. Studies of employment of the handicapped have shown that when intelligent accommodation of the handicapped person is applied, there is little absenteeism, low utilization of health care plans, and usually top productivity. The examining physician should not be the one to decide to hire or not to hire; this is an employer decision.

Visiting the Workplace

Plant visitations by the physician to the patient's place of employment are encouraged and necessary. The immediate value of these visits to the physician is that they provide a more thorough knowledge of work conditions and job requirements on a first-hand basis. Added bonuses are that (1) the patient will realize that the physician cared enough to make the extra effort, and (2) the employer will be satisfied that the physician is really interested in the workplace environment and his employees. The employer's satisfaction may result in new patient referrals by the company and a better working arrangement between the company and the physician, and the monetary rewards will more than compensate for the time spent on the initial visit.

TREATING THE INJURED/ILL WORKER

Evaluating the Disability

The primary care physician may be called upon to evaluate the injury or illness of a worker for the purpose of documenting a worker's compensation claim. This task can be difficult, because most physicians know little about worker's compensation regulations. The laws differ from state to state, but the concept on which all the laws are based is that of "impairment evaluation," and definite principles and guides about this are available.[10, 14, 1] Certain basic terms must be understood:

Impairment—any anatomical or functional abnormality or loss.

Disability—actual or presumed activities curtailed because of "impairment" which in turn may or may not be combined with other factors.

Permanent—maximal medical rehabilitation has been achieved, and the abnormality or loss is considered to be stable or nonprogressive at the time of the evaluation. No fundamental or marked change can be expected in the future.

Partial—anything less than total.

Permanent impairment can be measured with a reasonable degree of accuracy and uniformity, as it is evidenced by loss of structural integrity, loss of functional capacity, or persistent pain that is substantiated by clinical findings. The evaluation of permanent impairment is a function that physicians alone are competent to perform. The American Medical Association's *Guides to Evaluation of Permanent Impasirment* contains recommended percentage values related to the criteria provided and covers 13 organ systems.[10]

Workers' compensation regulations cover much more than impairment evaluation. The laws of all of the states require that complete medical care for the patient sustaining a work-related injury or illness be paid for by the employer or a third-party payer who has contracted with the employer for the financial responsibilities.[5] The employee must receive two thirds of his or her base wages, up to a maximum dollar amount or time; and in many states, rehabilitation, either to the previous work level or to some other gainful occupation, must be accomplished. This rehabilitation may take the form of physical therapy, occupational therapy, prosthetic devices, and/or retraining through added educational endeavors. The state workers' compensation board should be contacted for the particulars in each state.

It is strongly recommended that if a physician is going to undertake impairment disability evaluations, then the expertise and guidance of a fellow physician who is knowledgeable and willing to share his expertise should be sought. Lacking this, the state workers' compensation board can be helpful in giving guidance. A third mechanism is to seek aid from a reputable lawyer who is noted to be fair and knowledgeable in these cases.

Evaluations always have a certain amount of subjectivity involved, and it is paramount that the physician keep an unbiased attitude at all times, making sure that the patient receives what he or she is entitled to under the laws of the state, but no more. These evaluations must be objective and accurate.

Controlling the Cost of Disability

Disability costs to employers are usually spoken of in terms of billions of dollars and may mean little or nothing to most of us because of their magnitude.[5] More is revealed when one looks at individual patient costs to employers when the employee is not producing: The workers' compensation daily reimbursement is usually two thirds of the worker's normal wages and is not subject to taxes. Workers' compensation begins three to seven days after the injury, depending on individual state laws, but if the patient is still away from work after a certain period, the initial waiting period is also paid for. These financial benefits help to explain why some patients are reluctant to improve or return to work when all signs so indicate, although these patients may not admit to this motive.

As far as physicians and employers are concerned, "disability control" is the issue causing the greatest disagreement. The employer, of course, wishes to reduce disability costs as much as possible. Often, the company would like to use the experience of the employee, even if his or her disability requires liberal accommodation although many labor-management contracts do not allow any type of accommodation—placement is solely on the basis of seniority. Unfortunately, as is often seen, physicians want to deny any part in disability certification by saying they are "only interested in the health" of the employee. However, the third-party payer and the patient-employee will usually not let them take this stance—they must fill out the disability section of the health form or they will not be paid. The hardest step, but, professionally and honorably, the only one to take, is to accumulate a series of facts: What are the patient's limitations and abilities? What accommodations to the employee's condition can be made? Discuss the findings or lack of them with the patient, stressing the advantages (psychosocially) of returning to the work force as soon as it is safe, and stressing, where appropriate, that recovery may not be complete and discomfort may be present but that proper placement by the company and avoidance of harmful activities will allow this early return. This places some of the responsibility for the cure on the patient.

In disability control, never assume the role of "insurance policeman." These activities are administrative functions. Do make valid, thoughtful decisions about the patient's abilities and be flexible enough to say "yes" or "no" as the employee's situation changes.

Getting the Patient Back to Work

Derebery and Tullis[8] say that the patient needs to return to work as soon as possible, because otherwise his recovery may be delayed by the "reinforcers" of his illness: the disability income, the sympathy and attention from his family and community, the escape from responsibility, and/or the use of his illness as a tool of revenge against the company or as a method of resolving internal conflicts. The practice of prescribing additional rest and inactivity for the patient experiencing delayed recovery following, for example, a musculoskeletal injury, further reinforces the delaying process and adds physiologic deterioration to the trauma.

The patient whose physical recovery is delayed, for whatever reason, learns to be psychologically disabled as well, and the physician who offers to speed the recovery is sometimes seen by the patient as a threat, since the physician is challenging the patient's image of himself as a disabled person. Bearing this in mind, it is important that the physician respond with compassion, understanding, and firm therapeutic goals, rather than returning the patient's hostility.

Treatment of this type of patient is best carried out by the primary care physician, but psychiatric assistance may be required. The best prescription would be an early return to some form of work, and it is essential that the physician work with the employer to achieve this. Inactivity should be kept to a minimum. The patient might also be helped to recovery by relaxation training, perhaps with biofeedback techniques taught by appropriate professionals. Psychologic problems that might have contributed to the delay in recovery should be corrected, if possible. By stopping narcotic medications and substituting anti-inflammatory drugs and other nonnarcotics, the physician may remove another chief "reinforcer" of the patient's illness.

Communicating With the Patient's Employer

Effective communication with the patient's employer can be the key to the successful reintroduction of the recovering worker to the workplace. For example, "ability" forms are probably the most common method of communication between the physician and the employer or other third party on behalf of the patient. The form may be a prescription blank with a terse "may not work" (Fig 3–2) or a more elaborate form (Fig 3–3); but whatever the form, it is the content that matters (Figs 3–4 and 3–5). These forms should be filled out in such a way that the recipient may properly evaluate the ability of the patient to perform in the workplace without causing further damage to himself or to his fellow employees or to company property. A frequently heard excuse for poor communication is, "I didn't know a doctor or nurse was going to get this." Therefore, the physician should ask the patient-worker if the form will go to a company doctor or nurse. If a structured medical department at the workplace does exist, write a note that gives complete information, one that you would like to receive when you do a consultation, not one that may diminish your stature in the eyes of the recipient. Remember to discuss only the patient's ability to work and get the patient's permission before you send the note. If there are no medical personnel at the workplace, it is all the more important to be specific in laymen's terms as to "ability."

The Business and Industry Health Group

Name John Smith Date 2/6 1984

Address 10470 Point Drive KCMO

Rx

May not work.

[signature] M.D.

Substitution Permitted — M.D. Dispense as Written

Refill ______ Times DEA Reg. No. ______

2316 E. Meyer Kansas City, MO 64132 (816) 276-4411	Admiral Blvd. at Oak Kansas City, MO 64106 (816) 842-1146	6300 Enterprise Rd. Kansas City, MO 64120 (816) 231-3611	10000 W. 75th Shawnee Mission, KS 66204 (913) 362-3687

Form No. 21-E22-001 **PRESCRIPTION BLANK**

FIG 3–2.
This form and note provides minimum information; even the physician identification remains unclear, making further clarification difficult.

The Business and Industry Health Group

Name John Smith Date Jan. 10 1984

Address 10470 Point Drive, Kansas City, MO

Rx
Acute anterior wall myocardial infarct 10/15/83.
Coronary angiography 11/17/83.
Anterior vessel 90% occluded.
Coronary angioplasty 11/18/83 with occlusion reduced to 40%.
Treadmill stress test to 80% of maximal capacity with no S-T segment or T wave changes 1/4/84.
Return to full activity 1/11/84.

Substitution Permitted — M.D. [signature] Dispense as Written — M.D.

Refill ______ Times DEA Reg. No. ______

2316 E. Meyer Kansas City, MO 64132 (816) 276-4411	Admiral Blvd. at Oak Kansas City, MO 64106 (816) 842-1146	6300 Enterprise Rd. Kansas City, MO 64120 (816) 231-3611	10000 W. 75th Shawnee Mission, KS 66204 (913) 362-3687

Form No. 21-E22-001 **PRESCRIPTION BLANK**

FIG 3–3.
Sample of an ideal short form and report. It communicates that the treating physician realizes that another physician will be making decisions for the employer and gives all the medical information needed, as well as a personal opinion as to the patient's availability for work.

The Business & Industry Health Group

Research Medical Center
2316 East Meyer Boulevard
Kansas City, Missouri 64132

816/276-4411

Name ____________________

Employer ____________________

Chart No. ____________________ Date ____________________

Time Arrived ____________________ Time Released ____________________

Diagnosis ____________________

☐ Scheduled for appointment on ____________ at ____________

☐ Return to regular work on ____________

☐ Return to work on ____________ with the following restrictions:

- ☐ No exposure to cold, heat, water, dampness, chemicals, oil, solvents, paint, dust, welding, coolants. (Circle appropriate restrictions)
- ☐ No climbing of stairs or ladders
- ☐ No work above ground or surface level
- ☐ No work around high speed or moving machinery
- ☐ No operating of mobile equipment
- ☐ No lifting over ____________ lbs.
- ☐ No working requiring repetitive waist bending
- ☐ No repetitive shoveling
- ☐ No push or pull over ____________ lbs.
- ☐ No kneeling or squatting
- ☐ Should be sitting ________% of time
- ☐ No reaching above shoulder level
- ☐ No use of ____________
- ☐ Should be considered permanent
- ☐ Unable to work on ____________

☐ Other: ____________________

If the above restrictions constitute light duty and such is not available, it is assumed that the patient will be sent home rather than allowed to work.

Form 12-E00-020 ____________________ MD

FIG 3–4.
An "ability form" of this nature provides the physician with an easy method to convey to another medical or a nonmedical supervisor the patient's ability to perform within restricted circumstances. It is better for the physician to spell out physical capabilities and allow management to make a decision on work availability. Otherwise, the physician, who is poorly equipped to know of such availability, may be depriving the employee of gainful employment and the company of a useful employee.

Once a worker's abilities are defined, he or she may say, "No work exists for me," or "We don't have such jobs (that fit the abilities you describe)," or "My boss would rather not have me if I can't do my regular job." If this occurs, the physician should simply ask the patient-employee for his or her supervisor's phone number and talk with the supervisor about altering the patient's job. In this day and age, with industries trying to reduce their nonproductive costs (disability and worker's compensation), managers are much more receptive to creating new job situations to accommodate the patient's ability.

Determining 'Work Relatedness'

There are times when a worker-patient presents with an illness or injury whose cause has not been clearly established, and the physician may have to decide whether the patient's work is the cause or is a contributing factor.

How does one go about determining the work relatedness of injury and illness other than by asking the patient what he thinks? Perhaps a more basic question the physician has to ask is, "How do I even begin to think through a 'work relatedness' decision?" A screening, self-administered history should be taken on all patients of working age. A practical and useful form is shown in Figure 3–6 and should be reviewed when seeing a worker for a new complaint. If the physician does not care for this added paperwork, then, as a minimum, each patient should be asked what his job is and be asked to describe what the job entails. The physician should not be afraid to show ignorance by asking questions of the patient. Most jobs have a language peculiar to the job. For instance, a patient may say, "I run a Michigan press," which means the press was made by the Michigan foundry but tells you nothing about what kind of press it is and how it is run, until you ask further questions. As in any other part of the history, ask enough questions and get enough details about the job and its requirements and the worker's environment so that you feel you can see how the patient's work fits in with the overall health history. Once this has been done, you can start thinking of the work-relatedness of the patient's problem.

There are some very good criteria[3, 11, 12, 20] that one can apply in the determination of work relatedness decisions which should allow the primary care physician to arrive at a reasonable conclusion with a comfortable certainty. These are the following:

1. Are the symptoms consistent with the diagnosis?
2. Are the signs consistent with the diagnosis?
3. Is the temporal relationship of exposure and disease clear?

ATTENDING PHYSICIAN'S RETURN TO WORK RECOMMENDATIONS RECORD

Company Name

Patient's Name (Last) (First) (Middle Initial) | Date of Injury/Illness

TO BE COMPLETED BY ATTENDING PHYSICIAN—PLEASE CHECK

DIAGNOSIS/CONDITION (Brief Explanation)

I saw and treated this patient on ____________ (Date) and based on the above description of the patient's current medical problem:

1. ☐ Recommend his/her return to work with no limitations on ____________ (Date).
2. ☐ He/She may return to work on ____________ (Date) with the following limitations:

CHECK ONLY AS RELATES TO ABOVE CONDITIONS

☐ **Sedentary Work.** Lifting 10 pounds maximum and occasionally lifting and/or carrying such articles as dockets, ledgers, and small tools. Although a sedentary job is defined as one which involves sitting, a certain amount of walking and standing is often necessary in carrying out job duties. Jobs are sedentary if walking and standing are required only occasionally and other sedentary criteria are met.

☐ **Light Work.** Lifting 20 pounds maximum with frequent lifting and/or carrying of objects weighing up to 10 pounds. Even though the weight lifted may be only a negligible amount, a job is in this category when it requires walking or standing to a significant degree or when it involves sitting most of the time with a degree of pushing and pulling of arm and/or leg controls.

☐ **Light Medium Work.** Lifting 30 pounds maximum with frequent lifting and/or carrying of objects weighing up to 20 pounds.

☐ **Medium Work.** Lifting 50 pounds maximum with frequent lifting and/or carrying of objects weighing up to 25 pounds.

☐ **Light Heavy Work.** Lifting 75 pounds maximum with frequent lifting and/or carrying of objects weighing up to 40 pounds.

☐ **Heavy Work.** Lifting 100 pounds maximum with frequent lifting and/or carrying of objects weighing up to 50 pounds.

1. In an 8 hour work day patient may:
   a. Stand/Walk
   ☐ None ☐ 4-6 Hours
   ☐ 1-4 Hours ☐ 6-8 Hours
   b. Sit
   ☐ 1-3 Hours ☐ 3-5 Hours ☐ 5-8 Hours
   c. Drive
   ☐ 1-3 Hours ☐ 3-5 Hours ☐ 5-8 Hours
2. Patient may use hand(s) for repetitive:
   ☐ Single Grasping ☐ Pushing & Pulling
   ☐ Fine Manipulation
3. Patient may use foot/feet for repetitive movement as in operating foot controls: ☐ Yes ☐ No
4. Patient may:

	Not At All	Occasionally	Frequently
a. Bend	☐	☐	☐
b. Twist	☐	☐	☐
c. Squat	☐	☐	☐
d. Climb	☐	☐	☐
e. Reach	☐	☐	☐

OTHER INSTRUCTIONS AND/OR LIMITATIONS <u>INCLUDING PRESCRIBED MEDICATIONS</u>

3. ☐ These restrictions are in effect until ____________ (Date) or until patient is reevaluated on ____________ (Date).
4. He/she is totally incapacitated at this time. Patient will be reevaluated on ____________ (Date).
5. Referred To: ☐ None ☐ Private physician ____________ (Doctor)
   ☐ Return Here ____________ (Date & Time) ☐ A Consultant ____________ (Doctor, Date & Time)

Physician's Signature | Date

AUTHORIZATION TO RELEASE INFORMATION

I hereby authorize my attending physician and/or hospital to release any information or copies thereof acquired in the course of my examination or treatment for the injury identified above to my employer or his representative.

Patient's Signature | Date

SMSSI (6/84) DISTRIBUTION: *WHITE—Employer* *CANARY—Doctor* *PINK—Employee*

FIG 3–5.
The attending physician's return-to-work recommendations record prepared by the Committee on Environmental and Occupational Health of The State Medical Society of Wisconsin and endorsed by the Society's Liaison Committee on Health Care Costs. The form is not copyrighted and may be reproduced without restrictions. The Wisconsin SMS Services, Inc., has printed the form in three-part sets, which are available on request for a nominal cost. (From *Wis Med J,* June 1985; 84:98. Used by permission.)

SUGGESTED OCCUPATIONAL EXPOSURE HISTORY
Part I

Please answer the following questions. Begin with your present job and list all jobs or military service you have held in order of date whether full or part time.

TODAY'S DATE NAME SOCIAL SECURITY NUMBER JOB CLASSIFICATION(S)	List potential hazards exposed to: (examples)				Work related illnesses or injuries	
	Physical	Chemical	Biological	Psychological	YES	NO
	Noise Radiation Vibration Electrical shock Temperature extremes Repetitive motion Heavy lifting	Mercury Lead Dust Gases Fumes Acids Solvents Caustics	Viruses Bacteria Parasites Fungus Animal bites Etc	Boredom Work shift fatigue Risk of falling Risk of being buried Repetition		
COMPANY NAME CITY, STATE JOB TITLE FROM: TO: AVERAGE HR/WK	HAZARDS: COMMENTS:					
COMPANY NAME CITY, STATE JOB TITLE FROM: TO: AVERAGE HR/WK	HAZARDS: COMMENTS:					
COMPANY NAME CITY, STATE JOB TITLE FROM: TO: AVERAGE HR/WK	HAZARDS: COMMENTS:					
COMPANY NAME CITY, STATE JOB TITLE FROM: TO: AVERAGE HR/WK	HAZARDS: COMMENTS:					

FIG 3–6.
A two-part form for taking a patient's occupational health history. (From *Wis Med J*, December 1981; 80:21.)

SUGGESTED OCCUPATIONAL EXPOSURE HISTORY
Part II

SECONDARY WORK (examples)	List potential hazards exposed to: (examples)				Work related illnesses or injuries	
Firefighting Civil defense Farming Gardening Civic activities Etc	**Physical** Noise Radiation Vibration Electrical shock Temperature extremes Etc	**Chemical** Mercury Lead Dust Gases Fumes Acids Solvents Caustics	**Biological** Viruses Bacteria Parasites Fungus Animal bites Etc	**Psychological** Boredom Work shift fatigue Risk of falling Risk of being buried Repetition Etc	YES	NO
ORGANIZATION CITY, STATE JOB TITLE FROM: TO: AVERAGE HR/WK	HAZARDS: COMMENTS:					
ORGANIZATION CITY, STATE JOB TITLE FROM: TO: AVERAGE HR/WK	HAZARDS: COMMENTS:					
ORGANIZATION CITY, STATE JOB TITLE FROM: TO: AVERAGE HR/WK	HAZARDS: COMMENTS:					
HOBBIES & ACTIVE SPORTS						
ACTIVITY CITY, STATE FROM: TO: AVERAGE HR/WK	HAZARDS: COMMENTS:					
ACTIVITY CITY, STATE FROM: TO: AVERAGE HR/WK	COMMENTS:					

Some chemicals have effects on the reproductive system. Have you or your present or former spouse had any problems with reproduction? If so, please indicate circumstances (e.g., stillborn, deformed, miscarriage, infertility).

EXPLAIN: ______________________________

____

4. Do fellow workers with similar exposure have similar problems?

5. Is workplace monitoring data available and indicative of suspected exposure?

6. Is the condition biologically plausible and confirmed?

7. Is there a lack of nonoccupational exposure to the toxic agent?

If the above criteria are met,[24] the physician is in a firm position to advise the patient, the employer, and any third-party payer about causation and fiscal responsibility, and, just as important, the physician can then take steps to *prevent further exposure of the patient and other members of the work force.*

Surveillance Examinations

In order to determine the work-relatedness of an employee's health problem or to monitor the occurrence of work-related health problems among a group of employees, a physician may be called upon to perform surveillance examinations. Surveillance examinations require that a physician know what type and amount of exposure may have occurred and what the specific and nonspecific bodily effects are produced by the substance(s) the employee is exposed to. The purpose of these examinations is to determine potentially harmful effects, both acute and chronic, from exposure to specific substances or environmental conditions. The physician needs to know the substance or substances involved, concentrations during the exposure, and the amount of time the employee is exposed. Accumulating "hard data" on exposures that prove harmless can be just as important to the general work force as discovering harmful effects, although "negative" results are seldom documented or reported in the literature. If harmful conditions *are* discovered, the physician should never suppress this finding or let political or social pressures influence his or her medical decisions.

Referring the Patient

Consultations and referrals in occupational medicine differ somewhat from those in private practice. In primary care delivery, there is a bond between the private patient and the physician which does not necessarily exist in the employee-patient-physician relationship. The patient may have no choice about seeing you, since he may have been sent by the employer or third-party payer.

Primary care physicians will find themselves referring cases they previously would have cared for themselves, since the financial burden on the patient is no longer there to influence a decision not to refer. Employers will often want the opinion of a specialist in addition to that of the primary care physician's, in order to strengthen their findings in court in case there is a legal dispute over compensation. In some areas, such as plastic surgery, the cost of the ultimate outcome (permanent disfigurement awards) will justify the added cost.

Consultants should not only be the best available in their subspecialty, but they also must be knowledgeable about the facets of occupational medicine discussed in this chapter. It is just as important for the consultant as it is for the primary care physician to know about ability evaluations, workers' compensation, work-relatedness determinations, disability control, ethics, and communications to a third party. Your ability to handle cases is judged by how well your consultants also manage the case and by the results they get.

Before any patient is referred however, (excepting an emergency) permission should be sought from the employer or "third-party payer." Even though your decision on a consultant may be correct, the third-party may want another consultant for some other reason (the company may have better communication or past experience with their consultant or he may be less expensive). As long as the third-party's choice is considered competent and ethical, I believe the primary physician should go along with it. However, you should have no qualms about disagreeing with the third-party's choice if the ultimate good of the patient is jeopardized. I have always prevailed in the need for referral or in the choice of consultant when I have presented my reasons to the employer or the third-party payer. Without prior approval for the consultant, you may find yourself in the position of trying to convince the company to pay the consultant's fee after the fact.

How well you and your consultant communicate is very important. You must give your consultant the benefit of all you know about the case, and he must reciprocate and be aware that you will have to relay his findings to the company. The consultant should give you frequent and timely reports, and both of you should have from the patient a signed release to transmit reports to the company, their insurance carrier, and legal representatives.

In the hope that this chapter has engendered a desire to know more about occupational medical practice, the reader is referred to Chapters 2, 5, and 8.

REFERENCES

1. Abrev BC: *Physical Disabilities Manual*. New York, Raven Press, 1981.
2. Adams R: *Occupational Skin Diseases*. New York, Grune & Stratton, 1983.
3. *A Guide to the Work-Relatedness of Disease*. NIOSH Publication #79–116. US Government Printing Office, Superintendent of Documents, Washington, DC 20402, 1979.
4. American Occupational Medical Association, 2340 S Arlington Heights Rd, Arlington Heights, IL 60005.
5. *Analysis of Worker's Compensation Laws 1983*. US Chamber of Commerce, 1615 H St NW Washington DC 20062.
6. Annas GJ: Legal aspects of medical confidentiality in the occupational setting. *J Occup Med* 1976; 18:537–40.
7. Casarett J, Doull J: *Toxicology: The Basic Sciences of Poisons*, ed 2. New York, Macmillan Publishing Co, 1980.
8. Derebery VJ, Tullis WH: Delayed recovery in the patient with a work compensable injury. *J Occup Med* 1983; 25:829–35.
9. *Federal Register*, Vol 45, #102, May 23, p 35277, 1980.
10. *Guides to the Evaluation of Permanent Impairment*. Chicago, American Medical Association, 1984.
11. Hamilton A, Hardy HL: *Industrial Toxicology*, ed 4. (Revised by AJ Finkel.) Boston, Publishing Sciences Group, 1983.
12. Hunter D: *The Diseases of Occupations*, ed 6. London, Hodden & Stroughton, 1978.
13. Karrh BW: The confidentiality of occupational medical data. *J Occup Med*, 1976; 18:137–40.
14. Kessler HS: *Disability Determination and Evaluation*. Philadelphia, Lea & Febiger, 1970.

15. Kuenssburg EV: A note on ethics and the part-timer in occupational health. *J Med Ethics* 1980; 6:197–98.
16. Key M, Key AL: *Occupational Diseases: A Guide To Their Recognition*. NIOSH Publication #77–181. Superintendent of Documents, US Government Printing Office, Washington, DC 20402, 1977.
17. Lotspeich vs Chance Vought Aircraft (Texas Civil Appeal 1963).
18. *Medicine and the Workplace*. Needham Heights, Mass, Damon Corporation, 1979.
19. New York Central Railroad Co. vs. Viler (NY 1931).
20. Proctor NH, Huges JP: *Chemical Hazards of the Workplace*. Philadelphia, JB Lippincott, Co, 1978.
21. Rosenstock L: *Ethical Dilemmas Facing Clinicians Who Provide Health Services to Workers*. Tucson, Ariz, Project Module, Arizona Center for Occupational Safety and Health, University of Arizona Health Science Center, 1983.
22. Sauer G: *Manual of Skin Diseases*, ed 4. Philadelphia, JB Lippincott, Co, 1980.
23. Tabershaw IR: Whose 'agent' is the occupational physician? *Arch Environ Health* 1975; 30:412–416.
24. *The Occupational & Environmental History*. Tucson, Ariz, Project Module, Arizona Center for Occupational Safety and Health, University of Arizona Health Science Center, 1980.
25. Wilcox vs Salt Lake City Corp (Utah 1971).

4

The Occupational Health Nurse

Florence Ebert, R.N., C.O.H.N.

HISTORY OF OCCUPATIONAL HEALTH NURSING

The American Industrial Revolution had progressed for more than a century before nursing and industry recognized a mutuality of needs and interests. Nursing and industry gradually became cognizant of the benefits of the nurse's professional skills in safeguarding worker health.

The earliest "industrial nurses" provided home nursing services for workers and their families, caring for "typhoid and obstetrical" patients as well as those with other prevailing illnesses. The concept of the "industrial nurse" as an in-plant service came about in the United States during World War I, when the proliferation of industry and its growing work force revealed problems in health, safety, and welfare, and national concern resulted in legislative remedies.[18]

In 1888, the U.S. Bureau of Labor was created, and in 1910, an investigation of the match industry by the Labor Commissioner resulted in the first major public act to control occupational disease. In 1911 in Wisconsin, the first workers' compensation law was enacted, based upon the British concept of a no-fault system of benefits provided to most workers who had incurred work-related illness or injury.

Workers' compensation was first enacted in Germany, around the latter part of the nineteenth century. Around the turn of the century, Great Britain adopted their own workers' compensation laws.

Prior to the enactment of workers' compensation, the common law governed, and an employee who was injured had to prove negligence on the part of his employer to recover. He also had to overcome three common law defenses known as contributory negligence, assumption of risk, and the fellow-servant rule.

The result was that when he sued his employer, it was a time-consuming, uncertain process, expensive to both parties, and usually extremely harsh on the employee. The no-fault system eliminated the need to prove negligence, permitting the employee to receive benefits for medical care and lost wages incurred through work-related injury and illness. The rapid increase in the employment of occupational health nurses can be attributed to the government's insistence that factories and shipyards working to fulfill World War I contracts also provide employee health services.

Given the ground swell for social legislation in the United States and the passage of the Occupational Safety and Health Act (OSHA) of 1970, labor and nursing came to have concomitant goals for the preservation of the health and welfare of the nation's most valuable resource, the work force.

In 1980, the U.S. registered nurse population was estimated to be 1,662,382 nurses. Hospitals continued to be the predominant employer of registered nurses. Of those employed in nursing, an estimated 835,647, or 65.7%, worked in hospitals. The second largest group of employers of nurses was nursing homes, where 8% were working. In rank order, the proportion of nurses employed in other employment settings was 6.6% in community health, 5.7% in physicians' or dentists' offices, 3.7% in nursing education, 3.5% in schools, and only 2.3% employed in occupational health settings.

However, this 2.3% use of available nurse resources represents the largest health specialty group that regularly works in industry.

OCCUPATIONAL HEALTH NURSING AS A SPECIALTY

Occupational health nursing is considered a nursing specialty and is highly differentiated from other areas of nursing practice.

The scope of occupational health nursing practice is largely determined by the nurse's educational background, the management's expectations, and the identified hazards of the workplace.

The occupational health (OH) nurse is no longer limited to practice in the industrial setting. A study by McKechnie found that over half of the nurses worked in manufacturing industries in 1983, with 20.8% in light manufacturing and 31.3% in heavy manufacturing. The next largest percentage of nurses (22.9%) worked in hospital employee health services. Approximately 15% were employed in office settings, such as insurance companies or corporate headquarters. The remaining nurses worked for a variety of companies, including those dealing with warehousing, transportation, utilities, and research.[9, 11]

The simple tasks of the early occupational health nurses have changed greatly, with expectations of greater change for the future. In order to practice effectively, the professional occupational health nurse of today must be aware of the complexities confronting this nursing specialty. The issues critical to the practicing nurse are relevant skills, continuing education, preventive health modalities, employee counseling, and the other functions and responsibilities expected by the employer.[13]

In the United States, occupational health nurses are represented by the American Association of Occupational Health Nurses (AAOHN). Founded in 1942, AAOHN now includes state, local, and regional associations. Officers and the board of directors are elected by the membership. Standing national committees that conduct research and service activities for the association are appointed by the president with approval of the board of directors. A full-time professional staff is also maintained under the supervision of the executive director.

The AAOHN defines an *occupational health nurse* as a registered professional nurse employed by business, industry, or an organization for the purpose of conserving, protecting, or restoring the health of workers. The nurse is also employed to prevent disease and injury among employed workers at and through their place of employment. The nurse has the additional responsibilities of making first-level diagnoses and assessing physical and emotional needs. In addition, the nurse may provide total patient care in conjunction with the physician. The nurse functions independently or under nursing supervision.

Although the exact number is unknown, some practicing occupational health nurses in the U.S. are not members of their professional organizations, so they do not receive the professional information available to member nurses.

Lee has estimated that approximately half of all employed occupational health nurses are sole health care providers at the work site.[10] They have few or no opportunities for collegial interaction.

NURSE/MANAGEMENT RESPONSIBILITIES

The foremost responsibility of today's occupational health nurse is to provide occupational health nursing services,[7] which may include preventive health education, emergency care, counseling, safety assessments, environmental hazards identification, record keeping, worker rehabilitation, employee referral to community health resources, OSHA medical surveillance monitoring requirements, program continuity, and strategies directed to employee needs and organizational goals.

Ideally, the occupational health nurse sets goals to provide an occupational health nursing program tailored to the individual workplace. The occupational health program's goal is the protection and maintenance of optimum worker health and efficiency.

Management has an obligation to recognize the expertise of the occupational health professional and provide the professional autonomy, authority, and resources necessary for the development, organization, control, and administration of the program. Considerations for future occupational health concerns should be anticipated, assuring that the program remains effective and dynamic.

The goals of the occupational health nurse's program are reviewed and discussed by management and nurse. The program's scope, implementations, and ongoing audits are the responsibility of the occupational health nurse, with management's support.

Of mutual benefit to the occupational health nurse and management is the continuation of the occupational health nurse's professional growth. Work environments differ greatly; competency in a former position does not guarantee the same competency in a current position. Management must encourage additional training. If specialized skills are required, e.g., for performing pulmonary function testing, audiograms, and vision screening, management must provide the nurse with the time and resources for training.[19]

WORKPLACE REALITIES

Although the escalation of health care costs is of national concern, most companies have shown little interest in cost containment.

The National Institute for Occupational Safety and Health (NIOSH) published a 1980 study addressing the costs and benefits of occupational health nursing services, citing the benefits of improved employee morale, increased efficiency and productivity, and reduced costs for lost-time and medical treatment.[3] However, at present, most companies do not differentiate between quality occupational nursing care and the health care provided by clericals and paraprofessionals, who still administer many company health programs today. The nonprofessional personnel are paid less, but this savings to the company is negated by the larger losses in employee benefits that are available from professionally administered occupational health nursing programs.

Lack of Autonomy.—Although the occupational health nurse is a licensed health professional and has attained certification in this specialty, most managements will be reluctant to permit the autonomy necessary for effective nursing practice. All professionals must have autonomy, defined, according to Webster's as "the right or power of self-government, undertaken without outside control and independent of external influence."

Many practicing occupational health nurses must repeatedly justify their "worth" to managers who know little or nothing about occupational nursing. Personnel managers or other members of management charged with the supervision of the professional nurse should familiarize themselves with the standards of occupational health nursing practice (Table 4–1).

Isolation.—The occupational health nurse is often isolated from participating in managerial discussions, and his or her attempted input is usually disregarded.

Role Conflict.—Role conflict is an ever-present stressor confronting most occupational health nurses when nonnursing duties are expected.

> Role conflict results when roles are incongruous with the individual's values and/or other roles held by the individual. Occupational health nurses are accountable to their profession, the workers, and the management for whom they work. The role set is large and diverse. Role conflict is likely if nurses are not allowed to define their professional practice.[12]

(I know of an instance where the occupational health nurse was made accountable for entrees submitted in a company-sponsored contest.)

TABLE 4–1.

Standards of Practice for Candidates Applying* for Certification by Examination:† American Board for Occupational Health Nurses, Inc.

Standard I
An OHN is one who applies nursing principles in conserving the health of workers in all occupations.

Standard II
The nurse has professional preparation commensurate with the purposes of and gives direction to the nursing care program.

Standard III
The nurse has a philosophy and objectives which reflect the purposes of and gives direction to the nursing care program.

Standard IV
The nurse provides safe, efficient, and therapeutically effective nursing care through appropriate planning of each worker's care and the effective implementation of the plan.

Standard V
An adequate system of records and reports is maintained for effective care of the employee.

Standard VI
The nurse helps and participates in promoting environmental health and safety.

Standard VII
The nurse helps promote health maintenance of the worker.

Standard VIII
The nurse coordinates nursing activities with community health programs and benefit plans of the employing agency.

*From Keefer MW: *Occupational Health Nursing* 1983; 31:12. Used by permission.

†The criteria for each standard may be obtained from ABOHN, Inc., 2210 Wilshire Blvd, Suite 771, Santa Monica, CA 90403.

Ambiguity.—When the role of the occupational health nurse is not defined as to behavior, performance, professional status, and managerial duties, ambiguity results. Unless management legitimizes their managerial role, occupational health nurses perform managerial duties without the compensation commensurate with such responsibilities accorded to other identified managers.[12] Occupational nurses are often told, "Your job is what your supervisor wishes you to do."

Inadequate Performance Evaluations.—Management is often ill-prepared to evaluate the occupational health nurse's performance, due to a lack of knowledge or understanding of the professional's responsibilities.

Much of the nurse's time and energy is diverted from the priority of "worker health" by nonnursing assignments, which results in psychosocial stress and inequitable performance evaluations.

THE OCCUPATIONAL HEALTH NURSE'S JOB DESCRIPTION

Conflicts, ambiguity, and unrealistic management expectations of the nurse can be avoided if management will provide a written job description that outlines expected duties and responsibilities. Specific education, experience, and qualifications should be clearly stated.[1, 10, 11] When duties and responsibilities change, the job description must be revised.

Management errs in hiring a health professional with the expectation of obtaining a clerical fill-in. Too often, the occupational health nurse receives requests to perform nonnursing tasks from all levels of management.

It is essential for management to specify who the nurse reports to, who the immediate supervisor will be, and, equally important, how and from whom medical and administrative direction is received. (The need for medical direction is a legal requirement, as mandated by each jurisdiction or state practice act.)

There must be agreement between nurse and management regarding organizational goals and policies.

The moral and ethical concerns of the practicing occupational health nurse regarding medical directives, professional liability, confidentiality, health and safety, as well as legal issues, also must be addressed.[1, 8]

Sample Job Descriptions for the Occupational Health Nurse

The following job descriptions may be helpful to management and nurses in defining the role of the OH nurse in various settings.

Occupational Health Nurse (Plant Level)

Objectives.—Provide a professional health resource at the plant site in order to protect, maintain, and assist in the rehabilitation of the employee's health.

Qualifications.—Have a valid, current professional nurse's license to practice in the state of employment, plus a professional nurse's education leading to an R.N., a background in public health, emergency medicine, or occupational health, and at least two years' experience.

Responsibilities of Management.—Conduct a walk-through inspection of the plant with the nurse to acquaint him or her with the jobs and their hazards. Introduce the nurse to supervisors and provide a list of their names and departments.

Refer all illness, injury, and health problems to the nurse and refer all previously absent and returning employees to the nursing unit.

Support the nurse's attendance at occupational health seminars, workshops, and conferences.

Responsibilities of Corporate Environmental Health/Industrial Hygiene Services.—Provide hazard data sheets as references for the nurse's information on possible adverse health effects of materials at the plant site.

Provide information, assistance, and support in occupational health matters.

Obtain consultant answers on health problems from the corporate occupational health physician.

Review the performance of nursing functions annually. (The corporate occupational health nurse, if there is one, should do the assessment.)

Responsibilities of the Occupational Health Nurse.—***Perform the following functions. Treating and educating the employee.***—Provide emergency care and treat illness and injury, referring major problems to the plant physician. Obtain standing orders from the plant physician as a guideline for treating employee illness and injury. (A procedure guide book will be provided by the corporate environmental health and hygiene department.)

Review with each employee his or her fitness for returning to work.

Establish periodic employee health programs, such as blood pressure screening or distribution of allergy information.

Know the area resources for counseling and referring employees with nonoccupational health problems, e.g., the Red Cross, welfare agencies, and the American Cancer Society.

Monitoring plant health and safety hazards.—Know the plant areas and the hazards pertinent to occupational health.

Remain current on occupational hazards and changes by reviewing data sheets for symptoms that may be presented by employee exposures.

Attend safety meetings and report health hazards observed during periodic walk-through observations.

Assist the plant physician with employee physical examinations.—Obtain the health history and fill in forms for the examining physician. Perform the nursing assessment: check blood pressure, temperature, pulse, and respiration, obtain specimens, and perform urinalysis, sight screening, and other tests, as indicated.

Assist in the scheduling of examinations. Bring to the attention of the physician any effects of exposures or health problems since the employee's last exam.

Review all results of the examinations. Bring all abnormalities to the attention of the plant physician and corporate consultant. Review the exam results with the employee.

Maintaining records.—Maintain the medical records system according to corporate directions. Make sure records are accurate and legible and suitable for legal purposes. Write, not type, information into the medical records, and sign each entry.

Maintain the OSHA log and workers' compensation records (Fig 4–1).

Establish and keep current an individual employee health record file for each employee, and retain records of each for the period, as required by OSHA. Record all absences of employees with health reasons for the absence.

Keep medical records in strict confidence and store them in a locked cabinet. Reveal medical information only to the employee, trained health professionals, and/or government agencies, as directed under OSHA standards.

Maintaining the medical unit.—Assess the area assigned and order equipment as needed for optimum efficiency. Make sure that the medical unit stays clean and properly equipped.

Coordinating, consulting, acting as a liaison.—Seek help as needed from management, the plant hygienist, and/or the safety director. Consult with the corporate occupational health nurse as a resource for OH nursing direction.

Maintain contact with the treating physician and employee concerning lost-time compensation claims due to occupational illness or injury. Apprise the employee's supervisor of progress made.

Establish, in coordination with the safety director, a group of employees trained in CPR and first aid.

Act as a liaison between other health professionals, employees, and management.

Occupational Health Nurse (Corporate Level)

The role of the corporate occupational health nurse is to assure that quality nursing care is provided to all employees within a corporation. The corporate occupational health nurse is a relatively new role for the occupational health nurse. No definition of this position exists at present. It is estimated that there are less than 50 corporate occupational health nurses in practice today in the U.S.

The following is a sample for the corporate occupational health nurse's job description.

Objectives.—To oversee and direct the occupational health nursing program in conjunction with health care professionals.

To set the corporation's OH health nursing care standards and assure that all the corporation's nurses are provided with the resources to fulfill the requirements of the standards.

To provide a professional health resource at the corporate level, for the benefit of both management and employee, to protect, maintain, and assist in the documentation and assessment of all the corporation's employee occupational health programs.

To ensure quality professional occupational health care be provided and made available for all employees of the corporation.

Qualifications.—Be registered and currently licensed in the state where the OH nurse will be practicing.

Be currently certified in the practice of occupational health nursing.

Have five to ten years of occupational health nursing experience.

Have evidence of participation in ongoing continuing educational programs in occupational health nursing.

Have, preferably, advanced degrees in nursing and administration.

Have an extensive knowledge of workers' compensation, OSHA regulations, and various state laws covering the specific corporate sites.

Be able to change the health care department as changes in medical technology, philosophies of health care, and organizational structures occur.

Responsibilities of Management.—Walk through all corporate sites with the corporate OH nurse to acquaint him or her with the jobs, hazards, and supervisory and nursing personnel at each location.

Introduce the corporate nurse to supervisors and provide a list of names and departments at each location.

OSHA FORM 200

U.S. Department of Labor

Bureau of Labor Statistics
Log and Summary of Occupational
Injuries and Illnesses

NOTE: **This form is required by Public Law 91-596 and must be kept in the establishment for *5 years*. Failure to maintain and post can result in the issuance of citations and assessment of penalties.** ***(See posting requirements on the other side of form.)***

RECORDABLE CASES: You are required to record information about every occupational **death**; every nonfatal occupational **illness**; and those nonfatal occupational **injuries** which involve one or more of the following: loss of consciousness, restriction of work or motion, transfer to another job, or medical treatment (other than first aid). ***(See definitions on the other side of form.)***

For Calendar Year 19 ____ Page ____ of ____

Company Name
Establishment Name
Establishment Address

Form Approved
O.M.B. No. 44R 1453

Case or File Number	Date of Injury or Onset of Illness	Employee's Name	Occupation	Department	Description of Injury or Illness
Enter a nonduplicating number which will facilitate comparisons with supplementary records.	Enter Mo./day.	Enter first name or initial, middle initial, last name.	Enter regular job title, not activity employee was performing when injured or at onset of illness. In the absence of a formal title, enter a brief description of the employee's duties.	Enter department in which the employee is regularly employed or a description of normal workplace to which employee is assigned, even though temporarily working in another department at the time of injury or illness.	Enter a brief description of the injury or illness and indicate the part or parts of body affected. Typical entries for this column might be: Amputation of 1st joint right forefinger; Strain of lower back; Contact dermatitis on both hands; Electrocution—body.
(A)	(B)	(C)	(D)	(E)	(F)
					PREVIOUS PAGE TOTALS →
					TOTALS (Instructions on other side of form.) →

Extent of and Outcome of INJURY

Fatalities	Nonfatal Injuries				
Injury Related	Injuries With Lost Workdays				Injuries Without Lost Workdays
Enter **DATE** of death. Mo./day/yr.	Enter a **CHECK** if injury involves days away from work, or days of restricted work activity, or both.	Enter a **CHECK** if injury involves days away from work.	Enter number of **DAYS** ***away from work.***	Enter number of **DAYS** of ***restricted work activity.***	Enter a **CHECK** if no entry was made in columns 1 or 2 but the injury is recordable as defined above.
(1)	(2)	(3)	(4)	(5)	(6)

Type, Extent of, and Outcome of ILLNESS

Type of Illness							Fatalities	Nonfatal Illnesses				
CHECK Only One Column for Each Illness ***(See other side of form for terminations or permanent transfers.)***							Illness Related	Illnesses With Lost Workdays				Illnesses Without Lost Workdays
Occupational skin diseases or disorders	Dust diseases of the lungs	Respiratory conditions due to toxic agents	Poisoning (systemic effects of toxic materials)	Disorders due to physical agents	Disorders associated with repeated trauma	All other occupational illnesses	Enter **DATE** of death. Mo./day/yr.	Enter a **CHECK** if illness involves days away from work, or days of restricted work activity, or both.	Enter a **CHECK** if illness involves days away from work.	Enter number of **DAYS** ***away from work.***	Enter number of **DAYS** of ***restricted work activity.***	Enter a **CHECK** if no entry was made in columns 8 or 9.
(7)												
(a)	(b)	(c)	(d)	(e)	(f)	(g)	(8)	(9)	(10)	(11)	(12)	(13)

INJURIES ILLNESSES

OSHA No. 200

Certification of Annual Summary Totals By ____ Title ____ Date ____

OSHA No. 200

POST ONLY THIS PORTION OF THE LAST PAGE NO LATER THAN FEBRUARY 1.

Instructions for OSHA No. 200

I. **Log and Summary of Occupational Injuries and Illnesses**

Each employer who is subject to the recordkeeping requirements of the Occupational Safety and Health Act of 1970 must maintain for each establishment a log of all recordable occupational injuries and illnesses. This form (OSHA No. 200) may be used for that purpose. A substitute for the OSHA No. 200 is acceptable if it is as detailed easily readable, and understandable as the OSHA No. 200.

Enter each recordable case on the log within six (6) workdays after learning of its occurrence. Although other records must be maintained at the establishment to which they refer, it is possible to prepare and maintain the log at another location, using data processing equipment if desired. If the log is prepared elsewhere, a copy updated to within 45 calendar days must be present at all times in the establishment.

Logs must be maintained and retained for five (5) years following the end of the calendar year to which they relate. Logs must be available (normally at the establishment) for inspection and copying by representatives of the Department of Labor, or the Department of Health, Education and Welfare, or States accorded jurisdiction under the Act.

II. **Changes in Extent of or Outcome of Injury or Illness**

If, during the 5-year period the log must be retained, there is a change in an extent and outcome of an injury or illness which affects entries in columns 1, 2, 6, 8, 9, or 13, the first entry should be lined out and a new entry made. For example, if an injured employee at first required only medical treatment but later lost workdays away from work, the check in column 6 should be lined out, and checks entered in columns 2 and 3 and the number of lost workdays entered in column 4.

In another example, if an employee with an occupational illness lost workdays, returned to work, and then died of the illness, the entries in columns 9 and 10 should be lined out and the date of death entered in column 8.

The entire entry for an injury or illness should be lined out if later found to be nonrecordable. For example: an injury or illness which is later determined not to be work related, or which was initially thought to involve medical treatment but later was determined to have involved only first aid.

III. **Posting Requirements**

A copy of the totals and information following the fold line of the last page for the year must be posted at each establishment in the place or places where notices to employees are customarily posted. This copy must be posted no later than ***February 1 and must remain in place until March 1.***

Even though there were no injuries or illnesses during the year, zeros must be entered on the totals line, and the form posted.

The person responsible for the ***annual summary totals*** shall certify that the totals are true and complete by signing at the bottom of the form.

IV. **Instructions for Completing Log and Summary of Occupational Injuries and Illnesses**

Column A – CASE OR FILE NUMBER. Self-explanatory.

Column B – DATE OF INJURY OR ONSET OF ILLNESS.
For occupational injuries, enter the date of the work accident which resulted in injury. For occupational illnesses, enter the date of initial diagnosis of illness, or, if absence from work occurred before diagnosis, enter the first day of the absence attributable to the illness which was later diagnosed or recognized.

Columns C through F – Self-explanatory.

Columns 1 and 8 – INJURY OR ILLNESS-RELATED DEATHS.
Self-explanatory.

Columns 2 and 9 – INJURIES OR ILLNESSES WITH LOST WORKDAYS.
Self-explanatory.

Any injury which involves days away from work, or days of restricted work activity, or both must be recorded since it always involves one or more of the criteria for recordability.

Columns 3 and 10 – INJURIES OR ILLNESSES INVOLVING DAYS AWAY FROM WORK. Self-explanatory.

Columns 4 and 11 – LOST WORKDAYS—DAYS AWAY FROM WORK.
Enter the number of workdays (consecutive or not) on which the employee would have worked but could not because of occupational injury or illness. The number of lost workdays should not include the day of injury or onset of illness or any days on which the employee would not have worked even though able to work.

NOTE: For employees not having a regularly scheduled shift, such as certain truck drivers, construction workers, farm labor, casual labor, part-time employees, etc., it may be necessary to estimate the number of lost workdays. Estimates of lost workdays shall be based on prior work history of the employee AND days worked by employees, not ill or injured, working in the department and/or occupation of the ill or injured employee.

Columns 5 and 12 – LOST WORKDAYS—DAYS OF RESTRICTED WORK ACTIVITY.
Enter the number of workdays (consecutive or not) on which because of injury or illness:

(1) the employee was assigned to another job on a temporary basis, or
(2) the employee worked at a permanent job less than full time, or
(3) the employee worked at a permanently assigned job but could not perform all duties normally connected with it.

The number of lost workdays should not include the day of injury or onset of illness or any days on which the employee would not have worked even though able to work.

Columns 6 and 13 – INJURIES OR ILLNESSES WITHOUT LOST WORKDAYS. Self-explanatory.

Columns 7a through 7g – TYPE OF ILLNESS.
Enter a check in only ***one*** column for each illness.

TERMINATION OR PERMANENT TRANSFER—Place an asterisk to the right of the entry in columns 7a through 7g (type of illness) which represented a termination of employment or permanent transfer.

V. **Totals**

Add number of entries in columns 1 and 8.
Add number of checks in columns 2, 3, 6, 7, 9, 10, and 13.
Add number of days in columns 4, 5, 11, and 12.
Totals are to be generated for each column at the end of each page and at the end of each year. ***Only*** the yearly totals are required for posting.

If an employee's loss of workdays is continuing at the time the totals are summarized, estimate the number of future workdays the employee will lose and add that estimate to the workdays already lost and include this figure in the annual totals. No further entries are to be made with respect to such cases in the next year's log.

VI. **Definitions**

OCCUPATIONAL INJURY is any injury such as a cut, fracture, sprain, amputation, etc., which results from a work accident or from an exposure involving a single incident in the work environment.
NOTE: Conditions resulting from animal bites, such as insect or snake bites or from one-time exposure to chemicals, are considered to be injuries.

OCCUPATIONAL ILLNESS of an employee is any abnormal condition or disorder, other than one resulting from an occupational injury, caused by exposure to environmental factors associated with employment. It includes acute and chronic illnesses or diseases which may be caused by inhalation, absorption, ingestion, or direct contact.

The following listing gives the categories of occupational illnesses and disorders that will be utilized for the purpose of classifying recordable illnesses. For purposes of information, examples of each category are given. These are typical examples, however, and are not to be considered the complete listing of the types of illnesses and disorders that are to be counted under each category.

7a. **Occupational Skin Diseases or Disorders**
Examples: Contact dermatitis, eczema, or rash caused by primary irritants and sensitizers or poisonous plants; oil acne; chrome ulcers; chemical burns or inflammations; etc.

7b. **Dust Diseases of the Lungs (Pneumoconioses)**
Examples: Silicosis, asbestosis, coal worker's pneumoconiosis, byssinosis, siderosis, and other pneumoconioses.

7c. **Respiratory Conditions Due to Toxic Agents**
Examples: Pneumonitis, pharyngitis, rhinitis or acute congestion due to chemicals, dusts, gases, or fumes; farmer's lung; etc.

*7d. **Poisoning (Systemic Effect of Toxic Materials)**
Examples: Poisoning by lead, mercury, cadmium, arsenic, or other metals; poisoning by carbon monoxide, hydrogen sulfide, or other gases; poisoning by benzol, carbon tetrachloride, or other organic solvents; poisoning by insecticide sprays such as parathion, lead arsenate; poisoning by other chemicals such as formaldehyde, plastics, and resins; etc.

7e. **Disorders Due to Physical Agents (Other than Toxic Materials)**
Examples: Heatstroke, sunstroke, heat exhaustion, and other effects of environmental heat; freezing, frostbite, and effects of exposure to low temperatures; caisson disease; effects of ionizing radiation (isotopes, X-rays, radium); effects of nonionizing radiation (welding flash, ultraviolet rays, microwaves, sunburn); etc.

7f. **Disorders Associated With Repeated Trauma**
Examples: Noise-induced hearing loss; synovitis, tenosynovitis, and bursitis; Raynaud's phenomena; and other conditions due to repeated motion, vibration, or pressure.

7g. **All Other Occupational Illnesses**
Examples: Anthrax, brucellosis, infectious hepatitis, and benign tumors, food poisoning, histoplasmosis, coccidioidomycosis, etc.

MEDICAL TREATMENT includes treatment (other than first aid) administered by a physician or by registered professional personnel under the standing orders of a physician. Medical treatment does NOT include first aid treatment (one-time treatment and subsequent observation of minor scratches, cuts, burns, splinters, and so forth, which do not ordinarily require medical care) even though provided by a physician or registered professional personnel.

ESTABLISHMENT: A single physical location where business is conducted or where services or industrial operations are performed (for example: a factory, mill, store, hotel, restaurant, movie theater, farm, ranch, bank, sales office, warehouse, or central administrative office). Where distinctly separate activities are performed at a single physical location such as construction activities operated from the same physical location as a lumber yard, each activity shall be treated as a separate establishment.

For firms engaged in activities which may be physically dispersed, such as agriculture, construction, transportation, communications, and electric, gas, and sanitary services, records may be maintained at a place to which employees report each day.

Records for personnel who do not primarily report or work at a single establishment, such as traveling salesmen, technicians, engineers, etc., shall be maintained at the location from which they are paid or the base from which personnel operate to carry out their activities.

WORK ENVIRONMENT is comprised of the physical location, equipment, materials processed or used, and the kinds of operations performed in the course of an employee's work, whether on or off the employer's premises.

FIG 4–1.
OSHA log.

Achieve a mutuality of agreement with the corporate nurse's goals.

Allow the corporate nurse access to management for discussion and decision-making concerning the occupational health program.

Responsibilities of Corporate Environmental Health/Industrial Hygiene Services.—Provide hazard data sheets as references for the nurse's information for each corporate site.

Provide existing medical surveillance plans for all of the corporation's locations.

Provide information, assistance, and support in occupational health matters and instruct the nurse as to specific physical examination protocols in effect at each corporation location.

Responsibilities of the Corporate Occupational Health Nurse.—Assess all site areas assigned for optimum efficiency.

Know the site areas and hazards pertinent to the practice of occupational health.

Perform an annual audit of OH nursing professionals' performance to determine their compliance with nursing standards.

Establish and maintain individual employee health record files for every employee, and retain records of each for the period as required by OSHA, at the corporate location.

Know the medical surveillance programs applicable to each corporation site.

Seek help as needed from management, hygienist, physician or safety resource.

Act as a liaison between other health professionals, the employee and management.

Maintain any medical information in strict confidence, releasing this information only to the employee, trained health professionals, and/or government agencies, as directed under OSHA standards.

Provide an annual workshop for the occupational health nursing professionals.

Originate medical/nursing forms, and/or review and update existing forms as the need occurs.

Functional Descriptions of Occupational Nurses

The practice of occupational health nursing is large and diverse. Levels of professional practice will differ, as will desired educational backgrounds. The following are some of the functional descriptions of the prevailing levels of occupational health nursing practice.[10]

A *staff nurse* functions under nursing supervision.

A *charge nurse* works alone and has responsibility for the nursing service.

A *supervisor* develops, administers, and implements the nursing service.

An *administrator* administers a nursing service with satellite supervisors and a nursing staff.

A nurse *consultant* works in a corporate structure, in an insurance industry, or in local, state, or federal governmental agencies, or is self-employed to advise, recommend, and provide consultation.

A nurse *educator's* principal function is the training and education of occupational health nurses.

A *part-time nurse* from an industrial clinic or a community health nursing service provides routine or special nursing services to a plant.

A *relief nurse* temporarily replaces a full-time nurse.

A *company-employed visiting nurse* provides some care, or follow-up, for an employee at his home.

OCCUPATIONAL HEALTH NURSING: STATE OF THE ART

Job Summaries

The following are sample job summaries provided by practicing professional occupational health nurses in the field.

Occupational Health Nurse (Plant Level)

Nature of Employer's Business.—Manufacturer of electronic equipment employs 1,000 workers who are approximately 60% female, 40% male, aged 30–40 years average, and engaged as assemblers, machine operators, maintenance and cafeteria workers, in-management, engineering, clerical, and security work. The majority have technical skills.

Nurse's Job Description.—None was available when the nurse's employment began, but management requested that the occupational health nurse provide a written job description soon after employment.

Administrative Supervision.—The nurse reports to the personnel manager.

Medical Directives.—These are provided by the physician, who is engaged by the company as an independent health care provider and visits the occupational health unit twice weekly, for periods of two hours or less. The physician's specialty is surgery. The nurse is the sole full-time health care provider at the plant.

Professional Responsibilities.—The OH nurse provides nursing services for both occupational and nonoccupational illness and injury, maintains OSHA records and employee health files, counsels employees, and refers them to community resources for additional health and social services as needed.

The OH nurse assists the physician with employee physical examinations by obtaining health histories, performing eye screening using a standard vision test device (orthorater), and performing venipunctures.

The OH nurse is also responsible for workers' compensation claims. She obtains medical direction for the treatment of occupational illnesses and injuries and arranges for employee transportation, monitors employee progress, and obtains releases for work. The nurse informs management of the incident and progress.

Salary Reviews.—The nurse's salary is reviewed annually.

Additional Responsibilities.—The occupational health nurse is a member of the plant safety committee and conducts an inspection of an assigned area. Monthly, the nurse participates in the discussion of corrections of observable hazards.

For the employees, the nurse provides periodic special programs at the worksite, e.g., instruction in cardiopulmonary resuscitation, blood pressure screening, and smoking cessation workshops.

The occupational health nurse at this manufacturing facility is permitted to practice with autonomy, encouraged to participate in continuing education offerings, and has gained respect as a health professional. Professional organizational membership is mandated and paid for by the management.

Occupational Health Nurse in a Nonmanufacturing Environment

The following are thoughts from a colleague concerning the practice of occupational health nursing at the present time in a large insurance company:

> "I have 17 years of experience in occupational health nursing, in addition to several years as a public health nurse. There are many similarities between public health and occupational health job responsibilities and qualifications. The only differences are those of focus (home or work site health care).
>
> "Over the years, my job responsibilities have changed considerably. In the beginning, I did little more than provide first aid and do routine screenings. While not minimizing that role, I believe there is now a movement toward an expanded role for a nurse in the nonindustrial setting.
>
> "In response to this, I have increased my knowledge and skill in diverse areas such as physical assessment, emergency care, and patient education. My company has shown its support of my efforts by providing financial assistance for continuing education and for my participation in professional organizations.
>
> "While I appreciate this support, there remain some serious roadblocks to occupational health progress. Far too many persons in upper management view health care as an expendable fringe benefit. They feel it's too costly to maintain a staff and feel that employees make too frequent use of occupational health care and thus impede productivity. In reality, studies show far more time is lost to preventable illness.
>
> "Another problem is that we nurses are not often treated as educated professionals and, in fact, rarely receive management training. However, since we are part of the problem, we must become part of the solution. Our professional organizations must provide training where possible, as well as initiate extensive lobbying and educational efforts with senior managers of corporations.
>
> "It is imperative that we be viewed as competent professionals, just as the salespersons, underwriters, and accountants are. We should not be deprived of opportunities for advancement within the company.
>
> "Another way we can help ourselves is to eliminate duplication of services and competition within the company. This may be accomplished by merging the medical department into the company's human resources group. This action would provide a career path for the health care professional."

Sample Program Originated by an Occupational Health Nurse

The OH nurse may have great influence over how a company responds to health problems, as demonstrated by this complete program originated by me in response to an OSHA proclamation, For the Emergency Temporary Standard Reducing the Permissible Asbestos Exposure Limit (48 FR 51086, Nov 4, 1983, 29 CFR, part 1910).

Management's Role

The following health information is to be provided to each employee prior to his/her work with asbestos:

The Occupational Safety and Health Administration is aware of no instances in which exposure to a toxic substance has more clearly demonstrated detrimental health effects on humans than has asbestos exposure. The diseases caused by asbestos exposures are in large part life-threatening or disabling.

Health Effects.—Diseases resulting from exposure to asbestos fibers can reach the incurable stage before they are detected and can cause either death or severe disability. The symptoms are delayed and may occur 20 to 30 or more years after exposure, with disease more likely to occur as a result of repeated long-term inhalation or ingestion.

Asbestosis.—Asbestosis is a progressive and disabling lung disease caused by inhaling asbestos fibers. These fibers become lodged in the lungs, causing inflammation of air sacs and tubes. As the inflammation heals, it leaves scar tissue. This causes the lining of the air sacs to thicken so that it is hard for oxygen to get into the bloodstream.

Strained breathing caused by a lack of oxygen can lead to heart failure. Asbestosis is irreversible, once scarring has begun, and can continue even if exposure ceases.

Symptoms of asbestosis are a shortness of breath, pain in the upper chest or back, and a dry sound (rales) during inhalation. As the ability to breathe becomes more limited, the fingers and toes become "clubbed"—rounded with flattened nails. A bluish discoloration of the skin and lining of the mouth and tongue also may appear.

Cancer.—Lung cancer exacts the highest mortality of any asbestos-related disease. Lung cancer has caused up to 25% of all deaths in some groups of individuals heavily exposed to asbestos, compared with a risk factor of 4–5% for the general population.

The action of asbestos fibers alone is multiplied by the presence of other cancer-causing substances. For example, exposure to asbestos in combination with *cigarette smoking greatly increases the risk of lung cancer*. The symptoms of lung cancer vary, depending on where the cancer occurs. If it starts in the air passages, known as bronchi, the cancer will cause partial obstruction and irritation, and the symptom probably will be a cough. The sputum may contain blood. However, lung cancer also can start in any other part of the lung. These cancers are not suspected until they show up on x-rays, or until late in their development, when pain and a shortness of breath appear.

Mesothelioma is an extremely rare cancer in the general population. Mesotheliomas involving cancer of the lining of the lungs or abdominal cavity, however, are frequent in asbestos workers. Mesothelioma is incurable and can cause death in six months to two years. Symptoms are a shortness of breath and chest or abdominal pain.

Asbestos workers also risk cancers of the digestive system—cancer of the esophagus, stomach, colon and rectum. These cancers are thought to be caused by swallowing asbestos fibers ("Asbestos Standard Management's Role," U.S. Department of Labor, Occupational Safety and Health Administration, 1980, OSHA 3070).

Required Medical Examinations for Workers Exposed to Asbestos

Annual Examination.—An annual examination shall be provided or made available to each employee exposed to an airborne concentration of asbestos fibers. This comprehensive medical examination shall include as a minimum:

1. Chest roentgenogram (posterior-anterior, 14 × 17 in/36 × 54 cm)
2. A history to elicit symptomatology of respiratory disease
3. Pulmonary function tests to include forced vital capacity (FVC) and forced vital expiratory volume at one second (FEV_1)

Termination of Employment—Physical Examination.—The employer shall provide or make available to each employee who is engaged in an occupation where there is exposure to an airborne concentration of asbestos fibers, within 30 days before or after the termination of employment, a comprehensive medical examination, including:

1. A chest roentgenogram (posterior-anterior, 14 × 17 in/36 × 54 cm)
2. A history to elicit symptomatology of respiratory disease
3. Pulmonary function tests to include forced vital capacity (FVC) and forced expiratory volume at one second (FEV_1).

Recent Examinations.—If adequate records indicate that the employee has been examined in accordance with requirements promulgated by the standard for "Occupational Exposure to Asbestos" within the past one-year period, no medical examination is required.

Content of Employee Occupational Health Record File With Regard to Occupational Exposure to Asbestos

An individual record for each employee who works with asbestos shall be initiated and maintained in an accurate and complete manner. Each employee record shall consist of:

I. Cover identification completed by the plant employee supervisor or personnel department
II. Form 96-40-750.
III. Employee health record for physician's assessment, including:
   A. Pre-placement examination records
   B. Annual medical examination records
   C. Termination medical examination records
   D. All periodic roentgenograms
   E. All pulmonary roentgenograms
   F. All medical records and supporting documents to be retained by employer for a period of 20 years
   G. Employee authorization form for medical record release (Fig 4–2)
   H. Evidence of providing employee information of the following:
      1. Health effects associated with asbestos exposure
      2. The relationship between asbestos and smoking in producing lung cancer (Fig 4–3)
   I. Asbestos work and personal history (Fig 4–4)
   J. Medical history as pertains to work with asbestos (Fig 4–5)
   K. Physician's written opinion as to employee's risk of impairment due to asbestos exposure (Fig 4–6)

Retention of and Access to Medical Records

Medical Records–Retention.—Complete and accurate records of all employee medical examinations as pertain to the OSHA standard for employee occupational exposure to asbestos shall be retained by the employer for at least 20 years.

Access to Employee Medical Records.—Contents of required medical records shall be made available for inspection and copying to:

1. Assistant Secretary of Labor for Occupational Safety and Health
2. The Director of NIOSH
3. Authorized medical consultants of either of the above
4. An employee or former employee, upon request to his physician

Any physician who conducts a medical examination as required by this standard shall furnish to the employer all of the information required as specifically cited, plus any other medical information for this employee as relates to his occupational exposure to asbestos fibers.

THE OCCUPATIONAL HEALTH NURSE: A LOOK TO THE FUTURE

Emphasis on the White Collar Worker

According to the U.S. Labor Department's Bureau of Labor Statistics, in 1990 the work force will be employed in capital-intensive industries, with a big increase in the percentage of white-collar workers as health professionals, computer specialists, managers, administrators, and clerical employees.

Based in part on those projections, NIOSH has tried to anticipate the occupational health needs of the work force by 1990 in a new five-year report:

> As the work force matures and moves into service-related occupations, the incidence of cumulative trauma, musculoskeletal disorders, cardiovascular diseases, and psychologic disorders can be expected to increase.
>
> With about 24 million clerical workers expected in the work force by 1990, more health problems related to office work will manifest themselves. For instance, there may be an increase in the number of people suffering from acute and chronic pneumonitis—of which a primary cause is poor ventilation of hazardous substances such as secondary smoke, formaldehyde, molds, accumulated dust, and infectious agents.

AUTHORIZATION FOR ACCESS

EMPLOYEE OCCUPATIONAL EXPOSURE TO ASBESTOS MEDICAL SURVEILLANCE RECORD

I ______________________ (Name) former/present employee of __________ Chemical Corporation hereby give my permission and authorize Dr. ______________________ of ______________________ (Address) to full access of my medical surveillance records for occupational exposure to asbestos as required by the Occupational Safety and Health Standard for Occupational Exposure to Asbestos.

Employee's Signature ______________________ Date __________

Employer Representative Signature ______________________ Date __________

FIG 4–2.
Employee authorization form for medical record release.

CHEMICAL CORPORATION
MEDICAL SURVEILLANCE PROGRAM

AIRBORNE CONCENTRATIONS OF ASBESTOS FIBERS
EMPLOYEE OCCUPATIONAL EXPOSURE

Name: ______________________ Date: ____________
Employee No: ______________________ Social Security # ____________
Plant Location: ______________________ Supervisor: ____________
Job Title: ______________________
Job Description: ______________________

Date of initial work with airborne concentrations of asbestos fibers ______________________
Termination date: ______________________

(Please check)
1. Physical examinations
   pre-placement ________ Date: ________
2. Annual ________ Date: ________
3. Termination ________ Date: ________

I have been informed by my employer (   ) of *the health effects of Asbestos exposure* and the *relationship between Asbestos and smoking in producing lung cancer.*

Informant's signature ______________________ Employee's signature ______________________
Date: ______________________ Date: ______________________

FIG 4–3.
Form stating employee has been informed of asbestos exposure and of the relationship between asbestos and smoking in causing cancer.

The increased number of women in the work force has implications for ergonomics and job design, especially with women taking jobs traditionally held by men. Issues of fitting such jobs to women workers can be significant, especially for jobs requiring more physical effort.

The length of a 'normal' work week, which has not changed significantly over the last 35 years, is not expected to change by 1990. The normal work week is now 41.8 hours.[14] Working Americans now spend 36% of their lives 'on the job.' Over one third of each adult's life is spent working, representing a significant possibility for exposure to occupational risks that cause disease or injury.

The occupational health emphasis will change from the workers in a manufacturing environment to workers of the office environment.

The occupational health nurse will require additional skills and education to cope with worker problems of stress and allergic responses, development of chronic diseases, ergonomics, eye strain, occupational dermatitis, and musculoskeletal problems.[17]

Movement of Hospitals Into Occupational Medicine

Of interest to the future of occupational health nursing practice is the distinct trend of shifting the occupational medical practice to hospital settings, as hospital facilities contract with medium and smaller sized companies for comprehensive health services.

The occupational health nurse who practices in a hospital-based service as a contract employee to industry will lose professional autonomy, and industry will suffer some loss of employee trust and rapport now existing through the present system.

Many hospitals have depended on government payments for up to 75% of their income in some cases. When that percentage shrinks to 35% or 40%, hospitals must look for other sources for survival. Offering occupational health services has been one answer for some, and many others are expected to join.[5]

Shortage of Occupational Health Professionals

In 1977, it was estimated that there were 84,850 persons working in occupational safety and health activities. While accurate statistics on projected needs are difficult to locate, the best current estimate is that the nation will need between 99,720 and 106,120 safety and health specialists in 1985.

The annual increase of qualified personnel, including people completing formal academic degrees in occupational safety and health, industrial hygiene, occupational medicine or nursing, is 956 per year. The annual need is estimated at 5,300.

ASBESTOS WORK AND PERSONAL HISTORY

Annual: ____________

Termination: ____________

Name: ____________ Date: ____________

Employee No.: ____________ Social Security # ____________

Location: ____________ Supervisor: ____________

In order to assist the Medical Division with your medical examination, please answer the following questions.

Since your last physical examination:

HAVE YOU EVER WORKED IN OR HANDLED ASBESTOS IN ANY OF THE FOLLOWING INDUSTRIES:

	Yes	No		Yes	No
During Manufacturing Asbestos			In Coal Mining		
In Spraying Asbestos			In Dusty Work		
Removal of Asbestos Insulation			In Foundry or Casting		
In Demolition of Structures			In Textile Industry		
In Construction Trade			With Chemicals		
As a Cement Worker			With Lead		

LIST YOUR HOBBIES AND NUMBER OF YEARS PURSUED

1. ____________
2. ____________
3. ____________
4. ____________
5. ____________

HISTORY OF TOBACCO USE

1. Do you use tobacco? ____________
2. In what form - cigarettes, pipe, snuff, chew? ____________
3. How many cigarettes or pipefulls daily? ____________
4. How long have you smoked? ____________
5. Have you stopped smoking? ____________
6. How long ago? ____________
7. Did you or do you smoke on the job? ____________

FIG 4–4.
Asbestos work and personal history.

MEDICAL HISTORY (AS PERTAINS TO WORK WITH ASBESTOS)

Name: ______________________ Date: ______________

Employee No.: ______________________ Social Security # ______________

Location: ______________________ Supervisor: ______________

In order to assist the Medical Division with your medical examination, please answer the following questions.

Since your last physical examination:

HAVE YOU EVER WORKED WITH OR HANDLED ASBESTOS? ______________

State when - where ______________________________

____

HAVE YOU EVER HAD OR BEEN TOLD YOU HAD:

	YES	NO
Hypertension		
Heart Disease		
Allergies/Asthma		
Bronchitis or Emphysema		
Difficulty Breathing		
Lung Disease/Pneumonia		
Pleurisy		
Heavy smoker		
Heavy Drinker of Alcohol		
Frequent Colds - Sinusitis		
Difficulty Using A Respirator		
Frequent Upset Stomach		
Stroke		
Stomach Problems or Ulcer		
Frequent Diarrhea		
Disease of the Colon		
Disease of the Rectum		
Frequent Cough		
Difficulty Sleeping		

Do you use regular medicine or take drugs?
IF YES, STATE REASON FOR TREATMENT

____

____

____

Have you ever had Cancer in any form?
IF YES, EXPLAIN ______________________

____

____

____

____

Have you ever had any serious illness?
IF YES, STATE DISEASE AND EXPLAIN

____

____

____

____

LIST ANY PRESENT HEALTH PROBLEMS

1. ______________________________
2. ______________________________
3. ______________________________

FIG 4–5.
Medical history of employee as pertains to asbestos exposure.

Examination Date: ____________________

Name: ____________________

Social Security # ____________________

Type of Exam - Please Check (X)

Pre-placement

Annual

Termination

ASBESTOS WORK HISTORY

PHYSICIAN'S WRITTEN OPINION

	YES	NO
Pulmonary Disease		
Cardiovascular Disease		
Gastrointestinal Symptoms		
Pulmonary Rales		
Clubbing - Fingers		
Other Cardiopulmonary Symptoms		

State your written opinion as to whether the employee has any detected medical conditions which place the employee at increased risk of material impairment of health from exposure to asbestos or inability to use a negative or positive respiratory.

____

____

____

Examining Physician's Signature: ____________________

Date: ____________________

Employee's Signature: ____________________

Date: ____________________

ATTACH RESULTS OF MEDICAL TESTING

FIG 4–6.
Physician's written opinion as to employee's risk of impairment due to asbestos exposure.

Perhaps the greatest need is for occupational physicians and nurses.[9, 15]

The occupational health nurse must look to the future, become a member of occupational health nursing's professional organizations, educate consumers as to the benefits of professional occupational health nursing programs, and continue to increase her knowledge of occupational health issues.

ACKNOWLEDGMENTS

My appreciation to Dr. Carl Zenz, for his assistance, understanding, and appreciation of the role of the OH nurse; Sheila D. Hammons, for her secretarial skills; and Patricia Smyrniotis, R.N., for her collegial sharing.

REFERENCES

1. Billauer BP: The legal liability of the occupational health professional. *J Occup Med* 1985; 27:3.
2. Clements M, Graeter CJ: Multiple skills required to meet corporate nurse's role. *Occup Health Saf* 1984; May, p44.
3. *Costs and Benefits of Occupational Health Nursing*. US Dept of Health and Human Services, Public Health Service, National Institute for Occupational Safety and Health, 1980.
4. *Facts about Nursing*. Kansas City, Mo., American Nurses' Association, 1985.
5. Fishbein GW (ed): Occupational medical practice shifting to hospitals. *Occup Health Saf Lett* 1984; 14:13. Washington, DC.
6. Illinois Industrial Commission: *Information Handbook Illinois Workers' Compensation Act and Illinois Occupational Diseases Act (amendment)*, 1980.
7. Keefer MW: More than an examination: The process of board certification. *Occup Health Nurs* 1983; 31:12.
8. LaDou J (ed): *Occupational Health Law—A Guide for Industry*. New York, Marcel Dekker, Inc, 1981.
9. LaDou J (ed): *Introduction to Occupational Health and Safety*. Chicago, National Safety Council, 1986.
10. Lee JA: *The New Nurse in Industry*. NIOSH Pub. #78–143, Washington, DC, US Government Printing Office, 1978.
11. McKechnie MR: A descriptive study of the scope of practice of occupational health nurses in one-nurse units. *Occup Health Nurs* 1983; 31:3.
12. Michaud PL: Role of occupational health nurses in management. *Occup Health Nurs* 1984; 32:4.
13. *Occupational Health Guide for Medical and Nursing Personnel*, ed 3, Zenz C (ed). State Medical Society of Wisconsin, 330 E Lakeside St, Madison, WI 53701, 1985.
14. *Programs Planned by Program Areas*, NIOSH Publication 84–107. USHH USPH CDC, Feb 1984.
15. *Protecting People at Work: A Reader in Occupational Safety and Health*. US Dept of Labor, 1980.
16. *Standards for Evaluating an Occupational Health Nursing Service*. New York, American Association of Occupational Health Nurses, Inc, 1977.
17. Stellman J, Henifin MS: *Office Work Can Be Dangerous to Your Health*. New York, Pantheon Books, 1983.
18. *The Nurse in Industry (A History of the American Association of Industrial Nurses)*. New York, American Association of Occupational Health Nurses, Inc, 1976.
19. *What an Occupational Health Nurse Can Do for You and Your Employees*. New York, American Association of Occupational Health Nurses, Inc, 1977.

5

Occupational Health Services for Small Businesses and Other Small Employee Groups

Marcus B. Bond, M.D.

Most persons employed in the United States work in small groups; that is, the employing organization has only a small number of workers or the employees are widely dispersed in small units. In both instances, provision of occupational medical services often has been difficult, uncertain, unreliable, and lacking in quality. There are reasons for these deficiencies, and these reasons reflect poorly on the medical profession, business managers and sometimes unions. It is definitely possible to have good occupational medical services for an employee group of any size, but for small units more effort and dedication are required on the part of all three groups involved.

WHAT SERVICES SHOULD BE PROVIDED?

The former Council on Occupational Health of the American Medical Association developed several reports in the 1960s that provided detailed advice on the types of medical services believed to be appropriate for employers to furnish employees.[14] These reports were published in pamphlet form and even today are good basic guides to occupational health services for small plants, although they are obviously lacking references to more recent and important developments such as the establishment of the National Institute for Occupational Safety and Health (NIOSH), the Occupational Safety and Health Act (OSHA), the Rehabilitation Act of 1973, and various new state laws and regulations.

The health services that employers furnish to employees are called occupational health programs and deal with the health of employees as related to their work. Ordinarily, care for illnesses and injuries developing away from and unrelated etiologically to work is not included in an occupational health program. (However, medical care for certain nonoccupational illnesses is reported to be particularly appropriate for occupational health programs.[1, 23]) Complete medical care is provided for job-related illnesses and injuries for which there is a legal requirement under workers' compensation and other laws to provide treatment. The primary orientation and activities of the health program are preventive medicine—examinations and evaluations of employees at various times during their careers, advice and counseling to employees, follow-up examinations of employees with chronic disease, health education activities, and immunizations and screening tests under certain conditions. Initial treatment and assistance are provided to employees for emergencies at work, whether work-related or not.

The number of employees at one location and the nature of the work performed should be the primary determinants as to whether a health facility can be maintained at the work site. For employee groups numbering less than 200–300, it rarely is practical to attempt a medical department. An exception might be found where the work involves much close contact with potentially hazardous materials, such as ionizing radiation, or highly toxic chemicals, such as mercury, lead, beryllium, insecticides, and others. Work sites with materials of this sort often are located in areas somewhat remote from population centers as a precaution against harm to the community. This isolation makes it expensive and time-consuming to send employees to a physician's office. In most instances in which toxic materials are handled, frequent health checks are made on employees to evaluate possible harm from work exposures. Thus, more health services per employee may justify an in-plant medical department for a smaller group than if there are no unusual hazards associated with the work.

Out-of-Plant Services

There are many business establishments where only 1–50 employees work. Restaurants, motels, retail shops of all kinds, automobile service stations and garages, sales offices, and a great variety of other enterprises are common examples. Proprietors of small businesses have the same responsibilities as other employers for providing a safe work place and medical care of those injured or made ill by their work. The federal Occupational Safety and Health Act applies to "all businesses affecting interstate commerce" except federal and state governments. This definition will include nearly all employers and undoubtedly will stimulate many proprietors of small businesses to acquire occupational health services.

Small Units of Large Organizations

If small employee groups are part of a large company with headquarters elsewhere, advice and instructions can be supplied from the corporate offices, where staffs of specialists exist. Lawyers, physicians, nurses, industrial hygienists, safety experts, and labor relations representatives can combine their knowledge and provide specific instructions to supervisors and local physicians in any location covering any type of work operation. Such instructions should, of course, be consistent with general company policies, insurance and benefit provisions, labor contracts, and the laws of the particular state.

Selection of a physician obviously is a key first step, because a local physician, licensed in the state, is required for examinations, treatment, or any other professional activities. It is best if local management and the company medical director share the responsibility for obtaining a physician's services. Usually local managers are acquainted with several physicians in the community through social, business, and civic activities, and they can recommend one or more physicians to the medical director. The medical director can check physicians' credentials by consulting the *Directory of Medical Specialists* for those who are certified in a specialty. It is common that the medical director will be personally acquainted with one or more physicians in the particular community or may know officials in the state or local medical society who can provide information concerning available physicians.

When a physician has been agreed on by the medical director and local management, the physician should be contacted to see if he or she is interested in doing the work. If so, the medical director should visit this physician personally, if possible, or write a letter and include the company physician's manual or other written policies and procedures, description of jobs, including possible hazards, and the necessary periodic tests or examinations for employees.

The local manager should arrange for the physician to visit the plant or place of work so that the physician can actually see the working conditions and become acquainted with at least some of the supervisors. The frequency of visits after the first visit should be determined by the nature of the work and major changes in materials or processes. If significant hazards exist in the work environment, the physician should tour the work area every one or two months.

Remuneration of the physician may be on a fee-for-service basis, including hourly charges for visits to the workplace. If the services provided are frequent, a retainer or salary may be desirable for both parties. Such an arrangement increases the physician's attention to the employer's business and provides him with certain fringe benefits associated with employment, such as health and life insurance, pension, Social Security, and others.

The practicing physician who agrees to provide service to a company or other organization should honor his commitment. A small amount of effort initially will save much time and obviate confusion for all concerned and will particularly save the physician's time. A visit to the work site should be made for an observation of the working environment and a frank discussion of what the employer thinks his employee health problems are. The wise physician will do more listening than talking and recognize that each employee group is unique in terms of employee policy and how the job is done. Most often employers are delighted to conduct the physician through the work site and share any information concerning the business.

By visiting with the employer, the physician will be able to see beforehand if he or she is the kind of employer who would misuse the physician by asking for a "cover-up" or denial of injuries or illnesses from work exposure, or who would not reveal to the physician the actual contents of certain materials used at work under the guise of protecting trade secrets. There can be no secrets from the physician if he is to perform his function properly. Employers who would misuse physicians should be advised that there can be no compromise with honesty in dealing with the health of people.

After the physician has become familiar with the work environment and company policies, he should advise the employer how and when to send employees to his office for such nonemergency conditions as applicant examinations, return-to-work checkups, and periodic tests or examinations, such as blood counts, or chest x-rays. Instructions for these and for emergencies should be written and provided to the employer so that they can be posted on bulletin boards, distributed to supervisors, and placed in first aid kits and in company trucks. The company medical director can assist with these instructions. Emergency instructions should also include where to send patients at different times during the day and on special days, such as weekends and days off, the name, address, and phone number of the hospital emergency room, and the name of an associate or colleague who should be contacted if the physician is not available.

The physician then must instruct his own nurses and assistants in his office as to what commitments have been made to the employer and provide them with company forms and instructions. Reference books or articles pertaining to the hazards in the particular working environment should be obtained. The company medical director may furnish these or can advise on them.

The local physician will have the advantage of working with another physician—the company medical director—on problem cases. This can be reassuring when an unusual illness or reaction occurs that possibly could be related to work exposure. The medical director should be familiar with products, materials, and processes in the company and be able to provide guidance even if at long distance.

Small Independent Employee Groups

Companies or organizations that are complete and independent have the same problems as, and should be handled in a fashion similar to, small units of large organizations, as just described. More responsibility is placed on the local management and local physician, because there are no staffs of experts at headquarters to establish policy and practices. However, there is an advantage in the small, independent business in that greater flexibility usually is present.

The responsibilities of the employer include knowing when and how to obtain medical services for his employees. There are several sources of information available to him, such as the previously mentioned pamphlets of the American Medical Association on specific areas of health services.[2, 13, 14 17] Also, on a national scale, the American Management Association and other trade associations present courses on occupational health programs each year for businessmen. The American Occupational Medical Association has reprints and pamphlets available, and an article has been prepared on occupational health programs by Felton.[15] Nearly all state and many local medical societies have committees on occupational health that can provide information on this subject to both physicians and managers and direct managers to physicians interested in this work.

The owner or president of a business should have interest in occupational health services for his employees and should participate in the selection of a physician and the determination of the scope of services for the company. A manager reporting directly to the president should have responsibility for personnel matters, insurance programs, safety programs, and health services. Obviously, the responsibility for health services must be a joint one with the physician, who is responsible for all of his or her own activities.

Responsibilities of the physician are those already described plus the necessity for developing rules and practices for his services to the employer. Many of the references already cited[13–15] provide adequate general information for the physician to use in establishing his relationships with an employer. Where there are specific hazards in the work place, more detailed information must be obtained. This is available in other chapters of this book, and it also is wise to consult with a colleague who specializes in occupational medicine for advice concerning a particular problem. Workers exposed to certain heavy metals and their compounds, silica, coal mine dust, ionizing radiation, asbestos, excessive noise, chemicals with systemic toxicity, and other comparable hazards require periodic examinations for evidence of harm. Written instructions concerning such periodic examinations should be provided to the company, including the frequency and type of examination required for various jobs. Other instructions should be furnished, as described in the preceding discussion.

Physicians performing services for an employer should be familiar with the state workers' compensation act and occupational disease law. They should also know the resources of the state and local health departments in order to get prompt advice on epidemics, other disease prevalence, food poisoning, and local pollution levels and standards.

In-Plant Services

There are several factors to be considered in determining whether a medical facility should be established at the work site. The most important of these are the number of employees and the nature of the work. For the sake of simplicity, the nature of the work can be divided into those jobs that require biologic monitoring and/or periodic medical examinations of the workers and those jobs that do not. The term "require" refers to accepted medical standards and/or regulations. Thus, asbestos workers must have periodic medical examinations because of OSHA regulations, although this was good medical practice prior to such regulation. The frequency of medical examinations or monitoring procedures on employees further influences the decision concerning a plant medical facility. Other factors of importance include the proximity of community health resources to the work site, the type of medical and disability insurance for employees, and the labor turnover.

Within the above framework, the following guidelines are offered. Numbers of employees refers to the total number of employees, even though not all are subject to periodic monitoring and medical examinations. For example, clerical and other nonexposed employees benefit from a medical department at the work site even though they do not have the examinations required for others. A work force of 300 that includes employees who require periodic monitoring and medical examinations can justify an in-plant medical department with a full-time nurse and part-time physician.[16] If employees number between 100 and 300, a work site health facility staffed with a part-time nurse may be appropriate in some instances. With a work force of 300 to 700–800, one nurse usually is sufficient, depending on adequate clerical help. A part-time physician is adequate for a group of this size, and the number of hours per week will vary with the actual procedures that must be done by a physician. A group of 800–1,000, including a substantial number who require examinations and monitoring, will justify a full-time physician and at least two nurses.

For employee groups in which there are no exposures that require periodic medical examinations, the activities of an occupational health program are somewhat different. Here, the philosophy and objectives of management play a bigger role, since there are no laws or regulations covering health programs, either in-plant or out-of-plant.

Nearly all businesses have employees who perform potentially hazardous work, the most common example being the operation of a motor vehicle on public roads. Drivers of cargo trucks who operate interstate must have periodic medical examinations under Department of Transportation regulations.[33] Although not required of other drivers, it is good preventive medicine for such employees to have at least a screening examination at intervals of about two years for younger persons and annually for those over age 50 or those with chronic disease.

Other examples of workers who encounter hazards include the operators of duplicating machines, building maintenance personnel, and craftsmen such as plumbers, electricians, and construction workers. These workers require stable musculoskeletal systems, good coordination, and good function of the special senses, yet there are no regulations requiring these employees to have periodic occupational health examinations, unless there also are one or more of the specific exposures covered by OSHA or other regulations. It is recommended that employees in such jobs be given screening examinations at two-year intervals for the young and healthy and annually for employees over age 50 and those with chronic disease.

A specially trained nurse or physician's assistant can perform screening examinations routinely, with physician examination of those with significant problems. A wallet-sized health record is a way of having important as well as routine information readily available in case of emergency. A suggested form is shown in Figure 5–1.

There are excellent articles describing various aspects of the small plant medical department, including its staffing and operation.[16] Other articles have explained the role of the nurse,[8, 9, 26 34] and still others have dealt with the role of the industrial physician and the family physician.[20, 21, 26 27] No attempt will be made here

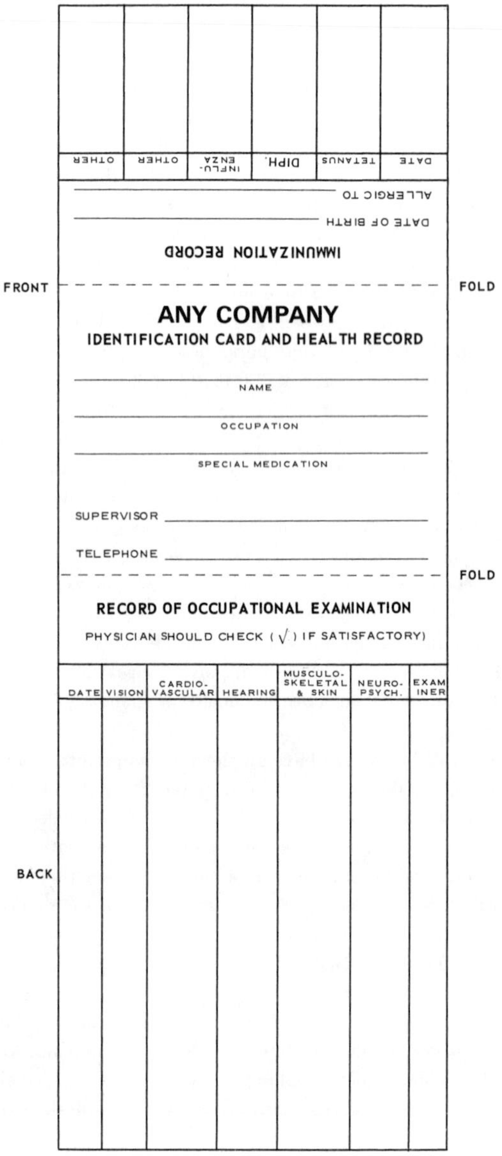

DATE	TETANUS	DIPH.	INFLU-ENZA	OTHER	OTHER

ALLERGIC TO ____

DATE OF BIRTH ____

IMMUNIZATION RECORD

FRONT — FOLD

ANY COMPANY

IDENTIFICATION CARD AND HEALTH RECORD

____
NAME

____
OCCUPATION

____
SPECIAL MEDICATION

SUPERVISOR ____

TELEPHONE ____

FOLD

RECORD OF OCCUPATIONAL EXAMINATION

PHYSICIAN SHOULD CHECK (√) IF SATISFACTORY)

BACK

DATE	VISION	CARDIO-VASCULAR	HEARING	MUSCULO-SKELETAL & SKIN	NEURO-PSYCH.	EXAMINER

FIG 5–1.
A wallet-size employee health record.

to review these articles; they should be read for complete information. The title of an article by Howe is "Small Industry: An Opportunity for the Family Physician."[21] The use of the word opportunity indicates that physicians in practice can expand their knowledge and their services to the community by getting out of their offices occasionally to see health matters in a more positive way—at the workplace.

Discussion

The physician who undertakes to provide his services to an employer must recognize that changes have occurred in the work setting as in all other aspects of American life. No longer may an employer have certain jobs for men only and others for women only. Discrimination because of race or age also is forbidden. For example, physicians will be required to determine if a particular woman is able to do a particular job that has always been considered a man's work. Also, it no longer is possible to have a rule that persons older than age 40—or some other age—may not do certain types of work. Each individual must be examined and a judgment given on the basis of findings in that individual. There are no scientifically established guidelines in many of these areas. Because of new and increasingly active federal agencies with rules against discrimination and more active promotion of individual rights by many organizations and individuals, physicians can expect more challenges of their advice to employers concerning when and under what conditions a person may work.

The federal Occupational Safety and Health Act became effective April 28, 1971. It states that all employers shall provide a safe working place for all employees—the "General Duty" rule. Standards for the permissible amounts of potentially harmful substances and conditions at work have been and will be established. Any employee may directly or through a representative report what he thinks is a dangerous condition in the work environment to the federal or state enforcing authorities. The latter will investigate and report their findings to both the employer and the employee. The employer may not penalize an employee who makes such complaints. Physicians will be increasingly called on to judge not only whether a particular condition at the work site is potentially harmful but also whether harm has occurred to an individual from such exposure. Many times this will be difficult, because the animal organism has a limited number of ways in which it can respond to insults of any kind. In other words, the pathology found may not provide proof as to the exact cause.

The activities that have been called safety-related generally have been easily distinguished from what are called health matters in industry. Safety has always meant such things as avoiding injuries by learning the proper physical methods of accomplishing a task, using protective equipment, including tools, safety shoes, and safety glasses, compiling statistics concerning injuries, and providing first-aid training. Many persons working in safety programs now are scientifically trained in that field. Formal undergraduate programs in safety as a scientific discipline have recently been developed.

Health programs in industry have been run by the licensed health professionals—physicians and nurses. Under the new federal laws, including the Coal Mine Health and Safety Act, however, safety and health activities merge, particularly in industrial hygiene and toxicology. Here is an opportunity and a responsibility for physicians to help by giving guidance and assistance to employers who must plan for a "safe" working environment. Small businesses are hard-pressed to find enough persons trained in control of the work environment. Certainly physicians cannot assume this role, but they can help by pointing out when an expert in industrial hygiene is needed and by being familiar with the resources, both public and private, in this area.

The Occupational Safety and Health Act requires employers to make and maintain more detailed records than has been the practice of most employers. For example, if there are "potentially toxic substances or harmful physical agents" in the work environment, periodic measurement of the actual concentrations of these substances to which workers are exposed must be made and the records maintained so as to be available to federal inspectors, who also may make their own measurements. Results of such tests made by the employer or inspectors must be made available to any employee working in that environment—a worker thus is entitled to know his own exposures. It is likely that physicians will be asked by their patients and by employers about the significance of certain exposures they have had; physicians should be prepared to answer such questions or at least know where to find the answers.

Under the Occupational Safety and Health Act, records of injuries and illnesses due to work must be kept in more detail than now is common. For example, injuries or illnesses due to work must be recorded if there is loss of work time, medical treatment (not first aid), loss of consciousness, limited work ("light duty"), or transfer to another job due to the injury or illness. This is the employer's responsibility and should not be a problem, since in most instances of this sort the same information is required for reporting to the state under workers' compensation or occupational disease laws.

It is a real asset for an employer to have a physician available to care for employees who are hurt at work and to provide certain other services, such as applicant examinations, health evaluation examinations, and advice on the many areas in which an employer now has responsibilities for the health of his workers. This can be an interesting and profitable experience for the physician. Physicians who engage in part-time occupational medicine should be honest, ethical, and interested in the health of the employee in relation to his work. The primary benefit is to the employee, who will feel reassured when he gets good-quality health services promptly and pleasantly when it is the responsibility of the employer to provide it.

ENVIRONMENTAL HEALTH & HYGIENE POLICY

As a responsible manufacturer of a wide variety of specialty chemicals and pesticides, Velsicol's plants, laboratories and offices shall be maintained as clean and healthful places of employment.

At all times, Velsicol's facilities shall be designed and operated in compliance with the spirit and letter of federal, state and local occupational health and hygiene regulations.

Velsicol acknowledges and shall satisfy its responsibility to promptly provide current, comprehensive information on potential adverse health effects and appropriate handling procedures for chemicals handled by both our employees and our customers.

It is a basic responsibility of all Velsicol employees to make the health and safety of fellow human beings a part of their daily, hourly concern. This responsibility must be accepted by each one who conducts the affairs of the corporation, no matter in what capacity he may function.

A goal of the Velsicol Chemical Corporation is to achieve and maintain a corporate occupational health & hygiene program which is a model for the Chemical Industry.

Chairman of the Board &
Chief Executive Officer

President & Chief
Operating Officer

FIG 5–2.
A sample policy statement.

BASIC OCCUPATIONAL HEALTH SERVICES

It was stated at the beginning of this chapter that good occupational health services can be supplied to an employee group of any size. The most important determinants are the energy, enthusiasm, and knowledge of the physician and a sincere desire by the employer to provide such services. This is especially true for employee groups so small that a medical department is unrealistic. The services and activities discussed here can be carried out either in the physician's office or in a medical department at the work site.

Standard Activities and Services

Policy

Small employee groups of large organizations usually will be covered by a policy statement applying to the entire organization. Except in very small organizations, a written policy statement describing the purpose and objectives of the occupational health program is desirable. Following the policy statement, a more detailed description of the program should be prepared and can serve as instructions to supervisors and employees as to how to use the services under different circumstances of employment (Fig 5–2).

Applicant and Preplacement Examinations

There is not complete agreement among occupational physicians concerning the type of examination for applicants or even if any medical examination is indicated.[11, 29, 30, 35] There is reasonable agreement that an examination is appropriate for candidates for certain jobs, whether they be applicants or employees proposing to transfer into other jobs. These jobs are those that are potentially hazardous to the employee or others or those that require a considerable amount of physical strength, stamina, coordination, and good function of the special senses.

It is recommended here that a screening procedure be given new applicants for jobs that are neither hazardous nor strenuous and that a more complete examination be given those who propose to work in other jobs. The screening examination should include a self-administered health questionnaire, pulse and blood pressure, a vision test, and a urinalysis for glucose and albumin. The screening examination should be performed in the medical department or physician's office and can be done by a nurse or specially trained physician's assistant.[8, 9, 19] The health history should be reviewed carefully with the applicant, and past and present health problems should be recorded in considerable detail. In addition to the screening tests, observations should be made concerning the general appearance and behavior, gait and posture, skin, and personal hygiene. When apparently significant abnormalities are detected by the screening procedure, the physician then should examine and evaluate the applicant or employee. For those applicants with a history of disease or defects that may be chronic or recurrent, it often is necessary to obtain, with the signed permission of the individual, reports from other physicians or institutions that provided care.

For persons who propose to work in potentially hazardous and strenuous jobs, a more thorough physical examination should be done. This type of examination can be done by a *specially trained* nurse or physician's assistant and those patients with significant abnormalities should be referred to the physician. Some companies have been carrying out complete examinations with specially trained nurses and report satisfaction with their experiences.[8, 11] The "special training" may be given by company physicians or by academic departments in a medical center. Many medical centers have programs for special training of nurses and physician assistants.[5]

Records of applicant and employee examinations should be kept in the plant medical department in locked files available only to medical department personnel. If there is no medical department, the records should be kept in the physician's office. In either instance, it is necessary to report to the company certain information resulting from medical evaluations. Ordinarily, the physician will report that (1) the applicant (or employee) has been evaluated only for nonhazardous and nonstrenuous work (complete examination recommended if later assigned to other work); (2) no medical condition has been detected which causes an increased risk of health impairment from the job; (3) the applicant is recommended with limitations (For example, the applicant should work with glasses only or with a hearing aid, or should not work above the surface, i.e., on ladders or scaffolds, or the person has a disease or condition that might cause sudden incapacitation—diabetes treated by insulin, epilepsy or certain cardiovascular diseases—and therefore is not recommended for work with certain machines, for operating vehicles, for work above the surface or for working alone for prolonged periods); (4) the applicant is not recommended for any job until correction is obtained, e.g., glasses or surgical repair of hernia; or (5) the applicant is not recommended for current placement because of active and progressive disease.

Special Examinations and Standards

There was an era when occupational medicine had a poor reputation among many workers and unions because of overly rigid health standards for new employees. This criticism was justified in some instances, particularly in those companies that refused to hire persons with even minor handicaps. Now, most occupational physicians strive to make their recommendations concerning work suitability as accurate as possible and to make use of handicapped persons' abilities. The important role for the physician in industry is to assess the capabilities of applicants and employees as accurately as possible and make his recommendations accordingly. This should contribute to a healthier and safer work force.

Applicants for hazardous and strenuous work should be evaluated with emphasis on the particular job requirements. For some jobs, physical coordination and acuity of special senses are important to prevent harm to persons or equipment and buildings. Certain jobs require greater muscular strength and stamina, and workers in such jobs must have a stable musculoskeletal system in order to remain on the job many years. For still other jobs, the physical demands are not great but the physiologic status must be measured before starting to work where there are toxic materials or radiation or noise or other harmful substances or conditions in the working environment. Specific types of examinations, x-rays, and/or laboratory tests are needed for workers exposed to ionizing radiation, toxic metals, certain dusts, solvents, and other toxic materials. These are discussed in the chapters relating to the particular hazardous condition or substances.

In assessing physical abilities, it is useful to have guidelines concerning recommendations for persons with some degree of disease or impairment. This will ensure general consistency among different physicians as to the significance of various conditions. The guidelines should be based on the opinions of several experts in the particular clinical area and, to the extent possible, based on validated opinions. The latter are scarce, for the simple reason that we do not recommend persons for jobs if clinical judgment indicates a significant chance for harm because of a certain handicap and, therefore, there rarely are controlled studies.

There are a few areas in which agreement is fairly good on guidelines for job placement of handicapped persons. Brief mention of a few, along with references, will be made for some not covered in other chapters.

It must be kept in mind that medical recommendations about placement and work limitations must always be based on specific evaluations of each individual, and not on whether a person is a member of a group, e.g., epileptics or diabetics.

Vision.—Visual tasks vary greatly and are influenced by illumination, reflectance, color, object size, and many other factors that are beyond the scope of this brief discussion. For most jobs, it is enough to consider simply near and far visual acuity, field of vision, and color vision. Employees who operate commercial passenger or cargo vehicles, including aircraft, must conform to federal standards,[27, 28] which should be obtained for ready reference. Vision testing of applicants and employees is best accomplished with one of the vision screening devices that screens acuity (far and near, each eye separately), color vision, phorias, and depth perception (stereopsis). The depth perception test alone is not considered accurate enough to use as a basis for work restrictions. (Orthorater, from Bausch and Lomb, Inc., Sightscreener, from the American Optical Company, and Vision Tester, from the Titmus Optical Company are examples of screening machines.) The results of such screening are entered on a card that is so arranged as to indicate those abnormalities that require referral to an ophthalmologist for detailed evaluation. The ophthalmologist is an important consultant to the occupational physician, and his services are needed frequently.

Safety glasses conforming to American National Standards Institute (ANSI) Publication Z87.1–1968 for industrial use should be required where eye hazards exist in the working environment. The term "eye hazards" must be interpreted with judgment after observing the work site to consider not only such routine potential hazards as dust and smoke but also the possible effects of a sudden disruption of the work process. For example, molten metal or irritating chemicals may splash into the eye because of an accident, and although the risk based on frequency of occurrence may appear small, the potential seriousness of the injury may be sufficient to recommend using safety glasses routinely.

The ANSI Standard Z87.1–1968 provides that spectacles must have nonflammable frames and lenses of plastic or heat-treated glass that are at least 3 mm thick in the center and able to withstand the impact of a 1-inch steel ball dropped from a height of 50 inches. There is another standard for dress glasses, ANSI Z80.1–1972, which provides that lenses must be at least 2 mm thick in the center and be able to withstand a ⅝-inch steel ball dropped 50 inches.

Contact lenses of the hard corneal type or the newer soft, large hydrophilic type are more and more common and the physician in industry must understand the potential problems related to such lenses. First, it is important to know if an individual with contact lenses tolerates them comfortably for ten hours or more each day. Second, where there are appreciable amounts of dust, smoke, or irritating fumes or liquid irritants that could splash into the eyes, contact lenses are not recommended by most ophthalmologists.[22] Often a judgment must be made, however, as to the degree of potential hazard, because some persons obtain better visual correction with contact lenses and therefore need them. These persons should wear the proper safety spectacles or goggles over their contacts when in an area where any degree of potential eye hazard exists. One little-noticed regulation under the Occupational Safety and Health Act prohibits the wearing of contact lenses if a respirator is to be used in a contaminated atmosphere.

Persons with long-standing monocular vision usually learn a degree of depth judgment that makes them able to work at any job except those covered by federal regulations for operating commercial vehicles, trains, or airplanes. However, individuals who are recently monocular may be at increased risk for a variable period of time in working with moving machinery or working at heights, and may need work restrictions.

Vision standards are used by the military and other federal government agencies, the Department of Transportation,[28] the Federal Aviation Administration,[27] and many companies. Although there is reasonable agreement among these standards, there is no single set of visual abilities that could be considered universal consensus standards. For example, the Department of Transportation requirements for interstate truck drivers are 20/40 (Snellen) in each eye and with both eyes, with or without correction, and a field of vision of at least 70° in the horizontal meridian in each eye, plus the ability to recognize the traffic signal colors, red, green, and amber. The American Medical Association Ad Hoc Committee on Medical Aspects of Automotive Safety published their recommendations in 1969.[8] This Committee recognized three classes of drivers: Class 1, professional drivers of passenger and emergency vehicles (fire engines, ambulances, etc.); Class 2, commercial taxi drivers and professional drivers of freight trucks; and Class 3, operators of personal vehicles. Visual acuity of 20/25 (Snellen) in each eye with spectacle correction of less than 10 D is required for Class 1. For Class 2, central visual acuity of 20/40 in the better eye and at least 20/60 in the worse eye is required, with a "special report" needed if spectacle correction is 10 D or more. Class 3 drivers must have 20/40 or better in one eye. These figures are given for quick reference, but the entire report should be read for a description and discussion of test methods and other factors. The AMA Committee, although now disbanded, reviewed their recommendations in 1972 and agreed that the central visual acuity recommendations are still valid and stated that certain other professional groups have adopted their standards.

Cardiovascular.—Applicants and employees should have an accurate diagnosis of any cardiovascular disease so that classification (status and prognosis) can be made by the American Heart Association Classification. This usually will be sufficient to determine suitable job placement. Those persons whose disease causes an increased risk of sudden incapacitation should not be recommended for strenuous or potentially hazardous jobs. Such judgments should be made carefully, because improved management of heart disease in recent years has made it possible for more and more cardiac patients to be productively employed. Unless the occupational physician is experienced or trained in cardiology, the advice of one who *is* should often be obtained in cardiac cases.

The confirmation of a diagnosis requires cardiac examination at rest and after exercise and should include a chest x-ray and ECG. Consultation with the treating physician and obtaining previous hospital records can yield valuable information as well. In some areas, the regional chapter of the American Heart Association maintains a Work Classification Unit, where a detailed appraisal of work capability can be obtained.

Accurate diagnosis is the key to establishing work guidelines at the time of employment and can aid in counseling with personnel and management as to expectations for the future.

Musculoskeletal.—Many labor-saving machines and devices have eliminated much of the physically difficult work in factories and warehouses. This is true to a lesser extent in the construction and service industries, where a stable musculoskeletal system is required for a career in many jobs. Preplacement medical assessment, if perfect, would predict all those whose backs, knees, ankles, shoulders and other structures will not withstand stressful exposures over many years. Such persons then could be oriented toward jobs more suitable. Our clinical abilities are not good enough to identify all those who will develop early degenerative arthritis, for example, but yet are sufficient to pick out some, and this is important enough to justify a careful examination in those with a history or findings of musculoskeletal abnormalities.

The physical examination should be done thoroughly and carefully, with the person undressed. A routine should be followed that tests for the symmetric strength and the range of motion of all extremities and the spine. This may be done by a specially trained nurse or physician's assistant, but significant abnormalities that are thus noticed should be evaluated by a physician. The recommendation by the physician that a person not work at a job applied for is a serious matter to the person concerned and should not be done casually.

Two of the most common difficult areas in preplacement examinations are the knees and the low back. Knee injuries are common in young persons, particularly in sports. Injury to the semilunar cartilage often requires its surgical removal, leaving the joint without the cushioning effect on the femur and tibia. Joint capsule and supporting ligaments often are injured at the time of the cartilage injury. The joint is "weakened" in the sense that degenerative changes usually appear by the age of 40 and often within a few years if stressful activities are pursued. For these reasons, many orthopedists and occupational physicians recommend that such persons not be assigned to jobs that require sustained severe stress on the knees, e.g., telephone linemen or certain foundry jobs. Those who have a full range of motion and normal strength and are asymptomatic a year or more postmeniscectomy usually can tolerate moderate activity, such as most craft jobs.

Low back pain is common in all populations and the relationship to activities at work is difficult to evaluate. The expense of caring for persons with back pain that is considered work-related under compensation laws, plus the difficulty of subsequent job placement, make low back trouble a serious problem for employers. Because of this, great efforts have been made by physicians in industry to examine the low back thoroughly to attempt to identify those persons who are more likely to develop low back pain. Success in this direction has been only modest but yet worthwhile.

A careful and thorough physical examination of the back is essential, but this will not permit identifying all those who will have low back trouble later. An individual with a moderate to severe increase in lumbar lordosis, thoracic kyphosis, and cervical lordosis, whose posture when viewed from the side reveals the head forward of the midcoronal plane and the lower abdomen sagging forward, and whose hamstring muscles are so tight that he can reach only to 12 inches above the floor—this person usually is prone to low back pain. This person probably will have episodes of low back pain no matter what his vocation is, but clinical judgment indicates that he should probably not be recommended for heavy physical work, particularly if there is a history of prior low back trouble. His back trouble will be less severe and less likely to be job related if his work is not stressful to the low back. Most persons do not have such exaggerated physical findings and milder degrees of abnormality require careful judgment as to selection and placement. A history of low back pain is helpful, but applicant health histories are not always accurate. A history of more than one disabling episode of low back pain or even one episode with sciatica would justify a recommendation against heavy lifting and other strenuous work.

X-rays of the low back have been used by many physicians to supplement the physical examination. Those who report their experiences do not agree on the value of this procedure.[18, 22, 23, 28] An ad hoc committee of the Industrial Medical Association reported in 1964 on recommended techniques and standards for using low back x-rays as a screening procedure but did not take a position on the value of this.[3] A compromise position is to give candidates for heavy work a careful history and physical examination. These procedures alone will detect some not suited for heavy work, and no x-ray is needed. Those with a history or findings suggestive but not definite enough for decisions concerning recommendations may be given a low back x-ray for a more thorough evaluation. Applicants with no history of low back pain and with normal physical findings need not be screened by x-ray. Not all experienced physicians will agree with this position concerning low back preplacement screening. It is hoped that someday a prospective study will be made in which all applicants are given low back x-rays but with the results not used in placement recommendations. Then, after several years, information would be available as to the significance of various abnormalities found only by x-ray. Such studies may never be done, simply because doctors who do preplacement back x-rays believe that abnormalities detected only by x-ray predispose to low back pain and therefore recommend against hiring or at least placement in strenuous jobs.

In January of 1973, a conference was sponsored by the National Institute for Occupational Safety and Health on the subject of low back x-rays as a preplacement technique. Present were orthopedists, radiologists, and occupational physicians experienced in this subject. The only conclusions that could be drawn were that (1) information in the literature does not prove or disprove that low back x-rays are a useful screening technique in preventing low back injuries and that (2) only a prospective study of adequate size and proper design can produce this information. The proceedings of this conference have been published.[36]

Mental Abnormalities.—The usual applicant examination will not detect most persons with psychoneuroses unless current or prior treatment is admitted. Perhaps this is proper, because psychoneurosis is so common and many such persons are good employees. The physician's role is, after all, to evaluate for employment and not to play God. Yet, it is known that many neurotic employees lose excessive time from work,[5] and it is a common experience among occupational physicians to see work schedules and production disrupted because of personality clashes between neurotic employees and supervisors and other employees.

Those applicants with a history of treatment for mental disease should be investigated carefully and written reports obtained from the physicians and institutions who provided treatment. Persons with symptomatic phobias or with certain psychophysiologic reactions, especially cardiac, may require special placement and may need psychiatric treatment either before or after employment. Applicants with personality disorders and any of the various sexual deviances should be referred for evaluation by a psychiatrist, and special attention should be given to their histories. Many of these persons will require recommendations against their working in job situations that might involve too much freedom and responsibility—in other words, these persons often do better in a small group with limited contact and responsibility with the public. Periodic follow-up visits are recommended, and this may permit many with mental abnormalities to remain useful and productive citizens.

Applicants with a history or presence of a psychosis often are unsatisfactory in the average work setting. Very careful investigation of the history must be made, and if all the factors appear favorable, such persons may be able to work successfully if placed in positions with limited responsibility, at least initially, hopefully with an understanding supervisor.[10] Follow-up of these persons on the job is indicated to ensure that they pursue proper treatment and to detect exacerbations of their disease.

Alcoholism and other drug abuse are important, and it is essential that the physician have a good understanding of the potential for helping many of these persons in the work setting.

Fitness Examination.—Fitness examination is a suitable term for health evaluations any time during the career of an employee. It simply means the evaluation of the fitness of an employee for his work, and it may be done on a regular periodic basis (these are also called occupational examinations) or on an episodic basis when there is or appears to be a health problem that might interfere with attendance or performance.

For certain jobs, fitness examinations that are done on a periodic basis are to ensure that the employee has continued special skills and abilities to safely continue his job or to evaluate whether the employee has suffered potential harm from work exposures. The latter examinations (to detect injuries due to noise, toxic substances in the environment, etc.) are covered in other chapters. Federal regulations require operators of passenger or cargo vehicles to be examined periodically. It is recommended that all employees in potentially hazardous work be given a fitness examination at intervals that can vary from one to two years, depending on age and type of work. Requirements for such examinations covering certain jobs are included in regulations of the Occupational Safety and Health Administration, and this list likely will be expanded.

Fitness examinations requested by the employer also are important. These would include those requested by the physician and nurse based on their knowledge of a particular health problem, those requested by the insurance or benefit department, and, most important, those requested by the supervisor. Personality change, increased absence from work or tardiness, or other factors in the appearance and behavior of an employee often permit the supervisor to identify the existence of a health problem early, when treatment may be most effective. When supervisors refer employees for a fitness examination, they should communicate in writing or verbally their observations and reason for concern. This is necessary for the physician to properly evaluate a possible health problem, and he or she must correlate what the supervisor says with the history obtained from the employee. This may permit uncovering a condition that the employee wishes to conceal, such as alcoholism or mental illness.

The physician is assisted in fitness examinations by having a prior medical history on the particular employee. Therefore, the examination need only be thorough enough to evaluate the problem and might consist of a brief office visit or a very thorough examination that includes referral to other specialists. A report to the supervisor is necessary and should include the following information: whether the employee is (or is not) able to work at his or her regular job, whether he is able to work at another job, whether the employee has (or does not have) a health problem, and if so, whether advice has been given for proper medical care. The report to the supervisor includes a general statement concerning prognosis, but no diagnosis or other detailed information should be revealed; this protects the confidentiality of information concerning the employee and contributes much to obtaining the respect of the employee.

Fitness examinations should be given on return to work after a sickness or disability leave of one week or longer. This permits confirmation that the employee actually is able to return to work or not. A return to lighter work or shortened hours initially often is helpful in rehabilitation. Fitness examination during a sickness absence sometimes is indicated if the return to work is delayed beyond that expected. In this instance, it may be discovered that the diagnosis or treatment is improper, and helpful recommendations can be made, especially if care is being given by quacks or cultists. It also may permit detection of the employee who would abuse the sickness disability payments plan by not returning to work when adequate recovery has been achieved.

Health Education and Health Counseling

Every time an applicant or employee visits a physician or nurse, there is some health education and/or counseling given. Medical departments in industry provide an ideal opportunity for these services, which constitute an asset for the employees and for the employer as well. Employers increasingly are paying the costs for health care for employees and their dependents. It is economically important for the employer that his employees have an entry into the health care system when needed and, further, that the care obtained is proper. Both physicians and nurses in industry play an important role in guiding employees to the proper health care resources. An almost equally important role is played when the need is for counseling rather than pills or surgery, and physicians and nurses experienced in occupational health programs generally are very skilled in the art and science of counseling. The education and counseling functions often are overlooked when assessing the costs and benefits of occupational health programs because of the difficulties in determining the units of service that can be defined.[6] This is unfortunate, because experience and common sense indicate that these activities are among the most valuable to both employer and employees. And these benefits are available to all employees, not just those exposed to potential hazards. This is an important point in justifying the costs of a health program in any sizable employee group.

DISCUSSION

Occupational medicine is a broad and fascinating field of medical practice. Not all of the problems that will confront a physician in industry can be covered in this or any other chapter. Most of the important subjects are discussed in this book. Specific exposures that may occur in the work place and cause harm are discussed in several chapters and should be consulted for information relating to them. It must be remembered that a physician in industry is first of all a highly trained professional who is licensed by the state to make judgments when facts are not clear enough to be definite. This judgment must be exercised frequently in occupational medicine as in any other field of medicine. It must be informed and honest.

REFERENCES

1. Alderman MH, Davis TK: Hypertension: Central at the work site. *J Occup Med* 1976; 18:793–796.
2. American Medical Association: *Guide to the Development of an Occupational Medical Records System,* ed 2. Chicago, American Medical Association, 1984.
3. American Medical Association: *Guides to the Evaluation of Permanent Impairment,* ed 2. Chicago, American Medical Association, 1984.
4. American Medical Association Council on Scientific Affairs: *Medical Evaluations of Healthy Persons*. *JAMA* 1983; 2249:1626–1633.
5. Bond MB: Mental disease in employed persons. *J Occup Med* 1969; 11:663.
6. Bond MB, et al: An occupational health program: Costs vs. benefits. *Arch Environ Health* 1968; 17:408.
7. Bond MB, et al: Low back x-rays: Criteria for their use in placement examinations in industry. *J Occup Med* 1964; 6:373.
8. Brogan MN: Utilization of nursing talents in Bell Canada. *J Occup Med* 1971; 13:511.
9. Cipolla JA, Collings GH, Jr: Nurse clinicians in industry. *Am J Nursing* 1971; 71:1530.
10. Cole NJ, Shupe DR, Allison RB: Work performance ratings of former psychiatric patients. *J Occup Med* 1966; 8:1.
11. Collings GH, Jr: The pre-employment examination—worth its cost? *J Occup Med* 1971; 13:422.
12. Committee on Medical Aspects of Automotive Safety: Visual factors in automobile driving and provisional standards. *Arch Ophthalmol* 1969; 81:865.

13. Council on Occupational Health, American Medical Association: A management guide for occupational health problems. *Arch Environ Health* 1964; 9:408.
14. Council on Occupational Health, American Medical Association: Scope, objectives and functions of occupational health programs. *JAMA* 1960; 174:533.
15. Felton JS: Organization and operation of an occupational health program. *J Occup Med* 1964; 6:25.
16. Fleming AJ, D'Alonozo CA, Zapp JA: *Modern Occupational Medicine*. Philadelphia, Lea & Febiger, 1960, p 31.
17. *Guide to Developing Small Plant Occupational Programs*. Chicago, American Medical Association, 1983.
18. Harley WJ: Lost time back injuries: Their relationship to heavy work and preplacement back x-rays. *J Occup Med* 1972; 14:611.
19. Howard DR: The physician's associate in occupational medicine. *J Occup Med* 1971; 13:507.
20. Howe HF: Relationship between plant physician and family physician. *JAMA* 1962; 179:975.
21. Howe HF: Small industry: An opportunity for the family physician. *Gen Pract* 1962; 26:166.
22. Kelley FJ: Pre-employment medical examinations including back x-rays. *J Occup Med* 1965; 7:132.
23. Kosiak M, Aurelius JR, Hartfiel WF: The low back problem. *J Occup Med* 1968; 10:588.
24. Logan AG, Milne BJ, Archer C, et al: A comparison of community and occupationally provided antihypertensive care. *J Occup Med* 1982; 24:901–906.
25. Novak JJ, Saul RW: Contact lenses in industry. *J Occup Med* 1971; 13:175.
26. *Occupational Health Guide for Medical and Nursing Personnel*, ed 3., Zenz C (ed). State Medical Society of Wisconsin, 3300 E Lakeside St, Madison, WI 53701, 1985.
27. Patterson RB: Problems faced by the less than full time occupational physician. *J Occup Med* 1971; 13:277.
28. Redfield JT: Low back x-ray as a screening tool in the forest products industry. *J Occup Med* 1971; 13:219.
29. Rodman MH: The pre-employment physical examination. Recent experiences at Massachusetts Institute of Technology. *J Occup Med* 1965; 7:608.
30. Schneider RF, McDonagh TJ: Experience data on university recruits hired without pre-employment examinations. *J Occup Med* 1971; 13:363.
31. *The Physician and Workers' Compensation*. Chicago, American Medical Association, 1983.
32. US Dept of Transportation: *Federal Aviation Regulations*, 1969, pt 67, chap III.
33. US Dept of Transportation: *Motor Carrier Regulations*, Sections 391:41 and 391:43, 1971.
34. Wagner SP: Role of occupational nurse in efficient worker utilization. *Arch Environ Health* 1962; 4:451.
35. Williamson SM: Eighteen years experience without pre-employment examinations. *J Occup Med* 1971; 13:465.
36. *X-Rays in Pre-employment Physical Examinations*. Conference on the Low Back. Chicago, American College of Radiology, 1973.

6

Investigating Environmental Health Hazards

James M. Melius, M.D., Dr.P.H.

While the customary approach to investigating possible occupational health hazards usually focuses on evaluating exposures in relation to environmental standards or criteria, the investigation of a reported occupational health hazard by the Health Hazard Evaluation Program of the National Institute for Occupational Safety and Health (NIOSH) often necessitates a broader approach. In addition to evaluating exposures, potential health effects must also be assessed. In conducting the investigation, the availability of potential sources of information on exposure and health effects for that working population must be ascertained. Then, an appropriate and efficient approach to evaluating the specific problem can be designed and implemented. The following approach is based on the experience and capabilities of NIOSH's Health Hazard Evaluation Program, but should be applicable to similar evaluations conducted by private industry, academic groups, or other governmental agencies.

EXPOSURE-RESPONSE RELATIONSHIP

The essence of evaluating and controlling occupational health hazards is knowledge of the association between exposure to a toxic substance and resulting adverse health effects. For some situations, extensive information will be available on this exposure-response relationship, while for others (e.g., mixed exposures or newly introduced chemicals) little will be known, and this information will have to be at least partially developed as part of the evaluation. Before discussing the methods used in evaluating occupational health hazards, it is important to review the general approaches used for determining the presence of an occupational health hazard in a specific workplace:

Environmental Criteria

Using environmental criteria is often the most direct and efficient method for evaluating and controlling occupational health hazards. One simply measures exposure to a toxic substance and then compares the result with environmental criteria or standards. These criteria are available from the Occupational Safety and Health Administration (OSHA), from the National Institute for Occupational Safety and Health Criteria Documents and other publications, and from other organizations such as the American Conference of Governmental Industrial Hygienists (ACGIH).[8,7,1] Exposures in excess of a criterion determine the presence of an occupational health hazard.

However, this approach is not always satisfactory. Exposure monitoring may be difficult to conduct for a variety of reasons (e.g., intermittent exposure or lack of an analytical method).

Available environmental criteria for a substance may not be appropriate for the situations encountered (e.g., there may be no criterion for short-term exposures). There may be exposures to multiple toxic substances or there may be a significant route of exposure not addressed by the criteria (e.g., dermal). In addition, the criteria may be outdated and not address recently documented toxic effects of a substance or delayed effects occurring at lower levels of exposure. Thus, while environmental monitoring may be quite important in the evaluation of an occupational health hazard, additional approaches are often necessary.

Epidemiologic Approach

In the epidemiologic approach, one determines the incidence or prevalence of a specific health effect in the exposed population as compared with the incidence or prevalence of the same health effect in an unexposed (or less exposed) population. While obviously very useful in identifying occupational health problems and in establishing environmental criteria to control these hazards, this approach is not always applicable for investigating specific occupational health problems. Determining a statistically significant excess of disease in a specific working population may be difficult for a variety of reasons, including inadequate population size, lack of adequate records, or changes in exposure over time. Another major detriment to using this approach is the long latency period between initial exposure and the appearance of many occupationally related illnesses. Thus, not finding an excess of disease in an exposed population at the present time does not mean that current exposures will not result in future disease. An epidemiologic approach should not be the sole determinant of the presence or absence of an occupational health hazard, but it can be a useful tool in evaluating specific occupational health problems. (Refer to Chapter 71 for a thorough discussion on occupational epidemiology by Hernberg.)

Health Effects Consistent With Exposure

Although there are very few diseases pathognomonic of particular occupational exposures, there are many diseases and symptoms known to be associated with specific occupational exposures.[10] In evaluating workers exposed to a toxic substance, determining the prevalence of symptoms or illness known to be associated with that exposure among the exposed population can be quite useful in determining the presence of a hazard in that workplace. In particular, this approach is useful for substances causing acute or subacute symptoms or illnesses in situations where industrial hygiene evaluation is difficult or where present exposure criteria do not exist or do not appear to be adequate for the substances involved. Certain other factors need to be taken into account in evaluating the results of this approach, including consideration of latency, the presence of other factors associated with these symptoms or illness, and the degree of association between the exposure and the health effect being monitored.

Although in specific situations any of these approaches may be used in determining the presence or absence of an occupational health hazard, one should consider all three in approaching any specific workplace evaluation. Most important, both exposures and health effects must be considered when evaluating a specific occupational health problem. Ignoring exposure may lead to an incomplete understanding of the cause of the occupational health hazard and, thus, difficulty in recommending appropriate controls for that problem. Ignoring potential health effects may lead to overreliance on exposure criteria which may be inadequate or inappropriate for the particular occupational health problem under consideration.

The course of the evaluation of a specific occupational health problem will depend on many factors. However, in deciding how to conduct the evaluation, a number of sources of information on both exposure and health effects must be considered.

EXPOSURE

In evaluating a specific occupational health problem, information on occupational exposures in the affected worksite can be obtained from a variety of sources. Often, much can be learned by reviewing available records on exposure monitoring and process information. This information can then be supplemented by appropriate industrial hygiene and biologic monitoring.

In considering these sources, a few important considerations should be kept in mind. First, the usual latency between exposure and chronic disease manifestation requires the assessment of both past and present occupational exposures. Second, both qualitative and quantitative information on exposures are usually required. This is particularly important in reviewing past exposure monitoring records. Due to limitations in available sampling and analytical methods, exposure to important toxic substances may be missed if past exposure is presumed to be limited to the monitored substances. Process information or samples may provide a more complete assessment of exposures in that workplace. Several sources of information on exposure are outlined below.

Exposure Records

There are usually several important sources of information on environmental exposures in a facility which may be reviewed both for information on past exposure and for defining an approach to current exposure monitoring. Examples include:

1. Industrial process records
2. Information from suppliers (Material Safety Data Sheets)
3. Environmental discharge data
4. Monitoring data from the company, their insurance company, or governmental agencies

For qualitative information, process records may provide important information on the substances used in the process, the pertinent physical parameters (e.g., heat), or important contaminants. This can be supplemented by information from suppliers and by Material Safety Data Sheets on substances used in the process to provide some assessment of the potential exposures in the industrial process.

This information, coupled with general knowledge on exposures in that particular industry, may provide the necessary basis to direct further environmental sampling. Occasionally, this can be supplemented by data on air and water discharges and waste products from the facility from the federal Environmental Protection Agency (EPA) or state or local environmental agencies.

For more quantitative information, available exposure monitoring information should be reviewed. This may include monitoring conducted by the company, by their insurance carrier, or by governmental agencies. Reports from the Occupational Safety and Health Administration (OSHA), OSHA consultation programs, NIOSH, and other monitoring groups may be available for that facility. For example, in conducting an evaluation of cancer risk among workers exposed to benzene at a plant in Ohio, NIOSH was able to estimate past exposures at that plant from records of monitoring conducted by the Ohio Industrial Commission.[9]

In evaluating this information, several important factors must be considered. Have there been any major changes in the process, in the substances used in the process, or in control technology for that process (including personal protective equipment)? Piecing together these changes and their impact on exposure from that process can be difficult, but it may be quite important for evaluating past exposures. Considerations in the evaluation of environmental and biologic monitoring information will be discussed below.

Environmental Monitoring

In reviewing environmental monitoring records and in developing an approach for environmental evaluation of a worksite, several important factors must be considered. These include:

1. Sampling and analytical method
2. Type of samples (area vs. personal breathing zone)
3. Timing of samples

4. Use of personal protective equipment
5. Other routes of exposure

The most important consideration is the sampling and analytical method used for the environmental monitoring. Since these methods have changed quite rapidly over the past several years, information on the sampling and analytical method must be reviewed when evaluating any environmental data. Such considerations should include the sensitivity of the method, its specificity, the presence of compounds known to interfere with the analysis, and the quality control on the analytical work. Many industrial hygiene sampling and analytical methods have been initially designed for the current occupational standards or criteria, and, thus, often are not sensitive enough for detecting much lower levels of exposure.

Another important consideration is the sampling protocol used. What types of samples were taken (area, personal breathing-zone) and what areas of the facility were sampled? Have recent modifications in the facility been made that would alter the interpretation of these results? Were long-term samples taken for a situation in which there were only short-term exposures? Was the sampling conducted under normal operating conditions? In the case of particulates, were respirable and nonrespirable particulates distinguished?

More general limitations of environmental monitoring must also be recognized. Environmental air monitoring considers only one route of exposure (respiratory). Other routes of exposure (dermal and ingestion) are not directly evaluated. Thus, other forms of environmental assessment must be considered in these situations. Although there are methods to determine skin exposure, these may not always provide an accurate assessment of skin absorption. The interpretation of wipe samples from workplace surfaces or skin is difficult. Respiratory protective equipment also affects the validity of the air samples. Only recently have we started to develop field methods to accurately assess concentrations inside a respirator.[6]

Exposure to complex mixtures of toxic substances also poses problems for environmental monitoring. Often, identification and quantification of all toxic substances in these mixtures can be quite difficult. Yet it is important to evaluate these exposures to develop appropriate exposure criteria. For example, the evaluation of the health hazards from exposure to the soot generated by a fire in a transformer containing polychlorinated biphenyl (PCB) required the identification of many of the substances in this complex mixture and the toxicity testing of this soot in animals in order to evaluate its toxicity.[15] Finally, usual approaches involve the monitoring of only a small number of workers. Extrapolation of these results to the entire workforce may be questionable, and individuals with routinely higher or lower exposures may not be identified.

Biologic Monitoring

Biologic monitoring has several advantages over air monitoring. First, it may take into account other routes of exposure, including dermal and ingestion. Second, the use of personal protective equipment poses less of a problem, since skin absorption (including that through protective clothing) and respiratory absorption (through a respirator) are assessed. Individual differences in exposure, due to personal factors or work practices, may be identified by these methods.

Some of the factors to be considered when assessing biologic monitoring are

1. Time course of absorption, metabolism, and excretion
2. Analytical techniques
3. Metabolism
4. Normal values
5. Other sources of exposure

The time course of absorption, metabolism, and excretion is most important. For some exposures, monitoring methods may address mainly chronic exposures (e.g., PCB), short-term exposures (e.g., benzene) or a combination of the two (e.g., lead). Second, as one is attempting to measure small quantities of a substance in a biologic sample, collection and analytical techniques are quite important, as are laboratory standardization and quality control.[11] Knowledge of the metabolism of the substance is important in determining what substance or substances to monitor and what type of specimen to obtain (e.g., blood or urine). "Normal" values may be difficult to obtain due to limited use of these tests in groups without occupational exposure. Thus, often a control or comparison group is important to evaluate results. In addition, the relationship between exposure to specific air levels of a substance and the resulting biologic levels may be poorly defined, limiting the interpretation of results relative to specific air levels. Finally, many of these measurements may be affected by other environmental or dietary sources of exposure (see Chapter 13 for a detailed discussion of biologic monitoring).

Estimating Exposure

Occasionally, there is very little environmental or biologic monitoring information available to assess past exposures accurately at a worksite. In those cases, the limited available information may have to be used to estimate past exposures for these workers. Often the available environmental monitoring can be combined with information on job or work assignments to provide at least a semiquantitative estimate of past exposure for use in analyzing health effects information.[4] Interviews with the worker can also be used to obtain some information on exposure. These interviews are particularly useful if estimating exposures for a single acute exposure. For example, in a study of fire fighters exposed at a fire at a chemical dump, questionnaire information on time spent at the fire, proximity to the fire, and use of protective equipment were used to estimate each fire fighter's relative exposure.[3]

MONITORING OF HEALTH EFFECTS

Potential health effects from occupational exposure must also be assessed in investigating a reported occupational health hazard.

While major emphasis should be on overt illnesses related to occupational exposures, early indicators of these health effects often provide valuable information on the potential development of diseases in a specific work force. Thus, ascertainment of symptoms or of physiologic or biochemical changes due to occupational exposures may be important in the assessment of an occupational health problem.

Occupationally Related Diseases

Evaluation of illness specific to occupational exposures (e.g., silicosis) is usually quite straightforward, although the accuracy of diagnostic methods and of the recording of these illnesses must be considered in evaluating populations exposed to these substances. However, most illnesses due to occupational exposures also may be caused by other factors.[10] Thus, in evaluating the occurrence of these illnesses, other risk factors, such as smoking for bronchitis or diet for colon cancer, must be considered and epidemiologic comparisons must often be made to determine the presence of an excess of these illnesses in the exposed population.

The methods used for evaluating the occurrence of an illness in a specific workplace will depend partially on the available health records. Examples of different sources to be considered for medical or death records include the following:

1. Company medical records
2. Insurance company records
3. Union pension or health fund records
4. Required injury and illness reporting forms
5. Other disease reporting systems, such as cancer registries or state health department reporting

As part of a pension or insurance plan, many companies or unions keep information on deaths among current and/or former employees. Often this information will include a copy of the death certificate. Insurance companies may also manage such benefit programs and may provide information on the cause of death. Such sources are preferable to the more complicated process of attempting to locate death records on all past employees by a search of vital statistic records.

Accurate records on medical illnesses may be more difficult to obtain, depending on the usual form of medical care for that illness and the availability of any systematic method to access this information. Company-maintained medical records and injury and illness logs may provide some information, depending on the illness and the type of medical care provided. Medical insurance claims can also be useful in ascertaining illnesses for which medical care would be sought. For example, in an evaluation of cardiovascular disease among welders, medical insurance records provided a good source of information on clinically confirmed coronary artery disease.[5] However, the usefulness of insurance records may be dependent on the type of insurance coverage and medical care usually provided. Occasionally, local hospital records, health department disease reporting records, or local or state disease or cancer registries may provide useful information for a specific workplace.

After collecting appropriate medical records, several factors must be considered in reviewing them. The degree of ascertainment is most important. If many cases of illness or death would be missed by the records, one would have difficulty basing any conclusions on this source. For example, medical conditions that would be treated by a personal physician rather than the company's medical department may not be recorded in the company's medical records. Insurance claims may be submitted to the insurance company for the worker's spouse and thus not be included in the company's records on that worker. Often this can be checked by comparing the reporting of individual cases in different record systems.

Latency between first exposure and the occurrence of illness must also be considered. Company medical records may not contain information on deaths occurring after retirement, which are quite common for diseases with long latency periods. As mentioned above, other risk factors must often be considered when evaluating specific illnesses. Some of this information may be available through other records systems at the facility. For example, smoking information may be available from medical records. Often a study can be designed to control for these other factors.[13] Diagnostic accuracy must also be considered in evaluating record systems. Lack of uniform or up-to-date diagnostic testing may lead to substantial underreporting of specific illnesses.[12]

In the absence of accurate records to ascertain the occurrence of illness among employees in a specific workplace, one can conduct medical diagnostic testing on the exposed workers (and, often, on a suitable comparison group). Often this study will be combined with the evaluation of other early indicators of the effects of occupational exposures. The factors outlined above should be considered when designing such a diagnostic study.

Other Indications of Toxic Effects

Given the usual long latency period between first exposure and the occurrence of many occupationally related illness, one often wants to evaluate earlier symptomatic or physiologic indicators of adverse health effects from occupational exposures. These indicators often have the additional advantage of being discernible in a relatively small population exposed to a toxic substance and may provide the opportunity to intervene prior to the occurrence of more permanent or clinically apparent health effects.

Symptom questionnaires often provide a relatively efficient approach to evaluate possible health effects from occupational exposures. At the same time, the investigator can collect information on disease occurrence, other risk factors, and exposures. Useful information can often be obtained for eye, skin, or respiratory irritants, for neurotoxic exposure, or even for specific occupational exposures (e.g., colic from lead exposure). In many situations, a control or comparison group is helpful in evaluating the response from the exposed population, although, in some situations, responses from just the exposed group will suffice.

Several factors need to be considered in designing a questionnaire for a specific evaluation. The time frame of the question is quite important. For acute symptoms that are quite prevalent among the general population (e.g., headache) a short time frame is appropriate (e.g., "in the past two days"). For chronic symptoms, reference to another standard questionnaire for such symptoms is often useful (such as the American Thoracic Society questionnaire for chronic respiratory symptoms).[2] Possible confounding factors such as smoking also need to be addressed in the questionnaire. However, in the initial approach to an occupational health problem, a rigid questionnaire may be an impediment to eliciting significant details on a problem. In these cases, a clinical interview approach may be more helpful.

Early physiologic or biologic indicators of the health effects of occupational exposure have become very important techniques in the evaluation of occupational health problems. These tests often provide an opportunity to elicit toxic health efforts prior to more clinically apparent damage. Such tests are available for a variety of toxic exposures, including lead (protoporphyrin levels), soluble uranium or cadmium (β_2 microglobulin), and some carcinogens (cytogenetic studies). For example, in the evaluation of workers exposed to soluble uranium, urinary amino acid and β_2 microglobulin levels provided an earlier indicator of renal tubular damage in a group of exposed workers with clinically normal renal function.[14] In evaluating the use of such tests, several factors should be considered. Comparison groups are often very important for the interpretation of test findings. Even for commonly used clinical tests, the clinical "normal range" may not be appropriate for an occupational group. Other factors which may affect the test (e.g., medications or diet) need to be ascertained and controlled for in the study design and analysis. Careful collection and analytical techniques need to be used. A laboratory with considerable experience with a given test and with good quality control should be used for the testing. Finally, many of these tests need to be carefully explained to the participating workers. Individual results are often difficult to interpret, and the long-range clinical implication of many of these tests is unknown.

DESIGNING A STUDY

In designing an occupational health hazard study, our usual approach at NIOSH is to first conduct an initial visit to a facility to gather information on a problem reported to us. This initial visit is designed to collect the necessary background information on exposure in that workplace, to review the available records systems for exposure and health information, to collect preliminary environmental sampling (usually qualitative), and to conduct medical interviews with exposed workers to define possible health effects better. Based on this initial information, we design a follow-up survey appropriate to the reported problem. This follow-up visit may include environmental monitoring, medical interviews and testing, and/or a more complete study of a particular health outcome using available records systems.

The follow-up visit is designed to determine whether or not there is an occupational health hazard in that workplace and what steps need to be taken to alleviate that problem. Based on our knowledge of the workplace, our study is designed to collect information relevant to determining whether there is an occupational health hazard based on environmental criteria, epidemiologic comparison, medical findings consistent with toxic exposure, or some combination of these. Several other factors help to determine the direction of our evaluation, including the type of problem being reported (acute vs. chronic), the known toxicity of the substances used in that workplace or for that occupational group, the size and work experience of the population, and practical considerations of cost and logistics.

CONCLUSIONS

The evaluation of occupational health problems is often difficult, particularly given the incomplete knowledge of the toxic effects of occupational exposures. In any evaluation, both exposure and health effects must be considered, and then an appropriate approach pursued. The results of this evaluation must provide the basis for correcting any problems found and for appropriate follow-up action to assure that similar problems do not recur. The general approach outlined in this paper has worked quite well for the NIOSH Health Hazard Evaluation Program and should be applicable to the evaluation of similar problems by other groups.

REFERENCES

1. American Conference of Governmental Industrial Hygienists: *Threshold Limit Values for Chemical Substances and Physical Agents in the Workroom Environment With Intended Changes for 1986*, Cincinnati, Oh, ACGIH, 1986.
2. Ferris B: Epidemiology standardization project. *Am Rev Respir Dis* 1978; 118:6 (pt 2).
3. Jannerfeldt E, Melius J: *Chemical Control Fire Interim Report*. NIOSH, 1981.
4. Landrigan P, Melius J, Rinsky R, et al: *Approaches to The Estimation of Exposure in Occupational Epidemiology*. Banbury Conference on Risk Quantification and Regulatory Policy, May 1984.
5. Melius J: HETA 79–088–768 US Steel, NIOSH Report, 1980.
6. Myers W, Peach M, Allender J: Workplace Protection Factor Measurements on Powered Air Purifying Respirators at a Secondary Lead Smelter—Test Protocol. *Am Ind Hyg Assoc J* 1984; 45(4):236–241.
7. National Institute for Occupational Safety and Health, US Dept of Health, Education, and Welfare: *NIOSH Publications Catalogue*, ed 6, 1985.
8. Occupational Safety and Health Administration: *OSHA Safety and Health Standards*. 29 CFR 1910:1100 revised, 1980.
9. Rinsky R, Young R, Smith A: Leukemia in benzene workers. *Am J Ind Med* 1981; 2:217–245.
10. Rutstein D, Mullan R, Frazier T, et al: Sentinel health events (occupational): A basis for physician recognition and public health surveillance. *APHA* 1983; 73:1054–1062.
11. Saltzman B, Yeager D, Meiners B: Reproducibility and quality control in the analysis of biological samples for lead and mercury. *Am Ind Hyg Assoc J* 1983; 44:263–267.
12. Silicosis—South Dakota, Wisconsin. *MMWR* 1983; 32:318–319.
13. Steenland K, Beaumont J, Halperin W: Methods of control for smoking in occupational cohort mortality studies. *Am J Epidemiol*, in press.
14. Thun M, Baker D, Smith B: *Health Hazard Evaluation Report 81–055–954: Cotter Corp*. NIOSH, 1981.
15. Turner J, Collins D: Liver morphology in guinea pigs administered either pyrolysis products of polychlorinated biphenyl transformer fluid or 2,3,7,8-Tetrachloro-p-dioxin. *Toxicol Appl Pharmacol* 1983; 67:417–429.

7

Organization and Staffing

Arthur L. Knight, M.D.

Carl Zenz, M.D.

Organization within the corporate environment for occupational medicine varies with the breadth of services offered and the responsibilities held. Examples of organization in small plants are given in Chapter 5. The manual, *The Industrial Environment—Its Evaluation and Control,*[10] by National Institute of Occupational Safety and Health (NIOSH) has suggestions on where the occupational physician fits into the corporation structure when he or she is utilized only as a medical expert.

"Occupational medicine" traditionally meant that branch of medicine practiced by physicians in preventing or treating health problems associated with people at work.[21] Occupational medicine began as industrial medicine, with programs for on-the-job treatment of injuries. Occupational medicine is one of the three subspecialties under the American Board of Prevention Medicine, along with public health and aviation medicine.

The basic ethics[8] of occupational medicine, which are outlined in the pamphlet, *Principles of Privileged Communication,*[18] are similar to those in other fields of medicine, except that the occupational physician, being a manager of the corporation, may be subject to bias, and is often so perceived.[16]

DEVELOPMENTS IN OCCUPATIONAL HEALTH SERVICE

Less Need for the Physician at the Worksite

Numerous changes are occurring on the "corporate scene" that are having an influence on the role of occupational medicine. The efforts of occupational medicine, safety, and industrial hygiene during the last several decades have greatly reduced the need for primary medical care by a physician at the worksite. The occupational health nurse is gradually being liberated and is assuming greater responsibilities for routine physical examinations, preemployment evaluations, health screenings, and employee counseling.[13]

The successful control of work environment hazards by safety, industrial hygiene, and biomechanical personnel has (combined with recessionary periods) reduced the physician-to-employee ratio in many companies. In the U.S., the more financially secure companies still have a physician for every 3,000 employees, while some large corporations have one full-time physician for every 15,000 employees and some companies of 15,000 employees have no full-time physician at all.

The managements of many of the larger corporations are taking a greater interest in health care costs, naively assumed decades ago,[26] that now have become a significant part of the corporation's operating costs.[5] Management is realizing that healthier employees with "low-risk life-styles" are more efficient and cost-effective employees. Therefore, the scope of corporate health services has broadened considerably.

The corporate health service now needs to encompass many disciplines, among which are biomechanics, psychology, ergonomics, health promotion, nutrition, industrial hygiene,[1] insurance evaluation, workers' compensation law, statistics, safety, epidemiology, data processing, cost analysis, and occupational medicine. In most of these disciplines, the occupational physician, part-time or full-time, has little or no expertise. Coordinating all the disciplines and programs requires primarily a skilled manager.[4, 19, 24] In general, medical schools have persisted in producing physicians trained mainly in primary care[3] so that, increasingly, nonphysicians are assuming leading roles in directing health services in the communities as well as in the corporations.[22] Some universities are training nonphysicians to be managers of industrial health service.

Diverse Occupational Health Service Systems

How should the complex task of safeguarding worker health best be handled? And who should be in charge of the task?

Japanese Model.—In Japan, this problem has been approached by establishing a medical school for occupational medicine, as a result of Japan's first occupational safety and health law, passed in 1972, which required an employer to undertake comprehensive safety measures to protect his work force from industrial injury and also to promote responsibility and health consciousness among employees. The law required more than just adherence to the minimum safety standards—it required the creation of a comfortable working environment and the appointment of a general safety and health supervisor for each workplace, whose responsibility, besides the routine medical examination and health maintenance of the work force, is to provide health and safety education and investigate industrial injuries. The law stipulated that enterprises employing more than 1,000 workers, or employing 500 who were exposed to hazardous environments, must employ one full-time industrial physician. Those employing more than 3,000 workers were to have more than one such physician.[6]

The Japanese University of Occupational and Environmental Health provides modern academic and clinical courses comparable to those in the United States, but includes courses in environmental health sciences, electronics, information science, human ecology, radiation biology and health, hospital and medical administration, industrial toxicology, ergonomics, engineering, and environmental health engineering. In 1982, the university established a school of occupational health nursing. Tuition fees are exempted if the graduate spends nine years in occupational medicine following graduation.

German System.—Since 1974, German law has called for a certain number of scheduled physician hours per number of employees based on perceived risk factors. The work force is divided into four risk categories. The first, and highest-risk, group consists of those working with dangerous substances; the second group includes shift workers, such as firefighters; the third group, blue-collar workers; and the last group, those working in stores and banks, etc.[20] Group 1 requires 1.2 hours of physician time per worker per year; group 2, 0.6 hours; group 3, 0.25 hours; and group 4, 0.2. This means that, for example, 50 bank employees would require from 2 to 12 hours of physician time per week. This system seems designed to use the occupational physician for primary medical care only, and would appear to be a waste of professional talent and a limit on the expansion and research of occupational health.

Government-Supported Systems.—In many countries with "socialized medicine," such as Australia, India, and some European countries, government supplies part of the occupational health care needs. In Örebro, Sweden, the occupational health clinic offers comprehensive services, including industrial hygiene and safety, and is funded by the government (40%) and local industry (60%).[9]

A Large Corporate Department.—Some large U.S. companies develop outstanding occupational health departments on their own initiative. While Japan's educational and organizational staffing is certainly a leading example for the world, another example of corporate responsiveness, described by Waggoner, is Garrett Corporation in Los Angeles, California.[25] In this "high tech," primarily aerospace manufacturing firm, which employs approximately 24,000 worldwide, with 24 divisions and subsidiaries at 25 U.S. locations and in 27 other countries, the corporate medical department is staffed by a medical director, 3 full-time physicians, 19 full-time registered nurses, 1 physician assistant, 2 certified safety engineers, 3 certified industrial hygienists, and 2 radiologic technologists, along with secretarial and clerical staff. At Garrett's locations, designated fee-for-service consultants are engaged.

Utilizing the Occupational Health Nurse.—The occupational health nurse can perform many of the functions necessary to a company health service. Admittedly, occupational health nurses have not yet met the challenge to move into the work environment[12] and have lost financially to the industrial hygienists, who have secured a place in those corporations with environmental hazards.[23] However, an industrial organization could utilize a nurse for each 250 to 500 employees if the nurse becomes involved in safety, industrial hygiene, counseling, "screening,"[13] wellness, biomechanics, employee health education, or other activities in addition to nursing.

HMOs, PPOs, and Emergency Clinics.—The emergence of "Health Maintenance Organizations" (HMOs) and "Preferred Provider Organizations" (PPOs), some with routine medical examinations and emergency care, has lessened the need for in-plant primary care, but most are not as yet staffed with occupational medical specialists. The small emergency clinics in industrial parks are increasing, but the quality of care and range of service is often unsatisfactory. These clinics are usually staffed by a general practitioner or general surgeon. Most of the necessary facets of occupational health are not met by these types of treatment centers.

Occupational Health Clinics.—A number of true occupational health clinics or organizations, staffed by physicians trained in occupational medicine as well as by industrial hygienists, are developing. These facilities have the expertise to assist in workers' compensation, provide testimony or advice to lawyers, make plant environmental inspections, determine the need for biologic monitoring, advise an industry on new legislation, help in employee education, make or arrange for expert biomechanic surveys, and offer other services for occupational health. This type of facility is an answer to the needs of the small plants, but also to the local plant of the large corporation. This trend should be supported by the large corporations who should use the local occupational health clinics as an extension of their corporation health services at the clinic's locality. This "externalization of services" seems to be increasing in the U.S., and offers advantages, not the least of which is a more "neutral" physician-worker atmosphere.

FUNCTIONS OF THE OCCUPATIONAL HEALTH SERVICE

Policy and Procedures.—Occupation health staffing of a company is varied because its composition and size depend upon the range of functions selected, from first aid to full control of the corporation's health care costs. Each corporation should have a written health services policy in the corporate policy manual. The occupational health services department should have its policy and the procedures for the staff in a manual; this manual should be loose-leaf, and a method should be developed for keeping it current. Several fine pamphlets have been written on occupational medicine programs and preparing a procedure manual.[7, 17, 23]

Records.—Records and reports are an important part of an occupational medicine program, since they reveal to management the type and amount of service that has been rendered, the costs of the program, the state of employee health, and the level of the standards of the facilities.

The records are the basis for statistics to help evaluate the occupational health program, to assist in accident prevention for epidemiologic investigations, and to increase knowledge of the relationship between work and health. (See Hernberg on occupation epidemiology in Chapter 71.)

For each employee there should be a separate file containing information on that employee's health (history, examinations, laboratory tests, vision, hearing, treatments given, counseling, illness record, workers' compensation reports, and copies of group insurance reports) and occupational environmental data, even if everything is "within normal." (Environmental data would include industrial hygiene reports, sound surveys, and information on environmental hazards, such as the amount and duration of any exposures.)

THE FUTURE OF OCCUPATIONAL HEALTH SERVICE

The challenges to occupational health services are many, not the least of which is overcoming the difficulty of keeping a personal and confidential service for the individual employee while the field becomes ever more technical and complex.

Occupational medicine needs to be more involved in the promotion of mental health, use of psychology, training of managers, education of employees, application of ergonomics, and research into employee motivation and satisfaction. These are the areas in which, in the future, the objectives of accident prevention, cost reduction, reduced absenteeism, and a lessened turnover can be more effectively achieved.[15]

Occupational health needs to bring its services into the very small company of 3–50 employees, including the neglected small branches of the larger corporations, which often have elaborate occupational medical departments in their main installations, in many instances to provide "executive health examinations."

There is a growing awareness and an increased competence among international labor groups, which have developed active programs and input in areas of occupational medicine, industrial hygiene, safety, and environmental health.

Developing efficient, low-cost methods of bringing electronic developments and biomedical information into the mainstream of occupational health is essential to a more scientific understanding of the natural history of work and health. A main responsibility for occupational medicine is to relieve employers of a major part of the burden of a country's health care costs, chiefly through sound preventive programs.[27]

REFERENCES

1. Ahmad I: The changing role of the industrial hygienist. *Am Ind Hyg Assoc J* 1977; 38:142.
2. Collings GH: Examining the "occupational" in occupational medicine. *J Occup Med* 1984; 26:509.
3. Cullen MR: Occupational medicine. *Arch Intern Med* 1985; 145:511.
4. Egdahl RH, Walsh DC: *Corporate Medical Departments*. Cambridge, Mass, Ballinger Publishing Co, 1983.
5. Egdahl RH: *Industry's Voice in Health Policy*. New York, Springer-Verlag New York, 1979.
6. Felton JS: Occupational medicine gets its own university. *World Health Forum* 1985; 6:18.
7. Felton JS: *Organization and Operation of an Occupational Health Program*. Chicago, American Occupational Medical Association, 1964.
8. Fletcher J: *Humanhood: Essays In Biomedical Ethics*. Buffalo, NY, Promethesis Books, 1979.
9. Heijman K: Personal communication to C. Zenz, July, 1984.
10. *The Industrial Environment—Its Evaluation and Control*. National Institute for Occupational Safety and Health, Dept of Health, Education, and Welfare, 1974.
11. Karrh BW: Occupational medicine. *J Am Med Assoc* 1984; 252:2274.
12. Knight AL: The problem of industrial nursing advancement in the USA. *Proc XIV Int Cong Occup Health*, 1963.
13. Knight AL: Let George do it. *NY State J Med* 1972; 2345.
14. LaDou J (ed): *Occupational Health Law—A Guide for Industry*. New York, Marcel Dekker, Inc. 1981.
15. LaDou J (ed): *Introduction to Occupational Health and Safety*. Chicago, National Safety Council, 1986.
16. Murray R: Ethics in Occupational Health Practice, in Schilling RSF (ed): *Occupational Health Practice*, ed 2. London, Butterworths, 1985.
17. *Occupational Health Guide for Medical and Nursing Personnel*, ed 3, Zenz C (ed). State Medical Society of Wisconsin, 330 E Lakeside St, Madison, WI, 53701, 1985.
18. *Principles of Privileged Communications*. New York, American Association of Industrial Nurses, Inc, 1970.
19. Schenke R: *The Physician in Management*. The American Academy of Medical Directors, 1982.
20. Schukmann F: Occupational Medicine As Practiced in the Federal Republic of Germany. Presented at the Annual AOMA Meeting, Kansas City, 1985.
21. *Scope, Objectives and Functions of Occupational Health Programs*. Chicago, American Medical Association, 1971.
22. Spiegel AD: Essay review of VWR and Ruth Sidel's *Reforming Medicine: Lessons of the Last Quarter Century*. *NY State J Med* 1985; 85: 45–46.
23. *Standards, Interpretations and Audit Criteria for Performance of Occupational Health Programs*. Akron, American Industrial Hygiene Association, 1978.
24. Vasquez MBZ, Schuman, BJ: The medical administrator in the occupational health setting. *J Occup Med* 1977; 19:5:327.
25. Waggoner JN: The operation of a corporate medical department. *Aviat Space Environ Med* 1985; 56:1115–1117.
26. Walsh DC, Egdahl RH: Payer, provider, consumer: Industry confronts health care costs. New York, Springer-Verlag New York, 1977.
27. World Health Organization: *Evaluation of Occupational Health and Industrial Hygiene Services*. Report on a WHO Working Group, WHO Regional Office for Europe, Copenhagen, 1982.

8

Clinical Aspects of Occupational Medicine

Harold R. Imbus, M.D., Sc.D.

Although occupational medicine is considered a type of preventive medicine, clinical problems arise frequently and are a major concern of most physicians working in this field. Occupational diseases, rehabilitation, and problems of placement of handicapped persons have not received the same attention from researchers and clinicians as the nonoccupational problems. Therefore, the physician working in this field often has difficulty finding information, either because relatively little has been written or because of an absence locally of available literature. Consultants experienced in occupational problems often are not available. Furthermore, although clinical problems often are simple for the treating physician, for the patient work requirements, psychologic factors, and interpersonal relationships at work can magnify them to major proportions. For these reasons, occupational clinical conditions can prove to be difficult and even burdensome; however, they provide the conscientious physician with one of the finest challenges of medicine, namely, the opportunity to influence an individual's adjustment, rehabilitation, or longevity in his work.

OCCUPATIONAL DISEASES

Problems in Diagnosis

Occupational diseases are caused by a pathologic adaptation of the patient to his working environment; therefore, in order to properly diagnose occupational diseases (or any diseases caused by environment for that matter), the physician must evaluate both patient and environmental exposure. Very few occupational diseases present with specific pathognomonic, clinical or laboratory findings. Thus, the anemia of benzene intoxication, the peripheral neuritis of acrylamide poisoning, the bronchitis of byssinosis, the fibrosis of asbestosis, the granuloma of berylliosis, the nodulation of silicosis cannot be adequately diagnosed as to etiologic agent from clinical and laboratory findings* alone. Only with knowledge of exposure, in addition to clinical factors, can an accurate diagnosis be made. Obtaining adequate environmental data and weighing their importance as causative factors can be an extremely difficult problem for the practicing physician, especially for one not experienced in this. Nevertheless, by applying the principles described herein, the practicing physician frequently can make an accurate diagnosis or, in more difficult cases, a preliminary evaluation prior to referral to other specialists.

The physician should recognize emotional factors that may complicate the diagnosis and treatment of the occupational disease patient. Depending on their feelings toward their employer, these patients may manifest hostility and anger, depression, concern for their ability to continue to work, or rejection. They may believe that they have given a great deal for an unappreciative and neglectful employer who is deserting them now that their work has caused them to become ill. The more enlightened and understanding the attitude of the employer, and the more positive the preexisting relationship has been, the less likely are these negative feelings to develop; nevertheless, they are quite common even in the best of circumstances. They may lead patients to arrive at illogical conclusions and to prediagnose their condition as occupational. These patients then may become quite suspicious of anyone who does not agree with their premises. These feelings are quite common, do not necessarily indicate malingering, and should not create a negative attitude on the part of the physician.

Unfortunately, in many cases there is a significant differential in indemnity between workers' compensation and other forms of insurance, resulting in a powerful economic motive for the disease to be designated occupational. Third parties, representing either the employee or the employer, may create pressure for their viewpoint, making objectivity even more difficult. Physicians should guard against a tendency toward bias. The personal physician of the employee may feel pressure to diagnose an occupational etiology, whereas the physician representing the employer may feel the opposite. The physician, although empathizing with either viewpoint, nevertheless must evaluate the facts as a true professional and detach himself from external pressures.

Manifestations of Occupational Diseases

Occupational diseases may affect any system of the body. The target organ or system may respond in a way that is quite specific or peculiar to that type of exposure. For example, silicosis and

*Lung biopsy, which may be of value in the last three, is discussed in Chapter 14.

coal miner's pneumoconiosis have pathologic findings that are reasonably specific for these diseases; these findings would enable a diagnosis by the pathologist from a biopsy or autopsy specimen. Exposure to other types of toxic substances may not result in characteristic pathologic findings but in reasonably specific clinical symptomatology and/or physiologic changes, which, when combined with laboratory findings indicative of exposure to the substance, create a specific set of manifestations. For example, in carbon monoxide intoxication, headache, weakness, and dizziness (characteristic but nonspecific responses) combined with a laboratory finding of carboxyhemoglobin of about 35% (specific laboratory finding) constitute a specific set of manifestations of carbon monoxide intoxication. In lead intoxication, headache, constipation, and colicky abdominal pains (nonspecific but characteristic responses) combined with a laboratory finding of blood lead concentration of 100 μg/100 ml (laboratory finding specific of exposure) constitue a reasonably specific set of manifestations of lead intoxication.

Of course, one must use care not to overlook exceptions; for example, abdominal colic and constipation can be a manifestation of many other conditions, and a level of lead concentration of 100 μg/100 ml blood can be seen without clinical intoxication. Therefore, it is possible, given this set of circumstances, that an individual could have had prolonged exposure to lead, resulting in a high level in the blood without clinical intoxication and an acute intestinal obstruction producing the abdominal colic. The clinician should be ever mindful of these exceptions.

Most occupational diseases have a set of manifestations that are not specific but are characteristic of the exposure. The organs of the body have a limited variety of responses to various external insults and may respond in a single way to a large number of agents. These responses usually take the form of inflammation, necrosis, or tissue proliferations, such as fibrosis, carcinoma, or granuloma, and these characteristic responses may be indistinguishable from those produced by a wide variety of other agents. For example, the chronic bronchitis produced by exposure to cotton dust is indistinguishable clinically and pathologically from that produced by cigarette smoke, and the toxic hepatitis produced by trichloroethylene is indistinguishable from that produced by alcohol. In chronic irreversible occupational disease, after removal from the agent, there may be no laboratory evidence of exposure, since such is indicative of acute exposure that has long since been removed.

Evaluation of Patient

History and Physical Examination

The physician should utilize the same process used in the diagnosis of any condition; namely, history of symptomatology, past history, family history and review of symptoms. The special occupational history will be discussed later.

The physical examination should include a general examination, with special emphasis on the organ system likely to be affected and specific physical findings likely to be seen in the disease under investigation; for example, the lead line in lead intoxication, the enlarged liver seen with overexposure to toluene, or the enlarged spleen in overexposure to benzene. The physician who omits general evaluation of the patient and proceeds only to those items in the examination pertinent to the exposure not infrequently will err in his diagnosis by failing to uncover nonoccupational disease.

Laboratory tests done in connection with the occupational disease work-up are in four categories:

Tests For General Assessment of Health and to Rule Out Other Conditions.—Evaluation in cases of suspected intoxication should routinely include complete blood count, chest x-ray, electrocardiogram, urinalysis, "Sequential Multiple Analyzer" (SMA 23), or similar laboratory procedures.

Nonspecific Tests of Exposure.—Some of these, already listed above, include such tests as mean corpuscular volume, mean corpuscular hemoglobin concentration in cases of exposure to hemotoxic agents, serum glutamic oxaloacetic transaminase (SGOT), serum glutamic pyruvic transaminase (SGPT) in exposure to liver toxins, a reduction in forced expiratory volume 1 second (FEV_1) during the course of the working day when the patient is exposed to pulmonary irritants, delta aminolevulinic acid in red cells in lead intoxication, a differential count or sputum test for eosinophils, as, for example, in suspected allergy to wood dust. It should be emphasized that these tests are not specific for a particular exposure but do indicate anatomical or physiologic alteration that may be present in a variety of conditions, including occupational exposure.

Tests for the Agent or Its Metabolite That Indicate Exposure.—There are a number of these based on a knowledge of metabolism of the substance involved. For example, it is known that gradual absorption of inorganic lead is characterized by increased lead in the blood. Exposure to toluene may be detected by analysis of hippuric acid in the urine and exposure to trichloroethylene by trichloroacetic acid in the urine and by breath analysis for the substance itself. Most of these tests only indicate absorption of the substance into the body and/or metabolism of it. Because of the variability of response by patients, they do not necessarily indicate intoxication. However, with some substances, such as carboxyhemoglobin, there are levels of concentration at which intoxication is expected. Some tests are not specific, such as trichloroacetic acid in the urine. Some, such as lead in the blood, generally indicate prolonged exposure, whereas others, such as detection of the substance on the breath, are associated with recent exposure of long or short duration. These tests not only can be quite helpful in determining that recent exposure has occurred but, in some cases, in establishing the degree of exposure.

Tests That Establish a Hypersusceptibility.—There are several tests that establish a hypersusceptibility to a disease condition that may be stimulated, precipitated, or aggravated by occupational exposure, described by Stokinger and Scheel[16] as follows:

1. Hereditary serum antitrypsin deficiency and chronic obstructive pulmonary disease.

2. Glucose-6-phosphate dehydrogenase deficiency and hypersusceptibility to hemolytic chemicals.

3. Test for hypersusceptibility to carbon disulfide.

4. Immunologic screening tests for hypersensitivity to organic isocyanates.

Not infrequently we are loath to explain the development of severe disease following relatively minor exposure. The tests mentioned above indicate hereditary predisposition to development of certain disease conditions that may be caused by or aggravated by occupational exposure. For example, serum α_1 antitrypsin deficiency may be associated with development of severe emphysema in an individual not exposed to pulmonary irritants. It is believed that relatively minor occupational exposure may accelerate the development of the disease or may confuse the picture in an individual who has developed a disease due to unrelated causes. Some industrial medical departments utilize these tests as screening examinations prior to employment. The number and usefulness of tests such as these probably will increase in the future.

Evaluation of Exposure

Evaluation of exposure, which is necessary in diagnosing work-related conditions, adds a dimension to occupational medicine usually not found in other clinical practice. Yet, many physicians are inexperienced and uncomfortable in this. The physician working with a large company with industrial hygiene services has an advantage here. However, most physicians do not have ready access to sophisticated industrial hygiene services. Nevertheless, application of several principles and knowing where to get help will result in a satisfactory diagnosis in most cases.

The nature of the exposure, namely, the generic name or the type of chemical, dust, or physical agent must be determined. In addition, the state of the substance or agent to which the patient was exposed is necessary knowledge. Was it a dust, vapor, fume, gas, or solid? Next, the physician should make a preliminary assessment of the toxic hazard by determining the site of action of the substance or agent and the likely contact that may have occurred under the circumstances. For example, an employee exposed to 100 decibels of noise is not likely to have continued deterioration of his hearing due to noise if he is wearing adequate protection in a satisfactory manner. Even though exposed to noise, harmful amounts would not reach the cochlea under these circumstances. Likewise, a substance that is toxic by contact with the respiratory system cannot make such contact unless it is in an inhalable form. For example, the metal beryllium would not be toxic if contacted by the skin in the metallic state; only if it is converted to a dust or a fume capable of being inhaled can it be toxic.

The physician also must ask, "What are the amount and duration of exposure?" He should have some idea of how much of the agent it generally takes to cause illness. How long does it take for illness to occur? He then will avoid the pitfall of misdiagnosing occupational illness after relatively minimal exposures of very short duration not sufficient to have caused disease. In occupational medicine, quantitative aspects of safe exposure are expressed in the concept of the Threshold Limit Value (TLV), a time-weighted average exposure. Details of TLVs are described elsewhere in this volume (see Chapter 29 and Appendix A).

How can the physician not practicing within a large corporation obtain the information described above? It can be difficult and time consuming; nevertheless, in most cases it is not impossible and can be most rewarding to the physician who is concerned with making adequate diagnoses. Information about occupational exposure generally is obtained from

1. The occupational history of the patient
2. Industrial hygiene data

Occupational History.—If the history is to establish exposure or lack thereof to the suspected substance or agent, it can be quite detailed and time consuming; however, for the busy physician, this often is not practical. Time can be saved by focusing on the questions that will be the most productive of information.

The physician should determine where the patient works and how long he has worked in this place. This alone may be helpful, especially in small communities in which physicians have general knowledge of the industries in the area. If the physician is not familiar with the company or plant, he should determine what the product is. It is important to be as specific as possible concerning this. For example, in textiles, it will make a great deal of difference whether the product is cotton textiles or one of the various types of synthetics. If the company makes castings, are these from iron or brass? If it makes metal products, does it merely assemble the products or does it actually mold the metal in question? Other general information that is helpful is that concerning the company's safety and hygiene practices—whether the company has an occupational health program and are the employees given periodic health examinations and pre-employment examinations?

The above information is helpful in formulating a general impression of possible exposures. Questioning then should become more specific to determine exactly what the patient's job is. Often he or she will use terminology to describe the job that may be quite foreign to the physician unless the physician has had experience with the particular type of trade in question. Although it often is quite difficult to determine specifically what the patient does without viewing the operation, much information often can be obtained directly from the patient by asking him or her to specifically describe the operation, perhaps to reproduce the motions involved and to describe the various materials with which he works. For example, if work is done on a conveyor line, the physician may assume that a great deal of lifting and pushing is involved. This may or may not be true. Specific questions concerning the size and approximate weight of objects, height above the floor level from which and to which they are lifted, distance carried, and the frequency of lifts will clarify these requirements.

Description of the job should include the materials with which the employee works. The employee may or may not know the materials with which he or she is in contact. Awareness on the part of the employee will increase with implementation of the Occupational Safety and Health Act (OSHA) hazard communication standards requiring labeling of containers and informing employees of toxic substances with which they are working. Often the patient will only know of a trade or slang name for the substance in question. If such is the case, the physician may be able to obtain more specific information from the employer, or, short of this, have the employee bring the specific trade name and the address of the manufacturer. Under the new standard, manufacturers are required to supply information concerning the contents of their products on the request of medical and industrial hygiene personnel.

The patient should describe the form in which the substance is and the type of contact that he or she has. Is it a liquid? If so, does it emit vapors that were inhaled? Was there a skin contact? Is any protection provided, and, if so, how effective does the protection appear to the patient? For example, if he or she is wearing a respirator, does the company have a program for its maintenance? Has there been instruction in proper cleaning and maintenance or is this provided? Is he or she able to smell the chemical through the respirator? Does the respirator appear to have a proper fit?

The employee should be questioned as to whether other employees are experiencing a similar problem. It is important to determine how the symptoms relate to work. With an occupational disease characterized by acute symptoms, one would expect exacerbations of symptoms in relationship to work and some degree of remission during weekends and vacation periods. Some exposures cause symptoms so acute that they are noticed shortly after the beginning of the workday. Others may result in acute but delayed symptoms that occur after the employee is home at night. Byssinosis is characterized by the former, whereas exposure to Canadian red cedar and zinc fumes may result in the latter. When chronic disease is the result of the exposure, symptoms may appear gradually during a period of weeks, months, or even years after beginning employment. They may or may not improve with temporary removal from employment. In this respect, it is important to determine whether there were any similar symptoms prior to employment. Quite often an occupational exposure will provide an aggravation to a preexisting condition or a latent but developing condition. This is especially true with exposure to pneumoconiosis-producing agents and pulmonary irritants when there is preexisting subclinical chronic obstructive lung disease.

Finally, the physician should determine what other stresses and exposures there are other than those that are job related. The role of smoking is a very important factor in many occupational lung diseases. Smoking provides an effect in addition to the occupational exposure. Noise exposure frequently results from hobbies or a second job. In my experience, many cases of noise-induced hearing loss have been seen in relatively young men who are coming into a noisy industry for the first time. Often the history of noise exposure in the military service, on the farm, from driving heavy mechanical equipment, or from shooting rifles can be elicited in these cases.

Industrial Hygiene Data.—The occupational history of the employee can give valuable insight into the possible etiology of his condition. However, a more precise indication of exposure can be obtained from industrial hygiene surveys of the work site. Details of this approach are provided in Chapter 2. The practicing physician should be familiar with ways to obtain these data. Large companies often have an industrial hygiene staff and, if so, they often are quite willing to supply the practicing physician with any necessary data.

More detailed information may be obtained through the company, which can supply the specific names and types of chemicals or physical agents and a rather detailed description of the process involved. Practicing physicians who are dealing with these types of cases will benefit themselves and their patients if they become familiar with the operations in the local industry. Many industries are happy to have physicians visit and learn operations and procedures. Quite often the smaller industry may have an industrial health problem that it is unaware of or about which it does not know how to obtain information. There are a number of private consultants who will do industrial hygiene surveys of various types. Experienced occupational physicians and industrial hygienists usually are aware of these, and information as to their whereabouts may be obtained by consulting one of them. Unfortunately, the great popularity of industrial hygiene surveys, brought about by the requirements of the Occupational Safety and Health Act of 1970, has resulted in a considerable number of partially qualified or unqualified persons conducting various types of occupational health surveys. Since there is no licensing requirement for these in most states and no actual standards that must be met, it behooves the physician or company resorting to such services to be very careful to select those of known reliability and competence. Industrial hygienists have a certification process similar to that for medical specialties. Although certification is not required, it may provide quality assurance when the hygienist is not known.

Many large cities have occupational health departments and can provide occupational health surveys on request. Likewise, on a state level, either the state health department or department of labor or industrial commission often has qualified industrial hygienists and industrial hygiene laboratories capable of conducting surveys. A number of states have assumed the industrial hygiene function for OSHA. Since an ordinary OSHA-related inspection can result in a citation, there are provisions for an on-site consultation. It is best to familiarize yourself with what services are available in this respect in your state.

The National Institute for Occupational Safety and Health (NIOSH) has industrial hygiene capability for a hazard investigation. They will conduct hazard surveys in industry where there are problems of special interest or unexplained health problems that cannot be investigated routinely. Likewise, OSHA has industrial hygienists; however, their inspections are usually done in conjunction with enforcement of the OSHA act. When an employer is cooperative and anxious to solve an employee health problem, a visit from an OSHA inspector may not always produce the best result. Nevertheless, any employee or, in fact, any interested individual, including an employee's physician, has the prerogative of making a complaint to OSHA regarding a health condition in a plant and requesting an inspection.

The Judgment or Matching Process

Once the physician has evaluated his patient, obtained the necessary laboratory studies, and obtained information regarding exposure, he or she then must exercise clinical judgment in making a diagnosis. In occupational conditions, this should not represent an undue problem to the practicing clinician, since there are many disease conditions for which precise diagnostic tests are not available. Johnstone and Miller[10] state, "In the matching process one must adhere to the law of specificity to the degree possible. The law of specificity requires that one ask and have answered such questions as:

Is the suspected substance known to have toxic problems?

Did the reaction in the case under study conform to known established reactions?

Is the suspected chemical capable of being absorbed? If so, what system or systems is it known to affect?

Did an undue exposure actually occur?

Are the laboratory data confirmatory of intoxication or systemic injury?

Since it often is not possible to make a precise diagnosis initially, the clinician working with occupational disease patients may, for practical purposes, establish a working diagnosis that will provide the basis for necessary recommendations for treatment and removal from exposure, if necessary. Later, a final diagnosis or medicolegal diagnosis can be made, based on the outcome of observations during the treatment. One pitfall in the diagnosis of occupational diseases is to make a diagnosis too quickly. In questionable cases, this may become a matter of contest between industry, physician, employee, insurance carrier, or labor union, leading quickly to an adversary situation. Such conditions are not conducive to optimal diagnosis and treatment. Practicing physicians who are going to be dealing with these types of cases will benefit themselves and their patients if they become familiar with the workers' compensation laws of their state.

Since there are many situations in which diagnosis is difficult and fraught with pitfalls, physicians should avail themselves of qualified consultants whenever necessary. This aspect appears to be more neglected by practicing physicians in diagnosing occupational conditions than other types of illness. Many physicians are not aware that there are qualified specialists who can assist them with these diagnoses. Physicians in the field of occupational medicine, even though often working full-time for a large industry, usually are ready and willing to provide information concerning sources of assistance for particular problems. Many of the large medical schools have competent staffs who will deal with special occupational disease problems. It is much better for the physician to obtain help, when in doubt, at an early stage in his contact with the employee. Such willingness to refer usually is interpreted by both patient and industry as a sign of impartiality, since referral often is made anyway after a questionable or inadequate diagnosis by the practicing physician. It is much better for the practicing physician to have referred in the first place.

Treatment of Patient

Treatment of occupational disease conditions follows the same principles of treatment of other diseases; however, removal or protection from exposure is an essential consideration in treatment.

As with other disease conditions, the physician first must determine whether there is a specific treatment. In some chemical exposures, such as carbon monoxide intoxication, methemoglobinemia, and lead intoxication, there are specific treatments aimed at neutralizing or eliminating the offending substance or restoring the body physiology to a normal state. These specific treatments are described elsewhere in this volume and also in standard books of clinical toxicology.

Unfortunately, since the manifestations of many occupational diseases are not specific, the treatment also will not be specific. Liver disease caused by chlorinated hydrocarbons is no different in treatment from that caused by ethyl alcohol. Chronic obstructive pulmonary disease caused by dust inhalation is treated the same as chronic obstructive pulmonary disease caused by cigarette smoking. Occupational contact dermatitis follows the same principles of treatment as nonoccupational contact dermatitis caused by poison ivy.

Control of exposure, of course, usually is necessary; however, a common mistake is to consider only one type of control of exposure; namely, removal from the job. Physicians should consider the fact that those who suffer from occupational diseases frequently have worked on a particular job for many years. This is the individual's trade and livelihood, and since the occupational disease manifestations, especially those that are chronic, may not appear until late years of life, removal from the job often presents a most difficult problem for the patient. Needless to say, it is not something that should be undertaken lightly; indeed, permanent removal should be a last resort, especially in the more highly skilled jobs.

This question should be answered: Is this individual highly susceptible to the exposure, making it unlikely that reasonable controls will effect the desired relief? If so, attempts to keep the person in the same job are likely to be unsuccessful. However, quite frequently the exposure of the individual is unwarranted and unnecessary, and adjustments in the environmental situation can bring about relief. If an industry has employees who are unduly exposed to a harmful agent, it should make every effort to control this to the degree necessary to bring exposure to levels acceptable by current standards. The physician may be able to assist the patient by discussing this with company officials so that exposure can be minimized. It has been my experience that, frequently, relatively minor and inexpensive changes can bring about a greatly reduced exposure. Principles of control, namely, ventilation, enclosure, shielding, or work practices, are discussed in other chapters.

The physician should consider the seriousness of the condition in the light of the consideration of removal versus environmental control. Obviously, an irreversible condition that will progress even with minimal exposure warrants a change in job; however, self-limited or acute conditions that usually are completely reversible may be handled by limiting future exposure. In these cases, the employee usually can be assured that no permanent damage has occurred and that if the exposure is brought under reasonable control, recurrences of the condition should not occur.

Protective devices are another means of control of exposure. There are problems in their use and they are not considered acceptable means of control of exposure over long periods of time when feasible engineering controls are available. Also, it is not infrequent that protective devices, especially respiratory protective devices, are most difficult to wear for those who need them most. For example, an employee exhibiting chronic obstructive pulmonary disease would be most affected by exposure to dust and would be in most need of wearing a respiratory protective device. However, resistance to respiration is increased by the respirator and since the employee already is impaired, additional resistance to respiration often is not well tolerated and is quite fatiguing.

Nevertheless, the use of protective devices can be most helpful in selected cases, especially where short-term or intermittent usage is required because of heavy intermittent exposure. For example, I once was asked to evaluate a textile employee who had worked all his life with dyes. The employee was a heavy smoker and had developed emphysema and chronic bronchitis. He also had noticed in recent years that his respiratory symptoms had been increasingly aggravated by his work with dyes. The dust from these dyes would produce cough, sputum, and shortness of breath. He was advised by his family physician to obtain work elsewhere. Since the employee was highly skilled in this area, he would have had to take a significant reduction in wages, leave a job that he thoroughly enjoyed, and, in middle age, learn another skill. He questioned management about any possible way in which he might stay in his present job. Careful questioning by me revealed that it was only occasionally that he sustained exacerbations of his cough and dyspnea when exposed to dye dust. This was in relation to the use of several very dusty dyes of an irritating nature. He indicated that this particular mixing process occurred only once or twice a week. Since his obstructive lung disease was not advanced, he was able to wear respiratory protection during the limited periods when he was mixing the offending dyes. This protection, combined with measures taken to treat his underlying condition, namely, cessation of smoking and administration of antibiotics, enabled him to continue working on this job without difficulty.

The employee suffering from an occupational disease needs whatever reassurance the physician can give. Disease, of course, is always a threat to most individuals. Occupational disease not only threatens one's health but, in particular, offers an ominous threat to one's ability to continue to provide for one's self and family. Since it was the job that caused the sickness, the employee often will jump to the conclusion that he or she no longer can perform on that job. These negative thoughts and concerns interfere with recovery and rehabilitation. Utilizing the principles described above, it quite often is possible for the physician to reassure the employee that returning to work is possible. A great deal, of course, depends on the employer's attitude, willingness to control the environmental conditions that created the condition, and overall attitude toward the employee. When the practicing physician has developed the proper rapport with employer and employee, he or she is in a very strong position to intercede and to produce a favorable climate for recovery and rehabilitation. Every care must be taken that the physician and the patient do not come to premature conclusions concerning the patient's inability to continue working. Where it is obviously apparent that the patient cannot continue on his present job but will be fully capable of engaging in other types of activity, he should be strongly reassured of this at an early stage in the treatment.

MEDICAL PLACEMENT

Preplacement Examination

The value of the preplacement examination is as follows:

1. To determine the individual's physical and emotional capacity to perform a particular job.
2. To assess the individual's general health.
3. To establish a baseline record of physical condition for epidemiologic and medicolegal purposes.

Determination of Physical and Emotional Capacity for Job Performance

This has been and should continue to be the primary purpose of performing the preplacement physical examination. Theoretically, individuals can be matched to specific jobs according to aptitude and physical and emotional capabilities. If the match is correct, presumably a happy, healthy employee will result; if incorrect, the employee will not succeed, because of a lack of physical or mental capacity, or perhaps some illness will develop or preexisting illnesses will worsen as a result of the work, or the employee will leave the job. Although there appears to be some theoretical basis and experience to substantiate the above, many previously held concepts are without adequate statistical validation. The necessity to evaluate physical capacity arose as a need to determine that individuals could do work that frequently required hard labor without harm to themselves or to others. Employers had a fear of the employee aggravating a preexisting condition, with a resultant workers' compensation case.

Although these points are valid, unfortunately there developed some cases of overapplication of rigid criteria of fitness. In times of a readily available workforce to do heavy, hard labor, the pre-employment examination sometimes became a "culling process" wherein those with a "slight blemish" or about whom there was a slight concern about ability to perform tasks were eliminated as prospects. Now federal laws do not permit rejection for employment because of conditions which do not have a direct bearing upon the person's capacity to perform that job.

Although many jobs involving considerable exposure to health hazards still remain, improved industrial hygiene, a general lessening of the physical demands of many jobs, automation and high turnover rates, with difficulty in obtaining skilled workers, appear to have diminished the physical fitness aspect of the preplacement examination for most jobs.

Nevertheless, jobs requiring exposure to heat, chemicals, dust, heavy labor, and other adverse conditions still exist. With the advent of OSHA standards delineating physical examinations requirements for certain jobs, namely, those characterized by exposures to chemicals and physical agents, the preplacement examination has assumed a new and increasingly important role.

In evaluating physical capacity for a particular job, the physician can categorize individuals with significant impairment as follows:

Stable Impairments.—These cause some limitations but are not likely to progress or be worsened by job activity, if the employee is placed properly. Amputations, ankylosis, spasticity, residual effects of polio, blindness, deafness, and cerebral palsy are examples of these. The major consideration here is: Can the employee perform the job in question with reasonable efficiency and safety and without undue stress to himself?

Impairments, Stable or Unstable, That May Be Made Worse by the Work Exposure.—Examples of these are: chronic skin disease, such as psoriasis, in an employee to be placed in a job requiring exposure of the skin to solvents, and liver disease in an employee being placed in a job involving exposure to solvents. With these conditions, careful evaluation of both the medical condition and the job requirements should be made to ensure that the employee's condition is not made worse by his work.

Progressive Conditions.—Chronic obstructive lung disease, congestive heart failure and ankylosing spondylitis are examples of this. Although placement in other than sedentary work may be possible, it should be recognized that progression of the condition may, in the near future, make necessary placement in less-demanding work.

Conditions of Intermittent Impairment That May Result in Incapacity.—Uncontrolled epilepsy, and poorly controlled diabetes subject to intermittent acidosis and insulin shock are examples of this. With these conditions, incapacity could result in the employee becoming suddenly unable to perform his job.

Guidelines for the employment of individuals with a variety of conditions have been outlined by the President's Committee on Employment of the Handicapped.[1]

The judgment of whether a person is physically qualified for a particular job is a serious responsibility for the examining physician. The physician should formulate a logical approach to this responsibility. Decisions then will be based on experienced clinical judgment in the light of knowledge of existing job conditions and the person's physical condition.

General Health Considerations

As work becomes less strenuous and various types of employment-related insurance and medical benefits are increased, especially in major corporations, increasing consideration has been given to evaluating an individual's general health status prior to employment. Unfortunately, many employers now are in the position of considering the prospective employee as an insurance risk. In my opinion, the evaluation of insurance risk is not a proper role for the occupational physician. When this is necessary prior to employment, it should be based on actuarial principles, according to previous criteria established by the insurance company. The responsibility for disqualification for insurance reasons should not fall on the occupational physician.

The employer has a right to expect reasonable regularity of attendance and reasonable longevity on the job. This is increasingly important in highly skilled jobs where expensive training and investment are required. In this respect, the health team performs a beneficial service to the employee and the employer alike. The preplacement examination affords an excellent opportunity to counsel with the employee regarding correction of medical conditions that later can lead to disability.

Present knowledge of coronary risk factors reveals the beneficial effect of treatment of even mild hypertension in preventing stroke and probably myocardial infarctions. The serious risks of smoking and overweight afford an excellent opportunity for the physician and/or nurse to counsel with the employee. Those conditions that are amenable to treatment should be referred to a private physician for further evaluation and care. It often is desirable to follow up in the medical department to determine that optimal effective treatment has been achieved. The physician who is on part-time duty in industry and has his own private practice should carefully avoid utilizing this opportunity as a means of building his practice.

Establishment of a Baseline Record of Physical Condition for Epidemiologic and Medicolegal Purposes

This aspect of the preplacement examination is becoming increasingly important, with legislative emphasis on prevention of occupational diseases. In the early days of occupational medicine, a number of well-defined occupational disease conditions were noted by practitioners. However, there now is increasing awareness that occupational disease conditions often are quite nonspecific and cannot be clinically or even pathologically differentiated from other conditions. Emphysema, bronchitis, and certain types of liver disease are notable examples. Adequate medical evaluation and follow-up of employees offer a splendid opportunity to develop comparative data of the incidence of a variety of disease conditions in the light of known occupational exposure. In addition, this provides a real protection to employees, since they can be alerted to any changes.

Some states allow the use of pre-employment data in computing disability for workers' compensation awards for occupational disease. Notable among these is the preplacement audiogram. In states with scheduled benefits for hearing loss from which is deducted preexisting hearing loss, accurate evaluation at the time of employment is imperative. Otherwise, the employer is in a position of paying for awards made for all of an employee's hearing loss, since he cannot document the preexisting condition. It is possible that this concept will expand into other areas; namely, in pulmonary disease. Likewise, many states have provisions for second injury and/or handicaps in their workers' compensation laws that allow the preexisting component of an occupational disease to be deducted from the employer's premium. A special fund has been established in some states that allows the employee to be awarded the full amount for his disability, but the payments for the preexisting component are taken from a general fund rather than directly from the employer's premium. Obviously, where such provisions exist, it is important for the employer to determine the health status of the employee at the time of employment.

Despite the above considerations, the preplacement evaluation has fallen into disrepute and disuse in a number of areas. Its benefit to either employee or employer often is questioned. In high-turnover, low-hazard industries there may be a very real question of adequacy of "cost-benefit ratio." Collings[9] found a favorable cost-benefit ratio, whereas Williamson[18] questions the value of the pre-employment examination. Some industries have approached this problem by utilizing a brief health history prior to employment and a more complete examination after the employee completes a period of several weeks or several months of employment. Other industries are using paramedical personnel, including nurses, to do the preplacement examination. These, in my experience and that of others,[6, 7, 15] seem to work quite well. Certainly, measurement of the cost-benefit ratio has to be a highly individualized thing, depending on the industry, and the responsible physician can make a contribution to this by documenting any significant benefits or lack thereof.

In hazardous job situations entailing exposures to chemicals and physical hazard, the preplacement examination certainly appears necessary. Perhaps some of the disrepute into which it has fallen is not so much a result of lack of benefit that it can afford but from poor quality, both of examination and application of the knowledge obtained therefrom.

If the physician is overly liberal in interpretation of physical capacity requirements, there is not only the risk of placing a number of individuals who cannot perform the job but the employee risks serious injury due to the preexisting problem. Examples are the placement of individuals with heart disease in hot or stressful environments and individuals with preexisting back conditions in situations involving frequent and heavy lifting. If this happens many times, the employer and, for that matter, the employee, too, lose confidence in the preplacement examination procedure of the physician involved.

On the other hand, overly rigid interpretation of criteria leads to the rejection of a large number of individuals who are perfectly well qualified medically for the job in question. The physician should not withhold recommendation for a particular job because of some remote possibility of incapacity for the job. Obviously, the seriousness of such incapacity and the probability of such occurring must be weighed in making this determination.

Because of the concern for providing equal opportunity, and also to provide uniformity, there is some merit in setting up physical standards for a job. This can be helpful; however, unfortunately, rigid physical standards do not take into account an individual's motivation and the remarkable ability of the human body to compensate for deficiencies. Therefore, standards are best stated in terms of needed capacity rather than in terms of impairment. For example, a standard should be stated, "Must have ability to do frequent heavy lifting" rather than "Must not have history of back injury in the past" or "Must have no likelihood of sudden loss of consciousness" rather than "Any past history of epilepsy is disqualifying." The physician should become familiar with any OSHA physical examination requirements for jobs involving certain exposures.

In the final analysis, judgment regarding job capacity must be a medical decision. Any attempt to eliminate this judgment factor will result in unnecessary rejections or poor placement. The physician should face the responsibility in making these judgments and not be unduly swayed by management or employee. Two experienced occupational physicians and I practiced together for a number of years in doing preplacement evaluations and applied the principles outlined above. It is remarkable how consistent our judgments were. Furthermore, the physician only *recommends*, based on knowledge of the individual's physical capacity and the job requirement. The physician should present his or her recommendations, stating whether the person is fully qualified or limited in any way. If limited, these limitations should be stated specifically. The final decision of acceptance or rejection rests outside the medical sphere.[13]

History.—The history is the most important single procedure in evaluating fitness for work. Past disease conditions, surgery, present complaints, and psychologic aspects are all determined by the history. There may be some question of the reliability of a history obtained in a pre-employment examination, especially if it is believed that positive answers may result in a prospective employee being denied the job.

The time spent and the skill of the interviewer are important factors in obtaining a reliable history. In my opinion, some self-administered questionnaires are quite unreliable. In a recent experience during a demonstration of obtaining a pre-employment history, I had occasion to interview a supervisor and ask him questions on a preplacement examination form. The employee gave positive responses to ten questions. It then was determined that several months previously he had himself completed the identical questionnaire prior to the institution of the direct-questioning technique. This questionnaire was taken from the files and indicated positive responses to only five questions. The supervisor was a very reliable employee with a good record, and the discrepancies were readily explainable by his lack of complete understanding of the questions. Although self-administered questionnaires appear to have some value in periodic automated health screening, in my experience, the average self-administered pre-employment questionnaire has marked limitations. Significant positive responses to the medical history should include diagnosis, place of treatment, name of attending physician, disability, and whether or not there are any residual impairments. A notation of the type of follow-up care is important also.

Physical Examination.—In most cases, a physical examination can be performed rather quickly and should consist of a basic general examination, with emphasis on an orthopedic examination and any other systems likely to be subject to strain, for example, the skin in the chemical industry or the cardiovascular system in hot industry. In my experience, one of the most neglected aspects of the preplacement examination conducted by the practicing physician performing this service for industry is the orthopedic examination and the most overemphasized is the evaluation of hernia. Simple range-of-motion examinations of the spine and the joints of the extremities are very helpful in determining any active orthopedic problem. These take only a few minutes and are quite valuable.

Evaluation and Placement of the Returning Employee

The occupational physician often is called on to evaluate an employee who has been absent for a serious illness. If the work is demanding, physically or mentally, and if there has been a serious disease capable of producing residual impairment, the employee and the employer want to know if the employee is physically able to return to his job. Physicians, if possessing access to management, often are in an excellent position to evaluate objectively the demands of the job and relate this information to their clinical knowledge of the patient. The occupational physician obviously should work closely with the treating physician, and every attempt should be made to reach a mutual agreement in questionable cases. The attending physician often is in a difficult position in that he or she may have pressure from the patient, either to return to work at the earliest possible date or to be absent longer than necessary. Without a knowledge of the working conditions, it is difficult for the physician to evaluate the job description objectively.

On the other hand, the employer, in the case of a highly important employee, may create pressure that could result in a premature return to work or, in the case of an "undesirable" employee, result in prolonged sick leave, permanent disability, or unnecessary transfer to another job. The attending physician's responsibility is to the patient. The occupational physician, in addition to his responsibility to the patient, also has a responsibility to protect the safety and health of other employees and, to a reasonable extent, the interest of the employer for whom he does the examination. Despite what may seem to be conflicting interests, I have found that seldom is it not possible for two reasonable physicians practicing with a high degree of professionalism to be able to reach agreement.

In general, the principles of evaluation for return to work are similar to those outlined above under evaluation of physical capacity, general health, and epidemologic and medicolegal considerations. The physician, however, cannot necessarily apply the same criteria to the skilled employee returning to work after an illness that he would to the new employee just beginning. Employees who have performed a certain job for many years are expected to be better able to compensate for impairments, since they already know the job and know how to do it with the least expenditure of energy and effort. Likewise, from the general health aspect, the occupational medical evaluation on return to work offers the opportunity to determine follow-up measures and to encourage the employee to take full advantage of the attending physician's recommendations for follow-up and also to offer the facilities of the occupational medical department, for example, in follow-up blood pressure readings or dressings where indicated and agreeable with the attending physician and company policy.

However, the occupational physician who stops at evaluation of the patient will miss many real opportunities for rehabilitation. There is an added element in return to work after illness beyond those of preplacement evaluation in that the convalescing employee has just been through a major physical and psychologic upheaval. Failure to consider this obvious fact may result in failure of a successful return to work. For practical purposes, rehabilitation can be considered in two phases:

1. Off-the-job rehabilitation
2. On-the-job rehabilitation

Off-the-job rehabilitation consists of all those efforts of the attending physician and rehabilitation specialist, such as physical therapy, vocational training, care in the rehabilitation center, sheltered workshop, specialized work capacity determinations, such as in the cardiac work evaluation center, to determine fitness to work in special situations. These specialized procedures of work evaluation are described elsewhere in this volume. Utilization of these in difficult cases will increase the percentage of employees who can be rehabilitated. However, in the majority of cases, even with significant residual impairments or emotional overlay, the occupational health team can accomplish rehabilitation on the job without utilizing specialized services.

On-the-job rehabilitation is a team approach utilizing the combined services of attending physician, occupational physician and/or occupational health nurse and employer. On-the-job rehabilitation is an extension of off-the-job rehabilitation. The two overlap; thus, rehabilitation by the treating physician and rehabilitation centers may continue after the employee has returned to work; on the other hand, on-the-job rehabilitation measures imply that they are coming from the place of work and begin even before the employee returns to work.

Necessary to on-the-job rehabilitation are the following:

1. Interest of the employer and the occupational health team during the illness.
2. Medical evaluation from an occupational viewpoint prior to return to work:
   A. Physical.
   B. Psychologic.
3. Job evaluation from the viewpoint of physical and emotional demands.
4. Employer's understanding of the employee's problem.
5. Motivation and reassurance of the employee.
6. Modified work and/or a gradual resumption of full duties.
7. Follow-up by the occupational health team.

Interest of the Employer and the Occupational Health Team.—The occupational health team should encourage the supervisor, personnel manager, and other key personnel to show an active and continued interest in the employee throughout his illness, beginning at the earliest possible date after his incapacitation. This interest should be sincere and helpful in nature, never threatening, not spying or demanding of premature return to work. Except in cases of overwhelming medical evidence to support it, the attending physician, the occupational physician, the nurse, and the employer do a great disservice by talking about retirement, altered work schedule, or requirements until the picture of recovery has become clear. Employers should be encouraged not to jump to premature conclusions, not to demand a quick prognosis of eventual rehabilitation, and to try to be patient in making a final determination of what the employee can do. The employer should encourage the employee about returning to work, emphasize the employee's value, and indicate willingness to take whatever reasonable measures are necessary to accommodate his rehabilitation.

Medical Evaluation From an Occupational Viewpoint Prior to Return to Work.—The attending physician has been in contact with the patient and has evaluated him, both at the time of illness and periodically during convalescence. The occupational health team should also participate in the evaluation prior to return to work. In many areas, the attending physician is a member of the occupational health team. This team should ascertain the nature of the patient's illness, any complications, any required medications that might affect performance, and any other important data, such as severe allergy to penicillin. Particular emphasis should be placed on ascertaining the state of recovery as it relates to the requirements of the patient's job. It is possible that special evaluation may be necessary in special cases; for example, in an employee recovering from a myocardial infarction who has to do heavy work. Such cases should be referred to a cardiac work evaluation clinic. This should be jointly agreed on by the attending physician and the occupational physician.

Physicians should not demand complete recovery prior to return to work. This often places the employee at a disadvantage and interferes with his rehabilitation, whereas to return him prior to the time that his natural defenses are able to cope with physical and chemical hazards in the job may cause recurrence or exacerbation of his illness. There is an optimal time for return to work after strength has returned but prior to complete recovery. Return to work should not be recommended before the diseased or injured organ or part is strong enough to withstand the demands placed on it. Guidelines of average periods necessary for strength to return to injured or diseased organs, for example, after a fractured radius, a hernia repair, or a myocardial infarction, can and should be established, based on the best current thinking of cardiologists, surgeons, orthopedists, and other specialists.

Nevertheless, the physician should always remember that it is a patient, not "a broken arm," "a heart attack" or "a hernia repair" that is returning to work. When the patient is ready may differ from when the arm, the heart, or the hernia is ready, and this determination still is very much an art. So many variables are involved—type of work, environmental conditions, skill of the patient in performance of the work, availability of modified work, previous state of health, the patient's attitude and motivation and the attitude of the employer—that a precise optimal time to return to work cannot be established scientifically. Experience, judgment, and a willingness to listen to and work with the patient will be of more help to the clinician than any inflexible approach.

Psychologic evaluation is a very important part of the medical evaluation by the occupational health team. The patient's attitude toward return to work—Is he confident that he can do the job? Is he afraid that he will not be able to do the job? How does he relate to his supervisor and other employees? Is he looking forward to return to work or would he prefer to retire?—are all important questions that, of course, have an extremely important influence, probably far more, in most cases, than actual physical capacity. Any physician knows that it is most difficult to deal with employees who have made up their minds that they will not be able to return to work.

Job Evaluation From the Viewpoint of Physical and Emotional Demands.—This includes the employee's physical capacity in the light of the work requirements. The physician, because of a lack of time, may be unable to do this personally; however, if at all possible, some member of the occupational health team—for example, the nurse—should view the work operation and make observations pertinent to the work capacity. A trained professional person can surmise valuable points about energy expenditures, body movements required, height to which and weight of objects to be lifted—actual on-the-job inspection. Short of this, a detailed description of the job by the employee and/or supervisor is helpful.

Employer's Understanding of the Employee's Problem.—The employer needs to know, in some detail, the employee's physical capacity and any limitations on the job that may be exhibited. Employers do not need to know the details of diagnosis and treatment, although, in my experience, they usually already have this information.

The physician and other members of the occupational health team should understand that in a production-oriented society in which departmental production is rewarded, supervisors often are hesitant about accepting a limited employee back into the department. In this respect, it should be pointed out to all levels of management that there are marked advantages in doing so. Aside from humanitarian considerations, continued payment of disability is costly, and an employee who has been properly rehabilitated by the employer often works with a greater degree of regularity and loyalty than many other employees. Therefore, although production by this employee may be reduced temporarily, in the long run it often is increased.

Motivation and Reassurance of the Employee.—The combined efforts of the occupational health team and the employer in motivating and reassuring returning employees have a powerful effect on their ultimate rehabilitation. When doubt is expressed by the attending physician, the occupational physician or nurse, or employer about the employee's ability to perform the job, it often is transferred to the employee, who then will anticipate complications. Employee and employer need reasonable assurance that a return to work can be achieved without difficulty. If there is serious doubt on the part of the physician, consideration should be given to modified work or a gradual return to work.

Modified Work and/or a General Resumption of Full Duties.—Abrupt return to strenuous activities after several months' pause, even for a person who has not been ill, will be extremely difficult, perhaps detrimental. This abrupt change in activities can be prevented by starting the patient on exercise, such as walking, to increase stamina. Nevertheless, if it can be arranged, a gradual resumption of full activity or temporarily modified work may be extremely helpful in the rehabilitation process. Gradual resumption can take the form of part-time work, gradually increasing to full-time, more strenuous activity interspersed with lighter activity or temporarily modified work involving a less strenuous activity. Request for a modification of work or part-time work with a gradual increase to full-time should be specifically stated by the physician. If a member of the occupational health team has reviewed the job, there is added assurance to the employee and management alike that medical personnel understand the job requirement. In this case, the physician can approve return to a specific job. If the physician does not fully understand the job, he should list specific limitations concerning number of hours to be worked, lifting, bending, stooping, or physical exertion. A note from the physician indicating that the employee can return to "light work" is not sufficient and often results in the employee not returning at all until approved for full work, or perhaps returning to a job that is just as strenuous or more so than previous jobs.

Follow-up by the Occupational Health Team.—In cases in which a gradual return to work or modified work is recommended, where proper placement is difficult or there is some uncertainty of rehabilitation, follow-up at appropriate intervals by medical personnel should be arranged. Depending on the nature of the condition, it can be arranged for the plant nurse, if available, the physician's nurse or the physician to see the employee, as necessary. This is a very important aspect that ensures that the "work prescription" is satisfactory and that the employee is progressing as anticipated.

PERIODIC HEALTH EXAMINATIONS

Details of periodic health examinations are covered elsewhere in this volume; however, they are discussed briefly here from the viewpoint of the clinician. Periodic health examinations basically are of two types: general and hazard-related. General examinations are done as part of a health maintenance program or where there is a possibility of some ill-defined, low-grade, or subtle hazard from a variety of working conditions. Hazard-related examinations are performed to monitor employee health in relation to specific health hazards. These can be complete examinations or isolated procedures appropriate to the hazard involved. Examples are: the blood lead determination in a brass foundry, liver enzyme studies for those exposed to chlorinated hydrocarbons, audiograms in a forge shop, and pulmonary function tests for employees exposed to dust. Ideally, it would be desirable to have a complete examination of all employees on an annual basis. Obviously, this is not practicable in all industries. Therefore, the physician then must determine the type of examination procedure appropriate to the hazard involved. Frequently, these types of examinations can be accomplished by trained paramedical personnel; however, the physician should always maintain the responsibility for the direction of the program and interpretation of the results.

REFERENCES

1. American Medical Association, Council on Occupational Health: Employability of workers handicapped by certain diseases—A guide for employers and physicians. *Arch Environ Health* 1968; 17:389.
2. American Occupational Medical Association Occupational Medical Practice Committee: Scope of occupational health programs and occupational medical practice. *J Occup Med* 1979; 21:497–499.
3. American Medical Association Council on Scientific Affairs: Medical Evaluations of Healthy Persons. *JAMA* 1983; 2249:1626–1633.
4. American Medical Association: *Guides to the Evaluation of Permanent Impairment*, ed 2. Chicago, American Medical Association, 1984.
5. Cullen MR: Occupational medicine. *Arch Intern Med* 1985; 145:511.
6. Bews DC, Baillie JH: Pre-placement health screening by nurses. *Am J Public Health* 1969; 59:2178.
7. Brogan MM: Utilization of nursing talents in Bell Canada. *J Occup Med* 1971; 13:511.
8. Calabrese EJ: *Principles of Animal Extrapolation*. New York, John Wiley & Sons, 1983.
9. Collings GH: The pre-employment examination—Worth its cost? *J Occup Med* 1971; 13:422.
10. Johnstone RT, Miller SE: *Occupational Diseases and Industrial Medicine*. Philadelphia, WB Saunders Co, 1960, p 90.
11. Karrh BW: Occupational medicine. *J Am Med Assoc* 1984; 252:2274.
12. Lauwerys RR: *Industrial Chemical Exposure: Guidelines for Biological Monitoring*. Davis, Cal, Biomedical Publications, 1983.
13. Lincoln TA, Hurt HB: Should the medical department give a "yes" or "no" answer to employability? *J Occup Med* 1971; 13:472.
14. *Occupational Health Guide for Medical and Nursing Personnel*, ed 3, Zenz C (ed). State Medical Society of Wisconsin, 330 Lakeside St, Madison, WI 53701, 1985.
15. Glaser W, Crocco J: The training of nurse-clinicians. *J Occup Med* 1971; 13:515.
16. Stokinger HE, Scheel LD: Hypersusceptibility and genetic problems in occupational medicine—A consensus report. *J Occup Med* 1973; 15:564.
17. *The Physician and Workers' Compensation*. Chicago, American Medical Association, 1983.
18. Williamson SM: Eighteen years' experience without pre-employment examinations. *J Occup Med* 1971; 13:465.
19. Your Body at Work: Human Physiology and the Working Environment, in Delin B (ed): *Arbetsmiljö/Föreningen for arbetarskydd* (Working Environment/The Environment Association). Stockholm, Sweden, Kungsholms Hamnplan 3, S-112 20, 1984.

Preparing the Employee for International Business Travel

William B. McClellan, M.D.

Foreign travel for business purposes differs from casual tourism in several ways. First, the business traveler has a definite business goal to reach; optimum utilization of mental faculties is necessary, and either physical illness or fatigue can defeat the purpose of the business trip. Second, business trips are often unexpected, and time to prepare for travel limited. Third, business trips often take the traveler far afield from the usual tourist routes. Fourth, the business traveler is often alone rather than with a travel group. Fifth, the business traveler usually has closer physical and social contact with local residents than does the casual tourist. All of these general facts—and the many individual eccentricities of individual businesses—make special preparation of the business traveler advisable.

PREPARING THE INTERNATIONAL BUSINESS TRAVELER

If the business traveler makes frequent, continued trips to the same destinations or has a semipermanent foreign base, personal medical preparation can also be made at regular intervals and should be made routine. If trips are infrequent, or not routine, or not to a semipermanent foreign assignment, individual medical preparation before the trip may take far longer and require greater planning for each trip. The needs of the individual business traveler in any business organization, therefore, should be anticipated by physicians, and appropriate procedures and facilities should be established well in advance of utilization.

In preparation for foreign business travel, the prospective business traveler should have an initial complete history and physical examination to determine the existing state of health, medication being used, and immunization history. After this examination, a schedule of medical immunizations can be established, and appropriate advice as to medication schedules can be prepared. From North America to Europe the traveler will move in a minimum of five time zones, and the traveler to the Orient seven or more. Instructions for adjusting the times of medication during travel are needed to ensure continuing accurate medication dosage. In some instances, travel to some foreign areas may be inadvisable if specific adverse health conditions and special health risks in the travel area combine to put the prospective traveler at high risk of serious illness; the pretravel history and physical examination are also useful for detection of such a combination and enables authoritative discussion of individual contraindications to travel.

CROSSING TIME ZONES BY AIR

The prospective traveler will have sleeping, eating, and working times changed dramatically by East-West travel. The North-South traveler, even in the same time zone may find great difficulties with humidity and temperature, and all travelers by air face changes in altitude. Airline schedules that take up most of the normal sleeping hours, the propensity of airlines to serve food and beverages at unusual hours, and the disturbance of rest during travel by crowding, immobility, in-flight movies, noise, and especially alcoholic beverages, make the temporary mild deterioration of physical and mental states during business travel inescapable.

The traveler in a jet airplane moves very rapidly through time zones when traveling in an easterly or westerly direction. When travel is in one of these directions and a number of time zones are passed, some bodily functions that display a daily rhythmicity are temporarily desynchronized, and, in the average traveler, variable vague symptoms appear. Mild gastrointestinal symptoms, loss of appetite, and poor and broken sleep are common complaints.

Physiologic changes in body temperature and endocrine, renal, cardiovascular, respiratory, and neural rhythms have been shown. Adaptation after varying periods of time in the new time zone have also been shown, and some studies have shown a greater effect in West-to-East travel. Outside of the discomfort felt, it is uncertain how important this is to the business traveler, since motivation is theorized to be important. In flight crews, after repeated time zone changes, little obvious impairment has been shown. Further, subjects allowed to exercise outside appear to adapt more quickly than subjects isolated in a hotel.[5] The combination of the effects of bodily changes, fatigue, and stress undoubtedly influences the business traveler's efficiency to some extent, but in an individual fashion and degree (see Chapters 68 and 69).

For these reasons business travelers should be advised to eat very sparingly, to drink no alcoholic beverages, and to rest as much as possible during air travel. The author's advice to business travelers has been to rest at least overnight after travel, before endeavoring to conduct any business.

EXPOSURE TO DISEASE IN FOREIGN COUNTRIES

Immunizations should be scheduled far enough in advance to allow recovery from acute reactions before travel, and the latest United States Public Health Service and World Health Organization schedules should be consulted for specific foreign area requirements.

Instructions for special precautions to be taken with food and drinking water are needed for most of the underdeveloped countries of the world and for some developed countries. Most of these recommendations can be found in the "Health Hints for the Traveler" section of the supplement to the Morbidity and Mortality Weekly Report (MMWR) entitled *Health Information for International Travel*.[2]

Travelers to the large cities of Western European countries and to Japan, Mexico, and Australia are unlikely to meet unusual diseases that are not recognized and controlled by local health authorities. This is also true for many of the other large cities and certain small countries, such as Israel, Singapore, and Hong Kong, particularly if the traveler stays and lives in accommodations established with the view of attracting foreign travelers. In tropical and subtropical areas and in poorer temperate areas, however, the traveler may meet diseases not transmitted in the U.S., Canada, and Western Europe, and the business traveler must be especially prepared medically when travel is to these areas.

Diseases that after World War II seemed quiescent or declining have recurred over wide areas and have affected great numbers in recent years. The single happy exception seems to be smallpox, which has been eliminated. Sleeping sickness due to trypanosomiasis is endemic in 25 African countries, and there are about 10,000 new cases every year.[7] Chagas' disease—South American trypanosomiasis—now affects 10 to 12 million people,[1] malaria resurgence worldwide may now account for 300 million cases per year, and in tropical Africa alone, there are more than 1 million annual malaria-related deaths.[8] Falciparum malaria is showing increasing resistance to antimalarials, and this drug-resistant malaria has spread rapidly. Approximately 200 million persons worldwide are infected with schistosomes,[6] and the disease is found in areas of Africa, Asia, South and Central America, and the Caribbean. The highest rates of hepatitis B infection are found in sub-Saharan Africa and East Asia.[4]

For the physician or occupational medical department in the United States needing information about the current status of these and other diseases present in other world areas, the Center for Disease Control in Atlanta, Georgia, and the local health department can usually provide the needed information quickly. Additional consultation can be obtained from the division of tropical and/or infectious diseases in medical schools and public health schools. The Tropical Medicine Center for the School of Hygiene and Public Health of Johns Hopkins University can often provide additional information about such diseases, on a current basis.

Throughout the world, physicians can seek up-to-date advice from local public health departments, selected clinics, and most academic centers, in addition to the regularly published bulletins and documents from the World Health Organization's Geneva and its Regional Offices.

MEDICAL CARE IN OTHER COUNTRIES

Medical care and hospital care around the world are quite variable. If the need for medical consultants and hospital care in foreign areas requires recommendation (because of recurring needs of business travelers) by the occupational physician, a personal visit to the area and inspection of available facilities may be required. Only in this manner can the necessary judgments be made and continuing competent care assured. Advice from colleagues familiar with the area may be useful, of course, but such advice is not routinely available at this time to most physicians. While the ability of a physician in a foreign land to speak English is important to communicate accurately with English-speaking business travelers, such a linguistic ability does not give any valid information about medical judgment and training.

MEDICAL SCREENING FOR THE RETURNING TRAVELER

The increasing worldwide incidence and prevalence of transmissible disease, coupled with the uncertainties of medical care while abroad, make medical screening for the returning traveler advisable. While travel to Western Europe carries far less health risk than travel to Southeast Asia, all business travelers to foreign areas should be medically screened on return, since contact with large mobile populations during travel will have occurred. The depth and content of the screening procedure should vary, of course, according to the areas visited. Travelers who have visited malarious areas, for instance, should be cautioned to report any fever that occurs within six weeks after their return, while travelers returning in good health from Western European travel need not be so cautioned.

MEDICAL TRAVELING KITS

Some large organizations give their traveling employees small kits containing first-aid supplies and some medication to be used during travel. There are several reasons for this. First, the availability of pharmaceuticals around the world is quite variable, and pharmaceutical names vary from country to country, making the correct filling of prescriptions unpredictable. Second, pharmaceuticals that are quite active pharmacologically are available in some parts of the world without prescription, and toxic reactions after self-prescription is possible. Third, in some areas of the world, pharmaceuticals may not be standardized, and obtaining exact dosage of the correct medication may be very difficult.

If the practice of using such kits is followed, the kits should be retrieved from each traveler immediately on return to the U.S. and all medications properly discarded. Very careful and explicit instructions for use must be included, and a letter from the physician included in the kit should state, for governmental authorities, that the drugs are specifically prescribed for the use of the person carrying the kit. Every precaution to ensure against misuse must be taken, and since such kits do pose potential problems, widespread use of such kits is unwise; such kits should be used only for travelers to areas where there are known problems that the use of the kits will solve.

REFERENCES

1. Brener Z: Recent Developments in the Field of Chagas' Disease. *Bull WHO* 1982; 60(4):463–473.
2. Centers for Disease Control, Morbidity and Mortality Weekly Report: *Health Information for International Travel*. Atlanta, Centers for Disease Control, 1985.
3. Doege TC, Bell JA (eds): *Traveler's Health Abroad: A Guide for Physicians*. Chicago, American Medical Association, 1982.
4. Francis DP: Selective primary health care: Strategies for control of disease in developing world, III. Hepatitis B virus and its related diseases. *Rev Infect Dis* Mar–Apr 1983; 5(2):322–329.
5. Minors DS, Waterhouse JM: *Circadian Rhythms and the Human*. Littleton, Mass, PST Publishers, 1981.
6. Nash TE, et al: Schistosome infections in humans, perspectives and recent findings. *Ann Intern Med* 1982; 97(5):740–754.
7. UNDP/WHO/World Bank: Control of sleeping sickness due to trypanosoma brucei, gambinese. *Bull WHO* 1982; 60(6):821–825.
8. Wyler DJ: Malaria—Resurgence, resistance, and research. *N Engl J Med* 1983; pt 1, 308(15):875–878; pt 2, 308(16):934–940.

9

Trauma

Dudley Briggs, M.D.

In 1982 accidents causing deaths or disabling injuries cost the nation at least $88.4 billion. Of that amount, $31.4 billion was attributable to work accidents. Although modern occupational medicine programs are comprehensive in approach, the primary duty of in-plant medical departments is to provide primary care for workers who have work-connected injuries and illnesses. The immediate and perhaps life-saving care of a worker injured in an industrial accident is given by the occupational health personnel. The magnitude of injuries suffered at work is reflected by the National Health Survey conducted by the U.S. Public Health Service. The survey shows an annual estimate of 11,377,000 work injuries, of which 2,779,000 were severe enough to confine the person to bed for more than half of the daylight hours on the date of the injury or some following day.

Accidents are the leading cause of death for all patients aged 1 through 38 years. For persons of all ages, accidents now are the fourth-ranked cause of death, surpassed only by heart disease, cancer, and stroke.

Accidental work deaths for 1982 totaled 11,200 from a work population of 98.9 million. The variability of accident rates for different industries is outlined in Table 9–1. The National Safety Council estimates that the cost to industry, per worker, for accidents during 1982 was $320. The total loss in man days for accidents that occurred in 1982 was 80 million days. Total cash and medical care benefits for workers' compensation were $13.36 billion in 1980.

Of the 1.9 million disabling work injuries in 1982, approximately 70,000 resulted in some permanent impairment. Table 9–2 shows the relative frequency of injuries to parts of the body, the percentage of all injuries, and the percentage of all compensation paid.

An overwhelming number of injuries treated in plant dispensaries are minor injuries—cuts, bruises, and strains of the extremities. It is evident from Table 9–2, however, that disabling injuries are predominantly low-back strains and injuries to the extremities.

The ensuing discussion of treating industrial trauma presumes general principles in handling traumatic events that may depend on the skill of the physician and the facilities available for treat-

TABLE 9–1.
Work Accidents, United States, 1984*

	DEATHS		
INDUSTRY GROUP	TOTAL NUMBER	RATE PER 100,000	DISABLING INJURIES
All Industries	11,500	11	1,900,000
Construction	2,200	39	220,000
Agriculture	1,600	46	180,000
Service	1,900	7	410,000
Government	1,400	9	250,000
Transportation and public utilities	1,500	27	170,000
Trade	1,200	5	330,000
Manufacturing	1,100	6	300,000
Mining, quarrying	1,400	60	50,000

*Courtesy National Safety Council, Chicago.

TABLE 9–2.
Part of Body Injured in Work Accidents, 1982*

PART OF BODY	CASES	PERCENT OF CASES	PERCENT OF ALL COMPENSATION PAID
Trunk	550,000	29	38
Fingers/Thumbs	280,000	15	7
Legs	250,000	13	13
Arms	170,000	9	8
General	170,000	9	20
Hands	130,000	7	3
Head	110,000	6	5
Feet	100,000	5	4
Eyes	100,000	5	1
Toes	40,000	2	1

*Adapted from *Accident Facts.* Chicago, National Safety Council, 1983.

ment. Sometimes it is advantageous in large industrial settings to segregate trauma patients from persons taking preplacement examinations and physical examinations for hazardous work so that the treatment of traumatic injuries is not delayed. As a general rule, if there is an in-plant medical facility, it should be centrally located in relation to the majority of the work population. Remote areas should be supplied with trained first-aid personnel and appropriate transportation to the main medical facility or to a nearby hospital. Obvious difficulties with airway problems, bleeding, or potential fractures are approached immediately.

AT&T NETWORK SYSTEMS, COLUMBUS, OHIO, WORKS PROCEDURES

When the patient arrives in the medical department, his or her medical record is obtained and a complete history of the injury is recorded while the vital signs are obtained and recorded by the nurse in attendance. It is customary in our plant to color code the charts of patients who have diabetes, hypertension, cardiovascular disease, and allergies so that it is immediately apparent if there is something special about the patient being treated. Our medical record contains a detailed list of allergies and previous tetanus immunization. A summary of previous sickness absences and the durations and reasons are also on a summary sheet available in the chart. If the patient urgently requires immediate physician attention, the physician is summoned if he or she is on the premises, or arrangements are made for transportation to a hospital while the patient is attended. A patient with multiple injuries presents a particular problem in treatment and in the establishment of priorities of treatment.

General Principles in Management of Soft-Tissue Wounds

The vast majority of wounds of ambulatory patients (as well as their subsequent follow-up) are treated in the dispensary. Any indication that major vessels, nerves, or tendons are involved in the wound would mandate application of a sterile dressing and moving the patient for definitive care.

The history of injury in soft-tissue wounds is important in order to ascertain the possibility of embedded foreign bodies. It should include the mechanism of injury and the time of injury.

Animal bites and human bites are wounds that need to be given special attention against the possibility of rabies and the predilection to secondary infection, which sometimes accompanies human bites.

An employee exiting from our plant threw his lunch sack into a garbage pail in which there was a large cat. The cat reached up and bit or scratched the employee as he removed his hand from the garbage can, and so the possibility of rabies exposure in the employee was raised. Proper preventive medical measures depended on the prevalence of rabies and the lack or presence of provocation with which the animal bite occurred, and the decision was made, in conjunction with the local public health officer, not to give rabies prophylaxis.

Human bites, as another special case, are never surgically closed. The wounds are cleansed and allowed to remain open. (Special emphasis will be given subsequently to soft-tissue wounds of the hand.)

The typical tray that we use for repair of soft-tissue wounds is shown in Figure 9–1. The wound is examined to determine loss of skin or evidence of damage to surrounding tissues; then the wound is cleansed by using normal saline to irrigate the depths of the wound and soap to cleanse the surrounding skin. This is performed gently. If the wound is jagged or beveled, the wound edges are trimmed to ensure sharp skin edges. Any foreign material is removed by irrigation or by sharp dissection, and significant bleeding vessels in the wound are ligated with 5-0 chromic catgut. After the wound has been prepped and draped, it is infiltrated with an anesthetic solution of (usually) 1% Xylocaine. If the wound is deep, deep structures are approximated with sutures of 5-0 chromic catgut and the skin with either an interrupted or continuous suture of monofilament plastic material. Suturing on the face or other cosmetic areas usually is done close to the skin edge and with sutures placed closely together. Sutures over the back or the lower extremities are placed farther apart and farther from the skin edge. Finally, a sterile dressing is applied. Compressive dressings and splints are applied if the wound is over a joint or an area where motion will disturb the healing.

Tetanus Prophylaxis

The number of tetanus cases has fallen from approximately 500 in 1951 to 75 in 1983. The primary reason for the decrease has been the ever-expanding general use of tetanus toxoid immunization. Since tetanus is a preventable disease, *a history of immunization should be obtained from every employee at the time of his preplacement examination*. Employees without active immunization are given a series. *There is no excuse for tetanus cases in our working population*. The causative organism is present throughout nature. There is no natural immunity to tetanus and no immunity in those persons who contract the disease and recover. The mortality rate from tetanus has been about 50% over the past 20 years. The schedule recommended by the Center for Disease Control for tetanus immunization is shown in Table 9–3.

Guides and recommendations for tetanus prophylaxis emphasize four basic concepts: (1) administration of tetanus toxoid when indicated, (2) immediate, meticulous surgical care for all wounds,

TABLE 9–3.
Recommendations for Tetanus Prophylaxis in Wound Management

HISTORY OF TETANUS IMMUNIZATION (DOSES)	CLEAN, MINOR WOUNDS		ALL OTHER WOUNDS	
	Td*	TIG	Td*	TIG
Uncertain	Yes	No	Yes	No
0–1	Yes	No	Yes	Yes
2	Yes	No	Yes	No§
3 or more	No†	No	No‡	No

*Adult tetanus toxoid and diphtheria toxoid in combination is preferred to tetanus toxoid alone.
†Yes, if more than ten years since last dose.
‡Yes, if more than five years since last dose.
§Yes, if wound is more than 24 hours old.

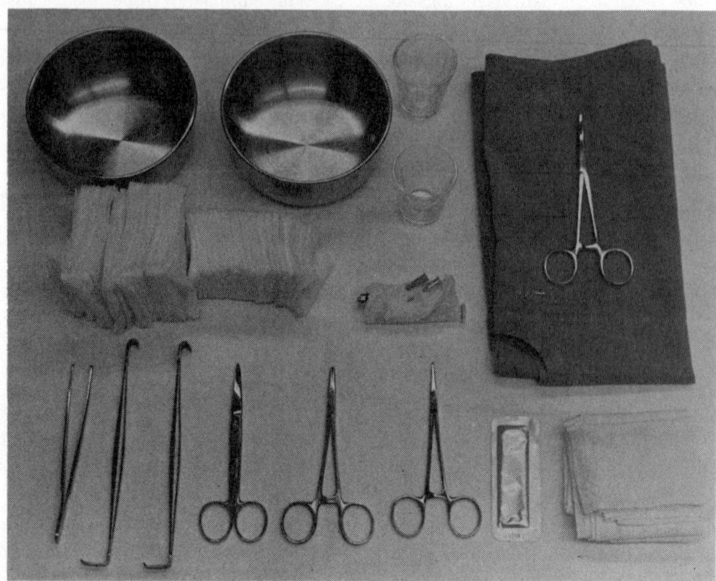

FIG 9–1.
Instruments and supplies used for repair of soft-tissue wounds.

(3) administration of tetanus immune globulin (human) when indicated, and (4) employment of emergency medical identification devices.

Electrical Injuries

Accidental death due to electrical injury causes more than 1,000 fatalities per year in the United States. Injury occurs when electrical current passes through the body. The nature and severity of electrical injuries are dependent upon (1) the type and voltage of the electrical current, (2) the resistance of the body at the point of electrical contact, (3) the pathway of the current through the body, and (4) the duration of current flow through the body or part.

Alternating current (AC) produces greater damage than a direct current (DC) of the same amperage. The AC flow at 60 cycles (Hz) that will produce a tingling sensation, the threshold of perception, is from 1–2 milliamperes (mA), and for DC, 5 mA. The maximum current at which a victim is still able to "let go" is 15 mA for AC and 75 mA for DC.

The effect of electrical injury may be immediate or life-threatening, causing cardiac or respiratory arrest which requires cardiopulmonary resuscitation (after cautiously breaking the victim's contact with the current source). Alternating current of 60 Hz at 110–220 volts traveling across the chest for less than one second is capable of inducing ventricular fibrillation at currents as low as 60–80 mA. Electrical injuries may visibly burn the tissue at the point of contact with the electrical source, as well as at the exit (or grounding) point. There is usually more tissue damage than is readily apparent. Current flow follows the path of blood vessels and muscles and may cause thrombosis and necrosis of tissues at sites remote from the apparent injury. There may be associated musculoskeletal injuries not only from the tetanic contraction of muscle, but also from the not uncommon fall of the electrically injured victim. Oliguria due to renal damage may be a sequela of electrical injury due to destruction of muscle and the production of myoglobin pigments in the urine. Because of this, some consider severe electrical injuries to be more like crush injuries than burns from a pathophysiologic standpoint. For this reason, it is recommended that intravenous fluid therapy include alkalization of the urine and osmotic diuretics to minimize acute tubular necrosis.

In summary, electrical burn victims may have more injury than is at first appreciated. There may be cardiac abnormalities, but they are usually transient. Because of the possibility of associated vascular, visceral, and musculoskeletal problems, severe electrical burns may require the attention of specialists from several disciplines. A period of close observation in the hospital may be necessary.

Head Injuries

Although injuries to the head comprise only 6% of work injuries, they stand at the top of the list, since seemingly minor trauma to the head with only transient loss of consciousness may signal the beginning of a course of events leading to permanent mental and physical defect—and even death if neglected.

Lacerations of the scalp pose a particular problem in soft-tissue wound care, inasmuch as the scalp has a rich blood supply and serious bleeding may occur from untreated scalp lacerations. Trauma to the head is in large part absorbed by the scalp. Lacerations that penetrate the galea aponeurotica must be closed in two layers to effectively control bleeding from the wound. If the galea is lacerated, particular care is paid to the wound to remove any foreign particles or devitalized soft tissue. I use interrupted 3-0 chromic catgut for repairing the galea and 4-0 silk for the scalp.

The principal concern in head injuries is the extent of injury to the brain itself. Because brain function is so critically affected by conditions of hypoxia, attention to an adequate airway should be the first matter of concern. After the airway is established, it is necessary to establish a baseline for subsequent observations and to determine the nature and type of injury sustained. A history of the accident is exceedingly important to ascertain whether there are other injuries present, particularly when the patient is conscious at the time of admission to the emergency facility. In regard to the history, it is important to know whether the patient was projected and landed on his head or had had force applied to his head externally, as from a falling object. The most important observations to be made early are the levels of consciousness. These observations should be made and recorded after noting the patient's response to painful stimulation, the ability to verbalize, whether speech is normal, and if the patient is able to make purposeful movements. These observations should be made at 15–30-minute intervals while the patient is under your care and recorded for the benefit of others who will be caring for the patient later. Attention should be given to the patient's pupillary size and reactivity. If both pupils are small and fixed (and the patient has received no medication), this may be indicative of pontine hemorrhage; if both pupils are dilated and fixed, this should be recorded. Both conditions are associated with a poor outcome. If both pupils are unequal but are not reactive, this is evidence of a local brain injury (usually involving the homolateral ocular motor system of the side with the dilated pupil). The degree of motor activity of the patient should be observed particularly in the extremities, and these objective observations later may help to determine whether the patient is demonstrating a progressive neurologic deficit. If there is an acute increase in the intracranial pressure subsequent to injury, the vital signs usually alter by (1) an increase in systolic pressure with a concomitant decrease or plateauing of the diastolic pressure, (2) a slowing of the pulse, (3) stertorous or irregular breathing, and (4) a rise in body temperature. In recording the vital signs, assessment of the deep tendon reflexes in the upper and lower extremities also should be recorded, along with a note concerning the presence or absence of a Babinski sign or clonus.

The history of the injury and the conscious level of the patient dictate whether x-ray studies are to be taken. If they are taken, it is well to *check for cervical spine injury;* this can be done effectively by a lateral x-ray of the cervical spine prior to taking skull x-rays to rule out cervical spine injury. If a linear skull fracture crossing a main vascular channel is seen on the x-ray film, we refer the patient for neurosurgical consultation and probable hospitalization whether or not there is evidence of an expanding lesion within the head. If the patient has suffered loss of consciousness and amnesia, we also have neurosurgical consultation and usually hospitalization for extended observation. In the absence of x-ray findings, but with cerebrospinal fluid issuing from the nose or the ears or with the presence of blood behind the drum, we also obtain neurosurgical consultation, since this is presumptive evidence of a basilar skull fracture.

Brain injury is the most important problem in a head injury that eventuates in loss of consciousness, loss of orientation, or other signs of altered brain function. The injury should be considered serious and be followed adequately with appropriate consultation until symptoms subside.

Facial Injuries

The common injuries to the face are those of the mandible and the nose and periorbital structures. Injuries to the bony parts of the face are delineated satisfactorily by Waters' projection of the facial bones (accomplished with the patient's chin on the radiographic plate in a 25° up position). Palpation of the rims of the orbit is a satisfactory clinical method of ascertaining zygomatic and orbital fractures. The presence of diplopia in a patient who has received a blow to the cheek should be a tip-off that there may be an orbital plate fracture, and this requires specialty consultation. Fractures in the maxillary area may result in entrapment of the second division of the trigeminal nerve and cause anesthesia below the eye. Similar contusions over the trigeminal nerve above the eye may cause some loss of sensation. Mandibular fractures present with pain on biting down, because of the resulting malocclusion. These fractures are a serious life-threatening injury only when both rami of the mandible are fractured, with posterior dislocation of the distal fragment resulting in airway obstruction, which is relieved by reducing the dislocation.

Eye Injuries

The occupational physician often has to provide emergency care for such conditions of the eye as foreign bodies, corneal abrasions, and chemical burns. The physician needs to be able to differentiate acute eye conditions, such as glaucoma, conjunctivitis, and iritis, from traumatic sequela.

Most eye injuries can be detected by careful attention to history, tests of visual function, and examination of the eyes with simple instruments. A history of hammering or grinding with subsequent loss of vision suggests an intraocular foreign body. These perhaps are the most likely overlooked injuries. The possibility of penetration or perforation of the eye by a foreign body is an indication for diagnostic x-ray examination of the orbit. In our medical department, our eye examination chair is opposite a Snellen eye chart, which is used routinely to evaluate visual acuity. A history of persistent discomfort in the eyes subsequent to trauma often is a symptom of superficial corneal abrasion.

Examination.—In carrying out the examination of the eye, care is taken in separating the lids to avoid pressure on the eyeball, particularly if there is any reason to suspect perforation or penetration of the eyeball. Figure 9–2 illustrates the proper method of separating the lids for examination of the eye by placing the thumb and forefinger opposite the lower and upper orbital margins respectively, compressing the lids against the bony rim of the orbit. Obliquely illuminating the corneal surface with a well-focused penlight is most likely to reveal a defect in the normally smooth surface of the cornea. It is helpful in delineating corneal abrasions as well as corneal opacities and foreign bodies. If fluorescein staining is done, we use sterile dry strips as illustrated in Figure 9–3, because solutions become contaminated.

The method of everting the upper lid for the discovery of a foreign body that may be present on the undersurface of the upper lid's tarsal fold is demonstrated in Figure 9–4. The secret of eversion is to grasp the upper lid and pull outward and downward while

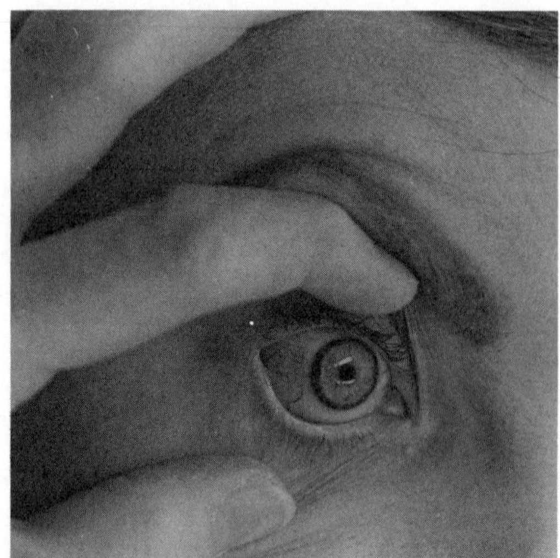

FIG 9–2.
Proper method of separating the lids for examination of the eye.

applying an applicator 1 cm or more from the lid margin to invert the tarsal fold.

Anesthesia.—We use local anesthesia for examination of the eyes in our dispensary; it consists of the topical instillation of proparacaine (Ophthaine). Removal of corneal foreign bodies, tonometry, and inspection of an abraded cornea and other superficial manipulations are readily carried out under topical anesthesia. The patients are warned not to rub their eyes, because it is easy for them to cause self-inflicted injuries to their corneal epithelium while their eyes are anesthetized. The duration of anesthesia usually is 10–15 minutes following the application of a topical anesthetic. It is well to remember that the healing of corneal epithelium is slowed by the use of topical anesthetics, and one should resist the temptation to relieve pain by the continued use of anesthetic drops.

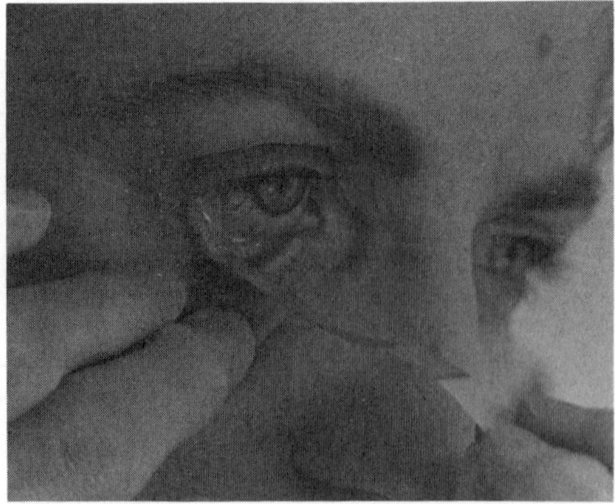

FIG 9–3.
Sterile dry strips used in fluorescein staining of the surface of the cornea.

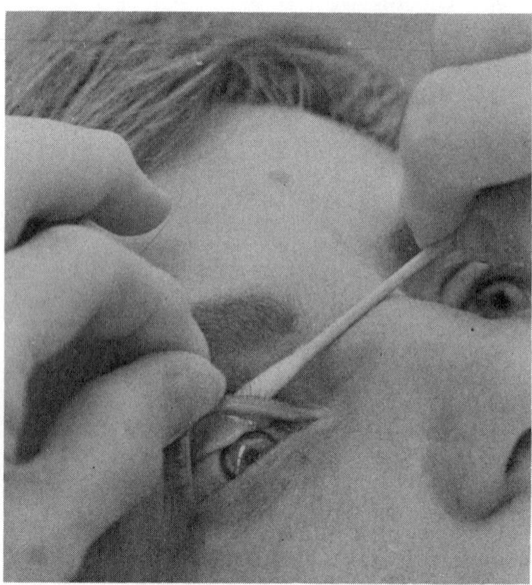

FIG 9–4.
Everting the upper lid for discovery of a foreign body.

Antibiotics.—The choice of antibiotics for either therapeutic or prophylactic use is based on the selection of an agent that will be efficacious for the bacteria present or likely to be present. We exclude the use of commonly used broad-spectrum antibiotics or penicillin, because they may expose the patient to the risk of sensitization, when there are other agents available that are equally as good. We customarily use gentamicin sulfate or a combination of neomycin, bacitracin, and polymyxin or sulfacetamide. We do not use antibiotic-cortisone preparations because of the several contraindications to the use of corticoid eye preparations (e.g., herpes ulcers or glaucoma).

Corneal Foreign Bodies and Abrasions.—Despite the wide use in industry of protective safety glasses, corneal foreign bodies and abrasions are among the most frequent ocular injuries. After application of a topical anesthetic, the eye is irrigated with a commercially available isotonic electrolyte solution (Dacriose), which is effective for removing foreign bodies from the conjunctival sac. Corneal foreign bodies are removed by using a sterile eye spud. It is well to have good illumination and good magnification by use of an eye loupe, and it is helpful to brace the hand against the cheek of the patient while removing the foreign body. This method is superior to using a cotton-tipped applicator, which, in itself, causes epithelial damage when one attempts to remove embedded foreign bodies. Because of the epithelial defect left by the removal of a foreign body, prophylactic antibiotics are used until there is complete healing of the defect, as evidenced by failure to stain with fluorescein, or complete disappearance of pain. Residual pain after 24 hours may be due to an undiscovered foreign body; on further examination, these usually are found on the tarsal surface of the mid upper lid or on the cornea. Foreign bodies found on the tarsal plate may be removed with a sterile cotton-tipped applicator. The patient is either patched, with instillation of antibiotic ointment, or is instructed in the use of antibiotic drops every three hours following removal of a foreign body, and examined at 24-hour intervals until complete healing has occurred. If there is a deep corneal abrasion, we add 5% homatropine drops and prescribe mild analgesics or sedation in addition to our other treatment.

Contusions of the Eye.—Injuries to the globe of the eye with blunt objects may produce hemorrhage, retinal detachment, rupture, or anterior or posterior dislocation of the lens. If finger tension of the eye is soft to palpation in comparison with the opposite side, rupture of the eye should be suspected, a Fox metallic shield placed over the eye, and the patient referred. The presence of bright red blood in the anterior chamber (hyphema) may occur following blunt trauma and is a signal for referral to an ophthalmologist regardless of the amount of blood.

Corneal Burns.—A great variety of agents are encountered in industry that, when splashed into the eye, cause damage to the cornea and adnexal eye structures. Regardless of the type of chemical, the emergency treatment is immediate, profuse, prolonged irrigation. The lids are separated widely and irrigation is carried out for several minutes. We customarily hang a bottle of Ringer's lactate solution or isotonic saline, usually 500 ml or 1 L, and use all of it in irrigating through sterile tubing. Any particulate matter is removed after topical anesthetic is introduced into the eye. Following copious irrigation, broad-spectrum antibiotics are placed in the eye and the patient is referred. Alkaline burns are treated with 0.15 M cysteine solution applied every three hours to prevent the production of collagenase, which could lead to a perforating corneal ulcer.

Burns of the eyes from ultraviolet light and welding arcs may cause a superficial keratitis of the corneal epithelium that characteristically becomes symptomatic a few hours after exposure and then causes severe eye pain. Fluorescein staining reveals a diffuse punctate keratitis. The topical antibiotics are used along with application of cold and the ingestion of analgesics and sedatives. The patient is examined at 24-hour intervals until there is complete healing of the corneal epithelium, as evidenced by lack of fluorescein uptake.

Differential Diagnosis of the Red Eye.—The main conditions to be differentiated among in evaluation of the red eye are acute *conjunctivitis*, acute *iritis*, and acute *glaucoma*. Visual acuity is not altered with acute conjunctivitis of a bacterial or allergic nature. Pain associated with a red eye would lead one to think of either corneal damage or, if associated with photophobia, acute iritis or, if the pain is severe, acute glaucoma. The cornea in acute glaucoma is cloudy, whereas it is not affected in the other two conditions. The pupil size in acute conjunctivitis is normal, whereas in iritis it is small and in acute glaucoma it is dilated. There is poor pupillary response except in acute conjunctivitis. The taking of ocular tension by a tonometer as illustrated in Figure 9–5 is one way of helping to confirm a diagnosis of glaucoma by showing an elevated intraocular tension. The importance of differentiating among the causes of red eye is that the prognosis may well be extremely serious without proper treatment if one is dealing with iritis, glaucoma, or the residuals of corneal ulcer or trauma.

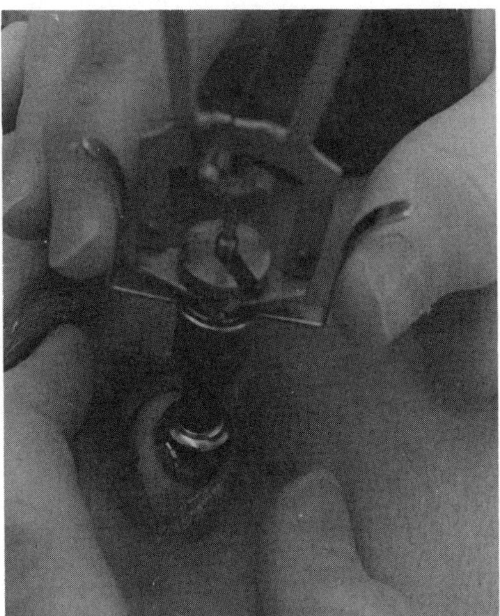

FIG 9–5.
Using a tonometer to evaluate ocular tension.

If treatment of red eye is undertaken with the presumption of acute conjunctivitis, one should expect the problem to clear within three to five days; if it does not, the patient should be referred for proper ophthalmologic evaluation.

Chest and Abdominal Injuries

Although the majority of thoracic and abdominal injuries are incident to auto accidents, a large number of such injuries are also attributed to falls and crush injuries that occur at work.

Fractured Ribs.—The most common injury of the thoracic wall is fractured ribs. In an uncomplicated simple fracture of ribs, the physical findings are definite. The patient usually has painful restricted respiration with limitation of motion on the affected side as well as sharp pain at the site of injury. On palpation, there may be crepitus present. By individual compression of adjacent ribs, the site of fracture usually is delineated by exquisite pain when the injured rib is compressed. Careful percussion and auscultation will reveal the presence or absence of additional signs of intrathoracic injury, such as pneumothorax, pleural effusion, or traumatic subcutaneous emphysema. It is unusual for there to be an intrathoracic injury when there is a simple rib fracture. The location of the injured rib can be ascertained by counting down from the second rib, which is the first rib palpable below the clavicle. If there is difficulty in clearly ruling in or out the presence of rib fracture, anteroposterior compression between the examiner's hands is helpful, particularly in obese or heavily muscled patients, in whom individual palpation of ribs is difficult. If anteroposterior compression is painless, lateral compression is tried also. Localized pain over the costochondral junction may reveal some discontinuity of the injured costochondral junction; fractures in this area are not revealed by x-ray examination.

If there is an injury causing fractures in adjacent ribs in two or more places, a condition of flail chest exists, in which there is paradoxical movement of the rib cage with regard to respiration. This condition requires prompt stabilization of the chest wall by application of either sandbags or an external device to fix the flail portion.

Complications of trauma to the chest include injury to the lungs as manifested by pneumothorax, hemothorax, bronchial rupture, contusion of mediastinal contents with cardiac tamponade due to pericardial effusion, and bleeding from or injury to the great vessels. To be aware of the likelihood of such lesions in severe chest trauma and to manage the patient effectively until referral, one has to be proficient at maintaining an open airway, treating shock, and getting the patient on his way to definitive care when the possibility of a serious intrathoracic injury is entertained.

Abdominal Injuries.—*Abdominal injuries* of a blunt nature sometimes are a complication of thoracic injuries, in which fractures of the lower ribs may cause injury to pelvic organs, the spleen, liver, and kidneys. Forces that produce fractures in the lower ribs also may injure underlying organs either by sharp trauma from broken ribs or from the blunt force of the trauma applied to the lower rib cage. If we suspect intra-abdominal injury because the patient has persistent pain, tenderness, or rigidity of the abdomen, we transfer the patient to the surgical center, where peritoneal lavage usually is carried out shortly after admission to rule in or out the presence of blood in the peritoneal cavity. Penetrating wounds of the abdomen from scribes, screwdrivers, and other sharp instruments raise the question of penetration of the peritoneal cavity. These cases, too, are referred for surgical consultation, unless it can be demonstrated by exploration of the wound that penetration has not occurred. The finding of blood in gastric aspirate or in the rectum, or blood in the urine, also dictates further investigation immediately posttrauma. Both the solid and hollow organs of the abdomen may be ruptured by blows that leave no mark or bruise on the anterior abdominal wall. Physical signs depend largely on the extent of peritoneal contamination. The key to discovering originally obscure injuries is frequently repeated examinations of the abdomen. If this cannot be carried out in the medical department, one is obliged, if the history suggests a significant force, to hospitalize the patient for these frequent examinations.

Trunk and Spinal Injuries

The trunk and spine constitute the most common region of the body that is injured in work accidents, being involved in 29% of all cases and representing 38% of all compensation paid.

Cervical Spine Fractures.—*Fractures and fracture-dislocations of the cervical spine* attend considerable violence or falls from a height. The proper transport and handling of these patients is a most critical factor, along with a history of whether there has been any movement of extremities following such an injury. The absence of movement and sensation will readily permit the recognition of a spinal cord laceration. If the patient is able to move the toes and legs, major cord damage has not occurred. If the legs are paralyzed and the patient is able to move the upper extremities, the lesion is below the cervical region. If there is impairment of arm function, the lesion is at the level of the sixth cervical vertebra or above. Adequate lateral x-ray studies that show all seven cervical vertebrae should be obtained to ascertain if there is dislocation of the vertebral bodies. With acute cervical trauma, it is not wise to move the patient until x-ray studies have excluded fracture or dislocation.

Compression Fracture of the Thoracic Spine.—Often the sequela of a fall, compression fracture of the thoracic spine is fairly common. It may cause intense pain, but it is not often associated with neurologic injury. The most common site is T-12 and L-1. Bed rest is usually all that is needed, although sometimes bracing is required.

Other Cervical Spine Injuries.—In the appraisal of *other lesions of the cervical spine that may cause pain,* we need to consider thoracic outlet syndrome, cervical ribs, and cervical disks. All of these conditions may be characterized by pain in the neck radiating to the shoulder or down the arm. The cervical rib is a supernumerary rib attached to the seventh cervical vertebra that may be bilateral or unilateral. On careful palpation of the neck, it may be found as a bony prominence in the supraclavicular space. In the other thoracic outlet syndromes, there may be compression of the brachial plexus or subclavian artery by the scalenus anticus muscle. Any motion that tenses the scalenus anticus muscle aggravates the pain in the upper extremity.

The diagnosis of *thoracic outlet syndrome* is made by demonstrating a nerve conduction deficit arising in the brachial plexus or by demonstrating vascular compression by suitable angiographic techniques. The treatment of these syndromes is removal of the first rib, the attachment of the scalenus anticus muscle, and/or removal of a cervical rib when it is present. Alternatively, these syndromes may be treated with exercises.

A *herniated cervical disk* may produce one of two syndromes, depending on whether the disk is herniated in the midline, producing signs of spinal cord compression, or whether herniation is lateral, producing nerve root compression. The history may be one of short duration of pain associated with frank herniation of the disk, or there may be a chronic history of pain that is associated with x-ray findings of narrowing of intervertebral foramina and hypertrophic changes on the vertebral bodies. Herniated cervical disks usually occur between the fifth and sixth cervical vertebrae, with involvement of the sixth cervical nerve root, or between the sixth and seventh, with involvement of the seventh cervical nerve root. With sixth-root involvement, there usually is diminished biceps reflex, and with seventh-nerve root involvement, diminished triceps reflex. Pain and paresthesia over the dermatomes corresponding to these nerve roots usually are present.

The Low-Back Problem

Pain in the low back is a major source of incapacitation among working people. Because low-back pain is such a complex medical problem, it is frequently difficult to relate the low-back problem to injury. In following workers with back problems, it is impressive how many have recurrent back problems and how difficult it is to diagnose low-back pain. It has been suggested that strength testing of individuals is an alternative to x-rays and history-taking for predicting which people will be capable of performing tasks with a minimum of low-back problems. Because of the importance of the low-back problem, I will describe what I consider to be a detailed examination, how the diagnosis of ruptured intervertebral disk is made, and what some of the signs of the low-back problem are.

Examination.—A detailed history of the patient with a painful back should include the onset and progression of symptoms, the type of pain and the area of radiation, a history of sensory deficit or motor weakness, and the factors that accentuate the pain and those that alleviate the pain.

With the patient disrobed, the stance and general habitus are noted. The patient is asked to walk on toes and heels and to walk flat to observe his gait. The presence or absence of scoliosis or kyphosis and the presence or absence of lordosis are noted also. With the patient standing, the musculature of the back is palpated for evidence of spasm. The patient is asked to stand alternately on the right and left foot to see if there is reciprocal relaxation of the paraspinal musculature. With the patient still standing, the mobility of the spine is tested by having him or her bend forward and backward from the waist and laterally to each side. With the patient either sitting in a chair or with hips held, rotational movements of the trunk are tested also. Any limitations or production of pain are noted during these maneuvers.

The patient then is asked to get on the examining table, and the manner in which this is done is noted. With the patient sitting, straight-leg raising is carried out with the knee fully extended and the patient relaxed. Straight-leg raising is carried to its limits on both sides and then both legs are raised simultaneously; individual excursion that is less than simultaneous indicates malingering. If there is complaint of pain, it could be attributed to hamstring tightness, and straight-leg raising is repeated, adding dorsiflexion of the foot at a level below the first indications of pain by the previous straight-leg raising test. Pain with dorsiflexion is indicative of sciatic irritation. Straight-leg raising tests again are performed with the patient supine. Following this, the patient is asked to flex the knees and pull both knees directly to the chest. This flexion is easily accomplished without pain in lesions involving the sciatic nerve.

The patient then is placed in the prone position and hyperextension of the hip is carried out. With the patient prone, the knees are flexed and the foot dorsiflexed. Complaints of pain in this position are indicative of malingering; this is called a positive Gordon sign. With the patient in the prone position, skin-rolling tests are carried out by rolling a segment of skin over the lumbar paraspinal area between the thumb and index finger. If pain is elicited in the back and down the leg, this is indicative of a functional problem. With the patient still in the prone position, palpation over the soft tissues of the back is carried out to detect lipomas, nodules of fibrositis, or fatty herniation, as well as tenderness over spinous processes and intervertebral spaces and laterally over the foramina.

The patient then is put in the sitting position again, and, with the legs hanging freely, deep tendon reflexes are obtained. Diminution of the knee jerk is compatible with involvement of the L-3/L-4 lumbar disk, whereas diminution of the ankle jerk is compatible with nerve root compression of the S-1 nerve root by L-5/S-1 disk protrusion. Sensory testing is performed with a pinwheel, with special emphasis on the anterior medial surface of the thigh for the L-4 nerve root syndromes, over the medial surface of the foot and great toe for L-5 nerve root compression, and over the dorsum and lateral surfaces of the foot and little toe for S-1 nerve root compression. Measurements for chest expansion and measurements of thighs equidistant above the patella and the calves at their point of greatest circumference are recorded. Limited chest expansion is an early sign of arthritis of the spine and is believed to be important. The true leg length is ascertained by measuring from the anterior superior iliac spine to the medial malleolus of each leg.

Diagnosis.—X-ray studies of the lumbar spine are of little aid in diagnosing acute ruptured disk but may show other causes of pain in the low back, such as spondylolisthesis, spina bifida, facet abnormalities, malignancies, disease of the hip joint, unilateral sacralization and transitional vertebrae, and sclerosis or fusion of the sacroiliac spine.

In *lumbar sprains and strains* there may be an alteration of the normal lumbar lordosis. There is splinting of the spine as the patient bends forward, usually bending from the hips rather than the waist. There may be restriction of the lateral motions of the lumbar spine, with pain referable to the spinal musculature on rotatory and lateral motion. There may be palpable and percussible areas of tenderness over the lumbar spine and the muscular attachments. Flexed-leg raising may produce pain and be markedly restricted with musculoligamentous injuries.

In *ruptured intervertebral disk* several manifestations are particularly important when associated with radicular pain. A lateral list of the lumbar spine may be present; this is the so-called sciatic scoliosis, with the list usually away from the site of the lesion. Besides pain and limitation of motion, the presence of positive sciatic stretch signs, measurable atrophy of calf and thighs, and a neurologic deficit and absent reflexes corresponding to the same level may indicate the level of extruded disk. Confirmation of the diagnosis of a herniated disk is by electromyography, myelography, computed tomography scanning, or magnetic resonance imaging.

Management.—The management of low-back pain includes bed rest, application of heat to the low back, back braces and muscle relaxant-analgesic combinations, and, occasionally, physical therapy in more refractory cases. Later in the recovery stage, William's exercises are prescribed to develop the flexor muscles of the spine and the abdominal musculature to help prevent recurrence. Conservative care is abandoned in extreme cases of back pain in which the neurologic deficit is rapidly progressive, and surgery is entertained. An alternative to surgery is chemonucleolysis. This procedure involves injecting a herniated disk with chymopapain. This procedure may offer an alternative to laminectomy and has the same indications.

The Shoulder Joint

Trauma to the shoulder girdle is a common occurrence in our experience. In examining for shoulder injuries, the patient should be disrobed so that both shoulders are exposed to allow comparison of one side with the other. The attitude of the patient in the way the arm and shoulder are held may be indicative of the underlying pathology.

Clavicular Fractures.—These are readily identified by palpation of the clavicles from the acromion to the sternoclavicular joint. Undisplaced fractures can be demonstrated by percussing gently over the clavicle on one side and then the other and eliciting pain at the fracture site.

Dislocation of the Acromioclavicular Joint.—This results in separation of the outer end of the clavicle, which is well demonstrated by having the patient hold a 5-lb weight in each hand and observing the elevated distal clavicle. This also is a good way of demonstrating it by x-ray examination.

Anterior Dislocation of the Shoulder.—In this common type of dislocation, the patient presents a flattened outer surface of the shoulder with lowering of the axillary fold.

Rupture of the Supraspinatus Tendon.—This is characterized by the patient's inability to initiate abduction of the arm. If the arm is elevated passively to 90°, the deltoid can contract and complete the movement. Short of 90°, the patient cannot control it; this is the "arm drop sign." In rupture of the rotator cuff, the supraspinatus tendon is the component involved most frequently; however, the infraspinatus and subscapular tendons may be involved also. Although it is almost impossible to rupture a normal tendon, most adults have degenerative changes, and any patient 50 years of age or older who reports a forcible strain or fall and an inability to abduct the arm and has no x-ray evidence of fracture, dislocation, or other abnormality most probably has a rupture of the rotator cuff. Orthopedic consultation for selection of treatment is indicated when the diagnosis is made.

Rupture of the Biceps Tendon or Muscle.—This usually occurs to the long tendon of the biceps. The force required to rupture a tendon is dependent on its condition, as it, like other components of the rotator cuff, undergoes attritional and degenerative changes, and the force required for its rupture depends on its strength. On physical examination there is noted a lump on the biceps with elongation and relaxation of the tendon and loss of biceps power. Proper treatment is operative repair.

Tenosynovitis.—Another common clinical syndrome that occurs in the shoulder is bicipital tendinitis or tenosynovitis. This usually presents in patients who engage in unusual exercises associated with a wide range of shoulder motion. There is pain over the anterolateral aspect of the humeral head, with pain increased by active and passive motion and tenderness located along the bicipital groove. Maneuvers that increase the tension of the tendon increase the pain. Rest, salicylates, and application of ice are beneficial in the acute stages. Injection of Xylocaine and locally acting corticoids also relieve the acute pain.

The Elbow

Elbow Fractures and Dislocations.—These important lesions in the elbow are readily diagnosed, except in the case of fracture of the radial head. Sometimes diagnosis of these fractures is made on clinical grounds and the arm is immobilized for a few days, then an x-ray is repeated, and visual evidence of fracture is seen on the x-ray film taken at that time. If there is much displacement of the radial head in the annular ligament at the elbow, sometimes it is necessary to remove the proximal fragment to effectuate good pronation and supination following radial head fractures.

Tennis Elbow.—Another important lesion of the elbow is that known as *epicondylitis,* which occurs in housewives, bench hands, plumbers, carpenters, executives, and even in tennis players and is commonly known as "tennis elbow." It is thought that the cause of tennis elbow is an overloading force at the aponeurosis of the extensor attachment on the lateral epicondyle of the humerus. The pathophysiology is a muscular contraction-stretch injury from repeated trauma to the elbow. The diagnosis is made by having the patient forcefully extend the hand at the wrist against resistance, producing pain over the lateral epicondyle. Treatment consists of rest, application of ice or local heat or ultrasound, plus oral anti-inflammatory medication, such as phenylbutazone. If response to this conservative treatment is not quick, an injection of Xylocaine and locally acting steroids into the common extensor attachment at the lateral epicondyle on one or two occasions usually affords relief. A few patients who are recalcitrant to all other therapies require surgical release of the extensor aponeurosis followed by an active rehabilitation program of exercises.

Olecranon Bursitis.—This sometimes may follow trauma to the bursa overlying the olecranon process. If there is hematoma with the acute trauma, application of a protective dressing with padding over the olecranon for ten days usually will produce subsidence of the swelling. If there is a chronic bursal effusion, aspiration of its contents and injection of a locally acting cortisone solution followed by a compressive wrap usually is curative. A few cases will be refractory to all treatment and will require surgical excision of the bursa.

The Wrist

When resulting from falls and other activities, wrist injuries usually are dismissed as being due to a sprain or ligamentous or capsular tear around the joint. To avoid the pitfalls of making a sprain diagnosis for something far more serious, x-ray studies are made of all wrist complaints associated with trauma.

Ganglions.—These may become manifest after acute flexion injuries of the wrist; however, it is naïve to suppose that they arise from single traumatic episodes. The treatment of ganglions ranges from surgical excision to neglect. I favor an intracystic injection of locally acting steroids and Xylocaine (1:1) of sufficient quantity to rupture the ganglion.

Fractured Navicular.—This may result from a fall on an outstretched hand and may even be obscure on the x-ray film. In cases such as this, where there is pain around the base of the thumb on the radial side of the wrist, we treat with a volar splint for ten days, followed by repeat x-ray if the patient still is symptomatic. If a fracture line is seen at this time, the patient is referred for orthopedic care, which usually consists of plaster immobilization for 10–12 weeks. If the second x-ray is negative and the pain persists, the patient is immobilized for another ten days and a repeat x-ray is taken. Radial styloid fractures produce similar pains, but if the x-ray studies reveal the correct diagnosis, immobilization for ten days, followed by active motion, usually is adequate.

Fractured Triquetrum.—The second most injured carpal bone is the *triquetrum*. This fracture usually is a dorsal avulsion fracture and should be suspected in patients whose recovery is delayed; it is characterized by prolonged discomfort over the dorsum of the wrist following a fall. Because of the possibility of obscure serious injuries to the wrist, such as scapholunate dissociation, we routinely refer all patients with prolonged wrist symptoms for orthopedic evaluation despite negative x-ray studies after two weeks of immobilization.

Carpal Tunnel Syndrome.—A compressive neuropathy of the median nerve at the volar carpal ligament in the wrist, carpal tunnel syndrome may be the result of trauma over the butt of the hand or may also be the result of a tenosynovitis involving the flexor tendons that pass beneath the volar carpal ligament. In addition to these causes, which may have some relationship to occupation, there are several other causes that are well to keep in mind, such as the connective tissue diseases (rheumatoid arthritis, systemic lupus erythematosus), acromegaly, pregnancy, a positive association with the taking of estrogenic hormones, hypothyroidism, or vibration. The diagnosis is suggested by numbness and tingling in the distribution of the median nerve, with weakness of the thenar muscles, and pain, predominantly at night, in the wrist, hand, and forearm. Diagnosis is made by finding an underlying cause and by prolongation of the nerve conduction velocity of the median nerve at the volar carpal ligament. Treatment is by section of the volar carpal ligament; the results are good when the operation is performed before permanent nerve damage has occurred.

The Hand

Perhaps 70% of the injuries seen at the electronics manufacturing plant at which I work are those of the hand. Proper care of hand injuries is most important from a surgical standpoint because of the frequency of injury and the adverse effects of improper treatment. We routinely x ray compressive or crushing injuries of hands to accurately diagnose any fractures, dislocations, or unsuspected foreign bodies. This is done after a careful sterile dressing is applied and bleeding has been controlled, if there are open wounds. We then carefully test for any sensory loss. Lack of motor function would indicate avulsed, ruptured, or lacerated tendons. *The assessment of sensory function and tendon intactness is carried out without disturbing the wound* and can be done adequately if one has a working knowledge of the anatomy of the hand.

If the hand trauma is a lesion that can be repaired in our emergency operating room, the hand is cleansed with soap and water, and anesthesia usually is 1% Xylocaine block. In treating trauma of the hand, I think that it is well to remember that the first operation is by far the most important one to the future functioning of the injured parts, and certainly if there is a competent hand surgeon in the community, it would be well to use him or her as a consultant in cases of flexor tendon injuries, fractures of metacarpals, and injuries to the hand that are complicated by severance of neurovascular bundles. There are many pitfalls to the treatment of deeper hand wounds and some of these are associated with rupture of the ulnar collateral ligament of the metacarpophalangeal joint of the thumb, pressure gun injuries involving paint or paint thinner or grease, and those wounds involving extensive loss of skin from the fingers or palm.

The common lesions of the finger that can be treated simply include the mallet injury, in which striking the end of the finger against a hard object (particularly when it is in flexion) causes avulsion of the extensor to the distal phalanx at its insertion to the base of the distal phalanx. There are many types of splints designed to treat this injury; however, any hyperextension of the distal phalanx slightly above the 0° level that is maintained for five weeks usually will give an excellent functional and cosmetic result in most cases. A mallet finger with an avulsion of a large part of the articular surface—usually more than one third of it—probably should be treated with open reduction.

De Quervain's Stenosing Tendovaginitis.—This involves the abductor pollicis longus and extensor pollicis brevis tendons. This disease is an inflammatory condition of the tendon sheaths. Similar conditions occur in other tendons in the hands, particularly the flexor pollicis longus and flexor sheaths of the fingers. It is thought that this is an inflammation occurring from repeated motion in aging fibrous tissues. The majority of the cases happen in people beyond the age of 30. However, an occupational connotation is not present in all cases, since the disease also occurs in infants. When this condition exists in the flexor tendons, the constricting area of the tendon sheath is incised through a small transverse skin incision. When it affects the tendon sheath of the thumb, incision is made just proximal to the anatomical snuffbox. The test for this condition is Finklestein's test, and it is performed by having the patient flex the thumb into the palm and make a fist over the thumb with the fingers, and then put the fist in ulnar deviation. This causes pain over the snuffbox and over the thumb's extensor tendon sheath at the wrist. Treatment consists of splinting the wrist, corticoid injections and, in cases refractory to the aforementioned, surgery.

Traumatic Amputation.—This leads to a special problem having to do with replantation. If a patient has a severed thumb or finger, it should be put in a plastic bag on top of iced saline and taken with the patient to the hospital. The part should be cool but not frozen. Although there is no deadline for finger replantation, the sooner the replantation is attempted the more likely it is that it will succeed. Even if replantation is not possible, at times defects can be closed with part of the skin from dismembered parts after appropriate preparation.

Hypothenar Hammer Syndrome.—This syndrome results from the use of the hand as a hammer, which is a common practice of auto mechanics and others who pound hard objects with their hypothenar eminence. The syndrome results from thrombosis or aneurysm formation in the superficial branch of the ulnar artery as it courses over the carpal bones just beneath the palmaris brevis muscle, subcutaneous tissue, and skin. Testing for occlusion of the radial or ulnar artery is possible in the office by use of the Allen test. The patient's wrist is held tightly between the thumb and forefinger. The radial artery is occluded along with the ulnar artery by digital compression. The patient then squeezes the blood from his hand by making a fist several times; on opening the hand, it is blanched. By first releasing the radial artery, its patency can be judged by rapid reddening and a return to normal color. Alternatively, the ulnar artery is first released, and if the hand returns to its normal color, this is evidence that the ulnar artery is patent also. This syndrome should be looked for in people who have cold sensitivity (Raynaud's phenomenon), those who have a painful lump or mass in the hypothenar region, and those who have numbness in the fourth and fifth fingers.

Vibration.—This can cause injury in the hand of a traumatic, vasospastic type, which is seen in chain saw operators. The vasospasms seem to be triggered not only by the cold handles of the chain saws but by the dominant frequency of vibration in the chain saw. Dominant frequency of vibration in the chain saw (125 Hz) falls in the same frequency region where the pacinian corpuscles are especially sensitive to vibration.

The Lower Extremities

Knee Injuries.—Diagnosing knee injuries according to the injured structure and the severity of the injury is the key to appropriate diagnosis and recovery. After the mechanics of the injury are reviewed and the areas of anatomical disruption or injury have been assessed, x-ray examination is carried out. However, x-ray examination of industrial knee injuries does not usually reveal evidence of trauma, since most such knee injuries are soft-tissue in nature. Presence of preexisting pathology or previous knee injury is important in worker injuries because the potential of injury to knees from sports is much greater than that at work. Understanding the presence of preexisting pathology is most helpful in understanding some knee injuries. Examination is carried out with the patient supine and with both legs exposed. The knees are inspected for the presence of swelling, redness, or deformity.

The *posterior capsule* of the knee can be tested for by lifting both heels off the table. A significant tear in the posterior capsule results in the knee curving backward.

A *dislocated patella* is readily apparent with the patient supine by the lateral posture and difficulty in extending the knee. The knee is palpated by putting pressure over the suprapatellar bursa and pushing downward and ballotting the patella with the other hand for the presence of fluid. Active flexion of the knees is carried out with the normal and the affected knee. Presence of fluid or blood within the knee joint may restrict flexion considerably. Even in acute injuries, the presence or absence of muscle atrophy is tested for by measuring a point equidistant from both patellas and over the calf at its greatest circumference.

Anterior cruciate ligament injury is tested for by having the patient put the knee into 90° of flexion resting the foot on the examining table and pulling just below the knee to see if there is an abnormal anterior laxity. The posterior cruciate ligament is tested for by pushing posteriorly with the knee in 90° flexion.

Collateral ligament laxity is demonstrated by having the patient's knee in about 20° of flexion and applying lateral and medial forces to ascertain the presence of laxity over the medial or lateral collateral ligaments. Pain over the collateral ligament without laxity would lead to diagnosis of sprain of the medial collateral ligament, and, indeed, this is the most frequent injury of the knee joint that I see.

With the knee flexed, palpation around the knee joint is carried out, looking for tenderness localized along the anterior edge of the articular surface of the tibia, which may be an indication of ligamentous or cartilage tear. With the patient prone, the foot is grasped and the knee flexed until the heel approaches the buttock and the foot is rotated outward as the knee joint is steadily extended. A click during this maneuver would be considered a positive test for meniscus injury.

Fractured patella is an obvious injury and is revealed by appropriate x-rays if physical findings reveal anterior knee compartment swelling.

Ankle Joint Injuries.—These are quite common and usually are treated lightly. However, inadequate and delayed treatment may result in an ankle subject to recurrent sprains and strains. Sprain of the ankle usually is an adduction injury, and the foot is inverted under the weight of the body, resulting in tears and strains of the external lateral ligaments. Exquisite tenderness usually is demonstrated by palpating the ankle around the bony landmarks of the malleoli. X-ray examination is carried out on all ankle sprains attended by excessive swelling, to rule out fractures in and around the ankle. Our initial treatment is ice, elevation, and a compression dressing, which is composed of sheet wadding and compressive elastic bandage. Reexamination is carried out 24 hours later, followed by the decision for further immobilization or ambulation.

Injuries to the Foot.—Fractures of the toes are extremely important and usually come about by compressive forces of considerable magnitude that are applied over ordinary (not safety) shoes. In simple transverse fractures of the phalanges of the toes not involving the big toe, appropriate soft-tissue care and taping of the toes adjacent is helpful. Use of fracture shoes affords some comfort by providing a firm sole that does not permit flexion or extension of the toes on walking.

Stress fractures or fractures of the midmetatarsal gradually arising are difficult to diagnose and at times are diagnosed only during the healing stage, as evidenced by the presence of callus. The diagnosis is thought of when the patient has some swelling over the dorsum of the forefoot, with pain on compression and on walking. Fractures of the proximal fifth metatarsal occur frequently in stepping off a curb or by lateral forces or contusions to the outer aspect of the foot. These, too, can be managed by fracture shoes if there is no great displacement of the fracture fragments.

Subungual Hematomas.—Subungual hematomas from contusions without fracture of the phalanges are handled by evacuating the pulsating hematoma. This is simply carried out by flaming the tip of a paper clip and gently burning a hole through the nail over the subungual collection. It escapes by itself and is attended by great relief.

Acknowledgments

Thanks to Patsy Strouse, R.N., Karl Kumler, M.D., Myron Smith, M.D., for their assistance.

REFERENCES

1. *Accident Facts*. Chicago, National Safety Council, 1983.
2. Armstrong TJ, Chaffin DB: Carpal tunnel syndrome and selected personal attributes. *J Occup Med* 1979; 21:481.
3. Artz CP: Changing concepts of electrical injury. *Am J Surg* 1974; 128:600.
4. Blaisdell FW, Trunkey DD: *Trauma Management, vol I, Abdominal Trauma*. New York, Thieme-Stratton, Inc, 1982.
5. Boyes JH: *Bunnell's Surgery of the Hand*, ed 5. Philadelphia, JB Lippincott, Co, 1970.
6. Bustrous GS, Bexton DG, Male JC, et al: Interference with the pacemakers of two workers at electricity substations. *Br J Ind Med* 1983; 40:462.
7. Cailliet R: *Neck and Arm Pain*. Philadelphia, FA Davis, Co, 1964.
8. Cailliet R: *Shoulder Pain*. Philadelphia, FA Davis, Co, 1966.
9. Dunphy JE, Botsford TW: *Physical Examination of the Surgical Patient*, ed 4. Philadelphia, WB Saunders Co, 1975.
10. *Early Care of the Injured Patient*, ed 3. Committee on Trauma, American College of Surgeons. Philadelphia, WB Saunders Co, 1982.
11. Eckert C: *Emergency Room Care*, ed 4. Boston, Little, Brown & Co, 1981.
12. Furste W: The Seventh International Conference on Tetanus, Copanello (Catanzara), Italy, editorial. *J Trauma* 1987; 27:1–99.
13. Goldwyn RM: The injured hand, a panel by correspondence. *Arch Surg* 1971; 103:691.
14. Havener WH: *Synopsis of Ophthalmology*, ed 6. St Louis, C V Mosby Co, 1984.
15. Hyvarinen J, et al: Vibration frequencies and amplitudes in etiology of traumatic vasospastic disease. *Lancet* 1973; 1:791.
16. Lampe EW: Surgical anatomy of the hand. *Ciba Clinical Symposia* 1957; vol 9, No 1, Jan–Feb.
17. Little JM, Ferguson DA: Incidence of hypothenar hammer syndrome. *Arch Surg* 1972; 105:684.
18. Nicholls RJ: Initial choice of antibiotic treatment for pyogenic hand infections. *Lancet* 1973; 1:225.
19. Schwartz GB: *Principles and Practice of Emergency Medicine*, 2 vols. Philadelphia, WB Saunders Co, 1978.
20. Shires GT: *Care of the Trauma Patient*, ed 2. New York, McGraw-Hill Book Co, 1979.
21. Vibration can cause injury, editorial. *JAMA* 1973; 223:683.
22. Wickstrom G, Hänninen K, Mattsson T, et al: Knee degeneration in concrete reinforcement workers. *Br J Ind Med* 1983; 40:216.
23. Worth MH: *Principles and Practice of Trauma Care*. Baltimore, Williams & Wilkins Co, 1982.
24. Zuidema GD, et al: *The Management of Trauma*, ed 3. Philadelphia, WB Saunders Co, 1979.

10

Occupational Dermatoses

C. G. Toby Mathias, M.D.

HISTORICAL ASPECTS

In 1700 A.D., Bernardino Ramazzini[99] called attention to diseases of workers in his classic text, *De Morbis Artificium.* This work contained explicit descriptions of a variety of occupational skin diseases which remain true even today. Examples included fissuring dermatitis of the hands from lye, leg ulcerations among salt miners, and grain mite dermatitis. As noted by Schwartz et al.,[109] this latter observation was remarkable, since Ramazzini was able to deduce the probable cause as an "invisible parasite" on the basis of his clinical observations alone, without the aid of a microscope.

In 1775, Percival Pott published the first detailed description of occupationally induced cancer of the scrotum in chimney sweeps, which he correctly attributed to soot penetrating through clothing and being rubbed into scrotal skin as the sweep descended within the chimney. The potent carcinogenic properties of tars were later verified by numerous authorities, and have proved to be an important research tool in the experimental induction of cutaneous neoplasm.

However, it was not until the Industrial Revolution that substantial medical attention was given to diseases of occupational origin. Robert Willan and Thomas Bateman described occupational contact dermatitis from shoe wax among cobblers and from sugar and spice among bakers. Thackrah noted contact dermatitis in tobacco handlers. Potton described dermatitis in silk winders. In 1859, Hespian reported dermatitis induced by coal tar. Becourt and Chevalier correctly identified chromate as an important cause of industrial dermatitis in 1859, and Halforto described mercury dermatitis in craftsmen. Occupationally acquired skin infections from fungus, vaccines, and anthrax were reported among animal and hide handlers by the distinguished French physicians Alibert, Rayer, and Ibresile.[109]

The first major treatise devoted solely to occupational skin disease, *The Dermatergoses,* initially published in 1915 and subsequently revised, was written by Robery Prosser White, an energetic English general practitioner.[98] The detailed clinical descriptions of a wide variety of skin disorders contained in this text remain remarkably accurate.

Following the dramatic growth and expansion of the chemical and petroleum industries in the United States after World War I, interest in occupational skin disease became so great that the U.S. Public Health Service organized the Office of Dermatoses Investigations in 1928. This effort culminated in the publication of *Occupational Diseases of the Skin* by Schwartz, Tulipan, and Peck in 1939.[107] The last revised edition of this excellent and comprehensive text was published in 1957.[109] Although dramatic technologic changes within industry since then have either made portions of this text obsolete or have created new causative agents, recent smaller texts provide excellent but limited supplemental information on these subjects.[2, 42, 74]

EPIDEMIOLOGY

Clinical Types

Occupational skin disease accounts for only a small portion (1%–2%) of all occupational injuries or illnesses. Excluding injuries, however, which account for 96%–97% of all cases, skin disease accounts for 40%–50% of all remaining occupational illnesses (Table 10–1).

Approximately 80%–90% of all types of occupational skin disease may be classified as contact dermatitis, while another 5% is due to infection. California data (Table 10–2) illustrate that only a small percentage of skin disease cases are due to disorders other than contact dermatitis or skin infection (e.g., urticaria, acneiform

TABLE 10–1.
Occupational Injuries and Illnesses, 1975*

TYPE OF CASE	TOTAL CASES	INCIDENCE†	PERCENT OF TOTAL
All	4,983,100	0.91	100
Injuries	4,819,000	0.88	96.7
Illnesses	163,000	0.03	3.3
Skin disease	74,400	0.014	1.5

*Adapted from Wang CL: The problem of skin disease in industry. Office of Occupational Safety and Health Statistics, US Dept of Labor, 1978.
†Rates per 1,000 full-time employees.

TABLE 10–2.
Types of Occupational Skin Disease (California, 1977)*

TYPES	PERCENT
Contact Dermatitis	92.2
Skin Infections	5.4
All Others	2.4

*Modified from California Department of Industrial Relations, Division of Labor Statistics and Research: *Occupational Skin Disease in California (With Special Reference to 1977).* San Francisco, California Department of Industrial Relations, 1982.

eruptions, or pigmentary disorders). Approximately 80% of all cases of contact dermatitis are believed to result from skin irritation rather than contact allergy.

Causative Agents

Causal agents of occupational skin disease are ranked in Table 10–3. The data probably reflect the large numbers of employees in the workforce who are exposed to these agents, more than any inherent risk from exposure to the individual causal agents themselves. The large percentage of cases attributable to poison oak is unique to California.

The most frequently identified solvents causing occupational skin disease in California have been acetone, chlorinated hydrocarbons (freon and methylene chloride), toluene, xylene, petroleum distillate, and alcohols. Fiberglass accounted for 70% of all cases attributable to dust, while rock wool (and other insulating materials), dried cement and plaster dust, paper dust, and sawdust accounted for most of the remainder. Fruits and vegetables caused almost two thirds of all cases of dermatitis attributable to food products. Epoxy resins accounted for the largest percentage of cases to various plastics and resins. Causal agents will vary in importance within various industry classifications. The most important causal agents within selected industries have been listed in Table 10–4.

TABLE 10–3.
Causal Agents of Occupational Skin Disease and Percent Distribution (California, 1977)*

CAUSAL AGENT	PERCENT
Poison oak	23.7
Soaps, detergents, cleaning agents	6.1
Solvents	5.0
Fiberglass and particulate dusts	4.7
Food products	4.2
Plastics and resins	3.9
Petroleum products (nonsolvent)	3.3
Plant and animal products (inedible)	3.3
Agricultural chemicals	3.0
Infectious agents	2.5
Metals and their salts	1.7
Cutting oils and coolants	1.3
Environmental conditions	1.1
Textiles, fabrics, materials	0.9
Rubbish, dirt, sewage	0.3
Miscellaneous chemical agents	17.9
All others	0.9
Unspecified	16.2
Total	100

*From California Department of Industrial Relations, Division of Labor Statistics and Research: *Occupational Skin Disease in California (With Special Reference to 1977).* San Francisco, California Department of Industrial Relations, 1982. Used by permission.

TABLE 10–4.
Important Causal Agents of Occupational Skin Disease by Selected Industry Classifications*

INDUSTRY CLASSIFICATION	PERCENT
Manufacturing	
Electronic equipment, components	
Solvents	12.8
Plastics and resins	10.2
Acids	8.8
Fiberglass	6.9
Metals and metallic salts	6.6
Machinery	
Cutting oils	14.2
Solvents	10.7
Petroleum products (nonsolvent)	10.7
Fiberglass	8.2
Plastics and resins	4.9
Fabricated metal products	
Petroleum products (nonsolvent)	17.1
Solvents	10.1
Metals and metallic salts	8.0
Acids	7.7
Cutting oils	5.9
Chemicals and allied products	
Solvents	12.7
Plastics and resins	8.4
Rubber and plastic products	
Plastics and resins	18.9
Fiberglass	14.9
Solvents	5.9
Stone, clay, glass products	
Fiberglass	8.7
Cement, mortar, plaster (wet)	8.7
Plastics and resins	8.4
Dusts	6.8
Solvents	5.0
Food products	
Fruits, vegetables, meats	32.2
Soaps, detergents, cleaning agents	8.2
Caustics	4.6

(continued)

TABLE 10–4. *Continued*

INDUSTRY CLASSIFICATION	PERCENT
Lumber and wood products	
Poison oak	39.7
Fiberglass	13.3
Glues, pastes, adhesives	7.3
Plants (inedible)	5.0
Agriculture	
Poison oak	35.5
Agricultural chemicals	16.2
Fruits, nuts, vegetables	11.8
Plant and animal products (inedible)	9.8
Construction	
Poison oak	54.3
Cement, mortar, plaster (wet)	8.8
Fiberglass and other dust	6.1
Hospitals/health services	
Soaps, detergents, cleaning agents	26.6
Infectious agents	16.7
Medicines, disinfectants	6.2
Restaurants	
Soaps, detergents, cleaning agents	48.6
Food products (miscellaneous)	10.6
Fruits, nuts, vegetables	4.8

*Adapted from California Department of Industrial Relations, Division of Labor Statistics and Research: *Occupational Skin Disease in California (With Special Reference to 1977).* San Francisco, California Department of Industrial Relations, 1982.

Rates and Risks

Because large surface areas of skin are directly exposed to the environment, this organ is particularly vulnerable to occupationally induced disease. Excluding injuries and accidents, the skin accounts for a disproportionately large percentage of all remaining occupational illnesses. Surveys conducted by the National Bureau of Labor Statistics (BLS) from 1972 to 1976 consistently demonstrated that the skin accounted for approximately 40% of occupational illnesses, with an incidence of 1.7 per 1,000 full-time employees in the private sector.[120] Although the proportion of occupational illnesses attributed to skin disease has remained relatively constant, the annual incidence figures have been steadily declining. By 1982, the incidence had fallen to 0.7 per 1,000 full-time private sector employees, a drop of over 50%.* With over 100 million people now employed in the private sector workforce,[115] one can conservatively estimate that there are at least 70,000 new cases of occupational skin disease annually.

The precise reason for this decline in annual incidence is unclear. Automation and new technology have almost certainly reduced the total numbers of individuals within industry directly exposed to potential cutaneous irritants and allergens, and they have contributed to a larger percentage of the workforce being employed in lower-risk, service-oriented occupations. However, there is reason to suspect that part of this decline has resulted from exploitation of a "loophole" in the Occupational Safety and Health Administration (OSHA) reporting system, from which the BLS statistics are derived. "Injury" is defined by OSHA as a condition resulting from a "one-time exposure," an unfortunately vague term. Injuries do not have to be recorded in the OSHA log unless they result in time lost from work, but regulations mandate that *all* illnesses be recorded, regardless of whether these cases result in lost work time. By considering an illness to have resulted from a "one-time injury," employers may be able to classify these as injuries, e.g., chemical burns. This is particularly advantageous if no lost work time has occurred, since the case would not have to be recorded in the OSHA log. In California's semiconductor industry, the annual incidence for occupational illness fell from 1.3 per 100 workers to 0.3, possibly due to this loophole.[69] Additionally, if an injury or illness is treated only with "first aid," the condition does not have to be reported. The employment of occupational health nurses and other safety personnel by large companies to administer "first aid" may not only reduce the overall costs of occupational disease, but also the incidence statistics.†

The difficulty in accurately determining the true incidence of occupational skin disease is compounded by the ultimate dependency of all reporting systems on reliable recognition by treating physicians, employers, or employees in the first place. Inadequate training in occupational dermatology and busy office work schedules may leave physicians unprepared to make a proper diagnosis or too busy to complete the proper reporting claims. Insufficient monitoring of the work environment and inadequate training of health and safety personnel may lead to underrecognition by management. If neither management nor physicians recognize occupational disease, the responsibility settles on the employee, who requires adequate job health education to do so. If a survey by Discher and associates[34] is correct, only 2% of occupational illnesses had been correctly diagnosed and entered into the BLS statistics. This observation led these investigators to conclude that the true incidence of occupational illness was probably 10–50 times greater than its reported incidence.

The incidence of occupational skin disease may vary from one geographic location to another. In 1977 skin disease accounted for 40% of all occupational illnesses in California, with an incidence rate of 2.7 per 1,000 full-time employees.[22] In South Carolina from July 1978 to June 1979, however, skin disease accounted for 83% of all the occupational illnesses, with an incidence rate of 1.1 per 1,000 workers.[62]

Manufacturing and agricultural industries have fourfold higher relative risks for development of occupational skin disease (Table 10–5). The incidence of occupational skin disease among agricultural workers is 4.1 per 1,000 employees, compared to an approximate average incidence of 1.3.

Disability

Bureau of Labor statistics from 1972 through 1976 indicate that approximately 23.7% of all occupational skin disease cases lost an average of 11 days from work.[124] Data from California and South Carolina have been similar, with 25% and 21.6% of all skin

*C. Wang, U.S. Dept of Labor, Division of Labor Statistics and Periodic Surveys: Personal communication.

†Joseph LaDou, MD, Peninsula Medical Clinic, Palo Alto, California. Personal communication.

TABLE 10–5.

Incidence Rates and Relative Risks for Occupational Skin Diseases by Major Industry Classification*†

INDUSTRY	ALL CASES	LOST WORKDAY CASES	LOST WORKDAYS PER LWC‡	RISK
Agriculture§	5.1	1.0	6.4	4.1
Manufacturing	2.6	0.6	11.7	4.1
Construction	1.0	0.3	7.3	0.8
Transportation	0.8	0.2	7.0	0.6
Services	0.7	0.2	6.5	0.5
Wholesale trade	0.5	0.2	20	0.4
Mining	0.4	0.2	7.5	0.3
Retail trade	0.4	0.1	15	0.2
Finance, insurance, real estate	0.1	<0.05	>18	0.1

*Adapted from Wang CL: *The Problem of Skin Disease in Industry.* Office of Occupational Safety and Health Statistics, US Dept of Labor, 1978.
†Rates per 1,000 full-time private sector employees.
‡Lost workday cases.
§Includes forestry and fishing.

TABLE 10–6.

Causal Agents of Occupational Skin Disease and Lost Workday Cases*

CAUSAL AGENT	LWC†	TOTAL	PERCENT
Poison oak	761	4,147	18.4
Soaps, detergents, cleaning agents	261	1,071	24.4
Solvents	161	880	18.3
Fiberglass and particulate dusts	127	780	16.3
Food products	219	739	29.6
Plastics and resins	146	681	21.4
Petroleum products (nonsolvent)	99	577	17.2
Plant and animal products (inedible)	108	575	18.8
Agricultural chemicals	136	526	25.9
Infectious agents	108	445	24.3
Metals and their salts	46	294	15.6
Cutting oils and coolants	24	235	10.2
Environmental conditions	36	189	19.0
Textiles, fabrics, materials	31	164	18.9
Rubbish, dirt, sewage	11	45	24.4
Miscellaneous chemical agents	645	3,113	20.7
All others	26	163	16.0
Unspecified	466	2,828	16.5

*Adapted from California Department of Industrial Relations, Division of Labor Statistics and Research: *Occupational Skin Disease in California (With Special Reference to 1977).* San Francisco, California Department of Industrial Relations, 1982.
†Lost workday cases.

disease cases losing an average of 9 and 10.2 days per lost workday case, respectively.[22, 62] Lost workdays are not normally distributed among these lost workday cases. In California, 25% of all lost workday cases lost more than one week (California Department of Industrial Relations). In South Carolina, 26% lost more than one week but accounted for 82% of all lost workdays; the median number of lost workdays was only 2.3.* Lost workday cases among female workers are not higher than among male counterparts, but there is a trend toward a greater number of lost workdays among women employed in manufacturing per lost workday case than among men.[22]

Lost workday case incidence and lost workdays per lost workday case are depicted in Table 10–5. Lost workday cases have been listed by causal agent from California data in Table 10–6.

Demographics

Data from California[22] indicate that, although more than 40% of the workers employed in 1977 were female, only 28% of occupational skin disease cases occurred among women. Excluding all cases among outdoor workers (primarily men), this figure rose to only 34%. This lower overall rate may be attributable to a larger proportion of women having been employed in occupations at lower risk for development of occupational skin disease. In manufacturing, the incidence rate for women was actually higher (4.7 per 1,000 women) compared to men (3.8 per 1,000 men). Whether this difference was due to an enhanced susceptibility of female skin to irritation or a relative inexperience among female workers has not been established.

Inexperience contributes to the development of occupational skin disease. California employers corroborate the opinion that recently hired employees are more likely to develop dermatitis than those with a longer period of employment. Approximately 25% of all disabling occupational skin diseases occurred within the first three months of employment, and 45% occurred within the first year. In contrast, only one out of six workers disabled for injuries or illnesses other than dermatitis had been employed for three months or less.[22]

The hands and wrists are the most frequent body sites on which occupational skin disease develops, while covered areas are involved in only a small percentage of cases. The hands were involved in one third of California cases,[22] while 80% of cases from South Carolina affected the hands.[112] Personal experience suggests that the latter percentage is a better estimate.

Costs

Reliable determinations of annual costs directly attributable to occupational skin disease are difficult to achieve, but some reasonable estimates may be obtained from published data. Assuming a private sector work force population of 100 million in 1984 and minimum incidence of 0.7 per 1,000 employees, there are at least 70,000 new cases of occupational skin disease annually. Based on South Carolina data, the average medical cost per case is $67.50 for an annual total of $4,725,000. The average compensation payments for lost wages are $1,590 per compensated case (i.e., only those cases losing more than seven workdays). Assuming 22.5% of all cases lose time from work and 25% of these lost-workday cases receive disability payments, the annual indemnity costs for compensated cases total $6,360,000.[85] Assuming 10.5 lost workdays per lost-workday case, an average eight-hour workday, and an average hourly wage of $8.28 in 1984, annual costs attributable

*Source: Ed Shmunes, Department of Dermatology, University of South Carolina.

to lost worker-productivity exceed $11 million. This brings the total annual costs of medical treatment, disability payments, and lost worker-productivity to $22 million. If the Discher report estimates of underreporting are correct (and there is good reason to believe they are), this figure needs to be inflated 10- to 50-fold, bringing annual cost estimates into the range of $220 million to $1 billion dollars annually.

STRUCTURE AND FUNCTION OF SKIN[41, 87]

The skin (Fig 10–1) is composed of two principal layers, the epidermis and dermis. Each layer contains structural elements which are important not only in regard to their function but also in regard to disease processes which may affect them.

The epidermis is approximately 100–200 μ thick. The innermost layer is composed of a thin layer of germinative basal cells, which reproduce every 14 days. The bulk of epidermal thickness is comprised of metabolically active squamous cells, which are connected to each other by numerous desmosomal junctions. Squamous cells synthesize keratinous filaments and keratohyaline granules, destined to become the principal structural proteins of the outermost protective stratum corneum as well as membrane-coating granules composed of complex lipids. As the squamous cells are pushed upwards by dividing cells from below, they enter a zone of transition (the granular layer) and undergo a process of maturation called *cornification*, in which cytoplasmic contents are condensed, nuclear contents disintegrate, and the membrane-coating granules are extruded into the intercellular spaces, where they contribute to the intercellular barrier. Intercellular tight junctions increase in number in the granular layer. The end result of this maturation process is a densely packed layer of relatively impermeable, cornified "dead" cells, the stratum corneum, which constitutes the principal protective barrier against penetration by exogenous chemical substances and microorganisms.

Some protection against exposure to alkaline substances is also afforded by virtue of the buffering action of lactic acid, amphoteric amines, and weak bases deposited on the stratum corneum surface by eccrine sweat, outward diffusion of carbon dioxide through the skin, or decomposition of the most superficial layer of cells. Free fatty acids, on the skin surface, derived from enzymatic degradation of sebaceous gland lipid, possess some antifungal and antibacterial activity, and offer further chemical protection against invasion by cutaneous microorganisms. Odd-numbered C5 through C13 fatty acids have more potent antifungal activity than even-numbered chains, while long-chain unsaturated fatty acids have limited bacteriostatic activity.

Melanocytes are located along the basal cell layer and synthesize a protective pigment, melanin. This pigment is packaged within melanocytes into granules (melanosomes). Under suitable

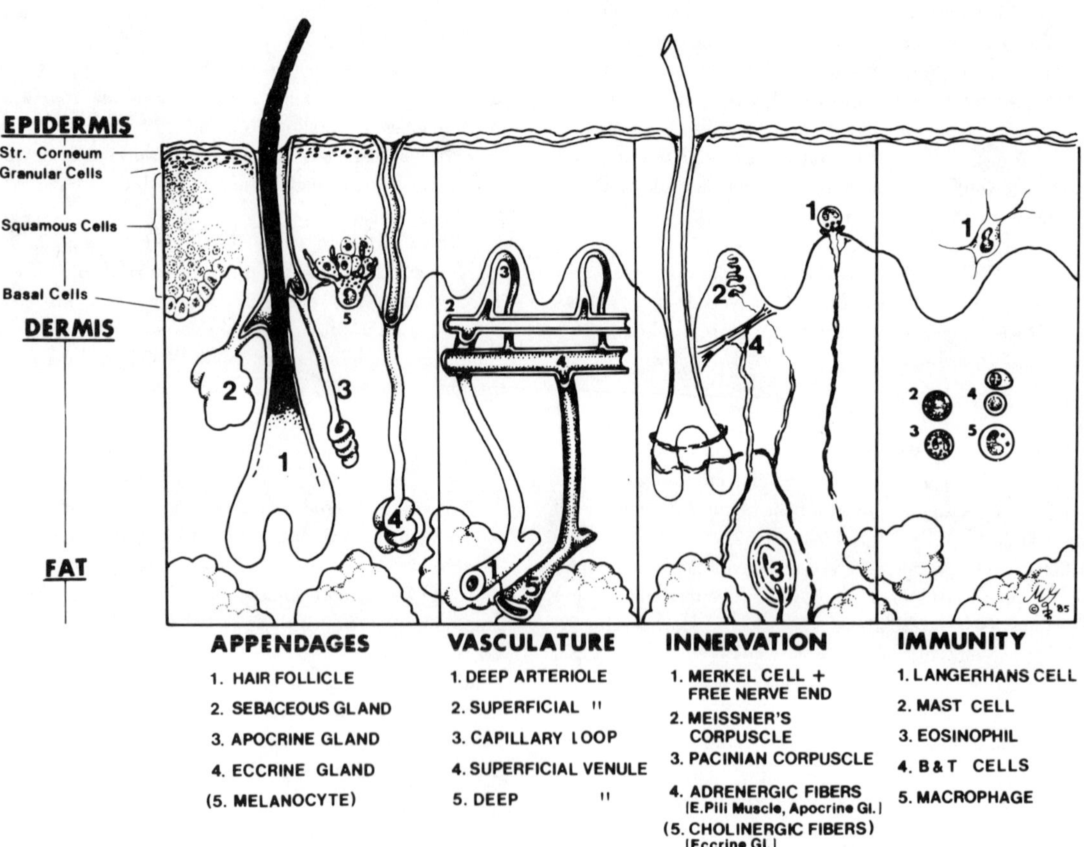

FIG 10–1.
Anatomical structures and components of skin. (Illustration courtesy of Dr. Marc Goldyne.)

stimulation from ultraviolet radiation, these granules are dispersed into neighboring keratinocytes through dendritic extensions of cytoplasm, resulting in the darkening of skin complexion and enhanced protection from ultraviolet radiation. The starting point of melanin synthesis is the amino acid tyrosine, which is converted by the copper-dependent enzyme tyrosinase into dihydroxyphenylalanine (dopa). Melanin synthesis subsequently proceeds through a number of intermediary steps before the final melanin polymer is formed. Melanocytes may be selectively inhibited or destroyed by the toxic effects of phenolic substances structurally resembling tyrosine, resulting in cutaneous depigmentation.

Langerhans' cells are present in the basal and suprabasal layers of the epidermis. These dendritic cells possess immunochemical surface markers similar to macrophages and histiocytes. Accumulated evidence strongly suggests that these cells actively participate in cutaneous immune regulation and surveillance and are responsible for antigen processing and presentation to circulating T lymphocytes. Selective uptake of simple contact antigens by Langerhans' cells has been demonstrated.[110] T lymphocytes subsequently circulate through dermal lymphatic channels to the paracortical areas of regional lymph nodes, where further antigen processing occurs.

Densely intertwined nerve tissue fibers, the dermal nerve network, transverse the superficial dermis and dermal papillae and function as the principal sensory receptors. Merkel cells, most numerous in the suprabasalar epidermis of fingers, oral mucosa, and outer sheaths of hair follicles, are closely associated with terminal neuroaxons derived from these myelinated cutaneous nerves. These cells contain densely cored cytoplasmic granules similar to monoamine-containing granules in other neuroreceptor cells and probably function as mechanoreceptors. Vater-Pacini corpuscles, which are found deep in the dermis of hair-bearing skin, are encapsulated, specialized nerve tissue organs responsible for the sensation of pressure. Other specialized nerve tissue elements found in the skin include mucocutaneous end organs, found most abundantly in superficial dermal tissue of mucous membranes, and Meissner's corpuscles, found only in the volar dermal tissue of the hands and feet. No specialized cutaneous sensation has been ascribed to these latter nerve endings.

Blood is distributed within dermal tissue through a highly developed, interconnected network of superficial and deep dermal vessels. Capillary loops extend from dermal arterioles to interface with the overlying epidermis within the dermal papillae. Cutaneous blood flow is regulated by constriction of metarterioles and precapillary sphincters, and a large volume of circulating blood may be brought close to the skin surface. The masses of interlacing small vessels function primarily for thermoregulation and tissue nutrition. Mast cells are often arranged around the walls of small vessels. These cells contain granules within which pharmacologically active substances (histamine, heparin, serotonin, and leukotriene precursors) are found. Upon appropriate physical, chemical, or antigen stimulation, mast cells release their granules, the contents of which participate in a number of diverse pathologic reactions resulting in vasodilation.

The bulk of perceptible skin thickness is due to a loose matrix of dermal connective tissue, composed of fibrous proteins (collagen, elastin, and reticulin) embedded in an amorphous ground substance. The tensile strength and elasticity of the dermis help protect the body from mechanical injury, while the permeability characteristics of ground substance allow diffusion of nutrients from dermal blood vessels to fibroblasts and other cellular elements of the dermis, as well as to the epidermis. Dermal connective tissue may participate in a number of pathologic reactions, including excessive scar tissue formation in response to cutaneous trauma.

Eccrine sweat glands are found on all cutaneous surfaces, but are most numerous on the palms and soles. The ducts of these coiled appendages transverse the epidermis and deposit their contents on the skin surface. Sweat glands are innervated by cholinergic nerve terminals and respond principally to thermal stimulation and emotional stress. Local heating of skin lowers the threshold response of sweat glands to cholinergic stimulation. Acclimatization of sweat glands to thermal stimulation also occurs, and repeated daily exposures to heat eventually produce a marked increase in the rate of sweating. Although the primary function of eccrine sweat glands is to provide evaporative cooling when the body is stressed by heat, secondary buffering of the skin surface against alkaline substances may be provided by lactic acid, amphoteric amines, and weak bases contained in sweat.

Sebaceous glands are intimately associated with hair follicles and share a common ductal opening, lined with stratified squamous epithelium, to the skin surface. The oily content of the sebaceous gland (sebum) is composed chiefly of triglycerides, wax esters, and squalene. Sebum production and secretion is principally due to androgenic stimulation. The glands are largest on the forehead, face, scrotum, and anogenital skin. In some locations, sebaceous glands may open directly onto the skin surface, for example, onto the meibomian glands of the eyelid margins and the glands of the areolae. In mammals, the general function of sebum is that of a sexual attractant (pheromone), but its function in man is unclear. The fatty acids derived from sebum have some bacteriostatic and fungistatic properties and may have a limited function in this regard once deposited on the skin surface. Apocrine glands, found in the axillae and anogenital skin, possess no known useful function in man, but their secretions may be responsible for sexual attractiveness in lower primates.

Hair follicles are found on all cutaneous surfaces except the palms, soles, and mucous membranes. The roots (bulbs) extend below the level of the sebaceous glands, with which they share a common duct. Hair grows cyclically, with alternating periods of growth (anagen phase) and quiescence (telogen phase); the transitional phase between growth and quiescence is termed catagen. The hair follicles of man grow and rest independently of one another, and some shedding of hair occurs continuously. Although the duration of the growth phase may be extremely variable, depending on the body regions in which the hairs are located, the quiescent phase generally lasts only one to three months. During this period, the hair bulbs shorten and retract, the outer root sheath in the bulb becomes detached, and "club" hairs are shed before new growth begins. Although hair has some protective and insulating functions in other animals, this function is relatively unimportant in man. Instead, the principal function of hair, with its richly innervated bulbs, appears to be that of a secondary sensory organ. Alterations in the hair growth cycle may lead to sudden and increased loss of hair.

The nail plates on the tips of the digits overlying the thickened, stratified epidermis of the nail beds are composed of tightly packed, keratinized cells. The germinal cells from which the plate is derived are found in the nail matrix, an oblique wedge of tissue located beneath the proximal nail fold. The cuticle, a cornified epidermal extension from the proximal nail fold over the nail plate, protects the nail matrix and underlying tissue of the proximal nail fold from exogenous chemical substances and microorganisms. Although man has adapted his nails for a number of uses, the primary function is to assist in the grasping and manipulation of small objects. The nail folds, matrices, and beds are susceptible to a number of environmental insults, resulting in dystrophic growth, infection, or separation of the plate from the nail bed.

The structure and function of the various cutaneous components, as well as their susceptibility to occupational disease, have been summarized in Table 10–7.

CLINICAL ASPECTS

Contact Dermatitis

General Considerations

Contact dermatitis is by far the most common occupational dermatosis. The term refers to the induction of cutaneous changes, usually accompanied by inflammation, from direct skin exposure to exogenous chemical or physical substances. Inflammation is provoked by either (or both) of two mechanisms, irritation or allergy. The end result of either reaction pathway is a progression of clinical changes inevitably accompanied by transudation of serum through the epidermis. These changes range from slight dryness, chapping, and redness of the skin surface to frank vesicles or blisters. At least 80%–90% of contact dermatitis cases are secondary to irritation rather than allergy, and the majority (another 80%–90%) are caused by chemical substances.

The inflammatory cutaneous changes that occur from skin irritation result from a direct, local, toxic effect on cellular elements in the skin, leading to cell death, release of lysosomal enzymes and soluble inflammatory mediators, recruitment of inflammatory cells, and further tissue destruction. Although substantial tissue destruction may quickly occur following relatively brief skin exposure to strong caustics or corrosives (i.e., chemical burns), the majority of cases of irritant contact dermatitis result from cumulative and repetitive exposures to "weak" irritants, substances which are not likely to produce visible cutaneous injury following only brief or limited exposure. Two points deserve repeated emphasis here: (1) virtually any substance, under the right set of circumstances, is potentially capable of causing irritant contact dermatitis,[66] and (2) clinical irritant contact dermatitis often results from multiple, cumulative exposures to several potential skin irritants, rather than from just a single substance. Irritant dermatitis generally remains confined to the primary areas of skin exposure and

TABLE 10–7.
Structure, Function, and Occupational Disorders of the Skin

STRUCTURE	FUNCTION	OCCUPATIONAL DISORDER
Stratum corneum	Barrier against chemical diffusion & microorganisms	Chapping from low humidity, chemical stains
Squamous and basal cells of epidermis	Cell regeneration, synthesis of stratum corneum, wound repair	Infection, contact dermatitis, neoplasms
Melanocytes and melanin	Absorption of ultraviolet radiation	Toxic vitiligo, melanoma, hyperpigmentation
Langerhans' cells, lymphatics, dermal macrophages	Immune regulation & surveillance	Delayed hypersensitivity reactions
Merkel cells, nerve tissue elements	Perception of environment	Toxic neuropathies
Blood vessels, mast cells	Thermoregulation, nutrition of tissue	Heat stroke, contact and systemic urticaria, flushing reactions, vibration "white" finger
Connective tissue	Mechanical protection against trauma, wound repair	Infection, granulomatous reactions, scleroderma, solar elastosis, scar
Eccrine sweat glands	Thermoregulation, buffering of skin surface	Miliaria, "rusting"
Sebaceous glands	Synthesis of skin surface lipids, chemical barrier against microorganisms	Oil acne, chloracne
Hair, follicles	Insulation and protection, secondary sensory organs, social appearance	Folliculitis, traumatic or toxic alopecia
Nails	Grasping & manipulation of small objects	Paronychia, dystrophy, oncholysis

does not spread to other parts of the body where the affected individual is not aware of direct exposure.

The factors which predispose to the development of cutaneous irritation are summarized in Table 10–8.[81] While the inherent caustic or corrosive chemical properties of a substance obviously influence whether cutaneous irritation will develop, other considerations are important. Physical properties such as molecular size, weight, ionization, and polarity affect the ability of a chemical substance to penetrate the protective barrier and provoke inflammation. Large (molecular weight greater than 1,000), polar, ionized molecules are poor penetrants in general, and thus are less likely to cause irritation. In the case of solid substances, the physical properties that determine the coefficient of friction against the skin are important determinants of frictional dermatitis. Quantitative aspects of exposure are modulated by the concentration of the potential irritant and the duration, frequency, or number of cutaneous exposures; the lower the concentration and the shorter or less frequent the exposure, the less likely cutaneous irritation will develop. The permeability of the protective barrier may be further compromised by other qualitative aspects of exposure. Occlusion or entrapment of chemical substances against the skin surface by water-impermeable membranes such as clothing increases the hydration and skin surface temperature of the stratum corneum, thus increasing its permeability; quantitative aspects of exposure may also be enhanced by preventing evaporation or wash-off of a potential irritant from the skin surface (Fig 10–2). When the temperature of the protective barrier is increased, it becomes more permeable; warm or hot potential irritants (such as dishwashing detergents) will transfer heat to the stratum corneum, enhance their own permeability, and increase their irritant potentials. If the potential irritant contacts the skin surface where the protective barrier is defective, as, for example, when the skin is dried or chapped, or there are traumatic scratches or lacerations or preexisting inflammatory skin disease, clinical irritation is more likely to develop. The anatomical skin site contacted by a potential irritant also influences the outcome; the eyelids, face, and genital skin (where the protective barrier is thinnest) are most susceptible to clinical irritation. Atopy is the single greatest risk factor determining host susceptibility to the development of clinical irritation, and the relative risk of developing occupational atopic dermatitis has been estimated to be 13.5%.[112] It is often stated that black

TABLE 10–8.
Factors Predisposing to the Development of Cutaneous Irritation

Potential irritant(s)
Chemical properties
Physical properties
Quantitative aspects of exposure
Concentration
Duration of exposure
Frequency and number of exposures
Qualitative aspects of exposure
Occlusion of substance against skin
Temperature of substance or skin surface
Preexisting skin damage to protective skin barrier
Anatomical skin site
Host susceptibility
Atopic disease
Race(?)
Sex(?)
Age(?)

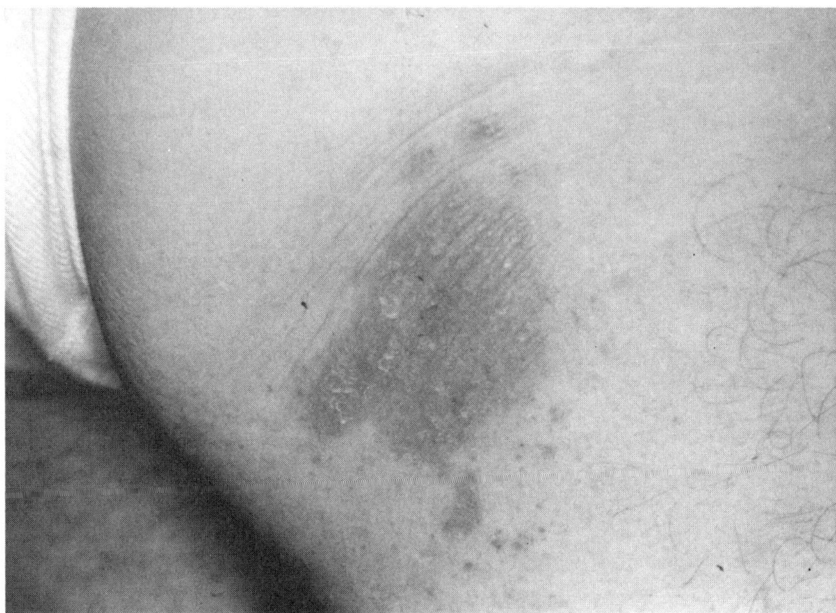

FIG 10–2.
Irritant contact dermatitis on the thigh of a machinist. The lesion developed from inadvertently placing a rag still moist with solvent in the pocket of work trousers.

skin is more resistant to irritation than white skin. Although this statement is supported by limited experimental data, there is no convincing evidence which indicates that these subtle differences are clinically important. Similarly, no strong body of experimental data supports the frequently alleged claim that women are more susceptible to cutaneous irritation than men. Increasing age may be an important determinant of susceptibility to cutaneous irritation, but this issue has not been thoroughly studied to date.

The development of allergic contact dermatitis requires that the affected individual first become immunologically sensitized to the offending substance. The sensitization process involves delayed hypersensitivity mechanisms, which require a period of one to three weeks following first exposure before sensitization can occur. Generally, the allergenic substance must first complex with skin tissue protein, following which this hapten protein conjugate is processed by cutaneous Langerhans' cells and subsequently transported by circulating T lymphocytes to regional lymph nodes, where further antigen processing and cell proliferation occur. Once sensitized, an affected individual will react within several hours to one or two days following cutaneous reexposure to extremely low concentrations of the offending substance. Unlike irritant contact dermatitis, allergic contact dermatitis frequently extends to other body surfaces remote from the primary site of direct skin contact with the allergen.

With the exception of poison oak, most potentially allergenic substances are relatively "weak" antigens and require either a damaged skin barrier (e.g., preceding irritant contact dermatitis) or repetitive skin contact to facilitate immunologic exposure. For these reasons, sensitization frequently occurs from long-standing exposure rather than exposure to a substance recently introduced into a worker's environment. Allergens that are also irritating are more likely to produce clinical sensitization. When the exposure to a potential allergen occurs only at low concentrations, there is often a history of preceding dermatitis suggestive of irritation. Unlike irritant contact dermatitis, however, where atopy is a clear predisposing risk factor, there do not appear to be any unique risk factors determining host susceptibility to allergic contact dermatitis.

As stated earlier, contact dermatitis accounts for most cases of occupational skin disease, and at least 80%–90% of all cases of contact dermatitis result from irritation rather than allergy. Excluding poison oak (where virtually all cases result from allergy) and skin infections, the list of causal agents in Table 10–3 becomes a reasonable rank order approximation of the most common cutaneous irritants. Possible exceptions to this rank order are plastic resins and metallic compounds, where many of these cases are probably allergic.

Common causes of occupational allergic contact dermatitis are listed in Table 10–9. Since exposure to many of these common sensitizers may occur from the domestic as well as occupational environments, the source of exposure should be clearly identified. Not uncommonly, a contact allergy in the workplace results from inadvertent sensitization from rubber gloves, first-aid cabinet preparations, or skin-cleaning preparations usually considered as preventive measures rather than causes of dermatitis.

Follow-up studies (lasting three to ten years) of occupational contact dermatitis indicate that only approximately 25% experience complete resolution of dermatitis and are symptom-free, while 50% are improved but continue to have periodic flares; the remaining 25% develop chronic, persistent eczema which is as severe (or worse) as the initial dermatitis.[20, 43, 54] Almost 30%–40% of persons with occupational contact dermatitis have their jobs changed or modified, but surprisingly only 25% experience complete clearing despite a job change. The prognosis is slightly, but not strikingly, better for allergic than for irritant contact dermatitis. The factors influencing prognosis are not well understood.

Contact dermatitis must be differentiated from endogenous inflammatory dermatoses, particularly atopic dermatitis, dyshidrotic eczema, and psoriasis, with which it may be confused by the unwary. Regardless of type (irritant or allergic), the principles of management include minimization or elimination of the causative exposures and liberal use of topical corticosteroid preparations. Allergic contact dermatitis usually requires complete elimination of exposure to the allergen. For extensive contact dermatitis (more than 20% of the body surface) or limited but severe involvement of the face, genitalia, or palms, systemic corticosteroid therapy is

TABLE 10–9.
Common Causes of Occupational Allergic Contact Dermatitis

*Poison oak/ivy**
Metallic Compounds
- Nickel*
- Chromate*
- Gold
- Mercury

Rubber products
- Accelerators*
- Antioxidants*

Plastic resins
- Epoxy resin,* hardeners, reactive diluents
- Phenolic resins
- Formaldehyde resins
- Acrylic resins
- Rosin (colophony)*

Organic dyes
- Paraphenylenediamine*
- Numerous others

Topical first-aid medications
- Neomycin*
- Thimerosal*
- Benzocaine*

Biocides and germicides
- Formaldehyde*
- Parabens*
- Quaternium-15*
- Formaldehyde releasers
- Isothiazolin-3-one derivatives

Miscellaneous product ingredients
- Fragrances*
- Ethylenediamine*
- Antioxidants

*These substances commonly produce sensitization from exposure in the domestic environment as well as the occupational environment.

preferred. A usually successful regimen is an initial dose of 70 mg of prednisone, tapering 5 mg per day over a two-week period. If 5 mg tablets are dispensed (total number of 105), the patient may be conveniently instructed to take 14 tablets on day 1, then to take one less tablet per day for the next 13 days.

Chemical Burns

Chemical burns may be considered as a special form of irritant contact dermatitis in which substantial skin necrosis and inflammation result from a one-time, usually brief, exposure to a chemical substance. Chemical burns may be divided into first-, second- or third-degree chemical burns, depending on the degree of tissue destruction, and are analogous to thermal burns. Some of these are of special interest either because of unique challenges of management or the potential threat of systemic toxicity from percutaneous absorption.

Chemical burns most frequently result from accidental exposure to a diverse number of organic and inorganic acids and alkalies. Acids generally damage tissue by coagulating protein through oxidation, reduction, desiccation, or salt formation mechanisms. Alkalies not only coagulate tissue protein by desiccation or salt formation, but they also saponify fats and cause liquefaction necrosis. In all cases, management includes copious lavage of the affected skin surface with water, debridement of necrotic skin, and application of a topical antibiotic preparation (usually silver sulfadiazine) followed by a nonadherent surgical dressing. Although neutralization of acids (dilute solutions of sodium bicarbonate, aluminum hydroxide gel, or milk of magnesia) or alkalies (dilute solutions of vinegar) have been recommended by some authorities immediately following water lavage, most consider this unnecessary.[59]

Burns from hydrofluoric acid (HF) (used as a rust remover, metal surface cleaner, etching agent in the semiconductor industry, and a reagent in numerous fluorination processes) typically cause intense pain and erythema which may not become clinically apparent for several hours following cutaneous exposure. Clinical symptoms tend to correlate with the concentration of the acid; signs and symptoms are likely to be immediate if the strength of the acid is greater than 20%, but are often delayed in onset when the exposure is less than 20%. Extensive tissue destruction occurs in part from the high affinity of the fluoride ion for calcium, and extensive destruction of underlying bone may occur from burns on the fingers. Following copious water lavage, treatment is directed at inactivation of the fluoride ion. The affected skin may be soaked with iced 25% magnesium sulfate (Epsom salts), 1%–2% benzalkonium chloride (Zephiran) or 1%–2% benzethonium chloride (Hyamine) solutions. Alternatively, 10% calcium gluconate gel may be applied repeatedly over burned skin. If pain persists, local injection of 10% calcium gluconate into the burned tissue is recommended.[59, 111] For HF burns of the fingertips, the nail may have to be avulsed to facilitate injection of calcium gluconate. If skin burns are extensive, potentially fatal decreases in serum calcium and magnesium concentrations may occur and require supplemental intravenous administration.

Alkyl mercury compounds, used as disinfectants, wood preservatives, and fungicides, are strong skin irritants and may cause second- or third-degree chemical burns. They are extremely toxic to the central nervous system, and fatal neurotoxicity may develop from continued absorption of the alkyl mercury compound still present in blister fluid or necrotic tissue. Blisters and necrotic tissue should therefore be debrided as soon as possible.[11] Despite the paucity of information on chemical burns from other substances which have important systemic toxic effects, immediate debridement of blisters and necrotic tissue should be considered in all similar situations (e.g., chemical burns from methyl bromide).

Phenol (carbolic acid) is highly corrosive to skin and is absorbed rapidly into the body. Systemic toxicity associated with phenolic burns has included cardiac arrhythmias, cardiopulmonary arrest, convulsions, and coma. Lavage with water is not particularly effective in removing residual phenol from the skin surface, and polyethylene glycol (PEG) 300 or 400 in 2:1 mixtures of PEG and alcohol have been recommended for skin decontamination.[17]

Among all chemical burns, white phosphorus is unique in that it ignites upon contact with air and may cause thermal burns if it is in contact with the skin. Used in the manufacture of munitions, explosives, and fireworks, white phosphorus is usually stored under water in underground holding tanks. In order to minimize the risk of continuing thermal burns, the skin surface should be kept wet while mechanical debridement of residual white phosphorus particles is performed. Irrigation of the skin surface with 1%–2% aqueous solutions of copper sulfate has been recommended, since copper sulfate combines with white phosphorus and forms a colored complex which facilitates the visual location of residual particles to be debrided.[32]

Chromic acid is widely used for surface treatment of metals, electroplating, etching, glass cleaning, photoengraving, and a variety of other industrial processes. It is a strong tissue-oxidizing agent and may produce small, usually painless ulcers ("chrome holes") of the fingers and hands. Inhalation of its vapors has produced ulceration and perforation of the nasal septum. Management includes frequent rinsing with a fresh aqueous solution of 10% ascorbic acid, which reduces the hexavalent chromate.[105]

Solvents

Dermatitis from solvents almost always results from contact irritation rather than allergy. Exceptions to this general rule are the naturally derived solvents, such as turpentine. Although most solvent vapors are irritating to the mucous membranes and respiratory tract, frank dermatitis from exposure to solvent vapors alone is extremely rare. Dermatitis most commonly results from repeated, direct skin contact with solvent rather than just an occasional brief exposure. Based on chemical and physical properties alone, the ten most potentially irritating solvents have been listed in Table 10–10. The irritant action of solvents is based on the dissolution of skin surface, stratum corneum, and cell membrane lipids. In general, an inverse correlation between the boiling point of a solvent and its irritant potential has been observed, with lower boiling point solvents generally being more irritating.[64] The ability of any solvent to produce clinical irritation may be modified by other circumstances or conditions of exposure, as discussed above. A more detailed description of dermatitis from specific solvents may be found elsewhere.[2]

Soaps and Detergents

Excluding poison oak, the second most common cause of occupationally acquired dermatitis in California, ranking only behind

TABLE 10–10.
The Ten Most Potentially Irritating Solvents, in Decreasing Order of Severity*

Carbon disulfide
Petroleum distillates (diesel, gasoline, kerosene)
Coal tar solvents (xylol, toluol)
Turpentine
Chlorinated hydrocarbons (methylene chloride, trichloroethylene, Freon)
Alcohols (methyl, ethyl)
Glycols (propylene glycol)
Esters (methyl acetate, butyl acetate)
Ketones (acetone, methylethyl ketone)
Dimethyl sulfoxide

*Adapted from Pirila V, et al: Legislation on occupational dermatoses of the International Contact Dermatitis Research Group. *Acta Derm Venereol* 1971; 51:141–150.

solvents, is soaps, detergents, and other industrial cleaning agents. Contact dermatitis may result not only from excessive or inappropriate exposure associated with the correct use of such products but also from incorrect or inappropriate use of these agents to clean skin.[83]

Soaps and detergents are usually dispersed in water for the purpose of removing dirt and stains from a variety of surfaces. The first step in the cleansing process is the wetting of the surface to be cleaned. All detergents contain surface active agents which lower the surface tension of water and facilitate its spread. Second, a layer of detergent must be absorbed at the interface of the cleaning solution and the soiled surface. Detergent molecules generally have hydrophobic ends which solubilize into the soiled surface. Third, the stain or soil must be removed from the surface to be cleaned and dispersed into the water. This is facilitated by mechanical agitation, heating the wash solution, and the addition of foaming agents to the cleaner. For special cleaning purposes, such as removal of proteinaceous stains or burned organic material, other additives such as enzymes or sodium hydroxide are required to facilitate surface cleaning. Finally, the removed soil or dirt must be prevented from redepositing on the cleaned surface. This is usually accomplished by addition of emulsifiers or antiredeposition agents. Most industrial detergents also contain builders (usually salts of phosphate or silicate) to prevent scum buildup. Liquid soap solutions containing organic compounds will have a biocidal preservative added. Formaldehyde is still sometimes used as a preservative in industrial liquid soaps marketed for skin cleaning.

Depending upon the cleaning task, a variety of special additives may be contained. Detergents which also disinfect inert surfaces usually contain phenolic substances (e.g., p-tert-amylphenol) which may occasionally sensitize. "Waterless" hand cleaners, marketed for cleaning the skin of mechanics, contain 15%–20% petroleum distillates. These are not truly waterless, since the solvent is formulated into a water washable cream base with a mild detergent action. They remove oil and grease stains reasonably well from most skin surfaces except the palms and palmar fingers, where the deep skin creases make the stains less accessible to the cleaning action of these agents. Since they contain a substantial amount of petroleum distillate, waterless hand cleaners may cause irritant contact dermatitis if used excessively.

Abrasive soaps contain inorganic minerals (borax, sand, pumice) or hard plant material (sawdust, ground vegetable matter) which produce mechanical friction and agitation on the surface to be cleaned, assisting in the removal of difficult dirt or grease stains. Abrasives may be found in scouring powders, but are also popular in powdered soaps marketed to clean mechanics' skin. Mechanics often prefer abrasive soaps to waterless hand cleaners, particularly for cleaning palmar skin. Excessive use of abrasive soaps may cause frictional dermatitis of the forearms or dorsal hands, but the palms (where the stratum corneum is thickest) tend to be resistant.

Contact dermatitis from soaps and detergents usually results from the irritating effects of alkalinity and delipidization of the skin surface, rather than sensitization. On those infrequent occasions when dermatitis results from sensitization, the biocidal preservative (e.g., formaldehyde) or germicidal disinfectant (e.g., p-tert-amylphenol), or lanolin (cream soaps) is usually responsible. Rarely, some other additive (optical whitener, dye, perfume) may sensitize.

Some general guidelines apply for prevention of dermatitis from soaps and detergents. Cleaning agents designed for inert surfaces, which are generally much harsher than toilet soaps and workplace solvents, should never be used to clean skin. Protective gloves should be worn whenever cleaning with industrial detergents; gloves should be removed and the skin immediately rinsed if detergent accidentally enters the gloves. The temperature of any wash solution should be kept at the lowest possible level that will get the job done. Waterless hand cleaners should be rinsed off the skin surface with mild soap and water following each use and should never be used on inflamed skin. The use of abrasive soaps should generally be restricted to palmar skin cleansing.

Cement

Cement is a mixture of mineral-like oxide compounds, similar in composition and structure to the naturally occurring silicates. It is made by burning together limestone (calcium carbonate) and a natural carrier of silicates and aluminum oxides (clay or shale) in a fired kiln, to which iron is usually added. The resulting kiln product ("clinkers") is subsequently cooled and ground into fine particles. Gypsum (calcium sulfate) is added at this stage to retard the setting time. The resultant mixture (cement) derives its industrial properties from the ability of its anhydrous compounds to react with added water to form hydrates, which increase in strength as the amount of free water decreases by progressive hydration and evaporation. The strength of cement can be further increased by the presence of inert fillers such as sand and rock (e.g., concrete).

Severe burns and ulcerations can result from prolonged skin contact with wet cement, and onset of symptoms is typically delayed several hours after exposure. Burns usually occur on the knees from kneeling on wet cement or on the ankles from cement splashing inside workboots. They probably result from the extreme alkalinity of calcium hydroxide in cement formed when water reacts with calcium oxide, combined with the effects of pressure and occlusion against the skin.[102]

Contact dermatitis from cement usually results from skin irritation secondary to the alkaline, hygroscopic, and abrasive properties of cement, and typically presents as a dry but only slightly inflamed dermatitis of the hands and arms. Occasionally, dermatitis results from allergic sensitization to water-soluble chromate present in cement. Chromate is not normally present in the raw materials used in cement, but it is inadvertently added when these materials are processed and fired in the kiln. The primary source of contamination is felt to be the bricks lining the kiln.[23] In such cases, the dermatitis usually has a more pronounced inflammatory component than is seen with irritant cement dermatitis. Cements manufactured in the United States have generally been found to contain only very small amounts of water soluble chromate (less than 5 ppm) compared to European cements, and true contact allergy from chromate in cement is correspondingly rare.[95] Nickel and cobalt, implicated in some European cases of cement dermatitis, are not present in American cements.

Water-soluble hexavalent chromate may be reduced to trivalent chromate by the addition of ferrous sulfate to cement[44] and is felt to reduce the risk of having contact allergy develop from chromate. Although this practice is now being followed in some European countries, it has not been adopted in the United States.

Fiberglass

Fiberglass has extensive application in thermal and acoustic insulating material, industrial textiles, and reinforcement fillers for plastics. The popularity of fiberglass is due to its virtually total resistance to thermal, chemical, or microbial degradation.

Spicules of fiberglass may produce a mechanical irritation which results in severe skin itching. The intensity of symptoms is inversely proportional to fiber length and directly proportional to fiber diameter; short fibers, less than 3.5 μ in diameter, are least likely to produce any symptoms.[53] Pinpoint excoriations are the principal clinical findings, although occasional inflamed papules may be present. Frank eczematous dermatitis is unlikely to be due to fiberglass. Individuals with underlying dermographism (i.e., skin that urticates following scratching, pressure, or friction to the skin surface) are most likely to be severely affected. Although strands of fiberglass may be coated with various plastic resins which may theoretically sensitize, allergic contact dermatitis from fiberglass does not appear to be a serious concern.[97] Dermatitis from fiberglass must be differentiated from scabies, which it may resemble.

Plants and Vegetation

The oleoresins found in poison oak *(Toxicodendron diversilobum)* and poison ivy *(Toxicodendron radicans)* are powerful skin sensitizers. The active sensitizing principle is a substituted catechol with a 15-carbon (pentadecacatechol in poison ivy) or 17-carbon (heptadecacatechol in poison oak) unsaturated side chain. The resin dries quickly on skin, clothing, shoes, or tools, and will maintain its allergenic potency for long periods of time unless oxidized. Partially oxidized resin appears black, and black stains may occasionally be detected on the skin or clothing of affected patients (Fig 10–3). Clinical dermatitis is usually characterized by areas of linear or streaked eczematous patches, where portions of the crushed or broken plant were dragged or pulled across the skin surface. Dermatitis may be spread or exacerbated following repeated exposures to fomites contaminated with resin, as work clothes or tools. Blisters of poison oak/ivy dermatitis do not contain any allergenic oleoresin, however, and skin contact with blister fluid from an affected individual will not precipitate dermatitis in another sensitized person.[65]

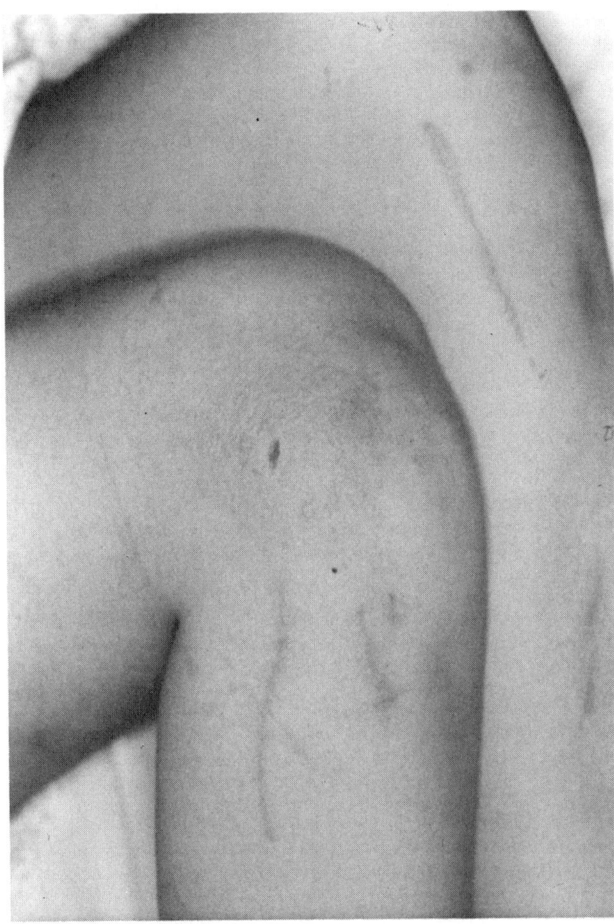

FIG 10–3.
Poison oak dermatitis, showing typical linear eczematous streaking where plant contacted the legs. A small black stain, representing dried oleoresin, is present near the knee.

Poison oak and ivy are members of the *Anacardiaceae* plant family, many of which contain identical or similar cross-reacting antigenic oleoresins. Individuals allergic to poison oak/ivy may inadvertently develop contact dermatitis when exposed to these other plant species or their products. Important members of this family include the mango tree, cashew nut tree, Japanese lacquer tree, and the Indian marking nut tree. A resinous oil derived from cashew nutshells has had extensive utilization in plastic resins and coatings, brake linings, and miscellaneous lubricants and occasionally precipitates dermatitis in exposed individuals previously sensitized to poison oak. Varnishes or lacquers derived from the Japanese lacquer tree, or objects coated with them, can cause similar occurrences of dermatitis.

Skin cleaning with soap and water following contact with poison oak/ivy is generally unsatisfactory in terms of removing oleoresin from the skin, unless it is performed within the first few minutes. Recent interest has centered on the possible prophylactic use of protective creams containing polyoxypropyleneamine salts of a linoleic acid dimer, which seem to bind to the resin and inactivate it.[92] Hyposensitization through oral administration of oleoresin extracts is effective experimentally in animals and under rigidly controlled conditions in man.[40] The efficacy of hyposensitization at a practical clinical level, unfortunately, is far from convincing. Variations in antigenic potency of extracts by different manufacturers (or between lots from the same manufacturer), problems of patient compliance, accidental reexposure to the plant before the recommended course of immunotherapy is complete, and side effects (e.g., perianal itching) all limit the likelihood of successful induction of tolerance. Hyposensitization treatment must begin three to four months prior to anticipated exposure, and maintenance dosages may have to be continued indefinitely.

Dermatitis from most other plants and woods is usually secondary to irritation from essential oils or juices in the stems, leaves, flowers, fruit, or wood. Important plants and woods which may occasionally sensitize the skins of forestry workers, gardeners, nursery workers, or wood workers are listed in Table 10–11. Next to poison oak/ivy, chrysanthemums and other *Compositae* species probably cause the greatest number of cases of contact allergy, particularly in nursery workers. In many instances of dermatitis from woods among forestry workers, contact allergy results from liverwort or lichens on the bark rather than from the wood itself. Exposure to potentially allergenic substances in the heartwood occurs when the wood is cut or sawed. Clinical dermatitis frequently occurs on exposed surfaces of the body indirectly exposed to allergens in pollen or sawdust (e.g., the face and neck) and may mimic photodermatitis. A characteristic dry, fissured dermatitis of the fingertips may occur among nursery workers or gardeners as a result of handling tulip or hyacinth bulbs.

TABLE 10–11.
Important Plants and Woods That May Cause Allergic Contact Dermatitis, Excluding Poison Oak/Ivy*

PLANTS	WOODS
Compositae (sesquiterpene lactones)	Cedar (thymoquinone)
Chrysanthemums	
Ragweed	
Sagebrush	
Feverfew	
Liverwort	
Lichens (usnic acid)	Cocobolo (dalbergiones)
Algerian/English Ivy (helenin)	Ebony (naphthoquinine)
Primrose (primin)	Mahogany (anthothecol)
Tulips (tulipaline A)	Pine and Fir (Δ-pinene, 3-carene)
Hyacinths	Rosewood (? quinone)
Garlic (diallyldisulfide)	Satinwood (?)
Onions	Teak (deoxylapichol)

*Sensitizing agent, where known, is included in parentheses.

Metals and Metallic Salts

Nickel is the most frequent metal which induces allergic contact sensitization and accounts for approximately 10% of all positive patch tests in North America. Occupational exposures occur mainly from metallic alloys or electroplating solutions containing nickel. In the case of solid metals, prolonged skin contact is generally required; heat, moisture, sweating, and friction probably facilitate the leaching of nickel from the metal and its subsequent absorption by the skin. Occasionally, sensitization occurs from contamination of industrial fluids (e.g., cutting fluids) with nickel leached from metal surfaces contacting the fluids. Sensitization is much more frequent in women, who tend to wear costume jewelry and to have pierced ears, than in men, who are more likely to be sensitized through occupational exposure.

Water-soluble hexavalent chromate may be both an irritant and a sensitizer. Alkaline solutions are more caustic to skin than acid solutions and typically cause "chrome ulcers" (see Chemical Burns). Occupational exposures occur from metals alloyed with chrome, electroplating solutions, tanning agents, paint and printing ink pigments, and industrial solutions or products to which chromate has been added as a corrosion inhibitor. Trivalent chromate has extremely low water-solubility, is poorly absorbed through the skin, and does not usually contribute to the development of clinical contact dermatitis. Trace amounts of chromate in cement probably do not contribute to cement dermatitis in the United States (see Cement).

Cobalt hypersensitivity frequently accompanies nickel or chromate allergy. Presumably, this occurs because cobalt is closely associated with these other metallic elements in the periodic table, and one metal is almost always contaminated with the other. Independent sensitization may occur from occupational exposures to cobalt in electroplating solutions, paint driers or cobaltous pigments, catalytic reagents, or hard metal grindings (containing approximately 90% tungsten and 10% cobalt).

Gold and its salts are strong potential experimental sensitizers, but clinical allergy is relatively rare. Metallic gold resists attack by water and oxygen and is virtually insoluble except in aqua regia; hypersensitivity from metallic gold objects is correspondingly and exceedingly rare. Soluble gold salts may occasionally produce allergic sensitization, but many are extremely irritating to the skin as well, such as gold potassium cyanide salts used in electroplating solutions.[80]

Beryllium salts are irritating and may cause painless skin ulcerations similar to chrome ulcers. Allergic contact dermatitis has also been reported. Both beryllium and zirconium salts, when inoculated into the skin, have produced allergic, delayed hypersensitivity granulomas. Awareness of severe respiratory disease from beryllium has led to the implementation of preventive measures to eliminate exposure, and clinical skin disease from beryllium is now exceedingly rare.

Inorganic arsenicals and platinum salts may occasionally cause allergic contact dermatitis, but sensitization from other metals is extraordinarily rare.

Rubber Products

Rubber products are manufactured from natural rubber latex or synthetic polymers of styrene-butadiene (SBR rubber), acrylonitrite-butadiene (ABR rubber), neoprene, isobutylene-butadiene (butyl rubber), polysulfides, polyurethanes, or silicone. With the exception of silicone and polysulfide rubbers, the other types all require addition of accelerators to speed the rate of cure and antioxidants to preserve the elasticity and flexibility of the rubber product. Other additives may include pigments, reinforcers, fillers, softeners, plasticizers, and phenolic resins (used as tackifiers).

In the manufacture of rubber, irritant contact dermatitis may occur from a variety of acids, alkalies, detergents, and solvents used in the process. Allergic contact dermatitis occurs not infrequently and is almost always due to an organic accelerator or antioxidant. While the list of potential sensitizing accelerators and antioxidants is enormous, common allergens include tetramethylthiuram disulfide, mercaptobenzothiazole, zinc dimethyldithiocarbamate, n-isopropyl-n-phenyl-p-phenylenediamine (IPPD) analogues, phenyl-β-naphthylamine, diethylthiorurea, and other related thiurams, mercapto compounds, p-phenylenediamine analogues, carbamates, naphthyl compounds, and thioureas.[2]

Clinical dermatitis from finished rubber products generally results only when the rubber item contacts the skin for long periods of time. Wearing apparel, especially protective gloves, rubber workboots, and facemasks, accounts for most of the occupational cases. Heat, sweat, and moisture are important cofactors, since the sensitizing accelerators or antioxidants must first be leached out of the solid rubber item. Preceding irritant dermatitis is common in cases of contact allergy to rubber gloves or boots. Often, the worker has ignored the wearing of appropriate protective gloves or boots until clinical irritant dermatitis has developed. The subsequent wearing of gloves or boots over inflamed, dermatitic skin may predispose to contact sensitization.

Germicides and Biocides

Industrial solutions or products that contain water and organic compounds generally require the addition of a biocidal agent to prevent decomposition of the product and prolong its shelf life. Examples include cutting fluids and emulsions, latex paints, liquid industrial hand soaps, first-aid creams, and water-based adhesives. When encountered in sufficient concentrations, virtually all biocides may be irritating or caustic, and most may sensitize. The likelihood of sensitization increases as the concentration of the biocide increases, and individuals who handle undiluted biocides (e.g., formulation of industrial products) are at greatest risk. Important biocidal agents are listed in Table 10–12. Formaldehyde and organic mercurials were formerly the most important causes of contact allergy in this group, but they have largely been replaced by other less-toxic agents; many of these may still release small amounts of formaldehyde or cross-react, causing dermatitis in formaldehyde-sensitive individuals. Formaldehyde may still be found, somewhat paradoxically, in industrial liquid hand soaps at up to 0.1% concentrations, although its use as a biocide in other industrial products has substantially decreased. Isothia-

TABLE 10–12.
Important Biocides Which May Irritate or Sensitize

TRADE NAME	CHEMICAL NAME
Formalin, Formol	Formaldehyde solution
Grotan BK*	Hexahydro-1, 3, 5-tris (2-hydroxyethyl) -sym-triazine
Grotan HD-2	2-chloro-N-hydroxymethylacetamide
Grotan K	Chloro-2-methyl-4-isothiazolin-3-one
Proxel CRL	1, 2-benzisothiazolin-3-one
Bioban p-1487	4-(2-nitrobutyl) morpholine and 4, 4-(2-ethyl-2-nitrotrimethylene) dimorpholine
Kathon CE, Kathon 886 MW	5-chloro-2-methyl-4-isolthiazolin-3-one and 2-methyl-4-isothiazolin-3-one
Skane M-8	2-N-octyl-4-isothiazolin-3-one
Quaternium-15,* Dowicil 75,*	1-(3-chloroallyl)-3,5,7-triaza-1-1-azoniaadamantine chloride
Tris Nitro	2-(hydroxymethyl)-2-nitro-1,3-propanediol
Dowicide 1, Dowicide A	O-phenylphenol
Sodium or Zinc Omadine	Sodium or zinc 2-pyridylthio-N oxide
Preventol D-2	Benzyl hemiformal
Preventol D-3	Chloromethylacylaminomethanol
Benzytol, Dettol, Ottasept Extra	Chloroxylenol, p-chloro-m-xylenol
Ottafact	Chlorocresol
Merthiolate	Thimerosal
Phermernite	Phenylmercuric nitrate
Captax, Dermacid, Mertax, Thiotax	Mercaptobenzothiazole

*Formaldehyde-releasing biocides.

zolin-3-one derivatives are emerging as an important new class of sensitizers.

Pesticides

The term *pesticide* designates any toxic chemical used against rodents, insects, fungi, weeds, or other pests. Skin disease among agricultural workers is relatively common and frequently attributed to pesticide exposure, although a direct causal relationship may be difficult to establish. Pesticides commonly implicated as causes of occupational skin disease are listed in Table 10–13. Dermatitis is most often observed, although several other adverse reactions have been reported (porphyria, urticaria, chloracne, erythema multiforme). Chemicals used as pesticides may have industrial applications outside agriculture (e.g., thiurams are used as rubber accelerators) or are used as biocides in industrial products. Irritant dermatitis is the rule and may be due to the vehicle in which the pesticide has been formulated, while true allergic contact dermatitis is relatively rare. The following classes of pesticides have consistently been among the most common contact allergens, in those few instances where pesticide-associated dermatitis has been evaluated by appropriate patch testing: carbamates, thiurams, captans, organomercurials, triazines, and pyrethrums. Formerly, contact allergy from pyrethrums was common and was caused by sensitizing sesquiterpene lactones contained in the crude extract (derived from a chrysanthemum species). Today, the extraction and purification process is such that the active insecticidal principle (pyrethroids) present in modern pyrethrum-containing insecticides should not contain any sensitizing sesquiterpene lactone. Contact allergy from pyrethroids or synthetic pyrethrins (derived from petrochemical sources) has not been observed. Skin disease attributable to pesticides sprayed on vegetation must be distinguished from skin disease caused by the vegetation itself, with which it is frequently confused. Pesticide-associated skin disease has been extensively reviewed by Adams.[2]

TABLE 10–13.
The Most Common Causes of Pesticide-Associated Skin Disease (California, 1977–1981)*

Sulfur
Propargite
Creosote
Benomyl
Glyphosphate
Weed oil
Methyl bromide
Captan
Difolatan
Dyrene

*Courtesy of Dr. Michael O'Malley, National Institute for Occupational Safety and Health.

Plastics, Resins, and Coatings

A plastic is any substance, solid in its finished state, which has the capacity to be molded into various shapes. Plastic resins may be derived from either natural or synthetic sources. Contact dermatitis may occur when the plastic is in its liquid or unpolymerized state, but generally does not result from solid plastic products or coatings unless substantial, free, unpolymerized resin is still present.

Rosin (colophony) is the most important natural resin which may cause allergic contact dermatitis. Wood rosin is obtained by distillation of a crude extract from the wood of the pine tree *(pinus palustris)*, while distillation of turpentine yields a more highly purified gum rosin. Rosin is a brittle material which becomes sticky when heated, thus lending it to a number of adhesive applications, e.g., hot melt glues and adhesive tapes. Rosin is also hydrophobic, nonconductive, and noncorrosive, properties which make it extremely useful for electrical soldering operations. It is frequently combined with other synthetic resins or natural drying oils to form new plastic substances with a variety of physical properties. Rosin contains many potential skin allergens, the two principal ones being abietic acid and alcohol. With the exception of rosin and resinous products derived from plant species related to poison oak/ivy (see Plants and Vegetation), contact dermatitis from other naturally occurring resins is extraordinarily rare.

Epoxy resins are synthetic resins which all share in common a highly reactive epoxide group contained within the molecular structure. Over 90% of commercial epoxy resins are based on the reaction of epichlorohydrin and Bisphenol A, producing monomers or polymers of the diglycidyl ether of Bisphenol A. Other types of epoxy resins are formed by reacting epichlorohydrin with hydantoin or other phenolic compounds. Epoxy resins uniquely combine the physical properties of strength, adhesiveness, and electrical and chemical resistance. Thus, they are extensively used in industrial paints, coatings, adhesives, and laminates, and may also be used to modify other resins. Reactive diluents (usually monoglycidyl ethers of alkanes or phenolic compounds) are frequently added to decrease the viscosity of the resin and to increase its flexibility. Polymerization requires addition of a curing agent (hardener), usually a polyfunctional aliphatic or aromatic amine, polyamide, or acid anhydride. The aliphatic amines will produce curing at room temperature, but the aromatic amines and anhydrides require addition of heat before curing can occur. Although the diglycidyl ether of Bisphenol A is a potent skin sensitizer, the epoxy reactive diluents or hardeners are responsible for approximately 10% of allergic contact dermatitis caused by epoxy resins. Dermatitis may be particularly severe when the epoxy resin is either sprayed or heat cured, since extensive skin contact from aerosolized particles or volatilized vapors can occur. Although the extremely alkaline aliphatic amine hardeners are potential skin irritants, clinical dermatitis from irritation is not very common, possibly because skin contact with the hardener is seldom prolonged. In this author's experience, careful investigation of contact dermatitis due to epoxy resin almost always demonstrates sensitization to the epoxy resin, reactive diluent, or hardener.

Phenolic resins are manufactured by reacting phenol (or some other phenolic) with an aldehyde (usually formaldehyde). The most important commercial phenolic resins are phenolformal dehyde, melamine formaldehyde, resorcinol formaldehyde, parater tiarybutylphenol formaldehyde, furfuryl formaldehyde, and cardolite (the condensation product of formaldehyde and a phenolic extract of cashew nutshell oil). Phenolic resins find extensive applications in plywood laminations, binders for foundry sand, impregnation of wood or plastic to increase insulation, and combination with other adhesives (e.g., neoprene glue) to increase moisture resistance. Although phenolic resins release formaldehyde, morethan 90% of cases of allergic contact dermatitis to phenolic resins occur from the resin itself rather than released formaldehyde.[28] Since industrial processes employing phenolic resins are usually heat cured, exposure to the vapors may cause severe dermatitis in sensitized individuals.

Acrylic and methacrylic acid are strong solvents and potential skin irritants. A number of useful thermoplastic acrylic resins can be derived by esterification, modification, or copolymerization of these acids. These include Plexiglas (polymerized methyl methacrylate), latex paints, coatings, inks, dental or bone cement, anaerobic sealants, and floor polishes. Recently, polyfunctional acrylates that rapidly cure upon exposure to ultraviolent light have been employed in printing inks, dental adhesives, and miscellaneous coatings; these resins require addition of an ultraviolet light absorber such as benzophenone to effect cure. Irritant contact dermatitis may occur from prolonged skin contact with any acrylic resin; cyanoacrylate vapors are particularly irritating to the mucous membranes. An unusual form of delayed skin irritation caused by polyfunctional acrylates has been observed, the onset of which was delayed 12–24 hours but which was frequently bullous or painful.[77] Esters of methacrylic acid, particularly methyl methacrylate, are the most important skin sensitizers, but allergic contact dermatitis has been reported from polyethyleneglycol dimethacrylate in anaerobic sealants,[82] and polyfunctional acrylates and methacrylates.[38, 91]

Polyurethane resins are formed from the reaction of a polyalcohol with a diisocyanate (e.g., toluene diisocyanate). Although the volatile diisocyanates are extremely irritating to the skin or membranes, allergic contact dermatitis occasionally occurs from the diisocyanate or a polyamine curing agent.

Organic Dyes

Most organic azo dyes are potential skin sensitizers, the most important of which are paraphenylenediamine and its analogues. Water-soluble azo dyes are more likely to cause clinical sensitization than insoluble dyes. Beauticians exposed to paraphenylenediamine derivatives in hair dyes, workers dyeing textile resins, and photographic film developers exposed to color developing solutions not infrequently become sensitized to azo dyes. In addition to allergic eczematous contact dermatitis, color developing solutions have caused lichen planus-like eruptions.[46]

Cutting Fluids

Cutting fluids are used in virtually all industries that cut, grind, or machine metals. These preparations are formulated with vegetable or mineral oils, water, and high-pressure additives (sulfur and/or chlorine). Cutting fluids are used to cool and lubricate the cutting tool and parts, to flush away metal chips during the cutting or grinding operation, and to prolong the work life of the cutting tool. Neat oils are most commonly employed for low-speed grinding or honing operations, while oil-water emulsions are employed for high-speed cutting or grinding, where higher temperatures are encountered. Irritant contact dermatitis is most commonly produced by the cutting fluid emulsions, which contain water, detergents, and emulsifiers as well as potentially irritating sulfurated or chlorinated oils; it is more likely to occur in machinists who must continually immerse their hands in cutting fluids throughout the work shift. Machinists frequently complain that "used" cutting fluid is harsher to their skin than "fresh" fluid, pointing to the possible role of contaminants or breakdown products in the development of irritation. Allergic contact dermatitis occasionally develops, and it is usually due to the biocide contained in the water-based emulsion, although metallic salts from the machined metal (e.g., nickel) or other additives (dyes, perfumes) are rare causes.[100] Some industries have recently adopted the practice of purchasing full-strength biocides and requiring employees periodically to add small amounts of fresh biocide to recirculating cutting fluid, in order to preserve its work life. The potential for becoming sensitized is markedly enhanced when skin contact to an undiluted biocide occurs, as opposed to the dilutions of biocide normally encountered in commercially formulated cutting fluid concentrations; this author has already observed several such cases.

Photodermatitis

Photodermatitis requires activation of a chemical substance on the skin surface by ultraviolet radiation (290–400 nm wavelength) for its clinical expression. Chemical substances capable of causing photodermatitis generally contain aromatic rings in their molecular structure and absorb ultraviolet radiation emitted by the sun. Most compounds that can absorb sufficient ultraviolet energy can cause phototoxic reactions if exposure occurs at sufficiently high concentrations, and some of these may also produce allergic photosensitization. Substances that do not have an absorption spectrum in the ultraviolet wavelength range are not likely to cause clinical disease. In all cases, inflammation develops on body surfaces normally exposed to sunlight (dorsal hands, arms, neck, face), provided that the responsible photosensitizer also contacts those anatomical areas. Covered skin, the eyelids, submental chin, and upper ears covered by hair are characteristically spared.

Phototoxic reactions, analogous to irritant contact dermatitis, are typically accompanied by immediate burning, stinging, or "smarting" of the skin shortly following sun exposure, and clinical inflammation appears more like an acute sunburn than an eczematous dermatitis. Inflammation is the result of a toxic photodynamic effect and is not mediated by immunologic mechanisms. Coal tar, pitch, creosote, and other products derived from coal tar may cause severe stinging and burning ("tar smarts"), the wavelength of activation being 340–430 nm.[29] Once this reaction has been initiated, much smaller amounts of ultraviolet light exposure can reproduce the stinging and burning sensations for several hours, even though a larger exposure was required to initiate it.[33] Phototoxic reactions are common in outdoor workers exposed to coal tar or its crude extracts, such as railroad workers who must handle creosote-impregnated ties. Coal tar epoxies contain up to 25% crude coal tar, and phototoxic reactions in outdoor workers exposed to this coating must be distinguished from epoxy resin allergy.

Furocoumarins are phototoxic substances found in various members of the *Rutaceae* and *Umbelliferae* plant families which may cause severe, painful, bullous reactions in any worker who must handle or harvest these plants or their essential oils. Important species include limes, lemons, figs, celery, carrots, parsley, parsnip, dill, rue, bergamot, and the gas plant. Indoor workers who handle furocoumarin-containing fruits or vegetables are susceptible as soon as they leave their employment and are exposed to sunlight (e.g., bartenders who squeeze limes), but the cause may go undetected without careful questioning. Celery harvesters are particularly susceptible to severe reactions, since a common fungal parasite ("pink rot") dramatically increases the furocoumarin content in infested plants.[12] Postinflammatory hyperpigmentation characteristically follows furocoumarin-induced phototoxic reactions and may be the only clinical manifestation in mild cases.

True occupational photoallergic dermatitis is relatively rare and clinically presents as an eczematous dermatitis in sun exposed areas. Formerly, halogenated salicylanilides produced large numbers of cases as a result of their use as antibacterial agents in toilet soaps. Their use has been banned in toilet soaps for years, but they may be occasionally encountered in janitorial cleaning agents or first-aid creams. Pharmacists, nurses, physicians, veterinarians, or individuals employed in pharmaceutical manufacturing may develop phototoxic or photoallergic reactions from photosensitizing drugs. Photoallergic reactions may sometimes be followed by a persistent state of light reactivity (persistent light reactor) where clinical dermatitis recurs following exposure to sunlight alone, in the absence of exposure to the original photosensitizing chemical. This has typically occurred following topical reactions to halogenated salicylanilides or systemic reactions to chlorothiazides, but it has recently been observed following photosensitization to epoxy resin.[4]

Occupationally acquired photodermatitis must be differentiated from endogenous photosensitivity disorders, including porphyria cutanea tarda, polymorphous light eruption, solar urticaria, and systemic lupus erythematosus. Outdoor employment, however, may substantially aggravate an underlying endogenous photosensitivity disorder or precipitate a reaction in individuals taking potentially photosensitizing medication for some other medical problem. Rarely, porphyria cutanea tarda may be precipitated by exposure to chlorinated aromatic hydrocarbons (e.g., hexachlorobenzene).

Topical and systemic therapy is the same as for contact dermatitis. Preventive measures must include avoidance of the provocative agent or sunlight (or both), or the use of broad-spectrum sunscreens that effectively shield throughout the entire ultraviolet spectrum (e.g., sunscreens containing p-aminobenzoic acid esters or cinnamates combined with benzophenones, usually having a protection factor rating of 15 or greater).

Important causal agents of phototoxic or photoallergic reactions are listed in Table 10–14.

TABLE 10–14.
Some Important Causes of Occupational Phototoxic or Photoallergic Reactions

Coal tar products	*Drugs*
Crude coal tar	P-aminobenzoic acid and esters
Pitch	Chlorothiazides
Creosote	Diphenhydramine
Dyes	Phenothiazines
Acridine	Griseofulvin
Eosin	Nonsteroidal anti-inflammatories
Fluoroscein	Benzophenones
Rhodamine	Nalidixic acid
Rose bengal	Quinine
Plants	Tetracyclines
Carrots	Sulfonamides
Celery	*Antimicrobials*
Bergamot	Halogenated salicylanilides
Dill	Bithional
Figs	Hexachlorophene
Lemons	*Miscellaneous*
Limes	Saccharin
Parsley	Cyclamates
Parsnip	Optical whiteners
Rue	Epoxy resin
Gas plant	
Angelica	
Buttercup	
Mustard	
Goose foot	
Scurfy pea	
St. John's wort	
Essential oils and fragrances	
Angelica root oil	
Bergamot oil	
Lemon oil	
Lime oil	
Orange oil (bitter)	
Rue oil	
Cedarwood oil	
Sandalwood oil	
Lavender oil	
Musk ambrette	
6-methyl coumarin	

Pigmentary Disorders

Toxic Vitiligo

Depigmentation resembling idiopathic vitiligo (Fig 10–4) can be caused by cutaneous exposure to a variety of phenolic or catecholic derivatives which structurally resemble tyrosine, an amino acid precursor of melanin synthesis.[47, 76] At low doses, these substances simply inhibit melanin synthesis, but at higher doses they may be cytotoxic to melanocytes, resulting in irreversible pigment loss. Phenolic or catecholic derivatives are frequently employed as antioxidants or germicidal disinfectants and may be encountered in rubber products or manufacture, photographic developing solutions, lubricating oils, plastics or adhesive manufacture, and institutional or industrial disinfectant cleaning solutions. Depigmentation may be preceded by inflammation of the affected skin and is frequently associated with allergic contact sensitization to the same chemical responsible for the loss of pigment. Important causes of toxic vitiligo are listed in Table 10–15. The essential chemical requirement of melanocyte toxicity appears to be a nonpolar side chain in the para position on the phenolic or catecholic ring structure.[14, 48]

Postinflammatory Changes

Hyperpigmentation may follow any episode of cutaneous inflammation, but it is more likely to occur in darkly complexioned

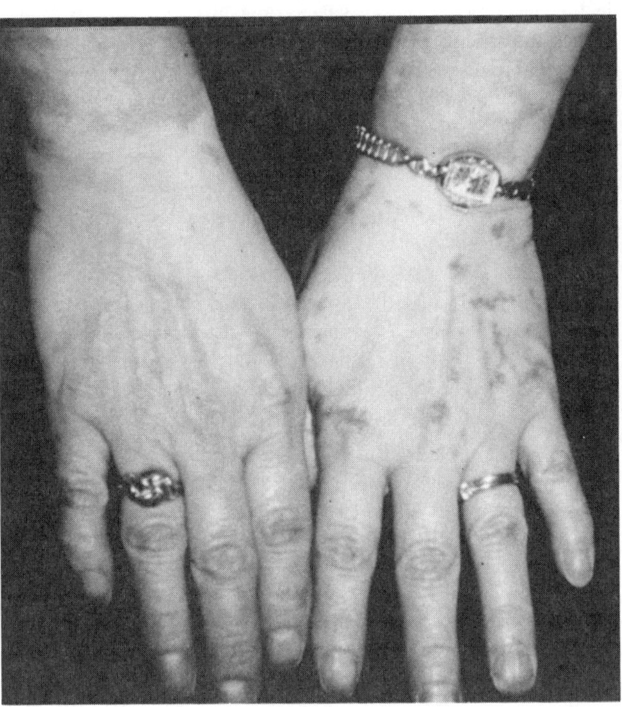

FIG 10–4.
Toxic vitiligo in a hospital custodial worker secondary to p-tert-amylphenol in a disinfectant cleaning solution.

individuals. Cutaneous darkening is due to accumulation of melanin from injured melanocytes or hemosiderin from extravasated red blood cells in dermal tissue. Pigment deposition may persist for years, particularly in black persons, although there is some tendency toward spontaneous improvement. Postinflammatory pigmentation may also follow reactions to photosensitizers (see Photodermatitis), but in these instances the increased pigment results from melanocyte stimulation (i.e., "tanning") rather than injury.

Loss of cutaneous pigment may occur when tissue injury is severe enough to destroy melanocytes, such as chemical or thermal burns.[108] This must be distinguished from toxic vitiligo.

TABLE 10–15.
Important Chemical Causes of Toxic Vitiligo

Hydroquinone
Monobenzyl ether of hydroquinone
Monomethyl ether of hydroquinone (4-hydroxyanisole, 4-methoxyphenol)
Paracresol
Para-tertiary butylcatechol
Para-tertiary butylphenol
Para-tertiary amylphenol
Ortho-phenylphenol
Ortho-benzyl-para-chlorophenol
4-Isopropylcatechol

Discolorations and Stains

Chronic intoxication from heavy metals, particularly silver, mercury, or arsenic, may produce diffuse slate-gray, blue-gray, or melanotic discoloration of skin. The nail beds may be similarly affected. Discoloration results either from metallic deposition within the skin or stimulation of melanin synthesis and is often accentuated in sun-exposed areas.

Numerous industrial substances may stain the skin. These stains serve as useful markers of cutaneous exposure and may be particularly helpful when symptoms of systemic toxicity are present without an obvious history of exposure. Nitrosylated compounds, including nitric acid, trinitrotoluene, dinitrophenol, and metaphenylenediamine, produce yellow to orange cutaneous stains. Many of these nitrosylated substances are initially colorless, and the characteristic stains appear only after oxidation occurs on the skin surface, or after nitration of the nuclei of various aromatic amino acids incorporated into cutaneous protein.[45] Explosive or abrasive forces may adventitially tatoo the skin with pigmented foreign particles.[3] "Coal miner's tatoo," produced by inoculation of coal dust into the skin, is such an example.

Acneiform Disorders

Environmental Acne

Preexisting acne vulgaris may be substantially aggravated by various occupational stresses. Heat and high humidity favor swelling of the keratinous ductal epithelium, with subsequent poral occlusion ("tropical acne"), which may precipitate substantial flares in acne-prone individuals employed in tropical climates or excessively hot work environments, such as foundries. Rubbing, pressure, or friction against the skin may provoke new acne lesions in susceptible anatomical areas ("acne mechanica"). Occupational causes of acne mechanica include face masks, belts, straps, tight-fitting work clothing, and pressure from seat backs.[86]

Oil Acne

Heavy, lubricating petroleum greases, oils, and pitch fumes may cause follicular plugging and pustular folliculitis (oil acne) and is seen not infrequently in machinists and automotive mechanics.[30] Lesions occur most frequently on body surfaces maximally exposed to the causative petroleum products, such as the dorsal fingers, hands, and extensor surfaces of the forearms, and may be particularly severe on parts of the body covered by oil-soaked clothing, such as the thighs. The mechanism of induction involves stimulation of follicular keratinization followed by ductal occlusion. Comedones (blackheads) are invariably present, but inflamed follicular papules and pustules are often numerous. The pustules of oil acne are usually sterile, but occasionally secondary bacterial infection may be present.

Chloracne

Chloracne (Fig 10–5) describes an acneiform disorder caused by either polychlorinated or polybrominated aromatic hydrocarbons, and the term "halogen acne" has been suggested as a more appropriate name.[30, 31] Chemical substances which may cause chloracne are listed in Table 10–16. Toxicity and acneigenic potential depend more on the stereoisomeric positioning of the halo-

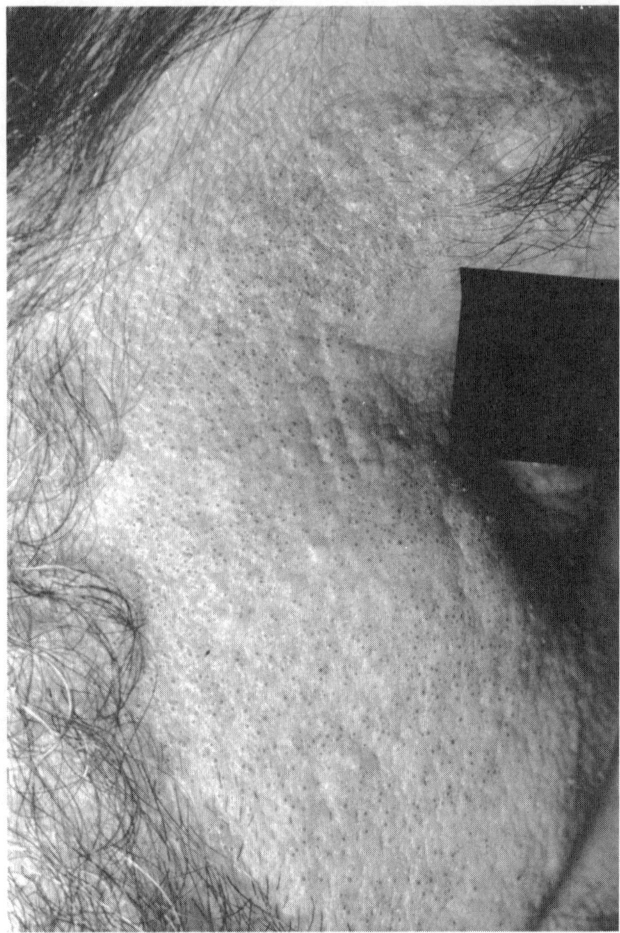

FIG 10–5.
Chloracne. Note preponderance of noninflammatory comedones and cysts. Sites of predilection are the malar crescents and posterior auricular folds. (Photo courtesy of Dr. James S. Taylor. Cleveland Clinic Foundation, Cleveland, Ohio.)

gen atoms than on the degree of halogenation itself.[2] The mechanism by which all chloracneigens produce disease involves induction of squamous metaplasia of the sebaceous gland ducts, followed by atrophy of the underlying sebaceous glands and subsequent formation of keratin-filled cysts.[115] The chemical responsible for inducing chloracne, however, cannot be detected in the cystic contents.[93] There is a rough correlation existing between acneigenic potential and ability to stimulate the aryl hydrocarbon hydroxylase microsomal enzyme system, with 2,3,7,8-tetrachlorodibenzodioxin being the most potent.[31]

TABLE 10–16.
Chemical Causes of Chloracne

Polyhalogenated biphenyls
Polyhalogenated dibenzofurans
Polyhalogenated naphthalenes
Polyhalogenated contaminants
  Dioxin (trichlorophenol, pentachlorophenol)
  Tetrachlorazobenzene and tetrachloroazoxybenzene (dichloroaniline and related chemicals)

The basic dominant clinical lesion is a small cystic swelling resulting from plugging of the pilosebaceous duct, ranging in size from a pinhead to a small pea. The follicular openings of many lesions become obscured, and the swellings begin to assume a characteristic pale yellow color ("straw colored cyst"). The locations in which lesions first begin to appear are the malar crescents (that is, the skin just lateral to the eyes) and the retroauricular folds, and in mild cases these may be the only areas involved. The nose is frequently spared. As the severity of the disease increases, cystic lesions become more numerous on the face, inflammatory lesions appear, and involvement spreads to the posterior neck, trunk, buttocks, and scrotum. The most severe cases may resemble cystic acne, although the number of inflammatory lesions is considerably less. Extensive scarring may occur as inflammatory lesions involute. Some degree of spontaneous improvement is the rule within a few months after cessation of exposure, and approximately 80% resolve completely within two to three years. In the most severe cases, residual lesions may persist for many years, but usually only in the malar regions and behind the ears.[31]

Dusky hyperpigmentation of the face may develop in chloracne cases as the severity of facial involvement increases. Meibomian gland swelling and a peculiar pigmentation of mucous membranes and nail beds occurred in the Yusho and Taiwan PCB (polychlorinated biphenyl) poisonings, where the route of exposure was by ingestion,[68, 126] but it has not been observed in cases caused entirely by cutaneous exposure. Erythema and dermatitis may develop following exposure to the sodium salts of chlorophenols,[31] but is not likely to occur from exposure to trace amounts of chloracneigens.

Chloracne must be distinguished from acne vulgaris, which may appear virtually identical in mild cases, solar elastosis with comedones (Favre-Racouchot syndrome), and other forms of environmental acne. The malar crescents and posterior auricular folds are almost always involved in chloracne cases. The occurrence of numerous, noninflamed, cysts outside the typical areas of distribution for acne vulgaris, documented substantial exposure to known chloracneigens, and absence of other external causes all favor a diagnosis of chloracne. Although histologic examination of chloracne cysts usually demonstrates squamous cell metaplasia and plugging of the infundibular ducts with atrophy of the underlying sebaceous glands,[30] its usefulness in establishing a diagnosis of chloracne has been questioned.[88] Treatment is generally unsatisfactory, but there is anecdotal evidence that topical or oral treatment with cis-13 retinoic acid has been helpful in selected cases.

Vascular Reactions

Urticaria

In comparison to occupational asthma, true occupationally induced urticaria is rare. The overwhelming majority of cases of generalized urticaria are either idiopathic in origin (almost two thirds) or are provoked by exposures outside the work environment (e.g., food or drug allergies). When caused by occupational factors, the route of exposure is almost always inhalation, and episodes of urticaria are invariably accompanied by other symptoms of inhalant allergy (asthma, rhinitis, or conjunctivitis). Some chemical sub-

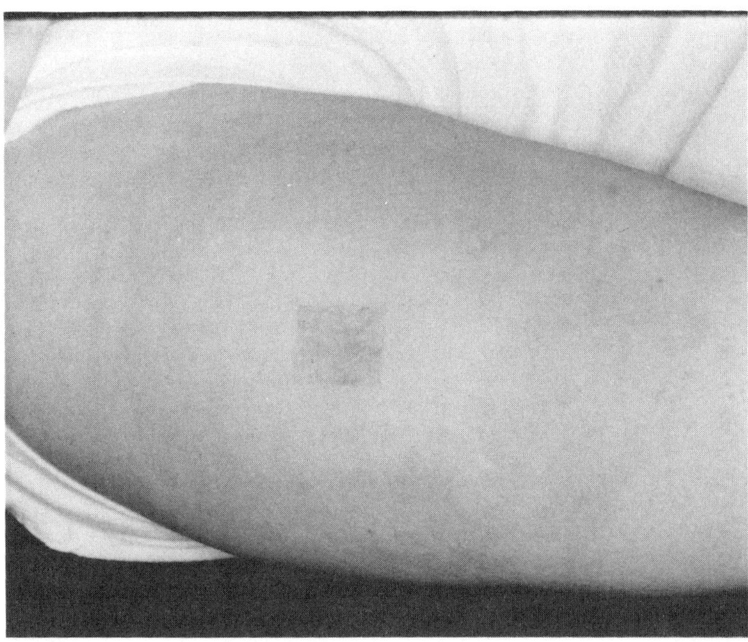

FIG 10–6.
Contact urticaria from carbon paper. The patient complained of swelling and itching of the fingers. A moistened piece of carbon paper produced this intense urticarial reaction after 20 minutes of occlusion against the skin.

stances are also capable of producing localized erythema or wheal and flare responses following skin contact, provided that sufficient penetration through the skin has occurred. This latter phenomenon has been dubbed "contact urticaria"[19] (Fig 10–6).

Urticaria may be provoked by either immunologic or nonimmunologic mechanisms, and its occurrence is not always synonymous with allergy. Urticaria from nonimmunologic mechanisms is caused by direct stimulation (chemical irritation) of the vasculature, indirect provocation of mast cell degranulation, or neural reflex vasodilation. Immunologic mechanisms generally involve IgE-mediated immediate hypersensitivity; more rarely, urticaria may be caused by immune complex-mediated vasculitis, due to activation of the complement cascade and generation of C3a and C5a anaphylotoxins.

Localized contact urticaria requires that the provocative agent first penetrate into the skin. In the case of small molecules, penetration may occur through intact skin. Vasoactive chemical substances capable of inducing localized erythema (rubefacients) have been employed medicinally for centuries as promoters of healing. Contact urticaria from immediate allergy to large proteinaceous molecules generally requires that the normally intact skin barrier be first compromised, since these large molecules would not normally be expected to penetrate intact skin. Atopic persons are more prone to develop immunologic contact urticaria, and they generally give histories of reacting to the provocative substance by inhalation or ingestion as well. Atopic persons who are employed in wet work occupations where skin irritation commonly occurs and who are simultaneously exposed to potentially allergenic proteinaceous molecules, are particularly susceptible, since the skin barrier is compromised by preceding contact dermatitis.[84] Occupations in which allergic contact urticaria is most likely to occur include gardening, food handling, and veterinary medicine, where the occurrence of clinical disease generally reflects a previously documented inhalant or food allergies.

The clinical eruption of urticaria consists of evanescent, pruritic, erythematous macules or wheals ("hives"), usually erupting within 15–60 minutes following exposure. Individual lesions usually subside within 24–48 hours after cessation of exposure. Contact urticaria, by definition, always occurs at the site of primary skin contact with the provocative substance; subjective stinging and burning suggest nonimmunologic mechanisms, while pruritus and swelling characterize immunologic contact urticaria. Generalized urticaria following a localized reaction is rare, but should also suggest IgE-mediated hypersensitivity. A peculiar clinical variant of contact urticaria, termed "protein contact dermatitis," may occur in food handlers or other workers with dyshidrotic or irritant hand eczema.[56] Immediate symptoms of itching, swelling, and redness are rapidly followed by increased vesiculation of the skin, which is more characteristic of delayed hypersensitivity reactions. Whether this biphasic response represents an interaction of humoral and cell-mediated immune mechanisms, or results from nonspecific accumulation of serum released by the urticarial reaction within preexistent microvesicles, has not been resolved.[19]

Causes of occupational urticaria are listed in Table 10–17. Outdoor workers are susceptible to ordinary inhalant allergies to grass, trees, or pollen, for example, which may be accompanied by generalized urticaria. With the exception of proteinaceous dust and molds, inhalant allergies with urticaria among indoor workers are extremely uncommon, and case reports attributing urticaria to chemical fume allergy are mostly anecdotal[63] and difficult to prove. One exception is "platinosis," a syndrome among workers exposed to fumes of platinum salts, consisting of conjunctivitis, rhinitis,

TABLE 10–17.
Some Common Causes of Occupational Urticaria

INHALANTS	SKIN CONTACTANTS
Dust	Dairy products
Molds	Fish
Grasses, trees, pollen	Citrus fruits
Castor bean pomace	Grains
Coffee bean dust	Meats
Platinum salts	Nuts
Penicillin	Spices
Formaldehyde(?)	Vegetables
Pesticides(?)	Medicinal rubefacients
Ammonia(?)	Animal hair and tissues
Sulfur dioxide(?)	Plants and grasses
Aliphatic polyamines(?)	Dimethylsulfoxide
	Alcohols
	Numerous other chemicals

asthmatic symptoms, urticaria, and angioedema.[15] This syndrome has been clearly demonstrated to involve IgE-mediated hypersensitivity to platinum compounds.

Diagnostic evaluation requires prick, intradermal, or epicutaneous provocative tests, with appropriately prepared extracts and sufficient numbers of controls; clinical challenge tests may be necessary in some cases. Confirmation of immunologic mechanisms involves RAST or passive transfer tests. Management consists of avoiding exposure to the provocative substances, and adequate doses of antihistamines. Care should be taken when the patient operates heavy equipment or machinery, since oversedation represents a safety hazard; antihistamines with the least sedating properties (e.g., tersenadine) should be selected in such circumstances. Nonsteroidal anti-inflammatory agents have benefited some cases of nonimmunologic contact urticaria.

Flushing Reactions

Flushing is a transient redness of the skin that occurs primarily on the face but occasionally on the neck and upper chest. It results from a temporary shunting of blood flow to the face into the superficial dermal blood vessels. In the occupational setting, exposure to several different chemical substances may trigger unpleasant flushing reactions.

Rubber industry workers exposed to tetramethyl- or tetraethylthiuram disulfide (disulfiram; Antabuse), which is used to accelerate rubber curing, may experience severe flushing reactions and headaches, along with nausea and vomiting, if alcohol is ingested shortly after work. In part, it was the observation of these unpleasant reactions in rubber workers in the 1920s and 1930s that led to the introduction of disulfiram as a treatment for chronic alcohol addiction.[13] Disulfiram inhibits the enzymic alcohol dehydrogenase, blocking the normal catabolism of alcohol, leading to an accumulation of acetaldehyde in the body, which is thought to be responsible for the reaction.

"Degreasers' flush" has been described in workers who subsequently ingested alcohol following exposure to trichloroethylene vapors.[10, 114] Trichloroethylene also inhibits the normal catabolism of alcohol.[89] Disulfiram-like reactions in industry workers have also been reported following exposure to N,N-dimethylformamide[73] and N-butyraldoxime.[72]

Rosacea is an acneiform disorder of the face characterized by erythema, telangiectasia, and a tendency toward papule and pustule formation. Connective tissue hypertrophy, particularly of the nose, may also occur. Flushing reactions are common in rosacea, may be accompanied by burning and stinging sensations in the skin, and are usually the earliest component of the condition to be identified. Although rosacea is generally considered to be an endogenous condition, transient flushing reactions may be triggered by a host of nonspecific environmental stimuli. These include sunlight, heat, alcohol, organic solvent vapors, and emotional stress. When these nonspecific stimuli are encountered in the workplace, considerable diagnostic confusion may result.

Connective Tissue Disorders

Vibration White Finger

Physiologic changes induced by vibration are reviewed in detail in Chapter 21. Operators of vibratory tools, such as chain saws, rock drills, chipping hammers, grinders, and many other power tools, may experience episodic numbness, tingling, and blanching of one or more fingers, identical to the cold-induced vasospastic changes of Raynaud's phenomenon. This disorder has been variably called "vibration-induced white finger disease," "traumatic vasospastic disease," or the hand-arm vibration syndrome. The latent interval between exposure to vibration and onset of symptoms is inversely related to the acceleration of the vibrating tool and the cumulative hours of daily exposure to vibration.[16] Frequencies above 60 Hz are capable of inducing vasospasms at threshold acceleration values in the range of 75 m/sec^2.[16] Since the Pacinian corpuscles respond most sensitively to frequencies in the 125 Hz range, reflex linkage of Pacinian corpuscles to the sympathetic innervation of the cutaneous vasculature has been suggested as a possible mechanism for induction of the vasospastic phenomena.[57] Other etiologic factors believed to be important are biodynamic forces involved in the holding or operation of the tool and individual host susceptibility (for example, smoking or preexisting vascular disease may increase susceptibility).[116]

The first symptoms consist of persistent numbness and tingling, developing within several minutes of commencing operation of a vibratory tool, followed by variable degrees of swelling of the fingers. With further exposure, blanching of the fingertips begins to occur and is generally most severe in the fingers exposed to the most intense vibration. At first, these symptoms may totally subside on weekends or vacations, but later they may be precipitated upon exposure to cold. The ischemia is followed by reactive hyperemia and cyanosis, and in advanced cases persistent cyanosis of the fingers is present. Ischemic ulcerations of the fingertips may develop, but the latter complication is fortunately rare. Paresthesias and neurosensory deficits are also the rule. The disease may be particularly severe in forestry workers operating chain saws who are simultaneously exposed to damp cold.[70]

Vibration-induced white finger disease must be differentiated from Raynaud's phenomenon that is associated with underlying connective tissue disease, occlusive vascular disease, brachial artery compression syndromes, dysglobulinemia, and neurogenic disorders. Spontaneous remission is not likely, except in mild cases, and moderately to severely affected workers must usually change occupations. Warm, protective clothing is necessary in cold climates. Pharmacologic therapy formerly consisted of vasodilatory agents such as reserpine, but recent interest has focused on calcium channel blockers. Although reportedly effective in the management of Raynaud's phenomenon associated with underlying collagen vascular disease, their effectiveness in vibration-induced white finger disease remains to be established.

Collagen Vascular Disease

Cutaneous changes similar to those observed in scleroderma or progressive systemic sclerosis have been reported in association with various occupational exposures,[52] which are listed in Table 10–18. Workers exposed to unreacted vinyl chloride monomer, used to manufacture polyvinyl chloride, have developed Raynaud's phenomenon, papular cutaneous sclerosis, sclerodactyly and fibrosis of the lungs, liver, and spleen, accompanied by lytic lesions of the middle distal phalanges (acroosteolysis).[78] These changes mostly revert to normal following cessation of exposures, but an increased incidence of angiosarcoma of the liver has been observed. Other than vinyl chloride disease, the vast majority of other reported cases of occupational scleroderma have occurred from exposure to silica dust (silicosis), but unlike vinyl chloride disease, the cutaneous sclerosis has been diffuse rather than papular.[101] A new sclerodermatous disorder has been recently described in Japanese workers exposed to epoxy resin, consisting of severe, diffuse cutaneous sclerosis and muscle weakness.[127] This latter disorder was attributed to a cyclohexylamine hardener (bis(4-amino-3-cyclohexyl)methane), which produced sclerodermatous skin changes, with increases in type 1 collagen, following intraperitoneal injections into mice. Reports attributing scleroderma to various solvent exposures are largely anecdotal and require further observation and confirmation.[104, 113, 128]

Peripheral Neuropathy

This subject is discussed in detail in Chapter 50. Although most cases are due to ingestion or inhalation exposures, the skin is an important potential route of exposure. Following absorption through the skin, peripheral conversion by the liver to a toxic metabolite may be necessary before neurotoxicity can develop (e.g., in exposures to n-hexane, methyl-n-isobutyl ketone). Occasionally, a few chemical substances which are directly neurotoxic may have a selective effect at the primary site of skin contact, such as acrylamide. Recently, synthetic pyrethroids have been shown to elicit cutaneous paresthesias in workers handling this insecticide.[67]

TABLE 10–18.
Occupational Causes of Scleroderma-Like Disorders

Vinyl chloride
Silica
Epoxy resin hardener (bis(4-amino-3-cyclohexyl)methane)
Perchloroethylene(?)
Trichloroethylene(?)
Miscellaneous organic solvents(?)

Neoplasms

Radiation

Considerable clinical, epidemiologic, and experimental evidence has established ultraviolet (UV) solar radiation to be one of our most potent and important environmental carcinogens. Despite the large number of individuals occupationally exposed to sunlight, and the relatively frequent occurrence of skin cancers in outdoor workers,[51] little effort has been expended to protect workers' skins adequately from carcinogenic UV radiation.

Squamous cell carcinoma (Fig 10–7), a neoplasm of epidermal squamous cells, occurs most frequently on areas of the body that are chronically exposed to sunlight, namely the head, neck, and dorsal hands and forearms. Within areas of chronic exposure, there is a further clustering on regions that receive the maximum amounts of UV exposure: the cheeks, nose, forehead, lower lip, and tops of the ears. Squamous cell carcinoma seldom arises spontaneously on normal appearing skin, and involved sites generally show other signs of extensive actinic damage. These latter changes include: thickened, yellowish, furrowed skin (solar elastosis); abundant cutaneous wrinkles; multiple, dilated, superficial cutaneous blood vessels (telangiectasiae); solar-induced lentigines (freckles); and flat, erythematous, scaling, premalignant actinic keratoses.

Basal cell carcinoma, a tumor of epidermal basal cells, demonstrates a similar, strong clinical predilection for anatomical areas chronically exposed to sunlight. Unlike squamous cell carcinoma, however, up to one third of basal cell carcinomas may develop within skin which is not chronically exposed, and there is a further tendency to cluster in periorbital skin and the nasolabial folds, which receive considerably less UV radiation than other facial sites, suggesting that additional factors other than sunlight contribute to its development.[120] Except for lentigo maligna melanoma, a clinical variant occurring in chronically sun-exposed skin of elderly individuals, the evidence linking malignant melanoma to chronic UV exposure suggests a complicated inter-relationship.[71]

Epidemiologic surveys have clearly demonstrated an increased risk for the development of squamous cell, basal cell, or melanoma skin cancers among white populations as one moves closer to the equator.[51, 119] When geographic locations at similar latitudes are corrected for the cumulative yearly amount of UV radiation actually reaching the earth's surface, the association becomes even stronger. Within any geographic location, a similar correlation between skin cancer incidence and cumulative individual exposure to UV radiation may be demonstrated. Host susceptibility and pigmentary skin differences also influence the development of skin cancer; while persons with Irish, English, or Scottish origins who sunburn easily have the greatest relative risks.[123]

Squamous cell carcinoma may be easily produced in hairless rodents by repeated exposures to artificial UV radiation, with the

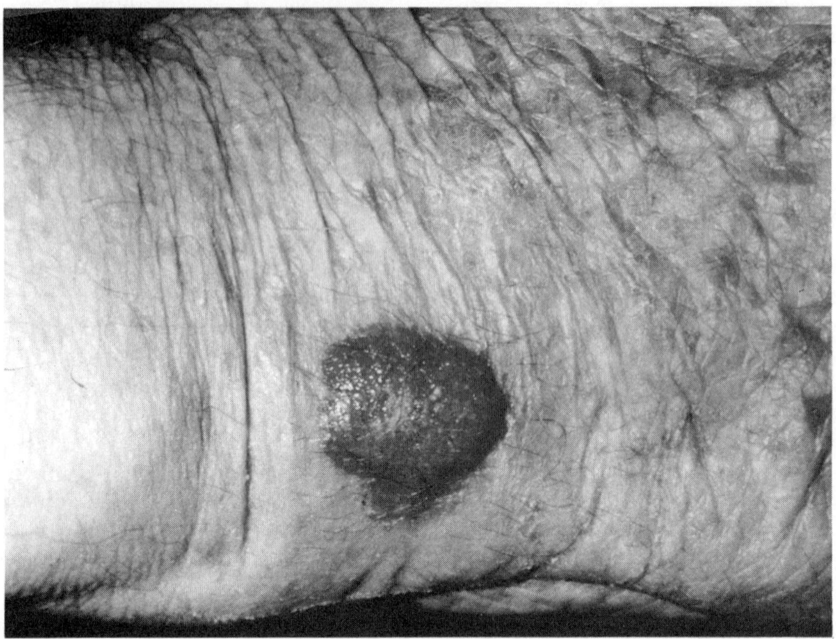

FIG 10–7.
Squamous cell carinoma arising within sun-damaged skin on the dorsal hand of a farmer.

primary carcinogenic wavelength being in the 290–320 nm range. Concomitant exposure to longer wavelength UV radiation, or environmental climatic changes induced by heat, wind, or excessive humidity, may augment carcinogenesis in the laboratory. Cutaneous chemical carcinogens, such as polycyclic aromatic hydrocarbons and nitrosourea compounds, have additive effect when combined with UV radiation. Furthermore, chemical irritants which are not primarily carcinogenic (e.g., croton oil) may promote the development of UV-induced squamous cell carcinomas. To date, neither basal cell nor melanoma skin cancer has been experimentally reproduced in laboratory animals following UV irradiation alone, but malignant melanoma has been reproduced following UV exposure only after benign melanocytic tumors have been first induced by topical application of dimethylbenzanthracene.[39]

Prevention of solar-induced skin cancers should be generally aimed at reduction or elimination of UV exposure. Hats and tightly knit clothing may substantially reduce sunlight exposure, but workers often cannot tolerate such protective clothing in hot climates. The most practical and efficient method of reducing UV exposure in outdoor workers should be the regular use of broad-spectrum sunscreens, preferably with a solar protection factor of 15 or greater. The selected sunscreens should also resist wash-off by sweating and should probably be reapplied several times during the work shifts.[94]

Cutaneous neoplasms may arise in areas of chronic radiodermatitis resulting from excessive exposure to ionizing radiation. Numerous cases have been observed in physicians, dentists, and other medical personnel who were inadvertently exposed while operating x-ray machines. The histologic types include squamous cell and basal cell skin cancers, with sarcomas or melanomas developing more rarely. Squamous cell carcinomas induced by ionizing radiation tend to be aggressive and metastasize early, compared to those of actinic origin.[25]

Polycyclic Aromatic Hydrocarbons

The role of polycyclic aromatic hydrocarbons in cutaneous carcinogenesis is well established. Squamous cell carcinoma of the scrotum of chimney sweeps was the first recognized occupational neoplasm and was later observed in mule spinners. Dimethylbenzanthracene and 3,4-benzyprine, found in coal tar and its derivatives (especially pitch, asphalt, creosote, and heavy mineral oil), are the most potent experimental carcinogens. After latent intervals of 6–20 years, keratotic papillomas ("tar warts") begin to appear on exposed surfaces. Sites of predilection include the face, forearms, hands, ankles, dorsal feet, and scrotum.[50] Other clinical signs of tar toxicity (oil acne, hyperpigmentation, phototoxicity) are usually present. Malignant degeneration into frank squamous cell carcinoma, however, probably occurs in only very few of the premalignant papillomas. Concomitant trauma and UV radiation exposure are generally considered important cofactors in tar carcinogenesis.[122]

Preventive measures are directed primarily at employee hygiene and education. Substitution of oils, free of carcinogenic polycyclic aromatic hydrocarbons, is desirable wherever possible and can substantially reduce the incidence of skin cancer.[37]

Arsenic

Despite the inability to induce experimental cutaneous tumor formation with arsenic, the circumstantial evidence implicating it as a cutaneous carcinogen is considerable. Numerous case reports have documented the development of arsenical keratoses and skin cancers in individuals who received Fowler's solution (sodium arsenite) for treatment of psoriasis. Taiwanese populations drinking water from artesian wells contaminated with arsenic have demonstrated a marked incidence of skin cancers compared to control populations.[117] One study of a group of factory workers exposed to inorganic arsenic demonstrated increased numbers of skin cancers in workers exposed to the highest levels of arsenic within the plant.[55]

Characteristic punctate, keratotic papules ("arsenical keratoses") develop on the palms and soles of individuals with chronic arsenic exposure. They generally range in size from 1 to 5 mm. Histologic examination usually shows varying degrees of nuclear atypia of the squamous cells, and degeneration into squamous cell carcinoma is sometimes observed. Arsenical keratoses must be distinguished from the punctate keratoses frequently seen on the palms or soles of black persons; these benign lesions remain confined to the palmar or plantar creases. Other signs of chronic arsenic exposure include a diffuse dusky pigmentation of the skin punctuated with white, slightly atrophic macules, giving the skin the appearance of "rain drops on a dusty road." Squamous cell carcinomas induced by arsenic exposure often occur on nonexposed skin surfaces; intraepidermal squamous cell carcinoma (Bowen's disease) is the most frequent clinical type and is associated with visceral malignancies. Basal cell carcinomas on nonexposed skin surfaces are also common.

Trauma

The role of trauma in cutaneous neoplasia remains controversial. Skin cancer arising directly within an area of cutaneous trauma has been documented on numerous occasions,[6, 35] but it should be considered a rare occurrence. Thermal burns with subsequent scar formation have been the most frequently observed form of associated trauma. In most cases, the skin fails to heal completely after the initial trauma, and malignancy develops after a variable latent period. If complete healing does occur, a causal relationship between the initial trauma and subsequent development of skin cancer should be suspected. Squamous cell carcinomas arising within burn scars on the legs from heating coals have been reported from India (Kangri ulcer) and Japan (Kairo ulcer), but they may be due primarily to polycyclic aromatic hydrocarbons in the coals rather than the actual trauma.[2] From a scientific viewpoint, evidence suggests that trauma is a co-carcinogen rather than a true carcinogen.[121]

Miscellaneous Neoplasms

A cutaneous T-cell lymphoma (mycosis fungoides) has been associated epidemiologically with work in construction and manufacturing industries and with pesticide and other miscellaneous chemical exposures.[106] Clinical observation suggests that in some cases, cutaneous T-cell lymphoma could develop from chronic bouts of allergic contact dermatitis and antigen stimulation, with subsequent malignant transformation of the stimulated clone of T cells.[120] These intriguing observations will require confirmation before definitive conclusions may be drawn.

Increased incidences of malignant melanoma have been observed in a number of occupations with diverse chemical exposures. At this time, no definite conclusions regarding causative exposures can be drawn on the basis of existing epidemiologic data.

Infections and Infestations

Individual workers employed in a diverse number of occupations may be exposed to a wide range of potentially infectious microorganisms. While virtually any kind of infection can occur as a result of some employment if conditions are favorable, some are considered to be specific risks for certain occupations and may have skin manifestations. Since a comprehensive review of infectious disease is well beyond the scope of this review, only those infections or infestations with primary or diagnostic cutaneous lesions will be considered here. Systemic infections with secondary skin manifestations will not be covered, although some (*e.g.*, brucellosis) may be specific for certain occupations.

Bacteria

Abrasions, burns, and lacerations, particularly when combined with poor skin hygiene, may nonspecifically predispose a worker to a number of bacterial skin infections. Atopic workers are most susceptible to bacterial skin infections, particularly *Staphylococcus*. Excessive heat and humidity may predispose to bacterial folliculitis or furunculosis ("boils"), especially when work clothing is constrictive.

The primary lesion of anthrax, caused by *Bacillus anthracis*, is a small papule which rapidly enlarges to form a boggy, gelatinous, painless mass topped with a hemorrhagic or necrotic vesicle or pustule; satellite lesions may surround the primary lesion. Infection almost always occurs on exposed surfaces of the body (face, neck, arms, hands) from direct, accidental inoculation of spores from contaminated animal hair or hides, particularly sheep and goats. Later, regional lymph nodes enlarge and signs of systemic illness (fever, malaise, leukocytosis, tachycardia) appear. In the United States, strict animal controls and vaccination programs have virtually eliminated this disease among ranchers and farmers, and workers at risk are now primarily dock workers or freight handlers who unload animal hides imported from foreign countries, where strict controls do not exist. Anthrax may be fatal unless adequately treated with intravenous penicillin (4–6 million units daily) or tetracycline (2 gm per day) for two weeks. This diagnosis is established on gram stain and culture of exudate from the primary lesion.

Erysipeloid occurs in fishermen, butchers, or other handlers of raw meat or poultry products. It is an acute infection of traumatized skin, and usually occurs on the hands or fingers following puncture or laceration of the skin on bones or cutting utensils. The initial lesion usually occurs within one week following cutaneous trauma and consists of a painful, sharply marginated, raised edematous plaque which expands peripherally without ulceration or desquamation. Low-grade fever and malaise may develop, but serious systemic illness or complications are rare. The untreated lesion usually resolves spontaneously within three weeks but may occasionally relapse. The causative organism, *Erysiplothrix insidiosa*, is difficult to demonstrate on either gram stain or culture of infected tissue, and the diagnosis is established primarily on clinical grounds. Erysipeloid must be distinguished from streptococcal cellulitis. The disease responds to oral penicillin (equivalent to 2–4 million units per day) or erythromycin (1 gm per day) for seven to ten days.

Mycobacteria

Primary tuberculosis of the skin may be caused by accidental inoculation of material from infected human or animal tissues into traumatized skin. In individuals with no preexisting immunity to *Mycobacterium tuberculosis*, the initial lesion is a generally painless papule arising within two to four weeks at the site of initial trauma, which slowly enlarges and ulcerates (tuberculous chancre). Regional lymphadenopathy develops within one to two months following the appearance of the primary lesion. The clinical lesion of primary inoculation tuberculosis occurring in individuals with some degree of previous immunity is a slowly expanding, hyperkeratotic, verrucous appearing plaque with a purplish inflammatory halo (tuberculosis verrucosa cutis); the regional lymph glands are usually not enlarged. In the past, primary inoculation tuberculosis was considered an occupational risk of physicians, pathologists, and morgue attendants, and was sometimes called "prosector's wart." It is a relatively rare disease today. The diagnosis is established by biopsy and appropriate culture of infected tissue. Treatment consists of isoniazid in combination with rifampin or other antituberculous drugs.

Atypical microbacterial infections of the skin occur through primary cutaneous inoculation. The most common occupational infection is caused by *Mycobacterium marinum* and occurs in persons who fish or other workers who clean fish tanks. The clinical lesion is a firm, granulomatous nodule of the dorsal hand or finger with a tendency toward central ulceration. Multiple lesions of the hand and arm, oriented along lines of lymphatic drainage, may occur and resemble those of sporotrichosis. Diagnosis is established by tissue biopsy and appropriate culture. Spontaneous healing of untreated lesions normally occurs within two to three years, usually with residual scar formation. Small lesions may be surgically excised. Treatment with conventional antituberculous therapy may be limited by drug resistance. Minocycline, 100–200 mg per day, has been reported as an effective alternative therapy.

Viruses

Primary or recurrent herpes simplex infections of the hand or fingers (herpetic whitlow) has generally been considered an occupational hazard of dentists, nurses, physicians, or other health personnel exposed to oral secretions. The clinical lesions are often excruciatingly painful, and extensive edema of surrounding tissues may occur, resembling cellulitis. Lymphangitic streaking and tender enlargement of epitrochlear or axillary lymph nodes may develop. Virologic examination of blister fluid from the lesions of a recent series of patients with herpetic whitlow have challenged an automatic presumptive relationship to oral secretions, since 11 of 13 patients grew type 2 rather than type 1 virus.[49] The usefulness of acyclovir in primary inoculation herpes simplex infections remains to be established. Conservative management consists of limb elevation, analgesics, and any one of a myriad of topical drying agents.

Orf (echthyma contagiosum) is transmitted to human skin following contact with infected sheep or goats, in whom the disease is usually present as a weeping, crusted eruption around the mouth. It is caused by the orf virus, a member of the poxvirus group, and occurs primarily on the hands of farmers, ranchers, or veterinarians tending to sheep. The clinical lesion is most often solitary and generally evolves through six stages, each lasting about six days: the papular stage (erythematous, firm papule), the target stage (a central nodule surrounded by a halo of normal skin and an outer periphery of erythema), the acute stage (red, weeping surface on the nodule), the regenerative stage (thin, dry crust over surface of nodule), the papillomatous stage (tiny papillomatous growths over surface of nodule), and the regressive stage (regression of papillomas and reduction in overall size of lesion). Diagnosis is confirmed by electron microscopic examinations of infected tissues or specific viral antibody titers in serum. Complete resolution of the lesion without therapy is the rule.

Milker's nodule is a viral skin infection caused by paravaccinia virus, acquired by direct skin contact with infected cows, where lesions occur on the teats. Thus, it occurs most commonly in farmers or other dairy workers responsible for milking cows. The clinical lesion bears a striking resemblance to orf, with the nodule passing through similar stages of evolution. The diagnosis is confirmed by electron microscopy or viral culture of infected tissue. Spontaneous resolution without treatment occurs.

Fungi

The majority of superficial fungal (dermatophyte) skin infections are not work-related. Work environments which are hot and humid, such as foundries, may predispose certain populations of workers to development of superficial dermatophyte infections in a nonspecific fashion, particularly the groin and feet, since the presence of moisture, sweat, and heat promotes fungal growth. Dermatophytes may infect the fingernails and hands of those employed in wet work occupations. *Trichophyton rubrum* typically causes a dry, scaling, sometimes painful eruption of the palms, which for unknown reason is characteristically present on only one hand of the affected individual, but spares the other (Fig 10–8); evidence of *T. rubrum* infection can usually be found elsewhere on the body, particularly the toenails and soles. Wet work dries the skin of the affected palm even further, exaggerating the symptoms, and the worker often notices improvement when not working. A scaling eruption confined to the palm of one hand should immediately prompt an examination of the feet and search for fungus.

Zoophilic fungi (i.e., those with animal reservoirs) may specifically infect farm workers, veterinarians, or other animal handlers. Zoophilic *Trichophyton mentagrophytes* may be carried by a wide range of animals and frequently produces an intense inflammatory cutaneous reaction with pustule formation. Lesions caused by *Microsporum canis* (dogs and cats) more typically have a "ringworm" appearance. *T. verrucosum* is acquired from infected cattle and may produce a deep inflammatory reaction of the neck, beard, or scalp. Diagnosis is established by demonstration of fungal hyphae on potassium hydroxide examination of scales or hair from infected skin. Superficial dermatophyte infections on the general body surface may be treated with topical imidazole antifungal preparations. Infections of the palms, soles, and nails, or deep inflammatory reactions on hair-bearing surfaces, do not generally respond well to topical agents, and oral therapy (250–500 mg of micronized griseofulvin or its equivalent, two times per day) is preferred. Oral ketoconazole also has been used for treatment of dermatophyte infections.

Sporotrichosis is acquired from accidental inoculation of the fungus *Sporothrix schenkii* from contaminated vegetation. Rosebush

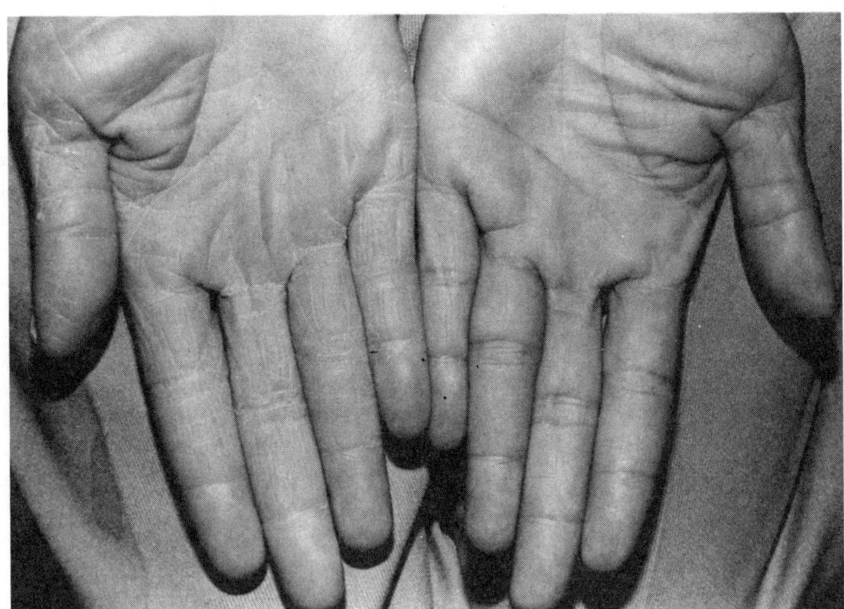

FIG 10–8.
Superficial dermatophyte infection of one palm, sparing the other, in a dishwasher.

thorns and sphagnum moss are favorite habitats of the organism, and the disease most frequently occurs in gardeners, florists, or nursery workers. The usual clinical presentation is an ulcerated nodule on the dorsal hand, followed by the appearance of similar cutaneous nodules spreading in a linear fashion along lines of lymphatic drainage. Definitive diagnosis by demonstration of the characteristic cigar-shaped organism in infected tissue is difficult, and culture is often required. Sporotrichosis must be distinguished from atypical mycobacterial infections caused by *M. marinum,* which it may mimic closely. The treatment of choice is 10–15 drops of a saturated solution of potassium iodide three times daily.

Warm, moist work environments may nonspecifically predispose to several clinical types of infection with *Candida albicans.* As with dermatophyte infections, *Candida* infections may develop in intertriginous body surfaces (the groin, axillae, and inframammary skin). Infection of the fingernail folds (paronychia) is perhaps the most frequent occupational infection caused by *Candida* and occurs in bartenders, beauticians, custodial workers, machinists, or virtually anyone else whose hands are constantly exposed to moisture while working. The clinical appearance is a red, swollen, mildly to moderately painful nail fold which does not suppurate, with local destruction of the cuticle. Erosive dermatitis from *Candida* infection occasionally occurs in the web spaces between the fingers. Treatment with topical mycostatin or antifungals is usually effective, but chronic paronychia may need to be treated for months.

Parasites

Outdoor workers are susceptible to a host of biting insects or other infestations which may present with cutaneous lesions. Hookworm (cutaneous larva migrans) and schistosome (swimmers' or clam diggers' itch) infections may develop in workers maintaining beaches, lakes, or streams. Scabies, caused by the mite *Sarcoptes scabiei,* may infect employees of hospitals, nursing homes, or chronic care facilities who attend infested patients. The intensely pruritic eruption of scabies may occur anywhere on the body surface below the neck, but typically includes the axillae, buttocks, genital and periumbilical skin, wrists, ankles, and web spaces between the fingers, where pathognomonic burrows are classically seen. Diagnosis is established by microscopic demonstration of the mite, eggs, or feces from skin scrapings of a burrow. The treatment of choice is lindane or malathion lotion, applied to the entire body and left on for 8–12 hours; treatment may be reapplied in one week. Alternatively, preparations containing 5%–10% precipitated sulfur or crotamiton may be used. Other mite infestations generally considered to be specific risks for certain occupations include the poultry mite *(Dermanyssus gallinae)* and the grain mite *(Pheomotes ventricosus),* which may cause pruritic papular eruptions in poultry workers or handlers of raw grain. The diagnosis must be established by demonstrating mites in the infected host, since they do not burrow or reside in human skin.

Disorders of Hair and Nails

Like the skin, the hair and nails are subject to a number of occupational afflictions, particularly infections, chemical discolorations, and abnormalities of growth.

Bacterial or fungal infection of hair follicles (folliculitis) has been previously discussed. Hair discoloration may result from accidental contact with industrial dyes and stains, but the cause is usually obvious. Workers with long hair who are employed around machinery with rapidly rotating parts are subject to traumatic hair loss (alopecia), if the hair accidentally becomes entangled in the machinery; the hair is literally pulled out by the roots, but complete regrowth in six to nine months is the rule and no treatment is indicated. When chemical or thermal burns severe enough to cause scarring and destruction of the hair bulbs occur on hair-bearing surfaces, permanent hair loss results.

Diffuse hair loss has been associated with toxic exposures (toxic alopecia) to thallium-containing rodenticides, boric acid, arsenic, and chloroprene,[36] and is virtually always seen in association with other signs and symptoms of systemic toxicity specifically related to the causative exposure. Hair loss usually begins within two to four weeks of an acute toxic exposure, but onset may be more insidious in the case of chronic intoxications. Microscopic examination of hair shafts in toxic alopecia usually reveals a characteristic narrowing or tapering of the shaft near the hair root, due to arrest or inhibition of mitotic activity, and hair loss is caused by breakage of the structurally weakened shaft at this point. When toxic alopecia is due to thallium exposure, the hair shafts will also show some pigment darkening near the root. Circumscribed patches of hair loss suggest a diagnosis of alopecia areata, an autoimmune disorder of hair, and should not be confused with toxic alopecia. Toxic alopecia is a reversible disorder, and hair regrowth commences within a few months, provided that exposure to the provocative toxic agent has ceased.

The nails are similarily susceptible to a number of environmental and occupational afflictions,[9] listed in Table 10–19. Individuals employed in wet work occupations are commonly subject to subungual or paronychial infection of the nails from yeast, bacteria, or fungi. *Pseudomonas* infections characteristically cause a greenish pigmentation beneath the nail plates. Topical therapy can be extremely difficult if the affected individual continues to immerse the hands in aqueous solutions. Topical liquid antibiotic preparations marketed for eye or ear infections are suitable for treatment of subungual or paronychial infections, provided the organisms are susceptible to the selected antimicrobial agent(s). *Pseudomonas* is not sensitive to most of the available topical antibiotics, but preparations containing tobramycin (one of the few topicals to which *Pseudomonas* is sensitive) may be effective.

The nail matrix, located beneath the cuticle and proximal nail fold, contains the germinative cells which form the nail plate. The matrix is vulnerable to a number of occupational insults, all of which can result in dystrophic, abnormal growth of the nail plate. Physical trauma, ionizing or microwave radiation, and mechanical vibration, may all damage the matrix and induce longitudinal ridgings (Beau's lines), brittleness, or thickening of the nail plates. Inflammation of the overlying proximal nail fold, whether bacterial or chemical in origin, produces ridging, stippling, or pitting of the nail plate. Direct absorption of potentially toxic chemicals into the nail folds may occasionally affect the matrix, without causing paronychial inflammation, and alter the growth of the nail plates.[8] Frequent exposure of the nails to solvents may partially dissolve and weaken the formed nail plate, and workers handling solvents frequently complain of thinness and brittleness of the nails.

Onycholysis (separation of the nail plate from the nail bed) most often results from accidental trauma and can be excruciatingly painful. If severe, the entire nail plate may be lost or shed within a few weeks, but complete regrowth ensues. Despite its apparent hardness, the nail plate is not a totally impenetrable barrier and chemical substances may penetrate through or beneath the nail plate, provoking inflammation (contact dermatitis) of the underlying nail bed, with onycholysis, without necessarily provoking inflammation of the paronychial tissue. Similarly, infection beneath the nail plate causes separation of the overlying nail plate.

Discolorations of the nails generally accompany dermatophyte infections of the nail plate, and range from varying shades of yellow and white to brown and black. *Pseudomonas* infections produce greenish subungual pigmentation. Organic dyes, such as hair dyes and photographic solutions, and coal tar derivatives can produce virtually any shade of discoloration, but yellow-brown to black is the most common. Nitrosylated compounds characteristically cause a yellowish discoloration of the nail plates, as well as the skin. Silver intoxication is associated with a characteristic blue discoloration of the lunulae, while PCB intoxication has been associated with brownish pigmentation of the nail bed, but this has occurred only in oriental populations. Horizontal white bands in the nail plate may be caused by repetitive occupational trauma to the nails; distinctive, transverse white bands (Mees' lines) have been classically attributed to arsenic intoxication.

TABLE 10–19.
Common Causes of Occupational Nail Disorders

Paronychial Inflammation	*Onycholysis*
Infection	Trauma
Staphylococcus	Contact dermatitis
Pseudomonas	Infection
Candida	*Discoloration*
Dermatophytes	Infection
Contact dermatitis	*Pseudomonas* (green)
Dystrophic Growth	Dermatophytes (white, yellow, brown/black)
Trauma	Chemical stains
Radiation	Nitrosylated compounds (yellow)
Vibration	Coal tar derivatives (brown/black)
Infection	Organic dyes (brown/black)
Dermatophytes	Chemical toxicity
Candida	Silver (blue lunulae)
Contact dermatitis	PCB (brown)
Chemical toxicity	Arsenic (white bands)
	Trauma (white bands)

Climatic Disorders

Heat and Humidity

Hot, humid environments, or dry environments which are hot enough to provoke copious sweating, may promote blockage of the eccrine sweat glands and a subsequent inflammatory papulovesicular eruption, termed miliaria rubra or "prickly heat." The precise factors which precipitate clinical disease are not completely understood, but the sweat ducts become plugged in the mid to lower epidermis. Lesions begin to appear within a few months of beginning work in a hot environment. The affected individual notes a prickling or stinging sensation, particularly on areas covered by clothing, which may become more pruritic and is often provoked immediately when activities that promote sweating are performed; symptoms subside when the worker moves to a cooler shelter. Miliaria rubra must be distinguished from folliculitis and other cutaneous pyodermas that are also promoted by hot work environments. Although miliaria rubra subsides spontaneously within one week, its disappearance may be aided by topical drying agents such as calamine lotion.

The combination of low humidity and low temperature promotes dryness and chapping of the skin, which quickly becomes pruritic ("winter itch"). When severe, frank eczematous changes develop, the extremities are the most frequently affected sites. Similar climatic conditions can be mimicked by refrigerated air conditioning systems and affect indoor workers during the summer time.[26] The condition responds to liberal use of topical moisturizers.

The combination of warm temperatures and low relative humidity (usually less than 35%) may produce subtle dryness of the skin and symptoms ranging from intense pruritic to low-grade eczema. Termed "low-humidity dermatosis,"[103] it may affect office workers exposed to warm, dry air from heating ducts, or employees engaged in manufacturing processes where low humidity is a necessary quality control measure, as in semiconductor manufacturing. The more vigorously the warm, dry air passes over the workers' skins, the more intense the symptoms. Urticaria has also been reported as an effect of low humidity, but it is unclear whether the phenomenon was simply redness secondary to the normal axon flare in response to scratching, or from underlying dermographism in a few affected individuals. Symptoms dramatically improve once the humidity is raised to 40% or greater and can also be ameliorated by topical moisturizers.

Rusters

A peculiar corrosive reaction of ferrous metals occasionally results from palmar sweat. Individuals capable of producing corrosion of metallic objects simply by touching their surfaces are known as "rusters."

The phenomenon occurs more frequently during the summer when sweating is greater, but it can also occur during winter months, since palmar sweating is also under emotional control. In addition to the unsightly cosmetic appearance of rusty fingerprints and blemishes, metallic products corroded by rusters may malfunction.

Once detected, such employees may lose their jobs. Most rusters give histories of excessive palmar sweating. Corrosion is generally thought to result from excessive concentrations of chloride ions in the palmar sweat of rusters,[18, 21] although this has been disputed;[60, 61] neither pH nor lactate concentrations in sweat appear to be of practical importance. Corrosion may be prevented by degreasing metallic objects in an appropriate solvent immediately after handling by rusters. Inhibition of palmar sweating with topical applications of aluminum chloride hexahydrate solutions has also been effective.[7, 61]

Percutaneous Absorption

Besides the lungs and the gastrointestinal tract, the skin may be an important route of entry for chemical substances that may produce systemic toxicity. For some exposures, such as chloracnigens and pesticides, the skin may be the principal or only route of exposure.[125] Chemical substances that are detoxified after first passing through the liver following intestinal absorption may be even more toxic when absorbed through the skin, since liver detoxification is bypassed.[5]

The development of signs and symptoms of systemic toxicity is determined not only by the inherent toxicologic properties of the chemical toxin, but also on its ability to penetrate through skin. Visible inflammation of skin is not a necessary prerequisite for significant percutaneous absorption, and many substances may produce serious systemic illness if enough is absorbed, without provoking clinical dermatitis. Obviously, a substance that may burn the skin or cause dermatitis, damaging the protective stratum corneum barrier, may enhance its own absorption and systemic toxicity. Factors that may promote percutaneous absorption include: prolonged skin contact with the potentially toxic substance; hydration of the stratum corneum beneath water-impermeable protective clothing, particularly when the potentially toxic substance is entrapped on the skin surface beneath the protective clothing; damage to the stratum corneum barrier from previous trauma (cuts or abrasions) or dermatitis; elevation of skin surface temperature, particularly from transfer of heat from warm or hot industrial liquids; and accidental contact with anatomical areas such as facial or genital skin, which are generally more permeable than the rest of the skin surface.[81]

Important occupational exposures that may produce serious systemic toxicity have been reviewed by Malkinson[75] and Birmingham.[12] Table 10–20 lists important exposures for which systemic toxic reactions have occurred as a result of skin absorption. Concerns regarding toxic exposures and percutaneous absorption have usually focused on relatively acute symptoms associated with exposure; long-term toxicities, particularly carcinogenicity, should also be considered.

ESTABLISHING THE DIAGNOSIS

History

In the course of taking the history from a patient who may have work-related skin disease, the following should be obtained: (1) an accurate chronologic sequence of events surrounding the onset of the skin disease, its subsequent clinical course, and associated work activities; (2) a description of the skin lesions and their initial anatomical locations and spread to other body sites; (3) disability caused by the skin disease; (4) identification of all relevant work exposures; (5) presence of similar skin disease in co-workers; and (6) response to previous medical treatment.

Work activities at the onset of skin disease often provide the most important clue for establishing the correct etiologic diagnosis since exposure to the responsible causal agent has likely occurred at that time. Note should be made as to whether the skin disease began while the patient was performing usual and customary work duties or while on modified assignment. Did the skin disease clear or improve while the patient was performing modified work duties or while not working, for example, during weekends, vacations, or lost work time due to illness? Did any specific activity or exposure exacerbate the skin disease? Care must be taken to distinguish clinical improvement that may be due to concomitant medical therapy from spontaneous improvement, which may occur when the worker is removed from the suspected causative work exposures.

While a clinical description of the skin lesions, obtained directly from the patient, is sometimes useful if no active lesions are present at the time of evaluation, this can be very unreliable, and

TABLE 10–20.
Some Chemical Substances That May Cause Systemic Toxicity Through Percutaneous Absorption

CHEMICAL	SYSTEMIC TOXICITY
Aniline, related azo dyes and derivatives	Methemoglobinemia, liver disease, bladder cancer
Arsenic	Malaise, weight loss, gastrointestinal disturbances, peripheral neuritis
Benzene	Aplastic anemia, myelofibrosis, acute myelogenous leukemia
Polyhalogenated aromatics (chloracneigens)	Gastrointestinal disturbances, liver disease, porphyria, cancer (?)
Cyanide salts	Diffuse cellular asphyxia, death
Mercury	Gastrointestinal disturbances, central nervous system intoxication, nephrosis
Organic solvents	Central nervous system depression
Organophosphates	Headache, diarrhea, increased urination, miosis and blurred vision, brachycardia, bronchorrhea and bronchospasm, muscle excitation and fasciculation, lacrimation, salivation, respiratory depression
Chlorinated hydrocarbons	Convulsion, delirium, central nervous system depression

a review of medical records (when available) is a preferable manner of obtaining a description of the initial clinical appearance. The initial skin site(s) to be involved are generally the areas of most direct skin contact with the causative agent; close attention should be paid to all potential exposures at the initial sites of cutaneous involvement. Dermatitis of the face and neck in a factory worker, for example, should suggest the possibility of an airborne exposure, such as a cutting fluid mist or overspray. The severity of the skin disease may be reflected in whether it has resulted in lost work time or job modification.

An accurate description of work duties and potential exposures is important, but it is not always possible to obtain reliable information directly from the patient; phone calls to supervisors or responsible health and safety personnel, as well as an occasional visit to the worksite, may be required. The evaluating physician should establish not only the identity of potential exposures, but also the quantitative and qualitative aspects of exposure. Have there been any new exposures introduced into the work environment prior to the onset of skin disease, or has there been an increase in amount or duration of skin contact with long-standing exposures, or a change in their circumstances? Protective clothing, such as gloves and work boots, and skin-cleansing products or techniques should be considered as potential causes of occupational dermatitis rather than solely as preventive measures. For example, did a potential irritant spill or splash inside work gloves, or were gloves put on before a potential irritant was properly cleansed from the skin? Environmental conditions, such as temperature and humidity in the workplace, should be established. All first-aid cabinet preparations used to treat the skin condition at the worksite should be identified as potential causes of, or contributions to, the skin disease.

The presence of similar skin disease in co-workers may provide another important clue to its occupational origin or etiology. Unfortunately, a history of similar skin disease based only upon the patient's account is notoriously unreliable. The physician is ill-advised to draw definitive conclusions regarding similar disease in co-workers unless he or she has personally evaluated them or reviewed appropriate medical records.

A thorough history should properly determine the presence of important risk factors, such as personal or family history of atopic allergies; antecedent skin disease or reactions, such as dermatitis from jewelry, cosmetic preparations, or hair dyes; and potential causative exposures in the domestic environment.

Physical Examination

Particular attention should be paid not only to the morphological appearance of individual skin lesions, but also to their distribution on the body surface. The search for a causative agent should be directed at chemical, physical, or biologic exposures actually occurring at the principal site(s) of involvement. Dermatitis that is confined only to palmar surfaces usually indicates that endogenous factors are probably operative.

The physical examination must help to differentiate occupational from endogenous dermatoses, principally psoriasis, atopic dermatitis, and dyshidrotic and various other forms of eczema. The entire skin surface should be examined for the presence of other characteristic skin lesions, particularly the feet. It is not unusual for an affected worker to deny the presence of skin lesions on covered parts of the body, especially if these other lesions are not asymptomatic. If the entire skin surface is not properly examined, the correct diagnosis may be overlooked.

Patch Testing

Although virtually any diagnostic procedure (blood tests, KOH examinations, skin biopsies) may be utilized in an evaluation of a suspected occupational dermatosis, the patch test is the most frequently employed. A great deal of confusion and misunderstanding surrounds this remarkably simple but useful test. The fundamental purpose of the patch test is to establish a diagnosis of allergic (not irritant) contact dermatitis. Interpretation of the patch test rests on the assumption that a suspected allergen will cause a localized eczematous reaction, resembling the clinical eruption under evaluation, when occluded against the skin of a sensitized individual; no reaction should occur on the skin of a nonsensitized person.

Details of the methodology may be found in appropriate textbooks on the subject.[28] All materials to be tested must first be standardized so that no false positive inflammatory irritant reactions (chemical burns) occur when occluded on the skin of nonsensitized, nonexposed individuals (controls). In most cases, this requires dilution of the test material in a suitable vehicle (usually white petrolatum) to a concentration below its irritant threshold. Test substances (already standardized) may be purchased commercially or prepared by the investigator according to published guidelines. Where no reliable guidelines exist (which is often the case for many industrial substances), the investigator must be prepared to establish the proper test concentration by running a sufficient number of controls (usually about 20). Table 10–21 lists the substances contained in the "routine" battery screening series of the American Academy of Dermatology. Evaluating physicians should not forget that at best the patch test procedure only indicates whether or not the tested individual is allergic to any of the tested substances. No conclusions can be drawn regarding allergies to substances which were never tested in the first place. "Routine" screening series are aimed primarily at detecting allergies in the domestic environment and do not contain other allergens more commonly encountered in the workplace.

The test procedure itself is as carefully standardized as to the test concentrations, and it should be stressed that any deviations from the procedure may lead to false negative or positive results. A small amount of test substance (at proper concentration) is placed on a metallic disc or filter paper disc backed with aluminum foil. The disc is attached to adhesive tape and placed on the upper back or upper outer arms. Both the metallic disc and aluminum foil are totally impermeable to water, thus providing total occlusion of the test substance against the skin surface and maximum skin penetration. Test strips are removed two days following application, and the test sites evaluated. An unequivocal positive reaction should demonstrate the presence of numerous papules or vesicles. Weaker reactions (erythema and edema without papules or vesicles) cannot be reliably distinguished from false positive marginal irritant reactions on the basis of morphology alone. Test sites must be reevaluated 72–96 hours following initial application, since 30%–40% of all positive reactions will be negative or equivocal at the 48-hour reading.[79] Incorrectly testing with only partially occlusive test materials, such as Band-Aids, or on the

TABLE 10–21.

Routine Patch Test Screening Series, American Academy of Dermatology, 1984–1985.

Medicaments		*Rubber Additives*
Benzocaine	5%	Thiuram mix 1%
Neomycin	20%	tetramethylthiuram monosulfide,
Metals		tetramethylthiuram disulfide,
Potassium		tetraethylthiuram disulfide,
dichromate	0.5%	dipentamethylenethiuram disulfide
Nickel sulfate	2.5%	Carba mix 3%
Resins		1,3-diphenylguanidine,
Epoxy (diglycidyl ether		zinc dimethyldithiocarbamate,
of bisphenol A)	1%	zinc dibutyldithiocarbamate,
Rosin (colophony)	20%	paraphenylenediamine
P-tert butylphenol		PPD mix 0.6%
formaldehyde	1%	n-phenyl-n-1-cyclohexyl-p-
Preservatives, germicidals		phenylenediamine
Formaldehyde*	2%	n-isopropyl-n-phenyl-p-phenylenediamine
Quaternium-15	2%	n, n-diphenyl-p-phenylenediamine
Thimerosal	0.1%	Mercapto mix 1%
Amidozolidinyl urea	2%	n-cyclohexyl-2-benzothiazole-sulfonamide
Vehicles, stabilizers		2,2-benzothiazyl disulfide
Wool lanolin		4-morpholinyl-2-benzothiazyl disulfide
alcohols	30%	Mercaptobenzothiazole 1%
Ethylenediamine		
HCl	1%	
Flavorings and fragrances		
Balsam of Peru	25%	
Organic dyes		
P-phenylenediamine	1%	
Antioxidants		
P-tert-butylphenol	1%	

*Aqueous vehicle. All other substances tested in white petrolatum vehicle.

wrong skin surface, such as the ventral forearm, or failure to perform a delayed reading, may invalidate the results.

If a valid positive patch test is obtained, the evaluating physician must then decide whether the result adequately explains the dermatitis under consideration. Positive reactions may simply represent past exposure and sensitization to the allergen or reflect exposure from the domestic environment, and do not necessarily mean that exposure to the allergen is actually occurring at the workplace.

The patch test should not be used to diagnose irritant contact dermatitis, since the conditions of the test (total occlusion against the skin for 48 hours) seldom approximate the actual conditions under which exposure is occurring. For example, induction of a third-degree chemical burn by patch testing a mechanic to undiluted diesel fuel to which he is only intermittently and briefly exposed does not definitely indicate that diesel oil is responsible for clinical dermatitis; a better explanation may be cumulative and repetitive exposures to some other solvent to which the mechanic is exposed for several hours a day. In the ultimate analysis, the diagnosis of irritant dermatitis is a clinical judgment resting on a knowledge of the physical or chemical properties of the exposures, familiarity with the actual conditions or circumstances under which exposure is occurring, and some personal experience with similar exposures.

The complications of patch testing include scarring, pigmentary alterations, infections, and accidental induction of sensitization which did not exist prior to the test procedure.

Conclusions

In most cases, a causal relationship between an observed skin disease and a work exposure will be accepted by a workers' compensation board if the condition has been primarily caused or substantially aggravated by employment. Virtually any skin disease may be aggravated by unfavorable work conditions or exposures; the term "substantial aggravation" leaves considerable latitude for interpretation on the part of the evaluating physician. If, in the opinion of the physician, the skin disease would not exist in its present state, or to its present extent, were it not for a specific occupational exposure or activity, then it may be properly considered a work-related disorder. When no signs or symptoms of a primarily endogenous skin disease, such as psoriasis or dyshidrotic eczema, were present prior to an occupational exposure or activity, it may be considered an entirely occupational disorder if the physician believes that the endogamous condition would not likely have spontaneously arisen at that point in time were it not for the occupational exposure or activity which appeared to precipitate it.

PREVENTION

Awareness of the various types of occupational dermatoses and the agents that may cause them is essential to any successful preventive program. Exposures which may cause occupational skin disease within various occupational settings are listed in the Appendix.

Prompt recognition and precise etiologic diagnosis are necessary not only for management of individual cases, but also for prevention of further outbreaks of dermatitis. Contact dermatitis may occasionally be prevented simply by replacing the offending allergen or irritant with a suitable alternative equal to the task of the removed substance.[1, 24]

Protective measures that contain the industrial process and reduce workers' exposures have been the traditional preventive measures for reducing the incidence of occupational skin disease. Protective clothing, such as gloves, boots, and aprons, are available in a number of fabrics or materials; these should be carefully selected with regard to chemical and physical resistance to workplace exposures, and workers should be cautioned concerning entrapment and occlusion of potentially noxious substances against the skin beneath protective clothing. Good skin hygiene and cleansing are other important measures, but workers must be instructed not to clean or wash excessively with harsh substances.[83]

Barrier creams have been highly touted as effective deterrents, but from a scientific viewpoint, hard evidence of efficacy is lacking.[27, 92] Commercially available barrier creams may be divided into four general categories: (1) vanishing creams that simply facilitate skin cleansing; (2) water-repellent barrier creams that contain film-forming, hydrophobic substances (silicone, stearates, waxes, oils); (3) oil- and solvent-repellent barrier creams, which contain beeswax or lanolin to repel oil, or tragacanth and acacia to repel solvent; and (4) ionic exchangers that contain acidic or alkaline bases to buffer the effects of acids and alkalies. In most situations, white petrolatum (Vaseline) is as effective as any other type of barrier cream. In situations where barrier creams have seemed anecdotally effective, their success is more likely due to the lubricating or moisturizing effect of the cream formulation and their ability to facilitate skin cleansing, thus minimizing the need for excessive or vigorous washing, which may cause secondary irritation.

REFERENCES

1. Adams RM: Allergen replacement in industry. *Cutis* 1977; 20:511–516.
2. Adams RM: *Occupational Dermatology*. New York, Grune & Stratton, 1983.
3. Agris J: Adventitious tatooing. *J Dermatol Sur* 1976; 2:72–74.
4. Allen H, Kaidbey K: Persistent photosensitivity following occupational exposure to epoxy resin. *Arch Dermatol* 1979; 115:1301–1310.
5. Ambrose AM, Christensen HE, Robins DJ, et al: Toxicological and pharmacological studies on Chlordane. *Arch Ind Hyg* 1953; 7:197–210.
6. Auster LA: The role of trauma in oncogenesis: A juridical consideration. *JAMA* 1961; 175:946–950.
7. Bang Pedersen N: Topical treatment of a ruster. *Br J Dermatol* 1977; 96:332.
8. Baran RL: Nail damage caused by weed killers and insecticides. *Arch Dermatol* 1974; 110:467.
9. Baran RL: Occupational nail disorders, in Adams RM: *Occupational Skin Disease*. New York, Grune & Stratton, 1983.
10. Bardodej Z, Vyskocil J: The problem of trichloroethylene in occupational medicine. *Arch Ind Health* 1956; 13:581–592.
11. Berkhart PG, et al: Treatment of skin burns due to alkyl mercury compounds. *Arch Environ Health* 1961; 3:106–107.
12. Birmingham DJ, Key MM, Tubich GE, et al: Phototoxic bullae among celery harvesters. *Arch Dermatol* 1961; 83:73–87.

13. Birmingham DJ: Cutaneous reactions to chemicals, in Fitzpatrick TB, Eisen AZ, Wolff K, et al (eds): *Dermatology in General Medicine*. New York, McGraw-Hill Book Co, 1979.
14. Bleehen SS, Pathak MA, Hori Y, et al: Depigmentation of skin with 4-isopropyl catichol, mercaptoamines and other compounds. *J Invest Dermatol* 1968; 50:103–117.
15. Boggs PB: Platinum allergy. *Cutis* 1985; 35:318–320.
16. Brammer AJ: *Exposure of the Hand to Vibration in Industry*. Ottawa, National Research Council of Canada, 1984.
17. Brown VKH, Box VL, Simpson BJ: Decontamination procedures for skin exposed to phenolic substances. *Arch Environ Health* 1975; 30:1–6.
18. Buckley WR, Lewis CE: The "Ruster" in industry. *J Occup Med* 1960; 2:23–31.
19. Burdick AE, Mathias CGT: The contact urticaria syndrome. *Dermatol Clin* 1985; 3:71–84.
20. Burrows D: Prognosis in industrial dermatitis. *Br J Dermatol* 1972; 87:145–146.
21. Burton JL, Pye RJ, Brookes DB: Metal corrosion by chloride in sweat. The problem of "rusters" in industry. *Br J Dermatol* 1976; 95:417–422.
22. California Department of Industrial Relations, Division of Labor Statistics and Research: *Occupational Skin Disease in California (with special reference to 1977)*. San Francisco, California Department of Industrial Relations, 1982.
23. Calnan CD: Cement dermatitis. *J Occup Med* 1960; 2:15–22.
24. Calnan CD: Studies in contact dermatitis, XXIII. Allergen replacement. *Trans St John's Hosp Dermatol Soc* 1970; 56:131–138.
25. Carnow DW, Worobec SM: Skin cancer in the workplace, in Drill VA, Lazar P (ed): *Current Concepts in Cutaneous Toxology*. New York, Academic Press, 1980.
26. Chernosky ME: Pruritic skin disease and summer air conditioning. *JAMA* 1962; 179:1005–1010.
27. Church R: Prevention of dermatitis and its medico-legal aspects. *Br J Dermatol* 1981; 105(suppl 21):85–90.
28. Cronin E: *Contact Dermatitis*. London, Churchill Livingstone, Inc, 1980.
29. Crow KD, Alexander E, Buck WL, et al: Photosensitivity due to pitch. *Br J Dermatol* 1961; 73:220–232.
30. Crow KD: Chloracne: A critical review including a comparison of two series of cases of acne from chloronaph—thalene and pitch fumes. *Trans St John's Hosp Dermatol Soc* 1970; 56:79–99.
31. Crow KD: Chloracne (halogen acne), in Marzulli FA, Maibach HI (eds): *Dermatotoxicology*. Washington, DC, Hemisphere Publishing Co, 1981, pp 461–481.
32. Curreri PW: The treatment of chemical burns: Specialized diagnostic, therapeutic, and prognostic implications. *J Trauma* 1970; 10:634–642.
33. Diette KM, Gange RW, Stern RS, et al: Coal tar phototoxicity: Characteristics of smarting reaction. *J Invest Dermatol* 1985; 84:268–271.
34. Discher D, et al: *Pilot Study for Development of an Occupational Disease Surveillance Method,* NIOSH publication 75–162, US Government Printing Office, 1975.
35. Downing JG: Cancer of the skin and occupational trauma. *JAMA* 1952; 148:245–252.
36. Ebbing FJ, Rook A: Hair, in Rook A, Wilkinson DS (eds): *Textbook of Dermatology*. Oxford, Blackwell Scientific Publications, 1979.
37. Emmett EA: Occupational skin cancer: A review. *J Occup Med* 1975; 17:44–49.
38. Emmett EA, Kominsky JR: Allergic contact dermatitis from ultraviolet cured inks—Allergic contact sensitization to acrylates. *J Occup Med* 1977; 19:113–115.
39. Epstein JH: Photocarcinogenesis, skin cancer, and aging. *J Am Acad Dermatol* 1983; 9:487–502.
40. Epstein WL, Byers VS, Frankart W: Induction of antigen specific hyposensitization to poison oak in sensitized adults. *Arch Dermatol* 1982; 118:630–633.
41. Fitzpatrick TB, Eisen AZ, Wolff K: *Dermatology in Internal Medicine*. New York, McGraw-Hill Book Co, 1979.
42. Foussereau J, Benezra C, Maibach HI: *Occupational Contact Dermatitis*. Copenhagen, Munksgaard, 1982.
43. Fregert S: Occupational dermatitis in a 10-year period. *Contact Dermatitis* 1975; 1:96–107.
44. Fregert S, Gruberger B, Sandahl E: Reduction of chromates in cement by iron sulfate. *Contact Dermatitis* 1979; 5:39–42.
45. Fregert S, Poulsen J, Trullson L: Yellow stained skin from sodium nitrite used in an etching agent. *Contact Dermatitis* 1980; 6:296.
46. Fry L: Skin disease from color developers. *Br J Dermatol* 1965; 77:456–461.
47. Gellin GA, Possick PA, Perone VB: Depigmentation from 4-tertiary butyl catechol—An experimental study. *J Invest Dermatol* 1970; 55:190–197.
48. Gellin GA: Occupational leukoderma: In vivo and in vitro studies, in Drill VA, Laza P (eds): *Current Concepts in Cutaneous Toxicity*. New York, Academic Press, 1980, pp 213–220.
49. Glogau R, Hanna L, Jawetz E: Herpetis whitlow as part of genital virus infection. *J Infect Dis* 1977; 136:689–692.
50. Goetz H: Tar keratosis, in Andrade R (ed): *Cancer of the Skin*. Philadelphia, WB Saunders Co, 1976.
51. Harber LC, Bickers DR: *Photosensitivity Diseases*. Philadelphia, WB Saunders Co, 1981.
52. Haustein UF, Ziegler V: Environmentally induced systemic sclerosis-like disorders. *Int J Dermatol* 1985; 24:147–151.
53. Heisel ED, Hunt FE: Further studies in cutaneous reactions to glass fibers. *Arch Environ Health* 1968; 17:705–711.
54. Hellier FF: The prognosis in industrial dermatitis. *Br Med J* 1958; 1:196–198.
55. Hill AB, Faning EL: Studies on the incidence of cancer in a factory handling inorganic compounds of arsenic. I. Mortality experience of the factory. *Br J Ind Med* 1948; 5:1–6.
56. Hjorth N, Roed-Petersen J: Occupational protein contact dermatitis in food handlers. *Contact Dermatitis* 1976; 2:28–42.
57. Hyvarinen J, Pyykko I: Vibration frequencies and amplitude in the aetiology of traumatic vasospastic disease. *Lancet* 1973; 1:791–794.
58. Iverson RE, Laub DR, Madison MS: Hydrofluoric acid burns. *J Plast Reconstr Surg* 1971; 48:107–112.
59. Jelinko C: Chemicals that "burn." *J Trauma* 1974; 14:65–72.
60. Jensen O: "Rusters." The corrosive action of palmar sweat: I. Sodium chloride in sweat. *Acta Derm Venereol* 1979; 59:135–138.
61. Jensen O, Nielsen E: "Rusters." The corrosive action of palmar sweat. II. Physical and chemical factors in palmar hyperhydrosis. *Acta Derm Venereol* 1979; 59:139–143.
62. Keil JE, Shmunes E: The epidemiology of work-related skin diseases in South Carolina. *Arch Dermatol* 1983; 119:650–654.
63. Key MM: Some unusual allergic reactions in industry. *Arch Dermatol* 1961; 83:3–6.
64. Klauder JV, Brill FA: Correlation of boiling ranges of some petroleum solvents with irritant action on skin. *Arch Dermatol* 1947; 56:197–215.
65. Kligman AM: Poison ivy (rhus) dermatitis. *Arch Dermatol* 1958; 77:149–180.
66. Kligman AM: Assessment of mild irritants in humans, in Drill VA, Lazar P (eds): *Current Concepts in Cutaneous Toxicity*. New York, Academic Press, 1980, pp 69–94.
67. Knox JM, Tucker SB, Flannigan SA: Paresthesia from cutaneous ex-

posure to a synthetic pyrethroid insecticide. *Arch Dermatol* 1984; 120:744–746.

68. Kuratsune M, Yoshimura T, Matsuzaka J, et al: Epidemiologic study of Yusho, a poisoning caused by ingestion of a rice oil contaminated with a commercial brand of polychlorinated biphenyls. *Environ Health Perspect* 1972; 1:119–128.
69. La Dou J: The not-so-clean business of making chips. *Technology Rev* 1984; 87:23–36.
70. Laroche GP: Traumatic vasospastic disease in chain-saw operators. *Can Med Assoc J* 1976; 115:1217–1221.
71. Lee JAH: Melanoma and exposure to sunlight. *Epidemiol Rev* 1982; 4:110–136.
72. Lewis W, Schwartz L: An occupational agent (n-butyraldoxime) causing reaction to alcohol. *Med Ann District of Columbia* 1956; 15:485–490.
73. Lyle WH, Spence TWM, McKinneley WM, et al: Dimethylformamide and alcohol intolerance. *Br J Ind Med* 1979; 36:63–66.
74. Maibach HI, Gellin GA: *Occupational and Industrial Dermatology*. Chicago, Year Book Medical Publishers, 1982.
75. Malkinson FD: Percutaneous absorption of toxic substances in industry. *Arch Ind Health* 1960; 21:87–99.
76. Malten KE, Seutter E, Hara I, et al: Occupational vitiligo to paratertiary butylphenol and homologues. *Trans St John's Hosp Dermatol Soc* 1971; 57:115–131.
77. Malten KE, den Arend JACJ, Wiggers RE: Delayed irritation: Hexanediol diacrylate and butanediol diacrylate. *Contact Dermatitis* 1979; 5:178–184.
78. Markowitz SS, McDonald CJ, Fethiere W, et al: Occupational acroosteolysis. *Arch Dermatol* 1972; 106:219–233.
79. Mathias CGT, Maibach HI: When to read the patch test. *Int J Dermatol* 1979; 3:127–128.
80. Mathias CGT: Contact dermatitis from cyanide plating solutions. *Arch Dermatol* 1982; 118:420–422.
81. Mathias CGT: Clinical and experimental aspects of cutaneous irritation, in Marzulli FA, Maibach HI (eds): *Dermatology*. Washington, DC, Hemisphere Publishing Co, 1983.
82. Mathias CGT, Maibach HI: Allergic contact dermatitis from anaerobic acrylic sealants. *Arch Dermatol* 1984; 120:1202–1205.
83. Mathias CGT: Contact dermatitis—When cleaner is not better. *Occup Health Safety*, 1984; 53(1):45–50.
84. Mathias CGT: Food substances may cause skin reactions among handlers. *Occup Health Saf* 1984; 53(9):53–56.
85. Mathias CGT: The cost of occupational skin disease. *Arch Dermatol* 1985; 121:332–344.
86. Mills OH, Kligman A: Acne mechanica. *Arch Dermatol* 1975; 111:481–483.
87. Montagna W, Parakkal PF: *The Structure and Function of Skin*. New York, Academic Press, 1974.
88. Moses M, Prioleau PG: Cutaneous histologic findings in chemical workers with and without chloracne with past exposure to 2, 3, 7, 8-tetrachlorodibenzo-p-dioxin, *J Am Acad Dermatol* 1985; 12:497–506.
89. Muller G, Spassowski M, Henschler D: Metabolism of trichloroethylene in man. III. Interaction of trichloroethylene and alcohol. *Arch Toxicol* 1975; 33:173–189.
90. National Institute for Occupational Safety and Health: Pilot study for development of an occupational disease surveillance method, NIOSH Publication 75-162. US Government Printing Office, 1975.
91. Nethercott JR: Skin problems associated with multifunctional acrylic monomers in ultraviolet curing inks. *Br J Dermatol* 1978; 98:541–552.
92. Orchard S: Barrier creams. *Dermatol Clin* 1984; 2:619–629.
93. Passi S, Nazarro-Porro M, Boniforte L, et al: Analysis of lipids and dioxin in chloracne due to tetrachloro-2,3,7,8-dibenzodioxin. *Br J Dermatol* 1981; 105:137–143.
94. Pathak MA: Sunscreens: Topical and systemic approaches for protection of human skin against harmful effects of solar radiation. *J Am Acad Dermatol* 1982; 7:285–312.
95. Perone VP, Moffett AE, Possik PA, et al: The chromium, cobalt, and nickel contents of American cement and their relationship to cement dermatitis. *Am Ind Hyg Assoc J* 1970; 31:12–15.
96. Pirila V, et al: Legislation on occupational dermatoses of the International Contact Dermatitis Research Group. *Acta Derm Venereol* 1971; 51:141–150.
97. Possick L, Gellin GA, Key MM: Fibrous glass dermatitis. *Am Ind Hyg Assoc J* 1970; 31:12–15.
98. Prosser White R: *The Dermatergoses or Occupational Affections of the Skin*. London, HK Lewis, 1934.
99. Ramazzini B: *Diseases of Workers (De Morbis Artificum)*. New York, Hafner Publishing Company, 1964.
100. Robertson MH, Storrs FJ: Allergic contact dermatitis from Portland cement. *Br J Dermatol* 1980; 102:487–489.
101. Rodnan GP, Benedek TG, Medsger TA, et al: The association of progressive systemic sclerosis (scleroderma with coal miners' pneumoconiosis and other forms of silicosis. *Ann Int Med* 1967; 66:323–334.
102. Rycroft RJG: Acute and ulcerative contact dermatitis from Portland cement. *Br J Dermatol* 1980; 102:487–489.
103. Rycroft RJG: Low humidity dermatoses. *Dermatol Clin* 1984; 2:553–559.
104. Saihan EM, Burton JL, Heaton KW: A new syndrome with pigmentation, scleroderma, gynecomastia, Raynaud's and peripheral neuropathy. *Br J Dermatol* 1978; 99:437.
105. Samitz MH, Scheiner DM, Katz S: Ascorbic acid in the prevention of chrome dermatitis—Mechanism of inactivation of chromium. *Arch Environ Health* 1968; 17:44.
106. Schottenfeld D, Fraumeni JF: *Cancer Epidemiology and Prevention*. Philadelphia, WB Saunders Co, 1982.
107. Schwartz L, Tulipan L, Peck SM: *Occupational Diseases of the Skin*. Philadelphia, Lea & Febiger, 1937.
108. Schwartz L: Occupational pigmentary changes in the skin. *Arch Dermatol* 1947; 56:592–600.
109. Schwartz L, Tulipan L, Birmingham DJ: *Occupational Diseases of the Skin*, ed 3. Philadelphia, Lea & Febiger, 1957.
110. Shelley WB, Juhlin L: Selective uptake of contact allergens by the Langerhans cell. *Arch Dermatol* 1977; 113:187–192.
111. Shewmake SW, Anderson BG: Hydrofluoric acid burns. A report of a case and review of the literature. *Arch Dermatol* 1979; 115:593–596.
112. Shmunes E, Keil JE: Occupational dermatoses in South Carolina: A descriptive analysis of cost variables. *J Am Acad Dermatol* 1983; 9:861–866.
113. Sparrow GP: A connective tissue disorder similar to vinyl chloride disease in a patient exposed to perchloroethylene. *Clin Dermatol* 1977; 2:17–22.
114. Stewart RD, Hake CL, Petersen JE: "Degreasers' flush": Dermal response to trichloroethylene and alcohol. *Toxicol Appl Pharmacol* 1974; 29:83.
115. Taylor JS: Environmental chloracne: Update and overview. *Ann NY Acad Sci* 1979; 320:295–307.
116. Taylor W, Brammer AJ: Vibration effects on the hand and arm in industry: An introduction and review, in Brammer AJ, Taylor W (eds): *Vibration Effects on the Hand and Arm in Industry*. New York, John Wiley & Sons, 1982.

117. Tseng WP, Chu HM, How SW, et al: Prevalence of skin cancer in an endemic area of chronic arsenicism in Taiwan. *JNCI* 1968; 40:453–463.
118. US Dept of Labor, Bureau of Labor Statistics: Employment and Earnings. US Government Printing Office, 1984 (May).
119. Urbach F, Epstein JH, Forbes PD: Ultraviolet carcinogenesis: Experimental, global, and genetic aspects, in Fitzpatrick TB, Pathak MA, Harber LC, et al (eds): *Sunlight and Man*. Tokyo, Tokyo Press, 1974.
120. Van der Harst-Oostveen CJGR, Van Vloten WA: Delayed-type hypersensitivity in patients with mycosis fungoides. *Dermatologica* 1978; 157:129–135.
121. Van Scott EJ: Basal cell carcinoma, in Fitzpatrick TB, Eisen AZ, Wolff K, et al (eds): *Dermatology in Internal Medicine*. New York, McGraw-Hill Book Co, 1979.
122. Vickers DFH: Industrial carcinogenesis. *Br J Dermatol* 1981; 105(suppl 21):57–61.
123. Vitaliano PP, Urbach F: The relative importance of risk factors in nonmelanoma carcinoma. *Arch Dermatol* 1980; 116:454–456.
124. Wang CL: *The Problem of Skin Disease in Industry*. Office of Occupational Safety and Health Statistics, US Dept of Labor, 1978.
125. Wolfe HR, Durham WF, Armstrong JF: Exposure of workers to pesticides. *Arch Environ Health* 1967; 14:622–633.
126. Wong KC, Hwang MY: PCB poisoning. Special issue. *Clin Med (Taipei)* 1981; 7:83–88.
127. Yamakage A, Ishikawa H, Saito I, et al: Occupational scleroderma-like disorder occurring in men engaged in the polymerization of epoxy resin. *Dermatologica* 1980; 161:33–44.
128. Yamakage A, Ishikawa H: Generalized morphea-like scleroderma occurring in people exposed to organic solvents. *Dermatologica* 1982; 165:113–116.

11

Ocular Responses to Chemical and Physical Injury

Jeffrey E. Coe, M.D.

Robert B. Douglas, Ph.D.

The effect of toxic substances on the eye has long been recognized as an important occupational health problem. Over one half of the substances on the current American Conference of Government Industrial Hygienists (ACGIH) list of hazardous chemicals have potentially deleterious ocular effects and, as new substances are introduced into manufacturing processes, this number will certainly increase. Thus, the setting and maintaining of occupational hygiene standards for ocular protection must continue to be among the primary goals of the occupational health specialist. This article will briefly consider some of the ways in which the eye responds to environmental agents, as well as the methods used to study the effects of these agents on the eye for the purpose of toxic substance control.

MEASURING METHODS

All of the methods currently used for determining the effects of environmental agents on the eye have major theoretical shortcomings. Ideally, such evaluation techniques would be simple, quantitative measurements made on human beings, thus eliminating concerns about intraspecies generalization and subjectivity in data collection and analysis. However, as will be seen, very few of the methods commonly used in ocular toxicology approach this ideal and, consequently, all are open to both criticism and improvement.

Liquids and Solids

The "Draize test" and its variants are the standard methods for determining the ocular injury potential of liquids and solids.[22, 29, 31, 40] At its most basic, this technique involves the application of a relatively large fixed dose (0.1 gm or 0.1 ml) of a test substance to one cornea of an albino rabbit, the untreated cornea being used as a control. After set periods of follow-up, both corneas are examined and graded according to specific criteria (Table 11–1) by trained observers.

The Draize test, then, involves both subjective interpretation and intraspecies comparison and, as may be expected, significant variability in results has been repeatedly documented.[3, 4, 6, 11, 12, 24, 48, 91] Of equal concern is that, even when used under optimal conditions, this technique has shown only fair correlation with known human ocular responses, most often overstating irritancy.[5, 17, 40] Whether this tendency is a function of the testing procedure or the rabbit eye is not clear. It is known that the structure of the rabbit eye is somewhat different from that of human beings (for example, rabbits are "lagophthalmic" with normal blinking rates much lower than those of primates). Draize-testing in nonhuman primates gives results closer to the human experience,[6, 11] but it has been considered unfeasible because of cost and the necessity for elaborate animal handling facilities.[40] Efforts to make the rabbbit eye lesion grading process more objective by use of slit-lamp examination or in vitro (postmortem) corneal thickness measurements have failed to gain general acceptance, and their results remain difficult to compare between laboratories and observers.[11] Alterations in the fixed-dose Draize protocol have also been suggested and, in one study, the use of smaller doses (0.01–0.03 ml) gave results more comparable with

TABLE 11–1.
Criteria for a Positive Reaction: FHSA Rabbit Eye Irritation Test[22,40]

Any of the following at any reading (24, 48, and 72 hr):
- Ulceration of the cornea (other than fine stippling)
- Opacity of the cornea (other than slight dulling of the normal luster)
- Inflammation of the iris (other than slight deepening of the folds or rugae or slight circumcorneal injection of the blood vessels)
- Obvious swelling of the conjunctivae with partial eversion of the lids
- A diffuse crimson-red with individual vessels of the conjunctivae not easily discernible

human observations.[40] However, even with this more "physiologic" approach, the questions of subjectivity in lesion grading remain to plague those requiring such data for setting occupational hygiene standards.

Gases and Vapors

The methods for evaluating the effects of gases and vapors on the eye are also far from ideal. Here, the testing procedures are less standardized and often do involve human subjects. In a commonly used technique, for example, subjects are exposed to test gases for five minutes at "eye ports" in the wall of a large gas mixing chamber. The subjects then grade their perception of eye irritation using one of a number of scaling methods.[28, 73] Clearly, the results from this type of exposure testing are highly subjective. This basic concern is further compounded by the wide range of "normal" responsivity to irritant gases and the rapid but individually variable rate at which tolerance develops.[47]

To eliminate the recurrent concerns of subjectivity and variability, two different directions have been taken. First, some investigators have abandoned the eye entirely, studying nonocular responses that can be objectively measured and that, emperically, correlate with known human ocular responses. Thus, rat pulmonary responses—bronchoconstriction[1] and respiratory rate[47]—have been used to measure irritant gas thresholds, as have the behavioral responses of rats conditioned to avoid irritants.[93] These varied techniques give useful results and often yield threshold limit values (TLVs) that approximate current standards. But, again, all involve extrapolation to man from other species and often necessitate arcane algorithms for final TLV estimation. Because of this, some doubt remains as to their utility in evaluating gases and vapors for which human TLVs have not yet been determined. As has been noted by an investigator in this field, the animal techniques are perhaps best considered methods for obtaining quick estimates of potentially dangerous levels for human exposure, rather than techniques for setting regulatory standards.[47]

Another approach has been to try to identify components of the human ocular irritant response that can be measured objectively. To this end, ocular surface temperature and blink rate have been studied but found either to be highly variable or difficult to instrument acceptably.[19] However, within narrowly defined experimental conditions, tearing has proved to be a quantifiable response. Preliminary studies measuring tearing in response to sulfur dioxide exposure have shown an ocular threshold of approximately 4 ppm (parts per milliliter).[20] This value is relatively close to the current sulfur dioxide TLV of 2 ppm and is well below the threshold for the subjective sensation of eye irritation (20–160 ppm in different sources[7, 27, 47]). Unfortunately, the technique involved (a modification of the Schirmer test) is somewhat invasive. Because of this, it is not acceptable to all subjects and, for the present, must be considered a research rather than a survey technique.

In summary then, a number of methods are currently used to evaluate the potential of chemicals to cause eye damage—their number, perhaps, indicates the dissatisfaction with each individual technique. The oldest and most widely used method, the Draize test, has attracted a large critical literature. But, in fact, no technique entirely avoids one or all of the basic design flaws and, for the foreseeable future, data from all of these methods will still be required to assist in the setting of hygiene standards.

MECHANISMS OF OCULAR RESPONSE TO INJURY

Because of the large number of oculotoxic substances, it will not be possible to provide a comprehensive listing in this section. For information on the ocular effects of specific chemicals, the primary resource remains W. M. Grant's *Toxicology of the Eye*, ed. 2 (Springfield, Ill., Charles C Thomas, 1974), while the effects of electromagnetic radiation on the eye are best surveyed in S. Lerman's *Radiant Energy and the Eye* (New York, Macmillan Publishing Co, 1980).

The focus of this section will be on the ways in which the human eye responds to chemical and physical injury. At the outset it should be said that the eye is, of course, a series of complex, interrelated structures—the ocular adnexa (lids, conjunctiva, lacrimatory apparatus), the cornea, the anterior chamber structures (iris, lens, ciliary body, and trabecular meshwork), the retina, and the associated neurologic and neuromuscular structures—each having its own distinct but related chemical and physical environments and each, occasionally, responding to toxic insult in a characteristic way. However, this complexity noted, it is possible to define three general types of ocular response to injury: (1) a primary response at the site of injury (for example, corneal changes following a burn or abrasion); (2) a later, more generalized ocular inflammatory response; and (3) the specific and often characteristic ocular response caused by certain systemically active substances (for example, the "optic neuritis" associated with methanol ingestion).

The Primary Ocular Response at the Site of Injury

Chemical Burns

Chemical burns of the eye represent the most common cause of serious toxic eye injury. Although no large-scale surveys of chemical eye injuries have been undertaken, several informal reports suggest that chemical burns comprise approximately 10% of all industrial eye trauma.[69, 74] Categories of chemicals causing direct ocular injury include alkalies, acids, organic solvents, pesticides, lacrimators (chloracetophenone, for example) and their intermediaries, vesicants (mustards and Lewesite), and ionic detergents. As would be expected with such a large and varied group of substances, the factors determining the extent of ocular injury are numerous. They include the substance's concentration, the final pH of the solution, the duration of exposure, the state of the ocular defense mechanisms (tearing, blinking), and the specific characteristics of the chemical (the anion and cation) itself.

The importance of the final factor, the chemical structure of the agent, cannot be overestimated and often can explain the clinically observed differences in the ocular toxicity of substances within the same group. Among the alkalies, for example, sodium and potassium alkaline salts are both fat- and water-soluble and quickly pass through all layers of the cornea, causing deep, progressive injury. Calcium alkaline salts, in contrast, tend to form stable, insoluble complexes with the corneal epithelial cell membranes. Because of this, they have only limited penetrating ability and their damage is usually confined to the superficial ocular structures.[74, 53] In contrast, ammonia, essentially a water-soluble gas, passes through the cornea most rapidly of all the alkalies and causes the most severe damage of any agent in this group.[53, 95]

Alkali Burns.—Because alkalies are so common and capable of causing such severe ocular injury, their effect on the eye has long been the subject of research. Contact with an alkali solution of pH greater than 11.5 results in the immediate destruction of corneal epithelial cell membranes with denaturation of intracellular enzymes.[35] The subsequent lysis of these epithelial cells loosens the connections of the epithelium to the deeper corneal layers, resulting in epithelial slough. Further penetration allows the alkali to enter the anterior chamber and directly damage the contiguous structures—the iris, lens, ciliary body, and trabecular meshwork.[68] A final, significant early change is a rapid (within 15 seconds of exposure) increase in intraocular pressure that has been linked to direct, alkali-induced shrinkage of the corneal and anterior chamber collagen.[78] This initial increase in intraocular pressure abates within one hour.[78] The most severely injured eyes may then go on to become hypotonic (phthisis bulbi) because of damage to the aqueous-forming structures.[69, 53] To all injured eyes there follows a characteristic anterior-chamber or panocular inflammatory response. The nature of the inflammatory response will be discussed later, but it should be noted here that an important component of the response is another, more profound and prolonged rise in intraocular pressure—a secondary glaucoma—related to an increase in the formation of aqueous humor and/or blockage of the aqueous drainage channels by edema and debris.[69]

These early phases of alkali injury to the eye also set in motion chemical changes that produce some of the late complications of these burns. The initial lysis of corneal cells is associated with the release of still unknown leukocyte-stimulating and chemotactic factors. The subsequent leukocyte infiltration and degranulation releases a variety of proteolytic enzymes, including collagenases, and superoxide radicals.[69, 53] Other important chemical alterations include a marked drop in ascorbate levels in the aqueous as well as the loss of activity of enzymes, such as superoxide dismutase, normally found in the anterior chamber.[95] Thus, the ability of the eye to scavenge free radicals is impaired, and these destructive agents, along with the collagenases, are thought to be the cause of the ongoing destruction that manifests itself as recurrent epithelial breakdown and ulceration. In alkali burns, this tendency toward ulceration is often quite prolonged and, unfortunately, may lead to ulceration, perforation, and loss of the eye months or even years after the injury.

Clinically, immediate pain is caused by the direct alkali stimulation of the corneal unmyelinated nerve endings and the rapid initial rise in intraocular pressure. However, these nerves are destroyed by the alkali, and the cornea rapidly becomes anesthetic. In appearance, the cornea becomes translucent or opaque due to corneal edema, the conjunctiva begins to swell and, depending on the nature, concentration, and extent of contact with the alkali, the perilimbal blood vessels may blanch or segment.[69] Because of the ongoing alkali damage, the immediate appearance of the burned eye is an uncertain indicator of the eventual outcome. However, the appearance of the eye after 24 hours has been found to be useful for prognostic estimation (Table 11–2). In grading alkali burns, a number of observers have noted that the condition of the perilimbal conjunctiva is more significant than that of the cornea, with perilimbal vascular changes or scleral translucency being highly predictive of later ulceration or perforation.[74, 53]

Acid Burns.—Acids generally tend to form insoluble complexes with the ocular surface structures they contact, limiting penetration and deeper ocular injury. Thus, although acid burns may cause ocular disability because of scarring of the lids, conjunctiva, and lacrimal apparatus, they are only rarely associated with the deeper, more prolonged changes seen with alkali burns.

Major exceptions to this pattern are the injuries caused by concentrated sulfuric acid (that produces a thermal-like burn) and hydrofluoric acid. In recent studies, for example, it has been shown that, for solutions of equal pH, the ocular damage caused by hydrofluoric acid is much greater than that from hydrochloric acid.[56, 88] From this observation, and studies of the effect of hydrofluoric acid on other tissues,[88] it has become apparent that the peculiar toxicity of hydrofluoric acid is related to its ability to rapidly penetrate tissue layers, producing deeper necrosis. Since this pathologic pattern is similar to that seen with alkali burns, it is not surprising that the clinical course of hydrofluoric acid burns is also similar to that of alkali burns. Here, too, healing is poor and prolonged, and the incidence of late complications (including ulceration and perforation) is high.[56]

Light Injuries

Thus far the external surfaces of the eye—the cornea, sclera, conjunctiva, and lids—have been considered the primary sites of ocular injury. However, because of the selective absorbtion (and

TABLE 11–2.
Severity of Alkali Burns[53]

GRADE	CORNEA	CONJUNCTIVA	PROGNOSIS
1	Epithelial damage	No ischemia	Good
2	Hazy, but iris detail seen	Ischemia less than one third at limbus	Good
3	Total epithelial loss; stromal haze, iris details observed	Ischemia of one third to one half at limbus	Vision reduced; perforation rare
4	Opaque; no view of iris or pupil	Ischemia affects more than one half at limbus	Poor; prolonged convalescence

transmission) of specific wavelengths by ocular structures, light (defined in the broadest sense as including ultraviolet through infrared, coherent and incoherent radiation) is capable of causing primary injury anywhere in the eye, from the corneal epithelium to the retina.

It is currently believed that light can produce three different types of ocular damage: (1) thermal injury (in effect, burning), (2) photochemical injury, and (3) structural damage from pressure-induced changes (sonic transients) associated with the operation of certain types of lasers.[18, 33, 41, 54] Although useful, however, this classification is an oversimplification. With light injuries, it is often impossible to clearly define the mechanism causing damage; at given wavelengths and power levels it is entirely possible to have all three mechanisms acting simultaneously.[32]

Experimental studies in rhesus monkeys have shown that any light source capable of raising the surface temperature of a pigmented portion of the eye—the retina or iris—by 10° C is capable of causing thermal injury. The cellular destruction associated with this type of deep primary injury appears immediately after exposure. Histologically, the increased local temperature causes an "explosive vaporization" of cells at the center of the lesion with less severe changes toward its periphery.[41, 90] After the thermal burn resolves, its central portion continues to show significant scarring.

Temperature increases sufficient to cause such thermal injuries to the retina or iris can be produced by some radiant, incoherent sources (xenon arc lamps, for example), but they are of particular concern with lasers. In one sense, however, the narrow, coherent laser beam may actually be protective of vision. The probability of a laser beam passing directly through the pupil and striking the macula is not great. Thus, although laser ocular injuries may be severe, they are not common, and generally tend to be small, discrete, retinal burns.[77] In a recent discussion of laser hazards, in fact, it was noted that it is precisely because many employees come to regard lasers as "safe", that they tend to disregard established ocular safety procedures—a common factor in laser eye accidents.[77]

Because it is avascular (and thus unable to rapidly transfer heat), the lens is also particularly susceptible to thermal injury. The most common source of lenticular thermal injury is radiation in the infrared and microwave portions of the spectrum. This type of radiation passes unimpeded through the cornea and aqueous before being absorbed and then concentrated on the posterior pole of the lens. The lesion produced after cumulative exposure is characteristic, consisting of a posterior opacification with lamellar splitting of the anterior lens capsule.[32, 41] Once common in employees working near hot furnaces, infrared cataracts of this type are relatively easily prevented by screening furnace openings as well as by the use of appropriate protective glasses. Lens damage from microwaves, however, is an ongoing cause for concern in telecommunications and defense workers, for example, who regularly work close to high-power, focused microwave sources.

Photochemical injury can be caused by ultraviolet radiation and visible light in the blue portion (400–550 nm) of the spectrum. Perhaps the most familiar photochemical ocular is ultraviolet keratitis ("arc eye"). The corneal epithelium strongly absorbs ultraviolet radiation shorter than 295 nm, and exposure to this type of radiation has been shown to cause direct photochemical changes in epithelial cell nucleic acids and aromatic amino acids, as well as indirect damage from the generation of free radicals. Histologically, inhibition of epithelial cell mitosis, nuclear fragmentation, and loosening of the epithelium can be seen. Clinically, following a latent period of 30 minutes to 24 hours, employees complain of pain, tearing, a "gritty" or "sandy" feeling in the eyes, photophobia and, occasionally, blepharospasm, while on fluorescein examination punctate corneal erosions can be seen. The delayed onset of symptoms in ultraviolet keratitis is insidious and accounts for much of the continued incidence of this condition in occupationally exposed workers. Although the lesions heal spontaneously, if the eye is frequently reinjured, corneal scarring and neovascularization can occur.[32]

Animal investigations have shown that the retina is also liable to photochemical injury, being particularly sensitive to blue (400–550 nm) light. Light in this portion of the visible spectrum, for example, has been linked to retinal lesions at power levels that do not significantly alter the retinal surface temperature.[41] Histologically, photochemical retinal lesions are quite different from thermal lesions. Recognizable change here does not appear until approximately 48 hours after exposure, and then consists of inflammation, macrophage infiltration, and depigmentation that is relatively uniform throughout the exposed area.[61] Again, in contrast to thermal lesions, the photochemical changes generally seem to resolve with only minimal scarring,[61] but the long-term effect of a single exposure or the cumulative effect of repeated photochemical injury is not currently known. Photochemical damage, rather than thermal injury, is now believed to be the cause of "solar" retinitis. Photochemical injury may also contribute significantly to the senile eye changes seen in welders, individuals working in bright environments or using instruments with narrow beams of bright light (ophthalmologists, for example), and those who have had lens extractions and, therefore, have lost the lens' protective filtering in the blue portion of the spectrum.[41]

The Ocular Inflammatory Response

Virtually any moderate to severe chemical or physical injury to the eye is capable of initiating a characteristic sequence of anterior chamber changes described as the ocular inflammatory response. Recognized clinically in human beings and also well illustrated experimentally in animals,[46, 94] this response, at its most extreme, consists of miosis, vasodilation, breakdown of the blood-aqueous barrier, protein infiltration into the aqueous, and increased intraocular pressure.[13]

Careful observation of the time course of these changes has revealed that the inflammatory response is actually biphasic, involving two related but different physiologic mechanisms. In studies of nitrogen mustard injuries to animal eyes, it has been shown that the first phase begins as early as one hour after injury. This early component of the response can be blocked by retrobulbar injection of alcohol or novocaine,[26] section of the ophthalmic division of the trigeminal nerve,[45] or experimentally induced herpes simplex keratitis,[45, 46] but not by prostaglandin inhibitors such as aspirin or indomethacin.[62] The second phase of the inflammatory response begins 3–12 hours after injury and can be blocked by systemic indomethacin, but not be denervation or other nerve-blocking techniques.[14, 15, 23, 67, 70] From such studies it has been concluded that the second, later phase of the inflammatory response is mediated by prostaglandins released from the anterior chamber, while the early phase represents a true neurogenic reflex.

Further investigation of the first, reflex phase of inflammation has shown that at least one (Substance P) and possibly any number of intermediate active transmitter substances are involved. Substance P-containing neurons have been identified in the human cornea,[85] as well as in the eyes of animals of a variety of species,[50, 60, 84] and appear to be derived from the trigeminal nerve[8, 10]—the sole corneal sensory afferent. In addition, Substance P has been shown to be released into the aqueous humor in response to eye irritation[8, 15, 46] and, in the rabbit eye, direct Substance P administration initiates inflammatory changes.[9]

Finally, from studies of herpes simplex keratitis in mice, it has been possible to relate corneal sensitivity to corneal Substance P levels.[59, 89] The implication of this finding is far reaching because it links Substance P to the cornea's rich supply of unmyelinated sensory nerve endings.[51, 52, 55, 87, 92, 96] Structurally, these nerve endings are quite similar to those previously identified as chemoreceptors in the nose and respiratory tract,[16] and it has recently been suggested that they probably are the actual ocular chemoreceptors.[21] Elegant ultrastructural studies have shown that the terminal portions of the unmyelinated axons are found in deep grooves in the surface of the corneal epithelial cells.[49, 92] This extremely superficial, exposed location—ideal for the perception of environmental changes—also may explain both the immediate pain noted with corneal chemical burns or irritation and also the rapid corneal anesthesia that follows as the superficial nerve endings are destroyed.

Ocular Responses to Systemically Active Toxic Agents

The variety of systemically active substances that can affect the eye is great, perhaps reflecting the large number of structures that must function in coordination to allow normal vision. The pathophysiologic mechanisms involved are also quite varied. It is possible, however, to divide the systemically active agents into several basic categories. Among others, these include chemical and physical asphyxiants, neuromuscular blocking agents, and specific neuroophthalmologic toxins.

The effects of chemical asphyxiants (carbon monoxide, cyanide) and physical asphyxiants (carbon dioxide, nitrogen, helium) on the eye are only one part of a clearly evident, broader pattern of central nervous system anoxia. Similarly, agents that block neuromuscular transmission, like the acetylcholinesterase inhibitors (organophosphorus insecticides and nerve gases), give recognizable ocular effects (pupillary constriction), that are, again, only one part (albeit highly recognizable) of a more generalized, characteristic syndrome.

It is the specific ophthalmologic toxins that are the systemic agents primarily responsible for permanent ocular changes. Of these agents, many—like methanol and carbon disulfide—have been known for over a century to cause ocular damage, but, in most cases, it has not been until relatively recently that their mechanisms of action have even begun to be understood. Undoubtedly, one reason for this slow progress is the lack of reliable human histopathologic information. Given these substances' toxicity, little detailed human pharmacokinetic data, (concerning, for example, dose-response relationships or receptor sites) are available, and the primary resources must remain either animal studies or reports of home and industrial exposures. Unfortunately, because the chemicals involved undergo metabolic transformation after absorption, animal data must here be looked on with even more scepticism than usual.

These problems notwithstanding, it can be said that no substance has yet been reported to directly injure the human ocular photoreceptors (the rods and cones),[72] although this has been demonstrated in rabbits with iodoacetate[65] and in rats with sodium malate.[39] Rather, the major primary sites involved in systemic oculotoxic injury are the optic nerve and visual cortex, and the agents affecting these sites can be further divided into those affecting central vision and those causing defects in peripheral vision.

Methanol

The most thoroughly studied and perhaps best understood of the systemically active chemicals is methanol—a substance primarily associated with loss of central vision.[72] It is currently believed that the ocular effects of methanol are confined to primates.[37, 71] Experimentally administered to monkeys, methanol is quickly metabolized to formic acid, producing a severe metabolic acidosis. The formate ion rapidly equilibrates in the blood and cerebrospinal fluid, after which the specific toxic effects on the eye begin.[42] Because the ocular effects of methanol are also seen in animals administered formic acid directly, as well as in animals in which the acidosis has been controlled, it is probable that formate is the actual toxic agent in methanol's optic neuritis.[34, 42] In monkeys, the appearance of the eyes in the first hours after methanol ingestion is quite benign, with some pupil constriction but no consistent fundus abnormalities.[42, 72] However, after 24 hours, most animals show fixed, dilated pupils with optic disc edema and hyperemia. These changes are similar to those associated with increased intracranial pressure, though this was found to be normal.[42] Fluorescein angiography and both light and electron microscopy of the retina show no abnormalities.[42] However, microscopic studies of the head and retrolaminar portions of the optic nerve show clear evidence of destruction, with loss of neurotubules and filaments as well as a variety of mitochondrial changes—general enlargement, loss of cristae, and accumulation in the area around the optic disc.[78]

This pattern of optic nerve ultrastructural changes has been interpreted as being consistent with axoplasmic flow stasis.[42] Nerve axoplasmic flow is necessary for electrical impulse conduction and is known to be an energy-dependent process.[34] Because formate blocks glycolysis—probably by inhibition of cytochrome oxidase[63, 64]—its rapid rise in blood and cerebrospinal fluid after methanol ingestion may interfere with the optic nerve's energy supply and electrical functioning. Although the logic of this explanation is attractive, it is worth noting that it has been derived entirely from postmortem studies of a relatively small number of rhesus monkeys and, consequently, should not be considered conclusive. However, of the systemically active toxic agents, methanol is virtually unique in that its mechanism of action can even be suggested in such detail. As will be seen, for other agents affecting central or peripheral vision, this is not at all the case.

Carbon Disulfide

The central vision defect associated with chronic carbon disulfide exposure ("retinopathia sulfocarbonica"), for example, has also been known for more than a century. Once seen in rubber and viscose rayon workers, retinal involvement as part of a more widespread carbon disulfide polyneuritis is still occasionally seen in Japanese[80] and Yugoslavian viscose rayon workers.[81] On ophthalmoscopic examination, pallor of the optic disc can be recognized, and fluorescein angiography reveals variable microvascular changes, including microaneurysms, dot hemorrhages, and small exudates.[81] It has been suggested that these vascular abnormalities may represent the basic ocular lesion in chronic carbon disulfide ocular toxicity.[81] Their similarity to the vascular changes seen in the retinopathy of diabetes mellitus has led to the speculation that carbon disulfide may, in fact, act by inducing a subclinical diabetic state.[81] A small study of Japanese viscose rayon workers has shown a significant number of abnormal prednisolone-augmented glucose tolerance tests, but the significance of this finding and its relation to the changes in ocular vasculature remain unknown.[79]

Methylmercury

Knowledge of the human ocular effects of methylmercury comes largely from the relatively recent cases at Minimata and Niigata in Japan[66, 82, 86] and Iraq,[2, 75] although the first report was as early as 1885[30] and the classic description remains that of Hunter, Bomford, and Russell.[43] Most victims show bilateral concentric constriction of visual fields with relative preservation of central vision.[86] Pupillary reflexes remain normal, but eye movements (recorded by electro-oculogram) are abnormal, with distinct muscular incoordination and "jerky pursuit."[44] On postmortem examination, lesions have been found to be widespread throughout the cerebral and cerebellar cortices, including the occipital visual cortex.[66, 82, 83] Histologically, the neurons in the anterior portion of the visual cortex seem to be selectively affected—a pattern that corresponds with the observed concentric peripheral visual field defect.[83] In the involved areas, neuron destruction is widespread and associated with glial proliferation, though other portions of the visual system, including the optic nerve and retina, are unaffected.[83]

The biochemical changes in the central nervous system caused by methylmercury remain unknown. Research on this subject has, again, been hampered by species differences. For example, recent electron microscopic studies in rats exposed to low doses of methylmercury have shown mercury accumulation in the retina,[38] and abnormal electroretinograms in these animals suggest that these mercury accumulations are functional. However, the significance of this finding is unclear, because retinal mercury accumulation has never been reported in human beings. Detailed studies in primates show ocular changes more similar to those seen in human methylmercury victims. But, histopathologic studies using ^{203}Hg in primates have shown that, although specific neurologic symptoms are expressed, the ingested mercury is actually widely distributed throughout the brain.[36, 76] This finding suggests that local factors (for example, differential rates of metabolism in the visual cortex) may be important in determining central nervous system neuron-tolerance to mercury, or it may be that some entirely different, as yet unknown, mechanism is involved.

Other Agents

Other systemic agents having oculotoxic effects include thallium, lead, quinine, nitrosocarbamates, and pentavalent arsenicals. However, as can be seen from the preceding examples, knowledge of the toxic effects of most of these substances remains primarily at the descriptive level, with more detailed understanding of pathophysiologic mechanisms being the exception. Clearly, ocular toxicology is a field with enormous research potential, and this research can not only be expected to explain the mode of action of specific agents, but also to reveal much about the basic mechanisms of vision.

CONCLUSION

For the occupational health specialist, the lessons to be learned from this brief survey of ocular responses to injury are clear. Loss of vision and lifelong disability can result from exposure of the eye to toxic substances. At present, even optimal treatment is often only partially successful and, with alkali burns in particular, late sequelae resulting in loss of vision are not uncommon. Implementation of an eye safety program—including posted warnings, personal protective devices (goggles, eye lavage stations), engineering controls for isolation of dangerous processes—is essential. With such a program and a thoroughgoing administrative commitment to its enforcement, the injuries considered here should no longer occur. They should be relegated to medical history rather than continue to be a source of tragedy for men and women at work.

ACKNOWLEDGMENTS

The authors would like to acknowledge the support of the following organizations: the European Coal and Steel Community, the Mason Medical Research Fund, the NATO Office of Scientific Affairs, the Republic Steel Corporation, and the TUC Centenary Institute of Occupational Health of the London School of Hygiene and Tropical Medicine.

REFERENCES

1. Alarie Y: Irritating properties of airborne materials to the upper respiratory tract. *Arch Environ Health* 1966; 13:433.
2. Bakir F, Damluji SF, Amin-Zaki L, et al: Methylmercury poisoning in Iraq. *Science* 1973; 181:230.
3. Ballantyne B, Swanston DW: Ocular irritation tests. *Br J Pharmacol* 1972; 46:577P.
4. Ballantyne B, Swanston DW: Screening tests for assessing the relative potency of sensory irritant materials. *Br J Pharmacol* 1973; 48:367P.
5. Beckley JH: Comparative eye testing: Man vs animal. *Toxicol Appl Pharmacol* 1965; 7:93.
6. Beckley JH, Russell TJ, Rubin LF: Use of the rhesus monkey for predicting human responses to eye irritants. *Toxicol Appl Pharmacol* 1969; 15:1.
7. Ben David A: *Sensory Receptors of the Eye as Initiators of Reflex*

Bronchoconstriction and Bradycardia, dissertation. University of London, 1977.

8. Bill A, Stjernschantz M, Mandahl A: Substance P: Release on trigeminal nerve stimulation, effects on the eye. *Acta Physiol Scand* 1979; 106:371.
9. Bito LZ, Nichols R, Baroody R: A comparison of the miotic and inflammatory effects of biologically active polypeptides and prostaglandin E_2 on the rabbit eye. *Exp Eye Res* 1982; 34:325.
10. Brodin E, Gazelius B, Lundberg J, et al: Substance P in trigeminal nerve endings: Occurrence and release. *Acta Physiol Scand* 1981; 111:501.
11. Buehler EV, Newmann EA: A comparison of eye irritation in monkeys and rabbits. *Toxicol Appl Pharmacol* 1964; 6:701.
12. Burton A: A method for the objective assessment of eye irritation. *Food Cosmet Toxicol* 1972; 10:209.
13. Butler JM, Hammond B: Neurogenic responses of the eye to injury. *Trans Ophthalmol Soc UK* 1977; 97:668.
14. Bynke G: Capsaicin pretreatment prevents disruption of blood-aqueous barrier in the rabbit eye. *Invest Ophthalmol* 1983; 24:744.
15. Camras CB, Bito LA: The pathophysiological effects of nitrogen mustard on the rabbit eye. 1. The biphasic intraocular pressure response and the role of prostaglandins. *Exp Eye Res* 1980; 30:41.
16. Canua H, Hinderer K, Wentges R: Sensory receptor organs of the human nasal respiratory mucosa. *Am J Anat* 1969; 124:187.
17. Carter RO, Griffith JF: Experimental bases for the realistic assessment of safety of topical agents. *Toxicol Appl Pharmacol* 1965; 7(Suppl 2):60.
18. Cleary SF, Hamrich PE: Laser-induced acoustic transients in the mammalian eye. *J Acoust Soc Am* 1969; 46:1037.
19. Coe JE: *The Objective Measurement of In Vivo Human Ocular Responses to Sulfur Dioxide*, dissertation, University of London, 1980.
20. Coe JE, Douglas RB: Objective measurement of ocular responses to chemical irritation. *J Physiol (Lond)* 1980; 308:53P.
21. Coe JE, Douglas RB: The effect of contact lenses on ocular responses to sulphur dioxide. *J Soc Occup Med* 1982; 32:92.
22. *Code of Federal Regulations*, Title 16, pt 1500.42. Washington, DC, US Government Printing Office, 1979.
23. Cole DF, Unger WG: Prostaglandins as mediators for the responses of the eye to trauma. *Exp Eye Res* 1973; 17:357.
24. Conquet P, Durant G, Laillier J, et al: Evaluation of ocular irritation in the rabbit: Objective versus subjective assessment. *Toxicol Appl Pharmacol* 1977; 38:129.
25. Cooper GP, Fox DA, Howell WE, et al: Visual evoked responses in rats exposed to heavy metals, in Merigan WH, Weiss B (eds): *Neurotoxicity of the Visual System*. New York, Raven Press, 1980, p 203.
26. Davson H, Huber A: Experimental hypertensive uveitis in the rabbit. *Ophthalmologica* 1950; 120:118.
27. Douglas RB: *Human Reflex Bronchoconstriction as an Adjunct to Conjunctival Sensitivity in Defining the Threshold Limit Values of Irritant Gases and Vapours*, PhD thesis. University of London, 1975.
28. Doyle G, Endow N, Jones J: Sulfur dioxide's role in eye irritation. *Arch Environ Health* 1961; 3:657.
29. Draize JH, Woodard G, Calvery HO: Methods for the study of irritation and toxicity of substances applied topically to the skin and mucus membranes. *J Pharmacol Exp Ther* 1944; 82:377.
30. Edward GN: Two cases of poisoning by mercuric methide. *St Bart's Hosp Rep* 1885; 1:141.
31. Edwards CC: Hazardous substances: Test for eye irritants. *Fed Reg* 1972; 37:8534.
32. Fischman A: Potential hazards of light toxicity from ophthalmologic devices, in Ernst JT: *1983 Year Book of Ophthalmology*. Chicago, Year Book Medical Publishers, 1984, p 231.
33. Fraunfelder FT, Vierstein LJ: Intraocular pressure variation during xenon and ruby laser photocoagulation. *Am J Ophthalmol* 1971; 71:1261.
34. Friede RL, Khang-Cheng H: The relation of axonal transport of mitochondria with microtubules and other axoplasmic organelles. *J Physiol (Lond)* 1977; 265:507.
35. Friedenwald JS, Hughes WF Jr, Herriman H: Acid-base tolerance of the cornea. *Arch Ophthalmol* 1944; 31:279.
36. Garman RH, Weiss R, Evans HL: Alkylmercurial encephalopathy in the monkey. A histopathologic and autoradiographic study. *Acta Neuropath (Berlin)* 1975; 32:61.
37. Gilger AP, Potts AM: Studies on the visual toxicity of methanol: V. The role of acidosis in experimental methanol poisoning. *Am J Ophthalmol* 1955; 39:63.
38. Gramoni R: Retinal function of rats exposed to organomercurials, in Merigan WH, Weiss B (eds): *Neurotoxicity of the Visual System*. New York, Raven Press, 1980, p 101.
39. Graymore CN, Tansley K: Iodoacetate poisoning of the rat retina. 1. Production of retinal degeneration. *Br J Ophthalmol* 1959; 43:177.
40. Griffith JF, Nixon GA, Bruce RD, et al: Dose-response studies with chemical irritants in the albino rabbit eye as a basis for selecting optimum testing conditions for predicting hazard to the human eye. *Toxicol Appl Pharmacol* 1980; 55:510.
41. Ham WT Jr: Ocular hazards of light sources: Review of current knowledge. *J Occup Med* 1983; 25:101.
42. Hayreh MS, Hayreh SS, Baumbach GL: Ocular toxicity of methanol: An experimental study, in Merigan WH, Weiss B (eds): *Neurotoxicity of the Visual System*. New York, Raven Press, 1980, p 35.
43. Hunter D, Bomford RR, Russell SD: Poisoning by methyl mercury compounds. *Q J Med* 1940; 9:193.
44. Iwata K: Neuroophthalmologic indices of Minimata disease in Niigata, in Merigan WH, Weiss B (eds): Neurotoxicity of the Visual System. New York, Raven Press, 1980, p 165.
45. Jampol AM, Neufeld AH, Sears ML: Pathways for the response of the eye to injury. *Invest Ophthalmol* 1975; 14:184.
46. Jampol AM, Axelrod A, Tessler H: Pathways of the eye's response to topical nitrogen mustard. *Invest Ophthalmol* 1976; 15:486.
47. Kane LE, Barrow CS, Alarie Y: A short-term test to predict acceptable levels of exposure to airborne sensory irritants. *Am Ind Hyg Assoc J* 1979; 40:207.
48. Kaufman H: If I can't measure it, what do I do with it? *Invest Ophthalmol* 1974; 13:412.
49. Kitano S: An embryological study of the human corneal nerves. *Jap J Ophthalmol* 1957; 1:48.
50. Laties AM, Stone RA, Brecha NC: Substance P-like immunoreactive nerve fibers in the trabecular meshwork. *Invest Ophthalmol* 1981; 21:484.
51. Lele P, Weddell G: The relationship between neurohistology and corneal sensibility. *Brain* 1956; 79:119.
52. Lele P, Weddell G: Sensory nerves of the cornea and cutaneous sensibility. *Exp Neurol* 1959; 1:334.
53. Lempe MA: Cornea and sclera. *Arch Ophthalmol* 1974; 92:158.
54. Marshall J: Thermal and mechanical mechanisms in laser damage to the retina. *Invest Ophthalmol* 1970; 9:97.
55. Matsuda H: Electron microscopic study on the corneal nerve with specific reference to its ending. *Jap J Ophthalmol* 1968; 12:163.
56. McCulley JP, Whiting DW, Petitt MG, et al: Hydrofluoric acid burns of the eye. *J Occup Med* 1983; 25:447.
57. McDonald TO, Shadduck JA: Eye irritation, in Marzulli FN, Maibach HL: *Dermatotoxicology and Pharmacology, vol 4, Advances in Modern Toxicology*. Washington, DC, Hemisphere Press, 1977, p 139.
58. McGuiness R: Ammonia in the eye. *Br Med J* 1969; 1:575.
59. Metcalf JF: Corneal sensitivity and neurohistochemical studies of experimental herpetic keratitis in the rabbit. *Exp Eye Res* 1982; 35:231.

60. Miller A, Costa M, Furness J, et al: Substance P immunoreactive sensory nerves supply the rat iris and cornea. *Neurosci Lett* 1981; 23:243.
61. Moon ME, Clarke AM, Ruffolo JJ Jr: Visual performance in the rhesus monkey after exposure to blue light. *Vision Res* 1978; 18:1573.
62. Neufeld AH, Jampol AM, Sears ML: Aspirin prevents the disruption of the blood-aqueous barrier in the rabbit eye. *Nature* 1972; 238:158.
63. Nicholls P: Formate as an inhibitor of cytochrome c oxidase. *Biochem Biophys Res Com* 1975; 67:610.
64. Nicholls P: The effect of formate on cytochrome aa^3 and on electron transport in intact respiratory chain. *Biochem Biophys Acta* 1976; 430:13.
65. Noell WK: The impairment of visual cell structure by iodoacetate. *J Cell Comp Physiol* 1952; 40:25.
66. Oyake Y: Pathology of organic mercury intoxication occurring in the Basin Agano. *Adv Neurol Sci* 1969; 13:108.
67. Patterson CA, Pfister RR: Prostaglandin-like activity in the aqueous humor following alkali burns. *Invest Ophthalmol* 1975; 14:177.
68. Patterson CA, Pfister RR, Levinson RA: Aqueous humor pH changes after experimental alkali burns. *Am J Ophthalmol* 1975; 79:414.
69. Pfister RR, Koski J: Alkali burns of the eye: Pathophysiology and treatment. *South Med J* 1982; 75:417.
70. Podos SM, Becker B: Comparison of ocular prostaglandin synthesis inhibitors. *Invest Ophthalmol* 1973; 15:841.
71. Potts AM: The visual toxicity of methanol: VI. The clinical aspects of experimental methanol poisoning treated with base. *Am J Ophthalmol* 1955; 39:86.
72. Potts AM: Duality of the optic nerve in toxicology, in Merigan WH, Weiss B (eds): *Neurotoxicity of the Visual System*. New York, Raven Press, 1980, p 1.
73. Renzetti N, Schuck E: Preliminary observations on the relation between eye irritation in synthetic systems and in the atmosphere. *J Air Poll Control Assoc* 1961; 11:121.
74. Roper-Hall MJ: Thermal and chemical burns. *Trans Ophthal Soc UK* 1965; 85:631.
75. Rustam H, Hamdi T: Methyl mercury poisoning in Iraq: A neurological study. *Brain* 1974; 97:499.
76. Shaw CM, Mottet NK, Body RL, et al: Variability of neuropathologic lesions in experimental methylmercurial encephalopathy in primates. *Am J Pathol* 1975; 80:451.
77. Sliney DH: Biohazards of ultraviolet, visible, and infrared radiation. *J Occup Med* 1983; 25:203.
78. Stern MR, Naidoff MA, Dawson CR: Intraocular pressure response to experimental alkali burns. *Am J Ophthalmol* 1973; 75:99.
79. Sugimoto K, Goto S, Hotta R: Studies on chronic carbon disulfide poisoning: A five-year follow-up study on retinopathy due to carbon disulfide. *Int Arch Occup Environ Health* 1976; 37:233.
80. Sugimoto K, Goto S, Taniguchi H, et al: Ocular fundus photography of workers exposed to carbon disulfide: A comparative epidemiological study between Japan and Finland. *Int Arch Occup Environ Health* 1977; 37:97.
81. Sugimoto K, Goto S: Retinopathy in chronic carbon disulfide exposure, in Merigan WH, Weiss B (eds): *Neurotoxicity of the Visual System*. New York, Raven Press, 1980, p 55.
82. Takeuchi T: Pathology of Minimata disease. *Adv Neurol Sci* 1969; 13:108.
83. Takeuchi T, Eto K, Okabe M, et al: Grade and distribution of pathological lesions in the nervous system in Minimata disease, from observations of 72 autopsy and 6 biopsy cases. *J Kumamoto Med Soc* 1977; 51:216.
84. Tervo K, Tervo T, Eranko L, et al: Immunoreactivity for substance P in the Gasserian ganglion, ophthalmic nerve, and anterior segment of the rabbit eye. *Histochem J* 1981; 13:345.
85. Tervo K, Tervo T, Eranko L, et al: Substance P immunoreactive nerves in the human cornea and iris. *Invest Ophthalmol* 1982; 23:671.
86. Tokuomi H, Okajima T: Clinical Minimata disease. *Adv Neurol Sci* 1969; 13:69.
87. Tower S: Unit for sensory reception in the cornea. *J Neurophysiol* 1940; 3:486.
88. Trevino MA, Herrmann GH, Sprout WL: Treatment of severe hydrofluoric acid exposures. *J Occup Med* 1983; 25:861.
89. Tullo A, Keen P, Blyth W, et al: Corneal sensitivity and substance P in experimental herpes simplex keratitis in mice. *Invest Ophthalmol* 1983; 24:596.
90. Unger WG, Cole DF, Bass MA: Prostaglandin and neurogenically mediated ocular response to laser irradiation of the rabbit iris. *Exp Eye Res* 1977; 25:209.
91. Weil CS, Scala RA: Study of intra- and interlaboratory variability in the results of rabbit eye and skin irritation tests. *Toxicol Appl Pharmacol* 1971; 19:276.
92. Whitear M: An electron microscope study of the cornea in mice, with special reference to its innervation. *J Anat* 1960; 94:387.
93. Wood RW: Determinants of irritant termination behavior. *Toxicol Appl Pharmacol* 1981; 61:260.
94. Worgul BV, Bito LA, Merriam GR Jr: Intraocular inflammation produced by x-irradiation of the rabbit eye. *Exp Eye Res* 1977; 25:53.
95. Wright P: The chemically injured eye. *Trans Ophthalmol Soc UK* 1982; 102:85.
96. Zander E, Weddell G: Observations on the innervation of the cornea. *J Anat* 1951; 85:68.

12

Determination of Fitness to Work

Mario C. Battigelli, M.D., M.P.H.

Testing for fitness may appear, on the surface, to be a simple and straightforward procedure: a subject is given a physical task pertinent to the job position under consideration, and the performance is assessed according to the obvious guidelines of adequacy: the "can" vs. "cannot" rule. This approach may be called a procedure a posteriori. The major drawback of this method stems from the risks associated with stress experienced by a worker-subject, faced by the full force of the task, particularly whenever impaired or elderly subjects are processed. The exercise testing needs to be both controlled and gradually developed in intensity, to afford a quantitative assessment within reasonable margins of safety. Furthermore, the assessment must be observed on an a priori, quantitative basis, in order to establish these margins of safety. After all, a major tenet of preventive care is to protect a worker from undue fatigue, since fatigue is strongly associated with loss of skilled activity and with injury.

Fitness and its reciprocal, disability,* intended as medical statements of reduced fitness, are complex entities, based on functional, anatomical, psychologic, and educational characteristics of the worker, since these factors relate to the mechanical and dynamic demands of a given job. It is precisely this relational characteristic of matching a person to a given task that is the essence of the fitness assessment process.

CLINICAL MEASUREMENTS

The whole process of determining fitness is a fact of measurement and, as such, is an exercise in relativity. The extent of fitness (or impairment) must be gauged in terms of the demand of a task to be performed, specified in type, intensity, and duration. Appropriate considerations for the specific environment and the structure in which the job takes place (e.g., ambient temperature, pressure, work schedule, and/or work-pause sequence) are equally important for this assessment. It follows that while the rules of measurements, taken individually, are quite simple, the overall interpretation of results, by necessity, seldom is a simple process. Obviously, the relation between the functional elements of a worker-subject and the physical tasks of a job position is influenced by the past medical experience of the examined individual, the motivation and preparedness, the rhythm of performance (speed and technique), and the basic stamina and physiologic endowment of the worker. Morgan et al. have given an elegant example of the importance of the actual load perceived by the subject (dyspnea on effort) by comparing applicants for compensation to hospital patients, matched by pulmonary capacity.[8]

As stated earlier, assessment of fitness and rating of disability are opposite and related facets of the same phenomenon. The techniques and principles used for one will similarly apply to the other.

Methods:

The Maximal Work Capacity

When the assessment of fitness is obtained in response to a general request for determining a worker's adequacy for the demands of heavy muscular tasks (i.e., manual labor), the measurement of maximal work capacity offers a rapid and convenient option, however preliminary. This measurement quantifies the maximum work intensity, sustainable by a worker, consistent with a steady state performance. Obviously, a full work capacity, which is that corresponding to the expected maximum for a given individual, qualifies an applicant for heavy muscular work without specific limitations. The same measurement may be used in screening for impairment (or disability), understood in the general terms of reduced fitness.

In its simplest format, the measurement of maximal work capacity may be obtained by imposing a controlled load, such as climbing, lifting, or pulling. The simplest procedure is the so-called *step test*. The subject is asked to step on and off a raised surface, repeatedly. A stepping device, preferably of variable height, a metronome, and a stop-watch are sufficient for the procedure.[11] If a pulse frequency recorder (or monitor) is available, the procedure is greatly facilitated. The work intensity (external work) may then be measured by the product of body weight, the height of the step, and the frequency of ascensions. The expression of kilogram-meters per minute (kgm/min) can be translated in watts according to the equivalence:

$$w = 9.8/60 \text{ kgm/min}\dagger$$

*Disability is a term with multiple connotations. In its administrative use, it assumes an exquisite economic meaning (i.e., employability) which significantly diverges from the medical rating of impairment.

†Note the watt is unit of power per second. For simplicity, a conversion factor of 6 (instead of 1/0.1633) is often employed in translating watt into kgm/min (kilogram-meter per minute).

The duration of this test is quite short, usually ranging from one to five minutes, with the pulse rate measured conventionally immediately at the end of the exercise period (in fact, 5–20 seconds after the exercise ends).

Table 12–1 reports the range of work intensity in relation to heart frequency.

The use of heart rate (HR) to monitor and quantify cardiorespiratory responses during exercise is buttressed by a wide body of published observations. The rationale is based on the fundamental relationship linking oxygen consumption to HR, which remains linear within a wide range of work ($\dot{V}_{O_2}$ = HR × stroke volume × atrioventricular difference). Work levels at top capacity correspond to maximal heart rates, which are commonly estimated by the predictive equation: HR MAX = 220 − age. The conventional value of 170 beats per minute (bpm) has been proposed and is used, particularly in Europe, to indicate standard maximal HR for the adult working individual.[13] Based on the linearity connecting HR to workloads, the frequency of 170 bpm is thus used to intercept the predicted maximal working capacity in a diagram relating load to heart frequency in a given individual. Figure 12–1 presents an example of this computation. The subject is a 50-year-old man, with a body weight of 75 kg, considered for a trucking job position as a dock loader. The worker is expected to lift boxes, with weight up to 30 lb, through a mean height of 1 m, from the bed of an utility cart, to a conveyor belt, at a maximum rate of five lifts each minute. Is this subject qualified for the task?

In lifting each box, the subject is considered to raise a third of his own body weight (the upper portion of his trunk, arms, and head) approximately through the same vertical distance of 1m. This results in a computed external work totaling 193 kgm/min (i.e., [25 kg body weight + 13.5 kg box] × 1 m × 5 lifts/min).‡

In order to establish the HR response of the subject, the worker is challenged at two mechanical loads, using the step test (three minutes at 468 kgm/min and at 656 kgm/min, respectively), monitoring the HR at the end of each exercise period. The two heart rates, after each exercise period, result in 98 and 130 bpm, respectively. Introducing these values in the diagram of Figure 12–1, the extrapolation to work capacity at 170 bpm (maximum work capacity) intercepts a maximum load of 860 kgm/min. It can be

TABLE 12–1.
Relationship of Heart Frequency to Exercise Intensity*

WORK	HR (BPM)
Light	up to 90
Moderate	90–100
Heavy	110–130
Very heavy	130–150
Extreme	150–170

*From Åstrand PO, Rodahl K: *Textbook of Work Physiology.* New York, McGraw-Hill Book Co, 1977, p 462. Used by permission.

‡This computation neglects the negative work done in bending down. This minor aliquot is roughly accounted for by the generous estimate of fractional body weight used.

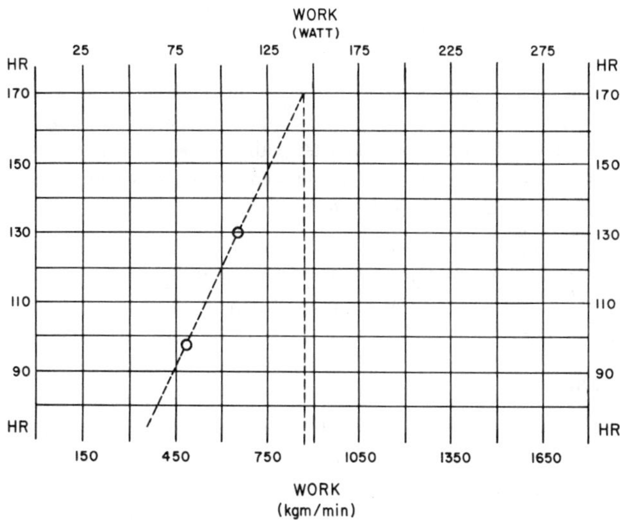

FIG 12–1.
Prediction of maximum physical work capacity.

seen that the projected mechanical demands imposed by the job for which the worker is considered remains well within the acceptable range of the heart rate.

More sophisticated items of equipment used to test work capacity include mechanically or electrically braked ergometers and variable-incline treadmills. With these devices, a subject is tested at progressively higher loads (step-wise), each applied for a duration between one and five minutes. The heart rate is monitored, and, since its increase is linear, in correspondence to increased loads, the extrapolation to maximal load can be obtained from submaximal tasks. In addition to HR, subjective perception of tolerance (i.e., fatigue) should be obtained to define better maximal limits. The continuous electrocardiographic (ECG) monitoring makes the assessment more informative. However, it should be remembered that minor abnormalities in ECG records may be noted during exercise in 75% of men and 50% of women older than 50 years, suggesting a limited specificity of this monitor in the general population.[7]

Oxygen Consumption and Aerobic Capacity

A more realistic and informative assessment of the physiologic cost of mechanical work is obtained with the measure of oxygen consumption. When this measurement is obtained at maximal work load, it is called maximum aerobic capacity or $\dot{V}_{O_2}$ MAX. Aerobic capacity and mechanical workload are directly related through the efficiency factor, both being linearly correlated with oxygen consumption. In fact, nomograms have been prepared for the estimate of oxygen consumption, indirectly, through the observation of heart rate response to the exercise with the step test.[6]

As additional convenience of the measurement of oxygen consumption is found in its ability to measure mechanical work. Since any muscular work operates on oxidative processes, the oxygen consumed during a given activity directly quantifies the work done. Different mechanical operation can, therefore, be estimated through the oxygen consumption, by the simple device of monitoring oxygen in expired air ($\dot{V}_{O_2}$ = $\dot{V}_{O_2}$ inspired − $\dot{V}_{O_2}$ expired).

A variety of predicted values for given age, body size, and sex have been published, providing reasonable estimates of maximal expected aerobic capacity. The observed/expected ratio obtained on this basis permits an assessment of the degree of fitness of a given individual. With the term of *functional aerobic impairment* (FAI), Bruce et al. estimate, with good reproducibility, the loss from expected maximal oxygen capacity in both patients and noncomplaining control subjects.[5]

$$\text{FAI} = \frac{\dot{V}_{O_2}\ \text{MAX predicted} - \dot{V}_{O_2}\ \text{MAX observed}}{\dot{V}_{O_2}\ \text{MAX predicted}} \times 100$$

Endurance Tests

Muscular endurance for demanding jobs can be similarly tested, through exhaustive trials of limited duration. Obviously, these demanding tests, of several minutes in duration, are acceptable and feasible only in selected persons who are well-endowed functionally, such as physical education students, athletes in training, military personnel, and workers selected for special tasks.

Outside of these special applications, testing for endurance remains based, conventionally, on the estimates of performance observed through one to five minutes' duration at submaximal loads. Physiologically, these estimates are quite justified, since steady-state conditions are reached soon after completion of one-minute exercise, for work levels up to moderate intensity. It is widely recognized that endurance largely rests on factors of motivation and training, while the traditional physiologic factors assume secondary importance.

A major limiting factor in using these tests for assessing endurance is the discrepancy found between the muscles used in walking, bicycling, and stepping, and the actual muscular groups that may be of importance in the job tasks, such as the arm muscles and the trunk muscles, which are not significantly engaged in the testing procedures. For these applications, the traditional measurement of individual muscle strength are more informative.

Strength Testing

Testing muscular strength in separate procedures involving the activity of limited muscular groups is an informative and often indispensable part of the fitness assessment. These estimates offer the additional information necessary to minimize injury associated with the strain experienced in lifting and related mechanical tasks. Example: a worker with the maximum ability to lift a 150-kg weight, will be taxed at 15% (utilization rate) of maximal capacity when requested to lift 25-kg weights.[3] Alternately, a worker with a maximum lifting ability of 40 kg, when requested to lift a 25-kg weight, will experience a utilization rate of 63%, which is commonly considered an excessive demand and is likely to cause injury. In measuring maximal strength, such as by weight lifting, a procedure of trial and error is followed, beginning with measuring the effects of moderate intensity and rapidly increasing to maximal efforts. Hand grip, arms, back, and leg strengths can be assessed separately, with excellent reproducibility, using simple equipment (dynamometers), which are quite suitable to the industrial dispensary. With these measurements, one needs to remember, however, the great variability of performance observed in normal subjects, a factor which greatly limits the estimates of loss. Furthermore, the rapid loss of strength that follows disuse, such as inactivity and bed rest, additionally complicates these estimates, such as may occur in the context of compensation procedures. It is recognized, in fact, that total inactivity may cause up to 5% loss of muscular strength per day.[9]

Flexibility Tests

In general, muscular strength is not the most important factor of fitness. Range of motion, dexterity, and speed of movement are probably more important for effective muscular work.

Measurement of the range of motion of a joint is the traditional objective of a physical examination. An additional element related to range of motion and used for the functional assessment of the trunk is technically known as a measure of *flexibility*. It is commonly measured by the *sit and reach test*.[12] The subject is asked to extend the arms forward, from the sitting position, with legs flat on the floor. In the normal young adult, the fingertips reach the toes and extend somewhat beyond them.

Perceived Efforts

Experience with patients presenting limited mechanical work endurance has disclosed an impressive correlation between the heart rate and the semiquantitative recording of subjective assessment of effort (i.e., perception). These observations have led to the formulation by Borg of a rating scale of perceived effort, called the Rating of Perceived Exertion (RPE).[4] Originally based on a 20-point range, this scale has been restructured on a ten-point range, with the option for extension beyond the extremes (Table 12–2).

In the words of Borg, "perceived exertion" is the single best indicator of physical strain, in quantitative terms.[4] Indeed, in subjects with significant cardiovascular limitations, such as angina patients, the RPE has been shown to be an accurate predictor of aerobic capacity.[10] In healthy workers, the RPE has provided convenient assessment of efficient lifting technique.[10]

We should conclude that the attempt to rate efforts through the "perceived" intensity by the subject examined ought to become

TABLE 12–2.
RPE: Rating of Perceived Exertion

RATING	PERCEPTION
0	Nothing at all
0.5	Very weak, just noticeable
1	Very weak
2	Weak (light effort)
3	Moderate
4	Somewhat strong
5	Strong (heavy effort)
6	
7	Very strong
8	
9	
10	Very, very strong
>10	Maximal effort

a more common part of an examination for fitness-impairment. With all due regard for the motivational outlook and personal bias that so often characterize the behavior of those who apply for compensation and related reasons, the examining physician ought to strive toward the definition and, if possible, the quantification of effort perception in the subjects examined, through the use of meaningful scales.

DETAILED ASSESSMENT OF DISABILITY

Several schemes available in the literature provide a general assessment of fitness to work without details as to the mechanism or cause of disability. For the precise assessment of nature, cause, and/or mechanism, differential diagnostic procedures are required.

A particularly useful device for disability evaluation in detail is to be found in the *AMA Guides to the Evaluation of Permanent Impairment*—indeed a valuable document.[1]

Again, it should be reiterated that the assessment of disability needs to consider the human person as a whole, with inclusion of attitudes, motivations, and education as integral parts of parameters to be estimated. No evaluation should be obtained out of context, but rather always in relation to a set of employment tasks that realistically match the individual's fitness and/or experience.

When the evaluation of fitness to work is done with the appropriate care and constraints, it is a rewarding professional accomplishment. Disability assessment, as stated, becomes in this way more than medical adjudication of compensation issues. Indeed, disability assessment is an application of quantitative medicine of invaluable importance in the optimal placement and management of people at work.

Fitness and disability need to be scrutinized in order to assess the value of the "whole person." For instance, in gauging the fitness of an individual for a given job, both positive attributes and limitations need to be accounted for in the process. Adequate dexterity and sensorial integrity by themselves are not sufficient in defining the risk of an operator of mobile equipment who has a coexisting seizure disorder. The latter, also, needs to be evaluated in its positive aspects, in respect to the disorder's response to treatment, the patient's compliance with treatment, and his or her social adjustment. Indeed, it has been demonstrated convincingly that any given medical "condition" is not a good predictor of "disability." The negative finding reflecting pathology or impairment must be evaluated in light of the individual's favorable qualities, educational resources, emotional stamina, and personal attitude toward work. In short, the evaluating physician cannot neglect to take an adequate social history and interpret it in regard to the patient's ability. In this endeavor, the assistance of social workers, rehabilitation experts, and an ergonomist engineer can contribute effectively to the physician's own assessment and management decisions.

REFERENCES

1. AMA Committee on Rating of Mental and Physical Impairment: *Guides to the Evaluation of Permanent Impairment*. Chicago, American Medical Association, 1971.
2. Åstrand PO, Rodahl K: *Textbook of Work Physiology*. New York, McGraw-Hill Book Co, 1977, p 462.
3. Ayoub M: Control of manual lifting hazards: III. Pre-employment screening. *J Occup Med* 1982; 24:751.
4. Borg GAV: Psychophysical bases of perceived exertion. *Med Sci Sports Exerc* 1982; 14:377.
5. Bruce RA, Kusumi F, Hosmer D: Maximal oxygen intake and nomographic assessment of functional aerobic impairment in cardiovascular disease. *Am Heart J* 1973; 85:546.
6. Magaria R: *Biomechanics and Energetics of Muscular Exercise*. Oxford, Claredon Press, 1976, p 39–42.
7. Morgan WKC, Seaton A: *Occupational Lung Diseases*, ed 2. Philadelphia, WB Saunders, Co, 1984, p 73.
8. Morgan WKC: Disability or Disinclination? Impairment or Importuning? *Chest* 1979; 75:712.
9. Müller EA: Influence of training and of inactivity on muscle strength. *Arch Phys Med Rehabil* 1970; 41:449.
10. Noble BJ: Clinical application of perceived exertion. *Med Sci Sports Exerc* 1982; 14:406.
11. Pollock ML, Wilmore JH, Fox SM: *Exercise in Health and Disease*. Philadelphia, WB Saunders Co, 1984.
12. Pollock ML, Wilmore JH, Fox SM: *Health and Fitness Through Physical Activity*. New York, John Wiley & Sons, 1978.
13. Shephard RJ: *Endurance Fitness*, ed 2. Toronto, University of Toronto Press, 1977, p 280.

13

Biologic Monitoring

Antero Aitio, M.D., Ph.D.

Jorma Järvisalo, M.D., Ph.D.

Vesa Riihimäki, M.D., Ph.D.

Sven Hernberg, M.D., Ph.D.

The goal of preventive occupational health is to reduce worker exposures to potentially harmful agents to levels which, to the best of our knowledge, do not cause any adverse or toxic effects. One step in this process is the assessment of exposure. Traditionally, this has been done through sampling and measurements taken from the workroom air. A deeper insight into the difficulties of relating external exposure parameters to the amount actually taken up, together with advances in analytical chemistry have, during the last 10–15 years, created a growing interest for developing measurements from the biologic media to be used along with environmental measurements for the assessment of actual personal exposure. The rationale is that an estimate of the amount of a chemical which has actually entered the body, the so-called internal dose, is likely to yield a better prediction of the potential toxic effects than mere measurements of the concentrations in the ambient air (Fig 13–1). This is no doubt a sound assumption, but we are merely at the beginning of a long road.

Monitoring was defined by a seminar sponsored by the European Economic Community (EEC), the National Institute of Occupational Safety and Health (NIOSH), and the Occupational Health and Safety Administration (OSHA)[5] as "a systematic or repetitive health-related activity designed to lead, if necessary, to corrective action." The same seminar defined biologic monitoring as "the measurement and assessment of agents or their metabolites either in tissues, secreta, excreta, expired air, or any combination of these to evaluate exposure and health risk, compared to an appropriate reference." This applies to the biologic monitoring of both workers and the general public. Monitoring is also a repetitive, *regular* activity, and it is important to include the assessment aspect in the concept. It is, furthermore, a *preventive* activity; it should not be confused with diagnostic procedures. (In the literature, the use of the term *biologic monitoring* has unfortunately not been consistent. Some have used this concept to cover also the measurement of physiologic responses, such as pulmonary function tests, and even tests for the early diagnosis of diseases, in addition to different biologic measurements.) We would also like to stress the distinction between monitoring and health surveillance, which is a wider concept encompassing several aspects of health screening and early diagnosis.[10] The EEC/NIOSH/OSHA working group[5] defined health surveillance as "the periodic medico-physiologic examinations of exposed workers with the objective of protecting health and preventing disease. The detection of established disease is outside the scope of this definition."

Meaningful biologic monitoring presupposes that four conditions be met:

1. The substance and/or its metabolites are present in some tissue, body fluid, or excretion suitable for sampling;

2. Valid and practical methods of analysis and sampling are available;

3. The measurement strategy is adequate (the samples are representative); and

4. The result can be interpreted in a meaningful way.

The feasibility of biologic monitoring is thus determined by two kinds of considerations: (1) a knowledge of the toxicology and kinetics of the substance; and (2) practical aspects. Even when there is sufficient toxicologic knowledge, the feasibility of sampling and the availability of simple, accurate, and inexpensive analytic methods have to be considered. It is also self-evident that the workers must accept the method, and that no risk to the worker is involved. It can be stated that few currently used biologic monitoring methods comply with all these criteria.

Before biologic monitoring can be generally recommended as the primary method of exposure assessment, much more must be learned about the toxicokinetics and metabolism of most of the toxic chemicals of concern. Dose-effect and dose-response relationships, based on dose estimates from the biologic media have

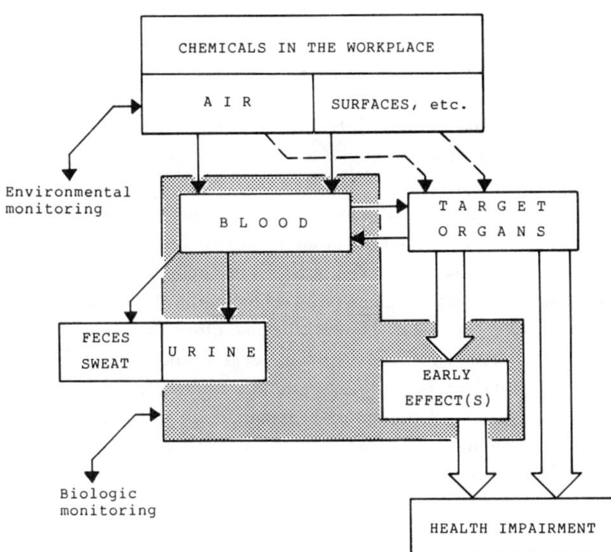

FIG 13–1.
The relationships between the kinetics, effects of chemicals, and environmental and biologic monitoring. The *thin arrows* indicate pathways of the chemicals; the *bold arrows,* the effects of the chemicals.

been elucidated for only a few of the substances for which biologic analyses are technically possible. Practical aspects, such as how to ensure the representativeness of the samples, must be further elaborated. Analytic sensitivity and accuracy must be improved and new methods must be developed for a great many substances. Because biologic monitoring at present is only evolving, one must always consider alternative ways—that is, environmental monitoring—of ensuring sufficiently accurate assessments of exposure.

No result is useful if it cannot be interpreted. Measurements from the ambient air can always be compared to hygienic standards, even when the latter are based on insufficient knowledge. For biologic measurements there are few regulatory standards. This leaves room for subjective judgment, either individual or collective, expressed in the form of various recommendations for biologic exposure limits. The better the dose-effect and dose-response relationships are known, the higher the likelihood for a correct judgment. Unfortunately there are only a few substances, mostly metals, for which enough quantitative toxicologic data are available. In most instances, the limits recommended are insufficiently documented. Sometimes they are based on direct, although insufficient observations on the relationship between levels in the biologic media and toxic effects. More often, they rely on indirect estimations based on, first, the relationship between biologic and ambient levels and, then, between ambient levels and toxic effects. Because ambient air concentrations poorly reflect the internal exposure, the latter approach is far from ideal. However, even if the dose-effect and dose-response relationships are insufficiently known, the presence of foreign substances in the biologic media indicates that exposure has taken place. This is rarely desirable, and especially the workers with the highest values should have their exposure reduced and they should be observed more closely, perhaps by means of medical examinations.

While knowledge on dose-effect and dose-response relationships is a prerequisite for the interpretation of the results of biologic monitoring whenever the prevention of *toxic* effects is concerned, the issue is fundamentally different when the aim is to prevent *cancer*. While toxic effects usually occur at a certain threshold level, no such level exists for carcinogens—at least not according to prevalent views. This implies that all exposure to carcinogens is undesirable and that, consequently, everything that exceeds "normal" levels in a biologic exposure test should be interpreted as "excessive."

One problem of biologic monitoring is whether this approach is ethically correct or not. It has been maintained that the worker must not be a walking sampling device, and that the mere idea of basing a monitoring program on absorption that has already occurred is unethical. Also, the drawing of blood samples has been criticized, since this procedure is not completely noninvasive and the sample can also be used for other purposes.

These viewpoints must be weighed against the advantages of biologic monitoring compared with environmental monitoring. Environmental monitoring does not account for skin absorption, internal accumulation, the use of personal protective devices, and differences in physical activity, working habits, and personal hygiene, nor for nonoccupational exposure, while biologic monitoring accounts for all of these. All these aspects justify biologic monitoring, we think, provided that biologic test results are used *only* to reduce the risk of toxic or carcinogenic effects on the exposed worker.

A biologic monitoring program requires the workers' informed consent. Biologic samples should be used only for the purpose for which they were meant, and if, for example, scientific research is combined with a monitoring program, the workers must be so informed and the research must be explained to them. Every action taken on the basis of the results of the monitoring must be in the interest of the worker, and the results must not be made public without the consent of every single worker involved. If these ethical rules are strictly adhered to, we think that there should be no objections to biologic monitoring as a means of preventing adverse health effects.

ENVIRONMENTAL AND BIOLOGIC MONITORING

The traditional approach for estimating the occupational exposure of workers to chemicals has been measurement of the chemicals in the ambient air, i.e., industrial hygiene measurements. This is, and probably always will be, the most important method for exposure estimation. The reasons are manifold and include analytic and legislative factors: The analytic methodology for air measurements is advanced; often the analyses are comparatively easy, because air is a homogenous and rather simple matrix. Also, even rather low concentrations may be measured, since the amount of air collected is not strictly limited. Practically all chemicals that are present in the workplace can be detected and analyzed. Because industrial hygiene measurements have been performed for such a long time, exposure-effect and exposure-response curves are available for many chemicals. Air measurements are traditional, and, in most countries, they are the sole basis of regulation.

TABLE 13–1.
Factors Affecting Uptake of Chemicals in the Body That Industrial Hygiene Measurements Are Not Likely to Account for

Variation in the concentration of the chemical at different locations
Variation in the concentration of the chemical at different points of time
Particle size and aerodynamic properties of particles
Solubility characteristics of the chemical
Alternative absorption routes (skin, gastrointestinal tract)
Protective devices and their efficiency
Respiratory volumes (workload-job energy demands)
Personal habits
Exposures outside the workplace

On the other hand, biologic monitoring in some cases has distinct advantages over air measurements, mainly because it is the *absorbed* chemical that is measured. Concentrations of a chemical in the air are not necessarily very closely related to the amounts absorbed, for many reasons (Table 13–1). Concentrations in the air are seldom stable but fluctuate with time and are different in different locations. The workload dramatically changes the inhaled volume of air, and, for many chemicals, the amount absorbed is directly related to the amount inhaled. One should also be aware of the possibility of coincident high-exposure peaks and increased workloads that are likely to be produced, e.g., by the malfunctioning of a closed (and presumably safe) process. Many chemicals are effectively absorbed through the skin, and this route of exposure is generally not at all related to concentrations of chemicals in the air. The particle sizes of various dusts profoundly affect their deposition pattern in the airways and thus their absorption. Personal working habits vary, and individuals may absorb different amounts of chemicals in superficially similar conditions. Protective devices may (or may not) affect the amounts absorbed. Traditional industrial hygiene measurements do not indicate the degree of protection afforded by masks, which may vary according to the different chemicals present, the condition of the mask, and the individual who wears it. It is thus quite evident that both industrial hygiene measurements and biologic monitoring may be used, most effectively in combination, in the estimation of the exposure and of the chemical body burden. These approaches complement, rather than compete with, each other.

EXPOSURE MONITORING

Kinetic Considerations and Sampling Strategies

In biologic monitoring, one may try to estimate the body burden of the chemical. An alternative approach is to ascertain the highest concentration attained in the body, especially in the target tissue. However, because the biologic monitoring of chemicals with mainly acute toxicity cannot be preventive, this approach probably is not equally rewarding.

The ease with which one can estimate the body burden of a chemical is very much dependent on the chemical, and especially on its kinetic properties in the body. For chemicals with long half-times—such as lead, cadmium, and mercury—the concentration in the blood (or even in the urine) reaches a plateau, which reflects the equilibrium between daily intake and excretion. In a stable exposure situation, the daily variation of the concentration is small, and an accurate picture may be obtained from even a single determination of the blood or urine level.

The situation is quite different for chemicals with short half-times. First, the concentration—especially in the blood—changes rapidly with time, and the concentrations found only reflect a very recent exposure. Very stringent standardization of the specimen collection time is needed in order to obtain meaningful results. Second, the representativeness of the value obtained may be very poor, since the concentrations of the chemical in the workplace air tend to change. Even if the working conditions are known, this gives only a rough idea of the most recent exposure. Thus, one may have to do the monitoring frequently in order to obtain a representative picture of the amounts absorbed. In practice, it is not possible to monitor effectively chemicals with half-times shorter than a few hours. However, many chemicals have several successive half-times, reflecting their distribution in different compartments of the body. Thus, lipid-soluble organic solvents, which have a very short half-time (on the order of minutes) in the blood and richly vasculated organs, tend to accumulate in the fatty tissues and are slowly released after exposure has ceased. The fat stores thus function as integrators, and exposure over whole days—and even several days—may be estimated from specimens collected approximately 16–18 hours after the end of the exposure. At this point, the half-times of, for example, lipid-soluble solvents are on the order of 10–20 hours. Excretion in the urine also functions as an integrator or buffer for a chemical, and the half-times are generally longer than those for chemicals found in the blood. Thus, excretion of a metabolite in the urine is often a kinetically preferable alternative in biologic monitoring.

Specimens in Use

Blood and urine are the main materials tested in the biologic monitoring of occupational exposures. Which one of these two is more preferable depends on the analytic and kinetic factors specific to the chemical in question. In some countries, an additional factor is the difficulty in obtaining the workers' permission to collect blood specimens. The use of hair has been studied rather extensively, mainly because of the ease of specimen collection and because hair might indicate exposures over a few months better than body fluids would. However, trace elements in the hair originate not only from several intrinsic sources, such as the matrix proper, sebum, and sweat, but also from extrinsic sources, such as dust, shampoos, and coloring chemicals. Determining the source of contamination of hair samples is practically impossible. Thus, hair cannot be recommended for biologic exposure monitoring.[16, 41, 50]

Some researchers have extensively used exhaled air in the biologic monitoring of exposure to volatile solvents. In experimental conditions, this has given good results. However, concentrations of solvents in exhaled air vary quite remarkably with the phase of expiration: they tend to be low in the air obtained from the dead space, and high in alveolar air. In practice, it is difficult to obtain specimens that represent true alveolar air. In addition, transportation and storage of exhaled air samples is problematic. Therefore, it seems that exhaled air specimens are not reliable for biologic monitoring. This may well change with the introduction—and reduction in price—of portable dedicated mass spectrometers that automatically correct the concentrations by the carbon dioxide content of breath specimens.

EFFECT MONITORING

Effect monitoring means that, instead of the substance itself or its metabolite, some specific or semispecific effect is measured. Monitoring of an early effect of the chemical would, in a way, be ideal for the prevention of the adverse health effects of a chemical: it would take into account even the individual differences in susceptibility, not just the amounts of the chemical taken up. However, the rationale of biologic monitoring is to *prevent effects*, and therefore effect monitoring is conceptually contradictory. On the other hand, the effect on which the monitoring is based could be nonadverse. Examples of effects that traditionally are considered nonadverse are the depression of the activity of 5-aminolevulinate dehydratase and the elevation of the concentration of zinc protoporphyrin in the erythrocytes. (However, increased excretion of proteins such as β_2-microglobulin and retinol-binding globulins in the urine in exposure to cadmium or other nephrotoxins is not reversible and has to be regarded as an adverse effect.)

Many effects monitored lack specificity: erythrocyte zinc protoporphyrin level is also elevated in iron-deficiency anemia, and microglobulin levels may be elevated in any tubular dysfunction and in certain immunologic disorders.

Measurement of effects should usually not be regarded as biologic monitoring, but as a part of health surveillance. In practice, biologic monitoring and health surveillance form a continuum in workers' health protection; all divisions in this continuum are artificial.

SOURCES OF ERROR AND QUALITY ASSURANCE

All laboratory analyses are prone to error: biologic monitoring is no exception. In fact, biologic monitoring suffers not only from all the weaknesses of clinical chemistry in general, but also from many other important failings.

The analytic error proper is beyond the scope of this text, but it should be stressed that in the majority of analyses in biologic monitoring, the analytic techniques applied are quite demanding, both with respect to the equipment involved and to the training and capabilities of the concerned personnel.

Much variation is generated by physiologic, kinetic, and environmental factors before the analysis proper and the variation associated with specimen collection forms a major part of the total variation.[14, 16] All such variations must be reduced by the health care personnel responsible for the sampling. The analyzing laboratory can do little to avoid them.

Physiologic and Environmental Sources of Variation

Body Posture.—Body posture markedly affects the concentration of chemicals in the circulating blood. In the upright position, water leaks from the blood vessels. Chemicals attached to cells or macromolecules show an apparent enrichment. In the recumbent position, the reverse takes place. The error thus generated may exceed 10% in a healthy person, but it may be many times higher in persons with various diseases. The same phenomenon is seen locally in the arm upon the application of tourniquet for specimen collection.

Diurnal Variation.—Many chemicals exhibit diurnal variation of the concentration. For example, concentrations of mercury in the urine are highest in the morning.

Volume of Urine.—The volume of urine excreted depends on the hydration state of the body. The effects of this variation on the concentration of different chemicals in the urine is largely unexplored. However, it is traditional to try to correct for the variation by standardizing the concentrations to a constant relative density (usually 1.018 or 1.024). The basis of correction chosen changes profoundly the figures obtained: correction to 1.024 gives values 33% higher than correction to 1.018. An alternative is correction to creatinine excretion, which remains rather stable irrespective of the hydration status. Another alternative would be the use of timed urine specimens, e.g., four-hour, eight-hour, or even 24-hour urines. This is not often achieved in routine biologic monitoring.

Diet.—Diet is an important source of many industrial chemicals. Urine concentrations of trace elements are related to their amounts in the diet—and thus, those in the soil. Even large amounts of organic chemicals, such as phenol, cresols, and hippuric and mandelic acids, may be derived from different items in the diet.

Environmental Contaminants.—Similarly, monitoring of occupational exposure to such widespread environmental contaminants as cadmium, mercury, chlorophenothane (DDT), and polychlorinated biphenyls from their concentrations in the blood requires a knowledge of local reference values for the nonexposed population.

Cigarette Smoking.—Cigarette smoke contains, among other things, carbon monoxide, hydrogen cyanide, and cadmium, and thus it is a significant source of error in the biologic monitoring of at least these chemicals when there are smokers among the worker population.

Individual Physiologic Variation.—The physiologic variation has to be dealt with by rigorous standardization of the specimen collection.[18] The sampling hour is to be standardized, preferably to the morning. This not only decreases the effect of diurnal variation, but it tends to decrease the effects of the preceding meal. The tested worker should avoid intensive physical stress for some hours before sampling. The subject should remain seated for 15 minutes before blood sampling. The tourniquet application time should be less than one minute.

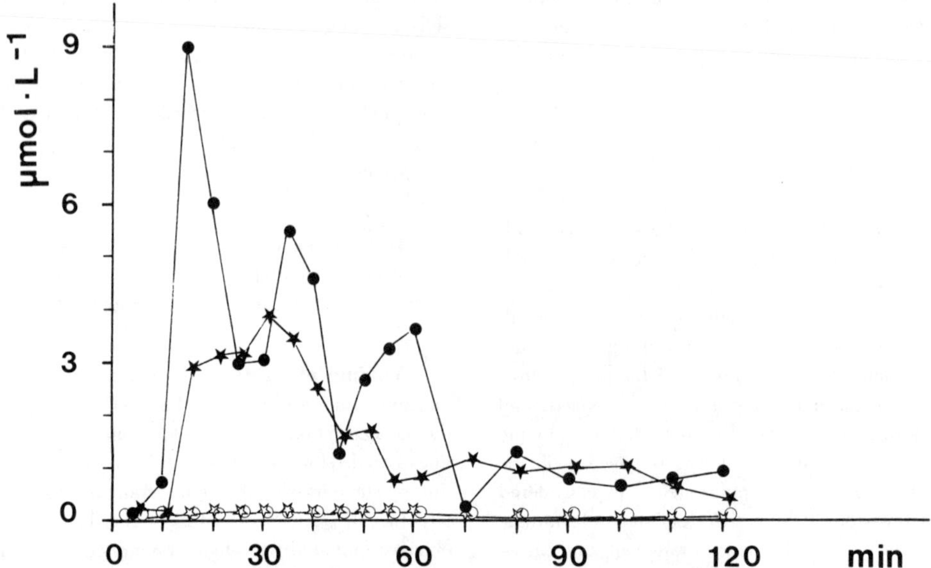

FIG 13–2.
Skin absorption of tetrachloroethylene and 1,1,1-trichloroethane. Blood concentrations of 1,1,1-trichloroethane *(stars)* and tetrachloroethylene *(circles)* in a volunteer who dipped one hand in the corresponding solvent. *Closed symbols:* blood from the exposed extremity. *Open symbols:* blood samples from the contralateral extremity. (From Aitio A, Pekari K, and Järvisalo J: Skin absorption as a source of error in biological monitoring. *Scand J Work Environ Health* 1984; 10:317. Used by permission.)

Kinetic Sources of Variation

The concentration of an exogenous chemical is seldom stable in body fluids but shows an exposure-related fluctuation. The time of collecting the specimen, therefore, is an important factor in the concentration found: the interpretation crucially depends on the timing (see Kinetic Considerations).

If a chemical is readily absorbed through the skin, this is usually regarded as a reason to prefer biologic monitoring over air monitoring. However, when an analysis of the concentration in the blood of the chemical itself is used in biologic monitoring, skin absorption may cause a substantial error. This is because the blood collected from a cubital vein does not represent the blood in the organism in toto, but rather a local concentration (Fig 13–2).

Variations Associated With Specimen Collection and Storage

The factors most likely to cause error in specimen collection and storage include contamination, chemical deterioration, evaporation, and precipitation and adsorption on vessel surfaces. Since the chemical nature of substances monitored is widely different, the relative importance of these processes also varies.

Evaporation.—Many organic solvents are volatile and may be lost even from closed containers.[32] Evaporation losses may be diminished by refrigeration. It is also advisable to fill the vials to the rim and make sure that they are tightly closed.

Chemical Deterioration.—This is a problem typical of organic chemicals. For each chemical, the storage stability has to be verified; refrigeration and, especially, freezing tend to improve the stability of many chemicals.

Precipitation and Adsorption.—Urine is often voided as an oversaturated solution of, e.g., uric acid or phosphates. These tend to precipitate upon storage. Trace elements may coprecipitate with the salts or may be adsorbed on surfaces of crystals. Acidification of urine usually decreases the precipitation losses of trace elements. Acidification decreases even adsorption of trace elements on vial (glass or plastic) surfaces; surface adsorption is usually of minor importance for urine or blood samples.[14]

Contamination.—This is by far the most important source of error in the analysis of trace elements.[14, 16] The magnitude of the problem is reflected, for example, in serum chromium values regarded normal in nonexposed people in different studies (Table 13–2): they have shown a precipitous fall during recent years. A similar table can be collected for many trace elements.

Contamination may come from the air in the workplace or the laboratory, from the worker's skin or clothes, from specimen containers, additives, reagents, or from the analyzing instrument.

Contamination from the workplace air causes the most dramatic analytic errors, since the concentration of the chemical (organic or inorganic) in the dust tends to be very high. Dust is found also on the worker's clothes, as well as on the skin. Because proper cleaning of the skin is not easy, it is better to use only venous blood, not capillary blood from the fingertip, in trace element analysis.

The risk of contamination in the collection of urine specimens is greater than for blood specimens. Urine specimens should be

TABLE 13–2.
Evolution of the Values Regarded as Normal Average Serum Chromium Concentrations in Nonexposed Men*

YEAR	AUTHOR	SERUM CHROMIUM (NMOLE/L)
1956	Monacelli et al.	3,600
1966	Glinsman et al.	540
1972	Behne & Diehl	198
1972	Davidsohn & Secrest	97
1974	Pekarek et al.	31
1974	Grafflage et al.	14
1978	Versieck et al.	3.1
1978	Kayne et al.	2.7
1983	Kumpulainen et al.	2.3
1984	Veillon et al.	2.1

*Adapted from Kumpulainen et al.,[60] Veillon et al.,[101] and Versieck and Cornelis.[102]

collected in a noncontaminated area only and only after the worker has taken a shower and changed clothes.

Nickel, chromium, manganese, and cobalt may leach to blood from disposable stainless steel needles.[103] The importance of this source of contamination has not yet been determined.[16] Meanwhile, if it is not possible to use platinum needles or plastic cannulae, it is best to discard the first 10 ml of blood.

Glass and various plastics contain varying amounts of many trace elements, and these may leach to water, urine, and blood.[84] It seems that no commercially produced container should be used for urine storage without a prior cleaning by acid soaking. General-purpose evacuated tubes are a notorious source of cadmium and lead, for example, and probably also of other trace elements. The special lead-free tubes seem suitable for lead analyses; for other trace elements, it still would seem preferable to verify the absence of contamination of the element analyzed before introducing a new brand of evacuated tube.

Quality Assurance

Quality assurance refers to all steps that may be taken to ensure that laboratory results are reliable.[113] A part of quality assurance is internal quality control, i.e., the procedures within the laboratory for assessing the analytical results in order to decide whether they are reliable enough to be released.[113] Internal quality control consists of analyses of control specimens within every analytic series. The results obtained are compared to predefined limits of acceptability. Without continuous internal quality control, a laboratory should not release any result.

External quality control is a system for the objective checking of laboratory performance by an external agency.[113] Although external quality control is a routine practice in clinical chemical laboratories, in many countries it is not yet the rule for laboratories doing biologic monitoring. At present, however, many national and international organizations have started external quality control programs (Center for Disease Control, NIOSH, Commission of the European Communities), and in the foreseeable future it is hoped that the currently rather weak quality of many occupational biologic monitoring laboratories[12, 38] will improve.

MONITORING OF EXPOSURE TO CARCINOGENS

The monitoring of exposure is an integral part of occupational genotoxicity, which is dealt with in this volume by Professsor M. Sorsa (Chapter 51). Only a short summary is given here.

Urinary Mutagenicity

Measurement of mutagenicity in urine has been the most widely used means of estimation of carcinogenic exposure by nonspecific means. Urine poses some problems in mutagenicity testing, notably the low concentrations of mutagens in the urine, the toxicity of urine against the indicator organisms, and the presence of the mutagen in the urine in an inactive form. The problem of sensitivity has been solved by applying concentration methods (generally XAD-resins) and by adopting very sensitive assay methods, most often the fluctuation modification of the classic Ames *Salmonella* microsome assay. In order to reactivate the chemicals in the urine, treatments with enzymes, such as glucuronidase and sulphatase, have been used. The toxicity of urine usually still sets limits to the sensitivity of the assay; toxicity should always be assayed together with mutagenicity.

Smoking is often the most formidable problem in the evaluation of mutagen/carcinogen exposures by mutagenicity assays: tobacco smoke contains a variety of chemicals that are excreted in the urine in a form that may be converted mutagenic. However, most of the mutagens in tobacco smoke are frame-shift mutagens, and in situations where the occupational exposures contain mutagens of other types, the smoking effect may be removed by using bacterial strains not sensitive to frame-shift mutagens.

One should not forget that only genotoxic carcinogens can be detected by mutagenicity assays. Also, it is possible that carcinogenic chemicals are excreted in the urine in a form that is not converted mutagenic by the standard techniques. In addition, it is possible that the concentration methods applied show very limited or even zero recovery for the mutagens in the urine. Therefore, negative results in urine mutagenicity testing should not be taken to indicate an absence of exposure to carcinogenic chemicals. Despite the problems involved, urinary mutagenicity monitoring has proven rewarding in the detection and follow-up of carcinogen exposure upon implementation of preventive hygienic measures.

Alkylation Products of Proteins, Peptides, Amino Acids and Nucleic Acids

Thioethers in the Urine.—The most widely applied assay has been analysis of thioethers in the urine. Urinary thioethers are mainly derived from the reaction of electrophilic chemicals with the tripeptide glutathione. After this alkylation reaction, glutathione thioethers are enzymatically degraded to yield N-acetyl-S-alkylcysteines, or mercapturic acids; these are excreted in the urine. Evaluation of carcinogen exposure from urinary mercapturic acid excretion poses several serious problems. A variable amount of mercapturic acids is derived from dietary sources. Because of the varying chemical structure of the mercapturic acids, their recovery in the purification steps of the analysis may be variable and low. The finding of urinary thioethers has to be regarded as a signal of exposure only, and the test for thioethers may be used in the follow-up of exposure in selected cases. The development of simpler methods for analyzing specific thioether compounds, at present too complicated for routine work, probably will overcome this problem in the future.

Alkylation of Hemoglobin.—This has also been used as an indicator of exposure to alkylating compounds. So far, the experience is rather limited, and the very high degree of sophistication required in the analysis limits wider application of this approach.

Alkylation of DNA.—As promising as this approach is, it is at present not yet applicable to routine biologic monitoring.

Chromosomal Damage

Most genotoxic chemicals are even clastogenic, i.e., they cause structural chromosomal aberrations that can be detected microscopically and, in addition, cause sister chromatid exchanges. There is also evidence that certain nonmutagenic carcinogens may cause chromosomal aberrations. Assay of chromosomal aberrations and sister chromatid exchange frequencies have been successfully used to indicate exposure to carcinogenic chemicals. Although, strictly speaking, these both represent effects rather than the absorbed amount of chemical, the relationship between these effects and the final carcinogenic outcome is obscure. Therefore, both chromosomal aberrations and sister chromatid exchanges at present have to be regarded as indicators of exposure rather than straightforward measures of risk. It is not yet known whether those individuals who show the highest frequencies of chromosomal aberrations or sister chromatid exchanges are at higher risk than the average. However, it is evident that groups with chromosomal damage have an increased risk of cancer development. Therefore, results from cytogenetic monitoring should not be evaluated on an individual basis, but rather on a group basis. Analysis of structural chromosomal aberrations is a very tedious task and requires highly skilled expertise. Evaluation of the morphologic changes is also, to some extent, subjective. Analysis of sister chromatid exchanges is technically less demanding and less time-consuming than that of chromosomal aberrations. However, the biologic basis of the phenomenon is less well understood, and the circumstances of cell cultivation have a remarkable effect on the frequencies of the sister chromatid exchanges detected. Therefore, at present, both chromosomal aberration and sister chromatid exchange examinations should still be regarded suitable for ad hoc studies only, not for routine monitoring programs. When they are used, a matched group of nonexposed people has to be studied concurrently.

IN VIVO MEASUREMENT OF BODY BURDEN OF CHEMICALS

Most chemicals are distributed in several different compartments in the body. For several, a tissue or organ may present considerable concentrations, i.e., a chemical is stored there. Thus, for example, lipid-soluble solvents are accumulated in body fat, cadmium in the liver and kidneys, methylmercury in the brain, and lead in the bones. Several dusts accumulate in the lungs, without in effect being distributed to the rest of the organism. Concentrations of chemicals in blood or urine do not necessarily reflect their body burden, and, recently, several approaches have been made to estimate directly the amount of the accumulated chemical at the site of accumulation. The most widely used method is neutron-activation measurement of cadmium in the liver and kidneys, but in vivo x-ray fluorescence also looks promising. In addition, use of magnetic properties in the magnetopneumographic studies for the measurement of iron-containing dusts in the lungs has developed rapidly in recent years. Reviews on these techniques have been recently published.[62, 68]

Neutron Activation

Neutron activation has been used to measure the cadmium content in the liver and kidneys, sites which show marked accumulation.[62] Portable devices for measurement have been manufactured. The sensitivity of the assay depends on the dose of radiation used. With a local skin dose of 5 mSv, levels occurring in the liver and kidneys of nonoccupationally exposed adults may be measured. Using these techniques, it has been shown that sensitive persons develop kidney damage when their kidney and liver cadmium concentrations reach approximately 215 and 30 μg/gm, respectively. It has also been shown that in nonexposed populations cigarette smoking doubles the body burden of cadmium.

X-ray Fluorescence

X-ray fluorescence has been used to measure the lead content of bones and the content of cadmium in the kidney.[62] For the determination of lead in bones, x-ray fluorescence is the only direct method available. The sensitivity of the method at present is sufficient to measure the lead concentrations in the bones of nonexposed adults. The radiation dose used is very small, and only small volumes of tissue are irradiated.

Magnetopneumography

Magnetopneumography is a technique in which iron-containing particles are magnetized, and the strength of the magnetic field thus generated—reflecting the amount of magnetic particles—is measured.[67] However, different iron-containing fumes differ greatly as to their magnetic properties, and the estimation of pulmonary dust amounts may be in error by a factor of 100. The recent introduction of a magnetic hardness sensor in the measuring device seems to have alleviated this problem at least to some extent. The problem with magnetopneumography is that it is iron, which is not the most toxic component of the fume, that is measured.

INTERPRETATION OF RESULTS

The results of biologic monitoring are evaluated by comparing them with relevant reference values. In biologic monitoring—as opposed to clinical chemistry, for example—two different sets of reference values may be discerned, those for occupationally nonexposed populations, and those for occupationally exposed populations. The former are much like clinical chemical reference values: they represent concentrations of chemicals found in normal healthy, nonexposed persons, living in circumstances otherwise comparable to those of exposed populations. It is important to note that these reference values may be markedly different in different populations, since most (toxic) chemicals are found in the environment and have access to the body, e.g., via the diet and beverages.

Reference values for the nonexposed have recently become more and more important, mostly because of increasing biologic monitoring of carcinogenic chemicals. Because no exposure to a carcinogen can be regarded as completely safe—even the smallest exposure increases the risk—it is very important to be able to assess even low levels of exposure and to discern exposed from nonexposed persons. Furthermore, reference values for trace elements in the general population given in the earlier literature are much higher than those regarded as correct now because of improvements in analytic techniques.

The reference values for occupationally exposed workers represent values regarded as acceptable under working conditions; thus, they rely on the acceptance of uptake of a certain amount of the chemical in the workplace. These reference values may be derived by two main approaches.

Health-Based Reference Values.—These are defined as levels in blood, urine, or other biologic media not giving rise to any detectable adverse toxic effects. They are based on exposure-effect and exposure-response relationships and do not consider technologic or economic feasibility.

Such values are difficult to obtain because of missing data, and only a few have been proposed. The World Health Organization (WHO) has recommended such values for lead, mercury, cadmium, a few solvents, and some pesticides. One should be aware that new toxicologic information may change our views even on these originally health-based values. For example, when the values for lead and cadmium were decided upon, their possible carcinogenicity was not known.

Administrative Standards.—These standards emerge as a joint consideration of health-based values and technologic, economic, administrative, and other nonscientific considerations. They inherently accept a certain risk, e.g., for the most sensitive segment of the population. Administrative standards usually do not exist for biologic monitoring. Lead is an exception, since several countries base their surveillance mainly on blood lead monitoring. Ideally, an administrative standard is not just a figure specifying the concentration not to be exceeded. Instead, it should also include guidelines on how, when, and how often to measure, and what should be done if the "action levels" are exceeded. Such an approach has been used in the blood-lead standard of the EEC.[91]

Most administrative biologic reference values are indirectly derived from workroom hygienic standards, such as threshold limit values. The average concentration in the biologic specimen that corresponds to an eight-hour exposure to the hygienic standard level is simply estimated. Compliance with the biologic standard may thus mean that about half of the workers have taken up more, the other half less, than the "acceptable" amount. Thus, although the biologic measurement usually more accurately reflects personal absorption, such reference values are profoundly different from the health-based values referred to above.

Reliability of Values.—The reliability of the reference values for biologic monitoring is not the same for all chemicals. Sometimes the relationship between concentrations in the biologic media are well known, sometimes not. Styrene is an example of the former case, n-hexane of the latter. Separate reference values should be worked out for chemicals in different physicochemical forms, because different chemical compounds of a single element behave completely differently in the organism. Thus, the relationships between the air and blood or urine concentrations become drastically different for different compounds (Table 13–3).

ANALYSIS OF SPECIFIC CHEMICALS

Sporadic reports on the levels of chemicals in the urine or blood of exposed people may be found for a rather large number of different chemicals. In this text, though, we deal only with those chemicals where experience has accumulated to such an extent as to allow meaningful interpretation of the results.

Metals

Aluminum

Aluminum is absorbed through both the oral and the respiratory routes, and it is mainly excreted through the kidneys. Exposure to aluminum in tungsten inert-gas welding or other processing of aluminum alloys leads to an elevation of aluminum concentration both in plasma and urine.[72, 92] The levels in serum, however, are much lower than those observed in dialysis encephalopathy. In newly hired aluminum welders, the concentration of aluminum in the urine rises rapidly and returns to control levels after a weekend

TABLE 13–3.
Relationship Between Concentrations of Nickel and Cobalt in the Air and Urine in Different Trades*†

TRADES IN WHICH COBALT IS USED	COBALT IN AIR (μG/CU M)	COBALT IN URINE (NMOLE/L)
Hard metal grinding	4.5	53–990
Porcelain factory	0.1 –1.4	10–95
Chemical factory	0.02–0.57	120–2,220
Smelter	0.1 –3.2	126–2,110
TRADES IN WHICH NICKEL IS USED	**NICKEL IN AIR (μG/CU M)**	**NICKEL IN URINE (NMOLE/L)**
Buffers/polishers	26 ± 48	70 ± 54
External grinders	1.8 ± 3.0	92 ± 41
Arc welders	6.0 ± 14.3	107 ± 70
Bench mechanics	52 ± 94	208 ± 232
Metal sprayers	2.4 ± 2.6	293 ± 167
Electroplaters	0.8 ± 0.9	179 ± 138
Nickel refinery workers	489 ± 560	3,780 ± 3,850

*Adapted from Bernacki et al.[26] and Hartung et al.[45]
†The different trades represent exposures to different forms of the metals.

rest with a half-time of eight hours. After several years of exposure, urinary aluminum concentrations are much higher and the values do not return to reference levels after a weekend.[91]

Urinary measurement of aluminum is the measurement of choice for occupational biologic monitoring. Due to the ubiquitousness of aluminum, the risk of contamination of the sample is very marked. Concentrations of aluminum in serum and urine in the nonexposed do not usually exceed 15 μg/L.[27, 72, 91, 92, 102] For occupationally exposed people, no reference limits can be set, but in tungsten inert-gas (TIG) welding of aluminum at total dust exposure levels of 5mg/cu m, the concentrations of aluminum may be increased more than tenfold[72, 91, 92] (see Chapters 45 and 65).

Arsenic

Arsenic (III) compounds have the tendency to accumulate in the organism, especially in the nails, hair, and keratinous layer of the skin. The accumulation of arsenic (V) derivatives is small. Arsenic is excreted in the feces, along with the dying skin cells, but mainly in the urine. Inorganic arsenic is methylated in the body to yield dimethylarsinic and methylarsinic acids, and in occupational exposure to trivalent arsenic, these methylated species, especially the dimethylarsinic acid, are the most abundant arsenicals excreted in the urine. The proportions of trivalent, pentavalent, and methylated arsenic species in the urine vary to some extent with the extent of exposure, and at different time points after exposure. It seems, however, that in moderate exposure, the methylation capacity of the organism is not exceeded.

An optimal method for the biologic monitoring of arsenic would be the measurement of arsenic (III), arsenic (V), methylarsinic acid, and dimethylarsinic acid in the urine separately. However, these analytic methods are time-consuming and rather complicated. Because, at present, even the kinetics of these different species are not very well known, it seems that measuring the sum of these would be the most practical and acceptable way, although the accuracy of the method is not 100%.[94, 100] Urinary total arsenic content—as measured after mineralization—cannot be used, since fish and shellfish contain very large amounts of organically bound arsenic, which are rapidly absorbed from the gastrointestinal tract, and excreted in the urine.

The concentration of arsenic in the urine in the nonexposed population depends on the content of arsenic in the drinking water, and reference values for the nonexposed thus have to be worked out separately for different geographic locations; the few published data indicate an approximate reference limit of 0.3–0.5 μmole/L (20–40 μg/L). An eight-hour exposure to an average air concentration of 50 μg As/cu m leads to urinary arsenic values of 2.2–3.0 μmole/L (150–250 μg/L) in an afternoon specimen.[28, 29, 82]

Cadmium

Cadmium is absorbed into the body through the respiratory and gastrointestinal tracts. In the blood, 70% of cadmium is in the erythrocytes. Cadmium strongly accumulates in the body, especially in the kidneys and the liver.

The excretion of cadmium from the body is very slow. The main excretion route is through the kidneys, but some excretion occurs also through the bile, saliva, hair, and nails.

For effective biologic monitoring of cadmium uptake, both the blood and urinary cadmium levels should be determined. However, depending on the body burden, and especially the kidney burden of cadmium, the interpretation of the results differs. Cadmium in blood reflects the exposure over some preceding months. At low levels of exposure, however, blood cadmium seems to reflect the body burden.[8, 44]

Before the cadmium-binding capacity of the kidney has been passed, urinary levels of cadmium mainly reflect the body burden. When the cadmium-binding capacity of the kidney is reached, the urinary excretion of cadmium increases dramatically. Simultaneously, signs of kidney damage (proteinuria, aminoaciduria, glucosuria) usually start to develop. At this stage, the urinary cadmium content is affected both by recent exposure and the body burden of cadmium.

Determination of urinary peptides like β_2-microglobulin, lysozyme, and retinol-binding globulin have been used to assess the effects of cadmium on the kidney. Of these, lysozyme or retinol kidney protein are preferable, because they are stable in urine.[48] However, only β_2-microglobulin analysis is at present widely available. As discussed earlier, these measurements, however, are not biologic monitoring in the strict sense—they indicate irreversible adverse effects—but are a part of health surveillance.

In nonsmokers, urinary cadmium is usually less than 15 nmole/L (1.5 μg/L), and cadmium in blood is less than 10 nmole/L (1 μg/L). Smokers may have blood cadmium levels up to 50 nmole/L, and urinary cadmium levels up to 10 nmole/L. The liver or kidneys of old cattle, horses, or deer may form an important source of cadmium.[56, 99]

The World Health Organization has recommended 5 μg/g creatinine (≃45 nmole/L) as a health-based limit for exposed workers.[11]

Deutsche Forschungsgemeinschaft[6] has issued administrative standards: 1.5 μg Cd/100 ml of blood and 15 μg/L of urine. The values suggested by Lauwerys[8] for cadmium in blood, 10 μg/L and in urine 10 μg/gm creatinine, fall between the WHO and German suggestions.

When the kidney cortex cadmium is increased close to the critical level, urinary cadmium is in the range of 50–100 nmole/L.

Chromium

Absorption, distribution, and excretion of chromium compounds vary markedly, primarily depending on the water-solubility of the compound and on the physical characteristics of the fume/dust. Certain chromates are rapidly absorbed and excreted. In contrast to the general belief, even some trivalent chromium compounds are absorbed rapidly.

Studies on biologic monitoring of chromium exposure in manual metal-arc welding have given quite uniform results: an eight-hour time-weighted average (TWA) exposure to 50 μg chromium/cu m results in urinary concentrations of chromium of 30 μg/gm creatinine (≃ 1 μmole/L) in an afternoon specimen. The first half-time of chromium in the urine is 10–40 hours; thus, values found on the next morning are somewhat lower. Chromium shows an accumulation in the body during the working week. In shielded gas welding, on the other hand, very little chromium is excreted in the welder's urine, and at present, welders of stainless steel using solely shielded-gas techniques may not be reliably monitored biologically. When the welder uses both metal-arc and shielded-gas welding techniques, urinary chromium values reflect mostly exposure in the arc welding. In arc gouging and flame cutting of stainless steel, urinary chromium values seem to reflect mainly the body burden of chromium.[15]

In chrome plating—where the exposing agent is chromic acid mist—levels of urinary chromium smaller than 100 nmole/L indicate time-weighted eight-hour exposures lower than 2 μg/cu m.[66] Urinary chromium values in the nonexposed seem to be below 10 nmole/L (0.5 μg/L).[19, 60]

Cobalt

Metallic cobalt and cobalt salts are readily absorbed from the lungs. Cobalt is concentrated in the liver and is excreted both in the urine and feces. Concentration of cobalt in urine is markedly increased in exposure to metallic cobalt and cobalt salts in different trades. Most of the cobalt is excreted rapidly, within 24 hours of the exposure. The relationship between cobalt concentrations and the risk of allergy, or chronic lung function impairment, is not known. Marked interindividual differences are seen in the relationship between air and urinary concentrations of cobalt; at present, no reliable quantitative estimation of exposure may be made from the urinary cobalt values.[45] The urinary concentrations of cobalt in the nonexposed are usually below 100 nmole/L (5 μg/L).[45, 71]

Lead

The main route of lead absorption in occupational settings is through the respiratory tract. Almost one half of the lead reaching the lower respiratory tract is absorbed. To a lesser extent, lead is also absorbed through the gastrointestinal tract. More than 90% of lead in the blood is in the red blood cells. Lead accumulates in bone, where about 90% of body lead is found. The half-time of lead in blood is 35–40 days; in bone around 20 years.[110]

Lead is mainly excreted through the kidneys (75%). Other routes include bile, sweat, and the keratinized tissues.

By far the best parameter to use in the biologic monitoring of lead is its concentration in blood. In a steady state, it reflects the concentration of lead in the rapidly exchanging soft-tissue pool.[49]

The concentration of lead in urine is variable and does not reflect the amount of lead in the body. On the other hand, urinary excretion of lead after administration of chelating agents has been suggested as an indicator of the mobilizable pool of lead in the body.[110] However, this method is not suitable for routine monitoring purposes.

Many parameters of heme synthesis have been measured as *lead effect*. These include red blood cell zinc protoporphyrin, urinary 5-aminolevulinate excretion, and the activity of 5-aminolevulinate dehydratase in red blood cells. For occupational biologic monitoring, erythrocyte protoporphyrin seems best; the erythrocyte 5-aminolevulinate dehydratase is too sensitive, and its instability upon storage also hampers its use. Urinary excretion of 5-aminolevulinate is less sensitive than the erythrocyte protoporphyrin and its accurate analysis is tedious. Measurement of the effects in the biologic monitoring of lead has two major drawbacks: it is by no means clear that the persons that show disturbances in the porphyrin metabolism are at greatest risk of the toxic lead effects, i.e., impairment of nervous system functions. Second, lead effects on porphyrin metabolism are not specific: diseases such as iron-deficiency anemia may simulate the effects of lead.

Now that reliable blood lead analyses are generally available, it seems that the primary approach in the biologic monitoring of lead is the measurement of blood lead; the monitoring of any of the effects adds little.

Lead in water and food markedly affect the level of lead in blood. Airborne lead from car engine exhausts, for example, may also elevate blood lead values. It is thus understandable that the levels found in occupationally nonexposed persons vary considerably in different countries.[99]

The World Health Organization has pondered the exposure-effect and exposure-response relationships of lead and has come to the conclusion that a health-based upper reference limit for men is 1.9 μmole/L (40 μg/100 ml), and for women of child-bearing age, 1.4 μmole/L (30 μg/100 ml).[11]

Manganese

Manganese is absorbed into the body both through the respiratory and gastrointestinal tracts. Manganese has an active absorption mechanism in the gut. Most of manganese in blood is in the erythrocytes. Manganese is mostly excreted in the feces; approximately 1% is excreted in urine. The half-time of manganese in the body seems to be in the range of 20–40 days.[114]

Manganese exposure in mild-steel welding seems to lead to an increased level of manganese in blood and urine. There is, however, a marked overlap in the values for the exposed and nonexposed people.[11, 23, 30, 114] In some (but not all) welders, the urinary manganese concentration showed a correlation with the ambient air manganese concentrations.[55]

The concentrations of manganese in the blood, serum, and urine of the nonexposed do not notably exceed 350, 20, and 50 nmole/L (20, 1, 3 μg/L), respectively.[8, 102]

At present it is not possible to set even tentative reference values for exposed persons.

Mercury

Metallic mercury evaporates at room temperature and is efficiently absorbed through the respiratory tract. Mercury vapor is oxidized in the body into mercury (II) ions, which bind to proteins. Mercury accumulates in the kidneys, liver, spleen, and bones. Metallic mercury is lipid-soluble and is transported through membranes without hindrance. Mercury is excreted slowly, mainly in the feces and urine. The half-time of mercury in the blood is approximately 70 days; there exists, however, a group of people with a slower clearance of mercury, with an approximate half-time of 120 days.

Exposure to mercury may be monitored from concentrations of mercury in the blood or urine. In equilibrium, the concentration of mercury in the blood reflects daily intake. Blood mercury is probably the single best indicator of mercury exposure. However, when blood mercury is quantified using the traditional analytic methods, even methylmercury will be measured. The amount of total mercury in the blood varies greatly in different populations, and it may be very high in fish-eating people, up to 200 nmole/L (40 μg/L), while it is generally below 50 nmole/L (10 μg/L) in non-fish eaters. Thus, if the concentration of mercury is high in the blood, a fractionating analysis, giving separate values for mercury salts and alkylmercuric compounds, should be performed. Various authors seem to be unanimous that approximately 125 nmole/L of inorganic mercury in the blood could be used as a reference value for the exposed.[8, 11]

Alkylmercury is not excreted in the urine; thus, measuring urinary mercury concentrations gives estimations not biased by simultaneous exposure to methylmercury. However, urinary mercury concentrations show marked diurnal variation, which cannot be fully compensated for by correcting to a common relative density or creatinine excretion. The urinary concentrations of mercury are highest early in the morning; the time of specimen collection for urinary mercury determinations should be standardized, preferably in the morning. Concentration of mercury in the urine of nonexposed is generally below 50 nmole/L (10 μg/L). The World Health Organization gives 50 μg/g creatinine, which is approximately 250 nmole/L, as the reference limit for the occupationally exposed.[11] Impairment of psychomotor performance has been reported in workers with urinary mercury values between 250 and 500 nmole/L.[85]

Nickel

Different nickel species differ remarkably in their kinetics in the body. Metallic nickel oxide and nonsoluble salts are only very slowly (within tens of years) cleared from the mucous membranes of the respiratory tract. Soluble nickel salts are rapidly cleared and are excreted in the urine.

Concentrations of nickel in the urine and plasma are elevated in workers exposed to a variety of nickel species in many different trades. Both urine and plasma—and even whole blood—analyses of nickel may be used in biologic monitoring. However, as the concentrations of nickel are generally much higher in the urine, this is to be preferred, although the risk of contamination during the sample collection may be more marked. Best defined is biologic monitoring of nickel exposure in electroplating, where only exposure to water-soluble nickel salts takes place. In these circumstances, an eight-hour TWA exposure to 100 μg nickel/cu m resulted in urinary nickel concentrations of 1.3 μmole/L after the exposure, and 1.0 μmole/L the next morning. The experience is similar in electrolytic nickel refining. In most trades, though, the exposure is more complex and may be mostly confined to slightly soluble nickel compounds. Then, urinary nickel concentrations are indicative of considerably higher exposures.[13]

In general, biologic monitoring of nickel may only give information on exposure, not on the risk of disease. However, in exposure to nickel carbonyl, it has been suggested that urinary nickel concentrations in excess of 8.5 μmole/L indicate severe poisoning and those between 1.7 and 8.5 μmole/L indicate a moderately severe case, whereas only mild symptoms are to be expected if the urinary nickel concentration during the first eight hours after the exposure remain below 1.5 μmole/L.[95]

At present there is general agreement on the values of nickel in the urine in nonexposed persons; average values reported from different parts of the world are generally 30–80 nmole/L (2–5 μg/L).[96]

Vanadium

Vanadium compounds are absorbed readily from the lungs; the absorption from the gastrointestinal tract is low. Vanadium accumulates in bones, liver, and kidneys. It is excreted slowly—with a half-time of several days—mainly in the urine.

Urinary concentrations of vanadium are high in vanadium-exposed workers. However, no data are available on the relationship between air and urinary vanadium concentrations. It is probable that this relationship is different in exposures to different vanadium compounds. Several recent studies have shown that the vanadium content in the urine of nonexposed persons is below 50 nmole/L (2.5 μg/L).[8]

Other Inorganic Compounds

Carbon Disulfide

Carbon disulfide (CS_2) may be absorbed into the body both through the respiratory tract and intact skin. There seems to be a great individual variation in the absorption of carbon disulfide through the lungs. At equilibrium, around 40%–50% of carbon disulfide is retained.[8, 111] Of the carbon disulfide in the body, 10%–30% is exhaled and 70%–90% is metabolized. Carbon disulfide carbon is exhaled in the form of carbon dioxide. Of the metabolites, 2-thiothiazolidine-4-carboxylic acid (TTCA) is excreted in the urine.[36, 87, 88]

Several measurements—carbon disulfide in the blood, thioethers in the urine, and iodide-azide positive derivatives in the urine—have been suggested as methods of biologic monitoring of carbon disulfide.[8, 111] Of these, the only promising one seems to be the determination of TTCA in the urine.[36, 87, 88] Blood carbon disulfide does not show any clear relationship to the daily exposure, and the urinary iodide-azide test is not sensitive enough at exposure levels below 100 mg/cu m. The level of TTCA in the urine increases during the working day even at carbon disulfide levels of 30–50 mg/cu m, and TTCA in a postshift urine specimen shows a relatively good correlation with the ambient air carbon disulfide concentration in personal samples.[88]

Carbon Monoxide

Carbon monoxide is easily taken up from the alveolar air. It is bound to hemoglobin with an affinity of about 240 times that of oxygen. Carbon monoxide in arterial blood declines biphasically after exposure. The first phase probably results from distribution in tissues, plus elimination through the lungs. The slower phase reflects the liberation of carbon monoxide from the tissues. The half-time of the slow phase of carbon monoxide elimination in sedentary men seems to be around four to five hours. Women seem to excrete it 30% faster than men.[61, 112]

Carbon monoxide exposure may be estimated from measurements of the blood carboxyhemoglobin mass ratio or the blood or alveolar air carbon monoxide concentrations. Of these, the determination of the carboxyhemoglobin mass ratio has been the most widely applied.

Due to the short half-time of carbon monoxide in blood, the time of specimen collection is very important. It would be best to collect the specimen immediately after exposure.

In nonexposed nonsmokers, the carboxyhemoglobin mass ratio is less than 0.015. In smokers, it is usually 0.03–0.08, but in chain-smokers, it may reach 0.15, and in cigar smokers, 0.20.

At levels in excess of 0.05, electrocardiographic and myocardial metabolism changes have been reported in patients with coronary heart disease. This corresponds to an eight-hour exposure to a carbon monoxide level around 30–40 ppm.

Fluorides

Fluorides are taken up through the respiratory and gastrointestinal tracts. Hydrogen fluoride may also penetrate the skin. Around 75% of fluoride in the blood is in plasma. The half-time of fluoride in plasma is four to nine hours. Most of the fluoride in the body is in the bone tissue.

The main excretion route of fluoride is in the urine. Some fluoride may be excreted in sweat. Fecal excretion amounts to 5%–10% of the daily intake.

Concentrations of fluorides in the urine of the nonexposed depend on the amounts of fluorides in the diet and beverages, which may vary markedly in different geographic locations. In Scandinavia, they seem to be 20–50 μmole/L (1.0–2.5 μg/L).[51] All laboratories should assess the local population for the reference ranges.

In arc welders of mild steel, an eight-hour time-weighted average exposure to 2.5 mg/cu m fluoride causes about 200 μmole/L (10 mg/L) concentrations of fluoride in postshift urine specimens.[90] In exposure to water-soluble fluorides only, a postshift level of fluoride in the urine of 500 μmole/L seems to correspond to 2 mg/cu m of fluorides in the air.[33, 51] The National Academy of Sciences[74] suggests 210 μmole/L as a health-based limit for urinary fluoride values; NIOSH[75] and the German Scientific Committee[6] suggest postshift urinary fluoride values of 7 mg/L (370 μmole/L) and 7 mg/gm creatinine, respectively.

Organic Chemicals

Aromatic Hydrocarbons

Benzene.—Benzene is effectively absorbed through the lungs. The retention after inhalation, at rest, is around 50%. Benzene also penetrates the skin. Benzene accumulates in tissues with high lipid content, and the half-time of benzene in those tissues is about 24 hours.[8, 24, 25]

Benzene is metabolized by the monooxygenase system to yield benzene oxide. This is further converted to phenol (the main metabolite, about 70% of the amount absorbed) or to dihydrodiol. The latter is further rearranged to cathecol. Also, hydroquinone and hydroxyhydroquinone are metabolites of benzene. Around 25%–50% of benzene is excreted in exhaled air. The shortest half-time of benzene is a few hours.[24]

Measurement of urinary excretion of phenol is the traditional method of biologic monitoring of benzene uptake. Only methods specific of phenol (e.g., gas or liquid chromatography) should be used. Phenol may be formed or taken into the body from sources other than inhaled benzene, such as cosmetics, drugs, or phenol. Therefore, on a time-weighted average exposure level of less than 5 ppm in eight hours, the urinary excretion of phenol correlates poorly with the air measurements. A better estimation of exposure may be obtained if values before and after the exposure are compared. Alveolar air measurements have long been used in the assessment of benzene exposure but have not found extensive use. Blood benzene concentrations might also serve as an alternative. However, the published methods lack sensitivity at exposure levels of a few parts per million of TWA exposure.

Concentrations of phenol in the urine are variable. An approximate upper reference limit for the nonexposed is 150 μmole/L. Time-weighted average exposure to 5 ppm benzene elevates the urinary phenol concentration (after-shift minus before-shift values) by approximately 200 μmole/L (20 mg/L).[8]

Toluene.—Toluene is readily taken up in the lungs (retention about 50%) and penetration through the skin may occur after prolonged contact with liquid toluene. About 80% of absorbed toluene is biotransformed to hippuric acid, which is excreted in the urine.

Cresol isomers are minor metabolites (about 1%) and traces of unchanged toluene may also be found in the urine. The rest is excreted, unchanged, in exhaled air.

The traditional method of estimating the uptake of toluene is an analysis of hippuric acid in urine. Exposure to the mean concentration of about 100 ppm of toluene is associated with 17–28 mmole/L of hippuric acid in spot urine samples voided at the end of the workday. In a nonexposed population, urinary concentrations of hippuric acid are usually in the order of 6 mmole/L; benzoates in the diet may increase this level two- to fourfold. (See Chapters 47 and 63, describing benzoic acid and related compounds.) Therefore, no firm conclusions about toluene exposure can be made from urinary hippuric acid, especially if the exposure is slight. Conflicting results have been published on how well urinary levels of o-cresol reflect toluene uptake,[20, 21, 81] but this method needs further validation.

Toluene uptake can also be assessed from toluene analysis of the blood. Blood samples taken during exposure can be used to roughly estimate the short-term uptake. Exposure to about 100 ppm of toluene at light or moderate workloads is associated with blood toluene levels in the range of 15–20 μmole/L.[21, 97] The Deutsche Forschungsgemeinschaft Biologische Arbeitsstofftoleranzwerte (BAT) value (which corresponds to an exposure of 200 ppm) is 37 μmole/L. On the other hand, a sample taken 16 hours after exposure, preferably before the onset of a new exposure on the last workday of the week, lends itself to an estimation of the toluene stored in the body. Exposure to TWA environmental toluene concentrations of 100 ppm correspond to about 2.0–2.3 μmol/L of toluene in a morning blood sample.[21, 58]

Ingestion of alcohol decreases the clearance of toluene and raises blood levels;[107] skin penetration involving the hands leads to misleadingly high local concentrations in the venous blood.[17] These factors are less likely to cause confusion in morning blood samples.

Xylene.—Xylene (isomers) are effectively absorbed through the lungs (retention about 60%–64%). Penetration of xylene through the skin is probably significant only after prolonged contact with liquid xylene. About 95% of absorbed xylene isomers are metabolized to corresponding methylhippuric acids (toluric acids) and about 1%–2% to xylenols (dimethylphenols). Less than 5% is eliminated unchanged in exhaled air. Xylene and methylhippuric acid are eliminated rapidly, with a half-time of about one hour during the first hours after exposure. Elimination from the storage sites (body fat) takes place more slowly, with a terminal half-time of about 2.5 days.

Uptake of xylenes can be estimated by analyzing urinary methylhippuric acids, which are specific metabolites. Urinary excretion of methylhippuric acid in a sample taken during, or at the close of, exposure indicates xylene uptake over a few preceding hours. At the end of a normal working day at exposure to about 100 ppm of xylene, urinary concentration of methylhippuric acid is about 12 mmole/L, varying between 8 and 15 mmole/L, depending mainly on the physical workload. One should note that technical xylene contains at least 15%–20% ethylbenzene. Alcohol interferes with xylene metabolism and thus leads to reduced formation of methylhippuric acid.[83]

Ethylbenzene.—Ethylbenzene is efficiently taken up in the lungs and significant penetration through the skin may occur after contact with liquid ethylbenzene. Ethylbenzene is primarily metabolized to mandelic (55%–65%) and phenylglyoxylic acids (20%–30%); several minor metabolites are also generated.[22, 40, 43] The initial elimination half-time of mandelic acid is three to four hours. Later, when ethylbenzene is slowly released from fat, the half-time is about 24 hours or longer. Only a few percent of unchanged ethylbenzene is excreted unchanged in exhaled air.

Uptake of ethylbenzene can be estimated from the urinary excretion of mandelic acid (see also Styrene, in this chapter). Mandelic acid in a urine sample taken at the end of a workday reflects the amount of ethylbenzene absorbed during the few preceding hours; 13 mmole/L of mandelic acid in urine roughly corresponds to an inhalation exposure at about 100 ppm of ethylbenzene in light work. Only negligible amounts of mandelic acid are detected in the urine of the nonexposed, provided that specific analytic methods (e.g., gas chromatography) are used. Simultaneous exposure to ethylbenzene and m-xylene results in inhibited metabolism of both compounds, and lowered amounts of urinary metabolites are observed.[3]

Styrene.—The uptake of styrene through the lungs is efficient (retention about 64%) and limited only by pulmonary ventilation. Noteworthy absorption through the skin occurs after contact with liquid styrene. Styrene is biotransformed almost exclusively to mandelic acid and phenylglyoxylic acids; these are excreted in the urine. Small amounts of vinyl phenol and phenyl ethanol are also formed. About 3% of absorbed styrene is exhaled, unchanged. The initial elimination half-time of mandelic acid is about four hours and that of phenylglyoxylic acid somewhat longer. Consequently, the ratio of these two metabolites is about 3:1 at the end of the workday and about 1:1 the next morning. From the next day onwards, metabolite excretion will be slower and governed by the slow release of styrene from adipose tissue.

Several methods may be used for the monitoring of styrene uptake. Since there is a wealth of information showing that a reliable assessment can be made on the basis of mandelic acid in the urine, other alternatives such as a supplementary analysis of phenylglyoxylic acid in the urine or analysis of styrene in the blood will not be dealt with here.

There is a fair correlation between styrene concentration in air and mandelic acid in urine. For practical reasons, spot urine samples voided at the end of a workday towards the end of the working week can be recommended. A person performing light work while exposed to levels of 50 ppm of styrene will have approximately 7 mmole/L of mandelic acid in an end-of-shift urine sample. In a specific analysis, for instance, gas chromatography, the urinary level of mandelic acid is negligible in the nonexposed; however, certain drugs may be metabolized to mandelic acid. Ingestion of alcohol inhibits the metabolism of styrene and thus renders the measurement of mandelic acid invalid.[108]

Halogenated Hydrocarbons

Dichloromethane (Methylene Chloride).—Pulmonary retention of dichloromethane is initially about 50%, but with time, and particularly with higher absorption rates, it decreases down to about 30%.[118] Skin absorption of dichloromethane may be more effective than for most organic solvents. At low rates of uptake, almost all dichloromethane is metabolized to carbon monoxide (30%–40% of the absorbed amount) and carbon dioxide, only some 5% is exhaled unchanged. At higher absorption rates, the metabolized fraction decreases due to saturation of the metabolism. Thus, exposure to 100 ppm of dichloromethane for more than 7.5 hours at rest resulted in a mass ratio of carboxyhemoglobin (COHb) of about 3.4%–5.7%; exposure to 200–250 ppm, 6.8%–9.6%;[34] but exposure to 500 ppm, only 11.4%.[93] Elimination of dichloromethane from the blood is rapid (half-time: one to two hours) during the first hours, but becomes slower later. Blood carboxyhemoglobin concentration reaches peak value at about the end of a workday's exposure and its decline exhibits an apparent half-time of eight to ten hours. This is a two-times slower rate than the disappearance of COHb after exposure to carbon monoxide and indicates the relatively slow release of dichloromethane from tissue metabolism.

Assessment of exposure to dichloromethane has been tried by measuring the parent compound in blood and the expired air and by an analysis of the carbon monoxide formed in the body (usually measured as carboxyhemoglobin in the blood). As carbon monoxide is probably of primary importance in the toxicity of dichloromethane, the latter seems preferable. However, this method of monitoring is confounded by carbon monoxide from other sources, notably smoking. Uptake of carbon monoxide from smoking has an additive effect on the COHb concentration.[35] Levels of COHb of 5% have been shown to impair the cardiac function at least in persons with coronary heart disease. Exposure to 100 ppm of dichloromethane raises the COHb mass ratio to about 5%–6% by the end of the workday. Since smoking may readily raise the COHb level to 5%, abstinence from smoking for about ten hours is required in order to obtain reliable results concerning dichloromethane exposure.

1,1,1-Trichloroethane (Methyl Chloroform).—1,1,1-Trichloroethane has a limited solubility in blood and tissues and a moderate solubility in fat, and its metabolism is slow. Consequently, its retention in the lungs is less (about 18%–25%) than that of most solvents and declines during the workday. Absorption through the skin from the liquid phase may occur to a limited extent. A small fraction of trichloroethane is metabolized to trichloroethanol and trichloroacetic acid, and about 90% is excreted unchanged in exhaled air. Elimination of 1,1,1-trichloroethane in the blood is at first rapid (elimination half-time less than one hour) but later mobilization from fat-rich tissues is relatively slow, and an elimination half-time of 53 hours has been observed.[76]

The best approach for the biologic monitoring of 1,1,1-trichloroethane is the measurement of its concentrations in the blood, preferably on the morning before new exposure, towards the end of the workweek. In such a sample 2 μmole/L of 1,1,1-trichloroethane corresponds to a continuous exposure to about 100 ppm. Deutsche Forschungsgemeinschaft gives a BAT value of 4.1 μmole/L, which corresponds to an exposure at 200 ppm.[6]

Trichloroethylene.—Trichloroethylene is effectively taken up through the lungs; a significant penetration of liquid trichloroethylene may also occur through the skin. About 70%–80% of absorbed trichloroethylene is biotransformed to trichloroethanol and trichloroacetic acid, and about 10% is exhaled unchanged. Elimination of trichloroethylene follows the usual pattern of lipid-soluble solvents: a rapid initial phase followed by one or two slower phases. Trichloroethanol is conjugated with glucuronic acid and eliminated in urine with a half-time of about 10–15 hours. The corresponding half-time for trichloroacetic acid is as long as 70–100 hours, mainly due to its extensive protein binding. Interestingly, women appear to excrete proportionally more trichloroacetic acid and less trichloroethanol than men in the context of identical exposures.

Several methods have been proposed for the assessment of trichloroethylene uptake. The most widely applied method is an estimation of urinary trichloroacetic acid alone or in combination with trichloroethanol. Due to differences in elimination kinetics, these two metabolites have a different relationship to a preceding exposure. Because excretion of trichloroacetic acid is delayed, there will be a clear increase over the workweek and a slow decline over the weekend. A urine sample taken at the end of a shift towards the end of the week will reflect the uptake over several preceding days.

Trichloroethanol excretion, on the other hand, peaks shortly after the end of daily exposure, and it will thus indicate the uptake over the same day. In an end-of-shift and end-of-work week sample from a worker exposed to about 50 ppm of trichloroethylene, the trichloroacetic acid concentration in urine is in the range of 460–760 μmole/L, and the sum of trichloroacetic acid plus total trichloroethanol is 1,300–2,100 μmole/L. The American Conference of Government Industrial Hygienists (ACGIH) biologic exposure index (BEI) value for trichloroacetic acid is 610 μmole/L, and for the sum of trichloroacetic acid and trichloroethanol, 1,900 μmole/L.[3] The World Health Organization has recommended 306 μmole/L of trichloroacetic acid in postshift urine as an occupational exposure limit on the grounds that, according to their assessment, most studies indicated adverse health effects when this value was exceeded.[115] There appears to be a large interindividual variation in the urinary excretion of metabolites, trichloroacetic acid in particular, whereas the variability is much smaller for blood trichloroethanol. Estimation of trichloroethanol in the blood at the end of shift towards the end of the workweek has been recommended by Deutsche Forschungsgemeinschaft (DFG) and ACGIH. The DFG BAT value is 33.5 μmole/L and the ACGIH BEI value 26.8 μmole/L, both corresponding to trichloroethylene exposure at 50 ppm.[3, 6]

Trichloroethanol and trichloroacetic acid are not specific metabolites of trichloroethylene. Other halogenated solvents are not, however, important confounders, because they yield only small amounts of these metabolites. In contrast, the occasional use of chloral hydrate (Neochloral) as a hypnotic drug needs to be taken into account. Ingestion of alcohol inhibits trichloroethylene metabolism, with a rise of the blood trichloroethylene concentration and a reduced urinary excretion of trichloroethanol and trichloroacetic acid as a consequence.

Tetrachloroethylene (Perchloroethylene).—Tetrachloroethylene is readily taken up in the lungs (retention is about 50%), and the liquid may also be absorbed significantly through the skin. About 95% of tetrachloroethylene is excreted unchanged in exhaled air. Only 2% has been recovered in the urine as trichloroacetic acid. The formation of trichloroacetic acid shows signs of saturation when the exposure level exceeds 50–100 ppm.[77] Elimination of tetrachloroethylene is rapid initially, but the terminal half-time is relatively long, about 70 hours. The slow elimination leads to a marked accumulation of tetrachloroethylene (in adipose tissue) during repeated exposures.

Assessment of exposure to tetrachloroethylene can be made by analyzing the compound in the exhaled air or in the blood. Analyzing urinary trichloroacetic acid has also been proposed for monitoring purposes, but at low levels of tetrachloroethylene exposure (of the order 20 ppm), its concentration is very low, even undetectable,[64] and at high exposures it is no more proportional to tetrachloroethylene uptake. Determination of tetrachloroethylene in the blood appears to be the best method for practical application. Continuous exposure to 50 ppm of tetrachloroethylene leads to about 6 μmole/L of tetrachloroethylene in a blood sample taken 16 hours after the workshift towards the end of the week.[64]

Polychlorinated Biphenyls (PCBs).—Polychlorinated biphenyl compounds are well absorbed through inhalation and ingestion and, to a minor extent, through the skin. They are carried in blood associated with serum lipids. Highly chlorinated PCB compounds have a tendency to accumulate in body fat tissue and the liver. Less chlorinated PCB compounds are also subject to biotransformation, which may comprise dechlorination, oxidation, and conjugation phases.

Due to the different behavior of various PCB compounds, the ratios of different PCB in fat and serum, as well as their half-times, vary.[89]

Measurement of the concentrations of PCB in blood has been used in biologic monitoring. The measurement strategy and the specimen used greatly depend on the type of exposure. For continuous exposures, such as occur in capacitor or transformer production, infrequent, routine monitoring may be used.[109] In capacitor accidents, there may be a need for frequent measurements just after the accident. When a simultaneous exposure to dibenzofurans or dioxins has occurred or seems probable, their determination would be preferable, even though analytic and economic considerations limit such measurements to a minimum. Because of the binding of PCBs to serum lipids, blood specimens should be collected after an overnight fast. In a nonexposed Finnish population, we found that serum concentrations of PCBs with 2, 3, 4, or 5 chlorine atoms did not exceed 3 μg/L.[69] Currently it does not seem possible to establish reference limits for exposed populations.

n-Hexane

Hexane shows a very limited solubility in blood, but is readily soluble in fat. Only 15%–20% of n-hexane is taken up through the lungs. Around 10% of absorbed n-hexane is exhaled, the rest is oxidated through the monooxygenase system to 2-hexanol, 2,5-

hexanol, γ-valerolactone and 2,5-hexanedione. With continuous exposure, hexane accumulates in the fat during the workweek.

Blood or alveolar air n-hexane and urinary metabolites all may be used in biologic monitoring.[79, 106] The urinary 2,5-hexanedione seems to be most applicable for routine biologic monitoring. Because of fat accumulation, a 2,5-hexanedione concentration in the urine increases for three to four hours after exposure; thereafter it decreases with a half-time of about 15 hours. The correlation of postshift urinary hexanedione concentration with the TWA exposure is reasonably good. An eight-hour exposure to 50 ppm has in different studies resulted in about 2–6 mg/L (20–50 μmol/L) of 2,5-hexanedione in postshift urine. The highest figures have been reported toward the end of the workweek.[53, 73, 79, 80]

Phenol

Phenol is readily absorbed through the skin, respiratory tract and gastrointestinal tract. Serious intoxications are generally due to skin absorption from splashes of liquid phenol. Phenol is conjugated with glucuronic acid and sulphuric acid; the conjugates are rapidly excreted in the urine.

Urinary concentration of phenol—as measured with a specific (gas or liquid chromatographic) method—reflects exposure during the preceding 24 hours. Exposure for eight hours to 5 ppm (19 mg/cu m) of phenol leads to an approximate 3,200 μmole/L (300 mg/L) urinary concentration of phenol. Extensive skin absorption makes biologic monitoring important as a means of exposure estimation. In the non-exposed, concentrations of phenol in the urine usually do not exceed 150 μmole/L.

However, drugs containing phenol or chemicals that are changed into phenol (such as certain antiseptic gargles) may lead to elevated urinary phenol concentrations.[8]

Chlorophenols

Chlorophenols are absorbed through the respiratory tract and the skin. Long-time, intensive skin exposure may lead to serious, acute intoxications. The chlorophenols differ in their rates of excretion: 2,4,6,-trichlorophenol (the most abundant of the trichlorophenols) has a half-time of 18 hours; that of 2,3,4,6-tetrachlorophenol, 5 days; and of pentachlorophenol, 16 days.[78]

Exposure to chlorophenols may be monitored from their urinary concentrations. Because of efficient skin absorption, biologic monitoring is probably superior to measurement of air concentrations. The proportions of different chlorophenols vary in different chlorophenol preparations and even in different lots of the same preparation. It is therefore best to analyse both tri-, tetra-, and pentachlorophenols.

The concentration of chlorophenols (sum of tri-, tetra-, and pentachlorophenol) is less than 0.5 μmole/L in the non-exposed. Recommendations for the exposed vary between 4 and 12 μmole/L.[4, 8]

Cyanides and Nitriles

Cyanides and hydrogen cyanide are readily absorbed by the gastrointestinal tract, lungs, and skin. Cyanides are detoxified to thiocyanates, which are excreted in the urine. Acrylonitrile, acetonitrile, and other nitriles are also, to a varying degree, metabolized to thiocyanates.

Exposure to cyanides may, in principle, be monitored from blood concentrations of cyanide or from urinary or plasma/blood concentrations of thiocyanates. Because of the short half-time, analytic problems, low concentrations, and instability upon storage, cyanide determinations are seldom used. Thiocyanate determinations are plagued by marked variations in the nonexposed: cabbage and other leafy vegetables contain large amounts of thiocyanate-producing chemicals; even dairy products and beer may contain thiocyanate-producing chemicals. The most remarkable source of variation in the thiocyanate concentrations, however, is smoking. The concentrations of thiocyanates in the plasma, and also in the urine, are on an average approximately 50 μmole/L in nonsmokers, with an upper limit of approximately 70–85 μmole/L, but may reach 250 μmole/L in smokers.[8, 53, 104, 105] Variation in the thiocyanate concentrations between individuals is much more marked than within the same individual over time; thus the difference in the thiocyanate concentrations on Monday morning and on Friday afternoon is the most reliable measure of cyanide uptake.

There has been only one study on the relationship between air cyanide concentrations and urinary thiocyanate excretion;[39] thus, no reliable quantitative estimations of uptake can be made at present.

In exposure to acrylonitrile, concentrations of thiocyanate in the urine were elevated in a group with an average exposure of 4.2 ppm but not in a group with an exposure of 0.5 ppm. On the other hand, concentration of acrylonitrile itself in the urine was elevated even at an exposure to 0.1 ppm. Concentrations of acrylonitrile in the air and urine also showed, on a group basis, a correlation with each other.[8] Thus, it seems that, because of the unspecificity of the thiocyanate assays, the better approach in the biologic monitoring would be analyses of the parent nitrile itself, instead of thiocyanates.

Dimethylformamide

Dimethylformamide (DMF) is absorbed both through the skin and by inhalation. It is extensively metabolized through demethylation and oxidation to formaldehyde and formic acid. Monomethylformamide is the main metabolite. The biologic half-time of dimethylformamide is around one hour.

For biologic monitoring of DMF uptake, n-methylformamide has been measured both in the blood and in the urine. Experimental human exposures suggest that monomethylformamide is rapidly excreted in the urine and its urinary half-time is around 12 hours. There is, however, a discrepancy between the published studies on the use of monomethyl formamide measurements in urine for biologic monitoring.[8, 59, 65, 117] Lauwerys suggests that monomethylformamide concentrations of less than 50 mg/g creatinine in postshift urine specimens proved safe with respect to the effects of both acute and long-term exposure of workers to DMF.[8]

4,4′-Methylenebis (2-Chloroaniline) (MOCA)

The most important route of exposure for 4,4′-methylenebis(2-chloroaniline) (MOCA) is skin absorption. Therefore, biologic monitoring is very important. In man, MOCA is excreted as such in the urine. However, in addition to this "free" MOCA, an equal amount may be excreted as an unknown conjugate that may be released by simply heating. The sum of the two, the "total" MOCA, is recommended for biologic monitoring.[41] On several occasions, urinary concentrations of MOCA in excess of 1 mg/L (3.7

moles/L) have been noted.[37, 86, 98] No reference values for urinary MOCA have been suggested, but it is evident that levels of less than 2 μg/L are rather easily attained. The Health and Safety Executive of the United Kingdom applies an "action level" for MOCA in urine of 10 μmole/mole creatinine.[7]

Pesticides

There are hundreds of chemicals on the market that are used as pesticides. It is thought that in most cases of normal handling and application of these chemicals the main route of uptake is via the skin. Thus, it is reasonable to think that biologic monitoring of exposure to pesticides should be regarded as an important activity. While there are many singular observations concerning the parent compound/metabolite concentration of active pesticide ingredients in biologic samples, only few acknowledged and validated methods are available. These relate mainly to organophosphorus compounds and organochlorines (for further information, see references 46, 63, and 70). A fair amount of experience has recently been gained on the biologic monitoring of exposure to chlorinated phenoxyacids.

Organophosphorus Compounds/Inhibition of Cholinesterases.—Many organic phosphorus esters are potent insecticides. They are readily taken up in the body by different routes, even the skin and the conjunctiva of the eyes, which, when unprotected, may receive a considerable exposure. Organophosphates are rapidly metabolized (many are at first metabolically transformed to active insecticides) and excreted.

It is possible to analyze the urinary metabolites of several organophosphorus compounds.[46, 63] The most commonly applied method of biologic monitoring is, however, based on the inhibitory effect of all organophosphates on blood cholinesterases, namely the plasma cholinesterase (butyrylcholinesterase) and the red blood cell acetylcholinesterase.[47] The acute toxicity of organophosphorus compounds is mainly due to inhibition of acetylcholinesterase in synapses of the nervous system and its end organs. Inhibition of blood cholinesterases is in principle parallel to the corresponding inhibition in target tissues, but the severity and time courses are not necessarily comparable, depending, for example, on the route and rate of absorption and on the characteristics of the compounds. Cholinesterase inhibition by organophosphates is to a large extent irreversible, and the recovery of the enzyme activities is slow, persisting up to several weeks. Furthermore, different rates of recovery have been observed for the two enzymes and for different, specific compounds. Consequently, it is common that cholinesterase inhibition accumulates when repeated exposures follow each other at short intervals. In cases of acute organophosphate poisoning, the inhibition of plasma cholinesterase is often more pronounced and occurs more rapidly than that of the red blood cell acetylcholinesterase; on the other hand, the latter enzyme may be more susceptible to certain organophosphates. While the plasma cholinesterase is more commonly assayed as a routine, it would be preferable to analyze red blood cell acetylcholinesterase as well.

Interindividual variation of cholinesterase activities is remarkable, and less but still significant variability occurs even within individuals. The baseline cholinesterase activities must therefore be measured at least once before the monitoring program for the season begins. The follow-up is then based on an observed decrease of activity attributable to organophosphorus exposure. A decrease of about 30% is an indication of a likely overexposure and an inhibition of 50% necessitates a removal of workers from further exposure to safeguard against symptoms of poisoning, until the activity has returned to about 90% of the normal individual value. A small proportion of the population has genetically determined variants of the plasma cholinesterase which exhibit very low activities. These persons appear not to be particularly susceptible to organophosphate toxicity, but their monitoring must be based solely on red blood cell acetylcholinesterase determinations.

Lindane (γ-Hexachlorocyclohexane).—Lindane is an organochlorine compound with insecticidal activity. Absorption of lindane is highly dependent on the carrier vehicle; it is readily absorbed from solutions of alcohol or other organic solvents, even through the skin. Lindane is lipophilic and it accumulates in adipose tissue, albeit to a much smaller extent than do organochlorine pesticides in general. In repeated exposures, blood lindane concentrations reach a steady state level within about a month or two. Lindane is biotransformed to several chlorinated phenols. Metabolic clearance and elimination are rather efficient; the half-time of lindane in blood is of the order of one week.

Lindane can be determined in whole blood or plasma, preferably with gas-liquid chromatography, utilizing electron-capture detection. The plasma lindane concentration is about two times higher than that in whole blood. Among workers occupationally exposed to lindane, plasma or whole blood concentrations have generally been less than 30 nmole/L, and in clinical cases of poisoning, the corresponding levels have been in excess of 1,700 nmole/L. The most sensitive indicator of an effect by lindane is thought to be enzyme induction. Induction has been observed when the plasma lindane concentration exceeds about 30 nmole/L. Thus, a concentration of 20 nmole/L of lindane in plasma could be proposed as a biologic guidance value on the grounds that it is about 100 times less than the level associated with clinical toxicity and because it would be just below the threshold for enzyme induction. The World Health Organization, however, has recommended that a whole-blood lindane concentration of 0.02 mg/L (70 nmole/L) be used in biologic monitoring as an individual maximum value.[116]

Chlorinated Phenoxyacids.—Several chlorinated phenoxyacid compounds are used as herbicides, such as 2,4-dichlorophenoxyacetic acid (2,4,-D), 2,4,5-trichlorophenoxyacetic acid (2,4,5-T), 4-chloro-2-methylphenoxyacetic acid (MCPA), 2,4-dichlorophenoxypropionic acid (dichlorprop), and 4-chloro-2-methylphenoxypropionic acid (mecoprop).

Chlorinated phenoxyacids are readily absorbed from the gastrointestinal tract and presumably also from the lungs. Absorption through the skin is relatively slow and incomplete; nevertheless, the skin is by far the main route of uptake in the occupational exposure. Chlorinated phenoxyacids are bound to plasma proteins, and their distribution to tissues is limited. They are eliminated unchanged in the urine with a half-time of one to three days.

Chlorinated phenoxyacids can be measured in the urine with gas chromatography. Among workers who have handled and sprayed these compounds, urinary levels at the end of the workday have ranged from about 0.2 to 70 μmole/L; higher concentrations have occasionally been found when extensive skin contamination has occurred.[57, 66] In the context of repeated, similar exposures over a work week or two, an even excretion of phenoxyacids in the urine was observed after the first few days; the highest levels tended to occur in morning samples. The relatively stable rate of excretion can probably be attributed both to a protracted absorption from the skin and to a delay in renal handling.

Occurrence of about 5–15 μmole of chlorinated phenoxyacids in a liter of urine towards the end of the week roughly corresponds to a daily uptake of a few milligrams. An exposure of this order of magnitude or less would indicate reasonable work hygiene. Furthermore, since the no-effect level of phenoxyacids in long-term animal experiments was about 3–10 mg/kg/day,[52] the proposed hygienic guidance values for human exposures offer a hundredfold margin of safety.

Conversion of Mass-Based Results to Molar Units

In Table 13–4, amounts are given in micromoles per milligram for many of the agents discussed in this chapter.

TABLE 13–4.
Conversion of Mass-Based Results to Molar Units

CHEMICAL	MICROMOLES PER MILLIGRAM
Aluminum	37.06
5-Aminolevulinic acid	7.626
Arsenic	13.35
Cadmium	8.896
Cobalt	16.97
Chromium	19.23
Fluoride	52.64
2,5-Hexanedione	8.761
Hippuric acid	5.581
Lead	4.826*
Mandelic acid	6.573
Manganese	18.20
Methylenebis (2-chloroaniline)	3.743
n-Methylformamide	16.93
Mercury	4.985
Methylhippuric acid	5.176
Nickel	17.04
Pentachlorophenol	3.755
Phenol	10.63
Tetrachloroethylene	6.030
Tetrachlorophenol	4.312
Thiocyanic acid	16.92
2-Thiothiazolidine (4-carboxylic acid)	6.127
Toluene	10.85
Trichloroacetic acid	6.120
1,1,1-Trichloroethane	7.495
Trichloroethanol	6.693
Trichlorophenol	5.064
Vanadium	19.63
Zinc-protoporphyrin	1.592

*The traditional unit for lead in blood is μg/100 ml; to convert to μmole/L, the figure is multiplied by 0.04826.

Amounts given in mass units per excreted creatinine, i.e., milligram/gram of micromole/mole creatinine, cannot be directly converted to volumetric units. The daily volume of urine is approximately 600–1,600 ml, and the daily excretion of creatinine is about 1–3 gm. Thus, values expressed in milligram/gram creatinine are roughly 0.5–1.0 times those expressed in mg/L.

The molecular weight of creatinine is 113.12; 1 gm is thus 8.84 mmole. Values expressed in mass/gram creatinine may be converted to mass/mole creatinine by multiplying by 113.12. Also, refer to Appendix B for SI units.

GENERAL REFERENCES

1. Aitio A, Riihimäki V, Vainio H (eds): *Biological Monitoring and Surveillance of Workers Exposed to Chemicals*. Washington, DC, Hemisphere Publishing, 1984.
2. Alessio L, Berlin A, Roi R, et al (eds): *Industrial Health and Safety. Human Biological Monitoring of Industrial Chemicals Series*. Luxembourg, Commission of the European Communities, 1983.
3. American Conference of Government Industrial Hygienists (ACGIH): *TLVs Threshold Limit Values for Chemical Substances and Physical Agents in the Work Environment and Biological Exposure Indices with Intended Changes for 1985–1986. Supplemental Documentation 1984*. Cincinnati, ACGIH, 1984.
4. Baselt RC: *Biological Monitoring Methods for Industrial Chemicals*. Davis, Cal, Biomedical Publications, 1980.
5. Berlin A, Yodaiken RE, Henman BA (eds): *Assessment of Toxic Agents at the Workplace. Roles of Ambient and Biological Monitoring*. The Hague, Nijhoff Publishers, 1984.
6. Deutsche Forschungsgemeinschaft (DFG): *Maximale Arbeitsplatzkonzentrationen und Biologische Arbeitsstofftoleranzwerte 1983*. Weinheim, BRD, Verlag Chemie, 1983.
7. Gompertz D: *Laboratory Methods for Biological Monitoring*, ed 2. London, Health & Safety Executive, 1985.
8. Lauwerys R: *Industrial Chemical Exposure: Guidelines for Biological Monitoring*. Davis, Cal, Biomedical Publishers, 1983.
9. Roi R, Town WG, Hunter WG, et al: *Occupational Health Guidelines for Chemical Risks*. Luxembourg, Commission of European Communities, 1983.
10. World Health Organization (WHO): Early detection of health impairment in occupational exposure to health hazards. *WHO Tech Rep Ser* 1975; 571.
11. World Health Organization (WHO): Recommended health-based limits in occupational exposure to heavy metals. *Tech Rep Ser* 1980; 647.

SPECIFIC REFERENCES

12. Aitio A: Quality control in the occupational toxicology laboratory, in WHO, Regional Office for Europe: *Health Aspects of Chemical Safety, Interim Document 4*. Copenhagen, WHO Europe, 1980.
13. Aitio A: Biological monitoring of occupational exposure to nickel, in Nickel in the human environment. *IARC Sci Publ* 1984; 53.
14. Aitio A, Järvisalo J: Biological monitoring of occupational exposure to toxic chemicals. Collection processing and storage of specimens. *Pure Appl Chem* 1984; 56:549. Also published in *Ann Clin Lab Sci* 1985; 15:121.
15. Aitio A, Järvisalo J: Levels of welding fume components in tissues and body fluids, in Stern RM, Berlin A, Fletcher J, et al (eds): Health Hazards and Biological Effects of Welding Fumes and Gases. *Excerpta Med 7th Congr Ser* 1986; 676:169–179.

16. Aitio A, Järvisalo J, Stoeppler M: Sampling and sample storage, in Stoeppler M (ed): *Trace Metal Analysis in Biological Specimens*. Foster City, Cal, Biomedical Publishers, in press.
17. Aitio A, Pekari K, Järvisalo J: Skin absorption as a source of error in biological monitoring. *Scand J Work Environ Health* 1984; 10:317.
18. Alström T, Gräsbeck R, Hjelm M, et al: Recommendations concerning the collection of reference values in clinical chemistry. *Scand J Clin Lab Invest* 1975; 35(Suppl 144):1.
19. Anderson RA, Polansky MM, Bryden NA, et al: Effect of exercise (running) on serum glucose, insulin, glucagon and chromium excretion. *Diabetes* 1982; 31:212.
20. Andersson R, Carlsson A, Byfält Nordqvist M, et al: Urinary excretion of hippuric acid and o-cresol after laboratory exposure of humans to toluene. *Int Arch Occup Environ Health* 1983; 53:101.
21. Apostoli P, Brugnone F, Perbellini L, et al: Biomonitoring of occupational toluene exposure. *Int Arch Occup Environ Health* 1982; 50:153.
22. Bardodej Z, Bardodejova E: Biotransformation of ethylbenzene, styrene and α-methylstyrene in man. *Am Ind Hyg Assoc J* 1970; 31:206.
23. Bencko V, Cikrt M: Manganese: A review of occupational and environmental toxicology. *J Hyg Epidemiol Microbiol Immunol* 1984; 28:139.
24. Berlin M, Gage JC, Gullberg B, et al: Breath concentration as an index of the health risk from benzene. Studies on the accumulation and clearance of inhaled benzene. *Scand J Work Environ Health* 1980; 6:104.
25. Berlin M, Tunek A: Benzene, in Aitio A, Riihimäki V, Vainio H (eds): *Biological Monitoring and Surveillance of Workers Exposed to Chemicals*. Washington, DC, Hemisphere Publishing, 1984.
26. Bernacki EJ, Parsons GE, Roy BR, et al: Urine nickel concentrations in nickel-exposed workers. *Ann Clin Lab Sci* 1978; 8:184.
27. Bertholf RL, Brown S, Remoe BW, et al: Improved determination of aluminum in serum by electrothermal atomic absorption spectrophotometry. *Clin Chem* 1983; 29:1087.
28. Buchet P, Lauwerys R, Roels H: Urinary excretion of inorganic arsenic and its metabolites after repeated ingestion of sodium metaarsenite by volunteers. *Int Arch Occup Environ Health* 1981; 48:111.
29. Carlson G: Korrelation mellan industriell exposition av arsenik och utsöndring i urin. Arbetarskyddsstyrelsens examensarbeten (mimeographed). Stockholm, Arbetarskyddstyrelsen, 1976.
30. Chandra SV, Shukla GS, Srivastava RS, et al: An exploratory study of manganese exposure to welders. *Clin Toxicol* 1981; 18:407.
31. *Council Directive (82/605/82) of 28 July 1982 on the Protection of Workers from Harmful Exposure to Metallic Lead and Its Ionic Compounds*. *Off J Eur Commun* 1982; L247:12.
32. Curtis CJ, Rein JE, Yamamura SS: Comparative study of different methods of packing liquid reagents. *Anal Chem* 1973; 45:996.
33. Dinman BD, Elder MJ, Bonney TB, et al: A 15-year retrospective study of fluoride excretion and body radiopacity among aluminium smelter workers. *J Occup Med* 1976; 18:21.
34. DiVincenzo GD, Kaplan CJ: Uptake metabolism and elimination of methylene chloride vapor by humans. *Toxicol Appl Pharmacol* 1981; 59:130.
35. DiVincenzo GD, Kaplan CJ: Effect of exercise or smoking on the uptake metabolism, and excretion of methylene chloride vapor. *Toxicol Appl Pharmacol* 1981; 59:141.
36. van Doorn R, Delpressine LPC, Leijdekkers Ch-M, et al: Identification and determination of 2-thiothiazolidine-4-carboxylic acid in urine of workers exposed to carbon disulfide. *Arch Toxicol* 1981; 47:51.
37. Ducos P, Maire C, Gaudin R: Assessment of occupational exposure to 4,4-methylenebis(2-chloroaniline) "MOCA" by a new sensitive method for biological monitoring. *Int Arch Occup Environ Health* 1985; 55:159.
38. Egan H, West TS (eds): *IUPAC Collaborative Interlaboratory Studies in Chemical Analysis*. Oxford, Pergamon Press, 1982.
39. El Ghawabi SH, Gaafar MA, El-Sahartti AA, et al: Chronic cyanide exposure: A clinical, radio-isotope, and laboratory study. *Br J Ind Med* 1984; 38:335.
40. Engström K, Riihimäki V, Laine A: Urinary disposition of ethylbenzene and m-xylene in man following separate and combined exposure. *Int Arch Occup Environ Health* 1984; 54:355.
41. Gibson RS: Hair as a biopsy material for the assessment of trace element status in infancy. *J Human Nutr* 1980; 34:405.
42. Gristwood W, Robertson SM, Wilson HK: The determination of 4,4-methylenebis(2-chloroaniline) in urine by electron capture gas chromatography. *J Anal Toxicol* 1984; 8:101.
43. Gromiec JP, Piotrowski JK: Urinary mandelic acid as an exposure test for ethylbenzene. *Int Arch Occup Environ Health* 1984; 55:61.
44. Hassler E, Lind B, Piscator M: Cadmium in blood and urine related to present and past exposure. A study of workers in an alkaline battery factory. *Br J Ind Med* 1983; 40:420.
45. Hartung M, Schaller K-H, Kentner M, et al: Untersuchungen zur cobalt-Belastung in verschiedenen Gewerbezweigen. *Arbeitsmed Soz Präventivmed* 1983; 18:73.
46. Hayes WJ Jr: *Pesticides Studied in Man*. Baltimore, Williams & Wilkins Co, 1982.
47. Health and Safety Executive: *Biological Monitoring of Workers Exposed to Organophosphorus Pesticides*, HSE Guidance Note MS 17. London, HSE, 1981.
48. Herber RFM: $Beta_2$-microglobulin and other urinary proteins as an index of cadmium nephrotoxicity. *Pure Appl Chem* 1984; 56:957.
49. Hernberg S: Lead, in Aitio A, Riihimäki V, Vainio H (eds): *Biological Monitoring and Surveillance of Workers Exposed to Chemicals*. Washington, DC, Hemisphere Publishing, 1984, pp 19–27.
50. Hilderbrand DC, White DH: Trace-element analysis in hair: An evaluation. *Clin Chem* 1974; 20:148.
51. Hogstedt CL: Fluorides, in Aitio A, Riihimäki V, Vainio H (eds): *Biological Monitoring and Surveillance of Workers Exposed to Chemicals*. Washington, DC, Hemisphere Publishing, 1984, pp 177–186.
52. International Agency for Research on Cancer (IARC): *IARC Monographs on the evaluation of the carcinogenic risk of chemicals to man*. Lyon, IARC, 1977, vol 15.
53. Iwata M, Takeuchi Y, Hisanaga N, et al: A study on the biological monitoring of n-hexane exposure. *Int Arch Occup Environ Health* 1983; 51:253.
54. Jarvis M, Tunstall-Pedoe H, Feyerabend C, et al: Biochemical markers of smoke absorption and self-reported exposure to passive smoking. *J Epidemiol Commun Health* 1984; 38:335.
55. Järvisalo J, Olkinuora M, Tossavainen M, et al: Urinary and blood manganese as indicators of manganese exposure in manual metal arc welding of mild steel, in Brown SS, Savory J (eds): *Chemical Toxicology and Clinical Chemistry of Metals*. New York, Academic Press, 1983, pp 123–126.
56. Kjellström T: Exposure and accumulation of cadmium in populations from Japan, the United States of America and Sweden. *Environ Health Perspect* 1979; 28:169.
57. Kolmodin-Hedman B, Höglund S, Åkerblom M: Studies on phenoxy acid herbicides. I. Field study: Occupational exposure to phenoxy acid herbicides (MCPA, dichlorprop, mecroprop and 2,4-D) in agriculture. *Arch Toxicol* 1983; 54:257.
58. Konietzko H, Keilbach J, Drysch K: Cumulative effects of daily toluene exposure. *Int Arch Occup Environ Health* 1980; 46:53.
59. Krivanek ND, McLaughlin M, Fayerweather WE: Mono-

methylformamide levels in human urine after repetitive exposure to dimethylformamide vapor. *J Occup Med* 1978; 20:179.

60. Kumpulainen J, Lehto J, Koivistoinen P, et al: Determination of chromium in human milk, serum and urine by electrothermal atomic absorption spectrometry without preliminary ashing. *Sci Total Environ* 1983; 31:71.
61. Kurppa K: Carbon monoxide, in Aitio A, Riihimäki V, Vainio H (eds): *Biological Monitoring and Surveillance of Workers Exposed to Chemicals*. Washington, DC, Hemisphere Publishing, 1984, pp 159–164.
62. Lauwerys RR: In vivo tests to monitor body burdens of toxic metals in man, in Brown SS, Savory J (eds): *Chemical Toxicology and Clinical Chemistry of Metals*. New York, Academic Press, 1983, pp 113–121.
63. Lauwerys RR: Occupational toxicology, in Doull J, Klaassen CD, Amdur MO (eds): *Toxicology. The Basic Science of Poisons*, ed 2. New York, Macmillan Publishing Co, 1980, pp 699–709.
64. Lauwerys R, Herbrand J, Buchet JP, et al: Health surveillance of workers exposed to tetrachloroethylene in dry-cleaning shops. *Int Arch Occup Environ Health* 1983; 52:69.
65. Lauwerys R, Kivits S, Lhoir M, et al: Biological surveillance of workers exposed to dimethylformamide and the influence of skin protection on its percutaneous absorption. *Int Arch Occup Environ Health* 1980; 45:189.
66. Libich S, To JC, Frank R, et al: Occupational exposure of herbicide applicators to herbicides used along electric power transmission line right-of-way. *Am Ind Hyg Assoc J* 1984; 45:56.
67. Lindberg E, Vesterberg O: Monitoring exposure to chromic acid in chromeplating by measuring chromium in urine. *Scand J Work Environ Health* 1983; 9:333.
68. Lippmann N: Magnetopneumography as a tool for measuring lung burden of industrial aerosols, in Stern RM, Berlin A, Fletcher J, et al (eds): Health Hazards and Biological Effects of Welding Fumes and Gases. *Excerpta Med 7th Congr Ser* 1986; 676:199–213.
69. Luotamo M, Järvisalo J, Aitio A: Analysis of polychlorinated biphenyls (PCB) in human serum. *Environ Health Perspect* 1985; 60:327.
70. Mercier M: Criteria (dose/effect relationships) for organochlorine pesticides. Commission of the European Communities. Oxford, Pergamon Press, 1981.
71. Molin Christensen J, Mikkelsen S, Skov A: A direct determination of cobalt in blood and urine by Zeeman atomic absorption spectrophotometry, in Brown SS, Savory J (eds): *Chemical Toxicology and Clinical Chemistry of Metals*. New York, Academic Press, 1983, pp 65–68.
72. Mussi A, Galzaferri G, Buratti M, et al: Behaviour of plasma and urinary aluminium levels in occupationally exposed subjects. *Int Arch Occup Environ Health* 1984; 54:155.
73. Mutti A, Falzoi M, Lucretini S, et al: n-Hexane metabolism in occupationally exposed workers. *Br J Ind Med* 1984; 41:533.
74. National Academy of Sciences (NAS/NCR) Committee on Biological Effects of Atmospheric Pollutants: *Fluorides*. Washington DC, NAS, 1971.
75. National Institute for Occupational Safety and Health (NIOSH): *Criteria for a Recommended Standard: Inorganic Fluorides*. US Dept of Health, Education, and Welfare, 1975.
76. Nolan RJ, Freshour NL, Rick DL, et al: Kinetics and metabolism of inhaled methyl chloroform (1,1,1-trichloroethane) in male volunteers. *Fundam Appl Toxicol* 1984; 4:654.
77. Ohtsuki T, Sato K, Koizumi A, et al: Limited capacity of humans to metabolize tetrachloroethylene. *Int Arch Occup Environ Health* 1983; 51:381.
78. Pekari K, Järvisalo J, Aitio A: Kinetics of urinary excretion of 2,4,6-tri, 2,3,4,6-tetra, and pentachlorophenol in workers exposed in lumber treatment. *Proc 26th Congr Eur Soc Toxicol*. Kuopio, Finland, June 16–19, 1985, p 183.
79. Perbellini L, Brugnone F, Faggionato G: Urinary excretion of the metabolites of n-hexane and its isomers during occupational exposure. *Br J Ind Med* 1981; 38:20.
80. Perbellini L, Brugnone F, Mozzo P, et al: Toxicokinetic aspects of n-hexane and 2,5-hexanedione in the biomonitoring of occupational exposure to n-hexane. *Int Symp Occup Exposure Limits*. Copenhagen, 16–19 April, 1985, in press.
81. Pfäffli P, Savolainen H, Kalliomäki P-L, et al: Urinary o-cresol in toluene exposure. *Scand J Work Environ Health* 1979; 5:286.
82. Pinto S, Varner MO, Nelson KW, et al: Arsenic trioxide absorption and excretion in industry. *J Occup Med* 1976; 18:677.
83. Riihimäki V, Savolainen K, Pfäffli P, et al: Metabolic interaction between m-xylene and ethanol. *Arch Toxicol* 1982; 49:253.
84. Robertson DE: Role of contamination in trace element analysis of sea water. *Anal Chem* 1968; 40:1067.
85. Roels H, Lauwerys R, Buchet J, et al: Comparison of renal function and psychomotor performance in workers exposed to elemental mercury. *Int Arch Occup Environ Health* 1982; 50:77.
86. Van Roosmaalen PB, Klein AL, Drummond I: An improved method for determination of 4,4-methylenebis(2-chloroaniline) (MBOCA) in urine. *Am Ind Hyg Assoc J* 1979; 40:66.
87. Rosier J, Billemont G, Van Peteghem C, et al: Relation between the iodine azide test and the TTCA test for exposure to carbon disulphide. *Br J Ind Med* 1984; 41:412.
88. Rosier J, Vanhoorne M, Van Peteghem C, et al: Preliminary evaluation of urinary 2-thio-thiazolidine-4-carboxylic acid (TTCA) levels as a test for exposure to carbon disulphide. *Int Arch Occup Environ Health* 1982; 51:159.
89. Safe S: Metabolism, uptake, storage and bioaccumulation, in Kimbrough RD (ed): *Halogenated Biphenyls, Terphenyls, Naphthalenes, Dibenzodioxins and Related Compounds*. New York, Elsevier North-Holland, Inc, 1980, pp 81–107.
90. Sjögren B, Hedström L, Lindstedt G: Urinary fluoride concentration as an estimation of welding fume exposure from basic electrodes. *Br J Ind Med* 1984; 41:192.
91. Sjögren B, Lidums V, Håkansson M, et al: Exposure and urinary excretion of aluminium during welding. *Scand J Work Environ Health* 1985; 11:39.
92. Sjögren B, Lundberg I, Lidums V: Aluminium in blood and urine of industrially exposed workers. *Br J Ind Med* 1983; 40:301.
93. Stewart RD, Forster HV, Hake CL, et al: Human responses to controlled exposures of methylene chloride vapor, Report No. NIOSH-NCOW-Envm-MC-73-7. Milwaukee, The Medical College of Wisconsin, 1973.
94. Stoeppler M, Apel M: Determination of arsenic species in liquid and solid materials from the environment and food, and in body fluids. *Fresenius Z Anal Chem* 1984; 317:226.
95. Sunderman FW, Sunderman FW Jr: Nickel poisoning VIII. Dithiocarb: A new therapeutic agent for persons exposed to nickel carbonyl. *Am J Med Sci* 1958; 236:26.
96. Sunderman FW Jr: Analytical biochemistry of nickel. *Pure Appl Chem* 1980; 52:527.
97. Szadkowski D, Pett R, Angerer J, et al: Chronische Lösungsmittelbelastung am Arbeitsplatz. II. Schadstoffspiegel im Blut und Metabolitenelimination im Harn in ihrer Bedeutung als Überwachungskriterien bei toluolexponierten Tiefdruckern. *Int Arch Arbeitsmed* 1973; 31:265.
98. Thomas JD, Wilson HK: Biological monitoring of workers exposed to 4,4-methylenebis(2-chloroaniline) (MBOCA). *Br J Ind Med* 1984; 41:547.
99. Vahter M: Assessment of human exposure to lead and cadmium through biological monitoring. Stockholm, National Swedish Institute

of Environmental Medicine, Department of Environmental Hygiene, Karolinska Institute, 1982.

100. Valkonen S, Järvisalo J, Aitio A: Urinary arsenic in a Finnish population without occupational exposure to arsenic, in Brätter E, Schramel P (eds): *Trace Element-Analytical Chemlstry in Medicine and Biology*. Berlin, Walter de Gruyter, 1983, vol 2, pp 611–621.
101. Veillon C, Patterson KY, Bryden NA: Determination of chromium in human serum by electrothermal atomic absorption spectrometry. *Anal Chim Acta* 1984; 164:67.
102. Versieck J, Cornelis R: Normal levels of trace elements in human plasma and serum. *Anal Chim Acta* 1980; 116:217.
103. Versieck JMJ, Speecke ABH: Contaminations induced by collection of liver biopsies and human blood, in: *Nuclear Activation Techniques in the Life Sciences*. Vienna, International Atomic Energy Agency, 1972, pp 39–49.
104. Vesey CJ, Kirk JC: Two automated methods for measuring plasma thiocyanate compared. *Clin Chem* 1985; 31:270.
105. Vesey CJ, Saloojee Y, Cole PV, et al: Blood carboxyhemoglobin, plasma thiocyanate, and cigarette consumption: Implications for epidemiological studies in smokers. *Br J Ind Med* 1982; 284:1516.
106. Veulemans H, Van Vlem E, Janssens H, et al: Experimental human exposure to n-hexane. Study of the respiratory uptake and elimination, and of n-hexane concentrations in peripheral venous blood. *Int Arch Occup Environ Health* 1982; 49:251.
107. Waldron HA, Cherry N, Johnston JD: The effects of ethanol on blood toluene concentrations. *Int Arch Occup Environ Health* 1983; 51:365.
108. Wilson HK, Robertson SM, Waldron HA, et al: Effect of alcohol on the kinetics of mandelic acid excretion in volunteers exposed to styrene vapour. *Br J Ind Med* 1983; 40:75.
109. Wolff M, Fishbein A, Thornton J, et al: Disposition of polychlorinated biphenyls among persons employed in capacitor manufacturing. *Int Arch Occup Environ Health* 1982; 49:199.
110. World Health Organization (WHO): *Environmental Health Criteria 3. Lead*. Geneva, WHO, 1977.
111. World Health Organization (WHO): *Environmental Health Criteria 10. Carbon Disulfide*. Geneva, WHO, 1979.
112. World Health Organization (WHO): *Environmental Health Criteria 13. Carbon Monoxide*. Geneva, WHO, 1979.
113. World Health Organization (WHO): *External Quality Assessment of Health Laboratories*, Euro Rep Stud 36. Copenhagen, WHO Europe, 1981.
114. World Health Organization (WHO): *Environmental Health Criteria 17. Manganese*. Geneva, WHO, 1981.
115. World Health Organization (WHO): Recommended health-based limits in occupational exposure to selected organic solvents. *WHO Tech Rep Ser* 1981; 664.
116. World Health Organization (WHO): Recommended health-based limits in occupational exposure to pesticides. *Tech Rep Ser* 1982; 677.
117. Yonemoto J, Suzuki S: Relation of exposure to dimethylformamide vapor and the metabolite, methylformamide, in urine of workers. *Int Arch Occup Environ Health* 1980; 46:159.
118. Åstrand I, Övrum P, Carlsson A: Exposure to methylene chloride. I. Its concentration in alveolar air and blood during rest and exercise and its metabolism. *Scand J Work Environ Health* 1975; 1:78.

PART II

Occupational Pulmonary Diseases

14

An Overview of Occupational Pulmonary Disorders

Stuart A. Levy, M.D.

The clinical and pathologic consequences that result from the inhalation of dust vary according to (1) the properties of the dust, (2) the intensity and duration of exposure, and (3) host susceptibility. The area of the respiratory tract affected and the response to the exposure depend on the dust's physical and chemical properties and its toxicity. The dust may be inhaled as a solid, fume, or mixture. Particles that measure 5 μ or less in diameter are capable of reaching the alveoli, and those that measure 1 μ have the highest probability of being deposited in the alveoli.[43] The sizes of various airborne contaminants are shown in Figure 14–1. The fate of the dust once it enters the alveoli depends on its solubility and reactivity. The more soluble reactive substances may evoke acute inflammatory reactions and pulmonary edema. Subacute and chronic reactions may be characterized by granuloma formation and interstitial fibrosis. Most of the dust that reaches the alveoli is engulfed by macrophages that migrate proximally to the airways and are expectorated or swallowed or may enter the interstitial tissues. The interstitial macrophages may enter the pulmonary lymphatics and be carried to the regional lymph nodes or enter the pulmonary capillaries and be deposited throughout the entire reticuloendothelial system. Some dust-laden macrophages may migrate through the interstitial tissues with little effect and incite an intense reaction when the pleura is reached. The alveolar clearance mechanism is highly efficient and capable of completely eliminating all particles smaller than 5 μ in diameter if the airborne concentration does not exceed 10 particles/cu cm. This mechanism can be overwhelmed,[27] and it is estimated that only 90% of the particles below 5 μ in diameter can be eliminated if the airborne concentration approaches 1,000 particles/cu cm.[70]

Individual susceptibility is difficult to assess. Workers exposed to the same environment for equal periods of time may develop different degrees of pulmonary disease. This may be due to the variation in the rate of clearance of dust from the lung,[185, 332] genetic factors,[168, 213] the effect of cigarette smoking, and coexistent pulmonary disease. One of the most important factors determining susceptibility to inhaled irritants is related to serum α_1-antitrypsin (SAT). This protein is a nonspecific inhibitor of trypsin, chymotrypsin, thrombin, elastase, collagenase, and various leukocyte proteases.[183] Inhaled irritants probably increase the rate of release of proteolytic enzymes from alveolar macrophages and leukocytes, which are capable of digesting human lung. Serum α_1-antitrypsin protects the lungs from the destructive action of these enzymes.[95] Individuals who are homozygous for SAT deficiency have approximately 15% of the normal SAT and are likely to develop emphysema at an early age if exposed to respirable dust or pollutants. The quantity of SAT in heterozygotes varies according to the phenotype, of which 20 have been identified.[297] The role of intermediate deficiency of SAT in heterozygotes has not yet been completely clarified.[57] Emphysema is associated with the ZZ and SZ phenotypes. A simple, reliable assay procedure has been proposed for the detection of SAT that has the potential for large-scale screening programs.[183] This would be particularly valuable in the selection and protection of potential employees who are genetically susceptible to the effects of most of the dusts described in this chapter.

Decades often pass between the onset of exposure and the emergence of disease. This long lag period may obscure the cause-and-effect relationship that is essential for adequate epidemiologic studies. It has been useful to consider the pneumoconioses to be caused by single agents. In reality, there are multiple etiologic factors, and mixed-dust exposure is encountered commonly. Unfortunately, there is very little currently known about the interaction of two or more inhaled dusts.

The chest roentgenogram is an indispensable aid in the evaluation of workers with pneumoconioses, but its limitations must be clearly recognized. The roentgenogram may be strikingly abnormal due to the presence of relatively inert dusts. There may be significant clinical impairment and extensive pathologic changes in the presence of a normal roentgenogram, as might occur in some of the organic pneumoconioses and in the early stages of asbestosis. Densities resulting from a pneumoconiosis may be localized to a small area of the lung, producing little clinical impairment. The nodular densities that characterize simple coal worker's pneumoconiosis may become less apparent if emphysema develops. The International Labor Organization (ILO) categorization of the degree and nature of abnormalities has represented a great advance in the standardization of the features of the chest roentgenogram,[64] which correlates with the indices of dust exposure and in many instances

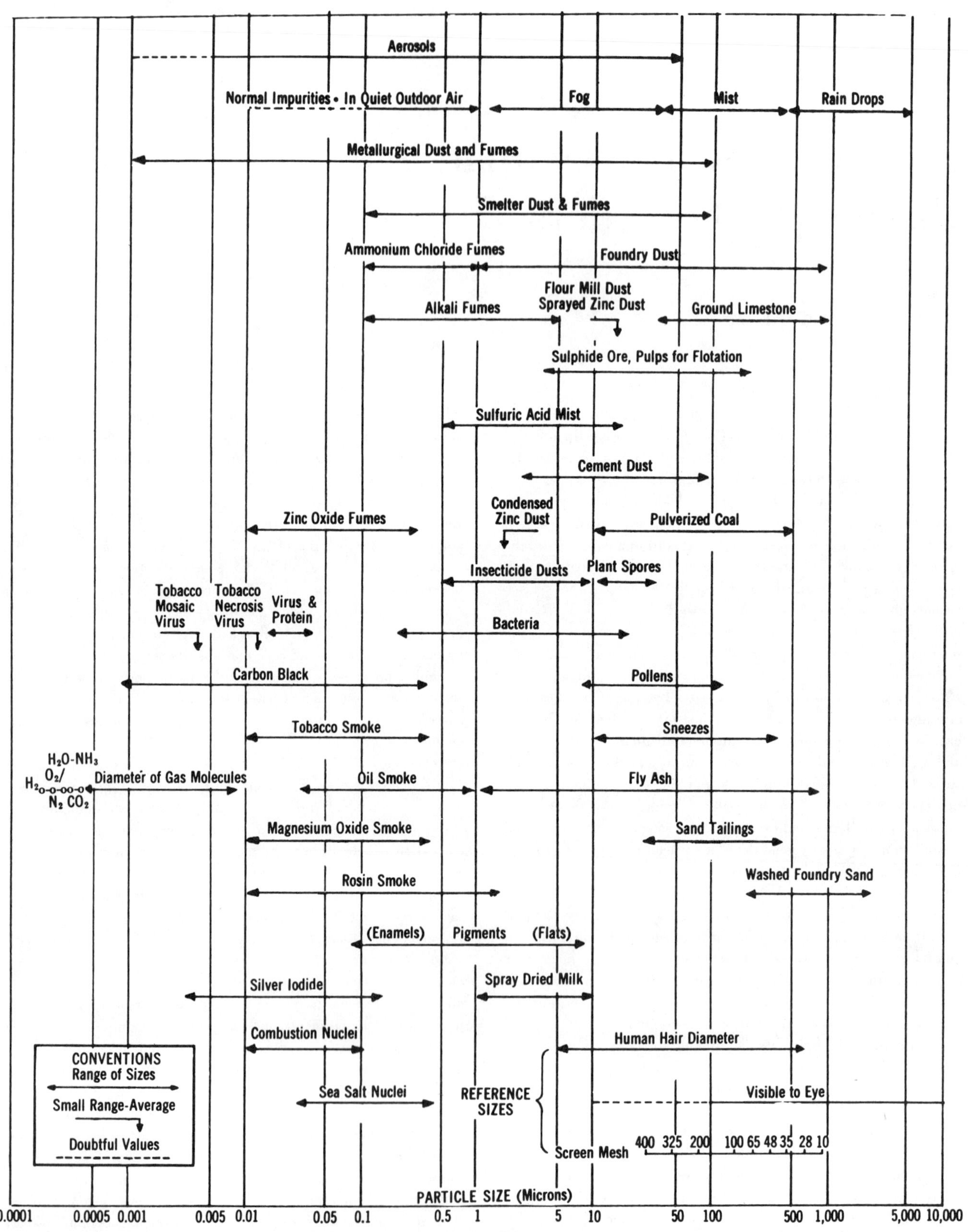

FIG 14–1.
The sizes of various airborne contaminants. (From Mine Safety Appliances Co, *Technical Information,* Section 10. Modified from *Fundamentals of Industrial Hygiene,* Olishifski J (ed). Chicago, National Safety Council, 1979.)

with pathologic and functional changes in workers exposed to silica, coal dust, and asbestos.[320] The chest roentgenogram should not be used to estimate the presence or extent of ventilatory impairment.

In many of the pneumoconioses, there is limited pulmonary function data, and occasionally conclusions have been reached, based on spirometry alone, that no impairment of pulmonary function exists at certain stages of disease. It should be emphasized that there may be profound alterations in gas exchange or pulmonary mechanics before the spirogram becomes abnormal.[167] Airway resistance, as conventionally estimated from the spirogram, reflects predominantly resistance to airflow in the large or central airways.[137] Small airways (less than 2 mm in diameter) are usually affected early in the course of most diseases that involve the alveolar wall and interstitial tissue, and obstruction of these small airways contributes little to the overall measurable resistance. New methods developed and refined to detect early functional impairment of the small airways are of research interest and not suitable for industrial screening purposes. However, the preventive diagnosis of occupational lung disease at an early and potentially reversible stage remains an obligatory goal.[81]

Objective criteria for the assessment of disability are essential. Claimants for disability benefits complain of more breathlessness than do patients with comparable ventilatory function who were referred for evaluation for other reasons.[94, 218] At present, spirometry remains the most suitable screening test for routine industrial applications, provided that the previously discussed limitations are recognized. The spirogram generally relates to morbidity as perceived by patient and physician when compared to other screening studies or tests for small airway disease.[81] Pre- and post-employment spirograms are necessary for the protection of workers in some industries; for example, in the prevention of byssinosis, where it is important to establish a baseline for future reference prior to exposure. There are many instruments available for mass screening applications.[334] Serious inadequacies have been found in several commercially available spirometers.[102] Minimum standards for spirometry have been established in an effort to assure acquisition of accurate data.[8] Additional pulmonary function tests are best performed at a referral center when a ventilatory impairment is suspected. They are of value in (1) determining the type and extent of any lung disease process, (2) following the progression of disease for changes in severity or in response to therapy, (3) developing further understanding between the functional, radiologic, and pathologic changes, and (4) legal and compensation purposes. A variety of pulmonary function tests are discussed briefly below. Other sources[19, 115] are recommended for more detailed information.

The vital capacity (VC) refers to the maximal volume of air that a patient can exhale after a maximal inspiration. If the exhalation is performed as forcefully as possible, the volume is referred to as the forced vital capacity (FVC). Changes in the vital capacity are more important than single determinations. An estimate of the flow rates can be obtained by measuring the volume exhaled during the first second (FEV_1). The maximal midexpiratory flow rate (MMFR) measures the average flow rate during the middle half of the FVC and often is referred to as the $FEF_{25\%-75\%}$ (forced expiratory flow between 25% and 75% of the FVC). A reduction in the VC indicates the presence of a ventilatory impairment that is obstructive in type if accompanied by a disproportionate reduction in the flow rates.

The residual volume (RV) can be determined by having the subject breathe through a spirometer circuit of constant volume for at least seven minutes. By measuring the dilution of helium, which is used as a tracer gas, the residual volume of air remaining in the lungs at the completion of exhalation can be calculated. Alternative methods are available for determining the RV, including the open-circuit nitrogen washout method and body plethysmography. The total lung capacity (TLC) is the sum of the VC and the RV. An increase in the RV when accompanied by an increase in the RV/TLC ratio reflects pulmonary overdistention and probable air-trapping. A reduction in the VC when accompanied by a decrease in the TLC reflects a restrictive ventilatory impairment.

The maximal ventilatory volume (MVV), formerly referred to as the maximal breathing capacity (MBC), is determined by measuring the volume of gas exchange during 12–15 seconds of maximal voluntary hyperventilation. The test is dependent on the motivation of the subject, muscle strength, fatigability, extent of air-trapping, and overall integrity of the respiratory bellows.

The pulmonary diffusing capacity (DL) is determined by measuring the amount of carbon monoxide that is transferred from the alveoli to hemoglobin in the pulmonary capillaries. Two methods are available: the single-breath method, during which the patient must hold his breath for ten seconds and then exhale, and a steady-state method, which requires less cooperation of the patient but is more sensitive to imbalances of ventilation and perfusion. The DL is dependent on the surface area available for transfer of gas, the size of the pulmonary capillary bed, and the amount of hemoglobin present. The percent predicted $FEV_{1.0}$, MVV, and RV/TLC correlate closely with dyspnea in subjects with obstructive lung disease. With interstitial disease, a combination of less than 50% predicted for the FVC or 40% predicted for the DL_{CO} is satisfactory criteria for the detection of subjects with disabling dyspnea.[94]

Arterial blood gases (Pa_{O_2} and Pa_{CO_2}) and pH often are normal at rest and become abnormal during exercise performed on a bicycle ergometer or on a treadmill. During exercise, the minute ventilation and oxygen consumption can be measured. The increased difference between alveolar and arterial oxygen tension [(A-a) O_2 gradient] at rest or after exercise often is an early indication of impaired gas exchange resulting from a mismatch in ventilation and perfusion.

Pulmonary compliance refers to the distensibility of the lungs and can be calculated by measuring the change in intrathoracic volume for a given change in intrathoracic pressure. The pressure change is determined by the use of an esophageal balloon. The compliance is reduced when the lungs become stiff and abnormally difficult to inflate.

ASBESTOSIS

Asbestosis is a general term used to describe lung disease resulting from the inhalation of six distinct varieties of fibrous mineral silicates. Chrysotile (white asbestos), a member of the serpentine family, consists of hydrated magnesium silicate and accounts for 95% of the world's asbestos production. Crocidolite (blue asbestos), amosite (brown asbestos), anthophyllite, tremolite, and actinolite constitute the amphibole family. Anthophyllite and chrysotile contain larger amounts of magnesium than does either crocidolite or amosite, both of which, in turn, have more iron than do the others. Chrysotile, composed of long, strong fibers that can be spun into fabrics, is found predominantly in Quebec; crocidolite and amosite, composed of fibers that are resistant to heat and acid, are found in South Africa; anthophyllite and tremolite are mined in Finland.

The risk from exposure to asbestos occurs most commonly in mining operations, asbestos textile operations—particularly carding, weaving, and spinning—and during the installation and removal of insulation on steam pipes and furnaces. The opportunity for exposure is widespread in other industries, since the material is also used for electric wire insulation, paint filler, and the manufacture of shingles, tile, and brake and clutch linings, and in plastics. In the United States, approximately 50,000 workers are involved in the manufacture of asbestos-containing products.[306] As with other dusts, the danger is greatest when finely divided particles are airborne. Consequently, the risk of miners developing asbestosis is not as great as for workers in the mills at the mine head or in the industries in which the processed fiber is handled. There are approximately 40,000 field insulation workers in the United States who are exposed to asbestos dust, and they cause secondary exposure to approximately 3–5 million other building and construction workers.[306] Usually, evidence of disease does not appear until more than 20 years after exposure. More than 70% of insulation workers have been shown to have an abnormal chest roentgenogram after 20–30 years' exposure;[276] however, a very brief exposure for as short a period as two to six months may produce asbestosis or pleural disease more than 20–30 years later.[75, 274]

The asbestos fiber is capable of penetrating deeply into the lung parenchyma despite its length, which may exceed 100 μ in some instances. Fiber diameter, not length, appears to be the major physical factor limiting asbestos penetration.[41] The precise pathogenesis of disease is not known. Multiple theories have been proposed which include the slow liberation of silicic acid or an immunologic reaction, with the protein-coated particle serving as the antigen in a mechanism similar to that discussed with silica (vide infra). It also has been suggested that the coating of the asbestos fiber with protein may be a protective mechanism rendering the fiber less fibrogenic.[318] The incomplete phagocytosis of asbestos fibers may result in the release of lysosomal enzymes from macrophages.[72] Most intriguing is the elaboration of reticulin and collagen at accelerated rates when chrysotile is added to fibroblasts in vitro.[134, 256] The biologic reactions of the different varieties of asbestos are remarkably dissimilar. Pleuropulmonary disease appears to be more prevalent in workers exposed to amosite,[327] and crocidolite presents a greater hazard than chrysotile.[2, 90, 302, 316, 323] There is conflicting evidence supporting the view that smoking does not appear to act synergistically in the development of asbestos-induced fibrosis,[262] in contrast to the clear association with pleural plaques.[326]

Pathology

In animal studies, asbestos particles are deposited at the bifurcation of alveolar ducts closest to the terminal bronchioles. Fibers are taken up by an early influx of macrophages, which exit by way of the mucociliary transport system, and type I epithelial cells, which are responsible for translocation of the fibers to the basement membrane and subsequently to fibroblasts and interstitial macrophages.[41] The uptake of asbestos by fibroblasts results in cellular proliferation and increased production of collagen. After ingestion of asbestos, macrophages release an unidentified substance that stimulates fibroblasts to produce more connective tissue. The fibrotic reaction is relatively acellular, with the occasional appearance of a few lymphocytes and plasma cells, particularly near the pleura. A positive gallium scan may reflect the inflammatory component.[25] Some alveoli may be completely obliterated by bundles of collagen. Asbestos bodies, which appear as brown or black fibers measuring up to 100 μ in length, are occasionally found in groups in both the fibrous connective tissue and the alveolar spaces adjacent to the areas of fibrosis. The bodies have a protein coat that is thicker at the ends, producing a drumstick appearance, and stains with Prussian blue. Asbestos is presumed to be responsible for the fibrotic reaction when asbestos bodies are seen; however, it should be recognized that these bodies may fragment[75] and become invisible by light microscopy. There is evidence that the smallest submicroscopic chrysotile fibrils are associated with the greatest degree of fibrosis[113] and examination of the lung by electron microscopy is necessary to identify these particles.[208] A nonspecific increase in fibrous connective tissue frequently causes thickening of the pleura, often obliterating the interlobar fissures. Fibrous plaques often develop on the parietal pleura, diaphragm, and pericardium. Pleural calcification is not seen commonly until 20 years after the onset of exposure. Occasionally, asbestos bodies may pass through the interstitial tissues and incite little reaction until they reach the pleura.

Chest Roentgenograms

Pleural thickening and pleural plaques are the most common abnormalities found on the chest roentgenogram.[105] The prevalence of pleural plaques is related both to cigarette smoking and the cumulative dose of exposure to asbestos.[242, 326] The plaques usually are bilateral and have to be relatively extensive or contain abundant calcium to be visualized.[139] They may be the only radiographic evidence of disease and often are seen without associated pulmonary fibrosis.[13] Although plaques are not always present, it is important to realize that approximately 85% of them seen at necropsy are not visible on the routine posteroanterior chest roentgenogram[139] even when calcified. There is a wide variation in the reported incidence of calcified plaques, ranging from 0%[286] to approximately 50%, and this may reflect exposure to different types of asbestos, observer variation, and radiographic technique. The calcifications commonly appear over the anterolateral regions of the lung and the central domes of the diaphragm. Bilateral calcified pleural plaques in the absence of a history of trauma or infection are strongly suggestive of asbestosis but not diagnostic, since they have been reported after exposure to mica, talc, bakelite,[286] and coal.[233] Calcification of the pleura, which may occur as a sequela of empyema, hemothorax, or tuberculosis, usually is unilateral.

The reticular pattern of interstitial fibrosis is seen in only 50% of the cases and initially appears in the lower lung fields. In the early stages, the intra-alveolar septa may be thickened 10–20 times its normal caliber without any radiographic abnormality.[13] Biopsy-proved interstitial pneumonitis due to asbestos has been reported without any radiographic abnormalities.[114] In some instances, evidence of fibrosis may be obscured by the presence of pleural plaques or pleural thickening.[13] The coarse reticular pattern extends to the mid and upper lung fields in the later stages of disease. The combination of parenchymal and pleural changes obscures the sharp cardiac borders, producing the "shaggy heart" sign. Radiographic progression has been documented after exposure ceases.[312] Hilar adenopathy is not as prominent as is silicosis in most cases[169] but occasionally may be massive even in the absence of tumor.[114] Pleural fluid may be present more often than has been recognized previously and may be either unilateral or bilateral.[114] The mixed-dust pneumoconiosis resulting from exposure to cement and asbestos is similar to classic asbestosis with regard to clinical and functional impairment and radiographic abnormalities. The magnitude of the abnormalities is generally less than would result from exposure to asbestos alone for the same period of time.[267]

Clinical Manifestations

The onset of symptomatic asbestosis is uncommon before at least 20–30 years of exposure.[276, 288] The most common initial symptoms are dyspnea and a nonproductive, irritating cough. As the disease progresses, both symptoms increase in severity and the cough may become productive of mucopurulent sputum. Auscultation of the chest may reveal basilar crepitant rales.[87, 162] Clubbing of the fingers and cyanosis usually are seen in the more advanced stages. Cor pulmonale is a frequent complication and a major cause of death. Pleural fibrosis may be sufficiently extensive to cause intense dyspnea and even death.[209] Pleural fluid was once thought to be a relatively uncommon occurrence and was the subject of case reports.[87] The annual incidence of pleural effusion is more common than previously recognized and is approximately 9 per 1,000 employees directly exposed and 4 per 1,000 employees indirectly exposed to asbestos. The prevalence of benign effusion is in excess of 3% of exposed workers.[93] Pleuritic pain commonly accompanies pleural fluid, but many patients have recurrent, short-lived pleuritic pain in the absence of pleural fluid. Unilateral pleuritic pain may precede the development of a mesothelioma by more than ten years[114] (vide infra). The demonstration of asbestos bodies in the sputum is not diagnostic of disease.

Pulmonary Function Tests

The decline of pulmonary function as a result of exposure to asbestos is dependent upon the type of exposure (mining, milling, etc.) and fiber type.[324] The mechanical properties of the lung may be altered before any abnormalities are detected on the chest roentgenogram. There is evidence that the earliest effects of the exposure to asbestos dust affects primarily the small airways[24, 148] and, therefore, may not be detected on routine pulmonary function studies.[114] The major abnormalities of lung function include a reduction in the vital capacity accompanied by impaired respiratory gas exchange. The diffusing capacity may be reduced and the alveolar-arterial oxygen gradient increased in patients with asbestosis who have no clinical evidence of disease.[114] Impaired diffusion is more strongly related to smoking than to intensity of exposure to asbestos.[242] The spirogram is sufficient to monitor the ventilatory impairment due to asbestosis and may be abnormal before the chest roentgenogram reveals any abnormalities.[324] It is also important to recognize that roentgenographic abnormalities may be extensive with little demonstrable impairment in the laboratory.[39, 288] The earliest abnormalities due to asbestos can be best detected by employing both screening tests.

Neoplasia

There is a unique association between asbestos and the development of pleuropulmonary malignancies and possibly neoplasms in other organs as well. The incidence of lung cancer of all cell types is increased,[75] but adenocarcinoma predominates.[132] The prevalence of lung cancer is higher in the asbestos textile industry than in the building products or friction materials industry.[91] This has been attributed to the higher level of dust exposure in the textile industry. A similar relationship between lung cancer and dust exposure has been found in mine and mill workers exposed to chrysotile.[194] The dimensions of the fiber, rather than the chemical composition, may be more critical in the development of tumors,[142] which may explain why crocidolite, which is long and thin, is the principal fiber associated with mesothelioma.[316] Peritoneal mesothelioma occurs only with exposure to amphibole asbestos.[67] There has been much speculation regarding the mechanism of action. Asbestos is a potent mutagen[56] and appears more likely to act as a tumor-promoter rather than as a classic chemical carcinogen.[67] The carcinogenic properties of crocidolite and amosite may be related to a macromolecular iron complex analogous to other known carcinogenic complexes of iron, of which iron-dextran is the most notable. The iron content of chrysotile is lower than crocidolite or amosite, but it may be present in sufficient enough quantities as a macromolecular complex to be carcinogenic.[131] Carcinogenic trace metals, such as nickel and chromium, are present in asbestos, particularly chrysotile,[69] but in amounts that, by themselves, probably are sufficient to cause cancer. Crocidolite and amosite contain small quantities of natural oils that are carcinogenic in animals in large doses.[131] It has been suggested that differences in physical properties may explain the varying carcinogenic potential,[44, 159, 295] and lastly, workers exposed to asbestos have been shown to have increased aryl hydrocarbon hydroxylase inducibility, which is an inducible microsomal enzyme system that may convert hydrocarbons to more potent carcinogens. In addition, asbestos has been shown to increase absorption and delay excretion of carcinogenic agents.[230] There is evidence that asbestos may be acting as a cocarcinogen with cigarette smoke, perhaps through the action of benzpyrene.[210] Death rates for lung cancer in asbestos workers who smoke are tenfold higher than in nonsmoking workers.[129] Possible mechanisms accounting for the synergistic carcinogenic effect of asbestos and cigarette smoke are summarized elsewhere.[67] The incidence of lung cancer is fivefold higher in exposed workers than in comparable nonsmokers not exposed to asbestos.[129] Pleural and peritoneal mesotheliomas are uncommon except in workers exposed to asbestos.[46] In one series of 144 cases, peritoneal mesothelioma exceeded the incidence of pleural mesothelioma.[46] The risk of developing a respiratory malignancy is enhanced by exposure to crocidolite.[322] The incidence of carcinoma of the gastrointestinal tract also appears to be higher than expected,[88, 166, 277, 278] although the carcinogenic potential appears to be low. In animal experiments, ingested chrysotile fail to induce neoplasm or any other lesion in the gastrointestinal tract.[127] There is conflicting evidence that transmigration of asbestos occurs through the gastrointestinal mucosa.[298] Generally a latent period of more than 20 years elapses before malignancies, including mesotheliomas, are detected;[275, 285, 316] however, the interval between first exposure to asbestos and death from mesothelioma has been reported to be as short as 3½ years.[124] Crocidolite is more fibrogenic than other types of asbestos[323, 324] and is also the principal fiber associated with mesothelioma,[316] although the intrapleural injection of many varieties of asbestos in animals can cause mesothelioma.[279, 315] A minimum intensity of exposure is necessary, regardless of duration, for the development of a mesothelioma. Some cases are reported with exposure as short as two days,[55] or several weeks.[45, 124] After this initial threshold is passed, the evidence for a dose response relationship is not as unequivocal as it is for lung cancer. Some reports have concluded that a definite dose relationship exists,[179, 232, 282, 330] while others have reached an opposite conclusion.[124, 194] Exposure to less than 100 fibers per year has not been shown to be associated with an excess risk of any respiratory malignancy.[322]

Environmental Recommendations

There is insufficient information at present to establish a definitive environmental standard for asbestos. More data are required regarding the various biologic effects of the different types of asbestos, as well as the possible variable effects of fibers of different sizes. It appears that dust control that is adequate to prevent asbestosis may not be adequate to prevent mesothelioma, since an exposure value of zero is impracticable to achieve.

Dose-response relationships (mppcf multiplied by years of exposure) are more meaningful than threshold limit values. The increase in mortality due to pneumoconiosis or cancer appears to be confined to workers with an exposure of 400[194]; however, "asbestosis" is more than ten times more common than in controls after 60 mppcf-year exposures.[224] Less exposure may not be associated with fibrosis.[324]

The United States Department of Health, Education, and Welfare classification of asbestos dust categories is outlined in Table 14–1 in terms of fibers greater than 5 μ in length per milliliter, with the warning that "conversion of data from mppcf to fibers/ml in all asbestos operations can only be done with considerable risk to the validity of the results."[306]

TABLE 14–1.
HEW Classification of Asbestos Dust Categories

DUST CATEGORY	CONCENTRATION AVERAGED OVER 3 MONTHS (FIBERS/ML)
Negligible	0– 0.4
Low	0.5– 1.9
Medium	2.0–10.0
High	>10.0

The Occupational Safety and Health Administration (OSHA) recommends that asbestos dust be collected with a personal sampling pump and that fibers be counted microscopically at 400–450 magnification using phase contrast illumination. The OSHA permissible level is 0.2 fibers/ml greater than 5 μ in length for an eight-hour time-weighted average airborne concentration. The National Institute of Occupational Safety and Health (NIOSH) recommended level is 0.1 fiber/ml, although current methods of measurement may not be capable of distinguishing between the two concentrations at these levels. The peak concentration recommended by NIOSH is 0.5 fibers/ml based on a 15-minute sampling period.

When it is necessary to work in "high dust" areas, an approved mask should be worn. Other work practices[306] should ensure that asbestos cement, mortar, coatings, grout, and plaster be mixed in closed bags or other containers. Asbestos waste and scrap should be collected and disposed of in sealed containers. Near the mines, roadways in open pits should be treated to reduce dust. Storage piles of ore should be moistened and waste dumps treated as well. In the mills, efficient exhaust ventilation and wet cleaning methods should be employed. In other industries, local exhaust systems at points of generation of dust, such as adjacent to hand-powered tools, is effective. The spraying of asbestos in building construction should be prohibited.[123] Well-made disposable overalls are acceptable and suitable for preventing contamination of work clothes.

COAL WORKER'S PNEUMOCONIOSIS

Coal worker's pneumoconiosis (CWP) is a disorder resulting from exposure to respirable dust generated in coal mining operations. The prolonged retention of dust in the lungs presumably is responsible for the ensuing tissue reactions.[177, 259] There are four ranks of coal found in the United States—lignite, subbituminous, bituminous, and anthracite—and essentially three mining methods: underground, strip mining, and augering.[270] Underground miners are exposed to the highest dust concentration, and the prevalence of pneumoconiosis and progressive disease is significantly higher in anthracite miners.[220] The dust is composed of a combination of carbon and varying percentages of silica (usually less than 10%). Little is known about the effects of other trace elements and organic constituents[104, 254] and nitrous fumes from explosives,[225] which are inhaled also.

Pathology

At necropsy, the lungs generally are gray-black. Discrete nodules can be seen and felt if the lungs are fixed in the inflated state. The cut surface of the lung reveals numerous pigmented foci 5 mm or more in diameter, which are referred to as the coal macule. They are often located in the vicinity of the respiratory bronchioles, which is of crucial importance and may explain some of the physiologic alterations described later. Microscopically, macrophages laden with black dust are seen enmeshed in fibrous tissue, predominantly reticulin with occasional strands of collagen, surrounding the respiratory bronchioles and adjacent alveolar structures.[158] The bronchioles become dilated as their walls rupture, pulmonary parenchyma is destroyed, and the percentage of lung tissue composed of abnormal air spaces increases, until there is complete disappearance of identifiable anatomical structures, and the capillary bed is reduced by the fenestrations. These changes have been termed "focal emphysema" and are not synonymous with the centrilobular (or, more appropriately, centriacinar) emphysema that occurs in other forms of emphysema not related to the inhalation of dust. Coal pigment can be seen between the bundles of smooth muscle in arteriolar walls, giving the appearance of vascular narrowing. The reduction in the capillary bed and hypoxia lead to pulmonary hypertension, right ventricular hypertrophy, heart failure, and cor pulmonale. Reduction of the pulmonary vascular bed alone does not lead to pulmonary hypertension until approximately two thirds to three quarters of the cross-sectional area is obstructed or destroyed. These are the pathologic changes that characterize "simple pneumoconiosis." At the time of death, approximately 30% of miners have more than one third of the lung involved with black dust amidst aggregates of stellate or spherical fibrosis. Of interest is the finding of distal focal and panlobular emphysema of equal incidence in miners and a control group of nonminers.[101] Lesions similar to silicotic nodules may be produced from exposure to mine dust containing a high quartz content,[73] but high quartz levels do not always produce silicotic nodules. In contrast to this, "complicated pneumoconiosis" is characterized by massive fibrosis, which usually is progressive and found predominantly in the upper lobes. These large masses are made up of irregular bundles of heavily pigmented black connective tissue and, unlike in silicosis, do not result from the aggregation of discrete micronodular tissue. In some cases, the silica content may be related to the development of progressive massive fibrosis (PMF),[73] although quartz was almost completely absent from the lungs of carbon electrode workers with PMF.[317] On the other hand, exposure to activated carbon alone for many years is not associated with the development of significant fibrosis even in the presence of radiographic evidence of dust.[319] Superimposed tuberculosis has been implicated in the development of PMF;[147] however, the reduction in the incidence of tuberculosis has not been accompanied by an expected reduction in PMF. Approximately 1%–2% of patients with simple pneumoconiosis still develop PMF each year,[177] the likelihood of which increases with age and rising radiographic category of simple pneumoconiosis.[283] There are animal studies suggesting that atypical mycobacteria can induce lesions similar to those seen in PMF.[118] Occasionally, the conglomerate masses cavitate due to ischemic necrosis,[301] and the cavity contains an ink-like, nonpurulent fluid of a maple syrup consistency.

Rheumatoid pneumoconiosis (Caplan's syndrome)[52] refers to the rapid development of nodules measuring 0.3–5.0 cm in diameter, distributed throughout both lung fields, in the presence of little or no radiographic evidence of pneumoconiosis (see below), associated with an elevated titer of rheumatoid factor or clinical rheumatoid arthritis. The nodules are characterized by concentric rings of active inflammation, necrosis, and coal dust. The severity and extent of the reaction are not related to the severity of the arthritis. There is recent evidence that rheumatoid factor, tuberculoprotein or another humoral factor in rheumatoid arthritis interacts with the dust in the lungs, producing the characteristic nodule.[26] The presence of autoantibodies in CWP may be a consequence of dust exposure and unrelated to the pathogenesis of PMF,[243] but a correlation exists between autoantibodies and age, extent of exposure,[260] and advancing radiographic category, which becomes more striking when the presence of rheumatoid factor is detected as well.[292]

Chest Roentgenogram

Extraordinary emphasis has been placed on the roentgenogram of the chest because of the fact that CWP cannot be diagnosed during life in the absence of radiographic changes. Categorization of the degree and nature of abnormalities has represented a great advance in standardization of the features of the chest roentgenogram in pneumoconioses.[64] Definite radiographic evidence of pneumoconiosis depends more on years underground than on age.[171] Little change is seen with less than ten years of exposure in the mine. The radiographic abnormalities usually correlate with the amount of dust in the lungs,[257] with postmortem anatomical measurement of dust macules and nodules, their silica and collagen content,[53, 228] and the duration and intensity of exposure.[141] In contrast to round opacities, the presence and extent of irregular opacities is associated with cigarette smoking, bronchitis, age, years worked underground,[3, 63] morbidity, and presence of emphysema.[180, 190] The percentage of working and retired miners with roentgenographic signs of pneumoconiosis is higher with anthracite miners (40%) than with bituminous coal miners (25%).[192, 193, 220] Only 40% of miners with pneumoconiosis are in category 3.[219]

The earliest roentgenographic changes consist of the appearance of a lace-like reticular pattern that later progresses to the micronodular stage of "simple pneumoconiosis." The nodules are between 1 and 10 mm in diameter and are not as distinct or homogeneous as those found in silicosis.

Many working miners have shortness of breath that occasionally is severe and is accompanied by pulmonary function abnormalities and a chest roentgenogram that reveals no evidence of a pneumoconiosis.[143] These miners may not have CWP, although it should be recognized that the shadow pattern of small opacities in CWP may not be seen in the presence of advanced generalized emphysema because of the increased lucency of the lung fields. There also is a great deal of observer variation in the interpretation of the chest roentgenogram in this disease.[5, 255]

The appearance of massive lesions, usually occurring in the upper lung fields and occasionally occupying an entire lobe, is characteristic of PMF. Cavitation usually is due to ischemic necrosis[301] or anaerobic infection[74]; however, superimposed tuberculosis, a fungal infection, or lung abscess should be considered also. Multiple areas of calcification may be noted throughout the large conglomerate mass when tuberculosis without cavitation is present. When the masses are unilateral, they may resemble bronchogenic carcinoma.

Involvement of the pleura is manifested by generalized thickening, obliteration of the costophrenic sulci and, occasionally, pleural plaques. Pleural calcification is a rare occurrence in CWP.[233]

Clinical Manifestations

Symptoms that miners and ex-miners develop are indistinguishable from those characteristically found in other chronic obstructive lung diseases, particularly chronic bronchitis. The prominent features include a chronic cough productive of mucoid, often coal-flecked sputum, frequent exacerbations of cough associated with purulent sputum, wheezing, and progressively worsening dyspnea. Clubbing and hemoptysis are not common, and their presence should suggest a coexistent disease.

Cigarette smoking is a cause of chronic bronchitis. When the cigarette-smoking miner with a chest roentgenogram compatible with CWP develops chronic bronchitis, it is impossible to determine whether the inhalation of dust or smoking is more responsible for the symptoms. This question is of importance for the purpose of compensation for occupational disability but it makes little difference as far as management is concerned. The symptoms are just as disabling for the miner, whether or not he had smoked cigarettes, as they are for any other patient with chronic obstructive pulmonary disease; however, a coal miner with emphysema may be eligible to receive disability benefits which are denied to other workers with comparable disability who never worked in a mine.[17] The occupational exposure is of importance in the interpretation of the chest roentgenogram and for anticipating complications (see below). The theme of compensation has assumed a prominent position in the whole subject of CWP and occasionally appears to be an end in itself.

In contrast to complicated pneumoconiosis, symptomatology and life expectancy in miners with simple pneumoconiosis is not significantly different from miners without pneumoconiosis.[135, 237] Simple pneumoconiosis rarely progresses if the worker is removed from the dusty environment.[103]

Dyspnea invariably is present in complicated pneumoconiosis, and its progression parallels the roentgenographic changes. The expectoration of sputum that resembles black ink is virtually pathognomonic of complicated pneumoconiosis and usually occurs when a large mass undergoes ischemic necrosis. Pulmonary tuberculosis or a lung abscess should be considered in the differential diagnosis when cavitary masses are seen on the chest roentgenogram. Eventually cor pulmonale ensues.[14] Miners have a higher than expected mortality due to emphysema, asthma, tuberculosis, and, surprisingly, carcinoma of the stomach. The relationship between lung cancer and CWP is controversial and inconclusive.[258]

Pulmonary Function Tests

Airway obstruction is the most frequently encountered abnormality of pulmonary function in coal miners.[143] It was mentioned previously that in simple pneumoconiosis, the pathologic changes occur predominantly around small airways; the physiologic effect of this is assuming increasingly greater attention. Because the early lesion in CWP is located in the small peripheral airways, the defect may not be detected by routine spirometric indices such as the FEV_1 and the FEV_1/FVC percent.[137] The residual volume is increased at an early stage, presumably due to small-airway closure rather than significant alveolar destruction, and increases with radiographic category.[178, 221, 234] The fall in pulmonary compliance with increasing frequency of respiration (frequency-dependent compliance) has been found in simple pneumoconiosis and appears to be the result of small-airway disease.[173] There is conflicting data as to whether lung mechanics is altered even up to category 2 CWP,[172, 223] but a reduction in the diffusion capacity has been demonstrated.[4] Exercise arterial blood gas analysis fails to detect a greater number of disabled workers than ventilatory studies alone.[218]

There is relatively good correlation between dyspnea, years spent underground, and the presence of airway obstruction,[143] and at virtually every level of cigarette smoking, an increasing number of years underground was associated with a decrease in expiratory flow rates. In simple pneumoconiosis, the chest roentgenogram does not reflect the magnitude of any ventilatory impairment.

Progressive massive fibrosis is accompanied by significant airway obstruction and large increases in the residual volume. The compliance is not altered in a predictable manner in each patient. As progressive fibrosis occurs, compliance may decrease, and as emphysema becomes significant, compliance may increase. In virtually all subjects with PMF, compliance still remains frequency dependent.

The diffusion capacity depends on many factors and can be reduced in simple pneumoconiosis, probably on the basis of a mismatch in ventilation and perfusion.[189] If the mismatch is severe enough, there may be a widening of the alveolar-arterial oxygen tension difference, and eventually hypoxemia may occur. Most miners with complicated pneumoconiosis have a reduction in the diffusion capacity. Pulmonary vascular resistance and pulmonary artery pressure during exercise are both increased in approximately half of miners with conglomerate nodules in the absence of airway obstruction. The magnitude of the increase is proportional to the loss of vital capacity.[266]

Treatment

The simple pneumoconioses are infrequently accompanied by symptoms, and treatment usually is not necessary. All workers with simple pneumoconiosis should be recalled for routine radiography. Occasionally a man is seen who shows widespread simple pneumoconiosis after only a short period in the mine (less than ten years). Such a man appears to be a hyperreactor to coal mine dust and should be advised to leave the industry.

Coal workers with PMF should be evaluated for active pulmonary tuberculosis with sputum smears and culture. Studies performed more than a decade ago reveal that only 2% of the workers with PMF had the tubercle bacillus in their sputum, and approximately 40% had the organism cultured at necropsy. Acid-fast bacilli were found on smear and culture in more than half of the patients when cavities were present in the large conglomerate masses.[301] Because of the difficulty in isolating the tubercle bacillus in PMF in the absence of cavitation, an argument can be made for treating all such tuberculin-positive miners for active tuberculosis. The outcome of treatment of tuberculosis in coal workers is as favorable as in the general population, particularly if the original regimen includes Rifampin.[150] Guidelines exist for the prophylactic use of Isoniazid.[7]

It is probable that the progression of simple pneumoconiosis to PMF may be averted by removing the miner from further exposure to coal dust.[177] Miners with a chest roentgenogram that reveals numerous small opacities that obscure the normal markings, e.g., category 3,[64] should be considered for work in areas that do not have high exposure to dust.

It is clear that miners who smoke cigarettes have more symptoms than do nonsmoking miners. The reduction of cigarette smoking is as important for the miner for the prevention of lung disease as ventilation and other environmental controls are in the mines. The failure to discontinue cigarette smoking once symptoms have developed is inexcusable.

The management of symptomatic patients with CWP is, in many respects, similar to that for other patients with chronic bronchitis and emphysema. Bronchospasm can be relieved with oral and topical bronchodilators. Bacteria are responsible for lower-respiratory infections in approximately half of the episodes, and the organisms most frequently responsible are *pneumoniae* and *Hemophilis influenzae*. When an antibiotic is required, ampicillin often is used because both of these organisms are sensitive to this agent. Approximately 5% of *D. pneumoniae* may be resistant to tetracycline.[122] If heart failure is present, the cautious administration of digitalis and diuretics is warranted with a low-salt diet. When hypoxemia is severe, low-flow oxygen can be administered using the established guidelines of the American College of Chest Physicians.[6] The effect of polyvinyl pyridine-N-oxide (PVNO) remains experimental in animals. When aerosolized in high concentration, fibrosis can be reduced.[329] The intravenous administration of PVNO in animals is of no therapeutic value once fibrosis occurs.[328]

Since treatment of coal worker's pneumoconiosis is not likely ever to be effective, prevention becomes the paramount concern.

Environmental Recommendations

Any program to prevent death and disability from CWP first requires identification of the high-risk areas in which workers are exposed to the highest concentrations of respirable dust. Dust-collecting techniques are not simple.[188] Ventilation and other environmental control measures then are employed to reduce the respirable dust to a standard that is in compliance with the Federal Coal Mine Health and Safety Act of 1969, which requires the operator of each coal mine in the United States to maintain an average concentration of respirable dust at or below 2 mg/cu m.

Respirator equipment is recommended for all persons exposed to concentrations of dust in excess of the levels required to be maintained by law; however, in view of the infrequency with which this type of equipment is used, it should not be substituted for environmental control.

In general, control measures that reduce respirable dust are limited to water and ventilation. Water infused into the coal seam has produced limited results. Water sprays are employed extensively throughout the coal mining industry to abate concentrations of total airborne dust as well as respirable dust. To reduce respirable dust, water sprays must produce a very fine mist to be effective on particles 1 μ or less in size. This procedure has not been completely successful. It has become increasingly apparent that the most significant parameter affecting the abatement of respirable dust is ventilation.[270]

All persons in the coal industry should have a preemployment medical examination, including a chest roentgenogram and pulmonary function studies. These examinations should be repeated at least at five-year intervals.

SILICOSIS

Pneumoconiosis resulting from exposure to silica may be the "commonest, best known, and most extensively studied of all occupational diseases of the lung."[48] Exposure to silicon dioxide sufficient to result in pneumoconiosis occurs in persons in a wide variety of occupations, including foundry workers,[195] granite workers,[128] miners of gold and silver,[203] workers in the ceramics industry[71] and in the manufacture of grinding wheels,[252] and in diatomaceous earth workers.[84] A mixed-dust pneumoconiosis may occur from the inhalation of silica and iron oxide, alumina, graphite, and possibly talc. The Occupational Safety and Health Administration estimates that in the United States, more than 1.1 million employees are exposed to the hazard created by the inhalation of silica dust. It is beyond the scope of this section to describe the prevalence of silicosis within each occupation in every industry. Suffice it to state that a careful occupational history is necessary to evaluate the hazard in each worker, recognizing that there are varying degrees of danger and dust in different jobs in the same industry and that the danger varies within the industry, depending on dust control methods and the length and intensity of exposure. Individual susceptibility may be genetically determined.[168]

Particles of silica larger than 5 μ in diameter are almost entirely eliminated by the nose, pharynx, trachea, and bronchi. Dust between 0.5 and 5 μ in diameter can float in the air and is likely to be retained in the lung if inhaled. Particles below 1 μ in size may present the greatest danger.

Pathology

At necropsy, pleural adhesions usually are found. The affected lung is gray and studded with white nodules. The cut surface often reveals total replacement of the normal architecture with hard, dense nodules predominantly in the upper lobes and perihilar regions. The nodules usually are 2–3 mm in diameter in the early stages. As the disease progresses, they coalesce, forming a continuous mass of fibrous tissue. This stage of massive conglomerate nodular silicosis differs from progressive massive fibrosis, which refers to a progressively enlarging mass, often occupying an entire lobe and not composed of discrete nodules. Cavitation of the massive lesions occurs occasionally and is due to ischemic necrosis, tuberculosis, or a superimposed lung abscess. The earliest lesions are seen in the region of the respiratory bronchioles. Local blood vessels and lymphatics become obliterated by infiltration with dust-laden macrophages and granulation tissue. Histologically, the silicotic nodule consists of a relatively acellular, avascular core of hyalinized reticulin fibers arranged concentrically and blending with collagen fibers toward the periphery, which has well-defined borders. The particles of silica responsible for the reaction are weakly birefringent and can be visualized under polarized light if they exceed 1 μ in diameter. Silica in the lung can be identified by x-ray defraction studies and by incinerating a portion of the lung and analyzing the ash. The silica content of the normal lung should not exceed 0.2% dry weight. The association between tuberculosis and silicosis occurs too often to be coincidental, and it now is generally accepted that silicosis predisposes to tuberculosis.[296]

A relatively new technique of scanning electron microscopy together with energy dispersive x-ray analysis has been used for the identification of fibrogenic metals[284] and silica.[107, 108, 110] This technique is of great value, because very small sections of lung tissue are required and the histopathology is not altered by the analytic procedure.

The classic whorled silicotic nodule occurs in the lungs of workers exposed to dust containing a high proportion of respirable free silica. For many years, it was believed that fibrosis in the lung could not be attributed to silica unless the classic nodule could be found on lung biopsy. There is substantial evidence that workers who inhale mixed dusts containing a small proportion (under 10%) of free silica may also develop a nodular fibrosis, but it does not resemble the classic whorled nodule. The reticular and collagenous fibers are arranged in a linear fashion, giving the nodule an irregular or stellate configuration. This type of reaction has been described in siderosilicosis,[96, 195] bauxite fume pneumoconiosis,[335] graphite pneumoconiosis,[186] and possibly talcosis[273] as well as coal worker's pneumoconiosis (see preceding section). In each of these abnormalities, silica and additional dusts are inhaled. They are discussed in subsequent sections in this chapter.

Pathogenesis

The initiating event in the development of silicosis appears to be the death of dust-laden macrophages, with the subsequent release of silica and an unidentified substance that stimulates fibroblastic activity.[133] This is associated with an increase in macrophage lipid peroxidase, which may injure lung tissue through a free radical mechanism.[112] The collagen is then hyalinized with a protein that is rich in gamma globulin; antinuclear antibody has been found in silicotic sandblasters and is related to the presence of large opacities on the chest roentgenogram;[151] and there is a higher than expected incidence of systemic lupus erythematosus in sandblasters,[15] suggesting that an immunologic process may be responsible for the propagation of fibrosis. The released silica particle may be ingested by another macrophage, self-perpetuating the process, although it appears that freshly deposited quartz presents the greatest hazard. There are practical implications if this theory is correct. If the magnitude of the initial event is sufficient, the fibrosis may proceed even when further exposure to silica ceases.[313] Recurrent bronchopulmonary infections enhance the development of silicosis,[61] and in animals, the addition of sodium glutamate to the drinking water favorably modifies the cytogenic action of quartz.[222]

Chest Roentgenogram

The duration of dust exposure before the development of radiologic evidence of silicosis is variable and may be as short as two years[48, 207] but usually is between 10 and 20 years.[241] There is evidence for a humoral phase of silicosis, which precedes by several years any radiographic abnormalities.[311]

The earliest silicotic nodules are not visible even with the best roentgenographic studies.[68] In most cases, the nodulation that characterizes the roentgenographic evidence of silicosis results from superimposition of small, multiple shadows 2–6 mm in diameter. The nodules are not uniform in size or shape and usually are very uniform in density but may be modified by infection or the presence of other dusts.[124, 244] Once nodulation appears, it usually will progress, even if the worker avoids further exposure to dust.[125] In some instances, the earliest detectable abnormality is a lace-like reticular pattern that may become coarser without demonstration of any nodulation as the disease progresses.[236] The reticular and nodular stages are referred to as "simple" silicosis. The large lesions (1–20 cm in diameter) that are seen in "complicated" pneumoconiosis usually result from the combination or coalescence of discrete nodules and generally migrate toward the hilum. Some of these massive lesions may involve an entire lobe or more than one lobe.[244]

The rapid development of soft nodulation, especially in the upper lobes, the appearance of massive densities (particularly with cavitation), and signs of endobronchial obstruction or pleural fluid may indicate superimposed tuberculosis;[38, 244, 289] however, as the prevalence of tuberculosis declines, the pathogenesis of cavitary silicosis often will be on an ischemic basis.[54] In silicotuberculosis, there is no relationship between radiologic appearance and bacteriologic status[38] unless cavitation is present. Calcification of massive lesions usually is regarded as evidence of tuberculosis.[244]

Hilar and paratracheal lymph nodes may be enlarged and occasionally contain calcium, which can be deposited in an irregular fashion or in such a way as to produce an eggshell appearance.[244] The eggshell calcification, which may occur in the abdominal lymph nodes also, is virtually pathognomonic of silicosis and is reported only as an extremely rare occurrence in sarcoidosis.[145, 198, 304]

Clinical Manifestations

The worker with simple silicosis usually is asymptomatic, and even the early stages of massive fibrosis are not associated with signs or symptoms.[174] The earliest symptom to appear is shortness of breath, which progressively worsens. Chronic bronchitis and airway obstruction are related to dust exposure at any level of cigarette smoking.[331] As massive fibrosis progresses, pulmonary hypertension develops and, eventually, cor pulmonale. Functional abnormalities may result which may not be clinically apparent,[227] but routine pulmonary function tests usually are normal until the onset of dyspnea, at which time an impairment may be found, with features of obstruction and restriction. Small airway obstruction independent of the radiographic extent of silicosis has been underestimated.[144] An elevation in the residual volume reflects pulmonary overdistention and possible air-trapping. The alveolar-arterial oxygen gradient may be widened and hypoxemia may be present after exercise and eventually at rest. Hypercapnia is a late manifestation.[20]

Silica has been shown to impair the ability of macrophages to inhibit the growth of tubercle bacilli,[289] explaining the higher than expected incidence of typical and atypical tuberculosis in sandblasters[15] and perhaps infection with other opportunistic organisms as well. Evaluation for pulmonary tuberculosis is indicated when suspicious radiographic changes are noted. Multiple sputum specimens are often necessary to confirm the diagnosis because of the high incidence of false negative smears and cultures attributed to inaccessibility of tuberculous foci to the airways because of fibrosis.[289] In addition to tuberculin skin testing, multiple sputum specimens should be obtained, the smears should be examined for acid-fast bacilli, and the specimens should be cultured. Tuberculosis should be highly suspected when cavitary lesions are seen on the chest roentgenogram. The lesions of silicotuberculosis progress very slowly and there may be little roentgenographic change over a period of years. There is no evidence that silicosis will impair the effectiveness of adequate chemotherapy for tuberculosis,[156] particularly if Rifampin is included in the regimen, but the degree of radiologic improvement is negligible in most cases. A one-year course of isoniazid is recommended for all tuberculin-positive individuals who do not have active tuberculosis,[7] although it may be less efficacious than with the general population. Occasionally, tuberculosis may reactivate in workers with silicosis after an adequate course of chemotherapy has been completed, and it has been suggested that the indefinite continuation of INH is justified.[215]

There is an acute form of silicosis that has several distinguishing characteristics. The duration of exposure necessary to produce an abnormal roentgenogram may be as short as nine months.[207] The onset of symptoms is abrupt rather than insidious and may occur after only 17 months' exposure.[48, 207] The clinical course is fulminating, strikingly short, and fatal, occasionally associated with massive proteinuria, renal failure,[119] and an autoimmune syndrome.[299] The histologic changes resemble alveolar proteinosis,[16, 48] and, if survival is long enough, typical silicotic nodules may appear.[119]

The management of the symptomatic worker with silicosis is similar to that outlined under Coal Worker's Pneumoconiosis. It should be emphasized that the hyperreactor to silica should be advised to leave the industry. Aerosols of aluminum chlorhydroxyallantoinate and, to a lesser extent, aluminum hydroxide protect animals against the fibrogenic action of quartz, perhaps by coating the particles with a protective layer or by preventing the quartz-macrophage interaction.[175]

Environmental Recommendations

The determination of a safe threshold limit value for silica is difficult because of the multitude of unknown variables—for example, the assessment of the pathogenicity of various kinds of silica, the effect of concomitant exposure to other dusts, and the variability of individual response. This is complicated by these facts: the rate of clearance of respirable silica is not known; the

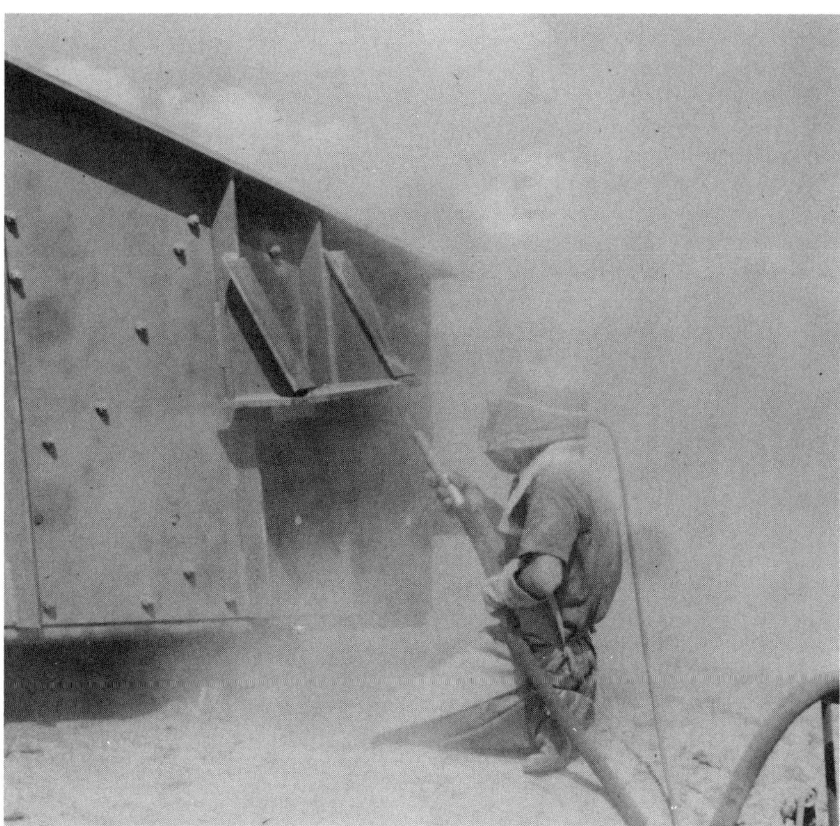

FIG 14–2.
Sand blasting rust and scale—a very dusty job. Generation of great quantities of silica dust requires complete respiratory protection using air-supplied respiratory equipment.

TABLE 14–2.
Crystalline SiO_2 in Various Materials*

MATERIAL	NORMAL RANGE CRYSTALLINE SiO_2 (IN PERCENT)
Foundry molding sand	50–90
Pottery ware body	15–25
Brick & tile compositions	10–35
Buffing wheel dressings	0–60
Road rock	0–80
Limestone (agricultural)	0–3
Feldspar	12–25
Clay	0–40
Mica	0–10
Talc	0–5
Slate and shale	5–15

*Courtesy of Julian Olishifski, National Safety Council, Chicago.

difference between a short, heavy exposure is not equivalent to a longer, intense exposure, although the total exposure may be identical; and, finally, the clearance of the quartz fraction that causes silicosis is negligible, as a result of which, fibrosis may progress perhaps for the rest of life even if exposure is terminated.[146] It is beyond the scope of this section to detail specific environmental control recommendations for each of the industries in which exposure to silica presents a significant hazard. In general, it is advisable to segregate operations in enclosed areas where silica is used. This should be coupled with efficient local exhaust ventilation. In the mining industry, wetting operations should be employed where feasible. In some instances, the substitution of other materials may eliminate the hazard, such as using steel shot or alumina grit in place of sandblasting (Fig 14–2). The Occupational Safety and Health Administration recommends measuring respirable silica using personal sampling pumps with filters. The collected dust then can be weighted for a given volume of air. For respirable quartz particles, both OSHA and the American Conference of Governmental Industrial Hygienists (ACGIH) in 1986 defined the threshold limit value (TLV) by the formula:

$$\frac{10 \text{ mg/cu m}}{\%SiO_2 + 2}$$

The percentage of crystalline SiO_2 in several materials is shown in Table 14–2.

SIDEROSIS AND SIDEROSILICOSIS

Siderosis is caused by the inhalation of relatively pure iron oxide, often as an extremely fine particulate fume produced during the cutting or burning of steel or iron. Welders, torch cutters, and sinterers constitute the majority of workers exposed to this dust. A finely divided form of iron oxide can be inhaled during the final polishing of silver.[196]

There is evidence that little if any pulmonary fibrosis is found at necropsy,[130] and virtually no pulmonary impairment develops clinically if the inhalation of iron oxide is not accompanied by silica or other elements. The roentgenographic abnormalities are largely a result of the fact that the iron oxide is opaque to the x-ray, and increased linear reticular markings and a fine stippling, mottling nodularity may be seen. The abnormalities on the roentgenogram actually may regress if the welder who has been working with an innocuous rod changes his or her occupation or the exposure to the fumes is reduced.[76] The presence of cough, wheezing, and abnormal small airway function is higher in welders than in controls and is enhanced by cigarette smoking. Smokers who do not weld have wheezing as often as welders who do not smoke.[238] Absence from work due to lower respiratory tract disease is higher in welders than in controls and is also enhanced by smoking.[97] Welders who smoke have abnormal spirograms twice as often as smokers who do not weld and 1½ times as often as welders who do not smoke. The cumulative effect of cigarette smoke and welding fumes thus is similar to that in other pneumoconioses.[140] It is difficult to believe that the lung can sustain deposition of unlimited quantities of iron oxide without incurring some demonstrable impairment. It was emphasized previously that the spirogram is relatively insensitive for the detection of small-airway disease, and more sensitive tests often are warranted, such as closing volumes and exercise arterial blood gas and compliance studies. Arc welders with dyspnea who had relatively normal spirometry were shown to have a reduction in both static and dynamic compliance.[294] During the sintering process, finely milled magnetite ore is converted to iron oxide by burning the ore with a small amount of powdered coal. Sinterers exposed for more than 25 years to low levels (5–10 mppcf) of predominantly iron oxide fumes (80% iron oxide, 8% silicates, 2% free silica) do not develop signs or symptoms of pulmonary disease nor could their pulmonary function studies be distinguished from controls.[163]

During the welding process, high temperatures cause metals to melt and boil, then unite at their points of contact. Electric arc welding has changed from using a base metal electrode on ferrous metals to using coated electrodes on alloy steels and nonferrous metals, such as aluminum, cupronickel, copper, brass, and bronze. The composition of the electrodes is a closely guarded trade secret and varies according to the metals being joined, but virtually all contain sodium silicate as a binding agent. As a result, the fumes created in the welding process contain the oxides of titanium, manganese, magnesium, aluminum, and copper as well as silica and ozone.[130, 206] Studies of welders' lungs have been concerned predominantly with the effect of iron oxide, but the inhalation of mixed dusts containing iron oxide and silica or iron oxide and other elements can lead to a mixed-dust pneumoconiosis characterized by pulmonary fibrosis.[12, 206]

It was emphasized previously that pulmonary interstitial fibrosis can result from the inhalation of iron oxide containing a small portion of silica, which might occur in workers who clean iron castings and in boiler scalers or in welders and torch cutters who work in foundries. Welding in a closed, poorly ventilated space is particularly hazardous.[106, 130, 217]

The ACGIH in 1986 has recommended that the total fume concentration should not exceed 5 mg/cu m in the breathing zone of the welder or others in the area.

Iron oxide and silica are also inhaled during the mining of iron ore. During the mining process, high-speed pneumatic drills produce a cloud of fine particles that is blown back into the miner's face. Blasting produces more dust, and since there is no gas problem, the men could return to work in an atmosphere so cloudy that a lamp could not be seen at a distance of 6 ft. In one study,[96] chemical analysis of the lungs of miners revealed high quantities of iron oxide (33%–39% of ash) and silica (5.5%–9.2% of ash). At necropsy, more than half the lungs revealed fibrosis, and in half of these there was coexistent tuberculosis. The degree of fibrosis was not related to the time spent underground nor to the amount of iron or silica present. Of considerable interest was that carcinoma of the lung was increased also. Subsequently, the radioactivity in the air in the mines was found to be elevated.[36] It still is not clear whether iron oxide is carcinogenic in man;[21, 181] however, there is evidence that inhaled iron oxide alone or in combination with other dusts causes lung cancer in mice.[49, 50, 51]

Long-term exposure to low levels of dust (5.0–7.5 mppcf) in magnetite miners also can produce a pneumoconiosis on the basis of sustained inhalation of iron oxide, free silica, and silicates.[163, 216]

GRAPHITE

Graphite, like diamond, is a crystalline form of carbon. Unlike diamond, it is quite soft, conducts electricity, has a melting point close to 4000° C, and is insoluble in all common solvents. Because of its inertness and infusibility, approximately 75% of the crucibles now made in the United States are composed of silicon carbide and graphite bonded with carbon. In the electrochemical industry, it is used for electrodes at which chlorine is to be liberated. Other conductors either interact chemically with chlorine or are too expensive for large-scale use. Nonconducting plaster casts are coated with graphite, giving them a conducting surface on which metals (copper or silver) can be deposited by electrolysis. The ease with which layers of atoms of the crystalline graphite can slide over one another makes it an excellent lubricant. Large quantities of graphite are used for foundry facings, recarburizing steel, and manufacturing paints, roofing compounds, and fuller brushes. It is the main ingredient in the high-grade carbon brushes of electric motors. When mixed with varying amounts of clay, it forms the "lead" in pencils. Natural graphite usually contains impurities, such as mica, silica, and iron oxide.

For many years it was believed that the inert properties of graphite extended to the lung, but now it is well recognized that safety precautions are necessary for all workers exposed to natural graphite, whether it be mined or processed. Further work is necessary to determine the prevalence of pneumoconiosis in graphite workers. With few exceptions, it was generally believed that silica was the offending agent for the pathologic changes in the lung caused by the inhalation of natural graphite. Of considerable interest is a report[180] of a worker who spent 17 years grinding synthetic graphite bars. He developed a pneumoconiosis, progressively worsening cough and dyspnea, and deteriorating pulmonary function tests; and eventually he died. At necropsy, the lungs revealed the typical findings of graphite pneumoconiosis reported by others.[245, 246] Of great importance was the fact that the ashed material from the lung contained no silica, only carbon (8.8%–9.5%) and very small quantities of iron (0.36%) and magnesium (0.027%). It seems reasonable to conclude that pure graphite can cause a pneumoconiosis and clinical impairment and that when free silica is present, the toxic action of the graphite is enhanced, or inhaled natural graphite enhances the toxic action of silica.

The roentgenographic findings resemble those in coal worker's pneumoconiosis and silicosis. The earliest change may be the disappearance of normal vascular markings, with the appearance later of pinpoint and macronodular densities in all lung fields. Massive lesions of the type seen in progressive massive fibrosis may appear, which can cavitate, occasionally as a result of coexistent tuberculosis. The pleura often is involved, and pleural fluid, pleural thickening, and pneumothorax may be seen.[246]

At necropsy, the lungs are gray-black to black and have the appearance of sponges that have been soaked in ink. Widely scattered spicules and plates of graphite can be seen often within intra-alveolar macrophages amidst diffuse interstitial fibrosis and occasional chronic pneumonitis. Massive fibrotic lesions, often with liquefaction of the center, resemble those found in CWP. There also are interwoven bands of collagen resembling those found in silicosis, which occasionally are the most prominent feature of the fibrotic lesion and may involve the bronchial lymph nodes as well.[246]

The symptoms resemble those described for CWP and include dyspnea, cough, expectoration of black sputum, chest tightness, and occasionally pain. It is important to recognize that the clinical symptoms are not in direct proportion to the extent of changes on the chest roentgenogram.

Aluminum

Pneumoconiosis may occur due to the inhalation of aluminum or aluminum oxide in combination with other substances. A potentially lethal disease is associated with the manufacture of corundum, an extremely hard abrasive. The process begins by first grinding bauxite and mixing it with iron and coke. The mix then is shoveled into large metal pots, carbon electrodes are lowered to the surface, and fusion occurs at a temperature of 2,000° C generated by an arc between the electrodes. Further mix is added to the pot as needed. During the process, dense white fumes are produced that contain aluminum oxide, silica, and several other substances. The silica constitutes 29%–44% of the fume, and alumina, 41%–62%. All fatal cases have occurred in furnace feeders or crane operators.[335] It is likely that the disease produced by the inhalation of these fumes is a mixed-dust pneumoconiosis. The modifying influence that various dusts have on one another was mentioned previously in connection with graphite and silica and iron and silica.

In fatal cases, on gross examination the lungs were gun-metal gray in color. Widespread induration could be palpated. Bullae, some of which reached enormous size, were particularly prominent in the subpleural region. Pleural thickening was found commonly, as well as adhesions at the site of previous pneumothoraces. Histopathologic examination showed diffuse interstitial fibrosis. It has been postulated that the initial lesion is septal edema followed by fibroblastic proliferation, infiltration of round cells, and, eventually, deposition of collagen.[280] Obliterative endarteritis was seen most frequently in the regions of greatest fibrosis. Emphysematous blebs were found in the midst of the overwhelming fibrous tissue and were likely to rupture spontaneously, producing a pneumothorax. The quantity of silica in the lungs has varied between 21% and 31%, and alumina, between 25% and 41%.

The chest roentgenogram in the early stages revealed a fine lace-like reticular pattern that gradually became coarser as the disease progressed and was more pronounced in the upper lung fields. Hyperlucent areas and linear shadows marking the borders of bullae or cysts were quite characteristic. Pneumothorax was a common finding. The diaphragm was irregular and tenting was seen frequently. In some cases, the mediastinum was widened and the hilar shadows were partially obscured.[280]

Dyspnea was the most prominent symptom, beginning insidiously and progressing rapidly. Sudden attacks of extreme shortness of breath were not uncommon. Most patients complained of a cough productive of frothy mucoid sputum. Other symptoms included substernal discomfort, tightness in the chest, pleuritic chest pain, weakness, and fatigue. Physical findings included tachypnea, cyanosis, and respiratory distress in the advanced stages. Wheezes, rales, and rhonchi were variable findings. Clubbing has not been described.[280] The clinical course is one of short industrial exposure and rapid development of disease, producing serious disability and death.

Pulmonary fibrosis also may occur in workers exposed to a very fine aluminum powder that is used for fireworks and aluminum paint. The powders are produced by pounding the cold metal, creating a fine flake. The pounding process lasts for approximately 12 hours to produce powder for fireworks (pyro) and 24 hours to produce paint powder. Exposure to high concentrations of dust occurs when the machines are emptied and filled and during certain weighing and screening processes.[212] At the end of a working day, the workers often look like metal statues.[86]

The pathologic changes consisted of generalized interstitial fibrosis, predominantly in the upper lobes. Ragged particles of aluminum were found interspersed throughout the fibrotic tissue. Pleural thickening and adhesions were not uncommon.[197, 211, 212]

The chest roentgenogram revealed a reticular pattern that progressively became coarser. In some instances there was a superimposed nodular component. Pleural adhesions were noted occasionally.[86]

The striking feature of this disease was the rapid progression from the onset of signs and symptoms to death. This transition can take place over a two-year period.[86, 211] The most common symptom was progressively worsening dyspnea. Other symptoms included weight loss, tightness in the chest, and cough. There is a report that the dyspnea may improve if the symptomatic worker leaves the dusty environment, despite the fact that the chest roentgenogram does not improve.[86] Inhalation of vaporized aluminum has been reported to cause interstitial fibrosis in an arc welder,[309] and crystalline aluminum silicate has been associated with diffuse interstitial fibrosis and granuloma formation.[226]

TALC AND MICA

Different forms of pneumoconiosis have been described, depending upon the composition of the commercial talc.[325] In addition, the ore in the talc mines may have between 1% and 17% free silica.[205] In the United States, talc is used in the paint, rubber, and ceramic industries and in the manufacture of asphalt products, insecticides, dusting powders, and cosmetics. Pneumoconiosis has been described in workers connected with the mining and milling of commercial talc deposits[161, 205] and those utilizing[273] or abusing[229] the mill products.

Pathologic changes in the lung consist of massive fibrosis, totally altering the normal architecture. In some areas, large, heavily pigmented masses of fibrous tissue can be seen containing numerous birefringent particles, often within macrophages. Some of these masses may show central necrosis. Bronchi and bronchioles usually are dilated, forming cystic spaces. The vasculature often is obliterated by diffuse fibrosis and accompanied by endarteritis with intimal hyperplasia.[273]

The early changes on the chest roentgenogram consist of a reticular abnormality, particularly in the mid and lower lung fields, which may become nodular later. Occasionally the nodules may coalesce. Multiple bullae are seen not uncommonly. Pleural involvement is frequent, evidenced by obliteration of the costophrenic sinuses and the cardiac border and the appearance of pleural plaques,[71, 205, 273] which occasionally may calcify and resemble the findings in asbestosis. Nearly one third of the workers with more than 15 years' exposure have pleural abnormalities.[116] Roentgenographic evidence of pleural or parenchymal disease is not likely to occur with less than 15 years' exposure.

The major symptoms of cough, sputum production, and shortness of breath are more prevalent in smokers.[116] Physical findings include decreased breath sounds, basilar rales, and clubbing of the fingers and toes in the more advanced stages.[161, 164] Cor pulmonale is a major complication. Approximately 10%–15% of the talc miners and millers with more than 15 years' exposure will succumb to this disease or a complication or both.[161] There is conflicting evidence as to whether the incidence of lung cancer is higher than expected,[154, 161, 261] and the difference may be due to the influence of cigarette smoking.

Pulmonary function abnormalities indicate a restrictive impairment (decreased vital capacity and total lung capacity) and, to a lesser extent, airway obstruction and a diffusion defect reflecting impaired gas exchange. Except for the diffusion capacity, the degree of ventilatory impairment demonstrated in the laboratory does not correlate well with the clinical or roentgenographic findings.[164]

The establishment of wet drilling techniques has been successful in reducing dust in the mines, but dust control still is needed in the mills and in mines not utilizing wet drilling. Concentrations of dust less than 20 mppcf is probably adequate to prevent pneumoconiosis, but prolonged exposure to lower concentrations is associated with an increase in symptoms suggestive of chronic bronchitis, i.e., cough productive of sputum and, to a lesser extent, wheezing.[100] The current TLV for talc is 2 mg/cu m.

Mica is a complex silicate of potassium, aluminum, magnesium, calcium, and fluoride. Pneumoconiosis is a rare complication of exposure to mica that is almost identical to the other silicoses, talcosis, and asbestosis.

KAOLIN

Kaolin is a form of hydrated aluminum silicate ($Al_2O_3SiO_22H_2O$) that is used in several industries: paper, plastics, paint, ceramics, rubber, adhesives, insecticides, and fertilizers.[39] The quarried material is removed from the mines in large, moist lumps, and refining varies according to the quantity of sand and mica that is present. In the United States, the clay is almost entirely free from grit, whereas in England the impurities are first removed by differential sedimentation using a high-pressure water jet. The suspension of clay in water is passed through filter presses, where the water content is reduced to approximately 30%. Further drying occurs in kilns. Once the kaolin is dry, it presents a dust hazard that is greatest in the bagging and car-loading operations. The prevalence of pneumoconiosis in these workers rises from 6% in workers with 5–15 years' exposure to 23% in those exposed for more than 15 years.[281]

The roentgenogram is characterized by fine, discrete micronodular densities throughout both lungs. These lesions rarely have been associated with clinical evidence of impairment of pulmonary function;[39, 157, 281] however, the vital capacity may decline slightly with increasing radiographic evidence of pneumoconiosis.[235] Fewer than 1% of the abnormal roentgenograms reveal confluent massive densities similar to the lesions seen in progressive massive fibrosis in silicosis and CWP. This stage is accompanied by progressively worsening dyspnea and eventually may be fatal. Since so few workers develop this advanced stage of disease, necropsy findings are limited. The basic pathologic findings are dense fibrosis with destruction of the normal pulmonary architecture, pleural adhesions, and emphysematous blebs.[85]

The miners of China clay are not at risk because the clay is wet, but dust control is necessary in the bagging process and during crude bulk storing and loading. A TLV of 30 mppcf or 10 mg/cu m for kaolin was adopted by the ACGIH in 1986.

TONOKO

Tonoko is a fine powder used in Japan in the furniture industry to impart a durable, smooth surface to protect wooden furniture. It is a mixture of clay and varying amounts of kaolin, mica, and feldspar, containing 50% quartz. Prolonged exposure in the order of 12–40 years can produce diffuse nodular densities on the chest roentgenogram and a minor ventilatory impairment.[155]

HARD METAL

Hard metal is manufactured by combining tungsten and carbon, with cobalt as a binder. The product, which has 90%–95% the hardness of diamond, is used for cutting edges of tools and drills. The cobalt, tungsten carbide, small quantities of titanium, tantalum, or vanadium carbide and carbon are mixed wet and then dried. The dried powder then is shaped into the desired forms and eventually heated in an atmosphere of hydrogen (sintering). Final grinding is accomplished with diamond or carborundum wheels. Pneumoconiosis may occur in workers mixing and shaping the powder and during the final grinding processes. Dust control measures usually are very effective, because the material is valuable and contamination is undesirable.

The pathologic alteration is one of diffuse interstitial fibrosis and hyperplasia and metaplasia of the bronchial epithelium,[22, 14] usually after many years of exposure.

The chest roentgenogram reveals a marked reticular and micronodular abnormality throughout all lung fields in the advanced stages.

Hard-metal disease may begin abruptly, with little or no preceding respiratory symptoms. There is considerable variation in the length of exposure before symptoms develop. The major symptoms include dyspnea, tightness in the chest, wheezing, chest pain, cough, which occasionally is productive, and, rarely, hemoptysis. In most workers, the symptoms are mild, and some individuals report more distress toward the end of the working day.[22] Some workers report disappearance of symptoms during weekends away from work or during vacation periods,[47] suggesting a hypersensitivity mechanism. Bech and his colleagues[22] summarized most of the previous work on this subject and presented evidence that although the agent responsible for the disease is not known, cobalt is highly suspected, based on its known irritating properties and its ability to induce a chemical pneumonitis in animals and man. Tungsten and tungsten carbide have been found to be relatively inert in animal experiments. Silicon carbide is capable of producing symptoms, radiographic and pathologic changes similar to tungsten carbide.[109] There is also evidence that titanium compounds may be fibrogenic in man.[89]

FELDSPAR

Nepheline rock consists mainly of feldspar, which is composed of a mixture of the silicates of sodium, potassium, and aluminum. There is no free silicon dioxide. In industry, the rock is milled to a fine powder that is used for producing glazes for pottery. The inhalation of this dust can produce fibrosis, which eventually can lead to respiratory failure and death.[18]

CEMENT

Cement dust contains calcium silicate and calcium oxide, and workers who bag the finished product often work in extremely dusty atmospheres. The chest roentgenogram may reveal a reticular and poorly defined micronodular abnormality,[264, 267] presumably on the basis of the presence of cement in the interstitial lymphatics. The fact that these calcium compounds do not cause a more dramatic change in the roentgenogram probably is attributable to their rapid clearance. The roentgenogram of the chest has been reported to be normal in baggers, some of whom have been working for more than 40 years in the same environment.[263] Pulmonary function tests reveal an obstructive impairment[267] that is accentuated by cigarette smoking[265] and may be missed unless small airway function is closely examined.[152]

PLATINUM

Chloroplatinic acid or one of its salts can cause dermatitis and asthma.[240] Some workers become sensitized after a few months of exposure and develop bouts of wheezing that can be relieved with bronchodilators and corticosteroids. Complete recovery can be expected if further exposure is avoided. Once a worker has been sensitized, minute quantities of the chloroplatinates can precipitate symptoms; for example, an asthma attack can be triggered simply by meeting people who have been in the platinum workshop. Workers with an atopic personal or family history should be excluded from occupations involving exposure to the chloroplatinates. Sensitized individuals can be detected by periodic postemployment skin tests.

IRON PENTACARBONYL

Iron pentacarbonyl [$Fe(CO)_5$] is a highly toxic flammable liquid that can form whenever carbon monoxide at a high partial pressure comes in contact with iron or steel, such as might occur in steel cylinders containing carbon monoxide. It has also been reported in gas manufacturing processes and may be formed in illuminating gases passing through iron pipes. Liquid iron pentacarbonyl has been used as an antiknock agent in some gasolines. The material is highly toxic, and exposed workers develop the immediate onset of dyspnea, headache, vomiting, and giddiness, which may be transiently relieved by removal to fresh air. Approximately 12–36 hours after exposure, the dyspnea returns, accompanied by cough, fever, and cyanosis. Death may occur 4–11 days after exposure, resulting from pulmonary consolidation and degenerative changes in the central nervous system. Highly sensitive sampling and analysis techniques are available.[37] The TLV of 0.1 ppm was recommended by the ACGIH in 1986.

COPPER SULFATE

A granulomatous pneumonitis (vineyard sprayer's lung) may result from exposure to bordeaux mixture, which is a 1%–2% solution of copper sulfate neutralized with hydrated lime. The solution is used in spraying vineyards to prevent the growth of mildew.[249] The onset of symptoms is characteristically insidious with progressive weakness, anorexia, weight loss, and dyspnea. Cough is a variable finding. The course varies with some workers experiencing gradual spontaneous improvement, while in others the disease progressively worsens. The chest roentgenogram characteristically shows a diffuse micronodular or reticulonodular pattern, predominantly in the lower lung zones. Massive opacities resembling those seen in PMF in CWP are seen in the chronic form of the disease. The diagnosis is made by finding copper either in the lung lesions or mediastinal lymph nodes. There is a high incidence of lung cancer in these workers.[314] The pathologic changes on lung biopsy resemble those of some of the organic pneumoconioses, and noncaseating hepatic granulomas containing inclusions of copper may be seen.[250]

MAN-MADE MINERAL FIBERS

Fiberglass may cause transient upper respiratory irritation,[126, 136, 231] but there is little conclusive evidence that exposure to fiberglass or mineral (slag) wool during manufacturing conditions is associated with excess mortality from lung cancer or nonmalignant respiratory disease.[92, 321] Detailed observations of experiences with fiberglass are described elsewhere in this book.

MEAT WRAPPER'S ASTHMA

The wrapping of meat and labeling of the packages is usually carried out in refrigerated rooms where there is little ventilation. Polyvinylchloride wrapping film is cut from a supply roll by using a wire heated to approximately 105° C. The folded ends are then heat-sealed under the package. The major emissions from the hot-wire cutting are di-2-ethylhexyl adipate and hydrogen chloride.[182] The pyrolysis products may be responsible for cough, chest tightness, wheezing, and shortness of breath,[42, 251] but it is not clear whether this is on the basis of direct chemical injury to the respiratory system,[149] an allergic sensitization process, or the induction of a state of bronchial hyperreactivity which is not on an allergic basis.[42] After the meat is wrapped, a label is heated to thermally activate an adhesive which is then affixed to the wrapped package. The temperature of the label heating element varies, depending upon the surface temperature of the meat package, and is usually between 200–210° C. The emissions from the thermal activation of price labels contain dicyclohexyl phthalate, the major ingredient in the adhesive, and its thermal decomposition products, which include phthalic anhydride.[182] Exposure to these fumes can also cause[10, 11, 290] or aggravate[42] asthma. There does not appear to be any long-term cumulative effect from exposure to polyvinylchloride pyrolysis fumes.[170] Most individuals who develop symptoms and demonstrate a fall in flow rate after exposure have preexisting chronic bronchitis or asthma and should avoid further exposure, particularly if the work environment is not well ventilated. (See Chapter 64 for detailed discussions.)

WOOD DUSTS

Exposure to crude oak dust, fine mahogany dust, and cedar wood dust is capable of producing both an immediate type I and delayed type III hypersensitivity reaction in woodworkers.[291] The prevalence of wheezing is low in workers exposed to Western Red Cedar dust, since most workers become symptomatic during the first two years of employment and leave the industry.

The etiologic agent has been shown to be plicatic acid,[59] but respiratory symptoms are higher and decline in pulmonary function more pronounced in workers who smoke than in nonsmokers with the same degree of exposure.[58] Approximately one half of workers with Red Cedar asthma develop persistent bronchial reactivity to methacholine and recurrent asthma even after further exposure ceases.[60] There is an excessive risk of developing cancer of the nasal cavity and sinuses among woodworkers in the furniture industry.[1, 333] It is not known which wood dusts are most carcinogenic.[9]

GRAIN DUST

Grain scoopers transferring grain from the holds of ships or workers in grain elevators develop a variety of respiratory complaints, the most common of which are cough, wheezing, and dyspnea.[79] Wheat appears to be the most irritating, but barley, corn, soybeans, and oats have been implicated as well. In most workers, symptoms disappear after exposure ceases. Although chronic bronchitis and airway obstruction may develop in nonsmokers,[82] smoking acts synergistically with grain dust and may be the most important predisposing factor for the development of chronic obstructive lung disease.[66, 79, 80] The adverse effect of grain dust on flow rates is related to the intensity and duration of exposure and can be ameliorated by wearing a mask,[65] but peak dust levels may be more important than time-averaged concentrations.[78]

The etiology of symptoms is not known, but there is a correlation between cutaneous reactions (positive prick test) and symptoms, implying that an allergen may be a factor in some cases; however, skin tests using grain and mold antigen cannot identify those workers who demonstrate a decline in pulmonary function during a workweek. The absence of specific precipitins makes an IgG-mediated reaction unlikely as well.[40] Other potential sensitizers in grain include fungal spores from penicillium and aspergillus, mucor, pullularia, thermophilic organisms, and insect debris from the wheat weevil. Grain handlers with a history of respiratory symptoms on exposure to durum wheat at work develop a significant fall in the FEV_1 only after inhalation of durum wheat extracts, but not to extracts of insects or mites.[77] Irritation of the skin, eyes, and nose is common,[79, 165] and the airways may be reacting to a substance which is capable of indiscriminately irritating mucus membranes. Similar respiratory symptoms develop in bakers and even housewives exposed to milled grain.[160]

Fever and chills (grain fever) may develop several hours after leaving work in as many as 20% of workers, after reexposure to dust following a two-week absence or after an unusually intense exposure.[303] (See Chapter 15 for complete listing.)

COTTON DUST (BYSSINOSIS)

Byssinosis is an occupational respiratory disease that occurs in the processing of cotton, flax, and hemp. Originally, the term *byssinosis* applied only to the disease in workers exposed to cotton dust, but an identical syndrome has been described in flax and hemp workers.[28–31, 287] In contrast, dust of polyacrylonitride synthetic fibers has very low biologic activity, but workers may still develop mild acute reduction in ventilatory function during a shift at the beginning of the workweek.[308] Since there are more than 800,000 workers in the United States exposed to cotton dust, the prevalence in this industry will be emphasized.

Incidence

Workers involved in operating cotton gin machines, baling cotton, and the initial stages of fiber processing (i.e., carders) are exposed to the highest concentrations of dust.[239] In most mills in the United States, the spinning machines are located in the same room as the carding machines, and, as a result, many "spinners" are at risk also. The disease may also occur in weavers and in cotton mill workers processing raw cotton into crude thick lint. The incidence of byssinosis in cardroom workers varies between 15% and 50%,[34, 201, 269, 272, 339] depending on the grade of cotton and dust exposure. The incidence in workers employed in the spinning rooms usually is less and depends on the distance of the spinning machines from the cards and the ventilation, as well as the above factors.

Pathogenesis

With the advent of automatic cotton-picking machines, large amounts of trash are added to baled cotton, including the brackets of the cotton boll. These leaves contain one or more low molecular weight agents that appear to be water-soluble and heat stable and cause bronchoconstriction probably by the release of histamine.[33, 83, 336] The biologic activity of the dust depends on the concentration of these agents.

Byssinosis may develop after a short exposure to the dust, and pulmonary function abnormalities (see below) are not necessarily related to length of exposure.[34] These observations mitigate against an immune response leading to bronchospasm, although the serum in cardroom workers with byssinosis has been found to contain high titers of antibodies to several constituents of the dry cotton plant compared to cardroom workers without byssinosis or to normal controls.[191] There is evidence to suggest that byssinosis and chronic bronchitis are frequent manifestations of cotton dust exposure and cigarette smoking and that the latter contributes more to the severity of these diseases than does work exposure.[201] Goblet cell and mucus gland hyperplasia are increased in cotton workers, but their relationship can be obscured by cigarette smoking. There is no correlation between exposure to cotton dust and the development of emphysema in both smokers and nonsmokers.[214, 253]

Clinical Manifestations

Byssinosis is characterized by the gradual onset of symptoms within hours of returning to work on Monday after a weekend absence from work. If exposure continues, the initial Monday symptoms of tightness in the chest, dyspnea, and cough recur throughout the week but still remain more severe on the first workday. A severe irreversible ventilatory impairment after exposure to cotton dust for at least ten years and usually more than 20 years is more likely to occur in those who experience characteristic Monday symptoms during the first year of employment.[30] This stage of the disease may be clinically indistinguishable from chronic bronchitis or emphysema,[32] although among workers with chronic cough, plasma IgG levels are higher in those with byssinosis than in workers with nonspecific chronic bronchitis;[153] however, it should be noted that there is no statistical evidence based on autopsy that emphysema results from chronic exposure to cotton dust.[214] Byssinosis was more common among heavy smokers than among nonsmokers.[204] Some workers who stopped smoking cigarettes without changing their work area noticed a disappearance of their symptoms;[201] however, the prevalence of chronic respiratory disease is high among workers at risk even if they have never smoked and exposure to hemp dust[29, 33, 35] and probably cotton dust[23] as well ceases.

Pulmonary Function Tests and Chest Roentgenogram

Abnormal spirometry is the most commonly reported defect in pulmonary function, both in symptomatic and asymptomatic workers,[34, 268] and the mid expiratory flow rate is the most sensitive index for detecting early airway obstruction.[338] Some workers may complain of tightness in the chest without any alteration in routine ventilatory studies, while others demonstrate marked hypoxemia with few symptoms and minor functional defects.[200] In the chronic stage, the findings are indistinguishable from those in any chronic obstructive pulmonary disease. The roentgenogram is usually normal,[28] and the finding of pulmonary overdistention is likely related to cigarette smoking rather than prolonged exposure to cotton dust.[253]

Environmental Recommendations

There is an inconsistent relationship between dust levels and the prevalence of byssinosis. A minimal amount of dust is necessary to cause symptoms and alter pulmonary function, but once this dust level is reached, the composition and biologic activity of the dust may be more important than the amount in the air.

The TLV for total cotton dust of 0.2 mg/cu m adopted by the ACGH in 1986 is not associated with acute loss of function.[138] To meet these requirements, all machines should be provided with exhaust systems, preferably at several locations on each machine. In addition, the spinning room should be provided with an overhead exhaust system and physically separated from the carding area. The worker must have an opportunity for a free physical examination. At the time of initial assignment, a standardized respiratory questionnaire and a spirogram should be administered, and a medical evaluation should be conducted annually, except in employees who have increased respiratory sensitivity, who should be monitored every six months. Preemployment screening of all workers should be used to exclude workers with preexisting lung disease. Workers with more than a 200 ml decrease in the FEV_1 during a Monday work shift or who have significant chest tightness should be considered for work away from the dusty areas. It would not appear advisable to permit cigarette smokers to work in areas of high exposure to dust. The airway response can be modified by disodiumcromoglycate and ascorbic acid,[336] and it has been suggested that preshift administration of these agents in workers with a large acute reduction in ventilatory function may be of value if they cannot be moved to another area.

Attempts have been made to reduce the pathogenicity of the dust. Washing cotton appears to eliminate the biologic activity. Unfortunately, the washed cotton does not process well. Steaming the cotton can reduce both the dust levels and the biologic activity of the dust, reportedly without altering the spinning qualities of the yarn,[202] and is worthy of further investigation.

TOBACCO DUST

During the manufacture of cigarettes, exposure to tobacco dust may lead to wheezing and tightness in the chest during a work shift which is unrelated to the duration or intensity of exposure. Chronic obstructive lung disease has not been reported.[120, 307]

COFFEE AND TEA DUST

Coffee dust[310, 337] and tea dust[305] contain components capable of directly constricting airway smooth muscle.

PESTICIDES

Approximately 20% of workers exposed to pesticides used in growing fruit have radiographic findings consistent with interstitial fibrosis. Fewer than 5% may present acutely ill with consolidating radiographic densities.[184]

PHENOL-FORMALDEHYDE

There is evidence to suggest that concentrations of phenol-formaldehyde resin fumes that are generally less than the current TLV can cause chronic airway obstruction, which is accompanied by a slight excess of respiratory symptoms.[271]

BAKELITE

Workers polishing furniture or appliances that contain the phenolic plastic, bakelite, are exposed to a dust that is capable of inducing a potentially fatal granulomatous pulmonary disease.[248]

FLY ASH

Fly ash, the solid residue remaining after coal combustion, has a high concentration of aluminum silicate and has been implicated in the development of interstitial fibrosis.[121]

SOOT

The inhalation of soot produced from coal-burning steam locomotives over a long period of time can produce pneumoconiosis in railway men.[62, 111]

FIREFIGHTERS

Firefighters may have hypoxemia for as long as ten hours after exposure to dense smoke from burning plastic materials.[117] The controversy as to whether recurrent exposure to fire and smoke will result in a diminution in ventilatory function[187, 247, 293, 300] may be related to the removal of the most impaired firefighters from active firefighting duties in those cohorts being studied.

RUBBER WORKERS

Rubber workers employed in the processing areas[99] and areas where there is exposure to heated rubber[98, 199] have a significant increase in respiratory symptoms. Cigarette smoking further enhances respiratory morbidity.[98, 176] The causative agents are not known, since there is exposure to many substances, including carbon black and a variety of organic and inorganic chemicals. In some areas, there is also exposure to talc.[100]

MISCELLANEOUS

There is a variety of substances that are radiopaque, are not fibrogenic in the lung, and cause little if any clinical respiratory impairment. However, striking changes can be seen on the chest roentgenogram when these substances are inhaled. Such abnormalities occur after the inhalation of the oxides of tin, vanadium, and antimony, and compounds containing barium and certain rare earth elements, including cerium, scandium, yttrium, and lanthanum. The occupational hazard of these substances is covered elsewhere in this text, as is berylliosis.

REFERENCES

1. Acheson ED, Cowdell RH, Hadfield E, et al: Nasal cancer in woodburners in the furniture industry. *Br Med J* 1968; 2:587.
2. Acheson ED, Gardner MJ, Pippard EC, et al: Mortality of two groups of women who manufactured gas masks from chrysotile and crocidolite asbestos: A 40 year follow-up. *Br J Ind Med* 1982; 39:344.
3. Amandus HE, Lapp NL, Jacobson G, et al: Significance of irregular small opacities in radiographs of coalminers in the USA. *Br J Ind Med* 1976; 33:13.
4. Amandus HE, Lapp NL, Jacobson G, et al: Significance of irregular small opacities in radiographs of coalminers in the USA. *Br J Ind Med* 1981; 38:313.
5. Amandus HE, Reger RB, Pendergrass EP, et al: The pneumoconioses: Methods of measuring progression. *Chest* 1973; 63:736.
6. American College of Chest Physicians: Recommendations for continuous oxygen therapy in chronic obstructive lung disease. *Chest* 1973; 64:505.
7. American Thoracic Society: Preventive treatment of tuberculosis. *Am Rev Respir Dis* 1971; 104:460.
8. American Thoracic Society Statement—Snowbird workshop on standardization of spirometry. *Am Rev Respir Dis* 1979; 119:831.
9. Andersen HC, Andersen I, Solgaard J: Nasal cancers, symptoms and upper airway function in woodworkers. *Br J Ind Med* 1977; 34:201.
10. Andrasch RH, Bardana EJ Jr: Thermoactivated price-label fume intolerance. *JAMA* 1976; 235:937.
11. Andrasch RH, Koster F, Lawson WH Jr, et al: Meatwrappers' asthma—An appraisal of a new occupational syndrome. *J Allergy Clin Immunol* 1975; 55:130.
12. Angervall L, Hansson G, Rockert H: Pulmonary siderosis in electrical welders. *Acta Pathol Microbiol Scand* 1960; 49:373.
13. Anton HC: Multiple pleural plaques, Part II. *Br J Radiol* 1968; 41:341.
14. Avila R, Villar TG: Suberosis. Respiratory disease in cork workers. *Lancet* 1968; 1:620.
15. Bailey WC, Brown M, Buechner HA, et al: Silico-mycobacterial disease in sandblasters. *Am Rev Respir Dis* 1974; 110:115.
16. Banks DE, Morring KL, Boehlecke BA, et al: Silicosis in silica flour workers. *Am Rev Respir Dis* 1981; 124:445.
17. Barclay WR: Black lung benefits. *JAMA* 1980; 243:2427.
18. Barrie HJ, Gosselin L: Massive pneumoconiosis from a rock dust containing no free silica. *Arch Environ Health* 1960; 1:109.
19. Bates DV, Macklem PT, Christie RV: *Respiratory Function in Disease*. Philadelphia, WB Saunders Co, 1964.
20. Ibid, pp 378–379.
21. Beaumont JJ, Weiss NS: Lung cancer among welders. *J Occup Med* 1981; 23:839.
22. Bech AO, Kipling MD, Healther JC: Hard metal disease. *Br J Ind Med* 1962; 19:239.
23. Beck GJ, Schachter N, Maunder LR, et al: A prospective study of chronic lung disease in cotton textile workers. *Ann Intern Med* 1982; 97:645.
24. Begin R, Cantin A, Berthiaume Y, et al: Airway function in lifetime nonsmoking older asbestos workers. *Am J Med* 1983; 75:631.
25. Begin R, Cantin A, Drapeau G, et al: Pulmonary uptake of Gallium-67 in asbestos-exposed humans and sheep. *Am Rev Respir Dis* 1983; 127:623.
26. Benedek TG: Rheumatoid pneumoconiosis. Documentation of onset and pathogenic considerations. *Am J Med* 1973; 55:515.
27. Bolton RE, Vincent JH, Jones AD, et al: An overload hypothesis for pulmonary clearance of UICC amosite fibres inhaled by rats. *Br J Ind Med* 1983; 40:264.
28. Bouhuys A: Byssinosis in textile workers. *Trans NY Acad Sci (Series II)* 1966; 28:480.
29. Bouhuys A, Barbero A, Lindell S-E, et al: Byssinosis in hemp workers. *Arch Environ Health* 1967; 14:533.
30. Bouhuys A, Barbero A, Schilling RSF, et al: Chronic respiratory disease in hemp workers. *Am J Med* 1969; 46:526.
31. Bouhuys A, Duyn JV, Van Lennep HJ: Byssinosis in flax workers. *Arch Environ Health* 1961; 3:499.
32. Bouhuys A, Heaply LJ Jr, Schilling RSF, et al: Byssinosis in the United States. *N Engl J Med* 1967; 277:170.
33. Bouhuys A, Nicholls PJ: Effect of cotton dust on respiratory mechanics in man and guinea pigs; in Davies CN (ed): *Inhaled Particles and Vapours*. London, Pergamon Press, 1966, vol II, pp 75–83.
34. Bouhuys A, Wolfson RL, Horner DW, et al: Byssinosis in cotton textile workers. *Ann Intern Med* 1969; 71:257.
35. Bouhuys A, Zuskin E: Chronic respiratory disease in hemp workers. *Ann Intern Med* 1976; 84:398.
36. Boyd JT, Doll R, Faulds JS, et al: Cancer of the lung in iron ore (Haematite) miners. *Br J Ind Med* 1970; 27:97.
37. Brief RS, Ajemian RS, Confer RG: Iron pentacarbonyl: Its toxicity, detection, and potential for formation. *Am Ind Hyg Assoc J* 1967; 28:21.
38. Brink GC, Grzybowski S, Lane GB: Silicotuberculosis. *Can Med Assoc J* 1960; 82:959.
39. Bristol LJ: Pneumoconiosis caused by asbestos and by other siliceous and non-siliceous dusts. *Semin Roentgenol* 1967; 2:283.
40. Broder I, Davies G, Hutcheon M, et al: Variables of pulmonary allergy and inflammation in grain elevator workers. *J Occup Med* 1983; 25:43.
41. Brody AR, Hill LH, Adkins B Jr, et al: Chrysotile asbestos inhalation in rats: Deposition pattern and reaction of alveolar epithelium and pulmonary macrophages. *Am Rev Respir Dis* 1981; 123:670.
42. Brooks SM, Vandervort R: Polyvinyl chloride film thermal decomposition products as an occupational illness. *J Occup Med* 1977; 19:192.
43. Brown JH, Cook KM, Ney FG, et al: Influence of particle size upon the retention of particulate matter in the human lung. *Am J Public Health* 1950; 40:450.
44. Brown RC, Chamberlain M, Griffiths DM, et al: The effect of fibre size on the in vitro biological activity of three types of amphibole asbestos. *Int J Cancer* 1978; 22:721.
45. Browne K: Asbestos-related mesothelioma: Epidemiological evidence for asbestos as a promoter. *Arch Environ Health* 1983; 38:261.
46. Browne K, Smither WJ: Asbestos-related mesothelioma: Factors discriminating between pleural and peritoneal sites. *Br J Ind Med* 1983; 40:145.
47. Bruckner HC: Extrinsic asthma in a tungsten carbide worker. *Ann Arbor Reports* 1967; 9:518.

48. Buechner HA, Ansari A: Acute silico-proteinosis. *Dis Chest* 1969; 55:274.
49. Campbell JA: Effects of precipitated silica and of iron oxide on the incidence of primary lung tumours in mice. *Br Med J* 1940; 2:275.
50. Campbell JA: Lung tumours in mice. Incidence as affected by inhalation of certain carcinogenic agents and some dusts. *Br Med J* 1942; 1:217.
51. Campbell JA: Lung tumours in mice and man. *Br Med J* 1943; 1:179.
52. Caplan A: Certain unusual radiological appearances in the chest of coal miners suffering from rheumatoid arthritis. *Thorax* 1953; 8:29.
53. Caplan A: Correlation of radiological category with lung pathology in coal workers' pneumoconiosis. *Br J Ind Med* 1962; 19:71.
54. Carpathios J: Cavitary silicosis. *Am Rev Respir Dis* 1961; 84:84.
55. Chahinian AP, Pajak TF, Holland JF, et al: Diffuse malignant mesothelioma. *Ann Intern Med* 1982; 96:746.
56. Chamberlain M, Tarmy EM: Asbestos and glass fibres in bacterial mutation tests. *Mutat Res* 1977; 43:159.
57. Chan-Yeung M, Ashley MJ, Corey P, et al: Pi phenotypes and the prevalence of chest symptoms and lung function abnormalities in workers employed in dusty industries. *Am Rev Respir Dis* 1978; 117:239.
58. Chan-Yeung M, Ashley MJ, Corey P, et al: A respiratory survey of cedar mill workers. *J Occup Med* 1978; 20:323.
59. Chan-Yeung M, Barton GM, MacLean L, et al: Occupational asthma and rhinitis due to western red cedar. *Am Rev Respir Dis* 1973; 108:1094.
60. Chan-Yeung M, Lam S, Koener S: Clinical features and natural history of occupational asthma due to western red cedar (Thuja Plicata). *Am J Med* 1982; 72:411.
61. Chiappino G, Vigliani EC: Role of infective, immunological and chronic irritative factors in the development of silicosis. *Br J Ind Med* 1982; 39:253.
62. Cochrane AL, Higgins ITT, Gibson JC: Yet another industrial pneumoconiosis? *Tubercle* 1958; 39:399.
63. Cockcroft A, Lyons JP, Andersson N, et al: Prevalence and relation to underground exposure of radiological irregular opacities in South Wales coal workers with pneumoconiosis. *Br J Ind Med* 1983; 40:169.
64. Cooperative Study by UICC Committee: UICC/Cincinnati classification of radiographic appearances of pneumoconiosis. *Chest* 1970; 58:57.
65. Corey P, Hutcheon M, Broder I, et al: Grain elevator workers show work-related pulmonary function changes and dose-effect relationships with dust exposure. *Br J Ind Med* 1982; 39:330.
66. Cotton DJ, Graham BL, Li KYR, et al: Effects of grain dust exposure and smoking on respiratory symptoms and lung function. *J Occup Med* 1983; 25:131.
67. Craighead JE, Mossman BT: The pathogenesis of asbestos-associated diseases. *N Engl J Med* 1982; 306:1446.
68. Craighead JE, Vallyathan NV: Cryptic pulmonary lesions in workers occupationally exposed to dust containing silica. *JAMA* 1980; 244:1939.
69. Cralley LJ, Keenan RG, Kupel RE, et al: Characterization and solubility of metals associated with asbestos fibers. *Am Ind Hyg Assoc J* 1968; 29:569.
70. Davies CN: The handling of particles by the human lungs. *Br Med Bull* 1963; 19:49.
71. Davies CN (ed): *Health Conditions in the Ceramic Industry*. London, Pergamon Press, 1968.
72. Davies P, Allison AC, Ackerman J, et al: Asbestos induces selective release of lysosomal enzymes from mononuclear phagocytes. *Nature* 1974; 251:423.
73. Davis JMG, Chapman J, Collings P, et al: Variations in the histological patterns of the lesions of coal workers' pneumoconiosis in Britain and their relationship to lung dust content. *Am Rev Respir Dis* 1983; 128:118.
74. DelCampo JM, Hitado J, Gea G, et al: Anaerobes: A new aetiology in cavitary pneumoconiosis. *Br J Ind Med* 1982; 39:392.
75. Demy NG, Adler H: Asbestos and malignancy. *Am J Roentgenol* 1967; 100:597.
76. Doig AT, McLaughlin AIG: Clearing of x-ray shadows in welders' siderosis. *Lancet* 1948; 1:789.
77. DoPico GA, Jacobs S, Flaherty D, et al: Pulmonary reaction to durum wheat. *Chest* 1982; 81:55.
78. DoPico GA, Reddan W, Anderson S, et al: Acute effects of grain dust exposure during a work shift. *Am Rev Respir Dis* 1983; 128:399.
79. DoPico GA, Reddan W, Flaherty D, et al: Respiratory abnormalities among grain handlers. *Am Rev Respir Dis* 1977; 115:915.
80. Dosman JA: Chronic obstructive pulmonary disease and smoking in grain handlers. *Ann Intern Med* 1977; 87:784.
81. Dosman JA: Preventive diagnosis in occupational pulmonary disease. Ann Intern Med 1975; 83:274.
82. Dosman JA, Cotton DJ, Graham BL, et al: Chronic bronchitis and decreased forced expiratory flow rates in lifetime non-smoking grain workers. *Am Rev Respir Dis* 1980; 121:11.
83. Douglas JS, Zuskin E, Bouhuys A: Relationship between in vivo bronchospasm induced by textile dust extracts and in vitro histamine release from pig lung. *Am Rev Respir Dis* 1974; 109:712.
84. Dutra FR: Diatomaceous earth pneumoconiosis. *Arch Environ Health* 1965; 11:613.
85. Edenfield RW: A clinical and roentgenological study of kaolin workers. *Arch Environ Health* 1960; 1:392.
86. Edling NPG: Aluminum pneumoconiosis. *Acta Radiol* 1961; 56:170.
87. Eisenstadt HB: Asbestos pleurisy. *Dis Chest* 1964; 46:78.
88. Elmes PC, Simpson MJC: Insulation workers in Belfast. A further study of mortality due to asbestos exposure. *Br J Ind Med* 1977; 34:174.
89. Elo R, Maatta K, Uksila E, et al: Pulmonary deposits of titanium dioxide in man. *Arch Pathol* 1972; 94:417.
90. Elwood PC, Cochrane AL: A follow-up study of workers from an asbestos factory. *Br J Ind Med* 1964; 21:304.
91. Enterline PE, Kendrick MA: Asbestos-dust exposure at various levels and mortality. *Arch Environ Health* 1967; 15:181.
92. Enterline PE, Marsh GM, Esmen NA: Respiratory disease among workers exposed to man-made mineral fibers. *Am Rev Respir Dis* 1983; 128:1.
93. Epler GR, McLoud TC, Gaensler EA: Prevalence and incidence of benign asbestos pleural effusion in a working population. *JAMA* 1982; 247:617.
94. Epler GR, Saber FA, Gaensler EA: Determination of severe impairment (disability) in interstitial lung disease. *Am Rev Respir Dis* 1980; 121:647.
95. Falk GA, Briscoe WA: Alpha$_1$-antitrypsin deficiency in chronic obstructive pulmonary disease. *Ann Intern Med* 1970; 72:427.
96. Faulds JS: Haematite pneumoconiosis in Cumberland miners. *J Clin Pathol* 1957; 10:187.
97. Fawer RF, Gardner AW, Oakes D: Absences attributed to respiratory diseases in welders. *Br J Ind Med* 1982; 39:149.
98. Fine LJ, Peters JM: Respiratory morbidity in rubber workers. *Arch Environ Health* 1976; 31:5.
99. Fine LJ, Peters JM: Studies of respiratory morbidity in rubber workers. *Arch Environ Health* 1976; 31:136.
100. Fine LJ, Peters JM, Burgess WA, et al: Studies of respiratory morbidity in rubber workers. *Arch Environ Health* 1976; 31:195.

101. Fisher ER, Watkins G, Lam NV, et al: Objective pathological diagnosis of coal workers' pneumoconiosis. *JAMA* 1981; 245:1829.
102. Fitzgerald MX, Smith AA, Gaensler EA: Evaluation of "electronic" spirometers. *N Engl J Med* 1973; 289:1283.
103. Fletcher CM: Epidemiological studies of coal miners' pneumoconiosis in Great Britain. *Arch Ind Health* 1955; 11:29.
104. Freedman RW, Sharkey AG Jr: Recent advances in the analysis of respirable coal dust for free silica, trace elements, and organic constituents. *Ann NY Acad Sci* 1972; 200:7.
105. Freundlich IM, Greening RR: Asbestosis and associated medical problems. *Radiology* 1967; 89:224.
106. Friede E, Rachow DO: Symptomatic pulmonary disease in arc welders. *Ann Intern Med* 1961; 54:121.
107. Funahashi A, Pintar K, Siegusmund KA: Identification of foreign material in lung by energy dispersive x-ray analysis. *Arch Environ Health* 1975; 30:285.
108. Funahashi A, Schlueter DP, Pintar K, et al: Value of in situ elemental microanalysis in the histologic diagnosis of silicosis. *Chest* 1984; 85:506.
109. Funahashi A, Schlueter DP, Pintar K, et al: Pneumoconiosis in workers exposed to silicon carbide. *Am Rev Respir Dis* 1984; 129:635.
110. Funahashi A, Siegusmund KA, Dragen RF, Pintar K: Energy dispensive x-ray analysis in the study of pneumoconiosis. *Br J Ind Med* 1977; 34:95.
111. Furlaneto JA, Anderson AE Jr, Foraker AG: Soot emphysema in a locomotive engineer. *Arch Environ Health* 1969; 18:1008.
112. Gabor S, Anca Z, Zugravu E: In vitro action of quartz on alveolar macrophage lipid peroxides. *Arch Environ Health* 1975; 30:499.
113. Gaensler EA, Addington WW: Asbestos or Ferruginous Bodies. *N Engl J Med* 1969; 280:488.
114. Gaensler EA, Kaplan AI: Asbestos pleural effusion. *Ann Intern Med* 1971; 74:178.
115. Gaensler EA, Wright GW: Evaluation of respiratory impairment. *Arch Environ Health* 1966; 12:146.
116. Gamble JF, Fillner W, Dimeo MJ: An epidemiologic study of a group of talc workers. *Am Rev Respir Dis* 1979; 119:741.
117. Genovesi MG, Tashkin DP, Chopra S, et al: Transient hypoxemia in firemen following inhalation of smoke. *Chest* 1977; 71:441.
118. Gernez-Rieux C, Tacqnet A, Devulder B, et al: Experimental study of interactions between pneumoconiosis and mycobacterial infections. *Ann NY Acad Sci* 1972; 200:106.
119. Giles RD, Sturgill BC, Suratt PM, et al: Massive proteinuria and acute renal failure in a patient with acute silicoproteinosis. *Am J Med* 1978; 64:336.
120. Gleich GJ, Welsh PW, Yunginger JW, et al: Allergy to tobacco: An occupational hazard. *N Engl J Med* 1980; 302:617.
121. Golden EB, Warnock ML, Hulett LD Jr, et al: Fly ash lung: A new pneumoconiosis? *Am Rev Respir Dis* 1982; 125:100
122. Gopalakrishna KV, Lerner PI: Tetracycline resistant pneumococci. *Am Rev Respir Dis* 1973; 108:1007.
123. Gorson RO, Lieberman MS: The prohibition of the use of asbestos spray in building construction. *J Occup Med* 1973; 15:260.
124. Greenberg M, Lloyd Davies TA: Mesothelioma Register 1967–1968. *Br J Ind Med* 1974; 31:91.
125. Greening RR, Heslep JH: The roentgenology of silicosis. *Semin Roentgenol* 1967; 2:265.
126. Gross P: The biologic categorization of inhaled fiberglass dust. *Arch Environ Health* 1976; 31:101.
127. Gross P, Harley RA, Swinburne LM, et al: Ingested mineral fibers. *Arch Environ Health* 1974; 29:341.
128. Grundorfer W, Rabes A: Progressive silicosis in granite workers. *Br J Ind Med* 1970; 27:110.
129. Hammond EC, Selikoff IJ, Seidman H: Asbestos exposure, cigarette smoking and death rates. *Ann NY Acad Sci* 1979; 330:473.
130. Harding HE, McLaughlin AIG, Doig AT: Clinical, radiographic, and pathological studies of the lungs of electric arc and oxyacetylene welders. *Lancet* 1958; 2:394.
131. Harington JS, Roe FJC, Walters M: Studies of the mode of action of asbestos as a carcinogen. *S Afr Med J* 1967; 41:800.
132. Hasan FM, Nash G, Kazemi H: Asbestos exposure and related neoplasia. *Am J Med* 1978; 65:649.
133. Heppleston AG, Styles JA: Activity of a macrophage factor in collagen formation by silica. *Nature* 1967; 214:521.
134. Hext PM, Richards RJ: Biochemical effects of asbestiform minerals on lung fibroblast cultures. *Br J Exp Pathol* 1976; 57:281.
135. Higgins ITT: Chronic respiratory disease in mining communities. *Ann NY Acad Sci* 1972; 200:197.
136. Hill JW, Whitehead WS, Cameron JD, et al: Glass fibres: Absence of pulmonary hazard in production workers. *Br J Ind Med* 1973; 30:174.
137. Hogg JC, Macklem PT, Thurlbeck WM: Site and nature of airway obstruction in chronic obstructive lung disease. *N Engl J Med* 1968; 278:1355.
138. Holness DL, Taraschuk IG, Pelmear PL: Effect of dust exposure in Ontario cotton textile mills. *J Occup Med* 1983; 25:26.
139. Hourihane D O'B, Lessof L, Richardson PC: Hyaline and calcified pleural plaques as an index of exposure to asbestos. A study of radiological and pathological features of 100 cases with a consideration of epidemiology. *Br Med J* 1966; 1:1069.
140. Hunnicutt TN Jr, Cracovaner DJ, Myles JT: Spirometric measurements in welders. *Arch Environ Health* 1964; 8:661.
141. Hurley JF, Burns J, Copland L, et al: Coal workers' simple pneumoconiosis and exposure to dust at 10 British coalmines. *Br J Ind Med* 1982; 39:120.
142. Hwang C-Y: Size and shape of airborne asbestos fibres in mines and mills. *Br J Ind Med* 1983; 40:273.
143. Hyatt RE: Pulmonary function in coal miners' pneumoconiosis. *J Occup Med* 1971; 13:123.
144. Irwig LM, Rocks P: Lung function and respiratory symptoms in silicotic and non-silicotic gold miners. *Am Rev Respir Dis* 1978; 117:429.
145. Jacobs LG, Gerstl B, Hollander AG, et al: Intra-abdominal egg shell calcifications due to silicosis. *Radiology* 1956; 67:527.
146. Jahr J: Dose-response basis for setting a quartz threshold limit value. *Arch Environ Health* 1974; 29:338.
147. James WRL: The relationship of tuberculosis to the development of massive pneumoconiosis in coal workers. *Br J Tuber Dis Chest* 1954; 48:89.
148. Jodoin G, Gibbs GW, Macklem PT, et al: Early effects of asbestos exposure on lung function. *Am Rev Respir Dis* 1971; 104:525.
149. Johnson CJ, Anderson HW: Meat-wrappers' asthma: A case study. *J Occup Med* 1976; 18:102.
150. Jones FL Jr: Rifampin-containing chemotherapy for pulmonary tuberculosis associated with coal workers' pneumoconiosis. *Am Rev Respir Dis* 1982; 125:681.
151. Jones RN, Turner-Warwick M, Ziskund M, et al: High prevalence of antinuclear antibodies in sandblasters' silicosis. *Am Rev Respir Dis* 1976; 113:393.
152. Kalacic IVO: Early detection of expiratory airflow obstruction in cement workers. *Arch Environ Health* 1974; 29:147.
153. Kamat SR, Kamat GR, Salpekar VY, et al: Distinguishing byssinosis from chronic obstructive pulmonary disease. *Am Rev Respir Dis* 1981; 124:31.
154. Katsnelson BA, Mokronosova KA: Non-fibrous mineral dusts and malignant tumors. *J Occup Med* 1979; 21:15.

155. Kawakami M, Sato S, Takishima T: Silicosis in workers dealing with tonoko. *Chest* 1977; 72:635.
156. Keers RY: The treatment of silicotuberculosis, in *Health Conditions in the Ceramic Industry*. London, Pergamon Press, 1968, pp 63–69.
157. Kennedy T, Rawlings W Jr, Baser M, et al: Pneumoconiosis in Georgia kaolin workers. *Am Rev Respir Dis* 1983; 127:215.
158. Kleinerman J: The pathology of some familiar pneumoconioses. *Semin Roentgenol* 1967; 2:244.
159. Kleinfeld M: Biologic response to kind and amount of asbestos. *J Occup Med* 1973; 15:296.
160. Kleinfeld M: A comparative clinical and pulmonary function study of grain handlers and bakers. *Ann NY Acad Sci* 1974; 221:86.
161. Kleinfeld M, Messite J, Kooyman O, et al: Mortality among talc miners and millers in New York State. *Arch Environ Health* 1967; 14:663.
162. Kleinfeld M, Messite J, Shapiro J: Clinical, radiological, and physiological findings in asbestosis. *Arch Intern Med* 1966; 117:813.
163. Kleinfeld M, Messite J, Shapiro J, et al: A clinical, roentgenological, and physiological study of magnetite workers. *Arch Environ Health* 1968; 16:392.
164. Kleinfeld M, Messite J, Shapiro J, et al: Effect of talc dust inhalation on lung function. *Arch Environ Health* 1965; 10:431.
165. Kleinfeld M, Messite J, Swencicki RE, et al: A clinical and physiological study of grain handlers. *Arch Environ Health* 1968; 16:380.
166. Knox JF, Holmes S, Doll R, et al: Mortality from lung cancer and other causes among workers in an asbestos textile factory. *Br J Ind Med* 1968; 25:293.
167. Knudson RJ, Burrows B: Early detection of obstructive lung disease. *Med Clin North Am* 1973; 57:681.
168. Koskinen H, Tiilikainen A, Nordman H: Increased prevalence of HLA-AW19 and of the phenogroup AW19,B18 in advanced silicosis. *Chest* 1983; 83:848.
169. Krige L: Asbestosis—with special reference to the radiological diagnosis. *S Afr J Radiol* 1966; 4:13.
170. Krumpe PE, Finley TN, Martinez N: The search for expiratory obstruction in meat wrappers studied on the job. *Am Rev Respir Dis* 1979; 119:611.
171. Lainhart WS: Roentgenographic evidence of coal workers' pneumoconiosis in three geographic areas in the United States. *J Occup Med* 1969; 11:399.
172. Lapp NL, Block J, Boehlecke B, et al: Closing volume in coal miners. *Am Rev Respir Dis* 1976; 113:155.
173. Lapp NL, Seaton A: Lung mechanics in coal workers' pneumoconiosis. *Ann NY Acad Sci* 1972; 200:433.
174. Leathart GL: Clinical aspects of respiratory disease due to mining, in *Medicine in the Mining Industry*. Philadelphia, FA Davis, Co, 1972, pp 83–98.
175. LeBouffant L, Daniel H, Martin JC: The therapeutic action of aluminum compounds on the development of experimental lesions produced by pure quartz or mixed dust, in *Inhaled Particles*. London, Pergamon Press, 1977, vol IV, pp 389–400.
176. Lednar WM, Tyroler HA, McMichael AJ, et al: The occupational determinants of chronic disabling pulmonary disease in rubber workers. *J Occup Med* 1977; 19:263.
177. Lee DHK: Coal workers' pneumoconiosis—state of knowledge and research needs. *J Occup Med* 1971; 13:183.
178. Legg SJ, Cotes JE, Bevan C: Lung mechanics in relation to radiographic category of coal workers' simple pneumoconiosis. *Br J Ind Med* 1983; 40:28.
179. Legha SS, Muggia FM: Pleural mesothelioma: Clinical features and therapeutic implications. *Ann Intern Med* 1977; 87:613.
180. Leigh J, Outhred KG, McKenzie HI, et al: Quantified pathology of emphysema, pneumoconiosis, and chronic bronchitis in coal workers. *Br J Ind Med* 1983; 40:258.
181. Levy SA, Margolis I: Siderosilicosis and atypical epithelial hyperplasia. *J Occup Med* 1974; 16:796.
182. Levy SA, Storey JD, Plashko BE: Meat workers' asthma. *J Occup Med* 1978; 20:116.
183. Lieberman J: Alpha$_1$ antitrypsin. *J Occup Med* 1973; 15:194.
184. Lings S: Pesticide lung: A pilot investigation of fruit-growers and farmers during the spraying season. *Br J Ind Med* 1982; 39:370.
185. Lippmann M, Albert RE: The effect of particle size on the regional deposition of inhaled aerosols in the human respiratory tract. *Am Ind Hyg Assoc J* 1969; 30:257.
186. Lister WB, Wimborne D: Carbon pneumoconiosis in a synthetic graphite worker. *Br J Ind Med* 1972; 29:108.
187. Loke J, Farmer W, Matthay RA, et al: Acute and chronic effects of fire fighting on pulmonary function. *Chest* 1980; 77:369.
188. Lynch JR: Instrumentation, in Key MM, Bundy M (eds): *Pulmonary Reactions to Coal Dust*. New York, Academic Press, 1971, pp 212–215.
189. Lyons JP, Clarke WG, Hall AM, et al: Transfer factor (diffusing capacity) for the lung in simple pneumoconiosis of coal workers. *Br Med J* 1967; 4:772.
190. Lyons JP, Ryder RC, Campbell H, et al: Significance of irregular opacities in the radiology of coal workers' pneumoconiosis. *Br J Ind Med* 1974; 31:36.
191. Massoud A, Taylor G: Byssinosis: Antibody to cotton antigens in normal subjects and in cotton cardroom workers. *Lancet* 1964; 2:607.
192. McBride WW, Pendergrass EG, Lieben J: Pneumoconiosis study of Pennsylvania anthracite miners. *J Occup Med* 1966; 8:365.
193. McBride WW, Pendergrass E, Lieben J: Pneumoconiosis study of western Pennsylvania bituminous coal miners. *J Occup Med* 1963; 5:376.
194. McDonald JC, Becklake MR, Gibbs GW, et al: The health of chrysotile asbestos mine and mill workers of Quebec. *Arch Environ Health* 1974; 28:61.
195. McLaughlin AIG: Pneumoconiosis in foundry workers. *Br J Tuberc* 1957; 51:297.
196. McLaughlin AIG, Grout JLA, Barrie HJ, et al: Iron oxide dust and the lungs of silver polishers. *Lancet* 1945; 1:337.
197. McLaughlin AIG, Kazantzis G, King E, et al: Pulmonary fibrosis and encephalopathy associated with the inhalation with aluminum dust. *Br J Ind Med* 1962; 19:253.
198. McLoud TC, Putman CE, Pascual R: Eggshell calcification with systemic sarcoidosis. *Chest* 1974; 66:515.
199. McMichael AJ, Gerber WS, Gamble JF, et al: Chronic respiratory symptoms and job type within the rubber industry. *J Occup Med* 1976; 18:611.
200. Merchant JA, Halprin GM, Hudson AR, et al: Responses to cotton dust. *Arch Environ Health* 1975; 30:222.
201. Merchant JA, Kilburn KH, O'Fallon WM, et al: Byssinosis and chronic bronchitis among textile workers. *Ann Intern Med* 1972; 76:423.
202. Merchant JA, Lumsden JC, Kilburn KH, et al: Preprocessing cotton to prevent byssinosis. *Br J Ind Med* 1973; 30:237.
203. Merchant JA, Lumsden JC, Kilburn KH, et al: Dose response studies in cotton textile workers. *J Occup Med* 1973; 15:222.
204. Merchant JA, Lumsden JC, Kilburn KH, et al: An industrial study of the biological effects of cotton dust and cigarette smoke exposure. *J Occup Med* 1973; 15:212.
205. Messite J, Reddin G, Kleinfeld M: Pulmonary talcosis, a clinical and environmental study. *Arch Ind Health* 1959; 20:408.

206. Meyer EC, Kratzinger SF, Miller WH: Pulmonary fibrosis in an arc welder. *Arch Environ Health* 1967; 15:462.
207. Michel RD, Morris JT: Acute silicosis. *Arch Intern Med* 1964; 113:850.
208. Miller A, Langer AM, Teirstein AS, et al: "Nonspecific" interstitial pulmonary fibrosis. *N Engl J Med* 1975; 292:91.
209. Miller A, Teirstein AS, Selikoff IJ: Ventilatory failure due to asbestos pleurisy. *Am J Med* 1983; 75:911.
210. Miller L, Smith WE, Berliner SW: Tests for effect of asbestos on benzo (a) pyrene carcinogenesis in the respiratory tract. *Ann NY Acad Sci* 1965; 132:489.
211. Mitchell J: Pulmonary fibrosis in an aluminum worker. *Br J Ind Med* 1959; 16:123.
212. Mitchell J, Manning GB, Molyneaux M, et al: Pulmonary fibrosis in workers exposed to finely powdered aluminum. *Br J Ind Med* 1961; 18:10.
213. Mittman C, Pedersen E, Barbela T, et al: Prediction and potential prevention of industrial bronchitis. *Am J Med* 1974; 57:192.
214. Moran TJ: Emphysema and other chronic lung disease in textile workers: An 18-year autopsy study. *Arch Environ Health* 1983; 38:267.
215. Morgan EJ: Silicosis and tuberculosis. *Chest* 1979; 75:202.
216. Morgan WKC: Magnetite pneumoconiosis. *J Occup Med* 1978; 20:762.
217. Morgan WKC, Kerr H: Pathologic and physiologic studies of welders' siderosis. Ann Intern Med 1963; 58:293.
218. Morgan WKC, Lapp NL, Seaton D: Respiratory disability in coal miners. *JAMA* 1980; 243:2401.
219. Morgan WKC, Petersens MR, Reger RD: The "Middling" tendency. *Arch Environ Health* 1974; 29:334.
220. Morgan WKC, Reger R, Burgess DB, Shoub E: A comparison of the prevalence of coal workers' pneumoconiosis and respiratory impairment in Pennsylvania bituminous and anthracite miners. *Ann NY Acad Sci* 1972; 200:252.
221. Morgan WKC, Seaton D, Burgess DB, et al: Lung volumes in working coal miners. *Ann NY Acad Sci* 1972; 200:478.
222. Morosova KI, Aronova GV, Katsnelson BA, et al: On the defensive action of glutamate against the cytotoxicity and fibrogenicity of quartz dust. *Br J Ind Med* 1982; 39:244.
223. Murphy DMF, Metzger LF, Silage DA, et al: Effect of simple anthrocite pneumoconiosis on lung mechanics. *Chest* 1982; 82:744.
224. Murphy RLH Jr, Ferris BG Jr, Burgess WA, et al: Effects of low concentrations of asbestos. *N Engl J Med* 1971; 285:1271.
225. Murray R: An international view of coal workers' pneumoconiosis. *J Occup Med* 1970; 12:474.
226. Musk AW, Greville HW, Tribe AE: Pulmonary disease from occupational exposure to an artificial aluminum silicate for cat litter. *Br J Ind Med* 1980; 37:367.
227. Musk AW, Peters JM, Wegman DH, et al: Pulmonary function in granite dust exposure: A 4 year follow-up. *Am Rev Respir Dis* 1977; 115:769.
228. Naeye RL, Dellinger WS: Coal workers' pneumoconiosis. Correlation of roentgenographic and postmortem findings. *JAMA* 1972; 220:223.
229. Nam K, Gracey DR: Pulmonary talcosis from cosmetic talcum powder. *JAMA* 1972; 221:492.
230. Naseem SM, Tishler PV, Anderson HA, et al: Aryl hydrocarbon hydroxylase in asbestos workers. *Am Rev Respir Dis* 1978; 118:693.
231. Nasr ANM, Ditchek T, Scholtens PA: The prevalence of radiographic abnormalities in the chests of fiberglass workers. *J Occup Med* 1971; 13:371.
232. Newhouse ML, Berry G: Predictions of mortality from mesothelial tumours in asbestos factory workers. *Br J Ind Med* 1976; 33:147.
233. O'Brien RJ: Pleural calcification in coal miners. *J Occup Med* 1972; 14:922.
234. Ogilvie C, Brown K, Kearns WE: Overinflation of the lungs in coal miners. *Br Med J* 1967; 3:10.
235. Oldham PD: Pneumoconiosis in Cornish China clay workers. *Br J Ind Med* 1983; 40:131.
236. Oosthuizen SF, Theron CP: Correlation between the radiographic and pathological findings in silicosis. *Med Proc* 1964; 10:337.
237. Ortmeyer CE, Costello J, Morgan WKC, et al: The mortality of Appalachian coal miners, 1963 to 1971. *Arch Environ Health* 1974; 29:67.
238. Oxhoj H, Bake B, Wedel H, et al: Effects of electric arc welding on ventilatory lung function. *Arch Environ Health* 1979; 34:211.
239. Palmer A, Finnegan W, Herwitt P, et al: Byssinosis and chronic respiratory disease in U.S. cotton gins. *J Occup Med* 1978; 20:96.
240. Parrot JL, Hebert R, Saindelle A, et al: Platinum and platinosis. *Arch Environ Health* 1969; 19:685.
241. Peterson JF: Silicosis in hardrock miners in Ontario: The problem and its prevention. *Can Med Assoc J* 1961; 84:594.
242. Pearle JL: Smoking and duration of asbestos exposure in the production of functional and roentgenographic abnormalities in shipyard workers. *J Occup Med* 1982; 24:37.
243. Pearson DJ, Mentneck MS, Elliott JA, et al: Serologic changes in pneumoconiosis and progressive massive fibrosis of coal workers. *Am Rev Respir Dis* 1981; 124:696.
244. Pendergrass EP: Silicosis and a few of the other pneumoconioses: Observations on certain aspects of the problem, with emphasis on the role of the radiologist. *Am J Roentgenol* 1958; 80:1.
245. Pendergrass EP, Vorwald AJ, Mishkin MM, et al: Observations on workers in the graphite industry, Part I. *Med Radiogr Photogr* 1967; 43:70.
246. Pendergrass EP, Vorwald AJ, Mishkin MM, et al: Observations on workers in the graphite industry, Part II. *Med Radiogr Photogr* 1968; 43:2.
247. Peters JM, Theriault GP, Fine LJ, et al: Chronic effect of fire fighting on pulmonary function. *N Engl J Med* 1974; 291:1320.
248. Pimentel JC: A granulomatous lung disease produced by bakelite. *Am Rev Respir Dis* 1973; 108:1303.
249. Pimentel JC, Marques F: Vineyard sprayer's lung. A new occupational disease. *Thorax* 1968; 24:678.
250. Pimentel JC, Menezes AP: Liver granulomas containing copper in vineyard sprayer's lung. *Am Rev Respir Dis* 1975; 111:189.
251. Polakoff PL, Lapp NL, Reger R: Polyvinyl chloride pyrolysis products. *Arch Environ Health* 1975; 30:269.
252. Posner E: Pneumoconiosis in makers of artificial grinding wheels, including a case of Caplan's syndrome. *Br J Ind Med* 1960; 17:109.
253. Pratt PC, Vollmer RT, Miller JA: Epidemiology of pulmonary lesions in non-textile and cotton textile workers: A retrospective autopsy analysis. *Arch Environ Health* 1980; 35:133.
254. Rawat NS, Sinha JK, Sahoo B: Atomic absorption spectrophotometric and x-ray studies of respirable dusts. *Arch Environ Health* 1982; 37:32.
255. Reger RB, Amandus HE, Morgan WKC: On the diagnosis of coal worker's pneumoconiosis. *Am Rev Respir Dis* 1973; 108:1186.
256. Richards RJ, Jacoby F: Light microscopic studies on the effects of chrysotile asbestos and fiberglass on the morphology and reticulin formation of cultured lung fibroblasts. *Environ Res* 1976; 11:112.
257. Rivers D, Wise ME, King EJ, et al: Dust content, radiology, and pathology in simple pneumoconiosis of coal workers. *Br J Ind Med* 1960; 17:87.
258. Rockette HE: Cause specific mortality of coal miners. *J Occup Med* 1977; 19:795.

259. Rogan J: Coal worker's pneumoconiosis: A review. *J Occup Med* 1970; 12:321.
260. Rom WN, Turner WG, Kanner RE, et al: Antinuclear antibodies in Utah coal miners. *Chest* 1983; 83:414.
261. Rubino GF, Scansetti G, Piolatto G, et al: Mortality study of talc miners and millers. *J Occup Med* 1976; 18:186.
262. Samet JM, Epler GR, Gaensler EA, et al: Absence of synergism between exposure to asbestos and cigarette smoking in asbestosis. *Am Rev Respir Dis* 1979; 120:75.
263. Sander OA: The nonfibrogenic (benign) pneumoconioses. *Semin Roentgenol* 1967; 2:312.
264. Sander OA: Roentgen resurvey of cement workers. *Arch Ind Health* 1958; 17:96.
265. Saric M, Kalacic I, Holetic A: Follow-up of ventilatory lung function in a group of cement workers. *Br J Ind Med* 1976; 33:18.
266. Scano G, Garcia-Herreros P, Stendardi D, et al: Cardiopulmonary adaptation to exercise in coal miners. *Arch Environ Health* 1980; 35:360.
267. Scansetti G, Coscia GC, Pisani W, et al: Cement, asbestos, and cement-asbestos pneumoconioses. *Arch Environ Health* 1975; 30:272.
268. Schachter EN, Maunder LR, Beck GJ: The pattern of lung function abnormalities in cotton textile workers. *Am Rev Respir Dis* 1984; 129:523.
269. Schilling RSF: Byssinosis in cotton and other textile workers. *Lancet* 1956; 2:261.
270. Schlick DP, Fannick NL: Coal in the United States, in Key MM, Bundy M (eds): *Pulmonary Reactions to Coal Dust*. New York, Academic Press, 1971, pp 13–26.
271. Schoenberg JB, Mitchell CA: Airway disease caused by phenolic (phenol-formaldehyde) resin exposure. *Arch Environ Health* 1975; 30:574.
272. Schrag PE, Gullett AD: Byssinosis in cotton textile mills. *Am Rev Respir Dis* 1970; 101:497.
273. Seeler AO, Gryboski JS, MacMahon HE: Talc pneumoconiosis. *Arch Ind Health* 1959; 19:392.
274. Seilikoff IJ: Widening perspectives of occupational lung disease. *Prev Med* 1973; 2:412.
275. Seilikoff IJ, Bader RA, Bader ME, et al: Asbestosis and neoplasia. *Am J Med* 1967; 42:487.
276. Seilikoff IJ, Churg J, Hammond EC: The occurrence of asbestosis among insulation workers in the United States. *Ann NY Acad Sci* 1965; 132:139.
277. Seilikoff IJ, Churg J, Hammond EC: Relation between exposure to asbestos and mesothelioma. *N Engl J Med* 1965; 272:560.
278. Seilikoff IJ, Hammond EC, Churg J: Asbestos exposure, smoking, and neoplasia. *JAMA* 1968; 204:106.
279. Shabad LM, Pylev LN, Krivosheeva LV, et al: Experimental studies on asbestos carcinogenicity. *J Natl Cancer Inst* 1974; 52:1175.
280. Shaver CG, Riddell AR: Lung changes associated with the manufacture of alumina abrasives. *J Ind Hyg Toxicol* 1947; 29:145.
281. Sheers G: Prevalence of pneumoconiosis in Cornish kaolin workers. *Br J Ind Med* 1964; 21:218.
282. Sheers G, Coles RM: Mesothelioma risks in a naval dockyard. *Arch Environ Health* 1980; 35:276.
283. Sheenan DH, Washington JS, Thomas DJ, et al: Factors predisposing to the development of progressive massive fibrosis in coal miners. *Br J Ind Med* 1981; 38:321.
284. Siegesmund KA, Funahashi A, Pintar K: The identification of metals in lung from a patient with interstitial pneumonia. *Arch Environ Health* 1974; 28:335.
285. Sluis-Cremer GK: Asbestosis in South Africa—Certain geographical and environmental considerations. *Ann NY Acad Sci* 1965; 132:215.
286. Smith AR: Pleural calcification resulting from exposure to certain dusts. *Am J Roentgenol* 1952; 67:375.
287. Smith GF, Coles GV, Schilling RSF, et al: A study of rope workers exposed to hemp and flax. *Br J Ind Med* 1969; 26:109.
288. Smith KW: Pulmonary disability in asbestos workers. *Arch Ind Health* 1955; 12:198.
289. Snider DE Jr: The relationship between tuberculosis and silicosis. *Am Rev Respir Dis* 1978; 118:455.
290. Sokol WN, Aelony Y, Beall GN: Meat-wrapper's asthma. *JAMA* 1973; 226:639.
291. Sosman AJ, Schleuter DP, Fink JN, et al: Hypersensitivity to wood dust. *N Engl J Med* 1969; 281:977.
292. Soutar CA, Turner-Warwick M, Parkes WR: Circulating antinuclear antibody and rheumatoid factor in coal pneumoconiosis. *Br Med J* 1974; 3:145.
293. Sparrow D, Busse R, Rosner B, et al: The effect of occupational exposure on pulmonary function. *Am Rev Respir Dis* 1982; 125:319.
294. Stanescu DC, Laurentiu P, Gavrilescu N, et al: Aspects of pulmonary mechanics in arc welders' siderosis. *Br J Ind Med* 1967; 24:143.
295. Stanton MF, Layard M, Teferis A, et al: Carcinogenicity of fibrous glass: Pleural response in the rat in relation to fiber dimension. *J Natl Cancer Inst* 1977; 58:587.
296. Steele RA: The pathology of silicosis: Morbid anatomy and histology, in *Medicine in the Mining Industry*. Philadelphia, FA Davis, Co, 1972, pp 20–38.
297. Stokinger HE, Scheel LD: Hypersusceptibility and genetic problems in occupational medicine—A consensus report. *J Occup Med* 1973; 15:564.
298. Storeygard AR, Brown AL Jr: Penetration of the small intestinal mucosa by asbestos fibers. *Mayo Clin Proc* 1977; 52:809.
299. Suratt PM, Winn WC Jr, Brody AR, et al: Acute silicosis in tombstone sandblasters. *Am Rev Respir Dis* 1977; 115:521.
300. Tashkin DP, Genovesi MG, Chopra S, et al: Respiratory status of Los Angeles firemen. *Chest* 1977; 71:445.
301. Theodos PA, Cathcart RT, Fraimow W: Ischemic necrosis in anthracosilicosis. *Arch Environ Health* 1961; 2:609.
302. Thomas HF, Benjamin IT, Elwood PC, et al: Further follow-up study of workers from an asbestos cement factory. *Br J Ind Med* 1982; 39:273.
303. Tse KS, Warren P, Janusz M, et al: Respiratory abnormalities in workers exposed to grain dust. *Arch Environ Health* 1973; 27:74.
304. Tsou E, Romano MC, Kerwin DM, et al: Sarcoidosis of anterior mediastinal nodes, pancreas, and uterine cervix: Three unusual sites in the same patient. *Am Rev Respir Dis* 1980; 122:333.
305. Uragoda CG: Tea maker's asthma. *Br J Ind Med* 1970; 27:181.
305a. United States Air Force Occupational and Environmental Health Laboratory, Aerospace Medical Division Report: Asbestos: An update of epidemiology and pathology since 1976. deTreville RTP, ed. Brooks Air Force Base, Texas, 1984.
306. US Dept of Health, Education, and Welfare: *Occupational Exposure to Asbestos*, HSM 72-10267, 1985.
307. Valic F, Beritic D, Butkovic D: Respiratory response to tobacco dust exposure. *Am Rev Respir Dis* 1976; 113:751.
308. Valic F, Zuskin E: Respiratory function changes in textile workers exposed to synthetic fibers. *Arch Environ Health* 1977; 32:283.
309. Vallyathan V, Bergeron WN, Robichaux PA, et al: Pulmonary fibrosis in an aluminum arc welder. *Chest* 1982; 81:372.
310. VanToorn DW: Coffee worker's lung. *Thorax* 1970; 25:399.
311. Velican C, Latis G, Popa M, et al: Investigations concerning the preradiological stage of silicosis. *Br J Ind Med* 1959; 16:40.
312. Viallat JR, Boutin C, Pietri JF, et al: Late progression of radio-

graphic changes in Canari chrysolite mine and mill workers. *Arch Environ Health* 1983; 38:54.

313. Vigliani EC, Pernis B: Immunological factors in the pathogenesis of the hyaline tissue of silicosis. *Br J Ind Med* 1958; 15:8.
314. Villar TG: Vineyard sprayer's lung. *Am Rev Respir Dis* 1974; 110:545.
315. Wagner JC, Berry G, Timbrell V: Mesothelioma in rats after inoculation with asbestos and other materials. *Br J Cancer* 1973; 28:173.
316. Wagner JC, Sleggs CA, Marchand P: Diffuse pleural mesothelioma and asbestos exposure in the North Western Cape Province. *Br J Ind Med* 1960; 17:260.
317. Watson AJ, Black J, Doig AT, et al: Pneumoconiosis in carbon electrode makers. *Br J Ind Med* 1959; 16:274.
318. Webster I: The pathology of asbestos, in *Medicine in the Mining Industry*. Philadelphia, FA Davis, Co, 1972, pp 39–55.
319. Wehr KL, Johanson WG, Chapman JS, et al: Pneumoconiosis among activated carbon workers. *Arch Environ Health* 1975; 30:578.
320. Weill H: Epidemiologic methods in the investigation of occupational lung disease. *Am Rev Respir Dis* 1975; 112:1.
321. Weill H, Hughes JM, Hammad YY, et al: Respiratory health in workers exposed to man-made vitreous fibers. *Am Rev Respir Dis* 1983; 128:104.
322. Weill H, Hughes JM, Waggenspack C: Influence of dose and fiber type on respiratory malignancy risk in asbestos cement manufacturing. *Am Rev Respir Dis* 1979; 120:345.
323. Weill H, Rossiter CE, Waggenspack C, et al: Differences in lung effects resulting from chrysotile and crocidolite exposure, in *Inhaled Particles*. London, Pergamon Press, 1977, vol IV, pp 789–798.
324. Weill H, Ziskind MM, Waggenspack C, et al: Lung function consequences of dust exposure in asbestos cement manufacturing plants. *Arch Environ Health* 1975; 30:88.
325. Weiss B, Boettner EA: Commercial talc and talcosis. *Arch Environ Health* 1967; 14:304.
326. Weiss W, Levin R, Goodman L: Pleural plaques and cigarette smoking in asbestos workers. *J Occup Med* 1981; 23:427.
327. Weiss W, Theodos PA: Pleuropulmonary disease among asbestos workers in relation to smoking and type of exposure. *J Occup Med* 1978; 20:341.
328. Weller W: Long-term test on rhesus monkeys for the PVNO therapy of anthracosilicosis, in *Inhaled Particles*. London, Pergamon Press, 1977, vol IV, pp 379–386.
329. Weller W, Ulmer WT: Treatment of pneumoconiosis caused by coal-quartz dusts with polyvinyl-pyridine-N-oxide. *Ann NY Acad Sci* 1972; 200:624.
330. Whitwell F, Scott J, Grimshaw M: Relationship between occupations and asbestos-fibre content of the lungs in patients with pleural mesothelioma, lung cancer, and other diseases. *Thorax* 1977; 32:377.
331. Wiles FJ, Faure MH: Chronic obstructive lung disease in gold miners, in *Inhaled Particles*. London, Pergamon Press, 1977, vol IV, pp 727–734.
332. Wilkey DD, Lee PS, Hass FJ, et al: Mucociliary clearance of deposited particles from the human lung: Intra- and intersubject reproductivity, total and regional lung clearance, and model comparisons. *Arch Environ Health* 1980; 35:294.
333. Wills JH: Nasal carcinoma in woodworkers. *J Occup Med* 1982; 24:526.
334. Wood M: Pulmonary function analyzers for mass screening. *Respir Ther* 1973; 3:53.

334a. World Health Organization: Recommended health-based limits in occupational exposure to selected mineral dusts (silica, coal). *Technical Report Series* 734, Geneva, World Health Organization, 1986.

335. Wyatt JP, Riddell ACR: The morphology of bauxite-fume pneumoconiosis. *Am J Pathol* 1949; 25:447.
336. Zuskin E, Bouhuys A: Byssinosis: Airway response in textile workers. *J Occup Med* 1975; 17:357.
337. Zuskin E, Duncan PG, Douglas JS: Pharmacological characterization of extracts of coffee dusts. *Br J Ind Med* 1983; 40:193.
338. Zuskin E, Valic F, Butkovic D, et al: Lung function in textile workers. *Br J Ind Med* 1975; 32:283.
339. Zuskin E, Wolfson RL, Harpel G, et al: Byssinosis in carding and spinning workers. *Arch Environ Health* 1969; 19:666.

15

Hypersensitivity Pneumonitis

Larry A. Lindesmith, M.D.

Jordan N. Fink, M.D.

Edward P. Horvath, Jr., M.D., M.P.H.

Hypersensitivity pneumonitis, or extrinsic allergic alveolitis, is a granulomatous interstitial lung disorder resulting from a reaction to repeated inhalation of organic particulate matter of 1–5 μ in size occurring in a predisposed host.[106, 112, 117, 122] Environmental exposure to these organic antigens and occasionally to inorganic haptene-albumin complexes in the affected worker results in an inflammatory host response located primarily in the alveolar-air exchange portion of the lung rather than the conducting airways. The response, therefore, is infiltrative rather than asthmatic, even though similar organic antigen in other hosts may produce extrinsic allergic asthma.[106]

Ramazini's description in 1713 of recurrent episodic cough and shortness of breath in workers exposed to the dusts of overheated cereal grains is considered to be the first report of hypersensitivity pneumonitis.[98] Campbell in 1932 presented the first modern description of farmer's lung disease,[16] followed by Dickie and Rankin's classic description of the clinical and pathologic finding of acute granulomatous interstitial pneumonitis in farmers in 1958.[25] They showed that the pathophysiology involved the production of an alveolar capillary block with abnormal gas distribution and was reversible with avoidance of occupational exposure to moldy hay.[100] Pepys et al. demonstrated that farmer's lung was associated with the development of precipitins against thermophilic actinomyces.[94] Emanuel and co-workers showed that the spectrum of pathologic findings depended on the time relationship to acute exposure, and they popularized the finding of serum precipitins to the thermophilic actinomyces in diseased farmers.[33] A study surveyed 1,045 dairy farmers in central Wisconsin for serum precipitating antibody to a panel of antigens, including thermophilic actinomycetes, *Aspergillus*, and pigeon serum.[78] Of this group, 8.5% had precipitating antibodies to one or more of the thermophilic actinomycetes, while 0.4% had precipitins to *Aspergillus*. The individuals with precipitins were further evaluated; 36% had a history suggestive of farmer's lung and 10% had a questionable history for the disease.

PATHOGENESIS

Farmer's lung is thus well-established as the prototypic disease representing hypersensitivity pneumonitis. There has been a recent rapid expansion of knowledge of both immunologic and pathogenic mechanisms and of various etiologic agents that may produce this response. Prominent among these descriptions is that of pigeon breeder's disease, estimated to occur in 6%–15% of the individuals who raise pigeons for a hobby or business.[103] There are about 75,000 breeders in the United States; therefore, as many as 10,000 of these individuals could develop hypersensitivity pneumonitis and potentially irreversible pulmonary damage. The serum protein antigen in this disease provided the opportunity to produce a similar disease in experimental animals and led to a more exact definition of the immunopathology. In a population similarly exposed to potential sensitizing antigens, the number of individuals with disease ranges from 3% to 15%.[84] Yet, approximately 50% of exposed but asymptomatic individuals in similar environments have detectable humoral or cellular immune responses to the antigen without clinical evidence of disease. Thus, other unknown factors are important in the genesis of hypersensitivity pneumonitis. These factors may include the following.

Genetic Factors.—Evidence has suggested that farmer's lung or pigeon breeder's disease may be under genetic control, with an increased frequency of the HLA haplotype in ill individuals.[44] Other evidence has been presented that pigeon breeder's disease is not associated with genetic immunologic responsiveness, as determined by HLA typing of ill and well pigeon breeders.[109]

Infection.—Evidence using animal models of hypersensitivity pneumonitis suggests that some inflammatory event must occur in the lung in addition to recurrent antigen inhalation exposure for disease to develop. Animals chronically exposed to pigeon antigens demonstrated an immune response, but only a transient pulmonary inflammatory response was evident until a traumatizing agent such as bacille Calmette-Guérin (BCG) or carrageenan was given.[40] Such agents, including infectious organisms, may stimulate the immune response by adjuvant action or by enhancement of antigen absorption through the inflamed respiratory mucosa.

Toxic Factors.—The induction, progression, and severity of hypersensitivity pneumonitis may be related to a variety of toxic exposures. Possible toxicants include tobacco smoke, air pollution, and industrial exposure. The occurrence of pigeon breeder's disease has been linked to the use of hexachlorobenzene as a disinfectant in pigeon lofts. The toxic factors may enhance absorption of antigens as a result of pulmonary inflammation. They may also increase local immune responses or may act as systemic adjuvants.

Immunologic Factors.—There is evidence that, while the majority of individuals exposed to an inhalant antigen develop either a cellular or humoral response, only a small percentage develop disease. Control or regulation of the inflammatory immune response by suppressor lymphocytes or helper mechanisms most likely determines the extent of healing or disease induction. Defects in suppressor found in the lung milieu of ill pigeon breeders could not be detected in the lungs of well breeders.

Many distinct occupational exposures have been implicated in this type of host response—bagassosis, for example. More than 600 cases of bagassosis are referred to in the literature. Although approximately 500 of these cases were detected in Louisiana, the disease is of worldwide distribution and occurs wherever sugar cane is processed. Cases of bagassosis have been reported in Louisiana, Texas, Missouri, Illinois, Puerto Rico, India, Cuba, Italy, Great Britain, and Peru.[93] Several cases have been seen in non-occupationally exposed individuals, such as those using the material as a garden mulch, housewives residing in homes several miles downwind from sugar cane fields and processing areas, and employees working in air-conditioned offices at or near sugar cane processing areas.

The spectrum of affected workers was further expanded by the description by Banaszak of hypersensitivity pneumonitis due to contamination of an air-conditioner with a mold which, upon dissemination, produced disease in office workers.[4] Thus, even workers in modern offices might become subject to the disease. The identification of an immune complex response to a chemical antigen-IGG antibody complex formation to inhaled diphenylmethane di-isocyanate widens further the classification of agents that may produce hypersensitivity pneumonitis.[77] A comprehensive list of organic and inorganic occupational putative antigens is presented in Table 15–1.

CLINICAL FEATURES

The presenting clinical history and findings vary through a spectrum of acute, subacute, and chronic features.[46] In approximately one third of the patients, the typical acute disease presents as an attack of chills, fever, cough, and shortness of breath occurring four to eight hours after exposure to the inciting agent. This is followed by malaise, gradual resolution of fever, and a harassing cough, headache, myalgias, and persisting dyspnea.[95] The temperature may often be as high as 104–106° F. Acute symptoms usually subside within two to five days.

Physical examination reveals a moderately ill appearing, dyspneic, occasionally cyanotic patient with characteristic fine bibasilar rales. Wheezing is rare.[33]

A significant proportion of patients present with a subacute syndrome characterized by gradually progressive dyspnea often associated with repeated low-grade exposures to the antigen. The symptoms of acute disease appear to become attenuated,[111] but the dyspnea is progressive. Anorexia and weight loss are frequently identified.

A smaller percentage of patients have chronic disease which is insidious in onset. It is characterized by progressive dyspnea with features of interstitial fibrosis and/or airway obstruction. This is described as occurring most commonly after multiple episodes of symptomatic exposure.[13] In the subacute and chronic patient, physical examination may reveal high pitched end-inspiratory muscle rales suggestive of bronchiolitis obliterans.[25] Death can occur at any stage. The overall mortality rate has been estimated to be between 9% and 17%.[13, 33]

PHYSIOLOGIC FINDINGS

Pulmonary function testing in acute and subacute hypersensitivity pneumonitis reveals early air trapping (elevated residual volume) and normal airway resistance. Restriction (decrease in vital capacity) and stiffness (decrease in compliance) then develop, and gas exchange becomes impaired, manifested by hypoxemia due to ventilation-perfusion imbalance. Fibrosis and membrane thickening result in a diminished diffusing capacity.[100]

In the immediate aftermath of exposure, as seen following bronchial provocation inhalation challenges, an acute drop in forced expiratory volume (FEV_1) and forced vital capacity (FVC) occurs in a biphasic or delayed manner[41] (Fig 15–1). Chronic hypersensitivity pneumonitis is indistinguishable physiologically from other entities of combined obstructive airways disease and diffuse interstitial fibrosis.

CHEST ROENTGENOGRAMS

Normal chest roentgenograms may be found even in the presence of extensive granulomatous interstitial pneumonitis confirmed by biopsy.[34] Commonly, however, during the acute and subacute stages, roentgenograms reveal interstitial reticulonodular densities measuring up to several millimeters in diameter, scattered diffusely, with a basilar predominance. A severe, acute, disseminated infiltration, or "white-out" of the lung can occasionally occur. The x-ray findings tend to clear gradually over a period of weeks to months. In patients with multiple exposures, however, fibrotic densities may clear slowly, if at all, as chronic disease becomes established.[25, 68] The honeycombing of advanced hypersensitivity pneumonitis is indistinguishable from that of other end-stage lung diseases.

TABLE 15–1.
Hypersensitivity Pneumonitis: Putative Agents

DISEASE	OCCUPATION	ANTIGEN SOURCE	MAJOR ANTIGENS
	Thermophilic Bacteria and Bacterial Products		
Farmer's lung	Agricultural workers	Moldy hay and grain	*Micropolyspora faeni* [94]
Mushroom worker's lung	Mushroom workers	Compost	*Thermoactinomyces vulgaris* and *M. faeni* [64]
Bagassosis	Bagass workers	Moldy sugar cane	*Thermoactinomyces sacchari*[54]
Sisal worker's disease	Bag and rope makers	Rope dust	*Thermoactinomyces* spp.[119]
Coffee worker's lung	Coffee workers	Coffee bean dust	*Thermoactinomyces* spp.[126]
Humidifier lung	Office workers, others	Water reservoirs (contaminated ventilation systems)	*T. vulgaris, T. Candidus, M. faeni* [4] *Bacillus cereus*[70] *Penicillium* spp. (fungal)[10]
Fertilizer worker's lung	Fertilizer workers	Dirt	*Streptomyces albus*[65] endotoxin[43]
Detergent worker's lung	Detergent workers	Detergent beads, wood dust	*Bacillus subtilis*[45, 63]
	Fungi		
Wood worker's lung (maple bark stripper's lung, Sequoiosis, wood pulp worker's lung)	Maple bark strippers Lumber barkers Redwood workers Loggers	Moldy bark dust Moldy redwood dust	*Cryptostroma corticale*[32] *Aureobasidium pullulans*[23] *Graphium* spp. *Alternaria tenuis*[66] *Saccharomonospora viridis*[50]
Summer-type hypersensitivity pneumonitis	Occupants of Japanese wood houses	Wood Dust	*Cryptococcus neoformans*[83]
Dry rot disease	Old-house inhabitants (Europe)	Infected old wood	*Merulius lacrymans*[85]
Suberosis	Cork workers	Moldy cork dust	*Penicillium frequentans*[3]
Malt worker's lung	Malt workers	Moldy malt and barley	*Aspergillus clavatus*[12]
Paprika splitter's lung	Paprika splitters	Moldy paprika pods	*Mucor stolonifer* [62]
Wheat weevils disease	Flour workers	Infected wheat flour	*Sitophilus granarius*[11]
Cheese worker's lung	Cheese workers	Cheese mold	*Penicillium caseii* [24] *P. roqueforti*[17]
Horseback rider's lung	Horsemen	Moldy barn straw	*Sporobolomyces* spp.[22]
Lichen picker's lung	Lichen pickers	Moldy lichen *(Cladonia alpestris)*	*Aspergilles* spp. *Rhizopus* spp. *Cladosporum* spp. *Penicillium* spp.[104]
Papermill worker's lung	Papermill workers	Moldy wood chips	*Aspergillus* spp.[61]
	Animal Proteins		
Avian protein diseases Bird fancier's disease Budgerigar-fancier's lung Pigeon breeder's lung Poultry handler's lung	Bird handlers	Parakeets Pigeons Chickens Turkeys Ducks	Avian proteins from serum, excreta or feather bloom[103, 129]
Furrier's lung	Furriers	Fox fur, other?	Animal hair protein[97]
Rodent handler's disease	Animal laboratory workers	Rats, gerbils	Urine, serum proteins[19, 71, 128]
Pituitary snuff-taker's lung	Snuff producers	Pituitary snuff	Porcine and bovine pituitary protein[55]

PATHOLOGIC FINDINGS

Histologic sections of open lung biopsies have been reported to show varying stages of the disease. Basically, an acute granulomatous interstitial pneumonitis is described with components of alveolitis, soft granulomas, intra-alveolar buds, interstitial fibrosis, and miscellaneous minor vascular and bronchial structural changes, including occasionally significant bronchiolitis obliterans.[67, 69, 115]

A mural alveolitis, with interstitial invasion of predominantly lymphocytes, is the most consistent and early finding. A luminal component of alveolitis, with foamy macrophages, is often present,

TABLE 15–1. *Continued*

DISEASE	OCCUPATION	ANTIGEN SOURCE	MAJOR ANTIGENS
	Chemicals		
Bathtub refinisher's lung	Tub refinishers	Vapors	Di-isocyanates[38, 132]
	Foundry workers	Epoxy resins	Phthalic anhydride
	Urethane foam workers	Paint catalyst	Trimellitic anhydride
Insecticide worker's hypersensitivity pneumonitis	Insecticide workers	Insecticides	Pyrethrum[18]
Thesaurosis	Beauticians	Hair spray	Dimethylhydration-Formaldehyde resin[8] Polyvinyl pyrolidone[120]
Red cedar worker's lung	Red cedar workers	Red cedar wood	Plicatic acid[21]
Chromatographer's lung	Pauli's reagent workers	Chromatography spray	Sodium diazobenzene-sulphonic acid[36]
Hard metal lung disease	Tungsten carbide workers	Cobalt in solvents	Ionized cobalt[116]
Berylliosis	Beryllium workers	Beryllium dust	Beryllium[35]
Bakelite worker's lung	Bakelite workers	Bakelite	Phenolic plastic dust[96]
	Medications		
Bleomycin hypersensitivity	Cancer patients	Bleomycin	Glycopeptides of *Streptomyces verticillus*[60]
Gold-induced hypersensitivity pneumonitis	Arthritis patients	Gold treatments	Gold salts[81]
Acebutolol-induced hypersensitivity pneumonitis	Heart patients	β blockers	Acebutolol[2]
Amiodarone-induced hypersensitivity pneumonitis	Heart patients	Amiodarone	Amiodarone[1]

especially in the early phases.[33, 67] Granulomas tend to develop as the acute phase begins to subside. Giant cells, predominantly of the Langhans' type, and soft epithelioid cell granulomatous accumulations are found along with macrophages, monocytes, and interspersed lymphocytes. In general, the granulomas occur within alveolar walls or adjacent to small vessels.[67]

Intra-alveolar buds[67] have been described as loose connective tissue masses located within alveolar air spaces and attached to the alveolar wall by a stalk. These contain mononuclear phagocytes, fibroblasts, and a connective tissue matrix of collagen. The surface of the buds is often lined by macrophages or covered by fibroblasts, myofibroblasts, or epithelial cells. These, combined with fibrosis, may be the early components of bronchiolitis obliterans described in some of the more chronic patients.[115]

The presence of interstitial fibrosis in the alveolar walls is variable but present in all cases. The most unique feature of this reaction is the presence of lymphocytic infiltrates scattered throughout the fibrotic area, which helps to differentiate and distinguish these findings from those of other interstitial fibrosis patterns.[67] Vasculitis and perivascular infiltration with lymphocytes is occasionally noted and rarely becomes intense.[5]

Liebow and Carrington placed hypersensitivity pneumonitis within a spectrum of other vasculitic and exudative pulmonary diseases.[75] With newer information obtained by bronchoalveolar lavage techniques, it may no longer fit within such a spectrum. The pathology of the cellular components obtained from bronchoalveolar lavage in hypersensitivity pneumonitis reveals a marked predominance of T-suppressor lymphocytes.[102] Similar findings have been described with various etiologic agents, including beryllium.[35]

IMMUNOLOGY

The immunopathogenesis of hypersensitivity pneumonitis is still incompletely known. Early studies of the disease found an association with humoral precipitins and implicated antigens identified by diffusion-in-gel methods in vitro.[88] This resulted in hypersensitivity pneumonitides being classified as typical type III immune reactions as described by Gell and Coombs.[48] This concept was popularized by Pepys and Jenkins and was thought to be the basic mechanism for a number of years.[95] Since the type III immune reaction was preceded by a type I reaction in many situations, it was proposed that this may be part of an allergic response. However, studies of patients with pigeon breeder's disease and farmer's lung did not reveal abnormal levels of IgE, although elevations were confirmed in allergy patients.[90] While basophil degranulation is thought to be a confirmatory test for the presence of allergy associated IgE,[7] mast cell degranulation is shown to occur in the absence of IgE following stimulation in experimental pneumonitis. Development of a classic type III antigen-antibody plus complement (Arthus's reaction) response to inhaled antigen as a mechanism of hypersensitivity pneumonitis was, therefore, called an oversimplification by Salvaggio and Lopez in 1976.[76] Fink had earlier shown that up to 50% of subjects exposed to an antigen may develop precipitins without necessarily developing associated symptomatology.[39]

The current concept of the role of precipitins (type III reaction) in hypersensitivity pneumonitis is that they have no significant pathogenic role in the disease process but may be of diagnostic help in identifying agents in the environment to which the patient has been exposed. However, a positive precipitin test does

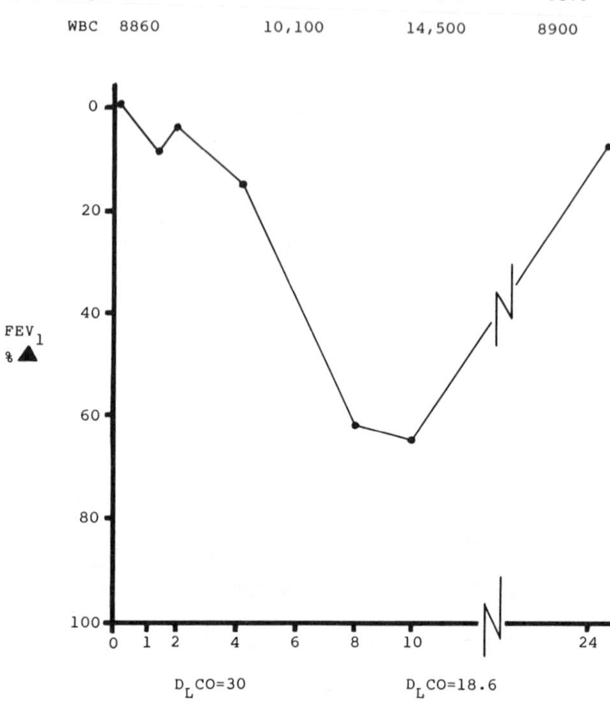

FIG 15–1.
Delayed drop in FEV (in hours) after inhalation challenge with pigeon serum in pigeon breeder. (From Fish JE: *J Occup Med* 1982; 24:379–386. Used by permission.)

not necessarily establish that these agents are, indeed, causative of the disease.[14] Since some patients have been identified with hypersensitivity pneumonitis in which no precipitating antibodies are found, a role for the activation of complement via the alternate pathway was proposed and confirmed experimentally by Edwards et al.[30, 113] and Marx et al.[78, 80] This mechanism has allowed for the proposal of endotoxins as playing a role in certain situations.[43] The current concept of the immunopathogenesis of disease in hypersensitivity pneumonitis is that of predominantly types II and III reactions.[73] The newer techniques that have led to this concept include: experimental model development with animal protein antigen injections,[15] broncheoalveolar lavage,[114] monoclonal antibody methods to help separate T-suppressor lymphocytes from other cells in lavage suspensions,[89] and lymphocyte transformation testing.[51, 52] The type IV hypersensitivity reaction is a cell-mediated, delayed, granulomatous mechanism that involves the T-lymphocytes becoming stimulated to clone. In addition, other immunologic mechanisms have been shown to develop in vitro in such reactions as that to trimellitic anhydrite-human serum protein complexes.[91] Successful development of animal models will facilitate further refinement of knowledge in these areas within the next few years.[107]

These explanations may be incomplete in that symptoms occur in few (3%–5%) exposed persons,[9] and more commonly in exposed relatives of diseased patients than in similarly exposed unrelated co-workers.[124] Host-factor difference is proposed as an explanation for this fact, centering in the past around the genetic HLA system.[44] However, such a relationship has not been confirmed.[42, 109] Further study has suggested that host factors involved with immune-response genes regulating the development of delayed hypersensitivity may play a role.[131] Hypersensitivity pneumonitis and the presence of precipitins in exposed workers is more common in nonsmokers,[127] perhaps due to more proximal deposition of antigens in smokers or perhaps because their hyperreactive macrophage population clears the antigen before it can exert an immunologic effect.

DIAGNOSIS

The diagnostic approach to the patient who presents with signs and symptoms of possible hypersensitivity pneumonitis is no longer as simple as previously thought. Several recent articles suggest approaches and criteria for identification of hypersensitivity pneumonitis.[31, 37, 49, 57, 108, 117]

The diagnosis is often suggested by a carefully taken clinical and occupational history.[27] Hypersensitivity pneumonitis should be suspected if dyspnea, cough, fever, and/or other symptoms are temporally related to exposure to sufficient antigen of appropriate 1–5 μ size distribution.[108]

The physical examination will usually reveal the presence of crepitant rales in a bibasilar distribution. Leukocytosis is often present, and the chest roentgenogram may demonstrate changes consistent with a diffuse interstitial and alveolar pulmonary response, but it may occasionally appear negative. Pulmonary function studies indicate a reduced vital capacity and/or total lung capacity, reduced compliance, usually reduced carbon monoxide diffusing capacity,[86] and reduced P_{O_2} with minimal airway obstruction.

The relationship of symptoms to an environmental or occupational exposure may need to be corroborated along several lines. Identification of exposure to agents known to cause hypersensitivity pneumonitis (see Table 15–1) is predominantly a matter of careful history taking and confirmation from the patient's employer. Observation of clinical and objective response to avoidance of exposure to the suspected antigen is usually a practical way to clinically confirm the relationship. Pulmonary function alteration and clinical responses to exposure at work may be determined by serial spirometry testing performed early in the week and again at the

TABLE 15–2.
Criteria for Diagnosis of Hypersensitivity Pneumonitis (in Order of Importance) When the Antigen Is Previously Known to Cause Hypersensitivity Pneumonitis*

1. History of exposure to antigen
2. Symptoms of cough, fever, dyspnea
3. Chest x-ray changes
4. Evidence of immunologic sensitization
5. Pulmonary function impairment
6. Pulmonary biopsy (selected cases)
7. Provocation inhalation challenge (selected cases)
8. Bronchial lavage (selected cases)

*Adapted from Emanuel DA, Kryda MJ: *Clin Rev Allergy* 1983; 1:509–532.

end of the work week. Similar testing performed serially through the day while at work may also be of value.

Precipitating antibodies that are reactive with the suspected organic antigen generally indicate antigenic response to exposure in patients with hypersensitivity pneumonitis.[29, 95] The enzyme-linked immuno absorbent serum assay (ELISA) may be used as a quantitative, rapid, sensitive, and less expensive replacement[31] for the double immunodiffusion approach of Ouchterlony.[88] In patients exhibiting characteristic symptoms after exposure to antigens in a typical environment, the finding of such antibodies may be all that is necessary to confirm the clinical impression of disease (Table 15–2). When unusual antigens or exposure circumstances exist, inhalation challenge with extracts of suspected antigens may become necessary using a modified Williams technique.[130] This should be done by an experienced challenge laboratory. Identification of the offending antigen may require careful collection of samples from the environment.[102] Extracts then must be made in the laboratory to be tested against the patient's serum.

When the diagnosis is uncertain or the antigen uncommon, bronchoalveolar lavage (BAL) may be helpful, though it is still regarded as experimental. In hypersensitivity pneumonitis, a very high lymphocyte percentage is found in the bronchoalveolar lavage cell population, with a decreased proportion of alveolar macrophages. There is an increase in total protein, IgG/albumin ratio, and often the presence of IgM and IgG antibodies.[105] The BAL fluid may be used also by looking for the presence of migration inhibitory factors.[84] These BAL findings help to distinguish hypersensitivity pneumonitis from other interstitial lung diseases, most of which reveal elevated granulocyte levels in the fluid rather than lymphocytes. Sarcoidosis, which is poorly distinguished by BAL since it too demonstrates lymphocytosis, requires the identification of typical granulomas in transbronchial and bronchial biopsies usually done at the same setting as the BAL.

When it is necessary to establish further immunologic mechanisms (Table 15–3), the finding of serum complement activation via the classic pathway may be identified by diminution in total complement or via the alternative pathway with conversion of C3 PA.[87] Blood lymphoblast transformation studies are helpful in indicating cellular hypersensitivity.[110] A rapid method for determining cell migration inhibition may also be of help.[47] Skin test reactivity is helpful in such forms of hypersensitivity pneumonitis as pigeon breeder's disease, but nonspecific components within the extracts may result in false positive results.[82]

TABLE 15–3

Criteria for Diagnosis of Hypersensitivity Pneumonitis When the Antigen Is Previously Unproven*

1. Exposure to sufficient antigen < 5 mm size
2. Dyspnea, cough, fever symptoms at 4–6 hours
3. Presence of bibasilar crackles
4. Chest x-ray changes, reticulonodular
5. Pulmonary function impairment appropriate
6. Immunologic response with humoral antibody to the antigen
7. In vitro lymphocyte response to the antigen
8. Provocation inhalation challenge positive
9. Pulmonary biopsy: Mononuclear cellular interstitial infiltrate with other compatible histopathologic features
10. Clinical change with manipulation of exposure
11. Bronchoalveolar lavage, apparent cellular and humoral responses

*Adapted from Roberts RC, Moore VL: *Am Rev Respir Dis* 1977; 116:1075–1090.

Transbronchial or open lung biopsies are necessary only in exceptional cases. Transbronchial biopsies may be helpful to exclude other specific diseases but generally yield insufficient material to establish hypersensitivity pneumonitis with certainty. An open lung biopsy through a limited thoracotomy will provide an excellent pathologic yield with low morbidity and no mortality.[101] The results should confirm the presence of a granulomatous interstitial pneumonitis to specifically distinguish the disease from other forms of interstitial pulmonary reactions that may be similar clinically, but not pathologically.[121, 125] For example, the clinical and x-ray findings of hypersensitivity pneumonitis may be duplicated in adverse reactions to Nitrofurantoin, but the lung biopsy findings reveal the subtle distinction of a nongranulomatous alveolitis.[59] A nongranulomatous alveolitis has also been reported in patients taking carbamazepine.[118]

In the differential diagnosis, one must take into consideration the possibilities of viral syndromes and fever (with cultures and acute and convalescent serum antibody titers), silo filler's disease (exposure to nitrogen dioxide within the first few days of filling a silo with fresh corn or hay), pulmonary mycotoxicosis, sarcoidosis, berylliosis, invasive fungal disease, and various forms of diffuse interstitial fibrosis.

TREATMENT AND PREVENTION

The cornerstone of treatment of hypersensitivity pneumonitis is avoidance of exposure to implicated antigens. In the acute and subacute forms of disease, complete resolution, usually within 12 months of clinical, physiologic, and roentgenologic abnormalities, can be expected without specific therapy.[100] Reversal of bronchoalveolar lavage findings may lag behind clinical improvement.

In the occasional patient with severe, acute disease, corticosteroids may be important to rapidly reverse a life-threatening hypoxemia.[74] In acute disease and patients with subacute progressive dyspnea, glucocorticoids (Prednisone 0.3–1.0 mg/kg/day for several weeks) may hasten the reversal of illness.[26, 53, 123]

Prevention of recurrence by avoiding antigens is not always feasible because of other factors involved in job or exposure changes.[106] In certain situations where the exposure to inhaled antigen can be kept relatively low, the use of disodium cromoglycate has been shown with inhalation tests to be protective in some patients.[92] The use of dust respirators is used but is not entirely protective.[58]

Changing environmental factors or altering engineering processes may help prevent exposure, and hence, disease. Successful alteration of the storage of bagasse resulted in a marked reduction of the incidence of bagassosis in recent years.[28] Recommendations to prevent office humidifier lung disease were recently published by the Center for Disease Control.[20] Multiple preventive measures on farms have proven effective in preventing farmer's lung disease.[31] These measures were initially identified predominantly by the victims rather than their physicians.

Acknowledgment

Supported by Asthma and Allergic Disease Center Grant AI 19104 from the National Institute of Allergy and Infectious Diseases, Grants HL 29390 and HL 29319 from the National Heart, Lung and Blood Institute, the Veterans Administration, and the Marcus Foundation, along with thanks to Ms. Catherine A. Walther (Dr. Fink).

REFERENCES

1. Akoun GM, Gauthier-Rahman S, Milleron BJ: Amiodarone-induced hypersensitivity pneumonitis. Evidence of an immunological cell-mediated mechanism. *Chest* 1984; 85:133–135.
2. Akoun GM, Herman DP, Mayaud CM, et al: Acebutolol-induced hypersensitivity pneumonitis, *Br Med J (Clin Res)* 1983; 286:266–267.
3. Avila R, Villan TG: Respiratory disease in cork workers. *Lancet* 1968; 1:620.
4. Banaszak EF, Thiede WH, Fink JH: Hypersensitivity pneumonitis due to contamination of an air conditioner. *N Engl J Med* 1970, 283:271–276.
5. Barrowcliff DF, Arblaster PG: Farmer's lung: A study of an early acute fatal case. *Thorax* 1960; 23:490–500.
6. Baur X, Dorsch W, Becker T: Levels of complement factors in human serum during acute hypersensitivity pneumonitis. *Allergy* 1980; 35:383–390.
7. Benveniste J: The human basophil degranulation test: An in vitro method for the diagnosis of allergies. *Clin Allergy* 1981; 1:1–11.
8. Bergmann M, Flance IJ, Blumenthal HT: Thesaurosis following inhalation of hairspray: A clinical and experimental study. *N Engl J Med* 1958; 258:471–476.
9. Bernardo J, Center DM: Hypersensitivity pneumonia. *DM* 1981; 27:1–64.
10. Bernstein RS, Sorenson WG, Garabrant D, et al: Exposures to respirable airborne penicillium from a contaminated ventilation system: Clinical, environmental, and epidemiological aspects. *Am Ind Hyg Assoc J* 1983; 44:161–169.
11. Bielory L: Hypersensitivity pneumonitis: Occupational exposure to *Sitophilus granarius* and *Thermoactinomyces vulgaris*. *Md State Med J* 1982; 31:25–26.
12. Blyth W, Grant IW, Blackadder ES, et al: Fungal antigens as a source of sensitization and respiratory disease in Scottish maltworkers. *Clin Allergy* 1977; 7:549–562.
13. Braun SR, Do Pico GA, et al: Farmer's lung disease: Long term clinical and physiologic outcome. *Am Rev Respir Dis* 1979; 119:185–191.
14. Burrell R, Rylander R: A critical review of the role of precipitins in hypersensitivity pneumonitis. *Eur J Respir Dis* 1981; 62:332–43.
15. Butler JE, Swanson PA, Richerson HB, et al: The local and systemic IgA and IgG antibody responses of rabbits to a soluble inhaled antigen: Measurement of responses in a model of acute hypersensitivity pneumonitis. *Am Rev Respir Dis* 1982; 126:80–85.
16. Campbell EJM: Acute symptoms following work with hay. *Br Med J* 1932: 2:1143–1144.
17. Campbell JA, Kryda MJ, Treuhaft MW, et al: Cheese worker's hypersensitivity pneumonitis. *Am Rev Respir Dis* 1983; 127:495–496.
18. Carlson JE, Villaveces JW: Hypersensitivity pneumonitis due to pyrethrum: Report of a case. *JAMA* 1977; 237:1718–1719.
19. Carroll K: Extrinsic allergic alveolitis due to rat serum proteins. *Clin Allergy* 1975; 5:443–456.
20. Center for Disease Control: Outbreaks of respiratory illness among employees in large office buildings—Tennessee, District of Columbia. *MMWR* 1984; 33:506–508.
21. Chan-Yeung M: Immunologic and nonimmunologic mechanisms in asthma due to western red cedar (Thuja plicata). *J Allergy Clin Immunol* 1982; 70:32–37.
22. Cockcroft DW, Berscheid BA, Ramshaw IA, et al: Sporobolomyces: A possible cause of extrinsic allergic alveolitis. *J Allergy Clin Immunol* 1983; 72:305–309.
23. Cohen HI, Merigan TC, Kosek JC, et al: Sequoiosis: A granulomatous pneumonitis associated with redwood sawdust inhalation. *Am J Med* 1967; 43:785–794.
24. DeWeck AL, Gutersohn J, Butikofer E: La Maladie des laveurs de fromage ("Käsewascherer Krankheit") une forme particuliere du syndrome du poumon du fermier. *Schweiz Med Wochenschr* 1969; 99:872–876.
25. Dickie HA, Rankin J: Farmer's lung: An acute granulomatous interstitial pneumonitis. *JAMA* 1958; 167:1069–76.
26. Dill J, Landrigan P, Ghose T: A study of the effects of systemic administration of adrenal glucocorticoids in an experimental model of hypersensitivity pneumonitis. *Clin Allergy* 1977; 7:83–92.
27. Dodson VN, Lindesmith LA, Horvath EP, et al: Diagnosing occupationally-induced diseases. *Wis Med J* 1981; 80(12):18–20.
28. Do Pico GA: Occupational lung disease in the rural environment, in Gee JBL (ed): *Contemporary Issues in Pulmonary Disease, Occupational Lung Disease*. New York, Churchill Livingstone, Inc, p. 152, 1984.
29. Do Pico GA, Reddan WG, Chmelik F, et al: The value of precipitating antibodies in screening for hypersensitivity pneumonitis. *Am Rev Respir Dis* 1976; 113:451–455.
30. Edwards JH: A quantitative study on the activation of the alternative pathway of complement by moldy haydust and thermophilic actimomycetes. *Clin Allergy* 1976; 6:19–25.
31. Emanuel DA, Kryda MJ: Farmer's lung disease. *Clin Rev Allergy* 1983; 1:509–532.
32. Emanuel DA, Lawton BR, Wenzel FJ: Maple bark disease. Pneumonitis due to coniosporium corticale. *N Engl J Med* 1962; 266:333–337.
33. Emanuel DA, Wenzel FJ, Bowerman CL, et al: Farmer's lung: Clinical, pathological, and immunologic study of twenty-five patients. *Am J Med* 1964; 37:392–401.
34. Epler GR, McLoud TC, Gaensler EA, et al: Normal chest roentgenograms in chronic diffuse infiltrative lung disease. *N Engl J Med* 1978; 298:934–939.
35. Epstein PE, Dauber JH, Rossman MD, et al: Bronchoalveolar lavage in a patient with chronic berylliosis: Evidence for hypersensitivity pneumonitis. *Ann Intern Med* 1982; 97:213–216.
36. Evans WV, Seaton A: Hypersensitivity pneumonitis in a technician using pauli's reagent. *Thorax* 1979; 34:767–770.
37. Fink JN: Evaluation of the patient for occupational immunologic lung disease. *J Allergy Clin Immunol* 1982; 70:11–14.
38. Fink JN, Schlueter DP: Bathtub refinisher's lung: An unusual response to toluene di-isocyanate. *Am Rev Respir Dis* 1978; 118:955–959.
39. Fink JN, Sosman AJ, Salvaggio EJ, et al: Precipitins and the diagnosis of a hypersensitivity pneumonitis. *J Allergy Clin Immunol* 1971; 48:179–181.

40. Fink JN: The use of bronchoprovocation in the diagnosis of hypersensitivity pneumonitis. *J Allergy Clin Immunol* 1979; 64:590–591.
41. Fish JE: Occupational asthma: A spectrum of acute respiratory disorders. *J Occup Med* 1982; 24:379–386.
42. Flaherty DK, Braun SR, Marx JJ, et al: Serologically detectable HLA-A, B, and C loci antigens in farmer's lung disease. *Am Rev Respir Dis* 1980; 122:437–443.
43. Flaherty DK, Deck FH, Cooper J, et al: Bacterial endotoxin isolated from a water spray air humidification system as a putative agent of occupation-related lung disease. *Infect Immunol* 1984; 43:206–212.
44. Flaherty DK, Hia T, Chenelik F, et al: HLA-8 and farmer's lung disease. *Lancet* 1975; II:507.
45. Franz T, McMurrain KD, Brooks S, et al: Clinical immunologic and physiologic observations in factory workers exposed to *B subtilis* enzyme dust. *J Allergy* 1971; 47:170–180.
46. Fuller CJ: Farmer's lung. *Dis Chest* 1962; 42:176–180.
47. Gauthier-Rahman S, Morlat JL, Leca G, et al: A rapid photoelectric method for reading cell migration from agarose microdroplets. *J Immunol Methods* 1982; 53:77–89.
48. Gell PGH, Coombs RRA: *Clinical Aspects of Immunology*. Oxford, Blackwell Scientific Publications, 1964, pp 320–337.
49. Grammer LC, Patterson R: Evaluation for hypersensitivity pneumonitis. *J Allergy Clin Immunol* 1982; 69:327–330.
50. Greene JG, Treuhaft MW, Arusell RM: Hypersensitivity pneumonitis due to *Saccharomonospora viridis* diagnosed by inhalation challenge. *Ann Allergy* 1981; 47:449–452.
51. Halpern B, Amache N: Diagnosis of drug allergy in vitro with the lymphocyte transformation test. *J Allergy Clin Immunol* 1967; 40:168–181.
52. Hanson PJ, Penny R: Pigeon breeder's disease: Study of the cell-mediated immune response to pigeon antigens by the lymphocyte culture technique. *Int Arch Allergy Appl Immunol* 1974; 47:498–507.
53. Hapke EJ, Seal RM, Thomas GO, et al: Farmer's lung. A clinical, radiographic, functional, and serological correlation of acute and chronic stages. *Thorax* 1968; 23:451–468.
54. Hargreave FE, Pepys J, Holford-Strevens V: Bagassosis. *Lancet* 1968; 1:619–620.
55. Harper LO, Burrell RG, Lapp NL, et al: Allergic alveolitis due to pituitary snuff. *Ann Intern Med* 1970; 73:581–584.
56. Haslam PL, Dewar A, Butchers P, et al: Mast cells in bronchoalveolar lavage fluids from patients with extrinsic allergic alveolitis, Abstract. *Am Rev Respir Dis* 1982; 125:51A.
57. Hendrick DJ: Bronchopulmonary disease in the workplace. Challenge testing with occupational agents. *Ann Allergy* 1983; 51:179–184.
58. Hendrick DJ, Marshall R, Faux JA, et al: Protective value of dust respirators in extrinsic allergic alveolitis. Clinical assessment using inhalation provocation tests. *Thorax* 1981; 36:917–921.
59. Holmberg L, Boman G, Bottiger LE, et al: Adverse reactions to nitrofurantoin. Analysis of 921 reports. *Am J Med* 1980; 69: 733–738.
60. Holoye PY, Luna MA, MacKay B, et al: Bleomycin hypersensitivity pneumonitis. *Ann Intern Med* 1978; 88:47–49.
61. Horvath EP: Unpublished data.
62. Hunter D: Devices for the protection of the worker against injury and disease. *Br Med J* 1950; 1:506.
63. Johnson CL, Bernstein IL, Gallagher JS, et al: Familial hypersensitivity pneumonitis induced by *Bacillus subtilis*. *Am Rev Respir Dis* 1980; 122:339–348.
64. Johnson WM, Kleyn JG: Respiratory disease in a mushroom worker. *J Occup Med* 1981; 23:49–51.
65. Kagen SL, Fink JN, Schlueter DP, et al: *Streptomyces albus:* A new cause of hypersensitivity pneumonitis. *J Allergy Clin Immunol* 1981; 68:295–299.
66. Kaplan RL: Hypersensitivity pneumonitis due to *Alternaria tenuis*. *Penn Med* 1982; 85:34.
67. Kawanami O, Basset F, Barrios R, et al: Hypersensitivity pneumonitis in man. Light and electron-microscopic studies of 18 lung biopsies. *Am J Pathol* 1983; 110:275–289.
68. Klein DL, Gamsu G: Thoracic manifestations of aspergillosis. *Am J Radiol* 1980; 134:543–552.
69. Klinge F: Die merkmale der hyperergischen entzundung. *Klin Wehnschr* 1927; 6:2265–2267.
70. Kohler PF, Gross G, Salvaggio J, et al: Humidifier lung. Hypersensitivity pneumonitis related to thermotolerant bacterial aerosols. *Chest* 1976; 69(suppl):294–295.
71. Korenblat P: Gerbil keeper's lung. A new form of hypersensitivity pneumonitis. *Ann Allergy* 1977; 38:437–450.
72. Kreutzer DL, McCormick JR, Thrall RS, et al: Elevation of serum chemotactic factor inactivator activity during acute inflammatory reactions in patients with hypersensitivity pneumonitis. *Am Rev Respir Dis* 1982; 125:612–614.
73. Leatherman JW, Michael AF, Schwartz BA, et al: Lung T cells in hypersensitivity pneumonitis. *Ann Intern Med* 1984; 100:390–392.
74. Levinson ML, Lynch JP 3rd, Bower JS: Reversal of progressive life-threatening gold hypersensitivity pneumonitis by corticosteroids. *Am J Med* 1981; 71:908–912.
75. Liebow AA, Carrington CB: Hypersensitivity reactions involving the lung. *Trans Stud Coll Physicians Phila* 1966; Ser 4. 34:47–70.
76. Lopez M, Salvaggio JE: Hypersensitivity pneumonitis. Current concepts of etiology and pathogenesis. *Ann Rev Med* 1976; 27:453–463.
77. Malo JL, Zeiss CR: Occupational hypersensitivity pneumonitis after exposure to diphenylmethane di-isocyanate. *Am Rev Respir Dis* 1982; 125:113–116.
78. Marx JJ, Emanuel DA, Dovenbarger WV, et al: Farmer's lung disease among farmers with precipitating antibodies to the thermophilic actinomycetes. A clinical and immunologic study. *J Allergy Clin Immunol* 1978; 62:185–189.
79. Marx JJ, Gray RL: Comparison of the enzyme-linked immunosorban assay and double immunodiffusion test for the detection and quantitation of antibodies in farmer's lung disease. *J Allergy Clin Immunol* 1982; 80:109–113.
80. Marx JJ, Motszko C, Roberts RC: Antibody-independent complement consumption by *Micropolyspora Faeni*. *Int Arch Allergy Appl Immunol* 1980; 62:133–141.
81. McCormick J, Cole S, Lahirir B, et al: Pneumonitis caused by gold salt therapy. Evidence for the role of cell-mediated immunity in its pathogenesis. *Am Rev Respir Dis* 1980; 122:145–152.
82. McSharry C, Banham SW, Lynch PP, et al: Skin testing and extrinsic allergic alveolitis. *Clin Exp Immunol* 1983; 54:282–288.
83. Miyagawa T, Ochi T, Takahashi H: Hypersensitivity pneumonitis with antibodies to *Cryptococcus neoformans*. *Clin Allergy* 1978; 8:501–509.
84. Moore VL, Pedersen GM, Hauser WC, et al: A study of lung lavage materials in patients with hypersensitivity pneumonitis. In vitro response to mitogen and antigen in pigeon breeder's disease. *J Allergy Clin Immunol* 1980; 65:365–370.
85. O'Brien IM, Bull J, Creamer B, et al: Asthma and extrinsic allergic alveolitis due to *Merulius lacrymans*. *Clin Allergy* 1978; 8:535–542.
86. Ogilvie CM, Forster RE, Blakemore WS: A standardized breath holding technique for the clinical measurement of the diffusing capacity of the lung for CO. *J Clin Invest* 1957; 36:1–17.
87. Olenchock SA, Mull JC, Major PC, et al: Activation of the alternative pathway of complement by grain. I. C3PA conversion and

quantification of complement consumption by rye. *Clin Allergy* 1978; 8:125–133.

88. Ouchterlony O: Diffusion-in-gel methods for immunologic analysis II. *Prog Allergy* 1962; 6:30–154.
89. Pacheco Y, Cordier G, Perrin-Fayolle M, et al: Flow cytometry analysis of T lymphocytes in sarcoidosis. *Am J Med* 1982; 73:82–88.
90. Patterson R, Fink JN, Pruzansky JJ, et al: Serum immunoglobulin levels in pulmonary allergic aspergiliosis and certain other lung diseases with special reference to immunoglobulin E. *Am J Med* 1973; 54:16–22.
91. Patterson R, Zeiss CR, Pruzansky JJ: Immunology and immunopathology of trimellitic anhydride pulmonary reactions. *J Allergy Clin Immunol* 1982; 70:19–23.
92. Pepys J, Hargreave FE, Chan M, et al: Inhibiting effects of disodium cromoglycate on allergen-inhalation tests. *Lancet* 1968; 2:134–137.
93. Pepys J: Hypersensitivity disease of the lungs due to fungi and organic dusts. *Monogr Allergy* 1969; 4.
94. Pepys J, Jenkins PA, Festenstein GN, et al: Farmer's lung. Thermophilic actinomyces as a source of farmer's lung hay antigen. *Lancet* 1963; II:607–611.
95. Pepys J, Jenkins PA: Precipitin (F.L.H.) test in farmer's lung. *Thorax* 1965; 20:21–35.
96. Pimentel JC: A granulomatous lung disease produced by bakelite. *Am Rev Respir Dis* 1973; 108:1303–1310.
97. Pimentel JC: Furrier's lung. *Thorax* 1970; 25:387–398.
98. Ramazini B: *DeMorbus Artificum Deatriba (Diseases of Workers)*. Wright WC (trans). Chicago, University of Chicago Press, 1940.
99. Rankin J, Kobayashi M, Barbee RA, et al: Pulmonary granulomatoses due to inhaled organic antigens. *Med Clin North Am* 1967; 51:459–482.
100. Rankin J, Jaeschke WH, Collies QC, et al: Farmer's lung. Physiopathologic features of the acute interstitial granulomatous pneumonitis of agricultural workers. *Ann Intern Med* 1962; 57:606–626.
101. Ray JF III, Lawton BR, Myers WO, et al: Open pulmonary biopsy. 19-year experience with 416 consecutive operations. *Chest* 1976; 69:43–47.
102. Reed CE: Measurement of airborne antigens. *J Allergy Clin Immunol* 1982; 70:38–40.
103. Reed CE, Sosman A, Barbee RA: Pigeon breeder's lung. *JAMA* 1965; 193:261–265.
104. Reijula K, Sutinen S, Tuuponen T, et al: Pulmonary fibrosis with sarcoid granulomas and angiitis, associated with handling of mouldy lichen. *Eur J Respir Dis* 1983; 64:625–629.
105. Reynolds HY, Fulmer JD, Kazmierowski JA, et al: Analysis of cellular and protein content of broncho-alveolar lavage fluid from patients with idiopathic pulmonary fibrosis and chronic hypersensitivity pneumonitis. *J Clin Invest* 1977; 59:165–175.
106. Reynolds HY: Hypersensitivity pneumonitis. *Clin Chest Med* 1982; 3:503–519.
107. Richerson HB, Suelzer MT, Swanson PA, et al: Chronic hypersensitivity pneumonitis produced in the rabbit by the adjuvant effect of inhaled muramyl dipeptide (MDP). *Am J Pathol* 1982; 106:409–420.
108. Roberts RC, Moore VL: Immunopathogenesis of hypersensitivity pneumonitis. *Am Rev Respir Dis* 1977; 116:1075–1090.
109. Rodey GE, Fink JN, Koethe S, et al: A study of HLA-ABC and DR specificities in pigeon breeder's disease. *Am Rev Respir Dis* 1979; 119:755.
110. Rom WN, Lockey JE, Bang KM, et al: Reversible beryllium sensitization in a prospective study of beryllium workers. *Arch Environ Health* 1983; 38:302–307.
111. Rylander R, Haglund P, Lundholm M, et al: Humidifier fever and endotoxin exposure. *Clin Allergy* 1978; 8:511–516.
112. Salvaggio JE, Karr RM: Hypersensitivity pneumonitis. State of the art. *Chest* 1979; 75(suppl 2):270–274.
113. Schorlemmer HU, Edwards JH, Davies P, et al: Macrophage responses to moldy haydust, *Micropolyspora faeni* and zymosan activators of complement by the alternative pathway. *Clin Exp Immunol* 1977; 27:198–207.
114. Schuyler MR, Thigpen TP, Salvaggio JE: Local pulmonary immunity in pigeon breeder's disease. A case study. *Ann Intern Med* 1978; 88:355–358.
115. Seal RM, Hapke EJ, Thomas GO, et al: The pathology of acute and chronic stages of farmer's lung. *Thorax* 1968; 23:469–489.
116. Sjögren I, Hillerdal G, Andersson A, et al: Hard metal lung disease. Importance of cobalt in coolants. *Thorax* 1980; 35:653–659.
117. Stankus RP, Salvaggio JE: Hypersensitivity pneumonitis. *Clin Chest Med* 1983; 4:55–62.
118. Stephan WC, Parks RD, Tempest B: Acute hypersensitivity pneumonitis associated with carbamazepine therapy. *Chest* 1978; 74:464.
119. Stott H: Pulmonary disease amongst sisal workers. *Br J Ind Med* 1958; 15:23.
120. Stringer GC, Hunter SW, Bonnbeau RC Jr: Hypersensitivity pneumonitis following prolonged inhalation of hair spray. Thesaurosis. *JAMA* 1977; 238:888–889.
121. Sutinen S, Reijula K, Huhti E, et al: Extrinsic allergic bronchiolo-alveolitis. Serology and biopsy findings. *Eur J Respir Dis* 1983; 64:271–282.
122. Symposium proceedings on occupational immunologic lung disease. *J Allergy Clin Immunol* 1982; 70:1–72.
123. Terho EO: Extrinsic allergic alveolitis-management of established cases. *Eur J Respir Dis* 1982; 123(suppl):101–103.
124. Terho EO, Heinonen OP, Mautyjarvi RA, et al: Familial aggregation of symptoms of farmer's lung. *Scand J Work Environ Health* 1984; 10:57–58.
125. Valenti S, Scordamaglia A, Crimi P, et al: Bronchoalveolar lavage and transbronchial lung biopsy in sarcoidosis and extrinsic allergic alveolitis. *Eur J Respir Dis* 1982; 63:564–569.
126. Van Toorn DW: Coffee worker's lung. *Thorax* 1970; 25:399–405.
127. Warren CPW: Extrinsic allergic alveolitis. A disease commoner in non-smokers. *Thorax* 1977; 321:567–569.
128. Warren CPW: Extrinsic allergic alveolitis due to rat serum proteins. *Clin Allergy* 1975; 5:443–456.
129. Warren CPW, Tse KS: Extrinsic allergic alveolitis owing to hypersensitivity to chickens—significance of serum precipitins. *Am Rev Respir Dis* 1974; 109:672.
130. Williams JV: Inhalation and skin tests with extracts of hay and fungi in patients with farmer's lung. *Thorax* 1963; 18:182–196.
131. Wilson BD, Sternick JL, Yoshizawa Y, et al: Experimental murine hypersensitivity pneumonitis. Multigenic control and influence by genes within the I-B subregion of the H-2 complex. *J Immunol* 1982; 129:2160–2163.
132. Zeiss CR, Kanellakes TM, Bellone JD, et al: Immunoglobulin E-mediated asthma and hypersensitivity pneumonitis with precipitating anti-hapten antibodies due to diphenylmethane di-isocyanate (MDI) exposure. *J Allergy Clin Immunol* 1980; 65:347–352.

16

Occupational Asthma

Ralph P. White, Jr., M.D.

Edward M. Cordasco, M.D.

Bronchial asthma is generally defined as a reversible bronchoconstriction characterized by exacerbations and remissions of wheezing, coughing, chest tightness, and dyspnea. Precipitating factors most commonly implicated in asthma are: significant weather changes, atmospheric pollution, tobacco smoke, respiratory infection, emotional stress, and several drugs, especially aspirin and β blockers.[12] Common extrinsic allergens are always sought, but occupational compounds precipitating asthma are frequently not considered. Several reasons for this exist. Months to years of exposure to many substances are required before sensitization develops, and during this latency period an individual may have no significant respiratory problems. Secondly, symptoms frequently occur several hours after one has left the work environment, making the association of symptoms with occupational exposure inconspicuous. Thirdly, exacerbations of asthma in atopic individuals are frequently attributed to common extrinsic allergens at home, such as animal dander, pollen, dust, or molds, despite no essential change in the home environment. Fourthly, those with an established diagnosis of chronic obstructive pulmonary disease may have their conditions erroneously labeled as progressive disease rather than superimposed asthma. Finally, since occupational asthma frequently presents with cough and dyspnea rather than wheezing, the recognition of asthma itself may be delayed.

The true prevalence of occupational asthma is difficult to estimate because of the difficulty in diagnosing asthma with atypical manifestations and relating it to the occupational environment. Some industries may be reluctant to report their total number of cases, as the incidence varies considerably among industries. It has been estimated that 5% of workers with Toluene di-isocyanate (TDI), 10%–20% of bakers, and 6% of those working with animals for scientific purposes will develop asthma.[12]

PATHOPHYSIOLOGY

There are three types of asthmatic reactions occurring in the occupational setting. First is the immediate or IgE-mediated reaction, also known as the type I immune reaction. The second is a pharmacologic reaction, with release of histamine, and thirdly, asthma may result from direct irritation of the tracheobronchial tree.

Several months to years of exposure are usually required to sensitize the individual to the substance in the immediate or IgE-mediated reaction. The antigen probably combines with a plasma protein or hapten, with T helper cells stimulating plasma cells to produce the IgE antibody, which then binds to mast cells.

When antigen binds to the IgE-mast cell complex, histamine, SRS-A, and eosinophilic chemotactic factor are released, producing bronchospasm. After the individual becomes sensitized, a very minute amount of antigen usually will produce symptoms, which generally occur within minutes after starting work or become manifest at the end of the day. There may be both immediate and delayed onset of illness. With continued exposure to the offending agents, symptoms worsen and atopic individuals are affected much more so than nonatopic individuals, although only a small percent of the total work force is affected. Immunologic memory or anamnesis will develop to the offending antigen. This means that an individual who has been sensitized to an IgE-mediated antigen may leave the work environment for a period of time, and, upon return to the same environment, experience a bronchospastic episode sooner than after the initial exposure.[34]

The hallmark of the IgE-mediated or type I reaction is an immediate positive skin test with the antigen. Other characteristics of the type I asthmatic reaction frequently present are elevated total serum IgE as well as an elevated antigen-specific IgE which is identified by the radioallergosorbent (RAST) test. Passive cutaneous transfer of the immune reaction from one individual to another by injecting serum from an affected individual into a skin site from an unexposed individual indicates a type I reaction.[18] Bronchial provocation testing with minute quantities of antigen promptly precipitates the asthmatic picture.

In the delayed reaction, symptoms may commence as early as one hour after exposure but usually peak four to eight hours thereafter, with recovery ensuing within 24 hours. This type was initially felt to be mediated by short-termed sensitizing IgG antibody or a type III immune reaction involving immune complexes.[28] However, current investigation favors an IgE-mediated mechanism. Serum precipitins and complement have been infrequently identi-

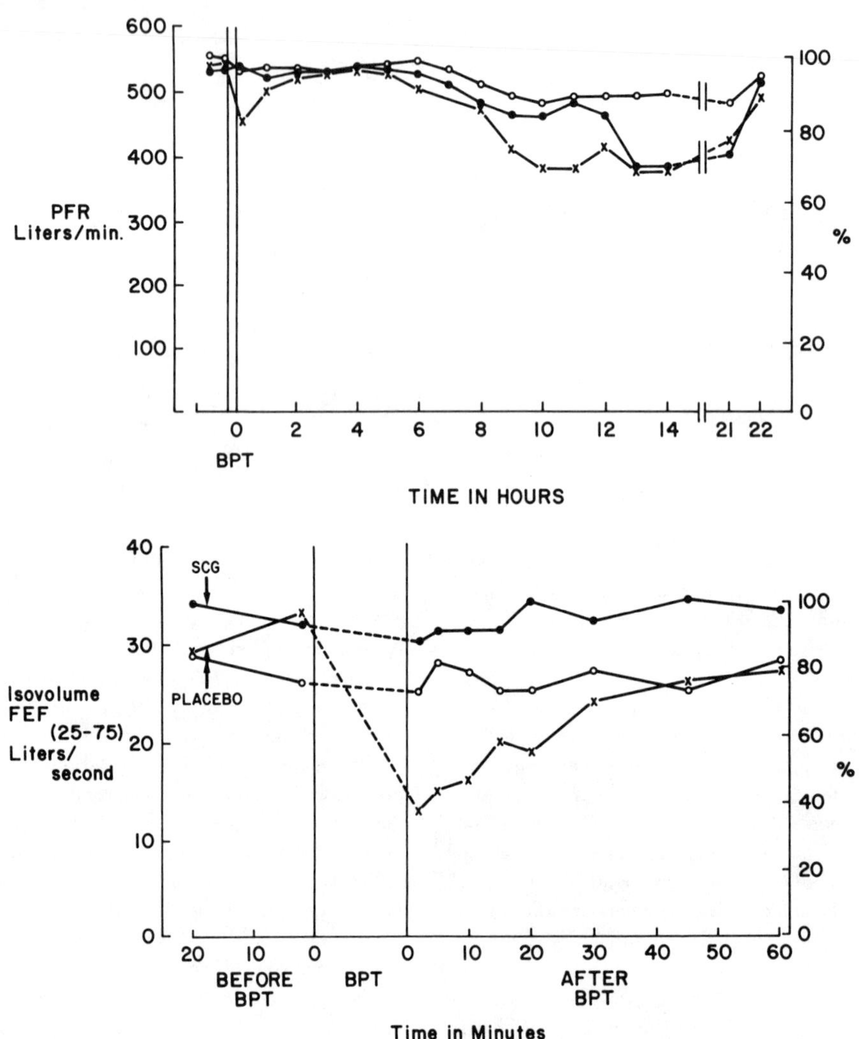

FIG 16–1.
Bronchial provocation testing with TDI. **Top,** influence of concentration on temporal pattern of response. All challenges in the exposure chamber lasted 15 minutes and were preceded by inhalation of lactose placebo. Exposure in a blind fashion to room air (saline) produced only minimal change in peak flow rate (PFR) over the following 24-hour period *(open circles).* There was no immediate change in PFR after exposure to TDI, 0.005 ppm; however, a peak 22% drop 12½ hours after challenge indicated the occurrence of a late reaction *(closed circles).* Challenge with TDI, 0.01 ppm, produced both immediate and late asthmatic responses *(crosshatches).* **Bottom,** effect of pretreatment with sodium cromolyn glycolate. All challenges in the exposure chamber lasted 15 minutes. No reaction occurred when the patient was treated with inhaled lactose placebo and then exposed in a blind fashion to the room air (saline) control *(open circles).* Subsequent exposure to 0.01 ppm TDI preceded by inhalation of lactose placebo resulted in an immediate 60% decrease in $FEF_{25\%-75\%}$ *(crosshatches).* Pretreatment with inhaled sodium cromolyn glycolate blocked the reaction with repeat exposure to 0.01 ppm TDI *(closed circles).* (Courtesy of R.M. Karr, M.D.)

fied and correlated with symptoms or a decrease in the FEV_1 and peak flow. Delayed or Arthus's skin reactions have been infrequently positive.[28] Bronchial provocation testing produces a delayed onset of symptoms (Figs 16–1, 16–2, and 16–3).

The second postulated mechanism of occupational asthma is that of direct chemical irritation of the tracheal bronchial tree with stimulation of irritant receptors and reflex vagal bronchoconstriction.[3] No latency period of sensitization is required, since symptoms may occur upon initial contact with a chemical or dust following a short exposure. Immediate and nocturnal symptoms may occur following a single exposure, as has been reported with TDI and formaldehyde asthma. Usually the increased concentration of the offending agent in the environment will determine the number of affected individuals. Immediate and delayed skin tests are negative. Serum total IgE has been normal and antigen-specific IgE has usually not been identified. One study reported elevated levels of IgE to a ptoyl-serum albumin complex which is thought to be the antigenic fragment of the TDI molecule.[23] Another study has

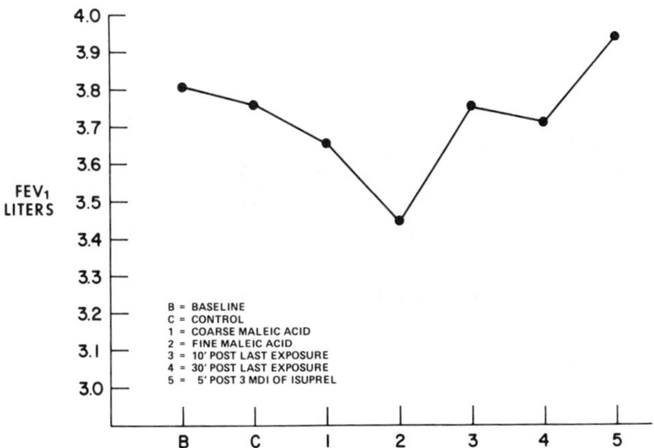

FIG 16–2.
Maleic anhydride BPT.

shown that isocyanates block the increase in cyclic adenosine monophosphates (cylic AMP) in blood lymphocytes to β-agonists and prostaglandins. This suggests that these substances may also produce asthma by blocking β- and prostaglandin-receptors, which is a pharmacologic mechanism. Therefore, more than one pathophysiologic mechanism may be operative in isocyanate-induced asthma.[7]

The final mechanism employed in occupational asthma is a pharmacologic mechanism. Byssinosis is the prime example of this type. Asthma is triggered by the release of histamine from mast cells, with symptoms most prominent on Mondays and disappearing by the end of the week as body histamine stores or prostaglandins are depleted. On the weekends the histamine stores are repleted. Upon return to work the first day of the week, contact with the antigen again stimulates the release of histamine from mast cells, with recurrent symptoms two to three hours thereafter. Immediate and delayed skin reactions with the antigen are negative, and serum total IgE is normal. Antigen-specific IgE has not been identified. Bronchial provocation testing will reproduce symptoms. Tables 16–1 to 16–6 list the most common compounds which have been reported to cause occupational asthma.

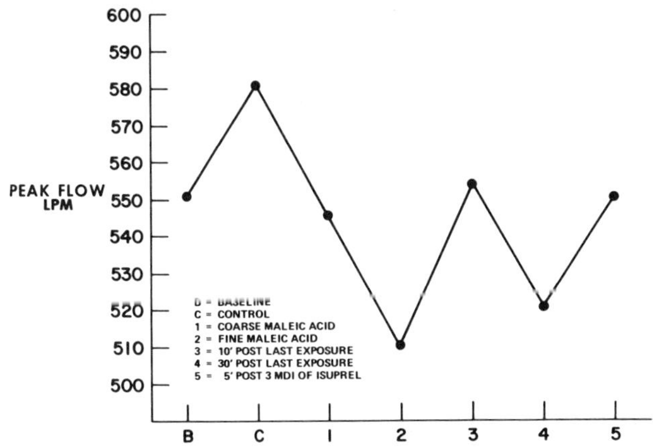

FIG 16–3.
Maleic anhydride BPT.

TABLE 16–1.
Common Agents Related to Occupational Ashthma

INORGANIC AGENTS
Ammonia
Nickel salts
Osmium oxide
Platinum salts
Tungsten salts
Phenyl glycine acid
Solder fluxes

TABLE 16–2.
Organic Dusts*

Cotton dust	Flour dust
Castor bean	Grain dust
Coffee bean	Wood dusts (e.g., cedar)

*Detailed discussion appears in Chapter 15.

TABLE 16–3.
Hydrocarbons

Ethylenediamine
Halogenated hydrocarbons
Trichlorethanes
Urea formaldehyde

TABLE 16–4.
Miscellaneous Causes

Ampicillin
Amprolium HCE
Enzymes (*Bacillus subtilis* [detergents])
Organophosphate insecticides
Piperazine
Spiramycin
Egg protein (inhaled powdered yolk and whole egg)

CLINICAL MANIFESTATIONS

Occupational asthma sometimes presents with atypical manifestations. Paroxysmal coughing, chest tightness, and dyspnea are frequently the most predominant symptoms. Wheezing is often less prominent. The cough is usually nonproductive or productive of small amounts of mucoid sputum, but occasionally, copious amounts of mucoid sputum are expectorated. Symptoms may commence in the late evening or awaken the patient in the early morning. This makes the association with the occupational atmosphere quite remote, so that individuals and physicians tend to implicate allergens and direct irritants in the home even when not readily identifiable. (See Figs 16–1, 16–2, and 16–3, which illustrate the immediate, dual, and late reactions.) Parkes has noted that although dyspnea is usually episodic in occupational asthma, it may progress for weeks or months without exacerbations and remissions. On withdrawal from exposure, recovery may not begin for ten days to months.[28]

TABLE 16–5.
Vinyl Plastic Derivatives

Polyvinyl chloride (PVC)
Polyvinyl acetate (VAC)
Polyvinylidene chloride
Polyvinyl alcohol
Polyvinyl butyrate
Polyvinyl formate
Propylene vinyl chloride copolymer
Ethylvinyl acetate
Polyvinyl carbazole
Phthalic anhydride
Trimellitic anhydride

As noted in the previous section, most substances which cause IgE-mediated or type I asthma may have a long period of sensitization during which the immunologic reaction develops. Improvement or complete disappearance of symptoms with improvement in peak flow and FEV_1 over the weekend together with recurrence of symptoms on the first workday with decline in the FEV_1 and peak flow is a strong point in favor of occupationally induced asthma. Improvement or disappearance of symptoms while on vacation away from home will not differentiate inciting allergens or irritants encountered at work from those at home. When patients with asthma triggered by occupational substances have an exacerbation of symptoms, the common precipitating factors of asthma such as extrinsic allergens, respiratory infections, and emotional stress should not be overlooked. It should also be recognized that an atopic individual may be exposed to common allergens in the work environment such as dust, molds, animal dander, and pollen.

Many industries check a baseline forced vital capacity (FVC) and a forced vital capacity at quarterly intervals in employees at risk because of an atopic history or occupational exposure.

A decreased FEV_1 and FEV_1 percent may be detected in an asymptomatic individual, who should then be further evaluated for obstructive airways disease. When patients manifest a restrictive ventilatory defect, hypersensitivity pneumonitis should also be considered. In individuals with an established diagnosis of chronic bronchitis and emphysema, symptoms may be attributed to polarization of these diseases. However, exacerbations and remissions of cough, dyspnea, chest tightness, and/or wheezing superimposed upon chronic cough and dyspnea, plus a strong index of suspicion, based on occupational exposure, should lead one to consider coexisting occupational asthma.

TABLE 16-6.
Plastics-Styrenics

Polystyrene resins
Acrylonitrile-butadiene-styrene
Styrene butadiene latexes
Styrene base polymers
Thermoplastic elastomers
Toluene diisocyanate

DIAGNOSIS

The difficulty in establishing the diagnosis of occupational asthma lies in recognizing this with atypical manifestations, then correlating it to the occupational environment, which may not be obvious. At the time a worker sees his physician he may be asymptomatic with normal physical examination. The forced vital capacity may show no significant improvement in the FEV_1 following inhalation of isoproterenol. In this situation a methacholine stimulation test to confirm the diagnosis of asthma and assess the degree of bronchial hyperreactivity should be performed. Occasionally, patients will have a negative methacholine stimulation test but have a positive chemical provocation test.[28] When symptoms occur after work, a careful history with detailed questions regarding current and previous employment and occupational exposure is of paramount importance. It is important to determine the chemical environment of the workplace. This information may sometimes be obtained from management, from material safety data sheets (MSDS) supplied by the chemical manufacturer, or from labels on the containers. Knowledge of the substances found to produce occupational asthma is absolutely essential. The knowledge that other workers have been similarly affected is extremely pertinent. A compilation of substances emanating from nearby factories should be obtained as well.[8] The inhalation of organic dusts or microorganisms in the environment or contaminating the ventilation system of the workplace can also result in occupational asthma or hypersensitivity pneumonitis. Thus culture of the workplace or ventilation system may detect relevant antigens such as *Thermoactinomyces candidus* or *Aspergillus fumigatus*. The chemical or cultured antigen may then be used in immunologic or bronchial challenge studies to clarify the relationship between the work environment and the symptoms.[35]

With typical asthma symptoms precipitated at work by a substance listed in Tables 16–1 through 16–4 documented to cause asthma, pulmonary function tests with bronchodilators, is recommended to establish reversible bronchospasm. A 15% improvement in the FVC following isoproterenol is significant. These compounds produce an IgE-mediated reaction, such as produced by phthalic anhydride or trimelitic anhydride, then a positive scratch test, elevated total IgE, and a positive RAST test lend strong support to the diagnosis. Many organic compounds similar to common environment allergens stimulate IgE antibody production. However, most small molecular weight chemicals, unless in combination in a hapten serum albumin complex, are not associated with IgE antibody formation.

Further pulmonary function testing is necessary with atypical manifestations and exposure to multiple compounds. A methacholine stimulation test should be performed in this instance to establish the presence and degree of bronchial asthma and a 15%–20% decrement in a FEV_1 is significant. Further documentation of illness involves the performance of a baseline FVC before work, repeating it at the end of the workday, or after the shift hours. Burge has recommended that workers be taught to determine their peak flows and record them every two hours from waking to sleeping.[6] A 25% decrease in the peak flow rate from baseline or a 15% decrease in the FEV_1 is consistent with asthma.[20] Peak flow determinations are most important in documenting the delayed asthmatic reaction occurring hours after work. Peak flow determination is subject to individual patient effort, and suboptimal results will invalidate the test. This pulmonary function test should be correlated with the FEV_1. Many asthmatics have a diurnal variation in peak flow which usually is lowest upon awakening in the morning and highest in mid to late afternoon. In order to recognize this diurnal variation, peak flow determination should be done daily for at least two weeks, including weekends and holidays. Changes in peak flow during and after work are critical only in comparison with baseline values after ascertaining diurnal variation.[6]

A more indirect and protracted way of diagnosing occupational asthma is to determine the FEV_1 or peak flow while the patient is symptomatic during or after work, and then to determine these tests after two weeks away from work.[6] This should show at least mild to moderate improvement and should be repeated in one to two weeks under identical circumstances for proper validation. The improvement away from the job with a significant decline after returning to work strongly suggests the diagnosis of occupational asthma.

To determine the substance or substances provoking asthma with exposure to multiple compounds or when atypical manifestations occur after work, bronchial provocation testing should be done. Agents which are fluid or soluble can be nebulized from a Wright's nebulizer through an oral nasal mask and a rebreathing bag with oxygen flowing though at 8 L/min.

Wood dust may be tested without dilution by having the subject tip the dust from one Petri dish to another. Certain chemical dusts such as platinum salts should be highly diluted with lactose, and piperazine can be tested in low dilution.[30] Toluene di-isocyanate has been tested by painting a surface with a resin used for polyurethane manufacturing or by burning a polyurethane-coated wire. Other isocyanates have been tested by heating the compounds at high temperatures.[30]

Bronchial challenge with chemical fumes or gases should be done at no greater concentration than is encountered at work, the precise levels of which can be determined by appropriate instruments. Following challenge, the forced vital capacity is initially determined and then subsequently every ten minutes for the first 90 minutes, and then when appropriate hourly during the waking hours.[20] Chemical challenge with fumes or gases may be extremely hazardous and this must be done only in safe, controlled settings. An industrial hygienist should be consistently available to monitor precisely the environmental atmospheric levels.

Delayed asthmatic reaction is detected by instructing the subject to measure his peak flow hourly at home until bedtime and following this if symptoms occur. A controlled challenge test must be done with the diluent to ascertain that the reaction is specific. Because of the need to assess the late reaction following this challenge, only one compound is tested on a given day. Although bronchial provocation is the most specific test in identifying the offending agent, it does not establish the pathophysiologic mechanism of the asthma.

There are important contraindications to bronchial provocation testing. When an individual has experienced severe symptoms or bronchospasm upon exposure to a solitary compound such as polyvinyl chloride, known to trigger asthma, bronchial provocation testing may induce severe bronchospasm. A physician must be available to promptly administer subcutaneous epinephrine and aerosolized isoproterenol if needed. Ideally, the test should be performed in the hospital laboratory. In a situation in which the offending agent is obvious, the test would be superfluous. Nebulizing a concentration that is greater than that to which one is exposed in the workplace could also result in severe bronchospasm not easily reversed. Testing individuals with severe chronic obstructive pulmonary disease (COPD) or severe chronic bronchial asthma with symptoms highly suggestive of occupational asthma may result in further decrease in the FEV_1 leading to severe respiratory distress and acute ventilatory failure. This may occur when the baseline FEV_1 is 40% to 60% of predicted. Under these circumstances the diagnosis can be made by a baseline FEV_1 and peak flow at the start of work and when symptoms arise immediately following work. These values can then be compared with those recorded after two weeks away from the occupation. Significant improvement in the FEV_1 of greater than 15% strongly substantiates the diagnosis of occupational asthma.

TREATMENT

When the diagnosis of occupational asthma is suspected, treatment with oral theophylline and/or β sympatomimetic agents and/or hand nebulizer therapy should be initiated. Tobacco smoking must be stopped completely. If the subject remains symptomatic on this regimen, cromolyn sodium (40 mg) inhaled before work has been shown frequently to diminish or completely prevent asthma. If possible, steroids should be withheld until the diagnosis is established, since they may obscure the asthmatic reaction. If symptoms persist despite the above program, the patient should be removed from the job immediately while the evaluation for occupational asthma is proceeding. Persistent severe symptoms requiring the individual to be treated in the emergency room or hospital, usually necessitates removal from the occupation. Pepys has shown that immediate IgE-mediated asthma can be blocked by inhaled bronchodilators and cromolyn sodium but not by systemic or inhaled steroids. Nocturnal occupational asthma has been blocked by steroids and cromolyn sodium, but only partially by inhaled bronchodilators. The persisting nocturnal reaction is the most difficult to treat, responding poorly to steroids and cromolyn sodium.[31]

After the diagnosis of occupational asthma is confirmed, with a specific substance or substances identified by bronchial provocation testing, the individual should be removed from further exposure to the offending agents. Many people who cannot find alternative employment prefer to keep their jobs if medication controls their symptoms, despite the risk of developing chronic bronchial asthma or even irreversible chronic obstructive pulmonary disease. These individuals should have quarterly determinations of forced vital capacity, before and after using bronchodilators. If there is a progressive decline in the FEV_1 without improvement following isoproterenol, they should be forced to transfer to a different work area or leave the company to avoid further exposure to these compounds. Respirator masks have provided little if any protection of inhalation of low molecular weight chemicals, which can evoke asthma at minute concentrations in susceptible individuals. However, in particulate emissions as with platinum, lead-zinc alloys, and tungsten carbide, these devices are usually protective.

Specific compounds causing the asthma must be identified. The first step is to obtain a list of the substances to which one is exposed from his or her foreman or from the industrial hygiene or safety departments of the company. The exact threshold limit value (TLV) of these agents should be available in the medical department. The affected individual often recognizes the substance only by code names and numbers. Some corporations are reluctant to release the list of chemical exposures. If many workers are afflicted by the same symptoms suggesting occupational asthma, OSHA officers will intervene to test and regulate the concentrations of the offending substances, as well as advising additional safety operations to industry. These methods may be costly to the industry, but will ensure the safety of the workers in reducing their susceptibility and disability from these irritating substances. They will also prevent or reduce frequent absenteeism from work, which would significantly reduce productivity and therefore increase the cost of medical care to the company.

PROGNOSIS

The prognosis of occupational asthma is highly variable, but generally favorable. After one leaves a particular job, symptoms may disappear within a few days or may persist indefinitely. Persistent nocturnal asthma following one exposure to TDI, grain dust, and formaldehyde have been reported. In such instances, it is well established that if one is not removed from the occupational environment despite prolonged adequate therapy, chronic bronchial asthma may ensue. Some evidence also exists that irreversible progressive obstructive airway disease may result from persistent exposure to compounds precipitating asthma.[28] Strong consideration should be given to removing those from significant occupational exposure who have symptomatic irreversible obstructive airway disease of undetermined cause with no history of smoking. This may result from chronic bronchitis or bronchiolitis secondary to their occupational dust or fume exposure, as has been reported from grain dust exposure.[28]

COMMON SUBSTANCES CAUSING OCCUPATIONAL ASTHMA

IgE-Mediated Reactions

Phthalic anhydride has been widely used in the manufacture of plasticizers, epoxy resins, and paints. Asthma has developed after several months of exposure, with both immediate and delayed onset of symptoms. Maccia and Bernstein have reported IgE antibody to a phthalic anhydride-serum albumin complex in vitro.[26] The immediate skin test has been positive, and bronchial challenge has provoked immediate and delayed reactions. Delayed reaction has been blocked by cromolyn sodium, suggesting that it is IgE-mediated, but the immediate reaction has not been blocked by cromolyn sodium on one study, suggesting that it may result from direct chemical irritation, at least in part, or from an IgE reagent.[10]

Trimellitic anhydride is a component of an epoxy resin that has three distinct syndromes. The first, which occurs after a latent period of months to years, is characterized by dyspnea, wheezing, and cough that occurs shortly after arrival at work. The RAST test, immediate positive skin test, and bronchial provocation test are usually positive. The second response also occurs after a latent period of several months to years, in which symptoms of cough, dyspnea, fever, arthralgias, and myalgias develop, approximately four to six hours after exposure. High titers of IgG antibodies have been found. The third response has occurred without a latent period after the first intense exposure, characterized by cough, dyspnea, and wheezing, with no signs of immunologic reaction. Finally, after two to three weeks' exposure to trimellitic anhydride fumes, a syndrome of cough, dyspnea, hemoptysis, anemia, severe hypoxemia, bilateral alveolar infiltrates, and decreased diffusion capacity has been reported. Identifiable antibodies reacting to a trimellite basement membrane conjugate and to erythrocytes are significant.

IgE asthma has been noted in workers who manufacture enzyme-containing laundry detergents. The enzymes derived from *Bacillus* asthma can occur promptly after exposure, wherein the patient will demonstrate a positive type I skin test and bronchial provocation test. Most of the patients from a large series in St. Louis were atopic individuals.

Ethylenediamine is a chemical employed in the rubber, lacquer, and shellac industries. In one study, atopic workers were affected. Symptoms were precipitated within 30 minutes by bronchial provocation testing and abated within two hours, and all patients had positive immediate skin tests.[19] In another study, the nonatopic status was demonstrated, with negative immediate skin test, and bronchospasm induced or precipitated four hours after bronchial provocation. Plasma histamine levels were elevated but did not correlate with bronchoconstriction.[24] Precipitating antibodies to ethylenediamine and Arthus's skin reaction were not found.[5]

Urea formaldehyde resin used in home insulation and as a bonding agent in particle and chip board components, has caused both immediate and late onset asthma. Most individuals, in our experience with 11 patients, have had negative chemical provocation tests as well as negative serum antibody studies,[8] except one patient.[27] Similar results have been recently published by Frigas and Filley.[17] Recurrent nocturnal asthma may persist for several days after exposure, as has been reported in TDI asthma.[11] It is felt that a component of the resin such as hexamethylene tetramine may be the cause of asthma.[32] Chronic bronchial airway irritation has been reported as dose-related in the working environment.[22]

Direct Irritation of the Tracheal-Bronchial Tree

Toluene di-isocyanate is a chemical used in the manufacture of polyurethane foam for insulation, varnish, paint, foam pillows, and cushions. Cough, wheezing, or chest tightness may occur shortly after the first exposure, and bronchial asthma may persist after exposure occurs. The pathophysiology of asthma related to TDI is still uncertain. One laboratory has demonstrated elevated IgE antibody to a p-tolyl serum-albumin complex thought to be an antigenic fragment of the TDI[23] molecule. Direct irritation of the afferent vagal receptors in the bronchial wall is postulated to be an important mechanism. There is recent in vitro evidence that TDI

TABLE 16–7.

Thermal Decomposition Products of Polyvinyl Chloride Meat-Wrapping Films*

Hydrogen chloride
Chlorobutane
Benzene
Toluene
1-chloro-2-ethyl hexane
2-ethyl-1-hexanol
Benzyl chloride
Diiso-octyl adipate (di-2-ethylhexyl adipate)

*Clinical factors discussed in Chapter 64.

blocks the increase of cyclic AMP from β agonists and prostaglandins by blocking beta and prostacyclin receptors.[7, 19]

Products of pyrolysis generated after polyvinyl chloride (PVC) wrapping is cut with a heated wire initiate "meat wrapper's" asthma. Hydrogen chloride is released, possibly producing irritation of the tracheobronchial tree. However, the concentration of hydrogen chloride is very minute, and therefore this is probably not a causative factor.[5, 37] Chemicals released in thermal decomposition of PVC meat wrappings are listed in Table 16–7. During the past few years, the employment of cooler cutting wires has decreased the number of pyrolysis products and lowered the incidence of meat wrapper's asthma. Phthalic anhydride and other products of the adhesive stamp label process may be significant. In one study of meat wrapper's asthma, 69% of those affected were also smokers. Symptoms occurred three to four hours into the work shift and tended to peak toward the end of the week, with definite improvement on weekends. Continued exposure may result in chronic bronchial asthma,[25] although we have not encountered this problem in a rather extensive clinical study.[14]

Styrene- and butadiene-induced asthma is also a clinical entity, probably resulting from degradation products, namely, mandelic acid and phenylglycoxylic acid. To our knowledge, no serum antibodies have been identified.

Pharmacologic Mechanisms

Byssinosis is seen in workers exposed to cotton dust in the initial processing stages and is the classic example of the pharmacologic mechanism characterized by histamine-induced asthma. Symptoms typically are worse on the first working day and disappear by the end of the week as body histamine stores are depleted. With continued exposure, bronchial asthma and irreversible chronic obstructive pulmonary disease may result.[2] The pathophysiology is postulated to be related to cotton bracts from the vegetable matter of cotton, which stimulate histamine release. Other hypotheses include endotoxin components of gram negative bacteria or fungal enzymes and chemical irritation by toxic compounds released from cotton dust, certain polymamines, or methyl ether compounds.[1, 28, 33] The immediate skin test and RAST test are negative, but the bronchial provocation test is usually positive. The examples of pharmacologic mechanisms are exemplified by TDI, which may block AMP or β_2-receptors and certain prostaglandins, hence stimulating a pharmacologic reaction.

Chan-Yeung and associates concluded that exposure to grain dust may cause asthma, most probably of an immunologic basis, as well as probable industrial bronchitis. Their conclusion was that asthma caused by grain dust is probably a type I reaction, since the immediate bronchial challenge reaction could be blocked by cromolyn sodium and the late reaction by inhaled beclomethasone.[9] Seeds, pollen, fungi, and insects in grain dust may be antigenic. Recurrent nocturnal attacks of asthma in one study were attributed to the grain mite, *Glycophagus destructor*.[15]

Immediate skin tests were negative in one study, but in another report they were positive. This correlated with an immediate reaction and positive bronchial challenge testing. doPico and colleagues found no correlation between immediate positive skin tests and positive bronchial challenge reactions to grain dust.[16] Most patients with asthma from exposure to grain dust have positive methacholine challenge tests, indicating nonspecific bronchial hyperreactivity. Chronic bronchitis has been manifested by chronic cough and dyspnea on exertion, and progressive obstructive pulmonary disease without significant improvement following isoproterenol.[13]

REFERENCES

1. Ainszworth SK, Newman RE: Chemotoxins in cotton mill dust: Possible etiologic agent(s) in byssinosis. *Am Rev Respir Dis* 1981; 124:280–284.
2. Beck GJ, Schachter EN, Maunder MA: A prospective study of chronic lung disease in cotton textile workers. *Ann Intern Med* 1982; 97:645–651.
3. Bernstein IL: Occupational asthma. *Chest Med* 1981; 2 (2):255–72.
4. Bernstein DI, Zeiss CR, Wolkonsky P, et al: The relationship of total serum IgE and blocking antibody in trimellitic anhydride-induced occupational asthma. *J Allergy Clin Immunol* 1983; 72:714–719.
5. Brooks SM, Vandervort R, et al: Polyvinyl chloride film thermal decomposition products as an occupational illness II. *J Occup Med* 1977; 19:192.
6. Burge PS: Could you be overlooking occupational asthma? *J Respir Dis* 1982; 3:97–112.
7. Butcher BT, Hedrick DJ: Occupational asthma. *Clin Chest Med* 1983; 4(1):43–53.
8. Carr RM, Davis RJ, Butcher BT, et al: Occupational asthma. *J Allergy Clin Immunol* 1978; 61(1):54–65.
9. Chan-Yeung M, Wong R, MacLean L: Respiratory abnormalities among grain elevator workers. *Chest* 1979; 75(4):461–467.
10. Chester EH, Schwartz HJ, Payne CB Jr, et al: Phthalic anhydride asthma. *Clin Allergy* 1977; 7:15–20.
11. Cockcroft DW, Hoeppner VH, Dolovich J: Occupational asthma caused by cedar urea formaldehyde particle board. *Chest* 1982; 82(1):49–53.
12. Cohen SH: Occupational asthma. *Compr Ther* 1982; 8 (3):27–34.
13. Cordasco EM, Lira R, Demeter S, et al: Industrial technology includes hazardous inhalants. *J Occup Health Saf* 1980; 49:42–45.
14. Cordasco EM, Kerkay J, Demeter S, et al: Newer aspects of polyvinyl chloride plasticizer related lung disease. Presented at the American Conference of Occupational Medicine, Washington, DC, April 1983, in press.
15. Davies RJ, Green M, Schoffield N: Recurrent nocturnal asthma after exposure to grain dust. *Am Rev Respir Dis* 1976; 114(1011).
16. doPico GA, Jacobs S, Flaherty D, et al: Pulmonary reaction to durum wheat. *Chest* 1982; 81 (1).
17. Frigas E, Filley WV, Reed CE: Bronchial challenge with formaldehyde gas. *Mayo Clin Proc* 1984; 59:295–299.

18. Fish JE: Occupational asthma: A spectrum of acute respiratory disorders. *J Occup Med* 1982; 24(5):379–386.
19. Gelfond HH: Respiratory allergy due to chemical compounds in the rubber, lacquer, shellac, and beauty culture industries. *J Allergy* 1963; 34:374–381.
20. Hendrick DJ: Bronchopulmonary disease in the workplace. Challenge testing with occupational agents. *Ann Allergy* 1983; 51(2):179–184.
21. Herbert FA, Orford R: Pulmonary hemorrhage and edema due to inhalation of resins containing trimellitic anhydride. *Chest* 1979; 76:5.
22. Horvath EP: The effects of formaldehyde in mucus membranes and airways in an industrial population. *Compendium of abstracts of XXI International Congress on Occupational Health*, 14.2, 109, 1984.
23. Ise CST, Chen SE, Bernstein IL: Induction of murine reaginic antibodies by toluene diisocyanate. *Am Rev Respir Dis* 1980; 120:89.
24. Krumpe PE, Finley TN, Martinez N: The search for expiratory obstruction in meat wrappers—studies on the job. *Am Rev Respir Dis* 1979; 119(4):611–618.
25. Lam S, Chan-Yeung M: Ethylenediamine induced asthma. *Am Rev Respir Dis* 1980; 121(1):151–155.
26. Maccia CA, Bernstien IC, Emmett EA, et al: In vitro demonstration of specific IgE in phthalic anhydride hypersensitivity. *Am Rev Respir Dis* 1976; 113(5):701–704.
27. McCarthy K, Kramer J: Personal communication, pulmonary laboratory, Cleveland Clinic Foundation, May 1984.
28. Parkes RW: Occupational asthma (including byssinosis), in *Occupational Lung Disorders*. London, Butterworth & Co., 1982.
29. Patterson R, Addington W, Banner AS, et al: Antihapten antibodies in workers exposed to trimellitic anhydride fumes: A potential immunopathogenetic mechanism for the trimellitic anhydride pulmonary disease-anemia syndrome. *Am Rev Respir Dis* 1979; 120:1259.
30. Pepys J: Challenge procedures in occupational asthma. *Bull NY Acad Med* 1981; 57(7):608–616.
31. Pepys J: Occupational asthma—An overview. *J Occup Med* 1982; 24(7):534–538.
32. Popa V, Teculescu D, Stanescu D, et al: Bronchial asthma and asthmatic bronchitis determined by simple chemicals. *Dis Chest* 1969; 56:395–404.
33. Schachter EN, Brown S, Zuskin E: Airway reactivity in cotton bract-induced bronchospasm. *Am Rev Respir Dis* 1981; 123:273–276.
34. Slavin RG: Occupational asthma. *J Hosp Pract* 1978; June, pp 133–46.
35. Smith AB, et al: Occupational asthma from inhaled egg protein. *Am J Ind Med* 1987; 12:205–218.
36. Wernfors M, Nielsen J, Schütz A, et al: Phthalic anhydride-induced occupational asthma. *Int Arch Allergy Appl Immunol* 1986; 79: 77–82.
37. White RP, Cordasco EM: Occupational asthma: A frequently overlooked entity. *J Intern Med Specialist* 1982; 3(5):90–100.

17

Establishing Causation and Evaluating Pulmonary Impairment

Larry A. Lindesmith, M.D.

There are four primary reasons for evaluating an employee's pulmonary capabilities. They are (1) the baseline determination of pulmonary capability for preemployment screening; (2) detection of disease; (3) back-to-work testing or determination of the capacity to perform a given job or a given level of work; and (4) determination of total or partial impairment of potential performance on the basis of damage to the respiratory system.

In the first situation, a biometric relationship exists between a measured breathing performance and groups of measurements of allegedly normal people used as reference values. The examiner has to make assumptions, such as the applicability of the reference values to the individual. Assumptions are made implicitly regarding the person's motivation, inclination, experience, endurance, and competence, thus making it difficult to assure an employer that a person with a given normal degree of pulmonary function can perform in a normal manner. In fact, in the screening for employment situations, the examiner commonly presents a disclaimer stating only that the given person has no evidence of being incapable of working. Here, a measurement of capability has been carried out, but it is not terribly important or germane except in relationship to the biometric fact that the person can perform within the boundaries of the norm for the tests of function examined.

Detection of disease also involves measurement compared to a healthy population. Standard principles should be followed.[46] A screening test should not be regarded as diagnostic, since further evaluation is usually necessary to establish a diagnosis and determine proper treatment.[10]

When testing for a patient's return to work or in determining his or her ability to perform a given job, a totally different approach in pulmonary evaluation is carried out, in that the results become more specific to the job. In this situation, if spirometry is abnormal, actual on-job measurement of oxygen consumption may need to be performed as an index of the amount of effort needed, or standard tables of metabolic costs of activities may be consulted.[8] The given employee's performance is then tested to determine the maximum level of oxygen consumption obtainable. Åstrand has shown that a given average activity level must require no more than 40% of a person's maximum oxygen consumption ($\dot{V}_{O_2}$ MAX) to be tolerated without fatigue or dyspnea during a 40-hour work week.[5] A biophysical relationship is thus measured, but the assessment falls short of predicting the ability to perform the job from other viewpoints, such as whether the patient has sufficient coordination ability or back strength.

In an evaluation for the determination of pulmonary impairment, still different presumptions and system demands come into play. In the first three situations above, the applicant or employee is most often desirous of working or returning to work and interested in performing well and so is highly motivated at the time of measurement. In contrast, in the case of an evaluation to determine workers' compensation, the employee is often motivated to show poor performance or, indeed, to emphasize symptoms of inability out of proportion to measured capabilities. A biophysical approach to the measurement of the employee's capability in relationship to his job requirement would again be most important. This is seldom feasible because of the expense and time involved. Also, the employee may have already ceased working and, in some cases, may feel that reexposure in the particular job may impair his or her lung function further and does not desire to be back in that job atmosphere. Here, the claimant believes his or her overall lung function is impaired. But, as Becklake has pointed out,[9] we are unable to measure "overall lung function." We are limited to our ability to measure size (lung volume), emptying rates (flow tests), functional surface area (diffusing capacity), and oxygen consumption at rest or with exercise. Even in recording oxygen consumption, we are measuring not necessarily what is most important. The $\dot{V}_{O_2}$ MAX by itself may not only reflect lung impairment or capability, but it is interrelated to heart function, diminishes naturally with age, and requires maximum effort and good muscle condition to demonstrate full capability. What is important, but not as easily measured, is the activity that is allowed by a person's oxygen consumption capability, and conversely, the activities, tasks, and jobs that can no longer be performed. We require a maximum oxygen consumption of 10 ml/min/kg as a minimum requirement for almost any activity. Most of us can attain 25 ml/min/kg and Olympic athletes can attain 50 ml/min/kg.

In seeking a measure of degree of impairment, it makes little difference whether we are evaluating an obstructive lung disease patient, one with restriction, one with chest wall problems from trauma,[32] or one with interstitial lung disease, whether for workers' compensation claim, private insurance disability claim, or social security disability claim. The difference among these variables is not the degree of impairment, but the standards upon which that degree of impairment is adjudicated into a determination of disability. While there has been a strong emphasis in the literature for a need for more standardized adjudication, this has not to date come about.[20, 24] Nevertheless, progress is being made toward improved standardization. As a result of publications such as that of Epler,[20] which show that the standards used in determination of disability by the Social Security disability evaluation systems in certain situations require that the patient be so disabled as to be near death, those standards have been recently reviewed by the Social Security administration. Another important step was a major conference held in Sweden in 1981 to review the relationship of pathophysiology to functional impairment.[6]

It is worth emphasizing that a distinction must be made between the terms of impairment and disability, and the following definitions, as presented by the American Thoracic Society, are used:

Impairment: this is purely a medical condition. It reflects a functional abnormality that persists after appropriate therapy and with no reasonable prospect of improvement. It may or may not be stable at the time the evaluation is made. If severe, it frequently precludes gainful employment. It is always a basic consideration in the evaluation of disability.

Disability: a term that indicates the total effect of impairment upon a patient's life. It is affected by such diverse factors as age, gender, education, economic and social environment, and the energy requirements of the occupation.

DIAGNOSIS AND CAUSATION

It is generally felt that the rating of health impairment should be within the province of a physician's expertise to quantitate, whereas the determination of disability is an administrative decision that requires consideration of many nonmedical as well as medical variables.[18] Nevertheless, in the case of work-related injury or illness, two additional factors must be considered by the physician and cannot be handed over to the administrators for determination of fact without appropriate physician comment: (1) the diagnosis of the disease thought to be responsible for the impairment; and (2) the evaluation of the probable cause of the impairment.

A severe degree of impairment alone is of material importance in disability determination under Social Security and some private insurance disability programs. However, the diagnosis and causation question becomes equally important and often difficult in determinations under the state's workers' compensation program and in civil litigation cases. The reasons for this difficulty revolve around the latency of disease and knowledge about causation of the disease.[7]

The latency period can be defined as the interval between the first exposure to a hazard and the manifestation of a resulting disease. Difficulties imposed by this latent period are due to impaired recognition of the connection between exposure and disease with impairment and to an often-diminished ability to gather pertinent evidence retrospectively. A third confounding influence of the latency period is its influence upon determining the employment-related aggravation of preexisting disease.

A complete, detailed occupational history is, of course, important in recognizing possible causal relationships. Good judgment of causality requires consideration of the latent period for certain agents. The known time-course of the disease process itself from inception until recognition may also have an impact on such judgment. For example, because of the known doubling times of cells in the maturation of adenocarcinoma of the lung to the point of being visible on x-ray, it would not be considered probable that an employee who has been exposed to nickel in a smelter for only one year at the time of diagnosis had a nickel exposure-related cancer.

The physician's opinion regarding causation is required as to medical probability to a reasonable degree. In arriving at an opinion, the physician must consider epidemiologic studies, patient exposure histories, and the presence or absence of preexisting disease.

Evidence regarding the use of protective equipment both from the standpoint of employers' policies and from the standpoint of the claimant's acknowledgment of such use can be helpful and should be sought. Industrial hygiene data regarding exposures can, of course, be very helpful but have seldom been available in the past. In addition, the opinion of the physician must be based also on workers' compensation law and, ever more importantly, on judicial interpretations of the law.[24, 42]

Guidelines regarding drawing inferences from epidemiologic studies have been published and should be incorporated into one's approach to the issue of causality.[31] For a sound basis for understanding and interpreting epidemiologic reports, refer to Chapter 71.

Three specific questions need to be resolved. First, is there a sufficiently established link known between an occupational exposure and a particular lung disease? In some situations, it may be well established in the scientific literature that such a relationship exists. In other situations, the judgment is less certain, because the connection has been shown to exist in animal studies but has not been necessarily confirmed in human studies. Here, the decision requires a public judgment utilizing the information at hand. In still other situations, the link is totally uncertain. This is often the case in alleged links popularized by the lay press and promulgated by external pressure opinions.

Second, does the claimant have the disorder being claimed? An examiner's decision often must be based on poor information and unsubstantiated opinion. Providing medical guidelines to the lay examiner through education may play a role in helping examiners to distinguish between opposing physicians' opinions. While legitimate differences of opinion between examining physicians may certainly exist, an increasing problem facing claim examiners today is one of physicians willing to disregard ethics in return for financial remuneration through their provision of unsubstantiated but impressive sounding opinions. While this is an even bigger problem in situations which proceed under tort law outside of the workers' compensation realm, it still is a problem within workers' compensation, because the long-term care afforded individuals by these physicians may be totally compensable under workers' compensation but only partially covered under other insurance coverage the employee may have available.

Third, did the alleged occupational exposure cause the claimant's illness? In some situations this is easily resolved by appropriate historic fact, but in many cases, uncertainty exists. To determine this requires addressing not only the question of whether sufficient degree or duration of exposure, indeed, could result in the disease condition, but also the question of whether nonoccupational exposure to a possible causative agent has been ruled out as a factor. It requires considering the existence of any minimal exposure-response relationship. It further requires considering the definitions of "aggravation," "by accident," and "in the course of employment" as used in workers' compensation law in a particular jurisdiction.[24] Even the common standard in most states that, to be compensable, the disease must not be an "ordinary disease of life," is altered by varying judgments in some jurisdictions that cloud this issue. For example, the "black lung law" has expanded the workers' compensation concept of providing a recompense for wages lost because of work-related impairment into virtually a retirement benefit for anyone who has worked in certain coal mining situations, even when the only evidence of any disease or impairment by medical judgment relates only to a past history of smoking cigarettes.[12] In an attempt to preclude this happening in the asbestos lung disease field, Mitchell has evaluated a large number of asbestos workers with and without a smoking history and has proposed a method of arriving at an appropriate medical judgment as to the relative impact of the person's cigarette smoking upon any total overall estimate of impairment.[39]

Attempts to discern causation may all become moot in the coming years. Increasingly, nonscheduled cases and judicial interpretations are reducing the dissimilarities between workers' compensation awards for impairment and disability and Social Security disability program awards, such that both programs are converging.[15] As employers find themselves holding more and more control over employee medical insurance as well as workers' compensation programs, a convergence of workers' compensation medical care coverage and company-provided general medical insurance could occur in such a manner (i.e., "no fault" insurance) as to eliminate any need for determination of causality in the provision of coverage for the medical care costs.

EVALUATION OF IMPAIRMENT

It has become accepted that the evaluation of impairment requires appropriate physiologic measurement. While very important in the establishment of diagnosis and causality, traditional data regarding occupational history, history of cardiopulmonary illness and trauma, general medical history, history of exposure to smoking and air pollution, general medication and allergy history, review of symptoms (especially dyspnea, cough, sputum production, hemoptysis, and wheezing) physical examination findings, and chest roentgenogram findings are all nondiscriminating in their predictive values regarding functional capability.

Dyspnea may be defined as a subjective feeling of shortness of breath or an uncomfortable feeling during breathing.[44] It is the basic subjective symptom of impairment and can be categorized as suggested by the Medical Research Council (Table 17–1).[37] While useful clinically, dyspnea needs to be evaluated objectively.[34] The complaint of dyspnea correlates poorly with the degree of physiologic impairment found, especially in patients seeking compensation.[20] It therefore becomes imperative that physiologic evidence of impairment be demonstrated to make plausible an alleged complaint of disability. Standard methods of evaluation need be used in order to validate the findings interdependently.[26]

TABLE 17–1.
Classification of Dyspnea

Grade I	Can keep pace on walking on the level with a normal person of the same age and body build but not on hills or stairs
Grade II	Can walk a mile at his or her own pace without dyspnea but cannot keep pace on the level with a normal person
Grade III	Becomes breathless after walking about 100 yards or for a few minutes on the level.
Grade IV	Becomes breathless while dressing or talking

Standards for equipment, techniques, and technician training have been agreed upon in recent years by the American Thoracic Society.[3, 4] These should be followed to assure technically reproducible and valid evaluations.[16]

Several classification schemes have been used over the years in attempting to define degrees of respiratory impairment.[18–20, 22, 23, 27, 30, 36, 38, 43, 49] Some schema utilize different physiologic measurements, depending upon whether the disease being evaluated was obstructive, restrictive, or fibrotic in character. Some schema utilize single physiologic tests, such as the maximal expiratory flow volume curve,[30] while others use a combination of several test results inserted into a complex formula.[47] Gaensler combined the use of a dyspnea index along with varying physiologic measurements of expiratory flow.[22] Different schemes have been suggested by the American College of Chest Physicians,[1] American Medical Association,[2] Department of Labor Employment Standards Administration,[17] Veterans Administration,[43] private insurance companies, and workers' compensation. Proposed evaluation methods utilize everything from subjective symptoms of dyspnea[43] only to complete investigation with treadmill testing.[36] Epler noted an especially wide variation of results in evaluations of interstitial disease.[20] He found that with the widely varied definitions of severe pulmonary impairment under different schemes, some patients would be called "severely impaired" by some methods but not be regarded as being impaired by other schemes.

The American Thoracic Society in 1982 developed a concensus of an evaluation approach.[3] This scheme, represented in Figure 17–1, is based upon a selection of tests in a stepwise manner that allows for cost efficiency as well as fairness to the claimant. This guideline, as well as some special exceptions to be discussed later, was subsequently adapted by the American Medical Association, modified slightly, and published in the *American Medical Association Guides to Evaluation of Permanent Impairment* in mid 1984.[2]

Pulmonary function tests for evaluating impairment should be performed after the patient has received full rehabilitation and therapy and is regarded to be in an optimal, stable condition. The

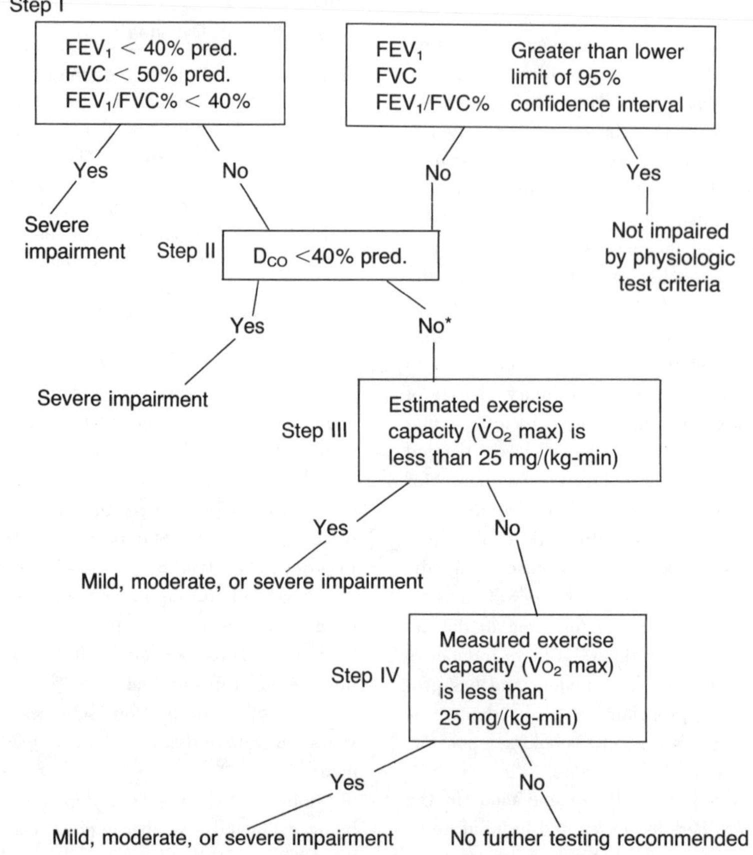

FIG 17–1.
Determination of impairment by physiologic testing. This test schema is proposed for determining whether an individual is impaired by respiratory disease. The reader should refer to the text for an explanation of the use of these tests. *If FEV_1, FVC, FEV_1/FVC%, and D_{CO} are above the lower cut-off limits and the patient continues to have complaints of breathlessness, continue steps III and IV. (Adapted from American Thoracic Society: Evaluation of impairment/disability secondary to respiratory disease. *Am Rev Respir Dis* 1982; 126(5): 945–951. Copyright 1982, American Lung Association.)

patient should be tested following the administration of a bronchodilator,[11] using acceptable techniques, and accepting the best test results. Biometric prediction equations should be utilized, such as those of Crapo et al.[13] The American Thoracic Society recommended the use of percent predicted values where ratings of impairment compared the individual's lung function with a comparable group of healthy individuals. The concept of a 95% confidence interval was used for the prediction of normal value limits below the predicted values.[10] The predicted values are acceptably obtained by the regression equations of Crapo for the FEV_1, FVC, and FEV_1/FVC percent (Table 17–2).[14] A percent-of-predicted approach as the limit of normal may also be used.[41]

In the first step, three measures of pulmonary function are included, i.e., FVC, FEV_1, and FEV_1/FVC percent, all based upon the best maximal forced expiratory maneuver. The individual is declared severely impaired if the results found in any of the three measurements are below the lower severe impairment limits, and then no further pulmonary function testing is deemed necessary for impairment purposes.

In the second step, the single-breath diffusing capacity[35] test should be performed when respiratory complaints persist to a greater degree than can be explained by the results of the forced spirometric measurement. The methodology is suggested to be that described in the 1978 Thoracic Society epidemiology standardization project,[21] and the predicted equations are those based upon Crapo and Morris,[13] normalized to standard hemoglobin concentrations for men at 14.6 gm/100 ml and for women at 12.8 gm/100 ml. If the subject has a diffusing capacity of 40% of predicted or less, he or she is considered to be severely impaired. The lower limit of value of normal is again regarded as that which is equal to the 95% confidence level value subtracted from the predicted value.

In the third step, maximal oxygen uptake estimation should be utilized to evaluate impairment when the values from the first and second steps fall below the 95% confidence intervals but above the severely limited values, and the patient still claims impairment. This approach limits the number of individuals for whom an exercise study is necessary. The estimated work capacity and oxygen consumption can be evaluated based upon the pulse rate measured during an exercise study on a bicycle or treadmill with knowledge of the power output generated during the study or by prediction tables.[28] If a $\dot{V}_{O_2}$ MAX of 15 ml/kg/min cannot be

TABLE 17–2.
Classes of Respiratory Impairment*

MEASURES OF IMPAIRMENT	CLASS 1 (0%, NO IMPAIRMENT)	CLASS 2 (10%–25%, MILD IMPAIRMENT)	CLASS 3 (30%–45%, MODERATE IMPAIRMENT)	CLASS 4 (50%–100%, SEVERE IMPAIRMENT)
Dyspnea	Grade I	Grade II	Grade III	Grade IV
Tests of ventilatory function†: FVC, FEV_1, FEV_1/FVC ratio (as percent)	Above the lower limit of normal for the predicted value as defined by the 95% confidence interval.	Below the 95% confidence interval but greater than 60% predicted for FVC, FEV_1, and FEV_1/FVC ratio.	Less than 60% predicted, but greater than 50% predicted for FVC, 40% predicted for FEV_1, 40% actual value for FEV_1/FVC ratio	Less than 50% predicted for FVC, 40% predicted for FEV_1, 40% actual value for FEV_1/FVC ratio, 40% predicted for D_{CO}
	or	or	or	or
$\dot{V}_{O_2}$ MAX	>25 ml/kg/min	20–25 ml/kg/min	15–20 ml/kg/min	<15 ml/kg/min

*Adapted from *AMA Guides to Evaluation of Permanent Impairment,* ed 2. Chicago, American Medical Association, 1984, p 98.
†FVC is forced vital capacity. FEV_1 is forced expiratory volume in the first second. At least one of the three tests should be abnormal to the degree described for Classes 2, 3, and 4.

reached, the participant may then be considered impaired for all types of labor, as a general guideline. Since it has been shown that when a person works at a self-adjusted pace the work output can be sustained for an eight-hour period if the worker does not exceed 40% of his or her maximum $\dot{V}_{O_2}$[5] (or for a shorter period of time 50% of achieved $\dot{V}_{O_2}$ MAX), then the worker can be more specifically considered severely impaired if 30%–40% of his or her observed $\dot{V}_{O_2}$ MAX does not meet the $\dot{V}_{O_2}$ costs of the occupational activities over an eight-hour period.[3]

In the fourth step, as opposed to estimated oxygen consumption, measured work capacity studies should be performed when one is not sure that the work capacity or maximum oxygen consumption was properly recorded under the third step. This may occur when the symptoms still outweigh the findings, or when inappropriate changes are observed in either the heart rate or ventilation measured. In this step, direct measurement is made of oxygen consumption during exercise, rather than estimating it based upon pulse rate and work load. Additional help may be obtained from arterial blood specimens during this exercise in certain situations. Alternative methods exist for studying the patient under steady-state work[28] or with an incremental work test.[45] The definition of severe impairment remains the same as in the third step.

In addition, in certain situations, a resting arterial blood gas showing a P_{O_2} of less than 50 mm Hg while breathing room air at sea level may confirm severe impairment, regardless of other studies not fitting appropriately. Care must be taken with this estimate, however, to make sure that no recent acute process has occurred, such as an upper respiratory infection, and that the patient remains in a stable, optimal condition.

The American Medical Association guidelines[2] consolidate the classes of respiratory impairment and present categories for determining partial impairment (see Table 17–2). Four classes were developed for categorizing results, using the test schema of the American Thoracic Society. The objective results are displayed in the table to correlate roughly with standard categories of subjective dyspnea.

This classification of respiratory impairment not only helps the physician to determine severe impairment and disability, but it is one of the first attempts since that of Gaensler[22] to classify partial permanent impairment. The concept of partial impairment remains controversial. If a worker is moderately impaired and, hence, unable to do heavy labor but can perform in a satisfactory manner at a desk job, but at less pay, should this imply partial disability? Is the worker stable at partial impairment but progressing to total impairment more rapidly than would be accounted for by the aging process, and should he or she be compensated differently? While these guidelines for partial impairment appear physiologically sound, experience with using them on a case basis is as yet limited.

SPECIAL SITUATIONS

Three categories of special situations exist in the process of the determination of pulmonary disability.

First, the patient may have significant pulmonary impairment but not be disabled. For example, the job may be sedentary and allow for a flexible work time in such a manner as to accommodate the employee's incapacity. The worker's previous experience and education may allow a satisfactory change of jobs to accommodate some impairment. The employee and employer may allow the use of therapeutic oxygen in the workplace to permit the employee's expertise to be used.

Second, the patient may be disabled without having impairment of pulmonary function by the measurements used. For example, in bronchiectasis, pulmonary function may be reasonably good, but the severity of coughing may preclude active regular employment, or excessive fatigability because of chronic infection may affect endurance. In sleep-related breathing disorders such as obstructive sleep apnea, chronic hypersomnia and the effects of chronic nocturnal hypoxemia, such as a reduced attention span and impaired reflexes, may combine to preclude the ability to work even though pulmonary function testing appears adequate. Other measures of impairment may be needed, such as the results of polysomnography evaluations. In lung cancer, the overall clinical condition of the patient should be measured to help determine impairment and, hence, disability, but the means for doing this are at times imprecise. An activities evaluation approach, first published in 1949,[29] remains in use clinically (Table 17–3), but is in need of modern objective reevaluation.[2]

The third special situation is that seen in severe asthma. Frequent severe attacks of bronchospasm requiring emergency treatment by a physician an average of at least six times per year, despite optimal therapy, and with the presence of chronic wheezing or rhonchi and prolonged expiration between attacks is the currently required guideline of the American Thoracic Society for severe impairment due to asthma. In the occupational setting, the determination of permanent impairment due to asthma caused by or aggravated significantly by documented workplace exposure requires an observation period away from the inciting agent of at least one to two years prior to making a determination of permanent impairment. During that period of time, patients may well find another type of job that they can perform quite adequately, even though they meet the basic asthma impairment criteria listed here. In this situation, patients may be disabled from the standpoint of return to the former workplace, but less than severely impaired by the standard criteria of impairment discussed in this chapter and sufficiently able to work in a different work environment on a full-time basis. Nevertheless, the employee should not return to exposure to the agent or agents alleged to induce the disease. Thus, the guidelines given by the American Thoracic Society may be misleading in some situations and require careful interpretation in relation to the individual case by the physicians and examiners involved.

Pulmonary hypertension, cor pulmonale, and increasing severity of hypoxemia with exercise are other situations where special consideration must be given because of the effects of these situations on endurance, even though transient measurements at rest may be within acceptable limits.

TABLE 17–3.
Functional Evaluation of the Patient With Lung Cancer*

PATIENT CONDITION	IMPAIRMENT (IN PERCENT)	FUNCTIONAL ASSESSMENT
A Able to carry on normal activity and to work	0	Normal, no complaints, no evidence of disease
	10	Able to carry on normal activity, minor signs or symptoms of disease
	20	Normal activity with effort, some signs or symptoms of disease
B Unable to work, but able to be at home, care for most personal needs, with varying degree of assistance needed	30	Cares for self but unable to carry on normal activity or to do active work
	40	Requires occasional assistance but is able to care for most of his or her needs
	50	Requires considerable assistance and frequent medical care
C Unable to care for self and requires equivalent of institutional or hospital care. Disease may be progressing rapidly.	60	Disabled, requires special care and assistance
	70	Severely disabled, hospitalization indicated
	80	Hospitalization necessary, active support treatment necessary
	90	Moribund
	100	Dead

*Adapted from Karnofsky DA, Burchenal JH: The clinical evaluation of chemotherapeutic agents, in MacLeod CM (ed): *Evaluation of Chemotherapeutic Agents.* New York, Columbia University Press, 1949, p 196. Copyright 1949, Columbia University Press.

PERIODIC FOLLOW-UP AND RE-EVALUATION IN IMPAIRMENT

It is an accepted phenomenon that pulmonary function progressively deteriorates with age in all its measurable parameters. At any given point in time, a given degree of impairment can be expected to worsen in the ensuing years. Since these aging effects are likely to affect us all, there is no reason to alter our usual interpretation of a given degree of impairment based upon what may happen in the future. Continued exposure to hazardous agents or substances, though, may bear consideration in making determinations. In obstructive emphysema, progression of functional impairment is hastened by continued cigarette smoking but can be slowed by cessation of smoking. In lung cancer, accelerated deterioration of function is likely whenever evidence of metastases is present, but functional loss may be no more than that anticipated for the general population once a five-year cure period has lapsed. In the process of determining disability, these non-aging-related considerations may play a role. In the process of evaluation of impairment, however, the measured degree of impairment at the moment should be used, provided the condition has been treated optimally and is thought to have stabilized and the patient remains on medications such as bronchodilators that optimize the condition at the time that functional measures are made.

Even though pulmonary impairment has not been worked into a schedule for workers' compensation along the lines that orthopedic impairments have, the use of guidelines such as outlined here will help standardize adjudications of disability in the future.

REFERENCES

1. ACCP Scientific Section Recommendations: The determination of static lung volumes. Report of the section on respiratory pathophysiology. *Chest* 1984; 86:471–474.
2. *AMA Guides to Evaluation of Permanent Impairment* ed 2. Chicago, American Medical Association, 1984, pp 85–101.
3. American Thoracic Society, Medical Section of the American Lung Association: Evaluation of impairment/disability secondary to respiratory disease. *Am Rev Respir Dis* 1982; 126:945–951.
4. American Thoracic Society: Snowbird workshop on the standardization of spirometry. *Am Rev Respir Dis* 1979; 119:831–838.
5. Åstrand P-O, Rodahl K: *Textbook of Work Physiology* ed 2. New York, McGraw-Hill Book Co, 1977, p 450.
6. Bake B (ed): Occupational Lung Disease. Pathophysiology and functional impairment. Congress of the Societas Europaea Physiologiae

Clinicae Respiratoriae, Gothenburg, Sweden, June 2–5, 1981. *Eur J Respir Dis [Suppl]* 1981; 113:1–198.

7. Barth P, Hunt A: *Workers' Compensation and Work Related Illnesses and Diseases*. Cambridge, Mass, Massachusetts Institute of Technology, 1980.
8. Battigelli MC: Determination of fitness to work, in *Occupational Medicine Principles and Practical Applications*, Zenz C (ed). Chicago, Year Book Medical Publishers, 1975.
9. Becklake MR: Respiratory impairment including assessment of disability. *Bull Eur Physiopathol Respir* 1975; 7:203–209.
10. Boehlecke B: Medical monitoring of lung disease in the work place, in *Occupational Lung Disease*, Gee JBL (ed). New York, Churchill Livingstone, Inc, 1984, p 225–232.
11. Cohen ER, Cohen BM: Routine use of metapoterenol sulfate aerosol in pulmonary disability evaluation. *Curr Ther Res* 1979; 25:641–649.
12. Comptroller General of the United States: Legislation authorized benefits without adequate evidence of black lung or disability. HRD 82–26, Jan 19, 1982.
13. Crapo RO, Morris AH: Standardized single breath normal values for carbon monoxide diffusing capacity. *Am Rev Respir Dis* 1981; 123:185–190.
14. Crapo RO, Morris AH, Gardner RM: Reference spirometric values using techniques and equipment that meet ATS recommendations. *Am Rev Respir Dis* 1980; 123:659–664.
15. Crum and Forster Insurance Companies: *Role of the State Workers' Compensation System in Compensating Occupational Disease Victims*. Morristown, NJ, June, 1983.
16. Detels R, Tashkin DP, Simmons MS, et al: The UCLA population studies of chronic obstructive respiratory disease. Agreement and disagreement of tests in identifying abnormal lung function. *Chest* 1982; 82:630–638.
17. Dept of Labor: Employee standards administration. *Federal Registry*, pt IV, pp 17722–17723, April 25, 1978.
18. *Disability Evaluation Under Social Security—A Handbook for Physicians*. US Dept of Health, Education, and Welfare, Publication #(SSA) 79–10089, Aug 1979.
19. Durnin JGVA, Passmore R: *Energy, Work and Leisure*. London, Heinemann, 1967.
20. Epler GR, Saber FA, Gaensler EA: Determination of severe impairment (disability) in interstitial lung disease. *Am Rev Respir Dis* 1980; 121:647–659.
21. Ferris BG: Epidemiology standardizations project. *Am Rev Respir Dis* 1978; 118:7–112.
22. Gaensler EA, Wright GW: Evaluation of respiratory impairment. *Arch Environ Health* 1966; 12:146–189.
23. Grimby G, Stiksa F: Flow-volume curves and breathing patterns during exercise in patients with obstructive lung disease. *Scand J Clin Lab Invest* 1970; 25:303–313.
24. Hadler NM: Occupational illness. The issue of causality. *J Occup Med* 1984; 26:587–593.
25. Hansen JE, Sue DY, Wasserman K: Predicted values for clinical exercise testing. *Am Rev Respir Dis* 1984; 129:549–555.
26. Horvath EP Jr (ed): National Institute for Occupational Safety and Health: *Manual of Spirometry in Occupational Medicine*. Atlanta, Centers for Disease Control, 1981.
27. Howard J, Mohsenifar Z, Brown HV, et al: Role of exercise testing in assessing functional respiratory impairment due to asbestos exposure. *J Occup Med* 1982; 24:685–689.
28. Jones NL, Campbell EJ: *Clinical Exercise Testing*, ed 2. Philadelphia, WB Saunders Co, 1982.
29. Karnofsky DA, Burchenal JH: The clinical evaluation of chemotherapeutic agents, in MacLeod CM (ed): *Evaluation of Chemotherapeutic Agents*. New York, Columbia University Press, 1949, p 196.
30. Knudson RJ, Slatin RC, Lebowitz MD, et al: The maximal expiratory flow-volume curve—Normal standards, variability, and effects of age. *Am Rev Respir Dis* 1976; 113:587–600.
31. Kusnetz S, Hutchison MK (eds): *A Guide to the Work-Relatedness of Disease*, revised. US Dept HEW, NIOSH, 1979.
32. Landercasper J, Cogbill TH, Lindesmith LA: Long-term disability after flail chest injury. *J Trauma* 1984; 24:410–414.
33. Lewis BM: Pitfalls of spirometry. *J Occup Med* 1981; 23:35–38.
34. Mahler DA, Weinberg DH, Wells CK, et al: The measurement of dyspnea. Content, interobserver agreement, and physiologic correlates of two new clinical indexes. *Chest* 1984; 85:751–758.
35. Make B, Miller A, Epler G, et al: Single breath diffusing capacity in the industrial setting. *Chest* 1982; 82:351–356.
36. McGavin C: Use of exercise testing in the assessment of respiratory disability. *Intern Med* 1983; 4:107–116.
37. Medical Research Council Committee on Research Into Chronic Bronchitis: *Instructions for Use of the Questionnaire on Respiratory Symptoms*. Devon, WJ Holman, 1966.
38. Miller WF, Scacci R: Pulmonary function assessment for determination of pulmonary impairment and disability evaluation. *Clin Chest Med* 1981; 2:327–341.
39. Mitchell RS, Chase GR, Kotin P: Evaluation for compensation of asbestos-exposed individuals. Detection and quantification of asbestos-related nonmalignant impairment. *J Occup Med* 1985; 27:95–109.
40. Morgan WKC: Pulmonary disability and impairment: Can't work? Won't work? *Basics RD* 1982; 10:1–6.
41. Sobol BJ, Sobol PG: Percent of predicted as the limit of normal in pulmonary function testing: A statistically valid approach. *Thorax* 1979; 34:1–3.
42. *The Bellmon Report*. *Soc Secur Bull* 1982; 45:3–27.
43. Veterans' Administration: *Schedule for rating disability*. Section 6600 for bronchitis, pp 72–3R; 6603 for emphysema, pp 75–2R; 6802 for pneumonitis, pp 78–3R. USGPO, Sept 1983.
44. Wasserman K: Dyspnea on exertion. Is it the heart or the lungs? *JAMA* 1982; 248:2039–2043.
45. Whipp BJ, Davis JA, Torres F, et al: A test to determine parameters of aerobic function during exercise. *J Appl Physiol* 1981; 50:217–221.
46. Wilson JMG, Jungner G: Principles of screening for disease. *WHO Public Health Papers*, #34, 1968.
47. Wilson RH, Hargis BJ, Honr R, et al: A clinical and laboratory method of determining degree of pulmonary disability with a proposed classification. *Am J Med* 1964; 37:251–262.

18

Pulmonary Function Testing in Industry

Edward P. Horvath, Jr., M.D., M.P.H.

The assessment of pulmonary function with a spirometer has become an increasingly common practice in industry and other outpatient settings. Spirometry is now properly regarded as an integral component of any respiratory medical surveillance program. During the preplacement evaluation, it can identify applicants with preexisting respiratory impairment to assure proper job placement and to assist in the selection of compatible respiratory protection. Periodic retesting of workers can detect pulmonary disease in its earliest stages, when corrective measures are more likely to be beneficial. Such intervention could include improvements in industrial hygiene control, job transfer, or medical treatment. Spirometry is also important in clinical medicine to facilitate diagnosis, determine the extent of impairment, and assess response to treatment. Pulmonary function tests assume a key role in epidemiologic studies investigating the incidence, natural history, and causality of environmental lung disease. The value of spirometry has not escaped the attention of governmental agencies. The Occupational Safety and Health Administration (OSHA) currently requires spirometry for employees exposed to asbestos, coke oven emissions, and cotton dust.[24] The National Institute for Occupational Safety and Health (NIOSH) recommends pulmonary function testing for exposure to several substances, including beryllium, cadmium, formaldehyde, nitrogen oxides, silica, sulfur dioxide, and toluene di-isocyanate.[22]

Until recent years, serious deficiencies had prevented the effective use of spirometry in the industrial setting. Poorly-trained technicians and nurses were performing and calculating tests incorrectly. Certain types of spirometers were technically unsatisfactory. Testing procedures and methodology lacked standardization. Recognition that these deficiencies impeded medical surveillance for occupational respiratory disease led to recommendations regarding the three essential components of proper spirometry: standardized methodology in performance and calculation of tests, minimum instrument performance standards, and technician competence. Professional groups and committees, including the American Thoracic Society (ATS),[9] the Epidemiology Standardization Project of the Division of Lung Diseases,[8] and the American College of Chest Physicians (ACCP),[31] have published documents outlining minimum requirements. The regulatory status conferred on the ATS standards by their incorporation into OSHA's cotton dust standard has led to their widespread acceptance in industrial and clinical settings. Concurrent with the formulation of technical standards, a model technician training course was developed by the U.S. Navy Environmental Health Center and the University of Cincinnati in cooperation with NIOSH. Completion of a NIOSH-approved course is required for spirometry technicians in the cotton dust industry and strongly recommended for all others.

PERFORMING THE FORCED VITAL CAPACITY MANEUVER

The maneuver in which the subject takes in a maximal inspiration and then rapidly, forcefully, and completely exhales is known as the forced vital capacity maneuver. To correctly perform this procedure, the subject must be properly prepared by a knowledgeable technician. The technician should explain the purpose of the test, know when to postpone spirometry, demonstrate the proper procedure, and position the subject for the forced expiratory effort. The subject should be questioned about the presence of any acute illness or recent respiratory infection that could influence test results. The patient may sit or stand, but the position should be indicated and remain consistent during subsequent testing. Adults may have significantly larger forced expiratory volumes standing as compared to sitting.[29] After the subject is positioned, he or she should be instructed to take the deepest possible inspiration from a normal breathing pattern, close the mouth firmly around the mouthpiece, and without further hesitation, blow into the instrument as hard, fast, and completely as possible. This particular method of eliciting the forced expiratory maneuver is referred to as the open circuit technique. It is the most common way of performing spirometry in the outpatient setting, and almost all subjects master this procedure with minimal explanation and practice. Some pulmonary physicians prefer the closed circuit technique, in which the subject establishes a constant tidal breathing pattern after insertion of the mouthpiece and performs the complete expiratory maneuver with the mouthpiece in place. As with the open circuit technique, the use of a nose clip is recommended. Regardless of which method is chosen, vigorous coaching is necessary throughout the entire forced expiratory maneuver.

Testing should continue until an acceptable spirogram is obtained. This consists of three acceptable forced expiratory curves that are free from (1) interruptions due to coughing, glotus closure, or an obstructed mouthpiece; (2) hesitant or false starts; (3) inconsistent or variable effort; (4) early termination of expiration; and (5) excessive variability. Tracings marred by cough, inconsistent effort, or false starts are usually readily apparent. Early termination of expiration occurs before the tracing becomes horizontal or "plateaus." The plateau of "end-of-test" occurs when there is no change in volume for at least 2 seconds with an exhalation time of at least 6 seconds or when the forced exhalation time is of reasonable duration (e.g., 15 seconds) in subjects with severe airway obstruction. To avoid excessive variability, the two largest FVCs and FEV_1s from acceptable curves should not vary by more than 5% or 100 ml, whichever is greater. Observance of the aforementioned standards will assure that maximal effort is obtained and values reported accurately reflect the individual's pulmonary function.

CALCULATING SPIROMETRIC MEASUREMENTS

Several parameters can be calculated from the forced expiratory maneuver. These include the forced vital capacity (FVC), forced expiratory volume in one second (FEV_1), forced expiratory volume in one second as a percent of the total forced vital capacity (FEV_1/FVC%), and the mean forced expiratory flow during the middle half of the FVC ($FEF_{25\%-75\%}$). The measurement of the FEV_1 is influenced by the point selected as the start of the test, the zero time point. The back extrapolation method is recommended as the most consistent and accepted technique for determining the zero time point.[9] Exceptionally hesitant expiratory starts may prevent accurate back extrapolation and determination of the zero time point. Any tracing with an extrapolated volume in excess of 5% of the forced vital capacity or 100 ml, whichever is greater, should be repeated. For purposes of reporting and interpretation, the largest observed FVC and FEV_1 should be used, even if they come from different spirometric tracings. However, practical experience has shown that the largest values usually do come from the same curve. Further, a recent study of over 1,800 subjects did not find a significant difference between selecting the largest FVC or FEV_1 result and using those from the single best curve.[28]

Using the BTPS Correction Factor

Before spirometric results can be properly interpreted, they must be converted to BTPS (body temperature, ambient pressure, saturated with water vapor). A constant BTPS correction factor is applied with the assumption that the subject's exhaled air (approximately 37° C) cools instantly upon entry into the spirometer to reach equilibrium with ambient temperature. Unfortunately, for most volume spirometers, this assumption is not correct, as the expired air fails to reach equilibrium with the ambient temperature during the early stages of the forced expiratory maneuver. The BTPS correction factor, and therefore also the FEV_1, will be falsely elevated.[14] At a room temperature of 22° C, the error in FEV_1 is about 2%. However, if the room temperature is approximately 15° C, the FEV_1 error (false increase) may be as high as 5%. The FVC is usually not affected because sufficient time elapses for thermal equilibrium to occur. Error introduced due to low ambient temperature is a particular problem in epidemiologic studies and medical surveillance programs. If ambient temperatures are significantly different between two comparison populations or if temperature fluctuates over the course of a work shift, any significant differences observed in FEV_1 could be due to the ambient temperature differences alone. The simplest solution to this problem is to maintain the ambient temperature at 23 ± 1.5° C. If this is not possible, the estimation of dynamic BTPS correction factors has been suggested.[14]

OTHER TESTS OF RESPIRATORY FUNCTION

Other more sophisticated tests of respiratory function, such as total lung capacity (TLC), functional residual capacity (FRC), and airways resistance (Raw) can be helpful in the diagnostic evaluation of selected workers. But these are generally too complex and expensive for routine use in medical surveillance programs. Instantaneous forced expiratory flow rates ($FEF_{50\%}$, $FEF_{75\%}$), closing volumes, and volume of isoflow are tests that appear to detect dysfunction in the small airways less than 2 ml in diameter. However, these tests require more sophisticated equipment and expertise. In addition, their utility in medical surveillance is limited by their greater variability. The maximum voluntary ventilation (MVV) is sometimes required by law in the evaluation of pulmonary disability, but is time-consuming and highly effort-dependent.

CHOOSING A SPIROMETER

The wide variety of available spirometers can be confusing. However, there are two general types: devices that measure volume directly and those that measure flow and derive volume indirectly by some other method such as integration of a flow signal. If the important indices are volume measurements, such as FVC and FEV_1, then an instrument that measures volume directly will generally be superior to an instrument that measures flow and derives volume.[13] The main advantages of flow-measuring devices are their portability and automatic correction to BTPS. However, they may be less accurate and more difficult to calibrate and maintain. The three most common types of direct volume-measuring spirometers are the water-seal, the dry-rolling seal, and the bellows. The three most common types of flow-measuring spirometers are pneumotachographs, hot wire anemometers, and rotating vanes.

Regardless of which type of instrument is selected, the purchaser should be certain that it meets ATS equipment recommendations.[9] The instrument should be accurate to ± 50 ml or 3% of the reading, whichever is greater, and be capable of measuring flows between 0 and 12 L/sec. It should be capable of measuring volumes up to 7 L and accumulating volume for 15–30 seconds depending on the parameter being measured. Fifteen seconds is deemed adequate for all tests except the untimed or "slow" vital capacity (VC). A paper record or graphic display is required. When waveforms (tracings) are to be hand measured, the time scale (paper speed) should be at least 2 cm/sec and the volume scale at least 10 mm per liter (BTPS). The instrument should allow the technician to use the back extrapolation method or an equivalent for determining the zero time point. Resistance to airflow from 0 to 12 L/sec should be less than 1.5 cm H_2O/L/sec. It should be capable of calibration in the field with a 3-liter syringe. Many commercially available spirometers meet the 1987 ATS equipment recommendations. However, before a user purchases a spirometer, it is advisable to review performance data provided by the manufacturer and results of spirometry testing from independent testing laboratories.

INTERPRETING SPIROMETRIC TESTS

Interpretation of spirometric tests is usually made by comparison with a set of published predicted normal values. One of the first reference standards was compiled by the Veterans Administration-Army Cooperative study,[20] but it contained a large proportion of smokers. The normal values reported by Morris and co-workers[21] were derived from healthy nonsmokers and are widely used in general pulmonary function laboratories. Unfortunately, they did not use the back extrapolation technique recommended by the American Thoracic Society. Crapo and associates[6] have recently developed reference standards using techniques and equipment meeting ATS standards. Their values for FVC and FEV_1 were almost identical to those of Morris when the latter were modified by the back extrapolation technique. The reference standards of Knudson[18] are required by OSHA for the cotton dust industry. To eliminate confusion from differences among currently used predicted values, the universal adoption of this set of reference standards has been advocated.[10]

Most regression equations have been calculated from populations that were exclusively or predominantly white. Several studies have documented that certain nonwhite racial groups have lung volumes that are lower than whites of the same age, sex, and height. This finding has been observed in blacks,[7, 26] Asian Indians,[5] Chinese,[2] East Indians[4] and various other racial groups.[23] In blacks, these differences have been attributed to a relatively smaller thoracic cavity and result in average lung volumes 10%–20% less than those of whites. It has therefore been recommended that predicted values derived from white populations be multiplied by a racial correction factor of 0.85 to adjust for these differences.[24] This procedure will facilitate proper interpretation of spirometry without inadvertently fostering discrimination in employment practices. It should be used until race-specific reference standards become generally accepted. This racial correction factor is not necessary for the FEV_1/FVC%, which is relatively less affected by ethnic differences.

The clinical decision of whether observed values for lung volumes in a given patient are normal or abnormal requires a definition of the limits of normality. One widely used method is setting the lower limits of normal at 80% of the predicted value. This approach has been used to develop spirometric guidelines for assessment of the degree of ventilatory impairment.[17] However, if the parameter being measured has a large coefficient of variation, setting the lower limit of normal at 80% of the mean may result in a proportion of the normal population being labeled "abnormal." A more recent method is to determine if the patient's value falls within the 95% confidence interval of the reference standard.[1, 6, 31] Although more statistically valid, in that it accounts for variability of a measurement within a normal population, the 95% confidence interval method has been in clinical use only for a relatively brief period. Another potential disadvantage of using the 95% confidence interval is that it assumes both a constant interval for all ages and heights and a normal distribution about the regression line.[15] This has not been found in all reference populations, which has led to yet another recommendation, that the lower 95th percentile criterion be used for defining the limit of normal.[19] Until a consensus develops, it is likely that all the aforementioned methods will continue to be used in clinical practice.

Although comparison of an individual's test results to a set of reference standards may be useful, an even more desirable approach is comparing a subject's observed value with his own previous studies. Because the coefficient of variation of a given test within a single subject is smaller than the population coefficient of variation, this approach should give better sensitivity.[15] Using the subject as his own control is the basis of longitudinal testing as conducted in occupational medical surveillance programs. Spirometry performed over the course of a work shift or from day-to-day can detect acute decrements in lung function, identifying workers who may be hypersusceptible to a particular airborne irritant. Longitudinal studies done over longer intervals, (e.g. annually) are designed to detect more insidious or chronic changes at the earliest possible stage.

FOLLOW-UP TESTING AND LONGITUDINAL STUDIES

The proper interpretation of longitudinal or follow-up studies requires the ability to distinguish lung function changes due to disease from other sources of variability. Adherence to recommended spirometry standards should minimize variability due to inconsistent technique, fluctuating patient effort, or instrument inaccuracy. The presence of circadian or diurnal variation over the course of a work shift has been found by some investigators[12, 16, 30] but not by others.[3] Large fluctuations in ambient temperature over the course of a work shift, which may not be completely compensated for by the usual BTPS correction factors, can also result in spurious changes in FEV_1. While the presence of diurnal variation and other factors can complicate the interpretation of pre- and postshift and day-to-day changes in pulmonary function, some guidelines are available to assist the physician in the decision-making process.

A significant change within a day's time has been defined as 5% or greater in FEV_1 and FVC and 13% in $FEF_{25\%-75\%}$.[25] A similar decline in these parameters has also been suggested as the acceptable limits of day-to-day variability.[27] The cotton dust standard considered a decrement in FEV_1 of 5% or 200 ml over the course of the working day to be potentially significant.[24] Follow-up clinical evaluation is warranted where a decrement in FEV_1 over a workshift is more than 5%, provided this decrement has been observed on more than one occasion.[15] Greater variability can be expected with small airways tests and among patients with airflow obstruction.

In longitudinal studies over a period of many years, the decline in pulmonary function due to aging must also be considered.

It has been commonplace in longitudinal monitoring to compare the annual change in lung function in a group of workers with that obtained from cross-sectional studies of normal populations. Annual declines from such cross-sectional reference groups average approximately 30 ml for FEV_1 and FVC. Given this rather small yearly decrement, the decline in pulmonary function in a given individual must be either very large or the subject must be observed over a long period of time. Further, the use of predicted annual declines derived from cross-sectional studies in the longitudinal monitoring of workers has been questioned. In one study, the age regression coefficient for FEV_1 and FVC determined cross-sectionally, was more than twice the longitudinal annual change computed from the same data.[11] The authors cautioned that this could lead to an underestimation of adverse effects from inhaled airborne substances and advised that in interpretation of annual changes in lung function, longitudinal observation should be compared only with longitudinal data derived from reference groups. However, until adequate longitudinal studies are available, the current practice of considering age regression coefficients as estimates of annual decline will necessarily continue.

In assessing longitudinal changes, a decline in FEV_1 or FVC greater than 10% (after correcting for aging) should be regarded as potentially abnormal. This is similar to the conclusion of others that significant week-to-week changes are 11% for FVC and 12% for FEV_1.[25] As has been observed during within-day testing, week-to-week variability in patients with airways obstruction is twice that of normal subjects. Circumstances permitting, abnormal results on either baseline or follow-up spirometry should be verified by repeat testing.

CONCLUSION

Regardless of which standards of normality are used, the final interpretation of spirometry remains the responsibility of the physician. It should be reemphasized that spirometric results must be correlated with other clinical information, including that derived from the medical history, physical examination, and chest x-ray. Similarly, clinical management in the occupational setting must be tempered by judgment. It is seldom, if ever, justifiable to deny an individual employment or transfer him or her to another job solely on the basis of minimally abnormal spirometry. Decisions regarding hiring or job transfer are oftentimes complicated by nonmedical issues such as economic considerations, legal constraints, and labor-management relationships. These factors, combined with lack of clear-cut medical guidelines, require the physician to maintain a measure of flexibility.

REFERENCES

1. Brooks SM (chairman): Surveillance for respiratory hazards in the occupational setting—American Thoracic Society Statement. *Am Rev Respir Dis* 1982, 126:952.
2. Ching B, Horsfall PAL: Lung volumes in normal Cantonese subjects: Preliminary studies. *Thorax* 1977; 32:352.
3. Cochrane GM, Prieto F, Clark TJH: Intrasubject variability of maximal expiratory flow volume curve. *Thorax* 1977; 32:171.
4. Corey RN, Ashley MJ, Chan-Yeung M: Racial differences in lung function: Search for proportional relationships. *J Occup Med* 1979; 21:395.
5. Cotes JE, Malhotra MS: Differences in lung function between Indians and Europeans. *J Physiol* 1965; 177:17.
6. Crapo RO, Morris AH, Gardner RM: Reference spirometric values using techniques and equipment that meets ATS recommendations. *Am Rev Respir Dis* 1981; 123:659.
7. Damon A: Negro-white differences in pulmonary function. *Hum Biol* 1966; 38:380.
8. Ferris BG (principal investigator): Epidemiology standardization project. *Am Rev Respir Dis* 1978; 118(pt 2):55.
9. Gardner RM (chairman): ATS Statement on Standardization of Spirometry—1987 Update. Approved by ATS Board of Directors. March 7, 1987.
10. Glindmeyer HW: Predictable confusion. *J Occup Med* 1981; 23:845.
11. Glindmeyer HW, Diem JE, Jone RN, et al: Noncomparability of longitudinally and cross-sectionally determined annual changes in spirometry. *Am Rev Respir Dis* 1982; 125:544.
12. Guberan E, Williams MK, Walford J, et al: Circadian variation of FEV_1 in shift workers. *Br J Ind Med* 1969; 26:121.
13. Hankinson JL: Instrument specifications, in Horvath EP (ed): *Manual of Spirometry in Occupational Medicine*. Cincinnati, US Dept of Health and Human Services, NIOSH, 1981.
14. Hankinson JL, Viola JO: Dynamic BTPS correction factors for spirometric data. *J Appl Physiol Respir Environ Exerc Physiol* 1983; 55:1354.
15. Hankinson JL: Pulmonary function testing in the screening of workers: Guidelines for instrumentation, performance, and interpretation. *J Occup Med* 1986; 28:1081.
16. Hruby J, Butler J: Variability of routine pulmonary function tests. *Thorax* 1975; 30:548.
17. Kanner RE, Morris AH (eds): *Clinical Pulmonary Function Testing*. Salt Lake City, Intermountain Thoracic Society, 1975.
18. Knudson RJ, Slatin RC, Lebowitz MD, et al: The maximal expiratory flow-volume curve. *Am Rev Respir Dis* 1976; 113:587.
19. Knudson RJ, Lebowitz MD, Holberg CJ, et al: Changes in the normal maximal expiratory flow-volume curve with growth and aging. *Am Rev Respir Dis* 1983; 127:725.
20. Kory RC, Callahan R, Boren HG, et al: The Veterans Administration-Army Cooperative study of pulmonary function. *Am J Med* 1961; 30:243.
21. Morris JF, Koski A, Johnson LC: Spirometric standards for healthy nonsmoking adults. *Am Rev Respir Dis* 1971; 103:57.
22. NIOSH recommendations for occupational health standards. *MMWR* 1983; 32:1S.
23. Oscherwitz M, Edlavitch SA, Baker TA, et al: Differences in pulmonary function in various racial groups. *Am J Epidemiol* 1972; 96:319.
24. OSHA Safety and Health Standards—General Industry, 29 CFR 1910. US Dept of Labor, OSHA, 1983.
25. Pennock BE, Rogers RM, McCaffree DR: Changes in measured spirometric indices: What is significant? *Chest* 1981; 80:97.
26. Rossiter CE, Weill H: Ethnic differences in lung function: Evidence for proportional differences. *Int J Epidemiol* 1974; 3:55.
27. Rozas CJ, Goldman AL: Daily spirometric variability. *Arch Intern Med* 1982; 142:1287.
28. Sorensen JB, Morris AH, Crapo RO, et al: Selection of the best spirometric values for interpretation. *Am Rev Respir Dis* 1980; 122:802.
29. Townsend MC: Spirometric forced expiratory volumes measured in the standing versus the sitting position. *Am Rev Respir Dis* 1984; 130:123.
30. Walford J, Lammers B, Schilling RSF, et al: Diurnal variation in ventilatory capacity. *Br J Ind Med* 1966; 23:142.
31. Zamel N, Altose MD, Speir WA: Statement on spirometry—Report of the American College of Chest Physicians Section on Respiratory Pathophysiology. *Chest* 1983; 83:547.

PART III

The Physical Occupational Environment

19

Biomechanics of Manual Materials Handling and Low-Back Pain

Don B. Chaffin, Ph.D.

When a person lifts, pushes or pulls on an object, forces are produced that can act in an adverse fashion on the musculoskeletal system. These forces are normally sensed by the person and maintained within the "safe" mechanical limits of the tissues involved. Unfortunately, however, either certain conditions can exist that increase the forces above what the person expected and normally could tolerate, or the mechanical properties of the tissues had deteriorated to a greatly reduced level, due to prior strains, disease, or lack of nutrition. It is the consideration of these conditions that is presented in this chapter. The occupational physician, by training and traditional authority, serves as a major contributor in protecting workers against the injury-producing physical stresses of the occupational environment. The newly emerging field of biomechanics can greatly assist the physician in understanding how specific forces operating on and within the body affect a person's health.

SCOPE OF CONCERN

The most general concern in this regard is: What can a person physically do that will not harm him? Reflection on that question often leads one to ask more basic questions regarding the person's health status and what tasks the person is being required to perform physically in a job. In the industrial setting, this means that the person's physical capabilities must be assessed along with the physical demands of a prospective job. In particular, one becomes most concerned with those physical attributes of the individual and job that have been found to produce either increased injury rates or a few severe injuries. In the past couple of decades, the medical statistics have resulted in a large emphasis being placed on understanding how the lifting, lowering, pushing, and pulling of loads adversely affects the health of a person's low back. This chapter is specifically oriented to this concern.

Three aspects of the relationship between manual materials handling and low-back pain will be discussed. These are, in order of presentation:

1. Biomechanics of manual materials handling
2. Job conditions that correlate with increased low-back pain incidence rates
3. Physical assessment of a person's ability to perform manual materials handling

BIOMECHANICS OF MANUAL MATERIALS HANDLING

It is a well-established fact that the stresses induced at the low back during manual materials handling are due to a combination of the load involved and the person's method of handling the load. In specific, the load held in the hands as well as the person's body masses when acted on by gravity create rotational moments or torques at the various articulations of the body. The skeletal muscles are positioned to exert forces at these articulations in such a manner that they counteract the torques due to the load and body weight. From the mechanical stress standpoint, it is unfortunate that the muscles are positioned as they are, since they act through relatively small moment arms. This means that they can produce large motions with small degrees of shortening, but any load operating on the body often produces exceedingly high muscle and joint forces. As an example, consider the major elbow joint flexor muscles, i.e., the brachialis and biceps brachii, as illustrated in Figure 19–1. Here, simply holding a given load in the hands requires about seven times greater muscle force than the weight of the load due to the mechanical disadvantage of the muscles.

As a numerical example, consider that a 200-N* object must be lifted with both hands (100 N in each) from the back of a shelf placed at about shoulder height. Figure 19–2 illustrates the posture. In this case, several biomechanic factors are worth noting. First, the elbow now is extended, which reduces the flexor muscle moment arm to about 25% of its former value (i.e., r_M now is about 1.2 cm for an average man). This means that the 100 N acting on each hand requires about 2,916 N of force in the elbow flexor

*The Newton designation (N) will be used throughout this chapter (1 N = 0.10 kg force ≈ 0.22 lbs of force).

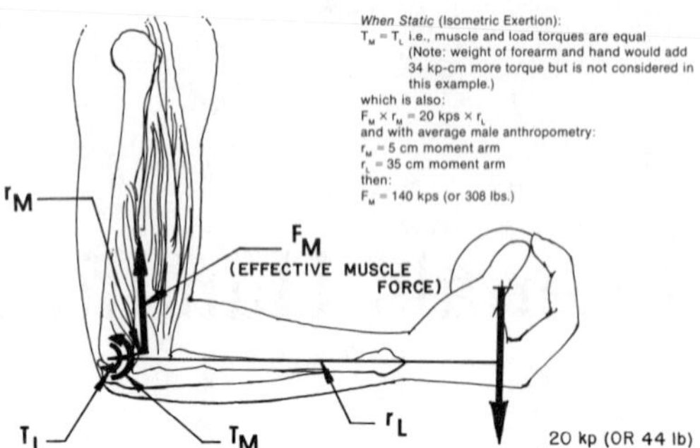

When Static (Isometric Exertion):
$T_M = T_L$ i.e., muscle and load torques are equal
(Note: weight of forearm and hand would add 34 kp-cm more torque but is not considered in this example.)
which is also:
$F_M \times r_M = 20$ kps $\times r_L$
and with average male anthropometry:
$r_M = 5$ cm moment arm
$r_L = 35$ cm moment arm
then:
$F_M = 140$ kps (or 308 lbs.)
r_M
F_M
(EFFECTIVE MUSCLE FORCE)
T_L
T_M
r_L
20 kp (OR 44 lb)

FIG 19–1.
Example of how an external load creates high internal muscle forces.

muscles, which does not include the extra load imposed by the forearm and hand weights. One might suggest that this muscle force may not be excessive, since muscles are stronger when contracting in an extended state. This is an important factor and does mean that the muscles may be capable of producing such high forces, but what about the bones, joint cartilage, and joint connective tissues? For instance, when the muscles pull across an extended joint, they compress the joint with about the same magnitude of force. As will be discussed, this coupling of the muscle and bone compression forces is an important concept when considering low-back biomechanics. In addition, high muscle forces inhibit blood flow, placing an extra stress on the heart and leading to early muscle fatigue.

Another biomechanic factor illustrated in Figure 19–2 is that the shoulder torques, and therefore shoulder muscle flexor forces are quite high due to the load acting through such a large moment arm. The average male arm length is about 63 cm to the center of grip. This means that the shoulder torque in the preceding example is about 6300 Ncm (i.e., 63 cm multiplied by 100 N). If one includes the weight and distribution of the masses of the arm, this value becomes closer to 7,340 Ncm, which empirical investigations have found to be more than what about 90% of the female population and about 40% of the male population could produce voluntarily in a similar posture.[16, 58] The major point, then, is that the shoulder joint is not well suited to withstand high forces when flexed or, as discussed by Tichauer[94] and Hagberg[40] when abducted.

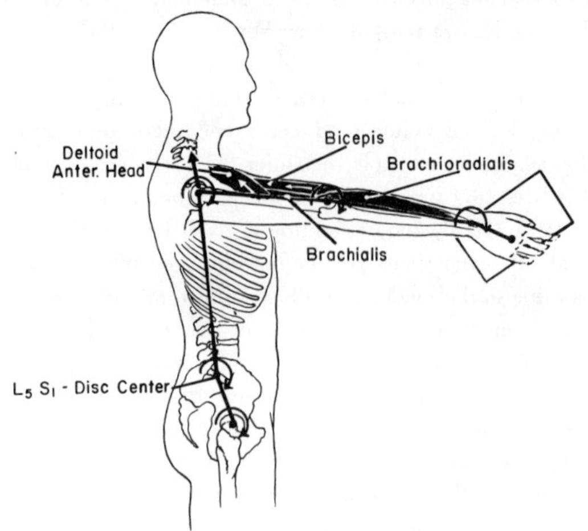

Deltoid
Anter. Head
Biçepis
Brachioradialis
Brachialis
L_5 S_1 - Disc Center

FIG 19–2.
Illustration of how leverage operates on shoulder, elbow, and lumbosacral joints.

One might suspect that such lifting requirements do not exist in industry today. Unfortunately, this is not true. One example of exactly the situation discussed here is shown in Figure 19–3. The layout of many machines, materials handling equipment, and storage devices often compels the operator to assume biomechanically awkward and potentially injurious postures. It should be noted in Figure 19–3 that because the required posture has caused the worker to be straining herself close to her expected arm and shoulder strengths, any sudden slip of the object either could cause an overstrain injury or cause the object to fall onto the worker's foot. This also illustrates how mutual the health and safety concerns are in most operational situations.

A final aspect of note in reference to Figures 19–2 and 19–3 is that when a 200-N (44 lb) load is held at arm's length, it also produces a high torque at the lumbosacral joint. If an average man's anthropometry is considered, such a load produces more than 12,000 Ncm of torque, which, in combination with the torso weight, produces a compression force at the L-5–S-1 disc that is equivalent to what holding about a 500-N (110-lb) load between the knees would produce. In other words, one does not have to "bend over" to produce high forces on the low-back structures. A person with strong arms and shoulders can position his body in ways that greatly multiply an external load's effect on the low back. The biomechanic means by which this occurs and the consequences to the low back are discussed in the following.

The lumbar spine can be thought of as a set of small links with flexible articulations (discs) between each. With proper geometric and physiologic data, the torques in each disc during a specific lifting activity could be predicted. Because the clinical and biomechanic data indicate the greatest problem to be at the lower lumbar spine, the L-5–S-1 disc (lumbosacral joint) has been used to represent the spinal stresses of lifting in earlier studies by Morris et al.[62] Tichauer[95] and Chaffin.[17] These models have clearly shown that during weight lifting, the bending moment at the lumbosacral joint can become quite large (on the order of 30,000 Ncm when lifting about 500 N from the floor). To counteract this torque, the muscles of the low-back region (primarily the erector spinae group) must exert correspondingly high forces, since they operate on small moment arms (about 3.8–8.5 cm, as referenced in an earlier work[15] and shown in Fig 19–4).

The high forces generated by the low-back muscles are the primary source of compression forces on the lumbosacral disc. These concepts are illustrated in Figure 19–5 for a person holding a variable load, designated F_H in the diagram. The graph at the bottom of Figure 19–5 displays the predicted compression forces at the L-5–S-1 disc for increasing loads held in four different positions depicted, using a man's 50-percentile anthropometric data and normative abdominal assistance values (as discussed in Chaffin and Andersson).[21]

The important concept in Figure 19–5 is that even when holding a load close, high compression forces are created in the disc.

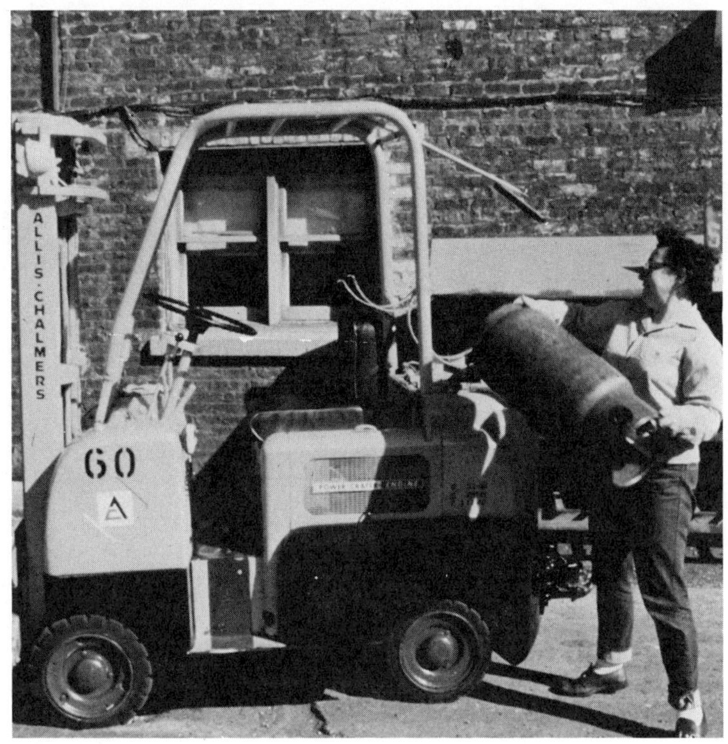

FIG 19–3.
Illustration of actual lifting situation requiring high arm and shoulder strengths where tank weight is 200 N (44 lbs).

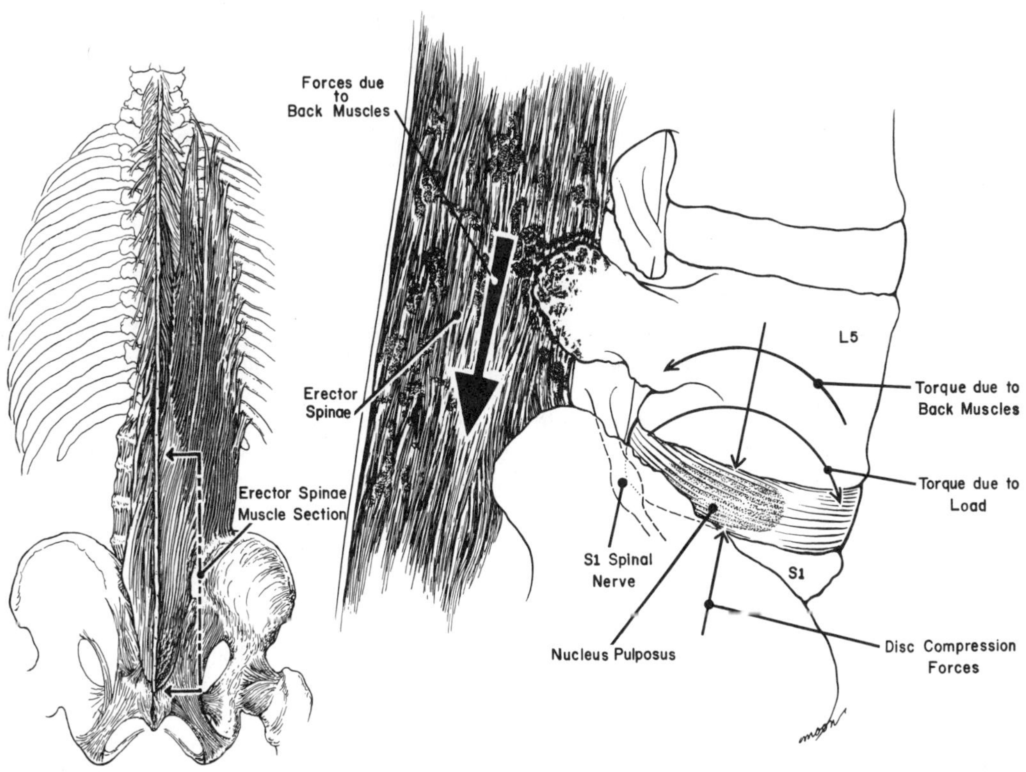

FIG 19–4.
Forces and torques operating during load lifting.

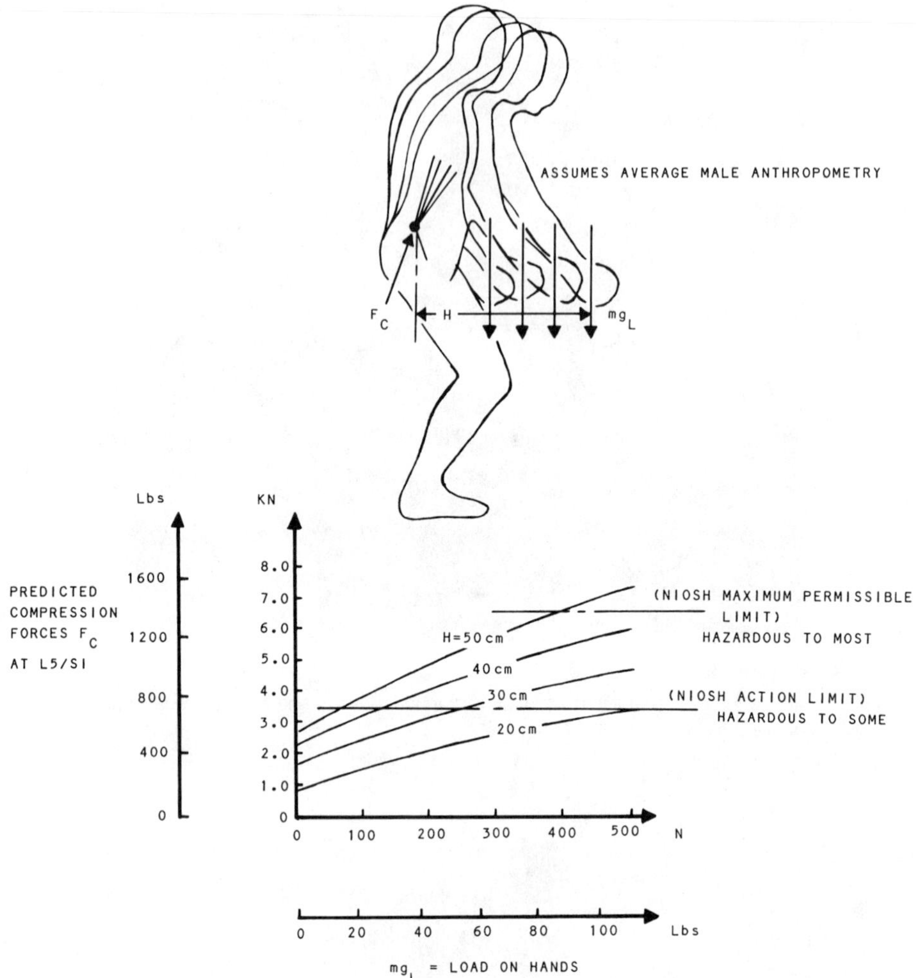

FIG 19–5.
Predicted L-5–S-1 disc compression forces for varying loads lifted in four different positions from body. (From Chaffin DB, Andersson GBJ: *Occupational Biomechanics.* New York, John Wiley and Sons, 1984. Used by permission.)

Direct pressure transducer measurements by Nachemson and Elfstrom[66] of the compression forces in the lumbar discs have confirmed the lower range of these predicted values.

The maximal amount of compression that can be tolerated by the lumbar spinal column has been estimated from axial loading compression tests on cadaver columns. Data from separate studies of this type by such researchers as Evans and Lissner[32] and Sonoda[86] disclose large biologic variations in the disc and its weight-bearing cartilage end-plates to withstand such stresses. A National Institute for Safety and Health (NIOSH) expert panel examined these and other data and suggested two "limits" be created. One is a lower limit, referred to as an *action limit,* wherein load and posture combinations would produce disc compression forces of about 3.4 kN (770 lb).[67] At these levels a significant number of discs showed microfractures in the cartilage end-plates and posterior annular fibers. Some epidemiologic data also confirmed that, at this compression level, an increased (about threefold) number of low-back medical complaints occurred, according to Chaffin and Park,[20] compared to a less stressed worker population. The NIOSH expert panel also recommended an upper limit, referred to as the *maximum permissible limit,* of 6.4 kN (1,430 lb). At this level, most people would be at risk of injury. Both of the NIOSH limits are shown in Figure 19–5. From inspection of the graph in Figure 19–5, it should be clear that even relatively light loads lifted away from the body can create injurious stress levels in the spine. These limits and their use will be further discussed later in this chapter.

Two additional observations are worth noting from the cadaver studies. First, the discs themselves, if healthy, do not appear to herniate. Instead, the cartilage end-plates that distribute the compression loads to the bodies of the vertebral segments fail, as described by Armstrong,[3] as well as the posteria elements of the annulus fibrosus, which develop small microtears. The large variation in strength of the cadaver columns may indicate that the spinal elements of some people already have been weakened by prior stresses, with resulting microfractures and scarring. If true, this could also contribute to the disc degeneration that now is acknowledged as being necessary before the more common and most serious discogenic low-back problems can develop. In other words, evidence indicates that repeated compressive stresses of life (and lifting in particular) can be sufficient to cause microfractures in the cartilage end-plates and annulus fibrosus, which then theoretically could alter the metabolism and fluid transfer to the disc. If this occurs, the capability of discs to withstand further compression loads would degenerate. The end result of this process is that the annulus fibrosus bulges or ruptures, later causing pressure on the adjacent nerve roots, as shown in Figure 19–6.

It is believed by Rowe[76] that 70%–80% of all chronic low-back pain will be diagnosed as discogenic after a period of repeated episodes. At the very least, degeneration, and the narrowing of the disc that results from it, will contribute to a more unstable spinal structure. Some evidence that disc degeneration is accelerated by physical stresses has been developed by Hult.[44] He reported that narrowing and osteophyte development of the discs and adjacent vertebral bodies were about two times greater in those people engaged in heavy physical labor than in sedentary workers.

The implications of this disc degeneration theory are far-reaching. Most important is that the assigning of low-back pain causation cannot simply be based on the immediate circumstances at the time when the pain first developed. In fact, most low-back episodes do not suddenly start with a "jabbing pain," although these cases are easily remembered and reported by patients and physicians alike. Rather, the symptoms more often are slow to develop, with stiffness, dull aching pain, and, finally, incapacitating discomfort, which occurs possibly hours or even days later. With this in mind, it is easy to rationalize why the statistics relating what a person physically does and the incidence of low-back pain generally are so poor. More will be said on this subject later in the chapter.

Returning to the biomechanic aspects of manual materials handling, several general concepts may need further definition. First, there remains the issue of how a person's posture affects the low-back stresses. It already has been shown that if the load is horizontally distant from the torso, large forces can result, even without bending over. Therefore, the number-one rule in materials handling is to ensure that the person is able to bring the torso as close to the load center of gravity as possible before lifting it. This often translates to having the person squat down beside the load with the legs straddling it when the load is on or near the floor and lift it between the knees. This assumes, of course, that the load is

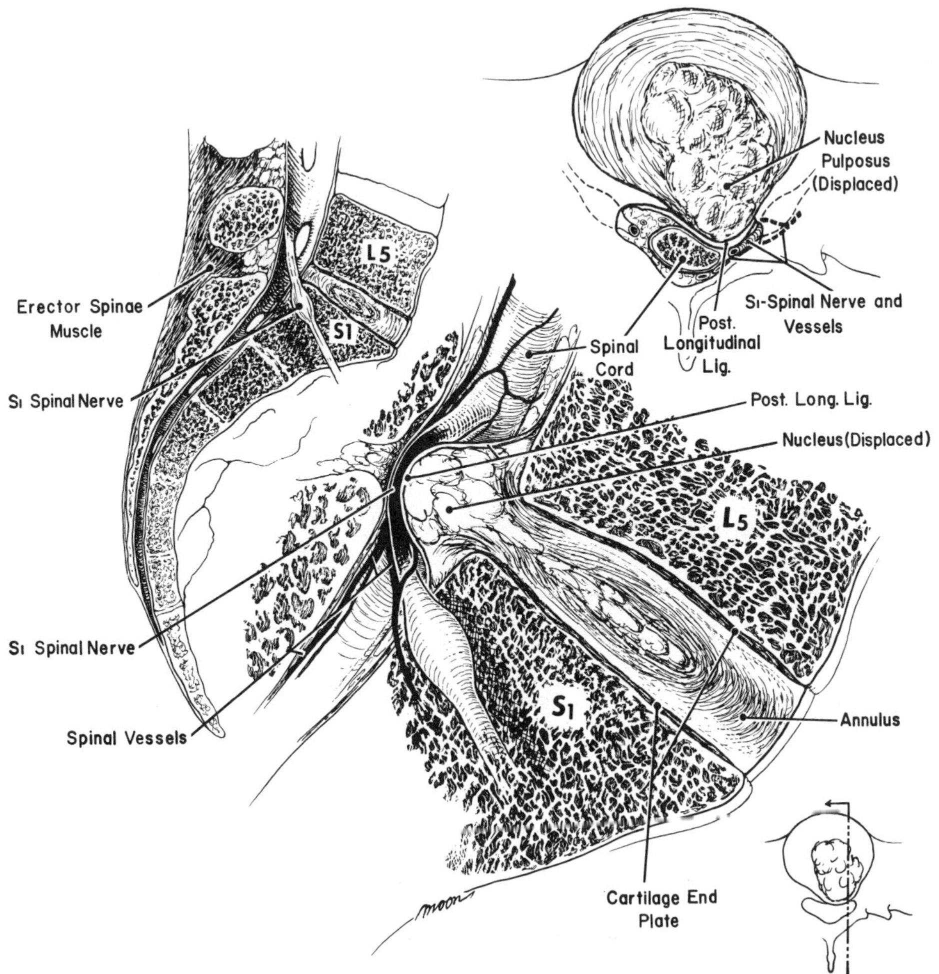

FIG 19–6.
Displaced degenerated disc exerting pressure on spinal nerves.

small enough to go between the flexed legs easily. If the load is small, the companion rule regarding keeping the back near vertical is biomechanically justified, since it reduces the stresses on the low back due to the torso weight. Unfortunately, lifting with the legs from a squatting position with the back vertical (i.e., the classic recommended posture) often is not possible, because the person so instructed does not have the quadriceps strength necessary to extend the knees and raise the body from such a position. In other words, most people, when lifting weights, lean their torso forward, thus reducing the torque on the knees. This is so common in lifting that the quadriceps muscles often are insufficiently developed to allow the person to "lift with the legs" when instructed to do so. Thus, the rule about "lifting with the legs while keeping the back vertical" must be qualified to include the physiologic fact that many people will not be able to perform such lifting without first building up their leg strengths. In addition, with some individuals, muscle-stretching exercises will be needed to provide the necessary range of motion in the knees, hips, and ankles.

A second, more complex qualification on the classic lifting rule must also be realized when lifting larger objects that cannot pass between the knees. A recent study by Park[68] disclosed that when a large object is lifted around the front of the knees, as required in the squatting type of leg lift just described, it necessarily causes the moment arm of the load about the low back to be large. This then causes the torque at the low back to be large and, hence, high spinal compressive forces and muscle forces result. In contrast, the more often-used stooped-back method of lifting allows the person to "move over and pull in" the weight to be lifted and thus reduce the load moment arm about the lower back. Figure 19–7 illustrates this concept. For the calculation of the forces in the example, a 130-N (30-lb) load is being lifted from a position that is 38 cm in front of the ankles and 38 cm above the floor. Nominal anthropometry and abdominal assistance values are assumed, as described by Chaffin.[19] It can be seen that the "stooped-over" position results in about one third less compressive stress on the low back than the squatting type of lift. It should also be evident that the stooped-over position allows the person to reduce the load moment arm of 35 cm about the low back even further by moving in over the load more than is shown, whereas the load moment arm of 50.9 cm for the squat lift is as small as possible due to the interference of the upper legs and the load.

A further limitation on lifting large objects with a squat lift arises from the fact that the arms must be extended farther in a more horizontal direction than with the stooped-over posture. As discussed earlier, such a position of the arms means that a high torque will be produced at the shoulders, which may not have the strength to move the load upward. Therefore, the person normally will lean forward more to lessen the load moment arm about the shoulders, and in so doing will cause greater stresses on the low back both by the effects of gravity acting on the torso mass and by hyperflexing the lumbar column. Such hyperflexion places a greater stress on the posterior portions of the annulus of the disc, thus distributing the compressive loads unevenly within the disc. This has led to the suggestion that lifting postures avoid a hyperflexed back. I agree with the suggestion that *hyper*flexion of the torso is contraindicated when lifting. As Troup[97] has described, moderated flexion of the torso does provide a more effective abdominal pressure assistance during lifting, thus reducing the low-back stresses. Therefore, some torso flexion appears to be acceptable, but extreme flexion could predispose the lower back to injury when the peak load occurs at the beginning of the lift.

Therefore, based on simple biomechanic concepts, one must conclude that instructions as to lifting postures must reflect concern for the person's strength and mobility as well as the size of

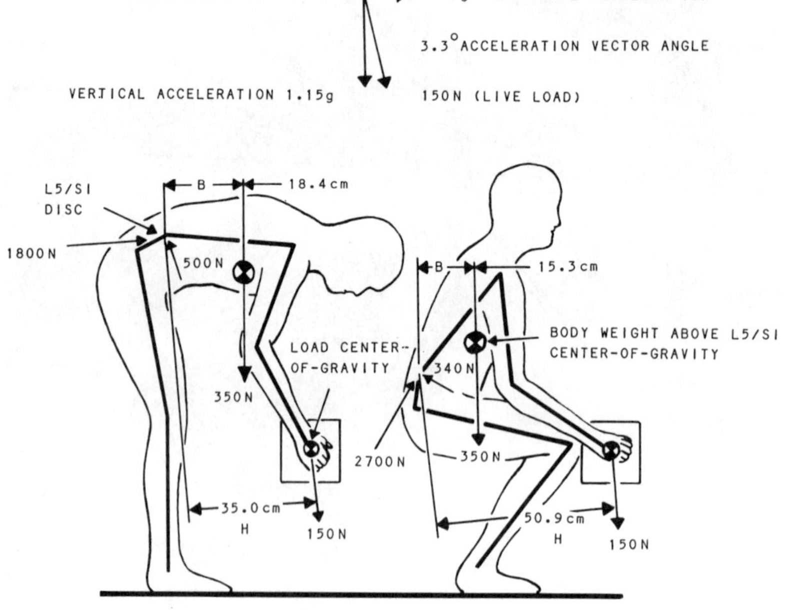

FIG 19–7.
Comparison of predicted reactive L-5–S-1 forces during lifting of large object weighing 130 N. (From Park KS, Chaffin DB: A biomechanical evaluation of two methods of manual lifting. *AIIE Trans* 1974; 6(2): 105–113. Used by permission.)

the object to be lifted. Lifting of objects that cannot pass between the legs should be done with the more traditional stooped-over torso and with legs slightly flexed. Where possible, however, loads should be reduced in size to allow them to come between the legs, or else two-person lifting should be required. When this is possible, a squatting leg lift with the back nearly erect and flattened by pretensing muscles is recommended. Unfortunately, these recommendations are based on biomechanic considerations only. Controlled field studies to determine the benefits associated with these have not been made. As Brown[12] and Jones[45] point out, much more research is necessary to establish the validity of any suggested lifting methods. For the present, however, biomechanically based recommendations certainly are worth serious consideration when counseling a person as to how a load should be lifted and carried safely.

Two additional observations perhaps are warranted at this point. The preceding biomechanics discussion has considered relatively symmetric and slow lifting of loads. Symmetric lifting, wherein the load is held with both hands in front of the body, is by far the most common method of handling a heavy load, since it equalizes the stresses bilaterally on the musculoskeletal system. There are situations, however, wherein moderate loads may be lifted asymmetrically. Unfortunately, the hazards of such lifting postures have not been documented in controlled field studies, but there are biomechanic reasons about which one must be concerned. An asymmetric lift, which has the person bring the load up along the side of the body, causes not only a lateral bending moment on the lumbar column but, because of lordosis of the column, it produces a rotation of each vertebra on its adjacent vertebra. One laboratory study by Farfan et al.[33] indicates that disc degeneration most often involves the annulus fibrosus, which is the structure that provides 40%–50% of the torsional resistance to twisting of the lumbar vertebrae. With disc degeneration, this torsional resistance can be reduced to less than one half its normal strength, thus providing a significant injury potential.

In addition, the asymmetric loading of the musculature of the back could produce a concentrated stress of sufficient magnitude to strain a specific muscle of the many muscles required to stabilize the column. In general, it must be concluded that lifting of loads to the side of the body are to be avoided. In general, a person's arm and shoulder strengths are not well enough developed to lift heavy weights in an asymmetric fashion, and therefore a person often faces the load and lifts in a reasonably symmetric fashion. Moderate load lifting, however, may be attempted using a side lift, and therefore instructions and job redesign often are indicated to avoid such lifting postures. Unfortunately, "safe" lifting levels have not been established for asymmetric materials handling. At present, this exists as one of the major areas of needed occupational biomechanics laboratory research and field investigation.

Another limitation regarding the present state of knowledge is the dynamics of load lifting. One investigation of Park[68] disclosed that the lifting of loads between 65 N and 23 N from the floor to an erect carrying position (load against the front of the upper legs) resulted in an acceleration effect that added 15%–20% to the static load at about 100–400 msec after the beginning of the lift. Furthermore, with fast motions, the ability of the somatic nervous system to coordinate the many muscles necessary to stabilize the spinal column is stressed. Electromyographic studies by Donish and Basmajian,[31] Tichauer,[92] and Morris et al.[63] have only recently begun to identify the temporal complexities involved in coordinating the recruitment of the back muscles. It has also been shown by Leskinen et al.[54] that the inertial effects of lifting moderately heavy loads can significantly increase the spinal compression forces. It is hypothesized also by Brown[12] that some low-back problems are related to muscle fatigue, which further inhibits coordination of the back muscles. Tichauer[95] suggests that unanticipated motions due to trying to catch falling or tossed objects cause low-back injuries. Clearly, dynamic actions that result in high inertial forces are more difficult to control. Therefore, it is reasonable to suggest to people who are engaged in manual materials handling that they move loads in a slow and deliberate fashion. Good foot traction and hand grips on the load should be sought and provided at all times.

Other suggestions regarding safe materials handling practices will be presented later in this chapter.

STATISTICAL DATA RELATING LOW-BACK PAIN AND MANUAL MATERIALS HANDLING JOBS

The preceding section has identified a few of the salient biomechanic factors involved when a person is lifting and carrying loads. These factors certainly must be considered when discussing the hazards and risks of manual materials handling with various managers and with patients. From the more pragmatic standpoint, one must also seek to find statistical evidence that will identify the socioeconomic dimensions of the problem, as well as to assist in further defining factors that contribute to the problem. This section presents some statistical data regarding the magnitude and potentially causal factors of low-back pain.

The seriousness of low-back pain in the work force, both in the United States and elsewhere, often has been stated. Estimates of the proportion of compensable medical claims that are low-back in origin range from about 15% for all U.S. industry (based on National Safety Council statistics) to as high as 30% for certain industries in Sweden.[44] Snook and Ciriello[80] report that the incidence rate appears to be increasing faster than the rates of other types of injuries. As an example, they cite the statistics for Wisconsin, wherein compensable back injuries increased from 7.7% of all claims in 1938 to 19.1% in 1965. Troup and Chapman[98] estimate that 30 million workdays were lost in Great Britain due to low-back pain in 1968. Hult[44] estimates that approximately 2 million workdays are lost annually in Sweden for similar reasons. Andersson[2] reports an average of 36 sickness absence days for each incident, which accounted for the highest absence rate for any disease category in Sweden. The average time lost per case for the more serious compensable back problems has been reported by the Department of Labor and Industries in the state of Washington to average more than 125 days. Similarly, Rowe[76] reported that the average time lost for all employees at Eastman Kodak due to low-back complaints was second only to upper respiratory ailments. In this same regard, it has been well documented that the length of incapacitation due to low-back problems is much greater (three to four times greater, according to Magora and Taustein[55]) if the person is engaged in heavy labor. Whether this is because the physician is reluctant to allow the worker to return to heavy labor or because heavy labor causes more extensive pathology has not been determined. In general, a person suffering a low-back incident appears to have about a 2%–4% chance of it becoming a permanent disability.

A recent survey by Brown[12] of compensable low-back incidents in Ontario disclosed a distribution as summarized in Figure 19–8. This indicates that once a case is referred for workmens' compensation, it is serious and probably will result in more than 30 days of lost work, depending on the diagnosis at the time. Also, for every compensable low-back case, perhaps there are ten or more nonserious (two to four days off work) cases that must be considered in the total problem.

The magnitude of the global medical problem perhaps is best illustrated by the following. Of 194 diagnostic groups classified by the Commission on Professional and Hospital Activities, discogenic problems ranked as the 11th reason for the days patients spent in the hospital for the total United States and was ranked as the number-one reason in 13 states.[42] The cost of treatment for low-back pain in the United States has been estimated at over $5 billion annually by Snook,[84] with another $10 billion paid for disability and indemnity.

Nachemson[65] estimates that 70%–80% of the world's population suffers from disabling low-back pain at some time in their lives. Furthermore, a majority of these episodes occur during the working ages (20–55 years), with the first medical episodes most often reported between the ages of 20 and 30.[44, 60, 65] The age distribution of the more serious compensable cases has been presented recently by Brown[12] and is reproduced in Figure 19–9.

It must also be recognized that low-back pain is recurrent in nature, with episodes occurring most often every three months to three years, according to both Hult[44] and Rowe.[76] Nachemson[65] believes that the frequency of repeated episodes peaks in the 40s. The fact that most low-back patients do not demonstrate consistent symptoms with time led Rowe and Morris to conclude that diagnosis greatly depends on following the progression of symptoms over time, with five years often being required to establish a good diagnostic classification. When such care is taken, Rowe believes that 70%–80% of all recurrent or chronic low-back cases will be diagnosed as discogenic.[76]

Therefore, it must be concluded that low-back pain is a major source of incapacitation, suffering, and cost to the world today. It tends to strike younger people and is recurrent in nature, although between episodes the person may be free from pain. Also, it must be recognized that causation is very difficult to establish because of the episodic nature of the symptoms. In fact, to refer to low-back pain as an "injury" is not doing justice to the complexity of the medical problem. Rowe believes that only about 4% of the low-back patients he reviewed could be classified as having "trauma-induced" symptoms, wherein a specific act was directly associated with the onset of injuries. The lack of a clear temporal relationship

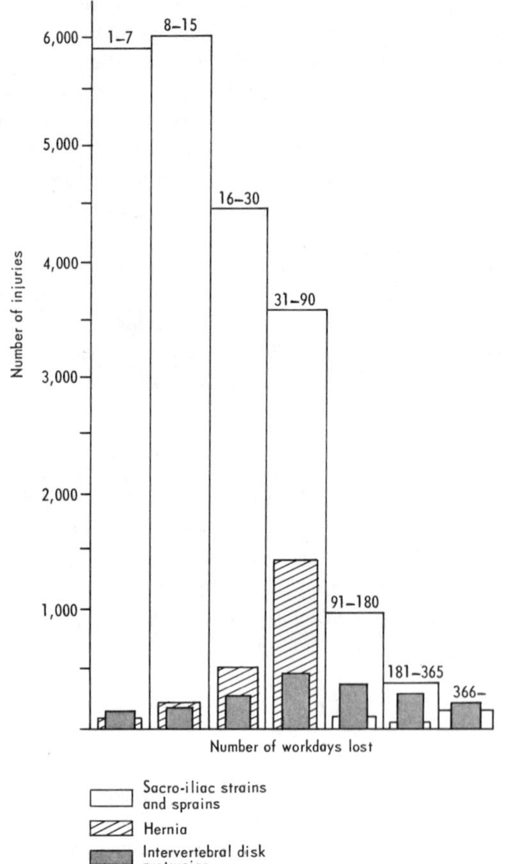

FIG 19–8.
Frequency distribution of low-back injuries.

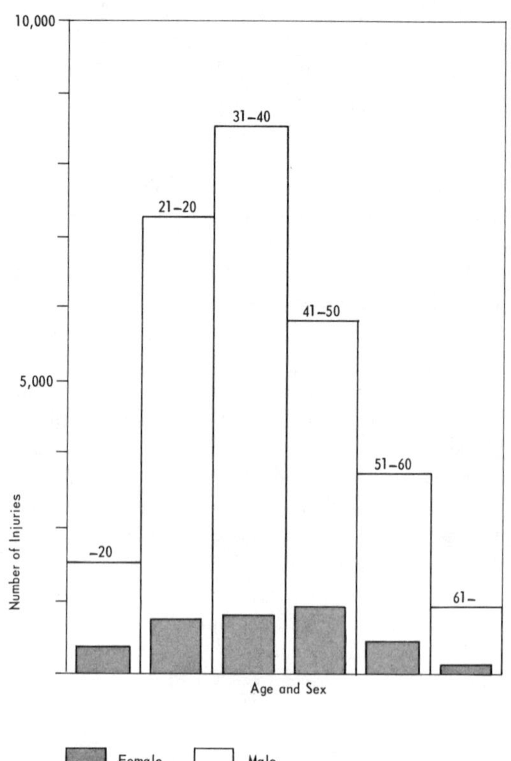

FIG 19–9.
Age distribution of compensable low-back injuries.

between a physical act and the onset of symptoms has made it difficult to acquire the statistics that might confirm hypothesized causation. Snook and Ciriello[80] discuss these statistics and conclude that neither retrogressive case studies nor cross-sectional studies clearly indicate the specific hazards associated with lifting activities. Despite these limitations, analysis of 26 state's workers' compensation cases of low-back pain by Klein, Jensen, and Sanderson[48] indicates that in occupational categories in which lifting of loads is prevalent, e.g., garbage collecting, construction, warehousing, and nursing, the incident rate was ten times the average number of claims (0.7 claims/100 worker-years). Much of the confusion in the results of past studies could have been avoided if the activities performed by the people were described with reference to the biomechanic factors presented earlier in this chapter. In other words, in the past studies, jobs have been simply classified as heavy, medium, or light work. When referring to low-back stresses, a job classified as light or sedentary by traditional criteria (i.e., in terms of the caloric cost of performing the job) still may require the person to lift a 10- or 20-kg tote box a few times during a work shift. Depending on body postures, these infrequent lifting acts could produce injurious mechanical stresses on the low back.

NIOSH MANUAL LIFTING JOB ANALYSIS

Because both the worker's posture and the load being lifted interact in a complex fashion to cause a lifting hazard for a person, NIOSH proposed a systematic method for evaluating such lifting acts. This method is described in detail in the document, *A Work Practices Guide to Manual Lifting*, published by NIOSH in 1981 and by the American Industrial Hygiene Association in 1983.[67]

From an epidemiologic perspective, the NIOSH guide cites studies revealing that musculoskeletal injury rates and severity rates increased significantly when

1. Heavy objects are lifted
2. The object is bulky
3. The object is lifted from the floor
4. Objects are frequently lifted

The four different criteria used in developing the guide—(1) epidemiologic; (2) psychophysical (strength); (3) biomechanic, and (4) physiologic (muscle fatigue)—indicate that no single task characteristic acts independently to influence the hazard level. All are interactive and often are multiplicative. This means that the recommendations that define a potentially hazardous lifting task should encompass the collective effects on each of the four criteria.

From population studies of strength anthropometry and aerobic work capacity, it is obvious that a large variation in lifting capability exists in any normal group of workers. Because of this, the NIOSH recommendations are based on two levels of hazard. The first level establishes an *action limit* (AL), in which an increased risk of injury and fatigue for *some* individuals exists if they are not carefully selected and trained for the lifting task found to exceed the limit. Specifically, the *action limit* is based on:

1. Epidemiologic data indicating that *some* workers would be at increased risk of injury on jobs exceeding the AL.

2. Biomechanic studies indicating that L-5–S-1 disc compression forces can be tolerated by most (but not all) people at about the 3,400-N level, which would be created by conditions at the AL.

3. Physiologic studies disclosing that the average metabolic energy requirement would be 3.5 kcal/min for jobs performed at the AL.

4. Psychophysical studies showing that over 75% of women and 99% of men could lift loads at the AL.

The second level of hazard in the NIOSH *guide* establishes a *maximum permissible limit* (MPL). This limit is based on:

1. Epidemiologic data indicating that musculoskeletal injury rates and severity rates are significantly higher for *most* workers placed on jobs exceeding the MPL.

2. Biomechanic studies indicating that L-5–S-1 disc compression forces cannot be tolerated over the 6,400-N level in most workers, which would be created at the MPL.

3. Physiologic studies disclosing that the metabolic energy expenditure rate would exceed 5.0 kcal/min for most workers frequently lifting loads at the MPL.

4. Psychophysical studies showing that only about 25% of men and less than 1% of women workers have the muscle strength to be able to perform lifting above the MPL.

Thus, the action limit (AL) and maximal permissible limit (MPL) permit lifting tasks to be classified into three hazard categories for control planning:

1. Those job lifting requirements *above the MPL* should be considered as unacceptable, and engineering controls should be sought to redesign the lifting conditions.

2. Those *between the AL and MPL* are unacceptable without administrative or engineering controls, thus requiring careful employee selection, placement, and training, and/or job redesign.

3. Those conditions *below the AL* are believed to represent nominal risk to most workers (i.e., a design limit).

This categorization is illustrated in the *guide* by considering the act of occasional (the frequency is less than 0.2/min) lifting of objects from a pallet height to carrying height. Figure 19–10 depicts the AL and MPL defined maximum weight values that can be lifted for varying object sizes. For such occasional lifts, fatigue avoidance is not of concern. Rather, as described earlier, the muscle strength and predicted L-5–S-1 back compression forces define the limits that are sensitive to the size of the object. Thus, if the person can maintain the load center of mass (or its effective load on the hands) close to the body, then a weight of greater magnitude can be lifted than if the load is located away from the body. Similarly, the initial vertical distance of the load from the floor, the vertical distance the load must be lifted, and the frequency of lifts will influence the weight maximum values for the task.

The following job factors must be measured and recorded to determine if a lifting hazard exists when using the NIOSH guide:

1. *Weight of the object lifted*, as determined by direct weighing. If this varies from time to time, the average and maximum weights are recorded.

2. *Position of load* with respect to the body. This is measured at *both the starting and ending points* of a lift in terms of horizontal and vertical coordinates. The horizontal location from the body *(H)* is measured from the midpoint of a line joining the ankles to the midpoint at which the hands grasp the object while in the lifting position. A rule of thumb is $H = (W/2 + 15)$ cm, where *W* is the width of the object measured along a horizontal axis (Figure 19–

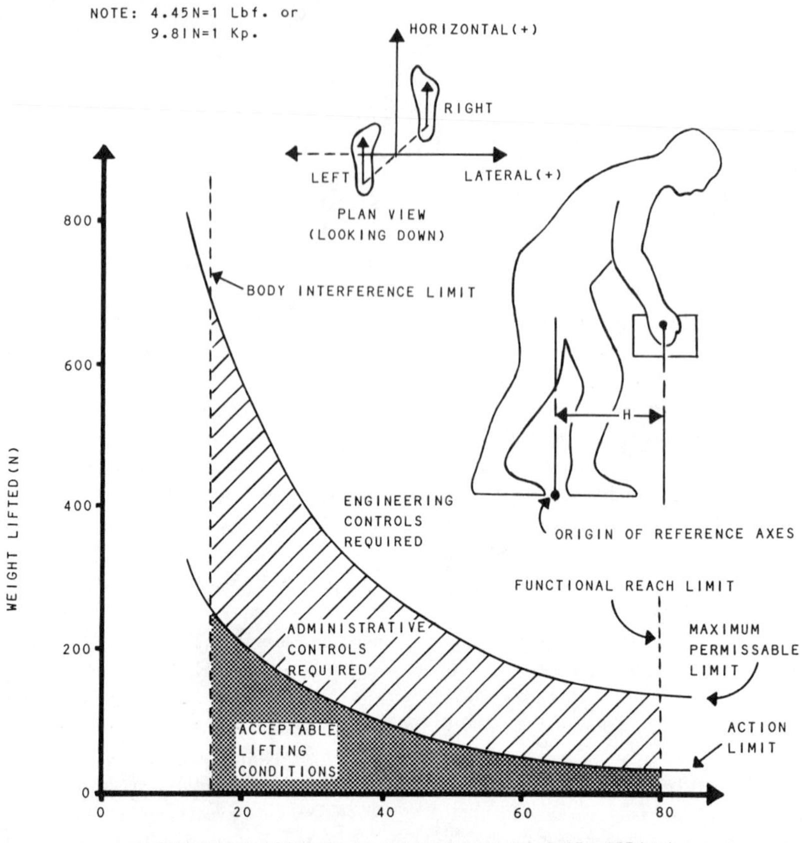

FIG 19–10.
Action limit and maximum permissible limit for different horizontal location of loads lifted from floor (V = 15 cm) to knuckle height (D = 60 cm) on an infrequent basis (F <0.2).

11 depicts this), assuming the object is lifted close to the front of the body. The vertical component *(V)* is determined by measuring the distance from the floor to the point at which the hands grasp the object. The coordinate system is also illustrated in Figure 19–12. If the four values vary from task to task (e.g., stacking cartons on top of each other), the job is separated into individual lifting tasks and each is evaluated separately.

3. *Frequency of lift*. This is recorded on the job analysis sheet in average lifts per minute for high-frequency lifting. A separate frequency should be entered for each distinguishable lifting task if performed at a frequency greater than once every five minutes.

4. *Period (or duration)*. The total time engaged in lifting is noted. This is defined as either being less than one hour or being more than one hour for the purposes of this procedure.

The resulting object weight and hand coordinate data obtained by such an analysis are compared with biomechanic and psychophysical strength limits. Data on lifting frequency and duration data are used to predict the metabolic energy requirements of a job, which are then compared to population work capacity norms.

To record job lifting data, a *Physical Stress Job Analysis Sheet* has been developed by NIOSH. It is shown in Figure 19–12, and filled in for a lifting task requiring a 200 N stock reel to be lifted once every shift to the top of a punch press, as illustrated in Figure 19–13. It is assumed that the lift is performed by grasping the object near the center and lifting it while standing in front of the

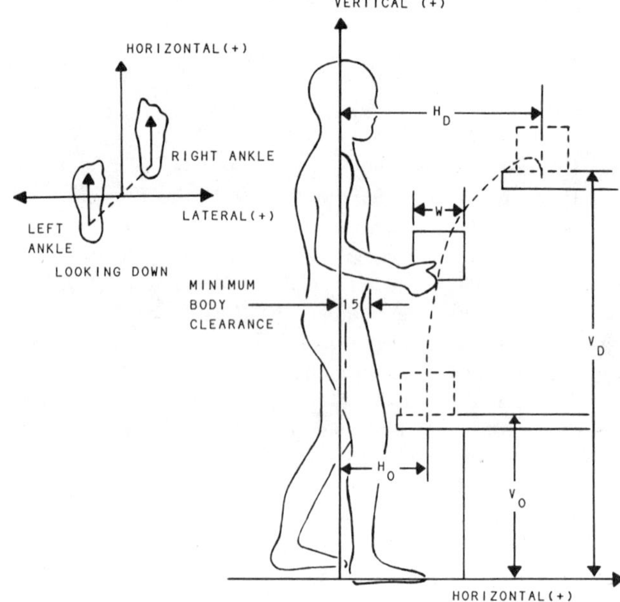

FIG 19–11.
Graphic representation of vertical and horizontal load coordinates that must be measured to determine NIOSH AL and MPL limits. (Adapted from NIOSH: *Work Practices Guide to Manual Lifting,* 1981).

PHYSICAL STRESS JOB ANALYSIS SHEET

DEPARTMENT FABRICATION DATE 6-7-86

JOB TITLE PUNCH PRESS ANALYST'S NAME JTL

TASK DESCRIPTION	OBJECT WEIGHT		HAND LOCATION				TASK FREQ	AL	MPL	REMARKS
			ORIGIN		DESTINATION					
	AVE (NEWTONS)	MAX	H cm	V cm	H cm	V cm				
LOAD STOCK	200	200	53	38	53	160	0			

FIG 19–12.
NIOSH job lifting analysis form, filled in for lifting task depicted in Figure 19–13. Note: the zero entry for task frequency denotes that the stock reel is loaded at a frequency of less than one every five minutes.

press. Both the dimensions of the stock reel and the press make this task difficult.

To allow consideration of the collective effect of the measured job variables, a prediction equation was defined by the authors of the NIOSH *guide*. To determine the maximum weight lifting value for a job at the *action limit*, the equation is

$$AL = 392(15/H)\ (1 - 0.004[V - 75])\ (0.7 + 7.5/D)\ (1 - F/F_{MAX})$$

and for the maximum permissible limit:

$$MPL = 3AL$$

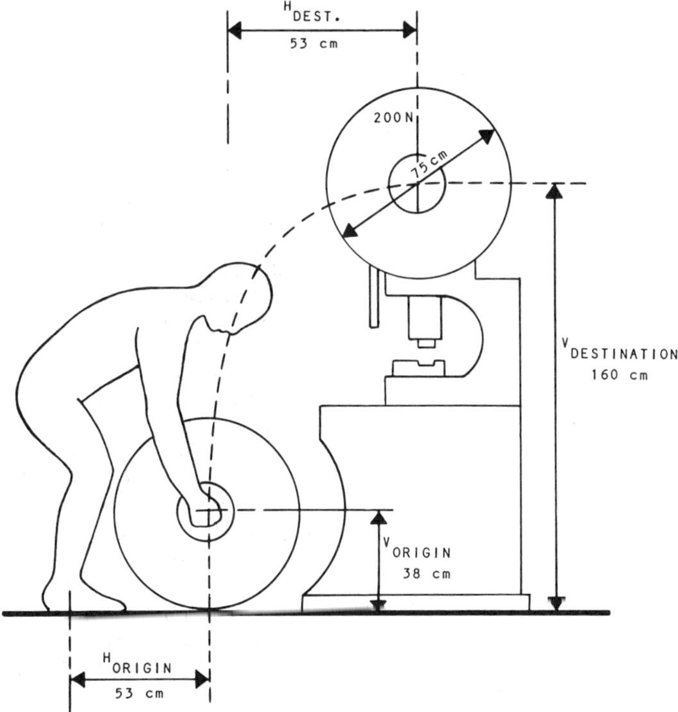

FIG 19–13.
Example of lifting stock onto punch press. It is assumed that the worker steps forward with the load to place it atop press, i.e., *H* remains constant, while *V* changes.

where *AL* and *MPL* are maximum weight lifting values (in Newtons) for the given job conditions; *H* is horizontal distance (cm) from the load center of mass at the origin of the vertical lift to the midpoint between the ankles, with a minimum value of 15 cm (body interference) and a maximum value of 80 cm (reach distance for most people); *V* is vertical distance (cm) from the load center of mass at the origin of the vertical lift measured from the floor, with no minimum value and a maximum of 175 cm (upward reach for most people); *D* is the vertical travel distance (cm) of the object, assuming a minimum value of 25 cm and a maximum of 200 cm minus the vertical V origin height. (Note: if the distance moved is small [D less than 25 cm], the effect is nominal, so D is set equal to 25 cm); and *F* is the average frequency of lifting (lifts per minute) with a minimum value for occasional lifts of 0.2 (once every five minutes) and a maximum value defined by both the period of lifting (less than one hour or for eight hours) and whether the lifting involves only arm work or significant body stabilization or movement. The maximal values F_{MAX} are given in Table 19–1.

Inspection of the prediction equation reveals that, under optimum conditions, 392 N can be lifted. This would occur for (1) occasional lifts (F less than 0.2), when (2) the load is held close to the body (H is 15 cm), (3) at carrying height (V is 75 cm), and (4) is not lifted far (D less than 25 cm). Any deviation from these optimal conditions results in a predicted decrease in predicted lifting capability. In essence, each lifting task parameter in the equation has a multiplicative discounting effect. Thus, the prediction equation can be expressed as

$$AL = 392(HF)\,(VF)\,(DF)\,(EF)$$

where: *HF* is a discounting factor due to the *horizontal* location of the load at the beginning of the lift; *VF* is a discounting factor due to the *vertical* location of the load at the beginning of the lift; *DF* is a discounting factor due to the *distance* the load is lifted; and *FF* is a discounting factor due to the *frequency* of lifts.

All of the discounting variables have maximum values of 1.0, which are achieved at the optimum conditions (above). The values of the discounting factors are given in Figure 19–14. Inspection of the graphs reveals that the horizontal location (H) and frequency of lift (F) factors can exhibit the greatest discounting effect. Thus, job evaluations must give these two factors careful consideration. The next most important factor is the vertical location of the load (V) at the initiation of the vertical lift, followed by the distance (D) that the load is moved.

NIOSH RECOMMENDATIONS TO CONTROL LIFTING HAZARDS

The NIOSH guide contains several examples of how jobs can be evaluated with reference to the MPL and AL values. Such an evaluation is the first phase of an effective control program. The guide continues by describing engineering and administrative controls which are often appropriate in reducing the hazard levels. The *engineering controls* involve either reducing the weight of the load lifted, or changing the workplace or container dimensions to optimize H, V, and D effects. Concomitant concern is required to minimize the frequency or period of lifting also.

Administrative controls advocated in the guide are of two

TABLE 19–1.

Maximum Frequency of Lifts Per Minute Allowed (F_{MAX}) for Different Postures (Hand Vertical Locations) and Lifting Periods*

DURATION OF LIFTING PERIOD	V > 75 CM (STANDING)	V > 75 CM (STOOPED)
1 hr	18	15
8 hr	15	12

*From National Institute for Occupational Safety and Health: *A Work Practices Guide for Manual Lifting,* NIOSH Technical Report No 81–122. Cincinnati, Oh, US Dept of Health and Human Services (NIOSH), 1981.

types: improved worker-selection and placement strategies and improved worker training. An objective assessment of a person's specific capability to perform heavy lifting is recommended. Worker training is also recommended to reduce lifting stresses. Such training requires that an individual have personal knowledge of (1) the risk of injury in the job due to lifting in a careless or unskilled fashion, (2) lifting methods by which one can reduce unnecessary stress, and (3) his or her own physical capacities to perform required lifts.

Such training involves several specific considerations, a few of which are listed in Table 19–2.

PERSONAL RISK OF LOW-BACK PAIN DUE TO MANUAL MATERIALS HANDLING

As indicated above, a major need in occupational medicine is to acquire the means to detect those asymptomatic people who are at high risk of a future low-back problem when given a job requiring manual materials handling. A second and somewhat related need is to develop the techniques necessary to diagnose accurately

TABLE 19–2.

Considerations in Developing a Manual Materials Handling Worker-Training Program*

Individuals involved in lifting loads above the action limit on a job should be made aware of

1. Past injury experience in the job or similar jobs within organization
2. Basic principles of biomechanics (e.g., use of levers, gravity, friction, and momentum) that would help in reducing stresses
3. Kinesiologic effects on the body (e.g., how muscles stabilize spine, move extremities, and create pressure within torso)
4. Individual body strengths and weaknesses (e.g., their own lifting capacity)
5. Importance of avoiding an unexpected situation (e.g., avoiding foot slipping, tripping, sudden loss of grip, and snagging clothing, and using foot guards)
6. Importance of developing lifting skills (e.g., keeping body close to load, not twisting with load, using smooth lifts, keeping the load within individual capacity, and planning the motion trajectory)
7. Importance of handling aids (e.g., how hoists, lifting platforms, conveyors, and hooks can be used to reduce stresses)

*Adapted from National Institute of Safety and Health: *Work Practices Guide for Manual Lifting,* NIOSH Technical Report No 81–122. Cincinnati, Oh, US Dept of Health and Human Services, NIOSH, 1981.

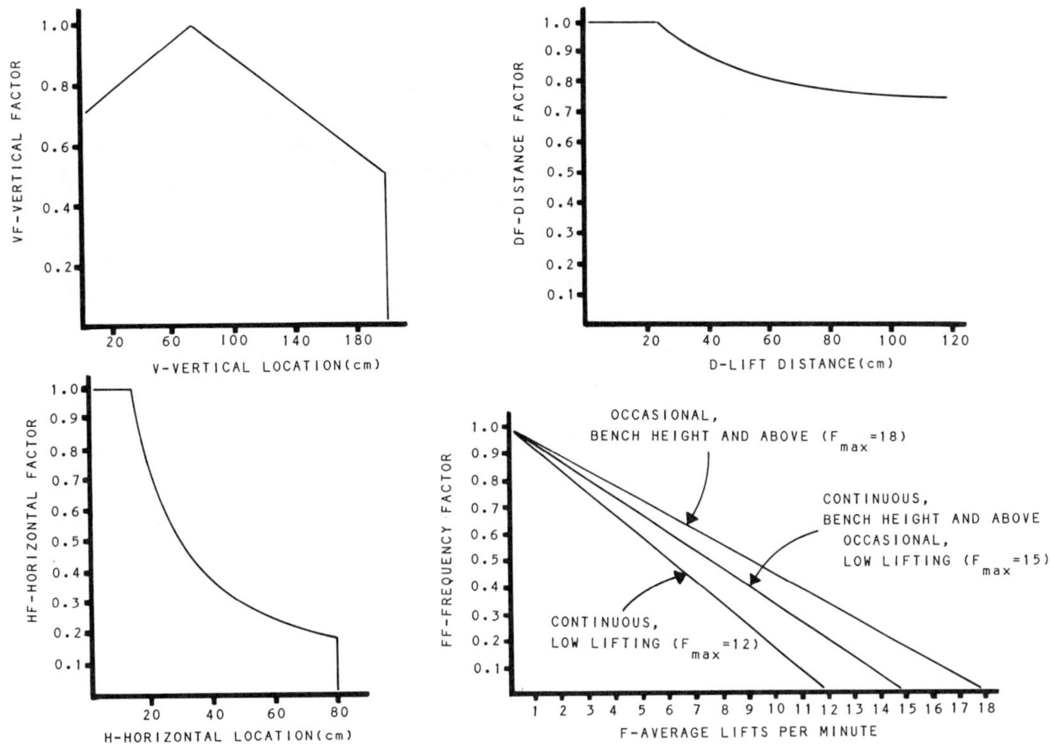

FIG 19–14.
Graphic depiction of discounting factors in lifting equation (From NIOSH: *Work Practices Guide for Manual Lifting*, 1981).

the organic cause of low-back pain. This latter topic is beyond the scope of this chapter. Some excellent discussions and analyses of the low-back diagnostic problem have been presented by Armstrong,[3] Spangfort,[87] Hult,[44] Rowe,[75] Nachemson,[65] and White.[100]

Physical Assessment for Lifting

As discussed in Chaffin and Andersson,[21] the most important part of the medical history deals with previous musculoskeletal problems. In fact, some physicians maintain that this is the only useful indicator of future risk in the medical history (Taylor,[89] Glover[37]). Low-back pain is probably the one condition most frequently discussed in the current literature regarding preemployment examinations. Recurrent episodes of low-back pain appear to be almost part of the natural history of the disease. Rowe[77] found that 83% of those with low-back pain had recurrent attacks, while recurrences in patients with sciatica were 75% (Rowe[78]). Similar findings were made by Dillane et al.,[30] Horal,[43] Hirsch et al.,[41] Leavitt et al.,[52] Gyntelberg,[38] Pedersen,[70] Troup et al.,[99] and Bierring-Sorenson.[10] Horal and Rowe found age to be a contributing factor; recurrences occurred more frequently at decades 20, 30, and 40.

Chaffin and Park[20] found a threefold increase in risk of having a back pain episode in subjects with previous history of back pain. Bergquist-Ullman and Larsson[9] report that 62% of a group of 217 workers with acute low-back pain had recurrences within a year, and 18% more in two years.

Bierring-Sorensen[10] performed a cross-sectional survey of 558 men and 583 women, aged 30–60 years. He found that subjects who in the year immediately before the study had either (1) many episodes of back pain, (2) many sickness absence days, (3) a short interval between episodes, or (4) an aggravated course of low-back pain, had significantly increased risk of low-back pain in the year following examination. Pedersen,[70] Troup et al.,[99] and Bierring-Sorensen[10] found a history of sciatica to be a risk indicator, while Dillane et al.[30] did not find this to be so. Magora and Taustein[55] found that persons who had experienced sciatica had more and longer sickness absence periods, a finding confirmed by Andersson.[2]

Pedersen[70] found that a history of more than three previous episodes of low-back pain indicated a poor prognosis should a new episode occur, in that the course of any new episode was both longer and more severe. Troup et al.[99] found that truly accident-related previous back pain was a negative prognostic factor in recurrences. Acute onset of low-back pain similarly appears to cause a longer duration of the pain episode (Bergquist-Ullman and Larsson,[9] Pedersen,[70] and Bierring-Sorensen[10]). Some optimism can be found in these studies, but Snook et al.[97] also report that simply obtaining a medical history for prior back pain is not enough to reduce back injury rates.

Physical Examination

The physical examination can reveal signs of dysfunction indicative of a risk of future problems. General observation of posture, ranges of motion and similar attributes do not seem to be reliable indicators; however (Andersson[2]) age and gender have some indirect influence on susceptibility; as discussed previously, the risk of musculoskeletal injury increases with increasing age, particularly from 20 through 40 years. The variability in individual risk is so great within age and gender groups, however, that to deny a person employment based solely on age or gender would be difficult to support.

Radiographic Examination

Preemployment x-rays of the lumbar spine are used widely. The usefulness of this approach is under debate, however. Further, there is serious concern about whether lumbosacral x-rays are safe. The correlation between most of the radiographic abnormalities identified on x-rays and the risk of low-back pain is weak. The exceptions are spondylolisthesis (an anterior displacement of one vertebra on the adjacent vertebra below, usually due to a skeletal defect) and severe degenerative changes, which have stronger risk prediction capabilities but are still debatable as the basis for denying a person a job. In general, there is disagreement on the importance of most radiographic defects and abnormalities (Splithoff,[88] Runge,[79] Hult,[44] Fullenlowe and Williams,[35] Fischer et al.,[34] Ross,[74] Bond et al.,[11] Connell,[26] Morton,[64] LaRocca and MacNab,[51] Wiltse,[101, 102] Torgerson and Dotter[96] and Magora and Schwartz[56, 57]). A number of studies have indicated a reduction in low-back sickness absence when using radiographic screening programs (Becker,[8] Kelly,[46] McGill,[59] Kosiak, Aurelius and Hartfield,[49] Redfield,[72] and Leggo and Mathiasen[53]).

All of these control programs, however, used preventive measures other than simply x-rays at the same time. Montgomery[61] in a review article questioned the evidence and advised against the use of preemployment back x-rays for determining future risk. LaRocca and MacNab,[51] Hadler,[39] and Rockey et al.,[73] came to a similar conclusion. In 1973, the American College of Radiology,[1] orthopedic surgeons, and the American Occupational Medical Association joined together in a conference to evaluate the effectiveness of such x-rays when compared to the potential radiation hazard. They concluded that the use of x-rays as the *sole* criterion for selection of workers was not justified and that more concern was needed to protect workers from unnecessary radiation in such examinations.

It is generally concluded that radiographs as a screening tool appear *not* to be indicated. At best, when a previous history of back pain is present, or clinical signs indicate possible disease, or where spondylolisthesis is suspected from clinical examination, radiographs are valuable to aid in determining further risk.

Anthropometry

It should be obvious from the preceding discussions that the worker must be matched to the work task in terms of reach and space requirements. In essence, if a specific reach requirement is documented for a job, it is necessary to evaluate the applicant's capability to perform such a reach.

Certainly, job requirements should be adjusted to the subject's normal range of motion. Preferably joints should not be bent or stretched to near their normal limits of motion and at least not held there for long periods of time, especially if under load. Abnormal mobility, as found on examination, is more often a sign of present or past illness (injury) than a future risk factor. Theoretically, a lack of mobility of one joint can cause comparatively greater stresses on another joint; for example, limited ranges of motion of the hips and knees can require more motion of the spine in a particular job. A rigid joint is also less well adapted to absorb shock.

It is a well-known fact that joint motion is impaired following injury. Bierring-Sorensen[10] found that a lesser range of spine motion in subjects with previous low-back pain was a sign indicative of increased risk of a future pain episode, while in previously healthy subjects, lesser spine mobility was in fact associated with decreased risk.

Strength Testing

The use of preemployment strength testing to reduce the incidence and severity of musculoskeletal problems has been met with considerable enthusiasm over the past decade or so. The obvious goal is to assure that only people with sufficient strength to perform a job safely will indeed be assigned that job. Muscle strength evaluation methods and equipment have been developed and are well described in Chaffin[23] and Chaffin and Andersson.[21]

There is some epidemiologic support that strength testing is a useful means of reducing back injury rates in particular. Chaffin and Park[20] found a threefold increase in the low-back injury rates in subjects performing jobs requiring strength that was greater or equal to their isometric strength-test values. A second longitudinal study was performed by Chaffin et al.[22] to further determine the value of strength testing, and again an almost threefold higher back-injury incidence rate was found in the overstressed group. In a later paper Chaffin et al.[25] suggested that specific placement and selection programs should be undertaken by industry based on strength performance criteria, a view echoed by Yu et al.[103] in a recent review article.

Another study by Keyserling et al.[47] involved the application of strength tests and a simultaneous biomechanic job analysis in the rubber industry. Subjects were strength tested, and jobs were biomechanically classified. The subjects were then assigned to jobs so that some were overstressed and others understressed. The medical records were followed for one year to determine musculoskeletal problems over that period. Although the follow-up period was short, a significant effect of job matching based on strength criteria was obtained. Troup et al.[99] in a prospective study found reduced dynamic strength of back flexor muscles to be a consistent predictor for recurrence or persistence of back pain.

It appears that strength testing can be a preventive approach, at least for low-back injuries. The testing procedure should be specific to the job being sought by the worker, however. It remains unclear whether a well-matched worker will develop a problem from a heavy physical job should the exposure period be extended beyond one year or more. Muscle strength and tissue resistance to future stress may not be directly related. In general, however, a worker should at least have the demonstrable strength required to perform a job for which he or she is employed prior to having to perform the job.

There is some evidence that individuals with a good state of general fitness have a lesser risk of chronic low-back pain than others and that recovery after a pain episode is faster in these subjects. Cady et al.[13] evaluated five strength and fitness measurements and recorded the occurrence of back injuries in 1,652 firefighters from 1971 to 1974. The prospective measurements included flexibility, isometric lifting strength, and cardiopulmonary tests. The firefighters were divided into three groups: least fit, middle fit, and most fit. A graded and statistically significant protective effect was found for added levels of fitness and conditioning. Although other factors could have contributed to the result, it is certainly worthy of note.

Choosing a Screening Method

In general, it is suggested that the following criteria be considered in choosing among methods of preemployment screening:

Is a test safe to administer?

Does it give reliable, quantitative values?

Is it related to specific job requirements?

Is it practical?

Does it predict risk of future injury or illness?

Each of these criteria is briefly discussed in the context of preemployment selection procedures.

As has been outlined, the current opinion is that the risk of having spine radiographs taken outweighs the possible advantage. Thus, radiographs should be considered only when indicated by the medical history and physical examination.

Various types of physical strength and endurance tests must be carefully evaluated to assure that they are safe. Previous history of musculoskeletal problems or cardiovascular problems may contraindicate testing of a specific person.

Reliability can only be determined by test-retest procedures, which should precede any new test program to be used. Specificity is important and requires a careful evaluation of the job's physical requirements to assure that a test is related to the job.

Practicality can vary from one workplace to the next. A history can always be obtained, but when quantitative testing is used, the following considerations should be met, as described in Chaffin:[24]

1. Hardware capable of simulation of different work situations
2. Minimal administration time
3. Minimal time of instruction and learning

The most difficult criterion is the last. Does the test predict risk of future injury or illness? To answer this requires careful evaluation of epidemiologic data that have been collected prospectively and for many years. It is hoped that such studies will be performed in the future to better validate the many varied procedures now being advocated.

FINAL COMMENTS

There should be no doubt that manual materials handling and, particularly, the act of lifting loads is potentially hazardous to many workers. The NIOSH guide is a recent effort to control one aspect of manual materials handling, namely, the simple act of lifting a load in the sagittal plane. It is an attempt to be more comprehensive than previous efforts relative to (1) job evaluation methods; (2) criteria used for the limits; and (3) control strategies.

It has been too short a time since its first publication in 1981 to discern the guide's effect on controlling musculoskeletal disorders in industry. Recent prevention programs advocated by Snook,[82] Chaffin and Park,[20] Tichauer,[93] Davis and Stubbs,[29] and Ayoub et al.[5] concentrate on setting upper limits to the load that can be lifted by most workers in various postures and with different lifting frequencies. In this sense, they advocate a maximum permissible limit. These proponents suggest, through reference to biomechanic, psychophysical, and retrospective epidemiologic studies, that reengineering of jobs to reduce heavy load lifting could significantly decrease both the incidence and severity of musculoskeletal disorders. The magnitude of such improvement in the injury and illness statistics has only been grossly estimated, however, and controlled, longitudinal, demonstration experiments have not been performed, though they are greatly needed.

The use of improved employee selection and training procedures, i.e., employment of an action limit with administrative controls, also has advocates (Davies,[28] Garg and Herrin,[36] and Keyserling et al.,[47] to name a few). Once again, however, longitudinal controlled experiments have not been performed to allow precise estimates of the impact of various types of administrative control programs.

In summary, one must conclude that the work practices advocated by NIOSH are another attempt to deal with a complicated and serious occupational health and safety problem. The NIOSH guide differs from past attempts in that it synthesizes data from many different studies and advocates both engineering and administrative controls. So far it appears to be well accepted.

Obviously, in the larger context of manual materials handling, control of manual lifting hazards is only one aspect. Research has indicated that many injuries result when one is pushing or pulling on objects or when carrying objects on a slippery or unstable floor. These matters are discussed further in Chaffin and Andersson.[21]

REFERENCES

1. American College of Radiology: Conference of Low-back X-rays in Preemployment Physical Examinations. Proceedings of Meeting, Jan 11–14, sponsored by NIOSH, contract HSM-00-72-153, 1973.
2. Andersson GBJ: Epidemiologic aspects on low-back pain in industry. *Spine* 1981; 6(1) 53–60.
3. Armstrong JR: *Lumbar Disc Lesions*. Baltimore, Williams & Wilkins Co, 1965, pp 42–45.
4. Asmussen E, Heebll-Nielsen K: Isometric Muscle Strength of Adult Men and Women. *Communications from Danish National Association for Infantile Paralysis* 1961; NR II.
5. Ayoub MM, Mital A, Bakken GM, et al: Development of strength and capacity norms for manual materials handling activities: The State of the art. *Human Factors* 1980; 22(3):271–283.
6. Badger DW, Dukes-Dobos FN, Chaffin DB: *Prevention of Low-Back Injury in the Industrial Work Force, A NIOSH Symposium Report*. Cincinnati, Oh, NIOSH Ergonomics Branch, 1972.
7. Becker WF: Prevention of back injuries through preplacement examinations. *Ind Med Surg* 1955; 24:486.

8. Becker WF: Prevention of low back disability. *J Occup Med* 1961; 3:329. 1961.
9. Bergquist-Ullman M, Larsson U: Acute low back pain in industry. *Acta Orthop Scand [Suppl]* 1977; 170–183.
10. Bierring-Sorensen F: *The Prognostic Value of the Low Back History and Physical Measurements,* unpublished doctoral dissertation. University of Copenhagen, Copenhagen, 1983.
11. Bond MB, et al: Low back x-rays, criteria for the use in placement examinations in industry. *J Occup Med* 1964; 6:373.
12. Brown JR: Lifting as an industrial hazard. *Am Ind Hyg Assoc J* 1973; 34:292.
13. Cady LD, Bischoff DP, O'Connel ER, et al: Strength and fitness and subsequent back injuries in firefighters. *J Occup Med* 1979; 21:269–272.
14. Caldwell LW, et al: A proposed standard procedure for muscle strength testing. Presented at the American Industrial Hygiene Association national meeting, May, 1972.
15. Chaffin DB, Moulis EJ: An empirical investigation of low-back strains and vertebrae geometry. *J Biomech* 1969; 2:89.
16. Chaffin DB, Baker WH: A biomechanical model for analysis of symmetric sagittal plane lifting. *AIIE Trans* 1970; 2:16.
17. Chaffin DB: A computerized biomechanical model-development of and use in studying gross body actions. *J Biomech* 1969; 2:429.
18. Chaffin DB: Human strength capability and low back pain. *J Occup Med* 1974; 16:248.
19. Chaffin DB: Low-back stresses, during load lifting, in Dhanjoo NG (ed): *Applications of Biomechanics*. New York, Marcel Dekker, Inc, 1975.
20. Chaffin DB, Park KS: A longitudinal study of low-back pain as associated with occupational weight lifting factors. *Am Ind Hyg Assoc J* 1973; 34:513.
21. Chaffin DB, Andersson GBJ: *Occupational Biomechanics*. New York, John Wiley & Sons, 1984.
22. Chaffin DB, Herrin GD, Keyserling WM, et al: *Preemployment Strength Testing,* NIOSH Technical Report. Cincinnati, Oh, NIOSH Physiology and Ergonomics Branch, 1977.
23. Chaffin DB: Ergonomic guide for the assessment of human static strength. *Am Ind Hyg J* 1975; 36:505–510.
24. Chaffin DB: Functional assessment for heavy physical labor, in Alderman MH, Hanley MJ (eds): *Clinical Medicine for the Occupational Physician*. New York, Marcel Dekker, Inc, 1982.
25. Chaffin DB, Herrin GD, Keyserling WM: Preemployment strength testing. *J Occup Med* 1978; 20:403–408.
26. Connell MA: Bony abnormalities of the low back in relation to back injury. *South Med J* 1968; 61:482.
27. Damon A, Stoudt HW, McFarland RA: *The Human Body in Equipment Design*. Cambridge, Mass, Harvard University Press, 1966.
28. Davies BT: Training in manual handling and lifting, in Drury CG (ed): *Safety in Manual Materials Handling,* NIOSH publication No 78–185. Cincinnati, Oh, US Dept of Health and Human Services, National Institute of Safety and Health, 1978.
29. Davis PR, Stubbs DA: Performance capacity limits. *Appl Ergon* 1978; 9:33–38.
30. Dillane JB, Fry J, Kalton G: Acute back syndrome—A study from general practice. *Br Med J* 1966; 2:82–84.
31. Donish EW, Basmajian JV: Electromyography of deep back muscles in man. *Am J Anat* 1972; 133:25.
32. Evans FG, Lissner HR: Biomechanical studies on the lumbar spine and pelvis. *J Bone Joint Surg* 1959; 41-A:218.
33. Farfan HF, Cossette JW, Robertson GH, et al: The effects of torsion on the lumbar intervertebral joints: The role of torsion in the production of disc degeneration. *J Bone Joint Surg* 1970; 52-A:468.
34. Fischer FJ, Friedman MM, van Denmark RE: Roentgenographic abnormalities in soldiers with low back pain: A comparative study. *Am J Roentgenol* 1958; 79:673–676.
35. Fullenlowe TM, Williams AJ: Comparative roentgen findings in symptomatic and asymptomatic backs. *Radiology* 1957; 68:572–574.
36. Garg A, Herrin GD: Stoop or Squat: A biomechanical and metabolic evaluation. *AIIE Trans* 1979; 11(4):293–302.
37. Glover JR: Back pain and hyperaesthesia. *Lancet* 1960; 1:1165–1169.
38. Gyntelberg F: One year incidence of low back pain among male residents of Copenhagen aged 40–59. *Den Med Bull* 1974; 21:30–36.
39. Hadler NM: Legal ramifications of the medical definition of back disease. *Ann Intern Med* 1978; 89:992–999.
40. Hagberg M: Workload and fatigue in repetitive arm elevations. *Ergonomics* 1981; 24(7):543–555.
41. Hirsch C, Jonsson B, Lewin T: Low back symptoms in a Swedish female population. *Clin Orthop* 1969; 63:171–176.
42. Holtz CL, Keyes MA: Regional differences in the use of hospital days. *PAS Reporter* 1971; 9:9.
43. Horal J: The clinical appearance of low back pain disorders in the city of Gothenburn, Sweden. *Acta Orthop Scand [Suppl]* 1969; 118:1–109.
44. Hult L: Cervical dorsal and lumbar spinal syndromes. *Acta Orthop Scand [Suppl]* 1954; 17:1–102.
45. Jones DF: Back strains, the state of the art. *J Saf Res* 1971; 3:28.
46. Kelly FJ: Preemployment medical exam including back x-ray. *J Occup Med* 1965; 4:132.
47. Keyserling WM, Herrin GD, Chaffin DB: Isometric strength testing as a means of controlling medical incidents on strenuous jobs. *J Occup Med* 1980; 22:332–336.
48. Klein BP, Jensen RC, Sanderson CM: Assessment of workers' compensation claims for back strain and sprain. *J Occup Med* 1984; 26(6):443–448.
49. Kosiak M, Aurelius JR, Hartfield WF: Backache in industry. *J Occup Med* 1966; 51:51–58.
50. Koyl LF, Hanson PM: *Age, Physical Ability, and Work Potential,* Report of National Council on Aging. US Manpower Administration and US Dept of Labor, February, 1969.
51. LaRocca H, MacNab I: Value of pre-employment and radiographic assessment of the lumbar spine. *Can Med Assoc J* 1969; 101:383.
52. Leavitt SS, Johnston TL, Beyer RD: The process of recovery: Patterns in industrial back injury, pt 1. Costs and other quantitative measures of effort. *Ind Med Surg* 1971; 40(8):7–14.
53. Leggo C, Mathiasen H: Preliminary results of a preemployment back x-ray program for state traffic officers. *J Occup Med* 1973; 15:973–974.
54. Leskinen TPJ, Stalhammar HR, Kuorinka IAA, et al: The effects of inertial factors on spinal stress when lifting. *Eng Med* 1983; 12(2):87–89.
55. Magora A, Taustein I: An investigation of the problem of sick-leave in the patient suffering from low-back pain. *Ind Med* 1969; 38:80.
56. Magora A, Schwartz A: Relation between the low back pain syndrome and x-ray findings. 1. Degenerative osteoarthritis. *Scand J Rehabil Med* 1976; 8:125.
57. Magora A, Schwartz A: Relation between the low back syndrome and x-ray findings. 2. Transition vertebrae (mainly sacralization). *Scand J Rehabil Med* 1978; 10:135–145.
58. Martin JB, Chaffin DB: Biomechanical computerized simulation of human strength in sagittal-plane activities. *AIIE Trans* 1972; 4:19.
59. McGill CM: Industrial back problems: A control program. *J Occup Med* 1968; 10:174.
60. Mirabile MP, Simons GR: An analysis and interpretation of industrial medical data. *J Occup Med* 1972; 14:227.

61. Montgomery CH: Preemployment back x-rays. *J Occup Med* 1976; 18:495–497.
62. Morris JM, Lucas DB, Bressler B: Role of the trunk in stability of the spine. *J Bone Joint Surg* 1961; 43-A:327.
63. Morris JM, Benner G, Lucas DB: An electromyographic study of the intrinsic muscles of the back in man. *J Anat* 1962; 96:509.
64. Morton RD: So-called normal backs. *Ind Med Surg* 1969; 38:46–49.
65. Nachemson AL: Low-back pain—Its etiology and treatment. *Clin Med* 1971; 78:18.
66. Nachemson A, Elfstrom G: *Intravital Dynamic Pressure Measurements in Lumbasr Discs*. Stockholm, Almqvist & Wiksell, 1970, pp 20–32.
67. National Institute for Safety and Health: *Work Practices Guide to Manual Lifting*, NIOSH Technical Report No 81–122. Cincinnati, Oh, NIOSH, 1981, and Akron, Oh, American Industrial Hygiene Association, 1983.
68. Park KS: *A Computerized Simulation Model of Postures During Manual Materials Handling*, PhD dissertation. The University of Michigan, 1973.
69. Park KS, Chaffin DB: A biomechanical evaluation of two methods of manual lifting. *AIIE Trans* 1974; 6(2):105–113.
70. Pedersen PA: Prognostic indicators in low back pain. *J Royal Coll Gen Pract* 1981; 31:209–216.
71. Poulsen E, Jorgensen K: Back muscle strength, lifting, and stooped working postures. *Appl Ergon* 1971; 2:133.
72. Redfield JT: The low back x-ray as a preemployment screening tool in the forest products industry. *J Occup Med* 1971; 13:219–226.
73. Rockey PH, Fontal J, Omenn GS: Discriminatory aspects of preemployment screening: Low-back x-ray examinations in the railroad industry. *Am J Law Med* 1969; 5:157–214.
74. Ross E: Ergebnisse einer Rontgen-Reihenuntersuchung der Wirbelsaule bei, 5 000 Maanlischen Judendlishen. *Fortschr Rontgenstr* 1962; 97:734–751.
75. Rowe LM: *Backache at Work*. Fairport, NY, Perinton Press, 1983.
76. Rowe LM: Low-back disabilities in industry: Updated position. *J Occup Med* 1971; 13:476.
77. Rowe ML: Preliminary statistical study of low back pain. *J Occup Med* 1963; 5:336–341.
78. Rowe ML: Disc surgery and chronic low back pain. *J Occup Med* 1965; 7:196–202.
79. Runge CF: Preexisting structural defects and severity of compensable back injuries. *Ind Med Surg* 1958; 27:249.
80. Snook SH, Ciriello VM: Low-back pain in industry. *ASSE J* 1972; 17:17.
81. Snook SH, Ciriello VM: Maximum weights and work loads acceptable to female workers. *J Occup Med* 1974; 16:527.
82. Snook SH: The design of manual handling tasks. *Ergonomics* 1978; 21:963–985.
83. Snook SH, Campanelli RA, Hart JW: A study of three preventive approaches to low back injury. *J Occup Med* 1978; 20:478–481.
84. Snook S: *The Perspective of Industry*. Proceedings on Industrial Low-back Pain, University of Vermont Orthopaedics Department, 1983.
85. Snook SH, Irvine CH: Maximum acceptable weight of lift. *Am Ind Hyg Assoc J* 1967; 28:322.
86. Sonoda T: Studies on the compression, tension, and torsion strength of the human vertebral column. *J Kyoto Prefect Med Univ* 1962; 71:659.
87. Spangfort EV: The lumbar disc herniation: A computer-aided analysis of 2,504 operations. *Acta Orthop Scand [Suppl]* 1972; 142:1–95.
88. Splithoff CA: Lumbosacral junction. Roentgenographic comparison of patients with and without backaches. *JAMA* 1953:152:1610–1613.
89. Taylor PJ: Personal factors associated with sickness absence. *Br J Ind Med* 1968; 25:106–110.
90. Tichauer ER, Miller M, Hathan IM: Lordosimetry—A new technique for measurement of postural response to materials handling. *Am Ind Hyg Assoc J* 1973; 34:1.
91. Tichauer ER: The efficiency of the human machine in work situations. Presented at the Research Conference on Applied Work Physiology, Sterling Forest Conference Center, Tuxedo Park, New York, April 10–11, 1968.
92. Tichauer ER: A pilot study of the biomechanics of lifting in simulated industrial work situations. *J Saf Res* 1971; 3:3.
93. Tichauer ER: *The Biomechanical Basis of Ergonomics*. New York, Wiley-Interscience s, 1978.
94. Tichauer ER: Industrial engineering in the rehabilitation of the handicapped, in *Proceedings of 18th AIEE Convention*. May, 1967, pp 171–180.
95. Tichauer ER: The biomechanics of the arm-back aggregate under industrial working conditions. American Society of Mechanical Engineers 65-WA/HUF-1. September 1966.
96. Torgerson BR, Dotter WE: Comparative roentgenographic study of the asymptomatic and symptomatic lumbar spine. *J Bone Joint Surg* 1976; 58A:850–853.
97. Troup JDG: Relation of lumbar spine disorders to heavy manual work and lifting. *Lancet* 1965; 1:857.
98. Troup JDG, Chapman AE: The strength of the flexor and extensor muscles of the trunk. *J Biomech* 1969; 2:49.
99. Troup JDG, Martin JW, Loyd DCEF: Back pain in industry—A prospective study. *Spine* 1981; 6:61–69.
100. White AH: *Your Aching Back*. New York, Bantam Books, 1983.
101. Wiltse, LL: Lumbar strain and instability. *Proceedings of the American Academy of Orthopaedic Surgeons Symposium on the Spine*. 1969; pp 54–83.
102. Wiltse LL: The effect of the common anomalies of the lumbar spine upon disc degeneration and low back pain. *Orthop Clin North Am* 1971; 2:569–582.
103. Yu T, Lewis H, Wise RA, et al: Low back pain in industry. *J Occup Med* 1984; 26(7):517–524.
104. Vetenskaplig Skriftserie: *10th International Congress of Biomechanics, Umea, June 15–20, 1985* (abstract book). Arbete och Hälsa 1985; 14.

20

Occupational Hearing Loss, Noise, and Hearing Conservation

Julian B. Olishifski, P.E., C.S.P.

OCCUPATIONAL HEARING LOSS

Occupational hearing loss can be defined as a partial or complete hearing loss in one or both ears arising in, or during the course of, and as the result of one's employment. This includes acoustic traumatic injury as well as noise-induced hearing loss. *Noise-induced hearing loss* is generally used to denote the cumulative, permanent loss of hearing that develops gradually after months or years of exposure to high levels of noise. Noise-induced hearing loss usually affects both ears equally in extent and degree.

Occupational hearing loss arising out of traumatic injury, such as explosions or a blow to the head, is compensable under the workers' compensation acts in all states. Noise levels much lower than those producing acoustic trauma may produce hearing loss if the exposure is sufficiently intense and prolonged. This type of hearing loss is termed sensorineural loss.

It has been acknowledged for well over 100 years that noise exposure of sufficient magnitude will produce a sensorineural type of hearing loss. However, the subject has been given serious study only in recent years. In spite of this recent effort, much remains to be learned about the relation of hearing loss to noise exposure.

Sensorineural hearing impairment cannot be assessed in terms of the loss of sensory cells and neurons; instead, some change in hearing function must be measured. The changes in function that are commonly measured are (1) the hearing threshold sensitivity for pure tones; and (2) some index of the ability to hear and understand speech. The determination of hearing threshold sensitivity for pure tones in a quiet environment is a standard procedure. Methods for assessing the ability to understand speech have not been well standardized, because the understanding of speech is affected by such variables as vocabulary, education, intelligence, and the nature of speech test material, in addition to hearing ability.

Factors Involved

Noise exposure can produce a permanent loss of hearing in exposed individuals, and whether it does is dependent upon a number of factors, including (1) the sound intensity; (2) the length of time an employee is exposed to the noise; and (3) individual susceptibility to noise-induced hearing loss. The more intense the given noise, the more it will produce hearing loss—also, the longer an employee is exposed to a particular noise, the greater the probability of injury to the auditory system from that noise.

Individuals vary a great deal in terms of how much hearing loss they will develop from exposure to a particular noise level for a particular length of time. If a group of workers were exposed to the same noise level over their working lifetime, some would have their hearing affected more rapidly and to a much greater extent than others. At present, there is no way to determine which employees are most susceptible to auditory system damage.

Populations at Risk

The National Institute for Occupational Safety and Health (NIOSH) has stated that 1.7 million workers in the U.S. between 50 and 59 years of age have compensable noise-induced hearing losses. According to NIOSH estimates, 14% of the working population are employed in environments where the noise level exceeds 90 A-weighted decibels (dBA) (Table 20–1). If individuals work in an environment where the predominant noise level exceeds 90 dBA for a number of months or years, some workers will develop hearing impairments. The number of workers exposed to noise hazards on the job far exceeds the number exposed to any other significant occupational hazard.

Safe Noise Exposures

It is impossible to establish any clear-cut distinction between "safe" and "unsafe" noise exposures. Criteria for noise exposure that have been proposed are based generally upon the results of studies involving exposures to continuous noise. Whether these predictions will also hold true for intermittent exposures to both continuous and impulse noise is somewhat controversial.

It is generally agreed that after repeated excessive noise exposure, some individuals can incur a hearing loss. There is a con-

TABLE 20–1.
Noise Exposures Above 90 dBA in Manufacturing*

CODE	NUMBER OF PLANTS IN SAMPLE	TOTAL NUMBER OF EMPLOYEES IN SAMPLE	NUMBER LOCATED IN AREAS 90 DBA AND ABOVE	PERCENT OF WORK FORCE EXPOSED	TOTAL WORK FORCE	NUMBER PROJECTED TO BE LOCATED IN AREAS 90 DBA AND OVER
Textile mill products	23	12,764	5,634	44.1	963,300	424,815
Petroleum and coal products	16	20,493	5,875	28.6	192,800	55,140
Lumber and wood products	14	5,654	1,460	25.8	601,000	155,058
Food and kindred products	17	23,690	5,959	25.1	1,898,600	476,549
Furniture and fixtures	11	10,374	1,849	17.8	465,400	82,841
Fabricated metal products	56	41,371	7,079	17.1	1,335,000	228,285
Stone, clay and glass products	5	2,502	416	16.6	643,800	106,870
Primary metal industries	51	71,208	11,001	15.4	1,190,000	183,260
Rubber and plastic products	4	7,671	1,105	14.4	589,500	84,888
Transportation equipment	46	199,212	23,445	11.7	1,705,500	199,543
Electrical equipment and supplies	7	8,790	973	11.0	1,778,100	195,591
Chemicals and allied products	8	3,081	324	10.5	1,014,400	106,512
Apparel and other textile products	1	50	5	10.0	1,353,100	†
Paper and allied products	21	14,997	1,385	9.2	687,400	63,240
Ordnance and accessories	12	39,403	3,480	8.8	193,900	17,063
Instruments and related products	6	3,254	193	5.9	433,800	25,594
Machinery except electrical	38	25,016	1,144	4.5	1,768,000	79,560
Printing and publishing	5	5,597	237	4.2	1,085,900	45,607
Total	341‡	504,427	71,564	14.1	16,999,500	2,533,416

*From NIOSH Criteria Document.
†Insufficient data for projection
‡2,709 questionnaires were sent to the manufacturing industries listed, of which 1,559 were returned. 341 of these respondents answered this question.

siderable difference of opinion among the acoustics experts as to the boundary that separates the harmless from the harmful noises. Because of the normal variation in susceptibility between individuals, it is not possible scientifically to set a realistic standard for exposure to noise that will protect everyone who is exposed. Generally, limits are set with the intention of protecting 90% or more of an exposed population.

Assessing the amount of hearing loss in employees due to noise exposure in the workplace has always been a difficult task. Outside of working hours, workers often engage in recreational activities in which noise intensity reaches hazardous levels. Generally, the hearing damage due to off-work activities is considered to be negligible when the noise exposure of these activities is low compared with that at the workplace. In such cases, compensation is awarded on the assumption that all the hearing loss due to noise is work-related. The question is how to determine whether the noise exposure from activities such as hunting, snowmobiling, and motorcycling, which are unrelated to work, is significant.

Another complicating factor is the difficulty, if not the impossibility, of determining what portion of an employee's hearing loss is due to the normal aging process, medications, life-style, and diseases capable of producing sensorineural pathology. Presbycusis is the loss of hearing that takes place with increasing age. Such a loss occurs even for persons who are otologically normal and have not been exposed to high occupational noise levels.

Determining that a hazardous level of noise exists at the workplace is one element in proving that a hearing impairment is work-related. The degree of noise exposure can be determined from noise-monitoring records—if available. Problems arise when no previous noise measurements have been taken. If present noise levels are below 90 dBA, it is difficult to determine what the earlier exposures were, particularly in cases where the work environment has been modified. For example, in a given workplace it may be that (1) different, modified, or rebuilt machines are now being used; (2) operating characteristics of the machines have been changed by wear and tear; or (3) some other change has been made in the working conditions.

NOISE AND ITS MEASUREMENT

Airborne sound consists of small, rapid, local fluctuations in atmospheric pressure that are capable of being detected by the human ear. Because of the large range of pressure fluctuations to which the ear responds, it is convenient to utilize the *decibel* (dB) scale, which is logarithmic, to express the magnitude of these pressure fluctuations.

The word *sound* can be used to mean a physical pressure oscillation (alternate increases and decreases in the normal static atmospheric pressure) or the resulting, subjective auditory sensation that occurs when the hearing mechanism is stimulated.

A vibrating sound source produces rapid pressure fluctuations that spread outward in the same way ripples do on water after a stone is thrown into it. The result of the movement of the air molecules is a fluctuation in the normal atmospheric pressure, or sound waves. These waves may radiate in all directions from the source and may be reflected and scattered. When the sound source stops vibrating, the sound waves disappear almost instantaneously.

The ear is extremely sensitive to these pressure fluctuations, which it converts into auditory sensations in the ear.

The term *sound* is usually applied to that form of energy that produces a sensation of hearing in humans; *vibration* usually refers to the nonaudible acoustic phenomena that are recognized by the tactile experience of touch or feeling.

Sound may be described in terms of three variables: (1) amplitude (perceived as loudness); (2) frequency (perceived as pitch); and (3) time pattern.

Amplitude, or Sound Level

Amplitude is the extent of the pressure fluctuations or the difference between static atmospheric pressure (with no sound present) and the total atmospheric presure with sound present. Sound pressure level (SPL) measurements are based upon the average amplitude of the pressure changes constituting the sound stimulus and are directly related to the intensity or energy characteristics of the sound (Fig 20–1).

The decibel scale is a logarithmic scale, not a linear one. The logarithmic scale is used because the range of sound intensities is very great. It is convenient to use logarithms to compress the scale to encompass all the sounds that need to be measured. The human ear has an extremely wide range of response to sound levels.

Another property of the decibel scale is that the sound pressure levels of two separate sounds are not directly (that is, arithmetically) additive. For example, if a sound of 70 dB is added to another sound of 70 dB, the total is only a 3-decibel increase (to 73 dB), not a doubling to 140 dB.

The 1983 hearing conservation amendment of the Occupational Safety and Health Administration (OSHA) requires employers to monitor noise exposure levels in a manner that will accurately identify employees who are exposed to noise at or above 85 decibels (dB) averaged over eight working hours, called an eight-hour time-weighted average (TWA). The exposure measurement must include all noise within an 80 dB–130 dB range and must be taken during a typical work situation. This requirement is performance oriented, since it allows employers to choose the monitoring method that best suits each individual situation.

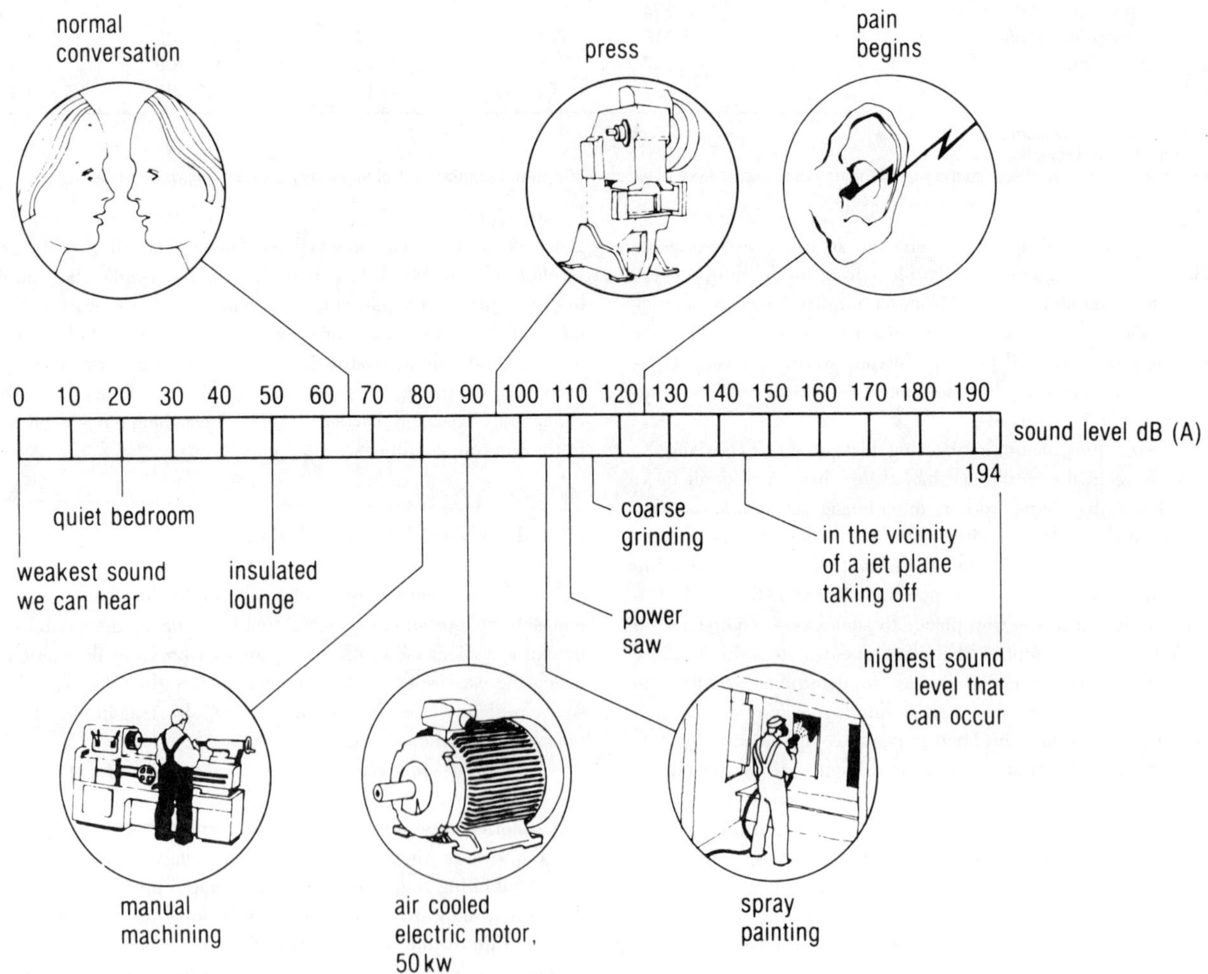

FIG 20–1.
Typical sound levels (dBA). (Courtesy U.S. Department of Labor.)

Frequency

The rate at which the sound pressure fluctuates determines frequency. The unit of time is usually one second and the term *Hertz* (Hz) is used to designate the number of fluctuations or cycles per second. The frequency range of audible sounds for healthy young ears is usually considered to extend from 20 to 20,000 Hz. The simplest type of sound, called a *pure tone,* consists of a very regular oscillation at a single frequency. This sound may be produced by a tuning fork. In contrast, music, speech, and noise, each containing a collection of many different frequency sounds, are called complex sounds (Fig 20–2).

The pattern of distribution of acoustical energy at the various frequencies is referred to as the *spectrum* of the sound. The frequencies of sound comprising speech are found principally between 250 and 3,000 Hz. To describe the spectrum of a noise, the audible frequency range is usually divided into eight frequency bands, each one octave wide, and SPL measurements are made in each band. A wide-band noise is one where the acoustic energy is distributed over a large range of frequencies.

Narrow-band noises, with most of their energy confined to a narrow range of frequencies, normally produce a definite pitch sensation. For a true narrow-band noise, only a single octave band will contain a significant amount of energy. The noise caused by a circular saw, planer, or other rotating devices is occasionally of the narrow-band type, but usually there is some spreading of the acoustic energy to several of the octave bands.

Time Pattern

Sound may be described in terms of its pattern of time and level: continuity, fluctuation, impulsiveness, and intermittency. Continuous sounds are those produced for relatively long periods at a constant level. Intermittent sounds are those which are produced for short periods, such as the ringing of a telephone or aircraft takeoffs and landings.

Continuous noise is normally defined as broad-band noise, of approximately constant level and spectrum, to which an employee is exposed for periods of up to six to eight hours per day, 40 hours per week, 50 weeks per year. A majority of factory workers work in this kind of noise environment.

Most damage-risk criteria are written for continuous noise exposure because it is the most common as well as the easiest to define in terms of amplitude, frequency content, and length of noise exposure. An example of damage-risk criteria for a continuous noise exposure are the levels set by the Department of Labor

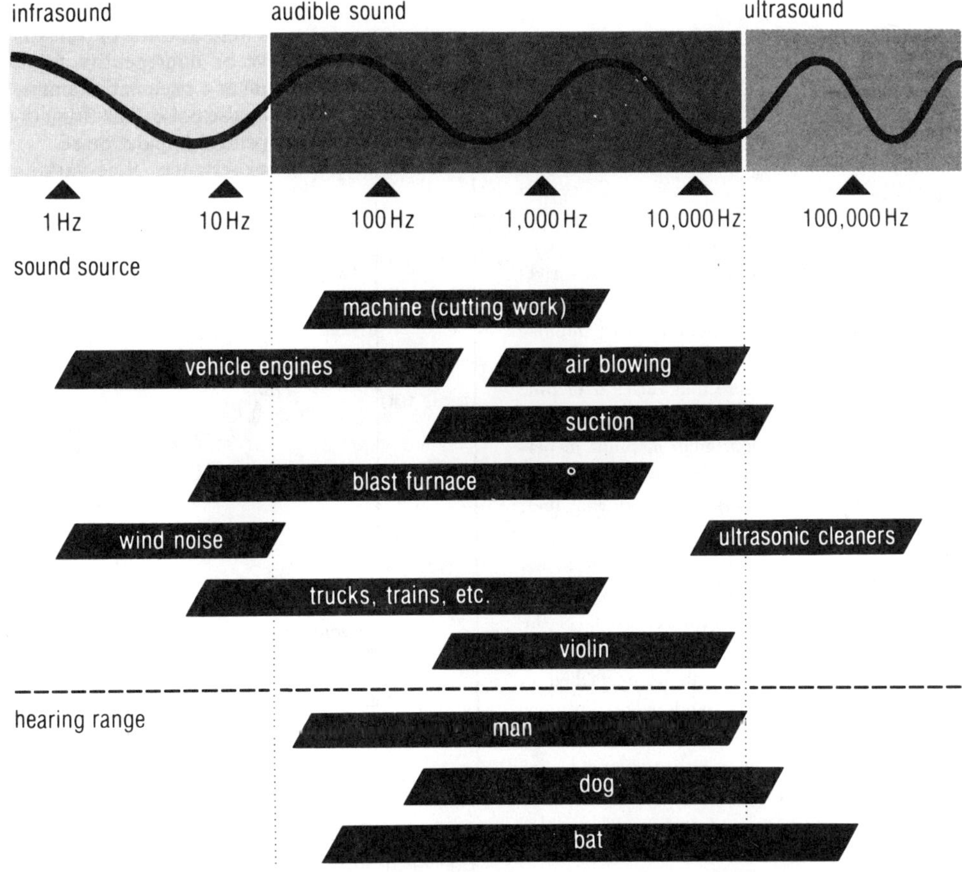

FIG 20–2.
Noise is a disorderly mixture of many different tones at many different frequencies. (Courtesy U.S. Department of Labor.)

TABLE 20–2.
Permissible Noise Exposure*†

DURATION PER DAY HOURS	SLOW RESPONSE dBA
8	90
6	92
4	95
3	97
2	100
1½	102
1	105
½	110
¼ or less	115

*From Occupational Safety and Health Administration: 29 CFR 1910, 1981.
†When the daily noise exposure is composed of two or more periods of noise exposure of different levels, their combined effect should be considered, rather than the individual effect of each. If the sum of the following fractions: $C_1/T_1 + C_2/T_2 \ldots C_n/T_n$ exceeds unity, then, the mixed exposure should be considered to exceed the limit value. C_n indicates the total time of exposure at a specified noise level, and T_n indicates the total time of exposure permitted at that level.

shown in Table 20–2. These figures specify allowable A-weighted noise levels that, in effect, permit the noise level to be increased by five dBA if the exposure time is cut by half.

Impact and Impulse Noise

The impulse type of noise consists of transient pulses, occurring in repetitive or nonrepetitive fashion. The operation of a rivet gun or a pneumatic hammer usually produces repetitive impulse noise. The firing of a gun is an example of nonrepetitive impulse noise.

Most workers experience noise exposure that varies over time because noise is cyclical or varies unpredictably at their work station or because they move around the department or plant in performing their job. Noise exposure codes provide for summing the series of partial exposures that such workers receive during their work period.

Nonsteady noise, such as impulse noise and impact noise, must be evaluated in terms of its temporal character as well as its sound level. Both the short-term and long-term variations of the noise must be described.

Individual impulse and impact sounds can be described in terms of their rise time, peak sound level, and pulse duration. Data from temporary threshold-shift studies indicate that ear tolerance to impact peak sound pressures is greatly reduced by increasing the rise time or burst duration of the sound. The rate and number of such impact sounds within an exposure period are also factors that should be considered when making hazard judgments for these types of sound.

It is not easy to measure accurately the sound levels of rapidly varying staccato noises. The meter movements of sound level meters cannot follow sudden peaks in sound pressure accurately. Consequently, the meter may systematically distort and misrepresent the sound pressure levels reached by the noise. This is particularly true with impact noises; for example, the noise of a drop forge.

The primitiveness of measuring techniques is one reason for the lack of a reliable method of studying the additional risk posed by the level of pulsing noise. In some recommendations, noise is defined as impulse noise if there is a difference of at least 20 dB between sound peaks and background noise. However, this definition lacks an unambiguous basis in either physics or medical science. Lahti et al.[25] began a study in 1979 into the causes, measurement, harmful effects and combatting of impact noise. To determine the effect of time weighting, a number of different readouts were produced of the same sound sample measuring in different ways. Sound levels and peak forms varied according to whether results were produced using fast and slow time weighting or an expression of the peak value.

The more clearly the principal sound was distinguishable from other noise, the greater was the difference between peak-value and time-weighted levels. For example, a sledgehammer produced a 19 dB difference between peak-value and slow time-weighted readings while grinding showed a 14 dB difference (Fig 20–3).

This finding led to a proposal for a new definition of the im-

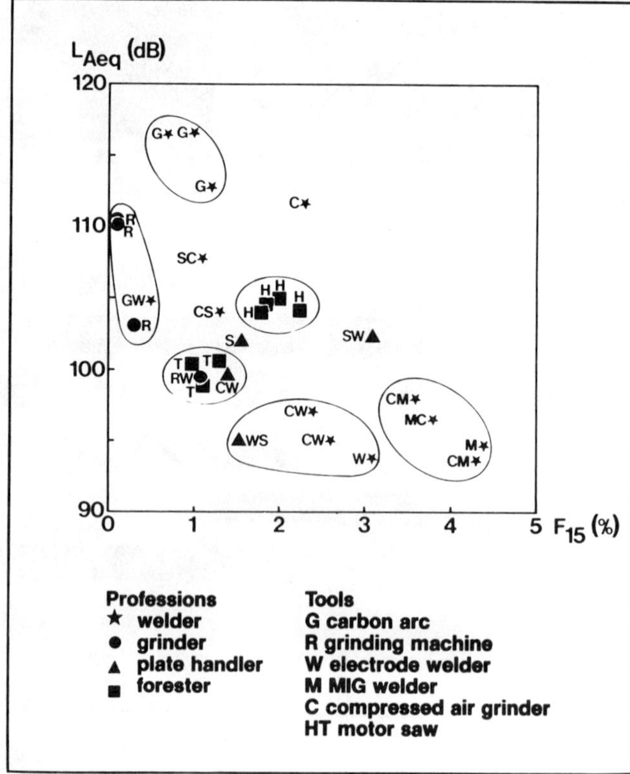

FIG 20–3.
Equivalent levels and impulse levels of noise by occupation and tool. F_{15} is the proportion of time that the impulse level is greater than 15 dB. (Courtesy Thelma Aro, Institute of Occupational Health, Helsinki, Finland)

pulse level of noise. In this definition it is defined as the difference between the peak value (L_{AP}) and the root mean square of the slow time-weighted value (L_{AS}).

The advantage of this definition is that it has a clear basis in physics. The impulse rating can be measured using a conventional decibel meter. A reading can be produced from a single impulse, but the definition also gives the possibility of measuring varying impulse noise and using more developed output functions. It was also proposed that the criterion for impulse noise should be a 15 dB difference between the peak level and the root mean square of slow time-weighted levels. Noise is defined as impulse noise if $L_{AP} - L_{AS} \geq 15$ dB.

A-Weighted Sound Level

A person's ability to hear a sound depends greatly on the frequency composition of the sound. People hear sounds most readily when the predominant sound energy occurs at frequencies between 1,000 and 6,000 Hz. Sounds at frequencies above 10,000 Hz, such as high-pitched hissing, are much more difficult to hear, as are sounds at frequencies below about 100 Hz, a low rumble, for example. To measure sound on a scale that approximates the way it is heard by most people, more emphasis must be given to the frequencies that people hear more easily.

The most commonly used scales on sound level meters are the C scale, which gives a flat, equally weighted response across the entire spectrum, and the A scale, which gives less emphasis to low-frequency sounds. The A scale is often used in noise measurements, since it provides more weight to the annoying high frequencies (Fig 20–4).

A sound level meter's A-weighting network is thought to rate most industrial broad-band noises much the same as the human ear does. Because of its simplicity and accuracy in rating hearing hazards, the A-weighted sound level has become the method recommended for measuring noise exposure by the American Conference of Governmental Industrial Hygienists (ACGIH) as well as the U.S. Department of Labor as part of the Occupational Safety and Health regulations.

Instruments

There is a wide variety of instrumentation available for the evaluation of noise exposure, from very simple equipment to extremely sophisticated equipment used by acoustics engineers and consultants. Noise level measurements for steady-state or continuous noise should be made with a sound level meter set to an A-weighted slow response or with an audiodosimeter of equivalent accuracy. For the measurement of impact noise (such as that from a drop hammer), an impact-noise meter with peak hold capability should be used. Sound level measuring instrumentation should be calibrated using an acoustical calibrator, preferably before and after the noise measurements. Instruments used for monitoring employee exposures must be carefully checked or calibrated to ensure that the measurements are accurate. Calibration procedures are unique to specific instruments. Employers have the duty to assure that the measuring instruments they are using are properly calibrated. They may find it useful to follow the manufacturer's instructions to determine when and how extensively to calibrate.

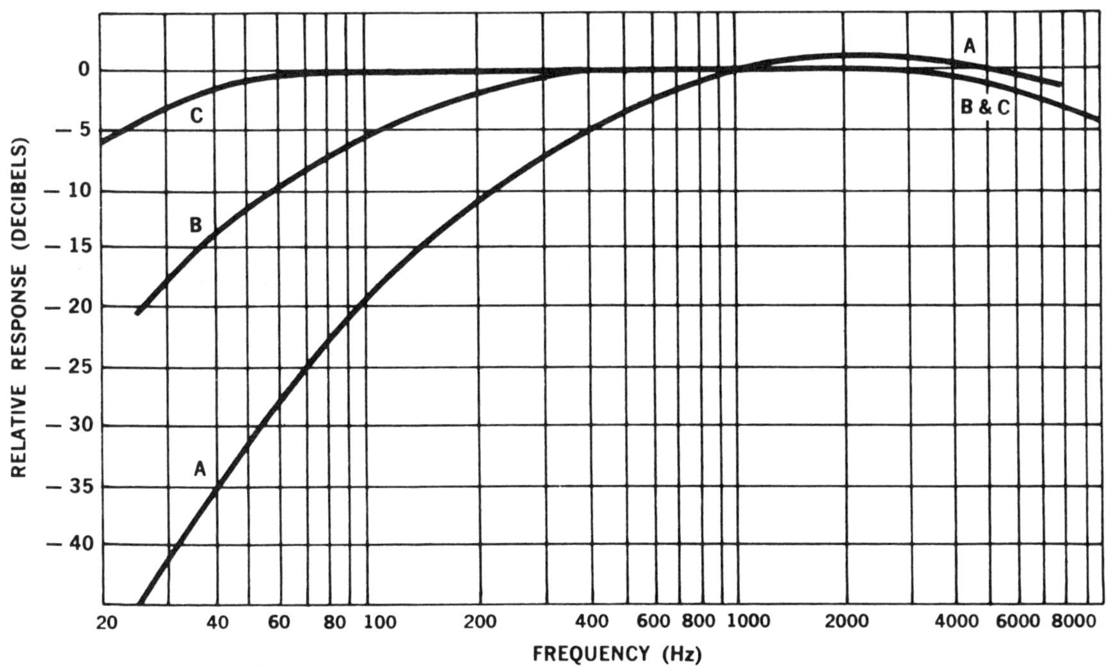

FIG 20–4.
Shown here are the frequency response attenuation characteristics for the A, B, and C networks. (From ANSI S1. 4–1971)

Sound Level Meters

The basic noise-measuring instrument, the sound level meter (SLM), is little more than an "electronic ear"; it changes noise into an electrical signal and displays it on an indicator. Thus, the sound level meter reads the noise level directly, and it displays it in terms of the decibel.

The American National Standards Institute (ANSI) has defined several classes of SLMs. Type 1 meters are precision laboratory devices, requiring skilled operators. These must be accurate to within ± 1 dB from 10 to 10,000 Hz. Type 2 meters must have A-, B-, and C-weighting networks, with both fast and slow settings. Accuracy must exceed ± 2 dB between 30 and 3,000 Hz. Type S2A SLMs feature similar accuracy specifications, but need only A-scales and slow settings. Type 3 instruments must also have three weighting networks and two sampling intervals, but accuracy specifications are relaxed to ± 3 dB between 30 and 3,000 Hz. There is also a Type S3A, which has only an A-scale and a slow setting.

The sound level meter contains a microphone, an amplifier with a calibrated attenuator, a set of frequency response networks (weighting networks), and an indicating meter. The sound level meter is a sensitive electronic voltmeter that measures the electrical signal from a microphone attached to the instrument. The alternating current (AC) electrical signal from the microphone is amplified so that, after conversion to direct current (DC) by means of a rectifier, the signal can deflect a needle on an indicating meter. An attenuator controls the overall amplification of the instrument. The response-vs.-frequency characteristics of the amplified signal are controlled by electrical circuits called weighting networks.

Microphone.—This responds to sound pressure variations and produces an electrical signal that is processed by the sound level meter.

Amplifier.—In a sound level meter, the amplifier must have a high available gain to measure the low voltage signal from a microphone in a quiet location. It should have a wide frequency range, usually 20 to 20,000 Hz. The range of greatest interest in noise measurements is 50 to 6,000 Hz.

Attenuator.—Sound level meters measure sounds that differ greatly in level. A small portion of this range is covered by the relative deflection of the needle on the indicating meter. The rest of the range is covered by an adjustable attenuator, which is an electrical resistance network inserted in the amplifier to produce known ranges of signal level. To simplify use, it is customary to have the attenuator adjustable in steps of 10 dB.

Meter System.—After the electrical signal from the microphone is amplified and sent through the attenuators and weighting networks, it is used to drive a metering circuit. The meter face displays a value proportional to the electrical signal applied to it.

Noise levels are seldom steady, so meter damping is adjustable to alter the response of the instrument to fluctuations in signal level. "Slow" response smooths the readings and is used for measuring factory environments and most machine noise. "Fast" response follows short-term variations in noise level.

Octave Band Analysis

Although the A scale on the sound level meter is used to determine compliance with acceptable limits set by OSHA, a full octave band analysis can be very helpful in identifying noise sources. In order to characterize a noise, it is often desirable to make a frequency analysis, which indicates how the sound energy is distributed over the audible range of frequencies. In such an analysis, the sound-pressure level can be measured for each of a number of different frequency bands. As an example, in an octave band analysis, filters are used to cause the sound-pressure level measuring apparatus to "hear" only a band of frequencies one octave wide (Fig 20–5).

Noise Dosimeters

Sound level meters can be used to measure an instantaneous noise level, but they are not designed to electronically sum up the noise exposures of mobile individuals exposed to changing noise levels during their work shift.

When a person moves away from a sound source, the sound level at his ears usually decreases. That is why the microphone of the sound level meter must be held near the person's ears if it is to measure accurately the sound that actually reaches the ear. A sufficient number of measurements would be required to develop a sound level map of the area. Then, to estimate an employee's noise exposure, a time and motion study would be required to determine just how long the employee spent in each sound level area during each day.

This problem is minimized by use of the noise dosimeter. The cumulative sound level measured by the dosimeter differs from that measured on a sound level meter—this depends on the relative positions of the microphone, the employee, and the noise source, and is due in part to body shielding and reflection. The use of dosimeters, although inviting, presents certain problems. It is not

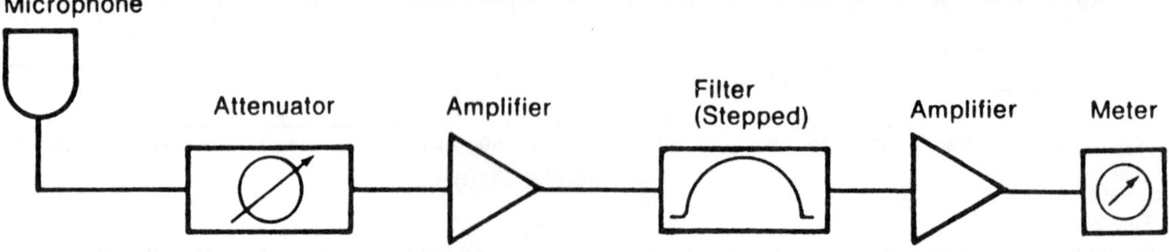

FIG 20–5.
The basic components of an octave-band analyzer.

as easy as it would appear to be to translate directly from summation of decibel levels to actual noise exposure over a period of time. Thus, dosimeters should be used with caution and a recognition of their limitations.

Noise dose is the conversion of fluctuating noise levels, measured within a certain time, to a measure of accumulated noise exposure. This conversion takes place in such a way that a 5-dBA change in level corresponds to a factor of two in time. For example: 90 dBA for eight hours provides the same noise dose as 95 dBA for four hours, or 100 dBA for two hours, and so on. This way of weighting noise with respect to time is described in the OSHA standards. In order to evaluate the risk, it is, therefore, necessary to measure the noise dose during a typical working day—if the dose exceeds the allowable level, the risk is present and precautions must be taken.

Consider two noises that have the same overall sound-pressure level but which have their acoustic energy distributed much differently over the audible range of frequencies. Specifically, one noise may consist chiefly of low frequencies, while the other noise is composed mainly of medium-to-high frequencies. Although these two noises do have the same sound-pressure level, they probably would not be equally loud, equally annoying, equally disturbing, or equally "noisy" to most people.

Annoyance from noise is strongly dependent on its energy content in each octave band. It is important to remember that sound meters cannot measure the qualities of noise to which humans respond. We hear "loudness" and "pitch," while meters measure sound-pressure levels and frequencies, so we would not expect a direct correspondence between meter readings and annoyance or disturbance. Although loudness depends primarily upon the sound pressure of the noise, it also depends upon the frequency. Similarly, although pitch depends primarily upon the frequency of the sound, it also depends upon the sound pressure.

Noise control techniques are dependent on the energy level in each octave band. The identification of pure tone components is an extremely useful diagnostic tool for finding and quieting the noise source. If a noisy machine is to be used in a room, the acoustic characteristics of the room as a function of frequency, and the radiated sound power level in octave bands must be known in order to estimate the noise level that would be produced by this machine.

Noise Exposure Evaluation

The best evidence to determine the actual exposure of a worker to noise includes measurements of noise levels obtained at the worker's job stations, past and present. When evaluating the noise measurements, one should consider both the location of the measurements and the number of measurements made.

Number of Noise Measurements.—In most cases, a few (two or three) noise level measurements, covering only a small portion of a working day, are not sufficient to establish the degree of noise exposure. Generally, measurements should be obtained covering most of a complete working day; covering several nonconsecutive workdays is even better.

Location of Noise Measurements.—The best location for taking noise measurements is in the hearing zone (within a few inches) of the ear of the employee or a worker doing an identical job, under conditions identical to those under which the employee worked. Measurements obtained at a stationary point in the work environment (area samples) can give an indication of possible exposure but can also be very misleading. For example, measuring noise levels a few inches from a noisy machine when the worker is located several feet away may indicate erroneously high exposures.

MECHANICS OF HEARING

To understand the causes of hearing loss, it is necessary to become familiar with the anatomy of the human ear and the functions of each part of the ear in the hearing process. The ear is a complex mechanism. There are many aspects of how the ear functions, particularly the workings of the inner ear and the pathways to the brain, that are not fully understood.

The peripheral auditory mechanism enables an individual to detect sound waves within a range of 20 to 20,000 Hz (hertz or cycles per second) and convert them into electrical impulses that are transmitted to the brain for interpretation.

Anatomy

The ear consists of three major divisions: (1) the outer ear, which collects the sound and converts it into vibratory motion of the eardrum; (2) the middle ear, which mechanically couples the eardrum to the fluid-filled inner ear; and (3) the inner ear, within which the nerve signals originate before transmission to the brain via the auditory nerve.

Outer Ear

The outer (external) ear is divided into two sections—the portion seen attached to the outer surface of the head (called the auricle or pinna), and the external auditory canal (Fig 20–6).

Pinna.—The pinna is a delicately folded cartilaginous structure, with a few small muscles, covered by subcutaneous tissue and skin.

External Auditory Canal.—Also termed the meatus, this is a skin-lined pouch about 1½ inches (3.8 cm) long, supported in its outer one third by the cartilage of the pinna and in its inner two thirds by bone of the skull. At its innermost end lies the tympanic membrane, or eardrum, that separates the external from the middle ear.

Middle Ear

An air-filled cavity, approximately 1–2 cu cm in volume, lying between the eardrum and the bony wall of the inner ear, is called the middle ear or tympanum (Fig 20–7).

Eardrum.—This membrane separates the external ear canal from the middle ear. The eardrum consists of an inner layer of mucous membrane and a middle layer of fibrous tissue. It is spiderweb in form, with radial and circular fibers for structural sup-

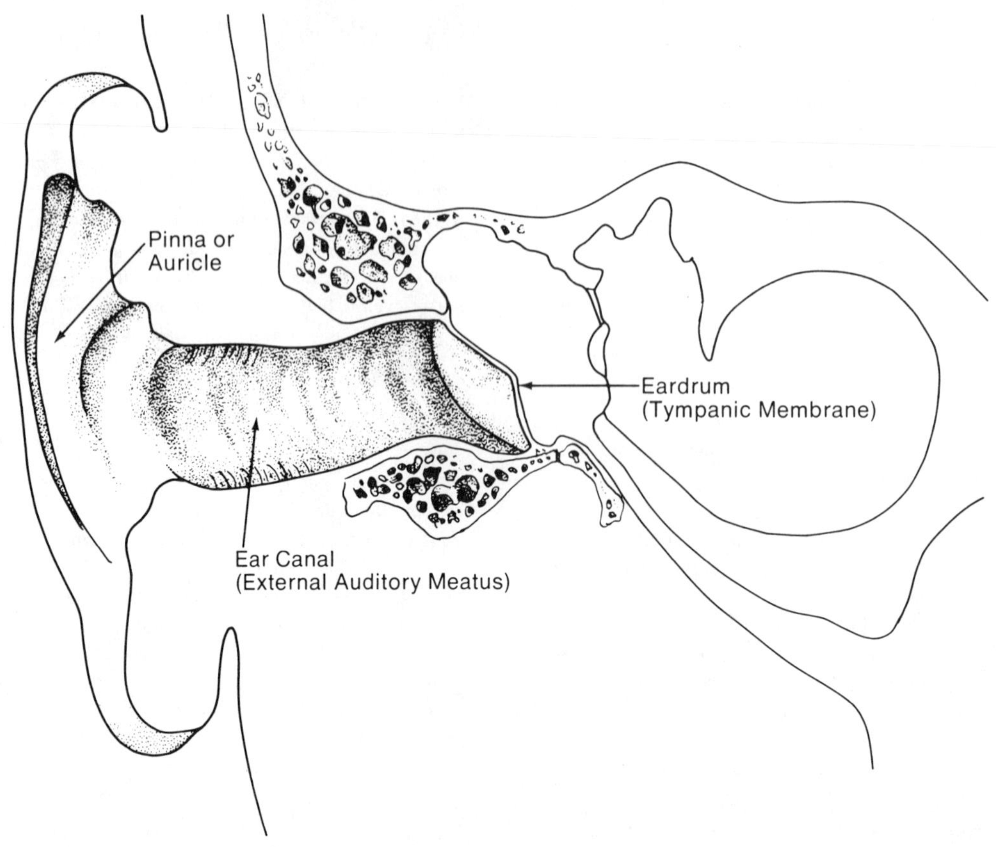

FIG 20–6.
The outer ear shown here can be divided into the auricle (or pinna) and the external auditory canal. (Courtesy Alliance of American Insurers.)

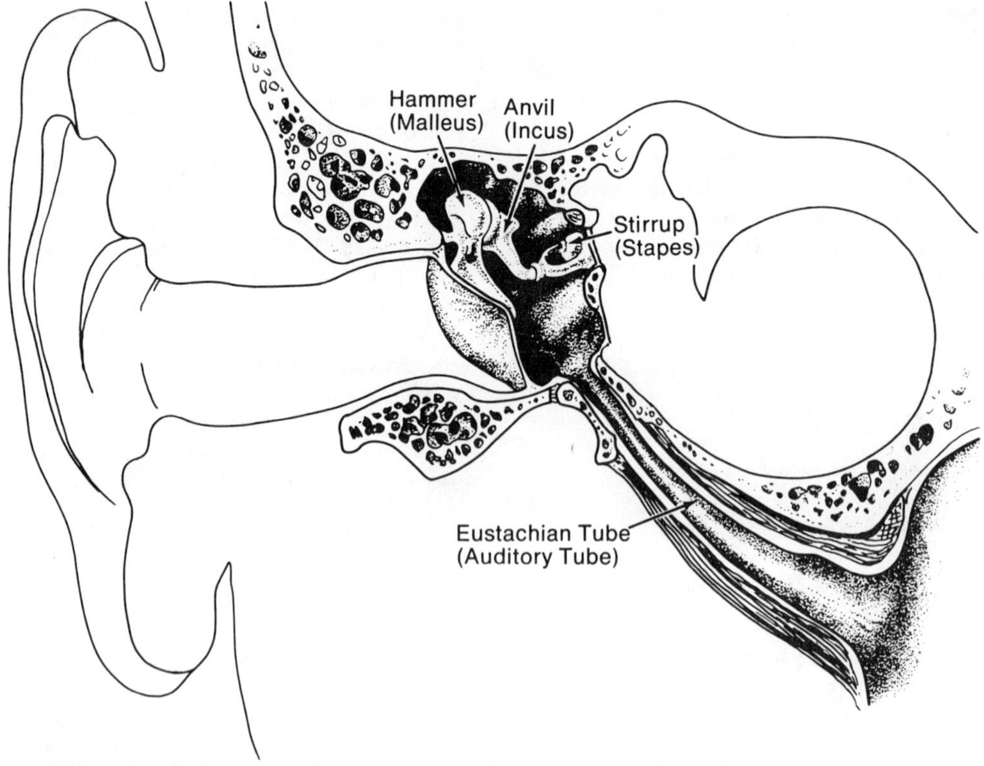

FIG 20–7.
The middle ear shown here is contained within the temporal bone and is made up of the eustachian tube, the middle ear space, and the mastoid air cell system. (Courtesy Alliance of American Insurers.)

port. Pressure on the two sides of the membrane is equalized by the eustachian tube, which opens from the middle ear into the throat.

Hammer, Anvil, and Stirrup.—The middle ear contains a series of three bony levers; the hammer, anvil, and stirrup, or malleus, incus, and stapes, with their associated supporting muscles. Their function is to transmit the vibrations of the eardrum to the inner ear and to transform them to a vibration or wave motion in the liquid which fills the inner ear (Fig 20–8).

Oval Window and Round Window.—The oval window and the round window are located on the inner wall of the middle ear. The round window is covered by a very thin membrane that moves out as the footplate in the oval window moves in. As the action is reversed and the footplate is pulled out, the round window membrane moves inward.

Inner Ear

The inner ear contains both hearing and equilibrium or balance mechanisms. A bony labyrinth, called the osseous labyrinth, the inner ear consists of a series of tiny canals and cavities hollowed out of the compact temporal bone. This labyrinth is filled with a fluid called perilymph in which a tubular membrane, the membranous labyrinth, floats. The inner ear is divided into the cochlea and the vestibular system (Fig 20–9).

The nerve fibers for hearing terminate in the cochlea. The basilar membrane is a fibrous, flexible membrane which runs the length of the cochlea and along which is distributed the nerve excitation mechanism. The basilar membrane is set into motion hydraulically by acoustic energy. The stimulation of the nerve endings involves a complex structure on the basilar membrane known as the organ of Corti. The inner and outer hair cells are the components of the organ of Corti that are critically involved in the nerve stimulation process. Damage to these hair cells appears to be related to noise-induced hearing loss. Damage from repeated noise exposures is not a result of the physical limits of the affected structures being exceeded, but rather, the primary mechanism for chronic noise damage appears to be physicochemical, metabolic stress exerted on the maximally stimulated cells.

The Hearing Process

The outer ear collects acoustic energy which the eardrum converts to mechanical energy. The middle ear transfers sound energy from the outer ear to the inner ear. As the eardrum vibrates, its motion is transferred to the attached hammer. Because the bones of the ossicular chain are connected to each other, the movements

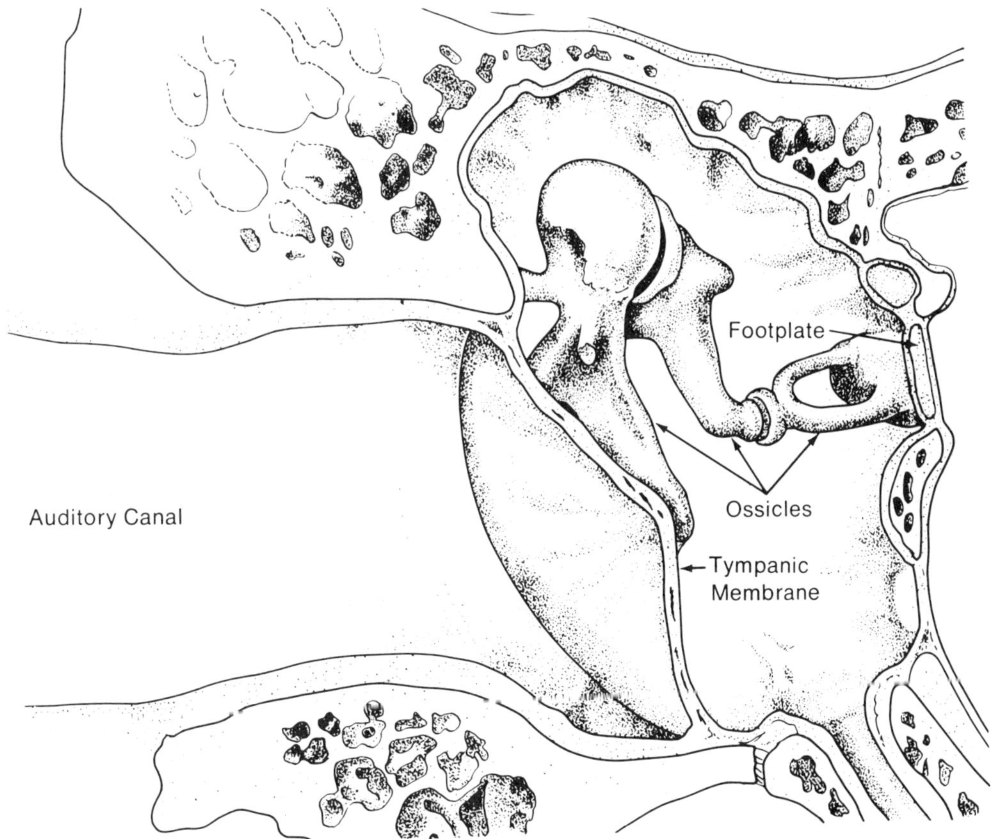

FIG 20–8.
The ossicles, located within the middle ear cavity, link the eardrum to an opening in the wall of the inner ear (the oval window). (Courtesy Alliance of American Insurers.)

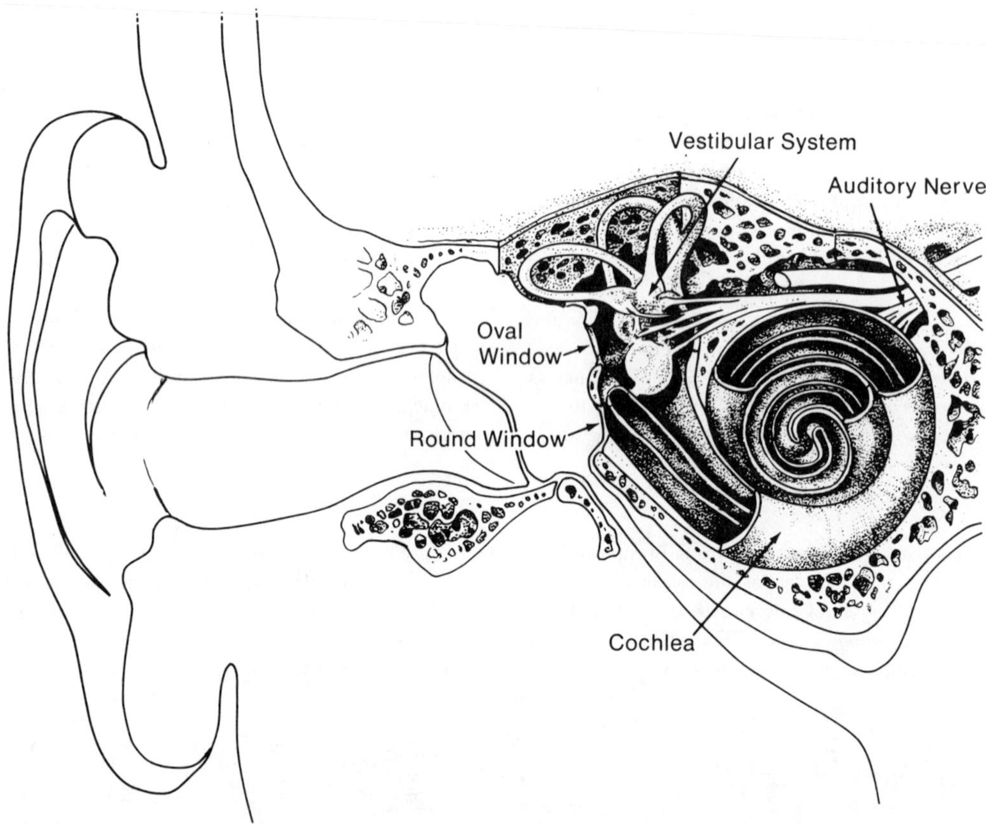

FIG 20–9.
Shown here are the major components of the inner ear, including the vestibular system and the cochlea. (Courtesy Alliance of American Insurers.)

of the hammer are passed on to the anvil, and finally to the stirrup, which is imbedded in the oval window. The movement of the footplate of the stapes within the oval window transforms this mechanical energy into hydraulic energy, setting the perilymph within the inner ear in motion (Fig 20–10).

The manner in which the hydraulic energy is transformed into electrical impulses to be sent by the auditory nerve to the brain is unclear. According to one hypothesis, the hair fibers from the hair cells embedded in the tectorial membrane permit the shearing action of the hair fibers to transfer varying amounts of energy to the hair cells. The hair cells then stimulate the hearing nerve-endings.

Threshold of Hearing

The threshold of hearing for a specified sound is the minimum sound pressure level of the sound that is capable of evoking an auditory sensation. The hearing threshold for an individual is not a sharp boundary but is defined in terms of the probability that a sound will be heard. The threshold depends on the characteristics of the sound, on the manner in which it is presented to the listener, and on the point at which the sound pressure level is measured (for instance, it can be measured at the entrance to the ear canal or in a free field in absence of the listener). To describe a hearing threshold, all of the above factors must be specified.

Threshold shifts, expressed in decibels, is the difference between the hearing threshold levels measured before and after noise exposure. If this shift is reversible (i.e., if the ear recovers completely after noise exposure, so that the threshold shift is reduced to zero), the threshold shift is said to be temporary; if the ear does not recover completely, the threshold shift is said to be permanent. If threshold shift is temporary, the hearing threshold returns to its values measured before exposure. The magnitude of temporary threshold shift depends on the time interval elapsing between the cessation of noise exposure and the measurement of threshold.

HEARING TESTS

Audiometry is the measurement of hearing. The results of such testing are recorded on an audiogram, a graph showing hearing (threshold) level as a function of frequency. Hearing (threshold) level is the number of decibels that the subject's threshold of hearing lies above the zero reference for that frequency. Thus, a pure-tone audiogram compares the hearing of the person being tested with a standard hearing level considered to be "normal" (i.e., the audiometric zero reference level).

Normal hearing is the median hearing level of a large group of young adults of ages between 18 and 25 years having no known

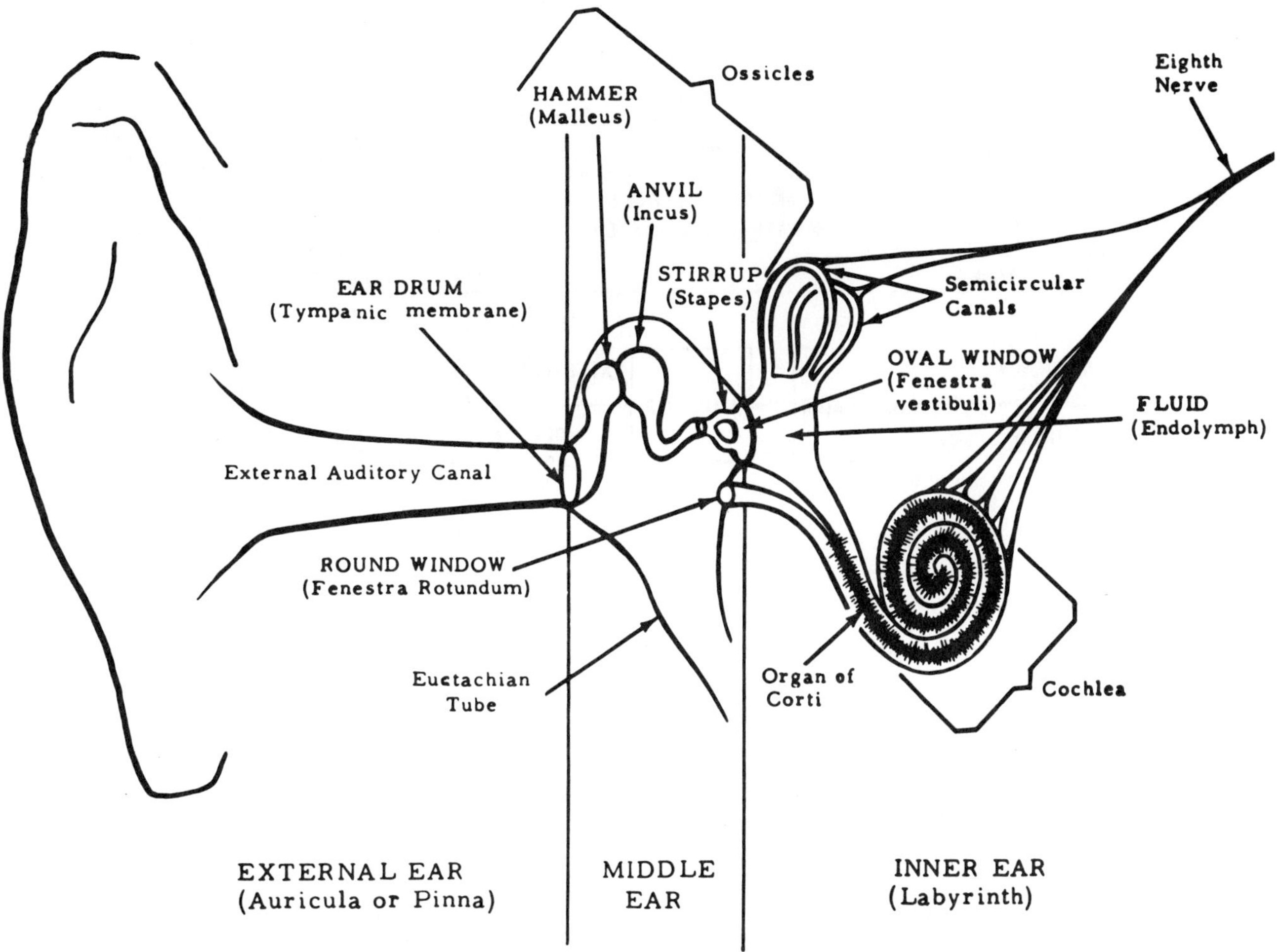

Fig 20–10.
How the ear hears. Wave motions in the air set up sympathetic vibrations which are transmitted by the eardrum and the three bones in the middle ear to the fluid-filled chamber of the inner ear. In the process, the relatively large but feeble air-induced vibrations of the eardrum are converted to much smaller but more powerful mechanical vibrations by the three ossicles, and finally into fluid vibrations. The wave motion in the fluid is sensed by the nerves in the cochlea, which transmit neural messages to the brain. (Courtesy American Foundrymen's Society.)

history of ear disease and no appreciable exposure to high-level noise. A set of sound pressure levels which represent the normal hearing threshold has been established as the zero reference level for audiometry.

A manual, pure-tone audiometer is an instrument in which the tester has control of the frequency and sound pressure level of the pure tones presented to the subject. The employee whose hearing is being tested responds to the test tone by raising a finger or hand or pushing a signal button. The technician selects a particular frequency, presents short tone pulses with a tone-interrupter switch, manipulates the hearing-level dial to determine the subject's hearing level, and records that level.

Audiometric testing not only monitors the sharpness or acuity of an employee's hearing over time, but also provides an opportunity for employers to educate employees about their hearing and the need to protect it.

Audiometers

The manual audiometer presents a variable sound level in an earphone. The audiometric technician measures at each frequency the minimum sound pressure level that the person can hear. The decibel difference between audiometric zero and the threshold is reported as the subject's hearing level, or hearing loss, at each frequency (Fig 20–11).

A pure-tone audiometer is essentially an electroacoustic generator that produces pure tones at predetermined frequencies and calibrated sound intensities. The frequency range is typically from 125 to 8,000 Hz and divided into discrete steps as described in Figure 20–10. The intensity is either continuously variable or variable in discrete 5-dB steps. Threshold measurement is done in 5-dB intervals on standard manual audiometers.

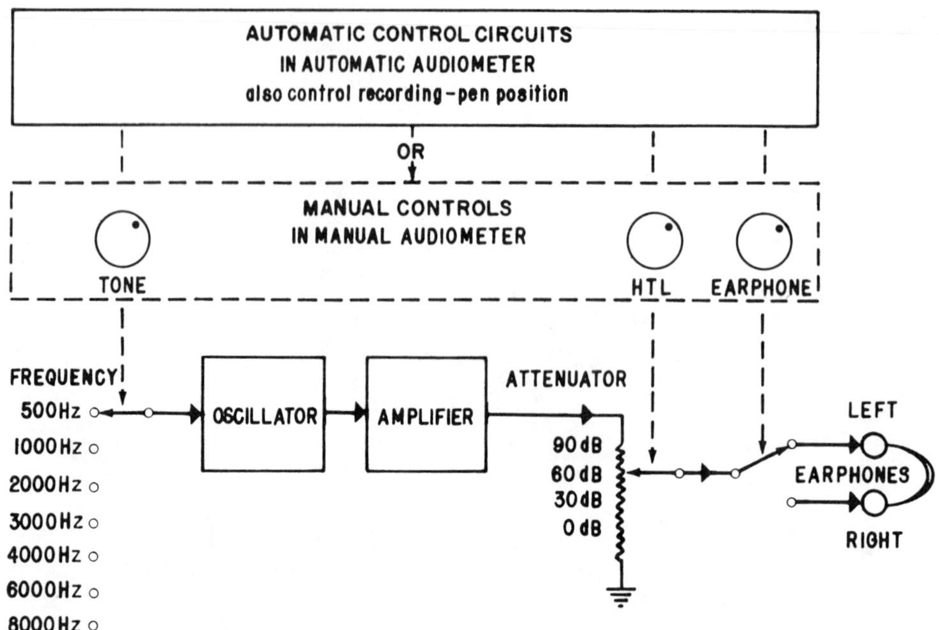

FIG 20–11.
Pure-tone audiometers differ widely in details but not in their basic makeup. An oscillator produces a signal at any one of the six or seven frequencies which is amplified and then applied to an attenuator to control its output level. From the attenuator it is applied to either the left or the right earphone. (Courtesy Alliance of American Insurers.)

Audiometric Zero

Zero hearing level in audiometry does not mean the absence of sound. The minimum sound pressure levels just audible to healthy young ears at different frequencies were assigned zero values and plotted on a chart, and a straight line was drawn to represent the standard audiometric reference threshold level or audiometric zero hearing level for human hearing.

There are two different decibel scales that must be differentiated. The scale for sound pressure level (SPL, or the "engineer's scale") has as its base of reference 20 micropascals (μPa) or 20 micronewtons (μN) per square meter, 20 μN/sq m (0.00002 N/sq m), or 0.0002 microbars (dynes per centimeter squared). This level of sound pressure is so faint that very few persons can hear it.

In contrast, the hearing threshold level (HTL) scale used in audiometry has as its base of reference a specific amount of sound pressure that is just audible to the average normal young ear; that is, the level at which the average normal-hearing person can just barely detect the presence of that sound. It ranges from 7 to 45 dB above the engineer's reference level, depending upon the frequency.

The zero decibel level reflects average normal hearing on both pure-tone and speech audiometers. If at any frequency it is necessary to amplify the sound above the zero decibel level, for example, by 20 decibels, for the subject to hear it, this amplified sound level is recorded as the subject's hearing threshold. This simply means that the subject's hearing acuity at the frequency being tested is 20 dB below the averge hearing level at that frequency, not necessarily that 20 dB of hearing ability has been lost.

Air-Conduction Threshold

The pure-tone air-conduction test measures the sound conducted to the eardrum through air (Fig 20–12). A pure-tone threshold for each tested frequency is determined by presenting a pure tone at the test frequency at intensities varied according to an established pattern. The threshold represents the lowest intensity at which a person is able to hear approximately 50% of the tone presentations. The subject's hearing thresholds are established at various octave intervals, usually from 250 through 8,000 Hz, with the interoctave interval of 3,000 Hz usually measured as well. Other interoctave frequencies available on the audiometer may also be measured, if the threshold level difference between octaves is 15 dB or more.

Bone-Conduction Threshold

Although the air-conduction test establishes the subject's hearing thresholds, it does not determine definitely whether the hearing loss, if any, is of a conductive or sensorineural type. To make this determination, the bone-conduction threshold test is made. In this test, sound vibrations generated by a bone vibrator held against the skull are conducted directly to the inner ear through the skull, bypassing the outer and middle ear (Fig 20–13). If a hearing loss is indicated by the air-conduction test, but normal hearing is indicated by the bone-conduction test, the hearing loss is conductive rather than sensorineural. Such a result indicates the loss is not due to prolonged exposure to noise.

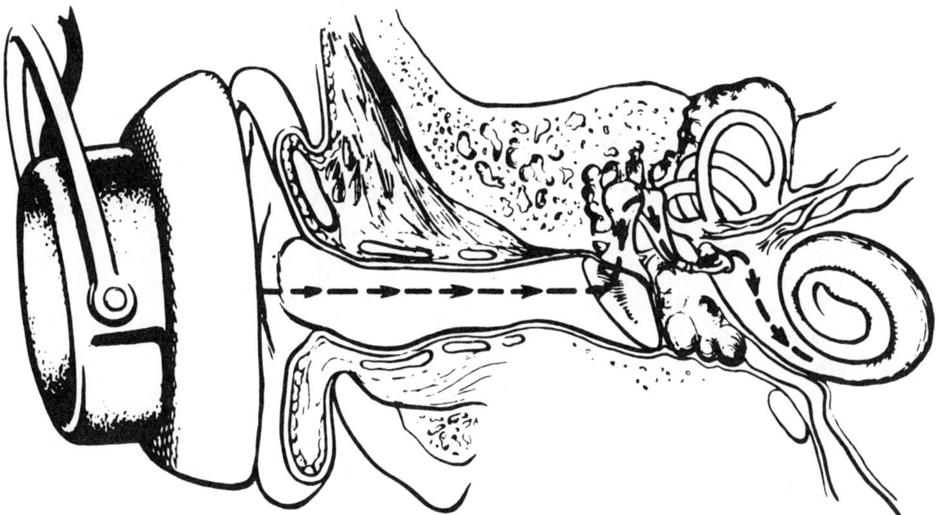

FIG 20–12.
An illustration of an air-conduction earphone. Note that the phone is placed directly over the external ear canal, and the sound waves are conducted (by air) to the eardrum and through the middle ear to the inner ear. (Courtesy Alliance of American Insurers.)

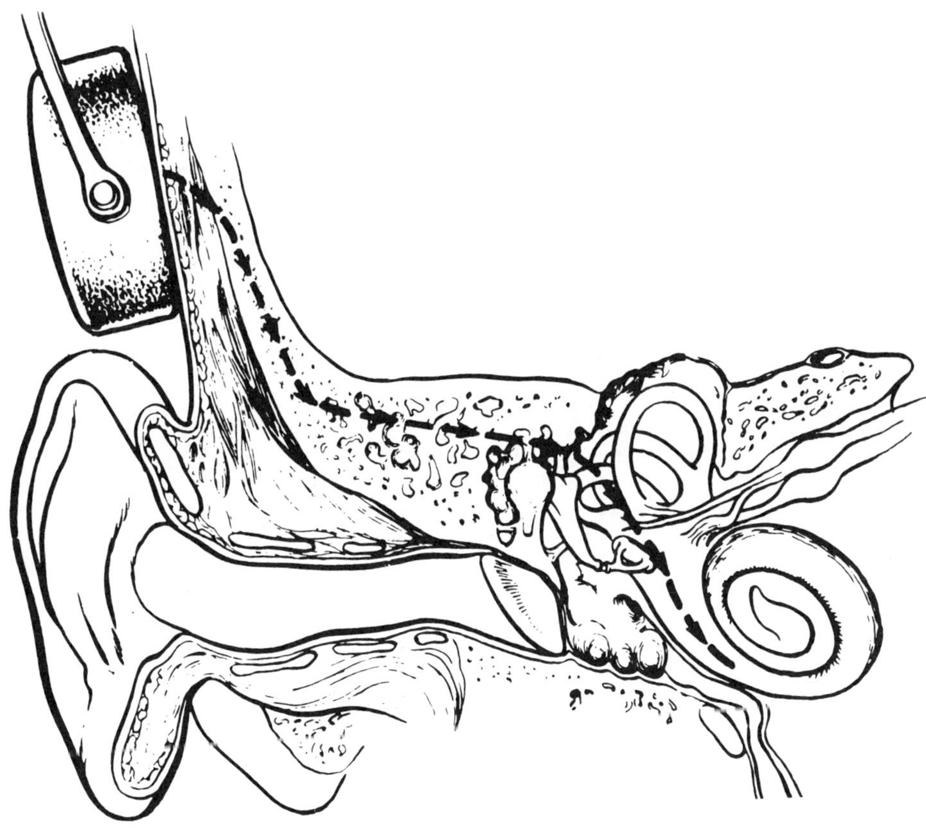

FIG 20–13.
Sound can be transmitted directly to the inner ear through the bones of the skull by means of a bone-conduction vibrator placed on the mastoid bone behind the outer ear. The *broken line* (with *arrows*) shows the path taken by the sound waves through the bony areas of the head to the inner ear. (Courtesy Alliance of American Insurers.)

Masking

Masking is the stimulation of one ear of the subject by controlled noise to prevent the subject from hearing, with that ear, the tone or signal given to the other ear. Since there is a chance that the test signal will cross over through the bones in the skull to the non-test ear, the non-test ear must be masked to eliminate it from the measurement process.

Unmasked bone-conduction thresholds indicate only that the better inner ear is functioning at the levels measured. No statement can be made about the other ear without masked thresholds, unless hearing in each ear is normal or the air-conduction threshold for each ear is equal and the unmasked bone-conduction threshold equals the air-conduction threshold. The examiner's skill is critical in obtaining bone-conduction thresholds. It is not uncomon for too much masking to be presented to the non-test ear. This masking then crosses back over the skull and interferes with the test ear results.

Audiograms

An audiogram basically consists of a graph with *frequency* indicated along the top or horizontal axis (abscissa) and *intensity* along the side or vertical axis (ordinate) (Fig 20–14).

Frequency.—The frequency scale across the top of an audiogram is expressed in either cycles per second (cps) or the newer, preferred term, Hertz (Hz). The frequencies used in a hearing test vary with the requirements of the hearing conservation program and federal and state laws. For many hearing conservation programs, the thresholds at 500, 1,000, 2,000, 3,000, 4,000, and 6,000 Hz must be measured. Some medical departments also call for tests at 250 and 8,000 Hz.

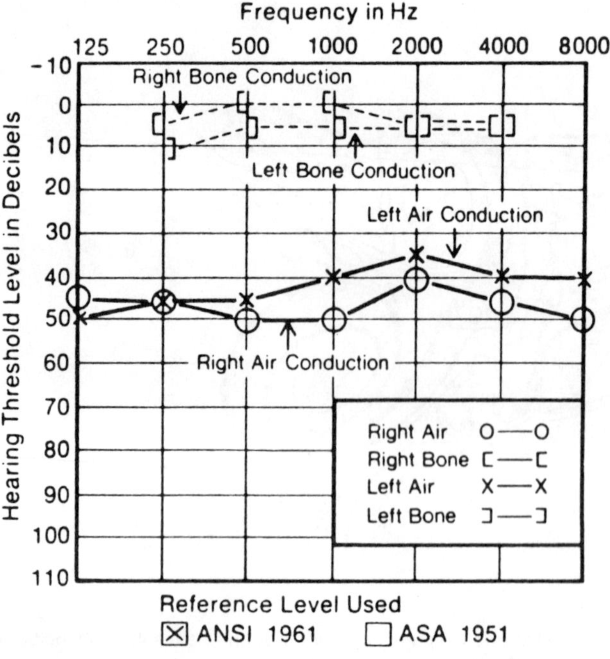

FIG 20–14.
A typical manual audiogram, indicating a conductive hearing loss.

For purposes of determining a compensable hearing loss, it is important to measure hearing at 8,000 Hz. This particular frequency is not usually included in the formulas for hearing loss due to noise exposure, yet it is a critical frequency for providing information concerning the possible relationship between the hearing loss and occupational noise exposure. The normal pattern seen in hearing loss due to noise exposure shows a rather precipitous reduction in sensitivity above 1,000 or 2,000 Hz, with stabilization or recovery between 4,000 and 8,000 Hz. Without an 8,000-Hz measurement, it is frequently impossible to distinguish high-frequency hearing loss resulting from a variety of other causes (including presbycusis) from hearing loss due to noise exposure.

Intensity.—The numbers on the left side of the audiogram indicate the intensity or loudness of the sound, which is measured in decibels. The smaller the number, the fainter the sound.

When a subject's hearing is measured, the threshold of hearing at each test frequency is established at the intensity level at which the sound can just barely be heard. The further a subject's threshold is below the zero line of the audiogram, the greater the loss of hearing. Generally, the pure-tone thresholds determined by air conduction for the right ear are recorded on the audiogram as circles, and those for the left ear are recorded as Xs (see Fig 20–14).

Accuracy of Audiograms.—Audiograms may not accurately reflect the true degree of permanent hearing loss. Several sources of variance may confound the estimate, including the testing environment, the skill of the person administering the test, the degree of temporary hearing loss resulting from a recent exposure to nonoccupational noise, and (since financial award is involved) attempts by the claimant to exaggerate the true loss.

Manual vs. Automatic Audiometers

Audiometers may be operated either manually or automatically. Using a standard manual audiometer, the examiner controls the presentation of tones and records the subject's responses. If an automatic audiometer is used, the intensity of the signal tone increases automatically. It is the subject who presses a button when he or she first hears the signal. This causes the sound to diminish. The subject releases the button when he or she no longer hears the sound. The results are recorded automatically on the audiogram form by a stylus that reverses as the subject presses and releases the button (Fig 20—15).

To explain it in other words, an automatic audiometer is an instrument that is programmed to present a pure tone in a predetermined sequence of frequencies, testing first one ear and then the other, and at the same time recording the subject's response on a chart. The subject alone controls the test with help of a handswitch, and the subject's hearing level is plotted continuously at each frequency. As long as the subject hears the tone, he or she holds the handswitch pressed and the intensity is decreased. When the subject no longer hears the tone, he or she releases the handswitch and the intensity increases again. This explains why an automatic audiogram curve is saw-toothed.

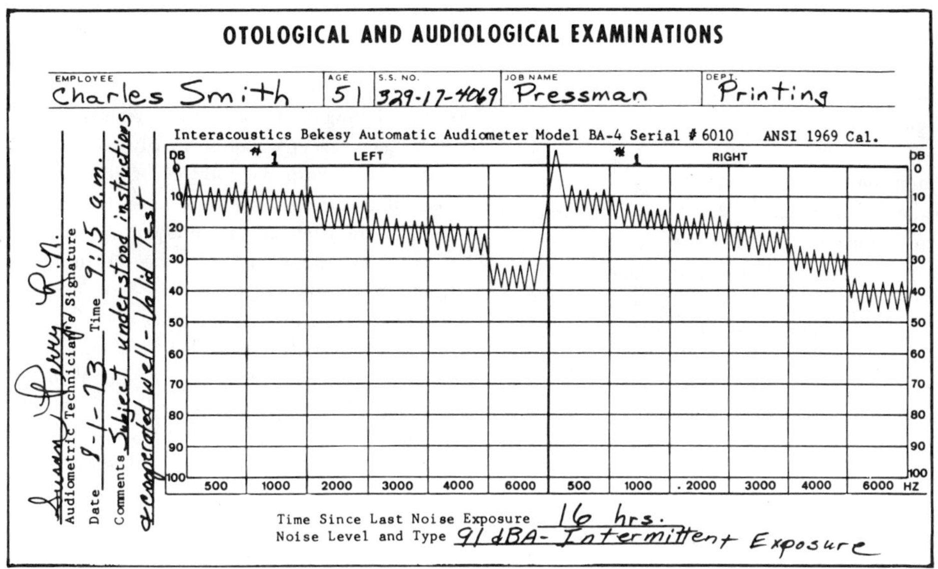

OTOLOGICAL AND AUDIOLOGICAL EXAMINATIONS

EMPLOYEE	AGE	S.S. NO.	JOB NAME	DEPT.
Charles Smith	51	329-17-4069	Pressman	Printing

Interacoustics Bekesy Automatic Audiometer Model BA-4 Serial # 6010 ANSI 1969 Cal.

Audiometric Technician's Signature Susan Perry R.N.

Date 8-1-73 Time 9:15 a.m.

Comments Subject understood instructions & cooperated well - Valid Test

Time Since Last Noise Exposure 16 hrs.

Noise Level and Type 91 dBA- Intermittent Exposure

FIG 20–15.

An automatic audiometer can be used to provide a graphic representation of a subject's hearing threshold. A pen is moved along the audiogram's horizontal axis (as a function of time) for each frequency.

Psychologic factors can have considerable influence on the subject being tested. Individuals might be less likely to feign a hearing loss for workers' compensation purposes if they feel their responses are being closely watched.

If both manual and automatic audiometers are routinely used in an industrial hearing-conservation program, it is recommended that, whenever possible, retests or follow-up tests be administered on the same type of audiometer that was used to obtain the baseline audiogram for that particular employee. This procedure avoids the basic problem of interpretation of threshold differences as a function of audiometer type (manual vs. automatic).

Speech Audiometry

Ability to hear speech is the preferred standard for rating hearing loss for compensation purposes. It has, however, been impossible to standardize speech test materials because of language difficulties and the differences in intelligence and educational levels of the persons whose hearing is being tested. Because of these variables, pure-tone threshold audiometry is recognized as the most reliable method available for establishing a quantitative measure of hearing acuity. Speech audiometry, which provides essential diagnostic information concerning the type and cause of hearing loss, is used to supplement pure-tone audiometry. Two commonly used speech tests are the speech reception test and the speech discrimination test.

Speech Reception Test

Equipment designed to control the volume of spoken words or sentences presented through earphones or loudspeakers is used to administer the speech reception test, which measures the subject's hearing threshold for speech. In determining the threshold, standardized lists of words (known as *spondee* words) are used; these words consist of two equally accented syllables, for example, baseball, birthday, or headlight. As in pure-tone audiometry, these words are presented at varying intensities until the lowest level at which the subject can repeat approximately 50% of the words is determined. This level is the subject's speech reception threshold (SRT).

The speech reception threshold is extremely valuable in validating pure-tone threshold results. There should be close agreement between the speech reception threshold obtained for a given ear and thresholds for pure-tones at 500, 1,000, and 2,000 Hz for the same ear. One of the most sensitive indicators of functional hearing loss is a discrepancy between the speech reception threshold and the pure-tone average.

The pure-tone average is calculated by averaging the pure-tone intensities recorded at 500, 1,000, and 2,000 Hz. If there is steep high-frequency hearing loss, only the intensities at 500 and 1,000 Hz may be averaged. If the speech reception threshold is 15 or more decibels better than the pure-tone average, there is strong evidence to suggest a functional hearing loss. On the other hand, a speech reception threshold that is significantly poorer than the pure-tone average may suggest hearing loss due to retrocochlear pathology.

Speech Discrimination Test

The speech discrimination test is administered after the subject's hearing threshold for speech has been established and is found to be about 35–55 decibels above the speech reception threshold. Here the standardized word lists consist of one-syllable words designed to test the subject's ability to discriminate among consonants. These phonetically balanced (PB) words include such words as deaf, fold, patch, and mop. The complete list is administered and the percentage of the words that the subject understands constitutes the speech discrimination score.

Special Diagnostic Procedures

Other diagnostic procedures are also used to assess hearing losses. These procedures include impedance measurement, tests for recruitment, and tuning fork tests.

Impedance Measurement

Recently, impedance measurement has become an integral part of some hearing examinations. A useful tool in supporting the presence or absence of conductive pathology, impedance measurement generally consists of two procedures: tympanometry, and acoustic reflex and reflex decay measurement.

Tympanometry.—This is used to assess the function of the conductive auditory mechanism. Tympanometry is a sensitive technique that does not require subject response. A probe tip is placed in the subject's ear. The probe tip is connected by rubber tubes to a manometer, which changes the air pressure within the external auditory canal, a probe tone generator, generally 220 Hz, and a condenser microphone, which measures the sound pressure level within the external canal. Simultaneously, the air pressure is changed and the compliance of the tympanic membrane, or eardrum, is recorded.

Maximum movement of the tympanic membrane in a normal conductive mechanism will occur when atmospheric pressure is created within the external auditory canal. If there is fluid or an adhesion within the middle ear cavity, the tympanic membrane will be stiff, and that stiffness will be reflected on the tympanometer. A perforated tympanic membrane or disruption or stiffening of the ossicular chain, as well as other middle ear pathologies, can be detected using this technique.

Acoustic Reflex.—The acoustic reflex is also used to detect conductive pathology. When a certain amount of sound pressure is generated within the inner ear, the muscle controlling the stapes contracts bilaterally. The sound intensity required to cause this contraction in the normal ear is generally from 70 to 100 dB above the threshold. The acoustic stimuli can be presented either contralaterally or ipsilaterally to the probe tip. The absence of an acoustic reflex, measured with the probe tip with the acoustic stimulus in the contralateral ear, is consistent with conductive pathology. The presence of an acoustic reflex is inconsistent with conductive pathology.

The acoustic reflex has been used in a battery of tests for functional hearing loss (see Tests for Functional Hearing Loss) and is particularly useful if a profound hearing loss is indicated. In a true organic profound hearing loss, no reflex would be anticipated. If a profound loss is indicated, yet an acoustic reflex is obtained at a level equal to, or softer than, the level the subject is admitting to hearing, it is almost certain that the subject is attempting to feign a profound hearing loss. The reflex decay test is often used in cases of suspected eighth-nerve tumors.

Tests for Recruitment

Recruitment of loudness, a condition that occurs in some partially deaf ears, is an increase in the subject's sensation of loudness that is out of proportion to the increase in the actual intensity of the sound. In other words, sound may be heard faintly or not at all by the subject at or near his or her threshold, while at some higher intensity level, the sensation of loudness may suddenly become much greater than that heard by a normal ear. Theories still being investigated suggest that a "recruiting ear" indicates pathology in the organ of Corti, which results in a sensory hearing loss, while recruitment is not ordinarily present when there is a lesion restricted to the nerve pathway, which results in a neural hearing loss. Because most cases of noise-induced hearing loss are believed to be centered in the organ of Corti, one possible outcome of these investigations might be the development of a test that would differentiate between noise-induced hearing loss and neural impairment due to other causes.

It is generally agreed that the loudness balance test (alternate binaural loudness balance vs. monaural loudness balance) is the only direct test of recruitment. Other tests whose findings are associated with recruitment are the short-increment sensitivity index (SISI), the reduced threshold of discomfort for pure tones and/or speech, and the reduced acoustic reflex.

Tuning Fork Tests

Tuning fork tests are not used in rating hearing impairments because they are qualitative rather than quantitative measurements. From a diagnostic standpoint, however, these tests do provide the physician with valuable preliminary information concerning whether the hearing loss is conductive or sensorineural in nature and whether one or both ears is/are involved. Generally, the otologist will make these tests to confirm audiometric test results.

Three tests are routinely employed: (1) the Rinne test compares the subject's ability to hear the tuning fork by airborne sound with his or her ability to hear it by bone conduction; (2) the Weber test determines which ear, if either, hears the tuning fork better by bone conduction, and (3) the Schwabach test compares the subject's ability to hear the fork by bone conduction with the ability of a listener with normal hearing to hear it in the same position. Usually, the otologist makes the comparison to his or her own hearing.

Tests for Functional Hearing Loss

Functional hearing loss implies an inter- or intra-test discrepancy. It is an umbrella term that includes malingering and psychogenic losses. In hearing health terms, *malingering* is defined as "a willful feigning of hearing loss." A *psychogenic loss* is an unconscious presentation of elevated hearing threshold. Unfortunately, there is no precise way to determine whether the person is malingering or presenting a psychogenic loss. Malingering is by far the more prevalent form of functional hearing loss.

Certain inconsistencies in response during the routine tests may suggest the possibility of malingering or psychogenic loss to the examiner. Probably the most sensitive indicator of functional hearing loss is a pure-tone/speech reception threshold discrepancy. If the speech reception threshold is 15 or more decibels better than the pure-tone average, there is strong indication of functional hearing loss. In cases of unilateral functional hearing loss, the pure-tone or speech Stenger test is often very helpful. Research has indicated that galvanic skin response audiometry and the Doerfler-Stewart test have limited reliability or validity when diagnosing functional hearing loss.

Because a particular pattern emerges, Bekesy audiometry is

often used in cases of suspected functional hearing loss. A modified version of the Bekesy technique that has also been used involves using an ascending, soft-to-loud, continuous tone and a descending, loud-to-soft interrupted tone (2.5 pulses per second). If the difference between the thresholds obtained for the two signals is 15 dB or greater (that is, the threshold for the continuous tone is 15 dB or more less than the threshold obtained for the interrupted tone), there is strong evidence of a functional hearing loss.

In a functional hearing loss, there are also other responses on the part of the subject which are apparent to the experienced examiner. These may include facial grimaces, absence of false positive responses, and one-half word responses to spondee word presentations.

HOW HEARING MAY BE IMPAIRED

Partial or total deafness may affect either or both ears. Hearing loss (Fig 20–16) may result from infection, obstruction, trauma, prolonged noise exposure, toxic agents, allergies, and many diseases.

Determining the cause of hearing loss involves a careful evaluation of the medical history, the occupational history, noise exposures, the medical examination, and the audiogram. The audiogram measures the loss of hearing but does not evaluate the cause. Because loss of hearing is only a symptom of damage in the hearing mechanism, multiple causes may exist. The differentiation of that part of the hearing loss due to noise exposure from that due to other causes sometimes is difficult and requires otologic consultation.

The following is an outline of the major causes of hearing loss and is not intended to be exhaustive or complete.

Infections of the Ear

Infections of the *external ear* (otitis externa) may cause swelling in the external auditory canal and result in obstruction and hearing loss.

Chronic infections of the *middle ear* (otitis media) may cause mild to severe conduction hearing loss. Acute infections may heal completely. The cause of the infection generally is secondary to infection elsewhere, usually in the respiratory tract.

Obstruction or Injury by Physical Agents

Impacted cerumen (wax) in the external canal is a frequent cause of hearing loss due to plugging of the canal.

Foreign bodies in the ear canal or, rarely, in the middle ear (insects, chewing gum, or other foreign materials), if not removed, may cause infection, with damage to the entire ear.

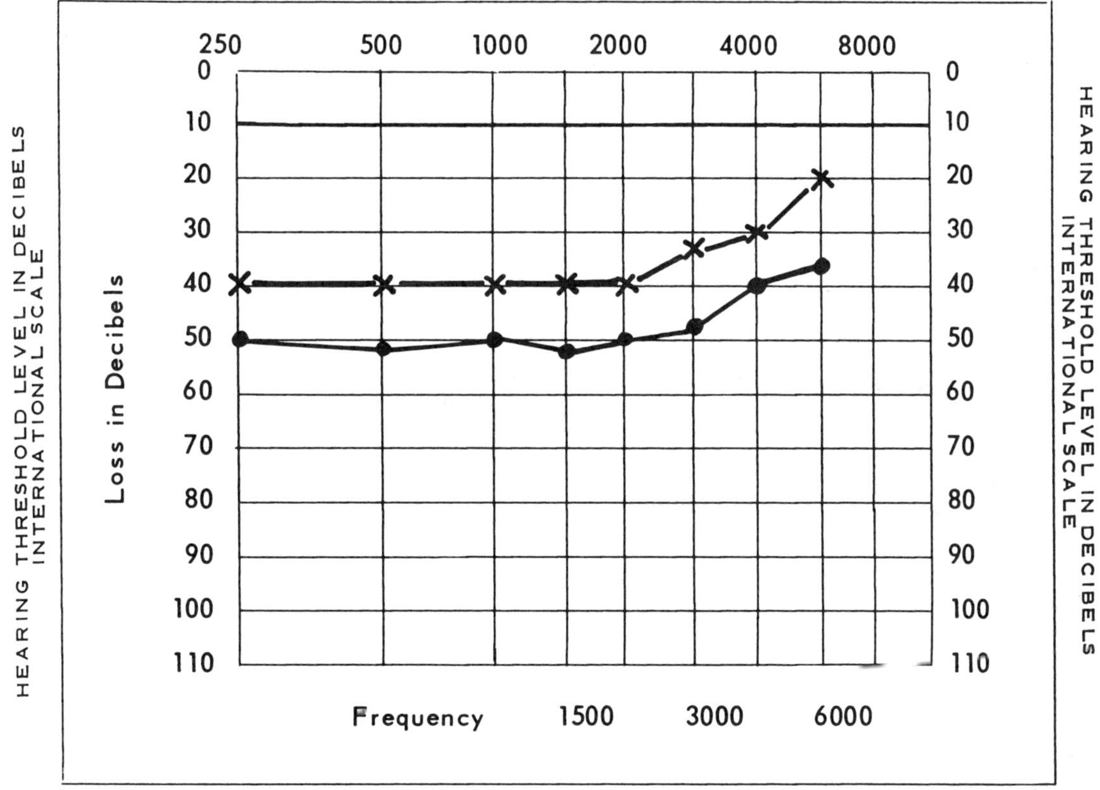

Fig 20–16.
Middle ear deafness occurs when there is wax accumulation in the ear canal or when some other part of the conductive mechanism breaks down. Eardrum damage, blockage of the eustachian tube, or bony growths prevent proper movement of the ossicles. In most cases, this type of deafness is correctable and we identify it as conductive deafness.

Trauma to the ear may cause serious hearing losses by rupture and/or dislocation of the drumhead and ossicles. The inner ear may be damaged by dislocation of the stapes or fracture of the temporal bone containing the cochlea. A sudden, intense pressure wave, such as produced by a blast, may cause hearing loss that may be partial or total, temporary or permanent.

Prolonged noise exposure may cause hearing loss. The intensity, vibration, frequency, duration of exposure to noise, as well as the age of the subject must be considered before causal relationship to hearing loss can be estimated.

Barotrauma (aerotitis) is middle ear damage due to rapid changes in altitude. This occurs most frequently in persons taking an airplane trip while they have a cold or sinusitis. The greatest difficulty arises during descent, when air cannot enter the eustachian tube from the throat to equalize the middle ear pressure.

Excessive lymphoid tissue (adenoids) in the nasopharynx must be considered an important cause of hearing loss in children.

Toxic Agents and Allergies

Quinine and its derivatives, tobacco (nicotine) and aspirin (salicylates), are possible causes of hearing loss in hypersusceptible patients. Discontinuation of the drug with the onset of ringing in the ears (tinnitus) or auditory nerve irritation reverses the process; continued use of the drug may cause permanent and irreversible hearing loss.

Widely used antibiotics may cause inner-ear hearing loss (nerve deafness) or labyrinthine disturbance (difficulty with balance). Some of these antimicrobial drugs are streptomycin, dihydrostreptomycin, neomycin, kanamycin (Kantrex), paromomycin (Humatin), rifampin (Rifadin, Rimactane), vancomycin (Vancocin) and viomycin (Vinactane, Viocin).

Numerous other drugs or materials may cause labyrinthitis or nerve deafness in individuals sensitive to these substances, or impaired hearing may result from the effects of allergy on the upper respiratory passages.

Diseases

Meningitis can cause hearing loss through involving any part of the hearing mechanism within the skull.

Tumors, hemorrhage, vascular disease or spasm, and certain neurologic diseases may involve the central auditory area, the auditory nuclei or the eighth nerve, with the production of hearing loss.

Many infectious diseases (mumps, measles, scarlet fever, diphtheria, respiratory infections) have been responsible for hearing loss in children. The effects may be due to direct infection in the middle and/or inner ear or as a secondary infection in the middle ear.

FACTORS IN HEARING LOSS CLAIM EVALUATION

Many complex acoustic, medical, and legal factors must be considered when determining the causal relationship between noise exposure and the resulting hearing loss. Those who investigate and adjust occupational hearing loss claims must understand the medical, acoustic, loss prevention, and legal aspects of the problem. Although it is difficult to predict the outcome of a hearing loss claim based upon a given set of circumstances, any conclusions must be drawn on the basis of knowlege of the applicable laws, regulations, and legal precedents of the jurisdiction involved.

The procedures and factors described here are intended to guide the development of methods for adjudicating claims of hearing loss that is allegedly due to a claimant's work environment. The decision of the person responsible for determining the causal relationship of occupational hearing loss must be based on an evaluation of the available information. When appropriate evidence is presented in a logical and orderly sequence, when major issues are identified, and when the basis for any presumption of cause is defined, then the decision-making process is facilitated, and as equitable a decision as possible is likely to result.

Unfortunately, information on a worker's past noise exposures is often unavailable, inadequate, or incomplete. All individuals are not alike and do not react in the same way to similar exposures to noise. Off-the-job exposures may contribute to or be a primary cause of hearing loss. These are but some of the factors that must be considered in the decision-making process.

Evidence of Hearing Loss

The first consideration in determining the probability of a cause-effect relationship between an occupational hearing loss and excessive noise at the workplace is to establish: (1) that a hearing loss does, in fact, exist; and (2) that the particular manifestations of the hearing loss appear to be the result of exposure to excessive noise at the workplace.

Occupational hearing loss can be defined as the loss of hearing in one or both ears as the result of one's employment. This last phrase is very important; the loss of hearing *must* be "as the result of one's employment." The loss may be the result of hazardous noise exposure or due to acoustic trauma.

Early Signs

Early signs of hearing loss include:

1. Difficulty in understanding spoken words in a noisy environment
2. Need to be near or look at the person speaking to help understand words
3. Familiar sounds are muffled
4. Complaints that people do not speak clearly
5. Ringing noises in the ears

Audiometric examination procedures

The degree of hearing loss can be determined by an audiometric examination, which tests the person's ability to hear pure tones at defined frequencies.

Audiometry is, in part, a subjective test—individuals vary in response during different tests made at different times. The resulting audiograms, as a result, may not accurately reflect the true degree of permanent hearing loss. Several sources of variance may confound this estimate: testing environment, the skill of the person administering the test, the degree of temporary hearing loss resulting from a recent exposure to either occupational or nonoccupational noise, and (since financial awards are involved) attempts by the claimant to exaggerate the true loss.

The audiometric examination should be administered only by skilled technicians who have received training in audiometry. In addition, a physician or audiologist should provide supervision to the audiometric testing program and set policies and procedures for its administration. For example, the program supervisor should spell out the criteria for referral, and specify how and when individuals should be informed of audiometric results and recommendations should be made concerning protection and/or placement of applicants or employees. Professional supervision of the audiometric testing program will support the acceptance of audiograms as evidence in legal proceedings.

It is important that the test be made in a room where the background noise is below certain specified limits. Excessive noise in the test room tends to mask the sound delivered by the audiometer to the earphones, thus producing a test record of some degree of hearing loss which does not actually exist. Ordinarily, room background noises are low in frequency; their masking effect is pronounced at frequencies below 1,000 Hz.

As assurance of reliable testing and consistency between tests, it is important that the audiometer be of a design that meets the specifications for audiometers approved and published by American National Standards Institute (ANSI 3.6–1969, R1973). It is also important that the calibration of the audiometer be checked frequently, because errors do occur through usage or abuse. Biologic monitoring should be done prior to using the audiometer.

Temporary Threshold Shift.—Hearing tests in compensation cases should be made after full recovery from any temporary threshold shift. Opinions differ among experts concerning the maximum period of recovery or stabilization of hearing after noise exposure in any given individual. Statements have been made that the *average* recovery time is about 16 hours—this is only an average figure and would not necessarily apply to any given individual. Also, this statement applies to relatively minor hearing losses; the higher the hearing loss, the longer the recovery time. Some authorities think that 48 hours' separation from noise is adequate for recovery; others estimate that the necessary recovery time to be spent away from the noise ranges from one to six months.

Accurate evaluation of permanent hearing loss may be difficult to establish if the claimant is working in a noisy environment at the time the audiometric tests are to be made. The physician must make sure that the worker has been away from noise for a sufficient period of time to eliminate any temporary threshold shift.

Base-line and Periodic Audiograms.—Base-line and periodic audiometric examinations made by the employer previously should be obtained and compared with present audiometric test results. The sensorineural hearing loss that results from noise exposure is similar to hearing loss caused by other less apparent factors. Without a base-line or preemployment audiogram, it is difficult to state what part of the employee's hearing loss was caused by the conditions at his or her present place of employment and what part of the hearing ability was already lost before he or she was hired.

A similar problem presents itself when the employee has worked for several companies and each one might have contributed to the total hearing loss—which employer should be held responsible for the hearing loss? Several states have enacted statutes that hold that the last employer is responsible for the entire hearing loss, unless there is competent audiometric evidence documenting the employee's baseline hearing level at the beginning of his or her employment.

If the hearing tests disclose a sensorineural loss, a carefully developed history of the loss is an important tool in objectively evaluating the cause. Once this type of loss has been diagnosed, there is no specific test that can either confirm or eliminate noise as the sole cause. In many cases, however, much can be learned by a careful examination of the subject's history and by the use of a battery of diagnostic tests. In some cases, it may be found that the hearing loss existed prior to the worker's employment but was not realized until disclosed by audiometric tests. In other cases, it may be disclosed that the worker's hearing was impaired by nonoccupational causes, such as otologic and infectious diseases, other noise exposure, or toxic drugs. A history of military service with exposure to gunfire or jet engine noise, for example, indicates that some hearing loss is to be expected regardless of industrial noise exposure. Having to pay compensation awards has alerted industry to the need for preplacement hearing tests to establish baseline audiograms.

Other Tests of Auditory Dysfunction.—There are many diagnostic procedures that may be used to assess auditory dysfunction. These include tests of the central auditory function—that is, the ability to process signals at the brain stem and cortical levels, brain stem-evoked response testing, and tone-decay measurements, to name a few.

Pure-tone threshold measurement is the procedure most critical to determining percent hearing loss. However, other measures, particularly speech audiometry and impedance measurement, are extremely important in arriving at a diagnosis which may or may not be consistent with hearing loss due to noise exposure.

Detailed descriptions of the tests that have been mentioned can be found in many textbooks on otology.

Differential Diagnosis

Noise-induced hearing loss is used to describe the cumulative loss of hearing, always of the sensorineural type, that develops over months or years of hazardous noise exposure. Noise-induced hearing loss usually affects both ears about equally in extent. In order to establish a diagnosis of noise-induced hearing loss and a causal relationship to employment, the physician must consider and report on a number of points of information.

Physician's Examination and Report

The cornerstone of the individual workers' compensation case is the physician's examination and report. A settlement that is fair to both the employee and the employer depends almost entirely on the adequacy and completeness of this report. In order to establish a diagnosis of noise-induced hearing loss and causal relationship to employment, the physician must consider the following factors (adapted from Glorig and House[16]).

Identification.—The report should include identification of the person whose hearing level is being evaluated and the date and place of the examination.

Chief Complaint.—The chief complaint of the patient, including the length of time the hearing impairment has been present, should be noted in the report.

Present Hearing Impairment.—The hearing impairment is described in the patient's own words. The physician records the patient's description of his or her hearing impairment as accurately and as simply as possible.

Occupational History.—The overall occupational history should include an accurate account of all jobs held by the patient, but it is best to question the patient first about the incident that the patient thinks caused the hearing impairment. Each account of noise exposure should include information about (1) overall noise level; (2) frequency composition of the noise; (3) time distribution of the noise during a typical workday; and (4) total duration of the noise exposure to date. In addition to a record of the total number of months in each job, the occupational history must include an estimate of the distribution of exposure during a typical workday.

Military History.—During military service, most persons are exposed to gunfire. Hearing loss at 4,000 Hz is found commonly in men who have had moderate to severe exposure to gunfire. Not infrequently, military noise exposures are severe enough to cause moderately severe hearing loss (Fig 20–17).

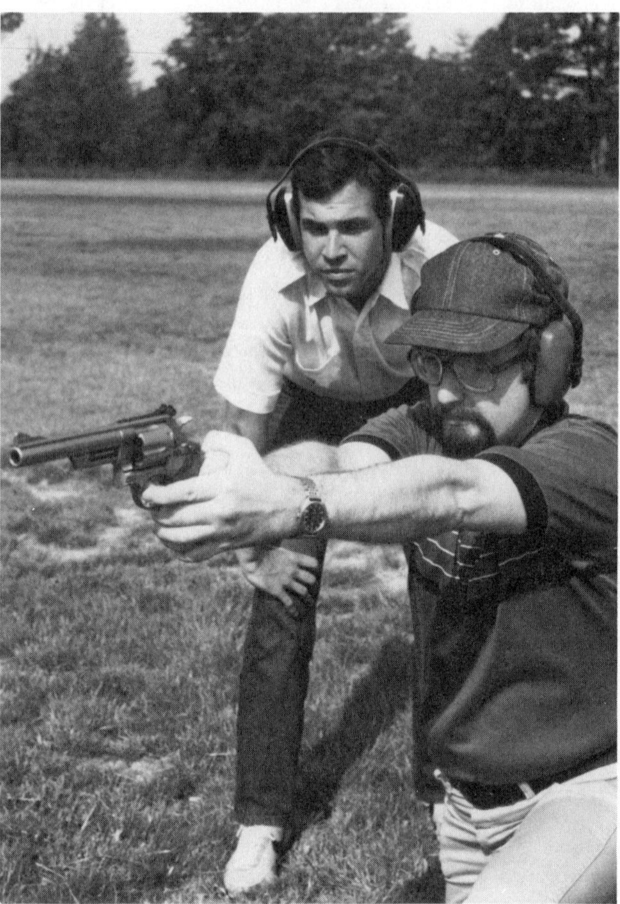

FIG 20–17.
Hearing protection is required when using guns for sport (and for police work).

Medical History.—There are many causes of hearing loss other than noise exposure. All possible reasons for the hearing loss must be thoroughly explored before causal relations are specified. When there is no preplacement audiogram, the physician must question the patient carefully about past illnesses and injuries. Childhood diseases, blows to the head or ears, and use of drugs such as quinine, streptomycin, and neomycin are all possible causes of hearing loss, and they must be considered and disposed of in every case before noise exposure alone can be blamed.

Family History.—The patient should always be asked if there is a history of hearing loss in his family. A negative answer is not significant, but a strong family history of hearing loss may be quite significant.

Physical Examination.—A careful, routine ear, nose, and throat examination should be made. Foci of infection may produce a generalized toxic condition which in turn may cause a hearing loss.

Audiometric Tests.—Hearing testing is a most critical part of the examination. Proper hearing tests imply use of adequate sound-treated hearing test rooms, carefully calibrated audiometric equipment, and trained technicians. Bone-conduction pure-tone tests, air-conduction pure-tone tests, speech reception thresholds, and speech discrimination tests may all be required (Fig 20–18).

Previous Medical Examinations.—Each patient should be questioned about previous examinations and particularly about previous hearing tests. Some patients may have had hearing tests at school or in the military services.

Importance of the History

A careful evaluation of the worker's medical, occupational, and family history is probably the most important step in the diagnostic procedure. The portion of claimant's medical history that pertains specifically to diseases and conditions of the ear and auditory nerve must be evaluated.

The following factors regarding past and present occupations should be evaluated:

1. Job titles
2. Type of work performed (complete listing, with actual dates)

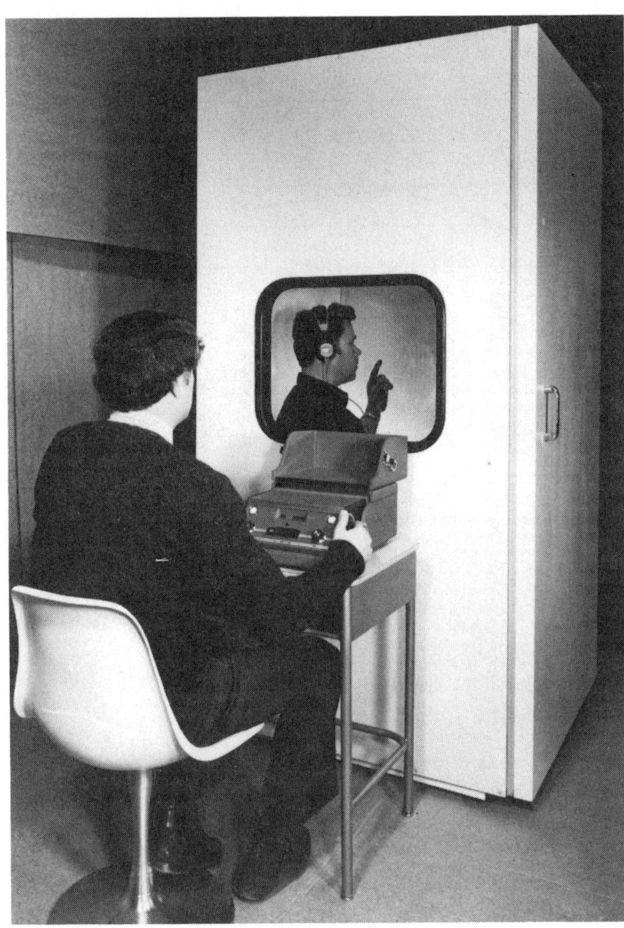

FIG 20–18.
A widely used audio booth. (Courtesy Eckel Co.)

3. Duration of each type of activity
4. Dates of employment and worker's age for each job activity
5. Geographic and physical location of employment
6. Product or service produced
7. Condition of personal protective equipment used (if any) and frequency and duration of periods of use
8. Nature of noise to which worker is or has been exposed, if known (include frequency and average duration of each noise-exposure situation)

Exposure to noise may also occur from a hobby or from off-the job activities. The following are examples:

1. Woodworking
2. Metal working
3. Loud music in any form from any source (Fig 20–19)
4. Auto repair
5. Operating tractors, lawn mowers, chain saws, and other loud equipment
6. Traffic
7. Pistol, rifle, or shotgun firing
8. Auto racing
9. Operating motorcycles, snowmobiles, or boats

Diagnostic Signals

Before reaching conclusions concerning the relation between the subject's hearing loss and noise exposure, the physician should make a complete ear, nose, and throat examination as well as administering the hearing tests.

A thorough clinical examination of the ear may include the following:

1. External ear examination for scars or malfunctions
2. Otoscopic examinations of eardrum (tympanic membrane) for any abnormalities
3. Examination of nose, throat, and nasopharynx for any abnormalities
4. Eye reflexes
5. Observation of nystagmus
6. Pure-tone air conduction audiometric examination
7. Pure-tone bone conduction studies
8. Speech reception testing for threshold and discrimination
9. Recruitment and tone-decay studies

The results of some specific tests may not be conclusive. In the final analysis, diagnosis is a matter of medical diagnostic acumen that is based upon all the known factors.

Employees who have sudden hearing loss may present problems to the consulting physician. A sudden hearing loss may occur as a result of acoustic trauma. However, sudden hearing loss does not result from exposure to typical occupational noise levels. Sudden hearing loss frequently occurs in the general population as the result of viral infection or vascular occlusion and from ruptured labyrinthine windows, leading to the escape of perilymph.

There are a number of indicators that will suggest the need for careful consideration of causes other than noise. Some of these are listed below and are based upon commonly expressed viewpoints by experts in this field.

1. A conductive loss is not caused by continuous exposure to noise. It may be occupational in origin, but in such cases it would be the result of a traumatic injury to the external ear, the eardrum, or the middle ear.

2. A mixed conductive and sensorineural loss indicates that exposure to noise is not the only cause.

3. Inconsistent responses during different tests suggest the possibility of malingering or functional loss.

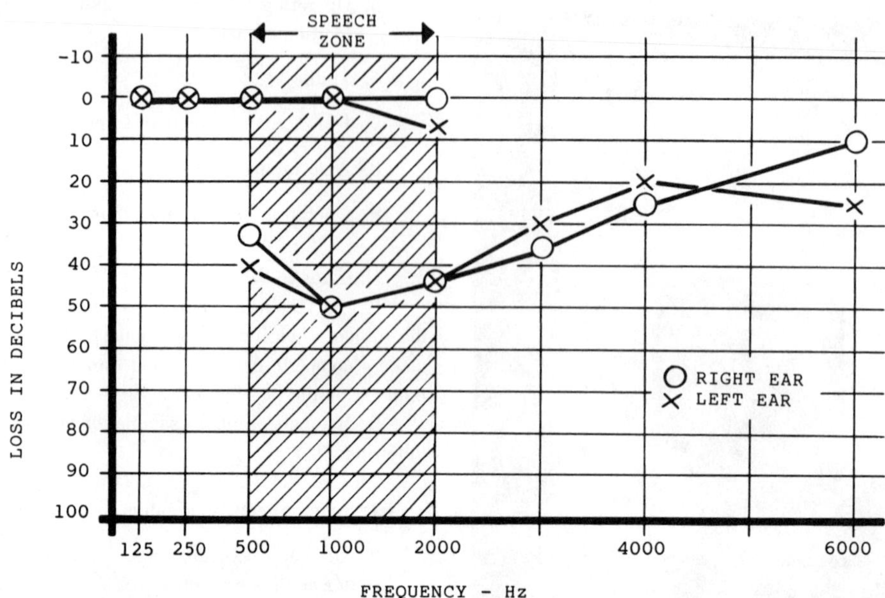

FIG 20–19.
A preemployment audiogram from a 20-year-old man with no history of any occupational exposures. His main hobby was "listening to music (nonclassical) with my stereo phones since I was 13."

4. If the speech reception threshold is 15 dB or more than the average of the pure-tone levels at 500, 1,000, and 2,000 Hz, a psychogenic loss or malingering should be suspected.

5. A pronounced loss in one ear, with the hearing in the other essentially normal, indicates ordinarily that the hearing loss is not due to noise exposure.

6. A record of exposure to gunfire or airplane engine noise in military service will indicate that significant losses, particularly at about 4,000 Hz, are to be expected regardless of industrial exposure.

7. Some hearing loss is to be expected among persons of advanced age, due to presbycusis and the common noise exposures affecting the entire population.

Assessing the Degree of Impairment

Impairment and Disability

The terms *hearing impairment* and *hearing disability* have been employed, often with the intention of conveying substantially the same meaning. However, some confusion has existed because of connotations attached to each of the terms. The definitions that follow are restated to coincide with those approved by the American Academy of Ophthalmology and Otolaryngology (AAOO) in 1979.

Permanent Impairment.—A change for the worse in either structure or function, outside the range of normal, is permanent impairment. The term is used here in a medical rather than a legal sense. Permanent impairment is due to any anatomical or functional abnormality that produces hearing loss. This loss should be evaluated after maximum rehabilitation has been achieved and when the impairment is nonprogressive at the time of evaluation. The determination of impairment is basic to the evaluation of permanent disability.

Evaluation of permanent impairment is an appraisal of the nature and extent of a person's illness or injury as it affects structure or function, and it lies within the scope of medical responsibility preparatory to the assessment of permanent disability. A permanent impairment is a contributing factor to, but not necessarily an indication of, the extent of a person's permanent disability under workers' compensation laws. *Impairment* need not imply an appreciable handicap and may be used in a more general sense to denote any deviation from normal.

Permanent Disability.—An actual or presumed inability to remain employed at full wages is a permanent disability. A person is permanently disabled or under permanent disability when the actual or presumed ability to engage in gainful activity is reduced because of impairment and when no appreciable improvement can be expected.

Evaluation of permanent disabilty is an administrative responsibility based, in part, on medical information. It is an appraisal of a person's present and probably future ability to engage in gainful activity as it is affected not only by the medical factor but also by other factors such as age, sex, education, and economic and social environment. Since many nonmedical factors have proven difficult to measure, permanent impairment often becomes the principal criterion of permanent disability.

Determination of disability is an administrative decision as to the worker's entitlement to compensation that should be based on a complete medical evaluation and an accurate assessment of function using standards that are uniform nationwide and that apply regardless of the manner in which the impairment was acquired.

It should be pointed out that the evaluation or rating of

permanent hearing impairment is a function of the physician alone. However, the evaluation or rating of permanent disability is an administrative and not a medical responsibility or function.

AMA Guides

A basis for rational evaluation of injury or disease is provided by the American Medical Association's *AMA Guides to the Evaluation of Permanent Impairment*. When first introduced in 1947, these guides provided the first generally accepted formulas for determining the percentage of hearing impairment. They provided a definitive method that could be easily applied and understood by judge, examiner, or jury and that makes provision for the establishment of the degree of hearing impairment in one or both ears.

Hearing Loss Formula

A formula for hearing loss compensation awards needs to be based on a reasonable cost of such a program to society. Damage-risk criteria involve psychophysical, political, and socioeconomic considerations. Generally, these decisions are compromises between providing total protection, at exorbitant cost, and providing a reasonable amount of protection to a given segment of the population at costs that can be absorbed by the government, industry, and ultimately by the taxpaying consumer.

Hearing impairment can be described by three parameters.

1. The first parameter is the selection of the hearing test frequencies that will be used to determine the severity of hearing impairment.

2. The second parameter is the "low fence," which can be defined as the minimum hearing threshold shift which has to be exceeded for legal hearing impairment to exist.

3. The third parameter is a scale for measuring the severity of hearing impairment based on a "multiplier" of decibels of hearing threshold shift above the "low fence."

The "multiplier" is used to convert decibels to dollars and determines the amount of the award payable as workers' compensation. Therefore, the selection of these parameters is of great importance to everyone concerned with hearing conservation, noise exposure, and workers' compensation (Table 20–3).

Procedure.—The following procedure is used to convert hearing threshold levels into percentages of hearing impairment, according to the 1979 AAOO formula:[19]

1. The average of the hearing threshold levels at 500, 1,000, 2,000, and 3,000 Hz is calculated for each ear.

2. The percent impairment for each ear is calculated by multiplying by 1.5% the amount by which the aforementioned average hearing threshold level exceeds 25 dB (low fence). A maximum of 100% is reached at 92 dB (high fence).

3. The binaural impairment assessment should then be calculated by multiplying the smaller percentage (better ear) by 5, adding this figure to the larger percentage (poorer ear), and dividing the total by 6.

Sample Hearing Loss Calculations.—Following are examples of the calculation of hearing loss:

A. Mild to marked bilateral hearing loss

	500 Hz	1,000 Hz	2,000 Hz	3,000 Hz
Right ear	15	25	45	55
Left ear	30	45	60	85

TABLE 20–3.
Hearing Loss Formulas Used in Various States (Current as of August 1981)*

FORMULA	AUDIOMETRIC FREQUENCIES USED (Hz)	METHOD OF CALCULATION	LOW FENCE (ANSI-1969)	HIGH FENCE	PERCENT PER DECIBEL LOSS	BETTER EAR CORRECTION	STATES THAT USE FORMULA†
AMA-1947	500, 1,000, 2,000, 4,000	weighted average	20 dB	105 dB	varies	7/1	KS
AAOO-1959	500, 1,000, 2,000	average	25 dB	92 dB	1.5	5/1	AZ, CT, GA, HI, MD, ME, MO, MT, NE, NH, NC, RI, VA, WA, WV
AAO-1979	Same as California	average	25 dB	92dB	1.5	5/1	CA
NIOSH Recommendations	1,000, 2,000 3,000	average	25 dB	92 dB	1.5	5/1	FL, CA, NY
CHABA‡ Recommendations	1,000, 2,000, 3,000	average	35 dB	92 dB	1.75	4/1	WI
California Formula (Now 1979 AAO)	500, 1,000, 2,000, 3,000	average	25 dB	92 dB	1.5	5/1	CA, IA, TX, OR
New Jersey	1,000, 2,000, 3,000	average	30 dB	97 dB	1.5	5/1	NJ
Illinois	1,000, 2,000, 3,000	average	30 dB	85 dB	1.82		IL

*From the Alliance of American Insurers: *Technical Guide No. 9,* ed 2. Chicago, Alliance of American Insurers, 1981, p 54.
†States with no formula formally adopted leave decision to examining physician (medical evaluation), who will probably now use the 1979 AAO.
‡Committee on Hearing, Bioacoustics, and Biomechanics of the National Academy of Sciences.

1. Calculation of average hearing threshold level:
   Right ear:

$$\frac{15 + 25 + 45 + 55}{4} = \frac{140}{4} = 35 \text{ dB} = 15\% \text{ loss}$$

   Left ear:

$$\frac{30 + 45 + 60 + 85}{4} = \frac{220}{4} = 55 \text{ dB} = 45\% \text{ loss}$$

2. Calculation of hearing handicap:

   Smaller number (better ear)

   15% × 5 = 75

   Larger number (poorer ear)

   45% × 1 = 45

   Total 120 ÷ 6 = 20% loss

   Therefore, a person with the hearing threshold levels shown in this audiogram would have a 20% hearing handicap.

B. Slight bilateral hearing loss

	500 Hz	1,000 Hz	2,000 Hz	3,000 Hz
Right Ear	15	15	20	30
Left Ear	20	20	30	40

1. Average hearing threshold level:
   Right ear:

$$\frac{15 + 15 + 20 + 30}{4} = \frac{80}{4} = 20 \text{ dB} = 0\% \text{ loss}$$

Left ear:

$$\frac{20 + 20 + 30 + 40}{4} = \frac{110}{4} = 27.5 \text{ dB} = 3.75\% \text{ loss}$$

2. Hearing handicap:

   Smaller number (better ear)

   0% × 5 = 0.00

   Larger number (poorer ear)

   3.75% × 1 = 3.75%

   Total 3.75 ÷ 6 = 1% loss (rounded off)

   Therefore, the hearing handicap is 1%.

C. Severe to extreme bilateral hearing loss

	500 Hz	1,000 Hz	2,000 Hz	3,000 Hz
Right ear	80	90	100	110
Left ear	75	80	90	95

1. Average hearing threshold level (use 92 dB maximal value):
   Right ear:

$$\frac{80 + 90 + 100 + 110}{4} = \frac{380}{4} = 95 \text{ dB} = 100\% \text{ loss}$$

   Left ear:

$$\frac{75 + 80 + 90 + 95}{4} = \frac{340}{4} = 85 \text{ dB} = 90\% \text{ loss}$$

2. Hearing handicap:

   Smaller number (better ear)

   90% × 5 = 450

   Larger number (poorer ear)

   100% × 1 = 100%

   Total 550 ÷ 6 = 92% loss

   Therefore, the hearing handicap is 92%.

Other Methods of Assessing Hearing

Veterans Administration Method.—While workers' compensation rules favor AAOO formulas, the Veterans Administration is one governmental agency that incorporates speech audiometry into a compensation scheme. The Veterans Administration has rated hearing impairment for many years, either by a combination of speech reception threshold (SRT) for spondee words and speech discrimination scores for phonetically balanced words, or by pure-tone thresholds. Normal limits of hearing are defined by an SRT of less than 26 dB (ANSI), a discrimination score of higher than 92%, *and* pure-tone thresholds of better than 40 dB (ANSI) for all audiometric frequencies from 250 to 4,000 Hz and better than 25 dB (ANSI) for at least four frequencies. Hearing losses that exceed these amounts are not necessarily eligible for compensation, even though they are no longer considered normal.

Social Security.—The U.S. Social Security Administration has national responsibility for the administration of both the Social Security program (Title II) and the newer Supplemental Security Income program (Title XVI). Title II provides coverage of cash benefits for those disabled workers (and their dependents) who have contributed to the social security trust fund through the FICA (Federal Insurance Contributions Act) tax on their earnings.

Under both programs, the definitions of disability are essentially the same. The programs define disability as "inability to engage in *any* substantial gainful activity by reason of a medically determinable physical or mental impairment which can be expected to result in death or has lasted or can be expected to last for a continuous period of not less than 12 months. . . ."

Substantial gainful activity is any work of a nature generally performed for remuneration or profit, involving the performance of significant physical or mental duties, or a combination of both. Work may be considered substantial even if performed part-time, and even if it is less demanding or less responsible than the individual's former work, and it may be considered gainful even if it pays less than the former work.

A *medically determinable impairment* is one which has medically demonstrable anatomical, physiologic, or psychologic abnormalities. Such abnormalities are medically determinable if they manifest themselves as signs or laboratory findings apart from symptoms. Abnormalities that manifest themselves only as symptoms are not medically determinable.

Symptoms are the claimant's own perception of his physical or mental impairments.

Signs are anatomical, physiological, or psychologic abnormalities that can be observed through the use of medically acceptable clinical techniques. In psychiatric impairments, signs are medically demonstrable abnormalities of behavior, affect, thought, memory, orientation, and contact with reality.

Laboratory findings are manifestations of anatomical, physiologic, or psychologic phenomena demonstrable by replacing or extending the perceptiveness of the observer's senses and include chemical, electrophysiologic, roentgenologic, or psychologic tests.

Conceptual basis of disability.—The determination of whether a person is disabled under the Social Security statute requires two separate judgments. One is an assessment of a person's remaining capacity to perform physical or mental activities. The second judgment is an assessment of the physical or mental capacity demands of a group of jobs which fall within a person's vocational spectrum. When the remaining capacity to perform is less than the demands of the job, the person is disabled. Such assessments require a quantification of both capacity to perform and capacity demands.

Medical evidence.—An individual who files an application for disability insurance benefits must provide a medical report signed by a duly licensed physician. Such a report should contain the applicant's medical history relating to the impairment or impairments which prevent work. The report should contain a description of a physical examination and supporting laboratory data needed to determine the nature and severity of the impairment. The evaluation criteria are helpful in determining the type of information needed. The medical report should not be limited to those clinical findings that are listed. All symptoms, signs, and laboratory findings that have a bearing on the person's impairment should be reported. Disability decisions cannot be made on the basis of clinical judgments relating to an applicant's diagnosis, prognosis, or remaining capacity to work unless the supporting signs or laboratory findings are also reported.

Hearing impairment.—Hearing ability should be evaluated in terms of the person's ability to hear and distinguish speech.

Loss of hearing can be quantitatively determined by an audiometer that meets the standards of the American National Standards Institute (ANSI) for air- and bone-conducted stimuli (i.e., ANSI S3.6–1969 and ANSI S3.13–1972, or subsequent comparable revisions) and performing all hearing measurements in an environment that meets the ANSI standard for maximal permissible backgrounds sound (ANSI S3.1–1977).

Speech discrimination should be determined using a standardized measure of speech discrimination ability in quiet at a test presentation level sufficient to ascertain maximum discrimination ability. The speech discrimination measure (test) used and the level at which testing was done must be reported.

Hearing tests should be preceded by an otolaryngologic examination and should be performed by or under the supervision of an otolaryngologist or audiologist qualified to perform such tests.

In order to establish an independent medical judgment as to the level of severity in a claimant alleging deafness, the following examinations should be reported: otolaryngologic examination, pure-tone air and bone audiometry, speech reception threshold, and speech discrimination testing. A copy of reports of the medical examination and audiologic evaluations must be submitted.

A patient who is not working can meet the Social Security definition of disability if he or she has an impairment or impairments with specific clinical findings that are the same as or medically equivalent to any set of findings under these evaluation criteria.

If the impairment is of lesser severity, in certain cases the patient may be found disabled if—considering the patient's impairment, age, education, and previous experience—he or she is unable to engage in substantial gainful work.

Other Factors in Hearing Loss Claim Evaluation

Tinnitus

There is a high incidence of tinnitus among employees in noisy industries. It is an important early sign usually associated with sensorineural hearing loss. One may, however, have severe tinnitus with little or no hearing loss, or the worker may complain of tinnitus and not of a severe or even noticeable hearing loss.

Evaluation of tinnitus is difficult because of the absence of objective signs or any recognized scientific criteria. Most jurisdictions provide compensation for tinnitus. It is a subjective symptom that is difficult to validate and impossible to quantify.

Transfer of the employee to quiet working surroundings may be recommended to prevent progression of hearing loss and tinnitus. Most employees are unwilling to make the change, because it may involve loss of seniority and a reduction in pay. Industry, as a rule, does not have enough quiet places to accommodate reassignment on a large scale.

Nonorganic or Functional Hearing Loss

Functional hearing impairment exists when there is no organic cause for the apparent hearing loss, and the inability to hear results chiefly from psychologic or emotional factors. Nonorganic hearing loss is frequently encountered in the evaluation of occupational hearing loss claims. *Nonorganic hearing loss,* as used here, indicates all abnormal auditory functions that cannot be accounted for by any anatomical or physiologic finding. It may take any of the following forms:

1. Stimulation of disease or impairment when there is no basis for the complaint

2. Exaggeration of the deficit, most often seen in hearing loss claims

3. False attribution—the worker blames the hearing loss on noise when it is actually due to other causes, such as otosclerosis or chronic otitis media

4. Malingering, which is the deliberate, conscious simulation of disease or impairment for a selfish motive—usually for financial gain

5. Neurosis, in which the motivation to simulate disease is unconscious and in response to emotional conflicts that have nothing to do with personal or financial gain (differentiation between malingering and neurosis may require psychiatric consultation)

Tests for nonorganic hearing loss are usually detection and proof tests. The evaluation of these nonorganic hearing loss cases, in many instances, remains largely an art. One should be aware of the complexity involved in detecting nonorganic hearing impairment. The claimant often manipulates the responses in order to increase the alleged loss. The best results are obtained from the synthesis of the claimant's history and otologic and audiologic studies.

Other Health Effects of Noise

It has been claimed that hazardous noise has a deleterious effect upon the health and general well-being of the worker. Although studies revealed that temporary physiologic changes can result from acute noise exposure, most of these changes are the result of stress reactions. Long-term studies of workers employed in noisy jobs will be required to establish a definite pattern and relationship of noise exposure to permanent health effects. The annoyance caused by noise depends primarily upon the worker who is being annoyed, personal motivation, and activities at the time of exposure. High-frequency intermittent noises from a hidden source tend to be most annoying. Noise that is annoying is not necessarily a health hazard.

Hearing Aids

Some of the state workers' compensation statutes provide for the cost and, in some instances, the maintenance of a hearing aid when it is medically and audiologically indicated. As a rule, no deduction is made for any help that may result from the use of a hearing aid. This is in accordance with the general policy of determining impairment of body functions without the use of a prosthetic device.

California, for example, has a rule stating that employers can ask that the claimant have a hearing test with a hearing aid. This test, and the "uncorrected" one, can be averaged to get a final figure. Yet, when the employer asks that the employee be tested with a hearing aid, the state will require the employer to provide lifetime replacement and maintenance of a hearing aid for the worker. This maintenance cost often exceeds that of the claim, and, naturally, few employers demand such a "corrected" exam.

Presbycusis, or the Aging Factor

The role of presbycusis (hearing loss due to the aging process) in hearing loss claims has received considerable attention. Research indicates that hearing loss increases due to aging, even for persons not exposed to occupational noise. Such studies show a gradual decline in the hearing sensitivity of the population. There is some disagreement as to how much of this loss is due to the aging process alone (presbycusis) and how much is due to environmental noise exposures (sociocusis). It is also not known how the aging process interacts with the growth of occupational hearing impairment. Usually, in workers' compensation, the entire impairment is compensable as long as an occupational factor in any way increases the impairment caused by the physical condition.

Several state compensation boards require a deduction for the hearing loss that accompanies age—for example, a deduction from calculated hearing impairment of one half decibel for each year of age over 40 years. The rationale for this is the desire to subtract the average amount of hearing loss from nonoccupational causes found in the population at any given age.

Date of Injury

The establishment of a "date of injury" within the meaning of the applicable law may have an important bearing upon the worker's eligibility to file a claim against the employer. The requirements, in this respect, have been established definitely in jurisdictions that have special occupational disease loss of hearing provisions.

In other states, the occupational disease provisions in the laws may relate the payment of benefits to the "last day of work," to the date of "incapacitation," or to "the beginning of disablement," caused by the injury being treated under the provisions applicable to accidental injuries. In such states, it may be important to determine the last date on which the employee was exposed to allegedly injurious noise and whether the exposure has ceased because of transfer to other work, termination of employment, strike, disablement, or any other cause. If the exposure has not ceased, it should be determined when the employee first visited a doctor and was told that he or she had a hearing loss that was presumably due to noise exposure.

Waiting Period

Otologists and compensation authorities have recommended various waiting periods in which the claimant must be removed from noisy employment before qualifying to file a hearing loss claim. It is important to eliminate any temporary threshold shift before testing persons for their permanent hearing threshold. There is scientific disagreement on how long this takes. The waiting time required varies with the extent of the noise exposure and individual susceptibility factors.

A waiting period does involve administrative advantages. When a worker terminates employment by retirement, his or her hearing status can be evaluated and the case closed. The six-month waiting period spreads out the filing of claims and protects the worker's right to establish a claim when no longer employed in a noisy occupation.

Validity of Testimony

Nonprofessional persons cannot be expected to collect and evaluate all of the information needed for a hearing loss compensation claim case. In most cases, physicians can provide testimony on medical conditions, plant managers will describe the operations involved, loss control representatives and safety engineers can provide information on the noise control measures, and industrial hygienists will testify concerning evidence of exposure. These professionals must consider all pertinent points in their area of expertise in order to present an accurate and meaningful evaluation of the available data.

An expert in a specific field is not necessarily competent to render judgment on an entire case but only on that portion which is within his or her area of expertise. No rigid rules for judging competency can be defined. The individual reviewing the hearing loss claim should verify (1) the professional qualifications of those testifying, and (2) the basis of the testimony, that is, the importance attributed to various pieces of the information reviewed, and the conclusions that were drawn.

It is desirable that the record should contain as much of the following information or evidence as is readily available or considered pertinent:

1. The employee's complete work assignment record, showing the positions held and, if possible, inclusive dates of work station assignments

2. A job description of the duties performed, the type of noise to which the employee was exposed, and the daily noise dose and the length of time of noise exposure on each job assignment

3. A description of the employee's work station, including a diagram showing the dimensions and layouts of the work area

4. A report of any sound level surveys made of the employee's work area

5. The safety precautions (such as providing earplugs or muffs) taken to eliminate or reduce noise hazards, a description of the safety devices, and the approximate number of hours per day and days per week they were used

6. A statement as to whether any other employees performing the same work under the same working conditions have made similar complaints

7. A copy of the report of the employee's preplacement medical examination and audiogram

8. All medical records in the possession of the employer and copies of all available audiometric tests

9. The date and time the employee was last exposed to noise on the job or a verification that the employee is still exposed

10. A statement indicating whether the employee had had any ear or hearing problems, including when they occurred and the names and addresses of all physicians who examined or treated the employee for hearing problems

11. Full details of any previous claim filed for workers' compensation or for similar benefits (e.g., Veterans Administration) because of this or any condition affecting the employee's ears or hearing, including the date of the claim, the name and address of the office where the claim was filed, and a description of any benefits received

To properly distinguish between an occupational and a nonoccupational loss of hearing claim, answers will have to be obtained to the following questions:

1. Has a hearing loss been clearly established?

2. Has it been shown that the hearing loss can result from excessive exposure to noise?

3. Has exposure to excessive noise been demonstrated (by work history, sampling data, expert opinion)?

4. Has exposure to the noise been shown to be of sufficient degree and/or duration to result in the hearing loss?

5. Has nonoccupational exposure to noise been ruled out as a causative factor?

6. Have all special circumstances been weighed? For example, were there any unusual events at work that reduced the effectiveness of hearing protective equipment?

7. Has the burden of proof been met? Did the evidence prove that the hearing loss resulted from, or was aggravated by, conditions at work?

If the answer to all of the above questions is "Yes," the decision can be made that the hearing loss is occupational in origin.

HEARING CONSERVATION

Reduction of Noise Exposure

Today, management, with some push from and direction of governmental agencies, finds that much can be done to curb excess noise and protect the hearing of workers, with the expense of doing so being well worth it in terms of increased machinery life and a quieter environment. Purchasing department personnel can be alerted to provide noise specifications when considering the replacement or addition of machinery. Designers of machinery know that their product has a better chance of being sold if they can utilize noise-control principles to reduce the decibel output. It behooves management to explore every noise source in terms of its complete correction or significant reduction, remembering that methods for controlling noise for a particular situation or machine depend on many factors. Usually it is to the employer's distinct advantage to engage qualified, experienced consultants to come into the plant, appraise the problem and specify what can be done and how much it will cost. There are some general methods for reducing noise levels, including some examples of specific measures taken by industry in the past with considerable success.

The most effective method of controlling noise is to reduce the noise at its source with good engineering design. This usually will be the responsibility of the manufacturer. In some instances, it is possible to modify existing equipment. This may be accomplished by changing the type of drive, installation of mufflers or applying damping materials to vibrating surfaces.

Good maintenance will help reduce some unnecessary noise caused by loose guards, worn gears, bushings, or bent shafts. For example, in one instance, automatic screw machines were found to produce a deafening roar. Investigation revealed that the operator had left off the guides, thus allowing the bar stock to whip. Replacement of the guides limited the excessive noise. Sometimes it may be necessary to use inserts of rubber, hardwood, or other material. Stock tubes that reduce bar stock noise are available for almost all conventional screw-machine turret lathes.

A high-speed, circular saw was found to produce a loud high-frequency type of noise while idling. The saw blade was returned to the manufacturer and, on the drilling of several holes and slots, the high-pitched characteristic of the noise was greatly reduced. One source of noise in metal-stamping plants is the flow of air through the orifices of ejectors. The ejectors often are left turned on for long periods when presses are not operating. By turning them off promptly when presses are not operating, noise can be reduced. In many cases, air ejection noise can be eliminated through control of airflow and mufflers that now are available. Hydraulic "jackhammers" are replacing the extremely noisy air hammer.

Sometimes it is possible to substitute a less noisy operation or material for one producing excessive noise:

Flame welding could be substituted for riveting in many operations.

The extremely noisy pneumatic riveting on frame assembly in a motor truck manufacturing concern was studied and corrected by replacing the riveting with rivet pressing.

Finished screw machine products were continuously ejected from a plant's machine into a noisy metal chute and tray. This disturbing noise was easily controlled by the use of fiber chutes and neoprene-lined metal trays.

Frequently, noise can be isolated so that its disturbing effect will be encountered by fewer people. A noisy machine or operation may be removed or walled off from a room containing many people so that only the personnel necessary for the job will be exposed. This relatively small number of employees then should be provided with effective ear protection, making supervision of the wearing of protection much easier. Well-insulated partitions and tightly closing doors should always be provided between a noisy room and adjoining areas.

In a small drop forge plant that makes forged hand tools, the actual forging, cleaning, and buffing operation was isolated in a small building removed from several hundred other workers who had such tasks as sorting, packing, or shipping. Previously, all of the employees were under one roof, and more than 300 employees were exposed to harmful and dangerous noise.

Total or partial enclosures for automatic and semiautomatic machines would prevent airborne noise from spreading throughout the surrounding area (Fig 20–20). Where it is not practicable to enclose the entire machine, it may be possible to provide small enclosures to cover just the points of operation, gears, or other noisy parts of the machine. The important design factors in the construction of enclosures include an impervious barrier, such as sheet metal or plywood, lining with sound-absorbing material inside the enclosure to prevent build-up of noise, and rubber-like material to seal the edges of panels of doors (Figs 20–21 and 20–22).

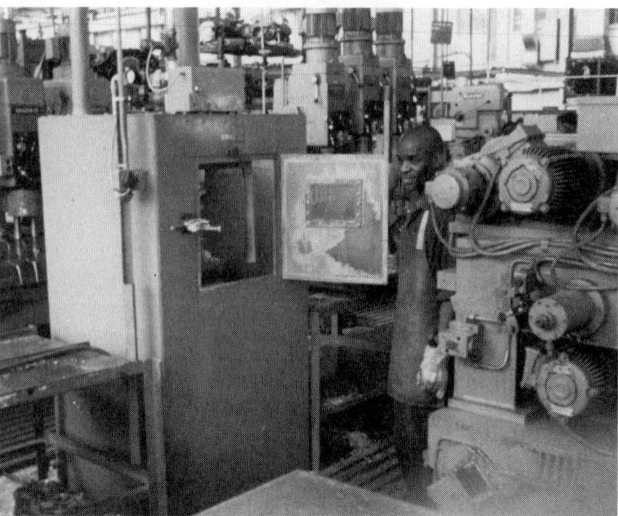

FIG 20–20.
The ideal method for control—completely isolating the noisy machining operation with a sound-proof enclosure (1976).

Other methods of controlling noise include the use of resilient mountings and the use of sound-absorptive materials. However, a "do-it-yourself" or trial-and-error approach to these methods of noise control often is time-consuming and proves ineffective in the end. One approach is to find a company that has solved a problem similar to yours. Years of experience have proved conclusively that where a precedent has not been set, skilled and experienced engineering consultants to work with local plant personnel usually are worthwhile. To make the most progress possible, it is recommended that one person in the plant organization be appointed to coordinate the work of noise exposure control and to report the progress and problems directly to top management. Noise control seminars are offered by many colleges and universities, and plant personnel should be encouraged to attend these. Excellent sources of information for those interested in pursuing practical information on noise control possibilities are available.

Personal Hearing Protection

It should be made clear that even though the possibilities of controlling noise are promising, some machines, for one reason or another, such as expense, reduced efficiency, or the awkwardness created in the handling of raw materials and finished product, cannot be quieted, despite the enthusiastic statements of the governmental agencies in regard to noise control (Figs 20–23 to 20–25).

Federal and state regulations now require that each employer provide personal hearing protection devices and require that employees use these faithfully and continually while on the job. The average worker, unfortunately, accepts noise as a normal part of his occupation. He soon adapts to it and seldom complains about it. This is why safety personnel, physicians, and nurses say the promotion of personal hearing protection devices is their most frustrating task (Figs 20–26 to 20–28).

Employees must always be told after the initial fitting to come back after several days' trial of one device just to be sure every-

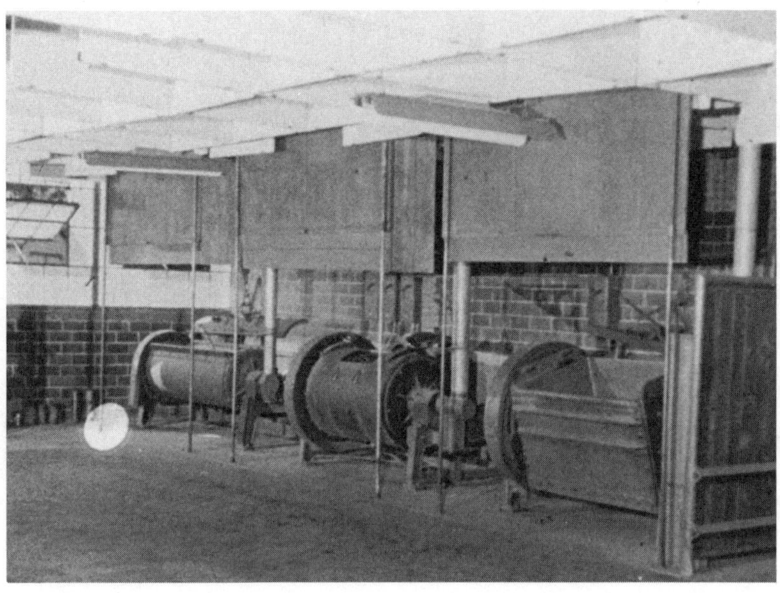

FIG 20–21.
Vibration mounts were installed under all tumbling barrels, which were coated with sheet metal deadener. This deadener is commercially available and is similar to undercoating material sprayed on automobiles.

thing is going well. Then, if the employee expresses dissatisfaction with the type or brand tried initially, he or she can try another and still another until satisfactory protection is found that will be worn every day. Many plants have learned that it helps considerably to have a variety of ear protectors. Unfavorable reactions are bound to occur when a person is told, "This is the kind that we have decided you should wear." Employees will have a far different attitude when they are told, "Try this type and come back in a week and let us know how it works. You are welcome to try other available kinds until you believe that you have the one that suits you best."

Types of Hearing Protectors

Insert Devices.—Probably the most popular of all protective devices designed to save hearing are the ear insert types of "earplug." These devices are relatively inexpensive in comparison to

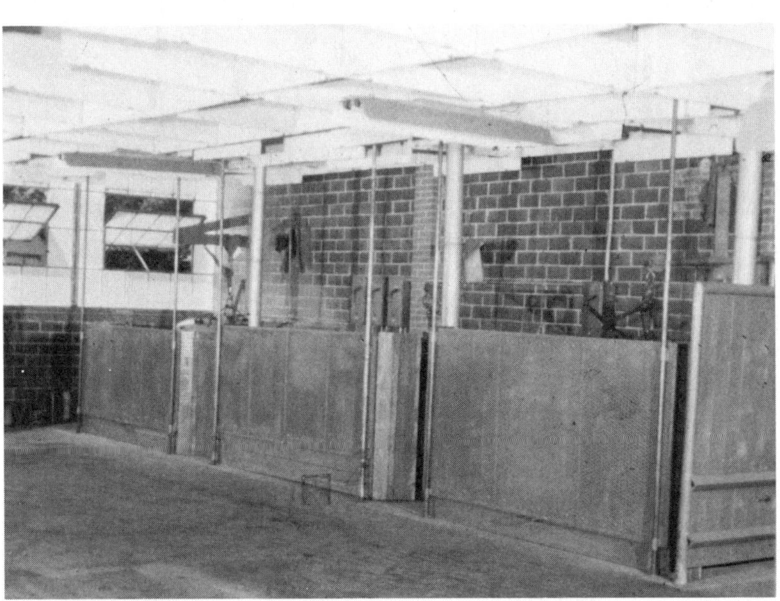

FIG 20–22.
The guards in front of the tumblers are fitted with sound barriers consisting of ¾-inch-thick spruce planks, which were sprayed with deadener. These barriers change the direction of the sound waves emanating from the tumblers.

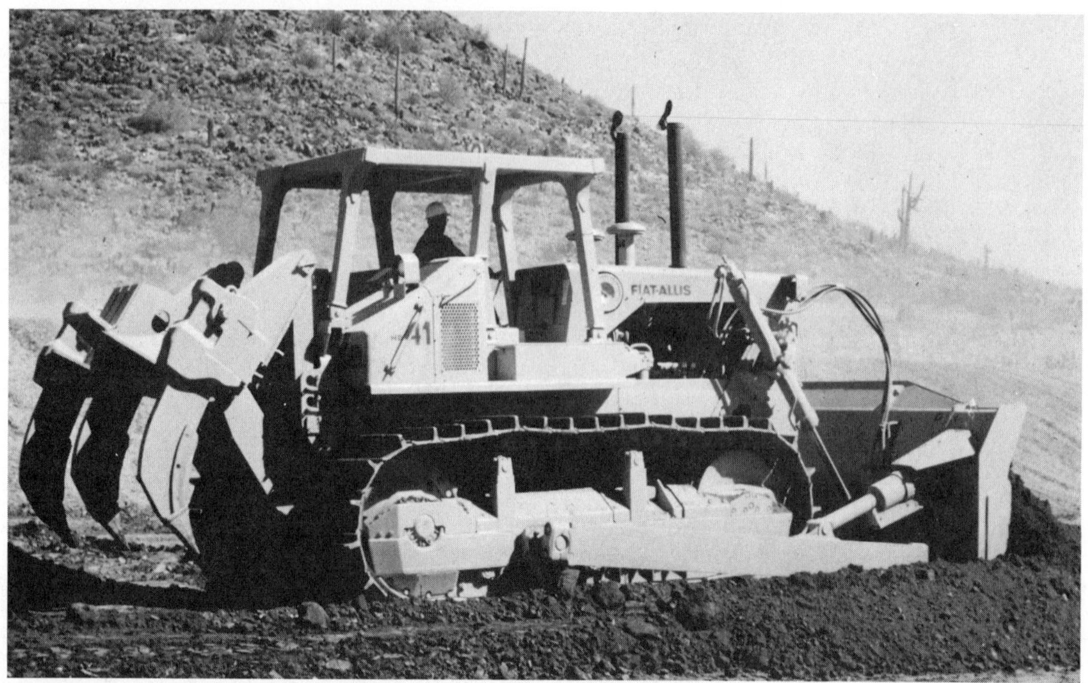

FIG 20–23.
Nearly all types of construction machinery can produce high noise levels. Although engineering techniques to reduce sound levels are applied by manufacturers, actual working conditions, such as type of terrain and use by operators and contractors, are beyond the control of the manufacturer. Operators can wear protective equipment, and sometimes cab enclosures are installed.

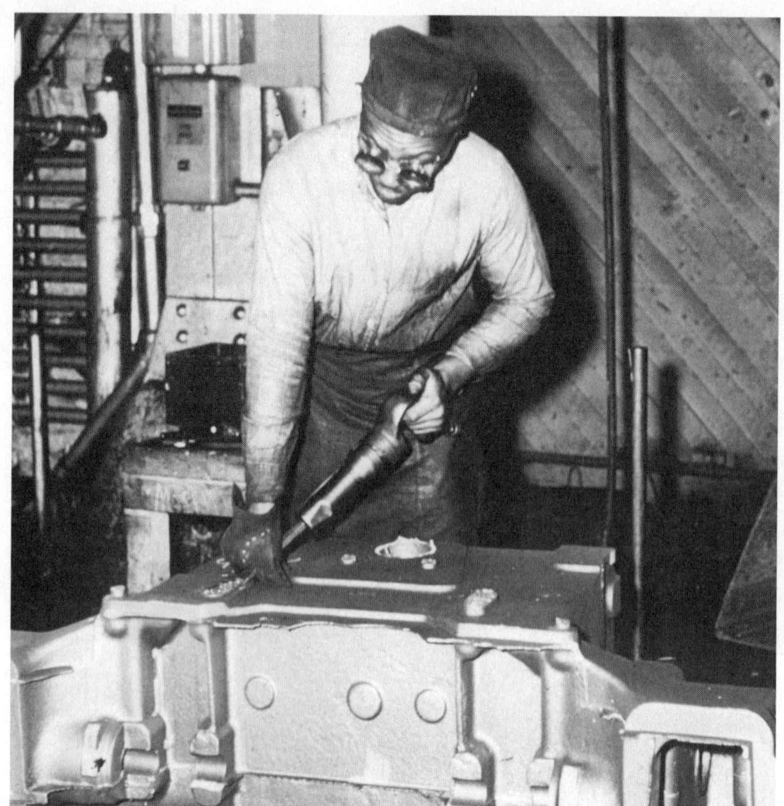

FIG 20–24.
Chipping on a large iron casting. This very noisy job demands individual hearing protection in the form of earplugs or similar devices.

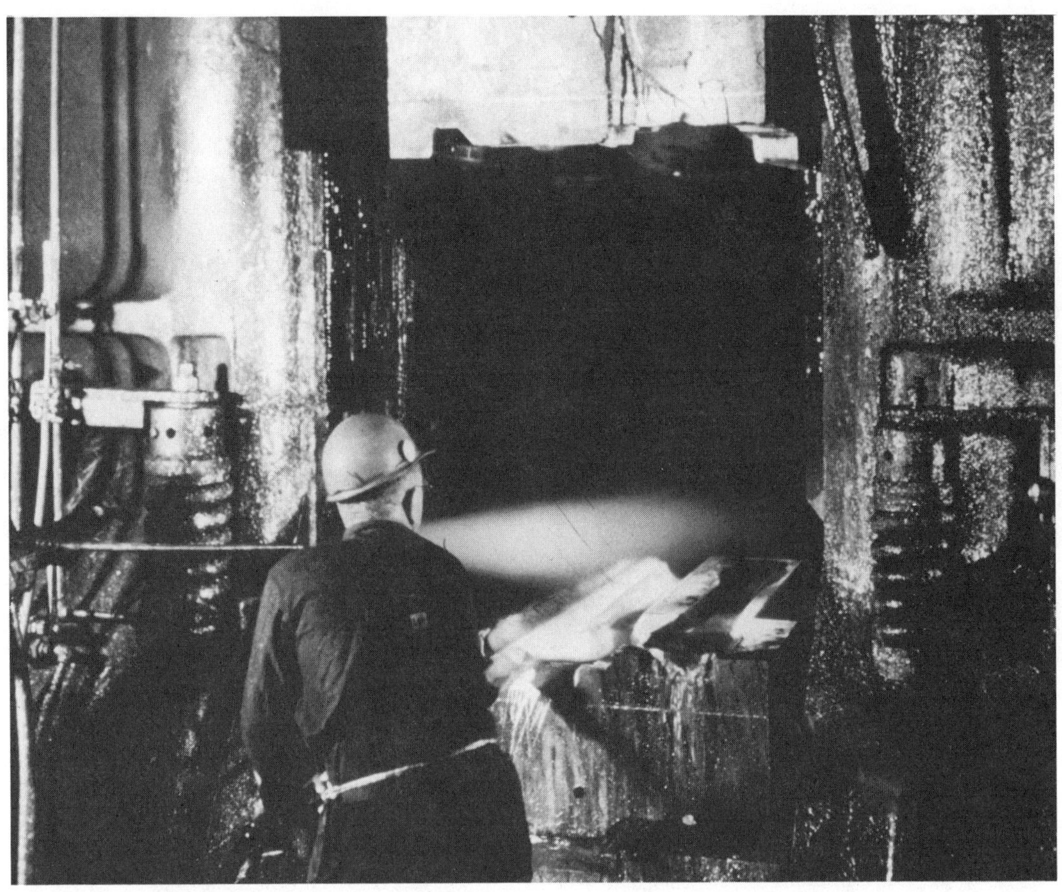

FIG 20–25.
A large forging press or "drop hammer." This is an extremely noisy process along with much radiant heat exposure.

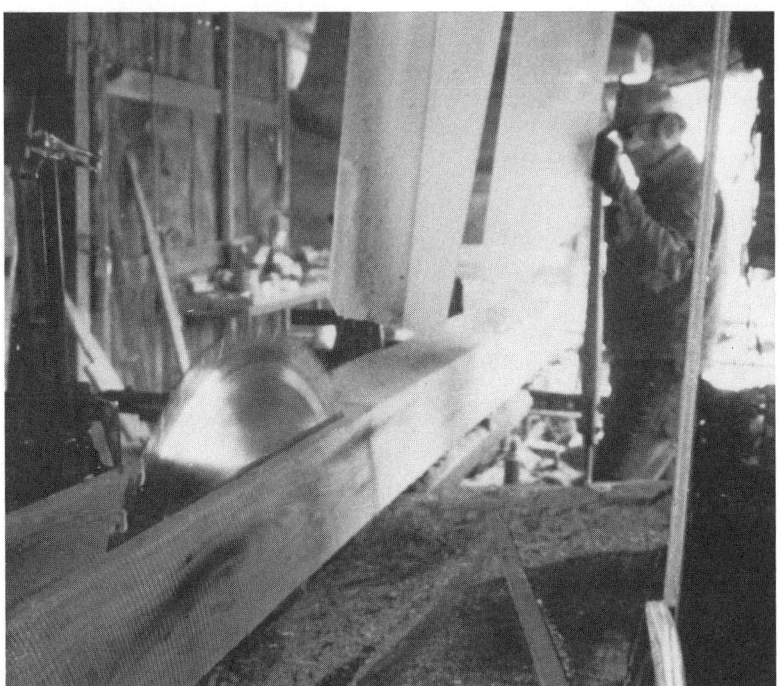

FIG 20–26.
A typical saw mill scene. Cutting cherry, oak, maple and walnut woods creates high noise levels. Earplugs or muffs seldom are used by these owner-operators and their employees (1985).

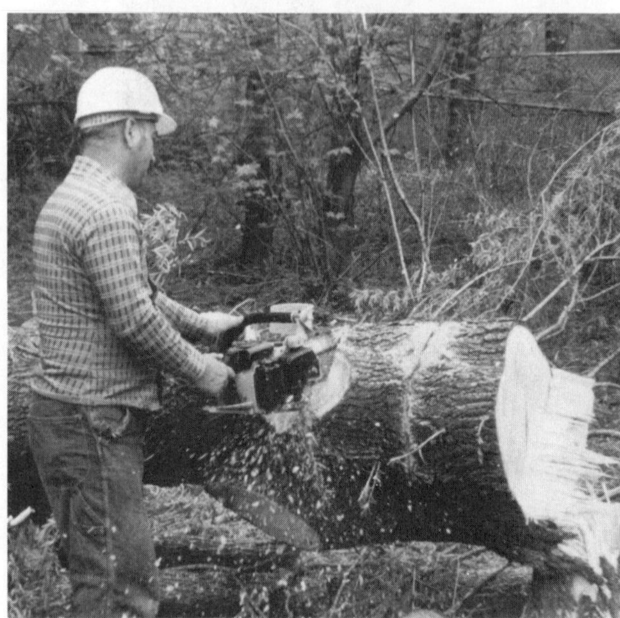

FIG 20–27.
Commercial tree cutter. Note lack of proper protective equipment (1985).

earmuffs and custom-molded devices and are completely comfortable to wear. Some insert plugs are attached to nylon cords or strings to hang around the neck when not in use to prevent loss and to remove easily when one wishes to converse or to take out during rest or lunch breaks. There are many varieties to choose from (Figs 20–29 and 20–30).

Do you remember walking through a noisy workplace and observing pellets of dry cotton in workers' ears? Unfortunately, dry cotton or wool, unless impregnated with a soft wax, are useless. The device most worn today is a rubber or neoprene bullet-shaped affair, sometimes flanged and sometimes smooth or plain, with a tab at the base used for withdrawal. Devices in the past have come in a variety of sizes, from extra small to extra large, since ear canals vary from 3 to 14 ml. However, the trend seems to be in the reduction of a many-sized product to a "fit all" that accommodates most ear sizes except the very small, but even these types now come in two general sizes.

A very popular device, which has the appearance of cotton but has excellent attenuation properties, is "Swedish wool," a nontoxic material of extremely fine glassfiber (less than 3 μ in diameter), which is available in preformed plugs. Workers say that they are comfortable to wear and reduce the noise sufficiently. It should be remembered that 92% of all industrial noise exposure in the United States seems to be below 105 dBA, making this product most acceptable. If there is a disadvantage, it is the cost, because the insert becomes soiled and usually must be discarded after eight hours of use.

Expandable-type ear protectors are a most recent invention. This material, shaped like a pellet or a bullet, is squeezed together and placed into the ear canal. In a matter of seconds, the expansion of this material fills the ear canal and shuts out the sound energy almost completely. It has one distinct advantage over the other disposable types in that it can be used over and over again until it becomes too soiled and dirty. Some users like such inserts very much. Others say that they are uncomfortable. Again, remember—the most successful protector is the one that is worn by the worker!

Earmuffs.—The primary arguments for the use of earmuffs in the past were the elimination of the usual fitting problems and the fact that they are so large and conspicuous that they are easily observed by supervisors to check on compliance. In addition, one should consider the potential loss of insert plugs and the fact that disposable types are expensive over a period of years. In these cases, the muff probably is a very good investment. Earmuffs tend to become uncomfortable in hot weather or with hot work (Fig 20–31).

Despite disadvantages that we hear from workers no matter

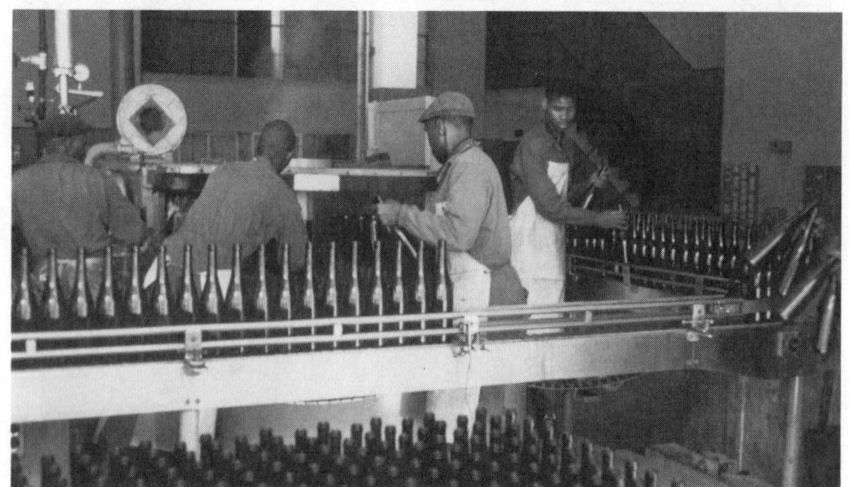

FIG 20–28.
A bottling line in a winery. A high noise level is produced; protective devices are indicated (1983).

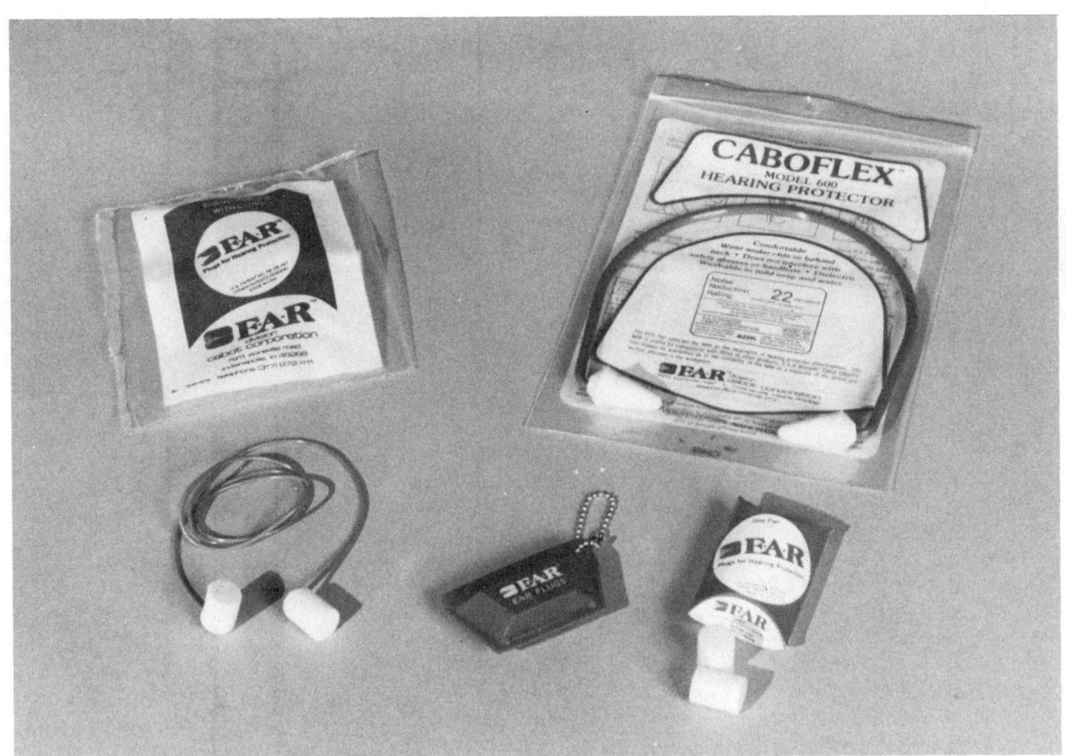

FIG 20–29.
Some of the different ear plugs available.

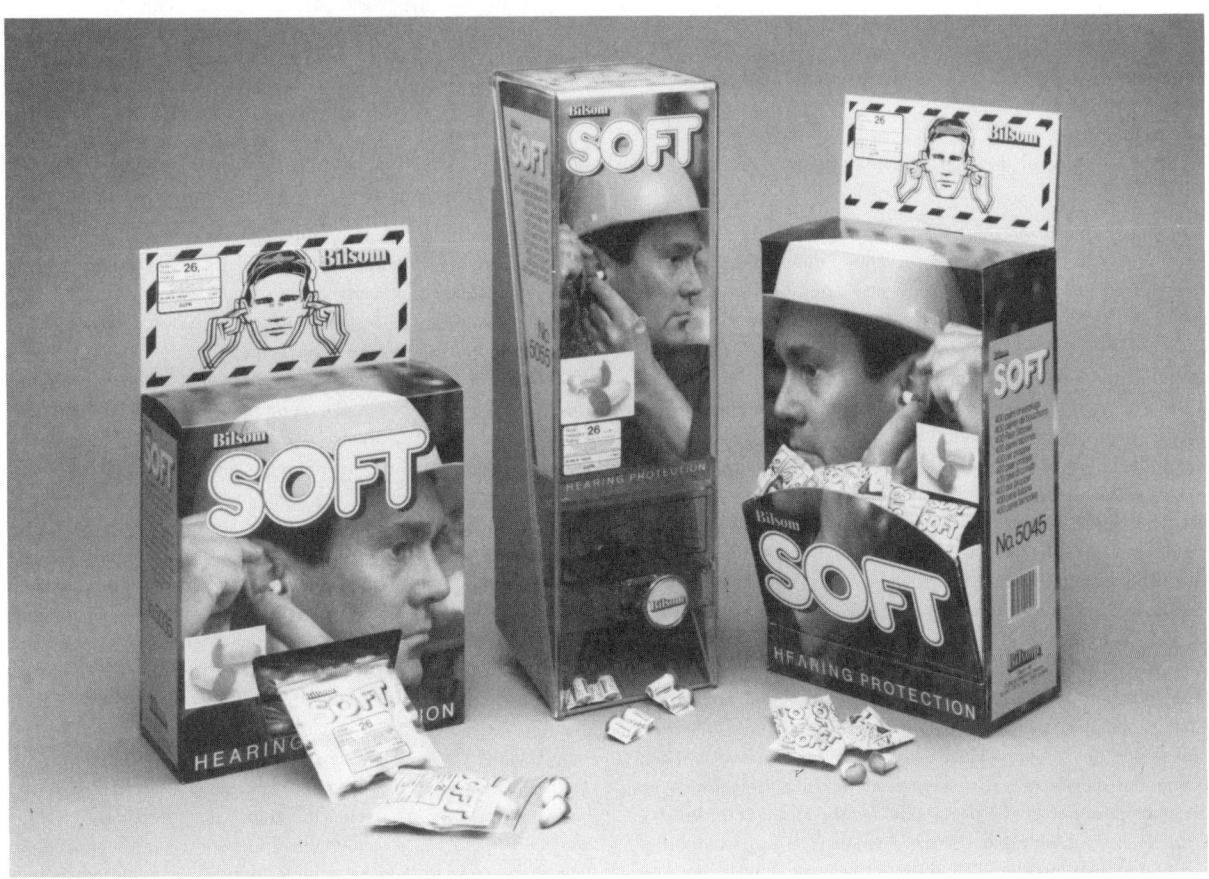

FIG 20–30.
Some of the different ear plugs available.

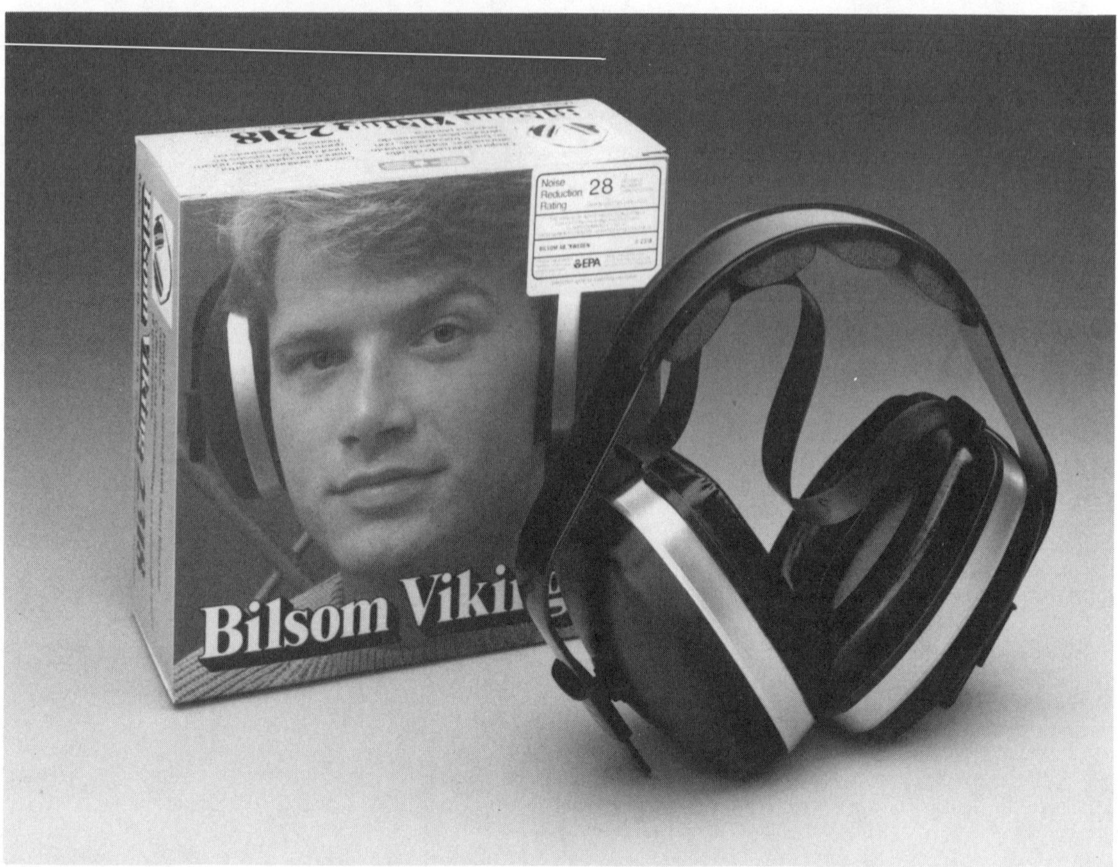

FIG 20–31.
One of many acceptable earmuffs in use.

what product they are wearing, safety directors believe that many workers prefer a muff over other types. They indicate that the complaints received are no different from those they have received in the past regarding *any* type of safety equipment required by management. Safety directors also seem to agree that it is not at all unreasonable to require earmuffs to be worn in any situation in which the worker is exposed to short-term and high-intensity noise (as in the case of air transportation ramp workers and maintenance personnel). It is the responsibility of the supervisor, *backed 100% by management,* to see that the regulation is carried out. Now, in the face of being fined or penalized because of government rules and regulations, management has no alternative but to say, "If you work for us, you must abide by our safety rules, which have been established for your own personal benefit."

Choosing and Fitting a Hearing Protector

The question often asked of hearing conservation specialists is "What is the best hearing protector?" The answer is *"The best protector is the one properly fitted and the one you wear."* When discussing the merits of various types of hearing protectors, the primary consideration of the physician, nurse, and safety director seems to be one of reduction or attenuation. Certain wearability factors need to be considered, including the ease of insertion and removal, durability, cost, ease of cleaning, and comfort. The great individual variation in attenuation of certain earplugs indicates that perhaps primary consideration should be given to the *selection* of an earplug *that fits properly* and *is comfortable*. It is indicated that if an earplug is *properly fitted* and properly seals the ear canal, it will attenuate to the degree anticipated.

One word of caution: *All insert-type protectors need some special attention when being placed into the ear canal*. The canal must be examined, preferably by a nurse. The device just cannot be "pushed" into the ear. The wearer must, of necessity, use a hand (from the opposite side of the head being fitted) to pull the outer ear *up* and *back* to enlarge the canal several millimeters. The device or material then should be turned at least one-half the circumference of the canal. *Only after this is done* should the user release the earflap or outer ear, which will hold the device or material securely. There should be a tendency to slightly "overfit" but not to the point of discomfort. If the fitting procedure produces undue discomfort, it must be repeated, but it should be possible to enjoy comfort and safety at the same time.

Usually, a protector can be checked for its efficiency by the wearer, noting if his voice sounds are distorted or if it sounds as if he is talking into a barrel. This shows that the sound energy created by the moving air molecules is not entering the ear canal and that the wearer is hearing sounds internally or through bone conduction. It would be a safe rule to say that if you are fitted with hearing protectors and you engage in limited conversation and you hear satisfactorily with no strange or different effects, the protector is doing little good.

Another good test is to note, when withdrawing the plug or material, if the canal is holding the plug just enough so that a slight "tug" is necessary to pull it out, but not to the point of discomfort. Usually, the first symptoms of discomfort disappear within the first day of use. Again, the initial "fit" is for trial and exploration only. The wearer should be encouraged to come back in a few days to report on his experience with the device. If discomfort or "fullness" is felt, perhaps a smaller size is indicated or the plug needs readjustment in some way. Ordinarily, the soft rubber premolded plugs are not uncomfortable once workers make up their minds that they will take the time necessary to get used to them. The physician, nurse, or safety director should explain fitting and wearing procedures thoroughly and not overlook any objections that workers may make.

Audiometric Examination of Employees

The audiometric examination is vital to the total hearing conservation program. It is the method by which we gauge the effectiveness of noise reduction and engineering controls. It becomes the final test of the effectiveness of personal hearing protection, and good audiometric examinations are, at present, the best way we have to detect an individual's susceptibility to noise. By comparing internal audiometric records, we are able to evaluate a person's adjustment to the strain of a noisy working environment. If hearing acuity continues to decrease despite noise-reduction measures and personal hearing protection devices, the matter becomes a grave problem for both the physician and the personnel director. However, in most cases, the worker with proper ear protection can work in almost any noisy environment. Early noise-induced hearing losses usually are indicated at the 3,000–4,000-Hz frequency range long before they are noticed by an individual and long before they may cause a communication or speech problem (Figs 20–32 and 20–33).

The Audiogram as an Educational Tool

By showing the worker his personal record of hearing sensitivity, the nurse or physician has a most effective device for the promotion of hearing protection. If the audiogram is used to explain the status of the worker's hearing at the time the hearing protector is being fitted for the first time, success almost invariably is ensured. The wearer now knows that his hearing is so good that it must be preserved at all cost. If the audiogram indicates that his acuity is deteriorating in the higher frequencies, the need to do all humanly possible to save the amount remaining is imperative. Utilization of the graph type of audiogram (Fig 20–34) is reported to be the physician's and nurse's most useful tool in obtaining 100% successful protection in the plant or workplace.

Too often the "why" and "how" of hearing protection are com-

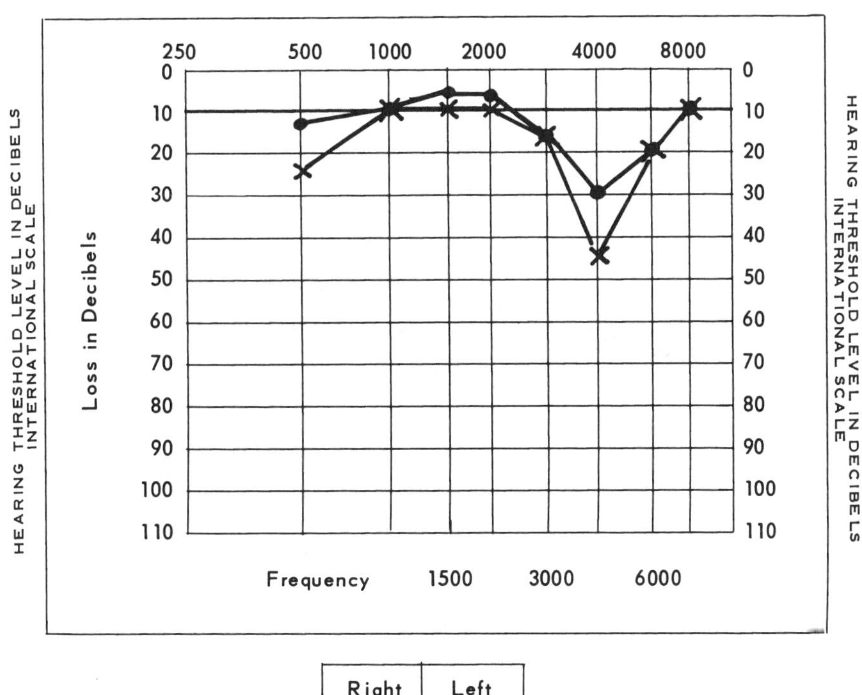

Right	Left
Red	Blue
●	X

FIG 20–32.
This notch at 4,000 Hz possibly could be early noise-induced deafness. The worker would not notice that he has this deficit at this stage, but without protection, it can only grow worse. The subject would not notice this loss.

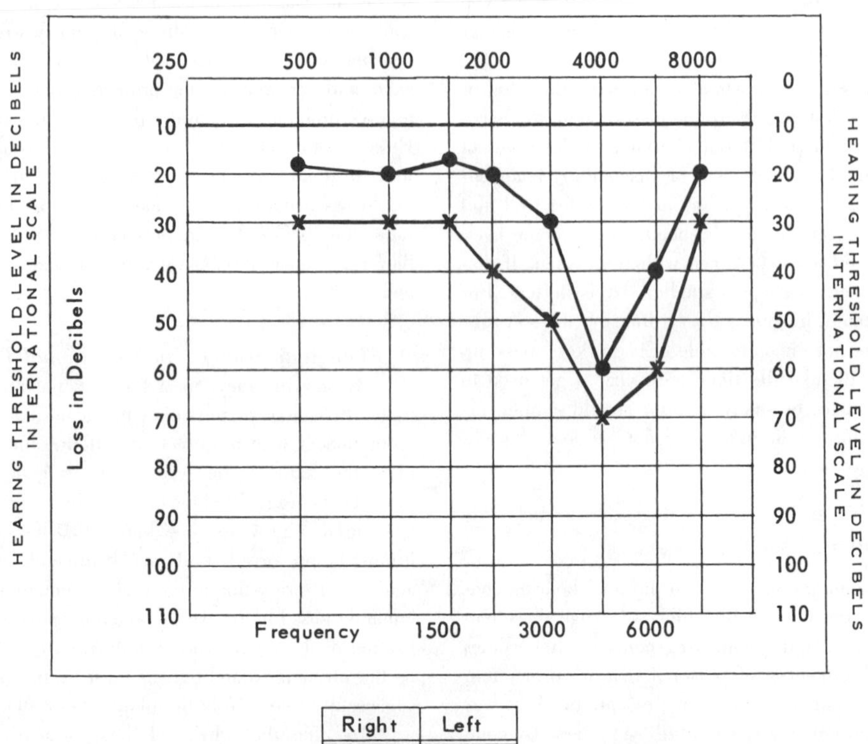

Right	Left
Red	Blue
●	X

FIG 20–33.
The notch at 4,000 Hz and return to improved hearing probably indicates more advanced noise-induced hearing loss. The notch will widen unless the employee is given ear protection, which he should wear in all noise situations.

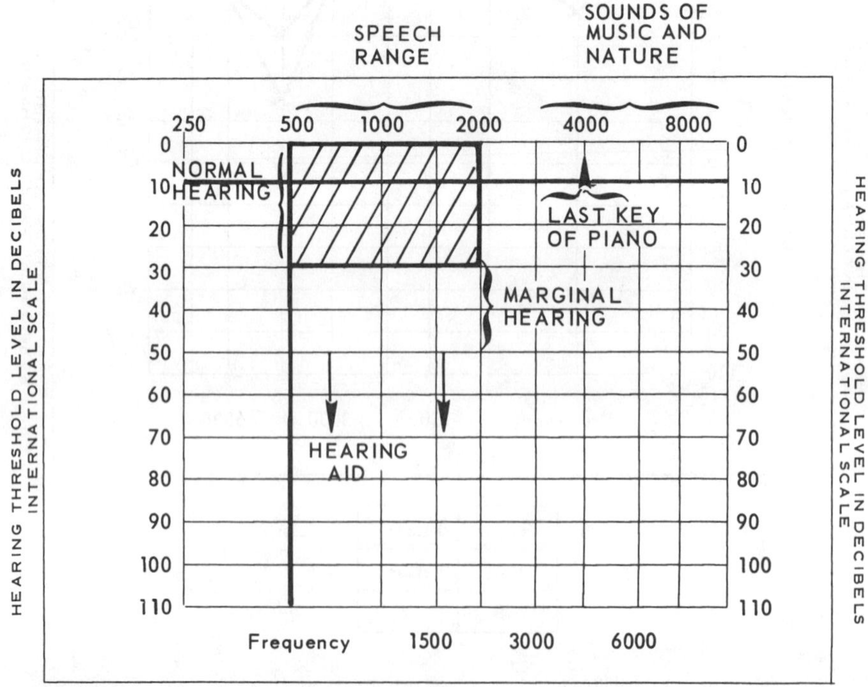

FIG 20–34.
This graph-type audiogram helps patients understand the results of their audiometric tests.

pletely ignored. It is only assumed that the worker should be delighted to wear protective devices. Hearing protection is a matter of *counseling* the worker and this requires *time*. For instance, in the course of an audiometric examination or a fitting for a protective device, employees should be alerted to and advised about "off-the-job" noise exposures as well as noise hazards at the workplace.

Detection of Nonoccupational Hearing Defects

An abnormal audiogram might be the key that could open the door to the correction of a defect or the rehabilitation of damaged ears (Fig 20–35). Even though occupational deafness is nerve deafness and is irreversible (Figs 20–36 and 20–37), in many cases there are instances of conditions that can be corrected through surgery and effective medical management. Other examples of abnormalities shown on audiograms are depicted in Figures 20–38 through 20–41.

When I first came into this specialized area nearly 20 years ago, the physician of one large company having 1,600 employees and without a noise problem urged management to include audiometric examinations as part of the regular periodic physical examination program. At the end of the year, more than 120 employees were referred to an otologist for specialized examinations. Needless to say, the management of this company did not need to be sold on the benefits of its hearing conservation program, because surgery and rehabilitation measures were of help to a large number of workers. Through the establishment of hearing conservation efforts, we not only are guarding our economic welfare but we are also contributing to the health and happiness of our workers.

Criteria for Making Referrals

When should workers be referred to an otologist for a specialized examination? The following "Otologic Referral Criteria for Occupational Hearing Conservation Programs" were devised by Robert A. Dobie, MD, Chairman of the Medical Aspects of Noise Subcommittee of the American Academy of Otolaryngology Head and Neck Surgery, 1101 Vermont Ave., NW, Washington, D.C. 20005:

> The Subcommittee on the Medical Aspects of Noise of the American Academy of Otolaryngology—Head and Neck Surgery recognizes that with the establishment of increasing numbers of occupational hearing conservation programs, there is a need for referral criteria. Workers screened by these programs frequently present problems requiring medical attention which the directors of the programs are not prepared to render. When the director is a physician, he recognizes what can be treated locally, and what needs to be referred to an appropriate specialist. This is not always true when the director is not a physician.
>
> In an effort to assist program directors of occupational hearing conservation programs, the following referral criteria were formulated. Because medical referrals are both costly and time-consuming, they should be held to a minimum. In cases of doubt, however, it is better to refer someone who did not need to be referred than not to refer someone who should have been referred. Communication between the

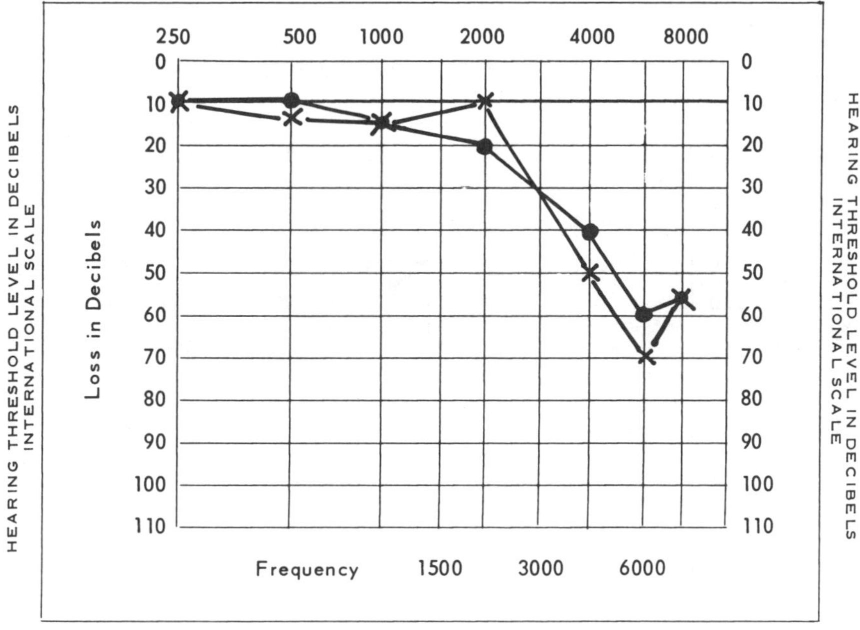

Right	Left
Red	Blue
●	X

FIG 20–35.
Beginning stages of bilateral sensorineural loss, speech range intact.

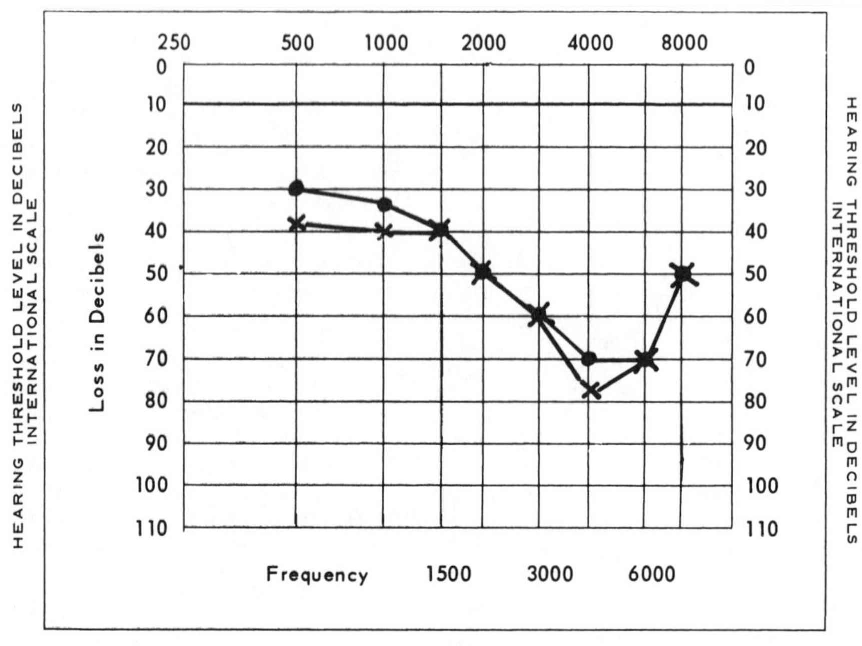

Right	Left
Red	Blue
●	X

FIG 20–36.
This audiogram indicates what could happen to a worker after 25–30 years of exposure in an extreme noise situation without hearing protection. The speech range, unlike that shown in Figure 20–35, shows beginning impairment.

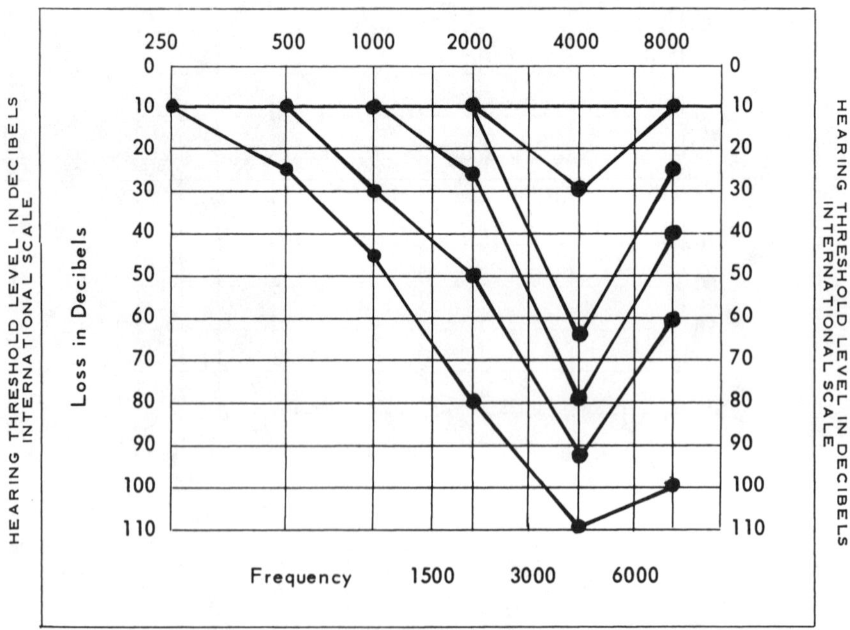

FIG 20–37.
This represents the results of many employees who worked in the hazardous noise of sawmills for a period of 25–30 years. The drop or notch at 4,000 Hz deepens after ten years of exposure. As time passes, and without hearing protection, the notch grows wider and the hearing impairment greater, finally interfering with the employee's ability to understand speech sounds.

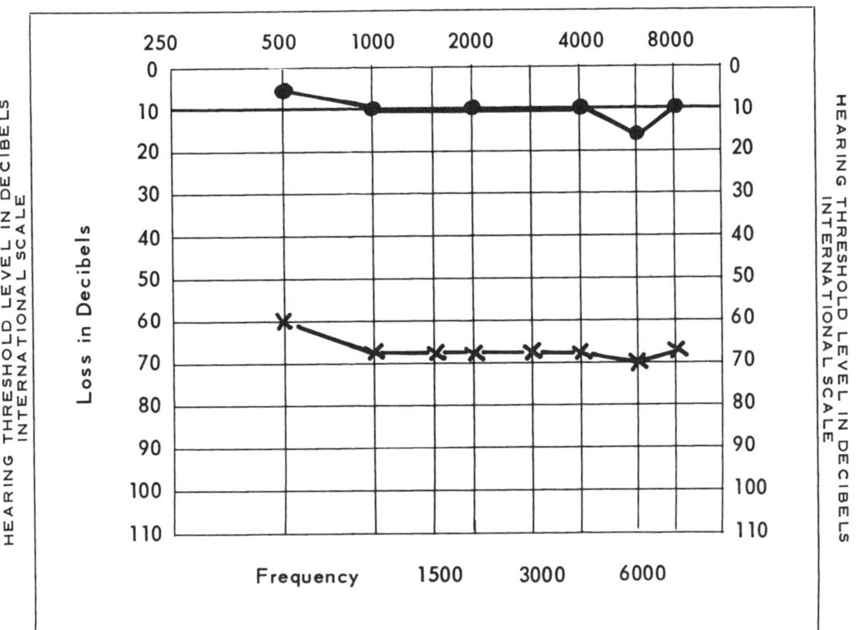

FIG 20–38.
This audiogram could be most deceivng. The discrepancy between right and left ears is great enough to question whether the subject is hearing much of the sound through his better right ear as the skull transmits the sound from the left side of the head to the more acute right ear. This type of audiogram requires a bone conduction test given by a qualified audiologist or otologist. If the readings are correct as shown, the hearing impairment could be caused by a previous mumps infection.

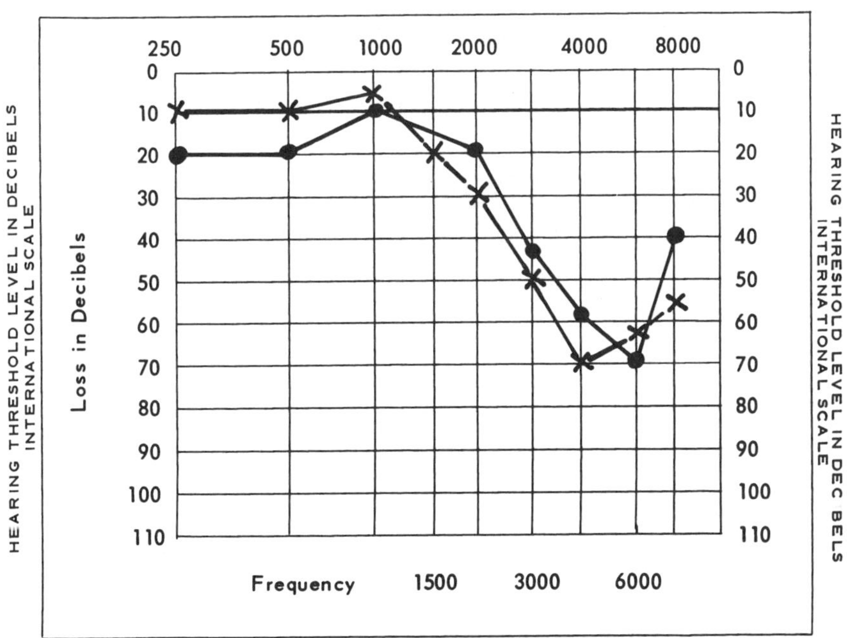

FIG 20–39.
Typical pure tone findings for a patient with nerve loss. Sensorineural deafness can be caused by noise, head injuries, such childhood diseases as mumps or measles, old age, and antibiotics. This is the person who hears people talk but finds it difficult to understand. Speech range still is intact.

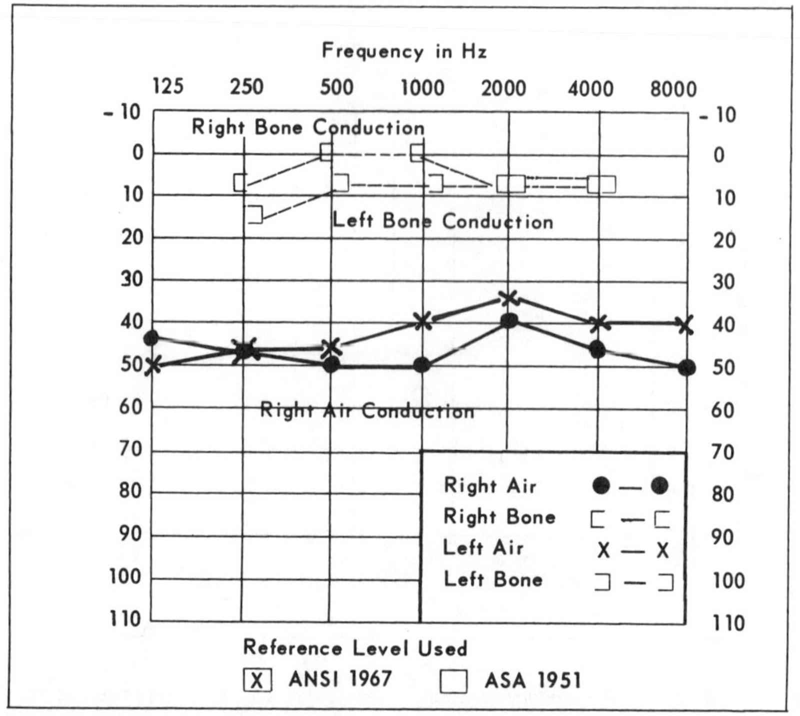

FIG 20–40.
A typical audiogram revealing a conductive loss. The dotted lines at the top show that when the middle ear mechanism is bypassed and the nerve pathway to the brain via the cochlea is measured, sound is easily transmitted, indicating collapsed ear canals or hardened wax in the ear canal. Only bone-conduction evaluation methods can give us this information.

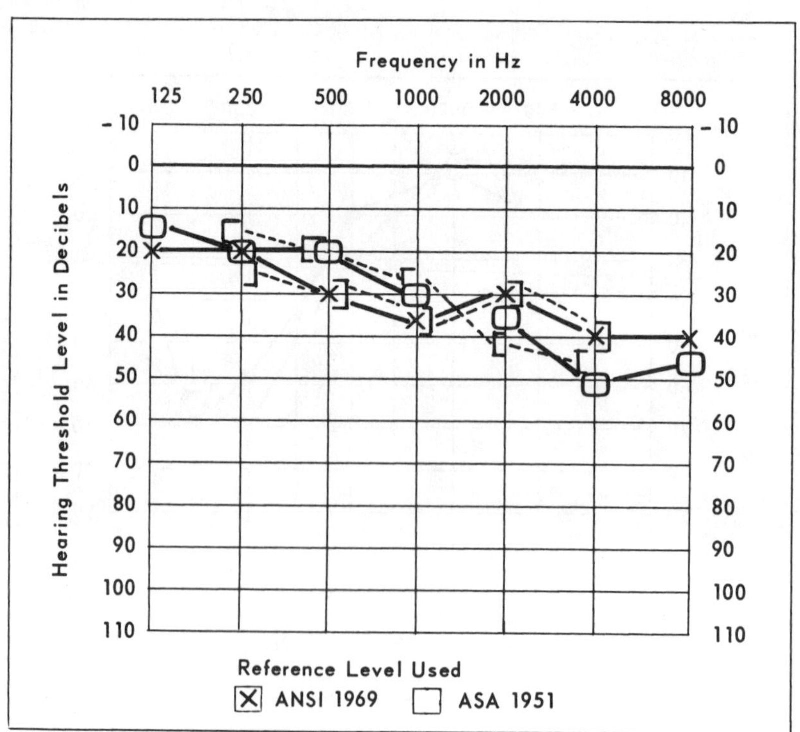

FIG 20–41.
An audiogram revealing sensorineural or nerve-type hearing loss. This person's bone-conduction and air-conduction levels are the same, indicating that there is damage in the cochlea or eighth cranial nerve. Ear surgery would be of no value.

person referring and the physician is urged in cases of doubt.

There are two sections to the following referral criteria: audiological and medical. Workers should undergo screening audiometry by a physician, an audiologist, or an accredited occupational hearing conservationist, on properly calibrated equipment that meets ANSI standards (ANSI S3.6-1969) in a proper test environment. If the test results indicate that the worker should be referred for failure to meet the audiometric standards set forth here, the hearing conservation program director may wish to refer the worker to an audiologist or an otolaryngologist for confirmation. If the audiologist confirms that the worker's hearing level does not meet these criteria, the worker should then be referred to an otolaryngologist for evaluation or treatment.

If a worker has any of the medical problems listed, that worker should be referred directly to an otolaryngologist.

AUDIOLOGICAL CRITERIA

There are two types of audiological criteria, to be applied to baseline and periodic audiograms, respectively. A baseline audiogram is the first audiogram performed; in some cases, this will be a preemployment audiogram. Periodic audiograms, performed yearly, are to be compared to the baseline. The criteria for referral for threshold shifts seen on periodic audiograms (Section B, below) should be clearly distinguished from criteria for threshold shift used to trigger "in-house" action by the hearing conservation program, such as refitting of hearing protectors, or counselling.

The Occupational Safety and Health Administration currently defines a "standard threshold shift" as a shift of 10 dB or more, in either ear, for the puretone average of 2, 3, and 4 kHz; this is intended to detect small changes in hearing so that preventive action can be taken. The criteria for threshold shift listed below, on the other hand, are intended to detect larger changes which are more likely to be significant, both medically and in terms of communicative difficulties.

Program directors may choose to have repeat audiograms done to verify apparent threshold shifts prior to taking action; this should be done within 90 days of the periodic audiogram in question. The criteria should then be applied to the repeat audiogram.

If a periodic audiogram (or retest as described above) demonstrates a "standard threshold shift" as defined by OSHA, this audiogram becomes the new baseline, to which subsequent periodic audiograms will be compared. However, for purposes of otologic referral, the original baseline should continue to be used. Otherwise, a slowly progressive hearing loss could become severe over a period of years: a series of small threshold shifts would occur, each triggering "in-house" action and resulting in a new baseline, but none large enough to result in otologic referral.

In addition to the quantitative criteria listed below, workers showing variable or inconsistent responses or unusual hearing loss curves should be referred.

A. Baseline Audiogram

1. Average hearing level at 0.5, 1, 2, and 3 kHz greater than 25 dB, in either ear.
2. Difference in average hearing level between the better and poorer ears of:
   a. more than 15 dB at 0.5, 1, and 2 kHz, or
   b. more than 30 dB at 3, 4, and 6 kHz.

B. Periodic Audiograms

1. Change for the worse in average hearing level, in either ear, compared to the baseline audiogram of:
   a. more than 15 dB at 0.5, 1, and 2 kHz, or
   b. more than 20 dB at 3, 4, and 6 kHz.

MEDICAL CRITERIA

1. History of ear pain, drainage, dizziness, severe persistent tinnitus, sudden, fluctuating, or rapidly progressive hearing loss, or a feeling of fullness or discomfort in one or both ears within the preceding 12 months.
2. Visible evidence of cerumen accumulation or a foreign body in the ear canal.

If a person has received otologic evaluation previously on the basis of failing the foregoing criteria, he should be re-evaluated if he develops ear pain, drainage, dizziness, disequilibrium, imbalance, or severe persistent tinnitus or shows significant change in hearing levels as defined in Section B above.

In patients with puzzling ear symptoms, such as diplacusis, fullness, and inconsistent audiometric findings, it is better to refer than possibly overlook a significant problem.

Communication between the referring individual and the otolaryngologist is essential.

GLOSSARY

This glossary defines words and terms often used in industrial noise measurements and audiometry. Many definitions were taken from sources listed in the References at the end of this appendix.

A

Accuracy. A statistical measure of the agreement between a quantitative observation and the observed phenomenon—the relationship of the measured value to the actual value.

Acoustic neuroma. Tumor or growth on or of the auditory nerve.

Acoustic trauma. A hearing injury produced by exposure to sudden intense acoustic energy, such as from blasts and explosions or from direct trauma to the head or ear. It should be thought of as one single incident relating to the onset of hearing loss.

Acoustics. Acoustics is the science of sound, including its production, transmission and effects.

Acusis. Normal hearing ability.

Adaptation. A hearing impairment characterized by an inability to hear a tone at threshold level and at uniform intensity. (Also called PATHOLOGIC FATIGUE or ABNORMAL TONE DECAY.)

Air-bone gap. The difference in decibels between the hearing levels for sound at a particular frequency as determined by air-conduction and by bone-conduction threshold measurements.

Air conduction. The process by which sound is conducted to the inner ear through the air in the outer ear canal utilizing the tympanic membrane and the ossicles as part of the pathway.

AMA hearing impairment formula. The American Medical Association formula for hearing impairment.

Ambient noise. The all-encompassing noise associated with a given environment, being usually a composite of sounds from many sources near and far.

American Academy of Ophthalmology and Otolaryngology (AAOO). A professional organization of medical specialists who establish standards pertaining to hearing.

Amplitude. The maximum displacement to either side of the normal or "rest" position of the particles of the medium transmitting the vibration.

ANSI. The American National Standards Institute is a standards-making body.

Aphasia. Loss by the brain of its ability to interpret the input received from the eyes and ears and to send out directing impulses for speaking and writing. It is not due to a mechanical defect in the hearing, speech, or other organs.

Articulation, percent, or Percent intelligibility. Percent articulation or percent intelligibility is the percentage of the speech units spoken by a talker that is understood correctly by a listener.

ASA. American Standards Association, now called ANSI, American National Standards Institute.

Attenuate. To reduce in strength or force. In sound, to reduce the intensity as expressed in decibels.

Audible range. The frequency range over which normal hearing occurs (approximately 20 through 20,000 Hz). For frequencies above 20,000 Hz, the term "ultrasonic" is used; for frequencies below 20 Hz, the term "subsonic" is used.

Audiogram. The chart or table relating hearing level (for pure tones) to frequency. A record of hearing level measured at several different frequencies. The audiogram may be presented graphically or numerically. (Also called a PURE-TONE, AIR-CONDUCTION AUDIOGRAM or a THRESHOLD AUDIOGRAM.)

Audiologist. A hearing specialist who holds a master's or doctorate degree in audiology and is concerned with the complete evaluation of auditory function and the rehabilitation of persons with hearing impairment.

Audiometer, pure-tone. An electroacoustical generator that provides pure tones of selected frequencies and of calibrated output, for the purpose of determining an individual's threshold of audibility.

Audiometric reference level. That sound pressure level (ASA, ISO, or ANSI) to which the audiometer is calibrated. A reference value, at a particular frequency, of the threshold of hearing for normal persons within a given age range, normally 18 to 25 years.

Audiometric room. A room that is intended for testing of hearing, insulated against outside noise.

Audiometric technician. A person who is trained and qualified to administer audiometric examinations for hearing-conservation programs.

Audiometry. 1. The science of dealing with the measurement of the sense of hearing. 2. The testing of the sharpness of hearing.

Auditory. Pertaining to, or involving, the organs of hearing or the sense of hearing, as in the *auditory* nerve.

Auditory acuity. The sharpness of hearing, as in *auditory acuity* test.

Auditory center. The group of nerve cells and structures in the brain concerned with the reception and interpretation of hearing impulses received from the ear; the nerve center concerned with hearing.

Auditory system. The auditory system consists of all parts of the ear and of the auditory nervous system that have to do with the process of hearing.

Aural. Pertaining to, involving, or used for, the ear.

Automatic (recording) audiometry. This method for determining hearing threshold allows the subject to control manually a mechanism that indicates on a graph when the sound is first heard and when the same sound disappears.

A-Weighted sound level. Sound pressure level in decibels as measured on a sound level meter using an A-weighted network. This network attempts to reflect the human ear's decreased sensitivity to low frequency sounds. (See dBA.)

B

Barotrauma. Injury to the ear caused by a sudden alteration in barometric pressure.

Baseline. A measurement of parameters at a specific point in time in order to define existing conditions and especially variations with time.

Basilar membrane. The basilar membrane is the membranous portion of the spiral lamina, which separates the scala media from the scala tympani.

Bel. A scale unit used in the comparison of the magnitudes of powers. The number of bels, expressing the relative magnitudes of two powers, is the logarithm (to the base 10) of the ratio of the powers. (See DECIBEL.)

Bias. Consistent error; a fixed difference between the average, in a set of experimental results, and the true value.

Binaural. Binaural listening is listening with both ears.

Biologic calibration. An audiometric test performed by the technician on a normal-hearing adult who has not been exposed to noise and has no history of ear disease. The results are then compared with the baseline audiogram to see if there is any change in the output level of the audiometer.

Bone conduction. Bone conduction is the process by which sound is conducted to the inner ear through the cranial bones.

Bone conduction hearing level. A measured threshold of hearing by bone conduction excitation, expressed in decibels.

Bone conduction test. A special test conducted by placing an oscillator on the mastoid process to determine the nerve-carrying capacity or efficiency of the cochlea and the eighth cranial nerve leading to the brain.

Bone vibrator. An electromechanical transducer intended to produce the sensation of hearing by vibrating the bones of the head.

Bony labyrinth. The outer hard shell of the inner ear filled with a fluid called perilymph in which a tubular membrane floats.

Broad-band. A wide-frequency range. Sound whose energy is distributed over a broad range of frequency (generally, more than one octave).

C

Calibrate. To check an audiometer for uniformity or accuracy. The two methods of doing this are biologic and electronic.

Cerumen. Earwax.

Cerumenous glands. Glands in the external auditory canal which produce cerumen (or earwax).

CHABA. Committee on Hearing, Bioacoustics, and Biomechanics of the National Academy of Sciences.

Cholesteatoma. A tumor of the middle ear in which the mucous membrane becomes inflamed.

Cochlea. The cochlea is a snail-shell–like cavity in the temporal bone, comprising that part of the labyrinth which contains the essential receptor organs of hearing.

Cochlear duct (or Scala media). A closed passage that occupies the central portion of the interior of the cochlea and that houses the hearing organ or organ of Corti.

Compensation formula. The method of calculating the percentage of hearing impairment. It includes a low fence, high fence, method of averaging hearing levels at specific frequencies, calculation of percentage per decibel impairment and better-ear correction.

Complex tone. A complex tone is a sound wave produced by the combination of components of different frequencies.

Conductive hearing loss. Conductive hearing loss is produced by interference with the conduction of sound in the conducting apparatus, for example, the external or middle ear.

Congenital. Existing at or before birth.

Consonant. Consonants are those speech sounds that involve the obstruction or impeding of the air stream by the articulation of two surfaces. (See VOWELS.)

Continuous spectrum. The spectrum of a wave, the components of which are continuously distributed over a frequency region.

Contralateral. 1. Situated on the opposite side. 2. Acting together with a structure on the opposite side.

Cross-hearing or **cross-talk.** Takes place when sounds delivered to one ear are transmitted either around or through the bones in the head in sufficient quantity to stimulate the opposite ear.

Cycle. An interval of time during which a sequence of changes takes place.

Cycle per second (cps). A unit of frequency. The preferred terminology is hertz, abbreviated Hz.

Cyclic noise levels. Levels that change repetitiously during machine duty cycle.

D

Damage risk criteria. A suggested base line of noise tolerance that, if not exceeded, should result in no hearing loss due to noise.

dBA. Abbreviation for decibels measured on the A-scale of a sound level meter; used in OSHA noise regulations and most environmental noise regulations. (See *A-WEIGHTED SOUND LEVEL*.)

Decibel. A decibel is 1/10 bel. The abbreviation *dB* is commonly used for the term decibel, a unit for measuring the level of a sound. The decibel is based on a ratio expressing how much greater a sound level is above a specified reference level. Two powers P_1 and P_2 are said to be separated by an interval of n bels (or 10n decibels) when $n = \log_{10} (P_1/P_2)$.

Difference limen. A difference limen is the increment in a stimulus which is just noticed in a specified fraction of the trials. The relative difference limen is the ratio of the difference limen to the absolute magnitude of the stimulus to which it is related.

Diplacusis. A difference of perception of sound by the two ears, either in time or in pitch, so that one sound is heard as two.

Disability. Medicolegal term signifying loss of function and earning power.

Disablement. Medicolegal term signifying loss of function without loss of earning power.

Discrimination. The ability of the hearing apparatus to discern discrete, particular signals in a complex sound field.

Discrimination loss. Discrimination loss is the difference in percent between the normal discrimination score for the test and the score obtained for the ear under test.

Discrimination score for speech. The percent of items in an appropriate form of hearing test, usually repeated, written down, or checked by the listener.

Dispersion. The spread of values of a variable about the mean or the median.

Dizziness. An imprecise term commonly used to describe various peculiar subjective symptoms such as faintness, giddiness, lightheadedness, or unsteadiness. (See also *VERTIGO*.)

Dosimeter. A device worn on the person for determining the accumulated sound exposure with regard to level and time.

Dyne per square centimeter. Physical unit of sound pressure.

E

Eardrum. The eardrum (tympanic membrane) is a conically shaped membrane that is stretched across the end of the external auditory meatus. It marks the boundary between the external and middle ears.

Earphone (receiver). An earphone is an electroacoustic transducer intended in audiometry to be closely coupled acoustically to the ear.

Eighth cranial nerve. A composite sensory nerve consisting of the cochlear and vestibular nerves that transmit auditory signals to the brain for interpretation.

Electroacoustic transducer. A transducer for receiving waves from an electric system and delivering waves to an acoustic system, or vice versa.

Endolymph. A fluid which fills the membranous labyrinth and bathes the hearing and balance organs.

End organ. The end organ of a receptor system is the mechanism by which stimulus energy is transduced to nervous activity. In hearing, the end organ within the cochlea usually refers to the organ of Corti.

Etiology. The study of the cause of disease.

Eustachian tube. A tube approximately 2½ in (63 mm) long leading from the back of the throat of the middle ear. It equalizes the pressure of air in the middle ear with that outside the eardrum.

Evoked response audiometry. Refers to the use of the electroencephalogram with a summing or averaging computer. This makes possible the evaluation of slight changes in electrical activity of the brain in response to a sound stimulus.

External auditory meatus. The external auditory meatus is a canal that extends from the pinna, inward to the eardrum.

External ear. The external ear consists of the pinna and the external auditory meatus. (See *PINNA*.)

External otitis. Inflammation or infection of the outer ear.

F

Fatigue. Auditory fatigue is the difference (in decibels) between the threshold of audibility after acoustic stimulation and the threshold before such stimulation. The amount of fatigue must be stated for a given time, or as a function of time.

Fence. See *HIGH FENCE* and *LOW FENCE*.

Fenestration. An operation in which the oval window, which has been made inoperative through a fixation of the stapes, is bypassed and a window is created in the horizontal semicircular canal. The new opening is covered by a skin flap so that sound vibrations are able to reach the inner ear.

Filter. A device for separating components of a signal on the basis of frequency. It allows components in one or more frequency bands to pass relatively unattenuated.

Frequency. The rate of repetition of a periodic quantity. Frequency may be expressed in hertz (Hz), kilohertz (kHz), or megahertz (MHz). The rate at which a sound source vibrates or makes the air vibrate determines its frequency. The unit of time is usually one second and the term hertz (Hz) is used to designate the number of cycles per second. Frequency is related to the subjective sensation of pitch. In speech, consonants are usually high frequency sounds while vowels are low frequency.

Frequency bands. A division of the audible range of frequencies into subgroups for detailed analysis of sound.

Functional hearing loss (psychogenic). A hearing impairment due to nonorganic causes, that is, psychologic.

Fundamental frequency. The fundamental frequency is the lowest natural frequency. The normal mode of vibration associated with this frequency is known as the FUNDAMENTAL MODE.

H

Handicap. See *HEARING HANDICAP*.

Harmonic. A harmonic is a component of a complex tone whose frequency is an integral multiple of the fundamental frequency of the complex tone.

Headphone or **Head receiver.** An earphone attached to a head band which holds the earphone to the ear.

Hearing. The subjective response to sound, and the nervous and cerebral operations which translate the physical stimuli into meaningful signals.

Hearing aid. An electronic device, fitted to the ear, that amplifies sound.

Hearing conservation. The prevention or minimizing of noise-induced hearing loss through the use of hearing protection devices and the control of noise through engineering methods or administrative procedures.

Hearing handicap. The disadvantage imposed by impairment sufficient to affect one's efficiency in the situation of everyday living.

Hearing impairment. A deviation or change for the worse in either structure or function, usually outside the normal hearing range.

Hearing level. A measured threshold of hearing at a specified frequency, expressed in decibels relative to a specified standard of normal hearing. The deviation in decibels of an individual's threshold from the zero reference of the audiometer.

Hearing loss. An increase in the threshold of audibility, at specific frequencies, as the result of normal aging, disease, or injury to the hearing organs. It is the symptom of reduced auditory sensitivity, synonymous with auditory impairment, when a specific cause can be ascribed. Also used, in a general sense, to describe the process of losing auditory sensitivity. Types of hearing loss are as follows:

1. CONDUCTIVE. A hearing loss originating in the conductive mechanism of the ear.
2. SENSORINEURAL. A hearing loss originating in the cochlea or the fibers of the auditory nerve. (Formerly called PERCEPTIVE DEAFNESS.)
3. NOISE INDUCED. A sensorineural hearing loss attributed to the effects of noise.

Hearing loss (hearing level) for speech. The difference in decibels between the speech levels at which the average normal ear and the defective ear, respectively, reach the same intelligibility, often arbitrarily set at 50 percent.

Hearing threshold level (HTL). Amount (in decibels) by which the threshold of audibility for that ear exceeds a standard audiometric threshold.

Hertz (Hz). Synonymous term for CYCLES PER SECOND. Most standardizing agencies have adopted hertz as the preferred unit of frequency. (See *FREQUENCY*.)

High fence. Point of 100 percent hearing impairment, dependent upon the specific compensation formula.

High-frequency loss. A hearing impairment, starting with 2,000 Hz and upward.

Hyperacusis. Abnormal acuteness of hearing, due to increased irritability of sensorineural mechanism.

Hypoacusis. Hearing impairment attributed to deficiency in the peripheral organs of hearing; may be conductive or sensorineural.

I

Impact. A collision of one mass in motion with a second mass, which may be either in motion or at rest.

Impact noise. The noise resulting from the collision of two masses.

Impairment. See *HEARING IMPAIRMENT*.

Impulse noise. Impulse noises are usually considered to be singular noise pulses, each less than one second in duration, or repetitive noise pulses occurring at greater than one second intervals. Also defined as a "change of sound pressure of 40 dB or more within 0.5 seconds."

Industrial audiometry. The use of audiometric procedures in an industrial hearing-conservation program.

Industrial hygiene. That science or art which devotes itself to the recognition, evaluation, and control of those environmental factors arising in or from the workplace that may cause impaired health or significant discomfort among workers or residents of the community.

Instantaneous sound pressure. The instantaneous sound pressure at a given point is the total instantaneous pressure at that point minus the static pressure at that point. The commonly used unit is the microbar.

Intelligibility. See *ARTICULATION*.

Ipsilateral. Pertaining to or located on the same side; as in *ipsilateral* paralysis of the limbs, paralysis of the arm and leg on the same side of the body.

ISO. International Organization for Standardization. Publications are available through ANSI.

L

Labyrinth. The labyrinth is the system of intercommunicating canals and cavities that make up the inner ear.

Level. A quantity related to power. The ratio, expressed in decibels, of the magnitude of the quantity to a specified reference magnitude.

Localization (Auditory localization). When a listener is asked to localize a sound, he is expected to report the direction of the sound source, or its distance, or both. In physiology, localization is also used to refer to a place in the nervous or other systems where a certain process is mediated.

Loudness. Loudness is the intensive attribute of an auditory sensation, in terms of which sounds may be ordered on a scale extending from soft to loud. Loudness depends primarily upon the sound pressure of the stimulus, but it also depends upon the frequency and waveform of the stimulus.

Loudness level. The loudness level of a sound is measured by the sound pressure level of a standard pure tone of specified frequency which is assessed by normal observers as being equally loud.

Low fence. The hearing threshold level at which hearing impairment begins as defined in a specific compensation formula.

M

Malingerer. One who pretends deafness or other abnormalities.

Masking. Masking is the amount by which the threshold of audibility of a sound is raised by the presence of another (masking) sound.

Mastoid. The mastoid process extends downward from the temporal bone behind the external auditory meatus.

Meniere's disease. The combination of deafness, tinnitus, and vertigo.

Method of adjustment (Method of averaging error). The method of adjustment is a procedure for measuring either the differential or the absolute hearing threshold. The observer controls the independent stimulus-dimension and sets it according to experimental instructions; for example, "just audible," "just noticeably different," or "just intelligible."

Method of constant stimuli. The method of constant stimuli is a procedure for measuring the differential or absolute hearing threshold. Stimuli are presented in discrete categories of the independent-stimulus dimension. The observer responds with a "yes" or "no," "same" or "different" after each stimulus presentation.

Method of limits (Method of serial exploration). A procedure for measuring the differential or absolute hearing threshold. In the method of limits, the experimenter gradually increases or decreases either a stimulus dimension or a difference between two stimuli and notes the change in the observer's response (for example, from audibility to inaudibility, or vice versa).

Microbar or **Dyne per square centimeter.** A microbar is a unit of pressure used in acoustics. One microbar is equal to 1 dyne/sq cm.

Microphone. A microphone is an electroacoustic transducer that responds to sound waves and delivers essentially equivalent electric waves.

Middle ear. The middle ear consists of the cavity containing the auditory ossicles.

Monoaural hearing. The perception of sound by stimulation of a single ear.

N

Narrow band. Applies to a narrow band of transmitted waves, with neither of the critical or cutoff frequencies of the filter being zero or infinite.

Neural. Of, or relating to, or affecting a nerve or the nervous system.

Neuritis. Inflammation of a nerve.

Neuroma. A general term indicating a tumor on or of the nerve. On the basis of newer knowledge, such tumors (or neoplasms) are now classified in more specific categories, for example, ganglioneuroma or neurinoma.

NIOSH. National Institute for Occupational Safety and Health—the federal research arm in safety and health.

NIPTS. Abbreviation of noise-induced permanent threshold shift.

Noise. Sound which is undesired by the recipient.

Noise exposure. A generic term signifying the total acoustic stimulus applied to the ear over a period of time.

Noise-induced hearing loss. This terminology is usually restricted to mean the slowly progressive sensorineural hearing loss which results from exposure to continuous noise over a long period of time.

Noise-induced permanent threshold shift. A permanent reduction in hearing level caused by noise.

Noise level. A level of noise, the type of which must be indicated by further modifier or context. The physical quantity measured, the instrument used, and the band width or other weighting characteristics must be indicated.

Normal threshold of hearing. The modal value of the thresholds of hearing of a large number of otologically normal observers between 18 and 25 years of age.

Nystagmus. An abnormal and involuntary movement of the eyes—side to side, up and down, or rotary.

O

Octave. An octave is the interval between two tones when they are separated either by a frequency ratio of 2:1 or by a musical interval of 12 semitones. An octave is the pitch interval between two tones such that one tone may be regarded as duplicating the basic musical import of the other tone at the nearest possible higher pitch.

Octave band. A division of the audible range of frequencies into subgroups such that in each division the upper frequency limit is twice the lower limit. The center frequencies used to designate the octaves are twice the center frequency of the preceding octave band.

Organ of Corti. An aggregation of nerve cells lying on the basilar membrane which picks up vibrations and transmits them to the brain, where they are interpreted as sound. The heart of the hearing mechanism.

Ossicles, auditory. Any one of the small bones such as the malleus, incus, or stapes which forms a chain for the transmission of sound from the tympanic membrane to the oval window.

Otitis media. Inflammation and infection of the middle ear.

Otogenous. Originating within the ear, especially from inflammation of the ear.

Otolaryngologist. A physician specializing in the practice of otology (ear disease), rhinology (nose disease), and laryngology (throat and larynx diseases).

Otologist. A physician who has specialized in surgery and diseases of the ear.

Otology. That branch of medicine that is concerned with the ear.

Otomycosis. An infection due to fungus in the external auditory canal.

Otorrhea. A discharge or running from the ear; said especially of a discharge containing pus.

Otosclerosis. Growth of bony tissue about the foot plate of the stapes and the oval window of the inner ear.

Otoscope. An instrument, usually provided with a lens and an illuminating system, for inspecting the ear, especially the external auditory meatus and the eardrum.

Oval window. The oval window is an opening in the middle ear. The stapes (third ossicle) is attached to a membrane that is stretched across this window.

P

Paget's disease. A generalized skeletal disease of older persons of unknown cause, involving a thickening and softening of the bones, as in the skull and ear.

Pain, threshold of. A sound pressure level sufficiently high to produce the sensation of pain in the human ear (usually above 120 dBA).

Paracusis Willisii. The sensation of a deafened person indicating that he can hear better in a noisy area.

Pascal. A unit of pressure. Unit symbol: Pa; 1 Pa = 1N/sq m or 10 dynes/sq cm.

Perceptive (nerve-type) hearing loss. The perceptive hearing loss involving pathologic conditions of the end organs or nervous system.

Perilymph. A fluid which fills the bony labyrinth, similar in composition to cerebrospinal fluid.

Permanent threshold shift. The component of threshold shift which shows no progressive reduction with the passage of time when the apparent cause has been removed.

Phonetically balanced list. A PB list is a list of monosyllabic words that contain a distribution of speech sounds that approximates the distribution of the same sounds as they occur in conversational "American English."

Phonetics. Phonetics is the study of the description and analysis of the sounds of speech.

Pinna (Auricle). The pinna is that portion of the external ear that projects outward from the side of the head.

Pitch. That attribute of auditory sensation in terms of which sound may be ordered on a scale related primarily to frequency.

Presbycusis. Deterioration in hearing caused by the aging process.

Pressure. Pressure is a measure of force divided by the area to which the force is applied. Usually measured in dynes per square centimeter.

Psychoacoustics. That branch of psychophysics that has to do with acoustic stimuli.

Psychogenic deafness. Deafness originating in or produced by the mental reaction of an individual to his physical or social environment. This is sometimes called FUNCTIONAL DEAFNESS and FEIGNED DEAFNESS.

Psychophysics. Psychophysics is the study of the relations between physical stimuli and the responses to which they give rise.

Pulse. A term more generic than impact and including impact and impulse.

Pure tone. A sound in which the sound pressure varies sinusoidally with time, characterized by its singleness of pitch.

Pure-tone audiogram. A record or chart that compares the hearing sensitivity of an individual in detecting faint pure tones. Usually shown as a graph or table depicting hearing thresholds in decibels at various frequencies.

Pure-tone audiometer. An instrument that provides pure tones for measuring hearing acuity.

R

Random noise. Noise due to the aggregate of a large number of elementary disturbances with random occurrence in time.

Receiver. See *EARPHONE*.

Recruitment. The condition where faint or moderate sounds cannot be heard while at the same time there is little or no loss in the sense of loudness of loud sounds. The condition in which an individual perceives an abnormally rapid increase in loudness as the sound pressure goes up. Usually characteristic of severe sensorineural deafness.

Repeatability. The ability of a transducer to reproduce an output reading when the same measure and value is applied to it repeatedly, under the same conditions, and in the same direction.

Response. The response of a device or system is a quantitative expression of the output as a function of the input under conditions which must be explicitly stated. The response characteristic, often presented graphically, gives the response as a function of some independent variable such as frequency.

S

Scala media. See *COCHLEAR DUCT*.

Semicircular canals. Organs of balance and space orientation located in the inner ear.

Sensation. A sensation is said to have occurred when an observer responds in an appropriate way after a stimulus has been presented.

Sensorineural. A hearing loss originating in the cochlea or the fibers of the auditory nerve.

Serous or **Secretory otitis media.** A condition in which fluid is present behind the eardrum. This can affect the ability of the middle ear to conduct sound to the inner ear.

Simple tone (pure tone). A simple tone is a sound wave, the instantaneous sound pressure of which is a simple sinusoidal function of the time.

Sinusoid. A sinusoid is any waveform that has the same shape as a sine wave, a graph relating the sine of an angle to the size of the angle.

Sociocusis. Hearing loss resulting from the cumulative effects of daily nonindustrial noise exposure.

Sound. Mechanical disturbance, propagated in an elastic medium, of such character as to be capable of exciting the sensation of hearing.

Sound level. A weighted value of the sound pressure level as determined by a sound level meter.

Sound level meter. An instrument designed to measure a frequency-weighted value of the sound pressure level. It consists of a microphone, amplifier, and indicating display, having a declared performance in terms of frequency response, rectification characteristic, and ballistic response.

Sound power of a source. The total sound energy radiated per unit time. The unit is the watt: symbol W.

Sound pressure. At a point in a sound field. The alternating component of the pressure at the point. The unit is the newton per square meter (N/sq m).

Sound pressure level. The sound pressure level of a sound, in decibels, is equal to 20 times the logarithm to the base 10 of the ratio of the sound pressure to the reference sound pressure. In case of doubt, the reference sound pressure should be stated. In the absence of any statement to the contrary, the reference sound pressure in air is taken to be 2×10^{-5} N/sq m (equals 2×10^{-4} dyne/sq m).

Sound propagation. The wave process whereby sound energy is transferred from one part of a medium to another.

Sound transmission. The transfer of sound energy from one medium to another.

Sound wave. A disturbance whereby energy is transmitted in a medium by virtue of the inertial, elastic, and other dynamic properties of the medium. Usually the passage of a wave involves only temporary departure of the state of the medium from its equilibrium state.

Spectrum. Spectrum is used to signify a continuous range of components, usually wide in extent, within which waves have some specified common characteristics; for example, audiofrequency spectrum.

Speech. Speech is one process by which human beings communicate with other human beings. (We have restricted the use of the term to those instances in which sounds are produced by a talker and are received by a listener.) The term may refer to physiologic, psychologic, or physical aspects of the hearing process.

Speech perception test. A measurement of hearing acuity by the administration of a carefully controlled list of words. The identification of correct responses is evaluated in terms of norms established by the average performance of normal listeners.

Speech reading. Also called lip reading or visual hearing. The interpretation of head, lips, and face as an aid to communication by speech.

Spondee words. Standardized word list composed of two-syllable words equally stressed on both syllables.

Stapedectomy. A corrective operation for otosclerosis. The stapes can be removed and replaced by a prosthetic device.

Stapedius. The small muscle connecting the rear wall of the middle ear cavity to the head of the stapes.

T

Temporary threshold shift. The component of threshold shift which shows progressive reduction with the passage of time when the apparent cause has been removed.

Threshold. The lowest level at which the subject can detect the presence of the test frequency at least 50 percent of the time.

Threshold of audibility (threshold of detectability). The threshold of audibility for a specified signal is the medium effective sound pressure of the signal that is capable of evoking an auditory sensation in a specified fraction of the trials. The characteristics of the signal, the manner in which it is presented to the listener, and the point at which the sound pressure is measured must be specified.

Threshold of feeling (or discomfort, tickle, or pain). The threshold of feeling (or discomfort, tickle, or pain) for a specified signal is the minimum effective sound pressure of that signal which, in a specified fraction of the trials, will stimulate the ear to a point at which there is the sensation of feeling (or discomfort, tickle, or pain).

Threshold of hearing. The value of the hearing threshold level which excites the sensation of hearing. The point at which a person just begins to notice the tone is becoming audible.

Threshold of intelligibility. The threshold of intelligibility for speech is the level at which the speech must be presented so that the listener will repeat correctly 50 percent of the test items.

Threshold shift. The deviation, in decibels, of a measured hearing threshold level from one previously established.

Timbre (musical quality). Timbre is that attribute of auditory sensation in terms of which a listener can judge that two sounds similarly presented and having the same loudness and pitch are dissimilar. (For example, one should be able to distinguish between the same notes played on a trumpet or a clarinet).

Tinnitus. A subjective sense of "noises in the head" or "ringing in the ears" for which there is no observable cause.

Tone. A sound that gives a definite pitch sensation. Sometimes, also, the physical stimulus giving rise to the sensation.

Tone deafness. The inability to make a close discrimination between fundamental tones close together in pitch.

Transducer. A device designed to receive oscillatory energy from one system and to supply related oscillatory energy to another.

Tympanic cavity. The space between the drum membrane and the bony capsule of the inner ear.

Tympanic membrane. Eardrum or drumhead.

V

Vertigo. The sensation of a person that objects are turning in circles around him. Sensation of movement causing unsteadiness.

Vestibular mechanism. The balance portion of the inner ear, consisting of the UTRICLE, the SACCULE and three SEMICIRCULAR CANALS. (See also *SEMICIRCULAR CANALS*.)

Vowel. A vowel, one of two types of speech sounds, is a continuous complex sound initiated by the vocal cords and modified by the nasal, oral, and pharyngeal cavities. (See *CONSONANT*.)

W

Wave. A wave is a disturbance that is propagated in a medium in such a manner that at any point in the medium, the displacement is a function of the time, while at any instant the displacement at a point is a function of the position of the point.

Waveform. The waveform of a sound is a graph showing the instantaneous amplitude, pressure, or intensity as a function of time.

Wavelength. Of a sinusoidal plane progressive wave. The perpendicular distance between two wavefronts in which the phases differ by one complete period.

White noise. A noise whose spectral density (or spectrum level) is substantially independent of frequency over a specified range. White noise need not be random.

Wide-band. Applies to a wide band of transmitted waves, with neither of the critical or cutoff frequencies of the filter being zero or infinite.

BIBLIOGRAPHY

American Industrial Hygiene Association (AIHA): *Industrial Noise Manual*, ed 3. Akron, Oh, 1975.

American National Standards Institute (ANSI): *Acoustical Terminology*, S1.1–1960.

Manual for Hearing Conservationist, Council for Accreditation in Occupational Hearing Conservation. Cherry Hill, NJ, Fischler's Printing, 1978.

Harris CM: *Handbook of Noise Control*, ed 2. New York, McGraw-Hill Book Co, 1979.

Newby HA: *Audiology*, ed 4. Englewood Cliffs, NJ, Prentice Hall, Inc. 1979.

Olishifski JB, Harford ER: *Industrial Noise and Hearing Conservation*. Chicago, National Safety Council, 1975.

Petersen Arnold PG, Gross Ervin E Jr: *Handbook of Noise Measurement*, ed 7. West Concord, Mass, General Radio Co., 1972.

Sataloff J, Michael P: *Hearing Conservation*. Springfield, Ill, Charles C Thomas, 1973.

Schmidt JE: *Paramedical Dictionary*. Springfield, Ill, Charles C Thomas, 1969.

Stedman's Medical Dictionary, ed 22. Baltimore, Williams & Wilkins Co, 1972.

Yerges Lyle F: *Sound, Noise, and Vibration Control*. New York, Van Nostrand Reinhold Co., 1969.

REFERENCES

1. *Acoustics Handbook*. Palo Alto, Cal, Hewlett-Packard Co, 1968.
2. American National Standards Institute, New York: *Criteria for Background Noise in the Audiometer Room*, S3.1–1960 (R–1971). *Specifications for Audiometers*, S3.6-1969 (R-1973).
3. *Analysis of Workers' Compensation Laws*. Washington, DC, Chamber of Commerce of the United States, 1984.
4. *Background for Loss of Hearing Claims*, ed 3. Schaumburg, Ill, Alliance of American Insurers, 1984.
5. Beranek LL (ed): *Noise and Vibration Control*. New York, McGraw-Hill Book Co, 1971.
6. Broch JT: *Acoustic Noise Measurements*. Cleveland, Oh, Burel & Kjaer, 1971.
7. Burns W: *Noise and Man*. Philadelphia, JB Lippincott Co, 1969.
8. *Criteria For a Recommended Standard—Occupational Exposure to Noise*, HSM 73-11001, National Institute for Occupational Safety and Health. Washington, DC, US Government Printing Office, 1972.
9. Davis H, Silverman SR (eds): *Hearing and Deafness*. New York, Holt, Rinehart, and Winston, 1970.
10. *Disability evaluation under Social Security—A handbook for physicians*, HEW Publication No. (SSA) 70-10089. Washington, DC, US Government Printing Office, 1979.
11. *Environmental Quality—The Tenth Annual Report of the Council on Environmental Quality*. Washington, DC, US Government Printing Office, 1979.
12. Fletcher H: *Speech and Hearing*. New York, D Van Nostrand Co, 1929.
13. Fox MS: Hearing loss statutes in the United States and Canada. *National Safety News*, October 1976, pp 48–54.
14. Ginnold RE: *Occupational Hearing Loss—Workers' Compensation Under State and Federal Programs*, US Environmental Protection Agency. Washington, DC, US Government Printing Office, 1979.
15. Glorig A: *Audiometry Principles and Practices*. Baltimore, Williams & Wilkins Co, 1965.
16. Glorig A, House WF: The importance of occupational and medical history of patients suspected of having occupational hearing loss. *Noise Control* 1958; 5:36.
17. Gosztonyi RE Jr, Vallallo LS, Sataloff J: Audiometric reliability in industry. *Arch Environ Health* 1971; 22:113–118.
18. Guide for conservation of hearing in noise, revised. *Trans Am Acad Ophthalmol Otolaryngol* 1959; March-April, pp 167–168.
19. *Guide for the Evaluation of Hearing Handicap*. American Academy of Otolaryngology Committee on Hearing and Equilibrium, and the American Council of Otolaryngology Committee on the Medical Aspects of Noise. *JAMA* 1979; 241:2055–2059.
20. *Guides to the Evaluation of Permanent Impairment*. Chicago, American Medical Association, Committee on Rating of Mental and Physical Impairment, 1979.
21. Harris CM (ed): *Handbook of Noise Control*. New York, McGraw-Hill Book Co, 1979.
22. Hutchison MK, (ed): *A Guide to the Work-Relatedness of Disease*, NIOSH Publication No 77–123. Washington, DC, US Government Printing Office, 1976.
23. *Industrial Noise Manual*, ed 3. Akron, Oh, American Industrial Hygiene Association, 1975.
24. Kryter KD: *The Effects of Noise on Man*. New York, Academic Press, 1970.
25. Lahti T, Pekkarinen J, Starck J: New noise level definition. *Work Health Safety* (Helsinki), 1984, p 24.
26. *Manual for Hearing Conservationist*. Council for Accreditation in Occupational Hearing Conservation. Cherry Hill, NJ, Fischler's Printing, 1978.
27. National Institute for Occupational Safety and Health: *The Industrial Environment—Its Evaluation and Control*. Washington, DC, US Government Printing Office, 1973.
28. Newby HA: *Audiology*, ed 4. Englewood Cliffs, NJ, Prentice Hall, Inc, 1979.

28a. Noise and Hearing Conservation Manual: Akron, Ohio, American Industrial Hygiene Association, 1987.

29. Olishifski JB, Harford ER: *Industrial Noise and Hearing Conservation*. Chicago, National Safety Council, 1975.
30. Paparella M, Schumrick DA (eds): *Otolaryngology*, vol 2, *The Ear*. Philadelphia, WB Saunders Co, 1973.
31. Petersen APG, Gross EE Jr: *Handbook of Noise Measurement*, ed 7. West Concord, Mass, General Radio Co, 1972.
32. Principles for the evaluation of hearing impairment. Council on Physical Medicine and Rehabilitation. *JAMA* 1955; 157:1408–1409.
33. Schuknecht HF: *Pathology of the Ear*. Cambridge, Mass, Harvard University Press, 1974.

34. Sataloff J, Michael P: *Hearing Conservation*. Springfield, Ill, Charles C Thomas, 1973.
34a. Ultrasound: Environmental Health Criteria 22, Geneva, World Health Organization, 1982.
35. Workers' compensation programs for hearing loss. *Sound and Vibration* October 1979; p 36.
36. *Your Body at Work: Human Physiology and the Working Environment*, Delin B (ed). Stockholm, Sweden, Arbetsmiljö/Föreningen för arbetarskydd (Working Environment/The Environment Association), Kungsholms hamnplan 3, S–112 20, 1984.

21

Occupational Vibration

William Taylor, M.D., Sc.D.

Donald E. Wasserman, M.S.E.E.

Noise and vibration in industry frequently emanate from the same source. The cause-effect relationship between noise and noise-induced deafness is clearly established—one can measure the level of noise at the workplace and determine how much hearing damage may be expected in employees. In the case of vibration, however, the relationship between exposure and the resulting health effects has not been fully established. Thus, vibration has been recognized relatively recently as a trauma-inducing physical agent.

Occupational exposure to vibration arises in many different ways, reaching the subject at levels that are disturbing to comfort, health, safety, and efficiency. In the case of *whole-body vibration,* transmission to the subject may be through supporting structures, such as the seat of a helicopter or the deck of a ship. Subjects often have their whole bodies vibrated in work processes that use vibration intentionally, such as in compacting or grading coal or in vibrating concrete molds (which prevents blow holes in the final castings).

In other industrial work processes, the route of entry to the human body is through the hands, wrists, and arms of the subject—so-called *segmental* or *hand-arm* vibration. The earliest hand-held pneumatic drills were used in France around 1840. Hand-vibrating tools were used for rock-drilling (jack-leg drills) by the turn of the century, for chipping and grinding in foundries in the 1930s, and in forestry operations (chain saws) in the 1950s. Because of the high vibration levels on the chain-saw handles and the new techniques in which chain saws were used for felling, debranching, and cross-cutting, all countries that produce timber reported an increasing incidence of segmental vibration effects in their sawyers.

Dividing the effects of vibration into the categories of (1) whole-body and (2) hand-arm or segmental is the approach already adopted in vibration research, in engineering vibration reduction programs, and in setting regulatory standards and recommended vibration limits. By international agreement, separate draft standards have been drawn up governing whole-body and segmental hand-arm systems. The purpose of this chapter is to acquaint the reader with the dose-effect relationships and to provide insight into the engineering aspects of draft regulations.[6, 18, 19] In addition, physicians who treat patients exposed to vibration need to know the general principles involved in the recognition, evaluation, and control of vibration as a health hazard.

THE MEASUREMENT OF VIBRATION

To define vibration, several parameters similar to those used in noise definition are universally used: frequency, amplitude, direction of application with respect to an anatomical axis, duration of exposure, and whether the stimulus is continuous or interrupted. The units that are interrelated are frequency (in Hertz or cycles per second), amplitude (displacement in meters), and acceleration (rate of change of velocity, in meters per second squared, m/s^2, and gravitational g units, where $1\ g = 9.8\ m/s^2$). Since the vibration impinging on workers is never a pure oscillation (a rare condition) but always complex, being composed of many frequencies at varying accelerations, spectrum analysis and averaging techniques are used universally (and increasingly so with the aid of solid state computers). These display, respectively, the vibration "finger print" impinging on workers and the root mean square (rms) levels over a known frequency band width. The signal fed into this instrumentation is initially obtained from the electrical output of an accelerometer (e.g., a small mass pressing against a piezo-electric crystal) mounted on the workpiece—for example, the handle of a chain saw or chipping hammer. Since vibration is a vector quantity (magnitude and direction), measurements in three mutually perpendicular directions are needed. Thus, three accelerometers are mounted mutually perpendicular on a cube to obtain the vector sum results.

The subject of units is, however, further complicated by the desire of instrument manufacturers for a single-figure unit for vibration. As in noise, the level (or acceleration) may be quoted in logarithmic units as decibels (dB), a particularly useful representation for quoting filtered or "weighted" levels when a single-figure unit is required for regulatory purposes. Vibration meters are now available for general-purpose vibration measurement and frequency analyses reading acceleration, velocity and displacement, rms function, and direct decibel measurement, which is useful for field work. Since the vibration dose depends on the operator's vibration exposure time, integrating vibration meters are also available, giving digital readouts of the percentage of permitted exposure according to International Organization of Standardization (ISO) Draft Recommendations (equivalent to the Leq Regulations in noise). In vibration work it is important to know in which directions the vibration forces are being applied. These are agreed upon internationally: fore and aft is the X axis; side to side, the Y axis; and vertical (cephalo-caudal), the Z axis.

Many scientists have difficulty with the acceleration unit, m/sec^2. At frequencies around 30–60 Hz, which coincide with the impacting frequencies of pneumatic, impulse, and rock drills, and foundry chipping hammers, high accelerations with peak values around 1,000–2,000 m/sec^2 are generated, with small displacements of the order of fractions of a millimeter. At frequencies around 1 Hz and below, which are found in large ships and semisubmersible oil exploration platforms, an amplitude or displacement of several meters is required to generate appreciable acceleration.

The human response to vibration depends to a marked degree on *resonance*, where maximum vibration energy is transmitted from the vibrating source to the person, who in turn actually amplifies this incoming energy, exacerbating the vibration effects. The characteristic frequencies and amplification factors will be determined by the *mass*, the *elasticity*, and the *damping* within the human body (Fig 21–1).

WHOLE-BODY VIBRATION

Many of the physiologic responses of human beings to vibration are frequency-dependent, limited to a narrow band reflecting the mechanical resonance of elastic structures within the body. Airborne noise of sufficient intensity and of low frequency below 100 Hz can also enter the body by direct absorption to excite nonauditory sense organs. The known frequency-dependent effects of both vibration and low-frequency noise are illustrated diagrammatically in Figure 21–2. Extensions of the horizontal lines by means of dots indicate extensions of the frequency ranges for which research evidence is meager. Where the response is largely psychologic, the autonomic nervous system reacts to noise and whole-body and segmental vibration through the so-called 'stress' reaction, the signs and symptoms of which have been extensively studied in the Soviet Union and East Europe.

In the past, research efforts concerning the effects of whole-body vibration on man both in the United States and in the United Kingdom have been mainly military-orientated, with studies conducted with fit, young, Army, Navy, and Air Force personnel. In the United States in the early 1970s, Wasserman and his colleagues[42] conducted a 45-plant walk-through survey and estimated that approximately 6.8 million workers were exposed to whole-body vibration (1.2 million to hand-arm vibration) in heavy equipment operations, trucking, farming, and bus driving. In the United Kingdom, nonmilitary, occupational research on whole-body vibration has been neglected, in contrast to the many publications (550) arising from the use of hand-held vibratory tools since the early 1900s.

In broad terms, human tolerance of whole-body vibration is lowest (in resonance) in the 4–8-Hz band, and the principal resonance of the seated, recumbent, or standing human body vibrated in the Z axis (cephalocaudal) occurs in the region of 5 Hz. Accordingly, current recommended limits for human exposure expressed in terms of acceleration, as a function of frequency (1–80 Hz), are set at their lowest in the 4–8-Hz band.[18] In contrast, when a subject is vibrated in the X axis (anteroposterior) or Y axis (lat-

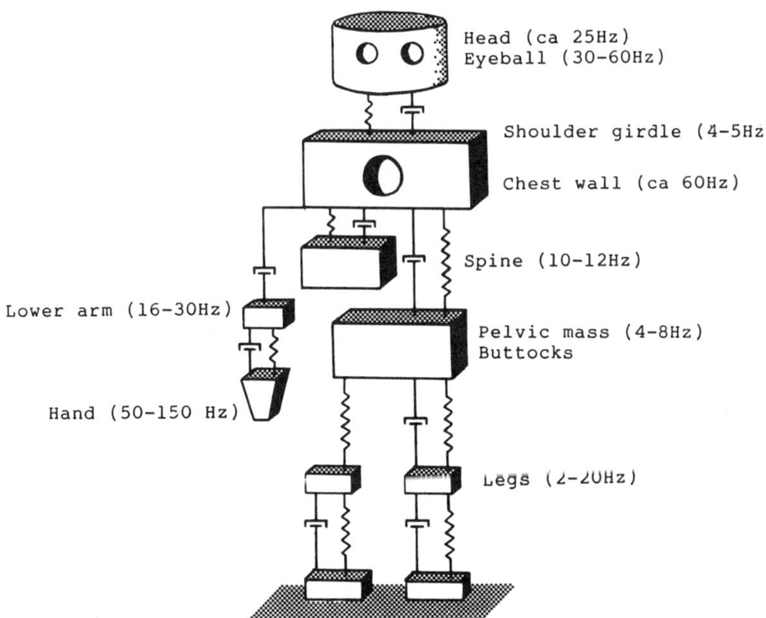

FIG 21–1.
Simplified mechanical system representing the human body. (From Brüel & Kjaer: *Technical Review,* No 1.)

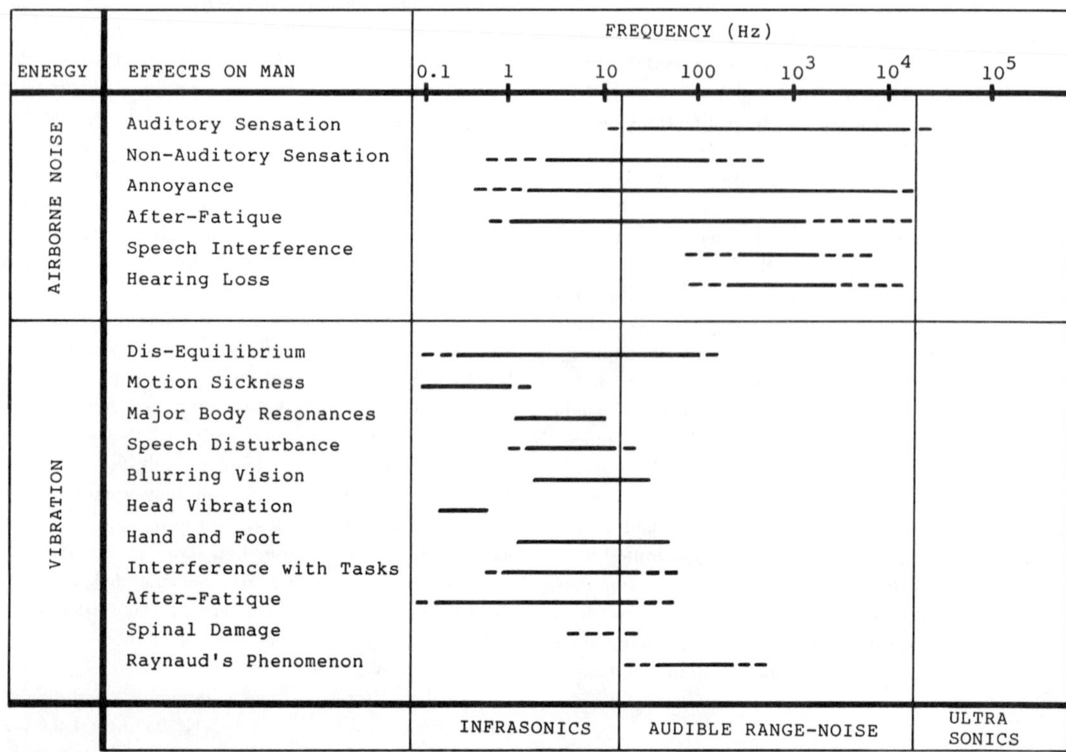

FIG 21–2.
Frequency-dependent effect of airborne noise and vibration on man. (Adapted from Guignard JC: Response to low frequency vibration. *Chartered Mech Eng* 1968; 399–401. Used by permission.)

eral), as in some railways, the principal mode of resonance occurs between 1 and 2 Hz.

Whole-body vibration in the range of 1–20 Hz, predominantly vertical, occurs in many types of commercial and earth-moving vehicles. The physiologic response is found in the cardiopulmonary system, with an increase in heart and respiratory rates, cardiac output, and oxygen intake. It is now known that these changes reflect a nonspecific response to mechanical vibration as a stressor. If the vibration level is high (up to 3 g), then gross interference with the hemodynamics of central and peripheral blood flow occurs in drivers,[7] which, in turn, could result in decreased work performance. Investigators in the Soviet Union in particular maintain that long-term exposure to whole-body vibration causes generalized debilitating effects mediated by the central nervous system. In addition, subjects exposed to long-term whole-body vibration suffer from disorders of the spine.[24, 30] The etiology has been difficult to establish with certainty, since the majority of surveys are poorly controlled and do not have appropriate age- and sex-matched control populations not subjected to vibration. Many surveys have indicated poor ergonomic design factors in the heavy equipment used, inefficient work methods, adverse climatic conditions, and in-built nonspecific stress. Therefore, it must be emphasized that the extent to which long-term exposure to moderate levels of whole-body vibration can injure normal subjects, as opposed to aggravating preexisting weakness, is an open question, at the present state of research.

Notwithstanding these general criticisms of many publications, occupational health physicians should be aware that long distance bus drivers, heavy equipment operators or trucker drivers,[12, 13] and, more recently, helicopter pilots undertaking long-duration commercial flights on double-rotor machines, may be more prone to spinal ailments, gastrointestinal disturbances, and venous, muscular, and joint disorders. In this research area, it has not proven possible by pure statistical methods to separate vibration per se from other variables, such as inefficient seating (which often amplifies vibration levels to the upper trunk and head), poor posture, long and irregular hours, and the general effect of both vibration and noise acting as a single stressor mediated centrally by neuroendocrinologic mechanisms. Nonspecific complaints such as headaches, lack of concentration, fatigue, vestibular signs, and even impotence, which lead to a reduction in working efficiency, have been commonly reported in the literature on vibration, but it has yet to be established by controlled studies that these complaints are *caused* by vibration. Furthermore, as in noise research, it is well known that initial signs and symptoms of stress disappear after prolonged exposure and that the human body adapts once the initial stress (which triggers the "fight or flight" stress reaction of our early history) has been recognized by the subject as unharmful.

Comparative data on the responses of women to whole-body vibration are lacking. Consequently, current standards on human exposure to vibration apply equally to both sexes. In many forms of transport in which both men and women are involved—for example, sea transport in ships—vibration energy below 1 Hz causes kinetosis (motion sickness), a disturbance which, if sustained, is a severe embarrassment to naval, army, and air force operations in peace and war. Although there is little information on subjective reaction below 1 Hz, motion sickness occurs between 0.25 and 0.5 Hz. In the "discomfort boundaries" illustrated by Allen[2] in Figure 21–3, the tolerance to motion falls rapidly from 1 Hz to around 0.3 Hz.

The draft International Standard *Guide for the Evaluation of Human Exposure to Whole-Body Vibration, 1978* has evolved from the early work of the pioneers in this research field—Reier and Meister (1931), Von Gierke (1965), Miwa (1967), and Von Gierke (1983).[19] These guidelines, together with the standardization of methods of vibration measurement, are incorporated in the International Standardization Organization in its draft standard ISO/DIS/2631. Because of the paucity of "hard data," this draft standard is being revised and upgraded (1986). The proposed vibration limits are tentative and cannot yet be applied as legal requirements or regulations, since, at this date, they provide only an approximation with the existing research information.

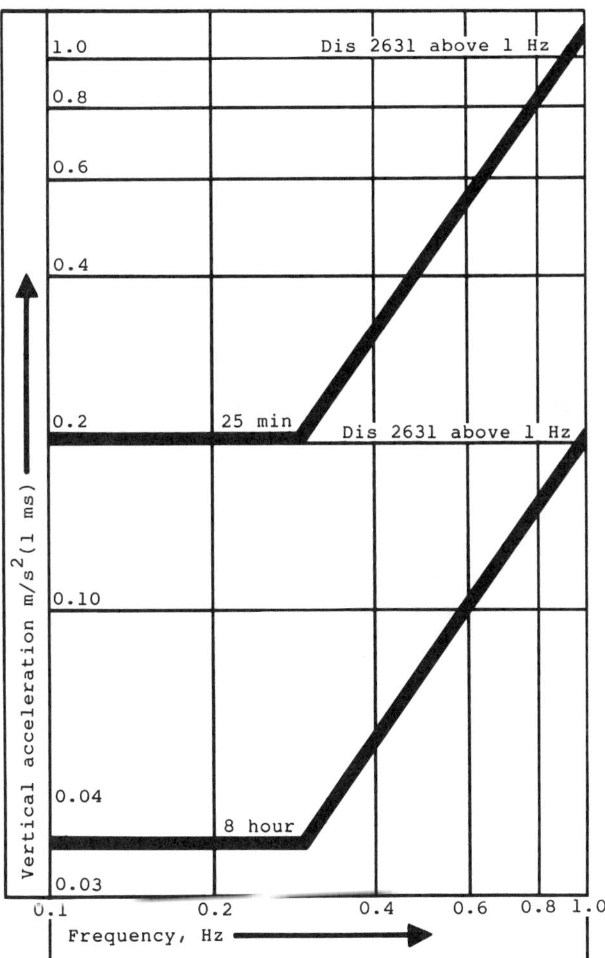

FIG 21–3.
Reduced comfort boundaries for frequencies 0.1 to 1.0 Hz. (Adapted from Allen G: *Proposed Limits for Exposure to Whole-Body Vertical Vibration 0.1 to 1.0 Hz.* AGARD Conference Report CPP 145, 1974.)

SEGMENTAL VIBRATION

Hand-arm or segmental vibration affects about 1.2 million workers in the U.S. alone, and the medical effects are more serious and more clearly defined than in cases of whole-body vibration. This is because much more basic information is known and published on all aspects of hand-arm vibration.

In the limestone quarries of Indiana, pneumatic, percussive tools replaced the mallet and hammer around 1900. By 1917, the air-operated hammer-drill was being used eight to ten hours per shift. In 1918, Dr. Alice Hamilton investigated an unusual "disease" in the stonecutters of Bedford, Indiana, who complained of "attacks of numbness and blanching of the fingers coming on suddenly under the influence of cold and then disappearing as in Raynaud's syncope." Dr. Hamilton's description[14] of the signs and symptoms of Raynaud's phenomenon of occupational origin have not been surpassed in the literature.

Vibration as a cause of Raynaud's phenomenon was first reported by Loriga in 1911.[23] Again, pneumatic drills were the source of vibration. The cause of the blanching of the fingers was correctly attributed to spasm or constriction of the digital arteries arising from the vibration of the rotary-percussive, air-driven drills used by the Indiana stonecutters and the Italian rock miners. It was also immediately recognized that the vascular signs and symptoms resembled the spontaneous vasoconstrictive phenomena induced by exposure to cold first described by Raynaud in 1862.[29] This clinical entity, unconnected with any physical stimulus except cold, is known to this day as primary Raynaud's disease. The etiology of this condition, which has been documented for 112 years, is unknown. Over the intervening years and with increasing medical knowledge, however, many more causes of "white fingers" have been recognized, including vibration. These other causes are collectively referred to as cases of secondary Raynaud's phenomenon and will be discussed under vibration-induced white finger differential diagnosis.

With increasing technologic development from 1900 to 1950, the use of vibrating hand tools expanded. Outbreaks of "white finger" arising from air-driven and electrically powered tools were reported by Seyring,[33] Hunt,[16] Telford,[39] Agate,[1] and others. The close association between the white finger attacks and the vibration entering the hands led to the introduction of a new descriptive term: vibration-induced white finger (VWF). This change in nomenclature did not recognize that vibration was affecting components in the hand-arm system other than the vasculature of the fingers. From 1950 it became clear that at least two other areas of degeneration were present. (1) degeneration of the peripheral nervous system, leading to sensory loss, loss of pain and temperature appreciation, and a general decrease in manual dexterity, and (2) the involvement of motor nerves and muscles of the hand-arm, resulting in the loss of grip strength.[8] At a recent symposium on the non-hand/arm effects of local vibration,[26] it was decided, for the future, to replace such terms as *vibration white finger* and *traumatic vasospastic disease* with *the hand-arm vibration syndrome*.

In 1960, Pecora[27] conducted a questionnaire survey in the United States and concluded that the hand-arm vibration syndrome was an uncommon occupational disease. In other countries, however, there was an alarming increase associated with the use of power-driven chain saws in forestry operations. Prevalences of the syndrome ranging from 40% to 90% in chain sawyers were reported from Australia,[11] Japan,[25] Sweden,[21] Finland,[40] Norway,[15] Czechoslovakia,[17] New Zealand,[3] and the United Kingdom.[36] In 1978 these authors, as part of a National Institute for Safety and Health (NIOSH) vibration study team, began onsite field testing of chipper and grinder workers and confirmed that, as in other countries, the prevalence of hand-arm vibration syndrome was of the order of 47% in foundries using pneumatic chipping hammers.[43] The evidence from these recent surveys indicates that these are the main factors involved in the hand-arm vibration syndrome.

1. The vibration level or intensity of the vibration, and its spectral content: The known hazardous frequency range is in the area of 6–1,000 Hz.

2. Extended vibration exposure time: Recent research surveys show a clear correlation between deterioration of the syndrome and increasing vibration exposure time.

3. Continuous vibration, as opposed to vibration interrupted with rest periods: Research data show the benefit of rest periods and the advantages of discontinuous vibration exposure with work breaks of ten minutes for every hour of continuous exposure.

4. Increasing grip force on tool handles: The greater the "coupling" at the hand-tool interface, the more efficient the transfer of vibration energy to the hand, and the greater the damage to arteries, nerves, tendons, joints, and muscles.

5. Lightness of the tool: The lighter the tool, the more energy is transferred to the hand, since there is less damping. Therefore, reduction in the weight of a hand-held vibratory tool, while reducing the workload on joints (elbow and arm), increases the vibration.

6. Inefficiency of gloves as protection from vibration: Tools generally produce vibration in the 6–1,500-Hz range. Wearing gloves does little to absorb the damaging frequencies from 6 to 500 Hz, although it is in this area that research teams are at present conducting investigations.[10] Conventional glove designs provide little attenuation below 500 Hz. Furthermore, gloves with built-in absorbent material are bulky and tend to reduce manipulative efficiency. There are at present three antivibration glove designs available, but they have not yet been evaluated for their ability to reduce vibration. In general, wearing gloves is advantageous because they maintain hand temperature and help prevent calluses on the skin of palms and fingers.

7. Individual susceptibility: Finally, as in other occupational hazards, susceptibility of the subject is a factor the occupational physician has to recognize. The so-called *latent interval* is the period between the first exposure to vibration and the appearance of the first white finger tip. The shorter the latent interval, the more hazardous the vibration. A person who has a very short latent interval compared to the mean of the vibration-exposed group has a particular susceptibility to vibration effects.

Segmental Vibration: Assessment of Disability

Occupational physicians have experienced difficulty both in quantifying the vibration stimulus and in assessing the disability, particularly for the purpose of worker compensation. The severity of the segmental signs and symptoms (clinical) and the extent to which the central nervous system is involved have been quantified by physicians in Japan by "levels," in the United Kingdom by "stages," and in Finland by a TVD (traumatic vascular disease) index. In all methods, the clinical assessment is based on the number of affected fingers that blanch during an attack, the number of attacks, the amount of interference with work and social activities, the reduction in grip force, the weather conditions necessary to provoke attacks, and the amount of interference with cold weather hobbies and outdoor activities, such as fishing, hunting, golfing, swimming, external house maintenance, and car maintenance. Outdoor workers exposed to low temperatures in the early morning are most prone to attacks, especially if they ride bicycles or motorcycles to work. This interference with work, home, and leisure activities has proven difficult to quantify but constitutes a definite reduction in the "quality of life." Furthermore, once the syndrome is at an advanced stage (stage 3 in the Taylor-Pelmear classification scale), then employment outdoors during the winter months is impossible.

Because of the reliance on the employee's own history of the attacks and subjective description of disability, it is not surprising that several different schemes for classification have been developed in different countries. Only the two most commonly used for medicolegal purposes will be considered here. The Taylor-Pelmear clinical grading into stages has been extensively used in the United Kingdom since 1968, since 1978 in the U.S.A., and, more recently, in Canada and elsewhere.[37] These stages are shown in Table 21–1.

In Japan, the U.S.S.R., and Eastern European countries, the classification is based on the Soviet work of Andreeva-Galanina and consists of levels, again emphasizing the person's own evaluation of his signs and symptoms.

In level I, there is numbness, intermittent pain of the fingers and forearm, and light sweating of the palms.

In level II, there is occasional secondary Raynaud's phenomenon with increasing numbness, pain, coldness, muscle pain, and joint stiffness in the fingers and forearm. A decline in muscle power of the upper arm and gripping force also appears. Dull headaches are frequent complaints and sweating of the palm increases.

In level III, there is frequent secondary Raynaud's phenomenon. There is muscle contracture and occasional appearance of ulnar nerve paralysis. Changes in the bones of the elbow joint are frequently detected. Extreme sweating of the palms occurs. Symptoms indicating neurosis and nervous instability appear. Nausea and vertigo occasionally appear.

In Level IV, secondary Raynaud's phenomenon is very frequent and prominent and may also appear in the legs. Muscle contracture, peripheral nerve paralysis, and changes in the bones of the elbow joint become apparent. Nervous instability and symptoms indicating neurosis increase further.

Clearly, there are substantial differences between these two classification schemes and in the interpretation of the dominant

TABLE 21–1.
Stage Assessment for Raynaud's Phenomenon*

CONDITION OF DIGITS	WORK AND SOCIAL INTERFERENCE	STAGE	
No blanching of digits	No complaints	0	No blanching
Intermittent tingling	No interference with activities	0_T	
Intermittent numbness	No interference with activities	0_N	
Both tingling and numbness	No interference with activities	0_{TN}	
Blanching of one or more fingertips with or without tingling and numbness	No interference with activities	1	
Blanching of fingers beyond tips, usually confined to winter	Slight interference with home and social activities, no interference at work	2	Blanching
Extensive blanching of digits: frequent episodes, summer as well as winter	Definite interference at work, at home, and with social activities, restriction of hobbies	3	
Extensive blanching of most fingers: frequent episodes, summer and winter	Occupation changed to avoid further vibration exposure because of severity of signs and symptoms	4	

*Complications are not used in this grading.

effects of vibration on the hand-arm system. In the Soviet Union and Japan, hand-arm vibration induces a systemic disease by causing damage to the autonomic centers of the brain—a neuropsychiatric component. Typical examples of the symptoms quoted in the Japanese and Soviet literature are fatigue, headaches, sleep disturbances, increased irritability, forgetfulness, nausea, vertigo, and muscular and joint pains. In advanced cases, these symptoms increase and may appear as the *diencephalic syndrome*.

At a 1983 symposium on the non-hand/arm effects of segmental vibration, it was concluded that "the generally accepted opinion, based on a critical review of the available literature and on physiologic and epidemiologic considerations, is that there are, at present, no data which confirm the hypothesis that hand-arm vibration causes damage to the autonomic nervous system of the brain." The interested reader is referred to this publication for further understanding of the complex interrelationships between hand-arm vibration exposure and the response of the human organism in terms of the central nervous system.

The United Kingdom stage classification, because of its essential simplicity, has proved to be valuable in medicolegal cases debated in the courts. However, some medical officers carrying out factory surveys have had difficulty relating the number and severity of blanching attacks with the employee's work, social, and hobby activities. To overcome this difficulty, the U.K. classification scheme II has been evolved (Tables 21–2 and 21–3). The numerical classification of blanching of the digits has been evolved by the Institute of Sound and Vibration Research, University of Southampton (ISVR Memorandum 632) (Fig 21–4).

Differential Diagnosis

Primary Raynaud's disease is distinguished by its early onset (60% of cases by age 30 years), the bilateral and symmetrical blanching of fingers provoked by cold, its familial association, and the absence of any predisposing disease or trauma. Secondary Raynaud's phenomenon is, in contrast, associated with many diseases, such as connective tissue diseases (scleroderma), occlusive vascular disease (arteriosclerosis, thrombosis), the dysglobulinemias (cryoglobulinemia), neurogenic diseases (poliomyelitis and syringomyelia), intoxication (acro-osteolysis, ergot, and nicotine) (Table 21–4). Simple trauma to the hands and fingers (lacerations, fractures) must also be eliminated in the differential diagnosis of vibration-induced secondary Raynaud's phenomenon. What these associated conditions have in common is that their pathophysiologic changes all affect blood flow, which, when reduced, produces white fingers through changes in pressure gradient, vessel diameter, and blood viscosity. Thus, in factory surveys, care must be taken in studying vibration-exposed populations to exclude all causes of secondary Raynaud's phenomenon unrelated to vibration, which may account for 15%–18% of the white finger cases reported.

In the search for degenerative changes due to vibration in the hand-arm system (blood vessels, nerves, bones, joints, connective tissue), it has proven difficult to differentiate between the effects of vibration and those arising from heavy manual work involving

TABLE 21–2.
Hand/Arm Vibration Stage Assessment by Signs and Symptoms, Scheme II (Rigby-Cornish)

CATEGORY	EXPOSURE TO VIBRATION	SIGNS AND SYMPTOMS
OO	None	None
O	Yes	None
I	Yes	Tingling and/or numbness
II	Yes	Episodic blanching* of digits on exposure, tingling and/or numbness
III	Yes	Acrocyanosis Permanent circulatory deficiency with sensory loss
IV	Yes	Tissue necrosis of any digit

*It is important to record if episodic blanching has been directly observed by the examining physician.

TABLE 21–3.
Subject's Assessment of Social Disability of the Vibration Syndrome, Scheme II (Rigby-Cornish)

CATEGORY	DISABILITY
A	No interference
B	No interference with work Interference with social and hobby pursuits
C	No interference with work Cessation of some activities both leisure and hobbies Loss of manipulative dexterity
D	Interference with work as well as social and leisure activities
E	Interference with work and social activities so severe that the subject requests change of occupation

constant repetitive movements of the hands and arms manipulating the hand-held vibratory tool. Recent evidence[28] appears to suggest that the vibration stimulus may be affecting each system separately and that, for example, the neurologic effects (on the mechanoreceptors of the skin) may be dependent on the spectral content of the vibration (i.e., the resonance phenomenon), and the loss of receptors may be independent of the pathologic changes seen in the digital arteries.

Objective Tests for the Hand-Arm Vibration Syndrome—Clinical Procedures

In order to provide an international stage classification for the hand-arm vibration syndrome, objective tests of impairment not dependent on the subject's own history of complaints will be required by all countries. Objective tests have to date been devised for the three systems known to suffer damage from vibration, namely, the circulatory, the sensory, and the motor-musculoskeletal systems. Hamilton, Rothstein,[31] and Leake[22] measured finger temperature, sensory loss, loss of pain sensation and temperature appreciation in the fingers of the stonecutters of Indiana. In the 1950s and 1960s provocative cooling of the hands (simulating the conditions necessary to produce blanching of the digits in a typical attack) was routinely used and the subsequent vasoconstriction measured by finger plethysmography.

TABLE 21–4.
Differential Diagnosis of Raynaud's Phenomenon or Vibration-Induced White Finger

Primary	
Raynaud's disease	Constitutional white finger
Secondary	
Connective tissue disease	Scleroderma Systemic lupus erythematosus Rheumatoid arthritis Dermatomyositis Polyarteritis nodosa Mixed connective tissue disease
Trauma	
Direct to extremities	Following injury, fracture, or operation Of occupational origin (vibration) Frostbite and immersion syndrome
To proximal vessels by compression	Thoracic outlet syndrome (cervical rib, scalenus anterior muscle) Costoclavicular and hyperabduction syndromes
Occlusive vascular disease	Thromboangiitis obliterans Arteriosclerosis Embolism Thrombosis
Dysglobulinemia	Cold hemagglutination syndrome Cryoglobulinemia Macroglobulinemia
Intoxication	Acro-osteolysis Ergot Nicotine
Neurogenic	Poliomyelitis Syringomyelia Hemiplegia

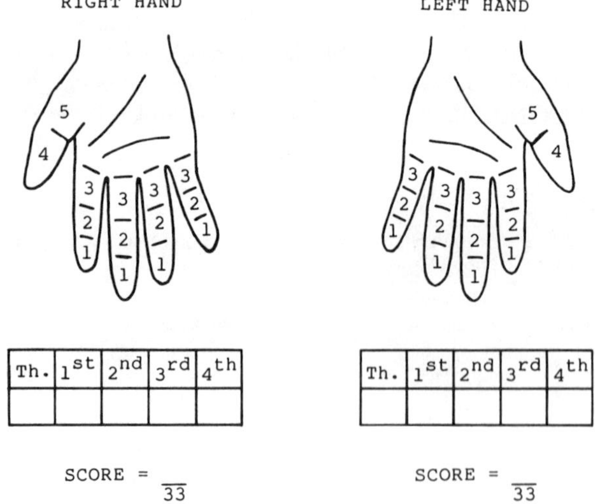

FIG 21–4.
Numerical values for digits affected by Raynaud's phenomenon, to be used for defining the stage of the condition. Each hand must be identified independently. This numerical system was devised by the Institute of Sound and Vibration Research, University of Southampton in England. (ISVR Memorandum 632).

More recently, the vibration perception threshold of the finger pulps has been measured, notably by Lidström. Although failing to relate directly vibrotactile sensory loss with stage assessments in a vibration-exposed population, Lidström gave vibration-exposed and control populations a provocative vibration dose and found significant differences in the temporary threshold shift of vibrotactile sensation.

Neurologic changes investigated include tactile discrimination tests (aesthesiometry), electroneuromyographic (EMG) measurements of the motor and sensory conduction velocities (MCV, SCV) of the median and ulnar nerve, and conduction velocity motor fiber tests (CVSP). Changes in the musculoskeletal system have been investigated with the following tests: grip force, pinching power (using the thumb and fourth finger), tapping ability, tonic vibration reflex (TVR), and urinary hydroxyproline excretion tests measuring collagen fiber breakdown. Unfortunately, the neurologic tests as devised at present have been found to be unspecific, in that they detect a range of polyneuropathies frequently found in industrial workers who are not exposed to vibration.

One further area extensively covered in recent years has been the cold pressor recovery tests (CPRI). These tests are based on the principle that if the digital arteries are damaged at the medial and intima coats and the vessel diameter has been reduced, then recovery times after provocative cooling should be prolonged. Such time changes in vibration-exposed and control groups should be detected by finger plethysmography. Pressure on a subject's nailbed—the Lewis-Prusik test—compresses the vessels in the finger pulp and measures the time required for the return of normal color. In normal subjects, even after cooling, the blood refills the compressed nailbed within five seconds. In subjects with the hand-arm vibration syndrome, this recovery time is substantially prolonged.

Despite the numerous claims made by investigators, no single objective test is yet available. Examination of the reported statistics indicates that the objective test evaluated succeeds only in demonstrating a significant difference between the vibration-exposed and the age- and sex-matched control group, but not between individuals. Furthermore, most of the objective tests described have not been correlated with stages (or levels).

Thus, it is not possible to make a precise objective assessment for an individual. It is likely, however, that the majority of tests described in the literature that would apply to individual cases were the base-line measurements available for that subject. Such prospective measurements are therefore necessary in the medical officer's surveillance of vibration-exposed employees. This principle of making preexposure measurements at preemployment medical examinations applies especially to plethysmography, in which it is difficult to control the variables regulating peripheral blood flow (vasomotor tone, core body temperature, emotional state). It is the experience of research workers in this field that blanching attacks cannot be triggered at will by cooling the extremities or even by reducing core temperatures by means of ice-cooled blankets over the thorax. The time of day in which plethysmography is carried out is another important variable. In neurologic testing it is essential to ensure that the subject be free from vibration exposure for at least 24 hours before any sensory testing. As with noise exposure, temporary threshold shifts must be eliminated prior to vibrotactile measurements.

A further complication, particularly in compensation claim evaluations, is that impairment, as measured by one or more of the standard objective tests, may reverse when the vibration stimulus is removed. Little is known about the reversibility of this syndrome. There is some evidence to support the view that stage 1 and early stage 2 syndromes will reverse, and the number and severity of the blanching attacks experienced by the subject in the winter months will lessen. A recent report contains evidence that even stage-3 cases may reverse to stage 0.[38] On this question of reversibility, age is an obvious crucial factor, since it is unlikely that reversible pathologic changes in digital arteries, for example, will occur in patients older than 45–50 years.

The early clinical tests for white finger—light touch (cotton wool), pain (sharp pin), temperature appreciation (probes)—are open to objection, because (1) there is observer bias, (2) the instrumentation is crude, and (3) there is usually inadequate preparation of the subject in terms of skin temperature and vibration exposure. Nevertheless, these fundamental tests from the data now available[43] are worthwhile, considering the large differences they usually reveal between vibration-exposed groups and controls.

For the physician confronted with the massive literature on the hand-arm vibration syndrome, the following summary of clinical testing is offered as a guide:

Screening Tests

Vascular Assessment.—Allen's Test (compression of vessels at wrist). Lewis-Prusik Test (nailbed compression). Brachial arteriography to outline artery in forearm, deep and superficial arches and digital arteries.

Thoracic Outlet Assessment.—Adsons Test (neck rotation on deep inspiration).

Carpal Tunnel Assessment.—Phalen's Test (wrist flexion). Tinel's Test (carpal tunnel percussion).

Nerve Impairment.—Aesthesiometry: two-point discrimination and depth-sense discrimination. Grip strength (dynamometer). Light touch, pain, and temperature.

Routine Laboratory Investigations

Blood.—Blood count, differential count, erythrocyte sedimentation rate, uric acid rheumatoid factor, antinuclear antibodies, cryoglobulins, serum protein electrophoresis.

Urine.—Proteinuria, hydroxyproline.

X-rays.—Hands, wrists, cervical spine, ribs (to exclude costoclavicular syndrome), cystic changes in bones of fingers and wrist (bone cysts).

Objective Tests

These include cold provocation tests, with or without finger plethysmography; electromyography; and vibrotactile sensitivity measurements.

DOSE-RESPONSE RELATIONS AND STANDARDS

To assess the hazards associated with vibration and its effect on human beings, standardization work began in 1968[41] within the International Standards Organization (ISO), with the objectives of (1) preventing the medical hazards of shock and vibration exposure, (2) guiding tool manufacturers in the design and development of safe tools, (3) developing uniform measurement methods and instrumentation, and (4) initiating research programs and methods to produce comparable research data.

Initially, four countries were involved, but by 1983, 20 countries were active in the field, with eight additional countries as observers. In 1978, ISO 2631, a *Guide for the Evaluation of Human Exposure to Whole-Body Vibration,* was produced. In 1979, ISO/DIS/5349, *Guides for the Measurement and Evaluation of Hu-*

man Exposure to Vibrations Transmitted to the Hand, was produced (following three draft proposals). A later version (second draft) of ISO/DIS/5349 is in effect in the U.S. (as of November 1986). Recently, the ISO committee has decided that exposure limits are the responsibility of governments and regulatory agencies, and hence the second ISO/DIS/5349 contains procedures for measuring vibration exposure but avoids laying down vibration limits. Unfortunately, the dose-response relationships reported by Brammer[5] are contained in an appendix. There has been, since 1964, an urgent need for occupational health guidelines, and it is therefore not surprising that standards have been developed based mainly on subjective laboratory experiments involving human response to vibration stimuli. Ideally, physicians are looking for dose-response relations that are quantitative and permit both prediction of the development of the syndrome and identification of tolerable vibration exposures. Recently Brammer and Taylor, based on published dose-response relations, have proposed threshold limit values[4] for exposure of the hand to vibration (Table 21–5).

The threshold limit values in Table 21–5 provide combinations of frequency-weighted, root-mean-square (rms) component accelerations and durations of exposure to which it is believed most persons may be repeatedly exposed without persistent health effects. The values may be used as an interim guide. They should not be regarded as defining a boundary between safe and hazardous exposure, because of many biodynamic and individual factors such as the degree of mechanical coupling (influenced by hand grip force and push or pull forces), individual susceptibility, operator skill and work practices, tool design, and tool maintenance.

TREATMENT OF THE HAND-ARM VIBRATION SYNDROME

For patients with diagnosed hand-arm vibration syndrome, *no* treatment is currently available. Therapy is essentially palliative. The vast majority of stage-2 and stage-3 patients are given vasodilators when they report their complaints to their general physicians. The results of attempting to dilate the peripheral vessels by direct action through chemotherapy has been unsuccessful throughout the countries of the world, and chemotherapy is dangerous for many persons, owing to undesirable side effects that affect balance. The failure of chemotherapy is due to the absence of a therapeutic agent that acts specifically on the digital arteries. Vasodilatation of the digital vessels by sympathectomy is immediate but, as in surgical procedures for primary Raynaud's disease, the improvement in blood flow is temporary (three to six months) and the vasoconstrictive attacks return with the sympathetic nerve supply still blocked or severed. A recent report[34] claims success with serial plasmapheresis. Success has also been reported for biofeedback therapy.[20, 32] The most recent development concerns the prostaglandin group of compounds, of which epoprostenol (prostacyclin) has a strong inhibitory effect on platelet aggregation and the capacity to dissolve recently formed platelet aggregation. Arteriography of stage-3 cases shows sudden complete blockage in the digital arteries, suggesting thrombii formation in already constricted vessels. Experimental work is now proceeding with the prostaglandins, but the major obstacle to progress with this form of therapy is the short life of these compounds, which is measured in minutes.

In the absence of treatment, the occupational health physician is advised (1) to examine a vibration-exposed population at annual intervals; (2) to search for Raynaud symptoms in preemployment physicals so that workers with such symptoms may be excluded from using vibrating tools; (3) to monitor the progress of hand-arm syndrome in exposed workers by staging the employees; and (4) to remove from exposure any person whose condition deteriorates to stages 2 and 3. At the same time, the engineering or safety division of the firm should be aiming: (1) to reduce the vibration of all hand-held tools to safe limits; (2) to regulate the daily vibration dosage; and (3) to provide, whenever possible, antivibration gloves and to encourage improved work practices that would minimize vibration coupling to the hand. It is the duty of the plant engineer to identify those parameters which determine the severity of the vibration exposure.[35]

It is a matter of regret that many tools that produce unsafe vibration levels are still being used thorughout the world. The pneumatic percussive chipping hammers and drills, for example, have vibration levels that are often 500 times greater than the threshold limit values for prevention of the hand-arm syndrome, and their design has not altered for at least 80 years. It is hard to believe that the signs and symptoms of white fingers, sensory loss, and musculoskeletal changes, which were so admirably described by Dr. Alice Hamilton as long ago as 1918,[14] are still being reported today.

TABLE 21–5.
Threshold Limit Values for Exposure of the Hand to Vibration

TOTAL DAILY EXPOSURE DURATION TOTAL TIME VIBRATION ENTERS THE HAND PER DAY, CONTINUOUS OR INTERMITTENT	VALUES OF THE DOMINANT, FREQUENCY-WEIGHTED, RMS COMPONENT ACCELERATION WHICH SHALL NOT BE EXCEEDED a_k, $(a)_{eq}$ m/sec^2
4 hours and less than 8	4
2 hours and less than 4	6
1 hour and less than 2	8
Less than 1 hour	12

REFERENCES

1. Agate JN: An outbreak of cases of Raynaud's phenomenon of occupational origin. *Br J Ind Med* 1949; 6:144–163.
2. Allen G: *Proposed Limits for Exposure to Whole-Body Vertical Vibration, 0.1 to 1.0 Hz*. Agard Conference Report CPP No 145, 1974.
3. Allingham PM, Firth RD: The vibration syndrome. *NZ Med J* 1972; 76:317–321, 486.
4. American Conference of Governmental Industrial Hygienists: *Threshold Limit Values for Chemical Substances and Physical Agents in the Working Environment. Vibration TLV. Physical Agent under Study*, 1984.
5. Brammer AJ: Threshold limit for hand-arm vibration exposure throughout the work day, in Brammer AJ, Taylor W (eds): *Vibration Effects on the Hand and Arm in Industry*. New York, John Wiley & Sons, 1982, pp 291–301.
6. British Standards Institution: *Guide to the Evaluation of Exposure of*

the Human Hand-Arm System to Vibration. Draft for Development: DD43. London, 1975.

7. Edwards, RG, McCutcheon EP, Knapp, CF: Cardiovascular changes produced by brief whole-body vibration of animals. *J Appl Physiol* 1972; 32:386–390.
8. Färkkilä MA, Pyykkö I, Starck JP, et al: Hand grip force and muscle fatigue in the etiology of the vibration syndrome, in Brammer AJ, Taylor W (eds): *Vibration Effects on the Hand and Arm in Industry*. New York, John Wiley & Sons, 1982, pp 45–50.
9. Gemne G, Taylor W: Editors' foreword, in Gemne G, Taylor W (eds): *Hand-Arm Vibration and the Central Autonomic Nervous System*. Special Volume of *Journal of Low Frequency Noise and Vibration*. London, Multi-Science Publishing Co, 1984, p ix.
10. Griffin MT, MacFarlane CR, Norman CD: The transmission of vibration to the hand and the influence of gloves, in Brammer AJ, Taylor W (eds): *Vibration Effects on the Hand and Arm in Industry*. New York, John Wiley & Sons, 1982, pp 103–116.
11. Grounds MD: Raynaud's phenomenon in users of chain saws. *Med J Aust* 1964; 8:270–272.
12. Gruber, GJ: *Relationship Between Whole-Body Vibration and Morbidity Patterns Among Interstate Truck Drivers*. NIOSH Publication No 77–167. Cincinnati, Oh, US Dept of Health, Education and Welfare NIOSH, 1976.
13. Gruber GJ, Ziperman HH: *Relationship Between Whole-Body Vibration and Morbidity Patterns Among Motor Coach Operators*. NIOSH Publication No 75–104, Cincinnati, Oh, US Dept of Health, Education and Welfare, NIOSH, 1974.
14. Hamilton A: *A Study of Spastic Anaemia in the Hands of Stonecutters*. Washington, DC, Government Printing Office, 1918. *Bull US Bureau of Labor Statistics* 236 (Industrial Accidents and Hygiene Series, No 19) pp 53–66.
15. Hellström B, Stensvold I, Halvorsrud JR, et al: Finger blood circulation in forest workers with Raynaud's phenomenon of occupational origin. *Int Z Angew Physiol* 1970; 29:18–28.
16. Hunt JH: Raynaud's phenomenon in workmen using vibrating instruments. *Proc Roy Soc Med* 1936; 30:171–178.
17. Huzl F, Stolarik R, Mainerova J, et al: Damage due to vibration when felling timber by power saw. *Pracon Lek* 1971; 23:7–15.
18. International Standards Organization: *Guide for the Evaluation of Human Exposure to Whole-Body Vibration*. ISO 5349, 1986.
19. International Standards Organization: *Guide for the Measurement and the Assessment of Human Exposure to Vibration Transmitted to the Hand*. ISO/DIS 5349, 1984.
20. Jacobson AM, Silverberg E, Hackett T, et al: Treatment of Raynaud's disease. *Psychiatr Clin* 1978; 3:125–131.
21. Kylin B, Lidström I-M, Liljenberg B, et al: I Almänna Halsoundersökmingen. II Undersökning Över Vibration SS Kador Hos Skogsarbetare. III Undersökning Över Skogsarbetarens Arbetsmiljo Hälso-Och Miljöundersökning Blend Skogsarbetare. *Al Rapport*. 1968; No 5.
22. Leake JP: *Health Hazards from the Use of the AV Hammer in Cutting Indiana Limestone*. Government Printing Office, 1918. *Bull US Bureau of Labor Statistics* 236 (Industrial Accidents and Hygiene Series No 19) pp 100–113.
23. Loriga G: Il Lavoro con i Martelli Pneumatici. *Boll Inspett Lavoro* 1911; 2:35–60.
24. Matthews J: Ride comfort for tractor operators. Review of existing information. *J Agricul Eng Res* 1964; 9:3–31.
25. Miura T, Kimura K, Tominaga Y: On Raynaud's phenomenon of occupational origin due to vibrating tools. Institute of Science of Labour (Japan) 1966: No 65.
26. Non-hand/arm effects of local vibration, in Gemne G, Taylor W (eds): *Hand-Arm Vibrations and the Central Autonomic Nervous System*. London, Multi Science Publishing Co, 1984. (Supplement *Journal of Low Frequency Noise and Vibration*.)
27. Pecora LJ, Udel M, Christman RP: Survey of current status of Raynaud's phenomenon of occupational origin. *J Am Ind Hyg Assoc* 1960; 21:80–82.
28. Pyykkö I, Hyvärinen H, Färkkilä M: Studies in the etiological mechanism of the vasospastic component of the vibration syndrome, in Brammer AJ, Taylor W (eds): *Vibration Effects on the Hand and Arm in Industry*. New York, John Wiley & Sons, 1982, pp 13–25.
29. Raynaud M: *On Local Asphyxia and Symmetrical Gangrene of the Extremities*. London, The New Sydenham Society, 1888 (selected monographs).
30. Rosegger R, Rosegger S: Health effects of tractor driving. *J Agricul Eng Res* 1960; 5:241–275.
31. Rothstein T: *Report of the Physical Findings in Eight Stonecutters from the Limestone Region of Indiana*. Washington, DC, Government Printing Office, 1918. *Bull US Bureau of Labor Statistics* 236 (Industrial Accidents and Hygiene Series, No 19) pp 67–96.
32. Sedlacek K: Biofeedback for Raynaud's disease. *Psychosomatics* 1979; 8:538–547.
33. Seyring M: Diseases Caused by Working with Pneumatic Tools. *Arch Gewerbepath Gewerbhy* g 1930; I:359–375 (In German).
34. Talpos G, Horrocks M, White JM, et al: Plasmapheresis in Raynaud's disease. *Lancet* 1978; 1:416–417.
35. Taylor W, Brammer AJ: Vibration effects on the hand and arm in industry: An introduction and review, in Brammer AJ, Taylor W (eds): *Vibration Effects on the Hand and Arm in Industry*. New York, John Wiley & Sons, 1982, pp 1–12.
36. Taylor W, Pearson JCG, Kell RL, et al: Vibration syndrome in forestry commission (UK) chain-saw operators. *Br J Ind Med* 1971; 28:83–89.
37. Taylor W, Pelmear PL: Introduction, in Taylor W, Pelmear PL (eds): *Vibration White Finger in Industry*. London Academic Press, 1975, pp xvii–xxii.
38. Taylor W, Riddle HFV, Bardy DA: *Vibration-Induced White Finger in Chain-Saw Operators in Thetford Chase Forest, Norfolk, England*. Report to the UK Forestry Commission, 1980, unpublished.
39. Telford ED, McCann MB, MacCormack DH: "Dead hand" in users of vibrating tools. *Lancet* 1945; II:359–360.
40. Tülila M: A preliminary study of the white finger syndrome in lumberjacks using thermographic and other diagnostic tests. *Work Environ Health* 1970; 7:85–87.
41. Von Gierke H: Development and present status of standardization work on human vibration exposure, in Gemne G, Taylor W (eds): *Hand-Arm Vibration and the Central Autonomic Nervous System*. Special Volume of *Journal of Low Frequency Noise and Vibration*. London, Multi-Science Publishing Co, 1984, pp 145–151.
42. Wasserman DE, Badger DW, Doyle TE, et al: Industrial vibration—An overview. *J Am Soc Saf Eng* 1974; 19–38.
43. Wasserman DE, Taylor W, Behrens V, et al: *Vibration White Finger Disease in UK Workers Using Pneumatic Chipping and Grinding Hand Tools. vol 1. Epidemiology*. NIOSH Publication No 82–118. Cincinnati, Oh, Dept of Health and Human Services, 1982.
44. Wasserman DE: *Human Aspects of Occupational Vibration*. Amsterdam, Elsevier, 1987.
45. International Standards Organization: *Guidelines for the Measurement and Assessment of Human Exposure* to Hand-transmitted Vibration, ISO 5349, Geneva, 1986.

22

Physical Work and Heat Stress*

A. Johan Kielblock, D.Sc.

Petrus C. Schutte, M.Sc.

As homeotherms, human beings are well equipped to live in a wide range of environmental conditions. In a sense, therefore, we are free, within reason, to determine our own activities, rather than have them determined for us by our environment. The price that has to be paid is that, unlike poikilotherms, deep-body (core) temperature cannot be allowed to fluctuate beyond a relatively narrow range without risking serious consequences to normal functional efficiency.

Circumstantial evidence suggests that human beings evolved as tropical animals: we possess a well-developed sweat mechanism and our skin is practically devoid of insulative hair. Moreover, the evolution of a thermoregulatory system that has a greater reserve of heat elimination than heat conservation capacity indicates that heat presented a greater threat to our ancestors than cold. Although no longer true as a generalization, the argument nevertheless remains relevant, even in modern society.

The ramifications of human heat exposure are legion: they embrace social relationships, physical and mental well-being, and, ultimately, human productivity. This chapter addresses one particular facet, namely, physical work in heat; it considers the thermal environment, man's capabilities and limitations during work in heat, and, finally, strategies to resolve the problems associated with heat exposure.

THE THERMAL ENVIRONMENT

The character of the thermal environment is determined not only by its total thermal energy content but also by the flow of thermal energy as a result of temperature differences. Heat-transfer analysis is a specialist field, but the environmental heat load can be approximated by a set of simple measurements.

*This chapter is dedicated to the memory of Nicholas P. Strydom (1923–1982), formerly manager of industrial hygiene, Chamber of Mines, who was a leading expert in work physiology and an enthusiastic teacher. He will always be remembered.

Quantification of the Environmental Heat Load

The basic measurements are those which have a bearing on human beings, namely, air temperature and radiation. (Conduction is mostly negligible and can be ignored for practical purposes.) To these can be added humidity and air movement, since they modify the heat load experienced by humans.

The characteristics of sensors and measuring equipment are well described in several texts, but it is evident that complete consensus does not exist. In the main, however, the recommendations of the International Standards Organization (ISO) and of the American Conference of Governmental Industrial Hygienists (ACGIH) enjoy general recognition. Some of the major differences in these recommendations have been listed in Table 22–1: their respective applications are likely to be determined by statutory requirements and/or the prevailing conditions.

The instrumentation referred to in Table 22–1 is simple, relatively inexpensive and, with proper care and calibration, extremely reliable and accurate. However, the suggested instrument arrangement for determination of the wet-bulb globe temperature (WBGT) index (see Heat Stress Indices) is too cumbersome for use in areas with difficult access or terrain. Under such circumstances, portable instruments, such as the Reuter-Stokes 'Heat Stress Monitor' (Canada) or the Scitec 'Tempstress' (South Africa), could be employed. These instruments are capable of providing the dry-bulb, wet-bulb, and radiant temperatures individually or as a single reading (index).

The wet-globe thermometer (Botsball) is an extremely useful, single-reading instrument (see Heat Stress Indices). The major advantages are related to its small size, the lack of electronic components that may fail, and the absence of glass thermometers that may break.

For comparative purposes, a fair assessment of the environmental heat load can be obtained by other portable instruments, such as the whirling (sling) psychrometer or the aspirating psychrometer, both of which measure dry- and wet-bulb temperature.

TABLE 22–1.
Recommendations for Thermometry

MEASUREMENT/ CHARACTERISTIC	ACGIH	BODY	ISO*
Air temperature			
Sensor	Any sensor protected from radiation without impeding air flow		
Range	−5 to 50° C		10 to 60° C
Accuracy	±0.5° C		±1° C
Wet-bulb temperature			
Sensor	–		Cylindrical; 30 (±5) × 6 (±1) mm
Range	−5° to 50° C		5 to 40° C
Accuracy	±0.5° C		±0.5° C
Wick material	Highly absorbent, e.g., cotton		
Sensor cover	Wick to entirely cover bulb of sensor		
Wick wetting	Directly; 30 min before reading		–
Stabilizing period	25 min minimum		–
Radiant temperature			
Sensor	–		–
Range	−5 to 100° C		20 to 120° C
Accuracy	±0.5° C		±0.5° C (20–50); ±1° C (50–120)
Globe diameter	15 cm		150 mm
Globe thickness	–		Thin as possible
Emission coefficient	–		0.95
Globe material	Copper painted matt black		Matt black
Stabilizing period	25 min minimum		–

*Approved by Australia, Belgium, Brazil, Canada, Denmark, Egypt, France, West Germany, Hungary, India, Italy, Netherlands, Poland, South Africa, Spain, Sweden, Switzerland, and Thailand.

Experience in the South African mining industry suggests that thermometer gradations should not exceed 0.1° C divisions.

Air movement is determined by anemometers. A hot-wire anemometer is preferable, because it is more sensitive to low air movements and turbulence. Vane or propellor anemometers are suitable at air velocities in excess of 0.5 m/sec and where laminar air movement is present.

In the present context, the objective of heat load quantifications is health and safety and not primarily the efficacy of strategies directed at reducing the thermal load through engineering practices. For this reason, all of the above measurements should reflect conditions where physical work is actually taking place.

Heat Exchange Between Man and the Environment

Heat exchange takes place by convection, radiation, evaporative heat transfer, and conduction. Since the contact area between the skin and solid objects is usually very small, conduction is negligible, and it is discounted except in the case of body-cooling garments.

For normal body function, heat exchange between the body and its environment should be balanced. Detailed analyses of such heat exchanges are complex (Stewart,[83] Kerslake,[41] Grucza[28]) and fall beyond the scope and purpose of this chapter. Inasmuch as the factors that have bearing on the nature of heat exchange are of practical value, the respective equations will be considered only in qualitative terms.

Convection.—Convection is the exchange of heat between the body surface (skin and clothing) and the surrounding air. The basic equation is

$$C = h_c (t_s - t_a)$$

where C represents the rate of heat exchange (*W/sq m* body surface); t_s and t_a, the body surface and air temperatures, respectively; and h_c, the convection coefficient. The driving force is the term $t_s - t_a$, but this is modified, through h_c, by air movement and body surface area (and hence posture). It is of practical importance, however, to appreciate that when t_a exceeds t_s, convective heat gain takes place. Calculated upper limit equilibrium skin temperatures (for a probability of less than 10^{-6} that rectal temperature will exceed 40° C) range from about 33.7° C at a work rate of 280 W/sq m to 35.6° C at 120 W/sq m.[83] From a health and safety point of view, air temperatures of 33° C and above should be viewed with concern.

Radiation.—Radiation is the process by which electromagnetic energy is transmitted through space. The equation is

$$R = h_r (t_s - t_r)$$

where R represents the rate of radiant heat flow (W/sq m); t_s, the mean body surface (skin) temperature; t_r, the mean surface temperature of surrounding objects; and h_r, the coefficient of radiant heat exchange. The coefficient makes allowance for body surface area, but, obviously, it does not contain a term for air movement. The notion that radiant heat exchange is influenced by air movement is therefore devoid of substance.

Evaporation.—The process of evaporation of water from the skin takes place as a result of differences in water vapor pressure between the skin and the surrounding air. The evaporation of 1 gm of water dissipates about 2.4 kJ of heat. The equation is

$$E = h_e (p_{sk} - p_a)$$

where E represents the rate of evaporative heat loss (W/sq m); h_e, the evaporation coefficient; and p_{sk} and p_a, water vapor pressures at skin and ambient temperatures, respectively. The coefficient makes allowance for body surface area, air movement, and atmospheric pressure. It is complicated by the nature of sweating and subsequent evaporation. (In the latter respect three regimes can be identified: (1) evaporation from a fully wetted skin with no dripping of sweat, (2) dripping from a partially wetted skin, and (3) dripping from a fully wetted skin.)

Although evaporative heat loss is suppressed by high ambient humidities, it is a common fallacy to argue that evaporative heat loss cannot take place in a saturated atmosphere. The underlying principle is that the driving force is determined by the term $p_{sk} - p_a$. Thus, at a skin temperature of 35° C, the prevailing (saturated) vapor pressure of 5.6 kPa far exceeds the saturated vapor pressure of 3.2 kPa at an air temperature of 25° C.

Heat Balance Equation.—The exchange of heat between the body and its environment is described by the heat balance equation. All living organisms generate heat, and it is therefore necessary to incorporate metabolic heat (H) into the equation. (The consumption of oxygen 1 L/min corresponds to 4,825 C/min, 20,197 kJ/min, or 337 W.) The equation representing steady state thermal balance is

$$H \pm K \pm C \pm R - E = 0$$

where K represents conduction. The symbol M is often used to denote total energy liberation in the body. To obtain the value for heat production, it is necessary to subtract mechanical work rate (W). The term $M - W$ may therefore replace H.

In practice, the heat balance equation can be 'manipulated,' with due cognizance of physiologic limitations, to describe various combinations of metabolic and environmental conditions under which thermal equilibrium exists or could be achieved. This approach presumes a comprehensive knowledge of all of the relevant variables and assumptions. Within the scope of occupational health, this approach falls in the province of the specialist biophysicist or bioengineer. For this reason the serious practitioner who seeks more than a qualitative assessment is referred to the *ASHRAE Handbook*.[1]

Human Thermometry

The influence of the thermal environment on man can be assessed by a number of physiologic parameters. Of these, body temperature measurements are of fundamental importance, since they reflect the extent to which thermal balance is being maintained. It therefore follows that such measurements would not only attempt to estimate body heat content, but they would also seek to be representative of the so-called controlled variable, i.e., the entity (temperature?) to which the human thermostat is most responsive.

Measuring sites, interpretation, technique, and instrumentation are often the subject of considerable controversy. The guiding principle is to clearly define the objective(s) of a particular measurement or set of measurements and then to select the most appropriate course of action with due cognizance of the limitations imposed. Table 22–2 lists a number of sites as well as the respective advantages and disadvantages.

The interpretation of body temperature is usually based on comparing isolated measurements (e.g., rectal temperature) with norms or, from a thermoregulatory point of view, mean body temperature. According to Mitchell et al.[57] mean body temperature is a fair approximation of the controlled variable. The general calculation is

$$T_m = cT_r + (1 - c)\,\overline{T}_s$$

where T_m represents mean body temperature; T_r, rectal temperature; $\overline{T}_s$, mean skin temperature; and c, a weighting factor. For neutral environments, the value for c is 0.65,[11] and for hot environments, 0.80 or even 0.90.[84] $\overline{T}_s$ is calculated from a series of measurements according to the equation:

$$\overline{T}_s = c_1T_1 + c_2T_2 + c_3T_3$$

where T_1, T_2, and T_3 represent various skin sites and c_1, c_2, and c_3 weighting factors, respectively. In reviewing the literature, Houdas and Ring[33] propose the following sites and weighting factors:

Cheek	0.07
Mid-abdomen	0.175
Arm (upper/antecubital)	0.19
Back (lumbar)	0.175
Leg (popliteal area)	0.39

Changes in mean body temperature are converted into changes in body heat content. The specific heat of the body tissues is about 3.5 kJ/kg °C (0.83 C/kg °C), i.e., a rise in mean body temperature of 1° C would add 3.5 kJ of heat for each kilogram of body mass. This term is useful when comparing individual responses to heat.

PHYSIOLOGIC RESPONSES AND ADAPTATION TO WORK IN HEAT

Human thermoregulation remains the subject of intensive research, and in the present context, where the emphasis falls on health and safety administration, the reader is referred to excellent recent reviews, notably by Bligh,[8] Brengelman,[10] Gisolfi,[23] Bligh and Moore,[9] and Houdas and Ring.[33] It is of practical importance to appreciate that it is unnecessary to postulate a 'set-point hypothesis' for the control of body temperature but, rather, that body

TABLE 22–2.
Sites for Measuring Body Temperatures: Advantages and Disadvantages*

SITE	ADVANTAGE	DISADVANTAGE
Oral (T_o)	Accessible; nonembarrassing Suitable for routine estimate Approximates T_e under neutral and hot conditions during rest Useful and reliable under controlled conditions for comparative purposes	Affected by ambient temperature Affected by mouth breathing Overestimates T_r during work in heat Stabilization period should not be less than 8 minutes
Esophageal (T_e)	Closely related to arterial blood temperature and hence 'core' temperature Responsive to thermal transients	Patient discomfort Learning process Unsuitable for routine measurements
Tympanic (T_t)	Approximates hypothalamic temperature and hence the 'controlled variable' (?) Responsive to thermal transients	Technical problems Often painful May be influenced by head skin temperature
Rectal (T_r)	Representative of core during steady-state Ease of measurement Suitable for routine measurements under certain conditions	Embarrassing procedure Overestimates 'core' temperature during leg work
Skin (T_s)	Reveals core-skin gradients Reflects environmental thermal load	Multisite measurements required (minimum 4)

*Based on a review of the literature and authors' experience.

temperature will be regulated (within limits) at the lowest level consonant with the maintenance of homeostasis.

Although thermal balance can be achieved solely by physical means, at least in theory, physiologic control is invoked whenever thermal balance is challenged. In essence, physiologic thermoregulation is achieved through three main effectors: (1) an elevation in metabolic rate to counter heat loss during cold exposure, (2) vasomotor adjustments that either facilitate (dermal vasodilatation) or restrict (dermal vasoconstriction) heat loss from the body, and (3) sweating, which promotes evaporative heat loss.

Heat Exposure and Acclimatization: General Considerations

On the first day of work in heat, great strain is placed on the thermoregulatory system. The sweat mechanism fails to meet its thermoregulatory commitments fully. On the other hand, vasomotor control ensures adequate skin perfusion, but it does so at the expense of other tissues and organs. Cardiovascular strain, as evidenced by high heart rates and low blood pressure, is therefore a consistent finding during heat exposure of the unacclimatized individual, and it is often manifested in fainting (syncope).

The principal adjustments that have been found to occur during heat acclimatization are aimed at achieving sweat rates consonant with thermoregulatory demands, while cardiovascular function, as reflected by lowered heart rates, becomes directed more toward maintaining an adequate supply of blood to organs and tissues other than the skin. Typical manifestations of the acclimatization process are presented in Figure 22–1. Initial exposures are characterized by significant and rapid elevations in rectal temperature, most probably as a result of the poor sweat rates. Circulatory strain is reflected in extremely high heart rates, a manifestation of the simultaneous demands of active skeletal muscle and skin blood flow.

The ability to perform work that is easily done in cool environments is impaired because the initial demands of thermoregulation and skeletal muscle activity are competitive, and the resulting strain is manifested in high heart rates. If these conditions (work in heat) last for several days, there is a gradual return of the ability to work with little or no discomfort—heat acclimatization has taken place.

The primary adaptive response to heat exposures may be regarded as an increased capacity to sweat.[58] It is, therefore, not surprising that workers with an inherently high degree of heat tolerance also exhibit profuse thermal sweating (Fig 22–2). However, the concept that the attenuation of total physiologic stress can be explained solely by increased sweating appears to be an oversimplification; it is probably also related to an expansion of blood (plasma) volume following an increased tendency for protein to remain in the blood,[74] an event regarded as a secondary feature of acclimatization to heat.[30] It is nevertheless convenient to define heat acclimatization as the physiologic mechanism whereby thermoregulatory strain is transferred from the circulation to the sweat mechanism.

Determinants of Work in Heat

It is obvious that while most individuals would, in a qualitative sense, exhibit the response pattern outlined above, the actual response pattern for any given individual is a function of a variety of factors. These determinants could broadly be divided into two categories: (1) inherent determinants, i.e., those over which the individual has no control and (2) external determinants, i.e., those over which the individual has some control or which he voluntarily accepts. In the latter category, the most important are nutrition and hydration.

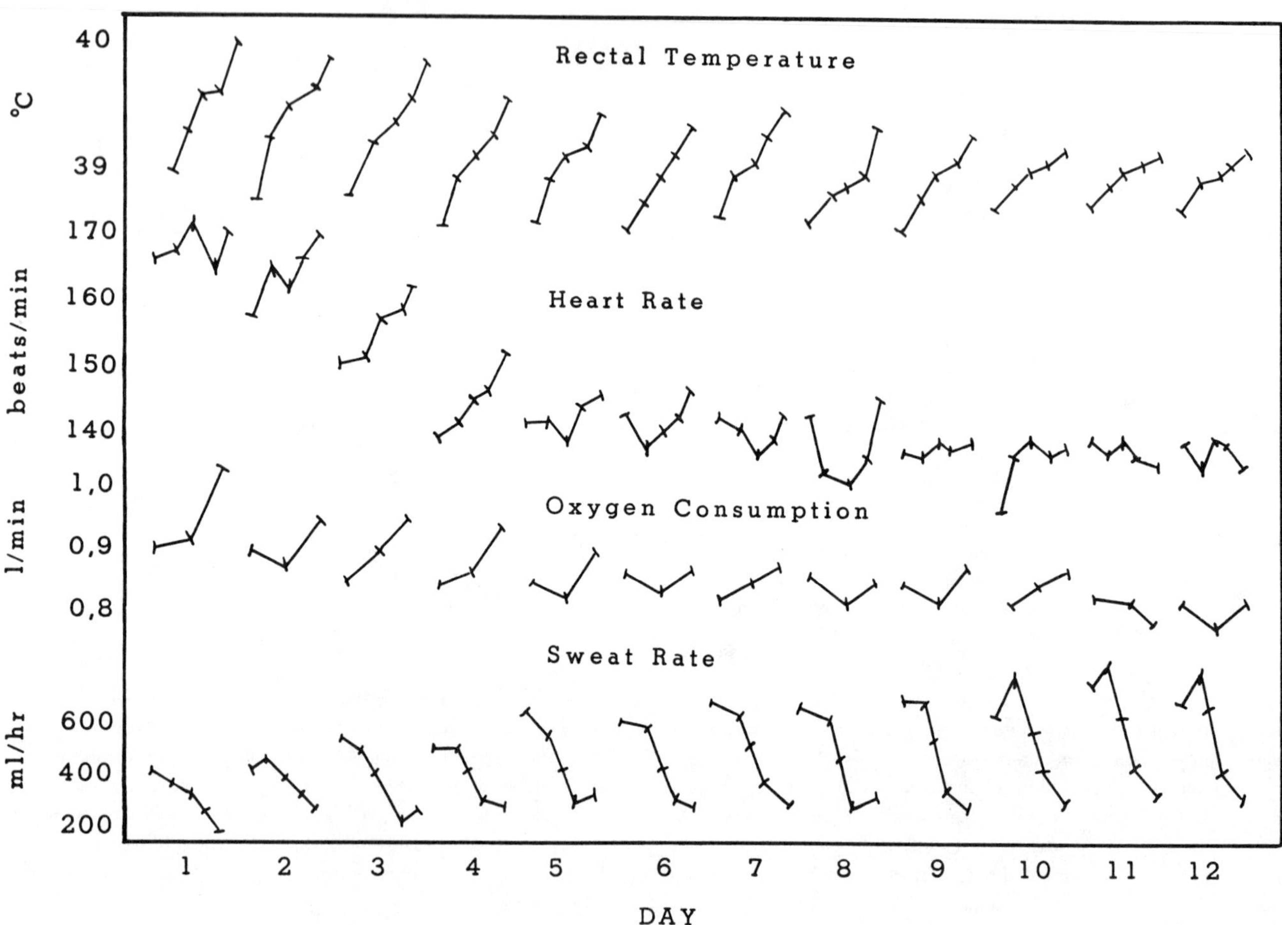

FIG 22–1.
Physiologic adaptation to hot, humid conditions (36.1° C dry-bulb; 33.9° C wet-bulb; air movement 0.75 m/sec) under laboratory conditions. An external work rate of 54 W was maintained for five hours a day over a 12-day period.

Maximal Work Capacity ($\dot{V}_{O_2 MAX}$).—The relationship between *maximal work capacity* ($\dot{V}_{O_2\ MAX}$) and tolerance to work in heat has been the subject of considerable research. There is general consensus that individuals with a high $\dot{V}_{O_2\ MAX}$ appear to be at an advantage in terms of exertional heat tolerance[63] and that a high $\dot{V}_{O_2\ MAX}$ could account for about 45% of the variability determining rectal temperature during prolonged exertion in heat.[62, 63, 81]

Of practical importance, however, is whether or not $\dot{V}_{O_2\ MAX}$ has sufficient predictive power to be used as a criterion of heat tolerance, especially when it concerns the health and safety of untrained workers performing strenuous manual labor in hot environments. On the basis of the above (i.e., $\dot{V}_{O_2\ MAX}$ accounts for about 45% of the variability determining rectal temperature), it is the authors' view that it would be morally indefensible in an industrial connotation to estimate heat tolerance in terms of $\dot{V}_{O_2\ MAX}$ (or parameters thereof) for the purpose of worker placement.

Age.—In the young, experimental evidence suggests that *age-related factors* associated with thermoregulation precludes the development of optimal heat acclimatization,[37] while in the aged the decline in heat tolerance is not primarily a function of age per se but rather of an age-related decline in $\dot{V}_{O_2\ MAX}$.[16, 17, 37] Older individuals are also more susceptible to contracting heat stroke,[85] and, once contracted, their chances of survival are less.[48, 85]

Sex.—Although Shapiro et al.[75] concluded that women exhibit a higher thermoregulatory setpoint than men, recent findings suggest that there are virtually no differences between the sexes when it comes to heat tolerance,[5] especially when age-matched for $\dot{V}_{O_2\ MAX}$.[5, 22, 31]

Ethnicity.—To demonstrate clear ethnic differences in heat tolerance is difficult. Based on a comparison between Arabs and Northern Europeans, it seems that any ethnic difference may be related more to differences in nutritional state and physical activity than to any structural adaptation to heat.[97]

Nutrition.—The turnover of certain key elements of nutrition is accelerated by strenuous physical labor, expecially when such tasks are performed in hot environments. For example, heavy ex-

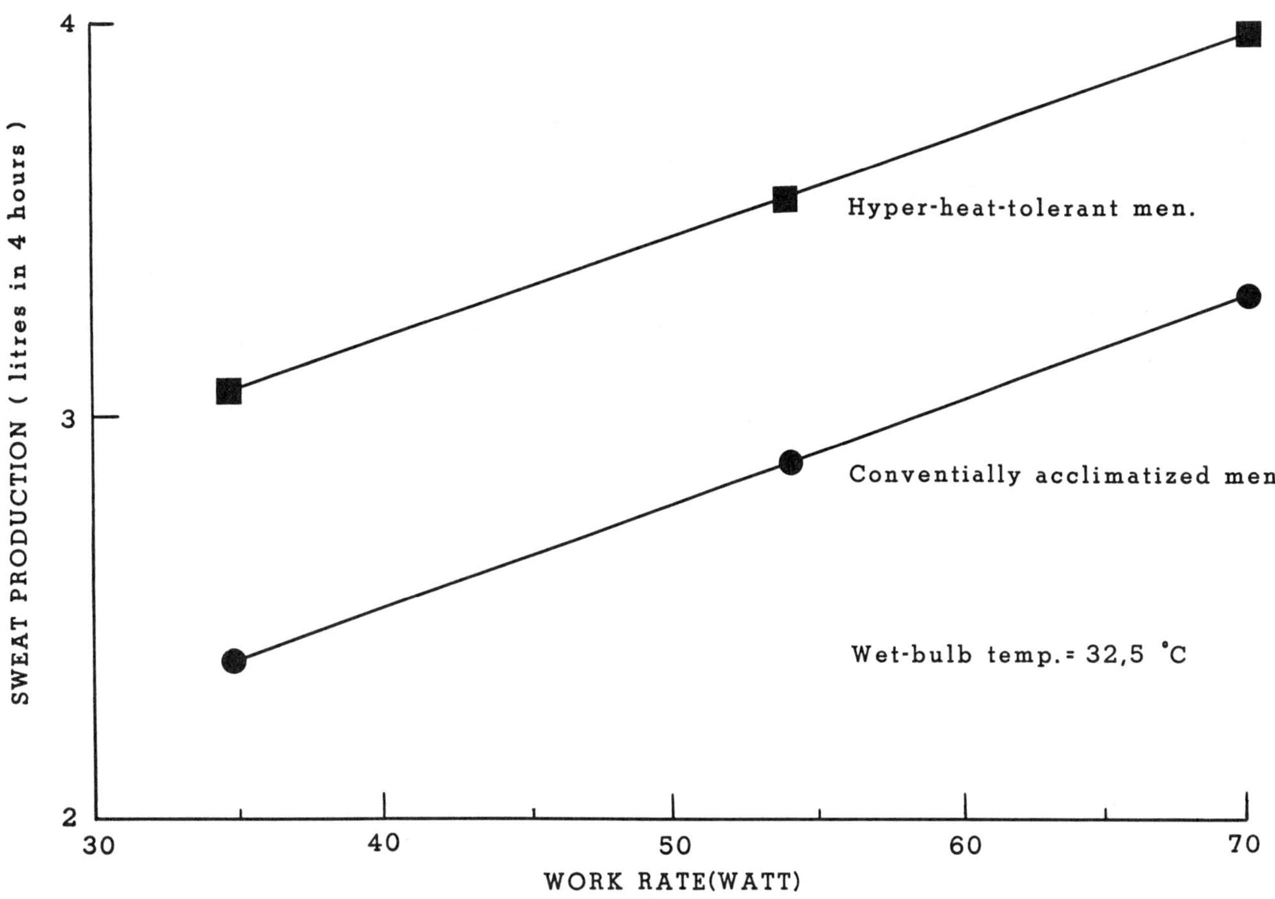

FIG 22–2.
Natural heat tolerance is associated with, amongst others, a more responsive sweat mechanism. For the general population, this can only be achieved through formal heat acclimatization.

posures could lead to a significant loss in zinc,[89] thus impairing normal growth, development, health, and ossification.[61] Potentially, the same applies to magnesium,[94] the relevance of which should be viewed against the relationship between deaths ascribed to ischemic heart disease and low magnesium intake.[52, 94] Prolonged, strenuous work is also likely to induce iron deficiency to the extent that supplementation becomes essential.[93] Iron deficiency leads to a measurable decline in work capacity; conversely, a significant increase in work productivity has been demonstrated following iron supplementation in iron-depleted individuals.[20] Similar studies by Viteri[91] have indicated clearly that undernourished groups worked at lower intensities and for shorter periods than supplemented groups, resulting in less work accomplished per time unit.

Perhaps the most dramatic turnover occurring during work in heat is that of vitamin C.[90] In a subsequent study, Strydom et al.[88] demonstrated that heat acclimatization in the South African gold mining industry could be accelerated by vitamin C supplementation and that the requisite level amounts to at least 250 mg per day. Inasmuch as Keren and Epstein[39] could not demonstrate any benefit of vitamin C supplementation on aerobic or anaerobic work capacity, the precise mechanism resides elsewhere. However, evidence does suggest that optimization of the vitamin C status of workers is essential when they are exposed to prolonged periods of work in heat.

Hydration.—One of the most profound determinants of continued work in heat is the state of *hydration* or, conversely, the prevention of dehydration. This applies not only to industrial workers, but also to defence force personnel and athletes. Symptoms include lassitude, anorexia, weariness, sleepiness, and apathy. Dehydration could result, in the short-term, from an inadequate supply of water and/or profuse sweating, while salt-depletion dehydration is a potential danger in the long-term. (The extent to which this is relevant in industrial societies, which are noted for their generally excessive salt intake, remains speculative.)

Fluid replacement strategies are primarily designed to counter dehydration (and possibly electrolyte loss) induced by profuse, sustained sweating. Although the fundamental approach of replacing exactly what is being lost at the same rate is quite simple in theory, the maintenance of an optimum state of hydration often presents practical problems:

1. Drinking water according to the dictates of thirst is insufficient to prevent a voluntary dehydration of up to 1% of body mass.[27] This is clearly illustrated in Figure 22–3.

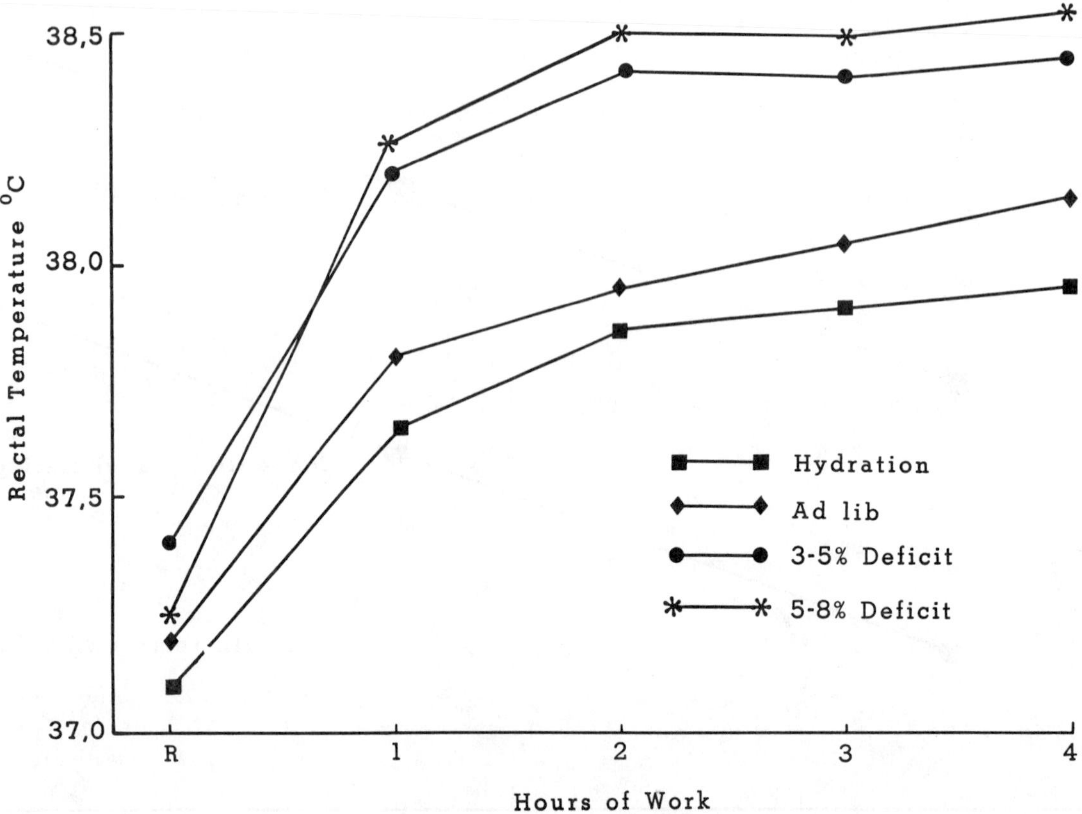

FIG 22–3.
The state of hydration has a profound effect on body temperature during work (external rate of 54 W) in hot, humid conditions (33.9° C dry-bulb; 32.2° C wet-bulb; air movement 0.5 m/sec).

2. Upon drinking water, a person's thirst is alleviated well before the fluid deficit is recovered, the attenuation of drinking subjectively being attributed to stomach fullness.[70]

3. Once dehydration has set in, the subsequent rate of water absorbtion from the gut will be reduced as a result of compensatory splanchnic vasoconstriction. This reflex, by which a redistribution of the cardiac output is achieved, occurs at dehydration levels approximating 1.5% of body mass.[71]

4. Sweat is a hypotonic fluid with an electrolyte content varying between 0.1 to 0.3 gm %. The most important constituent is sodium chloride (salt) which accounts for about 80% of the tonicity of sweat. On a balanced diet, or in the short-term (hours), the threat to continued well-being does not reside in salt depletion but in dehydration.

These considerations suggest that optimum hydration is best achieved by drinking relatively small amounts of water at relatively short intervals, e.g., about 250–300 ml every 20–30 minutes. Although the basic physiologic requirements are effectively met by ordinary tap water, there is no doubt that a cool, hypotonic beverage is preferable on the basis of palatability. Of further note is the availability of water: a man is less likely to drink regularly if it involves effort and time. Finally, it is evident that worker education is essential.

Obviously, the most important determinant of work in heat is the interaction of work rate, the duration thereof, and the environmental heat load. The fundamental restriction is not related primarily to heat gain from the environment but rather to the dissipation of heat from the body. This gives rise to the calculation of environmental cooling power (Fig 22–4), a concept which finds considerable application in the hot, humid South African gold mines.

Heat Illnesses: Recognition, Diagnosis, and Treatment

Attempts to classify heat disorders are complicated in view of the variety of causally related interactions associated with the physiologic stress of heat. However, an analysis of various classifications reveal that three conditions are of dominant importance: (1) heat cramps, (2) heat exhaustion, and (3) heat stroke. To this may be added the condition known as prickly heat.

Heat Cramps.—As a descriptive term, heat cramps is a complete misnomer. Exposure to heat per se does not elicit muscle cramps,[42] while the tetanic-like convulsions often observed during exposure to heat occur secondarily as a result of hyperventilation and the ensuing respiratory alkalosis.[36] Although oral salt therapy is widely held to bring about prompt alleviation of muscle cramp, it is unlikely that salt losses of such magnitudes are incurred, even

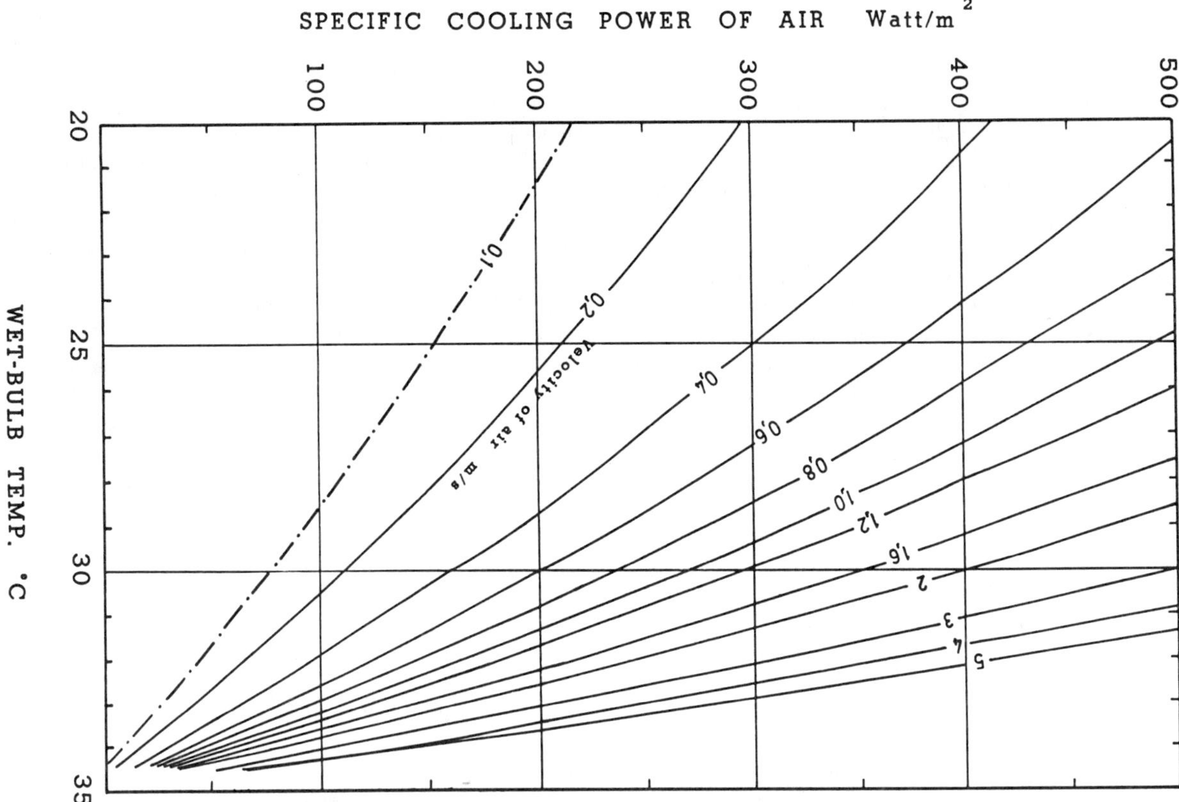

FIG 22–4.
Specific cooling power is defined as the cooling power of the environment with reference to a skin temperature of 35° C and equal dry-bulb and radiant temperatures 2° C higher than the wet-bulb temperature at a barometric pressure of 1,000 mbar. At a work rate of 300 W/sq m body temperature equilibrium will be possible at a wet-bulb temperature of 25° C and an air movement of 0.4 m/sec. At 30° C wet-bulb, the required air movement must be increased to 1.2 m/sec to maintain thermal equilibrium.

during profuse sweating. In view of the altered state of muscle tissue during prolonged exertion, e.g., electrolyte and acid-base changes,[42] in addition to the observation that plasma volume reduction is conducive to cramps and that cramps are alleviated by restoring plasma volume,[59] it is apparent that the cause of muscle cramp is far more complex than simple salt depletion. The fact that cramps may even occur in well-trained athletes supports this view and leads the authors to conclude that in general muscle cramp has its origin in an impaired microcirculation. Irrespective of the mechanism, and in agreement with Ryan,[72] we believe that the best cure for cramp is rest.

Heat Exhaustion.—Heat exhaustion is attributed to an inability of the circulation to meet simultaneously the demands of thermoregulation, i.e., by effecting a vast flow of blood to the skin, and those of vital organs such as the brain and active skeletal muscle.[6] This reinforces the concept that the primary strain of heat exposure is circulatory.[24] Chronic heat exhaustion, in contrast to the common acute version, may have its origin in salt depletion, i.e., dietary imbalance.

Heat exhaustion is more likely to occur during the unacclimatized state[6] and in individuals with some form of circulatory insufficiency. Obviously, the condition is aggravated by dehydration.[14, 42] However, it may also occur completely independently of dehydration as a result of an improper redistribution of the circulation.[6] Irrespective of the precise origin, it follows that the trigger mechanism is an effective reduction in circulating blood volume.[51]

Presenting symptoms of heat exhaustion are consonant with the underlying mechanism. Thus, weakness, a feeling of an inability to continue work, frontal headache, anorexia, nausea, faintness or actual fainting (heat syncope), and breathlessness are typical signs. Body temperature is normal or slightly elevated, sweating proceeds normally, and the skin is pale. Further investigation may reveal high heart rates and low arterial blood pressure, the signs of circulatory shock.

Heat exhaustion is self-limiting: either the victim is incapable of continued effort in heat or he faints. Subsequent treatment is directed primarily toward reinstatement of normal circulatory function. In uncomplicated cases of heat syncope, enforced cessation of muscle activity is sufficient to restore the circulation, and, other than rest and removal to a cooler environment, no further treatment is needed. On the other hand, dehydration-induced heat exhaustion, the more usual consequence of exposure to sudden increases in the environmental heat load and/or work rate,[51] should be treated by intravenous fluid infusions,[6] with care being exercised to prevent overloading the heart.[42] Moreover, dehydration-induced heat exhaustion, especially in highly motivated individuals (e.g., during sporting endeavors), probably constitutes the thin dividing line between primary dehydration and imminent heat stroke.[80]

Prickly Heat.—Prickly heat, or miliaria, is an acute, inflammatory disease of the skin. It occurs especially in the summer, in the tropics, and following prolonged sweating. The pathology is well-known: sweat gland ducts become blocked by a plug of keratinized cells and the accumulating sweat is forced through the wall of the duct into the surrounding tissues; an inflammatory reaction ensues due to irritants and infection.[19] In reviewing the literature,[51] three possible causes are listed: (1) excessive wasting away of the natural skin oils, (2) infection, and (3) electrolyte imbalance and the effect thereof on sweat composition. Of note is the observation that heat tolerance is compromised severely during such conditions.[64, 65] Treatment is symptomatic and preventive, but topical applications of corticosteroids may be used in some cases. Environmental controls and good personal hygiene, i.e., clean clothing, is most effective.

Heatstroke.—Heatstroke is regarded as one of the few true medical emergencies,[21] and if effective treatment is not instituted promptly, it carries a mortality rate of up to 80%.[42] Inasmuch as predisposing factors are often ignored through apathy, or not recognized as such because of inadequate training, the onset of heat stroke often seems mercurial and notoriously unpredictable.

By current definition, heatstroke represents a condition in which elevated body temperatures are causally related to tissue damage, often of an irreversible nature.[43] Although many tissues are damaged in heatstroke, the patient's outcome depends mainly on the degree of injury to the nervous system, kidneys, and liver, the latter two organs being damaged almost invariably.[45] The accurate diagnosis of heatstroke, by implication, therefore, rests solely on parameters of tissue damage, the most practical being the assay of tissue enzymes in serum.

Much of the current enigma of heatstroke is probably seated in earlier definitions of the affliction. From earlier reviews of the literature, Minard and Copman[56] and Leithead and Lind[54] set forth the view that heat stroke could be regarded as a "disorder of thermoregulation characterized by the total absence of sweating, body temperature in excess of 41.1° C (106° F), and severe disturbances in brain function." A major objection to such a definition is that sweat cessation is not always a cardinal sign, since heatstroke may occur not only from failure of the thermoregulatory system, as a result of impaired central nervous system function, but also from overloading its capacity.[43, 80] Moreover, the setting of apparently arbitrary temperature levels is equally unacceptable. At best, the older concepts describe a highly advanced degree of heatstroke.

While body temperature per se constitutes an invaluable guide to the severity of physiologic stress, the exposure time, often an unknown entity, is of equal importance.[34] This elementary observation obviates the need to define exactly when body temperature is too high.

While typical cases of heatstroke are diagnosed readily, adherence to the "classic" yardsticks (vide supra) invariably leads to an underestimation of the case, i.e., underdiagnosis. Indecision as to whether an individual has contracted heatstroke or is suffering some other affliction should under no circumstances be a consideration for withholding treatment. The initial treatment for heatstroke is completely noninvasive and, consequently, the patient cannot be harmed by it. The guiding principle should therefore be that whenever doubt exists as to whether an individual is suffering from heatstroke or any other affliction presenting similar signs and symptoms, *treat as for heatstroke*.

Treatment of heatstroke cases is directed primarily at a reduction of body temperature. The precise method, however, is controversial. Attempts to achieve a reduction in body core temperature by submersion in cold water, or packing the patient in ice, probably represents one of the most serious misconceptions regarding whole-body cooling.[95] Both these methods induce constriction of skin blood vessels, which in turn causes a diminished flow of blood through the skin. Inasmuch as this is tantamount to insulating the body core from the environment, heat dissipation is severely impaired. Although dermal vasoconstriction may be countered through whole-body immersion in lukewarm water (27–30° C), there are other disadvantages that render immersion techniques impractical, e.g., they make it difficult to administer oxygen and intravenous fluids, and a tub of water mixed with vomitus and excrement of comatosed patients is unhygienic to both the patient and his attendants. In fact, among others, these very shortcomings led to the development of the highly sophisticated Makkah Body Cooling Unit (MBCU), which is used extensively during the annual religious pilgrimage to Mecca, the Makkah Hajj.[46] Cooling rates of 0.06° C/min in body core temperature have been reported for the MBCU, which utilizes the principle of heat loss through evaporation.

Evaporative heat loss, in contrast, achieves a happy medium between the transport of heat to the skin by means of the circulation and its subsequent dissipation to the environment. This can be achieved in practice by the use of compressed air, a readily available commodity in most industrial settings, or by fans. The body surface should be wetted by splashing and spreading water over areas conducive to evaporative heat loss. Cooling rates of about 0.035° C/min can be achieved in this way which, although considerably less than the 0.06° C/min reported for Makkah Body Cooling Unit,[46] is nevertheless satisfactory during emergencies, according to our studies.[50]

It goes without saying that medical assistance should be summoned posthaste, and under no circumstances should body cooling be terminated unless an acceptable reduction in temperature has been achieved, i.e., a rectal temperature below 38.5° C.

On the basis of findings reported by Richards and coworkers[68] and Richards and Richards[69] on the treatment of heat-exhausted fun runners in the Sydney City-to-Surf Marathon, the role of intravenous fluid therapy may have been underrated thus far, not so much in reinstating normal circulatory function *per se*, but specifically in the maintenance of thermal homeostasis. This provides further support for the concept that the circulation bears the brunt of thermoregulation during work in hot environments.

In considering reports regarding the efficacy of various methods of reducing body temperature, it remains to be pointed out that experimental or clinical findings are seldom comparable in a direct sense, and, therefore, care should be exercised in paper evaluations of different methods.[50]

As stated earlier, the diagnosis of heatstroke, which is readily based on certain clinical findings, as well as a knowledge of the prevailing environmental conditions, is often complicated by the presentation of atypical symptoms. Although elevated serum enzyme levels in heatstroke have been reported by many researchers and clinicians, the significance of this has apparently been largely underrated. In 1967, however, Kew et al[44] proposed the use of serum enzyme estimations to enable a more accurate diagnosis of the affliction. Subsequent findings have amply supported this approach not only as being useful for diagnostic purposes, but also for establishing the severity and extent of tissue damage, as well as the general prognosis.

A review of the literature indicates that an elevation of serum enzyme levels is a consistent finding in heatstroke.[32, 79, 96] Of especial prognostic significance is the elevation of AST (aspartate aminotransferase) in that it is regarded as an indicator of the severity of tissue damage,[45] while an elevation in CK (creatine kinase) in cerebrospinal fluid may provide a good index of neurologic damage.[43] Furthermore, AST and LD (lactate dehydrogenase) levels are almost invariably increased in heatstroke.[45] Diagnostic procedures regarding heatstroke call for serum enzyme assays of LD, CK, AST, and ALT on admission and at 24 and 48 hours following admission. This diagnostic procedure should be followed in cases of overt heatstroke, and it should be applied also in atypical cases, suspected cases, or even when hearsay evidence suggests the possibility of heatstroke and the patient is asymptomatic. The emphasis on the inclusion of suspected cases in the diagnostic protocol may have an important medicolegal implication, namely, that a positive or, for that matter, an unequivocally negative diagnosis of heatstroke can only be made retrospectively.

In the final analysis, there is a clear distinction between serum enzyme elevations resulting from physical work in heat and heatstroke.[96] However, prolonged endurance events such as the 100-mile marathon are able to produce elevations which might approximate those encountered in heatstroke.[47] Experimental evidence even then suggests that a distinction between heat- and/or work-induced disorders can be better made by assessing both the level and pattern of enzyme release.[35]

Finally, evidence is accumulating that heat tolerance may be compromised severely following contraction of heatstroke.[40, 75] Unpublished case histories pertaining to heatstroke in the South African mining industry confirm these observations. The reassessment of heat tolerance following an incident of heatstroke is thus mandatory before heatstroke victims again attempt work in hot environments.

HEAT STRESS CRITERIA AND INDICES*

The most practical criteria of physiologic heat stress are body core (rectal) temperature and heart rate.[25] Qualitatively, both show a positive relationship to increasing work rates and heat loads (including combinations thereof), although the respective response patterns may differ significantly. For example, during prolonged work (54 W for four hours) in hot, humid conditions (33.2° C dry-bulb; 31.7° C wet-bulb), the increase in heart rate relative to rectal temperature for unacclimatized persons exceeds the value recorded for acclimatized persons. This implies that while dual upper limits certainly enhance safety precautions, care should be exercised to ensure that they are realistically adjusted to one another for set conditions.

For general industry there is the consensus that deep body temperature should not be permitted to rise above 38° C,[18] and accordingly this standard has been built into perhaps the most universally accepted heat stress index, the Wet Bulb Globe Temperature Index (see below). While the choice of 38° C may seem to be too conservative, especially to exercise physiologists, it should be borne in mind that it must serve for a considerable cross-section of the work force, workers who differ in age, sex, inherent work capacity, and fitness. On the other hand, for a youthful, healthy, all-male group in the South African mining industry, this value may be set at a much higher level, 39.5° C. This value is based on an analysis of Wyndham and co-workers'[98] findings, which clearly indicate that sweat production and physiologic heat conductance become "saturated" when rectal temperature approaches 39.5° C, i.e., sweat rate and conductance are at a maximum. Obviously, an upper limit rectal temperature criterion of 39.5° C can only be applied under conditions of strict individual supervision, where rectal temperature and heart rate are constantly monitored; it should under no circumstances be incorporated into 'indices' based on environmental conditions and estimated work rates.

Heart rate is not only related to work load (Table 22–3), but also reflects the influence of other factors, such as the environmental heat load. For sustained work (e.g., an eight-hour shift) there is general consensus that work rate should not tax more than 40% of an individual's maximal work capacity ($\dot{V}_{O_2\ MAX}$). For untrained men aged 20–60 years, an analysis of Shephard's data[78] reveals an average $\dot{V}_{O_2\ MAX}$ of 3.01 L/min (range: 2.27–3.90 L/min). This suggests that, *on average*, sustained work should not be performed at rates exceeding an oxygen consumption of 1.2 L/min, with a range of 0.9–1.6 L/min. Corresponding heart rates (see Table 22–3) are of the order of 110–130 beats per minute, the implication being that 110 represents an upper limit. Inasmuch as $\dot{V}_{O_2\ MAX}$ is systematically eroded with increasing heat loads, it follows that lower work rates are indicated to conform with this limit.

With training and heat acclimatization, when the individual is well capable of sustained work at much higher fractions of $\dot{V}_{O_2\ MAX}$, these restrictions are no longer relevant, and rectal temperatures approaching 38.5° C and heart rates of up to 135 beats/min are well tolerated (Table 22–4). In this context, Wenzel's[92] review is relevant.

From the above it is evident that considerable benefit could be derived in any given work situation, without sacrificing safety,

TABLE 22–3.
General Relationship Between Work Rate and Oxygen Consumption

CATEGORY	OXYGEN CONSUMPTION L/MIN	HEART RATE BEATS/MIN
Light	0.5–1.0	75–100
Moderate	1.0–1.5	100–125
Heavy	1.5–2.0	125–150
Very heavy	2.0–2.5	150–175
Extremely heavy	2.5	175

*For an excellent historical review of such indices, the reader is referred to an article by Lee.[53]

TABLE 22–4.

Rectal Temperature and Heart Rate Responses of Unacclimatized and Acclimatized Men* to Work in Heat†

PARAMETER	GROUP	N	MEAN ± SD	95% CONFIDENCE INTERVAL
Rectal temperature (°C)	Unacclimatized	104	39.07 ± 0.55	38.97–39.17
	Acclimatized	44	38.31 ± 0.34	38.20–38.41
Heart rate (beats/min)	Unacclimatized	104	166 ± 15	160–172
	Acclimatized	44	131 ± 14	127–135

*Healthy male recruits to the South African gold mining industry, aged 20–35 years.
†External work rate of 54 W maintained for four hours in hot, humid (33.2° C dry-bulb; 31.7° C wet-bulb) conditions.

from individual monitoring, if feasible. Unfortunately, in most instances, individual monitoring is impractical, and consequently, indices of the environmental heat load that correlate most closely with the physiological response to work in heat are applied. Of these, the Wet Bulb Globe Temperature Index (WBGT) is internationally recognized, especially where physical work is involved, while the Effective Temperature (ET) or Corrected Effective Temperature (CET) is intended as an index of comfort. However, irrespective of the particular index or its degree of sophistication, they all suffer a common shortcoming: metabolic rate is either omitted or estimated with no consideration of individual reaction. Of necessity, therefore, such indices are inaccurate and have to err on the side of conservatism.

WBGT Index

The WBGT Index and its use have been reviewed in several excellent texts, e.g., Ramsey,[66] and consequently only the essentials will be considered. The ACGIH version (Table 22–5) does not differ considerably from its ISO counterpart (Table 22–6). The main differences pertain to (1) number of work categories, (2) corrections for air movement, and (3) corrections for state of acclimatization (the ACGIH limits apply to acclimatized, fit individuals).

The WBGT can also be approximated by means of a so-called wet globe thermometer (WGT) or Botsball (BB). The relationship in degrees Celsius is

$$\text{WGBT} = 1.01\ \text{BB} + 2.6$$

or

$$\text{BB} = 0.905\ \text{WBGT} - 0.909$$

with a correlation coefficient of $r = 0.956$.[7] In view of its size, ruggedness, and ease of use, the BB has gained wide acceptance and threshold limit values have been developed (Table 22–7). Moreover, the natural wet-bulb (NWB) has a higher correlation coefficient with the BB than with the WBGT,[67] and the BB may therefore serve as a more reliable index of environmental conditions under conditions of high humidity.

When humidity levels of the environment are on the increase, the wet-bulb temperature is the predominant environmental condition to take note. From a physiologic point of view, a rise in dry-bulb temperature of 5°C can be equated with a rise in wet-bulb temperature of 1°C, i.e., a dry-bulb/wet-bulb environment of 45°C/30°C is tantamount to one of 33°C wet-bulb, saturated.[86, 99]

Effective Temperature

Effective Temperature is an index that combines into a single value the subjective thermal sensation resulting from air temperature (or globe temperature when radiant heat exceeds air temperature by more than 1°C), humidity, and air movement, i.e., a given ET exists for various combinations of temperature, humidity, and air movement (Fig 22–5). The index does not take into account metabolic rates other than for light or sedentary work and its use is therefore limited to an index of comfort or as a guide to analyze productivity. In summer, the maximum number of people should be comfortable at an ET of 21.7°C (range: 18–26°C), in winter at 20°C (range: 15–23°C). These values are subject to variation in different geographic regions. Although useful, the index does have a number of shortcomings: (1) it gives insufficient weight to the detrimental effect of air movement below 0.5 m/sec in hot, humid

TABLE 22–5.

Essentials of the WBGT Index (ACGIH)

1. Calculation

WITH SOLAR LOAD	WITHOUT SOLAR LOAD
WBGT (°C) = 0.7 WB + 0.2 GT + 0.1 DB	WBGT (°C) = 0.7 WB + 0.3 GT

WB = wet-bulb temperature, GT = globe temperature, DB = dry-bulb temperature (°C).

2. Threshold Limit Values

WORK-REST CYCLE (% OF EACH HOUR)	WORK RATE LIGHT	MODERATE	HEAVY
Continuous	30.0	26.7	25.0
75:25	30.6	28.0	25.9
50:50	31.4	29.4	27.9
25:75	32.2	31.1	30.0

3. Work Rate Categories

CATEGORY	METABOLIC RATE* O_2 L/MIN	C/HR	KJ/HR	W
Light	≤0.60	≤200	≤840	≤230
Moderate	0.70–1.0	201–300	841–1,250	231–340
Heavy	>1.0	>300	>1,250	>340

*Values have been rounded for convenience.

TABLE 22–6.
WBGT Threshold Limit Values According to ISO Specifications

METABOLIC RATE W	WBGT °C			
	ACCLIMATIZED		UNACCLIMATIZED	
<117	33		32	
117–234	30		29	
>234–360	28		26	
>360–468	25*	26†	22*	23†
>468	23*	25†	18*	20†

*No sensible air movement
†Sensible air movement

conditions; (2) it exaggerates the effect of high dry-bulb temperature at air movements in the range of 0.5–1.5 m/sec during physical work, and it underestimates the harmful effects of air movement in excess of 1.5 m/sec at dry-bulb temperatures of 49°C and higher; and (3) environmental conditions inducing the same physiologic stress, in terms of rectal temperature, heart rate, sweat rate, and tolerance, do not constitute the same ET, especially in severe heat stress.

PRODUCTIVITY

The competitive demands for adequate perfusion of active skeletal muscle and the skin impose a limit on work capacity, overall performance and, ultimately, productivity. Irrespective of the complexity of the task, human performance declines significantly in the ET range of 27–30°C. For strenuous physical work in gold mines, the decline is 5% at 29, 10% at 30, 17% at 31.5, and 30% at 32.5°C ET.[87] These figures were computed from data shown in Figure 22–6 and are representative of simulated mining conditions. Under actual conditions, the decline in performance is more severe. Using monthly production figures, Smith[82] recorded productivity losses on a typical deep-level mine in South Africa amounting to 1.08% at 26, 3.79% at 27, 7.86% at 28, 13.96% at 29, 22.76% at 30, 33.6% at 30, 50.54% at 31, and 70.19% at 32°C wet-bulb. These studies highlight the progressive decline in performance associated with increasing wet-bulb temperatures.

Smith's data[82] also reveal that "100% performance" can be maintained up to wet-bulb temperatures of about 25°C. This reinforces the view that relative humidity can be ignored in conditions where the wet-bulb temperature does not exceed 24°C, providing that the dry-bulb does not exceed 30°C.[86] However, it should be borne in mind that heat stress degrades mental performance well in advance of a deterioration in physical performance according to Hancock,[29] and that this may have an adverse effect on productivity, in that "a decrease in performance is more closely associated with the feeling of discomfort than with differences in physiologic strain."[55] Inasmuch as tasks requiring the acquisition of special skills or actions may be complicated by heat, despite partial heat acclimatization of the labor force,[15] this aspect deserves attention. At the time ET, the adverse consequences of humid conditions seem to be greater than in dry conditions.[77]

Increasing environmental heat loads ultimately also have a bearing on safety, and, although it is often difficult to link improvements to given interventions, there seems to be a close correlation between accident frequency rate and wet-bulb temperature (Fig 22–7).

STRATEGIES TO COUNTER HEAT STRESS

The strategies to counter the deleterious consequences of physical work in hot industrial settings are

1. Proper engineering design to achieve adequate cooling, ventilation, and shielding from radiant heat sources and/or to achieve a reduction in work rate through mechanization

2. Administrative control of personnel, whereby the number and duration of exposures are modified by work-rest cycles or the provision of cool rest areas

3. Personal protection by means of body cooling garments (microclimate cooling)

4. Physiologic control through selection and acclimatization

The obvious strategy to pursue first is engineering control, followed by administrative control. In most instances, these strategies provide adequate control; in others they are ineffectual because of economic and practical considerations. In view of possible social and morale implications, personal protection and physiologic control should be regarded as a last resort, to be used when the primary strategies (engineering and administrative control) have failed.

TABLE 22–7.
Threshold Limit Values for Botsball Units Related to WBGT*

METABOLIC RATE C/HR	WORK-REST CYCLE (% OF EACH HOUR)							
	CONTINUOUS		75:25		50:50		27:75	
	WBGT†	BB†	WBGT	BB	WBGT	BB	WBGT	BB
200	30.0	26.2	30.6	26.7	31.4	27.5	32.2	28.3
350	26.7	23.2	27.8	24.2	29.4	25.7	31.1	27.2
500	25.0	21.7	25.8	22.5	27.8	24.2	30.0	26.2

*Adapted from Beshir MY, Ramsey JD, Burford CL: Threshold values for Botsball: A field study of occupational heat. *Ergonomics* 1982; 25:247–254. Used by permission.
†In degrees Celsius.

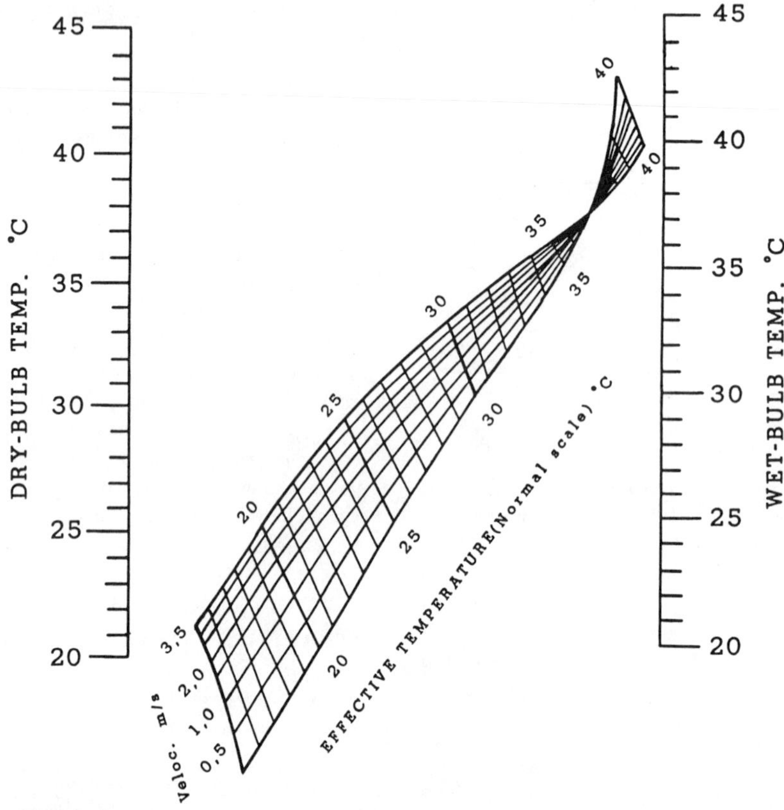

FIG 22–5.
Effective Temperature nomogram for lightly clothed men.

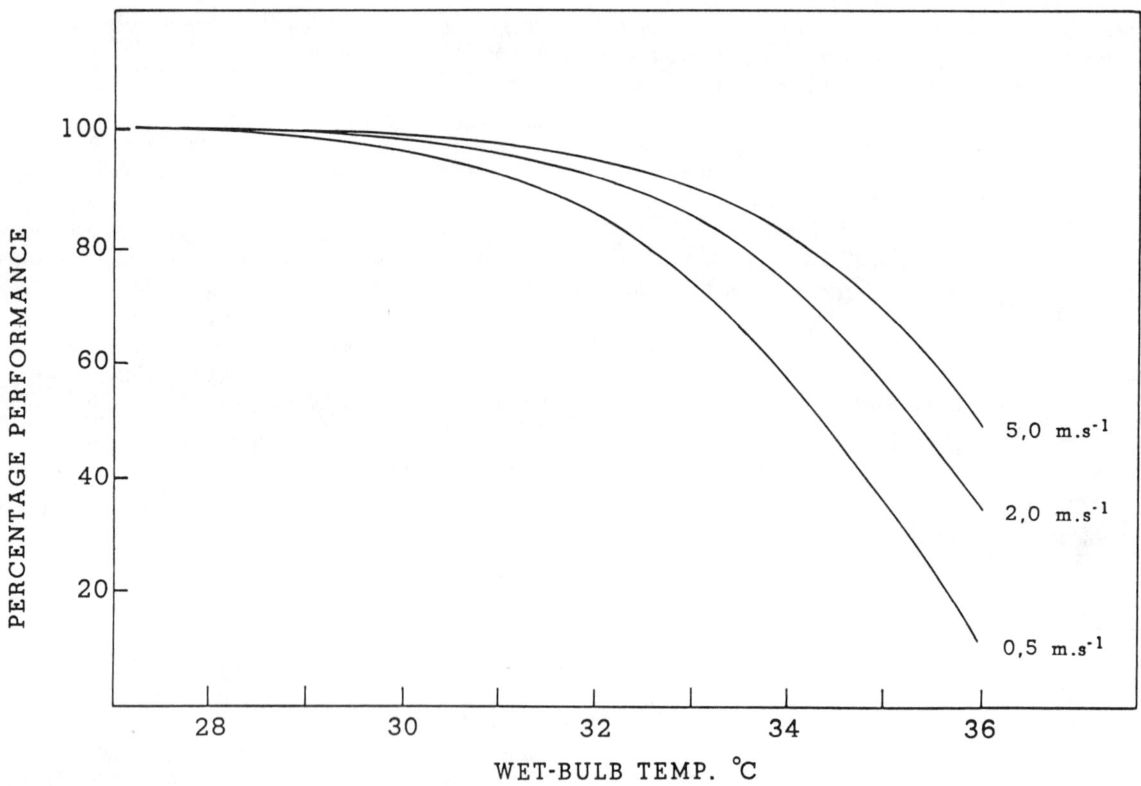

FIG 22–6.
The influence of air movement (0.5, 2.0, and 5.0 m/sec) and wet-bulb temperature on work performance. At 33° C wet-bulb performance declines by about 25% and 15% of the respective air velocities.

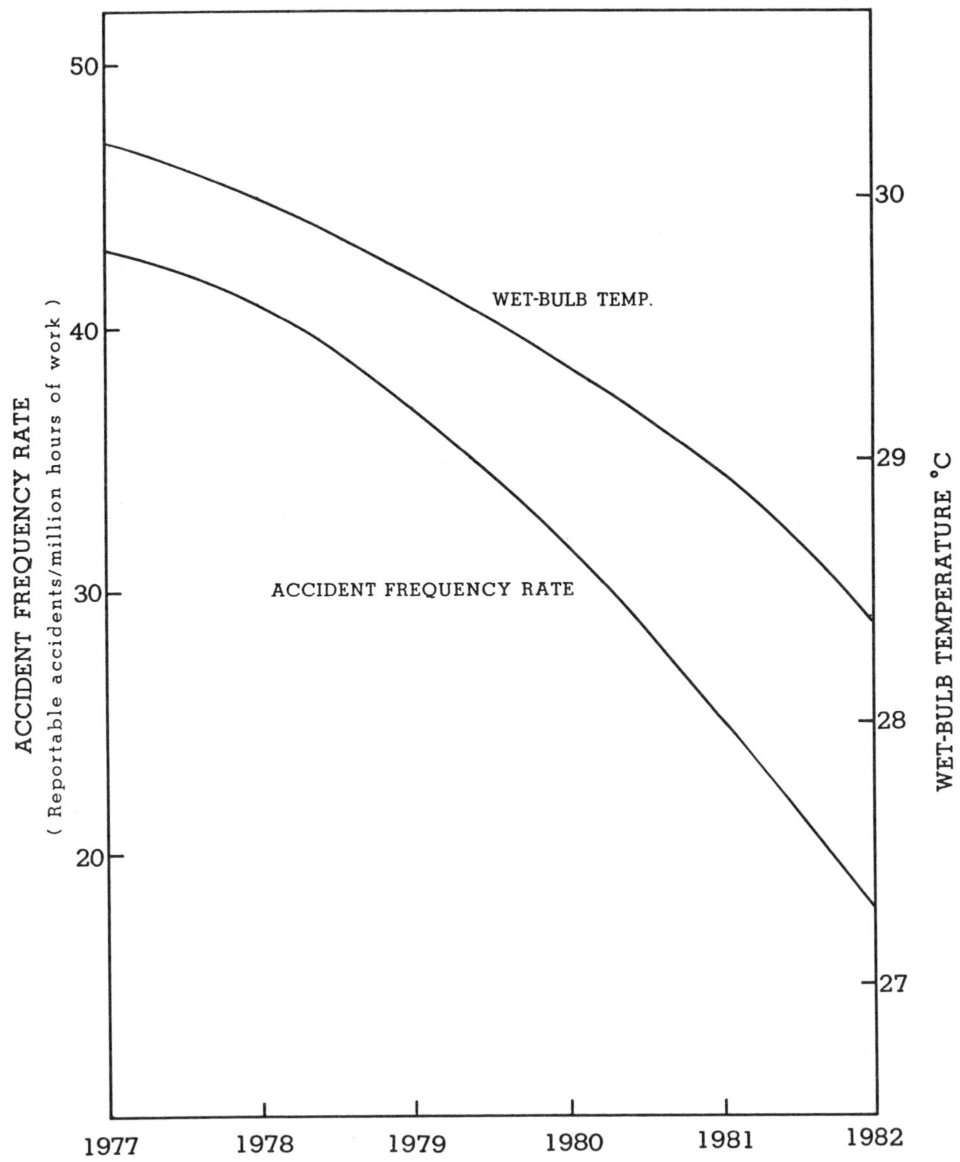

FIG 22–7.
Improved thermal conditions are not only associated with higher productivity, but also with a decrease in accidents. The findings apply to a South African gold mine and have been adapted from Smith (1984).

Inasmuch as engineering control falls outside the scope of this chapter (or indeed, can be assumed to have failed), and administrative control is adequately covered by the recommendations pertaining to the WBGT index, further discussion will be restricted to physiologic control and personal protection.

Physiologic Control

Physiologic control embraces (1) selection on the basis of natural heat tolerance and (2) heat acclimatization. The net result, irrespective of the means, is the availability of a physically superior labor force. Inasmuch as "normal" limits are likely to be exceeded, thereby reducing prevailing tolerances, the estimation of risk, in contrast to specifying a universally acceptable safe upper limit (e.g., core temperature of 38°C as per the WBGT index), becomes the fundamental health and safety consideration.

For given conditions (environment, work rate, and exposure), an unacceptable health risk may be defined in terms of the probability norm for the development of dangerously elevated core (rectal) temperatures. In the South African gold mining industry, a "dangerously elevated core temperature" is regarded as 40°C. The choice of this limit has its origins in the observation that a rectal temperature of 40°C represents the safe upper limit in terms of the likelihood of heatstroke developing.[80, 96] Further, the risk is regarded as excessive when the probability of reaching such body temperatures or higher exceeds a one-in-a-million chance, i.e., one-in-a-million acclimatized workers. In practice this means that 99.9999% confidence limits are applied. An example of such estimates is provided in Figure 22–8, and it follows that safe upper limit body temperatures and probability norms could be modified for given conditions and population sizes. However, mean responses should under no circumstances be used for the purpose of setting limits.

For continued work in heat, the health risk for unacclimatized men becomes excessive at wet-bulb temperatures of 25°C and above. On the basis of heatstroke statistics for the South African gold mining industry, heat acclimatization becomes mandatory at 27.5°C wet-bulb (Fig 22–9), irrespective of the dry-bulb temperature and air movement. (It should be borne in mind that unacclimatized men are not fully capable of taking advantage of increased air movements in view of their relatively poor sweat abilities.)

Heat accclimatization is achieved by repetitive exposures to the stress imposed by a given combination of environmental heat load, work rate, and exposure duration. The number of exposures required is proportional to the overall stress ultimately to be faced. To achieve this, a progressive increase in work rate may be indicated so that the risk of developing dangerous levels of hyperthermia remains "acceptable" on each occasion. For example, to achieve a satisfactory degree of heat acclimatization to perform physical tasks generally associated with gold mining in the wet-bulb temperature zone of 30–32.8°C, a five-day regime of four hours per day is required. The increase in work rate, which amounts to a daily average of about 15%, is shown in Table 22–8.

In theory, a satisfactory degree of acclimatization can be achieved by manipulating both the environmental heat load and work rate. However, inasmuch as the accurate control of climatic conditions to within narrow, specified limits is difficult in practice, the desired increase in stress is best achieved by manipulating only work rate. This approach could be used for the concurrent acclimatization of labor destined to work in lower wet-bulb temperature zones (see Table 22–8).

Experience in the South African mining industry suggests that a rectal temperature of 38.5°C represents an upper limit for the maintenance of thermal equilibrium for extended periods of time. Conversely, this suggests that a satisfactory degree of acclimatization is represented by equilibrium rectal temperatures that do not exceed 38.5°C over periods in excess of four hours of sustained effort.

Heat acclimatization is specific. There are no real shortcuts

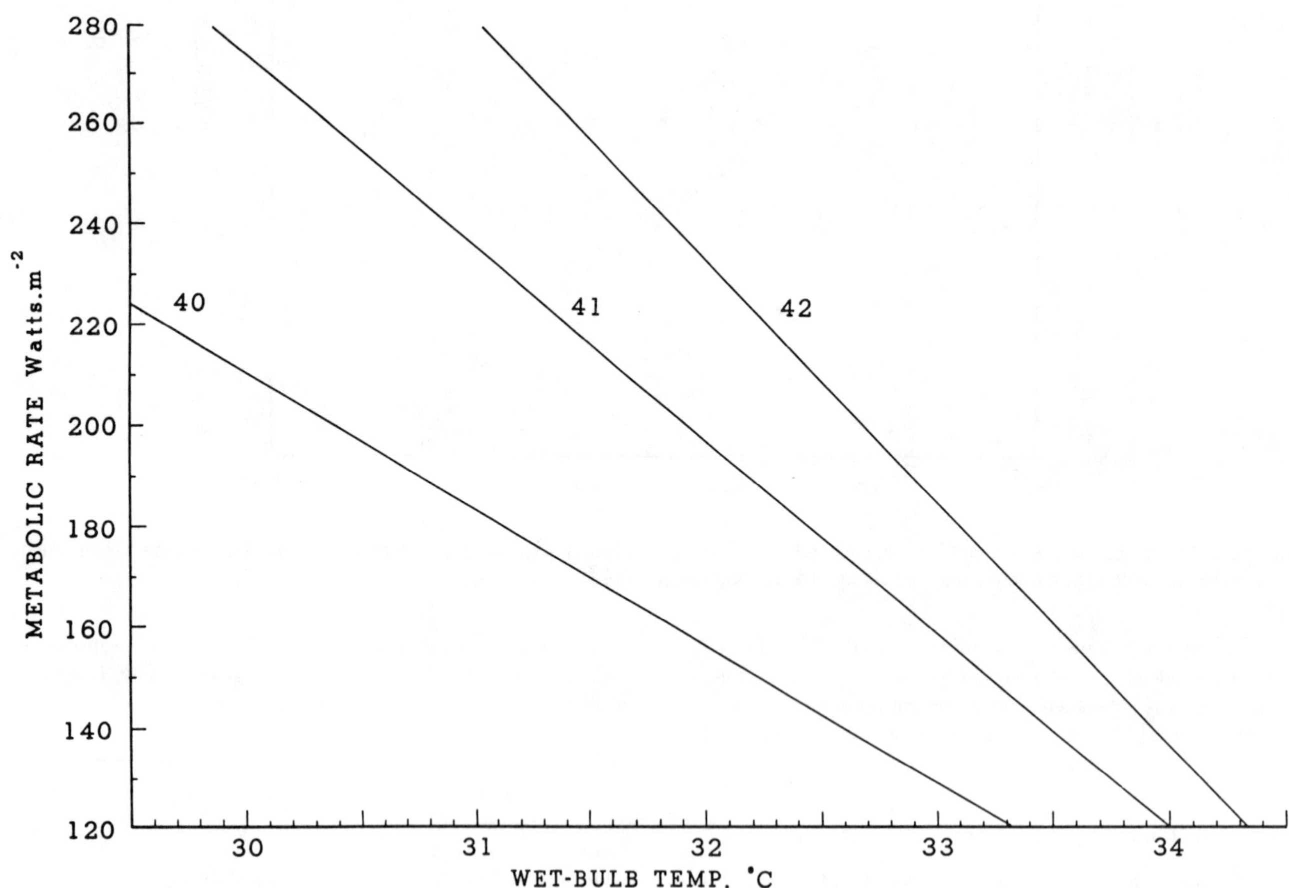

FIG 22–8.
Metabolic rate/wet-bulb temperature combinations required to ensure probability norms of less than a one-in-a-million chance that rectal temperature will reach various levels after four hours of work in hot, humid conditions (33.2° C dry-bulb; 31.7° C wet-bulb; air movement 0.5 m/sec).

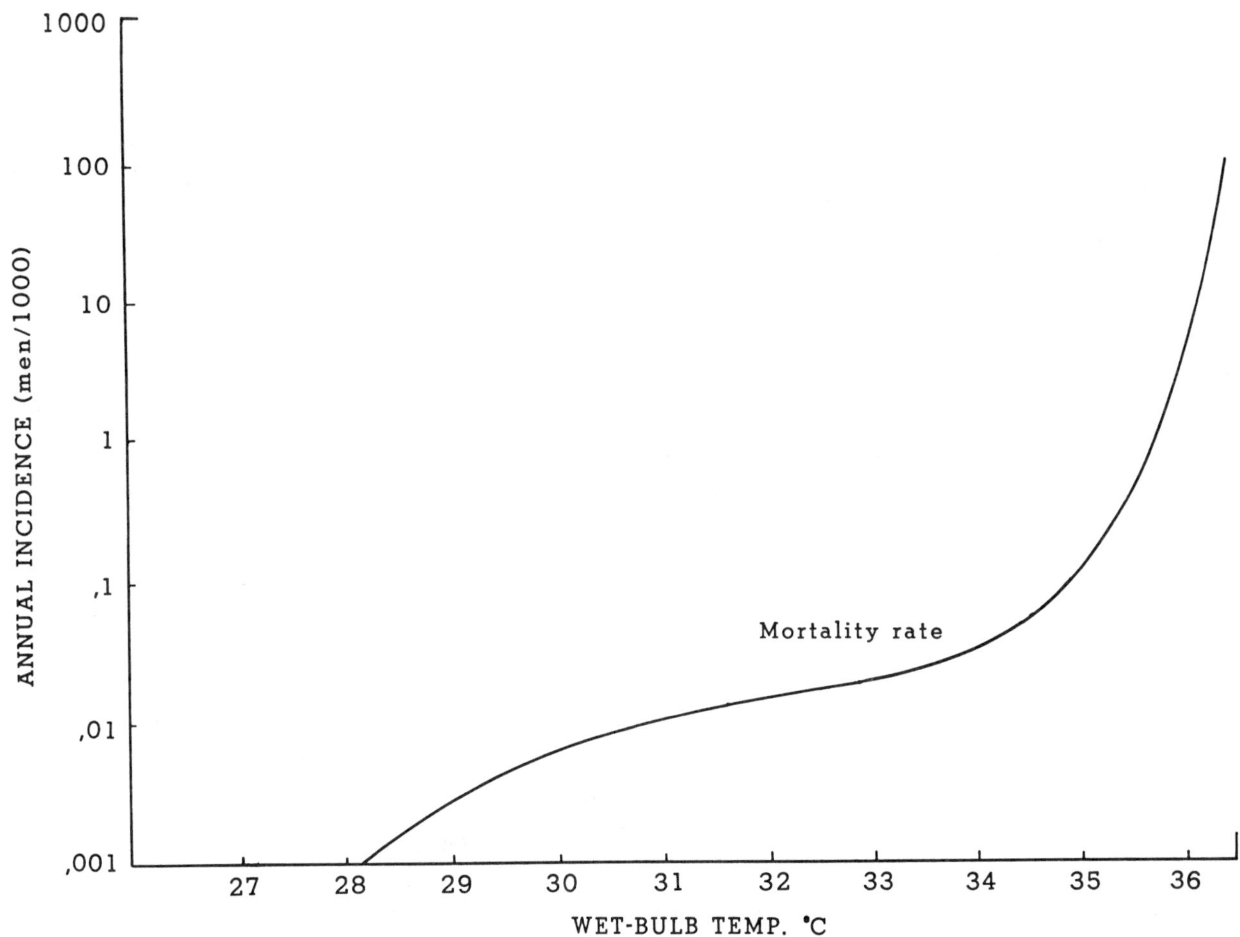

FIG 22–9.
Heatstroke mortality related to wet-bulb temperature. Statistics are based on a period of 11 years and represent a sample of 39 fatal cases which occurred in the South African gold mining industry. The mortality risk is less than one per 100,000 workers.

in achieving a satisfactory degree of heat acclimatization. Similarly, overacclimatization confers no special physiologic advantage. For example, Figure 22–10 illustrates the danger (in terms of elevated rectal temperature) of an inadequate daily exposure despite identical environmental conditions and work rate. However, data from the same experiments reveal that a daily exposure period of one hour prepares a person as well for work of one hour's duration as a four-hour exposure period for work of four hours' duration under identical environmental conditions and work rates (Fig 22–11).

TABLE 22–8.
Recommended Acclimatization Regime for Continued Work at Moderate to Hard Levels in the Wet-Bulb Temperature Range of 30 to 32.8°C*

ACCLIMATIZATION DAY	WORK RATES (W) FOR EACH 30-MINUTE INTERVAL								
	0–30	31–60	61–90	91–120	121–150	151–180	181–210	211–240	AVERAGE
1	35	35	35	35	35	35	70	35	39
2	35	35	70	35	70	35	70	35	48
3	35	70	35	70	35	70	70	70	57
4	35	70	70	70	70	70	70	70	66
5	70	70	70	70	70	70	70	70	70

*Environmental temperatures are 33.2°C dry-bulb and 31.7°C wet-bulb, with an air movement of about 0.5 m/sec. This corresponds to 32.15°C WBGT and 28.89°C ET. The same environmental conditions could be retained to achieve optimum acclimatization for work in lower wet-bulb temperature zones with slight modifications in work rate, e.g., in a wet-bulb temperature zone of 27.5–29.0°C, the work rate schedule shown for days 1, 2, and 3 could be followed. In work areas with wet-bulb temperatures greater than 29°C but less than 30°C, day 1, 2, 3, and 4 work rate schedules could be followed.

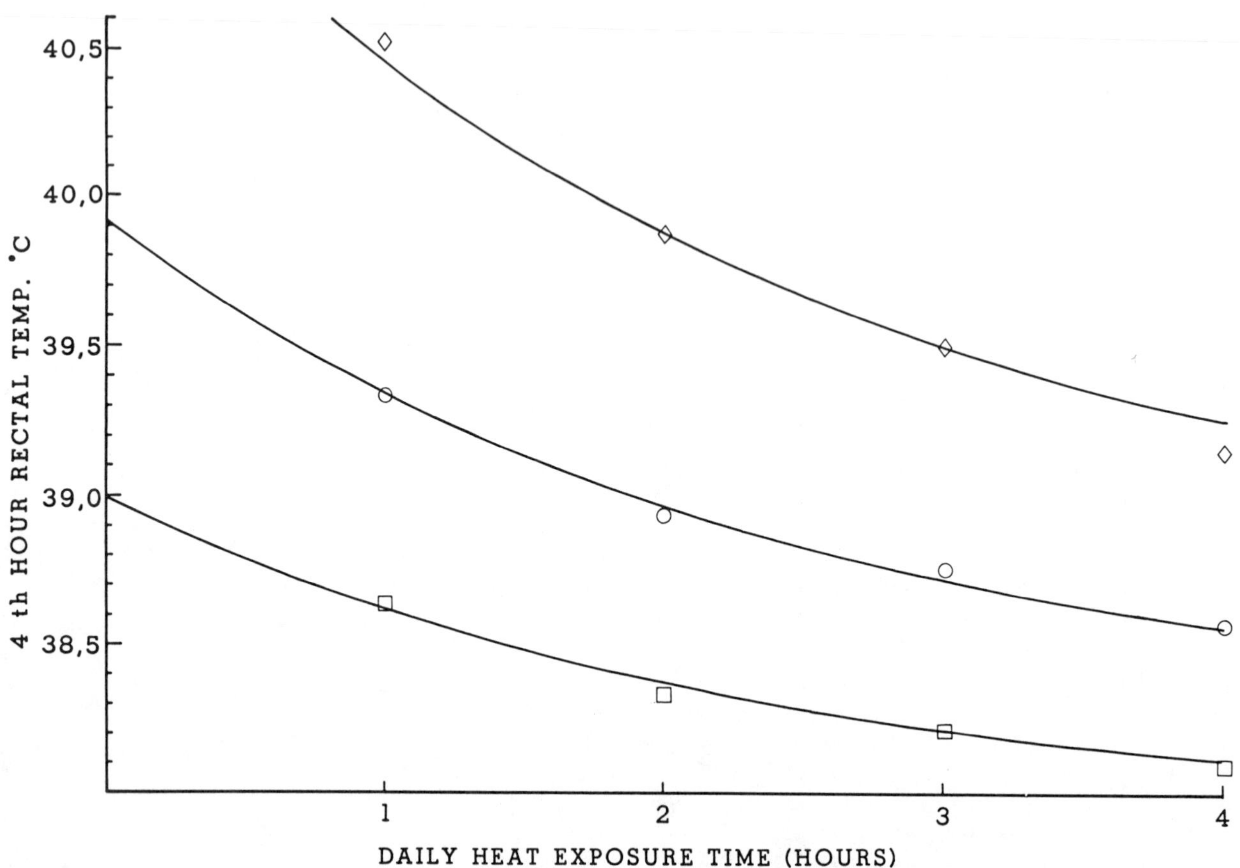

FIG 22–10.
The influence of variations in daily exposure on the degree of heat acclimatization. Four groups of men were acclimatized over a five-day period. External work rate amounted to 54 W at dry- and wet-bulb temperatures of 33.2 and 31.7° C, respectively. Daily exposures were one, two, three, and four hours, respectively. The results show fourth-hour rectal temperatures (with 95% confidence limits) for the respective groups on the sixth (test) day under the same conditions outlined above.

Natural tolerance to heat varies tremendously from one person to another. This observation can be applied in the design of a heat tolerance test (HTT) to identify individuals with a degree of natural heat tolerance sufficiently high to obviate formal heat acclimatization. The fundamental principle is that a naturally heat-tolerant individual should always be defined as one who does not stand to benefit from formal heat acclimatization. Using the same risk criterion outlined earlier, heat tolerance for an anticipated exposure of four hours' duration (33.2°C dry-bulb; 31.7°C wet-bulb; work rate at 54 W) is signified by rectal temperatures of 38.5°C or lower, and for two hours' duration, under the same conditions, 38.8°C. Oral temperatures of 37.5° and 37.8°C, respectively, could be substituted, although the discriminatory power is reduced toward a more conservative estimate.

Despite the advantages associated with climatic room acclimatization (CRA), e.g., control of climatic conditions, individual monitoring, and the availability of facilities for immediate treatment, it remains unproductive in terms of lost shifts. Thus, in the South African gold mining industry, where these aspects are extremely relevant, research was challenged with the development of a method of heat acclimatization without the attendant negative features of CRA. Subsequent research demonstrated that with coolant in contact with about one third of the body surface area, the rise in body temperature during work in heat is controlled to the extent that heat acclimatization occurs in a normal way: a rise in body temperature, a prerequisite to the development of heat acclimatization, is not prevented; it is only prevented from rising excessively, as shown by Schutte et al.[73] and Kielblock et al.[50] This method, microclimate acclimatization (MCA), is at present being phased into the South African gold mines as an alternative to conventional climatic chamber procedures (Fig 22–12).

The choice of coolant for MCA will be determined by factors such as exposure period, work rate, and environmental condition. For relatively short exposures (two to three hours), frozen-water jackets are quite sufficient, but for longer periods, frozen carbon dioxide (dry ice) is preferable. Obviously, economic considerations will also influence the final decision.

Procedures currently in use in the South African mining industry are summarized by way of a flow diagram in Figure 22–13. Although applicable to a large labor force (in excess of 300,000

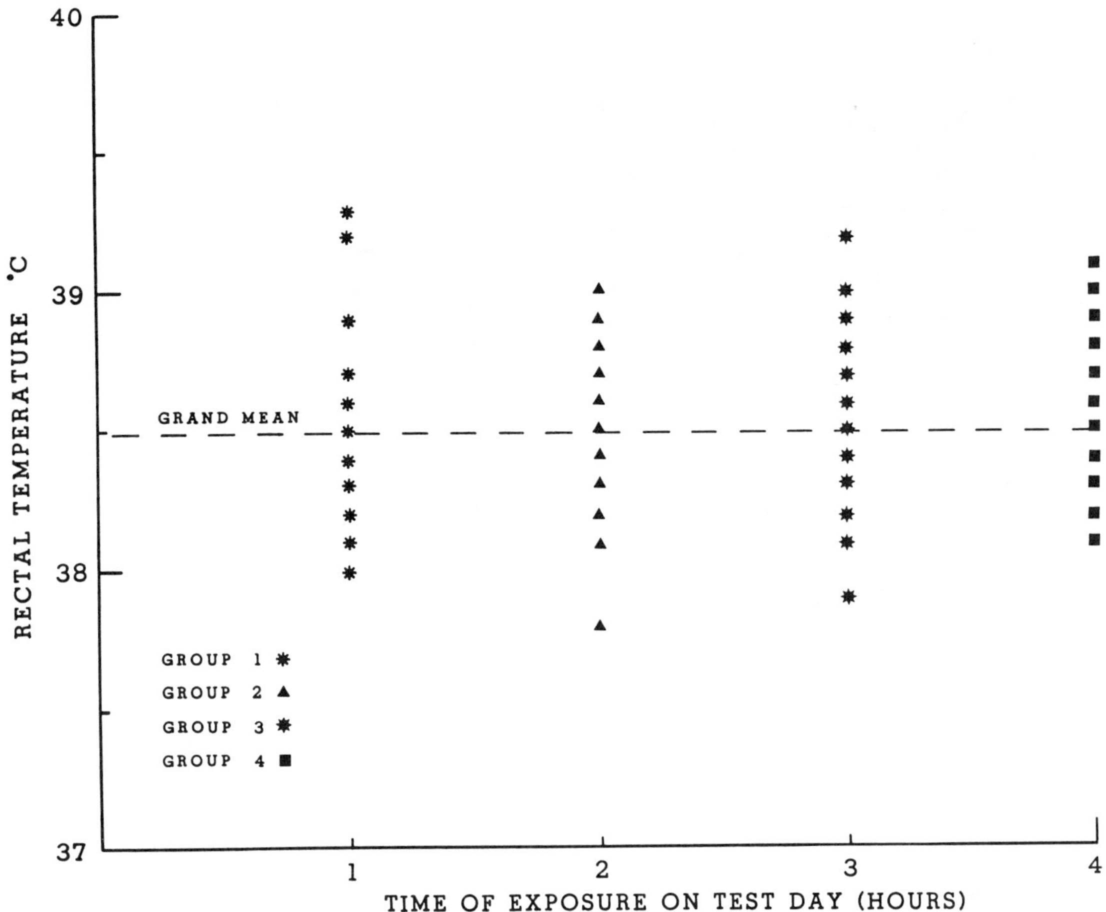

FIG 22–11.
Over acclimatization confers no special physiologic benefit. The data (see Figure 22–10 for experimental details) reveal that group 1 is as well acclimatized for one hour's work in heat as group 4 for four hours' work in heat. Thus, four hours' acclimatization is wasteful if the intended exposure amounts to only one hour.

workers), the general approach nevertheless remains relevant to any industry that has to rely on physiologic control as a strategy of "bearing the heat."

Personal Protection

Personal protection through body cooling garments is indicated as an alternative to physiologic control (selection based on heat tolerance and heat acclimatization) or if conditions are such that human capabilities will be exceeded, irrespective of superior heat tolerance or maximal heat acclimatization. The upper limits of heat tolerance applicable to the South African mining industry are given in Table 22–9. The data may be recalculated in terms of degrees centigrade WBGT or ET and may also therefore be applied as a guide to the derivation of upper limits for other combinations of environmental conditions.

Body cooling by means of special garments can be achieved by several means. A synopsis of the major systems, coolants, special features and references to manufacturers and scientific documents are presented in Table 22–10. The ultimate choice should be based on the following principles:

1. Under conditions conducive to instantaneous harm, protection can only be achieved through full body coverage.

TABLE 22–9.
Limiting Wet-Bulb Temperatures* for Various Work Rates in Hot, Humid Conditions†‡

WORK CATEGORY	WORK RATE		WET-BULB LIMITS °C
	O_2 IN L/MIN	W/SQ M	
Light	0.68	133	33.9
Moderate	1.05	205	32.5
Hard	1.41	275	30.8

*Based on risk criterion of a probability that rectal temperature elevations of 40.0°C or more are less than 1 in 10^6 (see text).
†Dry-bulb exceeds wet-bulb by 1.5°C; air movement varies between 0.3 and 0.5 m/sec.
‡The data apply to a test sample of 200 acclimatized male recruits varying in age between 20 and 37 years.

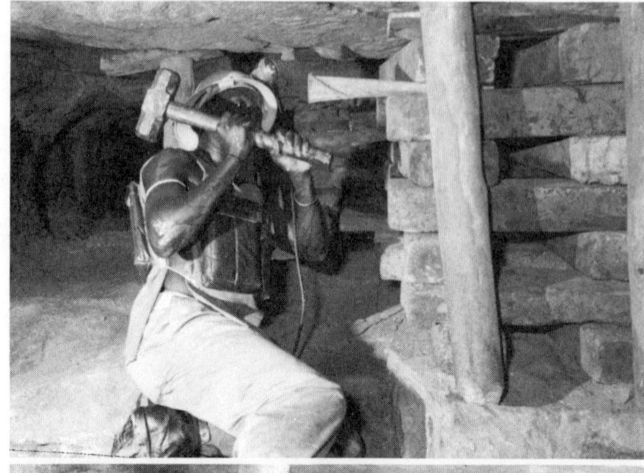

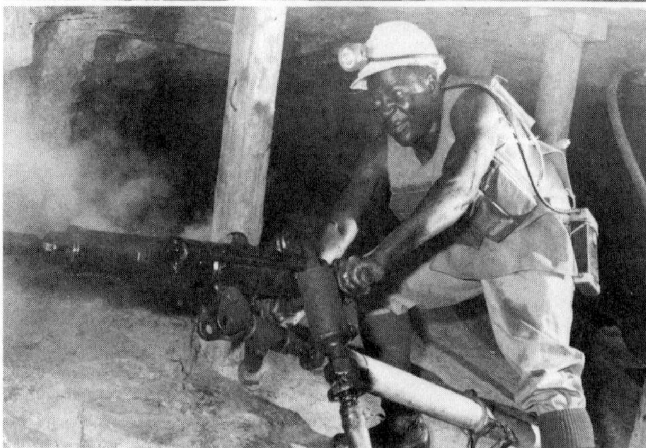

FIG 22–12.
Productive heat acclimatization in the South African gold mines. A body cooling jacket, containing four 1-kg dry-ice slabs, controls body temperature elevations sufficiently so that a satisfactory degree of heat acclimatization is achieved over a period of six consecutive shifts. The garment also finds application as a means of protection under abnormal conditions. The photographs were taken in a gold mine.

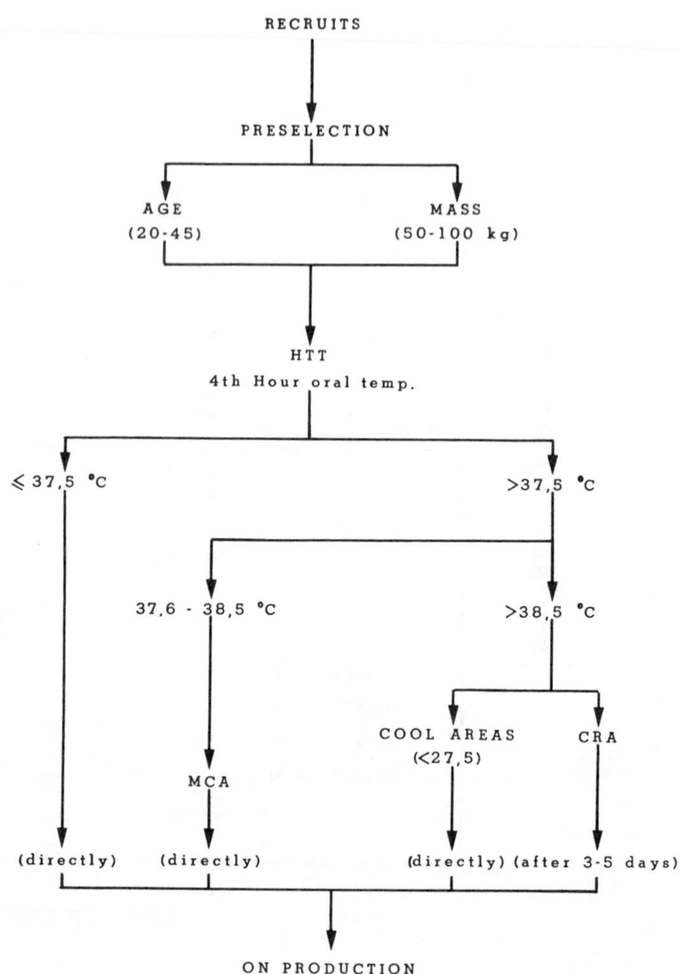

FIG 22–13.
Sequence of procedures for the allocation of labor for work in hot areas. Preselection is done on the basis of age and mass. The heat tolerance test identifies men with a degree of natural heat tolerance sufficiently high to obviate any further form of heat acclimatization and those eligible to undergo microclimate acclimatization (MCA). These men are productive from the outset. A third category will achieve full acclimatization only under rigorous climatic room conditions.

2. Roving tasks immediately rule out garments perfused by umbilical lines, unless the heat exchanger unit forms an integral part of the garment.

3. For stationary tasks, e.g., driving military or load-haul-dump vehicles, garments perfused by umbilical lines from remote heat exchangers are ideal, since restrictions imposed by garment bulk, mass, or cooling capacity do not apply.

4. More sophisticated, self-contained units are recommended for use in uncontaminated atmospheres, but they may be impractical in view of added bulk and mass if worn in conjunction with breathing equipment.

5. Head cooling garments should be worn, if practical.

6. Water-ice jackets are cheap and effective for short-term exposures (up to about two hours).

7. Dry-ice (carbon dioxide) jackets are extremely robust, and the cooling capacity is sufficient to provide protection for extended periods (up to about eight hours).

8. The cooling garment should be acceptable to the wearer.

9. The garments should be cost-efficient.

For conditions in the South African gold mines, the system of choice is a jacket containing dry ice (Fig 22–14). The system is economically viable, since the infrastructure exists. Moreover, the jacket is sufficiently robust to withstand the harsh work conditions, and the cooling capacity of about 17 W/sq m (1.5 times that of water ice), which is quite adequate to provide the necessary protection (Fig 22–15). Dry ice will also last an entire shift, which is an important consideration in work areas that are several kilome-

TABLE 22–10.
Body Cooling Garments: General Design, Coolant Type, and References

GENERAL DESIGN	TYPE OF COOLANT			
	AIR	WATER/LIQUID	ICE	DRY ICE
Full suit		Dräger, West Germany; ILC Dover, United Kingdom		
Jacket/vest	Shapiro et al.[76]	ILC Dover, United Kingdom; Nunneley and Maldonado[60]	Dräger, West Germany	Gard-Rite, South Africa; Schutte et al.;[73] Kielblock et al.[50]
Hood		ILC Dover, United Kingdom; Nunneley and Maldonado[60]		
Umbilical line	Essential	Essential, in conjunction with remote heat exchangers	Not required	

ters removed from the main shaft or central facilities. By sublimation, the initial mass of the frozen carbon dioxide of at least 4 kg is reduced to less than 1 kg at the end of the shift. This represents a meaningful bonus under such taxing conditions of work.

Personal Protection in Conjunction With Selection

The strategies described in the latter two sections (Physiologic Control and Personal Protection) have been based largely on prior knowledge of the environmental conditions workers are destined to enter. Proper planning is therefore possible. However, in the circumstances dictated by special operations, the environmental heat load likely to be encountered often is not known or cannot be predicted with certainty. Workers may therefore enter excessively hot environments and they may nevertheless be expected to complete certain tasks. Prime examples are rescue and firefighting operations, especially in mines and forest fire control.

In considering this uncertainty, it should be remembered that the workers at risk often constitute an elite group, specially selected on the basis of a variety of attributes of which heat tolerance, although important, is not the only criterion. Under these circumstances, the objective of selection places emphasis solely on the identification and rejection of grossly heat-intolerant individuals who, as a matter of course, constitute a weak link in an operation relying heavily on teamwork. It is assumed that, by virtue of good instruction, training, experience, and more than a modicum of common sense, the risk to the remaining team members would be minimized despite entering environments not normally suited for routine tasks.

The above approach has been implemented in the South African mining industry, where gross heat-intolerance for rescue brigadesmen is defined as an elevation in rectal temperature in excess of 39.0°C following a standard heat tolerance test of one hour's duration conducted at a dry-bulb temperature of 33.2°C, a wet-bulb temperature of 31.7°C, an air movement of 0.4 m/sec and an external work rate of 54 W (Chamber of Mines Application Report No. 8, 1985).[12]

In conjunction, the procedure described above includes the provision of special dry-ice cooling garments, designed to last a

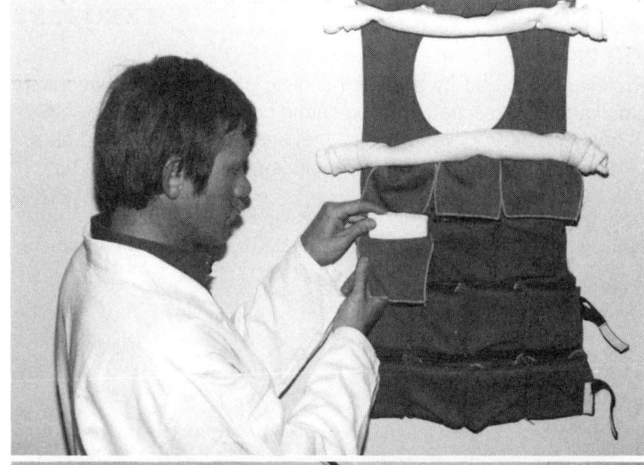

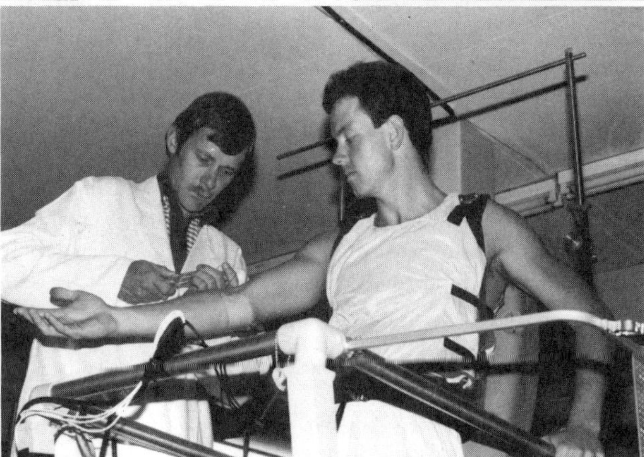

FIG 22–14.
A dry-ice jacket to afford protection for rescue operations. The particular design ensures unrestricted movement and does not interfere with breathing equipment. The photographs were taken during laboratory simulation.

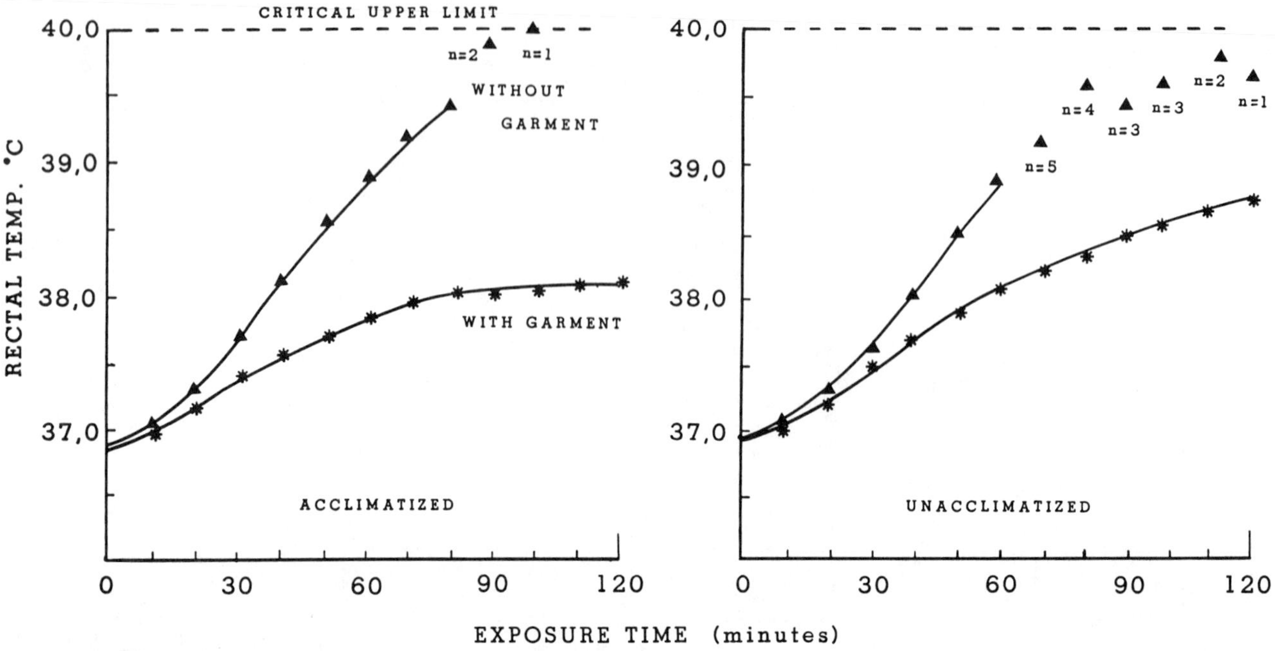

FIG 22–15.
Protection afforded by a dry-ice cooling garment under laboratory simulation of a rescue operation during hot, humid conditions (35.5° C dry-bulb; 34.0° C wet-bulb; air movement 0.5 m/sec) and an external work rate of 54 W. The benefit is significant in terms both of body temperature elevations and tolerance time. The results also indicate that body cooling could be employed as an extension of heat acclimatization, and not merely as an alternative.

minimum of two hours, for operations taking place in environments with wet-bulb temperatures in excess of 27.5°C.

CONCLUSION

In a sense, this chapter could be viewed as an attempt to apply the principle of ergonomics, i.e., "fitting the task to the man,"[26] in reverse order. Obviously, such an approach can be justified on the basis of economic and practical considerations. The perspective to retain, however, is that such considerations should not detract from industry's responsibility to provide a suitable thermal environment for workers. Therefore, it should be emphasized that the major strategies for preventing heat stress are, in order of priority, proper engineering design and construction, worker protection through the imposition of realistic stress indices, and, only as a final resort, "fitting the man to the task."

REFERENCES

1. American Conference of Governmental Industrial Hygienists: Threshold limit values. Heat stress, in *Threshold Limit Values for Chemical Substances and Physical Agents with Intended Changes for 1978*. Cincinnati, Oh, ACGIH, 1978.
2. American Society of Heating, Refrigeration and Air-conditioning Engineers: *ASHRAE Handbook. 1981 Fundamentals*. Atlanta, Ga, ASHRAE, 1981.
3. Ansari A, Burch GE: Influence of hot environments on the cardiovascular system. *Arch Intern Med* 1969; 123:371–378.
4. Åstrand P-O, Rodahl K: *Textbook of Work Physiology*. New York, McGraw-Hill Book Co, 1977.
5. Avellini BA, Shapiro Y, Pandolf KB: Physiological responses of men and women to prolonged dry heat exposure. *Aviat Space Environ Med* 1980; 51:1081–1085.
6. Belding HS: Resistance to heat in man and other homeothermic animals, in Rose AH (ed): *Thermobiology*. New York, Academic Press, 1967.
7. Beshir MY, Ramsey JD, Burford CL: Threshold values for the Botsball: A field study of occupational heat. *Ergonomics* 1982; 25:247–254.
8. Bligh J: Temperature regulation: A theoretical consideration incorporating Sherrington principles of central neurology. *J Therm Biol* 1984; 9:3–6.
9. Bligh J, Moore R (eds): *Essays on Temperature Regulation*. New York, Elsevier North-Holland, Inc, 1982.
10. Brengelman GL: Circulatory adjustments to exercise and heat stress. *Ann Rev Physiol* 45:191–212.
11. Burton AC: Human calorimetry II. The average temperature of the tissues of the body. *J Nutr* 1935; 9:26–27.
12. Chamber of Mines of South Africa: *Rescue Brigadesmen: Physiological Selection and Protection*, Application Report 8. Johannesburg, Chamber of Mines of South Africa, 1985.
13. Christensen EH: Physiology of work, in Parmeggiani L (ed): *Encyclopaedia of Occupational Health and Safety*, ed 3. Geneva, International Labour Organization, 1983, vol 2, pp 1698–1700.
14. Collins KJ: Heat illness: Diagnosis, treatment and prevention. *The Practitioner* 1977; 219:193–198.
15. Curley MD, Hawkins RN: Cognitive performance during a heat acclimatization regimen. *Aviat Space Environ Med* 1983; 54:709–713.
16. Drinkwater BL, Horvath SM: Heat tolerance and aging. *Med Sci Sports* 1979; 11:49–55.

17. Drinkwater BL, Bedi JF, Loucks AB, et al: Sweating sensitivity and capacity of women in relation to age. *J Appl Physiol* 1982; 53:671–676.
18. Dukes-Dobos FN: Rationale and provisions of the work practices standard for work in hot environments as recommended by NIOSH, in Horvath SM, Jensen RC (eds): *Standards for Occupational Exposures to Hot Environments*, pp 27–42. US Government Printing Office, 1973, pp 27–42.
19. Dukes-Dobos FN: Hazards of heat exposure. A review. *Scand J Work Environ Health* 1981; 7:73–83.
20. Edgerton VR, Gardner GW, Ohira Y, et al: Iron-deficiency anaemia and its effect on worker productivity and activity patterns. *Br Med J* 1979; 2:1546–1549.
21. Eichler AC, McFee AS, Root HD: Heat stroke. *Am J Surf* 1969; 118:855–863.
22. Frye AJ, Kamon E: Responses to dry heat of men and women with similar aerobic capacities. *J Appl Physiol: Respir Environ Exerc Physiol* 1981; 50:65–70.
23. Gisolfi CV: Temperature regulation during exercise: Directions—1983. *Med Sci Sports Exerc* 1983; 15:15–20.
24. Gold J: Development of heat pyrexia. *JAMA* 1960; 173:79–86.
25. Gonzalez RP, Berglund LG, Gagge AP: Indices of thermoregulatory strain for moderate exercise in heat. *J Appl Physiol* 1978; 4:889–895.
26. Grandjean E: *Fitting the task to the man. An ergonomic approach.* London, Taylor and Francis Ltd, 1980.
27. Greenleaf JE, Brock PJ, Keil LC, et al: Drinking and water balance during exercise in heat. *J Appl Physiol* 1983; 54:414–419.
28. Grucza R: Body heat balance in man subjected to endogenous and exogenous heat load. *Eur J Appl Physiol* 1983; 51:419–433.
29. Hancock PA: Heat stress impairment of mental performance: A revision of tolerance limits. *Aviat Space Environ Med* 1981; 52:177–180.
30. Harrison MH, Edwards RJ, Graveney MJ, et al: Blood volume and plasma protein responses to heat acclimatization in humans. *J Appl Physiol* 1981; 50:597–604.
31. Haymes EM: Physiological responses of female athletes to heat stress: A review. *The Physician and Sports Medicine* 1984; 12:45–59.
32. Herman RH, Sullivan BH: Heatstroke and jaundice. *Am J Med* 1959; 26:154–166.
33. Houdas Y, Ring EFJ: *Human body temperature. Its measurement and regulation.* London, Plenum Press, 1982.
34. Hubbard RW, Bowers WD, Matthew WT: Rat model of acute heatstroke mortality. *J Appl Physiol* 1977; 42:809–816.
35. Hubbard RW, Criss REL, Elliot LP, et al: Diagnostic significance of selected serum enzymes in a rat heatstroke model. *J Appl Physiol* 1979; 46:334–339.
36. Iampietro PR: Heat induced tetany. *Fed Proc* 1963; 22:884–886.
37. Inbar O, Bar-Or O, Dotan R, et al: Conditioning versus exercise in heat as methods for acclimatising 8- to 10-year-old boys to dry heat. *J Appl Physiol: Respir Environ Exerc Physiol* 1981; 50:406–411.
38. International Standards Organization: *Hot Environments—Estimation of the Heat Stress on Working Man, Based on the WBGT-Index (Wet Bulb Globe Temperature)*, ISO 7243, ed 1. Geneva, ISO, 1982.
39. Keren G, Epstein Y: The effect of high dosage vitamin C intake on aerobic and anaerobic capacity. *J Sports Med* 1980; 20:145–148.
40. Keren G, Epstein Y, Magazanik A: Temporary heat intolerance in a heatstroke patient. *Aviat Space Environ Med* 1981; 52:116–117.
41. Kerslake D McK: Effects of climate, in Singleton WT (ed): *The Body at Work.* London, Cambridge University Press, 1982.
42. Knochel JP: Environmental heat illness. *Arch Intern Med* 1974; 133:841–864.
43. Kew MC: Temperature regulation in heatstroke in man. *Isr J Med Sci* 1976; 12:759–766.
44. Kew MC, Bersohn I, Peter J, et al: Preliminary observations on the serum and cerebrospinal fluid enzymes in heatstroke. *S Afr Med J* 1967; 41:530–532.
45. Kew MC, Bersohn I, Seftel H: The diagnostic and prognostic significance of the serum enzyme changes in heatstroke. *Trans Roy Soc Trop Med Hyg* 1971; 65:325–330.
46. Khogali M: The Makkah body cooling unit, in Khogali M, Hales JRS (eds): *Heat Stroke and Temperature Regulation.* Sydney, Academic Press, 1983, pp 139–148.
47. Kielblock AJ, Manjoo M, Booyens J, et al: Creatine phosphokinase and lactate dehydrogenase levels after ultra long-distance running. *S Afr Med J* 1979; 55:1061–1064.
48. Kielblock AJ, Schutte PC, Strydom NB: Heat acclimatization: Perspectives and trends. *J Mine Ventil Soc S Afr* 1982; 7:53–58.
49. Kielblock AJ, Schutte PC, van der Walt WH: Development of microclimate acclimation in the South African gold mining industry, in Hales JRS (ed): *Thermal Physiology.* New York, Raven Press, pp 483–486.
50. Kielblock AJ, van Rensburg JP, Franz RM: Body cooling as a method for reducing hyperthermia: An evaluation of techniques. *S Afr Med J* 1986; 60:378–380.
51. Ladell WSS: Disorder due to heat. *Trans Roy Soc Trop Med Hyg* 1957; 51:189–216.
52. Leary WP, Reyes AJ, Lockett CJ, et al: Magnesium and deaths ascribed to ischaemic heart disease in South Africa. *S Afr Med J* 1983; 64:775–776.
53. Lee DHK: Seventy-five years of searching for a heat index. *Environ Res* 1980; 22:331–356.
54. Leithead CS, Lind AR: *Heat Stress and Heat Disorders.* London, Cassell, 1964.
55. Mackworth NH: Researches on the measurement of human performance. Medical Research Council Special Report Serial No. 268, London.
56. Minard D, Copman L: Elevation of body temperature in disease, in Herzfeld CM (ed): *Temperature. Its Measurement and Control in Science and Industry*, New York, Reinhold Publishing Co, 1963, vol 3, pt 3.
57. Mitchell D, Atkins AR, Wyndham CH: Mathematical and physical models of thermoregulation, in Bligh E, Moore R (eds): *Essays on Temperature Regulation.* New York, Elsevier North-Holland, 1972, pp 37–54.
58. Nadel ER, Pandolf KB, Roberts MF, et al: Mechanisms of thermal acclimation to exercise and heat. *J Appl Physiol* 1974; 37:515–520.
59. Neal CR, Resnikoff E, Unger AM: Treatment of dialysis-related muscle cramps with hypertonic dextrose. *Arch Intern Med* 1981; 141:171–173.
60. Nunneley SA, Maldonado RJ: Head and/or torso cooling during simulated cockpit heat stress. *Aviat Space Environ Med* 1983; 54:496–499.
61. Olhaberry JV, Leary WP, Reyes AJ, et al: Biochemistry of zinc. *S Afr Med J* 1983; 64:894–895.
62. Pandolf KB, Burse RL, Goldman RF: Role of physical fitness in heat acclimatization, decay and reinduction. *Ergonomics.* 1977; 20:399–408.
63. Pandolf KB: Effects of physical training and cardiorespiratory physical fitness on exercise-heat tolerance: Recent observations. *Med Sci Sports* 1979; 11:60–65.
64. Pandolf KB, Griffin TB, Munro EH, et al: Persistence of impaired heat tolerance from artificially induced miliaria rubra. *Am J Physiol* 1980a; 239:R226–R232.
65. Pandolf KB, Griffin TB, Munro EH: Heat intolerance as a function of percent body surface involved with miliaria rubra. *Am J Physiol* 1980b; 239:R233–R238.
66. Ramsey JD: Threshold limits for workers in hot environments, in Hemp R, Lancaster FH (eds): *Proceedings of the International Mine*

Ventilation Congress. Johannesburg, The Mine Ventilation Society of South Africa, 1975, pp 249–253.

67. Ramsey JD, Beshir MY: How good is NWB as a simple heat stress indicator? American Industrial Hygiene Association Conference, Portland, Ore, 1981.
68. Richards R, Richards D, Schofield PJ, et al: Management of heat exhaustion in Sydney's The Sun City-to-Surf fun runners. *Med J Aust* 1979; 2:457–461.
69. Richards R, Richards D: Exertion-induced heat exhaustion and other medical aspects of the City-to-Surf fun runs. *Med J Aust* 1984; 141:799–805.
70. Rolls BJ, Wood RJ, Rolls ET, et al: Thirst following water deprivation in humans. *Am J Physiol* 1980; 239:R476–R482.
71. Rowell LB, Bringleman GL, Blackman JR, et al: Splanchnic blood flow and metabolism in heat stressed man. *J Appl Physiol* 1968; 24:474–484.
72. Ryan AJ: Muscle cramps during running, editorial. *Physician Sports Med* 1982; 10:38.
73. Schutte PC, Rogers GG, van Graan CH, et al: Heat acclimatization by a method utilizing microclimate cooling. *Aviat Space Environ Med* 1978; 49:710–714.
74. Senay LC: Plasma volume and constituents of heat-exposed man before and after acclimatization. *J Appl Physiol* 1975; 38:570–575.
75. Shapiro Y, Magazanik A, Udassin P, et al: Heat intolerance in former heatstroke patients. *Ann Intern Med* 1979; 90:913–916.
76. Shapiro Y, Pandolf KB, Sawka MN, et al: Auxiliary cooling: Comparison of air-cooled vs. water-cooled vest in hot-dry and hot-humid conditions. *Aviat Space Environ Med* 1982; 53:785–789.
77. Sharma VM, Pichan G, Panwar MR: Differential effects of hot-humid and hot-dry environments on mental functions. *Int Arch Occup Environ Health* 1983; 52:315–327.
78. Shephard RJ: World standards of cardiorespiratory performance. *Arch Environ Health* 1966; 13:664–672.
79. Shibolet S, Fisher S, Gilat T, et al: Fibrinolysis and hemorrhage in fatal heatstroke. *N Engl J Med* 1962; 226:169–173.
80. Shibolet S, Lancaster MC, Danon Y: Heatstroke: A review. *Aviat Space Environ Med* 1976; 47:280–301.
81. Shvartz E, Shapiro Y, Magazanik A, et al: Heat acclimation, physical fitness, and responses to exercise in temperate and hot environment. *J Appl Physiol* 1977; 43:678–683.
82. Smith O: Effects of a cooler underground environment on safety and labour productivity, in Howes MJ, Jones MJ (eds): *Proceedings of the Third Mine Ventilation Congress (Harrogate)*. London, The Institution of Mining and Metallurgy, 1984, pp 363–368.
83. Stewart JM: Heat transfer and limiting physiological criteria as a basis for the setting of heat stress limits. *J S Afr Inst Min Metall* 1981; 81:239–251.
84. Stolwijk JAJ, Hardy JD: Partitional calorimetric studies of responses of man to thermal transients. *J Appl Physiol* 1966; 21:967–977.
85. Strydom NB: Age as a causal factor in heat stroke: *J S Afr Inst Min Metall* 1971; 72:112–114.
86. Strydom NB: The wet-bulb/dry-bulb gap controversy. *J Mine Ventil Soc S Afr* 1980; 33:54–55.
87. Strydom NB, Wyndham CH, Cooke HM, et al: Effect of heat on work performance in the gold mines of South Africa. *Fed Proc* 1963; 22:893–896.
88. Strydom NB, Kotze HF, van der Walt WH, et al: Effect of ascorbic acid on rate of heat acclimatization. *J Appl Physiol* 1976; 41:202–205.
89. Uhari M, Pakarinen A, Hietala J, et al: Serum iron, copper, zinc, ferritin and ceruloplasmin after intense heat exposure. *Eur J Appl Physiol* 1983; 51:331–335.

89a. U.S. Department of Health and Human Services, National Institute for Occupational Safety and Health: Criteria for a Recommended Standard. Occupational Exposure to Hot Environments, Revised Criteria, The Superintendent of Documents, U.S. Government Printing Office, Washington, D.C. 1986.

90. Visagie ME, du Plessis JP, Groothof G, et al: Changes in vitamin A and C levels in Black mine workers. *S Afr Med J* 1974; 48:2502–2506.
91. Viteri FE: Considerations on the effect of nutrition on the body composition and physical working capacity of young Guatemalan adults, in Schrimshaw NS, Altschul AM (eds): *Amino Acid Fortification of Protein Foods*. Cambridge, Mass, MIT Press, 1971.
92. Wenzel HG: Indoor climatic conditions: Physiological aspects, evaluation and optimum levels. *Ergonomics and Physical Environmental Factor*, Occupational Safety and Health Series, No. 21. Geneva, International Labour Office, 1970, pp 287–322.
93. Wishnitzer R, Vorst E, Berrebi A: Bone marrow iron depression in competitive distance runners. *Int J Sports Med* 1983; 4:27–30.
94. Wolfswinkel JM, van der Walt WH, van der Linde A: Intravascular shifts in magnesium during prolonged exercise. *S Afr J Sci* 1983; 79:37–38.
95. Wyndham CH, et al: Methods of cooling subjects with hyperpyrexia. *J Appl Physiol* 1959; 14:771.
96. Wyndham CH: The psychological and physiological effects of heat, in Burrows JA, et al (eds): *The Ventilation of South African Gold Mines*. Johannesburg, The Mine Ventilation Society of South Africa, 1974, pp 93–137.
97. Wyndham CH, Mentz B, Munro A: Reactions to heat of Arabs and Caucasians. *J Appl Physiol* 1964; 19:1951–1954.
98. Wyndham CH, Strydom NB, Morrison JF, et al: Criteria for physiological limits for work in heat. *J Appl Physiol* 1965a; 20:37–45.
99. Wyndham CH, Williams CG, Bredell GAG: The physiological effects of different gaps between wet and dry-bulb temperatures at high wet-bulb temperatures. *J S Afr Inst Min Metall* Sept 1965b; pp 52–56.
100. Wyndham CH, Kew MC, Kok R, et al: Serum enzyme changes in unacclimatized and acclimatized men under severe heat stress. *J Appl Physiol* 1974; 37:695–698.

23

Work Under Low Temperatures and Reactions to Cold Stress

William B. McClellan, M.D.

When one visualizes working in the cold, a mental picture of the arctic appears. It is true that work under arctic conditions is especially demanding and requires special preparation of the worker and special medical care preparation, but it is essential to realize that severe cold can affect working conditions in virtually the entire United States, and injuries from damp cold have even been reported in the tropics.

Work in dry cold conditions at normal elevation is productive of pathophysiologic hazards that are different from those produced by cold work at sea, work requiring periods of limb immobility under cold, damp conditions, or work requiring (or subject to) total immersion in cold water.

Continual or sporadic cold working conditions are not limited to soldiers, trappers, petroleum workers, prospectors, and Canadian mounted police. Cold—and often wet—working conditions regularly occur for construction workers, service station attendants, firefighters, traffic police, postal workers, fishing crews, seafarers, airline maintenance crews, road crews, strip miners, loggers, lumberjacks, emergency ambulance crews, pipeline crews, dock and harbor crews, and many others. Cold injury in the more temperate regions usually occurs as a result of poor preparation, failure to recognize hazard, or unpredictable weather.

PHYSIOLOGY

The dominating metabolic need of the human body exposed to cold is maintenance of core body temperature. There are defensive physiologic responses that enable humans to maintain core body temperature successfully during exposures to mild or moderate degrees of cold, but these are limited and can be readily overwhelmed, and progressive anatomical damage and physiologic deterioration can follow. Since human physiologic defensive mechanisms to combat cold are protective only to a moderate degree, man must rely upon external protective measures to survive and work under very cold conditions. There is some evidence of physiologic adaptation and acclimatization in humans, but such changes are limited, and may vary with duration and severity of exposure.[6, 15, 16, 21]

It is stated in the literature that persons who repeatedly immerse their hands in cold water while fishing show shorter cycles of vasoconstriction-vasodilation-vasoconstriction in their hands than persons whose hands are not similarly repeatedly and periodically immersed.[5] The natives of Tierra Del Fuego seem to demonstrate a higher metabolism that may have developed over the long-term, and Australian aborigines apparently have a remarkable ability to sleep in the cold. These examples appear to demonstrate some degree of true adaptation or acclimatization to cold and are consistent with experimental physiologic findings.

The conscious detection of cold temperature by human beings depends on cold receptors found in the skin. These are cutaneous nerve endings, but they are not anatomically discrete, specialized organs. They function alone when cold is moderate, but pain receptors are triggered as cold becomes more intense, and pain receptors dominate peripheral cutaneous response altogether at very low temperatures.[16] Sensation is lost entirely when tissue freezes, and local anesthesia occurs in the frozen area.

This peripheral nervous response is fed to the hypothalamus, which maintains central control of core body temperature. The hypothalamus response to cold is directly affected by blood temperature and a multiplicity of other signals, in addition to those primary signals sent by the peripheral cold receptors. The hypothalamus, when stimulated by signals of a cold environment responds with feedback and triggers available body defensive mechanisms to cold. Hypothalamic control is lost, however, when core body temperature falls below a minimum point.

Bodily defenses capable of being triggered are either increased heat production by increasing metabolic activity or decreased heat loss by reducing peripheral blood flow. Superficial vasoconstriction occurs as temperature of the air in contact with the skin falls and heat loss is then reduced; as heat loss continues, shivering begins, and increased metabolic heat is generated by this intense muscular activity. The superficial circulation in the limbs is quite responsive to cold, and the regulation of core body temperature is both protected by and dependent upon the heat balance of the extremities. Core body temperature must be maintained for the limbs to be warmed, and increased metabolic heat resulting from exercise results in increased warming of the extremities.

Physiologically, this explains the observation found in the literature that workers in extremely cold conditions can safely remove their gloves,[6] for limited periods, to accomplish work requiring fine manual dexterity. (There is, however, a hazard of bare flesh freezing to metal, on contact, in conditions of extreme cold. It should also be noted that the tips of the fingers, the area over the styloid process of the radius, and the olecranon process, the patellar area, the anterior ridge of the tibia, the inner and outer processes of the ankle, and the heel are especially prone to freezing injury because of the lack of fatty covering.[20])

The caloric intake required by workers in cold environments is high. In the average person, taking a meal increases metabolism slightly, and the effect peaks at about two hours and lasts four to six hours. Therefore, eating at least every four to six hours will increase internal heat production. It has also been stated, although this is difficult to quantify, that a snack before sleeping in the cold results in increased lengths of sleep before being awakened by cold.[4]

HEAT LOSS

Bodily heat is lost in cold environments by conduction, convection, and radiation. When protective coverings are wet, heat may also be lost by evaporation. Evaporation loss through the skin is, therefore, limited to situations where clothing becomes wet through by sweating or by outside moisture in a cold environment, and conduction loss occurs only when there is contact with a conducting surface. Convective heat loss, however, occurs naturally as warmed air around the body rises, and there is *very efficient* forced convective heat transfer when there is wind. This effect has been designated wind chill factor. Radiant heat loss occurs when surrounding surfaces are cold, since the human skin absorbs heat from surrounding surfaces of higher temperature, and loses heat to surrounding surfaces of lower temperature. The most dangerous and rapid heat loss occurs, therefore, when clothing is wet, wind is high, and surrounding surfaces are cold; or when the human body is immersed in cold water.

Kaufman and Bothe[14] performed experiments, similar to those establishing the concepts of wind chill, with bare and "clothed" cylinders and with cylinders that had wet clothing at temperatures above and below freezing. Clothing prevented heat loss associated with increased wind velocity on the bare cylinder. With wet clothing, evaporation increased with increased wind speed, but heat loss did not, and putting raincoats on the cylinders or freezing the wet cloth on the cylinders markedly reduced wet heat loss. According to Kaufman and Bothe, the concept of wind chill applies only to unprotected objects (Fig 23–1).

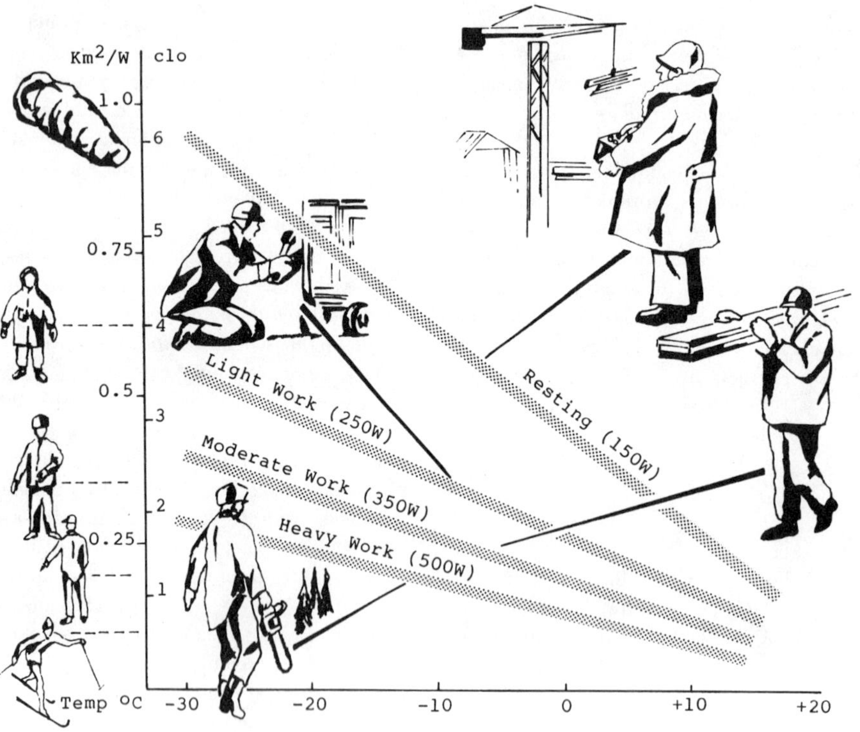

FIG 23–1.
Diagram points out the main features to consider when working outside during winter. Taken into account are work effort, temperature, and proper clothing (without wind). For example, with heavy work such as logging or snow shoveling, light clothes with an insulating value of 1.0 "clo" is suitable down to 0° C; 2.0 clo to −40° C. For standing, or little, or no physical activity such as a watchman, protective, well-insulated clothing is necessary: 3.1 clo (insulated coverall), good to −10° C.[24] See text for discussion and definitions; also Chapter 24. (Adapted from Magnus Gerne and Ingvar Holmér, Arbetarskydd no. 12, Arbetarskyddsstyrelsen, Solna, 1980.)

COLD INJURY

Cold injury occurs as a result of local tissue cooling with tissue anoxia and local tissue freezing or as a result of lowering of core body temperature.

Trench Foot

Trench foot (or immersion foot) occurs as a result of prolonged exposure of the extremity to cold and moisture, with the attendant depressed circulation and tissue anoxia, but without ice crystal formation in the tissues. Capillary walls of the extremity are injured, and there is edema, tingling, itching, and pain; blisters may form and be followed by skin ulceration and necrosis. In troops who have remained with the leg in a fixed position in cool damp areas, a lesser, but similar injury has been reported called "shelter leg."

Frostbite

Frostbite refers to the actual freezing of tissue, with formation of ice crystal in the tissue, resulting in disruption of cells. The depth of the frozen tissue is a critical factor in recovery. If blood vessels are frozen, necrosis follows, but even in those instances where freezing is very superficial, arterial spasm can occur, and blood viscosity can increase in the microcirculation. This blood viscosity may lead to local ischemia, but since the oxygen demand of the affected tissue is reduced by cold, immediate necrosis may be averted. As an injury of this kind occurs and progresses, the affected area of skin becomes red and then bluish red. There is burning pain in the affected area, then pain decreases, numbness occurs, and the area becomes waxy pale due to ischemia. The fingers, toes, cheeks, nose, and ears are usually first to be frostbitten, but areas over bone where there is little subcutaneous fat (these areas were described earlier) are particularly prone to superficial freezing injury. The fate of tissues that have been frozen usually cannot be determined immediately, and continuing observation is required.[5, 20]

Chilblains

A localized form of superficial freezing injury has been referred to as chilblains, pernio, or frost-nip. Although recovery is the rule, there may be small swelling of a dark bluish color (due to subcutaneous bleeding) which may go on to local ulceration and necrosis. The swelling may itch or be painful, and recovery may be slow. This injury, once sustained, is prone to recur with subsequent exposure to cold. The literature states[20] that some injuries of this kind may go on to generalized symptoms and easily recurring chilblains, which represent a change in the thermoregulatory mechanisms as well as local tissue damage. Therefore, workers who have had this injury of any degree should be carefully protected against future chilling.

Hypothermia

Hypothermia, or lowering of core body temperature, results when metabolic heat production of the body is not sufficient to replace heat lost by the body to the environment. Under ideal conditions, core body temperature is 98.6° F, with small individual variations. Clinical signs of hypothermia begin to appear when core body temperature has fallen to about 95° F. There is vasoconstriction, with pallor, incoordination, and muscular weakness, and dulling of mental abilities. As core body temperature falls, the pulse rate is slowed, breathing becomes shallow and slow, shivering diminishes, and consciousness is lost at core temperatures of 89.6° to 86° F. When core temperature has fallen this far, the skin may show blue mottling and breathing may be barely perceptible. At lower core temperature, there is danger of ventricular fibrillation. At a critical environmental temperature for each individual, defensive mechanisms of superficial vasoconstriction and shivering begins. Shivering consists of successive contractions in antagonistic muscles, and this intense muscular activity raises body heat production dramatically. The critical environmental temperature for activating these reactions in any individual depends on clothing, activity, general health, and environmental factors besides low temperature, such as moisture, wind speed, and radiant energy.

Immersion in cold water reduces core temperature very quickly and effectively. The thermal capacity of water to extract heat is more than 20 times that of air. Sudden immersion causes hyperventilation, and when submersion in water below 59° F (15° C) occurs, breath holding capability falls to 15–25 seconds.[8] The temperature of deeper tissues, including bone, may be chilled by immersion without surface tissue-freezing occurring, with subsequent evidence of deeper injury. Consciousness during immersion can be lost rapidly. It is apparent from these facts that seafarers, fishing crews, offshore oil workers, dock workers, and other workers in marine situations are at special risk of hypothermia, and preparation should always be made to protect these workers from immersion and to rescue them and treat hypothermia expeditiously if accidental immersion occurs.

It has been known for many years that the mental dulling that occurs as a result of hypothermia can lead to poor decisions, irrational behavior, and aberrant conduct. The net effects of these mental processes are actions that worsen the situation of the victim of hypothermia. During cold work, accidents and events that can produce hypothermia and subsequent mental dulling should be anticipated and provided for, as far as possible, so that the victim does not need to make critical decisions while hypothermic. Workers in isolated situations or involved in shipwrecks and other vehicle accidents are at particular risk in this respect.

TREATMENT

Medical treatment of cold injury, both local and hypothermic, consists of careful rewarming, general support, and treatment of sequelae.[5, 8, 10, 13, 17, 20]

Rewarming by either active or passive regimes in hypothermia requires close observation, intensive care, and—preferably—hos-

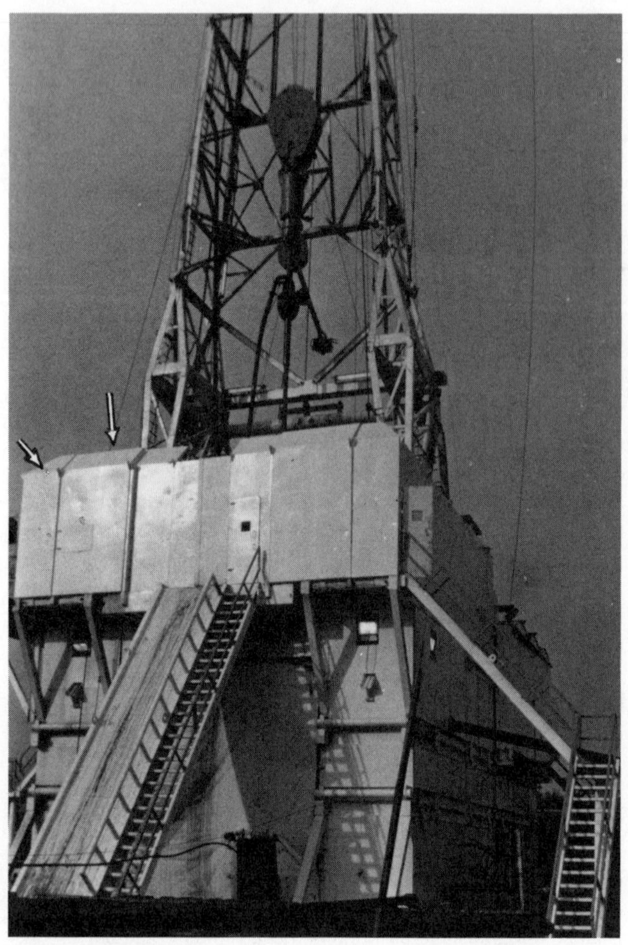

FIG 23–2.
An oil drilling rig specially equipped for the arctic. Heavily insulated sheathing throughout and wind deflectors *(arrows)* effectively aid in protecting the personnel on the rig's work platform.

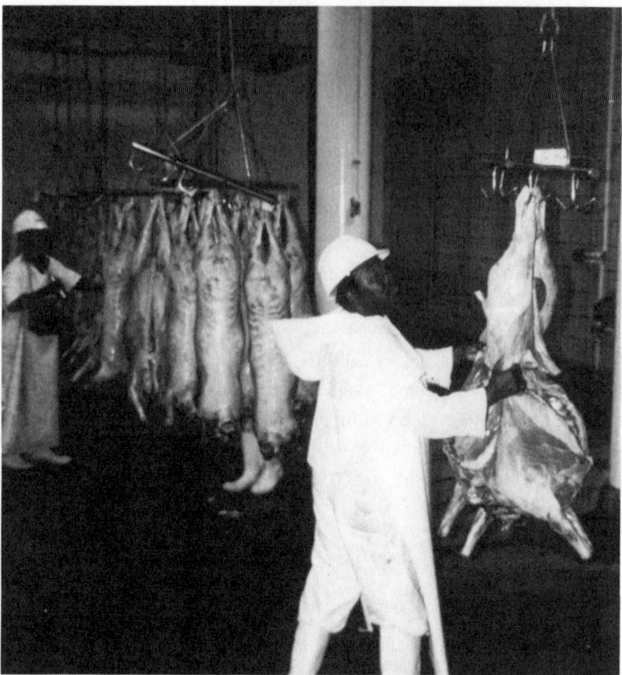

FIG 23–3.
Another example of work in low temperature-slaughter-houses (refer to Reference 2).

pitalization. The sequelae of hypothermia can be very serious and require extended treatment;[5, 8, 13, 17, 20] the lungs, kidney, vascular tree, blood electrolytes, and cells can be involved. The prognosis is very poor if the core body temperature has dropped below 77°–79° F, and the risk of ventricular fibrillation is increased. For all of these reasons the patient with hypothermia requires definitive treatment as quickly as possible. This requires preparation for emergency transportation, during which the patient should be protected from further chilling.

The patient with frostbitten extremities should have the extremities protected from further injury by cold or trauma when being transported for care, and this means that the patient should ride, not walk, to the clinical facility when the legs or feet become frostbitten. The rewarming of frozen limbs is extremely painful, and sequelae can be severe.

Details for treatment for these conditions can be obtained in other publications, some of which are listed in the bibliography at the end of this chapter. The literature on treatment is extensive, and, particularly in regard to treatment of hypothermia, it is not in complete agreement as to preferred methodology. Gentle, unhurried measures must be taken—rapid "rewarming" of extremities or body can lead to death of the hypothermic victim.[26]

PREVENTION

Prevention of hypothermia and local cold injury in workers depends upon providing adequate protection against cold and wet. Workers should have ready access to shelters that effectively shield them from the elements (Fig 23–2). Clothing design is of primary importance. Because of the critical tasks that must often be performed under these adverse climatic conditions, industry, and in particular the petroleum industry and the armed forces, as well as academic institutions have had a continuing interest in developing and utilizing efficient cold-protective garments. Even when persons are immersed in water, cold weather clothing provides some protection, and the development of wet and dry suits for divers that protect against cold has been a significant achievement. The insulating principle employed in design of effective cold weather clothing is the trapping of air between fibers, between layers of clothing, and in tiny pockets woven into cloth. A second principle of heat conservation of some of the newer survival blankets and space coats is reflection of heat radiated by the body back to the body through use of a reflectant material. A useful technique utilized in some cold weather clothing has been the use of closely woven material to reduce convective heat loss due to wind. Another useful practice has been to design clothing so that wetting of the clothing by perspiration during work can be minimized and so that external wetting from rain or wetting snow will be deflected by an impervious external garment.

In practical application,[1] clothing for terrestrial use in the cold should be layered, should be insulated, should have external layers impervious to wind, and (when necessary) to wetting. Layers should be easily removable to afford adaptability to varying degrees of body heat production during different levels of work, and external layers should be capable of being temporarily vented at waist, neck, and wrist, without removal, to reduce perspiration wetting. Clothing should be loose and nonconstricting to avoid circulatory obstruction (Fig 23–3).

Special footwear and gloves are needed for arctic conditions. Although the hands may be warm enough during exercise to temporarily remove outer gloves for work requiring dexterity, it must be repeated that severe local cold injury to the fingers can occur on contact with cold metal. For this reason inner net gloves should not be removed during work with the hands in very cold conditions, although they provide only minimal insulation. Shoes should protect against wetting of feet, should be insulative, should be loose, and should be large enough to wear layered socks. Obviously, different jobs in cold environments demand different designs of clothing to permit safe and effective working. The firefighter combatting a winter fire in Milwaukee needs different clothing from the worker on the Alaskan pipe line or the person fishing in waters off Labrador.

Health and Safety Education

Health and safety education of workers who will be exposed to cold should include information on the symptoms and causes of frostbite, immersion limb, and hypothermia. During the discussion of frostbite, workers should be expressly cautioned against rewarming frozen parts by cold soaks, massage, rubbing with snow, and other dangerous practices. The need for immediate rescue and speedy medical aid for victims of immersion hypothermia should be stressed, as should the value of drying off the victim, substituting warm, dry clothing, and placing the victim in a warm sleeping bag as first measures. Workers should know the absolute need for keeping hands and feet dry to prevent immersion limb, and the dangers of wet clothing from sweating and wet weather.

First-aid instruction for every worker in cold environments is necessary. In addition to the usual problems inherent in correct, immediate handling of trauma, the problems that arise when trauma is sustained under cold conditions are unique and require special handling. Bleeding may quickly result in shock; wounds open to the weather may freeze. Tourniquet application to a limb reduces warming blood flow, with the attendant increased risk of frostbite. Fractures requiring immobilization also impose a need for keeping the victim warm and dry, since metabolic heat formation declines with the decline in physical activity. Unconsciousness also reduces metabolic heating due to lack of physical activity, so special care must be taken to keep the unconscious victim warm and dry.

Carbon monoxide poisoning and fire are constant dangers under arctic conditions, and instruction in avoiding these hazards are appropriate for arctic workers.

An American Petroleum Institute booklet on arctic work[1] outlines some of the advantages of the "buddy system" while working in extremely cold environments. Partners can observe each other during work to spot early signs of frostbite of exposed areas and early signs of hypothermia. Lightly frostbitten extremities can be warmed by the partner's body. A worker's partner can apply first aid immediately when needed. Generally, individual isolation in cold environments is undesirable and should be avoided by proper planning. Possible accidents leading to isolation must be subjects of planning; and contingency rescue and medical evacuation equipment, personnel, and emergency supplies must be prepared and available constantly. Personnel who become the victims of transportation accidents should be instructed on appropriate survival techniques and be made aware of the dangers of faulty judgment due to hypothermia.

MEDICAL SELECTION OF WORKERS

Medical selection of workers for work under cold conditions requires evaluation of all of the usual medical qualifications for appropriate job placement, evaluation of the candidates' physical and emotional ability to work in a cold environment generally, and detection of specific diseases that might impair ability to work safely under specific cold working conditions. In persons who have exertional angina exposure to cold may precipitate an anginal attack. The exact reasons for this are unclear. Hattenhauer and Neill[19] have studied the effects of cold air inhalation on patients with coronary artery disease and found that coronary blood flow was not changed significantly. Changes in diameter of the large coronary vessels was not detected. They also found, however, that inhalation of air at $-20°$ C for four minutes provoked angina pectoris in 4 of 17 coronary disease patients at rest, and in 4 of 7 of the patients when they were paced at a heart rate level that was subanginal at room temperature. They report in an earlier study that cutaneous cold stimulation increased myocardial oxygen consumption and coronary blood flow. Study of the vital statistics of Minneapolis/St. Paul[3] showed that cardiovascular mortality is increased during times of winter temperature and snow, with the effect being most pronounced in persons with old myocardial infarction. During cold snaps in Toronto, sudden deaths among men younger than 65 years were increased. Deaths from ischemic heart disease in Boston increased 22% in the week following a blizzard. The possible adverse cardiac effects of work in the cold on persons who have coronary artery disease seem clear from this data. Whether cold unfavorably affects the incidence of stroke is not clear according to Caplan.[7] Deal et al.[9] investigated airway responsiveness to cold air inhalation of 35° C in 20 control subjects, 16 subjects with hay fever, and 44 asymptomatic asthmatics. They found no effect on lung function in normal subjects, a small but significant fall in forced expiratory volume in the hay fever group, but a much more marked fall in forced expiratory volume of the asthmatic group. Cold air in ventilatory amounts matching those associated with heavy work loads had no detected effect on the lung function of normal subjects. These authors concluded that cold air inhalation in unselected asthmatics is a potent stimulus for bronchoconstriction.

These studies show that persons subject to asthma, and, in some instances, persons with hay fever, and persons with coronary artery disease are at higher risk while doing work in the cold. Persons with peripheral vascular diseases affecting the extremities are at special risk of aggravating or precipitating attacks by cold exposure. Persons who have previously suffered with pernio or chilblains have been reported as being at increased risk during cold exposure. All of these conditions and a history of thermoregulatory disorders should be given special attention when acquiring a prework history from workers who will be exposed to low temperatures.

SUMMARY

There are many persons, even in temperate climates, who work in the cold. Pathophysiologic changes occur when bodily defense mechanisms are overwhelmed by cold, and these cold-induced injuries require careful treatment. Special protective clothing is needed for persons doing work at low temperatures. Health and safety education for workers at low temperatures should include special instruction in avoidance of injury due to cold exposure. Persons with cardiovascular, peripheral vascular, and asthmatic respiratory disease and with previous history of pernio are at special risk during cold work.

REFERENCES

1. American Petroleum Institute, Oregon Museum of Science and Industry: *Staying Alive in the Arctic*. Washington, DC, Plant Deck, Inc, Publishers, 1975.
2. Holmér I, Sundell J: Arbete i kallt klimat, Arbetarskyddsstyrelsens skriftserie Arbete och hälsa, Solna, Sweden, 1982.
3. Baker-Bloker A, et al: Winter weather and c.v. mortality in Minneapolis, St Paul. *Am J Public Health* 1982; 72:3.
4. Belding HS: Physiologic principles for protection of man living in the cold, in Fisher FR (ed): *Man Living in the Arctic*. Washington, DC, National Academy of Sciences, National Research Council, 1961.
5. Bouys C, et al: *Management of Wilderness and Environmental Injuries*. New York, Auberbach and Geer, 1983.
6. Burtan RC: Work under low temperatures and reaction to cold stress, in Zenz C (ed): *Occupational Medicine*. Chicago, Year Book Medical Publishers, 1975.
7. Caplan LR, et al: Cold related intracerebral hemorrhage. *Arch Neurol* 1984; 41:227.
8. Collins KJ (ed): *Hypothermia, The Facts*. New York, Oxford University Press, 1983.
9. Deal EC Jr, et al: Airway responsiveness to cold air and hyperpnea in normal subjects and those with hay fever and asthma. *Am Rev Respir Dis* 1980; 121(4):621–628.
10. Dembert ML: Medical problems from cold exposure. *Am Fam Physician* 1982; 25:99–106.
11. Douzou P: Developments in low temperature biochemistry and biology. *Proc R Soc Lond [Biol]* 1982; 217(1206):1–28.
12. Feldman RL, et al: Cold air exposure and angina pectoris. *Am Heart J* 1982; 104(1):73.
13. Felicetta JV, et al: Decreased adrenal responsiveness in hypothermic patients. *J Clin Endocrinol Metab* 1980; 50(1):93–97.
14. Kaufman WC, Bothe DJ: Wind chill reconsidered, Siple revisited. *Aviat Space Environ Med* 1986; 57:23.
15. Goldsmith K, Minard D: Cold, cold work, in *Occupational Health Safety*. New York, McGraw-Hill Book Co, 1971.
16. Guyton AC (ed): *Text Book of Medical Physiology*. Philadelphia, WB Saunders Co, 1971.
17. Harnett RM, et al: A review of the literature concerning resuscitation from hypothermia, pt 1. *Aviat Space Environ Med* 1983; 54:425–434.
18. Harnett RM, et al: A review of the literature concerning resuscitation from hypothermia, pt 2. *Aviat Space Environ Med* 1983; 54:487–495.
19. Hattenhauer M, et al: Effect of cold air inhalation on angina pectoris and myocardial oxygen supply. *Circulation* 1975; 51:1053–1058.
20. Key M, et al: *Occupational Diseases*. Dept of Health, Education, and Welfare, Public Health Service, US Government Printing Office, 1974.
21. Killian H (ed): *Cold and Frost Injuries*. New York, Springer-Verlag, 1981.
22. Nenzén B: Om du fryser om fötterna- Ta på dig mössan. Arbetsmiljö 2, Stockholm, 1986.
23. Radomski MV, et al: Hormonal response of normal and intermittent cold preadapted humans to continuous cold. *J Appl Physiol* 1982; 53:610–616.
24. Rätt klädd i jobbet, Arbetarskyddsnamnden. Solna, Sweden, National Board of Occupational Health and Safety, 1983.
25. Riggs CE Jr, et al: Metabolic effects of facial cooling in exercise. *Aviat Space Environ Med* 1983; 54(1).
26. Rapid heating fatal in hypothermia. *Work, Health, Safety*. Helsinki, Finland, Institute of Occupational Health, 1986, pp 28–29.

24

The Effects of Moderate Thermal Stress on Comfort and Productivity

Geoffrey B. Meese, B.Sc., M.Sc., Ph.D.

The moderate thermal stress zone can generally be thought of as a zone in which people can undertake normal activities without danger to health and without the need for abnormal protective measures. Extreme thermal conditions are in many ways easier to recognize and deal with; workers performing heavy manual work at a forge or packing food in a cold room are clearly at risk and the necessary protective clothing and rest periods can be prescribed and provided. Indoor environmental conditions, however, frequently fall between such extremes, and many additional questions arise. A factory worker at a lathe in an air temperature of 30° C is probably not subject to heat stress, nor is he likely to feel comfortable, but what effect do these conditions have on his productivity? The same questions arise for a worker assembling electronic components at a temperature of 15° C.

One of the objects of good building design is to create a structure that is not only an aesthetically pleasing and protective shell, but that promotes the activity or needs of the occupants. These needs may be for productivity, as in an office, factory, or school, or they may be for comfort, as in most parts of a home. Since it is usually not possible to provide a narrowly controlled indoor climate without considerable expense, it is likely that the indoor climate will vary within wide limits. The designer can usually predict these limits[116] but what penalty, in terms of loss of comfort or productivity, or both, will result?

In the case of commercial enterprises, the question may be one of cost effectiveness: "does the loss of 5% of performance for three months of the year justify the installation of heaters and insulation in a factory?" Indeed, there will be few buildings where the cost-effectiveness equation can be avoided.

Obviously, quantitative data will be more valuable than subjective feelings regarding the environment, although the latter may be important. If these data are required, then appropriate means must be devised for measuring the reaction of people to moderate thermal stress.

It does not follow that optimum comfort and optimum efficiency will occur under the same conditions. Most people would agree that they are optimally comfortable in bed but would agree that it does not produce the best working environment. In a study of factory workers in a climate laboratory by Kok et al.,[53] it was found that peak performance occurred at 32° C, about 10° C higher than the optimum preferred temperature.

Performance can be measured on real tasks in, for instance, a factory, school or ship, or the appropriate measurements can be made in a laboratory. The former usually implies a less controlled environment, while in the laboratory the task and its ambience may not simulate real life sufficiently well to allow the findings to be extrapolated. The validity of the measurements will depend on the nature of the tests or work tasks used; a laboratory test that proves to be temperature-insensitive may tell you little about the task it is intended to simulate if key factors are omitted. The problem of task suitability and techniques for improving task sensitivity has been discussed by Poulton,[93] who has suggested such methods as increasing the task difficulty, using an unfamiliar task, and measuring variability instead of mean performance.

Once the measuring criteria have been selected, allowance has to be made for the many factors that can influence these measurements, whether they be in a laboratory or in a field situation. Most of the modifiers of performance or subjective impressions of the environment will, of course, be due to differences in physiologic response; although age, sex, race, bodily conformation, and the level of acclimatization can all play a lesser or greater role. Other relevant features, such as the level of fatigue and motivation, are not so readily measurable.

A discussion of thermal stress usually concentrates on the dry-bulb temperature, but the total thermal environment is affected by six major variables:

1. The air temperature
2. The metabolic rate
3. The water vapor pressure of the ambient air
4. The thermal resistance of the clothing
5. The mean radiant temperature
6. The relative air velocity

(In this chapter, dry-bulb air temperature and radiant temperature are expressed in degrees Celsius. Humidity is expressed in terms of vapor pressure (in kPa) or naturally ventilated wet-bulb temperature in degrees Celsius. Effective Temperature is quoted when an original study has described the conditions in this way. The thermal resistance of clothing is expressed in the familiar "clo" or in sq km/W.)

The importance of these six factors will vary throughout the range of thermal stress conditions—some examples will illustrate this: The *Guidelines for Factory Building Design* in South Africa* recommends an upper limit of 30° C WBGT (Wet-Bulb Globe Temperature) for tasks with a light metabolic rate. These conditions could be achieved by a combination of 35° C dry-bulb and radiant temperature and 28° C naturally ventilated wet bulb or by a combination of 40° C dry-bulb and radiant temperature and 26° C naturally ventilated wet-bulb. The optimum thermal comfort at fixed clothing and air velocity levels of 0.5 clo (0.25 sq km/W) and 0.15 m/sec will occur at about 26° C if the metabolic rate is 58.2 W/sq m. If the metabolic rate increases to 140 W/sq m then the comfort temperature will fall to 18° C.[26]

This chapter will concentrate on the effects of moderate thermal stress on physiology and performance. Subjective thermal comfort cannot, however, be ignored, and due attention will be given to it, though for most enterprises the provision of optimum comfort conditions would be prohibitively expensive.

PHYSIOLOGIC RESPONSES TO MODERATE THERMAL STRESS

From the definition of moderate thermal stress used in the introduction it follows that extreme physiologic responses such as hypothermia and hyperthermia are unlikely to occur. Since the mechanisms that maintain body temperature in the cold and the heat are different, they should be considered separately.

Cold

The critical temperature, that temperature at which there is neither heat loss nor gain in the "modern, nonfasting European or American" when naked and inactive, is between 27° and 29° C.[82]

On exposure to temperatures below the thermoneutral zone, the body tends to lose heat, and in an attempt to maintain a stable core temperature it can (1) restrict heat loss, and/or (2) increase internal heat production. Heat loss reduction takes place mainly through the constriction of blood vessels, especially in the peripheral regions. This vasoconstriction can reduce heat loss by between one sixth and one third.[82] With decreasing temperature, involuntary muscular activity and possibly visible shivering will begin, which results in internal heat production. By this means a person can increase bodily heat production nearly three times.[82]

The relatively large surface area-to-volume ratio associated with the hands makes them particularly susceptible to cold, and the relationship between cold conditions and the resultant loss of finger sensitivity or dexterity has been extensively investigated. Early investigations by Lewis[61] described the effects of cold and the resulting vasoconstriction but also noted that if finger temperatures were between 10° and 14° C then vasodilatation could occur, with a subsequent rise in finger temperature. Mackworth[70] was responsible for initiating many of the studies on the effects of finger-skin temperature (FST) and finger sensitivity. Other studies (e.g., Stevens et al.[106]) have considered measures of numbness, pain, punctate sensitivity, and vibration sensitivity. The role of hand skin temperature (HST) and FST in the performance of simple manual dexterity tasks has also been considered. Most of the investigations have shown the expected deterioration in performance with cold, although the precise HST or FST at which this occurs depends on such factors as the tasks or techniques used and whether the subjects underwent whole-body cooling or hand cooling.[65, 97] One possible reason for the deterioration in manual performance in the cold was suggested by Hunter et al.,[46] who showed a reduction in finger flexibility at 12° C (FST) caused by increased resistance in the finger joints.

Modifications of the Cold Response

Age.—Age is one factor that could alter the response to cold. Because of their more inactive life-style, older people often have a poorer circulatory response. Collins and Hoinville[18] have shown that older people maintained their deep body temperature at a similar level to young adults but exhibited lower skin temperatures and poorer temperature discrimination. Suzuki et al.,[108] however, found a group of older men to have higher FSTs than young men. These different findings were in spite of great similarities in such features as bodily conformation and illustrate the difficulty of comparing findings where experimental techniques are not identical.

Acclimatization.—Another possible factor that could produce differences in reaction to cold is acclimatization. The cold defense mechanisms do not seem as amenable to modification as those used for the thermal control in the heat, but it seems logical to expect that continued exposure to cold would produce some adaptation. Brown and Page[12] showed that Eskimos had slightly higher skin temperatues and higher blood flow in the hands than a group of Canadian medical students. Wyndham[120] suggested that a form of acclimatization in Australian aborigines was their greater tolerance of cold discomfort. Acclimatization to cold has been described by Hellstrom.[42] He measured reductions in manual performance of between 28% (outdoor workers) and 46% (students) when the FST dropped from 25.5° to 15.5° C.

Sex and Ethnicity.—A further factor that requires consideration is whether different groups (variations in sex or ethnic origin) would show different levels of tolerance and sensitivity. Wyndham et al.[122] showed that in nearly naked supine subjects at 27° C air temperature, women had colder fingers than men but that these differences were not apparent at 5° C air temperature. Kok et al.[53] found women to have colder fingers and toes than men at temperatures below 24° C air temperature but these differences were not apparent or not significant at 6° C.

Wyndham et al.[124] showed that black men had colder fingers than white men between air temperatures of 27° and 17° C. The difference was 5° C at an air temperature of 27° C. Below 17° C,

*This publication, prepared by the National Building Research Institute and the Department of Manpower of the South African government, advises employers and employees on matters relating to thermal conditions.[83]

the black men still tended to have colder fingers but the differences were small and nonsignificant. Iampietro et al.[48] found no difference in FST between black and white men during whole-body cooling but during digital cooling the white subjects had warmer fingers and, after the cooling phase, required a shorter period for the onset of finger rewarming. More recently, Schiefer et al.[103] have shown significant FST differences between black and white, men and women between 18° and 6° C air temperature (Fig 24–1).

The general conclusion from these studies is that, between the thermoneutral zone and an air temperature that results in similar FSTs because of the extent of vasoconstriction, women tend to show lower skin temperatures than men, and blacks show lower temperatures than whites. The differences are not easy to explain; the greater obesity of females does not seem sufficient explanation for differences in peripheral temperature. Wyndham et al.[124] have suggested that black men show less insulation to heat flow than white men, that there are differences in vasomotor tone, and that dietary differences could cause dissimilar fat deposition. Further possibilities are differences in blood inflow to the digits or a different "set-point" temperature at which blood flow is reduced.

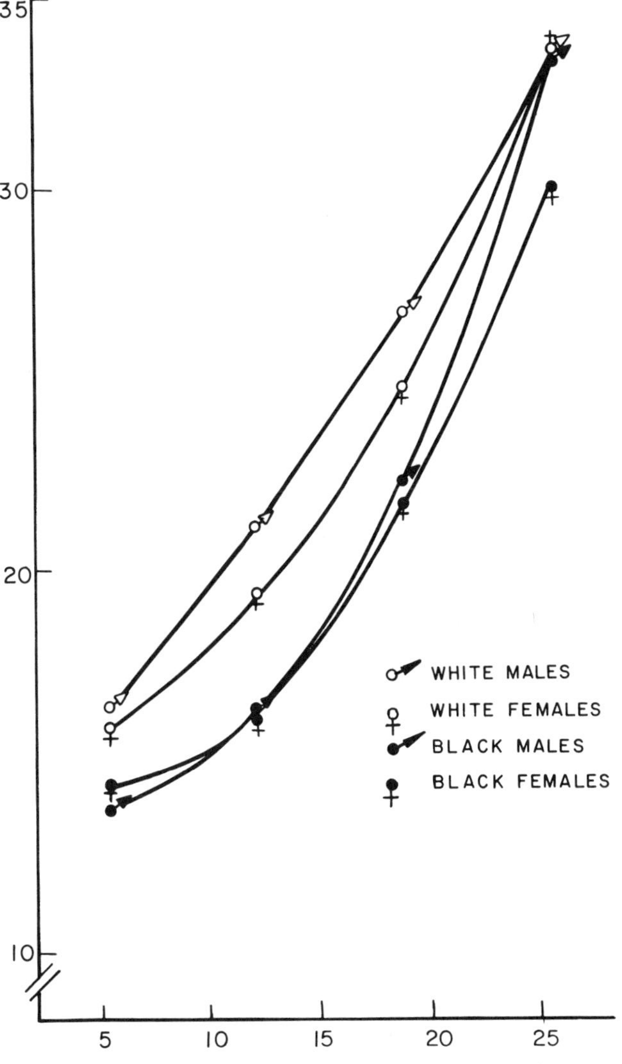

FIG 24–1.
Mean finger skin temperature *(FST)* for four groups of subjects versus air temperature. *X* = Air temperature (° C); *Y* = Mean FST (° C).

Effects of Cold on Performance

Finally, it is worth considering the possible performance consequences of these physiologic reactions to temperature. Obviously, a primary outcome will be a reduction in manual dexterity and sensitivity—this has already been noted and will be discussed in detail later. A further physical effect is that, as body temperature is reduced, there will be a lowering of muscle temperature, impaired neural conduction, increased muscle tension, and shivering. These factors will act against coordination and fine muscular control.

The second group of cold effects are nonphysical. Teichner[110] has suggested that cold has a distracting effect, so that a worker finds it difficult to concentrate on the task and can think only of the discomfort of being cold. This leads to changes in arousal; a measure of wakefulness. Provins[96] has suggested that a relationship exists between arousal and performance in that an optimum level of arousal exists for a particular task. When the arousal is above or below this level, then performance declines. In general, a boring task will require a higher optimum arousal level than will a complex one. Arousing factors in the environment could be, for instance, cold, heat, or noise. Incentives may also have an arousing effect. Arousal theory has led to the well-known inverted *U* relationship[19] which has proved so useful in explaining many confusing performance results (Fig 24–2). Unfortunately, there are as yet no independent measures of arousal, although Bell et al.[8] suggest that systolic blood pressure may be suitable. Although the arousal concept has many shortcomings, it has value as a means of examining data and needs to be taken into account where any potentially arousing conditions occur. (These remarks regarding the arousing effect of cold apply equally well for heat.)

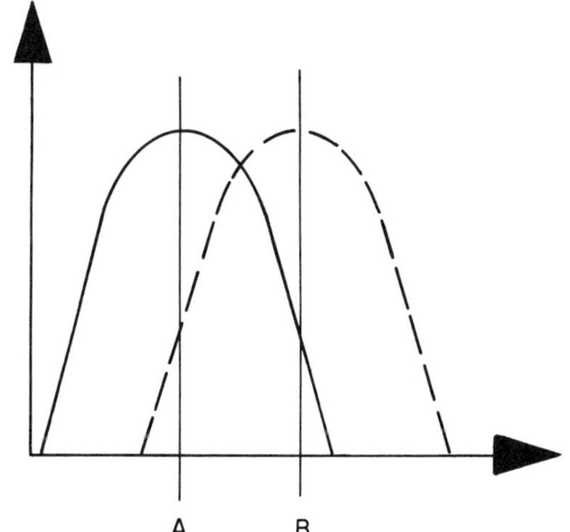

FIG 24–2.
The suggested relationship between performance and the level of arousal due to a factor such as cold or heat. *A* indicates the peak performance of a "complex" task for which a low level of arousal is optimal while *B* is the peak performance of a "simple" task. *X* = Level of arousal; *Y* = Performance.

Heat

In the heat, the body's physiologic systems are presented with a different problem. Exposure to temperatures above the thermoneutral zone means that the body will tend to gain heat, but the heat gain can be reduced by: (1) *a reduction in heat production*, i.e., work rate; and (2) *physiologic reactions* that will result in body cooling to prevent the core temperature rising.

Heat transfer to the surroundings can take place through the four channels of evaporation, radiation, convection, and conduction. Conduction is usually of little importance. As the temperature rises above the thermoneutral zone, there is a redistribution of the heat load via an increase in skin blood flow (vasodilation), particularly in the hands and feet, allowing the transfer of metabolic heat from deep tissue to the skin. There is a corresponding reduction in blood flow to the viscera and an increase in heart rate. As long as the air temperature and radiant temperature do not exceed the skin temperature, heat can be lost to the surrounding environment via radiation and convection. Skin temperature will, of course, vary with the environment and will show considerable variation over the body surface. As a general guide to expected skin temperature, Olesen and Fanger[86] showed that the mean skin temperature (MST) of 32 comfortable men and women averaged 33.5° C. Except for the significantly colder feet of the women—31.2° C as against 33.3° C—there was no difference between the sexes. At about 29°–30° C air temperature, an additional avenue of cooling, evaporative heat loss, becomes available, and when the air temperature and radiant temperature exceed the MST (about 35° C) this is the only way in which heat can be lost to the environment.

The body's thermoregulatory system acts to maintain the core temperature, also called the deep body temperature, at a constant level. If the core temperature reaches 39°–40° C heat stroke, or even death, may occur. The rectal temperature and the core temperature reflect the work rate and the thermoregulatory system acts to keep this constant, allowing for the fluctuations in air temperature. Skin temperature is to a large extent dependent on air temperature.[40] The sensitivity of the core temperature to the work rate once again underlines the interplay between the various factors making up the thermal environment and illustrates the way in which some safe conditions can become potentially unsafe if the work rate is increased, such as during an emergency.

The control of the sweating response is complex and has received intensive investigation. Controversy regarding the operation of the sweating response has centered around the relative roles of core temperature and skin temperature. Iwanga et al.,[49] for instance, have shown that the sweat rate has a negative linear correlation with the absolute value of the rectal temperature. Other workers, such as Benzinger,[9] have attributed a greater role to skin temperature. The amount of sweat that can be produced is considerable, and Kerslake and Brebner[50] found values of 2 kg/hr for subjects at rest. The precise heat loss benefit from the evaporation of sweat has not been entirely resolved, but an approximate value is that a sweat loss of 1 gm/min produces a heat loss of 41 W.[73] From estimates of known sweat rates and a knowledge of the metabolic rate associated with a task, it becomes possible to calculate the impact of the environment.

Another response to heat is an increase in the heart rate. Heart rate is primarily a response to workload,[100] but where a requirement for heat dissipation leads to vasodilation a greater strain is obviously placed on the heart. Krajewski[57] suggests 220 minus the person's age in years as the maximum number of beats per minute, Kok[52] suggested an upper limit of 110 beats per minute for an eight-hour shift, and Pandolf et al.[87] found increases of about one beat per minute per 1° C above 25° C. More recently, in a study by Kok et al.,[53] increases of about 20 beats per minute between 20° and 38° C were found for black and white men and women working at light tasks (about 60 W/sq m) (Fig 24–3). Increasing demand on the heart leads to heat exhaustion because of competition between skin and muscles for the available blood supply.

Modifications of the Heat Response

Just as with the physiologic reactions to cold, it is possible to determine a number of factors that modify the heat response.

Age.—Age may have a minor effect. Cleland et al.[16] found that a group of old people showed signs of greater heat strain than

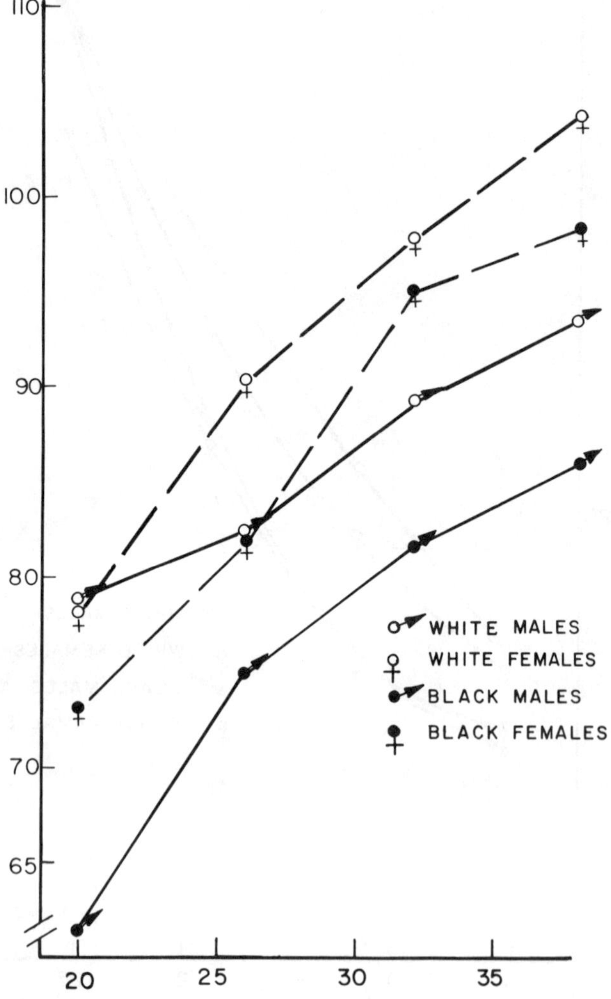

FIG 24–3.
Mean heart rates for four groups of subjects after exposure for 2.5–3.0 hours to one of four air temperatures, versus air temperature. *X* = Air temperature (° C); *Y* = Heart rate (beats per minute).

did a group about 40 years younger and suggested that it was due to poorer circulatory efficiency. Drinkwater et al.[22] have found that, contrary to expectation, the sweat rate does not decrease with age. One must conclude nevertheless that, with reduced circulatory efficiency and V_{O_2MAX}, the aged face a greater risk of heat stress.

Obesity.—Bodily conformation can alter the heat response. Vroman et al.[114] found that obesity alters blood flow between the skin and working muscle, and Epstein et al.[25] have shown that a high surface area-to-body mass ratio is a characteristic of heat-intolerant subjects.

Metabolic Rate Differences.—There is also a possibility of workers having different metabolic rates. Dieng et al.[21] have shown that African subjects have a lower metabolic rate change as they move from lying down to standing up than have European subjects, and it is now evident that differences of up to 40% in their resting metabolic rates can occur between individuals.[34]

Acclimatization.—Another major source of differences between individuals lies in their level of heat acclimatization, which produces physiologic adaptations that make an individual better suited to work in a hot environment. Acclimatization is a result of working at high temperatures and is not an inevitable outcome of fitness. The general conclusion from many acclimatization studies is that while physical fitness may confer some slight advantage, heat acclimatization will occur only if the deep body temperature, sweat rate, and heart rate are raised by work in the heat. This means that one cannot assume that people who live in hot countries will display much heat acclimatization unless their jobs regularly involve vigorous activity.

The major effects of acclimatization are: an increase in vasodilation, an increase in blood volume, a reduction in the heart rate, a lowering of the deep body temperature, earlier sweating, and an increase in the sweat rate.[56] Heat acclimatization is lost if work is not maintained under hot conditions, and the best indication of such a loss is an increase in the heart rate with temperature.[105]

Sex Differences.—Finally, the thermoregulatory response in men and women needs to be considered. Different reactions to the cold have been discussed, and variation in the response of men and women to heat has received an equal amount of attention. While there is disagreement over many details, there is general consensus that the response of women to heat is not as adaptive as that of men.[121] Interpretation of the results is often centered around whether these differences are due to fundamental physiologic factors or whether they are related to sex differences such as the generally lower body weight of women. Hertig and Sargent[43] found that women had higher rectal temperatures than men after walking in dry heat, and it is suggested that this is due to a poorer sweat response by the women. Burse,[13] in his review of sex differences in the thermoregulatory response, warns, "women generally are at somewhat greater risk of heat exhaustion, especially before acclimation."

Frye and Kamon[31] found that women had a less copious sweat response than men and as a result displayed higher skin temperatures. Fox et al.[29] have noted the importance of other factors, such as the women's lower basal metabolic rate, greater insulation, lesser heat acclimatization, and more extensive peripheral heat sink.

From the many studies that have been made, in spite of conflicting evidence, there are certain points on which there is agreement:

1. Women have higher skin temperature. This is illustrated in Figure 24–4, in which the mean chest skin temperatures of black and white men and women are shown.

2. Women have a poorer sweat response. This gives some long-term advantages in that it is less wasteful, but clearly it reduces their capacity for temperature control. Figures 24–5 and 24–6 contrast the chest temperatures of white men and women recorded at approximately half-hour intervals in a climate chamber. Both groups were identically clad and performed the same

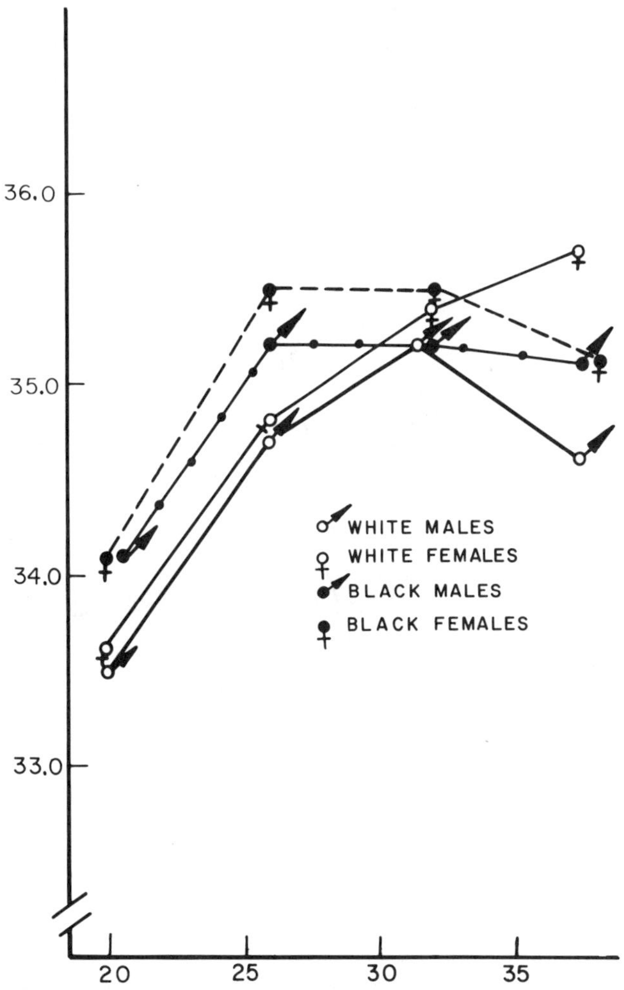

FIG 24–4.
Mean chest skin temperature for four groups of subjects after exposure for about two hours to one of four air temperatures, versus air temperature. *X* = Air temperature (° C); *Y* = Chest skin temperature (° C).

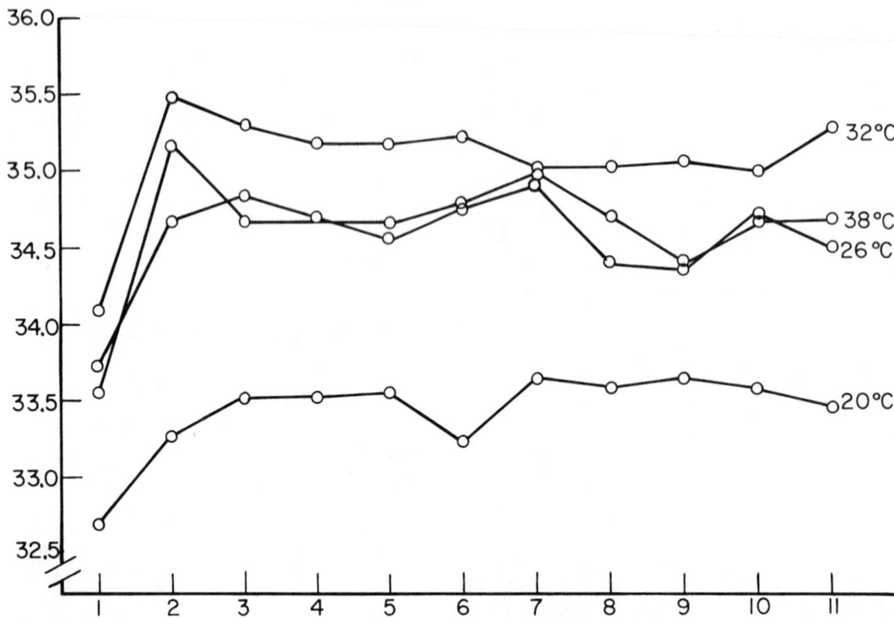

FIG 24–5.
White male mean chest skin temperatures recorded at intervals during the day at four air temperatures. *X* = Time (approximately half-hour intervals); *Y* = Chest skin temperature (° C).

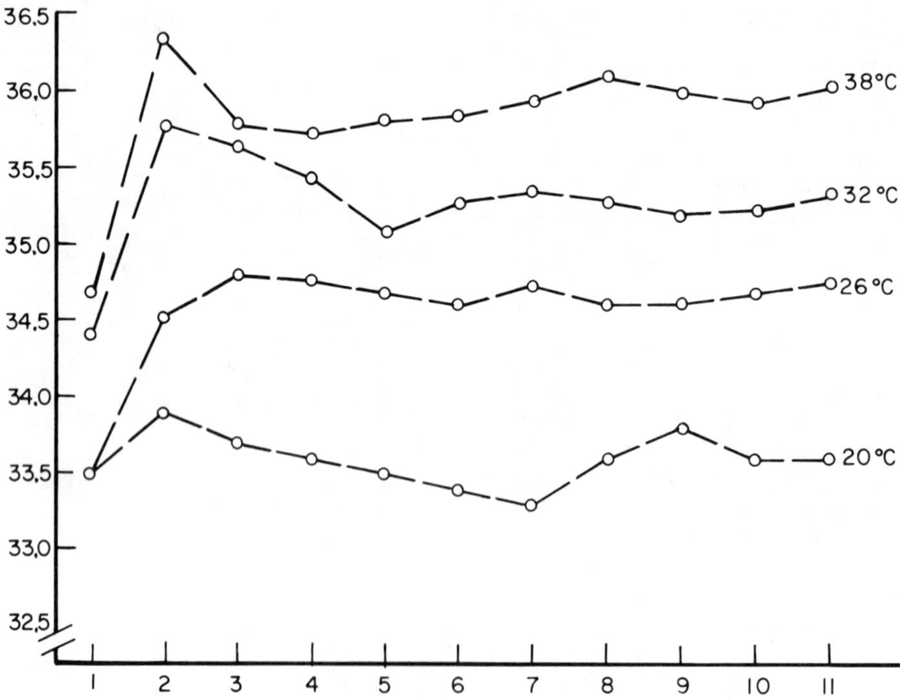

FIG 24–6.
White female mean chest skin temperatures recorded at intervals during the day at four air temperatures. *X* = Time (approximately half-hour intervals); *Y* = Chest skin temperature (° C).

work. The vapor pressure was low (1.0 kPa) during the exposure and the open-necked shirts allowed good evaporation of the sweat produced. The sweating inadequacy of the women is shown by their steady rise in skin temperature between 20° and 38° C, whereas the men were able to bring their chest skin temperature at 38° C air temperature below that at 32° C.

3. There are differences in male/female anatomy, such as the lower body-weight of females, their greater proportion of fat tissue, their proportionally greater surface area, and their lower aerobic capacity, which could affect thermal control. In the study described above (see Figs 24–5 and 24–6), the women were significantly more obese than the men when assessed on a ponderal index[11] (2.47 ± 0.27 for women vs. 2.34 ± 0.11 for men). The ponderal index is a measure of obesity and is defined as

$$\sqrt[3]{\frac{\text{mass in kilograms}}{\text{height in meters}}}$$

4. It is likely that the thermoregulatory set-point for women is higher than that for men.

5. The deep body temperature of women is higher than that of men. In the study of Kok et al.[53] core temperature was not measured, but women had consistently higher oral temperatures than men. (The relationship between oral and deep body temperature is not linear throughout the range, but Strydom et al.[107] found an oral:rectal temperature correlation of 0.83).

Ethnic Origin.—The final consideration in this section is whether ethnic origin has any modifying effect on the reaction to heat. Here the distinction must be made between people working in hot climates who have become acclimatized through their work and those who, because of their ethnic origin, have distinctive physiologic reactions which are appropriate to their environment. A further group requiring to be identified would be those whose behavior, tolerance, or diet conferred an advantage on them. The possibility of ethnic differences in thermal response is of interest to designers and legislators because account may need to be taken if a group of people are at a disadvantage under a particular set of circumstances.

Wyndham et al.[123] and Wyndham[120] found that unacclimatized black men had lower rectal temperatures than white men but that there were no significant differences in mean heart rate and sweat rate, although the latter was lower for black men. After acclimatization, there were no significant differences in rectal temperature, although the heart rate and sweat rate of the black men were still slightly lower. Wyndham et al.[123] suggest that these results indicate little inherent difference between the two groups. An earlier study by Robinson et al.[99] with black and white subjects matched for height and weight found the former to have lower sweat and heart rates and to be mechanically slightly more efficient. Kok et al.[53] showed that black men and women as judged by their chest temperature, were more prolific producers of sweat than white women. Black subjects also have lower heart rates on a within-sex comparison (see Fig 24–3).

The lower sweat rate of white women compared with men or black subjects was also shown by Hillyard and Dill.[44] Because of the many differences in technique, possible dietary differences, and unknown levels of acclimatization, it is difficult to compare results directly, although it would seem generally true that black subjects have a slight advantage in hot conditions, but this difference is too small to warrant attention.

Time of Day.—A final minor consideration is the time of day. The existence of day-night variations in deep-body temperature has been known for more than 100 years, and the investigation of these circadian rhythms has been extensively researched. A recent review of Aschoff[3] has shown that, for a person engaged in normal "activity" the rectal temperature is at a minimum (36.4° C) at about 6 a.m. to 7 a.m. and at a maximum (37.3° C) at about 6 p.m. Sleep deprivation, shift work, and personal characteristics will produce changes in these values and times. In terms of heat stress, these values will probably be of little relevance, but the relationship between circadian rhythm and such aspects of behavior as alertness[28] and performance[101] have been thoroughly investigated.

PERFORMANCE AND MODERATE THERMAL STRESS

A tremendous amount of research has been conducted into the effects of thermal stress on performance. However, because of the range of the work, from the collection of data in the field to carefully controlled laboratory experiments, it is difficult to comprehend the field as a whole. Much of the variability in findings, as already noted, is caused by the choice of tests and techniques. Poulton[94] has reviewed the general field of environment and performance and has suggested a theoretical relationship, similar to the inverted *U* relationship with arousal, where an optimum condition exists for the performance of a task. Therefore, selection of the range over which an experimenter has varied a parameter can have a marked effect on results. Poulton[95] has also shown in his reassessment of performance data that stressful conditions can often lead to improved output. He also underlines the necessity for objective measurement of performance data as opposed to the collection of subjective views and impressions, in spite of the difficulty of carrying out the former.

In this section we shall consider pertinent results obtained in four situations: (1) industrial studies, including work with military personnel; (2) school studies; and (3) office studies.

Industrial Studies

Most work involving thermal stress has been concerned with its effect on the performance of industrial workers or military subjects. It is convenient to consider field work and laboratory studies separately, with the early field studies providing evidence for continued investigation in the laboratory.

Field Studies

Some of the earliest work was conducted over 60 years ago in Britain by the Industrial Fatigue Board. Although the work was not solely concerned with thermal conditions, there were some relevant findings. Vernon[111] measured the seasonal variation in output from four tinplate factories and found that production was 10% lower in the hottest month than in the coldest. The difference rose to 30% in a poorly ventilated factory. The weaving of linen and cotton requires a humid atmosphere, but Weston[118] found a fall-off in the production of linen at wet-bulb temperatures above 23° C and Wyatt et al.[119] found lower cotton production when the wet-bulb temperature exceeded 21° C. There was also evidence for a reduction in the output from heavy physical work at about 31° C dry-bulb compared with 21° C.[113] Lifson,[64] however, failed to find an effect of heat (which often exceeded 38° C) on a heavy welding task. Production was recorded as daily output, which may have masked some variations in output that took place during the day, and, furthermore, the survey did not include any measure of the physiologic or psychologic cost of maintaining acceptable performance. Meese et al. (unpublished) found a positive correlation in two South African factories between production and dry-bulb temperature: (1) the daily output of hand-assembled electronic equipment increased by about 35% as temperature rose from 17° to 29° C, and (2) the production in a boot and shoe factory increased by nearly 40% between about 3° and 26° C (Fig 24–7).

There is also evidence to show a relationship between accidents and temperature, although, in practice, accurate data are very difficult to collect. Vernon[112] recorded accidents in a munitions factory and found them to be least frequent at 20° C; below 12° C and above 24° C the increase in frequency was more than 30%. In the cold both men and women were equally affected, but above 20° C the men appeared to be more prone to stress. (The higher susceptibility of men in the heat is a good example of the difficulty of analysis when a temperature effect is not a simple physiologic one, such as cold fingers; Wyon et al.[126] found that men felt subjectively hotter than women in a climate chamber at increasing temperatures while Beshir and Ramsey[10] reported higher levels of boredom and fatigue for women.) Vernon[113] and his colleagues also investigated accidents in coal mines and found them to be more frequent at 25° and 28° C than at 18° C. The accident rate increased with fatigue, and men older than 35 years were more likely to be affected by the heat.

In spite of the lack of control over conditions, work rate, motivation, supply of material, and clothing levels, there is sufficient information available from field studies to indicate that temperature has a measurable effect on performance—enough to justify laboratory investigation.

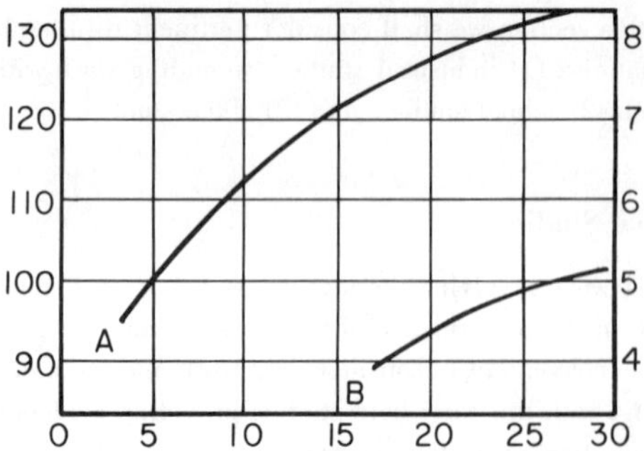

FIG 24–7.
Production (total units manufactured per hour) at two factories, A (n = 84, r = 0.26, $P < 0.02$) and B (n = 51, r = 0.39, $P < .01$), versus air temperature. X = Air temperature (° C); Y (left) = Production at A; Y (right) = Production at B.

Laboratory Studies

Because of the control that can be achieved in a laboratory, it is possible to consider cold and heat stress separately.

Cold Stress.—People are often required to work in cold conditions either outdoors, in deliberately chilled rooms, or in buildings that are inadequately heated during winter. The definition of moderate thermal stress quoted in the introduction would indicate that problems such as hypothermia and frostbite are unlikely to arise. Nevertheless, it is recognized that cold has a deleterious effect on performance. Studies in this temperature range, as we have already seen, have concentrated on the effects of cold on manual dexterity and on tasks in which the arousing effects of cold will lower performance.

Most investigations on finger-tip sensitivity and FST have used the *V* test of Mackworth,[70] a simple apparatus consisting of two rulers that are joined at one end, providing a gap of gradually changing width between the two edges. The subject is required to move his finger along the edges and say at what point it is impossible to determine the presence of a gap. The test was used by Mills,[80] Morton and Provins,[81] and Provins and Morton.[98] There is agreement that performance shows some deterioration below an FST of 25° C and falls off drastically below 10° C. Mackworth's[70] original apparatus has been modified by Wyon et al.[130] so that the subject places his forefinger on a block that is flat or has a gap and is required to say whether or not he can feel the gap. The subject cannot see the block and the gap is 4, 3, 2, or 1 mm wide.

The results of a study by Kok et al.[53] showed that the finger-tip sensitivity of black men and women fell off below an FST of 15°–16° C. Above this FST, the black group's performance was equal to or better than that of the white group. The fact that the white group did not show such a reduction in performance is because of differences in reaction to air temperature between the groups (see Fig 24–1). Schiefer et al.[103] have looked at the relationship between FST and manual dexterity as distinct from sensitivity. Performance was measured on four tasks: block threading, knot tying, a modified O'Connor peg test,[88] and a nut and bolt transfer task. Again, there was a major fall-off in performance at 15°–16° C FST, the reduction in performance was about 13% compared with that at an FST greater than 30° C (Fig 24–8). Other comparable critical values have been determined as: 8° C,[81] 15° C,[23] 12.8° C,[15] 10°–16° C,[66] and 10° C for severe loss and 20° C for some loss was measured by Stevens et al.[106]

Cold also affects finger flexibility, and the results obtained by Hunter et al.[46] and Hellstrom[42] have been discussed. In a study by Meese et al.,[75] results are given showing the effects of cold on finger flexibility and finger strength on a task where the worker was required to perform pencil rolling against different levels of retardation. The greatest percentage reduction was found when minimal retardation was applied, i.e., cold acts to reduce flexibility rather than strength (Fig 24–9).

The effects of cold and muscle strength have been investigated a number of times. Craik and MacPherson,[20] for example, found a reduction in hand strength and finger-thumb opposition

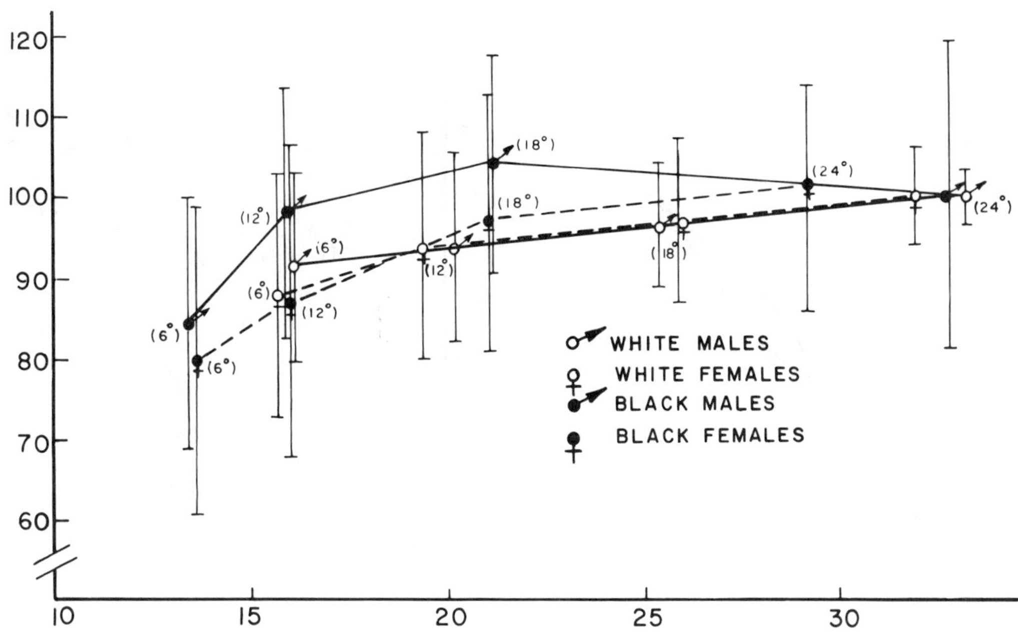

FIG 24–8.
Mean performance on a 2-mm gap test versus the mean FST for four groups (Performance is normalized against the within-group performance at 24° C. The air temperatures at which the tests were performed are shown on the graph.) *X* = Finger skin temperature (FST); *Y* = Normalized performance.

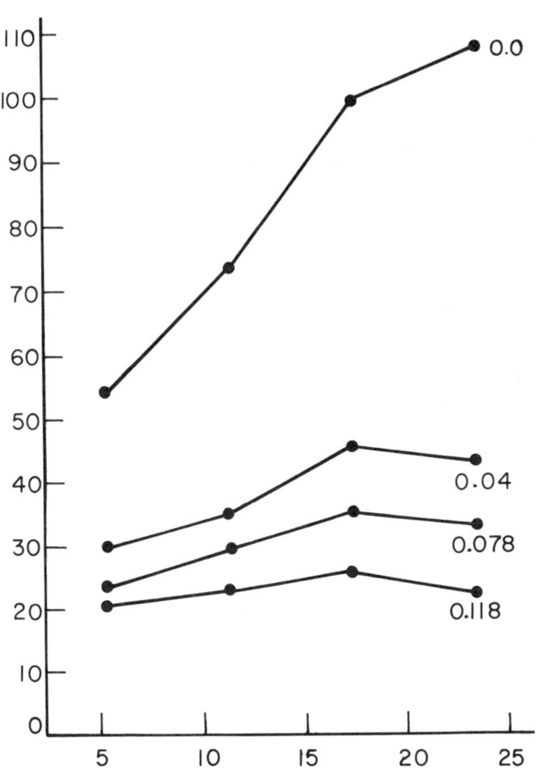

FIG 24–9.
Mean pencil rolling performance by a group of men versus air temperature at four levels of retardation; indicated in Newton meters. *X* = Air temperature (° C); *Y* = Number of revolutions in 30 seconds.

strength after immersion of the hand in water at 7° C for 15 minutes. Meese et al.,[75] however, found no reduction in grip strength at an air temperature of 6° C with workers who were normally clad for this temperature (0.9 clo [0.18 sq km/W] and 0.85 clo [0.17 sq km/W] for men and women respectively). It is unlikely that muscle temperatures ever get low enough to affect the muscle strength of appropriately clad workers in the moderate stress region.

A major study of the effects of cold on factory workers[53, 54, 63, 75–77, 129, 130] found reduced performance at low temperatures in a number of other manual skills, such as a simulated assembly line, where performance at 6° C was 15%–20% lower than at 24° C (Fig 24–10). Tasks requiring hand steadiness and arm steadiness, and presumably sensitive to shivering and increased muscle tension, were significantly affected by cold. Women, for example, showed a 73% increase in errors on the hand steadiness task at 6° C as compared with 24° C (Fig 24–11). A hand-eye coordination test and a rate control test, both of which one might expect to be performed worse in the cold, were not affected, possibly because the tests were too difficult. In a later study[62] with well trained subjects, the rate control task showed a 10% reduction at 6° C as compared with 24° C.

Studies of the effect of cold on mental tasks in which the distracting and arousing effects of cold might lead to reduced performance are less common. Teichner[109] concluded that cold does not reduce reaction time, although Meese et al.[75] found significant reductions in response rate with cold on a five-choice serial reaction task, hesitation errors (responses larger than one to five seconds) were affected for black men but for no other group. Black men and women also took longer in the cold to press a button

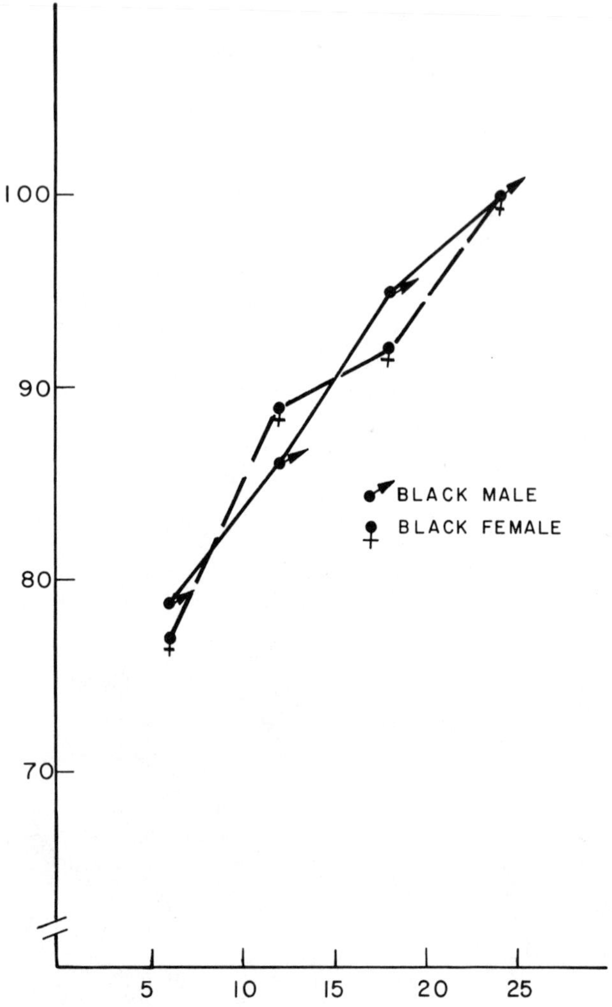

FIG 24–10.
Mean performance (within group, normalized against performance at 24° C) on a simulated assembly line task for a group of men and women, versus air temperature. *X* = Air temperature (° C); *Y* = Performance.

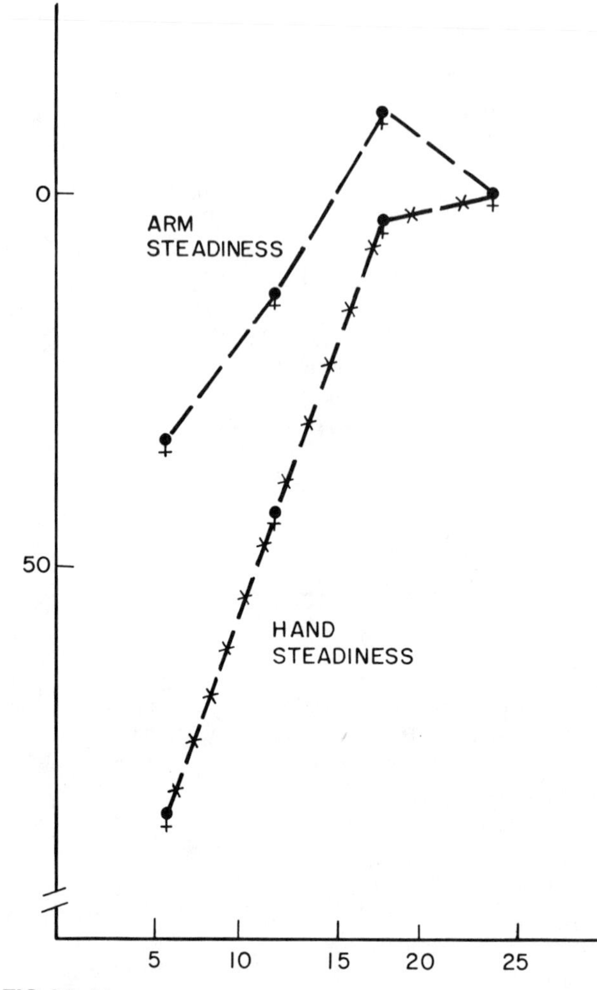

FIG 24–11.
Female performance (normalized against performance at 24° C) on two tracking tasks, versus air temperature. *X* = Air temperature (° C); *Y* = Performance, percent increase in errors per unit time.

registering that they had seen an introduced light delay. Ellis[24] found that reaction times on a serial reaction task were worse in the cold but that the effect was not significant.

Coleshaw et al.[17] found impaired memory and reduced speed of reasoning in subjects as their core temperature fell from 36.7° C to 35° C. Core temperatures between 36° and 35° C have been found in subjects after swimming, after diving in heated diving suits, and even with shift workers in the early morning. Kok et al.[53] found that, after about three hours' exposure at 6° C, about 70% of a group of black men had oral temperatures below 35° C.

Meese et al.[75] also looked at the effect of cold on a physically demanding task, a simulated spot welder (Fig 24–12), and found no effect on the response rate. However, the accuracy of the welds made by both white and black male workers was reduced in the cold.

It is wrong, however, to assume that environmental stress will inevitably lead to poorer performances, and Poulton,[95] in his review of environmental stressors, has drawn attention to the many instances where performance has *improved* under stress; particularly with heat and noise. Poulton[95] explains these improvements on the basis of arousal. Meese et al.[75] found that at 6° C white women significantly improved their rate of response on a serial reaction task—they were quicker, they hesitated less, and both black and white women made less incorrect delay detections. Those results suggest an arousing effect of cold, particularly with the white women whose heart rate increased below 18° C (Fig 24–13). Obviously, this improved performance as a result of adverse conditions is not something that workers would regularly accept.

In conclusion, the general effects of cold are the expected loss of dexterity, finger sensitivity, and muscle control. There is some evidence for the impairment of nonphysical tasks and for the arousing effects of cold. The work of Meese et al.[75] has shown that cold can begin to affect performance at a temperature of 18° C in spite of the fact that one normally expects conditions on the cool

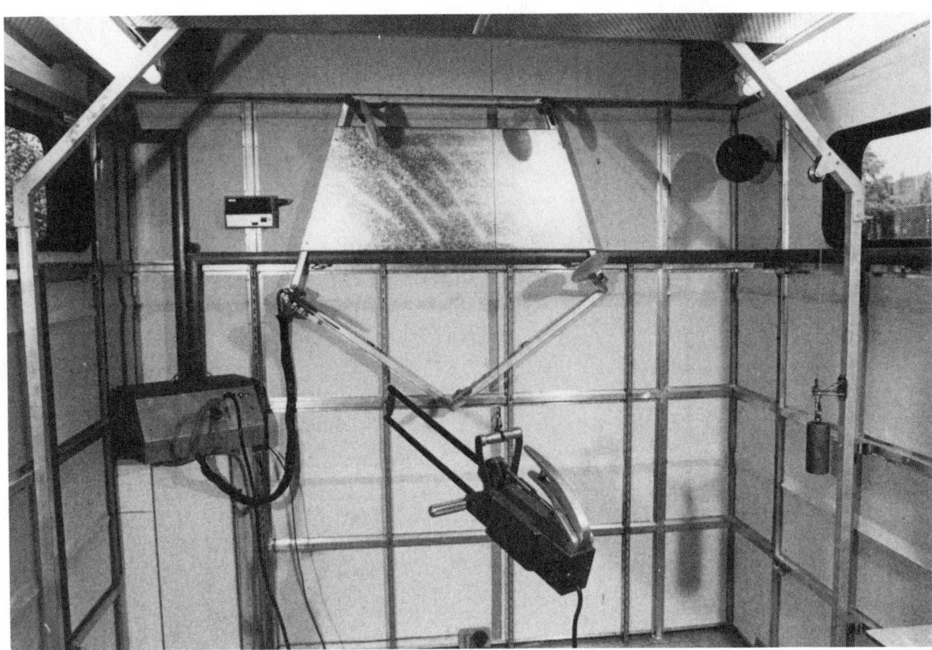

FIG 24–12.
Heavy pursuit task. A simulated spot-welder with five welding targets arranged at different angles in a pentagonal pattern.

side of comfort to aid performance. The effects of cold are widespread and considerable, and the size of the performance decrement between 24° and 6° C is highly specific but ranges between 5% and 70%.[77] It is likely that relatively simple modifications, such as insulation and the local heating of factory buildings, could easily pay for themselves in increased productivity.

Heat Stress.—Within the moderate thermal stress region on the hot side of comfort, it is unlikely that performance will be affected in as direct a physical manner as in the cold; the effects are more likely to be due to arousing and distracting factors. Grether[37] has reviewed much of the work that has been carried out on the effects of heat and has divided the studies into a number of categories.

Dexterity.—One of the very few studies of dexterity under hot conditions was that of Weiner and Hutchinson,[115] who found a significant deterioration in performance at 33° C (Effective Temperature) compared with a control temperature of 18.5°–20° C. Kok et al.,[53] however, found a number of tasks in which performance improved with mild heat stress. Working with black (B) and white (W), male (M) and female (F) subjects at 20°, 26°, 32°, and 38° C they found that for all groups except white women the peak in performance was usually at 32° C. This performance pattern was evident with a peg test (BM, BF) (Figure 24–14), a screw plate test (BM, WM), and an assembly line task (BM, BF).

Except for the presence of sweat on the fingers, it is difficult to accept that heat could produce any physical changes that could cause a reduction in performance on a dexterity task. It is more likely that, as Pepler[91] has suggested, heat reduced the "willingness" to work rather than the "capacity." Work with trained subjects[62] showed that they were able to overcome the drop in performance between 32° and 38° C, indicating that this reduction had neither a physical nor physiologic origin. The lack of a peak in performance at 32° C by the white women was probably a result of their poorer sweat response in this region, as noted earlier in the discussion of the effect of heat on physiology. White women usually had two peaks of performance: at 26° and 38° C. The latter was probably caused by the arousing effect of heat.

Reaction time.—Teichner[109] suggests that reaction time is unchanged over the range of −45° to +47° C but, as we have already seen, there is evidence for change in the cold. Does this also occur in the heat? Poulton[95] quotes two examples of improved reaction time in the heat, although Bell[7] found no significant effect of heat. In the major study of factory workers by Meese et al.,[75] there were few effects of heat on reaction time except for a peak at 32° C followed by a significant falloff at 38° C in a serial reaction task. Hancock and Dirkin[39] showed that an increase of 4.9° C in cortical temperature, achieved by using a heated helmet, brought about an increase in reaction time and a decrease in errors on a serial reaction task. In direct contrast to these findings, Nunneley et al.[85] found that elevated head temperature resulted in shortened reaction time and an increase in the number of errors.

There are many factors which have been shown to affect reaction time; age, the complexity of the task, the intake of alcohol, and a knowledge of the results. Grether[27] suggests that heat could reduce reaction time in simple tests but lengthen it in more complex tests. Nunneley et al.[85] point out the shortcomings of experi-

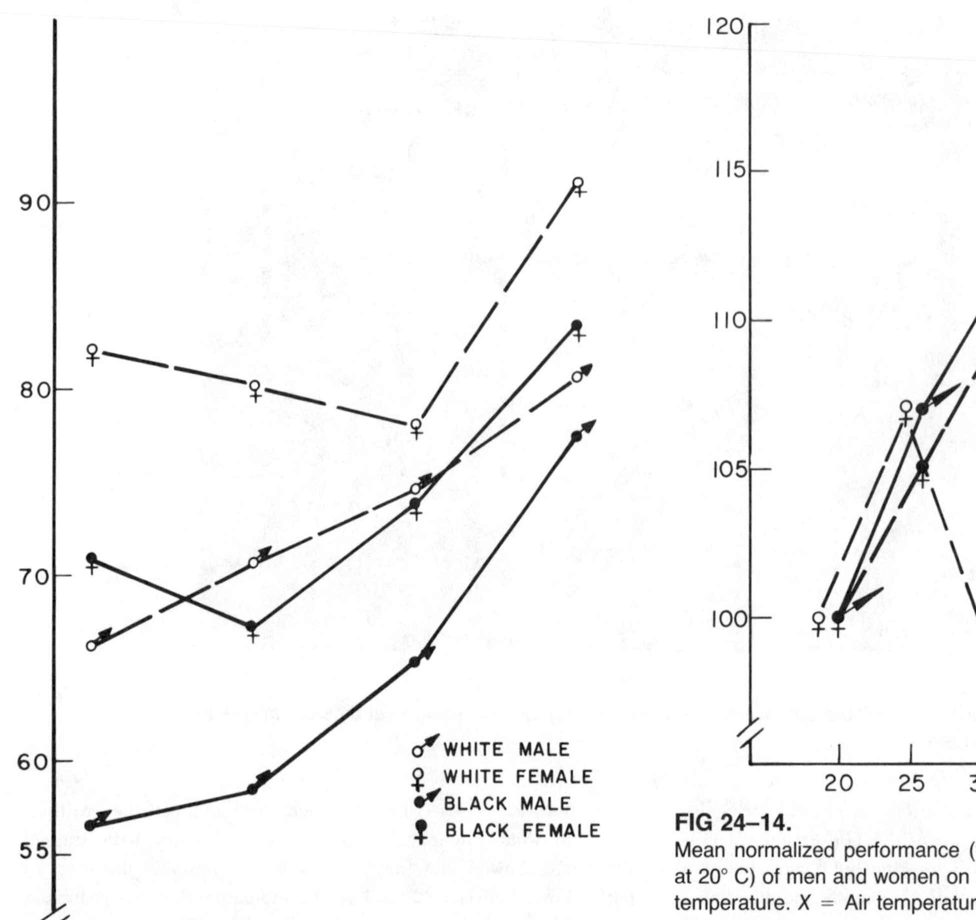

FIG 24–13.
Mean heart rates for four groups of subjects after exposure for 2.5–3.0 hours to one of four air temperatures, versus air temperature. X = Air temperature (° C); Y = Heart rate (beats per minute).

FIG 24–14.
Mean normalized performance (within-group, against performance at 20° C) of men and women on a manual dexterity task, versus air temperature. X = Air temperature (° C); Y = Performance.

mental methods and the difficulty of synthesizing the findings: poor measurement of the physiologic state of subjects, wide variation in the tasks used, possible learning effects, and subordination of the reaction time component to a control task in the test used. One cannot, therefore, at this stage conclusively state what the effect of heat is on reaction time; it is likely that the effect is specific to a particular task.

Mental and cognitive tasks.—Many investigations have been carried out on the effect of heat on mental work. The general conclusion would seem to be that there is some deterioration in performance at temperatures above about 29° C Effective Temperature. It is possible, however, that at particularly high temperatures there may be some improvement in performance caused by the arousing effect of heat; mild warmth is de-arousing and makes one feel drowsy and relaxed, but as the temperature rises, heat becomes a stimulus. Many tests have included some cognitive function as an aspect of the work, and Grether[37] has noted 16 relevant studies, half of which have shown little or no temperature effect on performance while the remainder have found effects only at the highest temperatures (e.g., Iampietro et al.[47]). Grether[37] concludes that at temperatures above 29.4° C Effective Temperature, which is equivalent to about 35° C dry-bulb and 26° C wet-bulb, performance shows little change. The only studies showing a considerable decline in performance under hot conditions are those of Mackworth[67] and Pepler.[89] Meese et al.[75] used a simulated inspection task in which cards were examined for similarities and errors, and they found few effects of temperature on either the rate of working or the errors made. In the same study, it was found that short-term memory tended to increase at high temperatures but that the effects were not usually significant.

Once again, the studies in this field have produced a range of conflicting evidence, and by careful selection one could deduce that heat resulted in either lowered or improved performance. The range of tests used and the variety of methods employed to bring about elevated temperatures mean that results are not usually comparable.

Vigilance and monitoring.—Vigilance tasks can be thought of as watching and/or listening for events to occur, usually at irregular, and often widely spaced, intervals. In warm conditions there is a conflict between the speeding up effect of heat and its distracting influence. Much early work grew out of the problems encountered in World War II, which required such people as wireless and radar operators to perform highly demanding tasks often under difficult circumstances. Some of the earliest studies were those of Mackworth,[69] who found with his clock test that detection was best at 26.1° C Effective Temperature and that morse code operators showed a severe reduction in performance above 30° C Effective Temperature. Mackworth[69] also showed that the poorer performers in the group showed the largest reduction at higher temperatures. This was an important demonstration that workers who are at their limit of ability have little "reserve" and are likely to be the most affected when conditions are not ideal. These studies used subjects clad only in shorts and with some acclimatization to hot conditions. In a later study, Pepler[89] confirmed that vigilance was best at an Effective Temperature of 27.8° C. Fraser[30] worked with coal miners on a vigilance task after they had completed heavy work in a hot saturated atmosphere and showed that prior exposure and work done could modify performance. Meese et al.[75] used a serial reaction task with a vigilance component: the detection of a 0.2-second delay in the extinguishing of a light. With the exception of white women, performance was best at 32° C 1.0 kPa (25° C ET) and was then reduced at 38° C 1.0 kPa (27.5° C ET). These findings confirm the general conclusions of Grether[37] that vigilance is reduced above an Effective Temperaure of 26.7° C.

As with most studies, cross-comparisons are difficult, but it is probably safe to conclude that performance is likely to deteriorate above conditions equivalent to 30° C at about 1.0 kPa (a relative humidity of just under 40%).

Tracking.—A wide variety of tasks can be considered under the general heading of tracking, and Grether[37] has concluded that with few exceptions they demonstrate a falloff in performance at temperatures beyond about 29.4° C Effective Temperature. Once more, the studies of Mackworth[68] and Pepler[89] are noteworthy, especially the demonstration of the role played by incentives.

The work of Bursill[14] is also important in this area in demonstrating the phenomenon of "tunnel vision." Bursill's subjects were required to perform a central tracking task while detecting occasional peripheral signals; in heat there was decreased ability to detect these signals and the effect was greatest on those signals farthest from the center. These results can be analyzed in terms of arousal theory and indicate that under conditions of high stress there is a reduction in ability to notice unexpected signals away from the central task. This finding is of importance to designers—for instance, a meter indicating danger should not be positioned far away from the central task, because it could be ignored under stressful conditions. Lewis et al.[62] used a rate control task and found that performance was unaffected with relatively untrained workers but that trained workers who had acquired considerable skill produced their worst performance under conditions of mild heat (32° C 1.0 kPa) and then improved as conditions became hotter (38° C 1.0 kPa or about 27.5° C Effective Temperature) (Fig 24–15). This would suggest that the low arousal conditions at 32° C were not favorable for the performance of this difficult task, although they resulted in good performance on a simple track-tracing task. On a heavy tracking task, Meese et al.[75] found, in general, more errors (missed targets and incorrect targets) for men at the higher temperatures, usually with the worst performance at 38° C 1.0 kPa.

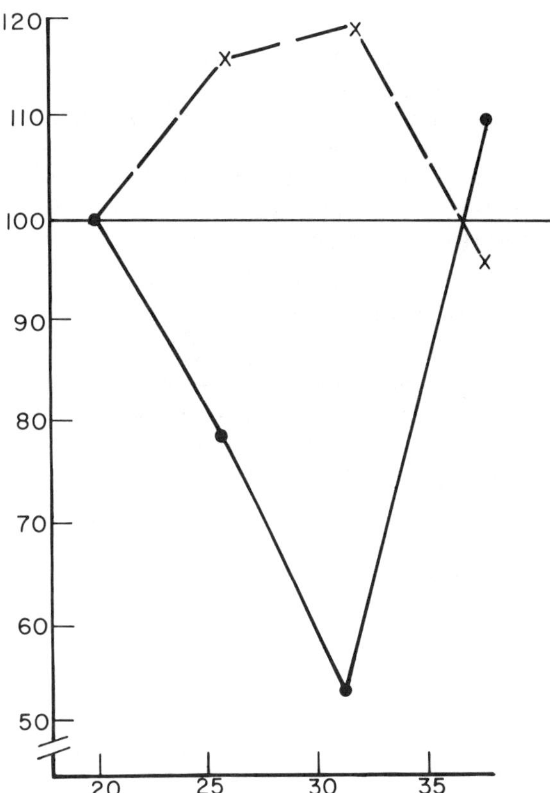

FIG 24–15.
Mean normalized performance (within group, against performance at 20° C) of trained *(solid line)* and relatively untrained *(broken line)* subjects on a rate control task, versus air temperature. *X* = Air temperature (° C); *Y* = Performance.

Factors modifying the behavioral response to thermal stress.—It is clear from the examples presented that analysis of performance data is most difficult because of the range of tests and techniques that have been used. There are a number of other features that can have a modifying effect on the response:

1. Age, sex, and ethnic origin have already been noted as factors to consider in regard to the temperature response.

2. The state of training for a task is important, and Lewis et al.[62] found that trained workers did not exhibit the falloff in performance at 38° C that had been evident with untrained workers, i.e., the trained workers by their skill were able to overcome the distracting effects of heat. This was not so, however, in manual dexterity tasks in the cold.

3. Motivation and incentives are of vital importance, and in Mackworth's[68] classic study, it was found that high incentives could compensate for the reduction in performance caused by heat so that work output under hot conditions and with high incentives was equal to that in cooler conditions with low incentives. One cannot assume from a level of performance that a worker is at the limit of his ability or is working well within his capacity. In some of Mackworth's studies the less effective workers were most affected by temperature, whereas in others it was the good workers.

4. Temperature is frequently not the only stressor present, and its effects may have to be considered in conjunction with other environmental factors, such as noise. The resulting effect of two or more stressors in combination is not easily predicted and studies have shown a number of outcomes. Pepler[90] found that the effects of heat and sleep were simply additive. Bell[7] found that noise and heat, which did not affect a primary task, did have an effect upon a secondary task. Certain combinations of conditions could cancel each other out, e.g., extreme heat and boredom.

5. The time of exposure is also important, particularly if the exposure period is spent on prolonged repetitive work.

6. Adequate acclimatization is known to be vital for heavy work in hot conditions but a lesser degree of acclimatization may play a role, and many studies have considered whether Europeans who have lived in the tropics for some time perform differently than those who have not. Results, however, are not conclusive.

7. A final consideration should be the relative roles of the six factors making up the thermal environment. Pepler[89] found that loss of performance in a pursuit motor task at two equivalent Effective Temperatures was greater at the higher humidity. Kok et al.,[55] however, increased the humidity at dry-bulb temperatures of 26°, 32°, 35°, and 38° C and found little effect on performance, even though the most extreme conditions were nearly 30° C WBGT. There were indications that those conditions were stressful; about 70% of a group of white women had heart rates exceeding 100 beats per minute at the end of a six-hour exposure while performing light tasks.

School Studies

Just as factories should be productive, efficient, and safe, so should schools provide the best possible environmental conditions for teaching and learning. This can be even more difficult to assess than performance in a factory, and most studies have concentrated on skills that are easily measured, such as reading speed, comprehension, and mathematical ability. Most of the work could be classified as field studies, although some has been conducted with small groups of children in a laboratory.

The effects of temperature on learning and test performance were investigated by Pepler and Warner,[92] who accepted "rate of change of performance" as a good measure of the impact of the environment. Their study used a programmed learning schedule lasting six weeks and determined significant effects of temperature on error rate, time to completion, and effort. The relationship was an inverted U-shaped curve, with best performance at 26.7° C, a falloff in performance at 16.7°–20.0° C and a lesser falloff in the warm conditions of 30.0°–33.3° C. There were few sex differences and no differences according to academic ability, and the optimum thermal comfort temperature was closer to 23.3° C than 26.7° C.

McNall and Nevins[74] summarized the findings from a comparison of the performance of children in air-conditioned and non-air-conditioned schools and found trends favoring the climate-controlled school, although the effect was often nonsignificant.

Langkilde et al.[59] found that at 4° C above thermal comfort (22.6° C) performance of a memory test was no better but was judged by the student subjects to be better, i.e., they were less critical. This the authors attribute to lowered arousal. Wyon and Holmberg[127] also used arousal theory to explain the poorer performance of 8 children aged 8 to 11 years at 27° C compared with their results at 20° and 30° C; a temperature just above comfort produced low arousal and inattentiveness. Wyon et al.[128] also found significant effects of heat on mental performance with older children (17 years old); their performance on memory and sentence comprehension tests was poorest at comfortable temperatures.

A different type of test has shown the effect of cold ambient conditions on the manual dexterity of schoolchildren.[117] Thus, 8-year-old children in a classroom during the winter at 7.6° C had lost about 20% of their performance at 25.5° C. Another approach is that of Schiefer et al.,[102] who analyzed the results of annual aptitude tests given to pupils aged 17 to 18 years and showed a small but significant effect of temperature on mathematics, a verbal skill, and both verbal and nonverbal reasoning. Cooler conditions favored a better performance.

Kevan and Howes[51] have reviewed much of the work on classroom environment and concluded that, in general, cool conditions appear to favor learning and that heat acts to reduce the willingness to work. They point out that precise temperatures will depend on such factors as local custom in regard to clothing. A further important point they note is that people working at their limit will tend to benefit most from improved conditions, which implies that children who are working well within their capacity will cope better with adverse conditions.

Office Studies

A number of studies have attempted to determine the effect of temperature on the performance of office workers. This work has its own set of specific problems: (1) the work is usually sedentary, so there is little opportunity to increase the metabolic rate; (2) the people employed cover a wide range of age and fitness, and some are handicapped; (3) productivity is often difficult to assess; (4) the occupants will have varying amounts of control over their environment in terms of clothing level, use of windows, fans, and heaters; and (5) the temperature range encountered in an office is usually narrower than in a factory building, so the effects of temperature are likely to be small and therefore more difficult to measure. Nevertheless, a number of studies have shown temperature effects of varying magnitude.

The largest project ever undertaken was that of the New York State Commission on Ventilation in 1914,[84] which included a typing test at 20° and 24° C with low motivation and no knowledge of results. The original analysis of the data concluded that there had been no effect of heat stress on performance, but a reanalysis by Wyon[125] using nonparametric statistics showed that the subjects at 20° C performed significantly better than at 24° C. The effect was considerable and Wyon[125] quotes values of 40%–50% reduction on average for a group. Langkilde[58] exposed 15 subjects to temperatures of 18°, 21°, 24°, 27°, and 30° C while they performed simulated office work and found a weak effect of temperature: subjects worked faster when they felt cool at 18° C and slower when they felt hot at 30° C than when they were comfortable at 24° C.

The general conclusion from office studies is that the effect of temperature on well-motivated staff, within the narrow temperature range normally encountered, is slight and that conditions on the cool side of comfort region are likely to produce the best results.

SUBJECTIVE THERMAL CONTROL

The preceding sections have shown the relevance of the moderate thermal stress region to performance, but subjective impressions of comfort cannot be ignored because of the possible consequences in terms of dissatisfaction. Thermal comfort has been defined as "that condition of mind which expresses satisfaction with the thermal environment."[2] There are two basic ways in which thermal comfort has been measured: (1) the subjects were able to adjust the temperature of an exposure chamber to their preferred level,[26] and (2) the subjects were requested to register their comfort vote on a rating scale, usually the Bedford scale.[5] The possibility of variation in the latter is legion. In a hot country, "comfort" may imply being slightly cool, thus allowing one to escape from the heat. The scale intervals are not equidistant, e.g., a vote of 3 (hot) on the ASHRAE[2] scale does not mean that one is three times hotter or more uncomfortable than when voting 1 (slightly warm). The range of temperatures over which the work is conducted will have a considerable effect on the votes recorded. For example, a group of subjects exposed at 20° C may vote "comfortable," but this does not mean that they would not record the same vote if exposed at 18° or 22° C. A further problem is in communication: in a country where many different languages are used, the terms may not be equivalent or the concept of thermal comfort may not even exist.

The methods of investigation outlined above have influenced the findings. (1) The more rigidly controlled laboratory experiments have stressed the fixed nature of the thermal comfort response and its predictability from a knowledge of the environmental and physiologic parameters, and (2) the approach in which subjects are able to vote has tended to show that subjective comfort impressions are more flexible.

The first approach has concentrated on temperatures close to optimum thermal comfort and is particularly associated with the studies of Fanger.[26] In addition to the ASHRAE[2] description of comfort, one can also consider comfort in terms of the physiologic requirements for that state. Benzinger[9] has defined comfort as the absence of signals that lead to thermal correcting behavior, while Fanger has defined three necessary conditions for comfort: (1) the body must be in thermal equilibrium, (2) the MST should be at an appropriate level for comfort, and (3) the sweat rate should be at a preferred level. Fanger[27] has suggested a skin temperature of close to 34° C as appropriate for comfort, while Gagge et al.[32] found that an MST of 33° C was necessary for comfort by a person engaged in sedentary activity.

From extensive studies in the laboratory Fanger[26] has developed his comfort equation and Predicted Mean Vote. This allows one to calculate the necessary conditions for comfort to be achieved and the thermal vote that would be recorded under any set of known circumstances. These two indices have proved useful and reproducible, with the proviso that most of the studies were conducted with sedentary, lightly clad subjects close to their optimum comfort temperature. As the activity level rises, the necessary physiologic conditions for comfort will, of course, change, and moderate sweating and a lower skin temperature will be required. Fanger's[26] work has stressed the essentially fixed nature of the comfort response and shown that it is not affected by such factors as age, sex, ethnic origin, or time of day. Fanger[26] has also shown that the preferred temperature of the individual is consistent, although McIntyre[72] has concluded that "the variability in warmth votes given by one person on different occasions is as high as the overall variability of votes."

The second approach to comfort has sometimes used laboratory conditions but has frequently been concerned with field surveys. Thermal comfort is a practical consideration, thermally uncomfortable conditions can be a source of immense dissatisfaction to occupants and therefore of great interest to the designers of buildings and heating and ventilating equipment. An advantage of field surveys is that they are relatively easy to conduct, and this approach has stressed the options open to people to adjust their thermal environment by changing their clothing, posture, or work rate. Findings by workers using this approach have shown effects of sex,[126] room size,[60] and circadian rhythm[4] on the comfort vote. A laboratory study by Meese et al.[79] found that two groups of workers under identical conditions and in similar physiologic states voted differently depending on the amount of time spent in the experimental situation. Workers who had attended the laboratory for only one day were less ready to express dissatisfaction at extreme temperatures than were a similar group who had participated in the experiment for three to four weeks. For example, at 6° C only 8% of the new workers voted that this condition was "much too cold" while 92% of the trained workers recorded this vote (Fig 24–16). The trained workers also had a much higher MST: comfort vote correlation than did the naive subjects: $r = 0.75$ and $r = 0.44$, respectively. Figure 24–16 shows that within the region of optimum thermal comfort there is little variation in voting behavior.

It is difficult to summarize such a wide field of investigation in which so many different techniques have been applied, but, in general, it would appear that the optimum temperature for sedentary, lightly clad individuals lies within a very narrow range for all ages and both sexes and is unaffected by ethnic origin. Outside the comfort region many other factors can play a significant role. This is further illustrated by Figure 24–17. Furthermore, it is suggested that the collection of field data on comfort votes would be more accurate if subjects were asked to vote on a number of occasions rather than only once.

Accepting the limitations of comfort-vote studies, it is worth considering their relevance to performance. Allan et al.[1] suggested that "performance correlates better with comfort than with any other single variable." Meese et al.,[78] however, working with about 500 subjects on a wide range of tasks, found that air temperature was a far better predictor of performance than comfort vote. For example, the correlation coefficient was $r = 0.611$ for air temperature and $r = 0.432$ for comfort vote with a group of women on a pencil-rolling task in the cold. Pepler and Warner[92] found that subjects performed least well at their preferred temperature, Meese et al.[75] found peak performance at 32° C and optimum comfort at 19°–22° C. Griffiths and Boyce[38] found optimum performance at a temperature similar to that of optimum thermal comfort, but, again, better correlations were found between performance and temperature than between performance and temperature assessment.

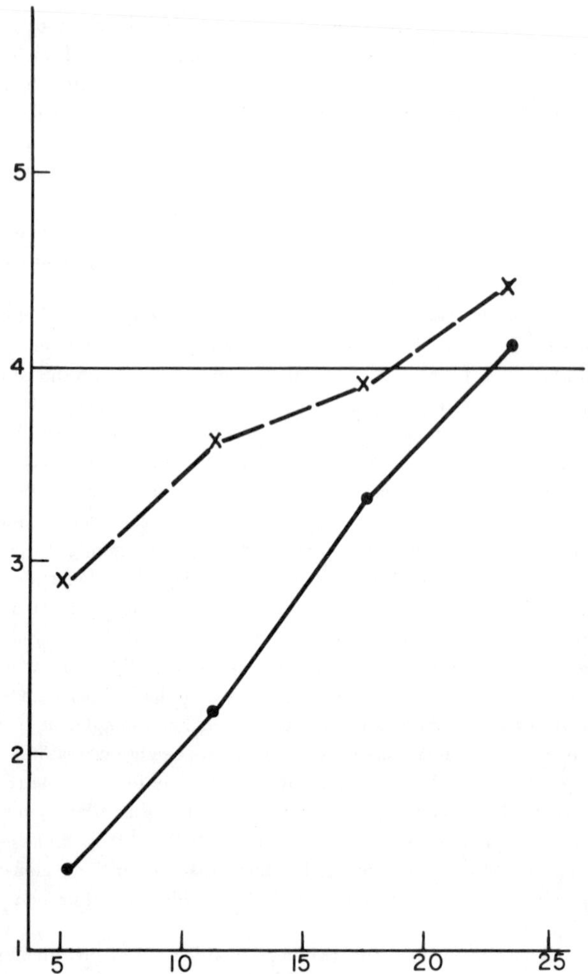

FIG 24–16.
Mean comfort vote on the Bedford scale (4 = comfort) of trained *(solid line)* and relatively untrained *(broken line)* subjects, versus air temperature. *X* = Air temperature (° C); *Y* = Comfort vote.

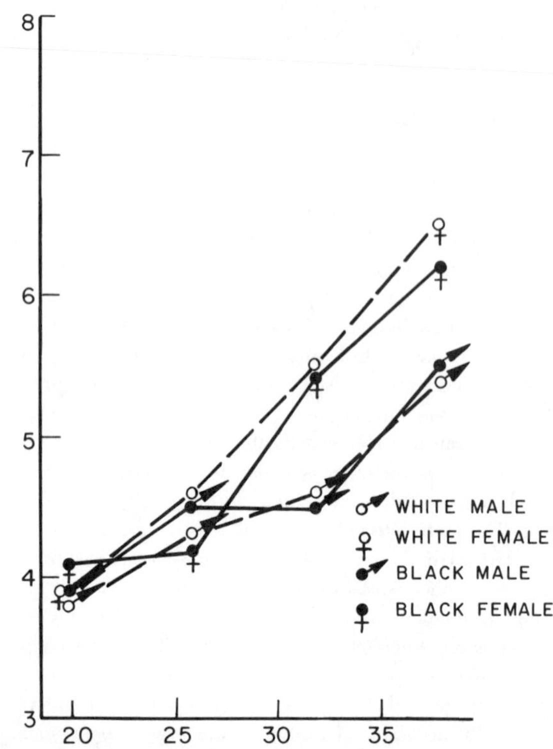

FIG 24–17.
Mean comfort vote on the Bedford scale (4 = comfort) versus air temperature, for four groups of subjects. *X* = Air temperature (° C); *Y* = Comfort vote.

Subjective thermal comfort also influences behavior. Harries and Stadler[41] have shown a high correlation between discomfort and aggressive behavior and a number of investigations have considered the relationship between antisocial behavior and thermal discomfort.

In conclusion, thermal discomfort can occur within the moderate stress region, and although well motivated people can tolerate this, it can be a source of great dissatisfaction. The provision of optimum thermal conditions is impossible because of variations in the perception of comfort by individuals, and in any case this may not even favor productivity. Control of the thermal environment is, however, of great importance to the individual, and it is recommended that people be given freedom to control their own microclimate through the use of fans, heaters, and modifications to their clothing. A change in clothing can lead to a dramatic change in comfort temperatures, an increase of 0.4 clo (0.08 sq km/W), for example, could lower the optimum comfort temperatures to 20° C from the currently accepted range of 22.2°–25.5° C.

ASSESSMENT OF THE THERMAL ENVIRONMENT

The factors making up the thermal environment have already been listed, but for many years a simple measure has been sought. A problem for industry or the armed forces is that if thermal conditions need to be assessed, then one must consider who is to do the assessing. A complex, accurate method that cannot be carried out on the shop floor is worthless. Consequently, many attempts have been made to develop an index that in a single value, gives a measure of the thermal stress of an environment.

One of the earliest measures of extreme heat stress was the Predicted Four-Hour Sweat Rate or P4SR[71] developed for use with military personnel; it was a measure of the amount of sweat secreted by fit, acclimatized young men exposed for four hours. The index has been confirmed as a very precise measure but is clearly of limited applicability. In 1955 Belding and Hatch[6] developed their Heat Stress Index (HSI) based on a heat exchange model that assumes a constant skin temperature of 35° C. These two indices were combined in the Index of Thermal Stress (ITS),[36] which owed its form to the HSI but used the sweat rate as a measure of strain. The most commonly used heat stress index, however, is the Wet-Bulb Globe Thermometer Index derived from the Corrected Effective Temperature (CET)[131] and defined as

WBGT (Wet-Bulb Globe Temperature) =

$$0.7\ t_w + 0.2\ t_g + 0.1\ t_d$$

where t_w is the temperature of a naturally ventilated wet-bulb, t_g is the globe (radiant) temperature, and t_d is the dry-bulb air temperature.

Both t_g and t_d are sensitive to air movement, so air speed plays a part in the final value of the WBGT. The measure is simple and well-proven, and has gained acceptance to the degree that small portable WBGT instruments are now available.

Other important indices that have been developed are the Effective Temperature,[45] which determined equal comfort lines as a function of air temperature and humidity. This became the standard index and has been used by air-conditioning engineers for about 50 years although it overemphasizes humidity under cool conditions and underemphasizes it in the heat. A number of other comfort indices were developed, but these have mostly been superseded by the indices developed by Fanger[26] and based on his comfort equation. His Predicted Mean Vote gives a measure of how uncomfortable an environment is when it is not at the optimum. A third index that is of immense practical value is the Predicted Percentage Dissatisfied (PPD). At the optimum thermal temperature, one cannot hope to satisfy more than 95% of a large sample and the PPD will increase as one moves further away from this point. The only other comfort index in common use is the Standard Effective Temperature,[33] which uses skin wetness and skin temperature to define the thermal state.

At the cool-to-cold end of the moderate stress region, air temperature and wind speed are of importance, and these have been combined into the Windchill Index,[104] but this only has relevance when outdoor conditions are being considered.

LIMITING CONDITIONS

Legislation has been devised in many countries to limit the exposure time and metabolic activity that can be undertaken in certain environments. Much of the development in this area arose out of work with military personnel, but is now applied throughout industry generally. South Africa, for instance, recommends an upper limit of 30° C WBGT for light continuous work and a lower limit of 10° C for light tasks.[83]

Goldman[35] has recently reviewed heat stress limitations and has suggested that the basis for recommendations should be on heart-rate criteria (a limit of 120 beats per minute for an eight-hour shift is suggested) and that greater emphasis be placed on individual fitness, genetically-based work capacity, and the state of acclimatization.

Limiting values are constantly under review, but in most industrialized countries, physically demanding tasks in hot conditions are less common in the workplace each year. It should not be forgotten, however, that a safe environment can become unsafe if one of the six major thermal variables changes. In an emergency, for example, a man may be required to work very hard in heavy protective clothing, thus exposing himself to danger.

A remaining problem in industry is exposure to high radiant temperatures, where legislation for this factor alone is negligible. Safety of the outdoor worker is also a problem, because the environment is changeable. Furthermore, because of loose organization, in agriculture for instance, legislation is more difficult.

REFERENCES

1. Allan JR, Belyarin CA, Flick CA, et al: *Detection of Visual Signals During Induced Cycles of Core Temperature,* Report 592. Farnborough, Hants, England, RAF Institute of Aviation Medicine, 1981.
2. American Society of Heating, Refrigerating and Air-conditioning Engineers: *Thermal Comfort Conditions,* ASHRAE Standard 55-66. New York, ASHRAE, 1966.
3. Aschoff J: Circadian control of body temperature. *J Therm Biol* 1983; 8:143–147.
4. Attia M, Engel P, Hildebrandt G: Thermal comfort during work. *Int Arch Occup Environ Health* 1980; 45:205–215.
5. Bedford T: *Basic Principles of Ventilation and Heating*. London, HK Lewis, 1964.
6. Belding HS, Hatch TF: Index for evaluating heat stress in terms of resulting physiological strain. *Heating, Piping and Air-conditioning* 1955; 27:129–136.
7. Bell PA: Effects of noise and heat stress on primary and subsidiary task performance. *Hum Factors* 1978; 20:749–752.
8. Bell PA, Loomis RJ, Cervone JC: Effects of heat, social facilitation, sex differences, and task difficulty on reaction time. *Hum Factors* 1982; 24:19–24.
9. Benzinger TH: The physiological basis for thermal comfort, in Fanger PO, Valbjorn O (eds): *Indoor Climate*. Copenhagen, World Health Organization, Danish Building Research Institute, 1978, pp 857–881.
10. Beshir MY, Ramsey JD: Comparison between male and female subjective estimates of thermal effects and sensations. *Appl Ergon* 1981; 12:29–33.
11. Broman B, Dahlberg G, Lichtenstein A: Height and weight during growth. *Acta Paediatr Scand* 1942; 30:1–66.
12. Brown M, Page J: The effect of chronic exposure to cold on temperature and blood flow of the hand. *J Appl Physiol* 1952; 5:221–227.
13. Burse RL: Sex differences in human thermoregulatory response to heat and cold stress. *Hum Factors* 1979; 21:687–699.
14. Bursill AE: The restriction of peripheral vision during exposure to hot and humid conditions. *Q J Exp Psychol* 1958; 10:113–129.
15. Clark RE: The limiting hand skin temperature for unaffected manual performance in the cold. *J Appl Psychol* 1961; 45:193–194.
16. Cleland TS, Bachman JC, Horvath SM: Tolerance of the elderly to moderate work—heat stress. *Int J Sports Med* 1981; 2:268.
17. Coleshaw SRK, Van Somern RNM, Wolff AH, et al: Impaired memory registration and speed of reasoning caused by low body temperature. *J Appl Physiol* 1983; 55:27–31.
18. Collins KJ, Hoinville E: Temperature requirements in old age. *Bldg Serv Eng Res Tech* 1980; 1:165–172.
19. Corcoran DWJ: Personality and the inverted U relation. *Br J Psychol* 1965; 56:267–273.
20. Craik KJW, MacPherson SJ: *Effects of Cold Upon Hand Movements and Reaction Times*. London, Military Personnel Research Committee, Military Research Council BPC, 43/196, 1943.
21. Dieng K, Lemonnier D, Bleiberg F, et al: Differences in the rate of energy expenditure of resting activities between European and African men. *Nutr Rep Int* 1980; 21:183–188.
22. Drinkwater BL, Bedi JF, Loucks AB, et al: Sweating sensitivity and capacity of women in relation to age. *J Appl Physiol* 1982; 53:671–676.
23. Dusek RE: Effect of temperature on manual performance, in Fisher RP (ed): *Production and Functioning of the Hands in Cold Climates*. Washington, DC, National Academy of Sciences, National Research Council, 1957, pp 63–76.
24. Ellis HD: The effects of cold on the performance of serial choice

reaction time and various discrete tasks. *Hum Factors* 1982; 24:589–598.

25. Epstein Y, Shapiro Y, Brill S: Role of surface area-to-mass ratio and work efficiency in heat intolerance. *J Appl Physiol* 1983; 54:831–836.
26. Fanger PO: *Thermal Comfort*. New York, McGraw-Hill Book Co, 1972.
27. Fanger PO: Thermal environments preferred by man. *Build International* 1973; 6:127–141.
28. Foret J, Benoit O, Royant-Parola S: Sleep schedules and peak times of oral temperature and alertness in morning and evening 'types.' *Ergonomics* 1982; 25:821–827.
29. Fox RH, Löfstedt BE, Woodward PM, et al: Comparison of thermoregulatory function in men and women. *J Appl Physiol* 1969; 26:444–453.
30. Fraser DC: In Pepler RD: *The Effect of Climactic Factors on the Performance of Skilled Tasks by Young European Men Living in the Tropics*. London, Applied Psychology Unit, Medical Research Council, 1953.
31. Frye AJ, Kamon E: Responses to dry heat of men and women with similar aerobic capacities. *J Appl Physiol* 1981; 50:65–70.
32. Gagge AP, Stolwijk JAJ, Hardy JD: Comfort and thermal sensations and associated physiological responses of various ambient temperatures. *Environ Res* 1967; 1:1–20.
33. Gagge AP, Stolwijk JAJ, Nishi Y: An effective temperature scale based on a simple model of human physiological regulatory response. *ASHRAE Trans* 1971; 77:247–262.
34. Garrow JS: Effect of obesity on human energy expenditure, in Angel A, Hollenberg CH, Roncari DAK (eds): *The Adipocyte and Obesity: Cellular and Molecular Mechanisms*. New York, Raven Press, 1983, pp 251–258.
35. Goldman RF: Prediction of heat strain revisited 1979–1980, in Dukes-Dobos FN, Henschel A (eds): *Proceedings of a NIOSH Workshop on Recommendation of Heat Stress Standards National Institute for Occupational Safety and Health*. Cincinnati, Oh, US Dept of Health and Human Services, 1980, pp 96–109.
36. Givoni B: *Man, Climate and Architecture*, ed 2. London, Applied Science, 1976.
37. Grether WF: Human performance at elevated environmental temperatures. *Aerospace Med* 1973; 44:747–755.
38. Griffiths ID, Boyce RR: Performance and thermal comfort. *Ergonomics* 1971; 14:457–468.
39. Hancock PA, Dirkin GR: Central and peripheral visual choice-reaction time under conditions of induced hyperthermia. *Percept Mot Skills* 1982; 54:395–402.
40. Hardy JD: Physiology of temperature regulation. *Physiol Rev* 1961; 41:521–606.
41. Harries KD, Stadler SJ: Determinism revisited. Assault and heat stress in Dallas, 1980. *Environ Behav* 1983; 15:235–256.
42. Hellstrom B: *Local Effects of Acclimatization to Cold in Man*. Norwegian monographs on medical science. Oslo, Universiteitsforlaget, 1965.
43. Hertig BA, Sargent F: II. Acclimatization of women during work in hot environments. *Fed Proc* 1963; 22:810–813.
44. Hillyard SD, Dill DB: Sweat rate and skin temperature in desert walks; blacks and whites, young and old. *Physiologist* 1981; 24:14.
45. Houghten FC, Yaglou CP: Determining equal comfort lines. *J Am Soc Heat Ventil Eng* 1923; 29:165–176.
46. Hunter J, Kerr EH, Whillans MG: The relation between joint stiffness upon exposure to cold and the characteristics of synovial fluid. *Can J Med Sci* 1952; 30:367–377.
47. Iampietro PF, Chiles WD, Higgins EA, et al: Complex performance during exposure to high temperatures. *Aerospace Med* 1969; 40:1331–1335.
48. Iampietro PF, Goldman RF, Buskirk ER, et al: Response of Negro and white males to cold. *J Appl Physiol* 1959; 14:798–800.
49. Iwanga K, Yasukouchi A, Yamasaki K, et al: Effects of body build and sweat rate on rectal temperature during acute heat exposure in man. *Ergonomics* 1982; 25:465–466.
50. Kerslake D McK, Brebner DF: Maximum sweating at rest, in Hardy JD, Gagge AP, Stolwijk JAJ (eds): *Physiological and Behavioural Temperature Regulations*. Springfield, Ill, Charles C Thomas, 1970, pp 139–151.
51. Kevan SM, Howes JD: Climatic conditions in classrooms. *Educ Rev* 1980; 32:281–292.
52. Kok R: Physiological changes during prolonged work on a bicycle ergometer, M Sc thesis. Dept of Physiology, Potchefstroom University for Christian Higher Education, Potchefstroom, South Africa, 1980.
53. Kok R, Lewis MI, Meese GB, et al: *The Effects of Moderate Cold and Heat Stress on the Potential Work Performance of Industrial Workers*. Pt 3: Effects of eight environmental conditions on skin temperature, oral temperature, heart rate and subjective comfort vote, BRR 587. Pretoria, South Africa, National Building Research Institute, CSIR, 1982.
54. Kok R, Lewis MI, Meese GB, et al: The effects of moderate cold and heat stress on factory workers in Southern Africa. 3. Skill and performance in the heat. *S Afr J Sci* 1982; 78:306–314.
55. Kok R, Meese GB, Lewis MI: *The Effects of Moderate Cold and Heat Stress on the Potential Work Performance of Industrial Workers. Pt 6: The Effects Increasing Humidity at Four Air Temperatures on the Performance and Physiology of White Females*. Pretoria, South Africa, National Building Research Institute, CSIR, in press.
56. Kok R, Strydom NB: *A Guide to Climatic Room Acclimatisation*, Research Report 41/70. Johannesburg, South Africa, Chamber of Mines of South Africa, Human Science Laboratory, 1970.
57. Krajewski JT, Kamon E, Avellini B: Scheduling rest for consecutive light and heavy work loads under hot ambient conditions. *Ergonomics* 1979; 22:975–987.
58. Langkilde G: The influence of the thermal environment on office work, in Fanger PO, Valbjorn O (ed): *Indoor Climate*. Copenhagen, World Health Organization, Danish Building Research Institute, 1978, pp 835–856.
59. Langkilde G, Alexandersen K, Wyon DP, et al: Mental performance during slight cool or warm discomfort. *Arch Sci Physiol* 1973; 27:A511–A528.
60. Levitt L, Leventhal G: Effect of density and environmental noise on perception of time, the situation, oneself and others. *Percept Mot Skills* 1978; 47:999–1009.
61. Lewis T: Observations upon the reactions of the vessels of the human skin to cold. *Heart* 1930; 15:177–208.
62. Lewis MI, Meese GB, Kok R: *The Effects of Moderate Cold and Heat Stress on the Potential Work Performance of Industrial Workers*. Pt 4: *Performance and Physiological Responses of Trained Workers in Relation to Eight Environmental Temperatures*, Research Report 589. Pretoria, South Africa, National Building Research Institute, CSIR, 1983.
63. Lewis MI, Meese GB, Kok R, et al: The effects of moderate cold and heat stress on factory workers in Southern Africa. 4. Effects on skin temperatures, oral temperature, heart-rate and comfort vote. *S Afr J Sci* 1983; 79:28–37.
64. Lifson KA: Production welding in extreme heat. *Ergonomics* 1958; 1:345–346.
65. Lockhart JM: Extreme body cooling and psychomotor performance. *Ergonomics* 1968; 11:249–260.
66. Lockhart JM, Kiess HQ: Auxiliary heating of the hands during cold exposure and manual performance. *Hum Factors* 1971; 13:457–465.
67. Mackworth NM: Effects of heat on wireless operator hearing and re-

cording Morse code messages. *Br J Ind Med* 1946; 3:143–158.

68. Mackworth NM: High incentives versus hot and humid atmospheres in a physical effort task. *Br J Psychol* 1947; 38:90–102.
69. Mackworth NH: Some recent studies of human stress from a marine and naval viewpoint. *J Inst Marine Eng* 1952; 64:123–138.
70. Mackworth NH: Finger numbness in very cold winds. *J Appl Physiol* 1953; 5:533–543.
71. McArdle B, Dunham W, Holling HE, et al: *The Prediction of the Physiological Effects of Warm and Hot Environments,* RNP Report 47/391. London, Medical Research Council, 1947.
72. McIntyre DA: Seven point scales of warmth. *Bldg Serv Eng Res Tech* 1978; 45:212–226.
73. McIntyre DA: *Indoor Climate*. London, Applied Science, 1980.
74. McNall PE, Nevins RG: Comfort and academic achievement in an airconditioned junior high school—A summary evaluation of the Pinellas County Experiment. ASHRAE Trans 1967; 73:III.3.1–III.3.17.
75. Meese GB, Kok R, Lewis MI, et al: *The Effects of Moderate Cold and Heat Stress on the Potential Work Performance of Industrial Workers*. Pt 2. Performance of diagnostic tasks in relation to air temperature at eight environmental conditions: Black and white male and female subjects: results and preliminary analysis, Research Report 381/2. Pretoria, South Africa, National Building Research Institute, CSIR, 1982.
76. Meese GB, Kok R, Lewis MI, et al: The effects of moderate cold and heat stress on factory workers in South Africa. 2. Skill and performance in the cold. *S Afr J Sci* 1982; 78:189–197.
77. Meese GB, Kok R, Lewis MI, et al: A laboratory study of moderate thermal stress on the performance of factory workers. *Ergonomics* 1984; 27:19–43.
78. Meese GB, Schiefer RE, Küstner PM, et al: Subjective comfort vote and air temperature as predictors of performance in factory workers. *Environ J Appl Physiol* 1986; 55:195–197.
79. Meese GB, Wentzel JD, Kok R, et al: Differences in subjective comfort votes between workers in similar thermal environments, in press.
80. Mills AW: Finger numbness and skin temperature. *J Appl Physiol* 1956; 9:447–450.
81. Morton R, Provins KA: Finger numbness after acute local exposure to cold. *J Appl Physiol* 1960; 15:149–154.
82. Mount LE: *Adaptation to Thermal Environment*. London, Arnold, 1979.
83. National Building Research Institute: *Guidelines for Factory Building Design. Part I: Thermal Conditions*. Pretoria, South Africa, National Building Research Institute, CSIR, 1982.
84. New York State Commission on Ventilation: *Report of the New York State Commission on Ventilation*. New York, Dutton, 1923.
85. Nunneley SA, Reader DC: Head-temperature effects on physiology, comfort, and performance during hyperthermia. *Aviat Space Environ Med* 1982; 53:623–628.
86. Olesen BW, Fanger PO: The skin temperature distribution for resting man in comfort. *Arch Sci Physiol* 1973; 27:A385–A393.
87. Pandolf KB, Gonzales RR, Gagge AP: Physiological strain during light exercise in hot-humid environments. *Aerospace Med* 1974; 45:359–365.
88. Parker JF, Fleishman EA: Ability factors and component measures as predictors of complex tracking behavior. *Psychol Monogr* 1960; 74(16):1–36.
89. Pepler RD: *The Effect of Climatic Factors on the Performance of Skilled Tasks by Young European Men Living in the Tropics*. London, Applied Psychology Unit, Medical Research Council, 1953.
90. Pepler RD: Warmth and lack of sleep: Accuracy of activity reduced. *J Comp Physiol Psychol* 1959; 52:446–450.
91. Pepler RD: Performance and well being in heat, in Hardy JD (ed): *Temperature: Its Measurement and Control in Science and Industry*. New York, Reinhold Publishing Corp, 1963, pp 319–336.
92. Pepler RD, Warner RE: Temperature and learning: An experimental study. *ASHRAE Trans* 1968; 74:211–219.
93. Poulton EC: On increasing the sensitivity of measures of performance. *Ergonomics* 1965; 8:69–76.
94. Poulton EC: *Environment and Human Efficiency*. Springfield, Ill, Charles C Thomas, 1970.
95. Poulton EC: Arousing environmental stresses can improve performance, whatever people say. *Aviat Space Environ Med* 1976; 47:1193–1204.
96. Provins KA: Environmental heat, body temperature and behaviour: an hypothesis. *Aust J Psychol* 1966; 18:118–129.
97. Provins KA, Clark RSJ: The effect of cold on manual performance. *J Occup Med* 1960; 2:169–176.
98. Provins KA, Morton R: Tactile discrimination and skin temperature. *J Appl Physiol* 1960; 15:155–160.
99. Robinson S, Dill DB, Wilson JB, et al: in Wyndham et al[123].
100. Roscoe AH: Stress and workload in pilots. *Aviat Space Environ Med* 1978; 49:630–636.
101. Rutenfranz J, Colquhoon WP: Circadian rhythm in human performance. *Scand J Work Environ Health* 1979; 5:167–177.
102. Schiefer RE, Meese GB, Wentzel JD: The magnitude of the effect of temperature on psychological test performance in standard 10 black pupils. *S Afr J Sci* in press.
103. Schiefer RE, Kok R, Lewis MI, et al: Finger skin temperature and manual dexterity—some inter-group differences. *Appl Ergon* 1984; 15:135–141.
104. Siple PA, Passel CF: Measurements of dry atmosphere cooling in subfreezing temperatures. *Proc Am Philos Soc* 1945; 89:177–199.
105. Stephens RL, Hoag LL: Heat acclimatisation, its decay and reintroduction in young Caucasian females. *Am Ind Hyg Assoc J* 1981; 42:12–17.
106. Stevens J, Green BG, Krimsley AS: Punctate pressure sensitivity: Effects of skin temperature. *Sens Processes* 1977; 1:238–243.
107. Strydom NB, Morrison JF, Booyens J, et al: Comparison of oral and rectal temperatures during work in heat. *J Appl Physiol* 1956; 8:406–408.
108. Suzuki K, Ijichim O, Matsuki T, et al: The hand and environment. *J Univ Occup Environ Health* 1981; 3:109–115.
109. Teichner WH: Recent studies of simple reaction time. *Psychol Bull* 1954; 51:128–150.
110. Teichner WH: Assessment of mean body surface temperature. *J Appl Physiol* 1958; 12:169–176.
111. Vernon HM: The influence of hours of work and of ventilation on output in tinplate manufacture, No 1, HMSO, London, Report of the Industrial Fatigue Research Board, 1919.
112. Vernon HM: *Accidents and Their Prevention*. Cambridge University Press, 1936.
113. Vernon HM, Bedford T, Warner CG: The relation of atmospheric conditions to the working capacity and the accident rate of miners, No 39 HMSO. London, Report of the Industrial Fatigue Research Board, 1927.
114. Vroman NB, Buskirk ER, Hodgson JL: Cardiac output and skin blood flow in lean and obese individuals during exercise in the heat. *J Appl Physiol* 1983; 55:69–74.
115. Weiner JS, Hutchinson JCD: Hot humid environment: Its effect on the performance of a motor coordination test. *Br J Ind Med* 1945; 2:154–157.
116. Wentzel JD, Page-Shipp RJ, Venter JA: The prediction of the thermal performance of buildings by the CR-Method, BRR 396. Pretoria, South Africa, National Building Research Institute, CSIR, 1981.

117. Wentzel JD, Meese GB: Influence of air temperature on the manual dexterity of schoolchildren. *S Afr J Sci* 1983; 79:67–68.
118. Weston HC: A study of efficiency in fine linen wearing, No 20 HMSO. London, Report of the Industrial Fatigue Research Board, 1922.
119. Wyatt S, Fraser JA, Stock FGL: Fan ventilation in a humid weaving shed, No 37 HMSO. London, Report of the Industrial Fatigue Research Board, 1926.
120. Wyndham CH: The adaptation of some of the different ethnic groups in Southern Africa to heat, cold and exercise. *S Afr J Sci* 1965; 61:11–29.
121. Wyndham CH, Morrison JF, Williams CG: Heat reactions of male and female Caucasians. *J Appl Physiol* 1965; 20:357–364.
122. Wyndham CH, Morrison JF, Williams CG, et al: Physiological reactions to cold of Caucasian females. *J Appl Physiol* 1964; 19:583–592.
123. Wyndham CH, Strydom NB, Morrison JF, et al: Heat reactions of Caucasians and Bantu in South Africa. *J Appl Physiol* 1964; 19:598–606.
124. Wyndham CH, Ward JS, Strydom NB, et al: Physiological reactions of Caucasian and Bantu males in acute exposure to cold. *J Appl Physiol* 1964; 19:583–592.
125. Wyon DP: The effects of moderate heat stress on typewriting performance. *Ergonomics* 1974; 17:309–318.
126. Wyon DP, Andersen I, Lundquist GR: Spontaneous magnitude estimation of thermal discomfort during changes in the ambient temperature. *J Hyg (Lond)* 1972; 70:203–221.
127. Wyon DP, Holmberg I: Systematic observation of classroom behaviour during moderate heat stress, in Langdon FJ, Humphreys MA, Nicol JF (eds): *Thermal Comfort and Moderate Heat Stress: Proceedings of the CIB (W45) Symposium, 13–15 September 1972, Garston*. HMSO, London, Building Establishment Report No 2, 1973, pp 19–33.
128. Wyon DP, Andersen I, Lundqvist GR: The effects of moderate heat stress on mental performance. *Scand J Work Environ Health* 1979; 5:352–361.
129. Wyon DP, Kok R, Lewis MI, et al: The effects of moderate cold and heat stress on factory workers in Southern Africa. 1. Introduction to a series of full scale simulation studies. *S Afr J Sci* 1981; 78:184–189.
130. Wyon DP, Lewis MI, Kok R, et al: *The Effects of Moderate Cold and Heat Stress on the Potential Work Performance of Industrial Workers*. Pt I. Background and experimental procedures, Research Report 381/1, Pretoria, South Africa, National Building Research Institute, CSIR, 1980.
131. Yaglou CP, Minard D: Control of heat casualties at military training centers. *Am Med Assoc Arch Ind Health* 1957; 16:302–316.

25

Medical Aspects of Commercial Diving and Compressed-Air Work

Eric P. Kindwall, M.D.

Certain types of construction and salvage work require people to work in an environment of increased ambient pressure. This pressure is necessary to counterbalance the increasing weight of water as the diver descends. In the United States alone there are more than 5,000 commercial divers and an estimated equal number of part-time divers, as well as hundreds of naval personnel engaged in underwater activities. More than 1.4 million amateur "scuba" divers in the United States and countless numbers of persons working under pressure in tunneling and sewer work must be taken into consideration.

In construction, work is done in pressurized environments in caissons used in building bridge piers and in pressurized tunnels. The caisson is simply an inverted box, open at the bottom, which is pressurized to keep water from entering. Compressed air is used in tunnels to dry out the working face and hold out water when digging through wet, porous ground or under rivers and lakes.

For every foot a diver descends below the surface, or the tunnel worker descends below the local water table, there is a linear pressure increase of 0.433 pounds per square inch (psi) for fresh water and 0.445 psi for salt water. Thus, a diver working in 100 ft of sea water would be subject to a pressure of 44.5 psi gauge (psig). Since the diver was already exposed to 14.7 psi absolute (atmospheric pressure) at sea level, the absolute pressure experienced at 100 ft is 59.2 psi. In the practical work situation, gauge pressures that show only the pressure differential from atmospheric are used. However, in calculating decompression schedules, absolute pressures are required.

Units of measure for pressure also need definition. One atmosphere equals 14.7 psi. This is equivalent to the weight of a column of sea water 33 ft high of 1 sq in cross section. Thus, for every 33 ft a diver descends, the pressure on his body increases by 1 atmosphere. At a depth of 99 ft, the diver is at 3 atmospheres gauge or 4 atmospheres absolute (ATA). It is usually customary when referring to pressure in atmospheres to mean atmospheres absolute, unless otherwise noted.

The metric system vastly simplifies diving calculations, since one kilogram per square centimeter (1 kg/sq cm) very closely approximates one atmosphere. Ten meters of seawater pressure is equal to 1 kg/sq cm. Thus. changes in atmospheres or meters in depth can be treated decimally. Nevertheless, the metric system is not used for diving or compressed-air work in the United States at this writing, although it is now commonplace in England, Canada, and the rest of the world.

THE EFFECTS OF COMPRESSED AIR ON THE BODY

Compressed air is the only gas used currently for the pressurization of caissons and tunnels, and despite great advances in mixed-gas diving technology, most diving operations are still carried out using compressed air. The effects of compressed air on the body can best be divided into mechanical effects and the effects of increased partial pressures of oxygen, nitrogen, and carbon dioxide.

Mechanical Effects

Increased pressure exerts no mechanical effect on the tissues of the body *per se,* since liquids and solids are incompressible except at pressures of hundreds of atmospheres, which are usually obtained only in the laboratory. Problems can occur, however, wherever there is a gas-tissue interface within the body, such as the middle ear, the paranasal sinuses, and the lung. The bowel also contains gas, which in rare instances can give rise to problems. As long as the air or gas pressure within these body cavities equals the pressure of air or water surrounding the body, no difficulties occur. If equalization is prevented for some reason, the body suffers damage, or *barotrauma,* as the ambient pressure is changed.

The Middle Ear

If the eustachian tube is obstructed by mucus, edema, or an overgrowth of tissue, equalization of the pressure in the middle ear cannot take place. The eardrum is forced inward during pressurization, with rupture of the healthy drum usually occurring at a pressure of 5–10 psig. This is accompanied by intense pain and a temporary decrease in hearing. Only rarely, however, does permanent hearing deficit and tinnitus develop. This may be due to tearing and leakage of the membrane at the round window and requires surgical exploration and repair if the deficit does not clear within two to three days. Rupture of the round or oval window on compression typically occurs only when Valsalva's maneuver is used too forcefully in combination with a blocked eustachian tube.

The degree of barotrauma to the tympanic membrane can be judged by its appearance. Wallace Teed, a United States Navy diving medical officer, devised a four-point scale for classifying middle ear injury. This scale is used by the U.S. Navy:[65]

Teed 1. Congestion in Shrapnell's membrane and along the handle of the malleus

Teed 2. Redness of the entire tympanic membrane with retraction

Teed 3. Hemorrhage into the tympanic membrane but not into the middle ear

Teed 4. Entire middle ear filled with blood, drum bluish in appearance and possibly ruptured

In uncomplicated barotrauma of the ear, even if the drum is ruptured, healing usually takes place in ten days to two weeks. Drainage of the middle ear can be improved by prescribing a decongestant, but no other treatment is usually necessary.

During pressurization, the individual may "clear" his ears by yawning, swallowing, or performing Valsalva'a maneuver. Sometimes it is helpful to stretch the neck away from the affected side by tilting the head and swallowing simultaneously. Equalization is more difficult if the diver is descending head first. It is easiest to clear the ears sitting up or standing. Decongestant nasal sprays or tablets may be used if desired. Pressurization is the only change that commonly causes difficulty, since during decompression, air escapes freely from the eustachian tube. However, the worker may experience a brief state of true vertigo ("alternobaric vertigo") before pressure begins to equalize in the middle ear.[66] This is usually of no consequence, but can panic an inexperienced diver.

Paranasal Sinuses

The openings to the sinuses must be patent or the application of increased pressure will force the capillaries lining them to distend and burst, filling the sinuses with blood. The most painful type of sinus squeeze involves the frontal sinuses. The maxillary, ethmoid, and sphenoid sinuses are less painful and also less commonly affected. If the worker's frontal sinus is blocked, the exquisite pain produced makes it impossible for him to compress deeper than a few feet.

If the sphenoid sinus is blocked, the pain is generally referred to the occiput or vertex of the skull. Decongestants and nasal sprays are the only readily available treatment for sinus blockage. In cases of severe sinus obstruction or eustachian stenosis, an otolaryngologist may be able to artificially widen the opening to the sinus or place a tiny polyethylene tube through the eardrum in the caisson worker. Divers not using dry suits cannot be helped by piercing the eardrum with a tube, since water would then enter the middle ear.

The Lungs

Except in breathhold or free diving, increase in pressure does not normally cause problems, since air can freely enter the lungs through the wide opening of the glottis.

Air embolism due to overexpansion of the lungs can result, however, if the glottis is held closed during decompression. The lungs tolerate only about 80 mm Hg intratracheal pressure or about 60 mm of mercury transpulmonic pressure before rupture.[59] Fatal air embolism can occur during decompression with fully expanded lungs from as little as 4 ft of water. With normal lungs, however, as long as the worker breathes in and out normally during decompression, this cannot occur. Air embolism is rare in caisson workers and tunnel workers because of the slow decompressions generally used. It is also quite unusual in deep sea divers who use the classic copper helmet and suit. When lung rupture does occur, the expanding air may either break through into the pleural space, causing a pneumothorax, or migrate medially to cause mediastinal emphysema, pneumopericardium, and subcutaneous emphysema in the area of the neck and clavicle, or rupture directly into the pulmonary capillaries. If air enters the pulmonary vasculature, it is carried by the pulmonary veins to the left heart, whence it is pumped directly into the brain. In this case, symptoms usually appear within 30 seconds to two minutes, and death may ensue within two to three minutes. As little as 0.4 ml of air-blood foam delivered to the brain stem via the arterial tree can be fatal. Rarely, symptoms may be delayed for more than a minute or two. If the victim does not die, convulsions, coma, or severe hemiplegia are the result. Scuba divers are statistically at greater risk for air embolism.

Mask Squeeze and Whole Body Squeeze

The diver's equipment may also play a role in the production of barotrauma. Goggles that do not communicate with the nose cannot compensate for the pressure changes and the eyes will be forced outward during descent, causing scleral hemorrhage. The mask can also produce ecchymoses and scleral hemorrhage if the diver forgets to equalize the mask through his nose. Treatment is benign neglect in the usual case.

Whole body squeeze can be a fatal complication of using the classic copper-helmeted deep-sea dress. If gas pressure in the helmet becomes less than the pressure surrounding the flexible dress, the entire body may be crushed and forced into the helmet.

The Intestines

If large amounts of gas are present in the gut, expansion during decompression may force an involuntary bowel movement. This is extremely rare, however. If gas is trapped in a loop of bowel extending through a hernia, its expansion during decompression could make the hernia irreducible, with disastrous results.

Effects of Increased Partial Pressures of Gases

Oxygen

Man is designed to breathe 20.93% oxygen at atmospheric pressure or 14.7 psi absolute. When the partial pressure of oxygen is increased, an unphysiologic condition results. Oxygen at partial pressures much greater than the 160 mm Hg experienced when breathing atmospheric air acts as a poison, and metabolism is actually slightly slowed. A profound vasoconstriction takes place, with striking blanching of the face and extremities, seen in experiments carried out with subjects breathing 100% oxygen at 4 ATA.[6] Although it affects all organs of the body, oxygen exerts its toxic effects primarily on the lungs and central nervous system.

Oxygen poisoning with damage to the respiratory system can occur at atmospheric pressure if the subject is permitted to breathe 100% oxygen for longer than about 24 hours. After approximately this period of time, the first symptoms of respiratory difficulty appear, known as the "Lorraine-Smith effect."[44] These consist of dry cough, substernal pain, diminished vital capacity, and patchy atelectasis. A chest x-ray film might be typical of early pneumonia. If the pressure is raised from 1 to 2 ATA (equivalent to breathing oxygen at a depth of 33 ft of seawater), these same symptoms will appear within approximately six hours. With continued exposure, the edematous first stage proceeds to a microhemorrhagic second stage, with pulmonary fibrosis as the final phase. Pulmonary fibrosis secondary to oxygen toxicity is irreversible.[43]

At a pressure of 3 ATA (66 ft of seawater pressure), a grand mal seizure will result in almost everyone after approximately three hours. This is termed the "Paul Bert effect."[10, 11] Individual susceptibility to oxygen poisoning varies widely and may change grossly in the same individual from day to day. Factors that promote the onset of oxygen convulsions are exercise, carbon dioxide buildup, cold, lack of sleep, fear, the use of certain drugs, and water immersion. Oxygen breathing can be tolerated by most people for periods up to 90 minutes at 3 ATA with little difficulty if they are at rest and recumbent in a dry chamber breathing oxygen by mask. However, actual tests show that a diver working in water at a depth of 50 ft (2.5 ATA) may suffer convulsions within 10–30 minutes.[71] Water immersion, of course, presupposes some exercise and, most commonly, chilling. Exercise and carbon dioxide buildup are the two most important factors. Because of the above factors, 100% oxygen must never be administered at pressures greater than 3 ATA (29.4 psig) in the dry chamber. Even with the subject recumbent, comfortably at rest, and well-ventilated, exposure time should not exceed 90 minutes. In the water, the U.S. Navy permits oxygen breathing up to ten minutes at a maximum depth of 50 ft (2.5 ATA) in decompressing resting divers in a closed, dry, diving suit. In active swimmers, oxygen breathing is only permitted to a maximum depth of 25 ft. Other navies specify an 18-ft maximum depth for long underwater swims by attack divers breathing 100% oxygen. For obvious reasons, scuba divers must never charge their tanks with 100% oxygen.

Even when oxygen is diluted, current U.S. Navy regulations stipulate that the partial pressure of oxygen at any depth in any mixture must not exceed 1.6 ATA effective for more than 30 minutes.

Often, there may be premonitory signs before actual seizure occurs. The symptoms in order of their likelihood of occurrence are:

1. Muscular twitching, usually around the lips or face
2. Nausea or vomiting
3. Light-headedness or dizziness
4. Tunnel vision and/or tinnitus
5. Air hunger or inability to take a full breath
6. Anxiety and confusion
7. Unusual fatigue or tiredness
8. Incoordination or clumsiness

I have also noted profuse sweating in many individuals breathing oxygen at 2.5 and 3 ATA.

If any of these symptoms are noted, other than sweating, it is best to immediately take off the mask (in the dry chamber) or otherwise diminish the partial pressure of oxygen the patient is breathing. The British have reported the so-called "off phenomenon" in which the patient may show only a few mild premonitory signs but as soon as the oxygen mask is removed, he sustains a grand mal seizure. This phenomenon, if it indeed exists, has been difficult to explain, but work by Ackles[1] has demonstrated that with a mass spectrograph catheter placed in muscle tissue, the amount of oxygen measurable increases many-fold as soon as oxygen breathing is discontinued. This may be due to the fact that when the oxygen-induced vasoconstriction is stopped, the tremendous amounts of oxygen dissolved in the blood and plasma then reach the tissues suddenly.

The actual mechanism of oxygen toxicity is still unknown. Present data indicate that oxygen poisoning occurs at the cellular level by direct poisoning of the enzyme systems involved in aerobic and anaerobic metabolism and electron transport. Oxygen behaves like a free radical under pressure and ruptures sulfhydryl bonds. Gamma aminobutyric acid metabolism is also disrupted.

Thus, it becomes clear that oxygen must be diluted with another inert gas when diving to any appreciable depth. The most common source of diluted oxygen is compressed air, which brings us to the subject of nitrogen.

Nitrogen and Other Inert Gases

Practical considerations usually limit the maximum pressure in tunnels and caissons to about 50 psig (3.4 kg/sq cm). Within this pressure range, the physiologic effects of breathing increased partial pressures of nitrogen are minimal. Only divers, therefore, are liable to the effects of "nitrogen narcosis," "rapture of the deep," or "the narks," as it is called by the British. In practical terms, this phenomenon will be encountered only at depths greater than about 100 ft (30 m). The first symptom is usually a barely perceptible circumoral numbness, which may be distressing to the inexperienced diver. As pressure is increased, the diver may feel giddy or light-headed at 6 ATA or 165 ft (50 m). At this pressure, there are definite symptoms of narcosis present in almost everyone, and the subject may be more talkative and appear slightly drunk. Individual reaction to increased nitrogen pressure is quite variable, and some persons are barely affected at pressures of up to 6 ATA while others appear quite drunk. Motor skills are not seriously affected, however, and coordination remains good down to depths of about 300 ft (90 m). However, intellectual processes and motivation become severely impaired; some individuals becoming unconscious between 325 and 350 ft (98–106 m). But a few divers in experiments carried out by Adolfson[2] remained conscious in compressed air at pressures equivalent to 400 ft (120 m) of seawater.

The U.S. Navy considers 190 ft (57 m) to be the practical limit for compressed-air diving, and all naval work carried out at depths greater than 190 ft is done using helium rather than nitrogen as the diluent for oxygen. The depth limit for air diving in the North Sea is set at 165 ft (150 m) by British law. Helium does not cause the severe narcosis seen with nitrogen and does not exert any appreciable effect on the central nervous system until depths of 550–600 ft (167–180 m) are reached. Helium is quite expensive, and those countries which do not have ready access to helium, therefore, find it necessary to use compressed air for diving to depths of 300 ft. Three hundred feet is about the absolute limit for diving using compressed air and at this depth only the most simple tasks of very short duration can be carried out. Only extremely experienced divers who have learned to concentrate on their work despite the effects of nitrogen narcosis can accomplish anything of value at these depths.

In experiments carried out by Adolfson at depths in excess of 300 ft, subjects reported symptoms of hallucinations and auditory disturbances resembling those seen in certain forms of mental illness.[2]

The mechanism of nitrogen narcosis has been the subject of controversy. At first, it was thought the simple mechanical effects of pressure were responsible. Later hypotheses cited impure air, carbon dioxide buildup due to decreased ventilation of the lungs secondary to increased density of the breathing mixture, histotoxic hypoxia, oxygen poisoning, and even latent claustrophobia. In 1935, Behnke et al.[7] identified nitrogen *per se* as the main cause, with carbon dioxide buildup and increased ventilatory difficulties as being only contributory. It was theorized for many years that nitrogen molecules in some way plugged the interstices in the neuron cell membrane, blocking ion transport. Water molecules were thought to be stabilized by nitrogen molecules in a loose bond, and this supposedly caused the relatively small nitrogen molecule to become more effective in blocking ion transport. This was called the "iceberg" theory. A corollary, called the "clathrate theory" involving a mechanism of "protein binding," was advanced by Pauling. Other mechanisms were studied also.[8]

However, work by Bennett[8] In the 1960s presents rather convincing evidence that the reverse is true and that a high partial pressure of nitrogen causes edema of the neuron cell membrane and actually facilitates ion transport across the membrane.

There appears to be no long-term ill effects from nitrogen narcosis and the diver's mental and physical status immediately reverts to normal upon reaching the surface.

Gases other than nitrogen also exert narcotic effects, generally in proportion to their oil-water solubility ratios. All the inert gases, including nitrogen, behave like aliphatic anesthetics when breathed at greater than atmospheric pressure.

The amount of narcotic effect closely follows the Meyer-Overton hypothesis (1899), which states that a parallel exists between the affinity of an aliphatic anesthetic for lipid and its narcotic potency.[46] Helium has the least affinity for lipids and, in practice, is found to be the least narcotic under pressure. It is followed in increasing fat affinity (and narcotic effect) by neon, hydrogen, nitrogen, argon, krypton, and xenon, in that order. Xenon has actually been used experimentally for anesthesia in the hyperbaric chamber and even at 1 ATA. Thus, hydrogen, which is the lightest of gases, is theoretically not the least narcotic. Crude neon, derived as a by-product of commercial oxygen production and actually a mixture of neon and helium, was investigated as a diving gas because of its availability but was found not to be cheaper than helium. Hydrogen may be more narcotic than neon and is explosive in mixtures of greater than 4% oxygen. Despite these drawbacks, however, hydrogen was used in experimental dives to 535 ft (160 m) by Zetterstrom[12] in 1945 and was reinvestigated again by Edel[25] and Fife.[33] Ornhagen of the Swedish Navy and the French diving company, COMEX, are continuing this work. Because it has half the density of helium, it makes the work of breathing much easier. In May of 1985, COMEX divers reached 1,500 ft (450 m) in a dry chamber while breathing 54% hydrogen and 45% helium. There was no evidence of high-pressure nervous syndrome (HPNS) and mouth breathing was not necessary, as it is with helium at that depth. The breathing mixture was dubbed "hydreliox"! This experiment confirmed that hydrogen has about 25% the narcotic potency of nitrogen, it has the capacity to counter HPNS, and that the divers felt "extraordinarily comfortable."

Nevertheless, helium is currently the most practical diluent for oxygen as extreme pressures are reached. The current pressure record for man is 2,250 ft (686 m) set in February of 1981 in a dry chamber dive at Duke University. Helium does not produce the usual narcosis even at extreme depths, but instead the extreme helium pressures can produce the high-pressure nervous syndrome, which consists of nausea and vomiting, uncontrollable shaking, and lack of coordination, an effect which begins to appear after rapid compression to depths in excess of 500 ft (150 m).[9] The HPNS can be minimized, however, by using extremely slow compressions (several days) to reach maximum depth or by adding 10% nitrogen, which counteracts HPNS. Because of the HPNS, practical diving at this time would appear to be limited to approximately 1,800 ft (550 m) with helium as the only diluent. Depths as great as 3,000 ft (900 m) may be possible with tri-gas mixes of helium, nitrogen, and oxygen, or helium, hydrogen, and oxygen.

Nitrogen and other inert gases also play an extremely important role during decompression even from modest pressures, since it is inert gas bubbles that appear to initiate the decompression sickness syndrome. This subject will be dealt with in a later section.

Carbon Dioxide

Normally, the air exhaled from the lungs contains approximately 4% carbon dioxide. Since metabolic rate is essentially unchanged by the application of pressure, the amount of carbon dioxide exhaled by a diver during the dive remains about the same as on the surface. As stated earlier, high partial pressures of oxygen slow metabolism slightly under extreme conditions, and, therefore, there could be a concomitant drop in carbon dioxide production basally. But divers are usually exercising, so carbon dioxide buildup poses difficulties.

The diver's chief problem with carbon dioxide is in obtaining adequate ventilation. As the density of the gas breathed increases due to increasing pressure, the carbon dioxide diffuses less efficiently from the alveoli with each exhalation and may contribute to nitrogen narcosis, as already discussed. It is extremely important that the diver have adequate ventilation of the helmet or breathing apparatus so that carbon dioxide buildup does not occur. If carbon dioxide buildup does occur, unconsciousness ensues when the level of carbon dioxide reaches a partial pressure of 70–80 mm Hg. At high partial pressures of oxygen (over 1.6 ATA) carbon dioxide control is especially important, since the normal carbon dioxide stimulus to breathe is blunted. The diver may become hypercapniac without air hunger and become unconscious from apnea and carbon dioxide intoxication without warning.

It is important that the diver's air supply be relatively free of carbon dioxide. About 3% effective is all that can be tolerated without discomfort (23 mm Hg). If 1% carbon dioxide is present in the air pumped down to the diver, it becomes 6% effective (46 mm Hg) at 6 ATA or a depth of 165 ft (50 m). This axiom also holds true for caisson workers. Carbon dioxide is 20 times as soluble in water or plasma as nitrogen and oxygen, and therefore, even small amounts may be liberated in bubble form at the beginning of decompression. These small carbon dioxide bubbles do not cause problems by themselves but may provide the bubble nuclei for later formation of nitrogen bubbles. This is so important that one commercial diving contractor insists that divers remain at absolute rest and ventilate for one minute after finishing work and before starting decompression.[34]

DECOMPRESSION SICKNESS

Decompression sickness was first observed in 1841 by Triger,[67] a French mining engineer who reported its appearance in coal miners working in compressed air. Apparently, the symptoms of pain in the limbs were treated with alcohol, both internally and externally, and the men returned to work the following day. The causes of decompression sickness began to be investigated more closely by the second half of the 19th century, and Pol and Watelle[52] were to write ironically "one pays only on leaving." In 1878, Paul Bert,[11] the French physiologist, wrote his monumental book, *Barometric Pressure,* in which he described nitrogen as the definite cause of decompression sickness and actually demonstrated that the bubbles appearing in the tissues of rapidly decompressed animals consisted mainly of nitrogen.

Schemes for decompressing workers exposed to compressed air were still haphazard and variable, however, and those who suffered decompression sickness were eliminated from the working force by self-selection. No rational decompression scheme was proposed until 1908, when J.S. Haldane, working on a commission from the British Admiralty, devised an empirical set of decompression tables based on scientific experiment.[15] The Royal Navy and most other groups involved in diving work (including the United States Navy) were quick to adopt Haldane's decompression tables and hypotheses. However, caisson workers and tunneling companies by and large remained ignorant of these new developments and continued with their own tables. There are few records as to the actual incidence of decompression sickness among caisson workers, since many workers would not report for therapeutic recompression unless the symptoms of decompression sickness were incapacitating or unbearable. Navies generally kept somewhat better records and also treated more true cases. It is important again to remember that people who were even normally susceptible to decompression sickness soon left compressed-air work in tunnels and caissons because of the shorter and less adequate decompressions used. Therefore, only individuals relatively resistant to decompression sickness remained in the population at risk.

Decompression sickness is also termed "caisson disease" or simply "bends." Reportedly, the word *bends* was first coined by the caisson workers building the piers for the Brooklyn Bridge. An affected posture or way of walking used by women of the era was called "The Grecian Bend."[45] Men suffering from decompression sickness were accused of "doing the Grecian Bend," a euphemism that was later shortened to "bends." There are synonyms for decompression sickness that should not be used, including the archaic *aero-embolism,* which is too easily confused with *air-embolism,* and *aeroemphysema,* and *dysbarism* (used by the U.S. Air Force), which is a term referring to all disorders resulting from a change in pressure.

The classical explanation for the disease is that gaseous nitrogen from the air breathed by the compressed-air worker is gradually absorbed into the tissues. This causes no difficulty so long as pressure is not reduced. However, should the worker decompress too rapidly to atmospheric pressure, nitrogen quickly bubbles out of solution, tearing tissues, plugging small vessels with gas emboli, and embarrassing circulation and even cardiac function itself.

Since the nitrogen bubbles can appear everywhere in the body, the symptoms are varied, and localization cannot be accurately predicted from one person to the next. The onset of the disease can be insidious or fulminating and may occur at any time starting during decompression to 24 hours postdecompression.

Symptoms range from a bothersome skin itch or skin rash to a vague soreness in an elbow, knee, or shoulder. As the disease progresses, the patient may suffer from extreme pain in the joints and muscles, vertigo ("staggers"), dyspnea ("chokes"), edema, blindness, paralysis ("diver's palsy") shock, and death. Should the afflicted compressed-air worker survive the acute attack, there may be permanent loss of sphincter control and paralysis. Another sequel to improper decompression is aseptic necrosis of the bone, coming on months or years later.

Hematologic changes also occur in decompression sickness, as demonstrated by End,[28] Swindle,[64] Cockett and Nakamura,[18] Ackles,[1] and Philp et al.[51] among others. In the decompression sickness syndrome, increased agglutination of red blood cells and platelets occurs, which can progress to sludging. Capillaries develop increased permeability, and patients may go into shock with extreme hemoconcentration and decreased circulating plasma volume. This was first described by Rudge in 1907.[57]

"Bubbles" and Their Relationship to Decompression Sickness

It has always been assumed that gases coming out of solution and entering a gaseous phase are responsible for the symptoms of decompression sickness. In air diving or caisson work this is primarily nitrogen. The reason for this assumption is that various gases can reach relatively high partial pressures in solution without offending normal physiology, but it is only when given the opportunity to assume a different form, i.e., a gas phase on decompression, that problems arise. Yet, "bubbles," which are macroscopic, tend to be a rather late finding in decompression sickness unless the decompression has been explosive or instantaneous. When bubbles are detected, they appear first in the veins. Bubbles are generally not observed in arteries, since the higher hydrostatic pressure there, of the order of 70–120 mm Hg, tends to prevent their formation. Experiments have shown that when intravascular bubbles do form, they appear first at the capillary venous junction. Thus, in typical decompression sickness, bubbles blocking the arterial supply to any area are probably nonexistent. Conceivably, venous return could be blocked in certain areas, but in my view, bubbles large enough to be seen or detected probably do not play a major role early in the usual case of decompression sickness.

The more likely possibility is that the "bubbles" are so tiny they are really macroaggregations of nitrogen molecules distributed all over the body. These are not visible to the naked eye but are large enough to have finite surfaces over which molecules of protein can be filmed and distorted or altered. One must make the assumption that the enormous surface area provided by these millions of macroaggregates could produce enough release of bioactive amines to drastically change tissue perfusion. Chryssanthou[16] has elegantly demonstrated that when biochemical reaction is blocked, gas buildup in the tissues cannot be demonstrated. Thus, when I refer to "bubbles" other than when giving "classic" descriptions of disease, I actually am referring to macroaggregates of nitrogen too small to be seen with the naked eye.

Derivation of Decompression Schedules

J. S. Haldane was the first to devise systematic decompression tables. Making measurements in both man and goats, Haldane estimated that the total time required for nitrogen saturation, i.e., no further uptake of nitrogen of all tissues of the body in man at any given pressure, was five hours. Using this as a base line, he exposed goats at progressively increasing pressures for saturation exposures followed by rapid decompression to 1 ATA. The goats did not experience bends until their exposure pressure exceeded 2 ATA pressure. From this observation and later observations of human volunteers, Haldane deduced that humans as well as goats could be decompressed from 4 ATA to 2 ATA or 8 ATA to 4 ATA. In other words, the organism should always tolerate a two-to-one reduction in absolute pressure without developing symptoms. In actuality, since microaggregates of nitrogen in the tissues probably initiate the decompression sickness syndrome, and air contains only 79% nitrogen, the expression "2:1 ratio" is not technically accurate. Decompression to the surface after a saturation exposure breathing air at 33 ft (10 m) produces a *nitrogen* tissue tension to *total ambient* pressure ratio of only 1.58:1. By stating that a 2:1 ratio was safe, Haldane was referring to total pressure—not the critical nitrogen-to-total ambient pressure ratio. Haldane thought that during such "safe" decompressions, all inert gas was held in supersaturation in the blood and tissues and then slowly eliminated. This has since proved not to be the case, as demonstrated by the work of Smith, Spencer, Walder, and others. Nevertheless, Haldanian theory with appropriate modification forms the basis of all commonly used decompression tables today.

Inert Gas Uptake and Elimination

Oxygen and carbon dioxide are physiologic gases, and therefore, there has been little evidence to implicate them in causing decompression sickness. However, when working or diving with compressed air, 79% of the gas breathed consists of inert nitrogen, which is the prime cause of difficulty during decompression. When pressure increases, an unstable situation results, and the partial pressure of nitrogen in the air breathed becomes greater than that of the tissues. The tissues take on additional nitrogen until saturated. When the ambient pressure is lowered, the tissues give up nitrogen, and desaturation occurs.

The rate at which nitrogen is taken up or eliminated depends on its solubility in the tissues, its molecular weight, the distance through which the nitrogen must diffuse, the partial pressure gradient for nitrogen across the diffusing surface, and the perfusion of the tissues involved. Perfusion of the tissues is perhaps the most important factor in saturation and desaturation, since the more vascular the tissue the greater will be the rate. On the other hand, fat that is poorly vascularized saturates and desaturates at a much slower rate. However, fat is able to absorb five times as much nitrogen as water. Haldane noted that the total body eliminated or absorbed nitrogen exponentially; that is to say, with any change in pressure, nitrogen was either eliminated or absorbed rapidly at first but then continued at a rate that slowed exponentially. Haldane found it expedient to refer to half-times in dealing with exponential curves, since a half-time is defined as the time it takes for the concentration of a gas to have changed to one half or, in the case of saturation, twice its original value. Since the total body is a spectrum of tissues, all saturating and desaturating at varying rates, no particular organ system or identifiable part of the body can be dissected free and labeled as a tissue that has a particular half-time. Haldane divided the body arbitrarily into five different half-time tissues for mathematical convenience. Although we have already stated that we cannot assign a particular tissue a specific half-time, the five- and ten-minute half-time tissues probably represent the blood and other vascular areas, while the longest half-time tissues probably are associated with poorly perfused fat or bone. Haldane demonstrated that goats became saturated with nitrogen in about three hours. He then extrapolated this work to man, using a comparison of alveolar diffusing area and body weight, and postulated that man would become completely saturated in five hours. This produced a theoretical "slowest" half-time of 50 minutes. Haldane assigned a 75-minute half-time to his slowest tissue as a safety factor. Later on, Behnke and Shaw studied nitrogen saturation in humans and concluded that man was 98% ± 2% saturated with nitrogen in six hours. In this case, the slowest tissue would have a half-time of 60 minutes. However, for practical purposes and as a safety factor, it was assumed that complete saturation occurs within 12 hours; and the standard U.S. Navy Decompression Tables are calculated using a 120-minute half-time tissue as the slowest tissue. Since the time the present U.S. Navy Standard Decompression Tables were calculated, further research with saturation diving has indicated that saturation may not be complete for periods of 24 hours or more. Hence, 240-minute half-times and greater have been used. Thus, with the body conveniently divided into different half-time tissues, it is theoretically possible to calculate "safe" decompression for short dives to great depths where the slow tissues never have an opportunity to saturate, or prolonged dives to shallow depths where the slow tissues saturate nearly completely. In each case, a "controlling tissue" is calculated for each decompression stop, and the specific *nitrogen*-to-*total* ambient pressure ratio for that tissue is never exceeded while undergoing decompression in stages. Over the years, empirical evidence has shown that the shorter half-time tissues can be assigned larger ratios of tissue nitrogen pressure-to-ambient pressure than the original 1.58:1. However, the slower tissues do not tolerate nitrogen tissue pressure-to-ambient ratios as large as 1.58:1 and appear to be as low as 1.1:1 for saturation exposures.

It must be borne in mind, however, that tissue half-times, tissue ratios, and calculated nitrogen partial pressures in tissues are only mathematical concepts. They do not necessarily represent what is going on within the human body, and the mere fact that tissue ratios and half-times have been altered over the years as experience dictated reveals that the mathematics were probably in error, since they had to be modified to match the observed results.

Haldane, in designing his tables, reduced pressure on the diver maximally during each stage of decompression in order to establish the greatest safe gradient from his tissues to ambient pressure. This was in order to produce the largest possible driving force for driving nitrogen out of the tissues. In doing this, he assumed that if the person remained symptom-free, no bubbles were formed in his tissues and all of the nitrogen was held in supersaturation. If this were the case, the maximum driving force would occur when pressure was reduced maximally but not sufficient to cause symptoms. Since Haldane's time, however, it has been demonstrated that bubbles do form during so-called "safe" decompressions and supersaturation does not actually persist. Also, more exact measurement in recent years has shown that saturation with nitrogen does not follow an exact exponential curve but is very slightly slower at the beginning slope of the curve and then crosses the exponential curve at approximately 90% saturation.[6]

Nevertheless, with all of its potential drawbacks, the Haldanian decompression theory has proved to be fairly practical and, when suitably modified, has formed the basis of most present-day decompression schemes. As the state of the art is in flux at the moment, a detailed description of the Haldanian method for calculating tables will not be given here. Most probably, future modifications will rely on digital computer models and more precise measurements of nitrogen elimination during actual decompression. As of this writing, there are several decompression computer models being tested or in operational use.

CAISSON AND COMPRESSED-AIR TUNNEL WORK

Caissons

Caissons are generally used for sinking bridge piers or structural foundations and furnish a means of removing mud and clay under water so that bedrock may be reached upon which to place the foundation. In recent times, the highest pressures used in caisson work reached 49 lb in the construction of Pier 3 for the Auckland Harbour Bridge in 1958.[56] As stated earlier, a caisson is simply an inverted box that forms the bottom of the bridge pier. The edges of the box are beveled so that they will cut into the clay or silt as weight is applied above. Usually the caisson and bottom of the pier are constructed as a unit in a graving or dry dock and later towed to the site, supported on their own buoyancy. The bottom part of the pier is heavier than the top, and thus, the center of gravity is below the center of buoyancy. When the caisson is approximately in place, work is continued, adding to the height of the bridge pier as the caisson sinks lower in the water. When it begins to touch bottom with rising and falling tide, the caisson is accurately positioned with theodolites, and this is planted firmly in place by pumping water into the lower compartments of the bridge pier above the caisson itself. Water is forced from the working compartment using compressed air, and the actual digging process can begin. When bedrock has been penetrated, digging is complete, and the working chamber is filled with concrete.

Two shafts are provided which extend from the working chamber to the surface—one for removing mud and other excavated material and one for the use of the working crew. A decompression chamber is placed at the top where the working crew can decompress at the end of each shift.

Decanting

Occasionally in caisson work the physical layout makes it difficult to provide a large decompression chamber for the working crew in physical continuity with the shaft from the caisson below. In such cases, "decanting" is used, wherein the workers decompress very rapidly from working pressure and then, within five minutes, move to a recompression chamber on an adjacent barge or platform and recompress to the original working pressure. A five-minute surface interval is all that is allowed in the decanting process and this corresponds to the maximum five-minute surface interval permitted by the U.S. Navy for surface-decompression of divers. However, decanting has the potential of producing a good deal of bubbling in the blood and tissues of the workers involved, and therefore is a process that should be discouraged. The present U.S. federal code does not provide for decanting as a means of decompression. Its inherent danger in tunneling or caisson work is that more than one individual is involved, so that it is hard to get a full gang moved from the exit lock or the working chamber to the recompression chamber within the five-minute interval. Dealing with a single diver, this becomes more practical. On the Auckland Harbour Bridge job, surface intervals as long as eight minutes were recorded despite every effort to keep the total surface interval below five minutes.[56]

Compressed-Air Tunneling

For economic reasons, contractors try to avoid using compressed air when digging tunnels. When tunneling through rock, compressed air is seldom necessary, since pumps are usually adequate to handle the water that may seep into the tunnel. In sand or mud, wells can frequently be drilled ahead of and in the immediate vicinity of the heading to locally lower the water table. In this way, water in the tunnel becomes manageable with pumps or with very low pressures of air. However, when the sand or muck becomes porous or the tunnel runs under a river or lake, there often is no practical way of keeping the water out except by putting considerable air pressure in the tunnel. To this purpose, an airtight bulkhead is erected across the tunnel so that pressure may be applied to the working face. Behind this bulkhead, a second bulkhead must be placed so that a decompression lock is created for the workers to enter and leave the work heading without having to drop the pressure on the heading itself. Under current U.S. tunnel regulations, tunnels of 14 ft or greater finished bore must have two entirely separate locks running parallel to each other, leaving the work heading.[68] One lock is for the exclusive use of workers for decompression (the man lock), and the other (the "muck lock") is for the removal of excavated material. In smaller tunnels, there is generally a single lock called a "combination lock" in which workers decompress and, between shifts, muck is removed. If digging is proceeding rapidly at high pressures in small tunnels, there is often difficulty "mucking out," since the combination lock is occupied for long periods of time by the workers coming off shift. On some large jobs, three decompression locks are connected in succession so that personnel can lock in past a shift undergoing prolonged decompression in the middle lock.

In tunnel digging, the general rule of thumb is that there must be at least 2 ft of earth above the tunnel for every pound of pressure used. Modern technology has greatly changed tunnel digging, in that mechanical "moles" have replaced a great deal of the pick and shovel technique of earlier years. In small tunnels and especially in soil of varying composition, pneumatically powered hand shovels ("air spades") are used to remove or loosen muck and boulders at the face, which are then scooped up by a 'mucking machine," a pneumatically powered scoop which loads the excavated material into muck carts which run on narrow gauge rails. On larger jobs, however, huge shields are used with cutting heads rotating the full circumference of the tunnel. These cutting edges deliver the excavated material to a conveyor belt which dumps it automatically into the muck carts. The shield is driven ahead by hydraulic rams. Depending on the type of ground being penetrated and its geographic location, the tunnel behind the shield is either faced with steel liner-plates for its entire circumference or with rings made of circular I beams. The rings are placed at 4–6-ft intervals, the space between them lined with heavy maple-heart planks. If planks are used, the bottom half of the tunnel must be tightly caulked with straw, oakum, or fiberglass to help keep out the water.

Pressure Recording and Gauges

The pressure in the working chamber, whether it be a caisson or tunnel, must be accurately recorded using a continuous circular recording graph with an aneroid-operated pen. Pressure gauges placed at the timekeeper's or lock attendant's station must also be extremely accurate so that the pressure in the working heading and the decompression lock can be instantly read. An error of as much as 1 lb in a gauge may cause decompression to take place on the wrong table. Since it is impossible to have an inspector in the tunnel at all times, the paper recording graph is a necessity to prevent a given shift foreman from "shorting" the decompression or to prevent unauthorized use of the decompression lock by some worker who does not wish to report having sustained decompression sickness.

Ideally, decompression from the long working shifts in tunnels or caissons should be handled by an automatic decompression valve that times the rate of depressurization through the use of tapes or cams. It is extremely difficult for a shift foreman or lock keeper to manually adjust the valves closely enough to adhere to the gradual decompressions required under the present federal code. Indeed, in the U.S., the Occupational Safety and Health Act (OSHA) of 1971 requires the use of automatic decompression controlling devices when pressures in tunnels or caissons exceed 12 psig.[68]

The present OSHA tables use continuous decompression or bleed-off pressure. Improved tables, now available, use stage decompression, which can be easily manually controlled; these tables should shortly be in general use (1987). The decompression controlling device and the recording graph should preferably be located at the same level as the working heading, but as in the case of caissons, if they must be located many feet above the working chamber or decompression lock, it is important that the air lines leading to them be free of water. A standing column of water 5 ft high in one of these lines would cause the gauge or graph to read over 2 lb lower than the actual pressure. Thus, remote gauges well above the chamber in which they are recording pressure should be checked periodically to be sure that water has not condensed in the line.

Air Masters

It is important that each shift working in a caisson or tunnel be supervised by an individual fully familiar with all aspects of work in compressed air. Frequently, this individual is called an air master, and normally he or she is the shift foreman. There must be one air master for each shift. The air master is responsible for compliance with all safety regulations and is responsible for each decompression. An error made by the timekeeper or lock tender is still the air master's responsibility. Additionally, the air master is responsible for educating each employee in regard to the hazards of working in compresssed air and how to avoid them. Ideally, the air master should be licensed by the state so that in the event an infraction of the rules becomes noticed, his license may be revoked.

Fire

Fires in modern caissons are rare because of their all-steel construction and lack of flammable materials within the caisson. There have been serious fires in older wooden caissons and in tunnels, however, stemming from the use of straw, hydraulic oil, and the wood planking used between steel rings. Welding and cutting are often carried on in tunnels, and this provides a ready source of ignition. For this reason, there should be a fire main extending to the working face with outlets spaced 200 ft apart. The fire hoses should be connected at all times, be 100 ft in length, and should be rot- and mildew-resistant. A fire fighting outlet should also be inside the manlock. If a tunnel fire is not extinguished soon after it starts, the hot steam generated when it is extinguished becomes unbearable to the men in the tunnel and the end result may be loss of the tunnel. There is a strict rule against smoking during decompresssion, but, nevertheless, this has frequently occurred. For this reason, oxygen decompression has not been met with enthusiasm in the United States because of the difficulty in supervising the workers. Oxygen decompression has tremendous advantages over air decompression, but there was a fire in Japan, resulting in the death of workers, where this has been attempted. At the present time, the U.S. federal code does not provide for oxygen decompression. When this is finally accomplished, however, some sort of overboard-dump system for exhaled oxygen will have to be used so that no oxygen buildup occurs in the decompression chamber itself. Oxygen decompression will be an economic necessity in light of our present knowledge of modern decompression requirements.

Ventilation

Even when oxygen is not used in decompression, it is important that ventilation be continuous while the lock is decompressed. In the past this was often overlooked, and carbon dioxide levels could reach 2% by the end of decompression. High carbon dioxide levels probably contribute to the incidence of decompression sickness. Most workers do not like the noise produced by a continuous supply of air to the decompression chamber, but with suitable air silencers on the inlet, it must be insisted upon. Current U.S. federal regulations require ventilation of the manlock during decompression.

Medical Supervision

Any construction company engaged in compressed-air, caisson, or tunneling work in the U.S. is required to retain a physician. The physician should be available at all times for emergencies and should be capable of entering the compressed-air environment in order to treat decompression sickness or air embolism. The physician also conducts physical examinations on all employees before they begin work and then at yearly intervals. He or she should be familiar with the basic physics and physiology of compressed-air operations. The physician is also responsible for first-aid training and seeing to it that proper first-aid equipment is maintained in the tunnel or caisson. Additionally, the physician should monitor the results of air sampling so that the proper air purity standards are maintained in the working environment. Good medical supervision can do much to increase the safety of compressed-air operations.

Instructions to the Workers

The following notice should be posted in the decompression lock and also in the change house so that compressed air workers may become familiar with additional steps they may take to avoid decompression sickness.

SUGGESTIONS FOR THE GUIDANCE OF COMPRESSED-AIR WORKERS

1. Eat a well balanced diet.

2. Be temperate. Avoid excessive alcoholic beverages the night before or within eight hours of going on shift.

3. Sleep at least seven hours daily.

4. Take extra outer clothing into the tunnel when going on shift and wear it during decompression to avoid chilling during that period.

5. Do not sit or rest in a cramped position during decompression.

6. Do not exercise during decompression. This does not mean you cannot move around to avoid sitting in one position.

7. Decompress according to the posted schedule, for this means safety and freedom from compressed-air illness or air pains. It also safeguards against damage to the bones.

8. Do not do hard exercise immediately after decompression.

9. Do not take a *hot* bath or shower within six hours of decompressing. A moderately warm bath or shower is permissible.

10. Do not go to sleep in a cramped position after decompressing.

11. Do not allow yourself to become chilled within six hours after decompression.

12. Report at once to the physician in charge if you suspect you are suffering from "air pains" or decompression sickness. Do not give workers who are suffering from compressed-air illness any alcoholic drink.

13. *If after decompressing, you develop "niggles" or air pains that persist longer than a half hour, call the medical lock at once!*

14. If you become ill away from the job site, communicate at once with the physician in charge, Dr. __________ , telephone __________ .

15. Wear your identification bracelet so it will be known what to do with you in an emergency.

16. Stay within a 30-mile radius of the recompression facility for at least one hour after locking out.

17. Do not re-enter the manlock if suffering from "air pains" or decompression sickness.

18. Do not engage in scuba diving at depths greater than 33 ft within 12 hours of coming off shift.

19. Do not engage in any scuba diving within 12 hours of going on shift.

20. Do not fly in any aircraft for at least 12 hours after coming off shift.

21. See that you are reexamined as required under the law.

Decompression Tables for Caisson and Tunnel Work (Table 25–1)

Prior to 1971, in the United States almost all decompression of caisson workers was carried out using modifications of the 1922 New York Code. When adhered to, this code used the so-called "split shift," wherein the workers spent two to four hours in com-

TABLE 25–1.

Standard Decompression Schedules Following Normoxic Nitrogen-Oxygen Saturation Exposures*†

DECOMPRESSION USING AIR AND OXYGEN SATURATION FROM 0 TO 100 FSW AT 5 FSW INTERVALS

	FIRST STOP			SUBSEQUENT STOPS		
SATURATION DEPTH RANGE (FSW)	DEPTH (FSW)	GAS	TIME AT STOP (HR:MIN)	DEPTH (FSW)	GAS	TIME AT STOP (HR:MIN)
96–100	80	Air	3:00	75	Air	4:00
91–95	75	Air	3:00	70	Air	4:00
86–90	70	Air	3:00	65	Air	4:30
81–85	65	Air	3:00	60	Air	4:30
76–80	60	Air	3:00	55	Air	5:00
71–75	55	Air	3:30	50	Air	5:00
66–70	50	Air	3:30	45	Air	5:00
61–65	45	Air	3:30	40	Air	5:00
56–60	40	Air	4:00	35	Air	0:30
				35	O_2	1:00
51–55	35	O_2	1:00	35	Air	0.30
				35	O_2	1:00
				30	Air	2:00
46–50	30	Air	2:00	30	O_2	1:00
				25	Air	0:30
				25	O_2	1:00
41–45	25	O_2	0:30	25	Air	0:30
				25	O_2	1:00
				20	Air	3:00
36–40	20	Air	1:30	20	O_2	1:00
				15	Air	0:30
				15	O_2	1:00
31–35	15	O_2	1:00	15	Air	0:30
				15	O_2	1:00
				10	Air	4:00
26–30	10	Air	2:00	10	O_2	1:00
				5	Air	0:30
				5	O_2	1:00
				5	Air	0:30
22–25	5	O_2	0:30	5	O_2	1:00
				30	O_2	0:30
0–21	No Decompression			Surface		

*Adapted from the *National Oceanic and Atmospheric Administration Diving Manual.*
†May be used safely with air saturation from 60 FSW

pressed air during the first half of their work shift and then decompressed to the surface for a period during the middle of the day. They then returned to the same compressed-air environment and worked an equal length of time for the second half of their shift, decompressing on the same schedule for the second half of the shift that was used on the first half. This procedure did not take into account that each man started his second half-shift of the day with large amounts of unreleased nitrogen still dissolved in his body, and so the second decompression of the day was very unphysiologic. In other words, a second exposure to compressed air within 12 hours amounts to a "repetitive exposure" because of the lack of desaturation from the first shift; and therefore, the decompression from the second shift should have been longer than the first. These tables produced an alarming incidence of aseptic necrosis. In my experience in Milwaukee, up to 35% of all the workers examined showed x-ray evidence of the disease.[47]

In 1963, the Washington State Tables were introduced, which, over their middle range, fairly closely approximate Naval decompression schedules. They use the continuous shift concept, with only one decompression per day. Naval schedules, of course, are based on Haldanian experience. The Washington State Tables were later adopted for use in California and Wisconsin and became the Federal Standard in 1971. These tables initially represented a vast improvement, in that not a single documented case of dysbaric osteonecrosis appeared in conjunction with their use from their introduction in 1963 until 1972. During that time these tables were used at pressures only up to 36 psig. In Milwaukee, from 1971 to 1973, the tables were used up to 43 psig, which we found to produce a 33% incidence of dysbaric osteonecrosis.[40] The decompression sickness problem was not completely solved either with the introduction of the Washington State Tables, since bends rates have varied between 1% and 26% for many shifts. For this reason, it is imperative that an appropriate recompression facility or medical lock be located adjacent to or in the immediate vicinity of the work area so that the inevitable cases of decompression sickness may be promptly treated. The specifications for an appropriate recompression chamber for treatment of decompression sickness are given in the Federal Code of 1971 for the United States.[68]

Our facility at St. Luke's Hospital, in conjunction with Peter Edel in New Orleans, recently completed a three-year test program using new computer-derived tables for caisson workers. It became clear that oxygen decompression was the only viable option commercially at higher pressures (over 18 psig) and that much more decompression is required for safety than was previously thought. The final version of the new schedules were tested in the laboratory and none of the subjects "bent." More important, the final new schedules had produced no bone lesions or positive technetium scans six months after the last exposure.[41] The new tables, labeled the Kindwall-Edel or Milwaukee Tables, in many cases take less decompression time when oxygen is used than do the present OSHA schedules.

In the United Kingdom, the split shift never gained favor, but continuous exposures of up to eight hours have been traditionally employed. The British 1958 Decompression Tables were shown to produce an alarming incidence of aseptic necrosis, as demonstrated by the Decompression Sickness Panel of the British Medical Research Council. For this reason, the so-called Blackpool Tables were created in the 1960s, which dramatically reduced the amount of aseptic necrosis seen to about 8% of the workers but did not completely eliminate it.[76] Even with the Blackpool Tables, decompression sickness proves to be a continuing problem.

Using the present tables, either British or American, it has been noted that in the early days of any project, there will be a very high incidence of decompression sickness before the workers become "acclimatized" or "habituated." Then, for some reason, the incidence drops off. The mechanism of this acclimatization, a very real phenomenon, is not understood at this time. Also, with any sudden increase in working pressure, though slight, there will be a rash of decompression sickness cases. When the men become acclimatized to the new working pressure, the incidence again drops off. Platelet decrease and other hematologic changes may explain acclimatization.

Emergency Decompression

In the event of serious injury to a worker which necessitates immediate decompression from the working heading or in the event of fire or flooding of the caisson or work shaft requiring the workers to be evacuated, an extremely serious problem is created. The only solution is immediate recompression in another chamber or the medical lock. If recompression can be accomplished within five minutes, this amounts to decanting, and decompression can probably be safely accomplished if the men are returned to their original working pressure and 10 or 15 minutes are added on to their calculated total actual exposure time at working pressure. However, if the five-minute surface interval is exceeded, as will often be the case in emergencies, it is mandatory to treat the individual or individuals in question as having decompression sickness on an appropriate oxygen treatment table. For surface intervals that only slightly exceed five minutes, the U.S. Navy Table 5 (described later) will probably be sufficient. However, for longer intervals after working at high pressures, it would be wisest to use the longer Table 6.

Experiments carried out by Edel demonstrated that divers completely saturated at a pressure of 23½ lb (53 FSW [feet of sea water]) could tolerate a surface interval without showing signs of decompression sickness for up to 15 minutes. At 19 minutes, one individual sustained severe neurocirculatory collapse.[24] In one of my cases I decompressed a man in four minutes from a six-hour exposure (98% saturation) at 28 lb followed by a 15-minute surface interval before recompression. The tunnel worker in question underwent emergency decompression because of a severe hand injury and was subsequently recompressed to 165 ft, breathing helium/oxygen for 15 minutes, before being returned to 60 ft over a four-minute period and placed on Table 6. He suffered no symptoms of decompression sickness at any time. During Table 6, the necessary surgery was accomplished. It is recommended that under no circumstances should a 15-minute surface interval be exceeded, since a danger of producing severe decompression sickness and/or neurocirculatory collapse becomes very great indeed. If neurocirculatory or severe symptoms of decompression sickness appear, or even if the patient complains of being very tired or sleepy, recompression to 165 ft should be carried out initially. Edel treated his experimental subjects decompressed from a 53-ft saturation at 60 ft on oxygen with success.

If a worker must be immediately removed from the work environment due to serious injury, it is sometimes possible to use a portable or one-man chamber to effect transfer to a medical lock where proper treatment can be initiated during decompression. In this way, the worker need never be exposed to ambient air pressure and risk bends during transfer. On one occasion, I successfully used a one-man portable chamber in this way to transfer a man with severe burns. The portable chamber can be carried into the heading and the patient can be placed in it, and then during decompression, the pressure in the one-man chamber can be held at 15 psig during the transfer. Later, the portable chamber is placed in the medical lock, the large chamber is pressurized until the pressure equals that in the portable one, and the patient is removed.

Air Supply for Caissons and Compressed-Air Tunnels

From the medical standpoint, the physician is concerned basically with the quality of the air supplied to the workers. Contaminants that must be closely watched are carbon dioxide, carbon monoxide, oxides of nitrogen, and oil vapor. Generally, large rotary compressors are used that produce the large volumes required for tunneling work. Smaller volumes of air are needed for caisson work as compared to tunneling. Since the caisson is sealed tightly except at the bottom, a good calculation is that 30 cu ft (0.85 cu ft) of free air per minute should be provided for each man working in the caisson. Air supply requirements for caisson work are much more predictable, and as long as sufficient allowance is made for air loss due to passing material through the muck lock and for decompressing work shifts, the volume requirements will be quite stable.

The air needs in compressed-air tunneling may vary greatly, depending on the porosity of the ground and the number of times the muck lock must be decompressed per shift, which, in turn, depends on the rate at which the mining is proceeding. Another factor that increases the requirement for ventilation is the production of carbon dioxide by rotting hay or microorganisms in the soil. If these conditions are severe, obviously much larger amounts of ventilating air will be needed to hold the carbon dioxide levels within acceptable limits.

A rule of thumb given by Richardson and Mayo[54] is that the volume requirement can usually be calculated by multiplying the square footage of the working face by 20 and adding 100 cu ft per man. This gives the number of cubic feet of free air required per minute. If this figure is used, it normally is enough to cover most practical contingencies. The metric equivalent is to multiply the area of the tunnel face in square meters by 6.1 and add 2.8 cu m per man. This gives the number of cubic meters required per minute.

The supply air must be distributed in such a way that no pockets of "dead air" are present. To this purpose, it is best to carry the supply air pipe as close to the tunnel working face as possible. A check valve should be provided at the end of the pipe so that, in the event of airline breakage or compressor failure, the tunnel will not immediately be decompressed and a worker could not be sucked traumatically into the end of the pipe. Smaller discharge ports with check valves should be provided at suitable distances down the tunnel to avoid carbon dioxide buildup in areas remote from the face. In the situation where one is dealing with a relatively "tight" tunnel and the ground is not porous enough to carry off the required volume of ventilating air, so-called "mop lines" may be rigged in the vicinity of the working face or elsewhere to ventilate off a portion of the air supplied. The "mop line" should be positioned in such a way that fresh air is carried through the general working area. A minimum figure, again, in a tight tunnel would be 30 cu ft (0.85 cu m) of free air per minute per worker.[54]

The best way, however, to determine whether the ventilation is sufficient is to make a determination of the carbon dioxide content of the tunnel at least once each shift. Mine Safety Appliances provides a sample pump with color-tube indicators which are fairly reliable for this purpose. However, personnel who do the sampling must be carefully instructed in the proper use of the equipment, and the sample pump must be inspected frequently to be sure it is operating within specifications. It quickly becomes fouled with mud in the usual case, and it will not pull a vacuum if the piston and cylinder are not properly lubricated. In the event that the carbon dioxide levels rise too high, more "mop lines" must be opened.

The large compressors providing make-up air for the tunnel itself are referred to as the "low air" compressors, whereas the compressors powering the pneumatic tools used in the tunnel provide "high air" for this purpose. It is important that the pneumatic tool air be checked for purity as well as the "low air" tool, since I have seen unfortunate incidents where contaminated pneumatic tool air produced serious problems. This is, of course, because the pneumatic tool air is discharged directly into the tunnel after passing through tools.

The "low air" compressors generally discharge their air into a large volume tank or receiver that is maintained at a pressure considerably in excess of that in the tunnel. A reducer valve downstream subsequently reduces the supply air to the desired pressure in the working area.

Of utmost importance from the standpoint of safety is that two separate sources of compressed air be available. Commonly, electric power is used to operate the main air compressors. In the event of power failure, however, there must be compressors *of equal capacity* that can immediately be started to keep the air pressure up. These emergency compressors are generally diesel-powered. Despite the cost of doubling the size of one's compressor plant, the standby compressors are a necessity, since an electrical failure could cause loss of the tunnel or severe decompression sickness in an entire shift.

I recommend that the minimal standards for air composition and purity set out in Table 25–2 be maintained in the tunnels.[78]

Carbon dioxide can increase the incidence of decompression sickness, as already discussed, and although 2,500 parts per million (ppm) is given as a maximum, it is highly desirable to maintain the carbon dioxide levels much lower.

FLYING AFTER DIVING OR EXPOSURE TO COMPRESSED AIR

It is sometimes necessary for people who have worked in compressed air to fly commercially after leaving the compressed-air environment. This is especially true in the case of a diver who may finish a job and have to be flown elsewhere for further work. Because further decompression to less than 1 ATA carries with it the risk of bends, certain precautions must be observed.

The normal maximum cabin altitude experienced by passengers flying in pressurized commercial aircraft is 7,500 to 8,000 ft at the maximum permitted operating altitude. This limit of 8,000 ft is mandated by the Federal Aviation Administration. In an effort to delineate safe parameters for commercial flight after diving, Edel et al. carried out a series of experiments in 1968. The results of their work indicated that it was probably safe to fly commercially after any dive which did not require decompression or was within the no-decompression limits if a two-hour surface interval was provided before flying.[23] This applied even to situations where repetitive diving had been carried out for not more than 12 hours and where there had been no decompression requirement for any of the dives. If, on the other hand, the subject has had exposures requir-

TABLE 25–2.
Minimal Standards for Air Composition and Purity in Tunnels

Oxygen	20%–22%
Carbon monoxide	Less than 20 ppm by volume
Carbon dioxide	Less than 2,000 ppm by volume
Oil or particulate matter	5 mg/cu m for environments between 1 and 2 atm gauge pressure
Methane	Less than 10% of lower explosive limit

ing decompression of any kind, the recommendation was to avoid commercial flight for at least 24 hours. Today experience has made us more conservative, and we currently recommend a 12-hour interval between diving and flying. If the individual has been doing saturation diving or high-pressure caisson work, 24 hours is usually observed.

Should a person on a commercial flight experience the onset of symptoms he believes may represent bends pain, he should *immediately* ask the cabin attendant for an oxygen mask. Preliminary data indicate that if delay occurs after bends pain appears and before oxygen breathing is started, inhalation of oxygen will have little, if any, benefit. Bends symptoms progress extremely rapidly at altitude. If symptoms progress despite oxygen, inform the aircraft captain and he or she may be able to raise the cabin pressure or descend to a lower altitude, or both.

COMMERCIAL DIVING

Types of Diving Gear

Scuba

The simplest type of underwater breathing gear for the commercial diver is the self-contained rig consisting of bottles of air strapped to the diver's back and a demand regulator that supplies air to the diver via hose and mouthpiece at whatever pressure the person happens to be diving. The action of the demand regulator is completely automatic and the only air that is consumed is that which the diver uses on demand. This unit is referred to as *scuba*, or *s*elf-*c*ontained *u*nderwater *b*reathing *a*pparatus.

The scuba is not a new idea; Jules Verne conceived of it in the 1860s. In the 1920s, LePrieur, a French naval officer, constructed a workable scuba; but as the air supply to the diver was continuous and not on demand during inhalation only, the time under water was impractically short before the tanks were exhausted.

It was not until 1943 that Emil Gagnon, a French engineer, and Jacques Cousteau, who is known to everyone in diving, devised a simple, rugged, demand-valve for use under water with scuba. Their original model was produced in secret in German-occupied France and became known in the United States and elsewhere only at the conclusion of World War II. The Cousteau-Gagnon patent was the basis for the principle of all demand regulators and was soon manufactured under license by the U.S. Divers Company in the United States. The orginal model was a "two-hose regulator" with all the reduction of air pressure from tank pressure to ambient pressure accomplished in a central unit affixed to the tank on the diver's back. Exhaust air was led from the mouthpiece back to the demand diaphragm to maintain the same pressure on the exhaust leg to prevent "free flow" or hard exhalation effort with the diver in most working positions. A few years ago, the "single-hose" regulator was introduced which placed the pressure-sensing diaphragm at the level of the diver's face next to the mouthpiece. Only first-stage reduction to pressure (to about 150 psi) was accomplished at the tank. The single-hose regulator has proved to be the more popular and the "double-hose" system is now obsolete.

United States and British underwater demolitions and beach clearance units did not use compressed-air scuba during World War II. Most of their work was accomplished by free swimmers. When scuba was a requirement, all navies used closed-circuit 100% oxygen rebreathers with the carbon dioxide removed by means of soda-lime cannisters. They left no bubbles, a necessity for clandestine military work, but had severe depth limitations because of the oxygen toxicity produced at depths greater than 25 ft. They have no place in commercial work.

The compressed-air demand-type scuba is now the most common rig used by sport divers. However, in commercial work, the compressed-air scuba has a very useful role for relatively shallow inspection jobs and for light work of short duration where decompression is not a requirement. Its advantages are easy portability, no requirement for a large, bulky compressor on the deck of the diving vessel, easy maneuverability underwater, and the rapidity with which it can be doffed and donned. Since this gear is used in the swimming mode, it is excellent for searching, since the bottom need not be disturbed if the diver is careful not to stir it up with his flippers. When using scuba, the diver wears a Mae West-type life jacket or "bouyancy compensator" which can be inflated with carbon dioxide, air from the tank or orally, a weight belt to adjust his buoyancy, flippers to make locomotion easy, and in cold water, a wet suit made of foam neoprene or some similar material. In extremely cold water, watertight dry suits are a necessity. In warmer water, long underwear may be worn to provide protection against cold, since it keeps a layer of warm air near the body and is quite satisfactory in this regard. Long underwear and coveralls also protect the diver against abrasions and injury from sharp objects. Usually, air is delivered to the diver using a mouthpiece held between the teeth and lips, and vision is afforded using a facemask that covers the eyes and nose. It is important that a facemask be used which includes the nose, since when pressure is increased, the pressure inside the mask must be equalized or a face squeeze would result. Non-pressure-compensated goggles are for this reason unsatisfactory for diving. Earplugs are never worn, since the pressure tends to drive them into the outer canal, damaging the eardrums as they are forced outward. When diving with scuba apparatus, it is generally wise to start the dive weighted 4–8 lb heavy, since the weight of air contained in the normal scuba cylinder of 72 or 80 cu ft at 2,200 to 3,000 psig is approximately 4 lb. If a two-tank unit is used, this becomes 8 lb. Starting heavy is useful, since it makes descent easier. As the air is used up in the bottles, the diver finds himself becoming lighter and, at the end of the run, will find he has 4–8 lb of positive buoyancy to assist him in his ascent. Another problem with diving using the wet suit and scuba gear is that, as pressure is increased, the air bubbles entrained in the foam wet-suit material compress, and the deeper the diver goes, the less buoyancy he has. Although quite buoyant close to the surface, he may find himself very heavy at depths in excess of 100 ft (30 m). Scuba is generally unsuited commercially for dives that require decompression, since the entire gas supply is carried with the diver. If decompression must be accomplished, extra gas bottles can be tied to the ascending line for use during decompression, but this is generally an unsafe practice and is to be avoided if possible. The U.S. Navy sets 130 ft (39 m) as the normal maximum limit for the use of scuba equipment. However, under certain circumstances, it may be used as deep as 150 ft (45 m) if operationally necessary. Deeper than this, the Navy prefers to use surface-supplied equipment or other specialized gear. Commercially, these limits are often ignored for short inspection dives; but under those circumstances, 190 ft (58 m) would be what I consider to be an absolute limit, since no suitable air decompression tables, which are not proprietory, exist for depths deeper than this. The only reason for permitting a dive to 190 ft with scuba gear would be for simple inspection and immediate return to the surface with appropriate decompression. A single-tank unit should never be used to depths in excess of 130 ft. Most scuba gear incorporates 80-cu ft (2.26-cu m) aluminum cylinders at 3,000 psig (204 kg/sq cm). However, double tank units of 180 cu ft (5.12 cu m) combined capacity at 3,000 psi are available.

A single 80-cu ft cylinder will last over an hour on the surface with the diver doing moderate exercise. At 33 ft (10 m), this time is cut in half due to Boyle's law. Thus, at 99 ft (30 m), the single-tank scuba diver finds his air exhausted in 10–15 minutes if physically active. There is a supposed "rule of thumb" that decompression sickness is not possible after a single dive using a single-tank 80-cu ft bottle, since the air is used up before any critical time-depth limit is exceeded. This is not true, because certain divers can "control breathe" to conserve air, and if depths deeper than about 50 ft (15 m) are exceeded, decompression sickness becomes a real possibility. The colder the water, the more air is consumed as shivering becomes manifest.

Diving Mask

Diving masks with air supplied from the surface have been used in one form or another for many years with good success. The first modern mask to gain wide acceptance in the commercial field was the so-called Jack Browne mask manufactured by the DESCO Corporation in Milwaukee, Wisconsin. This mask was invented by a civilian diver, Jack Browne, in 1945 and for many years was the U.S. Navy standard light-weight diving rig. Browne actually made a classified dive in a water-filled test tank ("wet pot") to 550 ft (167 m) on April 28, 1945, using this mask prior to its acceptance by the Navy.[29] Obviously, helium dioxide was used as the breathing gas for that dive. It was originally manufactured for use alone or in combination with a canvas suit ("Bunny Suit") equipped with a hood which had a rubber-lined opening around the face. The diver entered the suit through a back entry chute, which was closed with a clamp. The mask was then applied over the rubber edge of the hood around the face and held in place by straps. Communications were poor or impossible using this rig, and DESCO later created the "Harbor Suit," which incorporated the mask and the suit in one piece with a faceplate which opened in front. The faceplate contained a microphone, and an earpiece formed a receiver for diver communication.

In recent years, the Jack Browne mask has been used in combination with the wet suit or modern dry suits, and the heavy canvas "Bunny Suit" originally manufactured by DESCO has been discarded. This mask is still in wide use commercially and is still used occasionally in Gulf of Mexico diving. It was approved by the U.S. Navy for depths down to 90 ft (27 m), but found its chief use in hull inspections and minor jobs such as clearing screws or, in warm water, even changing screws. It is ideal in relatively shallow depths for jobs that require the diver to be on the bottom some time and where decompression may be required. However, in its present common form, voice communications are difficult, since there is usually no suitable method of providing an earpiece to the standard mask as used commercially. Should the mask be pulled from the diver's face, he is faced with the necessity of free ascent. Essentially, a mask may be the rig of choice in relatively shallow situations where the time required on the bottom precludes the use of self-contained equipment. Since the DESCO mask came into use, many other masks have appeared that have numerous improvements. Notably, the Kirby-Morgan Band Mask provides for communications and in many ways is safer and superior. It can be used to much greater depths and with mixed gas. Other very satisfactory masks are also available.

Deep-Sea Rig

Generally, when thinking of deep-sea diving, the average person envisions the picture of a diver wearing a copper helmet and breast plate sealed to a rubberized canvas suit with lead boots and belt to hold him on the bottom. The development of this first successful diving rig began with Augustus Siebe,[21] a German coppersmith working in London, who in 1819, built a copper helmet with glass view plates which was integral with a breast plate also made of copper. The margins of the breast plate were permanently riveted to a leather jacket which was open at the waist. The diver entered this rig through the waist opening with his arms being inserted into the sleeves and his head ending up in the helmet. The usefulness of Siebe's rig hinged principally on the force pump developed to supply it with compressed air and which was the first successful one built for this purpose. Air was forced down to the diver, and then the excess bubbled out around the waist. The diver had no control over the amount of airflow either on the inlet or the exhaust side. One unfortunate disadvantage of this early Siebe dress was that if the diver turned up-side-down, water completely filled the dress and the diver risked drowning. In 1837, Siebe revised his design and built the first closed dress.[21] This consisted of a water-tight flexible dress which was fastened to a removable helmet and breast plate by means of a rubber flange, clamps, and wing nuts. Air was supplied to the diver through a controllable air supply valve and released from the suit via an adjustable exhaust valve. The diver could thus work in any position without drowning, and he would also control his buoyancy and the amount of air he received for ventilation. Siebe's 1837 dress was copied by others and modified only slightly over the years. This basic design became the world's standard and was adopted by the British Admiralty as well as the United States Navy. Most commercial diving suits also followed the same basic pattern. During World War II, the United States Navy built its most recent version, the Mark V, and thousands of them were manufactured. Many of these rigs were later put into commercial use and are still in daily operation. Parts are readily available, since it has not been completely phased out by the Navy as yet.

The advantages and disadvantages of the standard deep-sea rig must be discussed. The reason it survived so long without basic modification was its obvious success. If the deep-sea rig is kept in a watertight condition, the diver can remain warm and comfortable working at extreme depths. If for any reason he should be knocked unconscious or become incapacitated, he will not immediately drown, since there is no mouthpiece to lose, and he will be surrounded by the bubble of air contained within the rig. The dress is quite sturdy and, therefore, is not liable to be damaged in hard service under water. These suits are often equipped with chafing pants so that the diver may kneel on the bottom or on a rough surface without damaging the suit. Buoyancy can be controlled by the diver himself so that he can make himself light to lift heavy objects, or he can let most of the air be exhausted from the rig to make himself heavy for working in place against a strong current. In the heavy condition, he can also manipulate heavy materials or tools without Newton's Third Law pushing him away from the object he is working on. Drilling, sawing, welding, and similar operations can be accomplished well with the heavy deep-sea dress. Communication can be good, since the helmet is equipped with microphone and receiver so that the diver may talk with the surface. If diving in extremely cold water, many suits of long underwear can be provided under the dress and three-fingered rubber gloves can be cemented to the cuffs to provide protection even to the diver's hands. All in all, the deep-sea diving rig has been an excellent diving apparatus, as its long successful record proves.

Its drawbacks, however, are notorious and must also be pointed out. The deep-sea diving suit is difficult and cumbersome to don and take off. It requires a lot of time to "suit up" for a dive, usually with the help of one or two tenders or dressers. The breast plate must be carefully mated to the flexible rubber collar of the dress to prevent leaks. The wing nuts must be then drawn down no more than hand tight with special tools. The weight of the dress before entering the water is bothersome; the Navy Mark V helmet and breast plate weighs 56 lb, the belt 84 lb, and the boots 15 lb apiece. On the heaving deck of a small workboat, it is hard for a diver thus encumbered to enter and leave the water. If he has to climb down a long ladder to reach the water, this is difficult and the problem is doubled when having to ascend the ladder. Carbon dioxide can build up inside of the helmet if the diver overexerts himself, and he may have to pause often and ventilate to bring the carbon dioxide down to acceptable levels. The carbon dioxide is heavier than air and tends to pocket in the bib or the area near the bottom of the helmet where it joins the breast plate. The diver often rebreathes his expired air from this area, so the carbon dioxide content can be high. When fogging of the faceplate occurs, most divers interpret this as being due to carbon dioxide buildup, but probably it simply implies inadequate ventilation, since it has nothing to do with the presence or absence of carbon dioxide. If fogging occurs, the diver may place his lips over the inside opening of the helmet petcock and obtain a mouth full of water by opening the petcock. He can then squirt this through his teeth at the faceplate to clear away the fog. The helmet is noisy, and for communications, the diver must often shut off his incoming air. (However, communicating with another hardhat diver underwater in a similar rig is easy, since the divers can put their helmets together with metal to metal contact and their speech is easily heard from one helmet to the other.)

Should for some reason the exhaust valve jam shut, the diver will find his rig suddenly overinflated, and he will "blow up" to the surface; a situation that can be fatal. If this shut-off occurs suddenly, the diver's suit will balloon out in such a way to cause him to be "spread eagled," and he will be unable to bend his arms inward to shut off his supply air. Once a blow-up has started, the diver will have great difficulty controlling it, since the farther he ascends, the more buoyancy he obtains as the air in his suit expands. Another problem that can be encountered with the deep-sea dress is that if the diver is lying on the bottom in a head-down position while working, air may pocket in the legs of the dress, causing a blow-up feet first. Since the exhaust valves are located in the helmet, there is no way to vent the air off the buoyant legs of the rig and there is no way for the diver to control his ascent. This problem can be minimized through the use of lacings on the legs to prevent pocketing of air in the lower half of the dress, but commercially, the use of these lacings is often ignored. If the diver blows up in a spread-eagled condition, he is utterly helpless as he approaches the surface. If he has been diving deep, he is subject to the effects of a sudden explosive decompression, or he may impact under the diving boat, crushing his helmet. If he is working with a closed rig, especially with sealed gloves, air may not be able to escape anywhere fast enough; and the rig itself may rupture, subjecting the diver to drowning.

Squeeze is one of the most dangerous possibilities with the deep-sea rig, since the rigid copper helmet and breast plate combined with the flexible dress afford an opportunity for an inequality of pressure to occur should the diver suddenly fall underwater, or if for some reason the pressure in the helmet is suddenly lost. If one takes the entire surface of the body in terms of square inches and subtracts the area represented by the rigid helmet and breast plate and then multiplies this number by the number of pounds per square inch exerted by seawater, one finds that about 4 tons is squeezing the flexible dress-covered portion of the diver's body at a depth of 10 ft (3 m). As long as the pressure inside the diving rig equals the sea pressure without, no problem occurs, but should the diver fall from the surface to 10 ft without admitting more air to the rig, a pressure of 4 tons will be exerted on the flexible portion of the rig, tending to drive the entire body into the helmet and breast plate. A minor whole-body squeeze will produce bruised clavicles, scleral hemorrhages in the eyes, and a sprained neck. A serious squeeze will cause the entire body to be crushed. In an accident reported in the East River at a depth of 30 ft (9 m), where the pressure in the helmet suddenly became equal with atmospheric pressure, the 12 tons of squeeze necessitated the diver's remains being dug out of the helmet with a spoon. Reportedly, in a similar accident following a fall off the bow of the wreck of the *Empress of Ireland* in the gulf of St. Lawrence, the diver was unable to reach his air supply in time and the softer parts of his body were found 12 ft (3.6 m) up the airline. It is helpful to remember that expansion or compression of air underwater is exponential, so that the deeper a diver is when he commences a fall, the less effect a whole-body squeeze will have. A fall near the surface is therefore much more dangerous than an equal fall 100 ft deeper. For example, a fall from the surface to 33 ft (10 m) with no additional supply of air will result in halving the volume in the diving rig, whereas a similar fall of 33 ft from 165 ft (50 m) to 198 ft (60 m) will cause only a one-seventh decrease in volume.

Over the last 40 years, some modifications and improvements have been made on the original Siebe design to better the diver's chances in case of accident. The first and most important is the nonreturn valve located on the helmet goose neck to which the diver's air supply is attached. This valve is a one-way valve that allows air to enter the dress but will not allow it to flow back out of the dress. In case the diver's air supply line is cut at the surface by accident or if the compressor fails, air cannot go back up the line, causing the pressure within the helmet to equalize to atmospheric pressure. This obviates squeeze in case of air supply failure. The nonreturn valve should be tested before every dive using the "smoke test," in which cigarette smoke is blown through the valve, but it should not be possible to blow smoke upstream through the valve.

A second extremely important improvement is the "chin button" exhaust control inside the helmet. If the diver suddenly finds that he is getting light, all he need do is hit the chin button to open wide his exhaust valve. Prior to the advent of the chin button, the diver had to reach his exhaust valve and manually screw it open. This was time-consuming and could often not be accomplished in an emergency. The diver can also seize the chin button with his teeth and hold the exhaust shut in the event of a fall. Another advantage is that the diver can temporarily and quickly change his buoyancy by use of the chin button as he works. Normally, the exhaust valve is set at 2½ turns open and left in that position, with the diver's buoyancy regulated by his air supply. Occasional ventilation can be quickly and easily accomplished by hitting the chin button. This is termed "taking a blow."

A third improvement has recently become available but has not as yet been widely used. This consists of the "LUAK," a method of collecting carbon dioxide from the bib area and delivering it directly to the exhaust port. The LUAK was developed by the Swedish Navy and is termed "the Stockholm exhaust" or the "Swedish Navy exhaust." Basically, it consists of a piece of flexible plastic tubing that picks up all of the exhaust air from the rig in the area of the bib so that more carbon dioxide is eliminated. There is an additional safety feature that prevents blow-up should the plastic tubing become kinked. This device is available commercially through the DESCO Company of Milwaukee, Wisconsin. With the LUAK, the diver's efficiency is increased 15%–30% while exerting himself in deeper water. It can be rigged in the field to any existing deep-sea helmet.

Depth limits for the conventional deep-sea rig are presently 190 ft in the U.S. Navy. Below that depth, helium-oxygen is used. However, the deep-sea rig has been successfully used to depths in excess of 300 ft on air. Frank Crilley holds the U.S. Navy record for depth on air in the deep-sea rig at 306 ft, set during salvage work on the F-4 off Honolulu in 1915. However, air decompression tables for depths greater than 190 ft (58 m) are particularly unreliable, even though the U.S. Navy has published the exceptional exposure air tables for depths down to 300 ft (90 m). As discussed earlier, nitrogen narcosis poses a formidable problem when breathing air, and helium-oxygen cannot be used in the conventional deep-sea helmet, since it is open-circuit and wastes tremendous quantities of helium. Therefore, helium diving with the standard deep-sea dress becomes economically unfeasible.

Modern Helmet Diving Suits

In recent years, especially with the advent of mixed-gas diving or diving using a breathing medium other than air, diving helmets have been developed which seal around the neck and which are used in conjunction with wet suits or hot water-heated wet suits. Mixed gas helmets with neck seals have been developed by Savoie, Lindberg, DESCO, Westinghouse, and others. All have certain advantages and disadvantages. All seem to have good communications and better visibility, and some have more than one mode of gas supply. The helmet basically is a more secure piece of equipment than a mask, and therefore, it is much safer at great depth. It also provides more physical protection to the head from projecting or falling objects.

In the Navy, the classic Mark V deep-sea rig is being phased out and replaced by the Mark XII helmet and suit, which is made of space-age materials, is lighter, easier to don, and can use more than one type of gas supply.

The trend today is toward greater flexibility in diving equipment so that a single type of helmet can be used either for shallow-water air-diving with surface supply, or very deep saturation work using a back-pack with a mixed-gas supply, or with a supply from a diving bell located at depth and the diver getting his gas from an umbilical leading to the bell. For diving at depths over 100 ft (30 m), even where umbilicals or backpacks are used, the diving apparatus is usually equipped with a so-called "bail out bottle" to enable the diver to reach the safety of the surface, bell, or habitat should his regular gas supply fail.

Another form of gas supply that may achieve commercial importance is the mixed-gas backpack that uses an oxygen sensor to keep the partial pressure of oxygen in the gas mix constant. Here, the entire gas supply is a closed circuit system with carbon dioxide being scrubbed out of the exhaust gas and oxygen metered in through an automatic valve as the sensor dictates. These rigs are complicated, requiring a good deal of maintenance. The complexities of breathing bags, redundancy of the oxygen sensor system which relies on electronics, and a very high initial cost have discouraged their use commercially. Decompression tables for constant partial-pressure-of-oxygen (P_{O_2}) rigs are specially calculated. Semiclosed circuits are already in wide use which do not rely on oxygen sensors but which recirculate gas through carbon dioxide scrubber cannisters. Make-up gas is then added to the breathing bag with a premixed oxygen partial pressure, and a certain percentage of gas is constantly exhausted to prevent inert gas buildup. The semiclosed rig uses only about 20% of the gas an open-circuit rig requires.

Air Supply Requirements for Divers

In the deep-sea diving rig, a great deal of air must be used to ventilate off the carbon dioxide produced by the diver, since there is a fairly large volume of air in the helmet to create an effective dead space. If the air supply is shut off to the standard Navy deep-sea rig, the diver has on the average about eight minutes of consciousness before the carbon dioxide level will overcome him. The diver doing a moderate amount of work produces about 0.05 cu ft/min carbon dioxide. If the object is to keep carbon dioxide content below 2%, then the helmet ventilation must be 50 times the amount of carbon dioxide produced per minute. In the case of moderate work, this would amount to 2.5 cu ft/min.[72] However, at a depth of 33 ft, to produce the same amount of effective ventilation, the volume required from the surface would be doubled; thus, 5 cu ft/min capacity of the compressor would be necessary. At 5 ATA, 10 cu ft would be required for this same amount of helmet ventilation. However, if a diver does extremely heavy work, he may produce twice as much carbon dioxide as when doing moderate work and then would require twice the ventilation. The *U.S. Navy Diving Manual* gives the following formula for computing an adequate air supply for a diver using the deep-sea rig:

$$S = 4.5 \times N \times \frac{(D + 33)}{33}$$

where *S* is air supply in cubic feet of free air per minute, *N* is number of divers, and *D* is depth in feet.

The metric equivalent of the above formula is

$$S = 0.127 \times N \times \frac{(D + 10)}{10}$$

where *S* is air supply in cubic meters of free air per minute, *N* is number of divers, and *D* is depth in meters. Even if it is only planned to use one diver, sufficient air should be available for a standby diver in an emergency.

With regard to the ventilation of the diving mask, the *U.S. Navy Diving Manual* states that the mask requires about the same amount of air as the deep-sea helmet.

In addition to volume, it is important to choose a compressor that will provide enough pressure to ventilate the diver adequately at the depth of his dive plus handle rapid descents and emergencies, such as falls. The U.S. Navy considers that a compressor should be capable of producing a pressure of 100 psig (6.8 kg/sq cm) over bottom pressure for dives deeper than 120 ft (36 m) and at least 50 psig (3.4 kg/sq cm) over bottom pressure for dives of less than 120 ft.

Most air compressors used in commercial operations are diesel- or gasoline-powered. The chief danger in the use of a compressor powered by an internal combustion engine is that exhaust fumes may be drawn into the compressor intake. In the case of a gasoline engine, this produces carbon monoxide poisoning, which may cause unconsciousness in the diver on the bottom. With diesel-powered equipment, the oxides of nitrogen may produce a severe pulmonary edema, which in turn can cause fatal decompression sickness, even though standard decompression schedules are observed.

The diving tender should always be careful to observe that the air intake is at sufficient distance from the exhaust of the driving engine so that no fumes reach it. If the diving vessel is moored to a single point moor, a shift in the tide could cause the positions of the intake and exhaust to move relative to the prevailing wind, and what was a safe situation at the beginning of the dive may become very unsafe later. *The physician should instruct tenders in this regard most carefully*.

Most compressors, with the exception of teflon-ringed or nonlubricated compressors, cause a certain amount of lubricating oil to be mixed with the compressed air. It is important that adequate removal filters are in the discharge line from the compressor and that these filters are either cleaned or replaced at intervals specified by the manufacturer. More than one diver has been made ill from lipoid pneumonia.

It is mandatory that every compressed-air system for a diver have a volume tank in the line. First, it provides an emergency reservoir of air to supply the diver long enough for him to reach the surface, should his compressor fail. Its second function is to prevent pulsations from the compressor from reaching the diver.

After the air has been compressed and cleaned, the Navy considers the following standards minimal for compressed air to be used for surface-supplied diving or charging open-circuit scuba cylinders:[72] Oxygen concentration should be 20%–22% by volume; carbon dioxide, not more than 0.05% (500 ppm); carbon monoxide, not more than 0.002% (20 ppm); oil vapor, not more than 5 mg cu m; and there should be no gross moisture, dust, or other foreign matter.

Regarding the matter of moisture, it is important to have water separators in the line, particularly in cold weather. Incidents have occurred where moisture has frozen in the air supply line and completely shut off the flow of air.[27] Although it cannot be dismissed as a possible cause, carbon monoxide is rarely produced by elevated cylinder temperatures or flashing of the lubricating oil within the compressor. If carbon monoxide is discovered in the breathing air, it is most likely from the exhaust of the compressor engine.

Mixed-Gas Diving

Mixed gas usually implies the breathing of helium-oxygen mixtures instead of air in order to attain greater depth without suffering nitrogen narcosis. More recently, there has been experimentation with other gases to replace nitrogen, but helium is still the one used commercially. Helium was first suggested as a diving gas by the physiologist Elihu Thompson in 1919 when in a letter to the U.S. Bureau of Mines, he suggested that previous depths could be doubled if helium-oxygen mixtures were used.[31] The Royal Navy first experimented with helium with the idea that helium gas would not produce bends. When it was found that helium did indeed produce decompression sickness, in some cases more severe than that seen with compressed air, they abandoned further efforts. The U.S. Navy, then working with the Bureau of Mines, did some preliminary experimental work with helium but came much to the same conclusion as had the British. In 1924, in Admiral Momsen's own words, experimentation with the use of helium as a diving gas was "put very much on the back burner."

It was not until 1937 that Edgar End, a 26-year-old intern at the Milwaukee County General Hospital, revived the idea of using helium-oxygen as a breathing medium for diving. Together with a diver colleague, Max Gene Nohl, who had designed his own self-contained deep-sea diving rig, End developed a set of decompression tables that he felt would be suitable for a rapidly diffusing gas such as helium. End and Nohl tested these tables on themselves in the medical recompression chamber at the County Emergency Hospital in Milwaukee and finally became satisfied that they had produced satisfactory schedules. Testing was then begun in the waters of Lake Michigan to see if both the decompression schedules and Nohl's self-contained rig would function under open-sea conditions. When they had passed the 295-ft (89 m) mark successfully, they felt that they were well within range of Frank Crilley's 1915 record of 306 ft (92 m) on air. In order to try for a new record, End developed a set of decompression tables which would enable Nohl to descend to 375 ft (114 m). The services of a coast guard cutter were procured, and in December of 1937, Nohl went down the descending line to break the world-record mark. After some difficulty with fouling his lines, Nohl surfaced and redescended; but instead of stopping at a preagreed 350 ft (106 m), he went all the way to the bottom at 420 ft (127 m). He spent some eight minutes on the bottom and then started decompression. End, not having prepared decompression tables for 420 ft, was faced with rapidly calculating them on the spot and trying to stay one decompression stop ahead of Nohl. Nohl surfaced without apparent ill effect.[29]

The fact that helium-oxygen had been demonstrated by End and Nohl to be useful as a gas for deep diving spurred the United States Navy to greater efforts to bring the gas into operational use. Under the aegis of Dr. Albert Behnke of the U.S. Navy, helium-oxygen tables were developed and ready for operational use with open-sea trials scheduled to take place off Portsmouth, New Hampshire, in the summer of 1939. It was then, while the new helium diving equipment was waiting in a warehouse at Portsmouth, that the submarine *U.S.S. Squalus* sank during sea trials in 240 ft (73 m) of water off the Isle of Shoals. The first dives made to the stricken submarine were made on air as a new downhaul cable had to be attached for the McCann Rescue Bell. After the 33 survivors had been removed from the boat, dozens of helium dives were made, making the first open-sea trials an actual operational exercise. The boat was successfully raised and subsequently recommissioned as the *U.S.S. Sailfish*.

The U.S. Navy was to be for 20 years the only organization to have helium-oxygen diving equipment in daily operational use. All submarine rescue vessels were equipped with helium-oxygen diving apparatus, and there was as yet no commercial use of this gas.

The Navy deep-sea helmet had been modified for use with helium as a semiclosed circuit recirculation hat by adding a carbon dioxide-removing cannister to the back and installing a venturi orifice to recirculate the gas. This system afforded an 80% savings in the very expensive helium gas, but the suit was quite bulky and clumsy. The helmet and breast plate alone weighed 103 lb. Electrically heated underwear was developed for use in this rig, but because of continuing problems with electrical failures, has not been used for many years. The Navy used Shell Natron to absorb carbon dioxide in its helium helmet, but after a fatal accident where water leaked into this caustic material and the resultant slurry was sprayed into the helmet, Baralyme was substituted. The original Navy helium rig was so large and bulky that it is amazing the amount of work that was accomplished with it, especially in the salvage of the *U.S.S. Squalus*. However, after that single operational accomplishment, the art of helium diving was not much further developed in the Navy; and all Navy First Class Divers were qualified only to a depth of 320 ft (97 m) to complete their training.

In all fairness to the Navy, however, it must be said that funding was not made available for further development of helium-oxygen gear, since the operational necessity for it could not be identified by those in charge of Navy budgeting. It was not until 1962 that helium-oxygen diving was begun again under civilian auspices. Meanwhile, the British had proceeded with helium diving and had reached a depth of 600 ft (180 m) off the coast of Norway in 1956.[21]

Because off-shore commercial oil drilling in California had already reached depths of approximately 250 ft (75 m), a need for civilian mixed-gas diving became a reality. Abalone divers had been contracting their services to the oil companies, but at 250 ft, breathing compressed air rendered them quite inefficient. In 1962, an abalone diver named Dan Wilson made a record-breaking mixed-gas dive to 420 ft (127 m) in the open sea using a demand-type breathing system and a modified Japanese abalone deep-sea diving suit. The following year, he was contracting mixed-gas diving services to off-shore oil companies, and commercial mixed-gas diving became a reality.[80]

On the West coast, the development of mixed-gas rigs centered mostly on modification of the deep-sea dress for semiclosed circuit use. On the Gulf Coast, however, mask diving had been popular for years, and masks were adopted for use with helium-oxygen. Helium-oxygen diving is now commonplace commercially, and British law requires that all dives in the North Sea deeper than 165 ft (50 m) be accomplished on helium.

Spurred on by economic necessity, civilian technology in the use of helium-oxygen quickly outstripped the U.S. Navy, and I know of one instance where a civilian diving company with only five years' experience in the field was able to perform a salvage job at extreme depth which the Navy had attempted but had been unsuccessful in completing. Only in the past few years has the Navy been funded to modernize their mixed-gas equipment, and this has resulted in the production of the Mark 1 and Mark 2 diving systems. The diving gear used is by and large based on original civilian designs; but with it, the U.S. Navy achieved a world record of 1,148 ft (350 m) in the open sea in June of 1975 during a saturation dive. The deepest working dive commercially was later carried out off Canada to over 1,600 ft (487 m) by the French diving company, COMEX.

Principles of Mixed-Gas Diving

Since the gas the diver breathes is an artificial one, the percentages of oxygen and inert gas (usually helium) must be predetermined. In very deep diving, it is important to avoid partial pressures of oxygen exceeding 1.6 ATA for longer than 30 minutes. The U.S. Navy formerly set this maximum at 2 ATA, but after a couple of unfortunate fatalities, lowered it to 1.6 ATA for 30 minutes. This means, for example, that if one were planning a dive to 450 ft (136 m) for 30 minutes, one would have to set a maximum oxygen percentage in the mix at 10.9%. This is because 450 ft of seawater equals 14.63 ATA, and 10.9% of 14.63 ATA equals 1.6 atmospheres of oxygen partial pressure. Needless to say, a complication is produced, because a gas mix containing only 11% oxygen is irrespirable on the surface and will not sustain life. For this reason, the diver starts out breathing 20% oxygen or air until he has passed at least 33 ft (10 m). Then, the gas mix must be changed as the diver descends to lean out the oxygen. The correct mixing of gas for deep diving involves a two-edged sword. As oxygen partial pressure is cut down to avoid oxygen toxicity, more inert gas is introduced, which lengthens decompression. If, on the other hand, the oxygen is enriched to shorten decompression, oxygen convulsions become a greater danger.

A very complete set of helium-oxygen decompression tables is included in the 1979 edition of the *U.S. Navy Diving Manual*. Instructions for the use of these tables are also clearly given there. However, these tables are based on a maximum helium tissue half-time of 70 minutes. This most probably is in error, and most commercial companies have found that Navy helium-oxygen tables produce an unacceptable incidence of bends at depths deeper than 250 ft for 45 minutes.[80] As a result, all commercial diving firms engaged in mixed-gas diving to great depths have developed their own helium-oxygen decompression tables and they appear to be superior. However, since these commercial tables were developed at private expense, they are proprietary and have not been published, nor are they available to the general public. If you are working for a particular diving company, you will become familiar with its own decompression schemes, which are trade secrets.

Most commercial companies switch from helium-oxygen to compressed air for decompression at depths between 60 ft and 100 ft, taking two to three hours for the switch. This has an immediate warming effect on the diver, and the amounts of nitrogen he absorbs during air decompression are minimal. Oxygen can later be substituted at very shallow depths. The Navy, on the other hand, decompresses its divers on helium-oxygen until the 50-ft stop, when the diver is shifted to oxygen. This involves an increased risk for oxygen convulsions, but the Navy has used this method more or less successfully for its mixed-gas diving since its inception in 1939. Civilian experience indicates that shifting to compressed air at 60 ft probably is more satisfactory, however, than coming all the way to 50 ft on helium-oxygen. Experiments done in our laboratory indicate no difference in helium washout using air or oxygen after the gas shift.

Occasionally, companies now use mixes of three gases for diving. This could be nitrogen, helium, and oxygen. Helium, neon, and oxygen was tried but abandoned as not being economical. Tri-mixes aid intelligibility of speech, decrease heating problems, and provide more economy. Again, decompression tables developed for use with these gases are proprietary and are not published.

Gas Standards for Mixed-Gas Diving

When one is delivering a breathable mixed-gas atmosphere to the diver underwater, pure gases will have to be purchased. Oxygen is now manufactured in only two grades: grade A, aviator's breathing oxygen, and grade B, for industrial or medical purposes.

The only difference between grade A and grade B oxygen is the permissible moisture content. In high-altitude flying, there is the risk of freeze-up of any moisture present in an oxygen system. However, in diving, a small amount of moisture present in oxygen that is 99.5% pure by law would pose no difficulty. Either grade A or grade B is suitable for diving work.[71] Actually, all commercial oxygen is produced by air reduction and is therefore free from water, which has been frozen out. Even welding oxygen is suitable for breathing.

The only producer of helium is the U.S. federal government, which sells it to gas suppliers. Four grades are described, but only grades A and D are currently being manufactured. Grade A helium is 99.999% pure and is oil- and moisture-free. Grade D is oil-pumped and, therefore, carries with it a risk of explosion if mixed with oxygen. Therefore, grade D is not suitable for diving work. If the other two grades, B and C, are ever produced, they would be suitable for diving.[71]

Nitrogen can be bought either water-pumped or oil-pumped. Oil-pumped nitrogen should not be used in mixed-gas diving. However, all grades of water-pumped nitrogen would appear to be suitable.

The mixing of gases for commercial diving use will vary, depending on the type of equipment in use. There are a number of automatic mixers that are available and they are extremely accurate, such as the Mix-Maker. However, gases are often premixed in cylinders for later use at specific depths. The usual method is to establish an approximate percentage by the "split and mix" method, in which one uses the changes in pressure in standard "H" cylinders to determine the percentage. For example, if one desires an 80%–20% mixture of helium-oxygen, one could start with a cylinder of helium at a pressure of 1,600 psig. The addition of pure oxygen to the cylinder to raise the total pressure to 2,000 lb should produce an 80%–20% mixture of helium-oxygen. However, during the transfer process, the adiabatic heat of compression will cause the gauge to read high, since warm oxygen is at greater pressure than cool oxygen, and one will later have to top off the tank to bring it up to specification. Furthermore, oxygen and helium do not necessarily mix immediately, and cylinders should be rolled in special rolling racks or allowed to equilibrate while stationary for at least 24 hours before analysis. When a mixture has been stable for 24 hours on reanalysis, it is suitable for use. It cannot be emphasized too greatly that analysis of gas for mixed-gas diving must be done with the greatest accuracy, since at extreme depth, an error of 1% could produce either convulsions or death from anoxia.

Helium Speech

When using helium-oxygen as the breathing gas, a great deal of difficulty is experienced in communications because of distortion of the diver's voice.

The resonance within the sinuses is a function of the density of the gas within them. Thus, with any gas lighter than nitrogen, a distinct change occurs in resonance. With extremely light gases, such as helium or hydrogen, the problem is at its worst. When Arne Zetterström, the late Swedish engineer, experimented with hydrogen-oxygen diving at depths in excess of 500 ft (151 m) his voice was so distorted that he had to resort to Morse code signals transmitted by tapping on his helmet.[12] Current helium divers suffer from the same difficulties, even though helium is twice as dense as hydrogen.

Attempts to electronically change the frequency of the helium diver's speech have been much more fruitful. The U.S. Navy and commercial firms now use various models of "helium unscramblers" which electronically change the frequencies into more understandable sounds. These helium unscramblers have undergone much improvement and are now in general use commercially where deep diving is carried out. Even so, helium speech is extremely difficult to understand, and all communications from the bottom must be as unambiguous as possible. Messages should be short and to the point. The diver must carefully choose his words and use opposites such as "open" and "shut," as opposed to "open" and "closed" which both contain the vowel "o." "Affirmative" and "negative" are probably better than "yes" and "no." Understanding helium speech takes practice, and it is best to have an experienced telephone talker on the phone when the helium diver is at work.

Diver Heating

Cold is one of the most formidable enemies the diver has to face underwater. Very seldom does the diver work in waters warmer than 86° F (30° C). If the temperature of the water is in excess of 86° F (30° C), the exercising diver faces eventual overheating.[71] However, most commonly, the water is much colder than this; and he or she must be protected against excessive heat loss. As the water circulates past an unclad diver, heat loss is extremely rapid, since warming the water that passes by requires about 3,000 times as much heat as warming the same volume of air.[71]

Obese people have a greater tolerance to cold water, because they conserve their body heat better due to a layer of fat which does not have a good vascular supply.

A person in water or air is comfortable if his average *skin* temperature is about 93° F (34° C). If the skin temperature falls below 88° F (31° C), he will eventually feel uncomfortably cold. At a skin temperature of approximately 86° F (30° C), shivering is initiated, producing heat. Shivering is the body's attempt to prevent a further drop in temperature. If the skin temperature of the hands falls below about 60° F (15° C), intolerable pain is produced. Even though a person may be able to think while affected by cold, the ability to accomplish work will drop off severely, due to loss of tactile sensation and to shivering. The 1970 *U.S. Navy Diving Manual* states that the average diver without protection can actively work in water between 70° and 80° F (21°–27° C) without discomfort. However, if the diver is resting, chills will develop within one to two hours. Below 70° F protection is usually needed, and simple diver's underwear may suffice down to temperatures of 60° F (16° C). Working without protection, a diver can tolerate about 3 hours of exposure at temperatures between 65° F and 70° F (18°–21° C), about 1½ hours between 60° and 65° F (16°–18° C), about 50 minutes at temperatures between 55° and 60° F (13°–16° C) and only about a half hour at temperatures between 50° and 55° F (10°–13° C). Generally, at water temperatures below 60° F (16° C), wet suits or dry suits are absolutely required.

In extremely cold water, around 36° F (2° C), such as found in the oceans at very deep depths, some form of diver heating is needed. The old Navy helium dress, which was devised in 1938 and in use through 1984, was notorious for causing extreme chilling, even though the diver remained dry within the suit with several suits of underwear. The helium surrounding his body conducted heat away at 13 times the rate experienced if he were surrounded by air. Thus, it never proved very satisfactory. Because commercial work requires long hours of exposure at deep depths, a better system had to be devised. The most practical method currently in use is the hot water-heated wet suit, in which hot water is pumped down to the diver and then distributed through a series of hoses to his limbs and trunk. The water then exits the wet suit through the cuffs and holes punched in the booties. Using wet suits of this type, the skin itself is not in contact with helium, so helium does not contribute to body heat loss except around the head and face and through the respiratory tract. At very deep depths, however, it has been found that heat losses associated with exhalation of the breathing mix are so great that heating of the inspired air must be provided for. Most commercial mixed-gas back-packs or "push-pull" units incorporate heating elements for the diver's inspired air by passing the hot water used to warm the diver's wet suit through a series of coils surrounding the incoming gas. On the first record-breaking U.S. Navy dive to 1,010 ft (306 m) in June, 1972, physiologists determined that the minimum inspired gas temperatures at 600 ft (180 m) had to be 31° F (0.5° C), 47° F (8° C) at 800 ft (240 m), and 56° F (13° C) at 1,000 ft (300 m). Should there be a failure of the diver's hot water heating system during the dive, the result could be fatal if the dive is not immediately aborted. This is because the inspired air will be unheated, and this alone may quickly cause death. Even at temperatures as high as 40° F (5° C) death may occur within an hour at shallow depths if the diver is not protected by some form of wet suit.

If a diver has been severely chilled during a dive (but not to the point of incapacitation), the best method of rewarming him is to have him take an immediate, warm (not hot) shower, and he should change into warm, dry clothes. *Hot* showers tend to cause or exacerbate decompression sickness.

Methods of Diving at Extreme Depths

Normally, most commercial surface-supplied or "over the side" diving is accomplished at depths of 100 ft (30 m) or less. However, this mode of diving may be used successfully to a maximum depth of 250–300 ft (75–90 m). At these extreme depths, the dangers of blow-up are serious; and if it occurs deeper than 300 ft, the chances of survival are almost nil. Also, handling the lifeline and gas-supply hose to the diver becomes quite a problem at depths approaching 300 ft. For this reason, if depths greater than 250 ft are considered, other means for getting the diver to the bottom must be used, such as bell diving, saturation diving, and one-atmosphere diving.

Bell Diving

The diving bell is not new; reportedly, it was first used by Alexander the Great. Von Treileben used a bell to depths of over 100 ft (30 m) in salvaging of the guns from the Swedish warship *Vasa* in the 1630s. Von Treileben's bell had no means of replenishing or cleansing the air, however. The first practical bell of note was invented by Haley in 1690. It consisted of a wooden truncated cone with a glass top and a heavy lead ballast plate hanging from the bottom. The bottom part of the bell was lined with lead to make it stable in water. Haley invented a unique air-supply system in which lead-lined barrels of air with attached hoses were lowered below the bell, and then the open end of the flexible leather hose was raised inside the bell above the level of the barrel to allow the air to escape into the bell. A hole in the bottom of the barrel permitted water to displace the air. Bottom times of one and a half hours were recorded using this equipment. Apparently it was used to depths of at least 60 ft (18 m). However, it was heavy and cumbersome, and there is no record of how much useful construction or salvage, if any, was accomplished with it.

Other diving bells have been developed which remained at atmospheric pressure, and so the occupants were not exposed to the hydrostatic pressure of the sea. Notable among these bells was the observation bell used in the salvage of the valuables from the wreck of the *Egypt* during the early 1920s. This bell operated to depths of 400 ft (120 m).[21] The most famous atmospheric pressure bell was that of William Beebe and Otis Barton, who descended to a depth of 3,600 ft (1,097 m) on a steel cable in 1934. However, these sealed bells will not be further considered, since they provide no method of egress for work at depth.

Modern bell diving came into its own in the United States in the 1960s, when it was found to be useful both in naval and commercial work to have a dry chamber at working pressure which the diver could readily enter should the need arise. Davis devised a submersible decompression chamber (SDC) in 1931, and it has since been used extensively by the British Admiralty. However, the SDC was usually employed only for the last 60 ft (18 m) of decompression to start oxygen breathing earlier and make the diver more comfortable.

On very deep diving jobs, especially in the commercial oil industry, bell diving is used to transport the diver to and from his workplace, and the bell is usually mated onto a deck decompression chamber where the diver can finish his decompression. The purpose of the modern diving bell is to provide an effective safety shelter immediately adjacent to the diver should something go wrong with his equipment. The second advantage is that it enables him to get out of cold water during decompression, and he may be safely transferred aboard the vessel to complete decompression without decanting. Another advantage is that should he wish to communicate with another diver at length, both divers can enter the bell for conversation or planning. The maximum depth commercially for the use of the diving bell when no saturation equipment is used is approximately 400–450 ft (120–135 m).[49] Obviously, at these depths, the divers breathe a mixture of gases other than air. Diving bells usually are spherical in shape for strength, carry a gas supply of their own, and have a number of view ports to enable the divers to view the scene of their work before making their egress. Important features of a commercial bell are sturdiness, its being built to ASME (American Society of Mechanical Engineers), Coast Guard, and Maritime Commission codes, and that it be equipped with an excellent carbon dioxide scrubber. Surface handling is a problem, especially in rough seas. Diving with the bell cannot normally be accomplished if the height of the waves is greater than 3–4 ft, unless special A-frame bell handling equipment is available or unless one is diving from a large platform. The bell is supplied with an umbilical cable to take the weight of the bell, plus wires and hoses for carrying electricity, make-up gas, and hot water for diving heating. It is normally slightly buoyant, with a ballast weight hanging below it. With the ballast weight on the bottom, the suspending umbilical can be slacked off and the bell is isolated from surface undulations.

The common mode in which the diving bell is used is that the divers enter the deck decompression chamber, which is pressurized to the approximate diving depth at which they will be working. The diving bell, which is mated onto the deck decompression chamber, is also pressurized to the same depth. After pressurization, the divers then open the bell and shut the hatch behind them. The bell is then detached from the deck decompression chamber and lowered over the side to the working depth. At depth, the divers then open the door in the floor and water is prevented from rushing in due to the pressure within the bell. At this point, the divers are free to finish donning their gear and swim out to accomplish the necessary tasks. They are connected with the bell by umbilical and now commonly use the "push-pull" equipment whereby they take their gas supply direct from the interior of the bell via a small compressor which supplies a demand valve on the side of their mask or helmet. For exhaust, they breathe out against another diaphragm that is compensated to whatever depth they are working, and the exhaust gas is then sucked back into the diving bell by a vacuum pump. With this system, the diver can work safely within 20 ft (6 m) either above or below the bell without having any difficulty in getting gas supplied to or exhausted from his rig. The atmosphere within the bell is constantly cleansed and kept at a constant partial pressure by appropriate monitoring equipment. When the job is completed, the divers reenter the bell and the door is closed. The bell is then immediately hoisted to the surface, maintaining the pressure of the first decompression stop, and mated onto the deck decompression chamber. When mating has been accomplished, the lower hatch of the bell is opened and the divers enter the decompression chamber to complete their decompression in dry comfort.

Saturation Diving

As stated earlier, simple "over the side" or surface-supplied diving should have as its maximum limit 300 ft (90 m), preferably 250 ft (76 m). From 250 to 450 ft (136 m), a diving bell or personnel transfer capsule (PTC) should be used which can be mated with a deck decompression chamber, but saturation facilities need not be used. However, for diving depths exceeding 450 ft, so-called saturation diving techniques must be employed because of the long decompression times involved.

The great advantage of saturation diving is that, once the tissues of the body have become saturated at any given depth with all the inert gas they can absorb, the decompression penalty from this exposure remains the same whether the diver remains 48 hours or three weeks. Thus, if he can live at pressure continuously, eight-hour shifts with no daily decompression requirement become theoretically and practically possible.

The first intentional saturation exposure of which the author is aware took place in the medical chamber of the Milwaukee County Emergency Hospital, Milwaukee, Wisconsin, on Dec. 22, 1938, when Edgar End, M.D., and Max Gene Nohl spent 27 hours at 101 ft (31 m) breathing air.[29] They decompressed fairly successfully, taking about five hours, with only Nohl experiencing some later discomfort. These symptoms of bends were treated with moderate pressures of air with complete relief.[29] Today five hours would be considered grossly inadequate decompression.

Practical saturation diving was first conceived of in 1957 by the late Cdr. George Bond of the United States Navy when working at the Submarine Medical Research Laboratory in New London. Cdr. Bond (later Capt. Bond) envisioned undersea laboratories located at various depths down to 600 ft (182 m) on the continental shelf. He calculated that scientists could work at full sea pressure in these laboratories studying physiology as well as submarine geology and marine biology for prolonged periods of time. Then they could be transferred to a shallower habitat where they could continue their studies while decompressing. Several habitats would be used, each one at a shallower depth, so that finally, the scientist could emerge with minimal decompression after completing his or her tour of study, which might go into weeks.[13]

It was first necessary to demonstrate that animals could tolerate saturation exposures. These research efforts were termed Project Genesis, and after further work at the Experimental Diving Unit in Washington under the direction of R. D. Workman, saturation decompression schedules were devised for human beings. These were later tested in the open sea on the Projects Sea Lab I and II. Meanwhile, in 1962, Ed Link saturated a diver for 24 hours at a depth of 200 ft (60 m) in the Mediterranean. Capt. Jacques Cousteau also established saturation habitats in the Conshelf series.

In 1965, commercial saturation diving was begun when Westinghouse, using their Cachelot diving system, worked on the Smith Mountain Dam in Virginia, U.S.A., to replace faulty trash racks at a depth of 200 ft (60 m). Divers were saturated for periods of up to five days on this job.

Saturation diving implies that the divers will be exposed to high pressures for long periods of time, and for this reason, the oxygen concentration is of the utmost importance. It is commonly accepted in the commercial world that no more than 0.6 ATA oxygen partial pressure should be maintained in the saturation complex and in the bell so that metabolic demands are met, but toxic levels are not exceeded. This is equivalent to breathing 60% oxygen on the surface. These exposures have proven safe for up to two weeks with regard to pulmonary oxygen toxicity, both in the North Sea and in air saturation in the Hydrolab habitat. Carbon dioxide removal equipment must also be provided, and this usually takes the form of open-ended canisters of Baralyme, through which air is circulated by means of fans. When it is necessary to introduce oxygen into the atmosphere to make up for metabolic losses, leakage or depressurization, oxygen is generally introduced into the scrubber system so that effective mixing takes place. All creature comforts must be accounted for, and these include comfortable bunks and adequate shower and toilet facilities. Controlling the temperature of the habitat is extremely important, since helium carries away 13 times as much body heat as does air. What could be a tolerable temperature in an air-filled chamber becomes intolerably cold if the chamber is filled mostly with helium. Normal temperatures in a helium saturation complex are usually held between 83° F (28° C) and 89° F (32° C) for the comfort of the occupants, with as low a relative humidity as possible.

Strict atmosphere control must be maintained with regard to the introduction of all volatile materials into the saturation complex. This includes pressurized aerosol cans that may implode under high pressure and contain freons with potentially toxic effects. Tinctures or medicinal alcohol should be avoided because of flammability, and it is my practice to use aqueous solutions of benzalkonium chloride for cleansing the skin prior to venipunctures. Cooking of food, which produces grease and smoke, is not permitted. Care must be exercised in the design of the chamber complex so that the sanitary facilities cannot inadvertently depressurize to atmospheric pressure. (In one tragic accident, a diver was disemboweled while sitting on the toilet when the sanitary tank was emptied.) All exposed wiring should be kept to a minimum. Lighting should be protected so that light bulbs cannot come into immediate contact with flammable materials. Nonflammable sheets and bedding should be used when possible, but extremely fireproof material, such as fiberglass, has proven to be very uncomfortable, producing urticaria.[3] Other substitutes are available.

After it has been thoroughly ascertained that none of the divers are suffering from upper respiratory infections, skin infections, or other diseases, pressurization can begin. When the door is closed, compressed air is admitted to the complex, raising the pressure to the equivalent of approximately 60 ft (18 m) of seawater. Further pressurization is stopped and the system is checked for leaks. Meanwhile, raising the pressure to approximately 29.4 psig has produced a partial pressure of oxygen of 0.6 ATA. Nitrogen should be less than 2%, because otherwise it can present complications during decompression. From this point on, no oxygen is admitted to the system during pressurization or during the dive except to make up for that used by the metabolism of the divers and that which might escape through leaks. Very accurate oxygen sensors must be used both within and outside the habitat to assure that the oxygen remains no higher than 0.6 ATA and there must be redundance in the event of failure of one or more sensors.

When it has been ascertained that no leakage is occurring and that all systems are functioning, further pressurization is carried out using pure helium. This is admitted through the blower duct of the carbon dioxide removal system, so that the fans will mix it thoroughly and no pockets of pure helium will develop that would asphyxiate the divers. Earlier systems relied on the diver's fanning the atmosphere vigorously with towels.[80] If the saturation dive is to be to a depth of 600 ft (182 m), it may be seen that the oxygen content of the chamber air will be only a little over 3% if the partial pressure of oxygen is kept at 0.6 ATA. It is therefore obvious that extremely accurate sensors must be used to maintain the correct oxygen partial pressures.

Carbon Dioxide Levels in Saturation Diving.—Carbon dioxide should be less than 0.5% surface equivalent. This means 0.5% "effective," or in other words, what the diver inhales with each breath should contain less than 0.5% carbon dioxide by volume. In the PTC, the carbon dioxide will probably be slightly higher, but every effort should be made to keep it down, since high levels of carbon dioxide tend to precipitate decompression sickness.

Cutaneous Infection.—One of the most troublesome medical problems that emerges while carrying out saturation diving operations is cutaneous infection. Because the divers are continuously exposed to wet conditions and high humidity, otitis externa and maceration of the skin with subsequent infection must be guarded against. Divers must be instructed to shower and thoroughly dry themselves after coming in from work, and boric acid solutions instilled into the ears will help to prevent otitis externa. Should it develop, the standard antibiotic remedies may be used. Intertriginous areas of the body should be well dusted with cornstarch or talcum powder to prevent maceration, and frequent clothing changes are mandatory. This seemingly minor problem can assume immense proportions and may even force the aborting of the dive should one of the divers develop a mass of open infected sores. Zinkowski[80] recommends that each diver provide himself with a personal "shorty" wet suit of one-eighth-inch thick foam wet-suit material for protection of the genitalia, and so that the hot water-heated suits which may be used by several divers will not carry cross contamination.

Decompression.—When the job is completed, depressurization takes place, usually at the rate of about 8 ft per hour deeper than 300 ft (90 m) with slowing to 4 or 3 ft/hr at the shallower depths. However, often parts of each 24 hours are spent resting or sleeping at specified stops so that the rate is not continuous. In emergencies, decompression has been as fast as 12 ft/hr from 210 ft (63 m) to 60 ft (18 m), and then 6 ft/hr and 4 ft/hr from 60 to 30 ft (18 m to 9 m) and 30 ft to the surface, respectively. As depressurization occurs, additional oxygen must be added to the system to maintain the atmosphere in the saturation complex at 0.6% ATA. At the shallower end of the dive, oxygen enrichment or oxygen breathing by mask is used by most companies.

Helium bends tend to come on more quickly than bends due

to nitrogen; the first signs of decompression sickness may often occur during depressurization from a saturation dive. Instruct the divers to report immediately any such symptoms, because further decompression will only worsen matters. (Refer to the section on Treatment of Decompression Sickness for additional information.) The diver should remain in the vicinity of the recompression chamber for at least 12 hours after emerging from a saturation dive. This will enable him or her to be immediately recompressed should decompression sickness develop.

One-Atmosphere Diving

There has been a very intense effort over the past five to six years to avoid the problems of pressure entirely when it comes to carrying out underwater work. Three methods have come to assume operational importance; the one-atmosphere suit, submarines, and remotely operated vehicles.

The One-Atmosphere Suit.—The idea of an armored diving suit is not new, the first successful one appearing about 1913 (Neufeldt and Kuhnke). The problem with this type of armored dress was that the joints tended to seize under heavy pressure, and they were too bulky and cumbersome to carry out much work, since the manipulator arms were primitive. In the late 1970s, the *Jim Suit* was developed, which, for the first time, overcame the problems of freely moving watertight joints at great depths (Fig 25–1). This suit has proved itself to depths of 900 ft (275 m) where useful work has been carried out in connection with the offshore oil industry. Follow-up designs quickly appeared, with the latest in the series being the *Mantiss* (Fig 25–2). In essence, this is a minisubmarine with arms that the occupant can move through movement of his own limbs and it allows the occupant to work directly on simple tasks on the bottom without having to be concerned about compression and decompression.

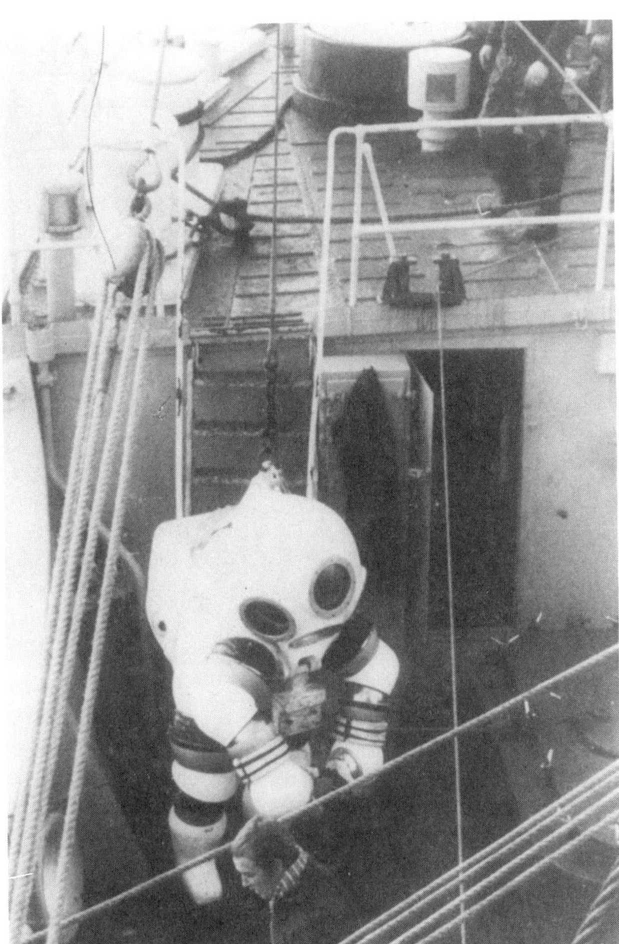

FIG 25–1.
Articulated armored diving dress, called *JIM.* Although weighing about half a ton on deck, this suit weighs only 60 lb underwater. Joints move freely under extreme pressure and the seals are pressurized so the suit cannot flood in the event of seal failure. (Courtesy Oceaneering International.)

Submarines.—Mini-submarines have been perfected to the point where they cannot only carry out inspection on submarine pipelines, but they are also able to accomplish simple tasks through the use of manipulator arms (Fig 25–3). These manipulator arms have become extremely sophisticated to the point of providing the operator with feedback so that he can actually feel how much pressure he is exerting on the object he is grasping through the manipulators. This makes it possible, for instance, to grasp an egg firmly with the manipulators without breaking it. A variety of tools are available that can be interchanged while the submarine is submerged at work. The advantage is that the human eye is very close to the task at hand and visual information such as depth perception is better than that achieved through TV.

Remotely Operated Vehicles (ROVs).—Pure technology has progressed so far that sometimes man no longer is required to enter the sea to get the work accomplished. The manipulator arms of a remotely operated vehicle can move its own arms and hands while television cameras are its eyes (Fig 25–4). Movement is provided by small thruster propellers, and the whole apparatus is in touch with the surface through a long cable, its umbilical. Prodigious amounts of work have been carried out by ROVs, including a dramatic rescue. In 1973, the small mini-sub *Pisces 3* sank in 1,475 ft of water off Southern Ireland with two men aboard. *CURV III* (Cable Controlled Underwater Recovery Vehicle), operated by the U.S. Navy, got to the men in a Force 6 gale and secured a lifting line to the sub. The sub was then hoisted to the surface, and the men were saved after 75 hours on the bottom.

It appears that remotely operated vehicles, submarines, and one-atmosphere suits or hybrids between submarines and the suits will achieve greater commercial importance as time goes on, because they make decompression unnecessary, with a resultant saving in time. Furthermore, the human being is not exposed to the risks of increased ambient pressure.

Medical Aspects of One-Atmosphere Diving.—When the diver or submarine operator is no longer exposed to sea pressure, the physician's concerns relate only to the adequacy of the life support system of an enclosed environment. Sufficient oxygen and carbon dioxide absorbent must be provided, not only to satisfy the requirements of the mission, but also for reserves in case of accidental fouling. Protection from cold must be provided as well.

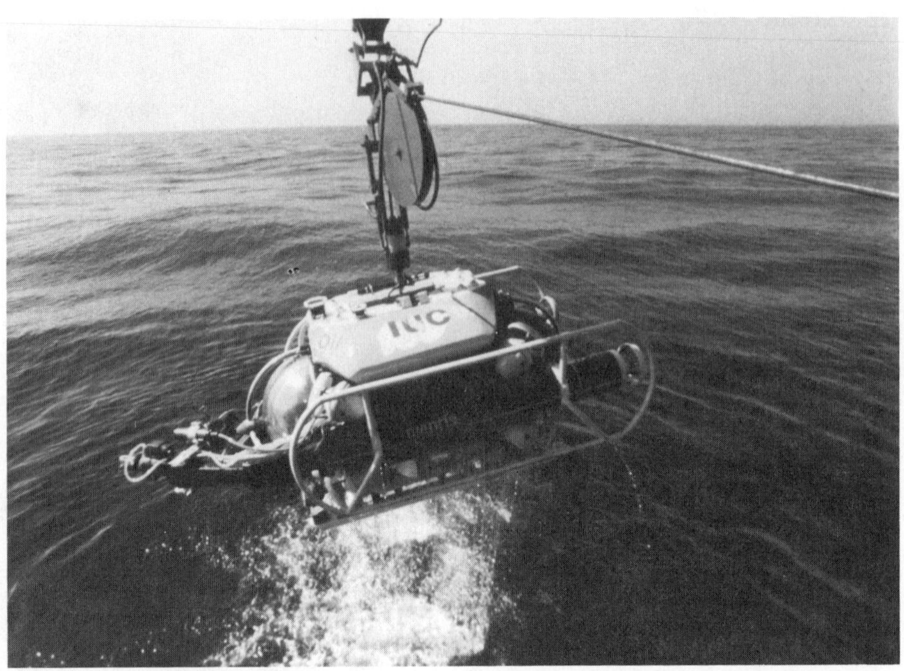

FIG 25–2.
MANTISS being removed from the water. Note the thruster propellers mounted at several different angles and the plexiglass dome for vision. This represents a combination of a tethered mini-sub and an armored suit. It can be used to depths of 2,300 ft (697 m). The most recent models can operate in three modes: (1) as an unmanned ROV; (2) with full pilot control; and (3) by pilot with topside assistance. (Courtesy International Underwater Contractors.)

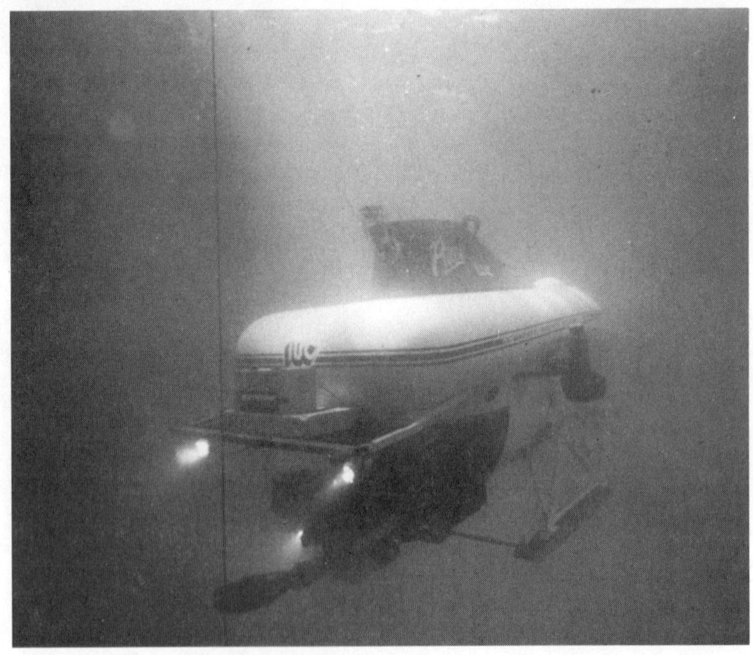

FIG 25–3.
Pisces VI. A mini-sub holding on to a vertical descending line with its manipulator arm. This submarine holds the world record for deep water exploratory drilling support at 4,876 ft (1,478 m). (Courtesy International Underwater Contractors.)

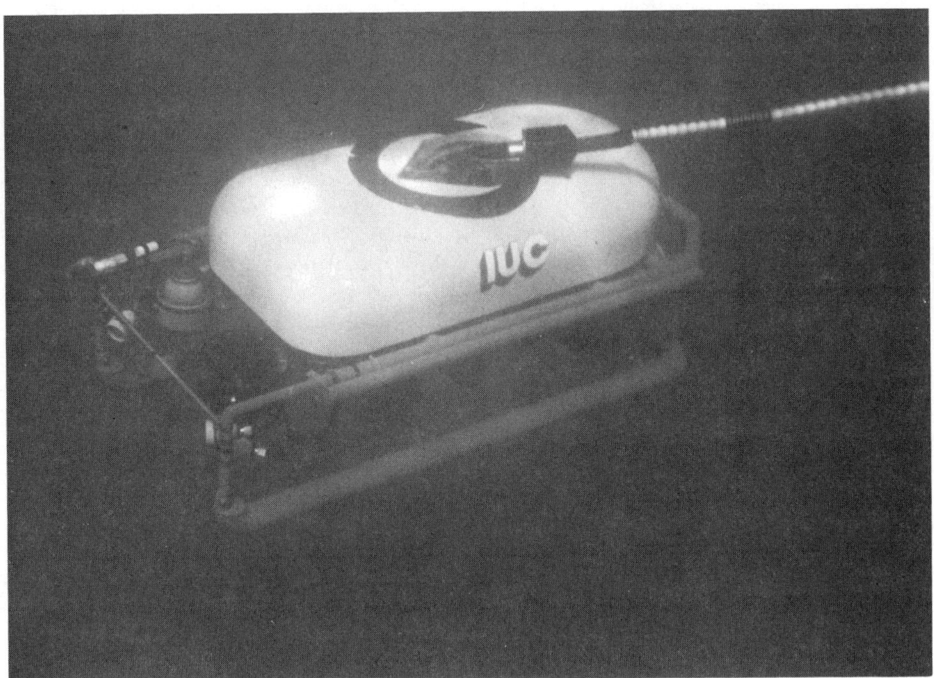

FIG 25–4.
Remotely operated vehicle, Recon IV. This unit is operable to 2,300 ft (697 m) where it can take pictures, do color video surveillance, provide cathodic protection to offshore structures and, with appropriate manipulator arms, can do installation, maintenance, repair, and salvage. (Courtesy International Underwater Contractors.)

Lithium hydroxide is much preferable to Baralyme as a carbon dioxide absorbent, since it will function well when cold—an important consideration should the submarine or armored suit be trapped at depth.

EMERGENCY MANAGEMENT OF PRESSURE-RELATED ACCIDENTS IN DIVING AND COMPRESSED-AIR WORK

The immediate management of a diver or compressed-air worker who is brought to the surface and develops symptoms of illness or injury can be divided into four phases. The first phase is immediate emergency care, the second is accurate diagnosis, the third is proper transportation to an appropriate medical facility, and the fourth phase is definitive treatment.

Immediate Emergency Care

Aside from a natural illness such as myocardial infarction, epileptiform seizure, pulmonary embolism, or cerebrovascular accident, the diver or compressed-air worker who becomes incapacitated or develops symptoms of pain or paralysis after returning to atmospheric pressure is most likely suffering from air embolism or decompression sickness. Air embolism is quite rare in tunnel workers and divers using the deep-sea rig, but quite common in scuba divers. Regardless of what symptoms the patient may have, immediately place him in the supine position. If the patient has symptoms related to the lungs (cough, hemoptysis) or central nervous system (unconsciousness, seizures, unequal pupils, blindness, paresthesias, or paralysis), he should be placed in the Trendelenburg position, since these symptoms and signs would point to air embolism. Since it will not be immediately known whether or not the patient may vomit, it is best to tilt him slightly to one side or the other to avoid possible aspiration. If embolism is *not* suspected, the patient can be returned to the horizontal position. Assure that the airway is patent. In the absence of spontaneous respiration, mouth-to-mouth resuscitation is indicated; and if a pulse is not detectable by carotid palpation, external cardiac massage should be instituted by a second person. Throughout the period of diagnosis and transport to the ultimate treatment center, the patient must be kept in very steep Trendelenburg position as much as possible, if embolism is suspected, and all measures should be undertaken to support cardiopulmonary function. Suitable blocks can be placed under the stretcher if the patient is transported in the ambulance, to maintain Trendelenburg. (Positioning of the patient is not critical in bends.) If the patient appears to be in shock, he should be wrapped in blankets to conserve heat.

The reason for the Trendelenburg position in air embolism is that lowering the head causes an increase in the hemostatic pressure in the head, with consequent vasodilatation. There are good experimental data to show that this vasodilatation facilitates the movement of air bubbles through the capillary bed in the direction of arterial flow and tends to restore circulation before irreversible damage occurs. Many divers have regained consciousness when this maneuver has been used, and some have even become asymptomatic before reaching the chamber. Trendelenburg should be maintained up to 30 minutes to an hour total.

First-aid personnel must be instructed not to give up any resuscitative attempts until the patient is pronounced dead by a licensed physician.

Diagnosis

It is important that diving and tunneling personnel be instructed in diagnosing the cause of the victim's difficulty at the scene so that the emergency recompression facility can be prepared in advance. In certain situations, the diagnosis may influence the choice of which facility is used.

Usually, cerebral air embolism is the most severe and immediately dangerous compressed-air or diving accident that will be encountered. Typically, the victim experiences onset of symptoms within seconds or minutes of surfacing. Personnel should be taught to recognize sudden unconsciousness, convulsions, paralysis, and/or bleeding from the mouth as signs of possible air embolism. Other signs that may not be noticed immediately are mottling of the tongue (Liebermeister's sign), unequal pupils, and subcutaneous emphysema above the clavicles and in the neck. Immediate examination should start with palpation for subcutaneous emphysema. There is occasionally a change in voice quality due to mechanical pressure on the larynx or the recurrent laryngeal nerves. The patient may complain of chest pain. Personnel should be taught to determine the presence of pneumothorax by observing the respiratory rate, the presence or absence of cyanosis, and asymmetrical respiratory movements. They can be told to place an ear against the chest wall to listen for a difference in breath sounds bilaterally. In cases where cerebral air embolism has not occurred but mediastinal emphysema is present, the patient will not have cerebral signs but will complain of fullness in the neck, chest pain, change in voice quality, and usually nausea. Personnel must become aware that diagnosis of cerebral air embolism carries with it the obligation to transport the victim as quickly as possible to a chamber which has the capability of recompressing the patient to 6 ATA. They should be instructed to attempt to reach such a facility, *no matter how far away it is!*

In the on-site differential diagnosis, decompression sickness is the next category to be considered. Except for obviously foolhardy "nonstandard dives" or in cases of accidental explosive decompression to the surface, decompression sickness usually comes on gradually, over a period of minutes to hours. After exposure to increased ambient pressure, most symptoms of decompression sickness will appear within three to four hours after returning to ambient pressure, but there have been instances where these symptoms have been delayed in onset for 12–24 hours. Beyond 24 hours after surfacing, it is extremely unlikely that any developing symptoms will be due to diving or compressed air. In Rivera's review of 935 cases of decompression sickness occurring in naval divers, 90% of all cases included pain.[55] The pain can appear anywhere in the body, but it is commonly located in the limbs. In divers it is more usual to find it in the arms, whereas in caisson and tunnel workers, the legs are more frequently involved. In saturation divers, the most common site is the knee. It tends to affect any part of the body that has been exercised a great deal during exposure to increased pressure and also tends to appear at the site of recent injury or sprain.

Rivera found that 25% of all cases of bends in naval divers involved neurologic symptoms. In commercial and sports divers, the incidence of neurologic symptoms tends to be much higher. These symptoms range from paresthesias and paralysis to vertigo, visual distortion, blindness, and unconsciousness. If the spinal cord is involved, the most common site is the upper lumbar or lower thoracic region which produces a paralysis from approximately T-10 down. The paralysis or numbness may be limited, however, to one extremity, even with spinal cord involvement.

In Rivera's series, 2% of the naval divers developed respiratory symptoms or "chokes." In divers, "chokes" may be a late manifestation, usually coming on five to six hours after surfacing. In tunnel and caisson workers, however, the incidence of "chokes" in the author's experience is 5%–6% and usually appears soon after returning to atmospheric pressure. This difference is probably due to contaminants in the air in tunnels and caissons, whereas divers usually breathe air or gas of very good quality. In the case of "chokes," even if the victim is a smoker, the inhalation of cigarette smoke will generally indicate a paroxysm of severe coughing (Behnke's sign). It is probably true that in the absence of chemical irritation of the lungs due to breathing contaminated air, approximately one third of the pulmonary capillaries must be blocked by bubbles or microthrombi to produce any respiratory symptoms.

It is important to instruct divers and compressed-air workers that all symptoms of decompression sickness, with the exception of mild skin itch or "skin bends" ("diver's lice"), be treated with immediate recompression. Skin itch may be a precursor to serious symptoms later.

The differential diagnosis between bends and air embolism may be difficult for the layman, but it is helpful to teach that decompression sickness usually occurs only after surfacing from depths greater than 33 ft and, then, only after sufficient bottom time has elapsed to permit enough inert-gas absorption. An exception is saturation exposure to air, in which the bends threshold is about 26 ft for most people. Air embolism is almost certainly the cause of any symptoms if the patient has been diving in less than 33 ft of water. Another differential diagnostic point is that paralysis due to decompression sickness is usually transverse if the spinal cord is involved and that it is from the waist down in one or both extremities. In air embolism, it usually produces a hemiplegia rather than a paraplegia. Except in extreme cases of blow-up or explosive decompression from saturation dives, cerebration is usually not affected in decompression sickness in divers and compressed-air workers. Curiously, cerebral signs and symptoms of decompression sickness with neurocirculatory collapse are much more common in aviation bends, perhaps because these decompressions are from "saturation" at one atmosphere and are usually rapid or explosive.

Transportation

Having observed the rules for positioning the patient during transportation, if he has air embolism, the most important factor in moving the victim becomes speed. In caisson and tunnel work, the recompression chamber is close at hand, so transportation normally is not a serious problem. However, in diving, the accident may have occurred far out at sea, where a number of hours must be spent in reaching shore. If this is the case, it would be wise to attempt radio contact with the shore to procure a Coast Guard helicopter or amphibian. The use of *low altitude* air transportation may easily mean the difference between life and death in the severely injured patient. If the patient is flown at high altitudes, any bubbles in his body become increasingly large, and the patient will deteriorate rapidly.

An important point to remember is that pressurized commercial aircraft are certified by the Federal Aviation Administration to maintain a maximum pressure of 9.4 psi across the pressure cabin hull. Most commercial airlines use 8.6 psi maximum as a matter of company policy. Using the 9.4 psi figure, a pressurized aircraft could simulate a seawater depth pressure in the cabin of 21 ft while standing on the runway at sea level. If the same plane were to fly at 5,000 ft and maintain the same pressure differential across its cabin, the corresponding simulated seawater depth would be about 15 ft. Thus, a diver could theoretically be transported at sea level or, in some cases, below sea level if a pressurized aircraft were used. In order to attain pressure in the cabin while on the ground or a pressure greater than sea level, an interlock in the cockpit must be disabled.

TREATMENT OF DECOMPRESSION SICKNESS

Pol and Wattele[52] were the first to note in 1854 that recompression of a caisson worker would relieve symptoms of decompression sickness. Since that time, recompression has been the standard remedy. Ideas have differed, however, as to what type of recompression should be used. It was held by some that the afflicted patient should be recompressed to his original working pressure. Others stated that he should be compressed to the depth of relief regardless of his working depth, and still others believed that recompression to the depth of relief plus 1 atmosphere was the most efficacious. In any case, treatment essentially stopped when the patient had reached maximum pressure, since there was no further compression of bubbles after that point. Once relief had been achieved, the next question was how to decompress the patient in such a way that he would not suffer an attack of bends again. There were many schemes devised for this also, but no one system seemed to be foolproof. An additional problem when treating decompression sickness in this manner was that, by recompressing the patient, one introduced an enormous amount of iatrogenic nitrogen into his tissues by simply taking him to depth, breathing air again. This extra nitrogen that entered during his treatment simply had to be released gradually to avoid further decompression sickness.

After reviewing all of the previous schemes for recompression therapy and testing new ones, the U.S. Navy promulgated the air recompression Tables 1 through 4 in 1945. These tables represented on the average a ninefold[35] improvement in the treatment of decompression sickness over previous methods and for years became the standard of the world (Table 25–3). The use of these tables embodied the principle that the patient should be taken to the depth of relief plus one atmosphere or, in any case, to a maximum depth of 165 ft (50 m). The reason that 165 ft was chosen as a maximum treatment depth was that it represented a trade-off between maximal recompression of offending bubbles and prolonging subsequent decompression. If an additional atmosphere is used to treat (as would occur at a depth of 198 ft), nitrogen narcosis becomes a formidable problem for both patient and inside tender. Additionally, not much reduction in the volume in the bubble is gained in adding this extra atmosphere, since the change in the bubble size is only from one sixth to one seventh of its volume on the surface. Its diameter change is even less. Once maximum pressure has been reached, and the patient has become symptom-free, it then becomes a problem of removing him from pressure without causing bends to appear again. For this reason, in serious cases, Tables 3 and 4 provide for a 12-hr "soak" at 30 ft (9 m) during decompression. The reasoning behind this is that it was believed that all tissues should equilibrate to 30 ft within 12 hrs and then (using Haldanian Theory), decompression to the surface without further signs of bends should be possible. As a safety factor, however, decompression from 30 ft is done in stages and very slowly, even after the 12-hour soak. When only air is used with these tables, they are inordinately long; the shortest one takes six hours and 13 minutes and Table 4, for serious symptoms, takes 38 hours. For reason of their length, these tables were necessarily not popular with divers and tunnel workers; but nevertheless, they did represent the only practical means for escape from unbearable pain or paralysis.

However, by 1964, a disturbing trend began to emerge. Taken as a whole, the incidence of failure of Treatment Tables 1 through 4 for initial recompressions was only 14.3% for the period of 1946–1964, but for the single year 1963, the failure rate was 21.9%. By 1964, it had climbed to 26.7%. Even more disconcerting was the fact that the failure rate on initial recompressions for serious symptoms on Tables 3 and 4 had jumped from 29.7% in the period 1946–1964 to 46.4% in 1963 and 47.1% in 1964.[35]

The increased failure rate was due to the fact that more and more sport scuba divers were being treated who had failed to follow any standard naval decompression schedule and, therefore, had made so-called nonstandard dives. As a result, the cases of decompression sickness which were treated on Table 4 were much worse than those previously treated.

The air decompression tables were inefficient because the major cause of the symptoms to begin with—nitrogen bubbles—were only reduced in size, and continued treatment actually added more nitrogen to the patient's tissues. Since one of the objects of treatment in the bends syndrome was absent in using the air treatment tables, i.e., the removal of nitrogen, oxygen suggested itself as an alternative.

However, oxygen cannot be used at great depths and indeed, 66 ft appears to be about the absolute limit for reasons of oxygen toxicity. Nevertheless, Yarbrough and Behnke tested oxygen treatment of decompression sickness in 1939 and suggested the use of oxygen at 60 ft, but after an initial 30 minutes of breathing air at 165 ft.[79] Dr. Edgar End, working in Milwaukee, Wisconsin, in 1947 began to routinely treat divers and tunnel workers stricken with bends with 100% oxygen by mask at a pressure of 30 lb for one hour without using a preliminary deeper excursion. His results were generally excellent, but he did not publish his findings, which represented experience with about 250 cases.[31]

TABLE 25–3.
Air Recompression Tables 1 Through 4*

STOPS	BENDS—PAIN ONLY		SERIOUS SYMPTOMS
Rate of descent—25 ft/min Rate of ascent—1 min between stops	Pain relieved at depths less than 66 ft Use Table 1A if O_2 is not available	Pain relieved at depths greater than 66 ft Use Table 2A if O_2 is not available If pain does not improve within 30 min at 165 ft, the case probably is not bends. Decompress on Table 2 or 2A	Serious symptoms include any one of the following: 1. Unconsciousness 2. Convulsions 3. Weakness or inability to use arms or legs 4. Air embolism 5. Any visual disturbances 6. Dizziness 7. Loss of speech or hearing 8. Severe shortness of breath or chokes 9. Bends occurring while still under pressure Symptoms relieved in 30 min at 165 ft, use Table 3; if not relieved, use Table 4.

POUNDS	FEET	TABLE 1†	TABLE 1A	TABLE 2	TABLE 2A	TABLE 3	TABLE 4
73.4	165			30 (air)	30 (air)	30 (air)	30 to 120 (air)
62.3	140			12 (air)	12 (air)	12 (air)	30 (air)
53.4	120			12 (air)	12 (air)	12 (air)	30 (air)
44.5	100	30 (air)	30 (air)	12 (air)	12 (air)	12 (air)	30 (air)
35.6	80	12 (air)	12 (air)	12 (air)	12 (air)	12 (air)	30 (air)
26.7	60	30 (O_2)	30 (air)	30 (O_2)	30 (air)	30 (O_2) or (air)	6 hr (air)
22.3	50	30 (O_2)	30 (air)	30 (O_2)	30 (air)	30 (O_2) or (air)	6 hr (air)
17.8	40	30 (O_2)	30 (air)	30 (O_2)	30 (air)	30 (O_2) or (air)	6 hr (air)
13.4	30	5 (O_2) (30 ft to surface)	60 (air)	60 (O_2)	2 hr (air)	12 hr (air)	First 11 hr (air) Then 1 hr (O_2) or (air)
8.9	20		60 (air)	5 (O_2) (20 ft to surface)	2 hr (air)	2 hr (air)	First 1 hr (air) Then 1 hr (O_2) or (air)
4.5	10		2 hr (air)		4 hr (air)	2 hr (air)	First 1 hr (air) Then 1 hr (O_2) or (air)
	Surface		1 min (air)		1 min (air)	1 min (air)	1 min (O_2)

*From *U.S. Navy Diving Manual,* Navships 0994-001-9010. Washington, DC, Navy Dept, Supt of Doctors, US Government Printing Office, 1970. These tables are now largely of historical interest.
†Time at all stops in minutes unless otherwise indicated.

The U.S. Navy Experimental Diving Unit again began researching the concept of oxygen treatment in 1963 under the direction of M. W. Goodman and R. D. Workman.[35] After two years of experimentation, two new treatment tables using oxygen at less than 3 ATA were developed. These were accepted by the U.S. Navy in August of 1967 and labeled Tables 5 and 6 (Table 25–4). The former is a shorter 135-minute schedule and is for type 1 or "pain only" bends. The latter is for pain that does not disappear within ten minutes at 60 ft on oxygen and for serious symptoms and recurrences. It is 285 minutes in length. In extremely serious cases, Table 6 can be lengthened by adding an additional 20-minute oxygen period at 60 ft, or another hour of oxygen at 30 ft, or both. If the table is lengthened or constitutes a repetitive exposure for the inside tender, he must breathe oxygen for the final 30 minutes of the table.

The disadvantages of oxygen treatment must be mentioned, however. Oxygen is toxic under pressure both to the lungs and to the central nervous system. Prolonged oxygen breathing can produce atelectasis, decreased vital capacity, and chest pain. Pathologically, a pneumonitis develops. Central nervous system toxicity with convulsions is a possibility. The interval before any of these symptoms develop is called the "latent period," and therefore, oxygen therapy must be interrupted or halted while the patient is still well within the latent period for oxygen toxicity.

Because the latent period is shortened the higher one raises the pressure, useful exposures must be limited to about 3 ATA. At this pressure, bubbles are reduced only to one third of their original size, as opposed to one sixth their original size at 165 ft while breathing air.

Oxygen under pressure constitutes a fire hazard. Even at at-

TABLE 25–4.

Oxygen Treatment Tables 5 and 6 for Treatment of Decompression Sickness and Table 6A for Treatment of Air Embolism*

STOPS	BENDS—PAIN ONLY			SERIOUS SYMPTOMS AND AIR EMBOLISM					
†	Pain relieved within 10 min at 60 ft If any pain persists after 10 min at 60 ft, use Table 6			Pain relieved after 10 min at 60 ft Serious symptoms include any one of the following: 1. Unconsciousness 2. Nervous system symptoms 3. Bends under pressure			Treatment of air embolism if symptoms moderate to a major extent within 30 min at 60 ft. If symptoms persist, use Table 4		
	TABLE 5‡			TABLE 6‡			TABLE 6A§‖		
DEPTH (FT)	TIME (MINS)	BREATHING MEDIA	TOTAL ELAPSED TIME (MINS)	TIME (MINS)	BREATHING MEDIA	TOTAL ELAPSED TIME (MINS)	TIME (MINS)	BREATHING MEDIA	TOTAL ELAPSED TIME (MINS)
165							30	Air	30
165 to 60							4	Air	34
60				20	O_2	20	20	O_2	54
60				5	Air	25	5	Air	59
60				20	O_2	45	20	O_2	79
60	20	O_2	20	5	Air	50	5	Air	84
60	5	Air	25	20	O_2	70	20	O_2	104
60	20	O_2	45	5	Air	75	5	Air	109
60 to 30	30	O_2	75	30	O_2	105	30	O_2	139
30				15	Air	120	15	Air	154
30	5	Air	80	60	O_2	180	60	O_2	214
30	20	O_2	100	15	Air	195	15	Air	229
30	5	Air	105	60	O_2	255	60	O_2	289
30 to 0	30	O_2	135	30	O_2	285	30	O_2	319

*From *U.S. Navy Diving Manual–1970.*

†The rate of ascent is 1 ft/min. Do not compensate for slowing of the rate by subsequent acceleration. Do compensate if the rate is exceeded. If necessary, halt ascent and hold depth while ventilating the chamber.

‡The time at 60 ft begins on arrival at 60 ft. The patient should be on oxygen from the surface.

§The time at 165 ft is total bottom time and includes the time from the surface.

‖Total time will vary as a function of this stop. The medical attendant should take enough time to accomplish a thorough physical examination, because the ensuing treatment is based on the patient's physical status.

mospheric pressure, an increase of 7% oxygen in the air will double the burning rate. In the hands of untrained personnel and in surroundings where dirt, grease, or oil may have accumulated or where any combustible materials may be present, it is potentially very dangerous. Constant monitoring of the atmosphere is essential to detect oxygen buildup before it reaches levels where a conflagration can develop without warning. One must never let the oxygen concentration exceed 23% in the chamber air.

The above limitations are quite real, but clinical experience demonstrates that even with these disadvantages, oxygen treatment at 60 ft (2.8 ATA) has proven much more efficacious than the old air Tables 1 through 4, especially in the more serious cases.

Severe decompression sickness, especially stemming from nonstandard dives, were often the very ones used in field-testing the new tables. By Nov. 15, 1965, a series had been amassed of 50 cases treated with adequate oxygen recompression at depths no greater than 60 ft. The failure rate for all initial recompressions in the experimental group was only 2%, as compared with 26.7% for Tables 1 through 4 in the year 1964. The failure rate in the serious-symptom or the type-2 cases was only 3.6% in the oxygen-treated group, as compared to 47.1% in the old tables. In comparing the data, the experimental caseload was composed of older divers who had been exposed to longer bottom time durations at deeper depths. The statistical validity of the results of treatment with the new tables as analyzed using the Fisher Test, the Chi-square estimation, and the Spearman rank correlation. The analysis showed the results to be statistically valid.[35] Thus, the new oxygen tables not only proved to be more efficient but tended to prevent recurrences which were even more time-consuming. An additional advantage of the new tables in terms of man-power management is that the inside tender can lock out with a minimum of decompression at any time. On the old tables, the inside tender was committed for the duration of the table.

Among the theoretical considerations that give the oxygen tables an advantage over Tables 1 through 4 are that at depths of 165 ft, where bubble size is reduced at the cost of additional inert gas uptake in tissue surrounding the bubble, persistent bubbles must grow in size to maintain both osmotic and dynamic equilibrium. This is based on Wyman's expression for rate of change of bubble radius based on the general gas law and Fick's first law of diffusion.[35] In addition, it must be noted that the rate of diffusion of gas from a bubble is dependent on its surface area. Compressing a bubble beyond one third of its original volume necessarily reduces its surface area.

Of equal importance is the tissue oxygenation that occurs. Tissues rendered hypoxic due to bubble embolus-induced ischemia are restored to function quickly under hyperbaric oxygen. With tissues adequately oxygenated, bubble shrinkage and immediate resolution are not overriding concerns. Another important point to remember is that high oxygen partial pressure decreases blood sludging, a major component of decompression sickness. Thus, it has become apparent that the most efficient therapeutic recompression tables currently in existence are the U.S. Navy Tables 5 and 6. At least these are the only tables that have statistical backing for their effectiveness.

There are some instances, however, in which low-pressure oxygen treatment cannot be used. There are cases where decompression sickness develops during gradual decompression following saturation diving at depths well in excess of 60 ft and in cases of accidental blow-up from depths greater than about 80 ft. In the latter case, especially if that diver has been on the bottom more than a few minutes, he must be immediately recompressed to his depth of relief, which will probably exceed his original working pressure. If blow-up occurs from a depth of greater than 165 ft, even U.S. Navy Table 4 will prove to be utterly inadequate. There are, unfortunately, well-documented cases where Table 4 was tried with fatal results in such circumstances.

In cases where decompression sickness develops during slow decompression from saturation work, the best technique[62] is to take the diver and the whole chamber complex back down 10–15 ft (3–5 m) and to enrich the oxygen content of his breathing gas delivered by mask. In enriching the oxygen mixture, one must be careful not to exceed critical oxygen toxicity limits. In the dry chamber, however, these limits are much greater than if the diver is immersed in water. The maximum enrichment of oxygen can be calculated by providing a mixture that is between 1.8 and 2.8 ATA oxygen partial pressure at the depth the patient is exposed for periods not exceeding 25 minutes. After 25 minutes of enriched oxygen breathing, the patient should breathe the chamber atmosphere for five minutes. Following relief and at least two periods of enriched oxygen breathing by *both* patient and tender, the diver may be again started on decompression at 1 ft/min to the original chamber depth or a scheduled stop, whichever comes first. If relief is not obtained in two oxygen periods, recompress a further 10–15 ft and continue enriched oxygen breathing for another couple of periods. Occasionally, recompression to depth of relief may be required. Do not continue decompression until the problem is under control.

In case of serious blow-up from depth between 80 and 165 ft after the diver has absorbed considerable quantities of nitrogen, recompression to at least 165 ft is indicated. The patient must be taken deeper if symptoms persist. However, if the patient becomes asymptomatic at 165 ft, decompression can be started on Table 3 or Table 4. Even if Table 4 is used, however, the *patient and inside tender* can be switched to Table 6 with all its extensions at 60 ft and decompression completed on oxygen. This takes only 11–12 hours instead of 38 hours and has proved quite satisfactory in my experience if the time at 165 ft is two hours or less. Helium-oxygen may be used instead of air at 165 ft, if available. I have used helium successfully in bends following air dives, even though the theoretical possibility exists that nitrogen bubbles might grow in size as helium diffuses into them. This has never proven to be a clinical problem, however. If both the inside tender and patient are breathing oxygen, it is sometimes advisable to have a third

TABLE 25–5.
Therapeutic Table COMEX 30

DEPTHS (M)	TIME (MIN)	GAS BREATHED: PATIENT	GAS BREATHED: ATTENDANT	TOTAL TIME (MIN)
30	40	50/50	Air	40
30 to 24	5	Air	Air	45
(Rate = 5 min/m)	25	50/50	Air	70
24	5	Air	Air	75
24	25	50/50	Air	100
24 to 18	5	Air	Air	105
(Rate = 5 min/m)	25	50/50	Air	130
18	5	Air	Air	135
18	25	O_2	Air	160
18	5	Air	Air	165
18	25	O_2	Air	190
18 to 12	5	Air	Air	195
(Rate = 5 min/m)	25	O_2	Air	220
12	10	Air	Air	230
12	45	O_2	Air	275
12	10	Air	Air	285
12	45	O_2	O_2	330
12	10	Air	Air	340
12	45	O_2	O_2	385
12	10	Air	Air	395
12 to surface	24	O_2	O_2	419
(Rate = 2 min/m)				

TABLE 25–6.
Therapeutic Table COMEX 30A: Only to Be Used Following a Hyperoxic Crisis or When Oxygen Is Not Available

DEPTHS (M)	TIME (MIN)	GAS BREATHED: PATIENT	GAS BREATHED: ATTENDANT	TOTAL TIME (MIN)
30	60	Air	Air	60
30 to 24				
(Rate = 1 min/m)	6	Air	Air	66
24 to 21				
(Rate = 20 min/m)	60	Air	Air	126
21 to 18				
(Rate = 22 min/m)	66	Air	Air	192
18 to 15				
(Rate = 24 min/m)	72	Air	Air	264
15 to 12				
(Rate = 26 min/m)	78	Air	Air	342
(2 tablets 5 mg valium on arrival at 12 m)				
12	10	Air	Air	352
12	40	O_2	O_2	392
12	10	Air	Air	402
12	40	O_2	O_2	442
12	10	Air	Air	452
12	40	O_2	O_2	492
12	5	Air	Air	497
12 to surface				
(Rate = 2 min/m)	24	O_2	O_2	521

person in the chamber breathing air in the event of sudden toxicity, i.e., a convulsion.

When a blow-up occurs from a depth greater than 165 ft, the diver should immediately be compressed to at least the depth of his original dive, and then after he is symptom-free or stable, he should be decompressed on a saturation table.

When the patient breathes helium-oxygen, it is easier to determine resolution of symptoms, since nitrogen narcosis will not mask persistent pain or neurologic signs. There is no guarantee that a saturation table will not produce decompression sickness at the shallower end, but on the other hand, liberal use of oxygen breathing after the 60-ft level has been reached may enable one to materially reduce the risk and manage symptoms if they recur.

Difficult Cases

For unusually difficult cases of decompression sickness that do not respond to Table 6, there are other alternatives, such as the use of COMEX Table 30 and 30a (Tables 25–5 and 25–6) or air saturation from 60 ft. The flow chart in Figure 25–5 was developed at the Undersea Medical Society Workshop on Treatment of Serious Decompression Sickness and Air Embolism at Duke University in 1979.[20] Although the principles of the flow chart are sound, the chart was not reproduced in the report, since it was believed people would feel obliged to follow it slavishly, considering it the only acceptable method. This is not the intent of the chart; its only purpose is to suggest *possible* alternatives.

Drug Therapy

In recent years, the art of treating decompression sickness has progressed beyond simply turning a valve and applying pressure with the patient breathing oxygen. There are numerous medical adjuncts to therapy which are very helpful. Since decompression sickness is initiated by bubble formation, gross hematologic

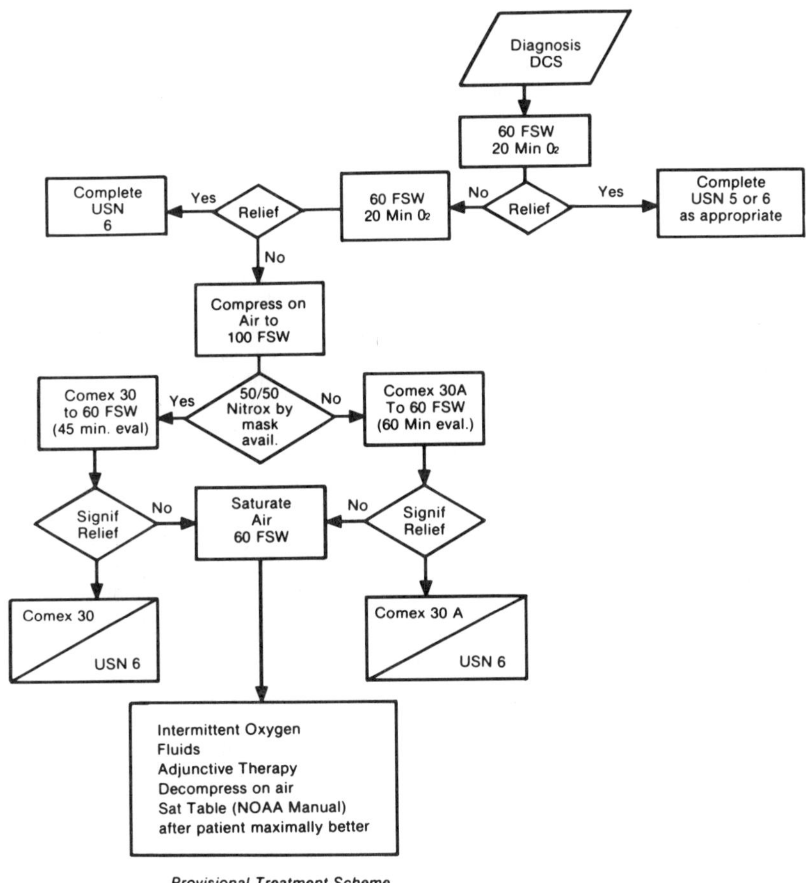

FIG 25–5.
Flow chart for treating decompression sickness, developed at the Undersea Medical Society Workshop on Treatment of Serious Decompression Sickness and Air Embolism, Duke University, 1979.

changes usually occur, consisting of platelet aggregation and blood sludging.

Philp[50] has demonstrated that heparin exerts a lipemia-clearing effect in obese rats and protects them from decompression sickness. Cockett[19] has also found in dogs that after severe decompression, a heparinized group survived, whereas an unheparinized control group died. Reeves and Workman, also in dog studies, found no demonstrable advantage to giving heparin to dogs with mild to moderate bends.[53] In severe cases, however, some clinicians feel that heparin may be indicated, especially in the presence of decompression sickness shock. A suggested dosage is 7,500 units of heparin intravenously to be followed by 5,000-unit doses at intervals later if necessary. When dealing with decompression sickness shock, enormous quantities of plasma are lost into the tissues from the vascular bed. I treated one such case where I had to administer 5½ L of plasma, saline, and other plasma expanders within the first eight hours to keep up with the plasma loss.[39] If the patient shows signs of shock, early digitalization has been helpful in my experience. Aminophylline appears to have little effect in "chokes" due to bends.

A word of caution is appropriate here regarding the use of medications in the chamber. Glass vials appear to withstand pressures up to 165 ft quite satisfactorily, but if forced to administer drugs to a diver who is saturated at a much deeper depth, implosion may result. It is suggested that all intravenous fluid bottles have a needle inserted into the stopper before pressurization is begun. During decompression, glass intravenous bottles that are not specially vented are a danger, since the entire contents of the intravenous bottle will be driven into the patient followed by a bolus or air as the gas above the fluid expands. Use only plastic bags for intravenous solutions. Most drugs can be given as usual under hyperbaric conditions without any particular change in their efficacy.

Another useful trick in the treatment of bends, which has been semihumorously termed "a Black Art" by Bennett, is the use of the well-inflated blood pressure cuff. This was used by Edgar End for many years. If, for example, you are treating a diver or caisson worker for a mild case of "pain only" or type 1 decompression sickness after a supposed adequate decompression schedule and only one sore spot persists in a knee or elbow, you may apply the blood pressure cuff over the sore spot and rapidly pump it up to 300 mm Hg, then immediately release it. Even after the cuff is removed, the pain may have permanently vanished and the patient will have complete relief. This is successful about 50% of the time, but sometimes either no relief is afforded or the sore spot moves either proximally or distally and more "cuff treatment" provides no further relief. It is worth trying in any case where the circumstances suggest it.

Signs and Symptoms

One of the most common errors in treating pressure-related diving accidents is that the physician fails to recognize the seriousness of the condition or misses important symptoms and signs. For example, a diver may fail to report an area of numbness or tingling in a leg but simply emphasizes that he has pain in the knee. If numbness or tingling are present, this indicates a spinal cord lesion and would mean that the patient should be treated on Table 6 even if he obtained relief within the first five minutes at 60 ft breathing oxygen. Thus, it is useful to refer to a checklist, since in an emergency situation, when much is going on, it is easy to forget to check all possibilities. Table 25–7 is a checklist compiled by Dick Clarke, an experienced diving medical technician, for use by a layman or physician in checking on the condition of a diver before and during recompression therapy. This checklist should be posted under a plastic cover both inside and outside the chamber.

A note I would add to the checklist is: never decompress a diver undergoing treatment while he is asleep. He may wake up later complaining of pain, and one will not know at what depth it started. Also, even if a man says he has complete relief of pain or other symptoms, have him walk the length of the chamber before decompressing.

There is occasionally a question as to whether a diver has bends or not. Mild symptoms of decompression sickness are often referred to as "air pains" or as the British call them, "niggles." Sometimes a diver or caisson worker may report he "feels the bubbles running," but has no particular discomfort—I have experienced the latter and although it is a vague term, is quite descriptive. Air pains or "niggles" that persist longer than 30 minutes

TABLE 25–7.

Recompression Chamber Checklist for Suspected Decompression Sickness/Air Embolism (To Be Used Prior to Treatment, for Relief of Symptoms, and Prior to Leaving and Upon Arrival At Stops)

I. Questions to ask the patient
   A. Is there any pain? Where and how severe?
      1. Is it sore to touch or pressure?
      2. Are there bruise marks in the area?
      3. Is the pain changed by motion?
   B. Any weakness, numbness or other peculiar sensations? Check his strength and compare his right side with his left by
      1. Normal hand grip
      2. Pushing and pulling strongly with both arms
      3. His ability to do deep knee bends
   C. Can the patient see clearly?
      1. Can he read a sentence from this checklist?
      2. Can he see a distant object?
      3. Are the pupils normal size and equal?
      4. Do the pupils close down when you shine a light in his eyes?
      5. Can he follow an object around normally with his eyes?

II. Appearance of the patient
   A. Can the patient walk normally? Is there any limping or staggering? Does he appear clumsy?
   B. Is his speech clear and sensible? Is there any alteration from his normal pitch?
   C. Can the patient keep his balance, with his eyes closed and his feet together?
   D. Does he appear mentally clear?
   E. Does he hear clearly?
   F. Is there any swelling around the base of the neck? If so, does it feel spongy?
   G. Is the Babinski reflex present or absent?

Should you suspect the presence of a serious symptom during this examination, a central nervous system disorder, unconsciousness/collapse, or the development of a symptom under pressure, discontinue the checklist and *recompress immediately.*

if mild. Often the niggles disappear within minutes of onset, and these, then, are not worth treating.

If a person surfaces from a dive or exposure to compressed air and complains of pain but says it might be due to a bruise or known sprain, the doctor is in a dilemma. If it is bends, treatment is mandatory; but if it is not, a lot of time will be wasted on Table 6 or some other schedule.

The correct procedure in this case is the "test of pressure." This used to be 100 ft on compressed air, but I prefer 20 minutes of oxygen at 60 ft. If, after breathing oxygen by mask at 60 ft for 20 minutes the pain is unchanged in *intensity, nature, position,* or *quality*, it is probably safe to assume one is not dealing with bends and proceed with decompression straight to the surface. Should the pain intensify or turn out to be true bends later, nothing has been lost and no more iatrogenic nitrogen has been introduced into the patient.

There is a case on record[69] of a civilian making multiple dives in a single day with no decompression and who felt pain at the end of the day. He handled this fairly successfully with copious amounts of alcohol but felt worse again the following day. On the third day, still feeling out of sorts, he consulted a physician who said he had a virus and prescribed aspirin. Still not feeling better, he saw a second physician who took a chest film, gave the same diagnosis, noted a temperature of 101° and prescribed penicillin. Then a friend suggested it might be bends and referred the patient to a nearby naval base. There, the patient complained of lower-back pain, partially relieved by moving around, and still had a temperature. He was examined by three submarine medical officers who all agreed the man did not have bends, but nevertheless, gave him a "test of pressure" because he had taken the trouble to come to the base. At pressure, his symptoms were dramatically relieved and his temperature returned to normal.

TREATMENT OF AIR EMBOLISM

In diving and compressed-air work, cerebral air embolism is caused by overdistention of the lungs, with subsequent rupture and passage of the gas into the pulmonary veins. From there the gas is carried to the left heart and then pumped directly into the brain. Cerebral air embolism may also occur as a result of air being introduced into the carotid arteries or aorta during surgery. In any event, the result is similar and the treatment the same: immediate recompression to 6 ATA or 165 ft. In treating air embolism secondary to diving, the victim will most commonly be a Scuba diver. Be certain that the patient does not have a pneumothorax, which can be a concomitant with rupture of the lungs. This will not immediately cause a problem during compression, but during decompression, if a tension pneumothorax has developed, the patient's respiratory embarrassment will be severe. If this is the case, a Claggett needle or McSwain dart should be inserted into the thoracic cavity and air evacuated using a syringe with a three-way stopcock. A Heimlich valve or a check valve fashioned from a condom can be attached, at a minimum. In the event one is treating cerebral air embolism secondary to surgery, if thoracotomy has been performed, the chest tube should have constant suction applied over a 20-cm water seal during the entire stay in the chamber. If lung rupture has resulted *only* in mediastinal emphysema, with or without pneumopericardium, the mediastinal air will usually be resorbed within a few days and chamber treatment is not indicated.

Cerebral air embolism due to ascending with a closed glottis has been recognized as an entity different from central nervous system decompression sickness only since the 1930s, when submarine escape began to be widely taught. When Tables 1 through 4 were promulgated in 1945, recompression therapy for cerebral air embolism always was undertaken using Table 3 or Table 4 because of the obvious central nervous system involvement. This was despite the fact that the etiology of cerebral air embolism was quite different from that of decompression sickness. Thus, 20–38 hours were wasted in the chamber after initial recompression to 165 ft.

In the middle 1960s, Waite became disillusioned with the results of treating air embolism patients with Table 4[75] and carried out a series of dog experiments in which he exposed the surface of the brain through plastic calvaria and then embolized the dogs by injecting air into their carotid arteries. The bubbles of air could plainly be seen circulating on the surface of the brain and when recompressed immediately, the bubbles were observed to disappear between 3 and 4 ATA. Waite took an experimental group of embolized dogs to 165 ft (50 m) and then immediately decompressed them on the standard navy air decompression table for ten minutes exposure at 170 ft. This "bounce dive" resulted in the amelioration of all symptoms of air embolism in the experimental group. The control group, which had not been recompressed, was left with severe neurologic residua if they survived. Waite was thus convinced that the long, slow decompressions required on Tables 3 and 4 were unnecessary in the treatment of air embolism, and the U.S. Navy Department was pursuaded to promulgate special air embolism tables labeled 5A and 6A (see Table 25–3) which required only a brief 15–30-minute stop at 165 ft, followed by decompression over four minutes to 60 ft. and then, continued treatment on the Low Pressure Oxygen Tables promulgated at the same time.[74] Table 5A has been abandoned, as it resulted in too many recurrences. Therefore, it is not included here.

In my experience, Waite's original hypothesis that Table 4 is unnecessary has been amply borne out. In our treatment of several cases of air embolism, some which were received after much delay, excellent results were achieved using only 9–30-minute bottom times at 165 ft followed by low-pressure oxygen treatment.[37] The reason for this is that once circulation has been reestablished, remaining for long periods at pressure probably has little further to offer.

It is advisable when transporting the patient to the chamber to place him in the Trendelenburg position, since the hydrostatic forces generated by the head-down position tend to dilate both the arterial and the venous sides of the circulation and enable bubbles to pass more freely through the capillaries. Atkinson showed that bubbles disappear in the direction of arterial flow.[4] Clinically, patients have been seen to wake up in the head down position even before pressurization.[37, 42] If, for some reason, a patient is taken to 165 ft while suffering from air embolism, and his condition is serious but still improving after 30 minutes at 6 ATA, one may still avoid the use of Table 4 by remaining at depth for up to two hours and then decompressing on the U.S. Navy Exceptional Exposure Air Tables to a depth of 60 ft. At this point, Table 6 is instituted, with both the doctor and the patient breathing oxygen to clear the iatrogenically introduced nitrogen.

The U.S. Navy Exceptional Exposure Air Tables are notoriously inadequate when used in their entirety, but if used only at the deeper stops, they do not appear to cause bends if oxygen is subsequently used shallower than 60 ft. Nemiroff [48] successfully used this schedule after having been exposed at 165 ft for 101 minutes. His embolism patient at that time had a dense right hemianopsia which failed to clear with pressurization alone, and it was decided to bring him to 60 ft for hyperbaric oxygen treatment. Decompression from 165 ft was in accordance with the Exceptional Exposure Air Table, which requires the use of the 170-ft-for-two-hour schedule. The first stop is 80 ft for two minutes, according to the schedule, but Nemiroff doubled the time at this stop. He then proceeded to 70 ft for ten minutes; and then, at 60 ft, shifted to hyperbaric oxygen. Within five minutes of reaching 60 ft and starting oxygen, the hemianopsia began to clear dramatically. The patient was asymptomatic on completion of the oxygen table.

In postsurgical patients, the after effects of anesthesia will mask any immediate improvement seen at 165 ft, and so, therefore, prolonging the stay beyond 15 minutes to a half hour is not warranted. The author has had excellent results in several cases treated with only brief exposures at 6 ATA.

If helium-oxygen is available, its use is suggested at 165 ft. Since approximately 79% of the patient's intracranial bubbles consist of nitrogen, it would seem foolish to add more nitrogen to the patient's tissues. Helium-oxygen provides a zero gradient for the nitrogen in the patient's intravascular bubbles to work against and probably speeds their elimination. But helium may theoretically diffuse into existing nitrogen bubbles faster than nitrogen can diffuse out, so that, theoretically, helium-oxygen could make bubbles grow in size if circulation is not reestablished. However, despite theoretical considerations, the author has encountered no difficulties with helium-oxygen in treating these patients. If the patient has breathed 80%-20% helium-oxygen for periods up to 40 minutes at 165 ft, decompression may be accomplished over a four-minute period to 60 ft without danger. However, if the patient remains at 165 ft for up to two hours, a seven-minute stop at 70 ft will be required before he can be brought to 60 ft for hyperbaric treatment with low pressure oxygen. If 50%-50% helium-oxygen is used at 6 ATA, no decompression stops will be required for 60 ft. In such case, this gas should be alternated with 80%-20% helium-oxygen for five minutes at 25-minute intervals to avoid oxygen toxicity.

Steroids were traditionally used liberally in the treatment of cerebral air embolism and I have used dexamethazone (Decadron) 20–40 mg intravenously upon arrival at the 30-foot stop. Postsurgical patients may already have had large doses of steroids when received at the chamber. Steroids may be continued for 48–72 hours and then may be discontinued without tapering. There is mounting evidence, however, that steroids may not be of value in embolism or other neurosurgical conditions. If symptoms remain in air embolism, and cerebral edema is suspected, daily retreatment with hyperbaric oxygen may be advisable over the following few days.

In any case, when one is dealing purely with a case of air embolism, Table IV is to be avoided, since it is an anachronism and never was developed for the treatment of this disorder. If a chamber capable of 6 ATA is not available, treatment with 100% oxygen at 3 ATA in the monoplace chamber may prove to be adequate alone.

UNDERWATER BLAST INJURY

Trauma due to an explosion is much more serious for a diver in the water than for a person exposed to a similar charge exploding at a like distance in air. On July 30, 1918, a diver working in the Hudson River 20 miles from Jersey City, suddenly asked to be hauled to the surface and inquired of his tender, "What gave me that terrible knock?" The tender on the surface was puzzled and completely unaware that anything unusual had happened. However, the newspapers the following day carried the headline that the Black Tom Ammunition Depot had exploded and 11 ships loaded with ammunition in the harbor had been destroyed. Thus, shock waves can travel great distances in water, while the force of a large explosion will be dissipated quickly in the air.

The pressure pulse of an underwater blast consists of an almost instantaneous rise to a maximum followed by a much more gradual falling off of pressure, the whole pulse lasting a few milliseconds. The pulse travels at about the speed of sound in water or 5,000 ft/sec. The smaller the charge, the shorter the pulse length. Because of the tremendous pressures in the immediate area of the charge, the shock wave may travel at varying speeds. Only at distances greater than 20 times the lineal dimensions of the charge does the wave travel at an orderly 5,000 ft/sec. The diver may be exposed to two impulses if he is between the surface and the bottom. The first one is direct, the second one from the reflection off the bottom. Thus, there can be two pulses that will damage tissues. Obviously, this situation is worse in shallow water with rock bottom, since a soft bottom can completely absorb the reflected impulse. When the sum of the direct and reflected pulse exceeds the critical value for the surface tension of water, the water surface breaks and the top layer is forced into the air or shredded to form the "dome." Further layers are torn off as spray while the remaining pulse pressure is spent. While this is observed on the surface, a diver submerged in the water even at some distance from the charge might sustain a positive pressure pulse and then, a pulse in a negative direction reflected back from the surface "dome." The air-water interface is elastic, however, and somewhat attenuates the reflected negative wave.

A depth charge, for example, when exploded, produces a gas bubble with a pressure of the order of 100,000 ATA. On the surface, a dome instantly appears, with shredding of the water-air interface. Later, as the gas bubble and explosion products themselves are forced up, the dramatic "plume" appears. The plume does little damage although it is spectacular in appearance.

The effects on the body vary depending on the distance from the charge and the depth of immersion. A completely submerged limb is subjected to little if any damage, since there is no gas-tissue interface. The tissues behave like the surrounding water, and no distortion is seen as the pulses pass through them. However, a limb that is partially submerged in water will be affected by direct blast pulses striking it at different times and pulses reflected from the surface. The pulse will be longest for the most deeply submerged part; for example, the foot and very short at the knee. This is a nonuniform application of pressure that tends to cause damage by squeezing the tissues upward.

The worst situation occurs when the whole body is submerged. The body has hollow, gas-filled organs—the sinuses, lungs, and gut. These provide gas-tissue interfaces. When the pulse passes, shredding occurs at the gas-tissue interface such as that occurring at the "dome" on the surface. Large displacements occur. A diver is best protected if he is wearing the deep-sea rig, and it is ballooned out at least to his waist. Then the shock wave will cause the shredding force to occur at the surface of the rig rather than directly on his lungs and gut.

The observed injuries from underwater blast fit well with the theories. The air- or gas-containing viscera are most damaged. The lungs are usually least damaged, and the damage to them is less likely to be fatal. The victim will usually have simple hemoptysis, but severe hemorrhage can occur. Abdominal injuries are the most severe, and these range from retro- and subperitoneal hemorrhage to rupture of the gut, usually on the antimesenteric side.

The most common site of injury is the lower abdomen, with the terminal loop of ileum usually involved. The second most common site is the cecum on the outer side just lateral to the longitudinal band. Gut perforations can seal over with omentum and simulate appendiceal abscess three or four days after the injury. Anyone who has been exposed to an underwater blast should be carefully watched for developing signs of an acute abdomen.

DYSBARIC OSTEONECROSIS OF THE BONE IN DIVERS AND COMPRESSED-AIR WORKERS

Dysbaric osteonecrosis, also known as aseptic necrosis or avascular necrosis, is a process whereby healthy bone breaks down and is destroyed due to lack of blood supply. This disease was first reported in compressed-air workers in 1912 by Bornstein and Plate.[14] The first description of it in divers appeared in the German literature in 1942. The overwhelming evidence points to inadequate decompression as the underlying factor.

It is presumed that bone, although supplied by nutrient vessels, does not have a large collateral circulation. If, during decompression, bubbles are formed in the veins which drain blood from the bone, or platelet aggregation occasioned by the formation of bubbles blocks some of the capillaries and veins, the flow through these vessels is stopped. Behind where the bubbles or emboli are lodged, the blood stagnates and sludges. If this blockage lasts for 12 hours or longer, all of the osteoblasts behind the blockaded point die from lack of oxygen and nourishment. When this occurs, nothing is seen on the x-ray study for a period of three to four months at a minimum. Then, the first changes that are noted are blurring of the trabeculae and a hazy thickening called "creeping substitution" or "creeping apposition" as used by Barnes.[5] The earliest signs that are seen on x-ray are not actually bone destruction but an attempt on the part of the body to infiltrate new bone into the affected part to strengthen an area which has become devoid of living bone cells.

If the area of bone destruction is in the shaft of a long bone, such as the femur, there is little to worry about. Most of these shaft lesions consist of saponified or calcified fat. Pathologic fractures due to lesions in the shafts of long bones do not occur.

If, however, the area of bone destruction happens to lie near the articular surface of a joint instead of the shaft, quite a different problem emerges. Here, when daily momentary loads that may be in excess of 300 lb are applied to the dead joint surface as the victim walks or manipulates heavy objects, the bone breaks down and begins to fragment, often with sequestrum formation. In such cases, there is no time for creeping substitution to take place, and once the articular margin of the joint has been compromised, its inevitable destruction occurs simply through the movements of the joint necessitated by daily living. It appears to be the severity of the insult that determines whether or not the joints or the shafts will be affected; the production of articular lesions seem to require a more severe decompression stress. The joints that most commonly cause trouble are the shoulder and hip joints. The wrists, ankles, and elbows have not been shown to be affected by aseptic necrosis due to occupational exposure to compressed air. An exception is a single report by El Ghawabi et al., who noted gross changes of aseptic necrosis in these joints and the knees among Egyptian tunnel workers engaged in construction under the River Nile.[26] However, El Ghawabi did not have a control group for comparison, so there is no way of knowing if other factors, such as high local incidence of schistosomiasis, may have played a role. In over 10,000 records of compressed-air workers employed in the British Isles, no lesions have been discovered in the ankles, wrists, or elbows. The knees are only rarely involved in aseptic destruction; three cases have been reported in the world literature in addition to the Egyptian report. Two of these cases were found in Milwaukee, Wisconsin.[47]

It is not known with certainty how much exposure is necessary to initiate aseptic necrosis in a given compressed-air worker or diver, but a single exposure followed by improper decompression from a pressure of 55 lb has been demonstrated to produce the disease. When the British submarine *Poseidon* sank in 1931 in the South China Sea at a depth of 125 ft, five men subsequently escaped. These five men were exposed to pressures which gradually approached 125 ft over a two- to three-hour period. Twelve years later, three out of the five survivors were found to have aseptic necrosis when surveyed in England by James.[36]

According to statistics maintained by the British Central Decompression Sickness Registry for caisson workers, the lowest pressure known to cause aseptic necrosis is 17 psig or the equivalent of 38 ft of seawater. The patient in question, a caisson worker, worked five shifts of eight hours at that pressure, coming directly to the surface at the conclusion of each shift. The patient did not undergo a decompression period, since this was not required under the 1958 British Tunnel Code.

Again, in commercial tunnel experience, the shortest experience known to produce bone necrosis has been two exposures on different days of two and one half and four and one half hours to a pressure of 35 psig or the equivalent of 79 ft of seawater. Two years after this exposure, both hip joints in the individual cited were affected. Again, decompression had been according to the 1958 British Tunnel Code, which called for 58 minutes and 91 minutes decompression for each shift respectively.

Thus, if British tunnel experience is applied to diving, a diver working at 38 ft all day in a harbor, using surface-supplied equipment, might not take any decompression and, accordingly, could be susceptible. If he were doing a simple job such as cutting off sheet piling, he would normally surface for lunch and then again at the end of the day, providing two embolizations of bubbles.

Increasing evidence implicates platelet and fat agglutination around the bubbles formed during decompression as being an important factor in producing the solid emboli which can permanently block the microcirculation.

One of the problems with aseptic necrosis in compressed-air workers or divers is that there may be a long period of delay before the disease becomes manifest on x-ray film. We do not have enough data yet to say what the longest interval is between exposure to compressed air or helium and the subsequent development of bone disease. However, drawing on experience from trauma and the use of systemic steroids as causes of aseptic necrosis, periods up to five years before the onset of roentgenologic evidence have been documented.

Divers who would be most apt to get aseptic necrosis are the ones who make so-called nonstandard dives. This means divers who habitually short themselves on decompression or do not adhere to recognized standard tables. The U.S. Navy undertook a formal survey of its divers and found several substantiated cases of aseptic necrosis. Most were only shaft lesions, however, chiefly in men who had done deep air or saturation diving. After a very complete survey, a 9% incidence of aseptic necrosis diagnosable by x-ray was found in Royal Navy divers. This does not mean that 9% of the divers surveyed were incapacitated, since in the Royal Navy series all of the lesions were shaft lesions, with the articular surface of the humeral head involved in only one case. Again, the Royal Navy divers who were found to have x-ray evidence of the disease had for the most part been engaged in deep experimental air diving or in helium saturation work.

Tunnel workers and caisson workers have for years followed schedules for decompression which were much shorter than the U.S. Navy and British Admiralty tables, and the incidence of aseptic necrosis in these people has been high: up to 35% in Milwaukee among workers following a modification of the New York decompression tables of 1922. On the other hand, compressed-air workers using the Washington State Decompression Tables for Tunnels and Caissons developed in 1963 showed a low incidence of the disease over the first 12 years of the tables' use.[60] These tables became the U.S. Federal OSHA Standard in 1971.

Sealey surveyed 86 workers who had used the OSHA table in Seattle at pressures up to 34 psig ten years previously and found a 6% incidence of shaft lesions.[60] I found, however, that when these tables were used in Milwaukee at pressures up to 43 psig, 33% of the men were affected, most with severe juxta-articular lesions.

As a result of these findings, our laboratory, working with Peter Edel of New Orleans, developed and tested new oxygen decompression tables (1983) and these now await approval by OSHA.

At this writing, there are not enough data to indicate what the incidence is among persons engaged in commercial helium saturation diving, but the disease has been found among commercial helium divers in the Gulf of Mexico and the North Sea.

So far, it has not been possible to demonstrate any direct relationship between the development of aseptic necrosis and a history of attacks of decompression sickness. The site of frequent attacks of bends bears no relationship to the area of the body later found to be involved in aseptic necrosis. Many individuals found to have aseptic necrosis never have had to request therapeutic recompression for decompression sickness. One reason for this, of course, is that there are a lot of phlegmatic individuals in the diving and compressed-air industry who elect to "walk off" symptoms of decompression sickness or treat them at home with the classic remedy of aspirin and a few stiff shots of whiskey. In other cases, it is possible that in divers or compressed-air workers with high pain thresholds, bubbles and microthrombi may be at work in their bones even though they do not have discomfort in their muscles and joints.

There are some 15–20 other diseases that can cause aseptic necrosis of the bone, and these must be ruled out in trying to determine whether or not the necrosis has been produced from working under increased ambient pressure. Common among these other conditions are chronic alcoholism; pancreatitis, which often accompanies alcoholism; sickle cell anemia trait, which affects 12%–15% of American blacks, but is occasionally found in white people; and a smaller number of more exotic diseases. However, if aseptic necrosis develops in a person who has been exposed to compressed air or helium, there must be strong evidence that the signs of the disease were present on x-ray before occupational exposure was undertaken to negate responsibility under the workers' compensation and Maritime laws. Most companies require that preemployment x-rays be done of the shoulders, hips, and knees in their divers and compressed-air workers, that special x-ray techniques be used, and that the films be carefully interpreted by experts intimately familiar with the early signs of the disease. These x-ray studies are then repeated at yearly intervals. Because of the high insurance premiums resulting from aseptic necrosis claims, companies are finding it necessary to go to the expense of taking x-rays even though it is not required as yet by federal law in the United States. As a responsible physician, one must insist on it.

Newer techniques for detecting aseptic necrosis early, or determining its activity if it is already present, have become available. The use of bone-seeking radioactive isotopes that are gamma-emitters has provided a tool to determine the activity of bone cells in suspected areas. If there is an increased concentration of isotope or hot spot in one area of the bone, it would appear that more than normal breakdown or repair is going on.

Technetium pyrophosphate Tc^{99} is extremely safe as well as inexpensive. It can show localized bone pathology within hours of a bad decompression, but is *too* sensitive for routine screening. Bruises and sprains show up on the scan, producing false positives, and even bone lesions due to decompression may spontaneously disappear without ever becoming positive on x-ray. If a scan on a diver proved to be positive, it would require removing him from diving until it could be determined whether or not the lesion were serious. In today's litiginous climate, this would produce an automatic lawsuit for damages.

With regard to the treatment for the individual who contracts aseptic necrosis, nothing need be done if the disease is in the shaft of a long bone, since the patient will be asymptomatic and there will be no disability or pain. If the disease is detected beginning at or near the articular surface of a joint before alteration of the articular margin has taken place, treatment consists of taking the weight off the joint until creeping apposition and strengthening can occur. In the case of the hip, this requires walking on crutches for many months with no weight bearing. When the shoulder is involved, the patient is advised not to do overhead work, not to raise a weight of greater than 10 lb above the shoulder nor to lift more than 25 lb from the floor with the affected arm. These patients are followed by x-ray at six-month intervals. In approximately 40% of the cases, the disease is present bilaterally. Thus, if both hips are involved, this would imply an almost "bed-to-chair" existence. In actual fact, this is not practical in young, vigorous persons; so in the usual case, the patient walks with canes or crutches and takes his chances.

The disease is, unfortunately, asymptomatic until actual disruption of the articular margin has occurred. At this point, when pain is noted for the first time, even putting the joint at rest will probably not prevent its eventual destruction, since the activities of daily living always cause some movement. Obviously, avoiding trauma or vigorous activity of the joint will prolong the period before the joint undergoes collapse. In those cases where actual destruction of the joint has taken place, surgery is the only treatment. Since the disease appears in young, physically active men, orthopedists try to delay surgery as long as possible or until the pain becomes intolerable. This is because, in the hips at least, the only practical solution has been complete replacement of the joint with a prosthesis.

Prosthetic joints have been used since about 1962 in England and began to be used in the United States about five years later, more or less on an experimental basis. Both the prostheses themselves and the surgical techniques for implanting them have improved markedly in the last few years so that now it is beginning to become permissible to operate on the patients in the younger age groups. However, no prosthetic joint has been produced which is as good as the natural one. Even though a prosthetic hip may be pain free, it is stiffer, less mobile, weaker, and subject to wearing out. The same is true for prosthetic shoulders, which are even less satisfactory. To date, prosthetic joints have been used largely in older patients who have not been physically active. It is too early to say how effective even improved versions of these prostheses will be in those who attempt to perform manual labor for a living.

PHYSICAL EXAMINATION STANDARDS FOR CAISSON AND COMPRESSED-AIR TUNNEL WORKERS AND FOR DIVERS

By and large, the criteria for physical qualification of persons employed in compressed-air work are little different from any group of workers who engage in hard physical labor. Certain very important exceptions exist. I will deal with each organ system and outline those areas that are important in this regard. If the examining physician is familiar with the principles of compressed-air physiology, he or she will not needlessly exclude workers who may have physical infirmities that will not be adversely affected by the compressed-air environment. From the insurance company's point of view, the greatest single risk is aseptic necrosis of the bone, because of the tremendous monetary losses which it can produce.

An additional consideration in *examining a diver* is the importance of knowing what kind of diving he or she is going to do. In general, the physical standards for diving are higher than those required for compressed-air caisson work, since the diver is usually working completely alone and is surrounded by water. The general level of intelligence of a diver should be higher and his or her overall knowledge of the physics and physiology of compressed air should be much greater. However, certain forms of diving are not very strenuous, may be to very shallow depths, and do not carry with them the long periods of enforced isolation away from medical help as does saturation diving. As an example, one can cite two extremes: the dredging foreman who once or twice a year must dive in 30 ft of water in a standard deep-sea rig to cut off sheet piling and the commercial oil field diver who must saturate on helium-oxygen mixtures to 600 ft for periods of many days. In addition, certain diving companies send their divers all over the world on short notice and it is incumbent on the examining physician to be sure that these persons are not suffering from diseases that could be incapacitating or have serious results if local medical help were not immediately available.

A diver must be a young, strong, healthy individual who should be able to swim and should be subject to generally higher physical standards than those required for caisson or compressed-air tunnel workers.

History

A routine medical history should be taken on each prospective candidate for compressed-air work or diving. This history would include the usual review of systems and inquiry into childhood and adult medical illnesses, surgical operations, and injuries. As a general rule, most diseases or disease processes are not adversely affected by the compressed-air or underwater environment unless they have to do with a hollow or gas-filled organ of the body. All other disease processes should be regarded as potentially disqualifying only if they interfere with normal hard physical labor.

Disqualifying Conditions

Below are a list of conditions that might disqualify a worker from compressed-air employment or from diving.

A History of Spontaneous Pneumothorax.—The chest x-ray films should be carefully examined for any signs of emphysematous bullae, lung cysts, or other pulmonary pathology. A history of spontaneous pneumothorax is automatically disqualifying under any circumstances. A history of traumatic pneumothorax is not necessarily disqualifying if there is complete healing and no evidence of air-trapping detected by x-ray or pulmonary function testing.

History of Ear Surgery.—Mastoid infections followed by mastoidectomy are not disqualifying. However, anyone who has had a history of surgery to improve hearing other than stapes mobilization should be potentially disqualified. If the patient has had a plastic procedure performed on his tympanic membrane or had a plastic strut inserted, the risk of disruption of his mechanical conductive mechanism is greatly enhanced by exposure to repeated compressions and decompressions. Simple partial deafness, a very common occurrence among persons who have worked for years with noisy pneumatic tools, is not disqualifying.

Active Asthma.—Active asthma is disqualifying. Many patients suffer from seasonal hay fever or have a history of childhood asthma. If the asthma is apparent during physical examination, the patient must be disqualified. Asthma is hazardous in that it prevents easy exchange of air from the alveolar spaces to the outside and promotes air-trapping that could result in dangerous emboli. It also may be brought on by exertion or breathing cold air—both likely to occur in tunneling. Many good workers, however, suffer from mild seasonal hay fever that can be controlled with "over-the-counter" decongestants. These persons may function well in the compressed-air environment. Seasonal hay fever should not be confused with asthma.

Chronic Alcoholism.—This illness not only is liable to be associated with excessive absenteeism, but it is well known to be a forerunner of aseptic necrosis in certain individuals. The aseptic necrosis produced is a result of fat emboli, but radiologically, it is indistinguishable from lesions produced by occupational exposure to compressed air. It will be very hard to elicit a history of chronic alcoholism from a would-be employee, but questions should be asked as to whether a patient has ever missed work because of being "hung-over"; and if there is any doubt, the former employer should be consulted. Examination may later reveal "liver palms," spider angiomata, an enlarged liver, or altered red blood cell indices.

Addiction to Narcotic or Stimulant Drugs.—This is disqualifying. Addicted patients are unreliable employees in compressed air or underwater, as well as in any other work environment; and because of their addiction, they are prone to steal from the employer. Physically, they are a bad risk for obvious reasons.

Epileptic or Convulsive Seizures.—If the patient has a history of epileptic or convulsive seizures, particular care must be taken. In the compressed-air environment or caisson, there is usually no serious immediate result of having a seizure. However, if the patient has had uncontrolled seizures, he is a poor candidate for compressed-air work; and a seizure during decompression will tend to predispose the individual to air embolism. In addition, tunnels and caissons are equipped with dangerous machinery, which could produce serious injury in a person who suddenly lost his ability to protect himself. Another disadvantage is that should a person have a seizure, immediate and appropriate first-aid measures would most likely not be available from his fellow employees. However, I did approve one man with a history of well-controlled epilepsy for continued work in a compressed-air tunnel. The man took Dilantin religiously and had not had a seizure in five years except after having taken three drinks of gin after a close friend was killed in a tunnel cave-in. Normally, he was an abstainer. The man had his seizure during nonworking hours, and since he normally did not drink, he was reinstated. He had already demonstrated his ability to work in compressed air without difficulty.

A history of epileptic or convulsive seizures, even if reasonably well-controlled, is an absolute contraindication in the diver, however. Underwater, a convulsion is extremely likely to be fatal.

Pancreatitis.—If a patient has a history of pancreatitis, it should be carefully determined whether he has concomitant gall bladder disease or a history of chronic alcoholism. Pancreatitis has been associated with the subsequent development of aseptic necrosis; and again, aseptic necrosis could falsely be attributed to compressed-air exposure if the two entities were associated in the same individual.

Psychosis.—If recurrent or if it has been present within the past five years, psychosis should be disqualifying. Patients with a history of psychosis are not more susceptible to compressed-air diseases but, in general, are not reliable employees. A patient who has to take phenothiazines on a maintenance basis to control psychosis should not be hired for work in tunnels or underwater. People with a history of hospitalization for nervous or mental disease should be carefully queried to determine whether or not they have a psychotic disorder such as schizophrenia or manic depressive psychosis.

Gross Obesity.—In general, a prospective employee should not be greater than 20% above the mean weight for his height for his age group. Obesity is a very real and statistically significant progenitor of decompression sickness. Body fat at 37° C absorbs five times as much nitrogen as does blood and lean tissues. As a result, obese persons absorb enormous quantities of nitrogen into their fat during the semisaturation exposures to which tunnel and caisson workers are subjected. The correlation between the number of attacks of decompression sickness and the thickness of the fatty skin fold over the triceps of the arm and area below the scapula on the back is very high. Extremely fat people do not generally apply for tunnel or caisson or diving work, in any case. Also, although it is puzzling to the statisticians, some quite obese persons do not seem to be subject to decompression sickness, while many lean and athletic ones suffer recurrent bends. It is perhaps best to have this concept in mind when examining prospective applicants. If a person has a history of being able to work successfully in compressed air despite obvious obesity, it would be unnecessary to disqualify him. Should an applicant who is obese subsequently demonstrate the expected susceptibility, he should then be disqualified.

The diver who is going to be making dives requiring decompression should be scrutinized especially carefully in regard to weight, because gross obesity can present formidable problems during decompression.

Advanced Age.—Increasing age has been well demonstrated to be correlated with an increasing incidence of decompression sickness. As a general rule, persons over age 50 should be discouraged from applying for shift work in compressed air. It may be, however, that experienced supervisors, tunnel engineers, and foremen will have to be examined for work in pressurized tunnels; and if they do not have an adverse history of decompression sickness, they may be cleared. Generally, persons engaged in hard physical labor, such as mucking and mining, should be in the younger age group. The reason for this is that even asymptomatic arteriosclerosis associated with aging seems to predispose to decompression sickness even though a worker may appear to be in excellent physical condition.

Age is a much more severe limitation in divers. Persons beyond the age of 45 should be considered as potentially over age for saturation diving. Deep diving should never be done by anyone over the age of 50, but there are a good many harbor divers in their 50s who are quite effective. On average, saturation divers, should be in their late 20s or 30s.

Conditions That Require Close Scrutiny

Below are listed certain maladies that may be detected in prospective applicants for compressed-air tunnel and caisson work or diving and that may require added scrutiny but are not *necessarily* disqualifying.

Diabetes.—A severe diabetic who takes large quantities of insulin and who has episodes of diabetic coma or insulin reaction should be immediately disqualified from compressed-air work. However, there is no harm in permitting a mild, nonbrittle diabetic under good control who has not had episodes of insulin coma or a diabetic acidosis to work in compressed air. Compressed air, *per se,* has shown no adverse effect on the course of the disease.

However, any diver who dives to deep depths and may be isolated for periods of time, who works in foreign countries, or who engages in saturation work should definitely be disqualified if he takes insulin. A mild diabetic who never has had an episode of acidosis or insulin coma and takes only small quantities of insulin might be qualified under certain circumstances for harbor diving.

Hypertension.—Many candidates examined for work in compressed-air will have elevated pressures. A reasonably healthy man in his early 30s or 40s, even though he may be suffering from hypertension, will have little likelihood of developing a stroke or blowing out an aneurysm while engaged in compressed-air work. Again, compressed air, *per se,* has no effect on hypertension, and one should consider such a patient on the same basis as one would consider any applicant for work in heavy construction.

Moderate hypertension might be tolerated in divers, but if diving in the North Sea, local regulations do not permit blood pressures greater than 140/90 in offshore commercial work.

History of Thoracotomy.—This should be subjected to close scrutiny. Thoracotomy for any reason raises the question of pleural adhesions or disruption of the air passages of the lungs. The reason for thoracotomy should be thoroughly investigated, and this may well be the determining factor as to whether or not a person works in compressed air or is allowed to dive. Patients who have had thoracotomy should be given a pressure test under carefully controlled conditions before being allowed to work in the pressurized environment if they have already not demonstrated an ability to do so in the past.

History of Fractures of the Humerus or Femur.—Aseptic necrosis has been known to follow fracture of the long bones, and if the fracture has been in the neck of the humerus or femur, the x-ray films should be carefully evaluated. Aseptic necrosis has been known to follow fracture as long as five years after the event. In any case, careful note should be made of the history of the occurrence of fracture so that it may be followed up on the yearly x-ray. Fracture of the distal humerus or femur is not as serious as fracture of the proximal shaft of the bone. Aseptic necrosis due to compressed-air work or diving has not been convincingly reported to occur in the elbow, wrist, or ankle, and only three cases have appeared in the world literature which involved the knee. The only joints commonly affected in aseptic necrosis are the shoulders and hips.

Migraine Headaches.—Migraine headaches may be adversely affected by employment in compressed air, being brought on by decompression. The reason for this is not known. If the patient has a history of absenteeism for severe and recurrent migraine headaches, it would be wise to consider not hiring him for economic reasons as well as medical ones.

A would-be saturation diver who has a history of migraine headaches and who may have to work at short notice outside the country might best be disqualified also.

History of Taking Systemic Steroids.—Systemic steroids, taken for any reason, have been associated with aseptic necrosis of the bone. Lesions have appeared up to five years after cessation of the drug. Local injection of steroids into a joint has *not* been associated with aseptic necrosis, so if a person has had a knee or shoulder bursitis treated with injections of steroids, there is not much cause for alarm. People who have taken systemic steroids should be closely scrutinized.

Physical Examination

Pressure Testing

A pressure test should be given to all candidates exposed to compressed air or to people with a history of potentially disqualifying sinus, ear, or lung conditions. An adequate pressure test consists of taking the candidates to 30 psig.

A candidate should not be excluded from compressed-air work simply because he fails to equalize pressure on a single occasion.

The diver's pressure test should be more severe than that required for the compressed-air worker, since the diver often has to make rapid descents. The standard U.S. Navy 50-lb Pressure Test (112 ft) usually is an adequate pressure test. Since the diver who is doing deep air of mixed-gas diving may be required to take oxygen decompression, thought may be given to requesting an oxygen tolerance test. In the U.S. Navy, this consists of breathing oxygen for 30 minutes at a depth of 60 ft in the dry chamber. However, the Royal Navy has abandoned this practice, since differences in susceptibility to oxygen toxicity vary so much from day to day in the same person that the test would appear to have little validity. One could only hope to screen out those who are idiosyncratically sensitive to oxygen poisoning. In my experience, there have been very few, if any, of these uncovered. Since operational oxygen decompression usually takes place in the dry chamber, a seizure is usually not fatal and I strongly believe this procedure has no economic validity.

An Examination Checklist

Height and Weight.—The patient's height and weight should be recorded *accurately*. It should be measured while the patient is disrobed, wearing only a hospital gown or shorts.

Ears.—Audiometric testing should be carried out initially on every prospective employee for work in compressed air. Testing should be done at 250, 500, 1,000, 2,000, 3,000, 4,000, and 6,000 Hz. Because tunnel and caisson workers are subjected to a very noisy environment due to the use of pneumatic tools and in-rushing air, it is important that any preexisting auditory impairment be documented to obviate future claims for occupational noise deafness. The employee's hearing should be at least 50% of normal in the human speech range. Old mastoid scars in the absence of other complications are not disqualifying. Perforated eardrums are not disqualifying in compressed-air workers but *are absolutely disqualifying* in divers. If the patient has chronic supperative disease of the middle ear with on-going infection, this should be treated and cleared up before employment under pressure. If the patient fails to clear his ears on pressure testing on three occasions, he should be disqualified.

Nose and Sinuses.—Acute or chronic supperative infection of the nose and sinuses will disqualify. Otherwise, the simple ability to pass a pressure test will be sufficient to qualify the person for compressed-air work.

Mouth and Throat.—Many men employed in compressed air have extensive caries and this is not disqualifying. A common source of difficulty is a *filled tooth,* which has a tendency to leak. Occasionally, during compression, such a tooth will be a source of intense pain to the worker, but it is uncommon for severely carious teeth that are unfilled to present any difficulty.

Eyes.—Vision at a distance should be 20/30 in at least one eye with correction. The ability to see in dim light is especially important. The patient should be able to read simple printed instructions at close vision with corrective glasses. It is not important that the employee have color vision. Fields of vision shall be grossly normal as measured by confrontation. The pupils should respond to light and accommodation, and, as a part of any compressed-air physical, retinal examination shall be carried out.

Cardiovascular System.—In examining the candidate for compressed-air work, the real point here is to determine whether or not he can be hired for a job requiring hard physical exercise. Auscultation of the heart should be performed. Severe valvular disease will usually be disqualifying. However, the presence of a murmur due to aortic stenosis of mitral insufficiency, if it is mild and not symptomatic, is not necessarily disqualifying. Because of nervousness about physical examination, the patient's pulse rate may often be found to be fast, but this should not be used as a basis for disqualification. If the patient has any suggestion of a cardiac problem in his history and he is older than 40, an electrocardiogram should be performed. In an otherwise healthy individual, even though he may be over 40, I usually waive the electrocardiogram. As mentioned previously, hypertension *per se,* if not very severe, should not be disqualifying.

In examining the diver, my criteria for qualification in regard to the cardiovascular system are somewhat stricter. A cardiologist's opinion should be secured before any saturation diver is qualified, if he exhibits a murmur due to aortic stenosis or mitral insufficiency, even if asymptomatic. An exercise electrocardiogram should be performed on everyone undergoing saturation diving, regardless of age.

Lungs.—On physical examination of the prospective compressed-air worker, the chest should be clear to auscultation and percussion. Any wheezes that persist after coughing should be carefully checked. Pulmonary tuberculosis, if active, will automatically disqualify. Chest x-rays are mandatory upon preemployment physical examination and should be repeated every other year while employed in compressed air. The radiologist should be particularly alert to rule out tuberculosis, bronchiectasis, emphysematous bullae, cystic disease, pneumothorax, or other air-trapping lesions. A Ghon complex or hilar adenopathy due to old tuberculosis that is inactive is not disqualifying unless it is severe or associated with air-trapping lesions. Pulmonary function tests are not necessary, except in doubtful cases where there is a question of air trapping.

A diver's lungs should be normal. This is because he is subject to more rapid ascents and much faster decompressions than compressed-air workers are exposed to and he may have to make a free ascent on occasion. Any diving candidate with hilar adenopathy or a Ghon complex should be considered for pulmonary function testing before qualification. The British offshore regulations require pulmonary function testing in any case.

Joint Mobility.—For compressed-air work and for diving, it should be ascertained that the patient can move all his limbs in every plane without pain. Carefully check to be sure the patient can stoop to the floor and bend his back without guarding or pain on moving the back.

Since diving involves very strenuous labor, often working in odd positions, it is especially important to ascertain that the patient is flexible.

Genitourinary System.—Venereal disease should be treated before the employee starts work. This is not because compressed air has a deleterious effect on venereal disease, but it is only good medical practice. Albumin in the urine is not disqualifying *per se* for the compressed-air worker but indicates some other pathology, which should be worked up thoroughly. If a patient is not clinically ill and does not have a disease process that would disqualify him from hard physical labor, there is no reason why he cannot enter the compressed-air environment.

However, any form of renal disease or albumin in the urine would disqualify a diver who is working with deep compressed-air or saturation.

Gastrointestinal System.—The prospective compressed-air employee should be evaluated in regard to his gastrointestinal system using the same standards one would use to determine the employability of anyone engaged in hard, physical labor. Gastrointestinal diseases that produce chronic illness or debilitation should disqualify. Hernia would naturally disqualify for any kind of hard, physical work, but, especially, if a gas-filled loop of bowel should exit the hernial opening, decompression could cause necrosis of the bowel.

Gastric or duodenal ulcer should be disqualifying in certain forms of diving. For instance, the patient may be on a saturation dive and the problem of hemorrhage might occur, or he might be subject to a sudden call to a foreign country for a diving job. Anyone with a history of gastrointestinal hemorrhage should be disqualified if he falls into this category. However, even a history of a gastrointestinal bleed would not necessarily disqualify a local harbor diver.

Nervous System.—The Romberg test should be used to determine the functioning of the vestibular system and the eighth nerve. When the mouth and throat are examined, the tongue should protrude in a midline. The extraocular movements should be noted, and the presence or absence of nystagmus should be recorded. The deep tendon reflexes should be examined, and if there is any inequality between sides, this should be carefully recorded. It should also be noted if the knee jerks and if plantar responses are extremely hypoactive. The presence or absence of the abdominal reflexes should be noted. It is important that this rudimentary neurologic evaluation be made, because if the employee later suffers from decompression sickness, it may be necessary to compare his preemployment neurologic exam with the physical findings he exhibits while suffering from bends. If the patient has a spinal cord lesion, there may well be a change in the neurologic status.

X-ray Studies

The following body areas are radiographed to determine involvement by aseptic necrosis: both shoulders, both hips, and both knees. Other areas may be examined if clinically indicated, but these other areas are optional and are not usually included in a radiographic survey.

Each of the above areas is radiographed individually to obtain the maximum radiographic and trabecular detail; i.e., each hip is radiographed separately; both hips are never included on the same film. The smallest focal spot available is employed to increase the radiographic detail. Adequate penetration (Kv) of the appropriate bone must be used, but a high Mas technique is employed to obtain the greatest contrast to the bone structures. The following table is recommended as an example of technique but may be modified according to the radiographic equipment available. All radiographs are done with a moving Bucky grid on 10 × 12-inch cassettes containing parspeed screens. It is important that gonadal shielding be used as well as shielding of the marrow-containing areas of the pelvis above the hip when hip radiographs are taken.

The following films are included in a radiographic survey. (When special detailed views are advisable, tomographic films are obtained of the suspected areas. Occasionally, stereoscopic views are useful.)

Shoulders.—Anteroposterior films should be taken with the shoulder in internal and external rotation (two films). The Grashey position is used because it affords an excellent view of the articulating surfaces of the glenoid of the scapula and the head of the humerus. Overlap of the glenoid, acromion, and humeral head are to be avoided. Technical factors: 40 Mas: 2 × (thickness of part in centimeters) plus 40 Kv. Example: 15 cm is the measurement of the shoulder joint—the calculation would be 15 × 2 = 30 + 40 = 70 Kv.

Hips.—Two films, anteroposterior and frog position lateral, should be taken. Technical factors: 60 Mas: 2 × (thickness of part in centimeters) + 50 Kv.

Knees.—Two films, anteroposterior and lateral should be taken. Technical factors: 30 Mas: 2 × (thickness of part in centimeters) + 40 Kv.

Laboratory Tests

A routine urinalysis should be done recording specific gravity and the presence or absence of sugar and albumin. A hematocrit and hemoglobin should be recorded and a test for sickle cell anemia trait should be performed on the first examination. Anyone with a positive test for sickle cell anemia trait should be excluded from compressed-air work and from diving. Sickle cell anemia trait alone has been associated with aseptic necrosis.

CRITERIA FOR THE EXAMINATION OF VISITORS TO THE COMPRESSED-AIR ENVIRONMENT

In general, visitors who are experienced in compressed air, such as consulting engineers, electricians, and equipment repairmen who intend to visit the working space on only one or few occasions, need not be subjected to a complete compressed-air physical examination. In lieu of this, they must complete a form required of all casual visitors to the compressed-air environment. The form is reproduced in Table 25–8. If any question on the form is answered in the affirmative, the visitor must be subjected to physical examination and/or clearance from a physician. If all the answers on the form are negative, the supervisor, licensed air master, or foreman may admit the visitor. In such cases, however, the visitor may not remain in the compressed-air environment longer than the times listed in Table 25–9. Beyond 40 psig, shorter exposure times are not practical, since compression time is always

TABLE 25–8.
Questionnaire for Visitors to the Compressed Air Environment

1. Do you have a history of spontaneous collapse of the lung (pneumothorax)?
   Yes ________ No ________
2. Have you ever had chest or thoracic surgery?
   Yes ________ No ________
3. Have you ever had ear surgery?
   Yes ________ No ________
4. Do you have any degree of deafness?
   Yes ________ No ________
5. Is your most recent chest x-ray more than one year old?
   Yes ________ No ________
6. Were there any abnormal findings reported to you regarding the chest x-ray?
   Yes ________ No ________
7. Do you currently have hay fever, asthma or sinus trouble?
   Yes ________ No ________

I certify that the above information is correct to the best of my knowledge.
Date ________________ Signature ________________________

TABLE 25–9.
Maximum Permissible Exposure Times for Experienced Visitors to the Compressed-Air Environment Who Have Not Had a Physical Examination

PRESSURE	MAXIMUM EXPOSURE TIME
0–12 psig	8 hr
13–16 psig	4 hr
17–22 psig	50 min
23–26 psig	30 min
27–31 psig	25 min
32–35 psig	20 min
36–40 psig	15 min

included in exposure time. If it is necessary for a casual visitor to enter such high pressures, he should have a current compressed-air physical examination.

Casual visitors who have had no previous experience in compressed air shall be required to have a physical examination, including a chest x-ray film. In such visitors, however, if they do not plan to work for periods of more than four hours, the caisson survey by x-ray, the audiogram, and the laboratory work may be omitted. If possible, a pressure test should be given to the visitor before he enters the work tunnel.

REFERENCES

1. Ackles K: Personal communication, 1972.
2. Adolfson J, Muren A: Air breathing at 13 atmospheres in naval diving personnel: Psychological and physiological reactions, in *Emotional Stress: Physiological and Psychological Reactions. Medical, Industrial and Military Implications*, Proceedings of an International Symposium Feb 5–6, 1965, Stockholm, Sweden. New York, Elsevier North-Holland, Inc, 1967, pp 267–273.
3. Angel T, Fluor Ocean Services: Personal communication, 1971.
4. Atkinson JR: Experimental air embolism. *Northwest Med* 1963; 62:699–703.
5. Barnes R: Caisson disease of bones. *Manitoba Med Rev* 1967; 47:547–551.
6. Behnke AR, Willman TL: Gaseous nitrogen and helium elimination from the body during rest and exercise. *Am J Physiol* 1941; 131(3):619–626.
7. Behnke AR, Thomson RM, Motley EP: The psychological effects from breathing air at 4 atmospheres pressure. *Am J Physiol* 1935; 112:554–558.
8. Bennett PB, Papahadjoupolos D, Bangham AD: The effect of raised pressures of inert gases on phospholipid model membranes. *Life Sci* 1967; 6:2527–2533.
9. Bennett PB, Elliott DH (eds): *The Physiology and Medicine of Diving*. London, Bailliere Tindall, 1982.
10. Bert P: *Barometric Pressure: Researches in Experimental Physiology*, Hitchcock MA, Hitchcock FA (trans). Columbus, Oh, Longs College Book Company, 1943, p 5.
11. Bert P: *La Pression Barometrique*. Paris, G Masson, 1878.
12. Bjurstedt H, Severin G: The prevention of decompression sickness and nitrogen narcosis by the use of hydrogen as a substitute for nitrogen (the Arne Zetterstrom method for deep sea diving). *Military Surgeon* 1948; 103:107–116.
13. Bond G: Personal communication, 1958.
14. Bornstein A, Plate E: Uber chronische Gelenkveranderungen, entstanden durch Presslufterkrankung. *Fortschr Geb Roentgenstrahlen* 1911–12; 18:197.
15. Boycott AE, Damant GCC, Haldane JS: The prevention of compressed air illness. *J Hyg* 1908; 8:342.
16. Chryssanthou C, Teichner F, Goldstein G, et al: Studies on dysbarism. III. A smooth muscle activating factor (SMAF) in mouse lungs and its increase in decompression sickness. *Aerospace Med* 1970; 41:43–48.
17. Clarke R: Personal communication, 1972.
18. Cockett ATK, Nakamura RM: A new concept in the treatment of decompression sickness (dysbarism). *Lancet* 1964; 1:1102.
19. Cockett ATK, Pauley SM, Roberts AP: *Advancement in Treatment of Decompression Sickness: An Evaluation of Heparin,* in Proceedings of the 3rd International Congress on Hyperbaric and Underwater Physiology, ed X. Paris, Fructus DOIN Editeurs, 1972.
20. Davis JC (ed): *Treatment of Serious Decompression Sickness in Arterial Gas Embolism*. Durham, NC, UMS Workshop, Duke University, UMS Publication 34 WS (SDS), 1979.
21. Davis RH: *Deep Diving and Submarine Operations*, ed 7. Chessington, Surrey, Siebe, Gorman and Co, Ltd, 1962.
22. De la Torre E, Meredith J, Netsky MG: Cerebral Air Embolism in the Dog. *Arch Neurol* 1962; 6:67–76.
23. Edel PO, Carroll JJ, Honaker RW, Beckman EL: Decompression sickness and flight after diving. *Aerospace Med* 1969; 40:1105–1110.
24. Edel PO: *Delineation of Emergency Surface Decompression and Treatment Procedures for Project Tektite Aquanauts*, Contract #NAS9-9176, NASA. Pasadena, Tex, J & J Marine Diving Co, Inc, 1969.
25. Edel PO, Holland JM, Fisher CL, et al: Preliminary studies of hydrogen-oxygen breathing mixtures for deep sea diving, in *The Working Diver*, in 1972 Symposium Proceedings, Salsbury D (ed). Washington, DC, Marine Technology Society, 1730 M S, NW, 1972, pp 257–270.
26. El Ghawabi SH, Nansour MB, Youssef FL, et al: Decompression sickness in caisson workers. *Br J Ind Med* 1971; 28:323–329.
27. Ellsberg E: *On the Bottom*. New York, Dodd, Mead & Co, 1937.
28. End E: The Physiologic Effects of Increased Pressure. *Proceedings of the 6th Pacific Science Congress* 1939; 6:91–97.
29. End E: Personal communication, 1956.
30. End E: The use of new equipment and helium gas in a world record dive. *J Ind Hyg Toxicol* 1938; 20.
31. End E: Personal communication, 1972.
32. Evans A, Barnard EEP, Walder DN: Detection of gas bubbles in man at decompression. *Aerospace Med* 1972; 43:1095–1096.
33. Fife WP: *The Use of Non-Explosive Mixtures of Hydrogen and Oxygen for Diving*, Hyperbaric Lab Report TAMU-SG-79-201. College Station, Texas A & M University, 1979.
34. Galerne A; President, International Underwater Contractors: Personal communication, 1972.
35. Goodman MW, Workman RD: *Minimal Recompression, Oxygen-Breathing Approach of Treatment of Decompression Sickness in Divers and Aviators*, BuShips Proj SF011 06 05, Task 11513-2, Research Report 5-65. Washington, DC, Bureau of Medicine and Surgery, 1965.
36. James CC: Late bone lesions in caisson disease. *Lancet* 1945; 2:6.
37. Kindwall EP: Personal observation, 1971.
38. Kindwall EP: Massive surgical air embolism treated with brief recompression to six atmospheres followed by hyperbaric oxygen. *Aerospace Med* 1973; 44(6):663–666.
39. Kindwall EP, Margolis I: Management of severe decompression sick-

ness with treatment ancillary to recompression: Case report. *Aviat Space Environ Med* 1975; 46:1065–1068.

40. Kindwall EP, Nellen JR, Speigelhoff DR: Aseptic necrosis in compressed air tunnel workers using current OSHA decompression schedules. *J Occup Med* 1982; 24(10):741–745.
41. Kindwall EP, Edel PO, Melton HE: *Safe Decompression Schedules for Caisson Workers*, Final Report, Research Grant 5R 01 0H 00947-03. Cincinnati, Oh, National Institute for Safety and Health, 1983.
42. Kruse CA: Air embolism and other skin diving problems. *Northwest Med* 1963; 62:525–529.
43. Lipton B, Dept of Anesthesiology, Mt Sinai School of Medicine, New York: Personal communication, March, 1972.
44. Lorraine-Smith J: The influence of pathological conditions on active absorption of oxygen by the lungs. *J Physiol* 1897–1898; 22:307.
45. McCallum RI (ed): *Decompression of Compressed Air Workers in Civil Engineering*. Newcastle-upon-Tyne, Oriel Press, Ltd, 1967.
46. Meyer HH: Theoris der alkoholnarkose. *J Arch Exp Pathol Pharmak* 1899; 42:109.
47. Nellen JR, Kindwall EP: Aseptic necrosis of bone secondary to occupational exposure to compressed air: Roentgenologic findings in 59 cases. *Am J Roentgenol Rad Ther Nucl Med* 1972; 115(3):512–523.
48. Nemiroff MJ: Unpublished data. Ann Arbor, Pulmonary Intensive Care Unit, University of Michigan, 1972.
49. Newbury H: Bell systems in *Proceedings of the 3rd Annual International Professional Diving Symposium, New Orleans, Nov 1972*. Washington, DC, Marine Technology Society, 1972.
50. Philp RB: The ameliorative effects of heparin and depolymerized hyaluronate on decompression sickness in rats. *Can J Physiol Pharmacol* 1964; 42:819–829.
51. Philp RB, Schacham P, Gowdy CW: Involvement of platelets and microthrombi in experimental decompression sickness: Similarities with disseminated intravascular coagulation. *Aerospace Med* 1971; 42:494.
52. Pol B, Watelle JJ: Memoire sur les effets de la compression de l'air. *Ann d'hyg Pub Med Leg* (Series 2) 1854; 1:241.
53. Reeves E, Workman RD: Use of heparin for the therapeutic prophylactic treatment of decompression sickness. *Aerospace Med* 1971; 42:20–23.
54. Richardson RS, Mayo HW: *Practical Tunnel Diving*, ed 1. New York, McGraw-Hill Book Co, 1941.
55. Rivera JC: Decompression sickness among divers: An analysis of 935 cases. *Milit Med* 1964; 129:314–334.
56. Rose RJ: *Survey of Work in Compressed Air During the Construction of the Auckland Harbour Bridge*, Special Report 6, Medical Statistics Branch, Dept of Health. Wellington, New Zealand, RE Owen, Government Printer, 1962.
57. Rudge FH: A case of caisson disease. *Lancet* 1907; 11:1675–1676.
58. Saper JR, Yosselson S: Raised intra-cranial pressure diagnosis and management. *Postgrad Med J* 1975; 57:89–94.
59. Schaefer KE, McNulty WP Jr, Carey CR, et al: Mechanisms and development of interstitial emphysema and air embolism on decompression from depth. *J Appl Physiol* 1958; 13:15–29.
60. Sealey JL: Aseptic bone necrosis survey in compressed air workers. *J Occup Med* 1975; 17(10):666–667.
61. Smith JP LCDR (MC) USNR: *The Use of Adrenocorticosteroids in the Central Nervous System Edema Due to Decompression Sickness*, unpublished monograph. Pearl Harbor, Honolulu, Submarine Escape Training Facility, 1966.
62. Spaur WH CDR (MC) USN: Personal communication, 1973.
63. Sukoff MH, Hollin SA, Jacobson JH II: The protective effect of hyperbaric oxygenation in experimentally produced cerebral edema and compression. *Surgery* 1967; 62(1):40–46.
64. Swindle PF: Occlusion of blood vessels by agglutinated red cells, mainly as seen in tadpoles and very young kangaroos. *Am J Physiol* 1937; 120:59–74.
65. Teed WR: Factors producing obstruction of the auditory tube in submarine personnel. *US Navy Med Bull* 1944; 42:293–306.
66. Tjernstrom O: Middle ear mechanics and alternobaric vertigo. *J Acta Otolaryngol* 1974; 78:376–384.
67. Triger M: Influence de l'air comprime sur la sante. *Ann Hyg G Publ* 1845; 33:463.
68. US Bureau of Labor Standards, Dept of Labor: Safety and health regulations for construction. *Federal Register* 1971; 36:7395–7404 (Apr 17).
69. US Naval Safety Center: *Navmed 816 file* (decompression accident reports). Norfolk, Va, US Naval Safety Center, 1966.
70. US Navy: *Oxygen Breathing Treatment for Decompression Sickness and Air Embolism*, Bumed Instruction 6420.2, Bumed 74, Aug 22 1967. Washington, DC, Bureau of Medicine and Surgery, 1967.
71. *US Navy Diving Manual*, Navships 0994-001-9010. Washington, DC, Navy Dept, Supt of Documents, US Government Printing Office, 1970.
72. *US Navy Diving Manual*, Navsea 0994-LP-001-9010. Washington, DC, Navy Dept, Supt of Documents, US Government Printing Office, 1979.
73. Van Genderen L, Waite CL: Evaluation of the rapid recompression-high pressure oxygenation approach to the treatment of traumatic cerebral embolism. *Aerospace Med* 1968; 39:709–713.
74. Waite CL: Personal communication, 1972.
75. Waite CL, Mazzone WF, et al: *Cerebral Embolism. 1. Basic Studies*. US Naval Sub Med Center Research Report no. 493, April 1967.
76. Walder D: Personal communication, 1971.
77. Willmon TL, Behnke AR: Nitrogen elimination and oxygen absorption at high barometric pressures. *Am J Physiol* 1941; 131:633–638.
78. Wisconsin Administrative Code: *Work Under Compressed Air*, Chapter Ind 12. Madison, Wis, Dept of Industry, Labor, and Human Relations, 1972.
79. Yarbrough OD, Behnke AR: The treatment of compressed air illness utilizing oxygen. *J Ind Hyg Toxicol* 1939; 21(6):213–218.
80. Zinkowski NB: *Commercial Oil-Field Diving*. Cambridge, Md, Cornell Maritime Press, Inc, 1971.

26

Ionizing Radiation

George L. Voelz, M.D.

Every occupational physician encounters questions or problems about ionizing radiation. These questions may result from the use of radiation in the workplace or in the practice of medicine; they may result from concerns about potential exposures in the environment or about some past experience that involved potential radiation exposure of unknown amount. Questions on radiation effects or medical management of persons after radiation exposure are often difficult because of the complex and seemingly infinite variations in which the questions or problems are presented.

The characteristics of ionizing radiation are defined by physical laws that permit measurement and evaluation with a degree of precision that is not available for most other biologic hazards. Acute radiation effects correlate well with physical measurements in a predictable way when accurate data are available. The risk of late health effects after radiation, such as cancer, is also known better than for other mutagens or carcinogens. Despite such knowledge, or perhaps because of it, there exists in most people a mysterious fear of radiation.

This fear has been termed the "radiation mystique" by some psychologists. Exposure to other chemical or physical agents usually does not create the same emotional response and exaggerated risk perception that is present after radiation exposure. Perhaps this comes from the fact that ionizing radiation cannot be detected by our normal senses. Maybe it rests on the history of radiation effects in early radiation workers and atomic bomb victims.

Proper management of radiation-exposed persons and correct responses to questions will do much to reduce the "radiation mystique." Unless physicians are knowledgeable about ionizing radiation and its health effects, the mystique may cause unnecessary and difficult problems for their patients even after minor events. Fear and anxiety are reduced when the patient possesses the facts to understand his or her situation. An important part of the physician's job is to provide that knowledge and understanding to the patient.

Radiation protection programs in industry have been highly successful in limiting radiation doses to workers. Modern radiologic techniques and procedures have also reduced radiation exposures to patients. Occupational physicians should assure that such protection programs are functioning successfully in the plants, workplaces, and medical offices under their medical supervision. Although consultants and radiation protection specialists will usually develop such programs, the physician knowledgeable in radiation can be especially effective in communicating with workers about potential risks and in planning for and delivering appropriate medical care for exposed persons.

BASIC CONCEPTS OF RADIATION PHYSICS

Interactions with Matter

Radiation refers to the complete process in which energy is emitted by one body or source, transmitted through an intervening medium or space, and absorbed by another body. The energy transfer occurs in the form of subatomic particles or electromagnetic waves.

Radioactivity is the phenomenon, exhibited by and being a property of certain elements, of spontaneously emitting radiation that results from changes within the nuclei of atoms of the element. The term *activity* is a common synonym for radioactivity. One must distinguish between radiation and radioactivity.

A *radionuclide* is an unstable or radioactive atomic species in which all atoms have the same atomic number and mass number. An *isotope* is any of two or more species of atoms of a chemical element with the same atomic number (same number of protons in the nucleus) but with different atomic mass. Isotopes may or may not be radioactive.

Ionizing radiation is any radiation consisting of moving particles or electromagnetic waves that carries sufficient energy to produce ions in matter. Ionization occurs when enough radiation energy is transferred to atoms in the material through which it is passing to displace an orbital electron, thus leaving these atoms as electrically charged ions. In tissue, the ionization of atoms within cells produces immediate biochemical changes that may result in immediate or late biologic effects. Except for extremely high doses, no immediate effects are perceived by the individual.

Ionization, shown schematically in Figure 26–1, occurs when a swiftly moving charged particle, such as an electron (β particle) collides with an orbital electron of an atom or, more frequently, as a result of the electrical attractive or repulsive force between the particle and the orbital electron. Electromagnetic radiation, such as x-rays or gamma rays, interacts with matter somewhat differently. Such radiation consists of a stream of electromagnetic energy waves called *photons* (or quanta). Photons have no electrical charge and pass through matter unimpeded until they collide with some

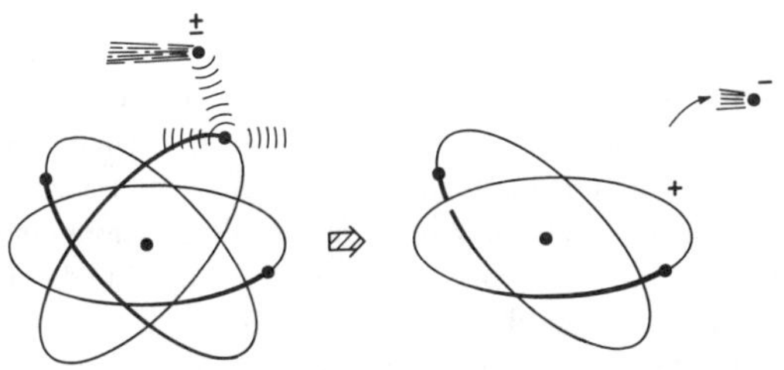

FIG 26–1.
Ionization by charged particle. Orbital electron of atom is given sufficient energy to eject it. In tissue, ionization produces free radicals or ionized molecules that react chemically with nearby atoms and molecules and results in altered cell physiology.

particle, either an orbital electron or the nucleus of an atom. Such a collision can either stop the photon or scatter it in another direction and also produce a secondary electron that can cause ionization. The interaction of photons with atoms and the transfer of photon energy to electrons is described by three reactions: photoelectric effect, Compton effect, and pair production. The probability of a given type of physical interaction depends on the energy of the x-ray or gamma ray and the density (atomic number) of the material. A description of these reactions can be found in basic radiation physics textbooks.[9, 62, 75]

The amount of energy present in radiation is measured in electron volts (eV). One *electron volt* is the kinetic energy that is acquired by an electron when it is accelerated in a vacuum through a potential difference of 1 volt. Multiple units, such as 1,000 eV (keV) or 1 million eV (MeV), are frequently used.

Each ionizing event results in a reduction of energy of the particle or wave. A typical value of the energy loss per ion pair produced in air is about 34 eV. Thus, a 1-MeV particle will produce about 30,000 ionizations (1,000,000/34) along its path before being brought to rest. The energy lost per micrometer of track length of the primary ionizing particle is called *linear energy transfer* or LET. It is determined by the charge and velocity of the ionizing particle. Biologic effects are influenced strongly by the LET of the radiation.

Penetrating power of ionizing radiation is related to the mass and charge of the particle as well as its kinetic energy. The more mass and electrical charge a particle possesses, the less penetration power it will have. Each ionizing event causes a fractional loss of kinetic energy (reduced velocity) of the particle and this process continues until the particle stops. A heavy, charged particle will produce more ionizations per unit length of its path, i.e., high LET, and as a result the particle slows down and stops more quickly. Thus, a 5-MeV α particle will traverse only about 3.5 cm in standard air and about 35 μ in water or soft tissue. An 8-MeV α particle has about twice these ranges in each. Note that penetration (track length) is shorter in denser material (water) than in light material (air).

The penetration of electromagnetic waves (photons) through matter is quite different from that of particles. Attenuation of photons occurs only as a result of random collisions with atomic nuclei or electrons in matter. Each photon continues to travel unimpeded until such an interaction occurs and thus the photons are stopped exponentially with distance rather than at a definite range. One may visualize this process as a complete or partial loss of energy of the photon involved in the collision, but the other photons are unaffected. The collision of the photon and an atom results in a high-speed electron being ejected from an atom. The electrons produce the ionizations. This process is why x-rays and gamma rays have much greater penetrating power compared with that of charged particles, such as α- or β-rays. The penetration of photons is decreased when they pass through heavy materials, such as lead.

Types of Radiation

Although many types of radiation have been described and studied by physicists, there are five main types involved in occupational health. They are x-rays, γ-rays, α particles, β particles, and neutrons. Their principal characteristics are summarized in Table 26–1.

X-Rays.—X-rays, also called *roentgen rays,* are penetrating electromagnetic radiation of short wavelength, 10^{-6} to 10^{-12} cm. The German physicist Wilhelm Roentgen discovered them in 1895 while studying the operation of vacuum tubes. X-rays are produced by bombarding a metal target with a stream of high-energy electrons. Modern x-ray tubes produce electrons with a heated filament in a vacuum and then accelerate them by means of a high positive voltage on a tungsten target. Peak voltages (kVp) of 100–150 kilovolts (kV) are commonly used in diagnostic medical x-ray units. Conventional x-ray therapy machines use voltages up to 300 kVp. Electron accelerators (betatrons) are used to obtain higher x-ray energies for deep therapy. It should be kept in mind that x-rays

TABLE 26–1.
Types of Ionizing Radiation Important in Radiologic Health

NAME	SYMBOL	CHARACTER	MASS*	CHARGE	SOURCE EXAMPLES
X-rays	(x)	Electromagnetic, energy <50–>1000 kVp	0	0	X-ray tube
Gamma	(γ)	Electromagnetic, energy <10 keV–>2 MeV	0	0	^{60}Co, ^{192}Ir
Alpha	(α)	Particulate, helium nucleus	4	+ +	^{239}Pu, ^{212}Po
Beta	(β)	Particulate, electron	1/2000	–	^{90}Sr, ^{3}H
Neutrons	(n)	Nucleus particle	1	0	^{235}U fission

*The atomic mass unit (AMU) is chosen so a neutral carbon-12 atom has a relative mass exactly equal to 12. This is equal to about 1 AMU for both a proton and a neutron.

are produced wherever high-voltage vacuum tubes are used, as for example, in Klystron tubes or television tubes.

Since x-rays are electromagnetic waves (photons), they have no mass and no electrical charge. The average energy of photons, and therefore their penetrating power, increases with the voltage applied to the tube. The energy of x-rays from a tube is expressed as the peak voltage, although the actual x-ray energies are a continuum from essentially zero up to the peak voltage. Filters, usually made of copper or aluminum, are used to remove the soft (less penetrating) x-rays.

γ-Rays.—The properties of γ-rays are identical to those of x-rays. The difference is simply their origin. Whereas x-rays are produced from electrons orbiting around an atom nucleus, γ-rays are emitted from reactions within the nucleus itself. γ-Rays are highly penetrating and frequently carry higher energy than x-rays. The most serious γ-ray exposures to man are from external radiation sources. γ-Ray-emitting radionuclides can also be taken into the body as an internal emitter, but the associated alpha or beta particles, having more intense ionization tracks, will usually present the dominant hazard. γ-Rays emitted from a specific radionuclide have discrete energies and thus can be identified by means of a γ-ray spectrometer.

α Particles.—Alpha particles are emitted from the nuclei of certain heavy-element nuclides, such as radium 226 and plutonium 239, during their radioactive disintegration. α Particles consist of two protons and two neutrons bound together. They have the largest mass (4 atomic mass units) and highest charge (+2) of the common radiation particles. These properties account for the very dense production of ionizations (30,000 to 100,000 ion pairs per centimeter of air) by an α particle. As noted earlier, the penetration or track length in tissue is about 50 μ, which means that only five or fewer cells are traversed by one particle. The short range of α particles explains why even a thin layer of moisture can easily prevent α particles from being detected by monitoring instruments. Surface alpha-monitoring is thus subject to considerable error. Alpha particles do not penetrate the horny layer of the skin and, therefore, are hazardous only if introduced internally into the body. Alpha particle-emitting radionuclides emit particles of discrete energies and can be identified by alpha spectroscopy.

β Particles.—These particles are speeding electrons that are emitted from the nuclei of atoms of certain radionuclides, such as strontium 90 or iodine 131. An electron has a small mass (about 1/1825 of an atomic mass unit) and a negative charge of 1. β Particles can traverse several centimeters of tissue, a path length that is about 1,000 times longer than that of an α particle. β Particles create up to 200 ion pairs per centimeter in air, a much less dense ionization track than that produced by α particles. Higher energy β particles can penetrate the skin and have produced serious β burns in some accidental exposures. β Particles emitted from radionuclides are not monoenergetic, but rather have a continuum of energies from essentially zero to a maximal value. The average energy, usually about a third of the maximum energy, is called the effective energy. For example, strontium 90 emits β particles with a maximum energy of 546 keV, but its effective β energy is 196 keV.

Neutrons.—Neutrons are nuclear particles with an atomic mass weight of 1 and no electrical charge. These particles are emitted from nuclei of atoms that are being disrupted either by fissioning of the nucleus or by impact from fast-moving charged particles, such as protons from an accelerator. Neutrons are very quickly absorbed by nuclei of other atoms in the vicinity and exist for only a fraction of a second. Therefore, they are found only near sources that can create these nuclear reactions—e.g., nuclear reactors, particle accelerators, nuclear fission devices, and neutron sources, such as californium 252, polonium-beryllium or radium-beryllium sources. Neutrons have a wide range of energies and usually are described as thermal (about 0.025 eV), epithermal or slow (up to 100 eV), intermediate (100 eV to 100 keV), and fast neutrons (more than 100 keV). The more energetic neutrons have a penetrating power that is nearly comparable to that of x-rays or γ rays. Neutron exposures result in high LET external radiation doses and can produce very significant radiobiologic effects.

Units of Radiation and Radioactivity

The units commonly used to describe radiation and radioactivity are listed and defined in Table 26–2. The following discussion gives some background information on these units and explains how they are used. There are currently two systems of radiation units in use: conventional and SI (Systeme International) metric units. In this chapter, both systems will be used by first giving the conventional unit followed by the comparable SI unit value in parentheses. The four areas of information described by these units are activity, exposure, absorbed dose, and dose equivalent.

Activity.—The basic measurement of radioactivity is the number of disintegrating nuclei per second. A disintegrating nucleus refers to the spontaneous transformation of the number or the internal arrangement of protons and neutrons within the nucleus of a radioactive atom. The basic SI unit, becquerel (Bq), is defined as one disintegration per second. The conventional unit, curie (Ci), was named for Marie and Pierre Curie for their discovery of radium. One curie is 3.7×10^{10} disintegrations per second. Common multiples of the curie and corresponding becquerels are listed in Table 26–3.

It should be noted that activity units relate to the number of nuclear disintegrations and not to the number of α particles, β particles, or γ-rays present. They also do not measure the mass. The mass associated with 1 Ci of activity is proportional to the atomic weight and the half-life of the specific radionuclide. Radionuclides with long half-lives require much more mass of material to make up 1 Ci of activity than those with short half-lives.

The *radioactive half-life,* commonly called the *physical half-life,* is the time required for disintegration of half the atoms of a given radioactive substance. Each radionuclide has a unique half-life. For example, ^{125}I and ^{131}I have a 60-day and an 8.1-day radioactive half-life respectively (Fig 26–2). It can be shown that the half-life ($T_{1/2}$) for a given nuclide is

$$T_{1/2} = 0.693/\lambda$$

The decay constant, λ, is the fraction of the number of atoms of a radioactive nuclide that decay (disintegrate) in unit time. The ra-

TABLE 26–2.
Units of Radiation and Radioactivity

UNIT DESCRIPTION	UNIT NAME	SYMBOL	DEFINITION
Activity	curie	Ci	3.7×10^{10} disintegrations/second (dis/s)*
	becquerel†	Bq	1 dis/s
	working level	WL	special‡ for radon/radon daughters
Exposure	roentgen	R	2.58×10^{-4} coulombs/kg of air§
	working level month	WLM	special¶ for radon/radon daughters
Absorbed dose	rad	rad	100 ergs/gm of absorbing material
	gray†	Gy	100 rad
	kerma‖	K	ergs/gm of absorbing material
Dose equivalent	rem	rem	rad × QF × DF × other factors**
	sievert†	Sv	100 rem

*Historical definition was the quantity of emanation (radon) from or in equilibrium with 1 gm of radium 226.
†Unit of the SI (System International) metric system.
‡One WL is 1.3×10^5 MeV of alpha energy from radon daughters per liter of air.
§Historical definition was the quantity of x- or gamma radiation that produces ions carrying 1 electrostatic unit of electrical charge of either sign in 1 cu cm of air under standard conditions. (1 r = 1.6×10^{12} ionizations/cu cm of air)
¶One WLM is an exposure to an average concentration of one WL for a working month of 170 hours. For members of the general population, a month is 730 hours.
‖An acronym that stands for *k*inetic *e*nergy *r*eleased in *ma*terial.
**QF = quality factors; DF = distribution factors

dioactive half-life is an unchangeable nuclear property that is unaffected by temperature, pressure, or chemical form.

A special unit called a *working level* is used only for measuring the concentration of radon and radon daughters in air. They present one of the more complex mixtures of radionuclides to be measured and this unit was derived to express the inhaled concentration in one number. The unit expresses the total amount of α energy present in a liter of air (see definition in Table 26–2). It has been a practical and useful unit, especially for use in mines or other work spaces where radon and radon daughters must be measured.

Exposure.—Exposure refers here to the measurement of a radiation level to which a person may be exposed. The principal unit of exposure is the *roentgen* (R). The roentgen defines a radiation field in terms of the amount of ionizations produced in air (see definition in Table 26–2). An exposure measurement in air must be distinguished from a dose to tissues. The amount of energy absorbed in air per roentgen is not the same as that absorbed in tissues. About 83 ergs/gm is absorbed in air per roentgen, whereas the absorbed energy in soft tissue is about 93 ergs/gm per roentgen. More dense tissue, e.g., bone, may have values up to about 100 ergs/gm per roentgen.

The roentgen measurement of x-rays and γ-rays can be expressed as an exposure rate, such as milliroentgens (mR = 1/1000 R) per hour. Roentgen is not commonly used today, because it is not easily converted to dose. It is impractical to use to measure

TABLE 26–3.
Multiples of the Curie (Ci) and Becquerel (Bq) Units

NAME	ABBREVIATION	EQUIVALENT VALUE	BECQUEREL* (DIS/S)
Megacurie	1 MCi	10^6 curies	3.7×10^{16}
Kilocurie	1 kCi	10^3 curies	3.7×10^{13}
Curie	1 Ci	1 curie	3.7×10^{10}
Millicurie	1 mCi	10^{-3} curies	3.7×10^7
Microcurie	1 μCi	10^{-6} curies	3.7×10^4
Nanocurie	1 nCi	10^{-9} curies	3.7×10^1
Picocurie	1 pCi	10^{-12} curies	3.7×10^{-2}
Femtocurie	1 fCi	10^{-15} curies	3.7×10^{-5}

*Prefixes may also be used. For example, 3.7×10^{10} Bq = 37 gigabecquerel (GBq).

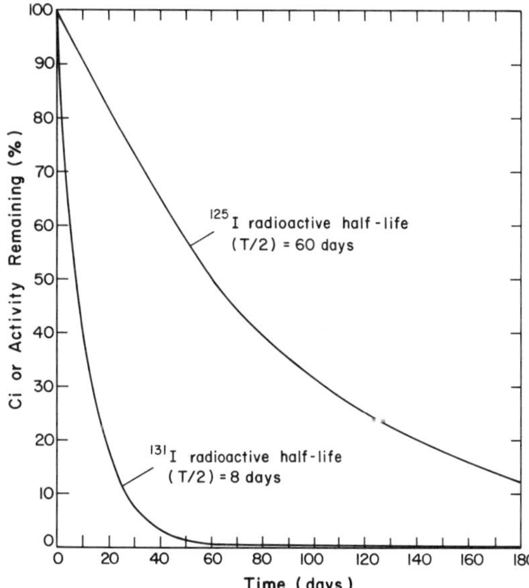

FIG 26–2.
Decay curves resulting from the physical radioactive half-lives of two iodine isotopes.

exposures from α or β radiation. Neutrons, which depend heavily on the composition of the irradiated material to produce ionizations or energy absorption, cannot be measured reliably in air. There is no SI unit comparable to the roentgen; however, expressing the exposure in coulomb per kilogram puts the result in basic SI units.

A special unit for inhalation exposure to radon and radon daughters in air is the *Working Level Month* (see definition in Table 26–2).

Absorbed Dose.—The conventional unit of absorbed dose is the *rad*. This unit, defined as 100 ergs/gm (or 0.01 joules/gm) of absorbed dose in any material, does away with the variation of energy absorption in different material compositions. For practical purposes, it should be noted that 1 roentgen exposure (about 93 ergs/gm) or 1 rad dose (100 ergs/gm) of x-rays or γ-rays delivered to soft tissue are approximately the same. The rad cannot be measured directly in tissue without specialized equipment. Many monitoring instruments are calibrated so that they read in rads or millirads per hour. The rad is the most common dosimetry term used in radiation protection work in the United States.

The SI unit for absorbed dose is the *gray* (Gy). One gray is equal to 100 rads. This unit is now used especially in England and Europe and may become more common in the U.S. in the future.

A special unit for absorbed dose used by dosimetry experts for some special purposes is the kerma (*k*inetic *e*nergy *r*eleased in *ma*terial). Kerma (K) is a unit of quantity that represents the kinetic energy transferred to charged particles by the uncharged particles per unit mass of the irradiated medium. The concept is closely related to the energy equivalent of exposure in an x-ray beam.

Dose Equivalent.—*Dose equivalent* (DE) is a quantity that expresses all types of ionizing radiation on a common scale for calculating the effective absorbed dose. It is defined as the product of the absorbed dose in rads and modifying factors. Although the rad specifies a known deposition of energy, it turns out that this does not always relate directly to observed biologic effects. Thus, 100 rads of x-rays do not have the same effect as 100 rads of neutrons. A *quality factor* (QF) is used in calculating a dose equivalent to adjust for such differences. The QF is a LET-dependent factor by which absorbed doses are multiplied to obtain (for radiation-protection purposes) a quantity that expresses the effectiveness of an absorbed dose on a common scale for all types of ionizing radiation. For most purposes, the QF can be taken as 1 for x-rays or γ-rays, 1 for electrons, 5 for protons, and 20 for α particles. The QF for neutrons varies significantly with energy. A value of 10 has been used up to now as a maximum value for neutrons, but this may be raised to 20 in the near future. *Relative biologic effectiveness* [RBE] is a term used by the radiobiologist. It is a factor used to compare the biologic effects caused by absorbed radiation doses in rads of a particular radiation under study with effects from the same doses of 250 kVp x-rays. *Relative biologic effectiveness* is a term used only in radiobiology and should not be confused with the QF.

Another modifier is the *distribution factor* (DF). This factor is used to account for differences in biologic effect resulting from nonuniform distribution of radionuclides deposited within an organ.

The conventional unit of dose equivalent is the *rem*. The rem is equal to the absorbed dose (in rads) times the QF times the DF times any other necessary modifying factors. It represents a quantity of radiation that is equivalent in terms of biologic damage (for purposes of radiation protection) to 1 rad of 250-kVp x-rays.

The SI unit of dose equivalent is the *sievert* (Sv). One sievert is equal to 100 rem.

RADIATION MEASUREMENTS

The physician in occupational medicine does not ordinarily become involved in monitoring radiation, but he or she should be able to interpret and evaluate the results. Of chief interest here is the measurement techniques that are used to determine exposure potential and absorbed doses. These are summarized briefly in four subject areas: radiation monitoring, personnel dosimetry, direct in vivo counting, and excretion sampling.

Radiation Monitoring

A fundamental way of measuring ionizing radiation is to count the amount of ionization produced in some suitable medium. Ionization of gases has been the most widely used method of detecting and measuring ionizing radiation; it is the principle used in ionization chambers, proportional counters, and Geiger-Muller (GM) meters. There are also a variety of crystals in which ionizing radiation produces a faint flash of light; these are called scintillation counters. The light flashes are measured with a photomultiplier tube that is directly coupled to the scintillating phosphor. The light intensity of each pulse is proportional to the energy of the radiation producing it; thus, the energy of the radiation can be measured in addition to the number of ionizing events. The radiation energies can be used to help identify the specific radionuclides producing the radiation. One of the more common phosphors in use is a sodium iodide crystal used in laboratory counting systems and whole-body counters. For detailed descriptions of these techniques, refer to texts[9, 62, 75] on radiation measurements.

Ionization chambers and GM meters are common portable instruments used for measurement of β, γ, or x-ray radiation. Discrimination against β radiation is made by use of a shield on the probe which is dense enough to stop β particles. Most β-γ instruments can be calibrated to read directly in milliroentgens per hour or millirads per hour. Some read in counts per minute (cpm). These readings can be converted approximately to milliroentgens per hour by dividing counts per minute by 2,500 (cpm/2500 = mR/hr).

A small-diameter end-window detector probe is a useful instrument for locating small β-γ particles on the skin and in wounds. It is helpful in final clean-up procedures to check areas that are difficult to decontaminate, such as around the nose, eyes, ears, and fingernails. The principal advantage of the small end-window detector is its ability to pinpoint the location as compared to larger GM detector probes.

Alpha radiation monitoring requires a special instrument designed with minimal absorbing material (a few milligrams per square centimeter at most) in the window of the detector. Because of the extremely low penetrating power of α particles, the survey must be made as close as possible to the surface being monitored. Fluids such as moisture or blood on the surface will preclude a reliable alpha survey. Alpha activity within a wound will not be detected by alpha monitoring instruments. The chance of misinterpretation or error of α monitoring is much greater than with β-γ radiation. Alpha readings are generally expressed in counts per minute (cpm). About half of the particles travel toward the detector, while the other half go in the opposite direction. A rough rule of thumb to obtain the number of nuclear disintegrations per minute is to double the cpm reading of the instrument.

For radionuclide contamination, it is helpful to know if the activity is transferable or not. This is done by taking swipes of the surface with a clean piece of filter paper and then counting the paper for radioactivity. This technique is widely used in surveying for radionuclides with low-energy β (e.g., tritium) or α radiation (e.g., plutonium).

Personal Dosimetry

Personal dosimeters are worn to determine the absorbed dose of penetrating (external) radiation. The common devices used for this purpose are pocket dosimeters, film badges, or thermoluminescent (TLD) badges.

The *pocket dosimeter* is a small ionization chamber about the size and shape of a fountain pen. It can be either a self-reading type or a type that requires a separate reader-charger unit. These are used primarily to obtain an immediate dose reading in the field. An important characteristic of these devices is that any failure or error results in high or off-scale readings. A zero or small reading is a trustworthy value, provided the device was in proper position on the exposed person.

The *film badge* uses photographic film to measure radiation dose. The badges are reliable dosimeters when properly calibrated, controlled, and processed. A good film dosimetry service should be able to measure x-ray, γ, and β radiation with an error of less than ± 30%. Film dosimetry has a dose range from about 10 mrad to nearly 1,000 rad (the high range does require special processing techniques). Special neutron film is sometimes included in personal dosimeters for measuring the dose from fast neutrons. The error for neutron dosimetry can be ± 100% or more. Note that if the neutron spectrum is unknown or does not contain a significant percentage of fast neutrons, neutron film results may be misleading. In recent years, film dosimetry has been frequently replaced by thermoluminescent detectors.

Thermoluminescent (TLD) detectors are crystals of various salts, such as lithium fluoride or californium fluoride, which can measure ionizing radiation by a phenomenon called thermoluminescence. Radiation that passes through the crystal displaces electrons into centers, or "traps," within the crystal lattice. On heating, these electrons are released with a simultaneous emission of light. The amount of light is proportional to the amount of the original radiation dose. Thermoluminescent detectors have advantages over photographic film because they are not influenced by heat, humidity, or aging. They can measure doses from about 10 mrad up to as much as a million rads.

Direct In Vivo Counting

Counting the γ radiation emitted from the body is a standard method for determining if there is radioactivity in excess of that from natural radionuclides found in everyone. Scintillation crystals are generally used for in vivo counting. These detectors are extremely sensitive and can measure the natural background activity present in each of us. The precision of measurement of γ-emitting radionuclides should be within about 30%. Both the quantity and specific energy of emitted γ-rays are measured. The quantities of each of the specific radionuclides present in the body can be determined. The sensitivity and precision is reduced seriously by external contamination, which is likely to be present after any recent contaminating accident.

There are several special types of in vivo counters designed for measurement of certain radionuclides, especially for the transuranium elements, which are those with atomic numbers above 92. These radionuclides, such as plutonium and americium, are α-emitters that also emit soft (low-energy) γ- or x-rays. Special detectors are designed to measure the low-energy γ- or x-rays. The α particles will not penetrate to the exterior of the body. These special counters are used especially for chest counting to detect the presence of these radionuclides in the lungs. Small versions of these detectors are also used as special wound counters.

Excretion Sampling

Collection and measurement of excreta, especially urine and feces, is a principal method for detecting the presence of internal emitters in the body, especially pure β- or α-emitters. The excretion rate can be used to estimate the quantity and type of radionuclide still present in the body. Such estimates are subject to considerable error because of individual differences as well as day-to-day variations in urinary excretion rates. The use of only one or two samples after an accidental intake has a significant possibility of error. A larger series of samples improves the accuracy of the estimate of the internal deposition, but the answer may still be in error by a factor of 3 or 4 for some radionuclides. For others, such as tritium or iodine, the accuracy is much better.

BIOLOGIC EFFECTS OF RADIATION IN MAN

General Concepts

Biologic effects in man after exposure to ionizing radiation result from the deposition of energy in tissue cells. The energy deposition in the form of ionization leads potentially to both immediate and long-term changes within cells. The immediate change after ionization is chemical, with formation of free radicals and excited molecules. In living tissue, the 60% or more water content is a major target of these reactions, in which OH and H radicals are formed. The reactions of these free radicals with biologically important molecules are called the "indirect" action of radiation. "Direct" action of radiation refers to an immediate interaction of ionizing radiation and critical biologic molecules. Either of these two mechanisms can damage critical molecules almost instantaneously (10^{-14} to 10^{-3} second) with the radiation exposure.

The effect of these primary events initiates a wide range of important radiation effects. Important types of radiobiologic damage are listed in Table 26–4.

The biologic effect of ionizing radiation in human beings is modified by different exposure conditions and several biologic factors. These are summarized here.

TABLE 26–4.
Selected Examples of Mammalian Radiobiologic Damage

LEVEL OF DAMAGE	IMPORTANT EFFECTS
Molecular	Damages macromoles, including DNA, RNA, and enzymes; interferes with metabolic pathways
Subcellular	Damages cell membranes, mitochondria, lysosomes, nuclei, and chromosomes
Cellular	Inhibits cell division, kills cells; causes carcinogenesis
Organ	Injures bone marrow, intestinal tract, cardiovascular and central nervous systems, with minor changes to acute deaths in severe exposures
Whole body	Death, cancer
Populations	Gene and chromosomal mutations in individuals can change genetic characteristics of offspring

Dose Rate.—The effect produced by a given dose of radiation will generally decrease as the dose rate is reduced. This reduction of effect has been termed the Dose Rate Effectiveness Factor (DREF). Biologic repair processes have a greater opportunity to be effective when more time is available. The reduction in biological effects per unit dose at high- vs. low-dose rates ranges from a factor of about 2 to 10; a most likely value is 3.[58] High dose rates would be over 5 rads/min (>0.05 Gy/min) as compared with low dose rates of the order of 5 rads/year or less (<0.05 Gy/year).

Dose Fractionation.—The division of a total dose into smaller fractions given at separate times causes less biologic damage than the same total dose given at one time. In effect, fractionation or protraction of dose is similar to a lower dose rate and gives time for more repair to occur.

Linear Energy Transfer.—The greater biologic effect of high LET radiation, such as α particles and neutrons, is taken into account by the QF value used to translate the absorbed dose (rad) into the dose equivalent (rem).

Tissue Sensitivity.—Tissues made up of rapidly dividing cells are markedly more sensitive to radiation than are tissues composed of slowly dividing cells. Tissues that are highly differentiated are composed of mature, specialized cells that are unlikely to undergo cell division, so they are likely to be less affected by radiation (radioresistant). Some radiosensitive tissues are germinal cells of the ovary and testis, bone marrow cells, and intestinal epithelial cells. Radioresistant tissues include liver, kidney, muscle, brain, bone, cartilage, and connective tissue.

Age.—Great radiation sensitivity is present during fetal development (discussed later) and to a much lesser extent in children.

Dose Distribution.—The effect of radiation is markedly changed by variation of dose to different parts of the body. For example, lower doses are delivered to bone marrow that is shielded, either by interposed tissue or by external shielding, or is located at a greater distance from the source than other portions of bone marrow. The cells in the lesser-exposed portion will provide an important salutary effect in maintaining the hematopoietic function in a heavily exposed individual. A person can survive much larger doses to limited portions of his body than a uniform dose to the entire body.

Individual Variations.—There is significant variation in the response of different individuals to a specific dose of radiation. The extent of this variation is not known, but some impressions are gained by looking at a postulated dose-lethality curve for normal man. Using this end point, it appears that differences of a factor of two or more can be anticipated between individuals.

Chemical Factors.—The presence of certain chemical factors at the time of radiation exposure can enhance or reduce the biologic effect. The most important chemical sensitizers are oxygen and the halogenated pyrimidines. The chemical radiation protective agents include a variety of sulfur-containing compounds, including cysteine, cystamine, cysteamine, glutathione (GSH), and S-(2-aminoethyl) isothiuronium bromide hydrobromide (AET).

Acute Radiation Syndrome

Exposure of the entire body to a large radiation dose, over 100 rems (1 Sv), in a single exposure, or within one or two days,

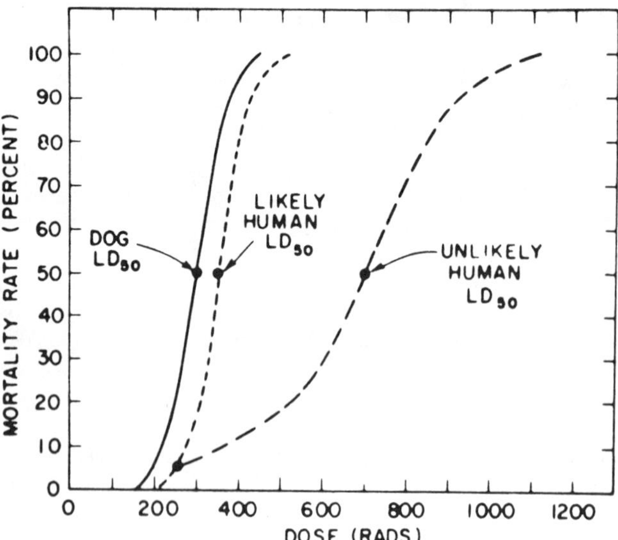

FIG 26–3.
Deduction of likely and unlikely radiation LD_{50} curves from human beings, assuming that human curve has the same slope as dog and that the lower end is established by Marshallese and clinical data. (From Lushbaugh CC: The impact of estimates of human radiation tolerance on radiation emergency management, in *The Control of Exposure to the Public to Ionizing Radiation in the Event of Accident or Attack.* Bethesda, Md, National Council on Radiation Protection and Measurements, 1982, pp 46–57.)

results in a progressive series of signs and symptoms known as the *acute radiation syndrome*. This syndrome has been observed in Japanese atom-bomb survivors; the Marshallese natives exposed to fallout radiation; reactor, accelerator, and criticality accident cases; persons exposed to lost radiography sources; and therapeutically irradiated medical patients. The clinical response and prognosis generally depend on the damage sustained by the hematopoietic system. The single dose that produces 50% mortality (LD_{50}) in healthy persons is estimated to be about 400–450 R or about 270–300 rads (2.7–3.0 Gy) to the midline of the body.[45] A dose-response curve postulated from the available data in man is given in Figure 26–3.

A summary of the principal clinical effects in relationship to acute whole-body doses of various magnitudes is shown in Table 26–5. As doses exceed about 200 rads (2 Gy), serious effects on the hematopoietic system become readily apparent. Andrews et al.[4] show the time relationships of the principal signs, symptoms, and hematologic changes (Fig 26–4) in a composite summary of five persons who received absorbed doses of 235–365 rads (2.35–3.65 Gy) as a result of a criticality accident. Using a QF of 2 for the neutron dose, the dose equivalent was calculated to be 298–461 rems (2.98–4.62 Sv). (For acute effects, the QF for neutrons is only 2 or less instead of a QF of 20 proposed for late effects.)

Initial or prodromal symptoms occur from about one to six hours after a significant acute exposure. The following symptoms can occur in some people as the indicated doses are exceeded: anorexia, 20 rads (0.2 Gy); nausea, 75 rads (0.75 Gy); vomiting, 100 rads (1 Gy); and diarrhea, 150 rads (1.5 Gy).[46] These doses assume an acute, one-time exposure and are midline whole-body doses. The severity of the symptoms may be variable and, therefore, their intensity is not very meaningful. The presence of diarrhea is an ominous sign. These initial symptoms subside within a few hours to several days if supralethal doses are not involved. There follows a relatively symptom-free latent period.

Another sign of interest after large doses is the presence or absence of skin erythema, which can appear within minutes to hours after a single large exposure. A positive response that correlates with a known exposure may suggest an exposure in excess of several hundred rads. Skin response to ionizing radiation is complex and is known to vary with dose fractionation, dose rate, radiation energy (LET), depth-dose distribution, area size, anatomical region, and the presence of other irritants or trauma.[39]

An early finding of more significance is the response of the peripheral lymphocyte count. If there are 1,000 or more lymphocytes per cubic millimeter at 48 hours after exposure, the likelihood of survival is very good. Lesser counts at this time suggest more serious doses and less than 500 lymphocytes/cu mm at 48 hours suggests a poor prognosis. During the first several days after exposure, a fluctuating leukocytosis will usually occur despite the lymphopenia.

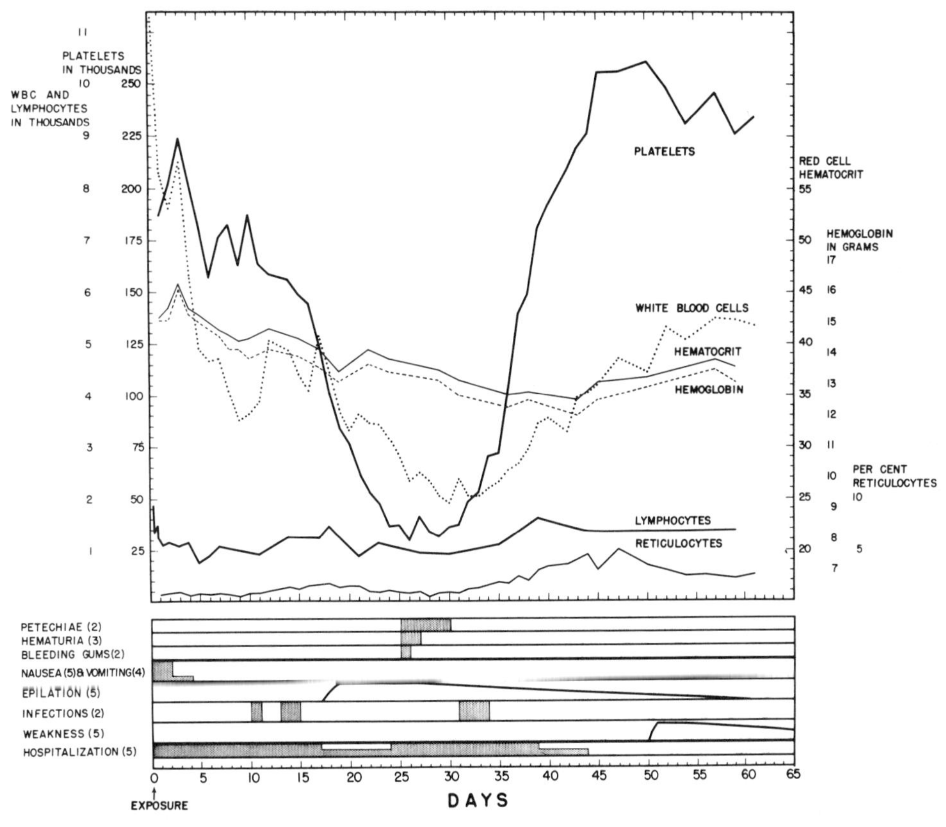

FIG 26–4.
Average hematologic values, clinical signs and symptoms of five patients exposed to 236–365 rads in the Y-12 criticality accident. (From Andrews et al: Criticality accident at the Y-12 Plant, in *Diagnosis and Treatment of Acute Radiation Injury*. Geneva, World Health Organization, 1960, pp 27–48.)

TABLE 26–5.
Dose-Effect Relationships Following Acute Whole-Body Irradiation (X- or Gamma)

WHOLE-BODY* DOSE (RADS)	CLINICAL AND LABORATORY FINDINGS
5–25	Asymptomatic. Conventional blood studies are normal. Chromosome aberrations detectable
50–75	Asymptomatic. Minor depressions of white cells and platelets detectable in a few persons, especially if baseline values established
75–125	Minimal acute doses that produce prodromal symptoms (anorexia, nausea, vomiting, fatigue) in about 10%–20% of persons within two days. Mild depressions of white cells and platelets in some persons
125–200	Symptomatic course with transient disability and clear hematologic changes in a majority of exposed persons. Lymphocyte depression of about 50% within 48 hours
240–340	Serious, disabling illness in most persons, with about 50% mortality if untreated. Lymphocyte depression of about 75+% within 48 hours
500+	Accelerated version of acute radiation syndrome, with gastrointestinal complications within two weeks, bleeding and death in most exposed persons
5,000+	Fulminating course, with cardiovascular, gastrointestinal, and CNS complications resulting in death within 24–72 hours

*Conversion of rad (midline) dose to radiation measurements in R can be made roughly by multiplying rads times 1.5. For example, 200 rad (midline) equal about 300 R (200 × 1.5).

Cytogenetic analysis of peripheral lymphocytes is the most sensitive laboratory test for detecting a clinical biologic response to ionizing radiation. The chromosome aberrations seen after radiation include inversions, translocations, deletions, dicentrics, and rings (Fig 26–5). The number of dicentrics and rings are used to estimate radiation doses. This technique is discussed in a later section on medical management of radiation cases.

Epilation occurs when doses in excess of about 300 rads (3 Gy) are absorbed by hair follicles. This sign occurs rather abruptly beginning about the 17th day after exposure.

The latent period after the prodromal symptoms may last up to about three weeks, depending upon the dose. A shorter latent period occurs with higher doses. After the latent period, the characteristic effects of radiation damage become evident—anorexia, fatigue, malaise, epilation, fever, infections, stomatitis, and hemorrhagic phenomena. The effects of bone marrow depression now dominate the clinical picture.[25] The peripheral lymphocyte count does not recover from its lows for many weeks. The leukocyte count decreases steadily after the first few days. For some unexplainable reason, there is an "abortive rise," or at least a leveling off, of the total leukocyte count at about 8–20 days after exposure. The lack of this "abortive rise" signifies a poor prognosis. Further depression ensues until the minimal values are reached at 25–45 days after exposure. Platelet values also reach their low at about 25–32 days after exposure. Fatal exposures will have accelerated schedules that reach minimal values in less than 20 days.

The red blood cells exhibit only a slow decrease during this entire period due to their longer cell life. Hemorrhage is the major factor that can produce a serious decrease in the red blood cell series. Otherwise, the radiation effects on the red blood cell series are not as serious as for leukocytes and platelets.

After the syndrome passes through the nadir of bone marrow depression, the blood elements begin to recover. The leukocytes and platelets recover completely within about six months or less; the lymphocyte recovery is slower and may remain at subnormal levels for several years. Clinical symptoms clear rapidly, with residual fatigue being the major complaint, and this may remain for many months. Temporary sterility for up to one or two years may be present at doses of about 250 rads (2.5 Gy) or more to the gonads. Although recovery of acute effects may be complete without sequelae, there remains the possibility of long-term or late effects of radiation exposures. Except for possible local sequelae that may result in regions of unusually high dose, the patient who has recovered from an acute whole-body radiation dose will appear surprisingly normal on medical examination.

The above description is based on whole-body midline doses in the range of about 200–500 rads (2–5 Gy) of x- or γ-rays. In this range the hematologic effects are the principal threat to the patient's life. At doses above 500 rads (5 Gy), ulcerations of the gastrointestinal tract and severe fluid loss occur within a few days up to two weeks and death occurs as a result of the gastrointestinal complications. At extremely high doses—several thousands of rads or more to the whole body—the individual experiences severe gastrointestinal symptoms immediately and is disabled within hours in a hypotensive shock. Severe loss of fluids from the intestinal tract and hypotension are progressive until death occurs in a few days. Severe burns of the skin at the regions of highest doses are likely in these cases.

Thoma and Wald[84] suggest a useful plan for the preliminary evaluation of clinical radiation injury after an acute whole body dose (Fig 26–6). A blood count profile rating system was also devised by them to classify radiation cases into the five broad injury categories as the blood count changes evolve.

Radiation Skin Burns

Local radiation skin burns can result from improper handling of β or γ sources or from heavy exposure to x-ray, neutron, or other particle beams. Development of radiation burn symptoms occurs much more slowly (days) than with thermal burns. Exposure to radiation may not be recognized; suspicion must be high if painful burn-like symptoms are a presenting symptom without known etiology.

Clinical classification of acute radiation burns is erythema (first degree), transepidermal injury (second degree), and full-thickness burns (third degree). Erythema, often difficult to identify in the first week, becomes more prominent in the second week.

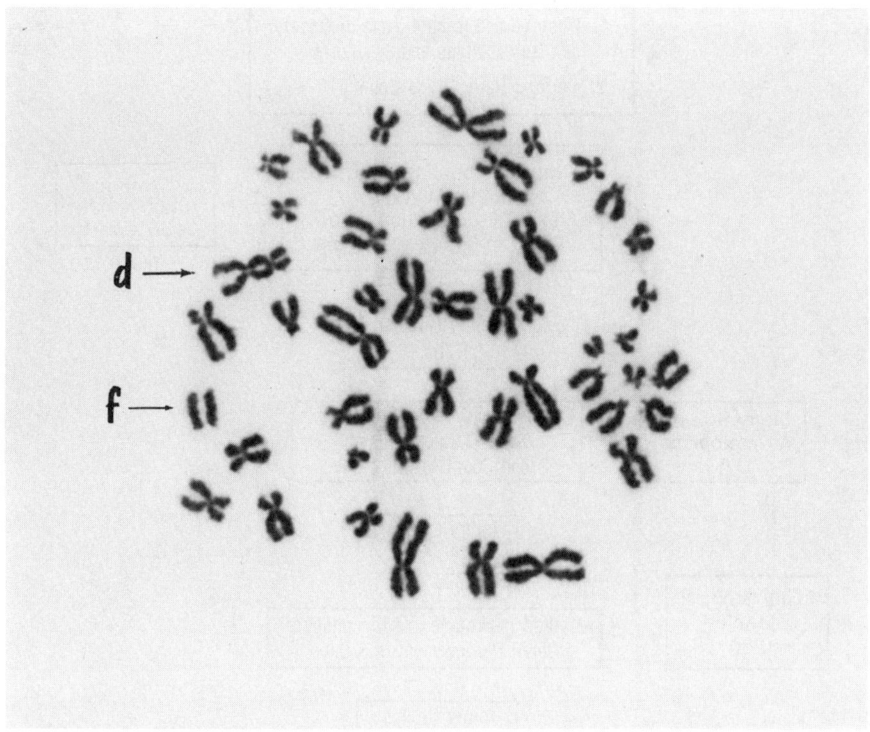

FIG 26–5.
Chromosome spread of a peripheral lymphocyte that contains a typical radiation-induced dicentric *(d)* and acentric fragment *(f)*. Dicentrics and rings are used in estimating radiation dose. (From Littlefield LG: The analysis of radiation-induced chromosome lesions in lymphocytes as a biological method for dose estimation, in *Proceedings of NATO Working Group Meeting on Assessment of Injury From Ionizing Radiation in Warfare.* Bethesda, Md, Armed Forces Radiobiology Research Institute, 1982, pp 351–387.)

Skin response is variable to the type and energy of the radiation as well as to the amount of surface area irradiated. Blistering from transepidermal injury occurs about three weeks after exposure. This usually heals without skin grafting if protected. The full-thickness burn results in moist desquamation and possible ulceration. Radiation damage in cases of full-thickness burns may produce an arteritis and result in a seriously decreased circulation to the underlying subcutaneous tissue and the involved skin. In the most severe cases, the arterial damage may result in necrosis and gangrene of the distal portions of fingers or extremities.

Threshold erythema and epilation begin at about 300 rads (3 Gy) and above for single doses of 100 keV x-ray. For higher energy x-rays (1,000 kVp), doses of 600 rads (6 Gy) or more may be absorbed with minimal erythema. Single acute doses of about 1,000 rads (10 Gy) or multiple doses over several weeks totaling 3,000 rads (30 Gy) will result in dry desquamation. Moist desquamation and ulceration will begin after acute doses in excess of 2,000 rads (20 Gy). Fractionation or protraction of the dose results in less skin damage for a given total dose.

Figure 26–7 shows local radiation burns on the fingers of a person who placed his hands near the beam port of an x-ray spectrometer. No burning was felt during a two- to four-second exposure period. About 15 minutes later, he discovered the machine was turned on. A radiation safety interlock circuit had been inactivated during recent modifications to the machine and resulted in this preventable accident.

Internal Radionuclide Exposures

Any radioactive material that enters the body, either through the lungs, gastrointestinal tract, wounds, or intact skin, becomes a so-called *internal emitter*. An internal emitter will continue to irradiate surrounding tissues until either it is excreted by some physiologic process, principally through the urine or feces, or it becomes inactive through radioactive decay.

The amount of absorption of radioactive material is dependent upon a number of factors. After inhalation of radioactive particulates, the absorption through the lung depends on the particle size and the chemical nature of the material. Absorption will be greater for small particles, under 5 μm, that can reach the nonciliated portion of the bronchial tree and alveoli where absorption can take place. Chemical forms that are relatively soluble in body fluids will be absorbed from the lung or gastrointestinal tract into the systemic circulation and redeposited in various organs. The complex processes of absorption and redistribution in the body are simulated by mathematical models[28] to aid in estimating uptake and organ doses for various radionuclides.

Each radionuclide has a physical half-life as well as an independent *biologic half-time* (biologic $T_{1/2}$), which is the time required by the body to eliminate 50% of an administered dose of any substance via the urine, feces, or other excreta. The *physical half-life* (physical $T_{1/2}$) is the time required for a radioactive substance to lose 50% of its activity by decay. The *effective half-life* is the time required for a radionuclide in the body to be diminished

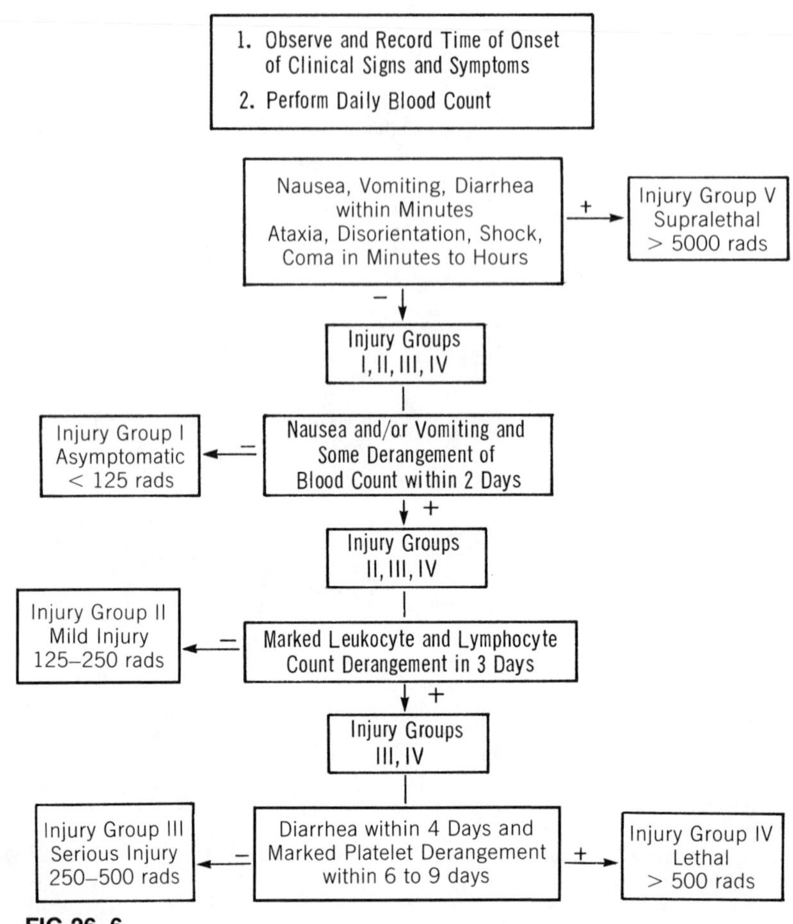

FIG 26–6.
Procedure for preliminary evaluation of clinical radiation injury. (Modified from Thoma GE, Wald N: Diagnosis and management of accidental radiation injury. *J Occup Med* 1959; 1:421.)

by 50% as a result of the combined action of radioactive decay and biologic elimination. Effective half-life equals

$$\frac{\text{biologic } T_{1/2} \times \text{physical } T_{1/2}}{\text{biologic } T_{1/2} + \text{physical } T_{1/2}}$$

An internal emitter will be metabolized according to its elemental chemical properties, just the same as its stable isotopes. Radioactive sodium 24 will be distributed to all tissues of the body just like the normal distribution of its stable isotope, sodium 25. Other radionuclides will concentrate in particular organs; for example, radioactive iodine 131 concentrates in the thyroid gland the same as stable iodine 127.

The internal dose is highly dependent on the physical properties of the radiation produced by the particular radionuclide. Alpha emitters are of particular importance as internal emitters due to the dense path of ionization produced by α particles, i.e., high-LET radiation. The dose rate to the organ is a function of the quantity of radioactivity per gram of organ tissue and the amount of energy deposited in organ tissue by each photon or particle produced. The total dose to the organ requires integrating the dose rate over time until the radioactivity has decayed.

The organ dose from internal emitters is delivered continuously and is thus protracted over time. As noted earlier, protraction of the dose permits more repair to occur and reduces the biologic effect to some extent in comparison to an acute radiation dose. It is not expected that internal emitters will result in an acute radiation effect unless the initial dose rate is exceedingly high.

The principal biologic effect of concern from occupational exposures to internal emitters is the induction of cancer. This potential late effect becomes manifest years later. The probability (risk) of an excess cancer from radiation is dependent on the radiation dose to particular organs and the radiosensitivity of those organs. This is discussed further in the section on carcinogenesis as a late effect of radiation.

Long-Term Effects of Ionizing Radiation

Some types of long-term effects of ionizing radiation occur from tissue damage only after doses exceeding a certain threshold level. Examples of such effects include chronic radiodermatitis, cataracts, and sterility. Below the threshold dose, these types of radiation damage are not apparent. Above the threshold, the radiation effect is roughly proportional to the dose.

Other types of long-term effects of ionizing radiation have

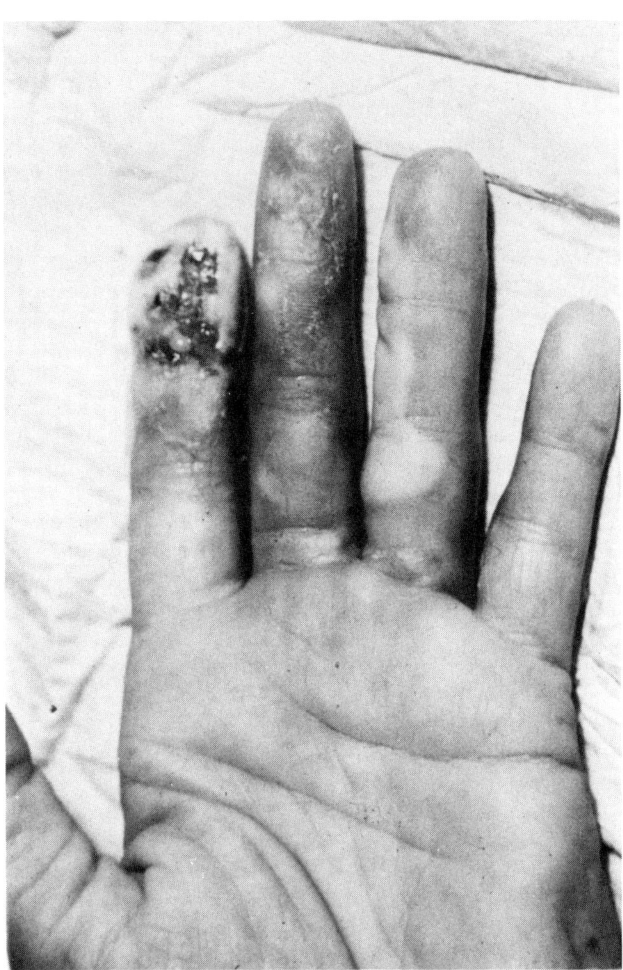

FIG 26–7.
Radiation burns 28 days after a single acute skin dose of 2,400–4,800 rads of 60-kVp x-rays. Dose to the palm was less that 1,000 rads. The employee suffered some loss of tissue and function of the left index finger. (Courtesy of Robert C. Ricks, Oak Ridge Associated Universities, Oak Ridge, Tenn.)

been observed to occur with an increased incidence that is proportional to the dose. Cancer induction and genetic effects are examples of this type of increased risk after exposure. It is the risk, i.e., the probability of an increased incidence of disease, that is proportional to the dose rather than the magnitude of the effect. For health protection purposes, it is assumed that such risk is present for any and all doses without regard to a threshold dose. These cancers and genetic effects have no diagnostic features that distinguish whether they are due to radiation or to other causes. The association with radiation is made by statistical analysis of dose effect relationships.

Chronic Radiodermatitis.—Chronic radiodermatitis results in a dry, hairless, red, atrophic skin that has numerous telangiectatic areas. The damaged skin cracks easily and has decreased resistance to trauma. Depigmentation was a prominent feature of the healed dermatitis seen in the Marshall Islanders after acute β-ray burns from fallout particles on the skin. Damaged areas may develop keratoses and malignancies at later times. Squamous cell carcinomas are the most common after irradiation, but basal cell carcinomas can also occur. It has been observed that the incidence of skin neoplasms may be enhanced by radiation without gross injury to the skin. Chronic skin changes may occur after subsidence of an acute radiodermatitis or may develop more gradually after multiple or protracted lower doses. Nevertheless, skin is not a particularly radiosensitive organ, and the risk of skin cancer after skin doses of a few hundred rads is apparently so low that it is not demonstrated in human epidemiologic studies. Doses required to produce late skin sequelae are in excess of 1,000 rads (10 Gy) to the basal cell layer of the skin.[39] Multiple exposures require substantially higher doses for the same effect. If high doses are protracted over periods of greater than 30 days, it is possible that chronic sequelae can occur without producing an acute skin reaction.

Cataracts.—The lens of the eye is especially sensitive to radiation when uniformly irradiated. Radiation cataracts have been studied in physicists exposed to neutrons during the operation of accelerators, in patients after therapeutic radiation, and in the Japanese atomic-bomb survivors. The extent of cataract opacity, as well as the incidence, is dose-dependent. Although minimum stationary opacities have been observed after single doses of 100–200 rads (1–2 Gy), progressive cataracts occur after doses of about 500 rads (5 Gy).[87] The lens is spared by fractionation of the dose. If the exposure is spread over 3–12 weeks, a dose of 1,000 rads (10 Gy) results in a 75% incidence of cataract and a dose of 1,500 rads (15 Gy) leads to 100% incidence.[87] The latent period varies from less than a year to 35 years, with an average of two to three years, although latency is also dose-dependent. Larger doses result in shorter latent periods.

Radiation cataracts form at the posterior pole of the lens as an initial subcapsular plaque and progress to opacification involving the nucleus of the lens. Most radiation cataracts do not progress beyond partial obstruction of vision. Although, in the early stage, this type of cataract can be readily differentiated from typical senile cataracts, the clinical appearance of a radiation cataract is indistinguishable from cataracts produced by other etiologic agents. Similar posterior subcapsular cataracts have been caused by intense, chronic infrared exposures, high-voltage electrical shocks or lightning shocks, radar and ultrasonic radiation, and certain drugs or toxic agents (e.g., nitrophenol, naphthalene, steroids, and MER-29). A particularly difficult differential diagnosis exists with complicated cataracts, which form in the posterior subcapsular area of the lens and are indistinguishable from radiation cataracts. These often occur without apparent cause, but may be associated with endogenous ocular and systemic diseases.

Under conditions other than gross accidental overexposure to radiation, it should not be anticipated that radiation will produce lens changes. However, the incidence of cataracts in later life may raise questions about a history of radiation exposure, and thus one must be prepared to document the radiation doses received at work.[89]

Sterility.—Although sterility is a well-known late effect of high doses of radiation to the gonads and is of more than ordinary concern to workers, it has not been a serious sequelae after accidental exposures. Accidental whole-body doses up to 300 rads (3

Gy), such as in the Marshall Islanders, exposed Japanese fishermen, and industrial accident cases, have not caused permanent sterility. Temporary periods of sterility do occur after such high doses for up to three years after exposure. Brief periods of sterility have been recorded after doses as low as 10–15 rads (0.1–0.15 Gy).[87] Conceptions after recovery have resulted in healthy children. In women, permanent sterility results from single doses of 320 to over 600 rads (3.2–6 Gy); in men, permanent aspermia occurs after doses in excess of 200 rads (2 Gy) up to 600 rads (6 Gy).[87] Radiation does not appear to have a long-term effect on potency or libido.

Prenatal Irradiation Effects.—An embryo or fetus is particularly sensitive to ionizing radiation injury. Malformations observed in experimental animals indicate that the sensitivity and the type of defect produced are markedly dependent on the stage of development at the time of irradiation. In the preimplantation period (nine to ten days after conception), death of the embryo is thought to be the only effect and is unlikely to be observed. Irradiation during the period of major organogenesis (second to sixth week of gestation in human beings) may induce all types of malformations after relatively large doses (50–200 rads [0.5–2 Gy] are used in experimental animals). After the sixth week, in humans, the susceptibility to malformations begins to decrease except for cerebral and gonadal developmental disturbances. A peak incidence of microcephaly and mental retardation was noted in Japanese children who were in the 7th to 15th week of gestation when their mothers were exposed within 1,200 m of ground zero of the Hiroshima atomic bomb blast.[50] The incidence was reduced in those exposed from 16 to 25 weeks postconception and no increase above the expected was noted for exposures after 25 weeks postconception. Their doses are estimated to be in excess of 50–100 rads (0.5–1 Gy). It has been estimated that 80% of malformed children with a history of irradiation in utero are microcephalics.[71]

For doses of less than 5 rads (less than 0.05 Gy) received at the period critical for the induction of any one specific type of maldevelopment, it is unlikely that an increase in this type of malformation could be measurable in human populations.[57] The possibility remains open that a dose of a few rads (5–10) at critical stages in human organogenesis can cause an increased incidence of developmental anomalies. The National Council on Radiation Protection and Measurements recommends that the maximum permissible dose equivalent to the embryo-fetus from occupational exposure of the expectant mother should be 0.5 rem (5 mSv) during the entire gestation period.[56] They note that any special restrictions that need to be imposed on potentially pregnant women depend on a number of circumstances. These include the amount and temporal distribution of radiation exposure and such matters as whether female employees agree to or are asked to disclose pregnancy to management and how soon after conception a pregnancy can be recognized.

Carcinogenesis.—Induction of cancer by ionizing radiation is the major late health effect and is the principle limiting risk on which guidelines for permissible radiation exposures to workers and to the public are based. Extensive discussions on the risk of cancer induction after low doses at low dose rates have dominated the subject of late effects of ionizing radiation in recent years. Three major reports from prestigious scientific committees have been published in the past decade. These reports are the 1977 report of the United Nations Scientific Committee on the Effects of Radiation (UNSCEAR),[86] the 1980 BEIR (Biological Effects of Ionizing Radiation) III report of the U.S. National Academy of Sciences,[65] and the 1985 radioepidemiologic tables report of the U.S. National Institutes of Health.[63] Several recent summary publications[7, 88, 93] are noteworthy within the vast literature on this subject.

Development of skin cancers on the hands of the early x-ray experimenters was reported by 1902, only seven years after the discovery of x-rays. Since then, many animal studies and human epidemiologic studies have shown that ionizing radiation causes an increased incidence of almost all types of cancers. The 1980 BEIR III report lists the following sites or tissues under the category of those in which radiation-induced cancer has *not* been observed: prostate, uterus and cervix, testis, mesentery and mesothelium, and chronic lymphocytic leukemia. Sites or tissues in which the magnitude of the dose-specific risk is uncertain are specified as: larynx, nasal sinuses, parathyroid, ovary, and connective tissues.[65] The relationship of ionizing radiation to the induction of malignant lymphoma is tenuous.[63] Major radiogenic cancers, together with references to a few supporting studies, are listed in Table 26–6.

Cancers induced by radiation are indistinguishable from those occurring naturally. Their existence can be inferred only on the basis of a statistical excess above the natural incidence. The latent period between radiation dose and clinical manifestation of cancer can be as short as two years for leukemias and bone cancers, but is typically ten years or more for solid organ tumors. The latent periods can be many years and have been observed to be as long as the periods of observation in man so far, i.e., about 35 years.

Another variable affecting the risk of radiogenic cancers is the age at exposure. Excess risk for radiogenic cancers appears to decline relative to base-line risk with increasing age at time of exposure. Base-line risk increases with age, and thus although the absolute excess risk will increase with increasing age at exposure, the risk relative to base-line incidence decreases.

The mechanism for carcinogenesis is not known; the principal theories involve gene mutation or an activation of a latent carcinogenic virus or oncogene. The process of carcinogenesis is traditionally viewed as occurring in three successive phases: initiation, promotion, and progression. Ionizing radiation can act as both an initiator and promoter of carcinogenesis. It appears that it is more potent as a promoter than an initiator. It is now thought possible that the long latent period that characteristically elapses between radiation dose and the clinical observation of cancer may result from the need for successive oncogenes to be activated or for other types of sequential promotional changes to take place.

The chief unknown about radiation carcinogenesis is whether a threshold dose exists below which cancer is not induced. That question still is not answerable. The risk of induction of excess cancers after radiation exposure is obtained from human epidemiologic studies. These studies in which a dose-effect relationship can be demonstrated usually involve radiation doses of 50 rads (0.5 Gy) and above. The projection of cancer risks at low doses and low dose rates is made by mathematical extrapolations from the data of these high-dose studies to low doses. Frequently a linear, nonthreshold assumption is made as a basis for extrapolation.

TABLE 26–6.
Radiation-Induced Cancers Observed in Human Epidemiology Studies

TUMOR TYPES*	EXPOSURE COHORT	TYPE OF RADIATION	KEY REFERENCES
Bone	Radiation dial painters	α: ^{226}Ra, ^{228}Ra	70
	Patients: tuberculosis, spondylitis	α: ^{224}Ra	49
	Patients: ankylosing spondylitis	X-ray	37
Breast	Fluoroscopy patients: tuberculosis	X-ray	8
	Radiotherapy patients: acute mastitis	X-ray	79
	Atom-bomb survivors	γ, neutron†	35, 85, 92
Colon	Atom-bomb survivors	γ, neutron†	35
Esophagus	Atom-bomb survivors	γ, neutron†	35
	Radiotherapy patients: spondylitis	X-ray	11
Leukemia	Atom-bomb survivors	γ, neutron†	24, 35
	Fetuses	X-ray	51, 83
	Radiotherapy patients: spondylitis	X-ray	81
	Early radiologists	X-ray	47
Liver	Thorotrast patients	α: thorium 232	48
Lung	Atom-bomb survivors	X-ray	35, 92
	Radiotherapy patients: spondylitis	X-ray	81
	Uranium miners	α: radon 222 daughters	5, 74
Kidney, bladder	Atom-bomb survivors	γ, neutron†	35
Salivary gland	Radiotherapy: thymus, head, neck	X-ray	22, 72, 78
Stomach	Atom-bomb survivors	γ, neutron†	35, 92
	Radiotherapy patients: spondylitis	X-ray	11
Thyroid	Atom-bomb survivors	γ, neutron†	68, 92
	Radiotherapy patients: tinea capitis	X-ray	69
	Fallout	β (iodines), γ	10

*Other cancer types that have been associated with radiation but whose risks are less certain include multiple myeloma, lymphoma, pancreas, brain, and skin.
†Japanese A-bomb neutron doses are being revised downward. Principal dose is from γ-rays.

This linear, nonthreshold relationship is shown as curve 'B' in Figure 26–8. In most cases, the linear hypothesis probably overestimates the risk from low-dose, low-LET radiation.[65] There is increasing evidence that a linear-quadratic dose-effect model estimates low dose effects more appropriately. This model is represented schematically by the S-shaped curve 'A' in Figure 26–8. In preparing the radioepidemiologic tables for the National Institutes of Health report,[63] the committee used the linear-quadratic model for all radiogenic cancers except for the thyroid and breast. They also noted that there is uncertainty about the carcinogenic effects of very low doses of radiation. The BEIR III committee was unwilling to make estimates of the carcinogenic effects of radiation for acute doses below 10 rads (0.1 Gy) or for continuing exposure to doses below 1 rad (0.01 Gy) per year.[65]

Based on human epidemiologic studies, animal experimental data, and use of mathematical models, risk coefficients have been calculated for the excess cancer incidence and mortality that is thought to be attributable to ionizing radiation. Examples of such risk coefficients for excess cancer incidence are listed in Table 26–7. Despite the uncertainties present in such numbers, it is noteworthy as a pioneering effort to quantify risk for specific doses and a few individual characteristics. The use of such risk coefficients in formulating health protection standards and in resolving litigation on alleged radiation health effects is in an experimental period. The standard-setting agencies will undoubtedly evaluate the societal opinion on risk-benefit decisions with better definition of risk coefficients than in the past. The courts are trying to figure out how to handle such data in expert testimony. Current discussions are considering if a calculated probability of causation in a specific case can provide a better basis for decisions than adversarial expert opinions.

It has been inferred[12] that as much as 75%–80% of fatal cancers in the United States result from the influence of life-style and other nonhereditary, or environmental, factors. Some major factors, according to epidemiologic studies, are smoking, alcohol consumption, and diet. Radiation, chemical pollution, occupational exposures, medical therapy, and infections are thought to contribute to a lesser extent. There are interactive effects between these various factors that are poorly understood. In evaluating the question of causation of cancer by a risk factor, such as radiation, one should consider the potential of multiple causes as well as the host-related characteristics.

Thus, the cancer risk from radiation at low doses and low dose rates is not known precisely. Nevertheless, it is better known than that for other carcinogens. The risk is small enough that, at current occupational exposure guideline limits, it is extremely unlikely that it will be observable by any current method of study. The presence of cancer in an individual who has had a history of radiation exposure, both occupational and medical, plus other possible additive and synergistic insults, provides an unsolvable prob-

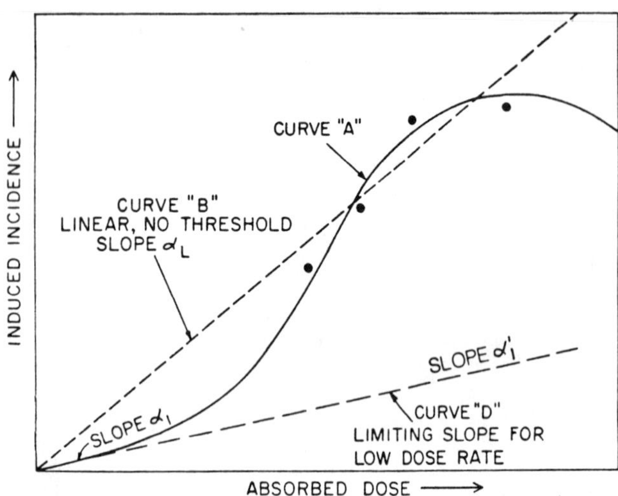

FIG 26–8.
Schematic curves of cancer incidence vs. absorbed dose showing four representative high dose/high dose rate data points. Curve *A* represents a linear-quadratic model; curve *B* is a linear model without a threshold.

lem. In case of litigation, the medical testimony will rest on opinions on the probability that the occupational radiation dose may or may not have been a major causative agent. The availability of risk coefficients for radiation should help form these medical opinions in the future.

Life Shortening.—A nonspecific life-shortening and aging effect has been claimed to be caused by radiation, based on gross experimental observations of irradiated animals. This concept is no longer considered to be valid. The UNSCEAR 1982 report[87] concluded, "while the presence of such an effect cannot be excluded for higher doses, there is no firm evidence that diffuse nonspecific mechanisms causing premature death in the irradiated animals may be operating at the low doses and dose rates of significance to the radiation protection of man." The report points out that the long-term radiation effects are essentially cancerogenic under these conditions and this explains the life-shortening seen in experimental animals. The same conclusion is noted for epidemiologic data in man, such as in the Japanese atom-bomb survivors study.

Genetic Effects.—Ionizing radiation can produce submicroscopic changes in individual genes (gene mutations) and observable damage to the chromosome structure (chromosome aberrations). If the involved gene is in a germinal cell of the testis or ovary, it can produce a heritable mutation. Mutations due to radiation were first noted in fruit fly studies during the 1920s. Most of our current information comes from experimental studies on animals, especially mice. There are very few data available on man. The largest study of genetic effects of exposed humans has been done on over 27,000 offspring of the Japanese atomic-bomb survivors.[73, 87] Two probable mutations have been observed in these children thus far; the number is far too small to provide a meaningful estimate of mutation rates.

The BEIR III committee estimated the increase from radiation exposure will be about 60 to 1,100 per million liveborn offspring per rem of parental exposure received in each generation before conception.[65] This expected incidence is reached only after a large number of generations of exposure because the disorders experienced in any given generation result both from newly induced mutations and from mutations transmitted from an earlier generation.

The UNSCEAR 1982 report[87] noted that data on experimental animals and man point to the possibility that the estimate for diseases falling under the category of chromosomal diseases may be lower than previously estimated. They estimated that when a population is continuously exposed to low doses of low-LET radiation at a rate of 1 rad (0.1 Gy) per generation (30 years is con-

TABLE 26–7.
Absolute Excess Cancer Incidence Per 100,000 Persons Per Year Per Rad (Organ Dose) for Low Levels of Low-LET Radiation*

TYPE OF CANCER	MEN EXPOSURE AGE (YEARS) 20–34	35–49	50+	WOMEN EXPOSURE AGE (YEARS) 20–34	35–49	50+
Leukemia†	.0846	.105	.156	.0538	.0670	.0990
Esophagus	.0052	.0084	.0224	.0052	.0084	.0224
Stomach	.0308	.0508	.134	.0308	.0508	.134
Colon	.0208	.0336	.0892	.0208	.0336	.0892
Liver	.028	.028	.028	.028	.028	.028
Pancreas	.018	.030	.0788	.018	.030	.0788
Lung	.056	.086	.120	.056	.086	.120
Breast‡	—	—	—	.49	.13	.08
Urinary	.0200	.0368	.0648	.0200	.0368	.0648
Thyroid	.05	.05	.05	.15	.15	.15

*From National Institutes of Health: *Report of the National Institutes of Health Ad Hoc Working Group to Develop Radioepidemiological Tables,* NIH Publ 85–2748. US Government Printing Office, 1985.
†All types of leukemia except chronic lymphatic.
‡Highest risk for female breast cancer (age 10–19) is 0.76. Risk coefficients for ages under 20 are not given.

sidered one generation) then the increment in genetic diseases is likely to be of the order of 20 cases per million births in the first generation and about 150 cases per million births at equilibrium.

The current incidence of human genetic disorder is approximately 107,000 cases per million liveborn.[65] Against this large background incidence of genetic disease, the small number of cases estimated from low doses of radiation will not be noticeable. It is also noteworthy that genetic effects are applicable primarily to doses that involve the majority of the population. Individual doses will of course be a concern to the individual, but the small number of such cases has no effect on population genetics. The estimated annual average genetically significant dose equivalent is 82 mrems/yr (0.82 mSv/yr) from natural radiation and 30–40 mrems/yr (0.3–0.4 mSv/yr) from man-made sources, mostly medical x-rays. The total is about 120 mrems/yr (1.2 mSv/yr). In a 30-year generation, the total dose is 120 mrems multiplied by 30, or 3,600 mrems (36 mSv) per generation. In view of the above genetic risk estimates and average population doses, one concludes that the genetic defects added by radiation exposure to the population are small indeed compared to the current incidence of genetic disorders.

SOURCES OF RADIATION IN THE WORKPLACE

The potential sources of ionizing radiation exposure in occupations are numerous. They include a large variety of man-made radioactive sources, radiation-producing machines and equipment, and special circumstances that enhance concentrations of natural radioactivity and exposures to natural radiation. Fixed apparatus can usually be well controlled by design, and thus the potential for sizable exposures is limited. Movable apparatus, portable radioactive sources, and intense radiation-producing machines present much greater potential for higher doses, especially accidental exposures.

Application of Radionuclides

A variety of radionuclides are used in industry to perform measurements or to do radiographic examinations. Radiometric techniques use an encapsulated radioactive source to irradiate an object to be investigated. A measurement of the transmission, reflection, or scattering of radiation gives information concerning the object. Examples of industrial uses of radiation and radionuclides are listed in Table 26–8.

Many radioactive sources are relatively small and are contained in well-designed source holders. The hazard potential is quite low. The sources of greatest hazard potential are used in field radiography. Radiography requires large γ-ray sources, usually ^{60}Co or ^{192}Ir (Figs 26–9, 26–10, 26–11). Careless technique or mechanical failure occasionally results in leaving the source in the guide tube outside the shield without recognizing it. Handling or approaching the cable under these conditions will result in large exposures in a few seconds. Loss or removal of a radiographic source from its shield has resulted in some of the worst radiation accidents recorded.

Accelerators and X-ray Machines

Particle accelerators are being used with increasing frequency in industry, universities, and medical radiotherapy departments. They include Van de Graaff accelerators, cyclotrons, betatrons, synchrotrons, synchrocyclotrons, and linear accelerators. Particles commonly used for acceleration are electrons, protons, and a variety of ions, such as hydrogen, deuterium, or helium. These de-

TABLE 26–8.
Industrial Uses of Radiation and Radionuclides

TECHNIQUE—PURPOSE	RADIATION SOURCES AND NUCLIDES COMMONLY USED
1. γ-ray transmission:	
a) Radiography—detect metal or weld defects, nondestructive testing	X-ray, ^{60}Co, ^{192}Ir
b) Thickness gauges—plate measurements in rolling mills	^{60}Co, ^{137}Cs, ^{192}Ir, ^{170}Tm, ^{90}Sr
c) Thickness gauges—paper, plastics, textiles, and foils	^{106}Ru, ^{90}Sr, ^{204}Tl, ^{85}Kr, ^{147}Pm
d) Density and concentration measurements in liquids	^{60}Co, ^{137}Cs
e) Level gauging in closed vessels	^{60}Co, ^{137}Cs
2. Back-scattering methods	
a) Thickness gauge for pipes and closed vessels, various coatings on metal	^{60}Co, beta emitters
b) Moisture gauges in soil, coal, sand, etc.	Neutron (RaBe) sources
c) Oil exploration	Neutron (RaBe) source, ^{252}Cf
3. Flow and flow pattern determination	^{38}Cl, ^{24}Na, ^{82}Br, ^{131}I, ^{51}Cr, ^{46}Sc, ^{134}Cs, ^{60}Co, ^{3}H
4. Leak detection from buried water, gas or oil pipes; telephone cables; tanks	Same as 3 above
5. Mixing efficiency, flow-through, and retention times	Radioactive tracers in process ingredients
6. Hydrologic measurements	^{3}H
7. Analytic measurements, including neutron activation	All
8. Wear measurements	^{60}Co, ^{59}Fe

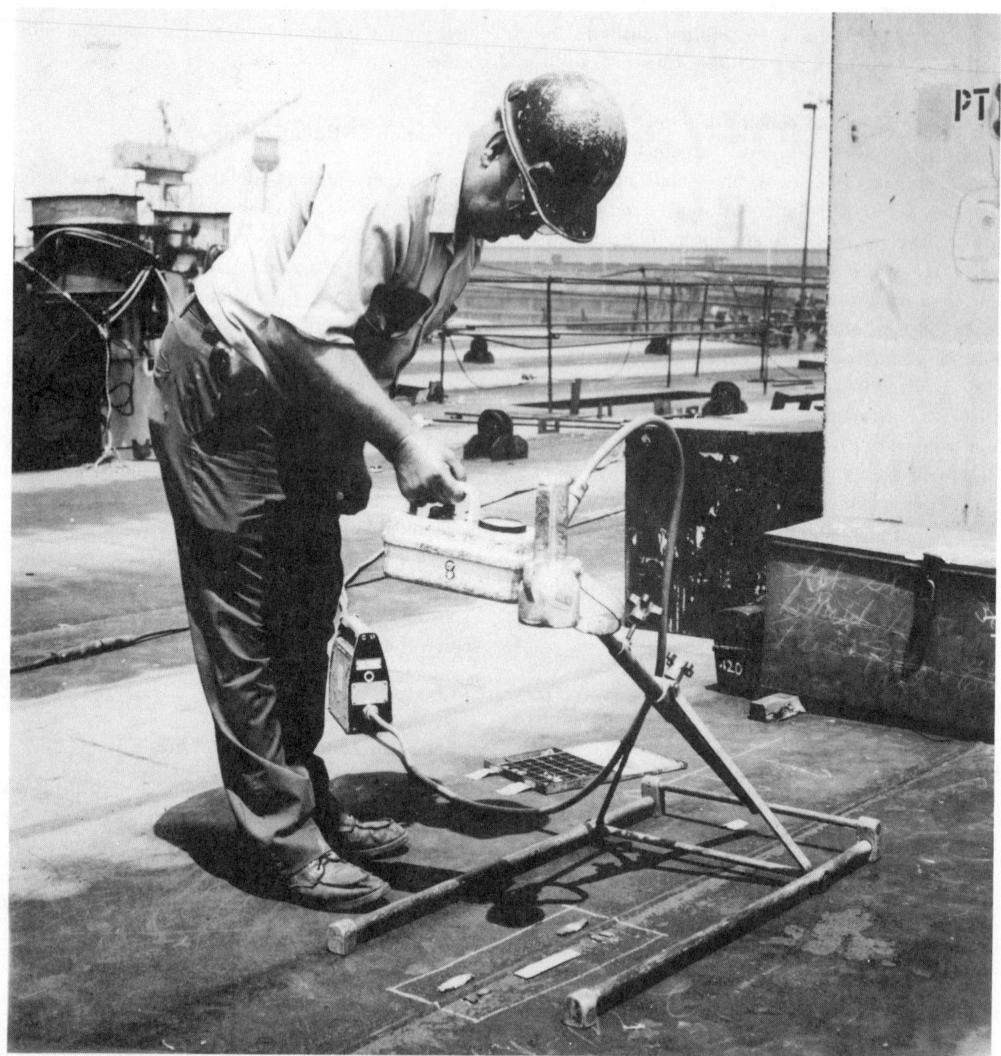

FIG 26–9.
Field γ-ray radiography using a high-level γ source, which is stored within the crank-out camera seen here near the technician's left knee. The technician, from a safe position, cranks the source out through a guide tube to its exposure position to make a radiograph. He is checking here to assure that the source is not out while he is setting up. (Courtesy of Stephen A. McGuire, U.S. Nuclear Regulatory Commission, Washington, D.C.)

vices produce a high-intensity beam of the particles moving at very high energy. The betatron, usually in the 5–25 MeV range, is used for radiographic examination of heavy metal objects (Fig 26–12). Accelerators are an important means of producing radiopharmaceuticals and other radionuclide sources. Particle beams from these machines produce secondary radiation of γ-rays, x-rays, and neutrons. Care is taken to have strict operating procedures and shielding arrangements to prevent radiation exposures. Accidental exposure of personnel from these beams can produce high doses in short periods.

X-ray machines for industrial applications are used most commonly for radiographic or fluoroscopic inspection of metal castings or welded metals. X-ray diffraction is a common technique employed to analyze the microstructure of materials. X-ray thickness gauging is used to monitor and control the thickness of moving metal sheets or strips during manufacture. The relatively fixed position of x-ray machines facilitates the use of well-designed and shielded facilities and thus the chance of accidental exposures is quite low. The experience in industry generally parallels the low incidence of accidental exposures in medical/hospital facilities.

Nuclear Reactor Industry

A nuclear reactor is a machine in which a controlled nuclear fission chain reaction takes place. Reactors are designed for several purposes: research, production of radionuclides, propulsion, and electrical power. They all operate with some type of fissionable fuel material, commonly ^{235}U or ^{239}Pu, usually in the form of pellets within rods. Reactors must have elaborate control mechanisms, cooling systems, and biologic shielding. The fuel produces

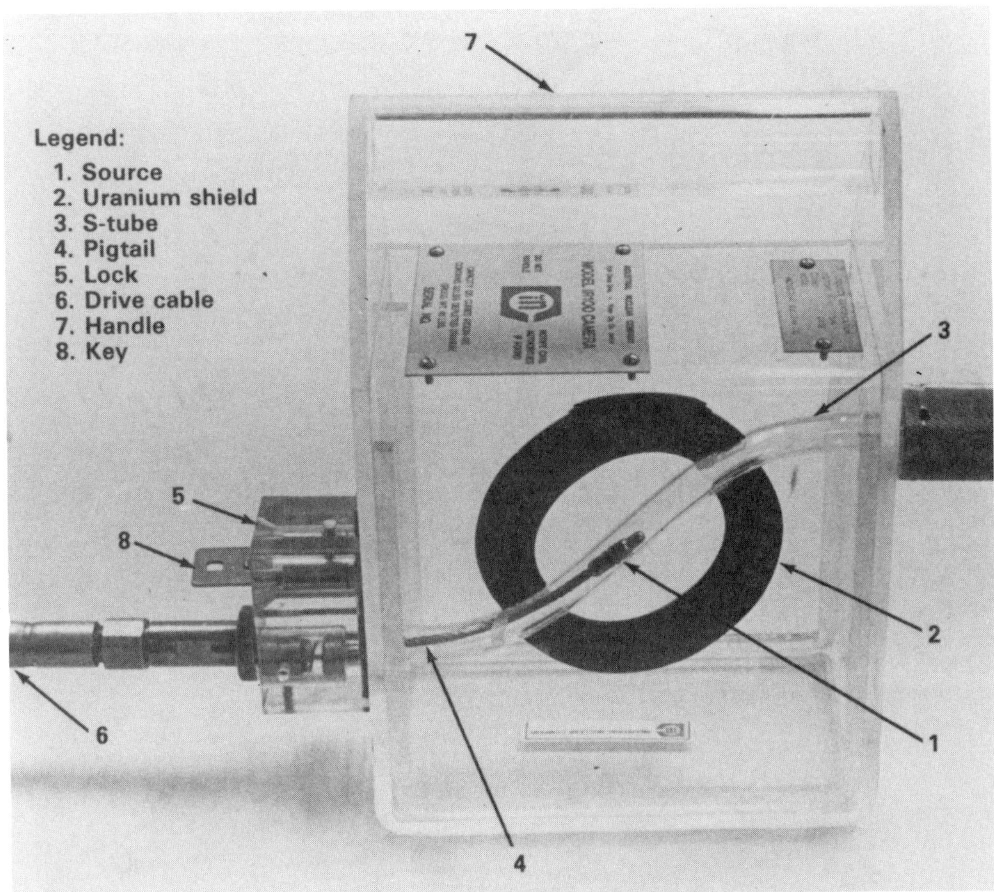

FIG 26–10.
Demonstration model of a portable crank-out camera for iridium 192. The drive cable *(6)* pushes the source *(1)* out of the shield *(2)* through a guide tube. Lost radiography sources have occurred because the fitting between the cable drive and the pigtail *(4)* disconnects. (Courtesy of Stephen A. McGuire, U.S. Nuclear Regulatory Commission, Washington, D.C.)

heat (energy) by means of a controlled, sustained fissioning of its atoms. Heat is removed via a coolant, commonly water, but sodium or potassium in breeder reactors and gases in air-cooled reactors.

The nuclear power program requires a series of industrial operations. The fuel is mined as natural uranium (0.7% ^{235}U, 99.3% ^{238}U) and is processed at a uranium mill. The natural uranium is enriched to various levels by separation at the large Department of Energy gaseous diffusion plants. The enriched ^{235}U is then fabricated into fuel elements within rigid specifications. Most U.S. reactors operate on uranium fuels enriched to about 2%–4% ^{235}U, but some require enrichment as high as 93%.

After the fuel has been used within a reactor, the highly radioactive rods are removed intact from the reactor and stored in water-filled basins at the reactor facilities. The current U.S. policy is not to process the fuel to recover the unused ^{235}U and other byproducts. The spent fuel rods are treated as high-level radioactive waste. Ultimately, this waste will be taken to a high-level waste repository for final disposition, but such a repository does not exist in the U.S. currently.

All persons working in reactor plants are classified as radiation workers. The biologic shields around a reactor reduce the radiation levels in the frequently occupied work areas to dose rates that are usually less than 1 mrad/hr (0.01 mGy/hr). The operators and technicians at reactors do not normally receive radiation doses approaching the current occupational radiation exposure guidelines. Maintenance craftspersons working around radioactive equipment and workers involved in refueling operations receive some of the higher radiation doses at reactor facilities.

In the industries supporting nuclear power, the chief radiation doses have occurred to underground uranium miners as a result of inhaling radon and/or radon daughters in mine air. Efforts to improve mine ventilation in the late 1960s resulted in much lower concentrations of radon and radon daughters as compared with earlier years. For example, air measurements in mines in the Grants, New Mexico, district indicate exposures to underground miners of 20–30 WLM/yr before 1967 and less than 2 WLM/yr after 1970. The uranium mill operators are also exposed to radon and radon daughters, but the mills historically have had much lower radon and radon daughters air concentrations than mines have had.

Radon and Radon Daughters in Air

Radon 222 is a gaseous decay product of ^{226}Ra, which is in the uranium chain of natural radioactivity. The parent radionuclide

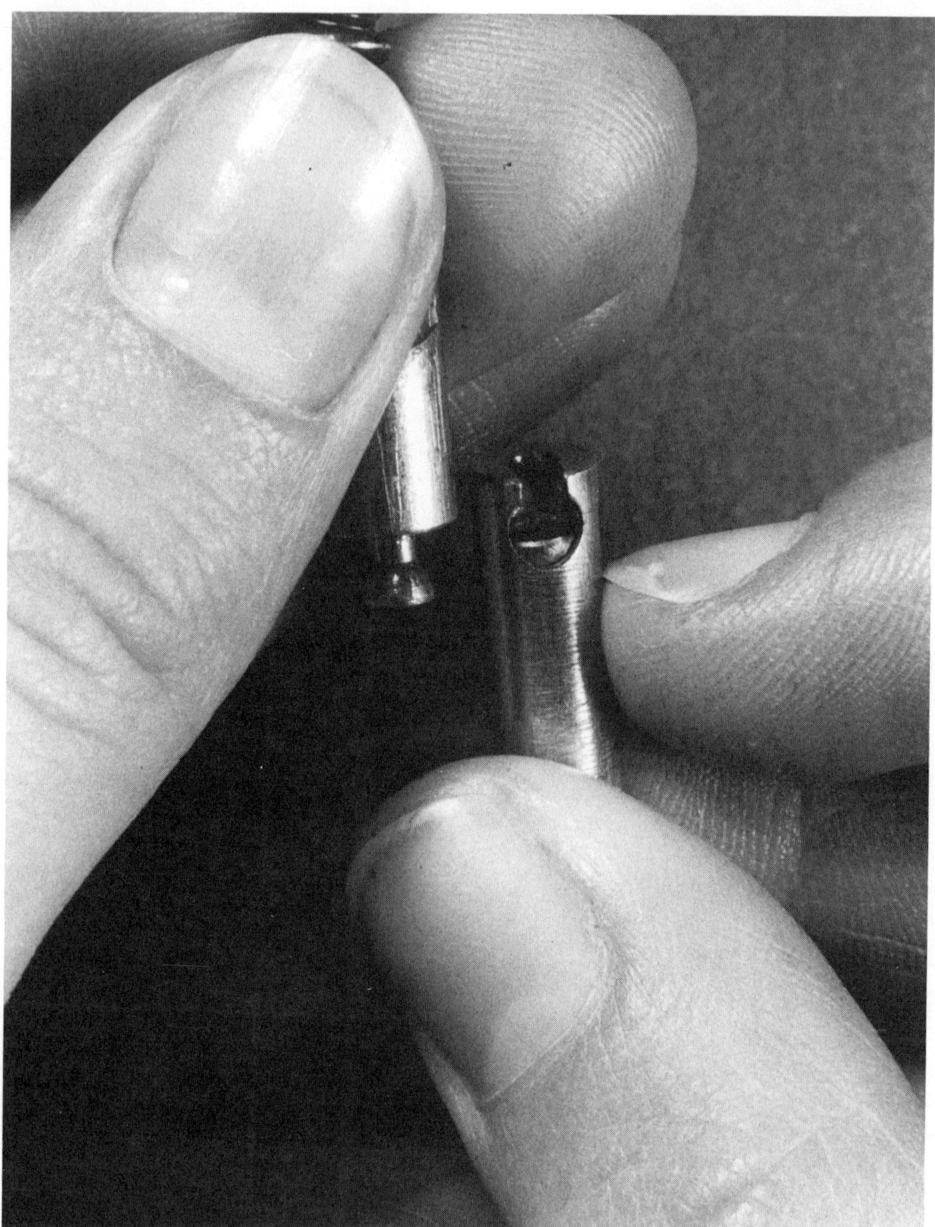

FIG 26–11.
New type of connector that attaches pigtail to drive cable securely. Note internal sleeve that slides up over knob to prevent an accidental disconnect. (Courtesy of Robert C. Ricks, Oak Ridge Associated Universities, Oak Ridge, Tenn.)

is ^{238}U, which is present throughout the earth's soils and rocks. Radon 220 (thoron) is a similar radionuclide but comes from the natural thorium decay chain. Radon gas diffuses out of the soil into the air. The radioactive half-life of ^{222}Rn is 3.8 days. It decays into a chain of short-lived radon daughters which attach to ambient dust particles in air. When inhaled, the particles are deposited on bronchial epithelial surfaces and the radon daughters irradiate the underlying basal cells, which are the target cells for the induction of bronchogenic carcinoma. The radiation dose comes from α particles given off during the first 20–30 minutes after inhalation. The radon daughters primarily responsible for the lung dose are two short-lived nuclides, ^{218}Po (with a half-time of three minutes) and ^{214}Po (with a half-time of less than one second). When radon is at or near equilibrium with its daughters, approximately 95% of the radiation dose to the bronchial epithelium comes from the radon daughters and 5% from radon itself. Irradiation of the lung is continuous because of continuing inhalation of radon and radon daughters.

The diffusion of radon from soil into a poorly ventilated space can result in an accumulation of the gas. This is especially impor-

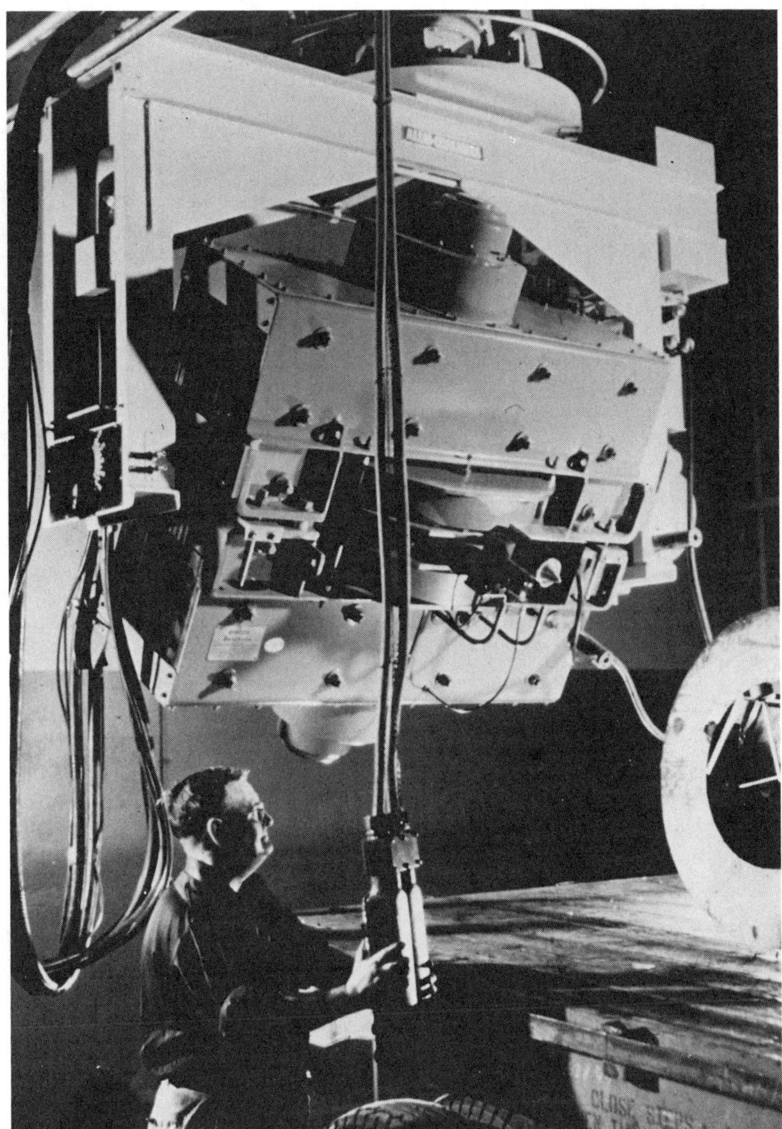

FIG 26–12.
A betatron produces high energy x-rays for radiography inspections. The technician is seen positioning the machine, but is behind heavy shielding during exposures.

tant if the soil has a higher than average content of radium. This mechanism accounts for the radon and radon daughter exposures of persons working in underground mines and in uranium mills. Worker exposures have also occurred in chemical plants that handle radium and in medical installations that prepare or use "radon seeds" for radiotherapy.

Radon and radon daughter exposures are also present outside the workplace. In recent years there is increased awareness that radon and radon daughter concentrations in some homes can be at levels similar to, or even above, those found in uranium mines. These occur especially in homes located on soil containing higher-than-average radium content. Radon and radon daughter concentrations in energy-efficient homes are also increased because of reduced ventilation rates. It is estimated[61] that the average environmental exposure in the U.S. of 0.2 WLM/yr could be responsible for about 20% of the natural incidence of lung cancer in nonsmokers.

Nuclear Power Sources

Heat produced by radionuclides during radioactive decay can be used for special energy sources on a small scale. Alpha particles emitted from a radioactive source, such as ^{210}Po or ^{238}Pu, travel only a few micrometers before colliding with other atoms. The loss of kinetic energy in the particles produces heat. The heat can be converted into electrical power with an efficiency of about

10% by a thermoelectrical conversion system. These generators are designed to produce up to several kilowatts of electrical energy. They are used for earth satellites, space exploration vehicles, navigational beacons, remote weather stations, and similar applications where dependable power is needed in difficult circumstances.

Space Flight

Cosmic radiation is the principal source of radiation doses to astronauts. High doses can result from the high particle radiation associated with solar flares.

Small doses are received by the crews of commercial or military aircraft. The doses are dependent on the altitudes and duration of the flight. A typical transcontinental commercial flight results in a whole body dose of about 3 mrem (0.03 mSv).

Transportation of Radioactive Material

Transportation of radioactive materials in commerce is a trivial source of radiation exposure to workers and the general public. Safety regulation in the transport of radioactive materials is vested in the U.S. Department of Transportation (DOT) and the U.S. Nuclear Regulatory Commission (NRC). Materials with specific activity of less than 2 nCi/gm (74 Bq/gm) are not subject to regulation in transportation but may still come under NRC licensing. Safety is achieved principally by proper and specified packaging according to the type, quantity, and form of the material and by limitation of the level of radiation from the material. Warning placards on the package indicate the amount of radiation present (less than 10 mrem/hr [0.1 mSv/hr] at 1 m unless shipped under special conditions). The regulations require that specific descriptive information must be included in shipping papers. The regulations, contained in the Title 49 of the Code of Federal Regulations, Parts 100-179, are summarized in *The Health Physics and Radiological Health Handbook*.[76]

PREVENTION OF RADIATION EXPOSURES

The term *health physics* was coined about 1942 at the Metallurgical Laboratory (University of Chicago), which was part of the Manhattan District Project effort to build the atom bomb. Health physics is the profession that provides radiation protection for people working with ionizing radiation. Since the initial operation of the first nuclear reactor at the University of Chicago, there has been a heavy demand on physics to evaluate and to anticipate any unique problems associated with ionizing radiation and nuclear energy. The health physicists have been impressively successful in reducing radiation doses to workers and in preventing adverse health problems. This finest example of preventive health work in industry owes its success to reasonable assessment of problems and timely application of scientific investigations plus the steady operational and research support by the federal government and industrial organizations.

Protective methods used to reduce worker exposures include combinations of several basic techniques. The successful application of these methods is dependent on the ability to assess and to predict the exposure potential in advance of the installation of a particular plant process or the performance of an operation or experiment.

These preventive methods are different for the two general classes of radiation exposure: (1) external or direct radiation, and (2) internal deposition of radioactive materials.

External Radiation Exposure Prevention

Time.—Limits on the time spent in a radiation area can control the dose to workers; this method requires the establishment of controlled areas if full-time occupancy is not permitted. It is not a desirable protection method, because it relies on careful administrative management of workers for success. Exposure-time control is useful occasionally in special situations involving higher radiation dose rates that are encountered for a limited time.

Distance.—Radiation dose rates are less as one moves away from the source. In the case of a discrete or "point" source, the radiation dose rate decreases inversely as the square of the distance from the source; this relationship is referred to as the "inverse-square law." If the distance from the source is doubled, the radiation level is reduced by a factor of 4. If the radiation source extends over large planar surfaces or if multiple sources exist, the inverse-square law is no longer valid. Common means of achieving distance are the use of long-handled devices, tongs, manipulators or remote operations in handling materials containing significant activity.

Shielding.—The absorption of radiation energy in shield materials is the most effective method for reducing doses to workers. The amount and type of material required for a particular application will depend on the source strength and type of radiation. Thus, β radiation can be shielded by relatively thin pieces of materials, such as plastic, aluminum, and thick rubber gloves. Against x-rays or γ-rays, a shield of high atomic number (i.e., high density) gives greater absorption than lightweight materials. Lead or concrete is frequently used for a permanent shield. The shield thickness needed for protection of personnel depends on the radiation source strength to be shielded. Neutron shields are designed according to the expected energy spectrum of the neutrons. Frequently, hydrogenous shields, such as water or paraffin, are used to slow down neutrons and they are captured in an outer layer of cadmium or boron, which has high-capture cross sections for low-energy neutrons.

Protection Against Internal Deposition of Radionuclides

The principal routes of deposition of radioactive substances into the body are by inhalation, ingestion, or absorption through intact skin or wounds. Preventive methods employed are similar to those used for toxic chemicals. These include ventilation, enclosed process systems, protective clothing, respirators of various kinds, and skin or wound decontamination procedures. Figure 26–13 illustrates the extensive use of the glove boxes and enclosed processes for containment of hazardous materials, such as ^{239}Pu. Nor-

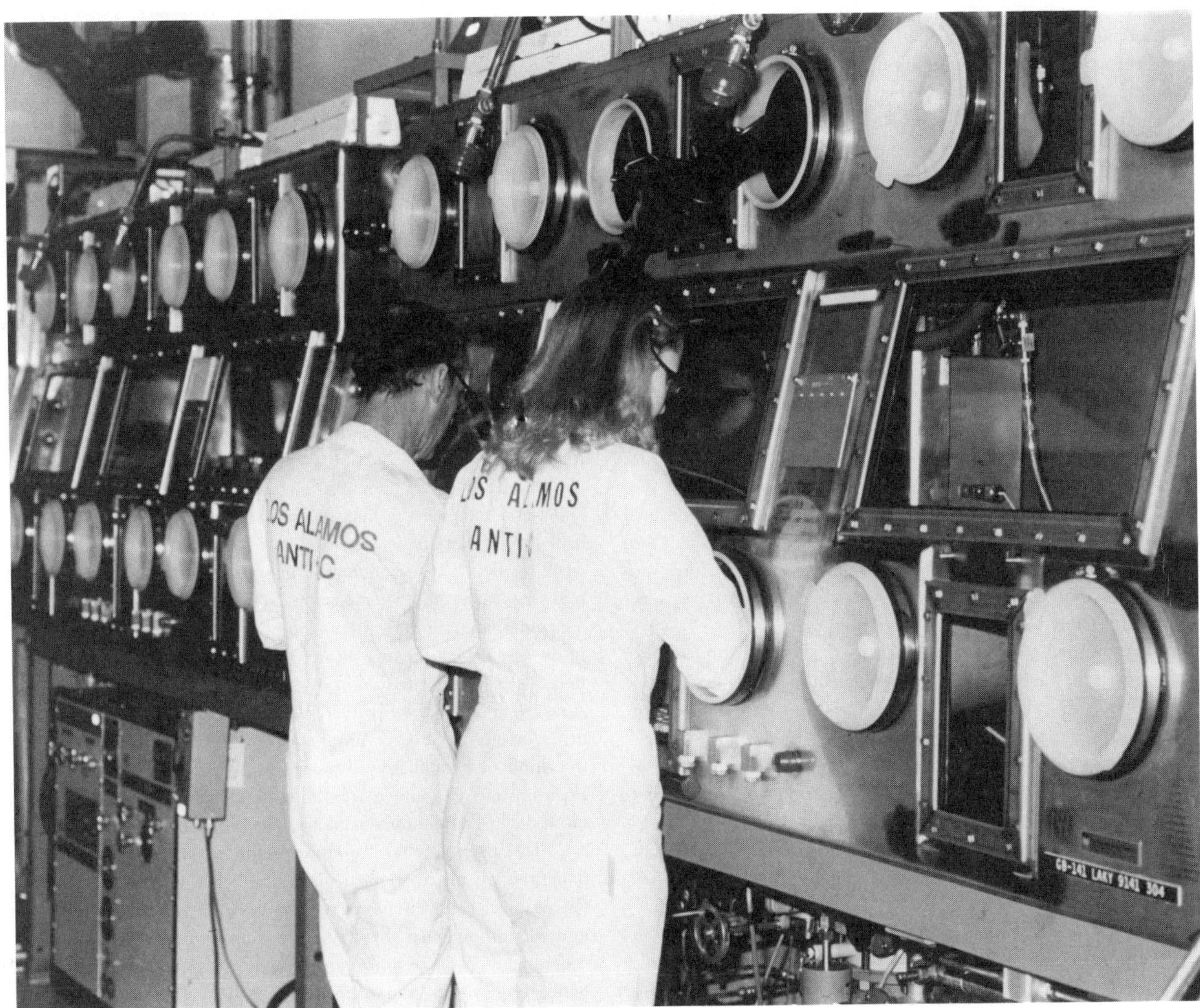

FIG 26–13.
Glove-box line used for handling plutonium is designed for maximum containment of radioactive materials. Note constant air-monitoring filter holders overhead along the line. (From the Los Alamos National Laboratory, Los Alamos, New Mexico).

mally the air in these rooms is free of radioactivity and respiratory protection is not needed. The use of respirators is not recommended for routine control of inhalation hazards, but rather is used for short-term protection, for special jobs in which exposure potential is higher than normal, or for emergency responses.

Control of radon and its daughters is accomplished generally by ventilation. Sufficient air changes per hour must be made to prevent the buildup of radon by emanation from mine walls or from mine water and also to prevent the buildup of the daughters toward an equilibrium condition. In some situations, simple ventilation provides inadequate control and must be supplemented by methods of reducing emanation of radon into workplaces by pressurizing the mine, closing off unused workings, or covering mine walls with a sealant. In some cases local removal of particles from the air by filters or electrostatic precipitators may be useful.

Many respirators are quite effective in removing radon daughters from the inhaled air, but they do not remove radon. Respirators are uncomfortable and their use is resisted by workers. Their use should generally be limited to exposures of short duration when it is not feasible to control the concentration of radon daughters and other radionuclides by containment or ventilation.

RADIATION EXPOSURE GUIDELINES FOR WORKERS

The first attempt to define radiation doses for practical control of occupational exposures was published in 1925; this work defined "tolerance dose" in terms of a numerical value. In 1928, the International Committee on X-ray and Radium Protection was formed for the purpose of adopting some interim protection regulations. In the same year, an effort to establish a United States position on radiation protection was organized through the National Bureau of Standards and resulted in the formation of The Advisory

Committee on X-ray and Radium Protection. These activities were the beginnings of the two principal organizations that make independent recommendations on radiation protection guidelines today, namely the International Commission on Radiological Protection (ICRP) and the National Council on Radiation Protection and Measurements (NCRP). The NCRP is chartered by the U.S. Congress to prepare recommendations and reports on radiation protection. Activities of both NCRP and ICRP have played a prominent role in allowing collective judgments of scientists to be developed, written, and published.

A recommendation that has been made by NCRP and ICRP is that radiation doses shall be kept "as low as reasonably achievable." This principle, called ALARA, is intended to assure that radiation doses occur only when necessary and will result in an overall benefit. This concept now plays a prominent role in occupational radiation regulations and takes precedence over the numerical guidelines given below.

In the United States, the federal government established the Federal Radiation Council (FRC) in 1959 to provide policy on human radiation exposure. The FRC was disbanded in 1970, and the responsibility for radiation protection standards was transferred to the U.S. Environmental Protection Agency, which still has that responsibility today.

Primary radiation protection guidance was established by the president in 1960 based on FRC recommendations.[16] These guidelines are listed in Table 26–9. They continue to be the basis for most current occupational radiation standards in the U.S. In addition, workers younger than 18 years are limited to 10% of these limits. The NCRP has recommended[54, 56] that pregnant women not be exposed in excess of 500 mrem (5 mSv) throughout the pregnancy in order to protect the fetus. This recommendation has not been formally incorporated in the occupational exposure guidelines up to now.

The dose for individuals within the general public is not to exceed 500 mrem (5 mSv) in a calendar year. For average exposure to the general population (when individual doses are not measured), the dose is to be limited to one third of the individual limit, or 170 mrem (1.7 mSv) per calendar year.[17] Current regulatory trends are to place off-site limits on specific categories of the neclear industry, e.g., 25 mrem (0.25 mSv) for air emissions from the nuclear fuel cycle facilities. The overall objective is to limit public exposure to below 100 mrem (1 mSv) per year.

Radiation dose guidelines to workers are similar for all workers, but the regulations for the Department of Energy contractors differ in some details from those of employers who have Nuclear Regulatory Commission (NRC) licenses to handle radioactive materials. The latter work under the Code of Federal Regulations (Title 10 of the Code of Federal Regulations, Part 20 or 10CFR20). The basic NRC limits are summarized in Table 26–10.

An NRC licensee may permit a dose not in excess of 3 rems to the whole body in any calendar quarter if two conditions are met: (1) the accumulated occupational dose to the whole body shall not exceed 5(N − 18) rems, where N equals the individual's age in years at his last birthday, and (2) the employer complies with the requirement to obtain all the necessary information on previously accumulated occupational doses received by the individual.

Control of radiation dose from internal emitters is based on limiting the intake. The NRC regulations (Tables in Appendix B of 10CFR20) give concentrations of various radionuclides in air and water that are the maximum permissible concentrations (average) for inhalation or ingestion for 40 hours per week for a 13-week period. These concentrations are used to judge whether the plant health protective measures are adequate. It should be recognized that under accident conditions short-term concentrations in excess of these levels do not necessarily result in excess radiation doses. Determination of overexposures is best made by in vivo measurements of the involved individuals and by measurements of urine or other biologic samples. The EPA issued a 1984 report[13] in which new radioactivity concentration guides for occupational exposure are calculated for radionuclides in air and water based on updated models for dosimetry and biologic transport.

The occupational radiation standards for radon and radon daughters in air are based on a limit of 4 working level months (WLM) per year, which was recommended by the FRC[18, 19] in 1969 and was promulgated by EPA.[14, 15] Conversion of WLM to rads to the lung is estimated to range from 0.5 to 1.2 rads per WLM, depending on age and exposure conditions.[60, 61] The estimate for miners is 0.5 rad per WLM.

The current trend in occupational radiation regulation is to use the concepts proposed in ICRP Report 26[26] and ICRP Report 30.[29–34] It seems likely that these concepts will soon be incorporated in regulations in the U.S. as they have in England and Eu-

TABLE 26–9.*

Primary Radiation Protection Guides*

TYPE OF EXPOSURE	CONDITION	DOSE
Whole body, active marrow, gonads, or lens of eye	Accumulated annual average	5 rem
Skin (whole body) or thyroid†	Annual	30 rem
Bone	Body burden	0.1 μg ^{226}Ra or its historical equivalent‡
Other organs	Annual	15 rem
Radon decay products	Annual	4 working level months

*Modified from Eckerman et al.[13] and the Federal Radiation Council.[16]
†Some Federal agencies use a 15-rem annual limit for thyroid.
‡ICRP calculates 50 rems/yr to the endosteal tissue lying within 10 μm of bone surfaces.[28] Some Federal agencies use a 30-rem annual limit for an average bone dose.

TABLE 26–10.
Exposure Limits for Workers in Radiation Areas (10 CFR 20.101)

BODY AREA	REMS/ CALENDAR QUARTER
1. Whole body; head and trunk; active blood-forming organs; lens of eyes; or gonads	1¼
2. Hands and forearms; feet and ankles	18¾
3. Skin of whole body	7½

rope. The maximum annual whole-body dose-equivalent limit for occupational exposure is 5 rems (0.05 Sv) in any one year. The whole-body dose-equivalent is derived by means of an effective dose-equivalent calculation. This calculation is to provide a value that represents equivalent health risks whether the whole body or only portions of the body are irradiated. Weighting factors are used that are ratios of the health risk of an organ or tissue dose to the total health risk when the whole body is irradiated uniformly. The weighting factors used by ICRP are: gonads, 0.25; breast, 0.15; red bone marrow, 0.12; lung, 0.12; thyroid, 0.03; bone surfaces, 0.03; and the remainder, 0.30 (or 0.06 for each of th e five organs or tissues with the highest dose equivalents in the remainder). The sum of the weighted mean organ dose-equivalents is called the effective dose-equivalent. The contributions of internal and external exposures are summed in determining the effective dose-equivalent. For control of internal emitters, the exposures are not to exceed an annual limit on intake (ALI). The ALI is that quantity of a radionuclide which, when taken into the body, commits the worker to a lifetime risk no greater than that associated with the annual whole-body dose-equivalent limit.

RADIATION DOSES TO MAN

Human populations are exposed to ionizing radiation from a variety of sources. Of the accumulated total dose to the population, over 90% of exposure in the U.S. is due to natural background, tobacco products, and medical exposures. Table 26–11 lists categories of exposure sources to the U.S. population. Additional description of the doses within each category is given in the following sections.

TABLE 26–11.
Annual Radiation Doses to the United States Population by Source in the 1980s

SOURCE	PERSON-REMS PER YEAR (IN THOUSANDS)	PERCENT OF DOSE BY SOURCE
Natural background	23,000	26.9
radon	46,000*	53.9
Medical/dental	12,300	14.4
Fallout	1,000	1.2
Nuclear fuel cycle	3	—
Consumer products	2,800	3.3
tobacco	(65,000)†	—
Occupational	190	0.2
Miscellaneous	120	0.1

*Dose to bronchial epithelium, calculated as the effective dose-equivalent.
†Dose to bronchial epithelium of the estimated 50 × 10^6 smokers.

Natural Sources

The two sources of natural radiation are cosmic rays and radiation from naturally occurring radioactive materials found in soil and rocks. The cosmic ray dose is variable with time and especially with altitude. For example, the dose rate at 1,800 m is about double that at sea level. Cosmic radiation also produces carbon 13 and hydrogen 3 (tritium) in our environment. Radionuclides that are principal contributors to our natural background are the nuclides in the uranium and thorium series and potassium 40. Exposures from these nuclides occur as direct external γ radiation and by internal deposition through air, water, and food. An approximate average whole-body dose in the United States from all natural sources is 80 mrem (0.8 mSv) per year. The contributions are about 29 mrem (0.29 mSv) per year from cosmic rays, 26 mrem (0.26 mSv) per year of external direct radiation from terrestrial radionuclides, and 27 mrem (0.27 mSv) per year from natural radionuclides within the body tissues.[65]

The radiation dose to the lung by radon and its daughters is now recognized as the largest contributor from natural sources to man. Doses to the bronchial epithelium on average are estimated to be about 2400 mrem/y (24 mSv/y.) Using the ICRP weighting factor for bronchial epithelium (0.08), the effective dose-equivalent for the whole body is about 200 mrem/y (2 mSv/y).

Medical/Dental

Radiation from practice of the healing arts results in the second major source of radiation exposure to the U.S. population. It is estimated that over 300,000 x-ray units are being used in the United States for medical diagnosis and therapy.[65] A 1970 survey by the Bureau of Radiological Health of the Food and Drug Administration indicated that about 65% of persons in the U.S. were exposed to x-rays for medical or dental purposes that year. The BEIR III report[65] estimated that the average person in the exposed group received about 103 mrem (1.03 mSv) per year for medical diagnosis and 3 mrem (0.03 mSv) per year for dental diagnosis. Averaging over the total population results in a medical/dental dose of about 78 mrem (0.78 mSv) per person per year. This average is now thought to be high; more recent estimates are about 55 mrem (0.55 mSv) per person per year.

Fallout

Large quantities of man-made radioactive materials were distributed to the environment throughout the world as a result of atmospheric nuclear weapons testing, especially during the 1950s and 1960s. Although much of this debris has since decayed, the remaining longer-lived radionuclides will continue to be a source of exposure for some time to come. The average whole-body dose-equivalent rate for the U.S. population is estimated now to be about 4–5 mrem (0.04–0.05 mSv) per year.[65]

Nuclear Fuel Cycle

The nuclear fuel cycle for nuclear power production in the United States consists of uranium mining, milling, uranium hexafluoride production, ^{235}U enrichment, uranium oxide fuel fabrication, power production, possible fuel reprocessing, and radioactive waste management. As shown in Table 26-11, the average radiation exposure from all processes is tiny compared to other sources; however, persons living close to such operations or near the rare nuclear accident will have greater exposure than others.

The core meltdown of the Three Mile Island Unit 2 reactor on March 28, 1979, released principally short-lived radioactive xenon and small quantities of ^{131}I. The maximum individual dose is estimated to have been less than 100 mrem (1 mSv). The population dose to persons within a 50 mile radius is estimated to be about 3000 person-rems (30 man-Sv). Containment of radioactive materials was very successful in this serious accident. By comparison, the release from the Chernobyl reactor accident is estimated to cause a collective dose of 200×10^6 person-rem (2×10^6) man-Sv over 50 to 70 years.

Consumer Products

The list of consumer and industrial products that result in low-level radiation exposure to the general population is extensive, e.g., television sets, luminous-dial watches, airport luggage x-ray inspection systems, dental prostheses, smoke detectors, high-voltage vacuum switches, electron microscopes, static eliminators, cardiac pacemakers, tobacco products, fossil fuels, and building materials. By far the most important of these products in terms of radiation exposure are tobacco products. The average whole-body dose-equivalent rate for the U.S. population is estimated to be about 4–5 mrem (0.04–0.05 mSv) per year.[65]

Occupational Exposure

In 1980, about 1.2 million U.S. workers were potentially exposed to ionizing radiation in their work.[38] Since 1960, the number of radiation workers has been increasing about 5% per year, that is, doubling in about 14 to 15 years. In 1980, the mean annual dose was 0.11 rem (0.0011 Sv) for all radiation workers and 0.23 rem (0.0023 Sv) for all workers with measurable doses. The mean dose to male workers was about three times that to female workers. Table 26–12 lists a summary of exposures in various occupational categories. Not listed in Table 26–12 are annual whole-body doses of 0.2 rem (0.002 Sv) average to 13,500 uranium miners, 0.15 rem (0.0015 Sv) average to 4,200 nonuranium miners, and 0.17 rem (0.0017 Sv) average to 97,000 flight crew members. The uranium miners also are estimated to have a mean annual exposure to radon and radon daughters of 0.5 WLM. This calculates to be about 0.25 rad (0.0035 Gy) or 5 rem (0.05 Sv) per year of α radiation to the lung and is in addition to the whole-body dose.

The distribution of the numbers of workers and their collective doses is shown for various ranges of annual dose equivalent (rem) in Figure 26–14. Since 1960, the distribution of doses above 1 rem (0.01 Sv) has changed substantially, with a large decrease in the fraction of workers approaching or exceeding 5 rems (0.05 Sv). Since 1965, the absolute number of workers exceeding 3 rems (0.03 Sv) has decreased, while the number exceeding 1 rem (0.01 Sv) has increased, and the number exceeding 2 rems (0.02 Sv) has remained relatively constant. Since 1970 the growth rate of collective dose was greatest for the nuclear fuel cycle.[38]

Lethal radiation doses are rare, on average less than one death per year worldwide.[20] Occupational radiation accidents resulting in acute lethal doses are even more rare. From 1945 to 1985, a total of 36 acute radiation deaths have been recorded from all circumstances. Twenty of these deaths resulted from exposure to sealed radiography sources. Sixteen of these 20 deaths resulted

TABLE 26–12.
Summary of Occupational Exposure of Workers to Radiation, 1980*

OCCUPATIONAL CATEGORY	NO. OF WORKERS (THOUSANDS)		MEAN ANNUAL DOSE EQUIVALENT (MREM)		COLLECTIVE DOSE EQUIVALENT (PERSON-REM, THOUSANDS)
	ALL	EXPOSED†	ALL	EXPOSED†	
Medicine (27% of collective doses)					
Hospital	126	86	140	200	17.2
Private	155	87	100	180	16.0
Dental	259	82	20	70	5.6
Other	44	21	40	90	1.9
Industry (25%)					
Radiography	27	18	290	430	7.8
Manufacture & distribution	29	12	110	270	3.2
Other users	249	126	110	210	26.5
Nuclear fuel cycle (37%)					
Power reactors	134	81	390	650	52.3
Other	18	11	145	200	2.2
Government (8%)	204	105	60	120	12
Miscellaneous‡ (3%)	76	31	70	160	5
All U.S. workers	1320	660	110	230	150

*Modified from Kumazawa S, Nelson DR, and Richardson ACB: *Occupational exposure to ionizing radiation in the United States,* EPA Report 520/1-84-005, 1984.
†Workers who received a measurable dose in any monitoring period.
‡Principally education and transportation.

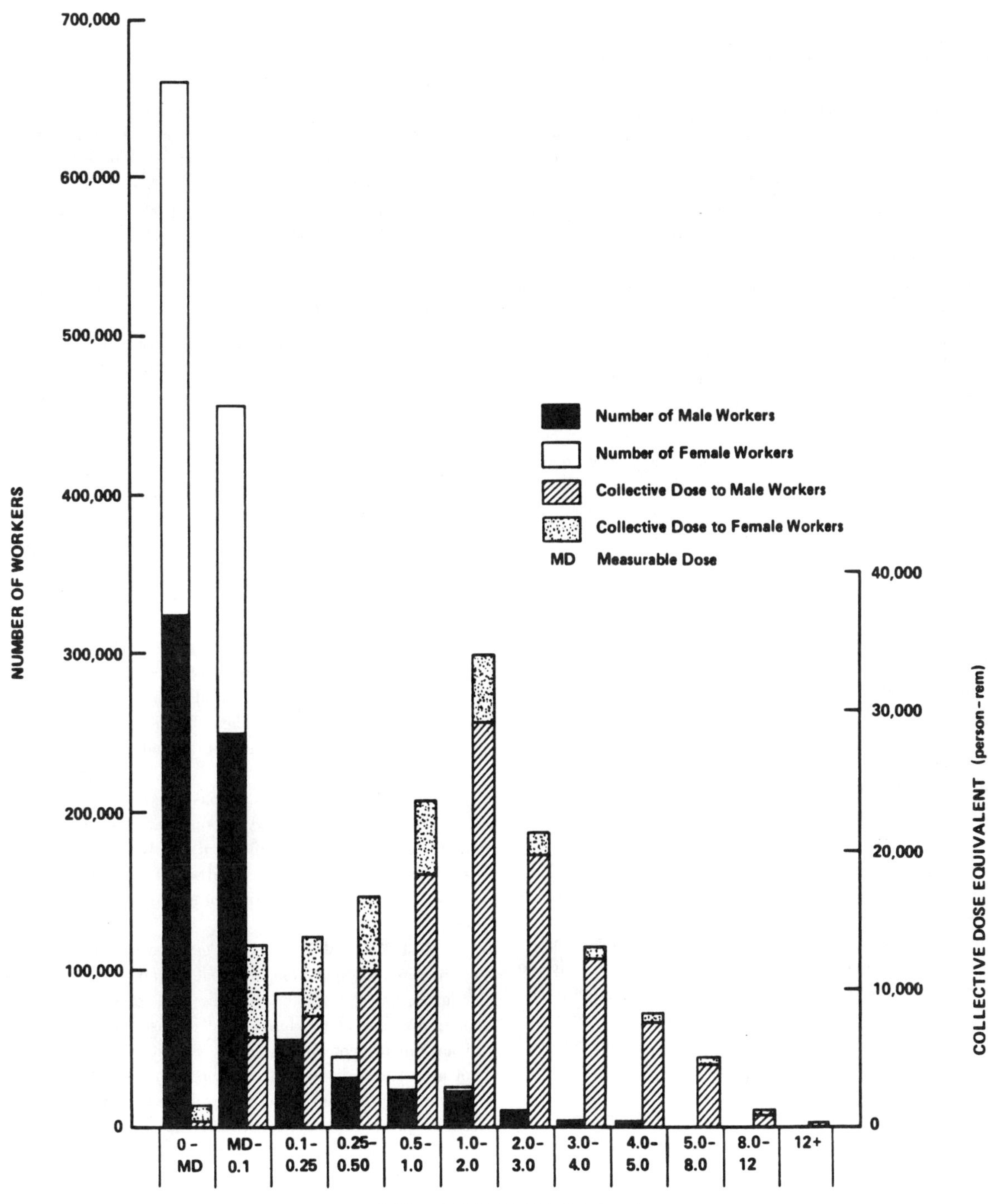

FIG 26–14.

Estimated numbers of U.S. workers who were potentially exposed to radiation in 1980 and their collective doses by dose range and sex. (From Kumazawa S, Nelson DR, Richardson ACB: *Occupational Exposure to Ionizing Radiation in the United States,* EPA Report 520/1-84-005. Washington, DC, Environmental Protection Agency, 1984.)

from the loss or theft of five sources. Two of the 20 cases were successful suicides, and two deaths resulted from accidental exposures within high-level irradiation facilities. Criticality accidents were the cause of six deaths in workers. Two of the six were exposed by criticality experimental assemblies, two by nuclear research reactors (none from power reactors), and two from chemical reprocessing of fissionable materials. (Not counted in this enumeration of acute radiation deaths are three individuals who died of traumatic injuries in the 1961 SL-1 reactor accident.) Seven deaths occurred as a result of medical misadministration of radionuclides in patients. Two persons died from handling tritium in uncontrolled circumstances. One person died acutely as a result of fallout from atmospheric weapons testing in the Pacific.

All the above history is overshadowed by the Chernobyl reactor accident in the U.S.S.R. on April 19, 1986. The reactor was a 3200 MW thermal, boiling-water pressure tube reactor. At the time of the accident, it was being deliberately operated in an unsafe mode and with important safety systems switched off in order to conduct an experiment. An explosive disassembly of the reactor core resulted from an uncontrolled nuclear power surge. The reactor building, which did not have a containment vessel, was blown open and set on fire. Release of fuel particles caused high radiation levels in the area. Power plant personnel and firemen responding to the accident shortly after the reactor disruption were heavily irradiated. Of about 300 persons admitted to hospitals, 203 had symptons of acute radiation syndrome. Whole body doses from 200 rads (2 Gy) up to 1600 rads (16 Gy) were reported. Thirty-one persons died of acute effects, most within 2 months of the accident. Thermal burns, beta radiation burns, and infections complicated these cases. No clinical symptoms of acute radiation syndrome were seen in the 135,000 people evacuated from the zone within 30 km of the plant.

Miscellaneous

Most of the exposure in this category is to airline passengers. It is estimated[65] that the average passenger dose equivalent is about 2.8 mrem (0.028 mSv) per year. The collective dose is about 100,000 person-rems per year. A small source is the dose due to transportation of radioactive materials. This source contributes about 15,000 person-rems per year for all forms of transportation—airplanes, trucks, vans, rail, and ships. Less than 500 person-rems per year is attributable to air emissions from nuclear facilities not related to the fuel cycle.

MEDICAL PROGRAM FOR RADIATION WORKERS

The number of factors to be considered for job placement in radiation work is actually small as far as potential radiation exposure is concerned. More important in the medical program is the evaluation of those factors that are necessary for effective performance of the particular job. This requires the physician to be thoroughly familiar with the job requirements to which the worker is to be assigned.

No standard medical criteria have been promulgated for radiation workers. Thus the physician may determine his own criteria or make decisions on an individual case basis. One exception to this is in the examination of nuclear power reactor operators. The NRC has accepted the recommendations in the American National Standards Institute's (ANSI) report on medical criteria for reactor operators.[2] Physicians responsible for such examinations should review these detailed recommendations before filing the necessary medical forms to the NRC.

The following considerations can be used in medical evaluations of workers who are assigned to work in radiation areas.

Preplacement Examinations

Past Occupational History.—Past radiation doses should be reviewed and evaluated, but work with or exposure to hydrocarbons, radiomimetics, and any other carcinogen or mutagen should also be determined. Work in medical x-ray departments should not be overlooked as a potential occupational exposure source. History of previous radiation exposures, both medical and occupational, should be documented in the medical record. Many companies request personal radiation dosimetry records from previous employers, but this information is usually not available at the time of preplacement medical examination.

Although radiation doses from medical diagnostic or therapeutic procedures are not included in a person's cumulative occupational radiation dose, they should be included in the medical history. Therapeutic radiation is of special interest, not only for the radiation doses involved, but also for the medical condition for which treatment was given. These factors may result in a determination that the individual is not a good candidate for radiation work.

If the applicant previously has worked with radioactive materials, particularly long-lived internal emitters such as plutonium, other transuranics, and radium, it is advisable to obtain a baseline radiochemical urinalysis and an in vivo count for the appropriate radionuclides at the time of employment.

Past Medical History.—Past medical problems of greatest interest include hematologic problems (anemia, granulocytopenia, or hemorrhagic disorder), skin diseases, diseases of the digestive tract, diseases of the lungs, and diseases of the eye, especially vision impairment and cataracts. A history of malignancy should not necessarily disqualify a person from working with ionizing radiation. Each person should be evaluated for the particular type of cancer, job requirements, and attitudes of the applicant, supervisor, and the employer. Findings should be carefully noted in the medical record as a preexisting problem.

In some positions, such as a reactor operator or chemical operator, a medical problem that could cause even momentary unconsciousness may be disastrous. A history of epilepsy, recurrent fainting, severe diabetes mellitus, and some forms of heart disease will be disqualifying for those critical jobs.

The physician should ascertain the job applicant's mental and emotional make-up during the medical history. A history of work or school performance, including reasons for change, absenteeism, accident record, and previous compensation claims may yield valuable information.

Medical Evaluation.—The examination of prospective radiation workers should consider the specific physical factors that are important for the performance of the specific job. Another objective is to disclose preexisting diseases, which may result from or be confused with radiation-induced disease at some later date. Some diseases of interest are neoplasms, blood dyscrasias, cataracts, and chronic dermatitis. These conditions are not unique to radiation and may be indistinguishable from similar pathology due to other etiologic factors.

Persons younger than 18 years and pregnant women come under special provisions of radiation exposure regulations, as noted earlier. As new hires, they would not normally be assigned to radiation areas. In general, occupational radiation exposures do not and should not exclude women from being radiation workers, because the doses and dose rates are expected to be low. The reduced radiation limits during pregnancy must be accommodated by the job assignments made during the pregnancy. Early notification of pregnancy should be required of employees.

The presence of chronic dermatosis should be noted. Some radiation jobs involve potential skin contamination with radioactive materials. These jobs usually require wearing rubber gloves and may require frequent hand-washing and occasional scrubbing with detergents or mild decontaminating chemicals. A diagnosis of eczema, and perhaps severe dyshidrosis, may disqualify the individual for these jobs. Examination of the skin for the telltale triad of chronic radiodermatitis—atrophy, hyperkeratosis, and telangiectasia—may help uncover a forgotten medical radiation therapy or unrecorded past radiation accident.

Each person should be given an ophthalmoscopic examination to determine the presence of lens opacities. This must be done in a darkened room using a +8 or +12 diopter lens setting. Slit-lamp examination of opacities will help to document any findings. Usually such findings will simply document the presence of opacities that do not impair vision and should not influence work assignments. The documentation may prove to be valuable for future reference and for use in case of subsequent litigation.

The minimum hematologic tests should include hematocrit or red blood cell count, hemoglobin, total and differential white blood cell count, and platelet estimate. Particular attention should be paid to findings of abnormal or excessive numbers of immature cells in the blood, abnormality in the quantity or characteristics of platelets, and instability or abnormal fluctuation of blood elements on repeat examinations. Refractory anemia, neutropenia, and thrombocytopenia, alone or combined, may constitute premonitory signs of leukemia months or years before a definitive diagnosis. They would weigh heavily against approving the individual for radiation work. It is less common to see megaloblastic and Coombs-negative hemolytic anemias as a preleukemic state.

In medical evaluations of radiation workers, there has been a tendency to place greater significance on minor blood count variations from "normal" than is warranted. The laboratory should determine standard deviations for its procedures on normal subjects. Values outside the 95% range should not be regarded as absolute reasons for disqualification but rather as levels at which additional evaluation and consideration should be given. Transient illnesses and physiologic variations as well as laboratory errors make repeated blood studies a necessity before a final decision on employability is reached.

Periodic Medical Examinations

Medical evaluations of radiation workers usually are not made more frequently than once a year, and, in many cases, longer intervals may be adequate. The interval between examinations should take into consideration the worker's general health, age, job assignment, exposure history, and the effectiveness of personnel and plant monitoring procedures. The minimal examination should include a careful history, physical examination, complete blood count, and urinalysis. Because biologic effects are observable only after acute radiation doses greatly exceeding annual occupational dose limits, the periodic medical examination or blood counts should not be used as a monitoring or radiation control procedure.

Items of special interest for radiation workers are: (1) review of occupational radiation doses, other possible physical or chemical hazards, and the accident record of the individual; (2) review of the interval medical radiation history; (3) examination of the skin, with particular reference to the fingertips, especially if radioactive materials or sources are being handled; (4) evaluation of blood counts; (5) evaluation of interval medical history and sick leave experience, especially a history of or suspected diagnosis of cancer; and (6) evaluation of emotional status.

The occasional person who undergoes medical radiation therapy may present problems in job placement upon return to work. The individual may have certain physical limitations, and restriction from additional radiation exposure at work may be justified. There are no predetermined answers to these problems, and each case must be decided on an individual basis.

An individual who has a blood profile characteristic of a possible preleukemic state should be considered for removal from a job that requires additional radiation exposures, but a current radiation worker who develops leukemia or other blood dyscrasia may be less disturbed if permitted to continue work as usual. Any legal liability the company may encounter as a result of his illness cannot be diminished at this time, and any additional occupational radiation exposure he receives will not affect his condition. The most important rule in managing such cases is good communication and rapport between employee and physician. This is true regardless of the ultimate decision, which must take the employee's attitude under careful consideration. The same philosophy can also be applied to other forms of malignancy that arise in radiation workers.

The need for special slit-lamp eye examinations in radiation workers appears to be limited to a few special circumstances in which radiation exposures are particularly difficult to monitor. Medicolegal problems may arise due to cataracts that are clinically similar to radiation-induced cataracts. Periodic physical examinations on all radiation workers should include an ophthalmoscopic examination, with particular attention to the lens, regardless of the radiation exposure history.[89]

An infrequent, but sometimes difficult, problem is presented by the individual with acute anxiety or other reactions focused on the potential radiation hazards in his work. Fortunately, such concerns are often minor, and simple reassurance or explanation may go a long way toward solving the problem. If several of these cases occur within a short time period, it may be a clue that there is a general uneasiness and possible misinformation operating within the work force. This is an excellent time to evaluate and improve indoctrination and training programs for the radiation workers. Improvement of these programs may be the answer. In rare instances, it may be necessary to recommend changing the individual's assignment to a nonradiation job to relieve emotional reactions.

Return-to-Work Examinations

The return-to-work examination after an illness will often determine changes in employee health status more promptly and effectively than periodic physical examinations. Company rules should be established that all persons using sick leave over an arbitrary period, usually about five workdays, shall report to the medical department before they return to work. At this time, the illness, any continuing disabilities, and future implications can be evaluated in light of the individual's normal job assignment.

Termination Medical Examinations

The employee's medical record should be reviewed at the time of termination from employment. Any known change in health status should be recorded as well as the status of any occupational injuries, illnesses, or exposures. Generally, a full physical examination is not warranted, unless a special problem exists; however, a brief termination health questionnaire is convenient, to complete the medical history for the full period of employment.

Medical Records on Radiation Workers

Unlike many occupational hazards that present acute or immediate effects, ionizing radiation doses may be claimed as an etiologic agent of late effects over many years. Most state workers' compensation laws provide that claims must be presented within a specified period (usually a year or two) after the onset or awareness of illness due to an occupational exposure. The key information needed to properly evaluate a claim will be the health physics information recorded during employment, personnel radiation dosimetry records, and the medical records. Therefore, these records for radiation workers should be preserved for periods of time that correspond to the normal life expectancy of the worker.

MEDICAL MANAGEMENT OF RADIATION CASES

Radiation cases can be classified into five categories according to the type of exposure. These categories are: (1) acute external (direct) radiation exposure to the whole body; (2) localized radiation skin burns; (3) radioactive contaminants on intact skin; (4) contaminated wounds; and (5) internal deposition of radioactive material. In practice, accident cases will often be combinations of two or more of the above categories. For example, localized radiation skin burns also result in some degree of whole-body exposure.

Nuclear facilities and hospitals should have a detailed emergency plan that includes management of radiation cases. The plan describes the emergency operating organization and defines the lines of authority, responsibilities, and functions of the assigned qualified individuals. The plan should describe prior arrangements made with physicians, hospitals, and ambulance services for medical assistance and transportation of contaminated, injured, and exposed individuals. The need for consulting services, such as health physics or waste management, should be considered and the necessary arrangements made. Details on preparing an emergency plan for radiation cases are available in other reports.[1, 40, 59, 76]

Acute External Radiation

Physicians are called upon occasionally to evaluate persons with minor radiation exposures or potential exposures. In some instances, an estimated exposure may only slightly exceed an administrative weekly limit, such as 100 mrem (1 mSv). A history of the circumstances should be preserved in the medical record, but examinations in these instances are of little value. They should be discouraged actually, because they may only lead to unnecessary anxiety in the workers. When such a referral is made, it is well to introduce some discussion on late effects. Generally, if the worker has concern about radiation-induced cancer, his notions about risk will be far too high. The physician should provide a realistic estimate of risk for the individual's circumstances, if possible.

The medical history of the radiation exposure should document the known circumstances of the exposure. The source of radiation should be described in terms of the type of radiation and source strength. Preliminary radiation measurements and estimates, if known, should be recorded. The position of the person relative to the source and the estimated length of exposure are important. Gastrointestinal symptoms (anorexia, nausea, vomiting, and diarrhea) during the first 6–12 hours are important to document since they may be related to a possible dose as described in the section on biologic effects.

The most useful early tests are blood counts and cytogenetic studies of peripheral lymphocytes, which contribute important information, even if normal. These tests should be considered when (1) a single acute whole-body exposure is estimated to be in excess of 3 rems (0.03 Sv); (2) a significant radiation dose is possible and where dosimetry or personal monitoring devices were lacking or possibly inaccurate; and (3) a request for tests is made by an employee after a documented incident, even if minor. An acute exposure of 3 rems (0.03 Sv) or more will occur only as a result of an accident or unusual circumstance. This suggests that with such an exposure there will very likely be some form of investigation and excitement surrounding the incident. Reassurance of the involved person(s) that his or her blood count is normal may be helpful. In an acute accident, a blood sample is usually taken immediately and repeated daily or several times a day over the first three days. The practical laboratory test available to all physicians is a complete blood count, from which the absolute lymphocyte count can be determined. As noted in the biologic effects section of this chapter, the lymphocyte count is an important test to assess during the first 48 hours after suspected high whole-body doses. For doses under about 100 rems (1 Sv), and surely under 50 rems (0.5 Sv), no lowering of the lymphocyte count is expected. The interpretation of lymphocyte counts must also take into account acute, transient decreases that are common with almost any form of stress, such as acute bacterial infections and traumatic injuries.

Analysis of chromosome lesions in peripheral lymphocytes is the most sensitive biologic test available for estimating a whole-body dose to penetrating external radiation. The lower limits of sensitivity are about 10–20 rads (0.1–0.2 Gy) for low-LET radiation and about 5 rads (0.05 Gy) for fission neutrons.[42, 44] A 10-ml blood sample, drawn in a sterile vacutainer containing sodium heparin, should be taken as soon after exposure as possible. Consultation with a laboratory familiar with special cytogenetic studies of radiation effects is necessary for proper transportation and analysis of the sample. Ionizing radiation typically produces dicentric chromosomes. Although many other agents can cause chromosome breaks, few induce dicentric chromosomes. The method requires about six to eight days for analysis, which means the results are more valuable for dosimetry than for immediate management of the patient.

The number of dicentrics and rings per 100 lymphocytes is counted by microscopic examination. Usually 300–500 cells are counted. Figure 26–15 displays two curves that show the relationship of the number of dicentrics and rings per 100 cells to the whole body dose. This type of calibration is best derived by each laboratory for its specific technique and procedures.

Chromosome analysis reflects an integrated dose to lymphocytes throughout the body and the result may differ from the dose recorded on a personal dosimeter located at one place on the body. Thus, this method may be especially valuable in cases in which there is nonuniform distribution of dose in different parts of the body. The presence of increased chromosome aberrations in an irradiated person does not provide a means for estimating the risk of malignancy or other clinical conditions.

Persons exposed to less than 100 rem (1 Sv) do not need to be hospitalized. They can be followed as outpatients and will normally require only counseling and minimal supportive therapy. For many persons, outpatient management is satisfactory up to about 200 rems (2 Sv) whole-body dose. In general, it is best to avoid hospitalizing patients, except in a sterile environment facility. The anticipated signs and symptoms of the acute radiation syndrome are described in the section on biologic effects, and a practical evaluation of clinical radiation injury after overexposure is outlined in Figure 26–6.

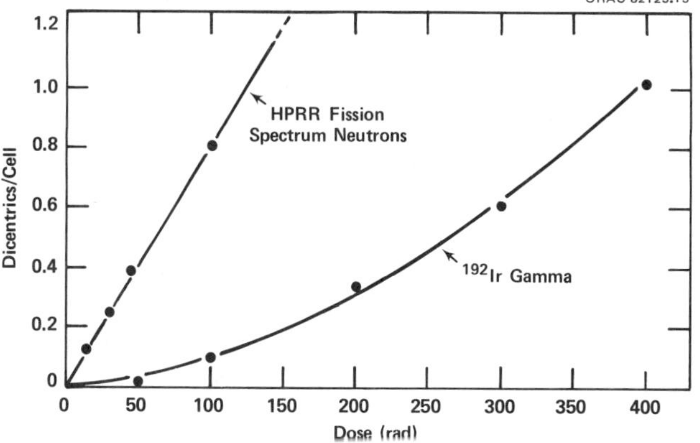

FIG 26–15.
Comparison of dose-response curves for dicentric induction in human lymphocytes after exposure to γ radiation from iridium 192 vs. fission neutrons from the Health Physics Research Reactor in Oak Ridge, Tenn. (From Littlefield LG: The analysis of radiation-induced chromosome lesions in lymphocytes as a biological method for dose estimation, in *Proceedings of NATO Working Group Meeting on the Assessment of Injury from Ionizing Radiation in Warfare.* Bethesda, Md, Armed Forces Radiobiology Research Institute, 1982, pp 351–387.)

Skin erythema can appear within minutes to hours after a single large radiation exposure, i.e., hundreds of rems. As noted earlier in the biology section, skin response to radiation is complex; thus, erythema is only a confirmatory sign and not diagnostic by itself.

Epilation is a late sign, being observed first on about day 17 to day 20 after exposure, and is of no value as an early clinical indicator.

Persons with doses estimated to be over 200 rems should be hospitalized. Persons with large doses, such as 300–1,000 rems (3 to 10 Sv), can be transported from a local hospital to a larger medical center with the necessary specialty services during the first few days after the initial prodromal symptoms have subsided and the initial dose estimates have been made.

Treatment techniques of special importance in the management of radiation cases with significant damage to the hematopoietic system are (1) prevention of infections by reverse isolation and "clean room" techniques, (2) antibacterial drug therapy, and (3) management of bone marrow depression by platelet and leukocyte infusions. Homologous bone marrow transplantation, performed as soon as possible but no later than ten days after exposure, should be considered for a person who has had a potentially lethal exposure, 600 rem (6 Sv) to about 1200 rem (12 Sv), and for whom a well-matched donor is available. The reader should refer to other publications[1, 3, 27] for additional details on patient management and therapy.

If a supralethal exposure of 5,000 rems (50 Sv) or more has occurred, the patient will survive only a few days, and medical treatment of these acute emergencies can be handled at the nearest hospital. Treatment will consist of pain relief, antiemesis medications, sedation, control of shock, and fluid balance management.

Localized Radiation Skin Burns

Sterile, protective dressings should be used on skin burns. No particular type of local ointment appears to be advantageous in treatment. The extent of whole-body radiation dose should be evaluated by means of history, dosimetry, possibly mock-up dosimetry measurements, and clinical evaluation, including blood counts.

For β-ray burns, early excision and skin grafting will spare the patient much discomfort and permit earlier restoration of function. Early surgical treatment is not advisable for skin burns produced by x-rays or γ-rays. The deeper penetration by such radiation does not permit one to make an early accurate evaluation of the extent of the burn and the future adequacy of the underlying circulation. Surgical repair and grafting of the area should be deferred until the lesion is well demarcated.

Areas of chronic radiodermatitis should be observed periodically for possible neoplasms. Keratoses and ulcerations should be excised and covered with split-thickness skin grafts as necessary.

Radioactive Contaminants on Intact Skin

Contamination of the normal skin by radioactive material is a common problem wherever these materials are being handled. The principal concern is usually not radiation dose to the skin or body, but rather to prevent uptake in the body by absorption, inhalation, or ingestion. Most radioactive materials are not absorbed through intact skin, but a few are, such as iodine, tritiated water, and soluble strontium compounds. Acidic and alkaline solutions may increase the permeability of the skin, especially if the integrity of the skin barrier is altered.

The treatment is to remove the radioactive material from the skin without injury. In most cases this involves simple washing of the skin with a mild detergent and water. Scrubbing with a soft cloth may be necessary. Scrub brushes should be used sparingly, if at all, because of the hazard of abrading the skin through overzealous scrubbing. It is important not to damage the skin by use of scrub brushes, scrubbing agents, or chemicals. The use of complexing or chelating agents, such as ethylenediaminetetraacetic acid (EDTA) or diethylenetriaminepentaacetic acid (DTPA), in decontaminating solutions has not been particularly helpful. If washing with detergent and gentle scrubbing is inadequate, use of 5% sodium hypochlorite (household bleach) will frequently be effective. It can be used full strength on the hands or forearms of most people. It should be diluted with about five parts of water for use on the face, neck, or around wound areas. Bleach is a skin irritant and some caution must attend its use. It may be preferable to leave low levels of contamination on the skin than to abrade or chemically injure the skin. Mild decontamination efforts performed on two or three occasions during the day or over several days are more effective than a single intensive effort. The use of an occlusive dressing (or rubber gloves, in the case of contaminated hands) between decontamination efforts may be helpful because of the sweating that is induced.

At times, the contaminant adheres to hair more than to the skin. Clipping hair is seldom necessary, but it may be considered if repeated washing does not remove sufficient radioactive material.

The reader is referred to other reports[1, 59] for additional details on decontamination of the skin.

Plans for emergency care of radiation accidents at nuclear facilities and in hospitals should devote attention to the problem of external contamination. One objective of the plan should be to prevent spread of loose radioactive material beyond the immediate work area where the patient is being treated. This work area should have good access to an outside entrance and be subject to only limited personnel traffic. The hallways should be monitored for radioactivity as soon as the patient is brought into the work area. Various decontamination rooms have been designed for either plant or hospital emergency plans.[23, 36, 59, 90] In hospitals, it is frequently possible to use rooms and facilities, such as physical therapy or cast rooms, that normally serve other functions. The essential features of the work area are good personnel traffic control, showers, hand sinks, washable floor covering, and adequate room for minor surgical procedures. The availability of a mobile x-ray unit is desirable for locating foreign bodies. Although a special hold-up tank is desirable for retaining contaminated water, such a specialized item may not be feasible for hospitals in view of their limited use. The radioactivity in water from personnel decontamination procedures will not ordinarily create problems in a domestic sewerage system because of large dilution factors and infrequent occurrences of this type of event.

Contaminated Wounds

In the event of severe injuries associated with radioactive contamination, the first consideration of the attending physician should be for the patient's general welfare. Emergency procedures to control hemorrhage, to restore respiratory and circulatory function, and to alleviate pain obviously are a first order of business, even if the contamination levels are high. For life-saving purposes it is suggested that whole-body doses to personnel up to 100 rems (1 Sv) are permissible.[54] In such circumstances, it is likely that even higher doses to the hands and forearms will occur. Competent health physics support should be obtained if high radiation doses to medical personnel are possible.

It is truly an exceptional case in which high radiation doses to the medical staff will be a concern. Most contaminated wounds, often relatively trivial injuries, will involve relatively low radiation levels. The first decontamination procedure should be an immediate rinsing of the wound with running tap water or saline irrigation in such a manner that the water flows away from the wound. Use of a pulsating water jet stream may be helpful. Application of a tourniquet frequently is mentioned as a useful procedure to reduce the uptake of radioactive materials, but in practice it is seldom used or needed. To the extent possible, the wound area should be treated using conventional aseptic techniques.

The progress of decontamination must be measured by means of some type of radiation instrumentation. For β-γ radiation, a portable survey meter is usually adequate. Alpha-emitters present more difficult monitoring problems and special wound counters are generally necessary. A person with monitoring experience should assist the medical team in radioactivity measurements.

Wound excision has been used primarily to remove long-lived α contaminants, such as ^{239}Pu. Small quantities of α contamination, such as 2 nCi (74 Bq) or less of ^{239}Pu, are usually not excised. Long-term problems have not occurred in these cases. If more activity is present, it is desirable to obtain complete removal of the contaminant from the wound, if possible. Excision of the area has been the only practical solution. The surgeon should complete the wound excision without creating functional disability if at all possible. Any significant sacrifice of function is not justified unless an unusually high contamination is present.

Beta-gamma-emitters in wounds will not usually present as much hazard as α-emitters. Excision has not been required often for β-γ contamination.

Internal Deposition of Radioactive Material

Medical management of persons exposed to radionuclides is designed to reduce the internal deposition of radionuclides in the body. The objective is to reduce the radiation dose to organs and hence also the risk of possible future biologic effects. This may be accomplished (1) by reduction of absorption and subsequent internal deposition of radionuclides and (2) by enhanced elimination of absorbed radionuclides. Both are achieved most effectively when therapy is begun immediately after exposure.

The decision to treat a person must be made as soon as possible after exposure. This period is also when the least information is available upon which to base medical decisions.

Information available immediately after an accident may consist of some scanty information on the details of the accident, probable identification of the major radionuclides by history of the operation, and perhaps a general idea of the level of contamination in the accident area by either initial monitoring surveys of surfaces or possibly air concentration measurements. Symptoms and signs in the exposed person(s) will relate to associated physical injuries, but none will be present from internal radiation doses. Nasal swipes are frequently used in nuclear facilities as an early indication of whether inhalation of radionuclides may have occurred. This procedure consists of swabbing the anterior nasal membranes with a moist cotton applicator or a moistened filter paper strip wound around a swab stick. Each nostril is swabbed with a separate swab in order to get a count on both sides. The applicator or filter paper is dried and then counted for radioactivity. To be meaningful, nasal swipes must be made within a few minutes of the accident and before showering of the individual.

Physicians cannot wait for better dosimetry if they are to start early therapy. Decisions to treat should be made and started at the plant's medical facility, if possible, rather than to refer the case to a hospital. There may be past experience with the radionuclide in question that will suggest whether treatment should be instituted or not. Although it is tempting to wait for initial results of whole-body counts or radioactivity measurements of a urine sample, the time lost in doing this cannot be regained. The risk from most treatments recommended for internally-deposited radionuclides is so small that it does not enter strongly into the initial decision of whether or not to treat. The underlying guideline for treatment is based on whether it is possible to obtain a significant dose reduction for the patient.

Table 26–13 contains a list of selected radionuclides and a limited amount of data on each that may assist in the initial appraisal of a potential internal exposure.

The following sections summarize some of the techniques and types of drugs available to either reduce the uptake of radionuclides or increase their elimination from the body.

Reduction of Uptake.—The procedures that may prevent or reduce uptake of radionuclides into the body include skin decontamination, proper management of contaminated wounds, reduction of gastrointestinal absorption, and treatment of inhaled radionuclides.

During the initial evaluation of an accident, such simple procedures as irrigation of the nose, mouth, and pharynx, removal of gastric contents, and the use of purgatives should not be overlooked. Any reduction in the residence time of the radioactivity in the gastrointestinal tract will reduce the dose to it and will reduce the time available for gastrointestinal absorption. The time for effective action for soluble compounds is only about 30–60 minutes.

The induction of vomiting by mechanical stimulation of the pharynx or passage of a stomach tube is the most effective means of removing the stomach contents. A less desirable procedure is the use of an emetic, such as ipecac syrup (15 ml) or an injection of apomorphine hydrochloride (0.1 mg/kg subcutaneously).

The administration of a laxative such as magnesium sulfate (15 gm in 100 ml water) will reduce the residence time of radioactive material in the lower segment of the large intestine. Magnesium sulfate may also produce relatively insoluble sulfate with some radionuclides such as radium or strontium.

Certain compounds can be used to reduce the gastrointestinal uptake of specific radionuclides. Most notable examples are Prussian Blue (1 gm in water three times per day) for cesium, thallium, and rubidium; aluminum-containing antacids (100 ml aluminum phosphate gel or aluminum hydroxide) for strontium; and barium or magnesium sulfate for strontium or radium. Phytates found in grains, especially oats and soybean products, form insoluble salts of calcium, magnesium, zinc, and iron.

Prussian Blue is not available in a pharmaceutical chemical grade and is not approved by the U.S. Food and Drug Administration as a drug. It has been well tolerated when given to persons. The longest period of administration has been three weeks. Constipation has been the only noted side effect. Preparation of a pure compound and approval for its use must be done as part of medical emergency preparedness.

Blocking and Diluting Agents.—A blocking agent saturates the metabolic processes in a specific tissue with the stable element and thereby reduces the uptake of the radioisotope. Stable potassium iodide, used to prevent the uptake of radioiodine in the thyroid, is an example of a blocking agent. To be effective, blocking agents must be administered in a rapidly absorbed form soon after exposure to the radionuclide.

Isotopic dilution is achieved by the administration of large quantities of the stable element or compound similar to the radionuclides being treated. The presence of a large quantity of the stable element dilutes the smaller quantity of the radioisotope. For example, forcing fluids reduces the biologic half-time of tritium (radioactive hydrogen) in the body due to dilution and enhanced turnover time of water.

Displacement therapy is a special form of dilution therapy in which a stable element of a different atomic number successfully competes with a radionuclide for uptake sites. An example is the use of calcium to reduce the deposition of radioactive strontium in the bone.

Other examples of blocking or diluting agents are strontium lactate or strontium gluconate for radioactive strontium; oral phosphate for ingested radioactive strontium; and oral or intravenous calcium for radioactive strontium or calcium. Oral administration of zinc and potassium is a diluting agent for their respective radioisotopes.

Mobilizing Agents.—Mobilizing agents are compounds that increase a natural turnover process and thereby induce a release of some forms of radionuclides from body tissues. This results in an enhanced elimination of the radionuclide from the body. These agents are also most effective if given soon after exposure, but some may still be effective if used several weeks later. An example is ammonium chloride, which acts as a mobilizing agent for radioactive strontium in the body.

Other examples of mobilizing agents are antithyroid drugs for radioactive iodine that is already deposited in the thyroid; diuretics for sodium, chlorides, potassium, and tritium (radioactive hydrogen); and parathyroid extract for calcium, phosphorus, and strontium. Antithyroid drugs should not be used when stable iodides are being used as a blocking agent, which is the preferred treatment.

Chelating Agents.—A number of chemical compounds are known that enhance the elimination of metals from the body by chelation, a process by which organic compounds (ligands) exchange less firmly bonded ions for other inorganic ions to form a relatively stable nonionized ring complex. This soluble complex is excreted readily by the kidney. A properly selected and administered chelating drug will enhance the excretion of some radionu-

TABLE 26–13.
Information on Selected Radionuclides*

NUCLIDE ($T½$) RADIATION†	LUNG CLASS‡	F_1§	ANNUAL INTAKE (μCi)¶	ORGAN‖	H_{50} (rem/μCi)**
^{241}Am (432 y) α,γ	W	5×10^{-4}	inh 5×10^{-3}	Bone surface	9.4×10^{3}
^{82}Br (35 h) β,γ	W	1	inh 2×10^{3}	Lungs	6.2×10^{-3}
^{14}C (5730 y) β	Gas		inh 2×10^{3}	Gonads	2.1×10^{-3}
^{252}Cf (2.6 y) α, γ, n	W	5×10^{-4}	inh 3×10^{-2}	Bone surface	1.8×10^{3}
^{38}Cl (37 m) β, γ	D	1	ing 5×10^{3}	Stomach wall	3.3×10^{-3}
^{60}Co (5.2 y) β γ	Y	5×10^{-2}	inh 1×10^{1}	Lungs	1.3
^{51}Cr (27.7 d) γ	Y	1×10^{-1}	inh 8×10^{3}	Lungs	2.0×10^{-3}
^{134}Cs (2.1 y) β, γ	D	1	ing 7×10^{1}	Gonads	7.6×10^{-2}
^{137}Cs (30 y) β, γ	D	1	ing 1×10^{2}	Gonads	5.1×10^{-2}
^{59}Fe (45 d) β, γ	W	1×10^{-1}	inh 3×10^{2}	Lungs	5.1×10^{-2}
^{3}H (12.3 y) β	Gas		inh 8×10^{4}	Soft tissue	6.3×10^{-5}
^{131}I (8 d) β, γ	D	1	ing 2×10^{1}	Thyroid	1.8
^{192}Ir (74 d) β, γ	Y	1×10^{-2}	inh 8×10^{1}	Lungs	1.9×10^{-1}
^{24}Na (15 h) β, γ	D	1	inh 3×10^{3}	Lungs	4.6×10^{-3}
^{32}P (14.3 d)β	D	8×10^{-1}	ing 2×10^{2}	Red active marrow	3.0×10^{-2}
^{147}Pm (2.6 y) α, β	W	3×10^{-4}	inh 1×10^{2}	Bone surface	3.8×10^{-1}
^{210}Po (138 d) α	D	1×10^{-1}	inh 2×10^{-1}	Spleen	8.0×10^{1}
^{238}Pu (87.7 y) α, γ	W	1×10^{-4}	inh 6×10^{-3}	Bone surface	8.1×10^{3}
^{239}Pu (24065 y) α, γ	W	1×10^{-4}	inh 5×10^{-3}	Bone surface	9.1×10^{3}
^{226}Ra (1600 y) α, β, γ	W	2×10^{-1}	inh 3×10^{-1}	Lungs	6.0×10^{1}
^{106}Ru (368 d) β, γ	Y	5×10^{-2}	inh 4	Lungs	3.8
^{46}Sc (83 d) β, γ	Y	1×10^{-4}	inh 9×10^{1}	Lungs	1.7×10^{-1}
^{90}Sr (29.1 y) β	D	3×10^{-1}	inh 4	Red active marrow	1.2
^{204}Tl (3.8 y) β	D	1	inh 1×10^{3}	Kidneys	1.1×10^{-2}
^{170}Tm (128.6 d) β, γ	W	3×10^{-4}	inh 1×10^{2}	Lungs	1.4×10^{-1}
^{235}U (7×10^{8} y) α, β, γ	W	5×10^{-2}	inh 3×10^{-1}	Lungs	5.5×10^{1}

*From Eckerman KF, Watson SB, Nelson CB, et al: *The Radioactivity Concentration Guides: A New Calculation of Derived Limits for the 1960 Radiation Protection Guides Reflecting Updated Models for Dosimetry and Biological Transport,* Federal Guidance Report 10, EPA Report 620/1-84-010. Oak Ridge, Tenn, Oak Ridge National Laboratory, 1984.

These data are highly selected and abbreviated; thus, they will serve for only the first cursory look at internal exposure potential. The dose will be highly variable with different chemical forms of the radionuclide and different particle size distribution of an aerosol. In most cases, the values selected should provide the more conservative (higher dose) values that may occur in an accidental exposure.

†The radionuclide symbol and atomic number are followed by its radioactive half-life in minutes (m), hours (h), days (d), or years (y). The type of radiation emitted is listed by its Greek letter designation.

‡If exposed by inhalation, the rate of lung clearance used to calculate the limiting annual intake and dose (H_{50} years) is indicated as days (D), weeks (W), or years (Y). Only one class is selected here as a sample case. Chemical properties of the involved compound must be considered in actual cases.

§This value is the fractional uptake from the small intestine to blood (f_1) after ingestion. Chemical properties of the involved compound must be considered in actual cases.

¶The mode of uptake used in calculating the annual intake and dose (H_{50} years) is indicated as inh (inhalation) or ing (ingestion). The limiting annual intake of the radionuclide in microcuries will result in a dose to the listed organ equal to its radiation protection guide in the 50th year of continuous intake. The numerical value is dependent on the chemical form of the inhaled or ingested material.

‖This is the organ receiving the highest radiation dose for the mode of intake and chemical properties assumed. Bone surface includes endosteal tissue within 10 μm of bone surfaces.

***H_{50}*: The committed dose equivalent per unit intake for the listed organ. Committed dose equivalent is the 50-year integral of the dose equivalent rate in a particular tissue after intake. The numerical value also can be interpreted as the annual dose-equivalent after 50 years of continued annual intake of unit activity, rem/μCi/yr.

clides and thus reduce their residence time in the body. Chelation therapy is most effective when it is begun immediately after exposure while the metallic ions are still in extracellular fluids and before their incorporation into cells.

The chelate that is principally used for removal of radionuclides is DTPA. It is effective for transuranium metals (plutonium, americium, curium, californium, and neptunium), the rare earths (such as cerium, yttrium, lanthanum, promethium, and scandium), and some transition metals (such as zirconium and niobium). Because of its usefulness in treating radionuclides, DTPA is discussed in more detail later.

There are other chelating agents that may be useful occasionally and are listed here without discussion. An example is EDTA, which chelates lead, zinc, copper, cadmium, chromium, manganese, nickel, and the transuranium metals. It is about one tenth as effective as DTPA for enhancing urinary excretion of the transuranium metals. Other chelating agents are dimercaprol or BAL (for mercury, lead, arsenic, gold, bismuth, chromium, and nickel), penicillamine (for copper, iron, mercury, lead, and gold), and deferoxamine or DFOA (for iron).

Two forms of DTPA are available for clinical use, the calcium salt (CaDTPA) and the zinc salt (ZnDTPA). The ZnDTPA is less toxic than CaDTPA in animal studies; therefore, ZnDTPA is recommended for longer-term treatment and for pregnant women.

However, CaDTPA is more effective than ZnDTPA in rats when given promptly after exposure to transuranium metals. This finding suggests that CaDTPA should be the preferred form of the drug to use during the first day or two after exposure.

No serious toxicity in man has been reported as a result of using CaDTPA or ZnDTPA in recommended doses. Long-term, low-dose administrations in man, 1 gm CaDTPA per week, caused no adverse effects after four years.[80] Also, CaDTPA binds trace metals present in the body, such as zinc and manganese. It is the reduction of these two metals that apparently accounts for toxicity seen after high doses in animal experiments. Doses over 2,000 mole/kg—the clinical human dose range is 10–30 mole/kg—can produce severe lesions of the kidneys, intestinal mucosa, and liver in animals. Teratogenesis and fetal death have occurred in mice when similarly high doses were given throughout gestation.

The effectiveness of DTPA in enhancing excretion of plutonium is affected markedly by the chemical form of the plutonium. After either contaminated wounds or inhalation of particles, the absorption of plutonium into the circulation may occur over many weeks, even years, when it is present as relatively insoluble plutonium compound, such as plutonium oxide. In these cases DTPA is not effective, because of the small amount of plutonium present in the blood and extracellular fluids soon after exposure. Soluble compounds of plutonium, such as the nitrate, have relatively rapid uptake and translocation, and in these cases more plutonium is immediately available for chelation. Data from persons treated with CaDTPA within about three hours of exposure indicate that about 60%–70% of soluble forms of plutonium are removed compared to the retention in cases without treatment.[21] Both CaDTPA and ZnDTPA are approved as investigational new drugs (IND) in the United States, but DTPA is not available from commercial sources. For physicians with a potential need for these drugs, DTPA can be requested from the Oak Ridge Associated Universities, REAC/TS Center, Oak Ridge, TN 37831-0117.

The recommended dose for DTPA is 1 gm once per day. The dose should not be fractionated, i.e., given in multiple doses per day. It can be given either intravenously or by aerosol inhalation. The intravenous administration of 1 gm DTPA in 250 ml normal saline or 5% glucose in water over 30 minutes has been the usual procedure. An alternate procedure, 1 gm diluted in 10 or 20 ml normal saline and injected intravenously by syringe over five minutes, is preferred by some physicians. In either case, care should be taken to avoid extravasation from the vein. Aerosol administration is done with 1 gm CaDTPA placed in a nebulizer and the contents inhaled over 15 to 20 minutes.

Because of its metallic taste, ZnDTPA is less suited than CaDTPA for aerosol administration. It is prudent not to use the inhalation route in persons with preexisting pulmonary disease. The drug is also contraindicated if significant leukopenia, thrombocytopenia, or kidney dysfunction exists. Clinical urinalysis should be normal prior to each treatment. A treatment protocol and follow-up reports are required under the terms of the IND agreement.

Lung Lavage.—Deposition of radioactive particles in the lung is a common mode of accidental exposure of humans to radionuclides. Insoluble particles, once inhaled into the lung, are dissolved slowly and translocated to other organs over many months and years.

Lavage of the tracheobronchial tree has shown promise in animal studies as a possible treatment technique for individuals who have inhaled relatively insoluble particles of radioactive material. The procedure requires placement of an endotracheal tube into the trachea and major bronchi under a general anesthesia and then the lung can be lavaged with isotonic saline.

Dogs treated after inhaling insoluble radioactive particles have shown reduction in their lung burdens from about 25% to 50% (average of 44% in eight dogs) after five lavages of each lung, ten total.[6, 52, 67] Radiation pneumonitis and early deaths were prevented in 75% of the treated dogs in contrast to the death of all untreated dogs. The same regimen of ten lavages removed 35% to 49% of ^{239}Pu and ^{238}Pu polydisperse aerosols of different chemical characteristics.[53] In baboons, 60% to 90% of the lung burdens of plutonium oxide was removed by ten pulmonary lavages.[66]

Possible use of this experimental technique in man requires a careful risk-benefit assessment. The risk lies primarily in the administration of a general anesthetic. The overall mortality risk appears to be 0.2%–0.5% for each procedure. Thus, this technique should be considered only in high exposures in which a reduction of 25%–50% of the dose could be expected to prevent acute or subacute effects, such as radiation pneumonitis or fibrosis. It should be recognized that the procedure's risk is immediate, whereas late effects of radiation dose to the lung may occur many years later.

Therapy for Selected Elements.—Brief comments are presented here as a treatment summary for a few elements that have important radioisotopes. This section discusses only certain drug therapy and does not go into other important aspects of medical management of radiation cases. For more complete information, the reader is referred to other reports.[41, 59, 91]

Americium: See Transuranic elements.

Californium: See Transuranic elements.

Cerium: See Rare earths.

Cesium: Prussian Blue (ferric ferrocyanide), 1 gm given orally with water three times daily, should reduce the biologic half-time from the usual 70 days to 35–50 days during the period of administration.

Curium: See Transuranic elements.

Iodine: Stable potassium iodide or sodium iodide (300 mg of iodide) should be administered orally as soon as possible and continued daily for 7–14 days to prevent recycling of the radioactive iodine. Success depends upon early administration of the drug, preferably within one to four hours of exposure. Little effectiveness is expected if given as late as 12 hours.

Lanthanum: See Rare earths.

Phosphorus: Aluminum hydroxide (100 ml) antacids will reduce gastrointestinal absorption. Phosphate (1 gm) will act as a diluting agent.

Plutonium: See Transuranic elements.

Radium: Magnesium sulfate (15 gm in 100 ml water) will reduce absorption of radium from the gastrointestinal tract. No effective therapy is available after absorption and deposition of the radium in bone. Administration of ammonium chloride and calcium may increase urinary excretion of radium slightly.

Rare earths: Chelation with DTPA should start as soon after exposure as possible. The IND protocol does not include rare earths for treatment by DTPA chelation, but animal experiments indicate that it is effective.

Strontium: Aluminum phosphate gel or aluminum hydroxide antacids (100 ml), if given shortly after ingestion, will reduce absorption from the gastrointestinal tract. Administration of strontium (500–1,500 mg strontium lactate orally each day or 600 mg strontium gluconate intravenously daily up to six days) or large doses of oral or intravenous calcium combined with oral ammonium chloride (1 to 2 gm four times per day) will enhance urinary excretion of strontium. This treatment needs to be started as soon as possible after exposure.

Transuranium elements: Chelation with DTPA should start as soon after exposure as possible, preferably within the first hour or two. Chelation therapy is not effective after inhalation of highly insoluble forms of these elements, high-fired plutonium oxide particles being the most notable example. A trial dose of DTPA, combined with monitoring of the urine for significant excretion of plutonium (or whatever element is involved), is a good way of determining the effectiveness of chelation therapy. Hall et al.[21] developed a model for plutonium excretion after DTPA treatment that suggests an optimal dosage schedule is provided with administration of DTPA on days 1 (immediately after exposure), 2, 4, 7, and 15 after exposure.

Tritium: Force fluids to tolerance of patient up to about two weeks. The length of treatment will depend on the estimated dose determined by measurements in daily urine samples. The normal 10–12-day biologic half-time should be reduced to six days or less.

ACKNOWLEDGMENT

This chapter is work performed under the auspices of the U.S. Department of Energy.

REFERENCES

1. American Medical Association: *A Guide to the Hospital Management of Injuries Arising From Exposure to or Involving Ionizing Radiation*. Chicago, Ill, American Medical Association, 1984.
2. American National Standards Institute, Inc./American Nuclear Society: *Medical Certification and Monitoring of Personnel Requiring Operator Licenses for Nuclear Power Plants*, ANSI/ANS-3.4-1983. La Grange Park, Ill, American Nuclear Society, 1983.
3. Andrews GA: Medical management of accidental total-body irradiation, in Hubner KF, Fry SA (eds): *The Medical Basis for Radiation Accident Preparedness*. New York, Elsevier North Holland, Inc, 1980, pp 297–310.
4. Andrews GA, Sitterson BW, Kretchmar AL, et al: Criticality accident at the Y-12 plant, in *Diagnosis and Treatment of Acute Radiation Injury*. Geneva, World Health Organization, 1961, pp 27–48.
5. Archer VE, Gilliam JD, Wagoner JK: Respiratory disease mortality among uranium miners. *Ann NY Acad Sci* 1976; 271:280–293.
6. Boecker BB, Muggenburg BA, McClellan RO, et al: Removal of ^{144}Ce in fused clay particles from the beagle dog by bronchopulmonary lavage. *Health Phys* 1974; 26:605.
7. Boice JD Jr, Fraumeni JF Jr (eds): *Radiation Carcinogenesis: Epidemiology and Biological Significance*. New York, Raven Press, 1984.
8. Boice JD Jr, Monson RR: Breast cancer in women after repeated fluoroscopic examinations of the chest. *J Natl Cancer Inst* 1977; 59:823–832.
9. Cember H: *Introduction to Health Physics*, ed 2. New York, Pergamon Press, 1983.
10. Conard RA, et al: *Review of Medical Findings in a Marshallese Population Twenty-Six Years After Accidental Exposure to Radioactive Fallout*, Brookhaven National Laboratory report BNL 51261. Springfield, VA, National Technical Information Service, 1980.
11. Court-Brown WM, Doll R: Mortality from Cancer and Other Causes after Radiotherapy for Ankylosing Spondylitis. Br Med J 1965; 2:1327–1332.
12. Doll R, Peto R: The Causes of Cancer: Quantitative Estimates of Avoidable Risks of Cancer in the United States Today. *J Natl Cancer Inst* 1981; 66:1191.
13. Eckerman KF, Watson SB, Nelson CB, et al: *The Radioactivity Concentration Guides: A New Calculation of Derived Limits for the 1960 Radiation Protection Guides Reflecting Updated Models for Dosimetry and Biological Transport*, Federal Guidance Report 10, EPA Report 520/1-84-010. Oak Ridge, Tenn, Oak Ridge National Laboratory, 1984.
14. Environmental Protection Agency: Underground mining of uranium ore, radiation protection guidance for federal agencies. *Federal Register* 1971; 36:9480.
15. Environmental Protection Agency: Underground mining of uranium ore, radiation protection guidance for federal agencies. *Federal Register* 1971; 36:12921.
16. Federal Radiation Council: *Background Material for the Development of Radiation Protection Standards*, FRC Staff Report 1. Washington, DC, US Dept of Commerce, 1960.
17. Federal Radiation Council: *Background Material for the Development of Radiation Protection Standards*, FRC Staff Report 2. Washington, DC, Supt of Documents, US Government Printing Office, 1961.
18. Federal Radiation Council: Radiation protection guidance for federal agencies. *Federal Register* 1969; 34:576.
19. Federal Radiation Council: Radiation protection guidance for federal agencies. *Federal Register* 1970; 35:19218.
20. Fry SA, Sipe A: DOE-REAC/TS Radiation Accident Registries: Serious radiation accidents worldwide, A selected bibliography, Unpublished report. Oak Ridge, Tenn, Oak Ridge Associated Universities, 1985.
21. Hall RM, Poda GA, Fleming RR, et al: A mathematical model for estimation of plutonium in the human body from urine data influenced by DTPA therapy. *Health Phys* 1978; 34:419.
22. Hempelmann LH, Hall WJ, Phillips M, et al: Neoplasms in persons treated with x-rays in infancy: Fourth survey in 20 years. *J Natl Cancer Inst* 1975; 55:519.
23. Holland RW: Planning a Medical Unit for Handling Contaminated Persons Following a Radiation Accident. *Nuclear Saf* 1969; 10:72.
24. Ichimaru M, Ishimaru T, Mikami M, et al: *Incidence of Leukemia in a Fixed Cohort of Atomic Bomb Survivors and Controls, Hiroshima and Nagasaki, October 1950–December 1978*, Technical Report 13-91. Hiroshima, Radiation Effects Research Foundation, 1981.
25. International Atomic Energy Agency: *Manual on Radiation Haematology*, Technical Report Series 25. Vienna, IAEA, 1971.
26. International Commission on Radiological Protection: *Recommendations of the International Commission on Radiological Protection*, ICRP Publ 26, Ann ICRP 1, No 3. New York, Pergamon Press, 1977.
27. International Commission on Radiological Protection: *The Principles and General Procedures for Handling Emergency and Accidental Exposures of Workers*, ICRP Publ 28, Ann ICRP 2, No 1. New York, Pergamon Press, 1978.
28. International Commission on Radiological Protection: *Limits for In-*

take by Workers, ICRP Publ 30, Pt 1, Ann ICRP 2, No 3/4. New York, Pergamon Press, 1979.

29. International Commission on Radiological Protection: *Limits for Intake by Workers*, ICRP Publ 30, Suppl to Pt 1, Ann ICRP 3, No 1–4. New York, Pergamon Press, 1979.
30. International Commission on Radiological Protection: *Limits for Intake by Workers*, ICRP Publ 30, Pt 2, Annals of the ICRP 4, No 3/4. New York, Pergamon Press, 1980.
31. International Commission on Radiological Protection: *Limits for Intake by Workers*, ICRP Publ 30, Suppl to Pt 2, Ann ICRP 5, No 1–6. New York, Pergamon Press, 1981.
32. International Commission on Radiological Protection: *Limits for Intake by Workers*, ICRP Publ 30, Pt 3, Ann ICRP 6, No 2/3. New York, Pergamon Press, 1981.
33. International Commission on Radiological Protection: *Limits for Intake by Workers*, ICRP Publ 30, Suppl A to Pt 3, Ann ICRP 7, No 1–3. New York, Pergamon Press, 1982.
34. International Commission on Radiological Protection: *Limits for Intake by Workers*, ICRP Publ 30, Suppl B to Pt 3, Ann ICRP 8, No 1–3. New York, Pergamon Press, 1982.
35. Kato H, Schull WJ: Studies of the mortality of A-bomb survivors. 7. Mortality, 1950–1978: Pt I Cancer mortality. *Radiat Res* 1982; 90:395–432.
36. Kelly FJ, Lemons BD: Radiation decontamination facility for the community hospital. *J Occup Med* 1972; 14:904.
37. Kim JH, Chu FC, Woodard HQ, et al: Radiation-induced soft tissue and bone sarcoma. *Radiology* 1978; 129:501.
38. Kumazawa S, Nelson DR, Richardson ACB: *Occupational Exposure to Ionizing Radiation in the United States*, EPA Report 520/1-84-005. Washington, DC, Environmental Protection Agency, 1984.
39. Langham WH (ed): *Radiobiological Factors in Manned Space Flight*. Washington, DC, National Academy of Sciences—National Research Council, 1967.
40. Leonard RB, Ricks RC: Emergency department radiation accident protocol. *Ann Emerg Med* 1980; 9:462–470.
41. Lincoln TA: Importance of Initial Management of Persons Internally Contaminated with Radionuclides. *Am Ind Hyg Assoc J* 1976; 37:16–21.
42. Littlefield LG: The analysis of radiation-induced chromosome lesions in lymphocytes as a biological method for dose estimation, in *Proceedings of NATO Working Group Meeting on the Assessment of Injury From Ionizing Radiation in Warfare*. Bethesda, Md, Armed Forces Radiobiology Research Institute, 1982, pp 351–387.
43. Livesey JC, Reed DJ, Adamson LF: *Chemical Protection Against Ionizing Radiation*, Lawrence Livermore National Laboratory report UCRL-15644. Washington, DC, Federal Emergency Management Agency, 1984.
44. Lloyd DC, Purrott RJ: Chromosome aberration analysis in radiological protection dosimetry. *Radiat Protect Dosimetry* 1981; 1:19–28.
45. Lushbaugh CC: The impact of estimates of human radiation tolerance upon radiation emergency management, in *The Control of Exposure of the Public to Ionizing Radiation in the Event of Accident or Attack*. Bethesda, Md, National Council on Radiation Protection and Measurements, 1982, pp 46–57.
46. Lushbaugh CC, Comas F, Hofstra R: Clinical studies of radiation effects in man. *Radiat Res* (Suppl) 1967; 7:398–412.
47. March HC: Leukemia in radiologists. *Radiology* 1974; 43:275.
48. Mays CW (ed): Biological effects of ^{224}Ra and thorotrast, proceedings of an international symposium. *Health Phys* 1978; 35:1–174.
49. Mays CW, Spiess H, Gerspach A: Skeletal effects following ^{224}Ra injections into humans. *Health Phys* 1978; 35:83.

49a. McGuire SA, Peabody CA: *Working Safely in Gamma Radiography*, report NUREG/BR-0024, US Nuclear Regulatory Commission. Washington, DC, US Government Printing Office, 1982.

50. Miller RW: Delayed effects occurring within the first decade after exposure of young individuals to the Hiroshima atomic bomb. *Pediatrics* 1956; 18:1.
51. Monson RR, MacMahon B: Prenatal x-ray exposure and cancer in children, in Boice JD Jr, Fraumeni JF Jr (eds): *Radiation Carcinogenesis: Epidemiology and Biological Significance*. New York, Raven Press, 1984, pp 97–105.
52. Muggenburg BA, Mauderly JL, Boecker BB, et al: Prevention of radiation pneumonitis from inhaled cerium-144 by lung lavage in Beagle dogs. *Am Rev Resp Dis* 1975; 111:795.
53. Muggenburg BA, Mewhinny JA, Miglio JJ, et al: The removal of inhaled ^{239}Pu and ^{238}Pu from Beagle dogs by lung lavage and chelation treatment, in *Diagnosis and Treatment of Incorporated Radionuclides*, IAEA Publ STI/PUB/411. Vienna, International Atomic Energy Agency, 1976, p 341.
54. National Council on Radiation Protection and Measurements: *Basic Radiation Protection Criteria*, NCRP Report 39. Bethesda, Md, NCRP Publications, 1971.
55. National Council on Radiation Protection and Measurements: *Review of the Current State of Radiation Protection Philosophy*, NCRP Report 43. Bethesda, Md, NCRP Publications, 1975.
56. National Council on Radiation Protection and Measurements: *Review of NCRP Radiation Dose Limit for Embryo and Fetus in Occupationally-Exposed Women*, NCRP Report 53. Bethesda, Md, NCRP Publications, 1977.
57. National Council on Radiation Protection and Measurements: *Medical Radiation Exposure of Pregnant and Potentially Pregnant Women*, NCRP Report 54. Bethesda, Md, NCRP Publications, 1977.
58. National Council on Radiation Protection and Measurements: *Influence of Dose and Its Distribution in Time on Dose-Response Relationships for Low-LET Radiations*, NCRP Report 64. Bethesda, Md, NCRP Publications, 1980.
59. National Council on Radiation Protection and Measurements: *Management of Persons Accidentally Contaminated With Radionuclides*, NCRP Report 65. Bethesda, Md, NCRP Publications, 1980.
60. National Council on Radiation Protection and Measurements: *Exposures From the Uranium Series With Emphasis on Radon and Its Daughters*, NCRP Report 77. Bethesda, Md, NCRP Publications, 1984.
61. National Council on Radiation Protection and Measurements: *Evaluation of Occupational and Environmental Exposures to Radon and Radon Daughters in the United States*, NCRP Report 78. Bethesda, Md, NCRP Publications, 1984.
62. National Council on Radiation Protection and Measurements: *A Handbook of Radioactivity Measurements Procedures*, NCRP Report 58. Bethesda, Md, NCRP Publications, 1985.
63. National Institutes of Health: *Report of the National Institutes of Health Ad Hoc Working Group to Develop Radioepidemiologic Tables*, NIH Publ 85–2748. Washington, DC, US Government Printing Office, 1985.
64. National Research Council, National Academy of Sciences: *Radiobiological Factors in Manned Space Flight*, Langham WH (ed). Washington, DC, National Academy of Sciences, 1967.
65. National Research Council, National Academy of Sciences: *The Effects on Populations of Exposure to Low Levels of Ionizing Radiation: 1980*. Report of the Committee on the Biological Effects of Ionizing Radiations. Washington, DC, National Academy Press, 1980.
66. Nolibe D, Nenot JC, Metivier H, et al: Traitement des inhalations accidentelles d'oxyde de plutonium par lavage pulmonaire in vivo, in *Diagnosis and Treatment of Incorporated Radionuclides*, IAEA Publ STI/PUB/411. Vienna, International Atomic Energy Agency, 1976, p 373.
67. Pfleger RC, Wilson AJ, McClellan RO: Pulmonary lavage as a ther-

apeutic measure for removing inhaled "insoluble" materials from the lung. *Health Phys* 1969; 16:758.
68. Prentice RL, Kato H, Yoshimoto K, et al: Radiation exposures and thyroid cancer incidence among Hiroshima and Nagasaki residents, in *Third Symposium on Epidemiology and Cancer Registries in the Pacific Basin*. Washington, DC, US Government Printing Office, 1982, pp 207–212.
69. Ron E, Modan B: Thyroid and other neoplasms following childhood scalp irradiation, in Boice JD Jr, Fraumeni JF Jr (eds): *Radiation Carcinogenesis: Epidemiology and Biological Significance*. New York, Raven Press, 1984, pp 139–151.
70. Rowland RE, Stehney AF, Lucas HF Jr: Dose response relationships for female radium dial workers. *Radiat Res* 1978; 76:368.
71. Rugh R: Radiology and the human embryo and fetus, in Dalrymple GV, Gaulden ME, Kollmorgan GM, et al (eds): *Medical Radiation Biology*. Philadelphia, WB Saunders Co, 1973.
72. Schneider AB, Vavus MH, Stachura ME, et al: Salivary gland neoplasms as a late consequence of head and neck irradiation. *Ann Intern Med* 1978, 87:160.
73. Schull WJ, Otake M, Neel JV: Genetic effects of the atomic bombs: A reappraisal. *Science* 1981; 213:1220.
74. Seve J, Kunz E, Placek V: Lung cancer in uranium miners and long-term exposure to radon daughter products. *Health Phys* 1976; 30:433–437.
75. Shapiro J: *Radiation Protection—A Guide for Scientists and Physicians*, ed 2. Cambridge, Mass, Harvard University Press, 1981.
76. Shleien B: *Preparedness and Response in Radiation Accidents*, US Dept of Health and Human Services Report FDA 83–8211. Washington, DC, US Government Printing Office, 1983.
77. Shleien B, Terpilak MS (eds): *The Health Physics and Radiological Health Handbook*. Olney, Md, Nucleon Lectern Associates, Inc, 1984.
78. Shore RE, Albert RE, Pasternack BS: Follow-up study of patients treated by x-ray epilation for tinea capitis: Resurvey of post-treatment illness and mortality experience. *Arch Environ Health* 1976; 31:21.
79. Shore RE, Hempelmann LH, Kowaluk E, et al: Breast neoplasms in women treated with x-rays for acute postpartum mastitis. *J Natl Cancer Inst* 1977; 59:813–822.
80. Slobodien MJ, Brodsky A, Ke CH, et al: Removal of zinc from humans by DTPA chelation therapy, *Health Phys* 1973; 24:327.
81. Smith PG, Doll R: Mortality among patients with ankylosing spondylitis after a single treatment course with X-ray. *Br Med J* 1982; 284:449–460.
82. Society of Nuclear Medicine, Inc: *Low-level Radiation Effects: A Fact Book*, Report of the Subcommittee on Risks of Low-level Ionizing Radiation. New York, Society of Nuclear Medicine, Inc, 1982.
83. Stewart AM, Kneale GW: Prenatal radiation exposure and childhood cancer. *Lancet* 1971; 1:42.
84. Thoma GE, Wald N: Diagnosis and management of accidental radiation injury. *J Occup Med* 1959; 1:421.
85. Tokunaga M, Land CE, Yamamoto T, et al: Breast cancer among atomic bomb survivors, in Boice JD Jr, Fraumeni JF Jr (eds): *Radiation Carcinogenesis: Epidemiology and Biological Significance*. New York, Raven Press, 1984, pp 45–56.
86. United Nations Scientific Committee on the Effects of Atomic Radiation: *Sources and Effects of Ionizing Radiation*, 1977 Report to the General Assembly, with annexes. New York, United Nations, 1977.
87. United Nations Scientific Committee on the Effects of Atomic Radiation: *Ionizing Radiation: Sources and Biological Effects*, 1982 Report to the General Assembly, with annexes. New York, United Nations, 1982.
88. Upton AC: The Biological Effects of Low-level Ionizing Radiation, *Sci Am* 1982; 246:41–49.
89. Voelz GL: Eye-survey study of nuclear reactor workers. *J Occup Med* 1967; 9:286.
90. Voelz GL: New equipment and facilities for radiation emergencies. *Arch Environ Health* 1967; 15:295.
91. Voelz GL: Current approaches to the management of internally contaminated persons, in Hubner KF, Fry SA (eds): *The Medical Basis for Radiation Accident Preparedness*. New York, Elsevier North Holland, Inc, 1980, pp 311–325.
92. Wakabayashi T, Kato H, Ikeda T, et al: Studies of the mortality of a-bomb survivors, Report 7. Pt III Incidence of cancer in 1959–1978, based on the tumor registry, Nagasaki. *Radiat Res* 1983; 93:112–146.
93. Webster EW: On the question of cancer induction by small x-ray doses. *Am J Radiol* 1981; 137:647–666.

27

Ultrawave, Microwave, Laser, Infrared, and Low-Frequency Radiation

Arthur L. Knight, M.D.
Julian Olishifski, P.E.
Carl Zenz, M.D.

Ultraviolet Exposures

Carl Zenz, M.D.
Arthur L. Knight, M.D.

Occupations potentially associated with ultraviolet radiation exposures, modified here, include aircraft workers, barbers, brick masons, burners (metal), ranchers, construction workers, cutters (metal), drug makers, electricians, farmers, fishers, food irradiators, foundry workers, furnace workers, gardeners, gas mantle makers, glass blowers, glass furnace workers, hairdressers, herders, iron workers, lifeguards, lithographers, metal casting inspectors, miners (open pit), nurses, oil field workers, pipeline workers, plasma torch operators, railroad track workers, road workers, seafarers, glass skimmers, steel mill workers, stockmen, stokers, tobacco irradiators, vitamin D preparation makers, and, especially, welders.

The International Commission on Illumination[8] has separated the ultraviolet spectrum into three different wavelength bands, 315–400 nm, 280–315 nm and 200–280 nm, for convenience in classification. These ranges, with slight variations, are also referred to as near, midrange, and far ultraviolet, respectively. Wavelengths below 200 nm are of little biologic significance, since radiation in this region (vacuum ultraviolet) is absorbed in very short pathlengths in air, with associated production of ozone.[43] (Ozone is produced principally at wavelengths less than 200 nm) (Figs 27–1 and 27–2).

The main areas of concern involving ultraviolet radiation exposure are possible damage to the eyes and skin irritation. With high-intensity ultraviolet sources, such as a sun simulator, skin irritation can occur in seconds. Clinical photokeratitis has been characterized by a period of latency that tends to vary inversely with the severity of exposure. The latent period may be as short as 30 minutes or as long as 24 hours, but it usually is 6–12 hours. Conjunctivitis follows, often accompanied by erythema of the facial skin surrounding the eyelids. There is a sensation of a foreign body or "sand" in the eyes and varying degrees of photophobia, lacrimation, and blepharospasm. These acute symptoms usually last 6–24 hours, with nearly all discomfort disappearing within 48 hours. The individual is visually incapacitated for varying periods of time. It is important to note that the ocular system, unlike the skin, does not develop tolerance to repeated ultraviolet exposure.

A common eye problem noted among welders, called "arc flash" or "arc eye," actually is conjunctivitis, generally caused by prolonged exposures.[13] The technical as well as practical aspects as a result of welding processes have been well described by Pattee et al.,[35] who stated that exact limits are difficult to define, because they depend on (1) the distance of the worker from the arc, (2) the angle at which the rays of energy strike the worker's eye, (3) radiation intensity, and (4) the type of eye protection worn by the worker. Bates[3] estimated that a safe exposure would be 20 seconds at 7 ft and 17 minutes at 50 ft (Fig 27–3).

In addition to the effect on the eyes, ultraviolet radiation can produce a skin burn very similar to sunburn,[24] such burns occurring on unprotected parts of the body that are exposed to radiation during welding. It has been pointed out that this type of radiation can be reflected from metal surfaces, walls, and ceilings of welding

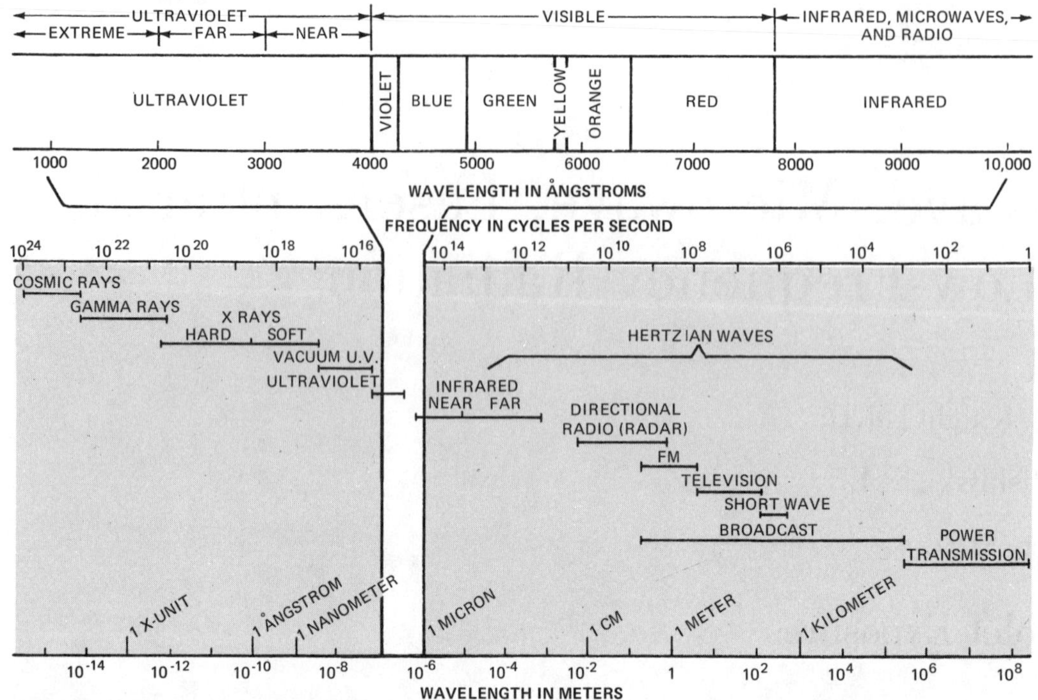

FIG 27–1.
The electromagnetic spectrum, encompassing the ionizing radiations and nonionizing radiations (expanded at left and right). A nanometer and a millimicron are identical units of length and each is equal to 10 Ångstroms.

1 centimeter	cm	10^{-2} meter
1 micrometer	μm (formerly micron)	10^{-6} meter
1 nanometer	nm (formerly millimicron)	10^{-9} meter
1 Ångstrom	Å	10^{-10} meter

(Courtesy of J. Olishifski, P.E.)

enclosures and from other surfaces. Of interest is that more ultraviolet radiation is produced when aluminum is welded than when stainless steel is welded. (Bright-rolled aluminum reflects almost 90% of the ultraviolet energy with a wavelength of 3,000 Å, whereas stainless steel reflects only about 30%.)

Kinsey et al.[22] studied the production of eye damage from arc-produced ultraviolet radiation and Rieke[40] considered it to account for 40% of all injuries in engineering shops. Grimm and Kusnetz[17] reported severe pain in workers several hours after a brief (ten-second) exposure to radiation from an arc torch that generated an intense flame 8–12 in long. Powell et al.[38] studied hazards from both laboratory and industrial plasma torches and found the output of these sufficient to cause eye and skin irritation on long exposure. Erythema on unprotected forehead and forearms developed within an hour after exposure began.

The photosensitizing ability of drugs and chemicals is mentioned in Chapter 10. The chronic effects of repeated ultraviolet exposure in individuals not adequately protected by pigmentation or other skin mechanisms are basophilic degeneration of the connective tissue, fragmentation of the elastic tissue (senile elastosis), and carcinogenesis.[11] Sunlight, but more specifically, wavelengths from about 290 to 325 nm,[5] is far more important than aging in producing skin changes.[23] Solar-damaged skin has markedly increased ground substance, increased elastic fibers associated with diminution of collagen,[34, 44] and epidermal atrophy with many abnormal cells in a disorderly pattern.[27]

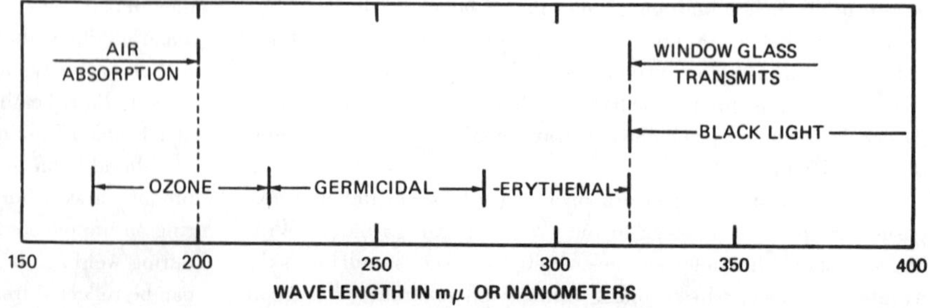

FIG 27–2.
The ultraviolet (UV) spectrum. One mμ or nanometer equals 10 Å.

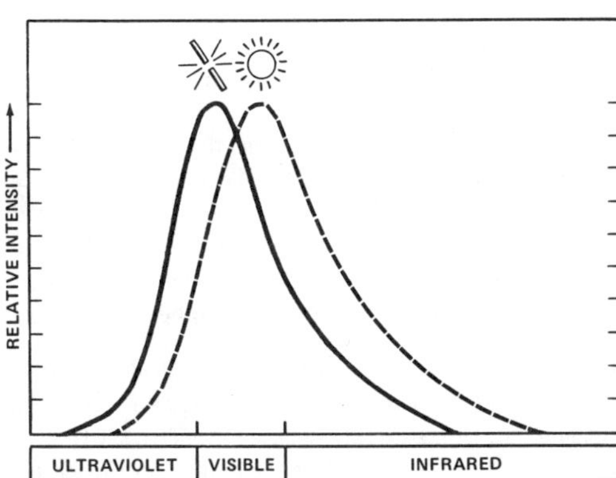

FIG 27–3.
Energy distribution in the radiation from a welding arc *(solid line)* and the sun *(dashed line).*

Epidemiologic, clinical, and tumor distribution studies have clearly implicated solar ultraviolet radiation as a factor in the etiology of human skin cancer. Brodkin et al.[7] present many early findings relating the incidence of basal-cell epithelioma to specific geographic regions, areas of the body, and complexion characteristics in individuals. The following arguments have been proposed to support the belief that sunlight is a causal factor in human skin cancer: (1) skin cancer occurs most frequently on exposed areas of the body,[46] (2) pigmented races have less skin cancer than do people with white skin,[10] (3) among white persons, those having outdoor work activities appear to have a greater prevalence of skin cancer than do those who work indoors,[4, 33] and (4) skin cancer is more common in light-skinned people living in areas where solar radiation is greater.[4, 28]

Considerable detail as to the histologic and cytologic changes induced by ultraviolet radiation may be found in the National Institute for Safety and Health (NIOSH) criteria document for occupational exposure to ultraviolet radiation.[47] This document describes a variety of environmental sources producing ultraviolet energy throughout the ultraviolet spectrum.

Low-pressure mercury vapor lamps emit several narrow bands; the lower the pressure of mercury vapor the fewer lines emitted. Much of this energy is of 253.7 nm wavelength, which is near the peak of germicidal effectiveness of 265 nm; hence, its usefulness in control of microorganisms in operating rooms,[18, 19] in control of airborne infection,[29, 41] in control of bacteria in meat processing,[31] in the prevention of product contamination in pharmaceutical houses and biologic laboratories,[36] in irradiation of air conditioning ducts,[32] and in making water potable.[30]

High-pressure mercury vapor lamps are used in photochemical reactions, in mineral identification, to produce fluorescence, and for diagnosis of dermal and scalp disorders and porphyria. Quartz-mercury arcs emit radiation over much of the ultraviolet spectrum and can cause erythema and conjunctivitis from radiation over the range of 200–320 nm.

Fluorescent-type ultraviolet lamps also emit germicidal radiation similar to low-pressure mercury vapor lamps. Although there is little evidence that they are significant sources of ultraviolet-induced injury, it is believed that they may cause skin and eye effects, since a small part of their output is below 320 nm.[2, 42] Fluorescent lamps used for general lighting purposes emit a negligible amount of energy below 320 nm. Although rare, skin photosensitization from these lamps has been reported.[6, 21]

High-pressure xenon arcs emit a spectrum like that of sunlight in a continuous spectrum. Carbon arcs emit a continuous spectrum from the incandescent electrodes on which a broad-band spectrum from the luminous gases is superimposed.

Incandescent sources emit very little ultraviolet energy except at temperatures above 2300° C.[25] Open oil and gas flames normally are less than 2,000° C. Oxyhydrogen and oxyacetylene flames are much hotter, so solids heated by these two flames may radiate ultraviolet.

The plasma torch can produce temperatures over 6,000° C, the temperature at the surface of the sun, and intense ultraviolet radiation can result. Exposure to radiation from plasma torches can result in sunburn and keratoconjunctivitis if skin and eyes are not protected.[38]

There are several important indirect effects of ultraviolet radiation produced in industry. It has been well known that ozone can be produced in substantial quantities near welding operations by the reaction of the atmospheric oxygen with the ultraviolet energy produced from the welding process. Ozone is known to be a powerful oxidizing agent, with a threshold limit value of 0.1 ppm (0.2 mg/cu m, considered highly toxic), irritating to the eyes and upper respiratory system, which, on prolonged exposure, can produce shortness of breath, coughing, pulmonary edema, and many other symptoms.

Lunau[26] reported that welders who were exposed to ozone concentrations of 9 ppm complained of respiratory or breathing difficulties as well as fatigue for as long as nine months after exposure. Pattee et al.[35] also stated that some ozone may react with the fume particulates. Of particular interest is the variation of ozone with the composition of various types of aluminum; the variation in ozone concentration may be attributable to the alloy content of the aluminum base metal or it may be attributable to differences in the surface characteristics of these alloys.

In studies conducted by another investigator,[15] it was noted that (1) more ozone was produced during the welding of aluminum than during the welding of steel, and (2) more ozone was formed when argon was used for shielding than when carbon dioxide was used.

Continuing with discussion of special work hazards in arc welding, Pattee and co-workers described limited investigations that had been conducted to collect and analyze the gases that are produced by the decomposition of chlorinated hydrocarbons used to clean and degrease metal parts. Although the chlorinated hydrocarbons are decomposed by both heat and ultraviolet radiation, most investigations have been concerned with the effects of ultraviolet radiation on these substances. The major decomposition products of such reactions are phosgene and dichloroacetyl chloride. These gases are classified as pulmonary irritants. Phosgene will produce dermatitis on contact with the skin. The inhalation of high concentrations of this gas will produce pulmonary edema, and death may result from respiratory or cardiac arrest. (The established threshold limit value for phosgene is 0.05 ppm [1974].)[39] The toxicity of dichloroacetyl chloride is not well known and a threshold limit value has not been established for it.

In early studies, Ferry and Ginther[14] attempted to relate the amount of phosgene in the atmosphere to the presence of various concentrations of trichloroethylene. High phosgene levels, much above 0.1 ppm, were measured. More phosgene was produced when argon instead of helium was used for shielding during gas tungsten-arc welding.

Dahlberg[9] also investigated the decomposition products of trichloroethylene as a function of ultraviolet radiation and made the following observations: (1) the main decomposition product was dichloroacetyl chloride and it formed three times as fast as phosgene, (2) the decomposition rate decreased rapidly as the trichloroethylene level decreased and the distance from the arc increased, (3) the decomposition rate appeared to increase when the gas metal-arc process instead of the gas tungsten-arc process was used for welding. With gas metal-arc welding in an area where the trichloroethylene concentration was 20 ppm, the dichloroacetyl and phosgene concentrations increased from 0 to 10 and 3 ppm, respectively, at a distance of 0.3 m from the arc.

The results of these investigations indicate that care must be exercised in the welding of metal parts that have been degreased in trichloroethylene and other chlorinated hydrocarbon cleaning agents. Also, welding areas should not be located near metal-cleaning facilities where such solvents are used, nor should they be located where fumes from cleaning facilities can be carried by natural or artificial convection currents. The odor of dichloroacetyl chloride is strong and disagreeable; it serves as an effective warning against phosgene.

The time of permissible exposure over an eight-hour period is determined by means of a formula that incorporates the relative biologic effects of ultraviolet radiation. It is this portion of the spectrum that poses the greatest threat of injury to skin and eyes. For that portion of the electromagnetic spectrum from 315 to 400 nm, the maximal limit of 1 mW (milliwatt) of ultraviolet radiation per square centimeter is recommended for exposures exceeding 1,000 seconds. For 1,000 seconds or less, the total radiant energy would be limited to 1,000 milliwatt-seconds (1 joule) per square centimeter. Technical problems in conducting accurate measurement of the broad-band ultraviolet energy are noted in the NIOSH document, and three approaches for determining compliance with the proposed standard are listed. Recommendations for protective clothing, medical examinations, work practices, labeling and warning considerations, and record keeping are included.[47]

REFERENCES

1. Andrews HL: *Radiation Biophysics*, ed 2. Englewood Cliffs, NJ, Prentice-Hall, Inc, 1974, pp 254–264.
2. Barnes R: An unusual hazard in forgery detection. *Med J Aust* 1970; 1:540.
3. Bates CC: The effects on the human eye of the radiant energy given off by various welding processes. *Sheet Metal Industries* 1952; 29:349.
4. Belisario JC: Effects of sunlight on the incidence of carcinomas and malignant melanoblastomas in the tropical and subtropical areas of Australia. *Dermatol Trop* 1962; 1:127.
5. Blum HF: *Carcinogenesis by Ultraviolet Light*. Princeton, NJ, Princeton University Press, 1959.
6. Bresler RR: Cutaneous burns due to fluorescent light. *JAMA* 1949; 140:1334.
7. Brodkin RH, Kopf AW, Andrade R: Basal-cell epithelioma and elastosis: A comparison of distribution, in Urbach F (ed): *The Biologic Effects of Ultraviolet Radiation with Emphasis on the Skin*. New York, Pergamon Press, 1969.
8. Commission Internationale de L'Eclairage (International Commission on Illumination): *International Lighting Vocabulary* ed 3. Paris, CIE Publications, 1970.
9. Dahlberg JA: *Formation of Dichloroacetyl Chloride & Phosgene in Welding Shops with Trichloroethylene Contaminated Atmosphere*, document VIII:296. Miami, International Institute of Welding, 1967.
10. Daniels F Jr: Man and radiant energy: Solar radiation, in Dill DB (ed): *Handbook of Physiology—IV, Adaptation to the Environment*. Washington, DC, American Physiological Society, 1964.
11. Daniels F Jr: Ultraviolet carcinogenesis in man, in Urbach F (ed): *Conference on Biology of Cutaneous Cancer*, Monograph 10. Bethesda, Md, National Cancer Institute, 1963.
12. Drinker P: The measurement and prevention of eye flash. *Welding J* 1944; 23:505.
13. Emmett EA, Buncher C, Suskind RB, et al: Skin and eye diseases among arc welders and those exposed to welding operations. *J Occup Med* 1981; 23:85.
14. Ferry JJ, Ginther GB: Gas produced by inert-gas welding. *Welding J* 1953; 32:396.
15. Frant R: Formation of ozone in gas-shielded welding. *Ann Occup Hyg* 1963; 6:113.
16. Gafafer WM: *Occupational Diseases—A Guide to Their Recognition*, Publ 1097, US Dept HEW, USPHS, 1966.
17. Grimm RC, Kusnetz HL: The plasma torch—industrial hygiene aspects. *Arch Environ Health* 1962; 4:295.
18. Hart D: Bactericidal ultraviolet radiation in the operating room—twenty-nine year study for control of infections. *JAMA* 1960; 172:1019.
19. Hart D, Nicks J: Ultraviolet radiation in the operating room—Intensities used and bactericidal effects. *Arch Surg* 1961; 82:449.
20. Industrial Medical Association: *Ultraviolet Radiation*. Chicago, IMA, Feb 15, 1973.
21. James APR: Sensitivity of the skin to fluorescent light. *Arch Dermatol* 1941; 44:256.
22. Kinsey VE, Cogan DG, Drinker P: Measuring eye flash from arc welding. *JAMA* 1943; 123:403.
23. Kligman AM: Early destructive effect of sunlight on human skin. *JAMA* 1969; 210:2377.
24. Koller LR: *Ultraviolet Radiation*. New York, John Wiley & Sons, 1952.
25. Leach WM: *Biological Aspects of Ultraviolet Radiation, a Review of Hazards*. BRH/ODE 70-7. USPHS, Bureau of Radiological Health, 1970.
26. Lunau FW: Ozone in arc welding. *Ann Occup Hyg* 1967; 10:175.
27. Lund HZ, Sommersville RL: Basophilic degeneration of the cutis—Data substantiating its relation to prolonged solar exposure. *Am J Clin Pathol* 1957; 27:183.
28. MacDonald EJ: The epidemiology of skin cancer. *J Invest Dermatol* 1959; 32:379.
29. McLean RL: The effect of ultraviolet radiation upon the transmission of epidemic influenza in long-term hospital patients. *Am Rev Respir Dis* 1961; 83:36.
30. Nagy R: Application and measurement of ultraviolet radiation. *Ind Hyg J* 1964; 25:274.
31. Nagy R: *Application of Ozone from Sterilamp in Control of Mold, Bacteria, and Odors*. Advances in Chemistry Series, No 21, American Chemical Society, 1959.
32. Nagy R, Mouromseff G, Rixton FH: Disinfecting air with sterilizing lamps. *Heating, Piping, Air Cond* 1954; 26:82.

33. Nicolau SG, Balus L: Chronic actinic cheilitis and cancer of the lower lip. *Br J Dermatol* 1964; 76:278.
34. Papa CM, Kligman AM: The effect of topical steroids on the aged human axilla, in Montagna W (ed): *Advances in Biology of Skin*. New York, Pergamon Press, 1965.
35. Pattee HE, et al: Arc radiation and heat. *Welding J*, May 1973; pp 297–308.
36. Phillips GB, Hanel E Jr: *Use of Ultraviolet Radiation in Microbiological Laboratories*. Library of Congress, Photoduplication Services, Publication Board Project, PB147 043, 1960.
37. Pitts DG, Gibbons WD: *The Human, Primate, and Rabbit Ultraviolet Action Spectra*. University of Houston College of Optometry, funded under NASA contract No NA39-10836, March 31, 1972.
38. Powell CH, Goldman L, Key MM: Investigative studies of plasma torch hazards. *Am Ind Hyg Assoc J* 1968; 29:381.
39. Report of the ACGIH Committee on Threshold Limits for the Air of Workplaces. Annual Meeting, American Conference of Governmental Industrial Hygienists, Miami, May 13, 1974.
40. Rieke FE: "Arc flash" conjunctivitis: Actinic conjunctivitis from electric welding arc. *JAMA* 1943; 122:734.
41. Riley RL, O'Grady F: *Airborne Infection—Transmission and Control*. New York, Macmillan Publishing Co, 1961.
42. Schall EL, et al: Hazards to go-go dancers from exposure to "black" light from fluorescent bulbs. *Am Ind Hyg Assoc J* 1969; 30:413.
43. Sliney DH: The merits of an envelope action spectrum for ultraviolet radiation exposure criteria. Presented at the 1972 AIHA Conference, San Francisco, May 18, 1972.
44. Smith JG, Lansing AI Jr: Distribution of solar elastosis (senile elastosis) in the skin. *J Gerontol* 1959; 14:496.
45. *The Welding Environment (A Research Report on Fumes and Gases Generated during Welding Operations)*. Miami, American Welding Society, 1974.
46. Urbach F: Geographic Pathology of Skin Cancer, in Urbach F (ed): *The Biologic Effects of Ultraviolet Radiation with Emphasis on the Skin*. New York, Pergamon Press, 1969.
47. US Dept of Health, Education, and Welfare: *A Recommended Standard for Occupational Exposure to Ultraviolet Radiation*, HSM Publ 73-11009. Rockville, Md, NIOSH, 1977.

Microwaves

Arthur L. Knight, M.D.

Carl Zenz, M.D.

During the past decade, new processes utilizing microwave systems have been developed and have become so economical that installations are found in home kitchens as microwave ovens. However, far greater use is found in industrial locations. Most industrial microwave equipment operates between 915 MHz and 2,450 MHz. Applications employing microwave energy are: drying purposes, including match heads, veneers, paper, plastic ceiling and pharmaceutical drying, and in the food industries for finish drying of potato chips, thawing frozen foods, and precooking chicken parts.

Microwave generators and radar are widely used in military service, navigation, tracking, communications, and other applications, such as medical therapy.

In referring to the electromagnetic spectrum, some authors refer to the frequency as megahertz and others refer to the wavelength in centimeters or meters. To convert these to one another, use the formula $\lambda f = c$, where λ = wavelength (meters), f = the frequency (cycles/second), and $c = 2.998 \times 10^8$ meters per second.

The electromagnetic spectrum runs from about 10^7 cm to 10^{-12} cm. The visible portion is a narrow band between 10^{-4} and 10^{-5} cm. Between 10^2 and 10^{-2} cm is a portion referred to as the microwave section (Fig 27–4), the large wave portion of which contains the ultrahigh-frequency radio waves; the median portion has radar, and in the small wave section are the microwaves that blend into the infrared section of the electromagnetic spectrum. The smaller microwaves that are near the infrared portion of the spectrum, such as the 10^{-1}-cm length, produce heat with little penetration and thus cause the tissue surface to be heated; on the eye, this means that the cornea is affected. At a wavelength of 10 cm, or at 3,000 MHz, the microwave penetration produces heat within the tissue; in the eye, the lens will be damaged, as may the iris. At 2 cm (10^2), the penetration and heat to the tissue are greatest, and damage can result to the internal organs.

The transmitted electromagnetic energy is absorbed by animal tissues and results in heat production. This heat production must be dissipated from the body to prevent a temperature rise. This is the basis for the use of microwave therapy. With increasingly higher power levels as well as potential leaks, one must be concerned with the potential health hazard to both the operating personnel and the general public.

It is known that, for man, frequencies above 15 MHz to 10^3 cm are in the biologically effective range. In this frequency, man may absorb anywhere from 20% to 100% of the incident radiofrequency (RF) energy without any proportional temperature rise.[3] As in bacterially induced fever, temperature rise of a limited amount will have no long-term sequelae. However, certain organs, such as the testes, are much more sensitive to a few degrees rise in temperature than is the body as a whole. The lens of the eye, having poor blood supply, has inadequate heat dissipation ability. A localized temperature rise can lead to serious protein denaturation as well as altering certain enzymes and other substances in the eye. More specific thermal effects are described by Westin.[10]

One should remember that the danger of absorption of certain microwave energy is that it causes internal heating with no forewarning of heating of the skin.

Investigations concerning other biologic effects of microwaves are being conducted, especially knowledge of whole-body cumulative effects from subthreshold exposures and effects from low-intensity irradiation.

In a recent commentary, Appleton[4] reviewed and discussed "microwave cataracts." He stated that experimental evidence is based largely on studies with rabbits and dogs, and it appears that the dose of microwaves that produces cataracts is so high that (except for the head) the animal's body must be shielded; otherwise, superficial burns and hyperthermic death would occur. (Also, mi-

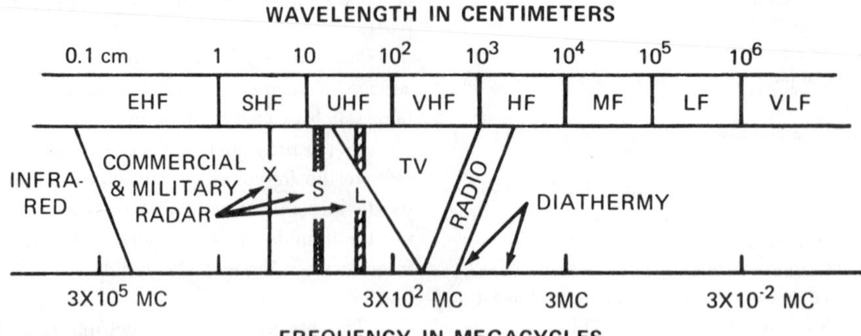

FIG 27–4.
Microwave spectrum.

crowave radiation at cataractogenic levels cannot be tolerated by these animals unless they have been previously anesthetized.) He noted that the cataractogenic dose of microwaves in rabbits is some 30 times as high as the maximal exposure allowed by our most permissive safety standards, and that there is no experimental evidence to support the hypothesis that subthreshold exposures have late cumulative effects.

Appleton reported results of a survey of workers who were exposed to microwaves as part of their occupation conducted by a team that included two ophthalmologists. Detailed examinations of the lenses of those individuals who had the greatest likelihood of exposure were carried out. Similar examinations were performed on personnel with minimal exposure, on the same military bases. Groups were matched as to age and sex. All subjects were examined in such a fashion that at the time of examination, no examiner was aware of which group the examinee represented.

Results of this survey (conducted during a five-year period) showed that biomicroscopically detectable physical signs in the lens, which are considered to be the components or precursors of cataract, occur equally in both groups, reasonably concluding that "*no lens damage was caused by occupational exposure to microwave energy*."

Based on the available evidence, both clinical and experimental, the following conclusions appear reasonable, according to Appleton: (1) lens damage probably has not occurred in humans from cumulative exposure to low levels of microwave energy; and (2) lens damage probably could not occur in a human from acute exposure to microwave energy without associated severe facial burns.

With present technology capable of installing very-high-powered radar aboard aircraft and spacecraft, it is becoming increasingly important to investigate the biologic hazard due to microwave radiation and to set meaningful and realistic limits. It is known that this hazard is an extremely complex situation, and the variables associated both with the human absorber (including thermal and nonthermal hazard, depth of penetration, standing wave formation, and dielectric coefficient of various tissues) and with the generator (pulsed versus continuous wave generation, and antenna rotation, for example) can be far-reaching. The need for further investigations of the problems is known, and until additional data are forthcoming, the present exposure criterion of 10 mW/sq cm must be adhered to.

REFERENCES

1. Andrews HL: *Radiation Biophysics* ed 2. Englewood Cliffs, NJ, Prentice-Hall, 1974, pp 270–281.
2. Anne A, et al: Relative microwave absorption cross sections of biological significance, in *Proceedings of the 4th Tri-Service Conference*, New York, 1960.
3. Anne A: *Scattering and Absorption of Microwaves by Dissipative Dielectric Objects: The Biological Significance and Hazards to Man*, Washington, DC, ONR TR #36, 1963.
4. Appleton B: Microwave cataracts. *JAMA* 1974; 229:407.
5. Cleary SF (ed): *Biological Effects and Health Implications of Microwave Radiation*, Proceedings of Symposium, Richmond, Va, Sept, 1969. Rockville, Md, US Dept of Health, Education, and Welfare, 1969.
6. Eure JA, Nicolls JW, Elder RL: Radiation exposure from industrial microwave applications. *Am J Public Health* 1972; 62:1573.
7. Odland LT: Observations on microwave hazards to USAF personnel. *J Occup Med* 1972; 14:544.
8. Salati OM, Anne A, Schwan HP: Radiofrequency hazards. *Elect Industries* Nov, 1962.
9. Suroviec HJ: Microwave oven radiation hazards in food-vending establishments. *Arch Environ Health* 1967; 14:469.
10. Westin JB: Microwave radiation and human tolerance: A review. *J Occup Med* 1968; 10:134.

Lasers

Arthur L. Knight, M.D.

Carl Zenz, M.D.

There has been an impressive growth of laser-generating equipment (light amplification by stimulated emission of radiation). There are at least 150 laser systems that have been reported and more than a dozen are available commercially.

Rockwell[12] has described how a laser operates. Put briefly, one can say that excitation energy is vigorously supplied to the active media to produce the specific condition called a population inversion. In this condition, one will find more atoms of the laser media in a specific excited-state energy level than are found in some lower level. This condition is contrary to the normal population of states in thermal equilibrium. One manner for an atom in an excited state to release excess energy is by the spontaneous emission of light in discrete units called photons. Due to population inversion, the energy release is accomplished by stimulated emission, which is unique to a laser device. In this case, a photon released by one excited atom will cause (stimulate) another excited atom it may encounter in its path also to release a photon of excess energy. The result of this interaction is the combination of two photons with identical coherence properties (phase relationship) so that they add completely together to produce a beam of greater intensity. As the beam progresses through the excited laser media, its amplitude will be rapidly increased, whereas its coherence properties remain unaltered. Frequently, mirrors within the laser system reflect the beam back and forth, increasing its intensity with each pass, until allowed to escape through a partially reflecting mirror or shutter. The escaping portion is the active emission from the laser. The process will continue for as long as sufficient pump energy is supplied to the laser media (Fig 27–5).

Rockwell also described "the pulsed laser" device, which creates a high-energy pulse lasting from a few hundred to several thousand microseconds. A high level of energy can be transmitted in the coherent beam produced by these devices. Terrill[15] stated that "a laser operating at 100 joules emits enough energy to burn a 100-W bulb for one second. But, by compressing the energy into one tenth of a millionth of a second, the laser can radiate pulses of 1,000,000,000 W. (In contrast, the sun radiates only 7,000 W/sq cm of surface.)" Obviously, this new device can be applied to many areas of use requiring high-energy densities.

Powell and Brown[9] estimated that 10,000–20,000 employees work in laser areas and may be potentially exposed to this energy. The largest class of workers potentially exposed to laser radiation are in the construction industries, comprising more than 40% of the workers in laser applications, which provide an exceedingly accurate technique to provide line and grade levels in sewer work, in pipe construction projects, such as erecting dams, tunneling, and even dredging, and also to delineate horizontal lines for installation of floors and use for mapping in distance measurements.

Because of the intense energy generated, the laser beam has been used to cut into extremely hard metals in seconds, including tungsten, and holes are drilled in diamonds that, in the past, took several days. Other laser applications are for medical treatment (ophthalmology), in dermatology to treat or decrease certain lesions, and in multiple simultaneous transmissions in communications.

Severe damage to the eye has been reported from accidental exposures to laser radiation. It is most important that workers using laser equipment be properly instructed in its safe use and cautioned never to look directly into a laser beam without proper eye protection. It should be remembered that smooth and reflective surfaces can redirect a laser beam and cause eye damage. Such things as glass-framed pictures and polished door handles should be eliminated around laser operations. A laser beam can damage either the cornea or the retina, depending on the wavelength of the laser.

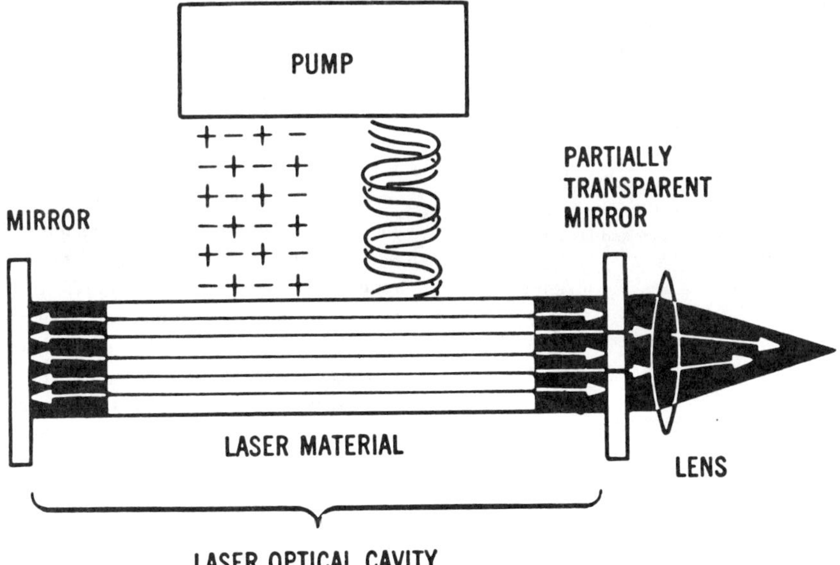

FIG 27–5.
Ordinary incandescent sources emit their light in all directions, at different frequencies, and at various amplitudes. The eye interprets light from these different wavelength mixtures as white or yellow-white. Laser light, on the other hand, is coherent, monochromatic, and highly collimated (concentration of light in a narrow beam for a long distance and in the same plane of polarization). The resulting light beams have extremely high intensity. (Courtesy of J. Olishifski, P.E.)

Protective eyewear cannot be relied on as the primary protective barrier, and adequate control measures, including enclosures, and remote viewing equipment are necessary. The safety eyewear protector for one type of laser likely will be useless for another laser with a diferent emission wavelength, since each type of laser is characterized by a single wavelength or closely related wavelengths, and the reflective plate in the protective eyewear is made to reflect only in that wavelength. The American National Standards Institute spells out the safety rules for lasers operating at essentially any wavelength or pulse duration, defining control measures for each of five classifications, and provides technical information on measurements, calculations and biologic effects. Included are hazard evaluation classification, criteria for exposure of the eye and skin, as well as the hazards of explosion, optical radiation, electrical hazards, medical surveillance and the administration of safety programs.[1] (The standard is designated as ANSI Z136.1-1973.)

REFERENCES

1. American National Standards Institute: ANSI Z136.1-1973.
2. Andrews HL: *Radiation Biophysics* ed 2. Englewood Cliffs, NJ: Prentice-Hall, 1974, pp 265–267.
3. Brownell AS, Parr WH, Hysell DK: Skin and carbon dioxide laser radiation. *Arch Environ Health* 1969; 18:437.
4. Goldman L: *Applications of the Laser*. Cleveland, CRC Press, 1973.
5. Goldman L, Rockwell RJ: *Lasers in Medicine*. New York, Gordon and Breach Science Publishers, 1971.
6. Griess GA, Blankenstein MF: Multiple-pulse laser retinal damage thresholds. *Am Ind Hyg Assoc J* 1981; 42:287–292.
7. Lund DJ, Beatrice ES: Ocular hazard of short pulse argon laser. *Radiat Health Phys* 1979; 36:7–11.
8. Marshall MJ: Hazard analysis on gaussian shaped laser beams. *US Army Environmental Hygiene Agency* 1980; 41:547–551.
9. Powell CH, Brown MC: Laser problems as related to the nation's health. *Arch Environ Health* 1969; 18:391.
10. Powell CH, Goldman L: Recommendations of the Laser Safety Conference. *Arch Environ Health* 1969; 18:448.
11. Powell CH, Goldman L: Review of Proceedings of the British Conference on Laser Safety. *Arch Environ Health* 1968; 17:286.
12. Rockwell RJ: Characteristics of laser radiation and laser instrumentation. *Arch Environ Health* 1969; 18:394.
13. Second International Laser Safety Conference, March, 1969. *Arch Environ Health* 1970; 20:145.
14. Sliney DH, Vorpahl KW, Winburn DC: Environmental health hazards from high powered infrared and laser devices. *Arch Environ Health* 1975; 30:174.
15. Terrill JG Jr: Microwaves, lasers, and x-rays—Adverse reactions due to occupational exposures. *Arch Environ Health* 1969; 19:265.
16. Wilkinson TK: Health aspects of laser use. *Arch Environ Health* 1969; 18:443.

Infrared Radiation*

Julian Olishifski, P.E.

Carl Zenz, M.D.

It is generally considered that the infrared region of the electromagnetic spectrum extends from the visible red light region (0.75 μ) to the 3000-μ wavelength of microwaves (Fig 27–6). Exposures to infrared radiation can occur from any surface that is at a higher temperature than the receiver.

Industrial applications include: (1) drying and baking of paints, varnishes, enamels, adhesives, printer's ink, and other protective coatings; (2) heating of metal parts for shrink-fit assembly, forming, thermal aging, brazing, radiation testing, and conditioning of surfaces for application of adhesives and welding; (3) dehydrating of textiles, paper, leather, meat, vegetables, pottery ware, and sand molds; and (4) spot and localized heating for any desired objective.

Infrared radiation may be used for any heating application where the principal product surfaces can be arranged for exposure to the heat sources. Transfer of energy or heat occurs whenever radiant energy emitted by one body is absorbed by another. The electromagnetic spectrum wavelengths longer than those of visible energy (0.75 μ) and shorter than those of radar waves are utilized for radiant heating. The best energy absorption of white, pastel-colored, and translucent products is obtained by using wavelength emissions longer than 2.5 μ. The majority of dark-pigmented and oxide-coated materials will readily absorb wavelength emissions from 0.75 μ to 9.0 μ.

Water vapor and visible aerosols, such as steam, readily absorb the longer infrared wavelengths.

Infrared radiation is perceptible as a sensation of warmth on the skin. The increase in tissue temperature on exposure to infrared radiation depends on the wavelength, the total amount of energy delivered to the tissue, and the length of exposure. Infrared radiation in the far wavelength region of 5–3000 μ is completely absorbed in the surface layers of the skin. Exposure to infrared radiation in the region between 0.75 μ and 1.5 μ can cause acute skin burn and increased persistent skin pigmentation.

This short wavelength region of the infrared is capable of causing injuries to the cornea, iris, retina, and lens of the eye. Excessive exposure of the eyes to luminous radiation, mainly visible and infrared radiation, from furnaces and similar hot bodies has been said for many years to produce "glass blower's cataract" or "heat cataract." This condition is an opacity of the rear surface of the lens and eye.

SAFE INFRARED EXPOSURE LEVELS

The available data indicate that acute ocular damage from the incandescent hot bodies found in industry can occur with energy

*Modified from *Fundamentals of Industrial Hygiene*, ed 2. J Olishifski (ed). Chicago, National Safety Council, 1979.

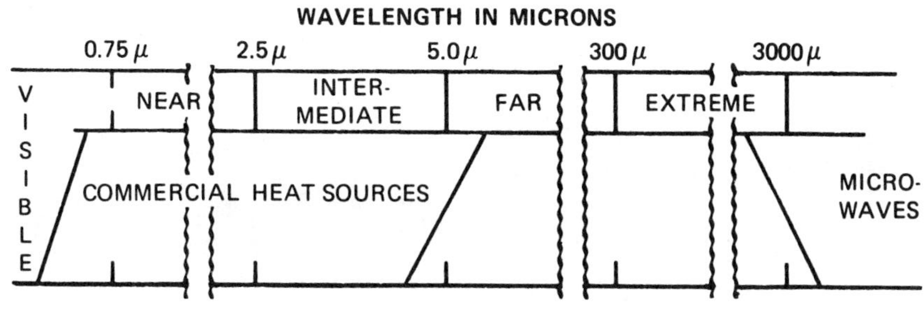

FIG 27–6.
Infrared spectrum.

densities between 4 and 8 Wsec/sq cm (1–2 cal/sq cm) incident on the cornea. The ocular tissues involved would depend on the wavelengths that are absorbed. As these relate to threshold phenomena, it would appear that a maximum permissible dose of 0.4–0.8 Wsec/sq cm (0.1–0.2 cal/sq cm) could limit the occurrence of these acute effects. A further reduction by a factor of 10 should prevent the more chronic effects of the intraocular tissues.

REFERENCES

1. Moss CE, Murray WE: Optical radiation levels produced by single-phase direct arc furnaces. *Am Ind Hyg Assoc J* 1981; 4:293.
2. Pollak VA, Romanchuk KG: The risk of retina damage from high intensity light sources. *Am Ind Hyg Assoc J* 1980; 4:322.
3. Sliney D, Wolbarshe M: *Safety with Lasers and Other Optical Sources*. New York, Plenum Publishing Corp, 1980.
4. US Dept of Health, Education and Welfare: *Research Report, Determination of Ocular Threshold Levels for Infrared Radiation Cataractogenesis*. DHHS Publ 80-121. Rockville, Md, NIOSH, 1980.
5. Suess MJ: *Nonionizing Radiation and Health*. World Health Forum, Vol 6, 1985.

28

Practical Ergonomics and Work With Video Display Terminals

O. Bruce Dickerson, M.D., M.P.H.

Walter E. Baker, Ph.D.

Ergonomics crosses the boundaries of several scientific and professional disciplines and utilizes data, findings, and principles from all of them. Zenz[46] depicts the scientific disciplines involved in ergonomics under the three general headings: (1) engineering and physical sciences; (2) biological sciences; and (3) behavioral sciences.

We[5, 13] and others[45] have emphasized that the application of good ergonomic design principles can result in improvements in worker health and safety, productivity, and work quality and satisfaction. Many studies[7, 11, 42] confirm that such results have indeed been realized.

The terms ergonomics and human factors engineering are often used interchangeably; but some authors believe that initially ergonomics was more physiology and health and comfort oriented, while human factors engineering was more oriented to the physical sciences. Chapanis[9] suggests a geographic bias with American professional societies in this field leaning toward the engineering approach while the European societies argue for a physiology-based approach.

However, not only is this difference fading, but with the adoption of a systems point of view, the scope of ergonomics has passed beyond the concern of the individual worker and his or her machine or workplace to include consideration of the total work environment. Chapanis[8] says, "What we do as ergonomists may have far reaching effects—on society, its productivity, and its economy." He urges us to consider several critical guidelines in dealing with this broadened scope.

Ergonomics is the linking together of various disciplines and resources such that we are able to favorably influence task-individual interfaces. Practical ergonomics shows how and what some of those limits are in our everyday practices and actions.

MODELS

To accomplish this, we believe it is important to understand the relationship between the individual, the tool, the physical environment or work station design, and the task, including its content and the organizational environment in which it is performed. Let us first understand what we mean by these terms.

We all use tools in our work: hand tools, power tools, machinist's tools, chemicals, and, of course, computer terminals. We use those tools at a work station, and the work station exists in both physical and organizational environments.

A work station might include a work bench and parts bins, an assembly fixture, or a control panel, equipment, table, desk, and chair. And, surrounding the work station, there are the physical environmental factors, which include lighting, ventilation, and other comfort requirements. The tool at a work station is used to perform the task. The task might be parts production or assembly, chemical process or control of a process, information processing, or data entry. Finally, using the tool at the work station to perform the task is the user or the operator. There are undeniable interactions and interrelationships among these three areas. What factors should be considered in each of these to help ensure the health, safety and productivity of the worker?

In the case of hand and power tools, there are many ergonomic and biomechanic aspects that must be considered: grip, weight, body and arm position, and movement.

In the case of instruments, control panels and terminals, many physical characteristics are necessary to ensure that visual information is presented in a way that avoids visual discomfort. We also need to consider the characteristics that ensure appropriate tactile feel and feedback, but first we must recognize and minimize potential hazards.

At the work station, too, there are biomechanic requirements to be satisfied, such as: position of parts, movements required, and the resulting physiologic effects.

Anthropometric requirements must also be considered:

Does the chair fit and satisfy the requirements of the user?

Are the work surfaces located in such a way that the body is in a comfortable, unstrained position?

Then, there are environmental conditions of the workplace such as lighting, noise, space, climate, and the control of hygiene factors of the environment—are all elements in control so that there is no hazard?

In any task, both job content and job context are important.[38] With regard to job content, several factors appear important in providing satisfaction and motivation.[22] For example, the variety of skills required, the identity of the task and its significance, the autonomy given to the operator, feedback, challenge, and opportunity are all factors that help make the job itself challenging and meaningful.

Job context includes management culture and tradition, management style and climate, support systems, opportunity for advancement, training, and worker involvement. The combination of job content and context factors relates to psychologic or psychosocial health.

Finally, there are the individual characteristics of the user that should be considered, such as experience, training level, physical characteristics, and personal needs.

Figure 28–1 shows a model of these factors. A satisfied and motivated worker is likely to be a healthy, safe, and productive worker. For this reason, the application of ergonomic principles to the workplace must be of interest to all of management and of particular interest to health and safety professionals.

Other models have been proposed and the following is from Sauter et al.[39] The variables involved and patterns of involvement or influence are shown in Figure 28–2, which depicts a conceptual framework for understanding on-the-job stress at a very basic level. Solid paths in the model denote potential primary effects of worker attributes and of workplace and job design characteristics. Broken paths reflect potential interactive effects. For example, physical

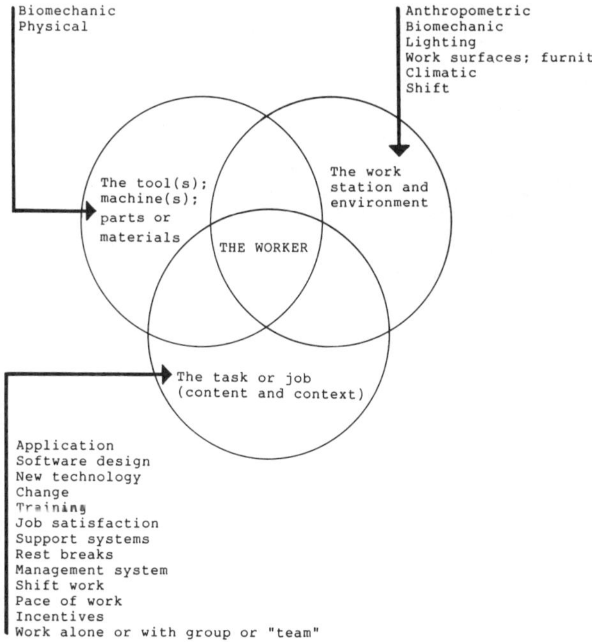

FIG 28–1.
Model of work: job factors involved.

environmental limitations, such as poorly designed chairs or work benches or visual display problems, may be of only modest consequence for workers with moderate production demands or for professionals or workers able to exercise control over the job regimen, but may be far more stressful for workers with stringent performance demands or lacking relief opportunities. The model also suggests causal relationships among the stress outcome parameters themselves. For example, visual or musculoskeletal discomfort may lead to anxiety over deteriorating health, and both may influence satisfaction with the job beyond effects more directly attributable to working conditions per se.

CUMULATIVE TRAUMA DISORDERS (CTD)

Musculoskeletal disorders rank first in frequency among alleged work-related injuries and diseases.[29] Cumulative trauma disorders resulting from repetitive movements and the cumulative work stress imposed by those movements occur far more frequently than do injuries from a single, sudden, infrequent overexertion. The cumulative effect of adverse muscle-loading resulting from improper position and inadequate body support also affects many workers. These conditions not only afflict manual workers but also workers in sedentary office occupations.

However, recognizing the cause does not always result in action. For instance, Figure 28–3 presents some important ergonomic components of an agriculture worker's activities in using the "short-handle hoe." In a study performed for the state of California, it was concluded that use of the short-handle hoe could result in permanent low-back disability. Subsequently, the California Supreme Court reached a decision eliminating its use by agriculture workers. The evidence pointing to permanent low back impairment with this type of work had existed for some time, but there were other factors that finally precipitated the change in work design.

A job analysis system has been described[3] that, by documenting several of the risk factors involved in CTD, enables tasks to be redesigned.

Hand Tools

The use of hand tools is an area that is receiving considerable attention recently. Tichauer and Gage[43] have described ergonomic principles basic to hand tool design. These authors state that the primary ergonomic consideration in designing hand tools is optimization of forces, that a tool should be designed to extend and reinforce the range, strength, and effectiveness of a limb, or limbs, performing a given task. To accomplish this function, designers in the past frequently followed only the rule to maximize the ratio of tool force output to hand force input. This obviously leaves much to be desired, since it does not take into consideration effective sensory feedback during the task or precise concentration of applied forces toward the desired location of the workpiece. For instance, the authors point out that without sensory feedback in a thread-tapping job, if the ratio is too large, the applied force may be excessive and result in stripped threads.

Distribution of contact pressures on surfaces of the hands and anthropometric characteristics are of extreme importance in designing hand tools. For example, longer handles which spread the

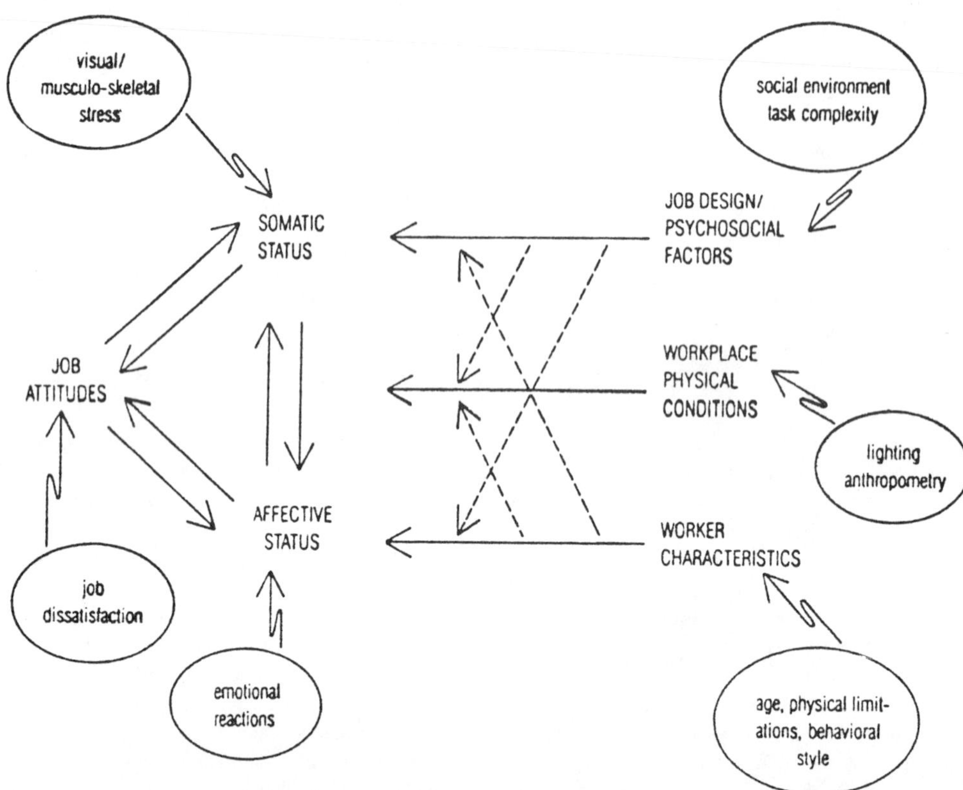

FIG 28–2.
A basic conceptual model of the stress process in office work.

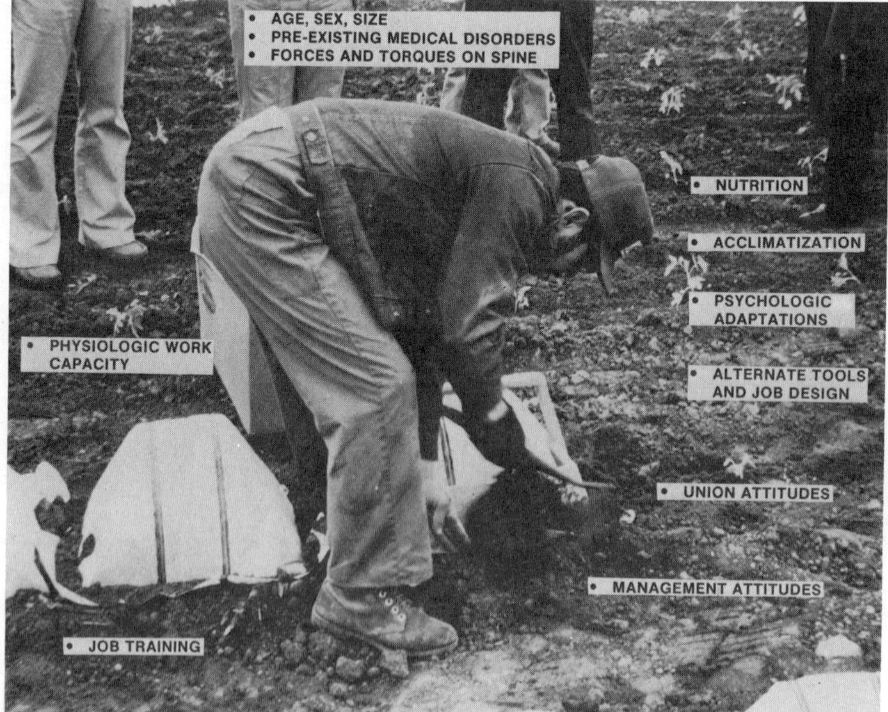
• AGE, SEX, SIZE
• PRE-EXISTING MEDICAL DISORDERS
• FORCES AND TORQUES ON SPINE
• NUTRITION
• ACCLIMATIZATION
• PSYCHOLOGIC ADAPTATIONS
• PHYSIOLOGIC WORK CAPACITY
• ALTERNATE TOOLS AND JOB DESIGN
• UNION ATTITUDES
• MANAGEMENT ATTITUDES
• JOB TRAINING

FIG 28–3.
Human factors in farm workers using the short handle hoe.

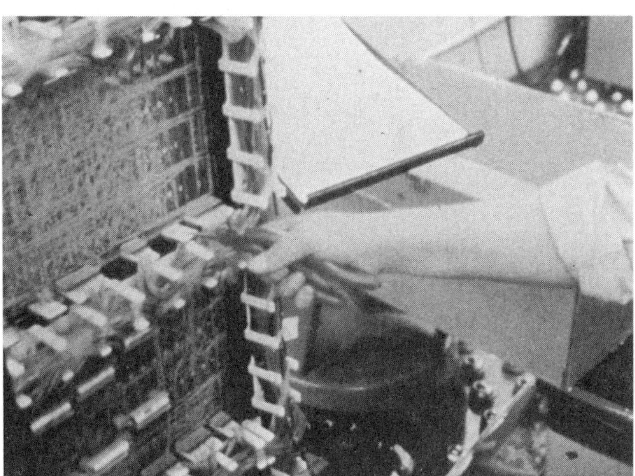

FIG 28–4.
Long-handle pliers for spreading pressure.

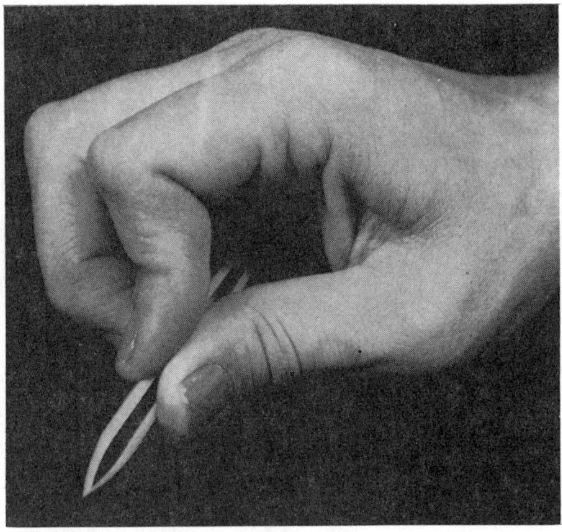

FIG 28–6.
Old-type tweezers caused finger and forearm pain.

pressure over a larger area of the hand are recommended (Fig 28–4). Tools and jobs should be designed so that they can be performed with straight wrists. Figure 28–5 shows how a deviated wrist, which would have been caused by the inappropriate use of a pistol grip tool, can be alleviated by using a vertical tool that is a better design for the task. Hands are stronger and less vulnerable to injury when the wrists are kept straight.

Garrett[20] has written of anthropometric and biomechanic variables in hands, and his data point to the need to design hand tools that are not restricted to the fit of the average hand but rather designed so as to fit the dimensions of the wide range of hands found throughout the working population. In many cases, hand tools for use by women should have dimensions different from those for use by men.

In practice in the electronics industry, one of us has encountered cases of tenosynovitis with prolonged use of a simple tool such as tweezers. Figure 28–6 shows the old type of tweezers used by a technician to handle hundreds of silicon wafers per day. Many employees using this type of tweezers complained of finger and forearm pains and a significant number experienced tenosynovitis. Numerous redesigns were attempted until the tweezers shown in Figure 28–7 were developed. Much less pressure was required to lift silicon wafers with the new tweezers, and symptoms disappeared with introduction of the newly designed tool into the work force.

New operations can lend themselves to new hand tool designs. For example, in a cable assembly operation the operators were supplied with plastic covers to sheathe the ends of large cables for protection during shipping and installation. But pressing the sides of the cover made the operators' fingers sore. A hand tool was designed that is light and spring-activated to stay open unless the grips are compressed or latched shut. Its jaws are angled at 45 degrees to reduce wrist strain. The device has greatly alleviated hand injuries and improved throughput.

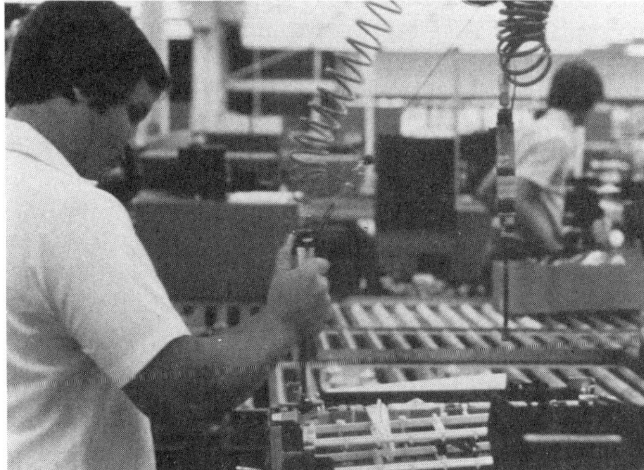

FIG 28–5.
Use of a vertical tool allows an undeviated wrist.

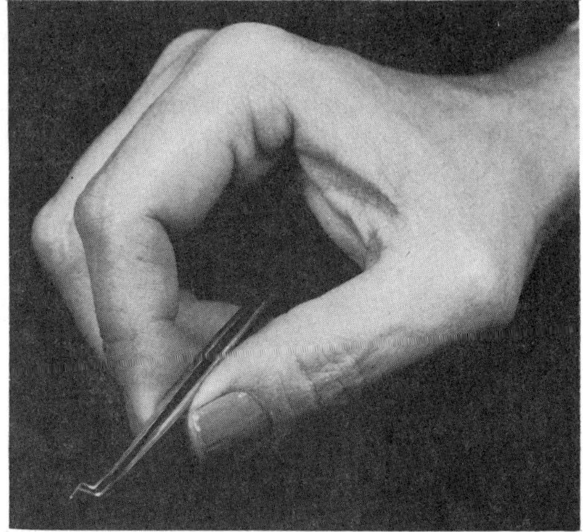

FIG 28–7.
Newly designed tweezers eliminated finger and forearm pain.

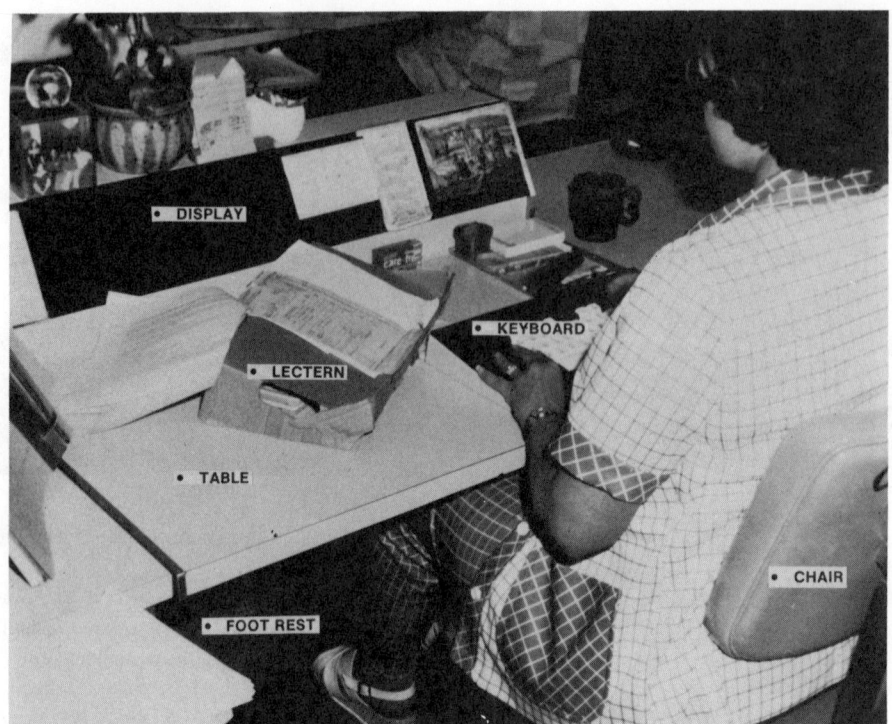

FIG 28–8.
"Human factors." Keypunch operator has constructed her own lecterns out of cardboard.

INFORMATION PROCESSING

The use of electronic data processing in a broad range of applications is growing rapidly. The application of ergonomics to the design, use, and application of information processing equipment for the user or operator would seem to be very important in view of this widespread use of such equipment.

Keyboards

Problems in the continuous use of keyboards have been with us for some time. Numerous articles[14, 18, 19, 28] have been written detailing conditions that can result from keypunch operations. Ferguson[18] describes "telegraphists' cramps and myalgia"; Duncan and Ferguson[14] and Kroemer[28] further expand on this subject with experimentally obtained results from individuals working with keyboards. Duncan and Ferguson[14] obtained medical results from faulty body positions versus keyboard operations and concluded that body positions of extended periods of shoulder abduction (elbow away from body), ulnar deviation of the wrist (palm down, hand turned outward) and wrist extension (palm down, back of hand turned upward) were important predictors of keyboard operators' medical symptoms (Fig 28–8).

Suggested keyboard designs[1] that could change these positions and reduce medical symptoms are as follows: (1) to correct the shoulder abduction, the keyboard should be positioned near the front edge of the table and be movable so that it can be turned in a horizontal plane; (2) to correct the ulnar deviation, again, having the keyboard in a movable horizontal plane is of prime importance; and (3) to correct the pronation and extension of the wrists, the keyboard should have a tilt.

Work Station

Today's information processing operator works at a visual display terminal (VDT). Conventional office furniture has been designed to suit the equipment and activities of a conventional office, most of which involve printed paper documents. Such office furniture was not, of course, designed with VDTs in mind. Although VDTs can be used to perform many conventional office tasks, such tasks are sometimes structured differently with a VDT. Neither the physical characteristics of the VDT nor the design of the tasks for which it is used were envisioned by the designers of conventional office furniture. As a result, VDT operators often find difficulty in using conventional office furniture comfortably. In order to minimize the stresses on the musculoskeletal system, attempts have been made to develop design guidelines[44] for video display terminal work stations. Figure 28–9 indicates some of the important VDT work station terms and dimensions that need to be considered. Evaluations of VDT work stations reveal that many of the discomfort problems experienced by operators might be attributed to awkward postures caused by lack of consideration of these guidelines. In other cases, it may be a matter of specific individuals not fitting "average" work stations. This has led to an increasing emphasis on designing adjustable work stations, which can be adapted to the individual worker's needs.

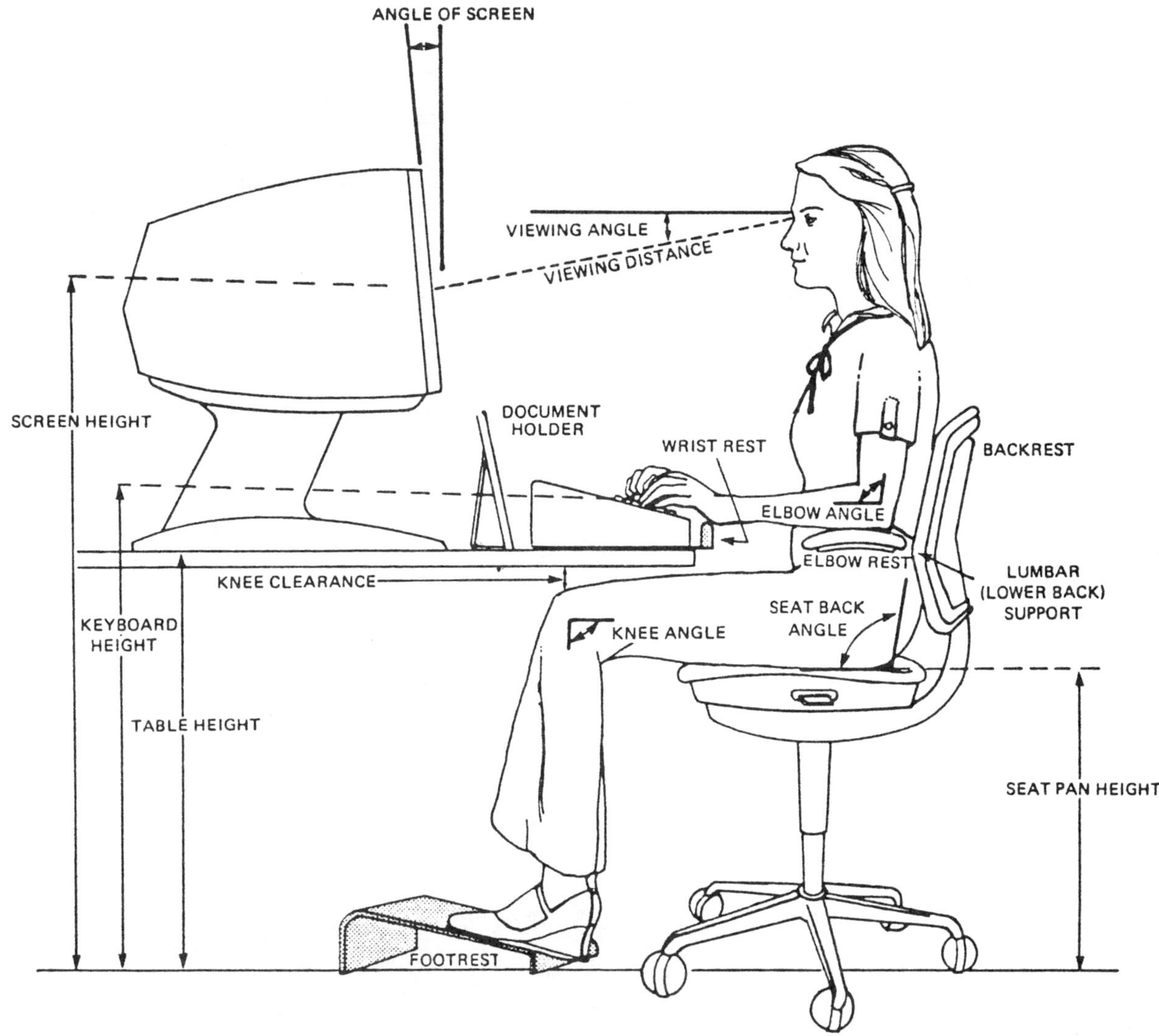

FIG 28–9.
Definitions of VDT work station terms.

Figure 28–10 is a diagram of such adjustable work stations. A recent review[4] of the postural musculoskeletal problems concluded that improvements could most certainly be made, but that the work tasks and worker preference[21] must not be overlooked.

Vision

Visual problems can be a major source of operator discomfort in information processing operations. Diffuse and specular reflections on the screen from glare sources such as overhead lighting fixtures, walls, and windows reduce the image to background luminance contrast ratio and so may reduce legibility. Appropriate design of the work environment can reduce these problems.[25, 44] Since the vision demands of this work may be different from other tasks, minor defects in the operator's visual function might be important. It is important to note that, because the viewing distance and viewing angle of the display screen are different from those for normal hard copy reading, different corrective lenses may be required. For example, normal reading bifocals require the operator to adopt an adverse head position when viewing a display screen, resulting in musculoskeletal discomfort. A single lens or a differently positioned reading segment will be required.

Of particular importance as we enter the age of electronic information processing is the way in which visually handicapped and older workers can perform with their eyes. If the average young adult is defined as having normal vision, all differences from this condition would be called abnormal. As in other areas in ergonomics, we must be careful not to design electronic equipment that favors one part of our population over another in the workplace. Normal aging is accompanied by changes in the physiology of the eye and visual system that reduce visual ability. Age markedly affects the accommodative ability of the eyes. The lens loses elasticity. The pupil also becomes smaller with age and this decreases the amount of light reaching the retina, which is one of the

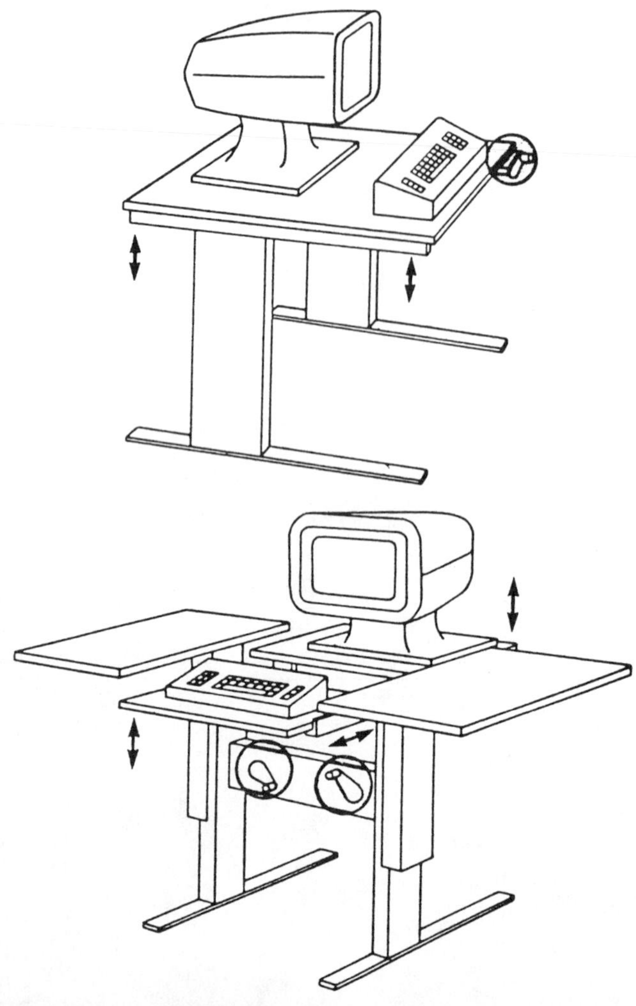

FIG 28–10.
Easily adjusted VDT tables. Any unassisted user can adapt the tables.

FIG 28–11.
Ergonomics involved in microscope work in the semiconductor industry.

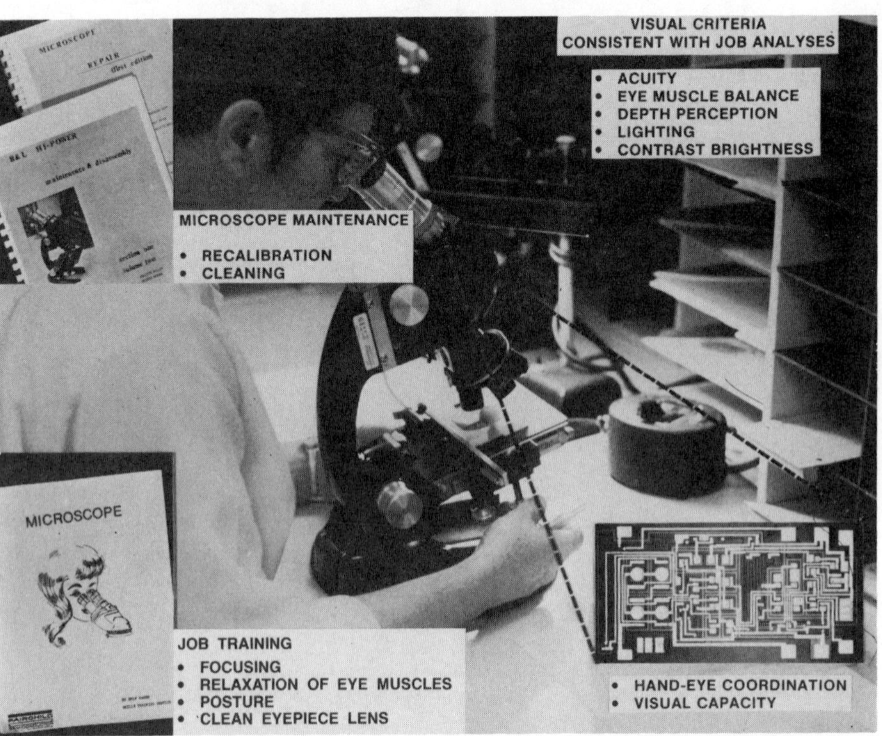

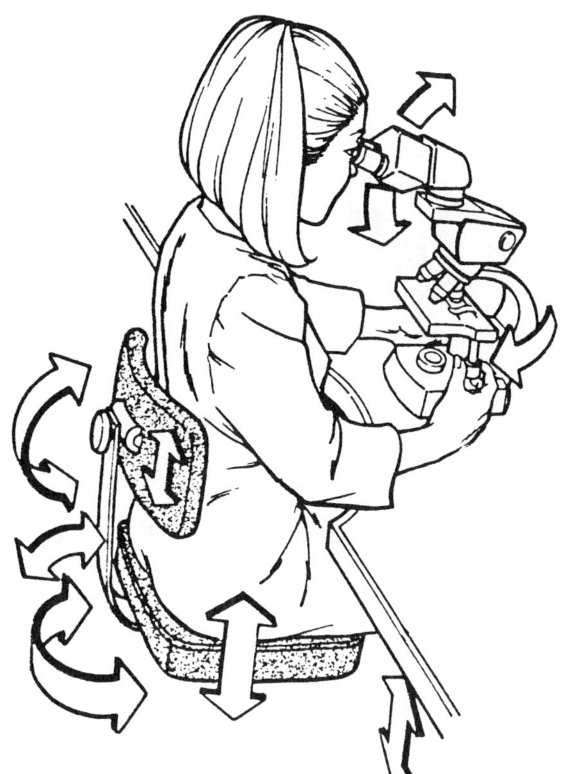

FIG 28–12.
Recommended work station adjustment possibilities for microscope work. (From the Swedish *Ordinance Concerning Work Posture and Working Movements,* 1983).

causes of loss of visual sensitivity, particularly at low luminance levels. Visual acuity declines with age, along with an increase in sensitivity to disabling glare as a function of age. Finally, there is a loss of contrast sensitivity. If we consider the vision of the young adult as normal, then that of those of us not young is not normal. Job designs in electronic information processing must allow for these changes, and individuals should be encouraged to have their vision checked at regular intervals.

Guidelines

Design guidelines for the installation and use of display terminals have been recommended or promulgated by various organizations, including governmental bodies. The Swedish directive[37] for work regularly involving reading display screens is an example. It covers such items as lighting intensity, position, and quality, luminance contrast, furniture adjustability, operator visual capability, and work organization. A highly instructive compilation of illumination for the most common jobs, ranging from typical office settings to different factory work areas, using color illustrations (depicting poor lighting and corrective lighting for each task), has been published by The Swedish Work Environment Fund.[6]

MICROSCOPE WORK

A similar vision-related task is microscope work. The worker in Figure 28–11 is performing microscope work in the modern semiconductor industry. She is viewing through a high-power lens the pattern shown at the bottom right part of the picture. Factors influencing the successful task-individual interface of a microscope worker are depicted. First, job analyses of various types of microscopes are performed. Applicants for microscope work are then vision tested, with vision profile results evaluated against visual criteria consistent with job analyses. Dickerson[12] has reported that in a specific sample studied, only 73% of employees were capable of full-time work with low- and high-power microscopes. Another 13% were capable of microscope work on a part-time basis of not more than four hours a day, preferably with low-power microscopes, and the remaining 14% were not recommended for microscope work. Of equal importance to job analyses and vision testing for proper placement of workers are proper microscope maintenance and job training. Microscopes often need recalibration and cleaning, especially if the job requires working with high-power magnification. Several factors are important in training individuals to use microscopes correctly. Methods of focusing microscopes are taught to individuals in the semiconductor industry with the realization that they may bring a field into focus hundreds of times a day. Training an individual to periodically relax his or her eye muscles by looking up from the microscope into the distance is an extremely important part of the orientation. Continual near-point accommodation can cause spasms of the ciliary muscles, which temporarily affect the vision of the microscope worker. During accommodation, the ciliary muscle contracts and, by contracting, relaxes the suspensory ligament. This permits the inherent elasticity of the lens to make the lens assume a more spherical shape, thereby increasing its refractive power and allowing it to focus on near objects. When viewing distant objects, the ciliary muscle re-

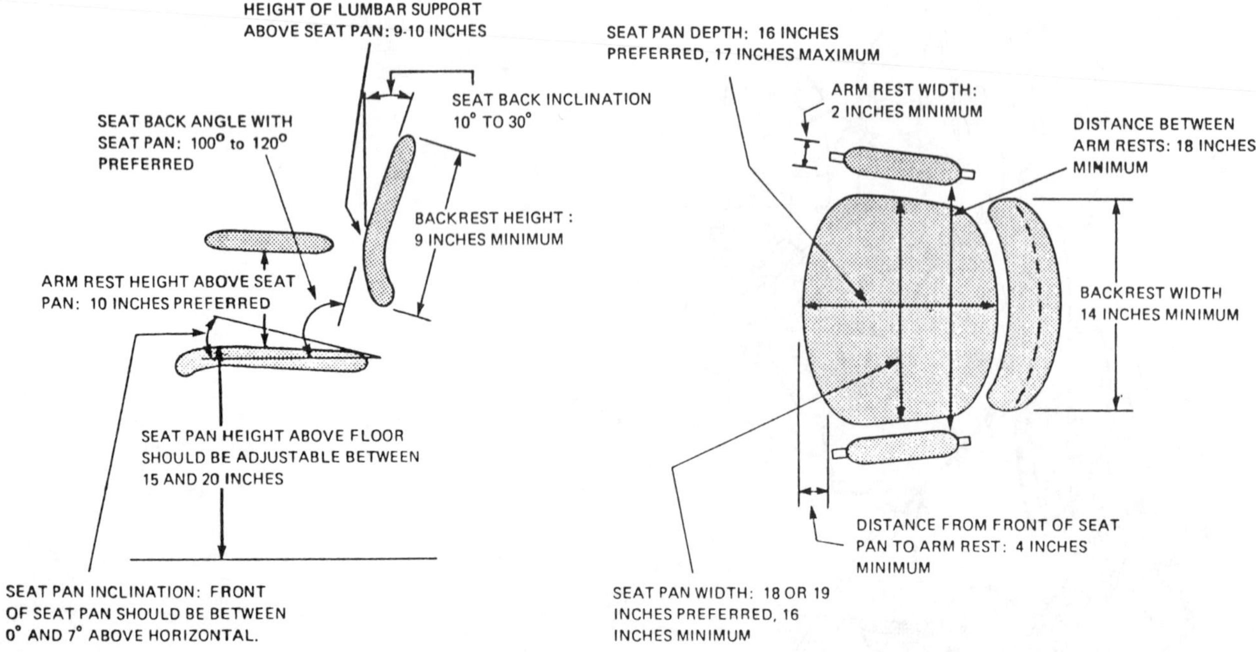

FIG 28–13.
Recommended dimensions for ergonomic office chair.

laxes and the lens flattens. MacLeod and Bannon[31] have contributed valuable suggestions to combat eyestrain while using the microscope.

In a study by Söderberg et al.[40] 80% of the operators who worked exclusively with microscopes reported various symptoms of visual discomfort, and statistical analysis showed a significant connection between visual discomfort and astigmatic refractive errors, quality of the binocular vision, and the duration of viewing time.

In addition to the visual requirements described, worker position demands attention to lessen discomfort and fatigue during prolonged microscope work. A recent study[30] using both objective (electromyography) and subjective (questionnaire) methods measured the musculoskeletal stress over time incurred by operators and found significant increases in stress over time. To combat this, adjustable work stations are recommended, and of considerable interest is the recent Swedish *Ordinance Concerning Work Postures and Working Movements* (1983) because of its generic nature (applicable to any type of work) and because its commentary specifically mentions the need for adjustability of the microscope work station (Fig 28–12). The ordinance spells out compulsory principles for workplace designs, and when these principles, for practical reasons, cannot be met, "the person doing the work must be given suitable disposed breaks."[35]

CHAIRS

Another item of interest in all work is the chair, since significant improvements in productivity as well as operator comfort and health can result from well-designed seating.[10, 35]

The seated person who is uncomfortable may or may not be constantly conscious of it. In either case, concentration spans are usually shorter and alertness may be diminished.

A well-designed chair (Fig 28–13) for the operator is one of the most important parts of a work station. It can favorably affect posture, circulation, the amount of effort required to maintain a position, and the amount of pressure on the spine.

The following recommendations should be followed:

The seat should adapt to the user, not vice versa.

Chairs should be stable and fully and easily adjustable from the seated position.

Seat pans and backrests should be upholstered and covered in a material which absorbs perspiration. They should be firm, with a compression of about 20 mm.

Seat pan height should be adjustable and should transfer the user's weight through the buttocks, not the thighs.

Backrests should adjust up and down and backward and forward for good lumbar support.

Where mobility is required, wheels or casters should be fitted to the chair (hard casters for soft floors and soft casters for hard floors). There are exceptions to this—for example, where a slippery floor makes it difficult to keep the chair in the desired position. Where wheels or casters are fitted, seats should preferably have five legs. This offers improved stability and reduces the risk of tipping over.

Seating should provide sufficient clearance for the flesh of the thigh in order to prevent reduction of blood circulation. The front of the seat should be of a "waterfall" design.

For tasks requiring frequent lateral movements, seats should swivel.

TABLE 28–1.
Indicators of the Need for Human Factors Engineering Evaluation

- ☐ Is absenteeism on this task too high?
- ☐ Is turnover on this task too high?
- ☐ Is production efficiency on this task too low?
- ☐ Is personnel assignment on this task limited by age, sex, or body size?
- ☐ Is the training time for this task too long?
- ☐ Is product quality too low?
- ☐ Have there been too many visits to medical?
- ☐ Does this task result in too much material waste?
- ☐ Is there excessive equipment damage on this job?
- ☐ Does the operator make frequent mistakes?
- ☐ Is the operator frequently away from his or her work station?
- ☐ Is this work station utilized on more than one shift per day?

The subject of the correct seated position or range of seated positions is still evolving, but the work of Mandal[32] and Grandjean and his associates[21] shows, in very different applications, that the classical orthogonal seated position may not be the optimum, and so they add further support to the above recommendations for a well-designed chair.

TABLE 28–2.
Indicators of the Need for Task Redesign

- ☐ Is the operator required to lift and carry too much weight?
- ☐ Is the operator required to push or pull carts, boxes, rolls of material, etc., that involve large break-away forces to get started?
- ☐ Is the operator required to push or pull carts and hand trucks up or down ramps and inclines?
- ☐ Does the task require the operator to apply pushing, pulling, lifting, or lowering forces while the body is bent, twisted, or stretched out?
- ☐ Is the work pace rapid and not under the operator's control?
- ☐ Does the operator's heart rate exceed 120 beats per minute during task performance?
- ☐ Do operators complain that their fatigue allowances are insufficient?
- ☐ Does the task require that one motion pattern be repetitively performed at a high frequency?
- ☐ Does the task require the frequent use or manipulation of hand tools?
- ☐ Does the task require both hands and both feet to continually operate controls or manipulate the work unit?
- ☐ Is the operator required to maintain the same posture, either sitting or standing, all the time?
- ☐ Is the operator required to mentally keep track of a changing work situation particularly as it concerns the status of several machines?
- ☐ Is the rate at which the operator must process information likely to exceed his or her capability?
- ☐ Does the operator have insufficient time to sense and respond to information signals that occur simultaneously from different machines?

TABLE 28–3.
Indicators of the Need for Workplace Redesign

- ☐ Do operators sit on the front edge of their chairs?
- ☐ Must the operator assume an unnatural or stretched position to see dials, gauges, or parts of the work unit or to reach controls, materials, or parts of the work unit?
- ☐ Is the operator required to operate foot pedals while standing?
- ☐ Does the operation of foot pedals or knee switches prevent the operator from assuming a natural, comfortable posture?
- ☐ Are foot pedals too small to allow foot position changes?
- ☐ Is a footrest necessary?
- ☐ Do operators frequently attempt to modify their work chair by adding cushions or pads?
- ☐ Are operators required to hold up their arms or hands without the assistance of armrests?
- ☐ Are dials and equipment controls difficult to operate or poorly labeled?
- ☐ Do the design and layout of equipment hinder cleaning and maintenance activities?
- ☐ Does the workplace appear unnecessarily cluttered?
- ☐ Is the operator required to use a nonadjustable chair?
- ☐ Can the operator be relieved of static holding work by providing clamps or supports for the work units?

PROBLEM IDENTIFICATION

There are methods available to assist in identifying problem job areas, and Tables 28–1 through 28–4 list the indicators one should look for in a typical manufacturing operation.[2] Table 28–5 shows the results from a study of an assembly operation of the recommended specifications of key factors. A complete work station design, including a modular and flexible work station with good parts accessibility, air tool delivery system (Fig 28–14), illumination, and chair (Fig 28–15), has shown excellent gains in productivity, health and safety, and worker satisfaction.[6, 41]

TABLE 28–4.
Indicators of Special Considerations in the Work Environment

- ☐ Could process noise cause hearing loss?
- ☐ Does process noise interfere with the reception of speech or auditory signals?
- ☐ Do the work tasks require special lighting?
- ☐ Do the operator's eyes have to move periodically from dark to light areas?
- ☐ Are there any direct or reflected glare sources in the work area?
- ☐ Do lights shine on moving machinery in such a manner as to produce stroboscopic effects or distracting flashes?
- ☐ Does task background coloration interfere with the color codes on knobs, handles, or displays?
- ☐ Is the air temperature uncomfortably hot or cold?
- ☐ Is the relative humidity uncomfortably high?
- ☐ Are radiant heat sources located near any work stations?
- ☐ Is the operator exposed to rapid thermal or visual environmental changes?
- ☐ Do hand tools or process equipment vibrate the operator's hands, arms, or whole body?
- ☐ Does process dust settle on displays, making them difficult to see?

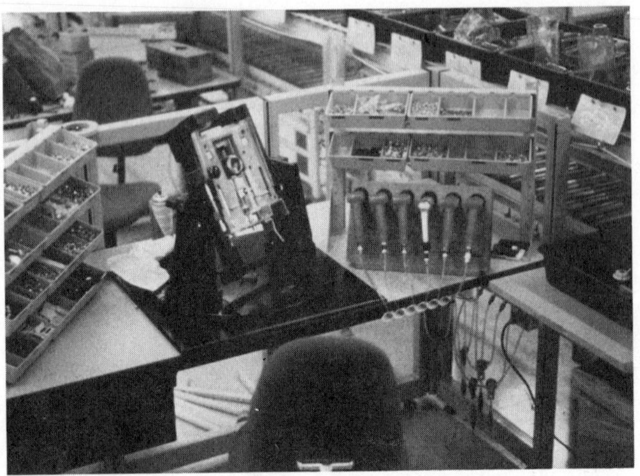

FIG 28–14.
Well-designed, flexible work station.

TASK DESIGN

Our review would not be complete without a brief comment on task design and environment. Stress is a factor in both job content and job context. Stress is a normal human condition and provides motivation for many human activities. Indeed, reasonable amounts of stress are essential for well-being. There are, however, many stressors in life. The 43 most stressful changes that might occur in a person's life have been identified,[36] and it has been found that it would be possible to predict the subsequent health of those assessed. Included on the list are: job security, job change, job responsibility, and management structure. A recent extensive study of stress and health concludes that individuals who experience a wide variety of stressful events or situations are at an increased health risk.[33] Events and situations in the work environment that contribute to stress include responsibility, work load, security, change, and interpersonal or role conflicts.

TABLE 28–5.
Comparison of Work Station, With Recommended Specifications

FEATURE	PRESENT WORK STATION SPECIFICATIONS	RECOMMENDED SPECIFICATIONS	PROPOSED WORK STATION SPECIFICATIONS
	Workbench		
Head tilt of worker	30–45 degrees	15 degrees maximum	0–10 degrees
Height of work station	34 in	27.5–34.5 in	26.75 in adjustable
Undersurface of work station	32.75 in	25 in minimum	25.75 in
Depth of work surface	28 in	*	31.5–34 in
Depth of surface area after setup	16 in	*	18.6–23.6 in plus cart area
Total surface area available after setup	680 sq in	*	1,680 sq in
Reach	16–24 in	23.3 in	22–29.5 in
	Chair		
Height of chair	24.6 in	13–18 in	17 in
Pan dimensions	16.5 in	15–19 in	17 in
Seat width	17 in	15.7 in minimum	17.5 in
Contour	none	front	front and rear
Backrest	4.5–10.7 in	4.2–9.5 in above seat pan	3.6–5.6 in
Width of backrest	14 in	15 in maximum	11–13 in
Movement	Seat does not swivel	360 degrees	360 degrees
Cushioning	2.5 in	0.75–1.5 in	1.5 in
	Visual aid		
Visual angles re: Character, height, and retinal image	9 min (1 mm) (using prints)	16 min minimum	20.8 min minimum (4 mm) (using microfiche)
Optimal visual zone (on the microfiche viewer)	32–45.9 in	32–45.9 in	33–44.5 in
Noise levels	72 dBA	66–80 dBA	80 dBA maximum
Illumination			
With overhead task lamp on	69 fc	100–150 fc	100–150 fc
With overhead task lamp off	40 fc	100–150 fc	100–150 fc

*Dependent upon the specific user group.
Abbreviations: in = inches; min = minutes; dBA = decibels on the A scale; fc = footcandles.

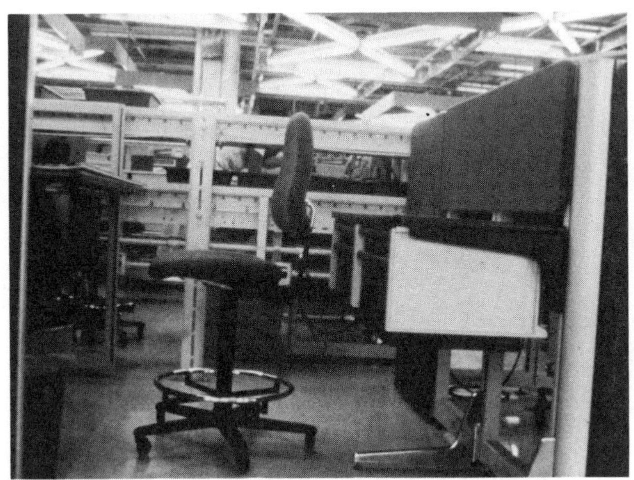

FIG 28–15.
Work station chair and good illumination.

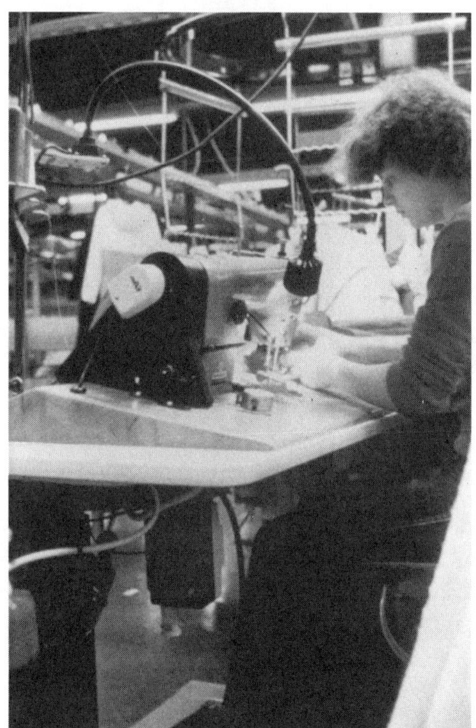

FIG 28–16.
Sewing, an ancient occupation greatly intensified by mechanization has been long known to cause distress among the countless workers. Neck and shoulder pains and tendinitis are common and the increasing pace of work has been enhancing ergonomic difficulties. Visual requirements and hand, finger, and eye coordination are necessary for all operators! Few studies have focused on this apparently nonglamorous work. In Finland alone about 32,000 garment industry workers will benefit from a newly-designed sewing table. The working surface has been illuminated and tilted to allow the worker to properly rest the forearms. (Courtesy of Thelma Aro, Institute of Occupational Health, Helsinki, Finland. Photo by Leena Frondelius-Kannus.)

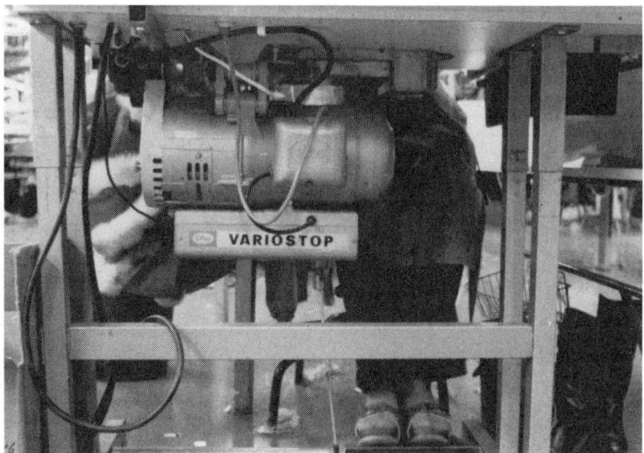

FIG 28–17.
The typical location for the drive motor. Note the cramped position of the legs. (Courtesy of Thelma Aro, Institute of Occupational Health, Helsinki, Finland. Photo by Leena Frondelius-Kannus.)

Other selected, but common, examples of ergonomic problem areas and some practical solutions are illustrated in Figures 28–16 through 28–26.

CONCLUSION

In summary then, the application of ergonomic principles to the design of tools, work stations and tasks may be the most significant contribution that can be made to improved worker health, safety, satisfaction, and productivity in this decade. We have explained the practical applications of some, but certainly not all, of those principles within the broader framework of the total work environment.

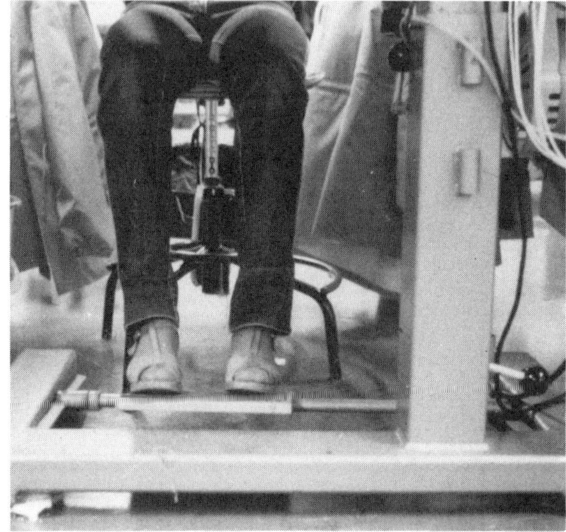

FIG 28–18.
The motor has been moved to one side offering improved leg room for the operator. (Courtesy of Thelma Aro, Institute of Occupational Health, Helsinki, Finland. Photo by Leena Frondelius-Kannus.)

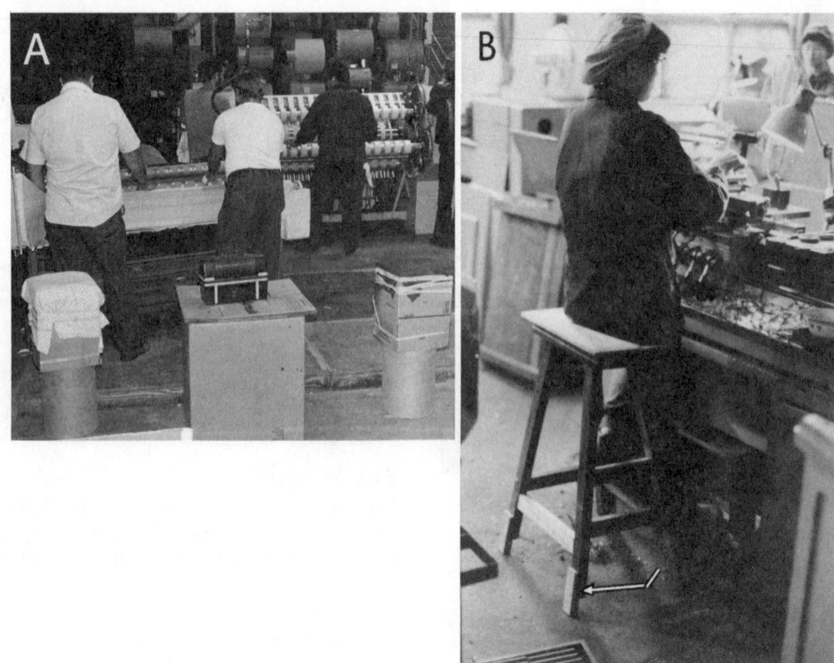

FIG 28–19.
A, tape manufacturing plant requiring attendants to stand almost constantly. Note the improvisations by employees for rest breaks. **B,** another example of practical ergonomic "self adjustment."

FIG 28–20.
A modern automotive plant with elegantly designed outside seating.

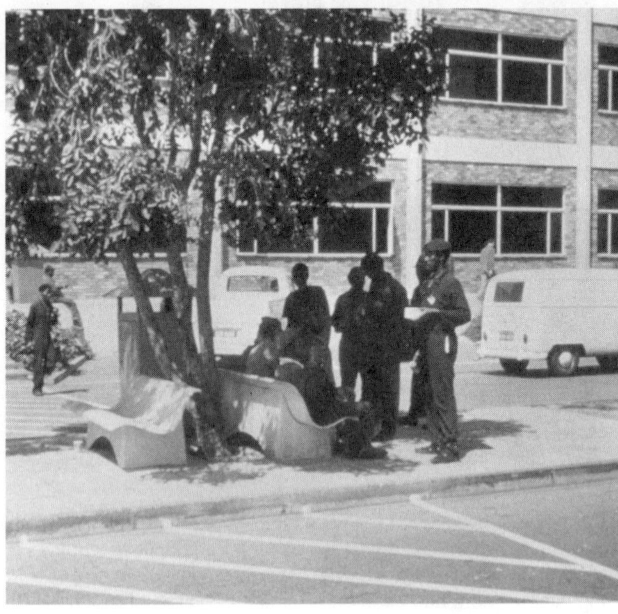

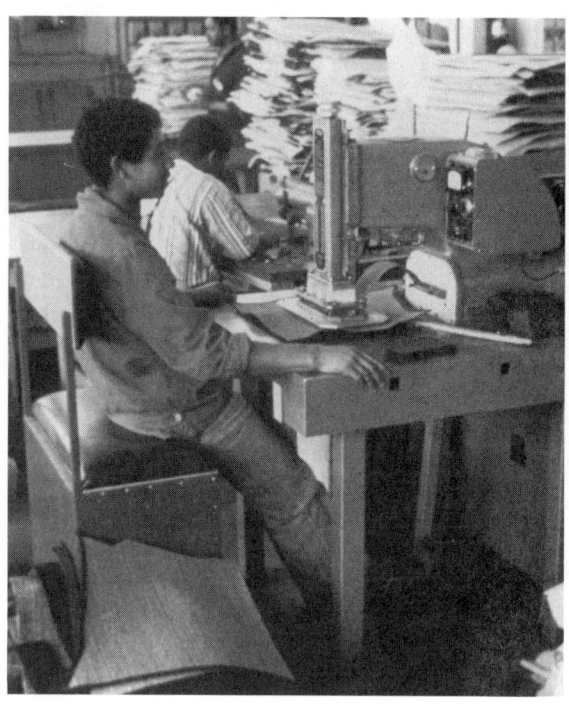

FIG 28–21.
Seating and foot pedal arrangement for embossing interior auto components (same plant as in Figure 1-20).

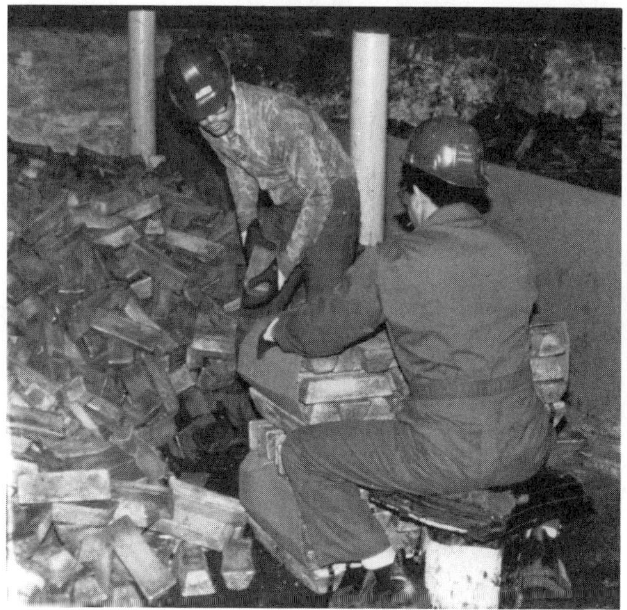

FIG 28–22.
Palletizing bronze ingots with worker-preferred positions (1984).

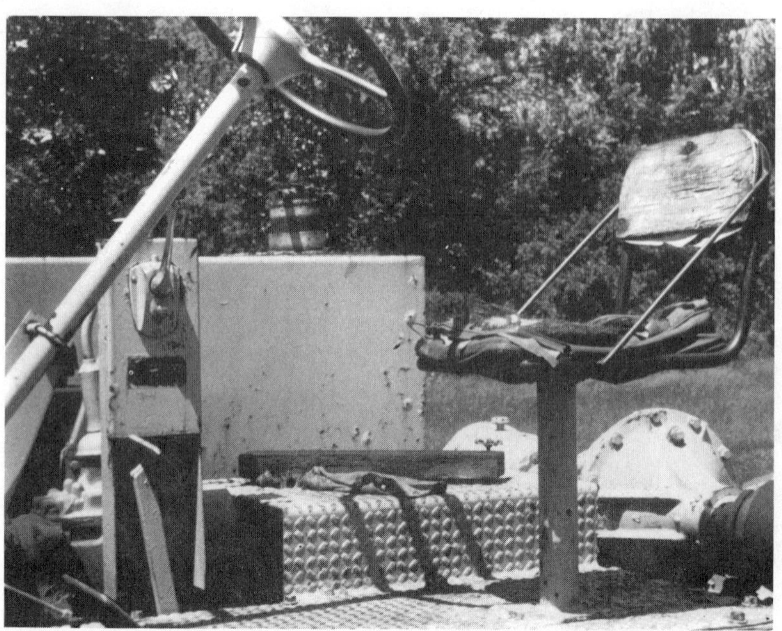

FIG 28–23.
Seating on road building machinery (1985).

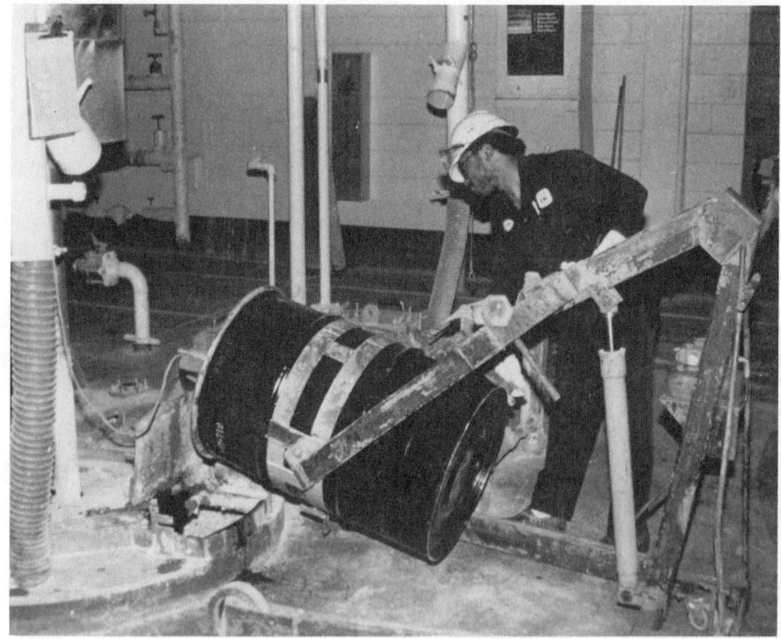

FIG 28–24.
Material handling of heavy drums in a modern and well run chemical industry (1985).

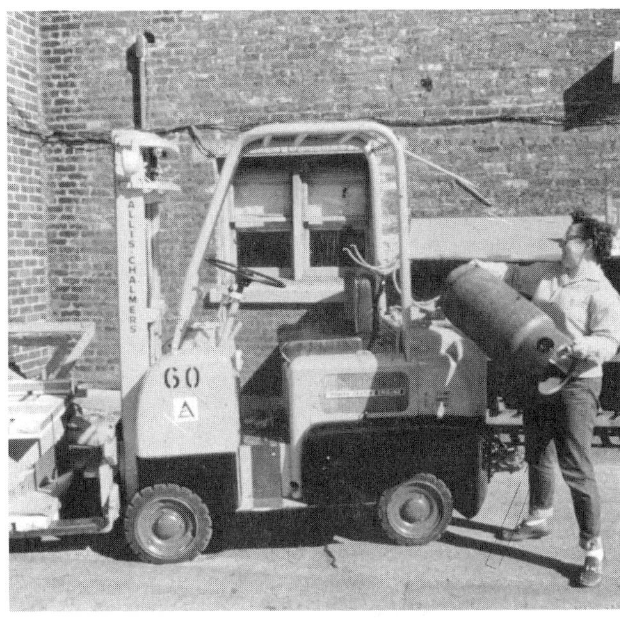

FIG 28–25.
A common method for refueling lift trucks by the driver.

The design and application of any tool must take into account: individual physiologic and anthropometric requirements in the design of the tool and the work station, the design of the task to meet employee needs, the appropriate management systems and practices, the careful and planned introduction and management of the change, and the use of the new system as a positive enhancement of our human capability.

We have indicated[5] that redesigned or new tools, work stations, and tasks need to be carefully integrated into the overall work system or else all our efforts at good ergonomic design may not achieve very much.[27]

Eventually, the responsibility of designing tools, work stations and tasks using ergonomic principles must be accepted by all parties involved and not be the sole province of ergonomists, who would then apply their technical expertise in the service of those accepted designs.

In addition to the specialized literature, excellent introductory guides are available today.[15, 16, 24]

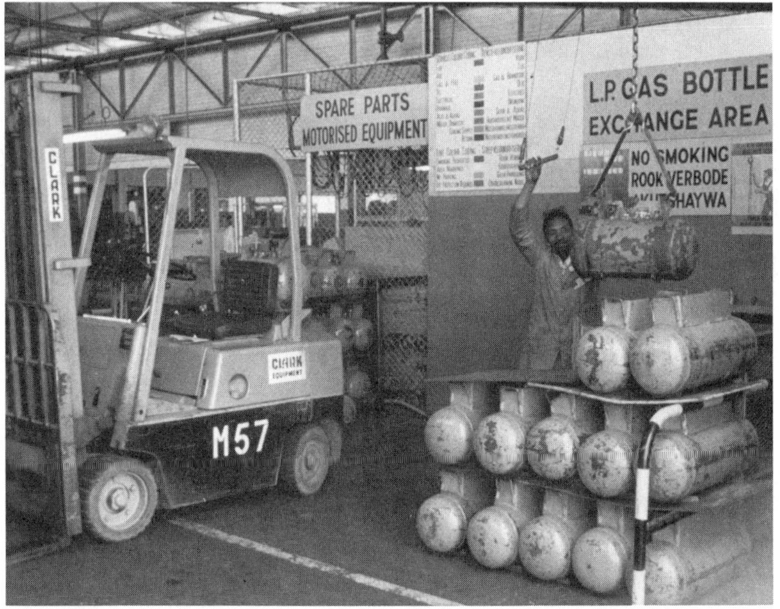

FIG 28–26.
Truck fuel tank changing station that uses mechanical aids to reduce work effort and decrease accidents.

REFERENCES

1. Alden DG, Daniels RW, Kanarick AF: Keyboard designs & operation: A review of the major issues. *Hum Factors* 1973; 14:275–293.
2. Alexander D, Smith L: Finding and fixing common design problems in manufacturing facilities. *Ind Eng*, June 1982; and *Manufact Ergon*, IBM 1/3 1983.
3. Armstrong TJ, Joseph BS, Wooley C: Analysis of jobs for control of upper extremity cumulative trauma disorders, in *Proceedings of the 1984 International Conference on Occupational Ergonomics*. Bowmemouth, England, Taylor & Francis, Sept 2–6, 1985, pp 416–420.
4. Arndt R: Working posture and musculoskeletal problems of VDT operations—Review and reappraisal. *Am Ind Hyg Assoc J* 1983; 44:
5. Baker WE: Positioning health and safety in the 80's. *Natl Saf News* 1984; May pp 40–44.
6. *Bra belysning på jobbet*, Arbetarskyddsfonden, Tunnelgatan 31, 11181 Stockholm, 1982.
7. Burri G: A practical ergonomics program in place and how it works, in *Cumulative Trauma Disorders and Ergonomics*. Chicago, National Safety Council, 1984.
8. Chapanis A: Perspective, in *Manufact Ergon*, IBM 1/2 1983, pp 2–3. Adapted from Quo Vadis Ergonomics, *Ergonomics* 1979; 22:595–605.
9. Chapanis A: Relevance of physiological and psychological criteria to man-machine systems: The present state of the art. *Ergonomics* 1970; 13:337.
10. Dainoff M: Visual, musculoskeletal, and performance differences between good and poor work stations: Preliminary findings, in *Proceedings of the Human Factors Society—26th Annual Meeting*, Seattle, Oct 1982. Santa Monica, p 144.
11. Derian J: Dunlop Company Redesigns Workstations, Boosts Productivity in High-Volume Inspection, *Manufact Ergon* IBM, 1/2 1983; pp 1–6.
12. Dickerson OB: Visual criteria aid in job placement. *Int J Occup Health Saf* 1976; 45:39.
13. Dickerson OB, Baker WE: Health considerations at the information workplace, in *Visual Display Terminals, Usability Issues and Health Concerns*. Englewood Cliffs, NJ, Prentice-Hall, 1984, pp 271–286.
14. Duncan J, Ferguson D: Keyboard operating posture and symptoms in operating. *Ergonomics* 1974; 17:651.
15. *Ergonomics Guidebook*, 5M1083. Chicago National Safety Council, 1983.
16. *Ergonomics Handbook*, IBM SV04-0224-00. Armonk, NY, International Business Machines, 1982.
17. Faulkner TW, Murphy TJ: Lighting for difficult visual tasks. *Hum Factors* 1973; 15(2):149–162.
18. Ferguson D: An Australian study of telegraphist's cramp. *Br J Ind Med* 1971; 28:280.
19. Ferguson D, Duncan J: Keyboard design and operating posture. *Ergonomics* 1974; 17:731.
20. Garrett JW: The adult human hand: Some anthropometric and biomechanical considerations. *Hum Factors* 1971; 13:117.
21. Grandjean E, Hunting W, Piderman M: VDT workstation design: Preferred settings and their effects. *Hum Factors* 1983; 25:161–175.
22. Hackman JR, Olham GR: Development of the job diagnostic survey. *J Appl Psychol* 1975; 60:159–170.
23. Hasselquist RJ: Increasing manufacturing productivity using human factors principles. *Proc Hum Factors Soc* 1981; 23:204–206.

23a. Helander M (ed): *Human Factors Ergonomics for Building and Construction*. New York, John Wiley & Sons, 1981.

24. Hopkinson RG, Collins JB: *The Ergonomics of Lighting*. London, MacDonald & Co, 1970.
25. *Human Factors of Workstations with Visual Displays*, ed 3. Armonk, NY, International Business Machines, 1984.
26. *Industrial Ergonomics*. Industrial Accident Prevention Association, 2 Bloor St East, Toronto, Ontario M4W3C2, 1982.
27. Keen PGW: The VDT as an agent of change, in *VDTs, Usability Issues and Health Concerns*. Englewood Cliffs, NJ, Prentice-Hall, 1984; and Information systems and organizational changes. *Communications of ACM* 1981; 24:66.
28. Kroemer KH: Human engineering the keyboard. *Hum Factors* 1972; 14:51.
29. Lahey JW: Bearing down on musculoskeletal disorders. *Natl Saf News* 1984; March pp 37–39.
30. Lee KS, Wu L: Physical stress evaluation of microscopists using electromyography, in *Proceedings of the 1984 International Conference on Occupational Ergonomics*, Toronto, Sept 12–17, pp 397–401.
31. MacLeod D, Bannon RE: Microscopes and eye fatigue. *Ind Med* 1973; 42:7.
32. Mandal AC: The seated man: Theories and realities. *Proc Hum Factors Soc* 1982; 24:520–524.
33. *NAS IOM Research on Stress and Human Health*, Publ IOM81-05. Washington, DC, National Academy Press, 1981.
34. Ong CN: Workplace design and physical fatigue: A case study in Singapore, in *Abstracts of International Scientific Conference on Ergonomic and Health Aspects in Modern Offices*, Torino, Italy, Nov 7–9 1983. London, Taylor & Francis, 1984, p 107.
35. Östberg O, Moss CE: Microscope work—Ergonomic problems and remedies in *Proceedings of the 1984 International Conference on Occupational Ergonomics*. Toronto, Sept 12–17, 1985, pp 402–406.
36. Rahe RH: Subject's recent life change and their near future susceptibility, in *Advances in Psychosomatic Medicine*. Basel, Switzerland, Karger, 1978, vol 8.
37. *Reading of Display Screens*, Directions No 136, ARBETARSKYDDSSTYRELSEN, Fack, S-100 26. Stockholm, Aug 2, 1978.
38. Rush HMF: *Job Design for Motivation*. New York, The Conference Board of New York, 1971.
39. Sauter SL, Gottlieb MS, Jones KC, Dodson VD, Rohrer KM: Job and health implications of VDT use. *Communications of the ACM* 1983; April.
40. Söderberg I, Calissendorf B, Elofson S, et al: Mikroskoparbete I. Utredning av ögonbesvar hos mikroskop-operatorer pa en elektronisk industri, Arb. och Hälsa 16, Stockholm, 1978.
41. Snyder KM: *The Design and Evaluation of an Ergonomic Workstation*, IBM Technical Report TR 54.265, and in *Manufact Ergonomics* IBM 1/3 1983; p 1–10.
42. Thompson T: Innovative assembly and modular materials handling. *Assembly Eng* 1980; 23:18–22.
43. Tichauer ER, Gage H: Ergonomic principles basic to hand tool design. *Am Ind Hyg Assoc J* 1977; 38:622.
44. *VDT's, Preliminary Guidelines for Selection, Installation and Use*. New York, AT&T Bell Laboratories, 1983.
45. van Wely PA: Ergonomics in a major European industry. *Am Ind Hyg Assoc J* 1971; 32:131.
46. Zenz C: Ergonomics: Work effort, determination of energy expenditure and fatigue, in Zenz C (ed): *Occupational Medicine: Principles and Practical Applications* Chicago, Year Book Medical Publishers, 1975, p 424.

PART IV

The Chemical Occupational Environment

29

Occupational Exposure Limits for Chemical Agents

R. L. Zielhuis, M.D., Ph.D.

A family of chemical quantity limits exists, e.g., for chemicals in workroom air, ambient air, drinking water, food, and also physical quantity limits exist, for noise and ionizing radiation, for example. In the 1975 edition of this book, the title of this chapter was: "Permissible Limits for Chemical Exposures." However, in 1977 the International Labor Organization (ILO) adopted the term "Occupational Exposure Limit" (OEL) which subsequently has also been used by the World Health Organization (WHO).[49, 50, 52, 53, 56] This quantity limit is discussed in this chapter.

ASPECTS OF DECISION-MAKING

Definitions

The threshold limit values (TLV) published by the American Conference of Industrial Hygienists (ACGIH) for several decades have served as the basis for OELs in many countries. The TLVs[2] refer "to airborne concentrations (in workroom air) of substances and represent conditions under which it is believed that nearly all workers may be repeatedly exposed day after day without adverse effect." The TLV-TWA is the time-weighted average concentration for a normal eight-hour workday and a 40-hour workweek; it refers to the whole working life. Threshold limit values are based "upon the best available information from industrial experience, from experimental human and animal studies and, when possible, from a combination of the three."

A few aspects should be emphasized. Threshold limit values refer only to *respiratory* exposure, although for substances that may penetrate the skin the notation "S" may be added for caution. The TLV-TWA is an arithmetic average concentration over a workday.

A TLV does *not guarantee* the absence of health risk; a "small percentage of workers may experience discomfort at concentrations at or below the limit, and a smaller percentage may be affected more seriously." It is never possible "to prove the negative." There always exists the possibility of an unknown hypersusceptibility. This statement is in contrast to that of the Occupational Safety and Health Administration (OSHA) standard,[11] which requires that "no employee shall be affected," a utopian statement that never can be guaranteed. The TLVs do not explicitly take into account reproductive hazards, for which criteria have recently been introduced in the Dutch, German, and U.S.S.R. definitions.

A Step-by-Step Approach

In 1977, the Dutch authorities set up a new procedure for deriving OELs, the Maximal Accepted Concentration (MAC),[57, 60] which envisages an "explicit process of systemic assessment of scientific data in the formulation of policy options,"[13] more so than in most other countries. This approach permits a better "balance of power" between those who create the working conditions (employers) and, consequently, occupational health risks, and those who actually run the risks (employees).

The Dutch authorities founded a Working Group of Experts (WGE), with members appointed à titre personnel. The task was to recommend a health-based (HB) OEL, or Maximal Accept*able* Concentration, after assessment of all relevant toxicity data; *only* health considerations were taken into account. A fully documented concept-report was distributed among other experts, designated by the Dutch organizations of employers and of employees, with a request to submit comments (within three months); subsequently, the WGE submitted a final *health-based* recommendation to the National MAC-Commission (NMC), and the advisory report was made public.

In 1978 the NMC was founded. The members are not appointed, but they are representatives of the organizations of employers and of employees, and of the government (Directorate General of Labor). The NMC takes both the HB-OEL as recommended by the WGE, and the socioeconomic and technologic constraints into account. The NMC recommends an *operational* OEL, the Maximal Acc*epted* Concentration. Finally, the Minister of Social Affairs and Employment decides upon the final OEL, after industries have had the opportunity to submit objections to the proposed OEL. When the operational OEL deviates from the HB-OEL, the reasons for this have to be explicitly documented in a public report.

This procedure explicitly permits full input by both employers and employees on the operational OEL. In addition, all documentation is open to the public. In 1984 the representative of the

Dutch Chemical Industry[28] strongly recommended to the European Economic Community (CEC) that this Dutch system be followed; the procedure had proven its use and feasibility since 1978. The Dutch chemical industry proposed to CEC to appoint an International Expert Group for establishing HB-OELs as an agreed-upon scientific basis. However, at least for the near future, an international MAC-Commission seems not yet to be realistic.

Health as Criterion

The OELs highly depend upon the definition of "health" chosen as criterion: does it mean preventing death and disease, forestalling early health impairment, even eliminating nuisance?

Health may be defined as "a nonstable condition of the human organism, of which the functional capacities leave nothing to be desired in the workers' own opinion and/or according to health experts; preexisting physical and mental capacities, depending on, e.g., age and sex, have to be taken into account; the functional condition should be comparable to that in nonexposed but otherwise similar groups of workers in the same society; allowance should be made for the present state of the art, present-day objectives of health care, social acceptability, and social habits."[57, 60] Therefore, OELs are meant to *preserve health* and not merely to prevent disease or death.

A distinction between "somatic health impairment" and "nuisance" should be rejected because (1) such a distinction is based upon a nonexistent dichotomy between soma and psyche; (2) with appropriate methods, subjectively perceived nuisance can be assessed objectively in groups of workers as signs of somatic impairment; (3) symptoms do not always occur before somatic impairment can be established; and (4) symptoms and signs may restrict "normal" functioning in the society and at work. Nuisance effects represent an intrusion on degrees of freedom, because subjects are hampered in their way of life. Stokinger[40] emphatically rejected the objections of those who state that "nuisance complaints from irritation are a labor relation matter." However, he referred particularly to such symptoms as co-inducers of disease, and still distinguished "health effects from merely nuisance."[42] This statement still leaves the distinction between signs and symptoms intact.

Assessment of health risks requires *operationalization:* a probable, causal, (semi)quantitatively expressed relationship between the incidence of health effects and the intensity, frequency, and duration of exposure should be demonstrated. This not only refers to the exposed workers themselves, but also to their offspring.

Total Exposure

Workers may be exposed to chemicals in workroom air. However, this constitutes only a part of their total exposure to chemicals. This chemical load again is only *one aspect* of the *total* environmental load.

Exposure to chemicals may induce impairment of health more or less *directly*, as, for instance, lead exposure leads to porphyrinemia, and anemia; cadmium exposure leads to proteinuria; and asbestos exposure to mesothelioma and asbestosis. However, exposure may also indirectly contribute to effects due to other factors. Most chronic diseases are caused by a variety of endogenous and exogenous factors, of which occupational exposure to chemicals is only one. In smoking asbestos workers, the lung carcinoma risk is greatly increased in comparison with the risk in nonsmoking employees. Workers with early cardiovascular impairment may be more susceptible to carbon monoxide. Smokers with an impaired respiratory tract may have a lower threshold for irritants. Smoking is one of the most important exogenous non-work-related factors, which, also, to a high degree, contributes to the health risk in exposure to many workroom pollutants. If smoking is socially accepted, then OELs may have to take into account this habit as a background variable. This aspect is more fully discussed by the author in the *Annals of Occupational Hygiene*.[66]

The Hygienic Rule

Man develops and maintains health only when certain essential conditions are adequate, i.e., human beings need physical and mental activity, nutrients, water, oxygen, sound, light, and human relationships. According to the *Ergonomic Rule*, such conditions of life should be of optimum duration, intensity, and frequency. Man requires an *optimal* load below an upper limit and above a lower limit. However, chemicals in workroom air have to be regarded as xenobiotic, i.e., as nonessential conditions. Exposure to chemicals at work should always be *minimized* as far as possible—this is the *Hygienic Rule*. Occupational exposure limits are never positive goals to be aimed at; the optimal goal is zero, or rather the lowest detection level.

Variability in Biologic Response

Within and between groups of "healthy " workers there is always a large variability; differences exist in genetic make-up, age, sex, past and present diseases, predispositions, food, beverage, and drug consumption, and smoking habits. A "standard" man or woman does not exist. The biologic basis of individual or group susceptibility has been discussed by Calabrese.[7] Within the healthy workers' population older than 40 years, one may expect 5%–10% without clinically manifest cardiovascular impairment, and 10%–15% with early respiratory impairment, both depending upon individual smoking habits. Therefore, one should not pay attention to average effects, as is usually done in animal experiments, but one should study the frequency distribution of responses to exposure. The tails of the distribution curve indicate vulnerable groups and individuals. The OELs should be geared to these special groups at risk and not to the fictitious "standard" worker.

The Toxicologic Data Base

Health-based occupational exposure limits are based upon assessment of all relevant toxicologic data. Reviews of the methodology of assessment have been published.[8, 37, 46, 47]

There exist at least four sources of data: animal experiments, human volunteer studies, casuistic observations, and epidemiologic studies.

Animal Experiments.—These elucidate mechanisms of action and exposure-effect/response relationships. The relative lack of respiratory exposure studies is a major drawback. Moreover, data on reproductive risks, which permit estimates of occupational risks, are very scarce. Too often, reliable data on toxicokinetics and on non-adverse-effect/response levels do not exist. This makes quantitative extrapolation from animal to man even more dubious than in the case of the Acceptable Daily Intake (ADI) of food additives. *Positive* decision-making procedures in the case of ADIs nowadays require a full set of toxicologic data *before* supplementation to food is permitted. The presence of xenobiotics in food is permitted up to a certain level; those that are not regulated are forbidden. However, OELs (and also quality limits for, e.g., drinking water and ambient air) are based upon *negative* decision-making procedures. For workroom air, only those chemicals that are regulated should not exceed a certain limit; for nonlisted chemicals no guidelines exist. In extrapolation from animal to man, safety factors have to be applied. At present there is a reasonable consensus in the application of safety factors for establishing ADIs, but for respiratory exposure no agreed-upon approach is available. A tentative proposal has been presented,[61] but much research and discussion is needed to establish a basis for consensus. For adult workers, (1) the individual variability in susceptibility will be smaller than for the general public, (2) the total duration of exposure is shorter, and (3) they are to a large extent exposed under supervised conditions. Therefore, the safety factor to be applied in deriving HB-OELs may probably be smaller than for ADIs, which are to be consumed by the general public for a whole lifetime.

Human Volunteer Studies.—These studies usually are carried out in small groups of relatively young, highly selected volunteers for short periods of time and under close supervision. They particularly provide information on toxicokinetics, irritation to mucosae, effects on psychoneurologic behavior, and performance. No conclusions can be drawn on health risks in long-term exposure. Volunteer studies may particularly be useful in establishing short-term exposure limits and for studies of methods of biologic monitoring.

Casuistic Observations.—These are usually limited to a few subjects. They often lack reliable data on exposure. The observations may provide useful hypotheses for further study and may serve as a warning signal.

Epidemiologic Studies.—These provide the most valuable source of information. They may either permit the establishment of increased relative risk ratios (RR) (positive studies) or they may indicate a low probability or even absence of such risks (negative studies). More important than the level of significance *(P)* is the range of the 95% confidence interval of the RR. In the case of RR = 0.9–7.0 the probability that, in practice, an increased risk may exist is higher than for a RR = 0.9–1.1, although in both cases the level of significance $P < .05$ is not achieved. It should be realized that it is much more difficult to establish the probable absence than the presence of adverse health risks.[23] Well-conducted studies, which permit the establishment of reliable HB-OELs, are rare.

The WHO[50] summarized some criteria to be used in the design and implementation of long-term exposure studies in workers in regard to (1) the assessment of exposure, e.g., environmental and biologic monitoring, the purity of the agent, and combined exposure; (2) the evaluation of exposure and effects in relation to age, size of group, socioeconomic status, ethnic status, duration of exposure, life-style, and obstetric history (the exclusion of confounders); (3) the methodologic aspects, e.g., design, interobserver variability, nonresponse, presence of adequate controls, validation of questionnaires, and statistical methodology; and (4) the evaluation of the non-adverse response levels.

Recently the WHO[55] published guidelines on studies in environmental (including occupational) epidemiology. Dinman and Sussman[13] concluded that policymakers too often do not apply critical judgment, or else they apply it inconsistently in critical evaluation of scientific data. To overcome this, they proposed a scoring procedure for assessing the quality of epidemiologic studies.

Expert committees, which have to propose HB-OELs, often are confronted with limited and/or poor epidemiologic data; nevertheless they have to propose at least a tentative OEL. When the data suggest an increased RR, then this cannot be ignored.

There is one major drawback in having to rely on epidemiologic studies: the aim of OELs is to *prevent* any increased health risk. Ideally speaking, workers should not be exposed when adequate assessment of risks has not yet been carried out in animal experimentation (*primary* prevention). In that case, epidemiologic studies still have to be carried out to assess the validity of the extrapolation from animal to man, possibly leading to corrective measures (*secondary* prevention).

Exposure Effect/Response Relationships

Exposure has to be related, at least semiquantitatively, to health effects. In occupational exposure, the "dose" is much more difficult to establish than in pharmacology; one speaks of exposure-effect/response relationships rather than of dose-effect/response relationships.

It is important to distinguish between exposure-effect and exposure-response relationships. The first describes the relation between exposure (intensity, duration, frequency) and effect (quality and quantity) in an individual subject or between exposure and the average graded effect in groups of animals or humans. Because a "standard" worker does not exist, the 95% confidence interval generally is much larger in humans than in experimental animals, which are usually of inbred strains, and tested under supervised uniform conditions. Some effects or events are stochastic or quantal: they either do or do not occur, e.g., death, abortion, malformation, or cancer. Quantal events cannot be averaged. From the viewpoint of health protection, not the average effect in groups of workers is important, but the relative frequency of exposed workers who experience more than the specified intensity of a specified graded effect or who suffer a quantal effect at specified exposure levels. This percentage is expressed in exposure-response relationships. These employees should first of all receive protection. Figures 29–1 and 29–2 illustrate how the same data can be expressed as exposure-effect and as exposure-response relationships. Figure 29–2 much more clearly than Figure 29–1 demonstrates the actual health risk within the group of workers.

Occupational exposures are difficult to establish accurately. The measured level of external exposure is subject to at least three errors:[16] (1) sampling and analysis, (2) selection of sampling place,

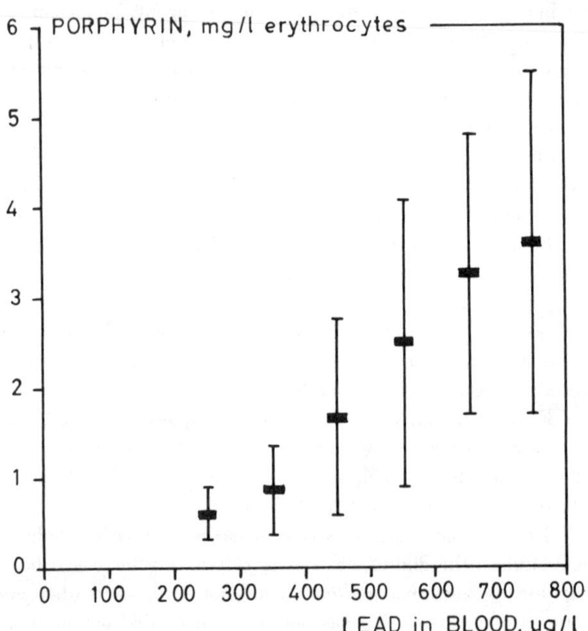

FIG 29–1.
Exposure of blood lead levels, average effect relationship. (Coronel Laboratory, study of 108 lead workers).

point of time, and averaging time, and (3) fractional uptake. Biologic monitoring better approximates the actual exposure than does environmental monitoring, because respiratory volume and dermal and intestinal resorption are also taken into account; moreover, individual deviations in toxicokinetics may be discovered.[59, 64] "Personal" sampling, again, approximates actual exposure better than "area" sampling. Many cohort studies are deficient in the assessment of actual past exposure, even when much painstaking effort has gone into measurement of the response. In most long-term studies, exposure probably is overrated because of inadequate monitoring strategies, too little attention paid to part-time exposures, use of respirators and other protective devices and clothing, distribution of exposure periods over time (seasonal effects), unusually hard work not monitored, and failure to take into account the effects of heat and humidity. This leads to *over*estimation of past exposure and consequently to *under*estimation of health risk.[43] In order to achieve valid exposure-response relationships it is necessary to have a file of all exposure data from the past to judge the validity of the exposure assessment.

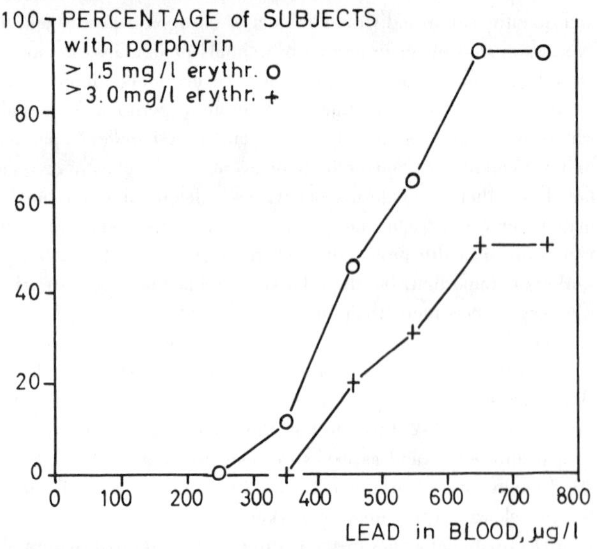

FIG 29–2.
Exposure of blood lead levels, response relationship.

The responses actually studied often present only the tip of an iceberg. There exists a continuum of workers' responses, from adjustment to the exposure, to a breakdown of the body's compensation abilities, then to health impairment, and on to disease and death.[21] Whether one observes an effect depends first of all upon the effects chosen for study and the sensitivity and specificity of the methods applied. Preconceived ideas about the potential effects may determine the design and outcome of a study.[9]

Exposure-response curves are derived from studies in animals and in employees. Figure 29–3 presents some highly simplified exposure-effect curves. The curves A, B and C may represent:

1. Three different effects caused by exposure to agent X

2. Effect X caused by exposure to three different agents

3. Average effect X caused by exposure to agent Y in three (groups of) workers, differing in capacity to cope with Y

4. Effect X caused by exposure to agent Y at three periods of life (e.g., age, state of health, pregnancy)

For many chemicals, reliable exposure-response curves are not available. One may have to rely on a few defined exposure data in relation to a few response data, i.e., on a few dots in an empty space.

The no-response exposure level in human studies can almost never be defined; rather, one speaks of *no detected* (observed) *response levels*, and then only for those responses that have been examined.

Adverse Effects

The biologic significance of specified effects is of paramount importance. It is still true what Stokinger[41] already stated in 1970:

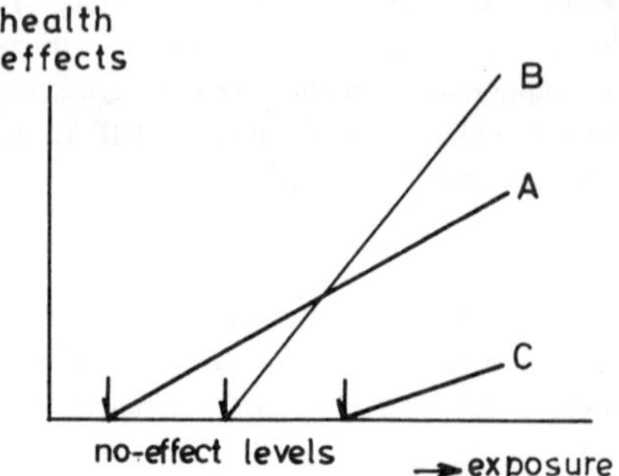

FIG 29–3.
Exposure-effect curves, nonessential chemical.

"It cannot be too strongly emphasized that if such highly sensitive tests as changes in enzyme and isoenzyme patterns or changes in behavioral response are used, follow-up studies must be made on a long-term basis to establish the toxicologic significance of such studies for a host. . . . Inhibited activity (of numerous enzymes) may be without toxicologic health significance and hence cannot serve as a health criterion." However, in a recent review of the present state of knowledge and future perspectives of the use of noninvasive assessment of microsomal enzyme activity in occupational medicine, Døssing[15] concluded that it seems justifiable to regard changes in microsomal enzyme activity as biologic changes with potential harmful consequences to the human organism. Reports from studies of drug-induced changes contain several observations of harmful short-term effects on the metabolism of hormones, vitamins, and other drugs. Whether long-term consequences occur in occupational exposure to chemicals still needs careful study.

An "effect" as such is a neutral concept: a biologic "change" is observed. It is a matter of decision by health experts *after* the study has been carried out to distinguish between "effects as such" and "adverse effects." Moreover, observation of a specified effect offers no guarantee that other relevant effects one has not looked for do not exist. New studies may discover previously unexpected hazards, just as recent studies have revealed the human carcinogenicity of vinyl chloride, or the atherosclerotic effects of carbon disulfide. In the study of exposure to asbestos, asbestosis was defined in the early years of this century, lung cancer in 1930–1940, and mesothelioma in 1950–1960.

The WHO[48] discussed at length the criteria for the "adverse" character of biologic effects. Some U.S.S.R. authors[36] called adverse "any effect which is: (1) significantly ($P < .05$) outside the limits of generally accepted 'normal' values; (2) significantly ($P < .05$) different from a control group, still within the 'normal' range, but persistent for a considerable time after the cessation of exposure; or (3) significantly ($P < .05$) different from a control group, still within the 'normal' range, but with significant departures from the generally accepted 'normal' values becoming manifest under functional or biochemical stress." However, these criteria too strongly rely on statistical significance, and therefore on, for example, the number of animals or humans examined. Moreover, generally accepted 'normal' values often are measured in selected patients, and progress of analytic and functional methods changes the 'normal' ranges.

The Committee for the Working Conference on Principles of Protocols for Evaluating Chemicals in the Environment in the U.S.A.[32] defined adverse effects as "those changes in morphology, growth, development and lifespan that (1) result in impairment of functional capacity or in decrement of the ability to compensate additional stress, (2) are irreversible if such changes cause detectable decrements in the ability of the organism to maintain homeostasis, (and/or) (3) enhance the susceptibility of the organism to the deleterious effects of other environmental influences."

Recently, the following definition was proposed:[39] "An adverse health effect is the causation, promotion, facilitation, and/or exacerbation of a structural and/or functional abnormality, with the implication that the abnormality has the potential of lowering the quality of life, causing a disabling illness, or leading to a premature death." This very much approximates the criterion of "health," as discussed earlier.

All criteria imply that effects as such do not necessarily indicate imminent health impairment at the time of examination. However, when these effects predict that health impairment may occur when exposure continues and/or that they may decrease the worker's capacity to cope with other environmental factors, then the effects should be considered "adverse."

It is not easy to distinguish between "nonadverse" and "adverse." One may distinguish four levels of consensus between experts:

1. A general consensus exists concerning the adverse character of an effect. A causal relation has been established between the exposure and the effect, based on firm biologic data.

2. One or a few studies suggest an increased risk of adverse effects at relevant exposure levels. The effect is in accordance with known working mechanisms. More research is still needed to put the suggested risk on a firmer basis.

3. A few observations indicate the probability of adverse effects, but contradictory evidence also exists.

4. Some authors suggest an increased risk based upon preliminary, perhaps poor, evidence.

An "adverse" health risk certainly should be accepted as a criterion for setting OELs in the case of 1 and 2 and maybe 3, depending upon the data available and the seriousness of the effect. Case 4 usually cannot be accepted as a criterion without further evidence.

Carcinogenic Effects

Establishment of OELs for carcinogenic chemicals raises more questions than answers.[62] Many regulatory authorities, e.g., OSHA,[34] apply "one-hit" linear extrapolation as a matter of principle: carcinogens are assumed to have no threshold dose—any exposure involves some risk. However, decisions about carcinogens may fall into the area of "transscience."[29] The present uncertainty in scientific risk assessment continues to be so great that the "regulatory processes must be considered principally political judgment rather than technical analysis."[45] Particularly, the discrepancy that results when comparing high-dose experiments in animals with low-dose exposure in workers and the lack of understanding of working procedures and mechanisms forces experts to assess risks far beyond the experimental dose-range and without a firm biologic basis.

Higginson,[24] former director of the International Agency for Research on Cancer (IARC), stated that, *in practice*, a threshold for carcinogenic risk often appears to exist, even when such cannot logically be derived from animal data. Apparently, *"operational threshold doses"* exist. He distinguished between a theoretical "apparent threshold," based upon the intake, and a "true genuine threshold," based upon the dose in the effector organ and the uptake. The Scientific Committee of the Food Safety Council in the U.S.A.[19] emphasized the inaccuracy of extrapolation: "human risk assessment is a very inexact science"—extrapolation indicates, at most, a "zone at risk." If four models for extrapolation (one-hit, multi-hit, multi-phase, and Weibull) are applied on the same animal data, then for some carcinogens the risk of 1.10^{-4} may differ even by a factor of 10.[5] Doll and Peto[14] even concluded that, at least in assessing carcinogenic risks, laboratory studies cannot be used for risk assessment, although they are useful for priority setting. The one-hit extrapolation, by definition, leads to an overestimate of the true risks; routine application of this model may even lead to a scientifically unwarranted overestimate. A *case-by-case* approach is needed.

Recent developments have elucidated that for cancerogenic chemicals that interact with DNA it may be more meaningful to relate tumor response to the concentration of DNA-adducts in the target organ rather than to the applied dose (intake): the toxicokinetics have to be taken into account. Although the relation between tumor response in the target organ may be linear, the nonlinearity of the dose-response curve for tumor production by initiator carcinogens may be due to the kinetic processes in the formation of such carcinogenic metabolite-DNA adducts.[25] The kinetic processes may show a nonlinear "hockey stick" behavior. Moreover, initiation may imply significant damage to genetic material, rather than a single-point mutation. In addition, some human carcinogens that were considered to be initiators have been shown to act rather as promoters or cocarcinogens, e.g., aflatoxin, DDT, and hormones.[24] Although OSHA[34] treats inorganic arsenic as an initiator, recent epidemiologic studies in workers[17, 44] suggest a promoter action.

Recent cancer research casts serious doubt on the feasibility of extrapolation from animal data to man. Ideally speaking, the particular workplace procedures and machinery should be understood and the dose levels and the route of administration should be appropriate to the actual conditions of exposure at the workplace, but few experiments fulfill these criteria.

Nevertheless, even in the presence of inadequate animal or human data, risk assessment involves a decision based on numbers, unless the use of a particular agent is completely prohibited in industry. Although one should always give the benefit of the doubt to the workers, this may lead to an extrapolation that is not considered scientifically warranted. In 1982, the IARC[27] concluded that, according to the present state of the art, seven industrial processes and 23 (groups of) chemicals, of which 12 are industrial carcinogens, are causally related to cancer in humans; 61 (groups of) chemicals or industrial processes are "probably" carcinogenic to humans; and 64 (groups of) chemicals or industrial processes could not be classified as to their carcinogenicity to humans.

As a first step, expert groups should present only the "virtual safe dose," or merely a list of risk estimates in exposure over working life; as a second step, the policy decision makers should determine the accepted risk.

Reproductive Effects

Chemical technology may have contributed considerably to increasing life expectancy, but at the same time may also have adversely affected fertility, pregnancy, and development of offspring.[18] In the last decade, studies of the reproductive risks incurred by male or female workers have opened a hitherto almost completely neglected field of research in occupational health. Various reviews have recently been published.[4, 10, 31, 33, 63]

Although some regulatory authorities have accepted the protection of offspring as a criterion for OELs, this still is largely a matter of well-meant intent than of guarantee, because of the paucity of data available. Few epidemiologic studies are conclusive. Too often, valid animal data are lacking; when high-dose experiments (usually with no respiratory exposure) indicate adverse reproductive risks, the no-adverse effect level has often not been established.

Reproductive risks may involve effects on libido and potency, fertility, menstruation, sperm, pregnancy, cancer induction, and fetal and postnatal development. Except in the case of genotoxic effects (which may exist already before conception), a threshold dose is usually assumed to exist.

In a critical review of epidemiologic data on occupational health risks to *female* workers, Zielhuis et al.[63] categorized the available evidence according to the degree or probability of the occurrence of detrimental effects, as shown in Table 29–1. This survey of available human evidence indicates that there still is a vast "terra incognita." For the majority of chemicals of the TLV list, no data are available at all.

Biologic OELs

Biologic monitoring may yield a bètter estimate of actual internal exposure (and consequently of health risk) than environmental monitoring. Biologic occupational exposure limits (BOELs) may also be applied, either in addition to the OEL for workroom air, or, in some cases, even in place of these.[2] The WHO[49, 50, 52] recommended biologic limits for individual or group exposure to cadmium (urine and blood), inorganic lead (blood), inorganic mercury (urine), toluene (hippuric acid in urine), xylene (methylhippuric acid in urine), trichloroethylene (trichloroacetic acid in urine), malathion and carbaryl (reduction of cholinesterase activity in blood), lindane (blood), and dinitro orthocresol (blood). Lauwerys[30] recently presented an extensive list of "tentative permissible limits."

There certainly is need for more research to develop new methods for biologic assessment of exposure and for increasing the validity of suggested BOELs. Recently, the ACGIH has added some Biologic Exposure Indices (see Appendix A).[2]

Value Judgments

Standard setting involves decision making, both in health-based assessment of health risks and when policy decisions have to be made. At least four types of choices have to be made by experts in the first step:[60] qualitative and quantitative choices and choices of tolerance times and subjects.

1. Qualitative choice.—Which type of effect is chosen to be relevant (A, B or C in Figure 29–3)? Should it be irritation of mucosa, slight reversible neurobehavioral changes, decrease of hemoglobin, or lung cancer? Does one also take "nuisance" into account? Should the OEL protect against the potential risk of traffic accidents after work in occupational exposure to solvents? What is considered "adverse"? The choices involve subjective judgments

TABLE 29–1.
Probability of Detrimental Effects to Female Workers From Occupational Exposures*†

COMPOUND	TLV-1982 (MG/CU M)	TO WOMEN GREATER THAN TO MEN	ESTABLISHED ONLY IN WOMEN	TO FEMALE REPRODUCTIVE ORGANS	TO PREGNANCY AND/OR OFFSPRING	TO INFANT DURING LACTATION
Category IA: Risks probably or even rather certainly existing around the TLV-1982 level of exposure						
Inorganic lead	0.15	xx		x	xx	xx
Cadmium	0.05	xx	xx		x	
Category IB: Suggestive but not conclusive evidence around the TLV-1982 level of exposure						
Carbon disulfide	30			x	x	
DDT	1				x	
Dieldrin	0.25				x	
HCH	0.5				x	
PCBs	0.5-1				x	
Formaldehyde	1-C			x		
Styrene	215			x	x	
Caprolactam	20			x	x	
Carbonmonoxide	55				x	
Arsenic	0.2				x	
Mercury, except alkyl mercury	0.05			x	x	
Alkylmercury	0.01				x	
Dichloromethane	360				x	
Chloroprene	45				x	
Category IIA: Suggestive but not conclusive evidence, groups of chemicals or work situations with moderate exposure						
Organic solvents				x	x	
PBBs					x	x
Operation room personnel				x	x	
Health care personnel				x	x	
Pharmaceutical industry				x	x	
Rubber industry		x			x	
Beauticians, hairdressers			x	x	x	

*Adapted from Zielhuis RL, Stijkel A, Verberk MM, et al: *Health Risks to Female Workers in Occupational Exposure to Chemical Agents.* Heidelberg, Springer-Verlag, 1984.
†x = suggestive, not conclusive; xx = probable or certain. Recent evidence and/or change in the TLV could have altered the conclusions, and to some extent, the numbers and the x's.

and may be biased due to prejudice about what is important.[9]

2. Quantitative choice.—Does one accept only a "minor" intensity of irritation of eyes, nose, and/or throat, or only a deviation of the forced expiratory ventilation (FEV) that is within the limits of physiologic variability in nonexposed controls?

3. Choice of tolerance subjects.—Should all subjects, including the most vulnerable ones, be protected, or should highly vulnerable subjects, e.g., the one person out of a hundred or a thousand, be excepted in the case of respiratory hyperreactivity? Does one exclude ambulant angina pectoris patients in considering an OEL for carbon monoxide exposure?

4. Choice of tolerance time.—Should a specified response "never" occur, or should it occur only a few times per day, or once a week?

In addition, experts have to decide upon the magnitude of safety factors in extrapolation from animal to man and from human volunteer studies to the work force at large. Moreover, what is the validity of the studies? What data should be rejected and, if so, why? Should the OEL for carbon monoxide and nitrogen dioxide protect only nonsmoking workers, disregarding self-inflicted exposure in smokers? Should social drinking habits after work be taken into account in setting OELs, e.g., for trichloroethylene or calcium cyanamide?

In the second policy-making step, other decisions have to be made based on factors such as economic and technologic constraints, international business competition, and national priorities in allocation of financial resources.

What is the risk to be accepted in the case of exposure to low-potency genotoxic carcinogens? Is the concept of "virtual safe dose" accepted? Is it ethically accepted to base the OEL on parameters of biologic monitoring only? Should one decide upon sex-dependent OELs, or should one set the operational limit at the lowest level, irrespective of sex?

Whatever limit is chosen as accep*table* (first step) or as accep*ted* (second step) is ultimately a matter of value judgment. The choices made should explicitly be stated and be made public.

Incompleteness of data does not permit the deferment of decisions; the importance of occupational health issues does not allow for a pause while the traditional sequence of experimentation, publication, peer review, and validation runs its course.[9] One may have to propose at least a tentative operational OEL.

All risks can never be avoided, for at least three reasons: (1) it is never possible to guarantee absence of any effect in any worker at any workplace, (2) available data are incomplete, and (3) there are neglected areas of research and new methodologies yet to be developed. The *periodic reappraisal* of OELs is essential.

An implicit acceptance of some risk has become an integral part of risk assessment and occupational health standard setting. "Objective" data-scoring systems may be very useful—although they should not be used for arriving at a judgment without thought—and they may illuminate the conceptual base of choices.[13]

Validity of OELs

Operational OELs should prevent impairment of health in workers and their offspring. However, how valid are the present OELs (TLVs, MACs)? Several deficiencies have already been indicated. The most important ones may be summarized as follows:

1. Man responds to a "dose," i.e., an amount of a chemical administered per unit of time, and not to a concentration, except maybe in the case of irritants. Occupational exposure limits are based upon an "assumed" respiratory volume, which may vary very much over place and time.

2. The choices underlying both health-based and operational OELs are often not clearly presented.

3. The criterion of "health" and of "adverse" often is not explicitly stated. Consensus on methods of extrapolation does not exist.

4. The toxicologic data base is often deficient. Many OELs have been based upon an assumed analogy with related compounds.

5. Too easily, OELs accepted in one country are regarded as also valid in other countries that have different cultural habits and living conditions.

6. The variability in susceptibility within and between groups of workers is insufficiently known.

7. Reproductive hazards have as yet hardly been studied.

In 1983–1985, the Dutch Working Group of Experts screened the available documentations of the ACGIH TLVs[1] and the DFG-German MAKs[22] in order to evaluate whether the TLVs of 1983–1985 appear to be reasonably well "underbuilt." The group could accept only about 10% of the present TLVs as possibly valid. This does *not* mean that the TLVs are too high; they may even be too low; the official documentations presented do not permit a conclusive answer.

Nevertheless, the present ACGIH TLVs have been proposed by a group of experienced occupational hygienists and physicians. The TLVs should be regarded as highly important guidelines. Occupational health protection is better served by relying on an experienced group of experts than by demanding a foolproof data base; an educated guess has more value than no OEL at all. On the other hand, the present state of the art forces occupational hygienists, physicians, and research workers to fill up the sometimes wide gaps of knowledge as soon as possible. The positive approach should ultimately replace the present negative approach.

Comparing the U.S. and the U.S.S.R.

Differences among countries in OELs are largely due to differences in definitions, criteria, technical feasibility, and sociopolitical judgments. Various papers[13, 26, 58] discussed particularly the differences between the TLVs from the U.S.A. and the MPCs (Maximum Permissible Concentrations) from the U.S.S.R. For several decades, both lists have served as guidelines for many countries all over the world.

Hatch[21] evaluated the different approaches in the U.S.A. and the U.S.S.R. very aptly; "neither position can be simply dismissed in favor of the other as being wholly unreasonable or contrary to established biological law." The differences in approach are schematically summarized in Table 29–2.

In previous years, U.S. TLVs and U.S.S.R. MPCs have widely differed. However, the discrepancy has become much smaller in recent years. The WHO[46–48] particularly has contributed much to the exchange of information and consequently to mutual understanding. Recently, various WHO study groups[49, 50, 53, 56] with members from the East and West have shown that, at present, international consensus on health-based recommended OELs has been achieved to a large extent for several widely used metals, solvents, pesticides, vegetable dusts, and respiratory irritants.

IMPLEMENTATION OF OELS

The Third Step

Occupational physicians and hygienists should realize that keeping exposure in workroom air below the operational OEL is *only one* of the measures to be taken in a preventive occupational health program, because: (1) respiratory exposure to one chemical refers only to one aspect of the total workload, (2) exposure through other routes, such as the skin or mouth, may also occur, (3) workers should periodically receive full information, health education, and instruction, and (4) vulnerable (groups of) workers may require special protective measures.

The OELs should never be regarded as *an optimum;* external exposure should always be below the OEL as far as possible (the Hygienic Rule).

Combined Exposures

Respiratory exposure to just a single chemical is more an exception than a rule:

1. The same compound may also be taken in by dermal and/or oral route. Particularly in the case of metals, workers may be exposed to a combination of different compounds of the same element, e.g., in ore smelting. It is not the metals as such but the

TABLE 29–2.
A Comparison of Occupational Exposure Limits in the United States and the Soviet Union*

TYPES OF DIFFERENCES	U.S. TLVS	U.S.S.R. MPC/MAC
Basic approach	Focused on the level of cell or organ	Organismic, emphasis upon control and integration through the nervous system (Pavlov)
Unit of measure	TLV: time-weighted average	MPC/MAC: maximum level, ceiling
Compensatory mechanisms	Accepted	Regarded as concealed pathology
Definition of health	Prevention of disease	Conservation of health
Choice of tolerance subjects	Most workers protected	All workers protected
Epidemiology	Much taken into account	Much less taken into account
Goal for worker	Freedom to strive onwards, to exploit one's own capacities	Freedom from unwanted stimuli
Operational use	Practicable in occupational exposure	Medical arguments overrule technical feasibility; goals to achieve†
Reproductive risks	Not included in definition	Included

*Adapted from Zielhuis RL: Differences in standards in East and West, in Grandjean PH (ed): *Standards Setting.* Copenhagen, Arbejdsmiljøfondet, 1977, pp 133–146.
†In the U.S.S.R. one also applies the so-called sanitary limits, which also take into account feasibility in practice.

metal compounds that determine the health risk. In the case of arsenic, environmental and biologic monitoring still is based largely upon measurements of arsenic as such, whereas workers may be exposed to both insoluble inorganic arsenic compounds, which may cause lung cancer, to soluble inorganic arsenic compounds, which may affect the nervous system, the liver, and the skin, and maybe also to organic noncarcinogenic arsenic from marine food.[65] Measurement of arsenic, chromium, or nickel in urine will not adequately assess the lung-cancer risk in exposure to nonsoluble or moderately soluble inorganic compounds. Methods of measurement should take into account the specific form of a metal used in a particular industry.

2. Exposure to other chemicals with a similar target organ may occur, as in the case of solvents, which are often applied in mixtures. When there is no evidence of potentiation or antagonism, one may assume an additive effect and one should calculate the sum of the following fractions (C = concentration in workroom air):

$$\frac{C_1}{OEL_1} + \frac{C_2}{OEL_2} + \ldots \frac{C_n}{OEL_n} = \leq 1$$

Scheffers et al.[38] developed somewhat more refined *effect-specific limit values* (ESLV) (no-adverse effect levels) for paint solvent mixtures. Effect-specific exposure indices (EI) with respect to mucous membrane irritation and to prenarcotic effects were taken from the literature. The EI is the sum of the ratios of the concentration in air and the corresponding ESLVs; this sum should not exceed unity, neither for the irritant nor for the prenarcotic potential.

3. Workers may also be exposed to chemicals that act on different target organs; in that case, each exposure should be treated as such, when there is no evidence of interaction.

4. Workers are also exposed to physical factors, such as noise, hot or cold climate, or work posture. Adherence to the OEL does not ensure absence of health risk from the total workload.

5. Life-style, home environment, use of pharmaceuticals (prescribed or abused), environmental climate, or nutrition may affect the toxicokinetics and/or dynamics of the agent in question. The WHO[51, 54] extensively discussed various examples of chemical exposure combined with these other factors.

6. In conclusion, OELs should always be geared to the *total actual work situation* in a department, and also take into account the socially accepted life-style of the workers in question.

Short-Term Exposure Limits

Occupational exposure limits usually are presented as time-weighted averages (TWA) per eight-hour work shift. However, the actual level in air will vary around the mean; the level often shows not a normal, but a log normal distribution. The upper accepted deviation of the mean should also be established.

The ACGIH[2] distinguishes various limits, specified according to time and frequency:

1. The "normal" TLV-TWA.

2. The short-term exposure limit (STEL), i.e., that concentration to which workers can be exposed for a short period of time without suffering from irritation, chronic or irreversible tissue damage, narcosis of sufficient degree to increase the likelihood of accidental injury, impair self-rescue or materially reduce work efficiency, provided that the TLV-TWA is not exceeded. Exposure at the STEL should not be longer than 15 minutes and not be repeated more than four times per day, within at least 60 minutes between successive exposures at the STEL. In some cases, TLV-STELs may be more relevant for health protection than the TLV-TWA, when the concentration is more important than the duration of exposure, as in the case of exposure to nitrogen dioxide.

3. *Ceiling values*, or TLV-C, which should not be exceeded even instantaneously, particularly in the case of highly irritating or

toxic substances. However, this requires continuous environmental monitoring with a signal that warns when the ceiling is going to be exceeded.

Some specific limits have been proposed to be used as a guide in abnormal work situations. *Emergency exposure limits* (EEL) refer to concentrations that can be tolerated without adversely affecting health during exposure for 5, 15, 30, or 60 minutes in an emergency; they can be used for planning preventive measures, e.g., escape routes.[3] *Emergency tolerance limits* (ETL) refer to inevitable peak exposures at planned points of time during the work period, e.g., during launching rockets.[35] *Maximum peak concentrations* limit exposures that occur more often under normal work conditions, e.g., during the opening of a reactor vessel.[42] Limits may also be expressed in exposure time: *time of useful function* (TUF) indicates the time available for safety measure in an airplane (e.g., acute decompression or rapid smoke development).[20]

Figure 29–4 illustrates various limits discussed in this paragraph.

Misuse of OELs

The implementation of OELs requires not only knowledge of the number value of the OEL but first of all expert understanding of measurement strategy, the toxicologic data base, and the underlying value judgments. Interpretation and application demand trained occupational physicians and hygienists. Too often, OELs are treated merely as numbers, whereas the same OEL for different chemicals may aim to prevent essentially different health hazards. Occupational exposure limits should never be casually manipulated with pocket calculators. The ACGIH[2] emphasized that OELs (TLVs) are *not* intended for the following uses:

1. As a relative index of toxicity (Example: the TLVs for hydrogen sulfide (10 ppm) and hydrogen cyanide (10 ppm-C) appear to indicate lower risk than the TLV for hydrogen chloride (5 ppm-C), although the first two aim at prevention of acute mortality, whereas the TLV for hydrogen chloride prevents irritation of mucosa
2. In the evaluation or control of community air pollution
3. In estimating the toxic potential of continuous, interrupted exposure or other extended work periods
4. As proof or disproof of an existing disease or physical condition
5. For adoption by countries whose working conditions widely differ from those in the U.S.A. and where substances and processes differ.

It might have been added that OELs also should not be applied as such in working conditions under high or low oxygen pressure (as in caisson work or at high altitudes) which demand an unusual workload.

Unlisted Chemicals

For many chemicals, no OEL is known. When the chemical is rarely present in air, an OEL is not necessary. The ACGIH 1986–1987 document[2] also lists a number of substances that are considered of low toxicity and are merely regarded as "nuisance" particulates, e.g., calcium carbonate, calcium silicate, glycerin mix, zinc oxide dust, and starch. The TWA is set at 5 mg/cu m of respirable dust. However, one should be aware of toxic impurities. Too easily, welding fumes are considered as inert nuisance dust; the composition, however, depends upon the alloy welded and the process and electrodes used. Welding fumes may even contain certain potentially carcinogenic chromium compounds. Moreover, inhalation of so-called inert dust may affect the elimination from the respiratory tract of other toxic dusts. In principle, completely inert dusts do not exist.

Novel Work Schedules

More and more novel work schedules are being introduced. In view of the high rate of unemployment, decreases of the total work week to 32 or 36 hours are considered and even beginning to be introduced. A 35–36-hour workweek may involve seven-hour days, five days a week, with two days off, but also 12-hour days, three days a week, with four days off. Another approach is to in-

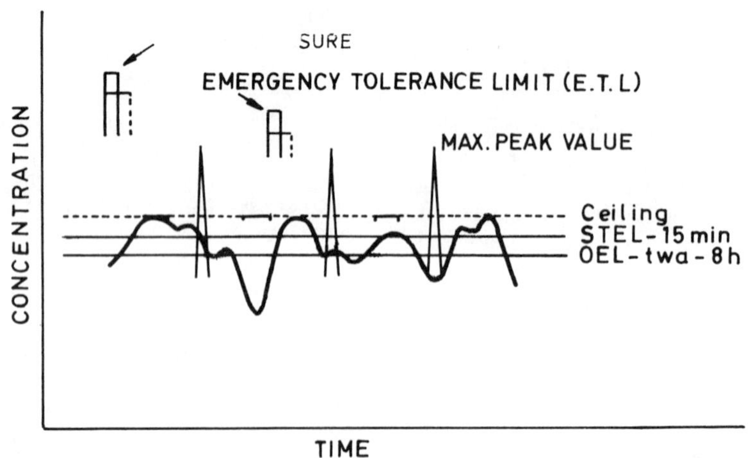

FIG 29–4.
Schematic presentation of various permissible limits.

crease the length of paid holidays. Do these new work schedules affect the OELs?

In view of the many uncertainties of the OELs, the biologic variability in response, and the warning that OEL numbers should not be misused for simple calculations, one should be very cautious about simply increasing the OEL by 20% in the case of a 32-hour workweek—all depends upon the specific toxicokinetics and toxicodynamics of the agent.

For those irritants whose concentration determines the OEL, no increase is permitted. The same may be true for narcotics and prenarcotics. For agents with a very long biologic half-life ($T_{1/2}$) and for which the effect depends upon the target organ burden, the equilibrium level, will increase with the concentration in air but not with the duration of exposure. For agents with a $T_{1/2}$ of 24 hours, the dose taken up in three workdays will have been eliminated after four days off. However, when the target organ burden exceeds the no-adverse effect level (NAEL), when the worker is on a 12-hour-day, three-days-a-week schedule, signs or symptoms may occur at an earlier date than when the same dose is taken up over a normal workweek.

Brief and Scala[6] offered a preliminary approach to take into account both the increased working hours per day and the decreased hours of recovery in the same 24-hour period, not taking into account the number of nonexposure days. They suggested that an OEL-Reduction Factor (RF) could be calculated as follows:

$$RF = 8 \times 24 - h$$

in which h is the number of working hours per day. With increasing h, RF decreases. This proposal should not be applied for work schedules with less than seven or eight hours a day or 35 hours per week. However, the authors did not take into account the $T_{1/2}$, the longer time off, and the significance of the target organ burden. They emphasized the need for a cautious approach, with good medical surveillance. It should be acknowledged that Brief and Scala discussed the need for reduction of the OEL in view of a longer working time per day, and not the possibility of increasing the OEL in view of the shorter work week. Although there may be reason to adapt OELs to normal working schedules, this should only be done after an expert reevaluation of the toxicologic data, and always case by case. For further review of this area of concern, refer to Paustenbach (in Patty's *Industrial Hygiene and Toxicology*, 1985, vol 3A, New York, John Wiley and Sons) concerning occupational exposure limits, pharmacokinetics, and unusual work schedules.

REFERENCES

1. American Conference of Governmental Industrial Hygienists: *Documentation of the Threshold Limit Values* ed 5. Cincinnati, ACGIH, 1980.
2. American Conference of Governmental Industrial Hygienists: *Threshold Limit Values and Biological Exposure Indices for 1986–1987*. Cincinnati, ACGIH, 1986.
3. American Industrial Hygiene Association: Emergency exposure limits. *Am Ind Hyg Assoc J* 1964; 25:578–579.
4. Barlow SM, Sullivan FM: *Reproductive Hazards of Industrial Chemicals*. London, Academic Press, 1982.
5. Breuer W, und Henschler D: Maximale Arbeitsplatzkonzentrationen: Analytische Bewertung von Durchschnitts- und Spitzenkonzentrationen. *Arbeitsmedizin, Sozialmedizin, Präventivmedizin* 1975; 10:165–170.
6. Brief RS, Scala RA: Occupational exposure limits for novel work schedules. *Am Ind Hyg Assoc J* 1975; 36:467–469.
7. Calabrese EJ: *Pollutants and High Risk Groups: The Biological Basis of Increased Human Susceptibility to Environmental and Occupational Pollutants*. New York, John Wiley & Sons, 1978a.
8. Calabrese EJ: *Methodological Approaches to Deriving Environmental and Occupational Health Standards*. New York, John Wiley & Sons, 1978b.
9. Carpenter RA: Scientific information, expert judgment and political decision making. *J Occup Med* 1976; 18:292–296.
10. Clarkson T, Norberg G, Sager PR: Reproductive and developmental toxicity of metals. New York, Plenum Publishing Corp, 1983.
11. Corn M: Regulations, standards and occupational hygiene within the USA in the 1980s. *Ann Occup Hyg* 1983; 27:91–105.
12. Dinman BD: Development of workplace environment standards in foreign countries: I Historical perspectives; criteria of response utilized in the USSR. II Concepts of higher nervous function in the USSR. III Procedures for development of MAC values in the USSR. *J Occup Med* 1976; 18:409–417; 18:477–484; 18:556–560.
13. Dinman BD, Sussman NB: Uncertainty, risk and the role of epidemiology in public policy development. *J Occup Med* 1983; 25:511–516.
14. Doll R, Peto R: *The Cause of Cancer*. Oxford, Oxford Medical Publications, 1980.
15. Døssing M: Noninvasive assessment of microsomal enzyme activity in occupational medicine: Present state of knowledge and future perspectives. *Int Arch Occup Environ Health* 1984; 53:205–218.
16. Drope E: Approaches to the evaluation of compliance. Paper read at the CEFIC-Symposium on Occupational Exposure Limits and Harmonisation in the Setting and Control of OELs for the Protection of Workers. Brussels, 1984.
17. Enterline PhE, Marsh GM: Cancer among workers exposed to arsenic and other substances in a copper smelter. *Am J Epidemiol* 1982; 116:895–911.
18. Fabro S: Reproductive toxicology: State of the art 1982. *Am J Ind Med* 1983; 4:391–395.
19. Food Safety Council: Quantitative risk assessment. *Food Cosmet Toxicol* 1980; 18:711–734.
20. Gaume JG, Bartek P: Theoretical determination of the time of useful function (TUF) on exposure to combinations of toxic gases. *Aerospace Med* 1969; 40:1353–1357.
21. Hatch TF: Criteria for hazardous exposure limits, *Arch Environ Health* 1973; 27:231.
22. Henschler D (ed): *Gesundheitsschädliche Arbeitsstoffe: Toxikologisch-arbeitsmedizinische Begründung von MAK-Werten*. Weinheim, Chemie-Verlag, 1981.
23. Hernberg S: "Negative" results in cohort studies: How to recognize fallacies. *Scand J Work Environ Health* 1981; 7[suppl 4]: 121–126.
24. Higginson J: The meaning of a "threshold," considerations applying to carcinogens in general. Paper read at the World Symposium on Asbestos, Montreal, Canada, Oct 5–9, 1982.
25. Hoel DG, Kaplan NL, Anderson MW: Implication of nonlinear kinetics on risk estimation in carcinogenesis. *Science* 1983; 219:1032–1037.
26. Holmberg B, Winell M: Occupational health standards: An International comparison. *Scand J Work Environ Health* 1977; 3:1–15.
27. International Agency for the Research on Cancer: *IARC Monographs of the Carcinogenic Risk of Chemicals to Humans*, suppl 4. Lyon, IARC, 1982.
28. Klinkert H: Some remarks by the chemical industry. Paper read at the CEFIC Symposium on Occupational Exposure Limits and Harmo-

nization in the Setting and Control of OELs for the Protection of Workers. Brussels, 1984.

29. Kotin P: Carcinogenesis: Problems and paradoxes. *J Occup Med* 1982; 24:290–294.
30. Lauwerys RR: Industrial chemical exposure: Guidelines for biological monitoring. Davis, Cal, Biomedical Publishers, 1983.
31. Mattison DR (ed): Reproductive toxicology. *Am J Ind Med* 1983; 4:393.
32. National Academy of Science: Principles for evaluating chemicals in the environment: A report of the Committee for the Working Conference on Principles of Protocols for evaluating chemicals in the environment. Washington, DC, NAS, 1975.
33. Nisbet ICT, Karch NJ: Chemical hazards to human reproduction. Park Ridge, Ill, Noyes Data Corp, 1983.
34. Occupational Safety and Health Administration (OSHA): *Federal Register* 1983; 48:1864.
35. Ricca PM: Exposure criteria for fluorine rocket propellants. *Arch Environ Health* 1966; 12:399–407.
36. Sanotzkii IV (ed): *Metody opzedelinija toksicnosti i opasnosti himicesckik vescestiv*. Moscow, Medicina, 1970, p 11–12 (in Russian). Quoted by WHO, 1978.
37. Sanotzkii IV, Ulanova IP: *Hygienic and Toxicological Criteria of Harmfulness in Evaluating Hazards of Chemical Compounds*. Moscow, Centre of International Projects, 1983.
38. Scheffers ThML, Jongeneelen FJ, Bragt PC: Development of effect-specific limit values (ESLVs) for solvent mixtures in painting. *Ann Occup Hyg* 1984; 28:386–398.
39. Sherwin RP: What is an adverse health effect? *Environ Health Perspect* 1983; 52:177–182.
40. Stokinger HE: Modus operandi of threshold limits, Committee of the ACGIH. *Am Ind Hyg Assoc J* 1964; 25:589–594.
41. Stokinger HE: Criteria and procedures for assessing the toxic responses to industrial chemicals, in International Labour Organisation (ILO): *Permissible Levels of Toxic Substances in the Working Environment*. Geneva, ILO, 1970.
42. Stokinger HE: Industrial air standards, theory and practice. *J Occup Med* 1973; 15:429–431.
43. Ulfvarson U: Limitations of the use of employee exposure data on air contaminants in epidemiologic studies. *Int Arch Occup Environ Health* 1983; 52:285–300.
44. Welch K, Higgins I, Oh M, et al: Arsenic exposure, smoking and respiratory cancer in copper smelter workers. *Arch Environ Health* 1982; 37:325–335.
45. Williams JR, Clark WL: Science and politics: The possible regulation of cancer promoters. *Environ Health Perspect* 1983; 50:351–354.
46. World Health Organization: *Methods Used in the USSR for Establishing Biologically Safe Levels of Toxic Substances*. Geneva, WHO, 1975.
47. World Health Organization: *Methods used in establishing permissible Levels in Occupational Exposure to Harmful Agents*, Tech Report 601, Geneva, WHO, 1977.
48. World Health Organization: *Principles and Methods for Evaluating the Toxicity of Chemicals*, Environ Health Criteria 6, pt I. Geneva, WHO, 1978.
49. World Health Organization: *Recommended Health-Based Limits in Occupational Exposure to Heavy Metals*, Tech Report 647. Geneva, WHO, 1980.
50. World Health Organization: *Recommended Health-Based Limits in Occupational Exposure to Selected Organic Solvents*, Tech Report 664. Geneva, WHO, 1981a.
51. World Health Organization: *Health Effects of Combined Exposures in the Work Environment*. Tech Report 662. Geneva, WHO, 1981b.
52. World Health Organization: *Recommended Health-Based Limits in Exposure to Pesticides*, Tech Report 677. Geneva, WHO, 1982.
53. World Health Organization: *Recommended Health-Based Occupational Exposure Limits for Selected Vegetable Dusts, Tech* Report 684. Geneva WHO, 1983a.
54. World Health Organization: *Combined Exposure to Chemicals. Health Aspects of Chemical Safety*, Interim Document 11. Copenhagen, WHO, European Region, 1983b.
55. World Health Organization: *Guidelines on Studies in Environmental Epidemiology*, Environ Health Criteria 27. Geneva, WHO, 1983c.
56. World Health Organization: *Recommended Health-Based Occupational Exposure Limits for Selected Respiratory Irritants. Tech* Report 707. Geneva, WHO, 1984.
57. Zielhuis RL: Standards setting for work conditions as risky behaviour, in Grandjean Ph (ed): *Standards Setting*. Copenhagen, Arbejdsmiljøfondet, 1977a, p 15–34.
58. Zielhuis RL: Differences in standards in East and West, in Grandjean Ph (ed): *Standards Setting*. Copenhagen, Arbejdsmiljøfondet, 1977b, pp 133–146.
59. Zielhuis, RL: Biological monitoring. *Scand J Work Environ Health* 1978; 4:1–18.
60. Zielhuis RL, Notten WRF: Permissible levels for occupational exposure: Basic concepts. *Int Arch Occup Environ Health* 1978/1979; 42:269–281.
61. Zielhuis RL, van der Kreek FW: The use of a safety factor in setting health-based permissible levels for occupational exposure. I A proposal. II Comparison of extrapolated and published permissible levels. *Int Arch Occup Environ Health* 1979; 42:191–201, 203–215.
62. Zielhuis RL: Occupational and environmental standard setting for metals: More questions than answers. *Toxicol Environ Chem* 1984; 9:27–40.
63. Zielhuis RL, Stijkel A, Verberk MM, et al: *Health Risks to Female Workers in Occupational Exposure to Chemical Agents*. Heidelberg, Springer-Verlag, 1984a.
64. Zielhuis RL: Biological monitoring, in Berlin A, Yodaiken RE, Henman BA (eds): *Assessment of Toxic Agents at the Workplace: Roles of Ambient and Biological Monitoring*. Boston, Nijhoff, 1984b.
65. Zielhuis RL, Wibowo AAE: Standard Setting and Metal Speciation: Arsenic, in Nriagen JOW (ed): *Changing Metal Cycles and Human Health*. Berlin, Springer-Verlag, 1984c.
66. Zielhuis RL: Total exposure and workers' health. *Ann Occup Hyg* 1985; 29:463–475.

30

Carbon Monoxide

Eric P. Kindwall, M.D.

Carbon monoxide poisoning is the most common of all poisonings in industry today and is responsible for over half of the poisoning fatalities reported each year in the United States.[12] Carbon monoxide is colorless and odorless and therefore gives no warning of its presence under any circumstances. In addition, almost any industrial item produced today involves the use of fire, oxidation, or combustion at some point during its manufacture. For these reasons, the possibilities of carbon monoxide poisoning are ubiquitous. Nearly all other industrial toxins have a characteristic odor, taste, or appearance, or produce some sort of irritation that warns the potential victim, a factor not present in carbon monoxide poisoning. Another reason that makes this form of poisoning particularly insidious is that the early symptoms can resemble other diseases. Nausea, headache, and dizziness are easily confused with the onset of a cold, stomach flu, or some other common disorder. Therefore, even though thousands of cases of carbon monoxide poisoning are reported annually, we can be sure that additional thousands are never recognized for what they are. It is incumbent on the occupational physician to be aware of this fact and have a high index of suspicion. The victim of an explosion with postconcussion syndrome or a man with the odor of alcohol on his breath may also have carbon monoxide poisoning. If the possibility of carbon monoxide poisoning is not considered, the correct diagnosis will never be made.

SOURCES OF EXPOSURE

Certain industries are recognized to be particularly hazardous with relation to carbon monoxide. These are iron and steel foundries, petroleum refining plants, kraft paper pulp mills, sintering mills, and facilities for the manufacture of formaldehyde and coke. Within these industries, the chief sources of carbon monoxide have been identified as the cupola in the iron and steel foundry, the catalytic cracking units in petroleum refineries, the lime kilns and the kraft recovery furnaces in kraft paper mills, and the sintering of blast furnace feed in sintering plants.[21]

Although these obvious and well-documented sources historically are known to produce large amounts of carbon monoxide, the greatest danger actually lies in such processes as welding, garage work, and forklift truck operation. Here, because the amounts of carbon monoxide produced usually do not create problems, carbon monoxide poisoning may strike without warning if either the source of carbon monoxide increases for some reason or ventilation is decreased. This chapter will consider both acute and chronic exposures to carbon monoxide, which produce different syndromes.

PATHOPHYSIOLOGY

Our understanding of the mechanism of carbon monoxide poisoning has recently undergone a rather dramatic change. It is true that carbon monoxide has an affinity for the hemoglobin moiety of the blood approximately 200–300 times that of oxygen, but most important, it enters the tissues and attacks the cytochrome system. This latter effect is what causes the clinical morbidity and eventual mortality. Most physiologists for the past 80 years have looked at the formation of carboxyhemoglobin as the main culprit. This has been because even small amounts (parts per million) of carbon monoxide could cause significant carboxyhemoglobinemia, and carboxyhemoglobin is incapable of carrying oxygen to the tissues. The explanation seemed quite straightforward, and it was not felt necessary to probe more deeply into the question of tissue toxicity.

However, beginning in 1926, Warburg noted that the action of the cytochromes was inhibited by carbon monoxide.[22] Haldane, in 1927, found that animals exposed to high concentrations of carbon monoxide under hyperbaric conditions developed a tissue toxicity despite adequate oxygenation.[6] In these tests, Haldane exposed animals to 3.1 atm of oxygen and then added an additional atmosphere of carbon monoxide. The carboxyhemoglobin levels rose to 98%, but while oxygen was present dissolved in the plasma, the rats sufferred no ill effects. However, when a second atmosphere of carbon monoxide was added, the rats promptly died. This indicated that carbon monoxide was having a direct effect on the tissues. Lewey and Drabkin noted that in dogs that had been chronically exposed to low levels of carbon monoxide so as to produce an 8.7% carboxyhemoglobinemia, the heart failed to extract lactate and pyruvate.[11] This was not explainable on the basis of an 8% or 9% relative anemia. In 1950, Chance demonstrated that mitochondria are inhibited and that the specific enzyme involved is cytochrome A_3 oxidase.[3] The situation was made more complicated by Ball, who in 1951 showed that carbon monoxide and oxygen compete for cytochrome oxidase but that cytochrome prefers oxygen in beef heart 9.2 to 1.[2] One was therefore initially led to think that the patient would have to be dead nine times over before any clinical effect could be seen from cytochrome oxidase inhibition.

Peirce et al. poisoned dogs with carbon monoxide and then compared treatment with hypothermia to treatment with hyperbaric oxygen.[15] The hypothermia was of sufficient degree to produce 4 vol % of dissolved oxygen in the arterial blood, but survivors were not obtainable. The failure of hypothermia suggested that hemoglobin binding as the sole cause of carbon monoxide toxicity needed reexamination.

Ingenito et al., in 1974, used an isovolemic heart preparation immersed in a hemoglobin-free perfusate to show that carbon monoxide affected myocardial metabolism.[7]

The most convincing study was done in 1975 by Goldbaum et al., who poisoned dogs with 13% carbon monoxide inhaled in air.[5] The dogs died within 15 minutes to an hour, with carboxyhemoglobin levels between 54% and 90%. The average was 68% carboxyhemoglobin. He then partially exsanguinated a second group of dogs and transfused them with plasma and colloid to maintain normal blood volumes. Even though 68% of the circulating red blood cells had been removed before volume was restored to normal, the dogs showed no ill effects. As a final demonstration, a third group of dogs was partially exsanguinated as was the second group. When the blood volume was restored to normal, using pack cells containing 80% carboxyhemoglobin from donor dogs, there were again no ill effects. This was despite the fact the circulating carboxyhemoglobin in the third group ranged between 57% and 64%, with an average of 60%. Goldbaum and co-workers concluded that it was tissue toxicity in the form of cytochrome A_3 oxidase poisoning which was the most important factor in carbon monoxide poisoning.[5]

These observations help explain my observations of the past 15 years that the carboxyhemoglobin levels reported by the laboratory frequently do not correlate well with the patient's clinical appearance.[9] Olsky and Wood found that in 100 patients admitted to Lutheran General Hospital in Park Ridge, Illinois, the carboxyhemoglobin level had no statistical prognostic significance (unpublished data).

A great deal has to be learned about the exact mechanism of cytochrome-monoxide binding, the stability and dynamics of this bond, and how it is affected by increased partial pressures of oxygen. Geyer et al. found that bloodless rats that had fluorocarbon substituted for their blood could survive 17 hours in a mixture of 10% carbon monoxide and 90% oxygen at 1 atm. Apparently, the 7.05 vol % freely available oxygen carried in physical solution by the fluorocarbon was sufficient to protect the cytochromes and prevented tissue toxicity.[4] Since carbon monoxide becomes dissolved in all the tissues of the body, it is even conceivable that other enzyme systems might be affected which have thus far escaped our attention. In summary, it can be said that carbon monoxide poisoning is highly complex and that a great deal more is involved than simple carboxyhemoglobin formation.

It is of interest to note that cyanide also attacks the same enzyme, cytochrome A_3 oxidase (although in its oxidized form), and that hyperbaric oxygen also ameliorates cyanide poisoning. Skene and Norman et al.[17] found that in mice that were poisoned with cyanide to produce a 96% mortality, treatment with hyperbaric oxygen at 2 atm reduced the mortality to 20%. Ivanov[8] was also able to restore electrical activity to the cerebral cortex of the mouse with hyperbaric oxygen after poisoning with cyanide. Several human cases have also been treated in the chamber with success.[20]

At any given level of carbon monoxide in the air the victim breathes, the rate at which his blood becomes saturated with carbon monoxide is directly proportional to cardiac output. Thus, a man working vigorously will note the onset of symptoms and signs much more quickly than will a man who is sedentary or at rest. From the practical standpoint, a man driving a forklift truck will have a much lower level of carbon monoxide in his bloodstream than will the man who is loading heavy barrels onto a pallet in the same environment. A person running around in a building seeking an escape route from a fire will be overcome more quickly than will someone quietly asleep.

When the tissues of the body become hypoxic, the heart must supply more blood by increasing both its rate and its ouput. Thus, the coronary arteries must supply more oxygen to the heart. Normally, the myocardium extracts 75% of the oxygen supplied to it via the coronary arteries. This is much more than the brain uses. Therefore, anyone with coronary heart disease soon will suffer from hypoxia of the myocardium, and the heart should be considered the first target organ in carbon monoxide poisoning because of the necessity for increased cardiac output. Normally, the myocardium extracts pyruvate and lactate from the coronary circulation for oxidation. When the carboxyhemoglobin reaches a mean of 8.7%, the myocardium fails to extract either of these two substances and actually produces both,[1] but this is probably due to cytochrome inhibition.

Chronic exposure to levels of carbon monoxide of various concentrations, but not immediately lethal, has produced changes in animals, both behavioral and histologic, that have proven to be extremely variable. On the basis of work from a number of investigators, it would be safe to say that it is presently impossible to state what levels of carbon monoxide in the blood will produce permanent pathologic changes in human beings. However, one investigator found that dogs exposed to 100 ppm carbon monoxide for 5¾ hours a day, six days a week, for 11 weeks, showed no electroencephalographic changes but did show psychomotor disturbances and cerebral cortical damage that tended to follow the course of the blood vessels. This same investigator also found that in one experiment, a diminished cardiac output was associated with more damage to the brain.

However, Meyer[13] found that the same pathologic anatomical changes occur after experimental cyanide poisoning. This supports the evidence that carbon monoxide disrupts cytochrome metabolism.

Brain damage can consist of infarction of the cerebral cortex, degenerative changes, formation of cysts, gliosis, paravascular infiltration, loss of myelin, and softening of the white matter. The basal ganglia show the most severe damage, with loss of cells and demyelination.[11]

In summary, carbon monoxide produces tissue hypoxia and, along with it, the expected changes in function and, if prolonged and severe, histopathologic changes that are associated with hypoxia.

DIAGNOSIS

Exposure to a known source of carbon monoxide, such as being in a closed garage or being overcome by smoke inhalation, is the primary diagnostic clue.

Textbooks classically refer to persons suffering from carbon monoxide poisoning as having a red flush with "cherry red lips." This may be true in some cases, but in my experience, the patient may well appear pale or of normal color, so coloration is of no diagnostic significance. As noted previously, the clinical picture in relation to a given blood level of carboxyhemoglobin is extremely variable and some persons may be profoundly unconscious with a carboxyhemoglobin percentage in their blood of lower than 20%. Others may be able to converse with levels as high as 58%.

The most common premonitory signs of carbon monoxide poisoning are headache, nausea and, occasionally, breathlessness. People with marginal coronary arteries may experience anginal pain as cardiac output is driven upward. A heavy smoker may be less tolerant to higher levels of carbon monoxide than a non-smoker, since he may have a "normal" level of 5%–6% carboxyhemoglobin. After these premonitory signs have appeared and the subject continues to remain in the carbon monoxide atmosphere, he may suffer from muscle weakness, dizziness, and confusion. This progresses on to stupor and eventual unconsciousness. It is important to note that there may be a phase in the poisoning where the victim is conscious and aware of his or her surroundings but is unable to move because of extreme muscle weakness. This phenomenon prevents some individuals who attempt suicide by means of carbon monoxide from changing their minds while still conscious.

When a person has been overcome by carbon monoxide and is brought to the emergency room or the clinic, a careful history gleaned from his rescuers generally will disclose the cause. However, in some situations, the presence of carbon monoxide in the person's work environment may be unknown and, then, the only definitive test is to quantify the amount of carbon monoxide present in either the blood or the breath. There are extremely accurate breath analyzers for carbon monoxide that are portable and will give an immediate indication if the person has been exposed. Other poisonous compounds do not interfere with an accurate carbon monoxide reading from these instruments, which use an electrochemical principle. The other very common test is to draw a blood sample, either venous or arterial, and to determine the amount of carboxyhemoglobin present. This can be done with a mass spectrometer but is accomplished more quickly and easily using the CoOximeter, manufactured by Instrumentation Laboratories, Cambridge, Massachusetts. It is important, however, that the CoOximeter be extremely well calibrated. A competent technician is necessary to keep this machine functional and have it provide data of any value.

In my experience, blood carboxyhemoglobin levels below 15% due to acute exposures rarely produce any symptoms. Between 15% and 25%, the patient may complain of headache and nausea. At levels above 25%, there may be electrocardiographic changes that show a depression of the S-T segment, especially in leads II, V_5 and V_6. If a level of 40% is encountered in the emergency room, the patient generally has a history of having been unconscious at the time he was removed from the exposure. I have seen prolonged exposures with blood levels of 36% and 38% produce death; on one occasion, I examined a victim who was dead on arrival with a level of 51%. However, relatively short exposures can produce carboxyhemoglobin levels that may run as high as 60% and 70%. Levels over 60%–66% usually are considered fatal. The highest carboxyhemoglobin levels I have encountered were 86% and 88% in victims who were dead on arrival. It would appear that 88% carboxyhemoglobin is about the maximum that the cardiovascular system can tolerate, even when it is in good condition, before function ceases.

The symptoms and signs do not correlate well with the absolute level in the blood. This usually can be explained on the basis of *length of exposure*. A carboxyhemoglobin level of 58% produced by a 15-minute exposure to extremely high levels of carbon monoxide has an infinitely better prognosis than a level of 38% in someone who has spent seven hours in a closed garage. In the latter case, the cytochromes have had time to be inhibited. When the unconscious patient arrives in the emergency room, in addition to getting a measurement of carboxyhemoglobin level from the blood, it is advisable to determine the state of the patient's electrolytes. Very frequently there is a profound acidosis despite adequate pulmonary ventilation. The arterial pH is the best indicator of clinical status and also correlates well with the prognosis. The acidosis should be corrected with intravenously administered bicarbonate as rapidly as possible. I treated one patient who required eight 44.6-mEq ampules of bicarbonate to bring the pH from 6.88 to 7.03. Often the potassium is low, and this must also be corrected. Other electrolyte functions usually are normal except that in certain cases of smoke inhalation, the carbon dioxide may be high due to pulmonary edema caused by chemical irritation.

TREATMENT

Carbon monoxide is eliminated exponentially, so it is useful to discuss the elimination rate in terms of half-lives. The normal elimination of carbon monoxide is quite slow because of its greater affinity for hemoglobin than for oxygen. If a person is taken from a closed garage and given country-fresh air to breathe, half of the absorbed carbon monoxide will be eliminated in five hours and 20 minutes. If the patient is given 100% oxygen to breathe by a tightly fitting mask, the actual measured elimination half-time is one hour and 20 minutes. This occurs only if the mask is exceptionally well-fitting. Most resuscitator units and anesthesia masks do not fit tightly enough to produce this curve. However, a good double-seal oronasal face mask usually can be relied on. If the patient appears to be in great respiratory distress or if his or her blood gases are extremely abnormal, one should consider intubation with an endotracheal tube. Our rule of thumb is that if the P_{CO_2} is greater than 60 mm Hg, the patient should be intubated immediately. There is danger in giving too much bicarbonate if the patient is not well ventilated, and in severe cases of smoke inhalation, the patient will require a volume-cycled respirator and competent pulmonary care.

In cases of smoke inhalation, a portable chest film is indicated early. Do not overlook the possibility that the patient may have aspirated while unconscious. The endotracheal tube should be well-suctioned to remove as much of the thick, black mucus or vomit as is possible. Laryngeal and subglottic edema are important dangers to be watched for, especially in small children. If the patient is a smoke-inhalation victim, burns about the face should immediately put the physician on the alert for laryngeal edema.

Treatment with 100% oxygen, either with or without a ventilator, is continued until the carboxyhemoglobin level is below 10%. At that point, the blood gases should be determined, and if the patient is well-oxygenated, oxygen treatment may either be discontinued or be continued at a lesser percentage. In cases of smoke inhalation, the use of 10 mg of Decadron intravenously, followed by 4 mg intramuscularly every six hours, is recommended. Do not give steroids prior to hyperbaric treatment, since this sensitizes the patient to oxygen toxicity of both the lung and central nervous system. Appropriate cultures should be taken in cases of smoke inhalation, and the patient should be placed on antibiotics. In cases in which aspiration pneumonia or chemical pneumonitis is anticipated, a suitable broad-spectrum antibiotic may be used before the cultures are returned.

Treatment With Hyperbaric Oxygen

If a hyperbaric chamber is available, this is by far the preferred method of treatment in severe carbon monoxide poisoning. Failure to refer severely poisoned patients for hyperbaric treatment, if available, has resulted in successful malpractice suits. Hyperbaric chambers may be either of the large walk-in type or small, monoplace chambers that are pressurized with pure oxygen. The large chambers are pressurized with compressed air and the patient breathes oxygen by mask for reasons of fire safety. Under hyperbaric conditions, the carbon monoxide is eliminated much more rapidly and other advantages are realized. The rationale for hyperbaric treatment is as follows:

1. Carbon monoxide is apparently displaced from cytochrome A_3 oxidase by a surfeit of oxygen and electron transport is restored.

2. If the patient is given oxygen to breathe at 3 ATA, the half-time for carbon monoxide elimination from the blood is reduced to 23 minutes.

3. As soon as the patient breathes oxygen at 3 ATA, 6.4 vol % of completely available oxygen are physically dissolved in the plasma—enough to support metabolism even in the complete absence of functioning hemoglobin. The arteriovenous difference in the cerebral blood flow is only 6.1 vol %. Thus, the patient's problem with oxygenating the brain and other tissues is immediately over on reaching 3 ATA.

4. Intracranial pressure secondary to cerebral edema is reduced of the order of 50% within one minute of the commencement of oxygen breathing. This has been documented by Sukoff, Hollin, and Jacobson[19] in animal and human studies.

At our facility, we have a large walk-in chamber where we routinely use 3 ATA as a treatment pressure, and we treat until the level of carboxyhemoglobin is 10%. As can be seen from the foregoing, if a person comes in with a 40% concentration of carbon monoxide, within 46 minutes the level will have been reduced to 10% with treatment at 3 ATA. We often treat for 46 minutes, or two half-lives, at 3 ATA and then drop to 2 ATA for the remainder of treatment or until the level is below 10%. In very severe cases where exposure has been prolonged and the patient is deeply unconscious, I may elect to use the U.S. Navy Decompression Sickness Treatment Table 6. This table starts at 2.8 ATA and provides a total of four hours of oxygen breathing at pressures of 2.8 to 1 ATA over a total chamber period of 285 minutes. The extra 45 minutes are used up in "air breaks" of 5–15 minutes interspersed in the schedule. (See Chapter 25.) The longest we have treated anyone in the chamber at 2 and 3 ATA in combination is approximately five hours. If the patient has not fully recovered at the end of treatment, additional treatments can be given on a daily or twice daily basis for two to four days. Myers has reported experience with patients whose first memory after poisoning occurred during the second hyperbaric treatment.[14]

Our basic rule of thumb is that if patients have a carboxyhemoglobin level of 25% or greater, they are routinely treated in the chamber even if they not particularly ill. This is because the symptoms will go away much sooner, and the patient will be spared the prolonged headache and nausea that usually follow carbon monoxide poisoning. This may also eliminate delayed aftereffects.

The electrocardiogram can be a good diagnostic tool in carbon monoxide poisoning. In our hospital, a routine electrocardiogram (ECG) is done immediately on admission to the emergency room; if the S-T segments are found to be depressed, the patient is taken immediately to the hyperbaric chamber even before the laboratory report is available. In other words, one can treat on the basis of the ECG alone.

In the event that one has only a one-person chamber and the patient is not breathing or has had cardiac arrest or is fibrillating on arrival at the emergency room, the patient should be treated with oxygen at atmospheric pressure first, and all ancillary aids, such as correction of electrolyte imbalance, along with defibrillation, should be carried out before placing the patient in the chamber. Particularly important here is the use of bicarbonate. When using a one-person chamber, it may be advantageous to place an endotracheal tube in the airway if the patient is unconscious before compressing him or her.

Occasionally, patients will experience ear discomfort during pressurization, and in the large walk-in chamber this may be alleviated by simple myringotomy. However, in the seriously monoxized patient treated in the one-person chamber, rupture of the eardrum perhaps is not too important, since spontaneous healing will take place within ten days. Aspiration pneumonia perhaps is not as likely in hyperbaric treatment, since during rapid decompression, vomitus tends to be forced out of the trachea.

Complications of Hyperbaric Treatment.—Rupture of the eardrums has already been discussed, but it must be kept in mind that oxygen toxicity can be extremely serious at pressures of 3 ATA. Within approximately three hours, even someone quietly at rest will experience a grand mal seizure. For this reason, exposure times at 3 ATA must be limited to no more than 90 minutes. If the patient is actively fighting or agitated, the likelihood of his having a seizure is much greater. For this reason, intravenously administered Valium, 10 mg, sometimes is used to calm a combative or agitated patient. With use of the one-person chamber, it is important that the patient be firmly lashed to the stretcher if he is combative. Very often, patients with carbon monoxide poisoning will be totally confused and believe that they are being hurt in some way by the physician.

Even at 2 ATA, oxygen poisoning can take place. This is in the form of the Lorrain Smith effect or oxygen toxicity to the lungs. Within approximately six hours of continuous exposure to 2 ATA, the patient will experience substernal pain, decreased vital capacity, and patchy atelectasis. If exposure is continued chronically, this can give rise to pulmonary microhemorrhage and fibrosis. We normally do not expose a patient continuously to 2 ATA of 100% oxygen for more than two hours.

FOLLOW-UP CARE

In cases of carbon monoxide poisoning uncomplicated by smoke inhalation, once the patient has been removed from the hyperbaric chamber, he or she generally is free to leave if there are no residual clinical symptoms. This is true even if the carboxyhemoglobin level has been as high as 55% or 60%. Obviously, if the patient remains sick even on removal from the chamber, further care must be provided. The most comon aftermath of severe carbon monoxide poisoning is cerebral edema. This can be countered with the use of steroids. Ten milligrams of Decadron is given intravenously on removal from the chamber, followed by 4 mg of Decadron intramuscularly every six hours. This may be continued for up to 72 hours and withdrawn abruptly. If steroid administration is carried beyond 72 hours, the steroids must be tapered. Steroid therapy is withheld until after the patient is removed from the chamber because it tends to exacerbate oxygen toxicity.

Patients treated with hyperbaric oxygen do not appear to develop cardiac or cerebral difficulties later. With nonhyperbaric treatment, arrhythmias two or three days after poisoning have been noted, along with elevated serum glutamic oxaloacetic transaminase, lactic dehydrogenase, and creatine phosphokinase. Patients also may develop confusion and other signs of mental deterioration after a delay of several days. In patients treated in the hyperbaric chamber, follow-up studies have revealed no change in the ECG and blood enzymes two to four days after treatment, or subsequent cerebral difficulties. For this reason, we do not hesitate to send clinically well persons directly home after hyperbaric treatment, but instruct them and their relatives that they should return if headache or other symptoms develop.

PREVENTION OF CARBON MONOXIDE POISONING

It is incumbent upon the industrial physician to identify potential sources of carbon monoxide poisoning and see to it that where a risk of carbon monoxide buildup exists, appropriate monitoring is undertaken. It should be remembered that there may be other causes of elevated carbon monoxide levels in the blood. Carbon monoxide can be produced endogenously in hemolytic anemia, and methylene chloride inhalation (200 ppm) has produced carboxyhemoglobin levels as high as 9.4% in eight hours.[16, 18]

Carbon monoxide poisoning tends to be seasonal, especially in the temperate climates. When an industrial process is started in the spring or summer, no one may suffer from overt poisoning, but when the doors and windows are closed during the winter months to conserve heat, unacceptable levels of carbon monoxide suddenly may appear. Thus, if there is any sort of combustion process going on in your plant, be especially wary as the cold winter months approach.

In an effort to prevent carbon monoxide poisoning, gasoline-powered forklift trucks have been replaced in many instances with electric trucks and propane-fueled trucks. Obviously, electric trucks are preferred. Irving H. Davis, regional chief of the Division of Occupational Health in Michigan, conducted some field investigations in 1970 that turned up interesting data supporting increased use of electric vehicles.[10] Contrary to popular opinion, propane-powered equipment may emit as much or more carbon monoxide than gasoline-fueled equipment. Propane users, believing themselves free from the carbon monoxide hazard, may neglect preventive maintenance and find themselves with critical problems. Others have relied on catalytic devices installed on internal combustion engine units to improve combustion and to lower emissions. Davis's investigations revealed that the devices were totally inoperative on 85% of the vehicles tested by the Michigan State Health Department. The industries regarded as particularly liable to carbon monoxide buildup from these units were auto assembly, appliance manufacturing, and auto parts manufacturing.

PERMISSIBLE THRESHOLD VALUES FOR CARBON MONOXIDE

A summary of the recommendations of the National Institute for Occupational Safety and Health (NIOSH) is as follows:

Employees are to be protected against acute carbon monoxide poisoning and deleterious myocardial alterations associated with levels of carboxyhemoglobin in excess of 5%. They are also to be provided protection from adverse behavioral manifestations resulting from exposure to low levels of carbon monoxide.

The recommended standard is designed to protect the safety and health of workers who are performing a normal eight-hour day, 40-hour week assignment. It was not designed for the population at large, and any extrapolation beyond the general worker population is unwarranted. Because of the well-defined relationship between smoking and a common exposure to carbon monoxide and inhaled smoke, the recommended standard may not provide the same degree of protection to those workers who smoke as it will to nonsmokers. Likewise, under conditions of reduced ambient oxygen concentration, such as would be encountered by workers at very high altitudes (e.g., 5000–8000 ft above sea level), the permissible exposure stated in the recommended standard should be lowered appropriately to compensate for loss in the oxygen-carrying capacity of the blood. In addition, workers with physical impairments that interfere with normal oxygen at liberty to the tissues will not be provided the same degree of protection as the general worker population. It is anticipated that the criteria and standard recommended in that document will be reviewed and revised as necessary.

Concentration

Occupation exposure to carbon monoxide shall be controlled so that no worker shall be exposed to a concentration greater than 35 ppm, as determined by a time-weighted reading, hopcalite-type carbon monoxide meter, calibrated against known concentrations of carbon monoxide, or by gas detector tube units certified under Title 42 of the Code of Regulations, Part 84.

No level of carbon monoxide to which workers are exposed shall exceed a ceiling concentration of 200 ppm.

Calibration, sampling, and analysis of carbon monoxide samples are to be in accordance with Appendix 1 of the Federal Regulations.

Medical Regulations

Each employer should provide medical surveillance for all workers who receive significant exposure to carbon monoxide as part of their work environment. Medical surveillance should include, but should not be limited to, the following:

1. Preplacement medical examination, including blood analysis for carboxyhemoglobin levels before and at the termination of the normal workday within one week of job placement, and determination of cholesterol and hemoglobin levels. The medical history should include the worker's smoking habits in terms of approximate number of cigarettes, cigars, or pipes smoked a day and number of years smoking has occurred. The medical history should also include some statement as to the presence or absence of disease symptoms in which hypoxia or increased oxygen demand is important, e.g., coronary heart disease, anemia, pulmonary heart disease, cerebrovascular disease, or thyrotoxicosis.

2. Medical examination on termination of employment must be carried out also.

Medical management may include recommendations ranging from job placement and improved work practices to specific therapy for individuals with one of the above diseases or its complications.

REFERENCES

1. Ayres SM, et al: Systemic and myocardial hemodynamic responses to relatively small concentration of carboxyhemoglobin (COHb). *Arch Environ Health* 1969; 18:699.
2. Ball EG, Strittmatter CF, Cooper O: The reaction of cytochrome oxidase with carbon monoxide. *J Biol Chem* 1951; 193:635–647.
3. Chance B, Erecinska M, Wagner M: Mitochondrial responses to carbon monoxide toxicity. *Ann NY Acad Sci* 1950; 174:193–204.
4. Geyer RP, Taylor K, Eccles R, et al: Survival of bloodless rats in 10% carbon monoxide. *Fed Proc* 1976; 35:828.
5. Goldbaum LR, Ramirez RG, Absalom KB: What is the mechanism of carbon monoxide toxicity? *Aviat Space Environ Med* 1975; 46:1289–1291.
6. Haldane JBS: Carbon monoxide as a tissue poison. *Bio Chem J* 1927; 21:1068–1075.
7. Ingenito AJ, Fiedler PC, Procita L: Negative inotropic action of carbon monoxide (CO) on the isolated isovolumic heart with a hemoglobin(HB)-free perfusate. *Fed Proc* 1974; 33:503.
8. Ivanov AP: Effects of increased oxygen pressure on animals poisoned by potassium cyanide. *J Farmakol Poksik* 1959; 22:468.
9. Kindwall EP: Carbon monoxide poisoning. *Hyperbaric Oxygen Rev* 1980; 1(2):115–122.
10. *Lead.* New York, Lead Industries Association, Inc, 1972, 35:10.
11. Lewey FH, Drabkin DL: Experimental chronic carbon monoxide poisoning in dogs. *Am J Med Sci* 1944; 208:502.
12. McBay AJ: Carbon monoxide poisoning (Law-Med Notes). *N Engl J Med* 1956; 272:252.
13. Meyer A: Uber Gehirnveranderungen bei Experimentelles Blausaurevergiftung. *Z Neurol Psych* 1933; 143:333.
14. Myers RAM, Snyder SK, Lindberg S, et al: Value of hyperbaric oxygen in suspected carbon monoxide poisoning. *JAMA* 1981; 246 (21):2478–2480.
15. Peirce EC II, Zacharias A, Alday JM, et al: Carbon monoxide poisoning: Experimental hypothermic and hyperbaric studies. *Surgery* 1972; 72:229–237.
16. Ratney RS, Wegman DH, Elkins HB: In vivo conversion of methylene chloride to carbon monoxide. *Arch Environ Health* 1974; 28:223.
17. Skene WG, Norman JP, Smith GP: Effect of hyperbaric oxygen in cyanide poisoning, in Brown I, Cox B (eds): *Proceedings of the Third International Conference on Hyperbaric Medicine*, Publ 1404. Washington, DC, National Academy of Science, National Research Council, 1966, pp 705–710.
18. Stewart RD, Hake C: Paint remover hazard. *JAMA* 1976; 235(4):398–401.
19. Sukoff MH, Hollin SA, Jacobson JH II: The protective effect of hyperbaric oxygenation in experimentally produced cerebral edema and compression. *Surgery* 1967; 62:40.
20. Trapp W: Massive cyanide poisoning with recovery: A boxing day story. *Can Med J* 1970; 102:517.
21. US Dept of Health, Education, and Welfare: *Criteria for a Recommended Standard for Occupational Exposure to Carbon Monoxide*. Rockville, Md, Health Services and Mental Health Administration, NIOSH, 1972.
22. Warburg O: *Biochem Z* 1926; 177:471.

31

Antimony, Arsenic, and Their Compounds

O. Bruce Dickerson, M.D., M.P.H.

Thomas H. F. Smith, Ph.D.

ANTIMONY AND ITS COMPOUNDS

Chemistry and Physical Properties

Antimony (Sb), like its relatives in Group V of the periodic table, is classified as an intermetal. It is closely related to arsenic in its chemical, physical, and physiologic properties. It has an atomic number of 51 and an atomic weight of 121.8. With a density of 6.7, it has a melting point of 631° C and a boiling point of 1750° C. It is primarily obtained from stibnite (antimony trisulfide, Sb_2O_3), which accounts for its Latin name and chemical symbol. The element is dimorphic, existing as a yellow, metastable form, composed of Sb_4 molecules as in vapor, and a grey metallic form that crystalizes with a layered rhombohedral structure. It conducts electricity more readily as a liquid than as a solid.[5]

In nature it occurs mainly as valentinite (Sb_2O_3), or cervantite (Sb_2O_4) or kermistite ($2Sb_2S_2O_3$). It is also found as ores of nickel (NiSb, breithauptite), nickel/sulfur (NiSbS, ullmanite), silver (AgSb, dicrasite) and numerous thioantimonates, such as pyrargyrite ($AgSbS_3$).

Antimony, like arsenic, is essentially a tervalent element, but *d* dihybridization enables antimony atoms to form pyramidal, bipyramidal, square pyramidal, and octahedral sets of bonds. Simple molecules containing tetrahedral bond, for example, gallium antimonide (GaSb) and indium antimonide (ISb), are of interest in the semiconductor industry. Soluble antimony compounds produce the gas stibine (SbH_3) when treated with zinc and sulfuric acid. This is a dangerously toxic gas, much like arsine. It burns with a green flame, decomposing to black antimony. Since it is no longer used industrially, there is no great risk of occcupational exposure.

Antimony ranks 28th in the elements found in the earth's surface, approximately 0.2 ppm. It is not considered an essential micronutrient. It can form inorganic and organic complexes, including combinations with other metals. More than 100 minerals contain antimony, but ores of any commercial value are limited to about a dozen.

Data on the daily intake of antimony are controversial. Values have been reported from 23 μg to 1,250 μg per week. Freshwater fish were found to contain on the order of 3 mg/kg of wet weight. Values reported for soil are 0.1—10.0 μg/Kg dry weight; for air, 1.4–55.0 mg/cu m; and water, 0.1–0.2 μg/L.

While environmental exposures are relatively low and the number of incidents of reported adverse health effects is small, the number of occupational incidents of exposure has always been significant. Only estimates can be made, because "hard" data are lacking, but a study of workers dying from lung cancer due to antimony exposures between 1925 and 1960 was considered to be inordinately high, based upon air levels ten times the threshold limit value (TLV) of 0.5 mg/cu m being measured, only after extensive control measures were put into place. By 1976, 18 years later, employees who started to work in the area after the new controls were put into place showed no lung cancer deaths.

Antimony in cigarettes has been studied by Nadharni and Ehman[8] who found that tobacco on the average contained 0.1 mg Sb/kg dry weight. Of this, 20% was inhaled in smoking.

In the past, the smelting of antimony liberated large quantities of arsenic and sulfur dioxide. This may account for some of the early occupational exposures and subsequent pathologies reported in the old literature. Today, improved refining processes have almost eliminated this problem. Levels of antimony now range from 0.12 to 5.6 mg/cu m, in most metal refining plants. Reves[10] reported levels of 4.7–10.2 mg/cu m in smelting works.

In the air, antimony oxidizes quickly. When heated, it reacts with halogens and it alloys in all proportions with lead. It will not react with boron or silicon.

Its uses are divided between metallic and nonmetallic applications. Rather interestingly, it is finding increasing use in the semiconductor industry because of its ability to combine with gallium and indium, being similar, in this way, to arsenic.

The hydride of antimony, stibine, has no current commercial use, and although highly volatile and very toxic, it is unstable and less readily formed accidentally than arsine. It is a hemolytic agent and is dangerous because it has no characteristic warning odor. Stibine has evolved during the charging of electrical batteries in which antimony was a component of the negative grid.

Absorption, Distribution, Metabolism, and Excretion

The absorption of antimony appears to be primarily limited to the inhalation route, unless it is ingested as a therapeutic agent, as it was from Roman times to the Middle Ages as an emetic and for parasitic infections. It manifests itself with characteristic "antimony spots" of the skin. These appear to be due to internal rather than external causes.

Antimony shows little tendency to store in the tissues, but rather distributes itself nonspecifically in all, with the exception of the liver and red blood cells. Thyroid and parathyroid glands retain the next greatest amount. Trivalent organic antimony is eliminated more slowly than the pentavalent form.

The metabolism of antimony is related, like arsenic, to a complexing with sulfhydryl groups of respiratory enzymes. In parasites, more so than in humans, it selectively blocks phosphofructokinase. This effectively blocks glycolysis, which is the main energy source for the parasite.

Older studies showed increased glutathione and nonprotein nitrogen content of blood, increased epinephrine in the adrenal medulla, and increased red blood cells in animals treated with organic antimony compounds.

The excretion of antimony is rapid. Some studies indicate small concentrations stored in the skin, adrenals, liver, and lungs.

Excretion from the lungs is about 80% in a few days. Pentavalent antimony leaves the body in the urine (80%); trivalent is similar. About 20% can be detected in the feces. For the most part, elimination by excretion is rapid.

Acute and Chronic Effects

The toxicity of antimony has been reviewed by Luckey[6] and also by Tucker.[13] It has some mysterious and potentially hazardous biologic properties. According to Ming-Hsin et al.,[7] it possesses unpredictable and sometimes fatal effects in the heart. Chopra[3] comments about its action on the liver.

Ming-Hsin et al.[7] reported a mortality of 50% from cardiac arrhythmias in a series of antimony poisonings between 1952 and 1953. Sudden death occurred after an interval of several hours, with no preceding symptoms and no distinctive postmortem signs of injury. This has been postulated to be due to a direct action of antimony on heart muscle.

Injury to the liver, manifested by gastrointestinal disturbance and mild jaundice, was reported by Chopra.[3] This could have been due to the ingestion of citric fruit juices (e.g., lemonade) prepared and stored in white enamelled jugs or buckets, which were commonly in use in the 1920–1930 era. These acidic juices leached antimony from the glaze.

Schroeder[11] reports that heavy exposure to antimony dusts causes severe irritation of the nasal passages, eyes, and lungs. These result mostly from occupational inhalation exposures. Irritation and soreness of the upper respiratory tract and severe pulmonary edema have been reported. Pneumococcinosis is a common chronic pathology.

Of more significant concern is a report from the Soviet Union[2] on higher rates of spontaneous late abortions (12.5% vs. 4.1%) and premature births (3.4% vs. 1.2%) and of neurologic problems (77.5% vs. 56%) among female workers exposed to antimony aerosers in a metallurgical plant. Teratogenic effects in animal studies are conflicting, but in the Soviet Union report, antimony was reported as passing through the placental barrier and being present in amniotic fluid, placental tissue, and umbilical blood.

Dermatitis from dust and salts has been observed. "Antimony spots," previously mentioned, are pustular eruptions, transient, and mostly confined to areas of sweating or increased body heat.

Reported chronic effects from inhalation of antimony dusts are obstructive lung changes and emphysema with increased pneumoconiosis. Electrocardiogram alterations may result from damage to the cardial musculature, which is reflected in the T wave.

Acute gastrointestinal effects can be vomiting, nausea, and diarrhea. Occasionally, elevated values for serum glutamic oxaloacetic transaminase and glutamic pyruvic transaminase will be observed.

At present the toxicologic significance of chromosomal alterations is debatable, but antimony tartrate has increased the incidence of human leukocyte chromosome breakage after a 48-hour treatment. No mutagenic data were found in a literature search for this article.

Carcinogenicity data are also scarce. However, lung cancer deaths have been reported in Great Britain[12] with 15 deaths in a workplace of 1,081 workers who were exposed to antimony for seven years or longer (average 22 years). Of these, three of the fatalities were "very heavy" smokers, three were "heavy," five "moderate," and only one a "light" smoker. Two did not smoke.

According to the Employment Medical Advisory Service this was about a twofold excess over expected values. The antimony exposures of workers dying of lung cancer from 1925 to 1960 can only be estimated, but with the possibility of the contamination levels being ten times the TLV (0.5 mgSb/cu m), even after 1963, they can be expected to have been inordinately high.

Further support is given to this by the evidence that no lung cancer deaths were reported for those first entering the workplace after 1958, when levels of antimony were between 0.5 and 1.0 mgSb/cu m, did not show evidence of lung cancer 18 years later [1976.].[12]

Stibine (SbH_3) should be assessed separately, since its physiologic effects are so similar to arsine. No fatality has been reported for human exposure, but this may be because it was masked by arsine or phosphine.

Stibine attacks the red blood cells and the central nervous system. Acute (sublethal) poisoning in man causes headache, nausea, weakness, vomiting, slow breathing and irregular pulse. Hemolysis of red blood cells causes the formation of "spine cells" (casts). An early symptom is hemoglobinuria.

Permissible Exposure

In the 1986–1987 edition of TLVs of the American Conference of Governmental Industrial Hygienists (ACGIH)[1, 4, 9] a level for antimony (CAS 7440-36-0) is given as 0.5 mg/cu m. The same value is advised for antimony trioxide (Sb_2O_3) (CAS 1309-64-4). The TLV for stibine (CAS 7803-52-3) is 0.1 ppm, or 0.5 mg/cu m with a short-term exposure limit (STEL) of 0.3 ppm or 1.5 mg/cu m.

Therapy

Therapy would be symptomatic and supportive to suppress or reduce the most adverse effects manifest. For stibine, treatment would be similar to that used for arsine.

Monitoring

Urinary monitoring has been employed as an "index of exposure." Usually more than 0.1 mg/L of urine is considered cause for concern. Work area monitoring is more useful and practical.

REFERENCES

1. American Conference of Governmental Industrial Hygienists: *Threshold Limit Values and Chemical Substances and Physical Agents in the Work Environment and Biological Exposure Indices for 1986–1987*. Cincinnati, ACGIH, 1986.
2. Balyaera AP (in Russian): Effect of antimony on reproductive functions. *Gig Tr Prof Zabol* 1967; 11:32–39.
3. Chopra RN: Experimental investigation of the constituents of antimony compounds. *Indian J Med Res* 1927; 15:41–45.
4. Donaldson HM, Cassady M: *Environmental Exposure to Airborne Contaminants in the Antimony Industry, 1975–1976*. Cincinnati, US Dept of Health, Education and Welfare, NIOSH, 1979, p 19.
5. Friberg L, Nordberg GF, Vouk VB (eds): *Handbook on the Toxicology of Metals*. New York, Elsevier North-Holland, Inc, 1980, Ch 16, pp 483–492.
6. Luckey TD, Venugopal B, Hutcheson D: *Heavy Metal Toxicity, Safety and Hormonology*. New York, Academic Press, 1975.
7. Ming-Hsin H, Smaoh-Chi C, Yu-Siu P, et al: Mechanism and treatment of cardiac arrhythmias in tartar emetic intoxication (in Chinese). *Chin Med J* 1958; 76:103–108.
8. Nadharni RA, Ehman ND: Antimony in tobacco. *Radiochem Radioanal Lett* 1970; 4:325–335.
9. National Institute for Safety and Health: *A Recommended Standard for Occupational Exposure to Antimony*, DHEW (NIOSH) Publ 78–216. Washington, DC, US Government Printing Office, 1979, pp 7.
10. Renes LE: Antimony poisoning in industry. *Arch Ind Hyg* 1953; 7:99–108.
11. Schroeder HA, et al: Zirconium, niobium, antimony and fluorine in mice. *J Nutr* 1968; 95:95–101.
12. Stockinger H: in Patty FA, Irish DD (eds): *Industrial Hygiene and Toxicology* ed 3. New York, Wiley-Interscience 1981, pp 1505–1517.
13. Tucker A: *The Toxic Metals*. London, Earth Island Ltd, 1972.

ARSENIC AND ITS COMPOUNDS

History

Arsenic has held the attention of chemists, physicians, authors, and doers of evil deeds since the time of the ancients. Its adverse properties have been characterized in the past by the symbol of the menacing coiled serpent, which was possibly devised by the Greek alchemist, Olympidorus, to represent it.

Agricola,[1] in his treatise *De Re Metallica*, published in 1556, wrote of the baneful behavior of arsenical cobalt, recognizing at that time the occupational relationship between the disease in the miners and smelters of Saxony and the smalite ($CoAs_2$) ore with which they were working. Because this naturally occurring form of arsenic yielded poisonous arsenical fumes, and no silver (as the miners expected it might from its shiny appearance), it was thought to house a "kobold" or goblin. In the course of time, this gave rise to the word *cobalt*.[18]

During the Middle Ages, arsenic enjoyed a widespread popularity as a medicinal, a suicidal, and a homicidal agent. By the nineteenth century, arsenic was widely prescribed in various forms as a tonic. Interestingly, the therapeutic dose was established by determining the threshold of the appearance of toxic symptoms. In the 11th edition of the *U.S. Dispensatory*[33] published in 1858, at least a half dozen "official" medicinal nostrums containing arsenic were included. (This may, as some authors have speculated,[4, 29, 32] indicate that Napoleon Bonaparte was being treated with arsenic rather than being deliberately poisoned by it, as has been proposed for many years.)

Writers Flaubert[6] (*Madame Bovary*) and Kesselring[13] (*Arsenic and Old Lace*) have capitalized on the public's fascination with arsenic as a poison. Flaubert described the death of Madame Bovary from arsenic poisoning in vivid clinical detail.

The sulfides of arsenic—realgar (AsS), which is a spectacular orange-red, and orpiment (As_2S), a brilliant lemon-yellow—were extensively employed as pigments in Chinese lacquers. Also used as pigments in the textile and paper industries were Scheele's Green (cupric arsenite, $CuHAsO_3$) and Paris Green (Cupraoacetoarsenite, $3Cu[AsO_2]$, $Cu[CH_3COO]_3$). Both of these brilliant green pigments were loosely incorporated into paper and cloth in such a way that considerable quantities of dust were generated in the cutting rooms. Artificial flowers were also coated with these substances, which provided both an occupational and a consumer health hazard. About 1880, a Committee of the Medical Society of London recognized this was a dangerous and unnecessary practice and recommended that it be discontinued.[10]

As early as 1888, Jonathan Hutchinson[11] described in great detail the dermatocarcinogenic propensity of arsenic. This condition resulted from the treatment of numerous illnesses with arsenicals. An interesting and as yet unexplained aspect of this malady is the appearance of the lesions many years after the treatment or exposure had ceased.[24]

Erlich's discovery of "606" (Salvarsan or arsphenamine) at the turn of the century gave rise to the synthesis of more than 32,000 compounds derived from arsenic that were examined for potential therapeutic purposes.

World War I saw the introduction of Lewisite (2-chlorovinyl dichloroarsine) as a powerful vesicant and incapacitating warfare agent. It produced extensive and insidious slow-healing blisters and lesions, violent sneezing, severe pain, and generalized terror. The search for antidotes led to investigations of the physiochemical actions of arsenic (which will be discussed elsewhere) and the development of BAL (British Anti-Lewisite, 2, 3-dimercaptopropanol) which, interestingly enough, is antidotal for most intoxications by arsenic derivatives but is not recommended for the treatment of arsine poisoning.

The cessation of hostilities brought about exploration of more peaceful and productive uses for arsenic compounds. Whorton[31] described the uses of arsenic derivatives in the agricultural industry between 1865 and 1938. While they are still in use, environmental concerns and the introduction of newer pesticides have diminished the use of these materials for this purpose.

Today, arsenic is employed in metallurgy, agriculture (as a cotton desiccant), animal husbandry (for sheep dip and growth promotion of swine and poultry) and in forestry (as a silvicide). These industrial applications account for the majority of the uses of inorganic and organic arsenic compounds.

The focus of the future and the new frontier of arsenic toxicology is more on the hydride of arsenic, arsine (AsH_3). This form of arsenic was first discovered by Scheele, in 1775. Little or no attention was given to it or its toxic properties until 1815, when a German chemist named Gehlen "inspired a small portion and at the termination of one hour was seized with continued vomiting, shivering, and weakness, which increased until the ninth day, when he died."

The possibility that poisoning might result from the action of water on arsenides of alkali metals was recognized in 1908.[9] In 1923, two cases of arsine (arseniuretted hydrogen) poisoning were reported in a dross factory in England. A thunderstorm flooded the floor where bags containing residues for the refining operation were stored. Two men were exposed at a distance of 10 ft. One died and the other was not affected, demonstrating the peculiar individual sensitivity to arsine.

Today arsine is vitally important and rapidly growing in use in the semiconductor industry. High purity arsenic (99.999%), produced by the reduction of purified arsenic compounds, is reacted with pure hydrogen to produce arsine gas. This is then combined with gallium to produce diodes and transistors. Some arsine finds use as a dopant in germanium and silicon devices (see sections on gallium and indium in Chapter 42).

With indium, arsine is used in infrared detectors and for Hall effect applications. Epitaxial gallium arsenide is a compound of arsine receiving increasing attention as a replacement for silicon chips.

Chemistry and Physical Properties

Arsenic (As) is an atmophilic metaloid or intermetal, which lies between germanium and selenium in the periodic table. It is a member of the Group V elements, with an atomic number of 33 and an atomic weight of 74.9. In any of its physiochemical properties it resembles phosphorus. It can exist in a bivalent (+2, −2), a trivalent (+3, −3), or a pentavalent (+5, −5) state.

Arsenic ranks 20th in abundance among the elements present in the earth's surface. It rarely, if ever, occurs as an isolated pure element. It is a major constituent of 245 mineral species, present as an alloy of 4, an arsenide of 27, a sulfide of 13, a sulfosalt of 65, an arsenate of 11, an arsenite of 116, a silicate of 7, and as three oxides. It is frequently present in the area of volcanic activity or geothermal exchange regions.

As an oxide it exists as a trioxide (As_3O_3), a tetroxide (As_2O_4), and a pentoxide (As_2O_5). The trioxide is of the greatest commercial importance. The pentoxide is mainly employed in the manufacture of insecticides, and the tetroxide is only of academic importance.

Arsenic trioxide exists as three allotrophic forms. There is arsenolite, which is composed of As_4O_6 molecules in which the four arsenic atoms occupy the corners of a tetrahedron and each pair is bridged by an oxygen atom. These As_4O_6 molecules are then arranged in a pattern so that their centers occupy the lattice points of a diamond structure. This crystalline form is stable below −13° C and melts at 272° C. At higher temperatures, claudite, a monoclinic form, exists. An amorphous glassy modification can also be prepared, and this forms melts at 313° C.

Arsenic trioxide is formed in nature by the weathering of arsenides.

Environmental and Occupational Exposures

Environmental exposures, being to a degree involuntary, should be viewed from a separate perspective. However, since the entry of arsenic into the body from environmental sources can contribute to the total body burden and thus impinge upon occupational measurements of exposure, they will be mentioned briefly.

Arsenic can be detected in most types of water. Most of the arsenic that is carried into the ocean is precipitated or adsorbed on marine clays. The amount measured probably represents 0.1% of the total. Household detergents contribute to the arsenic content of surface water. The lack of toxic symptoms is most likely due to dilution and self-purging. Levels of 1 to 73 ppm have been measured. Data on groundwater are sparse, but about 3% of the analyses conducted reveal less than 50 ppm.

A sampling of U.S. water of 727 samples showed less than 10 μg/L in 79%, higher than 10 μg/L in 21%, and 50 μg/L or more in only 2%. Inorganic forms of arsenic dominate most water samples.[5]

Trace amounts of arsenic are detectable in the atmosphere. There is currently no 24-hour maximal allowable concentration in the U.S.A. In the Soviet Union a limit of 3 μ/cu m is recommended. In general, in areas remote from industrial activity, concentrations of less than 0.02 μg/cu m are reported. A maximum level reported for the United States was 2.50 μg/cu m, in 1962 in Anaconda, Montana. It is not possible, from the evidence presented so far, to quantitatively assess the role of arsenic in ambient air as a possible contributor to lung cancer or arsenic poisoning in the community.

Industrial emissions from smelters, fossil-fueled power-generating plants, and geothermal power plants continue to be a source of air, water, and soil contamination. Coal contains arsenic, sometimes as high as 1,500 mg/kg. In the U.S., the average content of arsenic in coal is about 5 mg/kg.[4] Fossil-fueled smelters and power plants also co-generate sulfur dioxide, and this has been suggested to be a possible co-contributor to arsenic-induced respiratory cancer.[19]

Some agricultural areas show higher levels of arsenic in the soil due to heavy and repeated applications of pesticides. This has been detected by diminished plant growth.[19] At levels of 30 ppm of extractable arsenic, plant growth can be diminished by 50%.[19]

Waste disposal sites are and continue to be sources of arsenic contamination. These are being more carefully monitored and controlled at this time.

Arsenic is present in all living organisms. Marine fish contain as much as 10 ppm, freshwater fish about 3 ppm, and man and terrestrial animals usually less than 0.3 ppm, on a wet-weight basis. The average human body content is 3–4 mg but this varies with age and life-style. Urine varies normally between 0.1 and 1.0 ppm. Large daily variations can be expected, depending on diet and the type of food consumed. Most animals ingest food or water containing arsenic, and they in turn are eaten by man. Contaminated wine and beer have been cited as the cause of elevated levels if not frank poisoning. A history of arsenicals ingested years previously may not be detectable as arsenic in a patient, but it could serve as an index of suspicion when attempting to diagnose perplexing neoplastic diseases with evasive or ambiguous etiology.

An interesting observation is that during the 1950s tobacco often contained as much as 40 mg/kg of arsenic. Some tobacco in cigarettes may have caused the inhalation of as much as 100 μg of arsenic daily. A 30-year lag period has now intervened, and neoplatic activity could possibly begin to appear.

The preservation of life is perhaps dependent to a degree upon the "arsenic cycle" proposed by Frost.[7] This scheme perceives a closed system of sequential events in the geosphere. All members of the ecosystem are involved and actively participating. Arsenic is constantly being reduced, metabolized, and biodetoxified. It is everywhere in all living tissue and constantly changing. Man has modified the cycle only superficially by producing localized high concentrations. In the final analysis, a balance is established.

Numerous studies have been published regarding the effects of occupational exposure to arsenic. Eight appeared between 1969 and 1975. These concentrated on the occupations of smelting, orchard spraying, arsenical production, sheep dipping, and grapevine growing. The concerns of earlier investigators about dermal and other sites (organs) were addressed also.

Ott[21] demonstrated a positive carcinogenic dose-response relationship for respiratory cancer with estimated degrees of exposure among workers in a plant producing calcium and lead arsenates. Pinto and Bennet[23] statistically analyzed the data on workers from a copper smelting operation and found significant differences in 503 individuals (300 cancer cases vs. 160 expected). The smokers older than 65 years were calculated to be at five times the risk of cancer as were nonsmokers. Unpublished data by Rencher and Carter[25] indicated substantially higher cumulative exposure indexes for sulfur dioxide, sulfuric acid, copper, lead, and arsenic over a 29-year period as related to cancer deaths. Again, there was strong substantiation of the relationship between smoking and lung cancer in the exposed workers.

It has also been reported that increased mortality from both lymphatic and hematopoietic cancer has been attributed to high levels of inorganic arsenic in occupational situations of exposure.

The greatest occupational risk appears to be from inorganic rather than organic forms of arsenic. In spite of more than five centuries of having a reputation as a potent poison, it seems rather remarkable that arsenic remains still in need of further study and understanding.

Absorption, Distribution, Metabolism, and Excretion

The scope of this treatise does not include the biometabolism of arsenic in all forms of life. Those who are interested are directed to the National Research Council publication on arsenic[19], and the publication of the World Health Organization, *Environmental Health Criteria 18, Arsenic*.[34] These volumes provide multiple references and insights on this subject.

In the occupational setting, the respiratory tract provides the most common portal of entry for arsenic. Skin and the gastrointestinal pathways are possible, but less prevalent, routes, unless by accident or medication.

Airborne arsenic usually enters the body as the trioxide. Over 23% of the particles are usually larger than 4 μ. Particles of this size have a high rate of deposition in the upper respiratory tract. Because of the activity in the nasopharyngeal region and mucociliary clearance, much of the inhaled arsenic is dissolved and swallowed, thus entering the body through the gastrointestinal tract.

Frequently, perforation of the nasal septum, preceded by epistasis, irritation of the nose, crust formation, obstruction of nasal breathing, and necrosis, is caused by the transformation of the trioxide into the form of arsenous acid by the moisture of the mucous membranes. Smaller particles that find their way deeper into the respiratory tree produce irritation deeper in the bronchi and lung.

After absorption by the lungs or gastrointestinal tract, arsenic is transported throughout the body. Most of the arsenic in the blood clears from the plasma at a rapid rate.[14] Levels in the kidney and liver decrease with equal rapidity.

Approximately 80% of an ingested dose of dissolved inorganic trivalent arsenic is absorbed from the gastrointestinal tract. Limited animal studies indicate pentavalent arsenic behaves similarly. Compounds that enter the body in this fashion are subjected to the actions of bacteria and enzymes, and, after entry into the portal system, must pass through the liver before reaching the general circulation. The action of some microorganisms on arsenates is to reduce and methylate, thus converting them to dimethyl or trimethyl forms. This is equivalent to a detoxification, since methylated forms are less toxic compounds.

Organic arsenic appears to be absorbed by simple diffusion, not related to the size of the molecule, but probably due to its passing through the lipid portion of cellular membranes.

Causticity is a specific property of arsenic trioxide. Reports exist of local inflammation, skin irritation, vesiculation, folliculitis, and even sensitization. Systemic toxic effects have been reported from occupational accidents in which arsenic acid or arsenic trichloride was splashed on workers, indicating that the skin is a potential route of entry.

Once inside the body, arsenic compounds distribute themselves to all the tissues of the body, with the largest amounts migrating into muscle. It is interesting to note that the rat is an exception—it accumulates 79% of a given dose in its red blood cells. Arsenic in the human does not pass the blood brain barrier readily and is rarely found in spinal fluid.

Trivalent arsenic is converted to the pentavalent form in both humans and animals. Organic arsenic compounds, such as those found in seafood, are not biotransformed in the body but are excreted unchanged.

Studies on the excretion of arsenic in humans[17] indicate that clearance rates in the urine show a steady increase until the fourth day, at which point the pentavalent arsenic remains constant at 75%. By the sixth day, only traces remain, with none being detectable in feces.

Schrenk and Schreibis[26] gave the average arsenic concentration of the urine for individuals with no known exposure as 0.08 mg/L with a range of 0.02–2.0. Waltrous and McCaughey[30] determined levels of 0.04–3.8 mg/L (mean 0.44) in workers in a factory producing arsphenamine from arsanilic acid.

Urine concentrations have been used as an index of exposure, but multiple factors complicate these measurements. Hair analysis does not seem suitable for monitoring or assaying occupational exposures, since it is very difficult to differentiate arsenic adsorbed on the hair from external contamination from that incorporated into the hair shafts from the body burden. There is also little evidence to indicate that neoplasms have any ability to accumulate or store arsenic.[20]

Mechanism of Action

Arsenic was one of the first substances identified as acting through the formation of covalent bonds with the sulfur atom of mercapto-groups (also called sulfhydryl or thiol) in the body. This reaction is important because it is the only biologic pathway by which arsenoxides can enter a physiologic reaction. The reaction will take place even in the presence of a great excess of water. X-ray diffraction studies reveal that some organoarsenes (arsenobenzene) exist at a lower level of oxidation than arsenoxide. Actually, in the solid state, the former are trimeric pentavalent arsenic and do not act in the body until reduced. This leads to an understanding of the differences in toxicity between these two families of compounds.

The pyruvate oxidase system cannot be protected against trivalent arsenic, which under some circumstances can complex with two sulfhydryl groups in the same protein molecule. This forms a stable ring structure that cannot be easily ruptured by monothiols. The lipoic acid dehydrogenase of the pyruvate oxidase system is just such a thiol. It contains two cystine residues on different chains, kept adjacent by tertiary folding. Another sensitive enzyme is pyruvate oxidase, which uses lipoic (thiooctic) acid as a coenzyme. Arsenicals easily bridge and bind cystine-thiol groups, such as those found in lipoic acid.

The mechanism of the toxic action of pentavalent inorganic arsenic is less clearly understood. It is postulated that it must be reduced to a trivalent form before exerting its harmful effects. Whether this actually happens is a controversial issue. However, it does not appear to react directly with the active enzyme receptor sites. It has been postulated that arsenic competes with inorganic phosphate, in phosphorylation reactions, forming unstable esters, which then spontaneously decompose.[16] It has also been shown that arsenic uncouples oxidative phosphorylation by competing with phosphorus at one of the energy-conserving steps of the reaction. It has further been suggested that a nonhydrolytic mode of action inhibits mitochondrial energy-linked functions.

It is thought that dimercaptopropanol (BAL) counteracts arsenic poisoning, because the arsenic atom, unlike nitrogen, carbon, and oxygen, has a vacant d-orbital, which a lone pair of electrons from the sulfur atom of cystine can enter.[16] This leads to a higher valency transition complex having three sulfur atoms united to one arsenic atom (two supplied by the receptor and one by the attacking thiol). This complex is unstable and each arsenic-sulfur bond has a roughly equivalent chance of rupturing, giving a one-in-three possibility that the newly formed bond will survive. As the reaction continues, less arsenic is bonded to the receptors (a simple mass-action effect).

While the toxic effects of trivalent arsenic are potentiated by BAL in vitro, it is still employed with some degree of success as an antidote for various forms of arsenic overdose. It should be cautioned that BAL is, in fact, toxic in itself if the antidotal dose is exceeded.

Arsine has a mechanism of action entirely different from other arsenic compounds. It acts as a powerful hemolytic poison. Renal failure results from the blockage of the kidney tubules by hemoglobin casts and possibly some local irritation effects of the arsenic-hemoglobin degradation product. In acute cases, total kidney failure usually results in death.

Arsine appears to have an affinity for glutathione (a peptide composed of glutamic acid, cystine, and glycine). Reduced glutathione is necessary to support the integrity of the red blood cell membrane, by maintaining the erythrocyte-potassium pump mechanism. When this is impaired, sodium leaks into the cell, swelling and rupturing it, with subsequent hemolysis. All that remains is the "ghost cell" seen in peripheral blood. The strongly linked arsenic-blood complex is then excreted by the kidney, as mentioned previously.

Symptomatology

Acute Effects

Acute clinical symptoms from arsenic exposure will vary widely with the type and chemical state of the arsenic involved. The age, physical condition of the subject, duration of exposure and dose, as well as other factors, must be considered. Symptoms may appear in a matter of minutes or may be delayed for as much as ten hours before becoming apparent.[8]

Clinical signs range from acute abdominal pain with forceful vomiting to cramps in the extremities, restlessness, and spasms. Often a conspicuous stupor, convulsions, paralysis, and collapse will precede death in a comatose state. Arsenic is a capillary and epidermal poison which is usually reflected by accompanying exfoliative erythroderma as it migrates to the surface of the skin in subacute cases.

The most obvious clinical signs are profound gastrointestinal inflammation and cardiac abnormalities.

Arsenic trichloride has unique effects in the human. These include burns of the skin at the point of contact, "granulo-fatty" degeneration in multiple organs, and, at times, bronchopneumonia.

Arsine is the only known industrially used gas that causes massive hemolysis. (Stibine or antimony hydride, SbH_3, will also do this, but it is not used commercially.) Hematuria is profound within a few hours of poisoning. Jaundice and an unusual bronze color on the skin develop in about 12 hours. "Red wine" urine is confirmatory of acute arsine poisoning. The inhalation of 250 ppm of arsine gas is instantly fatal. Exposures of 25–50 ppm over 30 minutes are lethal, and 10 ppm can be, with longer periods of exposure. No mean lethal dose is known for man.

Arsine, unlike arsenic, preferentially binds to hemoglobin, producing hemolysis, hemoglobinuria, and subsequent renal failure. Like arsenic, it binds to the thiol groups; in this case, to those of hemoglobin. Damage to the other tissues is the result of the arsinohemoglobin complex.

Symptoms of low-dose exposure range from immediate to 36

hours after exposure. Giddiness, headache, light-headedness, vertigo, and hematemesis commonly occur almost immediately. Respiration and pulse are rapid, but blood pressure is normal. The skin becomes discolored and the abdomen boardlike, and electrocardiogram (ECG) changes occur, principally tenting and elevation of the T wave. Oliguria or anuria can develop quickly.

Treatment.—There is no specific antidote for arsine poisoning. Preservation of renal function is critical. Intravenous mannitol and bicarbonate will alkalize the urine. Hemodialysis may be required. This does not remove the nondialyzable arsine complex, but controls renal failure. Administration of BAL will not chelate arsine once it has complexed, but it will bind the gas before it enters the red blood cell. Some investigators have reported 10–15 more blood exchanges to be necessary to sustain life. Exchange transfusion has inherent dangers, but these are minimized by its value in this case.

While arsine is relatively new as an industrially used substance, it is interesting to note that 277 cases and 62 deaths between 1815 and 1950 were reported by Spoylar and Harger.[27] Further episodes have been reported more recently as use and interest in this substance increased.

Chronic Effects

Chronic arsenic poisoning develops gradually over a period of weeks or months, and unless the source of the poisoning is recognized as being related to occupational exposure, it may be difficult to diagnose the condition.

Currently reported in the literature are the chromatodermatologic changes which accompany chronic arsenicism. Facial edema is accompanied by a dusky red skin coloration. This follows an early erythematous blush and is always present in darker-toned skins. Desquamation often follows, and a pigmentation around scars, the neck, the armpits, and the nipples is discernible.

Keratoses on the palms and soles are apparent and often related to skin carcinomas. White striae in the fingernails, commonly called Mees' lines, are evident. Swelling and painful, hot, swollen feet that make walking difficult are also readily diagnosable symptoms.

In spite of liver enlargement, few liver function abnormalities are detectable. Since the liver does not store arsenic, biopsies proved to be of futile value. Portal cirrhosis has been reported from arsenic ingestion in food and medicine. Peripheral, symmetrical, and often painful neuritis, mainly affecting the extremities, is a common characteristic. Motor dysfunction and paresthesia (pins and needles) will be experienced.

Since arsenic in some form attacks the mucous membranes, keratoconjunctivitis, corneal necrosis, and rhinopharyngeal-tracheobronchitis have been reported.

The evidence for cardiac injury is clouded, but some myocardial damage has been apparent in the ECGs of affected individuals. In three cases, prolongation of the QT interval and abnormal T waves were attributed to direct myocardial damage. Some anemia has been observed, but is distinctly different from the severe hemolytic anemia caused by arsine.

From an occupational exposure aspect, two important characteristics of arsenic must be mentioned, relating to the actions or behavior of arsenic on the unborn. Kadowaki[12] reported increases in arsenic levels related to the length of pregnancy—these levels were two to four times higher in newborn infants than in seven-month-old fetuses. Earlier work showed that arsenic passes through the placenta in hamsters. This could be a consideration in fetoimmunologic or fetotoxicologic issues with female employees.

Equally important is a retrospective analysis and some probing introspective questions relating to arsenic and the developing immune system. Evidence suggests that arsenic is an immunosuppressant, if not an immunotoxicant.[19] An example is the correlation of herpes simplex and herpes zoster in both arsenic poisoning and cases of organ transplant where therapeutic presurgical immunosuppressant agents were used. The recurrent pulmonary infections of the children of Antopaoasta, Chile, may be indicative of a congenital immunodeficiency syndrome.[19] Arsenic, like certain steroids, reduces the lymphocytic count in leukemia, reflecting a selective and specific sensitivity of lymphocytes to arsenic. In this case, the children had to have had a prenatal exposure to arsenic which adversely affected their sensitive developing immune systems.[19]

Teratogenesis, Mutagenesis, Carcinogenesis.—The teratogenic effects of arsenic compounds have been recognized only recently. These actions have only been manifest and observed in animal species, but in light of the prenatal immunotoxic effects of arsenic, attention should be given to them. The defects reported may be individual species manifestations, but the chromosomal breakage in the lymphocytes of women workers exposed to arsenic may well predict other possibilities. Phytohemagglutinin-stimulated lymphocyte cultures of 34 patients were made by Petres, et al.[22] at the University of Freiburg Clinic to evaluate chromosomal aberrations. Of these, 13 had arsenic therapy and 20 did not; expressed as frequency per 100 mitoses, 49 secondary constrictions were seen in the experimental group compared to 3 in the control. "Other" lesions were 26, against 1 in the controls, and broken chromosomes were 65, against 2 in the controls. Aneuploidy was found at the expected frequency in the arsenic group. Lofroth and Ames examined the mutagenicity of arsenic on *Salmonella* in the Ames Test, but failed to show any positive effects for either trivalent or pentavalent arsenic.[15]

Monitoring and Workplace Control Levels

No direct-reading analytical instruments for determining arsenic levels exist outside the laboratory. Laboratory methods, after collection of the arsenic on filters, rely mostly upon atomic absorption spectrophotometry.

The National Institute for Occupational Safety and Health (NIOSH) recommended biologic monitoring for workers exposed to more than 5 µg As/cu m. Urinalysis is by far the most reliable procedure for this purpose. Pre-employment levels and a history of individual exposure and dietary habits should be obtained, to serve as a base-line value. Unexposed individuals normally show levels of about 0.05 mg/L.[28]

Hair and nails have been used for detection, but methods of analyzing both leave much to be desired and must be more thoroughly examined and standardized before they can become commonplace indicators.

Hygienic Standards.—The Threshold Limits Committee of the American Conference of Governmental Industrial Hygienists, recognizing the distinctly different health hazards associated with arsenic trioxide production and its handling and use, recommended in 1975 a TLV for arsenic trioxide production of 0.05 mg As/cu m with the carcinogenic classification of A1a, and with the proviso that antimony trioxide and sulfur dioxide be kept below a ceiling of 0.05 mg Sb/cu m and 5 ppm sulfur dioxide. The A1a designation refers to a carcinogenic classification for those substances proven carcinogenic for workers and for which a TLV has been assigned. For the handling and use of arsenic trioxide a TLV of 0.25 mg As/cu m was recommended.

A criteria document, issued in 1973, recommended especially the same limit as that for arsenic trioxide production, 0.05 mg As/cu m, for "arsenic." In 1975, a revised and updated NIOSH document recommended an air standard of 0.002 mg As/cu m, again making no distinction between health hazards associated with different types of exposure. The 1984–85 TLVs for chemical substances lists as soluble compounds arsenic at 0.2 mg/cu m (CAS 7440-38-2) and arsine (CAS 7784-42-1) at 0.05 ppm or 0.2 mg/cu m.

REFERENCES

1. Agricola G: *De Re Metallica*. Basel, 1556.
2. Albert A: The current bond in selective toxicity, in *Selective Toxicity*. New York, Chapman and Hall, 1979, Ch 12.
3. Brock R: Death of Napoleon. *Nature* 1962; 195:841–842.
4. Davis WF, et al: *National Inventory of Sources of Emissions as, Be, Mn, Hg,* V. Section I. EPA Report. Leawood, Kansas, WE Davis & Associates, 1971.
5. Durum WH, Hem JD, Heidel SG: *Reconnaissance of Selected Minor Elements in Surface Waters of the US Geological Survey, Circular 643*. Washington, DC, US Dept of the Interior, 1971.
6. Flaubert G: *Madame Bovary* (Paris 1857), Steegmuller F (trans). New York, The Modern Library, 1957.
7. Frost DV: Arsenicals in biology—Retrospect and prospect. *Fed Proc* 1967; 26:194–208.
8. Giberson A, Vazire MD, Mirahamadi K: Hemodialysis of acute arsenic intoxication with transient renal failure. *Arch Intern Med* 1976; 136:1303–1304.
9. Glaister J: *Poisoning by Arseniuretted Hydrogen or Hydrogen Arsenide*. Edinburgh, 1908.
10. Hunter D: In *The Diseases of Occupations*. Boston, Little, Brown & Co, 1969.
11. Hutchinson J: On some examples of arsenic-keratoses of the skin and of arsenic-cancer. *Trans Pathol Soc (London)* 1888; 39:352–363.
12. Kadowaki K: (In Japanese) *Osaka City Med J* 1960; 9:2083–2099.

12a. Kerr HD, Saryan LA: Arsenic content of homeopathic medicines. *J Clin Tox* 1986; 24(5):451.

13. Kesselring J: *Arsenic and Old Lace*. New York, Dramatists Play Service, 1968.
14. Lanz H Jr, Wallace PW, Hamilton JG: The metabolism of arsenic in laboratory animals. *Univ California Public Pharmacol* 1950; 2:263–282.
15. Lofroth G, Ames BN: Mutagenicity of inorganic compounds in salmonella typhimurim: As, Cr, Se. *Mutat Res* 1978; 54:65–66.
16. Lower OH, Hunter FT, Kip AF, et al: Radioactive tracer studies on arsenic. *J Pharmacol Exp Therap* 1942; 76:221–225.
17. Mealey J Jr, Brownell GL, Sweet WH: Radioactive arsenic in plasma, urine, normal tissues and intracranial neoplasms. *Arch Neurol Psychiat* 1959; 81:310–320.
18. Mellor JW: The origin of the word cobalt. *Inorganic and Theoretical Chemistry*. 1953; 14:419.
19. National Academy of Science: *Medical and Biological Effects of Environmental Pollutants—Arsenic*. Washington, DC, NAS, 1977.
20. Neubauer O: Arsenical cancer: A review. *Br J Cancer* 1947; 1:192–251.
21. Ott MG, Holder BB, Gordon HL: Respiratory Cancer and Occupational Exposure to Arsenicals. *Arch Environ Health* 1974; 29:250–255.
22. Petres J, Berger A: Zum Einfluss an organischen arsens auf die DNS synthese menschlicher lumphocyten in vitro. *Arch Derm Forsch* 1972; 242:343–352.
23. Pinto SS, Bennet BM: Effect of arsenic trioxide exposure mortality. *Arch Environ Health* 1963; 7:583–591.
24. Pinto SS, McGill CM: Arsenic trioxide exposure in industry. *Ind Med Surg* 1953; 22:281–287.
25. Rencher AC, Carter MW, McKee DW: A retrospective epidemiology study of mortality at a large western copper smelter. *J Occup Med* 1977; 19:754–758.
26. Schrenk HH, Schreibis L Jr.: Urinary arsenic levels as an index of industrial exposure. *Am Ind Hyg Assoc J* 1958; 19:225–228.
27. Spoylar LW, Harger RN: Arsine poisoning. *Ind Hyg Occup Med* 1950; 1:419–426.
28. National Institute for Safety and Health: Criteria for a Recommendation for a Standard of Inorganic Arsenic, New Criteria 1975, NIOSH Publ 75–149. Washington, DC, Dept of Health, Education and Welfare, US Government Printing Office, 1962.
29. Wallace DC: How Did Napoleon Die? *Med J Aust* 1964; 1:494–495.
30. Waltrous RM, McCaughey MB: Occupational exposure of arsenic in the manufacture of arsphenamine and related compounds. *Ind Med* 1945; 14:639–646.
31. Whorton JC: Insecticide residues and public health. *Bull Hist Med* 1971; 45:219–241.
32. Wilson DJ: Napoleon's Death. *Lancet* 1962; 1:428–429.
33. Wood GB, Bache F: Arsenic; preparation of arsenic compounds, in *The Dispensatory of the United States of America*, ed 11. Philadelphia, JB Lippincott Co, 1858.
34. World Health Organization: *Environmental Health Criteria 18, Arsenic*. Geneva, WHO, 1981.

32

Beryllium

Otto P. Preuss, M.D.

Beryllium, alloyed with copper, nickel, or aluminum, as ceramic oxide, or as the pure metal, is finding ever-increasing technical applications because of its unique physical characteristics. Its use also offers a good example of the impact a well-conceived environmental control program can have on the future of an entire industry.

The first adverse beryllium effects were published in the European literature during the late 1930s, but they failed to attract sufficient attention in the U.S.A.[13, 42] As a consequence, the increase in production of beryllium compounds during World War II resulted in the unmitigated exposure of a large number of American workers to extremely high concentrations and in acute respiratory reactions among many refinery employees, reported first in 1943.[38] Subsequently, cases of chronic beryllium disease (CBD) among fluorescent light bulb workers, characterized by granulomatous interstitial pneumonitis, were described in 1946.[15] After the identification of beryllium oxide as the offending agent and the discovery of numerous similar cases in other plants, the lamp industry agreed in 1949 to discontinue the further use of beryllium-containing phosphors. During the same year, the Atomic Energy Commission (AEC), then the prime consumer of beryllium metal, and the basic industry jointly developed data and recommendations for exposure controls, which were made binding for all AEC installations and for beryllium producers under contract. These controls were soon adopted by most industries processing and utilizing beryllium products and, by virtually eliminating further cases of the acute disease and reducing the occurrence of CBD to only a few isolated cases, permitted the beryllium industry to progress to its present technologically advanced stage.

PROPERTIES AND APPLICATIONS

The element beryllium (Be), discovered in 1797, is one of the lightest metals known, with an atomic weight of 9.015. It has a very high melting point (2341° F), stiffness-to-weight ratio, and dimensional stability. Its wide lattice and narrow cross section make it a good conductor for heat and electricity, make it radiolucent, and slow down and reflect neutrons without absorbing them. Because of these unique characteristics, the pure metal has readily found applications for structural components, guidance systems, and brakes in the aerospace technology, as control rods for nuclear reactors, and as γ-ray windows for diagnostic x-ray tubes and radiation detectors (Fig 32–1).

Beryllium oxide, or beryllia (BeO), a fine white powder, will form a strong ceramic material when compacted and sintered. Being a good electrical insulator and heat sink, it is used mainly in the electronic industry as a substrate for transistors and silicon chips, coil cores and laser tubes (Fig 32–2).

When alloyed with other metals, even in concentrations lower than 2%, beryllium will alter and significantly improve the properties of its parent metal. Beryllium copper, the most widely used alloy, is much stronger, more resistant to corrosion and fatigue than pure copper, and has good electroconductivity and excellent machining and casting characteristics. The electronics industry is its greatest user, mainly for connectors and current-carrying springs. Further common applications are molds for the plastic industry, bearing sleeves, spring fasteners, and repeater housings for underwater cables (Figs 32–3, 32–4, and 32–5).

PRODUCTION METHODS

The best known source for beryllium is beryl ore (beryllium aluminum silicate, $3BeOSiAl_2O_36SiO_2$) a pegmatite material found predominantly in South America, South Africa, and India. Known in its gem form as aquamarine and emerald, it contains 10%–12% beryllium oxide. Bertrandite, an amorphous beryllium silicate ($Be_4Si_2O_7[OH_2]$), contains less than 1% but requires less energy for its extraction than beryl and is found in large deposits in Utah, which has become an important domestic source. The extraction process is mainly chemical, involving hydrogen sulfide, hydrogen fluoride and hydrogen chloride, yielding beryllium hydroxide, the common feed material for the pure metal, alloys, and ceramic oxide.

Pure beryllium metal is obtained by heating beryllium hydroxide (BeOH) and ammonium fluoride (NH_4F) and reducing the resulting beryllium fluoride (BeF) with magnesium to metallic beryllium. Because of its brittle, crystalline structure, the metal then must be powderized and sintered under simultaneous application of heat, vacuum, and pressure before it can be fabricated. Beryllium copper master alloy, containing 4% beryllium, is produced in arc furnaces by adding beryllium hydroxide and carbon to copper. The final alloy contains 1%–2% beryllium and is either rolled into

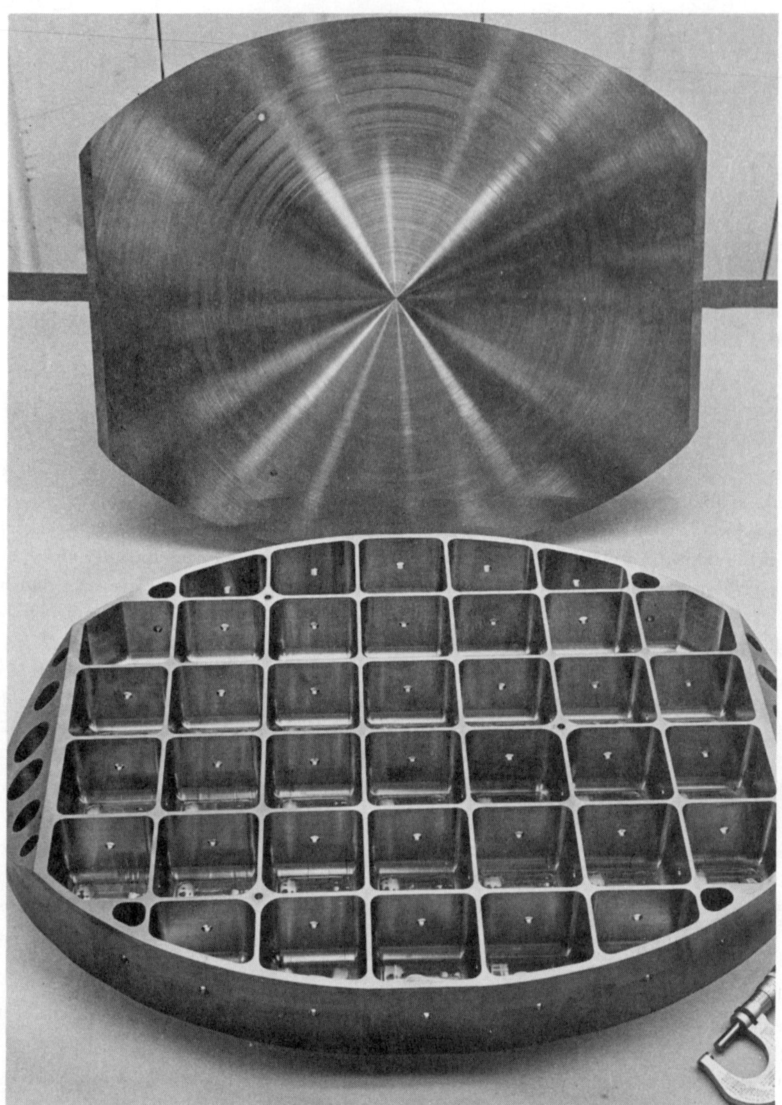

FIG 32–1.
Beryllium metal—space mirror.

sheets, extruded into tubes, bars, or rods, drawn into wire, or poured into castings.

Beryllium oxide (beryllia) is produced by calcining beryllium hydroxide, pressing the powder into the desired shapes, and sintering the green ware in ceramic kilns.

TOXICITY

Water-soluble beryllium salts, such as beryllium fluoride, beryllium sulfate, and beryllium chloride, as well as low-fired beryllium oxide are strong irritants and capable of causing dermatitis, acute inflammatory reactions of the respiratory pathways, and chemical pneumonitis.[38, 39] However, the importance of these acute disease forms for the present is greatly overrated. Being extraction and production intermediaries, water-soluble beryllium compounds are encountered in the basic industry only where, prior to the introduction of effective environmental control measures in the 1950s, they presented a definite problem. Thereafter, cases of acute chemical irritation occurred only sporadically due to inadvertently high exposures and none have been observed during the past 15 years.[22] Respirable particles from finished beryllium metal, oxide or alloys do not possess such irritant characteristics and therefore do not cause any acute chemical bronchitis or pneumonitis.

Cutaneous granulomata and ulcerations, described regularly in the older literature,[6] also ceased to be a problem with modern, significantly improved beryllium products. They were seen primarily with cuts from broken fluorescent light bulbs coated inside with a beryllium oxide containing phosphor but were also reported secondary to skin injuries caused by beryllium copper strip[34] and metallic beryllium. Fluoride impurities in the latter and beryllium

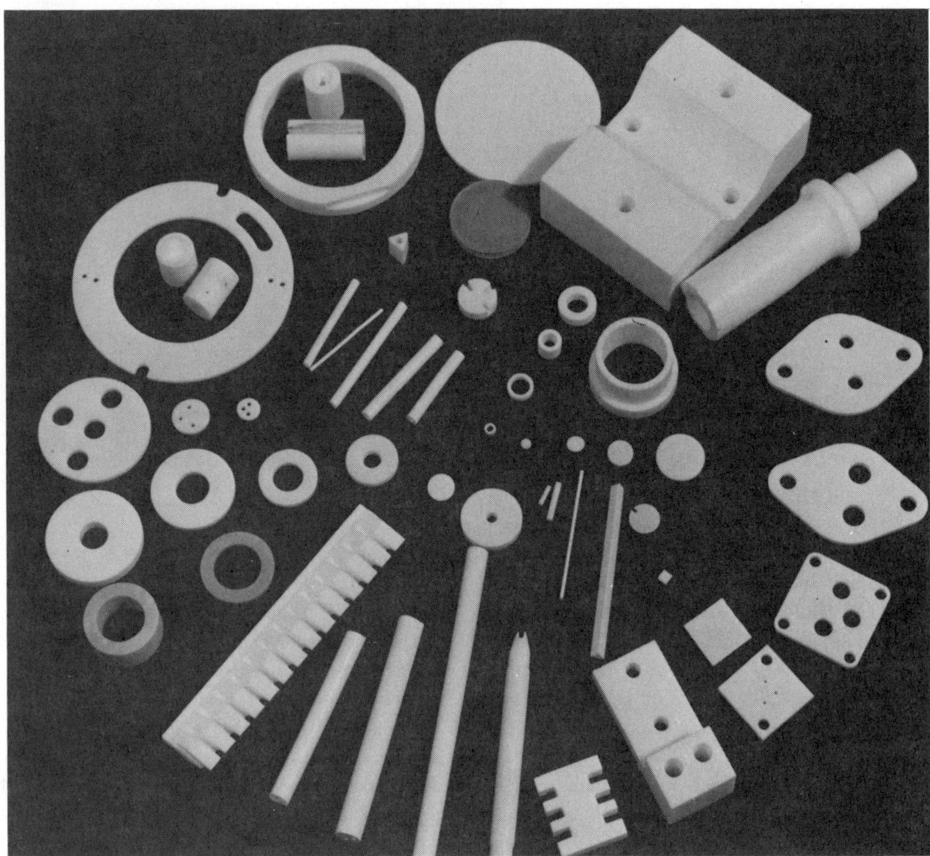

FIG 32–2.
Beryllium oxide—ceramic parts for electronic components.

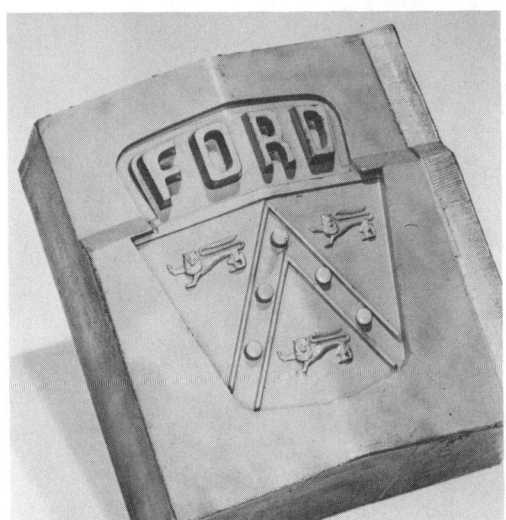

FIG 32–3.
Beryllium-copper alloy—mold for plastic automobile part.

oxide scale particles containing beryllium oxide on the surface of the copper alloys were mainly responsible for these cases until their potential sources were eliminated by continuous improvement of the product quality. Ten years' experience with cutaneous injuries from beryllium metal, alloys, or oxide at the dispensary of a major beryllium producer has shown that these lacerations, abrasions, cuts, or puncture wounds, if treated routinely and in the same fashion as injuries from ferrous metals, healed without delay or complications.[25]

Therefore, cutaneous and acute respiratory problems today are only of historic significance, especially as far as fabricating processes are concerned.

Chronic beryllium disease (CBD), however, must still be kept in mind as a potential hazard requiring constant vigilance whenever respirable beryllium particles may be encountered. The direct toxic mechanism of the beryllium ion is still poorly understood. It is known to interfere with the action of enzymes, such as alkaline phosphatase,[28] but this feature can certainly not be the cause of the chronic disease, since even among severely exposed workers never more than at most 4% were affected. Such striking selectivity and the demonstration of cutaneous hypersensitivity in CBD patients led some investigators as early as 1951 to suspect immune mechanisms as the principal etiologic factor.[35] Twenty years later, further proof of this theory was provided by accumulated evidence

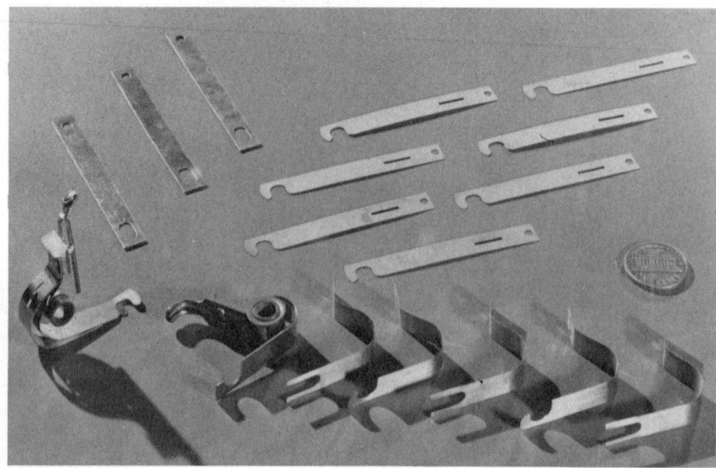

FIG 32–4.
Beryllium-copper alloy—ignition contact springs.

from animal experiments and the observations that lymphocytes from patients with CBD, if challenged with beryllium ions, will proliferate and produce a migration inhibition factor.[29] Today this theory has found universal acceptance. Since the beryllium ion is too small to possess antigenic properties of its own, but it is known to combine readily with proteins, so it is assumed that it acts by hapten formation. Although elevated gamma globulins have been found regularly in CBD, free-floating, humoral antibodies have never been demonstrated, and the beryllium-induced hypersensitivity therefore appears to be strictly cell-mediated.[29] The impression that the selectivity of CBD may be based on a generic determined predisposition was recently supported by animal experiments revealing the existence of CBD-susceptible and refractory guinea pig strains.[2] Investigations of the cellular profile found in the bronchoalveolar lavage fluid of CBD patients have shown a preponderance of lymphocytes with a high percentage of T cells and a high helper-to-suppressor cell ratio.[10] The principle deficiency of individuals predisposed to contract CBD therefore ap-

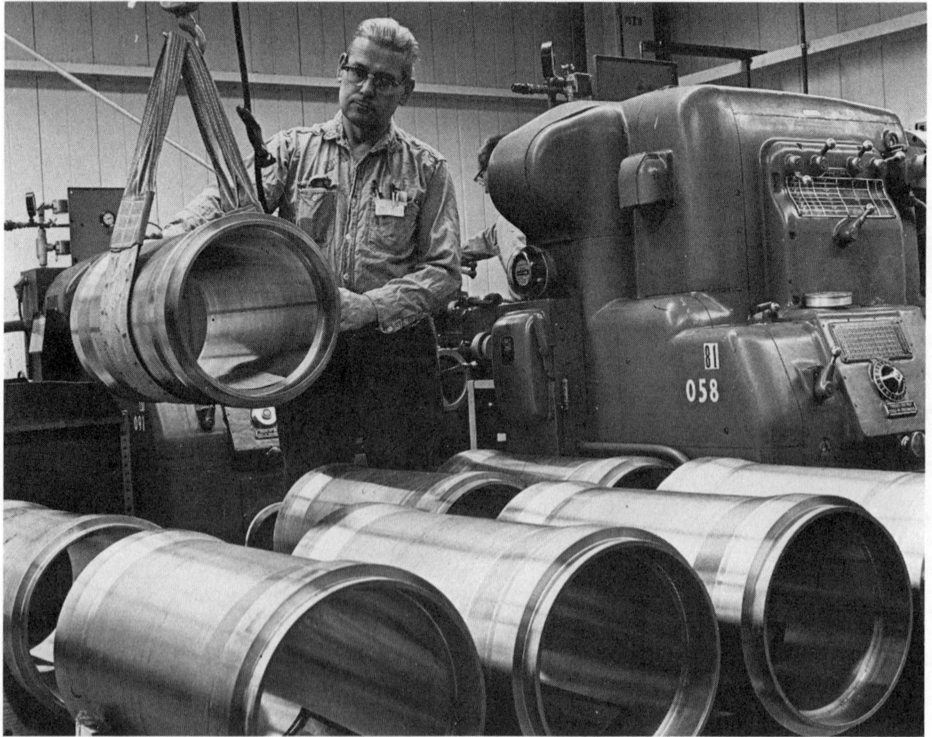

FIG 32–5.
Beryllium-copper alloy—repeater housings for transatlantic cables.

pears to be an inability to develop a sufficient number of suppressor cells to prevent the immune response from becoming excessive and destructive.

Beryllium oxide appears to be the molecule most likely to be responsible for causing CBD.[29] Entering the alveoli and interstitial lung tissue as solid particles—either directly as beryllium oxide powder, as precipitate from water-soluble beryllium salts, or on the surface of powderized pure beryllium metal—it will be phagozytized by alveolar macrophages and, in predisposed individuals, cause the formation of epithelioid cell granulomata, round-cell infiltration of the alveolar septa, and, eventually, fibrosis. Beryllium fluoride, known for a long time to be a strong skin sensitizer, has recently been found to produce a typical hypersensitivity alveolitis at concentrations exceeding the threshold limit value (TLV) significantly but below those capable of causing acute chemical pneumonitis.[27] This observation suggests that some of the acute pneumonitis cases described in the early literature as the insidious type could well have been hypersensitivity reactions rather than caused by the assumed direct chemical irritation.

The elimination of beryllium from the body proceeds very slowly and its presence in the lung tissues and urine can often be demonstrated many years after cessation of exposure. This feature is obviously one of the factors responsible for the long latent periods typical for CBD. However, what exactly triggers the disease at a certain point into its delayed development is still insufficiently explained. The fact that pregnancies, major surgery, or aging seem to have a precipitating effect and that corticosteroids can bring about improvement in the majority of cases suggests that depletion or insufficient production of the patient's own adrenocortical hormones may play a significant role. From the lungs beryllium gradually transfers to the bone, liver, and kidneys, which will excrete it slowly and without any tissue damage.

When ingested, neither beryllium metal nor its alloys or oxide will have any harmful effects on the intestinal lining nor will they be absorbed to any significant degree. Absorption through the skin is also minimal and has no clinical consequences.

DOSE-RESPONSE RELATIONSHIP

In contrast to the acute chemical pneumonitis, where sufficiently high concentrations of water-soluble beryllium compounds would affect almost every exposed worker, such clear-cut relationships have not been seen with CBD. Even by today's standards, astronomically high air levels of respirable beryllium oxide or beryllium metal particles failed to affect 96%–98% of all individuals working under such conditions. Furthermore, repeated lymphocyte proliferation tests on 537 healthy beryllium workers, of whom many had histories of long employment and high exposures in the past, showed less than 2% positive test results, with only slightly and inconsistently elevated stimulation indices. Those who did contract CBD had high stimulation indices and exposures which were at least 15 times higher than the present TLV of 2 μg/cu m but, in many instances, lasted only days or weeks.[25] From these observations, it becomes obvious that the development of CBD requires no prolonged exposure period but a predisposition for sensitization by beryllium ions and a minimum exposure of approximately 30 μg/cu m.

CARCINOGENICITY

Beryllium compounds have produced tumors in several animal species.[30, 40] Mutagenicity tests were negative with bacteria and yeasts but were positive in cultures of mammalian cells.[18, 30] Regarding teratogenic and reproductive effects, the presently available information is insufficient for any conclusions. No convincing evidence exists that beryllium is carcinogenic for humans. Two retrospective studies published in 1980[17, 41] reported elevated mortality ratios which appeared to be statistically significant but did not hold up under critical analysis. A much broader-based and better designed epidemiologic study is currently being undertaken by the National Institute for Occupational Safety and Health (NIOSH) and should be completed within the next two years.

PATHOPHYSIOLOGY AND CLINICAL SIGNS OF CHRONIC BERYLLIUM DISEASE

Chronic beryllium disease is characterized by a granulomatous, interstitial pneumonitis. Although some granulomata may be found in the liver, spleen, and lymph nodes as well, they do not cause any measurable functional impairment of these organs and the lung tissue is always the primarily affected site.

In newly developed, active cases, the histologic picture shows alveolitis and thickened alveolar septae with infiltration of the interstitial tissues by lymphocytes and plasma cells, nonnecrotizing, epithelioid cell granulomata, and giant cells with asteric and conchoid inclusion bodies (Fig 32–6). The pathophysiologic effects of these changes are a decrease of the vital and diffusion capacity associated with exertional dyspnea, substernal burning, and a nonproductive, dry cough. Chest x-ray films will reveal initially either a ground-glass appearance or more discrete, p-type, opacities with a disseminated, predominantly interstitial pattern. It must be emphasized, however, that early in the development of CBD, significant reductions in ventilatory and diffusion capacity may already

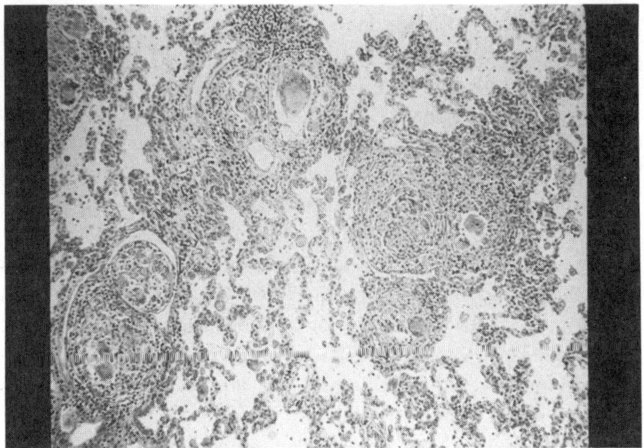

FIG 32–6.
Chronic beryllium disease—newly developed, active cases show alveolitis and thickened alveolar septae, with infiltration of the interstitial tissues by lymphocytes, plasma cells, nonnecrotizing epitheliod cell granulotoma, and giant cells with asteric and conchoid inclusion bodies.

be found prior to the appearance of obvious x-ray film manifestations. This was seen in nine out of ten employees who developed CBD while under periodic medical surveillance, in two cases of allergic alveolitis from beryllium fluoride exposure[25] and is also readily explained by the interstitial and alveolar histologic pattern seen with hypersensitivity pneumonitis in general. A moderate infiltration of the interstitium by small round cells alone will rarely produce the typical x-ray changes, which require a more intensive cellular infiltration and granulomatosis. These latter tissue changes develop gradually, generally over two to four years, and follow an asymptomatic interval which may extend from two up to 30 years after exposure.

Obstructive changes are not typical for the initial stages of CBD, but may be found in advanced cases, with granulomata and fibrosis encroaching upon small airways. Increased scarring from the latter will, in most cases, eventually result in contracted lungs, with raised diaphragms and permanent loss of airspace, which may reduce the ventilatory capacity by 50%–60%. Hilar adenopathy may occur but is hardly ever as pronounced and obvious as with sarcoidosis. In severe, progressive cases, the pulmonary arteries and cardiac shadow will become enlarged due to arterial hypertension.

DIFFERENTIAL DIAGNOSIS

The radiologic and pathophysiologic changes common in CBD are nonspecific and can be found in a variety of interstitial lung diseases of different etiologies. Of these, the most difficult to differentiate is sarcoidosis, since its clinical and radiologic appearance may be indistinguishable from CBD. Massive hilar adenopathy and extrapulmonary manifestations, such as uveoparotid fever, ocular granuloma, or peripheral neuropathy, are specific for the former[14] but do not occur frequently enough to be of much help in many instances. The histologic pictures have some statistical differences, with sarcoidosis tending toward more granulomatosis and CBD toward more interstitial infiltration,[12] but this has little meaning for the individual case, which, in general, shows both features together. An elevated beryllium concentration in urine and in lung tissues (more than 2 μg/100 gm tissue)[2] indicates exposure only, since high levels can also be found in workers with unaffected lungs.[19] Even if associated with granulomatous tissue changes, sarcoidosis must still be considered, because its occurrence among younger beryllium workers is not less likely than in the general population. The open lung biopsy—formerly done almost routinely—therefore offers very little actual assistance.

Since the patch test developed by Curtis[5] was also not consistent enough and entailed a potential risk of sensitization, considerable interest was directed toward in vitro tests.[7, 27, 47] Of these, the lymphoblast transformation test (LTT) proved to be the more reliable and easiest to perform. False positive tests were not a problem,[23] and a high stimulation index (1:4 or more) justifies a definite diagnosis. False negative and borderline positive test results still are prevalent, however, especially in older, nearly burned-out cases, or those under treatment with steroids. In these instances, the bronchoalveolar lavage may be of considerable assistance. Proliferation tests performed on lymphocytes obtained from the lavage fluid and peripheral blood of four patients with CBD revealed a significantly higher stimulation index among the lavage cells and thus confirmed the diagnosis of CBD by demonstrating the recruitment of beryllium-sensitized T cells to the lung tissue.[10, 31]

TREATMENT AND PROGNOSIS

Corticosteroids, with larger initial doses and maintenance doses of 5 mg t.i.d., may bring about improvement of subjective symptoms and pulmonary function without significant side effects. However, they seem not to alter appreciably the overall course of the disease which, in general, proceeds at one of the following three levels:

1. The initial radiological and functional changes regress, leaving minimal fibrosis and respiratory impairment.

2. The disease "burns out" at a more advanced fibrotic stage, leaving some definite, but relatively stable, ventilatory defect with little effect on the overall life expectancy.

3. There is continuous activity, with progressive inflammatory and fibrotic changes which will result in steadily increasing respiratory and circulatory disability, leading to cor pulmonale and decreased life expectancy. Steroids, even in larger doses, seem to have little effect on this category.

PREVENTION

Threshold Limit Value

In 1949 the Atomic Energy Commission adopted a tentative exposure standard with a TLV of 2 μg/cu m air as a time weighted average and a ceiling limit of 25 μg/cu m. Both values were successful in the virtual elimination of the acute chemical pneumonitis and a significant reduction of the chronic disease and were subsequently adopted by the American Conference of Governmental Industrial Hygienists (ACGIH), the American Industrial Hygiene Association (AIHA), the Occupational Safety and Health Administration (OSHA), and NIOSH in the 1972 *Criteria Document for Beryllium*.[21] Combined with an ambient air standard of 0.01 μg/cu m as a monthly average and the requirement that work clothing for extraction and production workers be issued and laundered at the plant site, they also prevented further occurrence of CBD among the general population living in the vicinity of beryllium production facilities. Thorough investigation had revealed that most "neighborhood" cases were caused primarily by beryllium dust carried into the workers' homes on their uniforms.

An OSHA proposal to lower the TLV to 1 μg/cu m because of suspected carcinogenicity[31] was debated during a ten-day hearing in 1977. Because of considerable controversy regarding materials submitted in support of the lower TLV, no decision was issued, and to this date the old standard has been maintained by OSHA under the following regulation:

1. The daily weighted average exposure during an eight-hour workday may not exceed 2 μg/cu m air.

2. Short-term exposures above 5 μg/cu m but not greater than 25 μg/cu m are permissible for a total of no more than 30 minutes per eight-hour workday.

The ambient air standard of 0.01 μg/cu m was adopted by the Environmental Protection Agency (EPA), which has added an emission standard of 10 gm/24 hr. For newly constructed facilities, the latter applies to the entire plant site and not to individual emission sources.[20]

New cases of CBD among production workers had shown a noticeable decrease in numbers, but continued to occur sporadically and brought questions about the threshold limit's effectiveness. The validity of the latter, however, was confirmed by the documented experiences of a major producer.[2, 22] These revealed that of 48 cases diagnosed between 1940 and 1975, only two had been hired after 1961, when the available control technology had made considerable progress, and were caused by well-identified, accidental exposure problems. Twenty-two cases were hired between 1940 and 1950, when technical control measures were virtually nonexistent and exposures were in the order of milligrams and grams. All of the remaining 24 cases were hired during shakedown periods occurring between 1950 and 1961, when the combination of new production processes and a large influx of inexperienced workers led to frequent and significant transgressions of the exposure limits. These observations, the fact that the accidental exposure concentrations exceeded 30 μg/cu m, and a recent epidemiologic review by Eisenbud and Lisson,[9] clearly support the effectiveness of the TLV.

Two papers from Japan[33] and Great Britain[3] report cases, which, in their authors' opinion, had exposures of less than 2 μg/cu m as weighted averages. Careful review of the reported data, however, revealed that all of the chronic cases were employed during periods when cases of acute chemical pneumonitis had occurred as well. Since the latter requires exposure levels above 100 μg/cu m,[8] one is justified in questioning the assumed low average exposure figures and, at least, must suspect that short-term peak exposure limits were exceeded significantly.

Technical Controls

Markedly advanced control technology today has made it much less difficult to maintain exposure levels at or below the threshold limits but does not eliminate the need for continued vigilance.

The extraction and basic production processes have the greatest inherent potential for excessive exposures. Among the fabricating processes, any operation likely to generate respirable particles, such as milling, drilling, and grinding of beryllium metal and oxide, and melting, welding, or buffing of beryllium alloys, requires close attention. However, effective venting devices installed directly at the source of such dusts or fumes (Fig 32–7) makes the achievement of safe worksite levels a relatively easy task. Sawing and machining with liquid coolants also keeps air beryllium levels sufficiently low but does require good housekeeping to prevent beryllium particles from drying out and becoming airborne.

Melting of beryllium copper alloys, in spite of their low beryllium content (1%–2%), makes good venting imperative, because its greater vapor pressure may lead to considerably higher concentrations in the escaping fumes. Thus, it is not the beryllium content but the potential for the generation of respirable particulates that will determine the extent of the preventive measures.

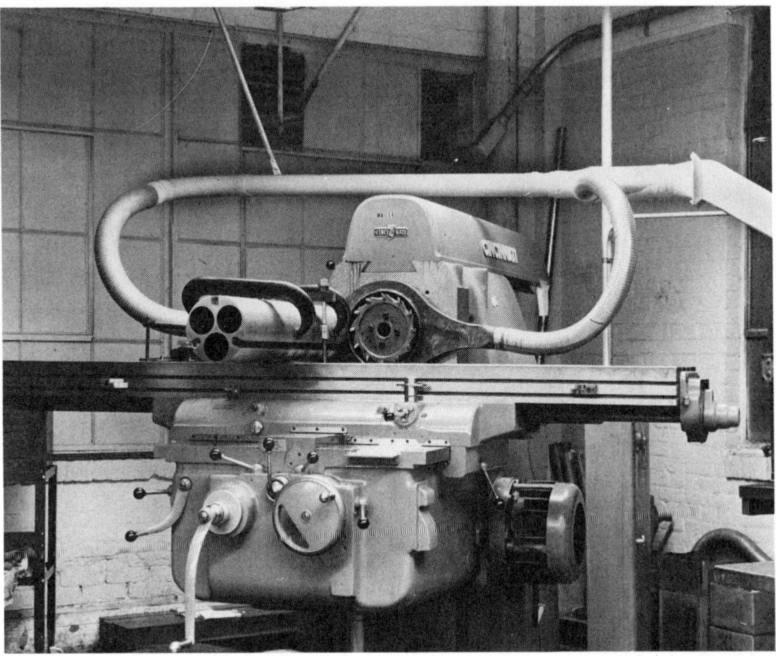

FIG 32–7.
Milling of beryllium metal. Note circular exhaust enclosure around cutting tool and high-powered collecting system.

Respirators should be used only for nonroutine, high-risk assignments, such as maintenance work on exhaust ducts or furnaces, or as an added precaution, as, for instance, during drum brakes.

Slitting, stamping, and cutting of beryllium alloys or laser scribing and trimming, ultrasound cleaning, and high-temperature firing of beryllia produce negligible amounts of fine particles and therefore, in general, do not require special venting. Mere handling and transporting of beryllium metal, beryllia, and beryllium alloys in solid form do not require any special precautions.

Air Sampling and Analysis

Whenever the initial assessment reveals ambient air concentrations at or above the threshold limits, worksite sampling must be performed at regular intervals. Samples should be taken from the operator's breathing zone and the general area, using both personal and high-volume sampling equipment.

Productions with significant emissions will require outplant monitoring by high-volume method for total suspended particulates.

Several analytical methods for beryllium have been worked out during the past three decades.[4, 16, 31, 37, 43] However, since these either lacked sensitivity or were too time-consuming, a rapid microanalytical method for measuring beryllium in biologic fluids has been developed recently.[36] It uses the formation of a trifluoroacetyl acetone derivative of beryllium and graphite furnace atomic absorption spectrometry for the most sensitive (1×10^{-5} μg/50 ml) final determination.

Preplacement Evaluation and Periodic Medical Surveillance

Currently, there exists no laboratory methods to screen out applicants who are predisposed to beryllium sensitization and the development of CBD. However, individuals with significant restrictive or obstructive lung disease should not be assigned to high-risk areas. For these, a superimposed CBD could severely compromise their already limited respiratory reserve.

Both preplacement and annual surveillance examinations should include:

1. A detailed pulmonary history
2. A 14″ × 17″ posteroanterior chest x-ray
3. Pulmonary function screening, including forced vital capacity (FVC) and forced expiratory volume (FEV_1) determinations
4. Additional measurement of pulmonary function parameters, such as diffusion capacity, and more frequent spirometry, for workers in beryllium extraction and basic production facilities where the exposure risk is significantly higher, as in fabricating processes

It is important to remember that a significant decrease of the vital capacity (15% or more) may have already occurred prior to the detection of distinct x-ray opacities. If repeat measurements at short intervals confirm the downward trend, or in case of suspicious symptoms and/or x-ray findings, a more detailed pulmonary function profile, including diffusion capacity and blood gas analysis, should be obtained. Definite reductions of the latter would call for a lymphoblast transformation test to rule out interstitial pneumonitis of different etiology.

REFERENCES

1. Barna BP, Deodhar SD, Chiang T, et al: Experimental beryllium-induced lung disease: I. Differences in immunological responses to beryllium compounds in Strains 2 and 13 guinea pigs. *Int Arch Allerg Appl Immunol* 1984; 73:42–48.
2. Cholak J: The analysis of traces of beryllium. *AMA Arch Ind Health* 1959; 19:205.
3. Cotes JE, Gilson JC, McKerrow CB, et al: A long-term follow-up of workers exposed to beryllium. *Br J Ind Med* 1983; 40:13–21.
4. Cucci MW, Neuman WF, Mulryan BJ: *Anal Chem* 1949; 21:1358.
5. Curtis GH: The diagnosis of beryllium disease with special reference to the patch test. *AMA Arch Ind Health* 1959; 19:150.
6. DeNardi JM, et al: Acute dermatitis and pneumonitis in beryllium workers. *Ohio State Med J* June 1949.
7. Deodhar SD, Barna B, VanOrdstrand HS: A study of the immunologic aspects of chronic berylliosis. *Chest* 1973; 63:309–313.
8. Eisenbud M: Origins of the standards for control of beryllium disease. *Environ Res* 1982; 27:79–88.
9. Eisenbud M, Lisson J: Epidemiological aspects of beryllium-induced nonmalignant lung disease: A 30-year update. *J Occup Med* 1983; 25:196–202.
10. Epstein PE, Dauber JH, Rossman MD, et al: Bronchoalveolar lavage in a patient with chronic berylliosis: Evidence for pulmonary hypersensitivity. *Ann Intern Med* 1982; 97:213–216.
11. *Federal Register* 202:48, 814 (Oct 17) 1975.
12. Freiman DG, Hardy HL: Beryllium disease. *Hum Pathol* 1970; 1:25.
13. Gelman I: Poisoning by vapors of beryllium oxyfluoride. *J Ind Hyg Toxicol* 1936; 18:371–379.
14. Hardy HL: Beryllium disease, a continuing problem. *Am J Med Sci* 1961; 242:150.
15. Hardy HL, Tabershaw IR: Delayed chemical pneumonitis occurring in workers exposed to beryllium compounds. *J Ind Hyg Toxicol* 1946; 28:197.
16. Klemperer FW, Martin AP: Determination of traces of beryllium in biological material. *Anal Chem* 1950; 22:828.
17. Mancuso TF: Mortality study of beryllium industry workers' occupational lung cancer. *Environ Res* 1980; 21:48–55.
18. Miyaki M, Akamatsu N, Ono T, et al: Mutagenicity of metal cations in cultured cells from Chinese hamsters. *Mutat Res* 1979; 68:259–263.
19. Metzner FN, Lieben J: Respiratory disease associated with beryllium refining and alloy fabrication. *J Occup Med* 1961; 3:341.
20. National Emissions Standards for Hazardous Air Pollutants, Regulation 40CFR61. *Federal Register* 38:8820 (April 6) 1973; amended (April 9) 1984.
21. National Institute for Occupational Safety and Health: *Recommendations for an Occupational Exposure Standard for Beryllium,* NIOSH Criteria Document TR-003-72, PB-210-806 NTIS. US Dept of Commerce, 1972.
22. Preuss OP: A contribution to the epidemiology of beryllium disease, in JBL Gee, et al. (eds): *Lung Diseases*. Raven Press, New York, 1984.
23. Preuss OP, Deodhar SD, VanOrdstrand HS: Beryllium disease, in Jones Williams W, Davies BH (eds): *Sarcoidosis and other Granulomatous Diseases*. Cardiff, Calif, Alpha-Omega, 1980.
24. Preuss OP: Statement presented at the OSHA Hearing on Beryllium Standards, August 1977.

25. Preuss OP: Unpublished, in preparation.
26. Preuss OP: Unpublished observation.
27. Price CD, Pugh A, Pioli EM, et al: Beryllium macrophage inhibition test. *Ann NY Acad Sci* 1976; 278:204–211.
28. Reeves AL: Beryllium, in Friberg L, et al (eds): *Handbook on the Toxicology of Metals*. New York, Elsevier North-Holland Biomedical Press, 1979.
29. Reeves AL, Preuss OP: The immunotoxicity of beryllium, in *Target Organ Toxicity*. New York, Raven Press, 1981.
30. Rosenkranz HS, Polrler LA: Evaluation of the mutagenicity and DNA-modifying activity of carcinogens and noncarcinogens in microbial systems. *J Natl Cancer Inst* 1979; 62:873–892.
31. Rossman MD, et al: The role of bronchoalveolar lavage in chronic pulmonary berylliosis. Presented at the International Conference for Bronchoalveolar Lavage, Columbia, Md, May 1984.
32. Sandell EB: *Colorimetric Determination of Traces of Metals*. New York, Interscience Publications, 1950.
33. Shima S: Beryllium poisoning and health care. *Sangyo Igaku J* 1980; 3(5):14–22.
34. Sneddon IB: Berylliosis, a case report. *Br Med J* 1955; 1:1448–1449.
35. Sterner JH, Eisenbud M: Epidemiology of beryllium intoxication. *Arch Ind Hyg Occup Med* 1951; 4:123.
36. Taylor ML, et al: *Anal Lett* 1968; 1:735.
37. Toribara TY, Sherman RE: *Anal Chem* 1953; 25:1594.
38. VanOrdstrand HS, Hughes R, Carmody MG: Chemical pneumonia in workers extracting beryllium oxide. *Cleve Clin Q* 1943; 10:10.
39. VanOrdstrand HS, Hughes R, DeNardi JM, et al: Beryllium poisoning. *JAMA* 1945; 129:1084.
40. Vorwald AJ, Reeves AL, Urban CJ: Experimental beryllium toxicology, in Stokinger HE (ed): *Beryllium: Its Industrial Hygiene Aspects*. New York, Academic Press, 1966.
41. Wagoner JK, Infant PF, Bayliss DL: Beryllium: An etiologic agent in the induction of lung cancer, nonneoplastic respiratory disease, and heart disease among industrially exposed workers. *Environ Res* 1980; 21:15–34.
42. Weber HH, Engelhard WE: Investigation of dusts arising out of beryllium extraction. *Zbl Gewerbehyg* 1933; 10:14–19.
43. Welford G, Harley J: Fluorimetric determination of trace amounts of beryllium. *Am Ind Hyg Assoc Q* 1952; 13:232.
44. Williams WR, Jones Williams W: Comparison of lymphocyte transformation and macrophage migration inhibition tests in the detection of beryllium hypersensitivity. *J Clin Pathol* 1982; 35:684–687.

33

Cadmium and Its Compounds

Otto P. Preuss, M.D.

Cadmium and its salts—especially cadmium sulfide and chloride—have found a great variety of industrial applications. Of its worldwide production, which now has reached approximately 20,000 tons yearly, about half is used for electroplating, since cadmium coatings provide good protection against atmospheric and galvanic corrosion. Other common uses are in brazing and soldering, and as a copper alloy for cables to improve strength and wearing capabilities and for bearing metals to reduce friction.

Cadmium is further used for cathodes in certain electrical storage batteries, as control rods in atomic reactors for neutron absorption, for fluorescent and photographic light sources, as pigment in paints (cadmium sulfate for yellow and cadmium selenide for red) and in antiseborrheic medications, antiseptics, and pesticides. Production and use of this quite toxic metal increase yearly by about 10%, and therefore attention has to be paid not only to its potential occupational hazards but to its potential as an environmental pollutant as well.

In nature, cadmium seldom occurs alone. Greenocktite, the only concentrated cadmium mineral, is quite rare, and most of the element is found as an impurity in zinc, lead, or copper ore. Accordingly, nearly all cadmium is obtained as a by-product from the extraction of these metals, and zinc ore, which may contain between 0.2% and 4.5% cadmium, provides its main source.[21, 30]

PROPERTIES

Cadmium is a malleable, lustrous, white-bluish metallic element that can be polished to a high gloss. When heated in air, it volatilizes and burns readily with a bright flame, producing a brownish-yellowish cadmium oxide fume (CdO). It is soluble in organic and inorganic acids and insoluble in water. (Atomic weight, 112.40; specific gravity, 8.6 at 20° C; melting point, 321° C; boiling point, 767° C.)

EXPOSURES

Occupational

The greatest number of acute intoxications have been reported from welding, brazing, and soldering operations, where the presence of cadmium in the alloy either was not known or was disregarded by the operator. Since the metal represents only a minor and often not specifically mentioned constituent in the majority of compounds, the same problem may occur in the chemical and pharmaceutical industries or wherever cadmium is being used. A classic example, just as with lead, is the blowtorch cleaning, cutting, or welding of metals that are cadmium plated or covered by paint containing cadmium pigments. Smelting and refining zinc ore, atomizing cadmium-silver alloys during the manufacture of brazing pastes, and spraying of cadmium pigment-containing paints also are potentially hazardous operations. A list of occupations with possible harmful exposures to cadmium is provided in Table 33–1.

Nonoccupational

Since cadmium is soluble in organic and inorganic acids, it can be leached into food from storage containers or cooking utensils coated with cadmium-contaminated zinc or even plated with pure cadmium. Severe intestinal intoxications of occasionally epidemic proportions have been reported from such sources.[2, 3]

Itai-Itai Disease.—Heavy stream pollution from zinc, copper, and cadmium refineries in Japan during World War II led to the accumulation of large amounts of cadmium in rice grown in the polluted water. Symptoms resembling severe chronic cadmium poisoning appeared among the population living on the rice from this area and were called "Itai-Itai-byo" (ouch-ouch-disease) because of the excruciating back pain and the—for many years—unknown etiology. Autopsies revealed, besides lead and zinc, high concentrations of cadmium in all organs. Although additional metallic pollutants obviously had also been present, it is believed that the cadmium content in the river water was mainly responsible for this disease.[15, 18, 26, 30]

TOXICITY

Metabolism, Storage, and Excretion[11]

In normal individuals, 2%–6% of ingested and 20%–50% of inhaled cadmium will be absorbed and transported to the liver. The liver detoxifies it by combining it with the low molecular weight protein, metallothionine. Elimination through the kidneys

TABLE 33–1.
Potential Occupational Exposures to Cadmium

Alloy making	Lithopone makers
Aluminum solder making	Lithopone working
Auto mechanics	Metallizing
Battery making	Paint making
Bearing making	Paint spraying
Brazers and solderers	Pesticide making
Cable and trolley wire makers	Pharmaceutical industry workers
Cadmium compound collecting-bag handling	Photoelectric cell making
Cadmium plating	Pigment making
Cadmium smelting	Plastic products making
Cadmium vapor lamp making	Sculptors, metal
Ceramics, pottery making	Small arms ammunition making
Copper-cadmium alloy making	Smoke bomb making
Dental amalgam making	Soldering
Electric instrument making	Solder making
Electrical condenser making	Storage battery making
Electroplating	Textile printing
Engraving	Torch-cutting, cadmium-covered metals
Glass making	Welding, cadmium alloy
Hobbyists, metal	Welding, cadmium-plated objects
Incandescent lamp making	Zinc mining, smelting, and refining workers
Jewelry making	Zinc refining
Lithography	

is very slow, since much of the cadmium-protein complex is reabsorbed and stored. Liver and kidneys contain approximately 50% of the total body burden, the balance being found mainly in the pancreas, salivary glands, thyroid, and intestinal mucosa. The estimated half-life ranges between seven and 30 years.

Inhibition of enzymes in various metabolic systems is presumed to be the basic mechanism of toxic cadmium action at the cell level. Many metallo-enzymes, such as carbonic anhydrase and several peptidases, are known to be inhibited by cadmium through displacement of their essential metals, especially zinc.[28]

Acute Cadmium Poisoning

Pathologic-Anatomical Changes.—It becomes obvious from the operations described that most occupational exposures may lead to the inhalation of cadmium, and, with inadequate environmental controls, to injurious effects on the respiratory pathways and the alveoli. There is general agreement that, in acute cadmium poisoning, the outcome depends on the severity of the respiratory involvement and that extrapulmonary effects play only a minor and prognostically insignificant role.[6, 13, 20]

Reactions in the upper pathways usually are not severe enough to force the worker to leave the area of exposure in time to prevent the cadmium from reaching the lower respiratory segment. Here, the injury response will produce three characteristic and often overlapping stages—edema, alveolar proliferation, and fibrosis.

The *edematous phase* usually begins during exposure, reaches its high point in anywhere from 4 to 48 hours, and generally diminishes after 72 hours. It represents a nonspecific inflammatory reaction not much different from any other deep lung irritation and results in rapid extravasation of fluid from the interstitial capillaries. Here, the fluid pressure can be so intense that entire sheets of alveolar epithelium may be separated from the stroma. As the fluid escapes into the alveoli, it will become more viscous due to precipitation of fibrin.

The second, *proliferative phase* represents a more specific response to the cadmium insult and leads to the picture of a "proliferative interstitial pneumonitis." It will involve thickening of the alveolar septa with cuboidal metaplasia of the epithelium, and proliferation of the reticular stroma with histiocytic infiltration, which may produce polypoidal lesions capable of obliterating the alveoli.

The third, *fibrogenic phase* represents a generalized pulmonary fibrosis with mainly peribronchial and perivascular distribution. This final stage, of course, can be observed only in those individuals who were able to survive the massive insult of the preceding two stages. It may result in some permanent, although generally minor, restrictive pulmonary disability.

Signs and Symptoms.—Initial symptoms involving the upper respiratory tract are rather minor or even completely absent.[3, 6, 7] Accordingly, they often fail to indicate the existing hazard and do not force the worker to remove himself from further exposure. The most common feature is dryness and fairly mild irritation of the oral and nasal mucosa, with some sneezing and coughing and frequently a peculiar metallic taste during or shortly after exposure. Cigarette smoking appears to intensify this taste. Often even these signs occur rather late, that is, four to eight hours after initial exposure. Eventually, after 8–12 hours, chills, headaches, nausea, vomiting, and weakness will occur and frequently are mistaken for a viral infection or, among welders and foundry workers, for metal fume fever or "brass chills." These premonitory, flu-like symptoms may persist, although they soon are overshadowed by the grave signs of pulmonary involvement which are commonly seen 24 hours after exposure. Of these, chest pains will be the first, followed by signs of respiratory impairment, and finally severe dyspnea. Due to the massive loss of fluid from the interstitial spaces and the often preceding additional dehydrating effect of severe vomiting, marked hemoconcentration may be seen. Despite the accumulation of exudates in the alveoli, auscultatory findings can be completely negative because of the precipitation of fibrin and subsequent cellular proliferation. In many instances, moist rales and rhonchi have been heard only with the onset of cardiac decompensation during the final hours before death. During the initial edematous stage there may be an ash-gray cyanosis with relatively little dyspnea. This is due to the variants in gas diffusion and the greater solubility of carbon dioxide, which still is able to escape into the alveolar fluid when the diffusion of oxygen already is impaired. During the second stage, after cell proliferation within the interstitial and alveolar spaces has set in, progressive interference with both gases will occur and will result in the typical signs of suffocation, namely, purple cyanosis and extreme dyspnea.[7]

Diagnosis.—In contrast to the rather late-appearing auscultatory signs, changes in the chest x-ray film may be seen relatively early, and the appearance of patchy infiltration throughout the entire lungs may be the first indication of severe injury to the pulmonary parenchyma.[3, 5, 7, 11]

Confusing the aforementioned symptoms with those of a flu or metal fume fever is quite common. However, marked chest pain, which rarely ever occurs with metal fume fever, and a history of exposure to fumes or dusts of a compound likely to contain cadmium should make the examiner sufficiently suspicious of possible cadmium poisoning.

Prognosis.—The fatality rate for severe acute cadmium poisoning lies between 15% and 20%. If premonitory symptoms, such as chill and chest pain, occur early (that is, much less than 12 hours after exposure), the prognosis for life is serious. Conversely, the longer the latent period between exposure and symptoms, especially pulmonary symptoms, the better the outlook for recovery.

Most fatalities occur within seven days during the edematous stage. Once this phase has been passed, the probability of a fatal outcome decreases, and rapid recovery, usually between the seventh day and the 11th day after exposure, is the rule. The chest x-ray film usually will clear completely within four weeks and complications are unlikely, except for some possible functional impairment in cases of excessive fibrosis.[6, 7]

Treatment[5]

1. Even in the absence of immediate symptoms, strict limitation of activities is required because of the time delay between exposure and the onset of pulmonary edema. Neglect of this rule may aggravate the toxic injury and result in needless death.

2. As soon as pulmonary symptoms are evident, a high concentration (70%–100%) of humidified oxygen at atmospheric pressure is indicated. Prolonged use of 100% oxygen, however, may have an additional injurious effect and should be avoided.

3. Tracheotomy as an early and elective measure may be preferable to an emergency procedure.

4. Nebulized bronchial dilators (Isuprel, epinephrine) together with nonirritating surfactants may relieve bronchial spasm and increase mucus excretion.

5. High doses of steroids intravenously and later by mouth may combat the edematous stage and prevent bronchiolitis obliterans.

6. Broad-spectrum antibiotics should be given with any signs of pulmonary infection.

7. Analgesics for severe chest pain may be necessary, but morphine and other respiratory depressants can be dangerous and are contraindicated.

8. The use of chelating agents is contraindicated (see chronic poisoning).

Chronic Cadmium Poisoning

Toxicology.—Accumulation of cadmium in the kidneys will occur even with relatively low but continuous exposure to cadmium dusts or fumes. It eventually will lead to damage of the renal tubules, with the excretion of low-molecule proteins as the first sign. Further symptoms, caused by progressive tubular deficiency, may take years to develop and are mainly the result of impaired reabsorption of protein, glucose, amino acids, calcium, and phosphorus and failure to concentrate and acidify the urine sufficiently.

Continuous inhalation of higher concentrations will injure the lung tissue first and result in generalized focal emphysema long before renal damage becomes evident. Dyspnea and oxygen diffusion impairment will be the leading findings in this instance. Chronic cough, bronchiospasm, and functional defects typical of obstruction may be absent, however, because of the different pathogenesis. In cases of severe chronic cadmium poisoning, a persistent nasal inflammation with watery discharge and loss of smell (anosmia), yellow rings on the teeth, pallor, and weight loss may be the most obvious symptoms. Increased destruction of red blood cells and bone marrow depression will result in mild to moderate hypochromic anemia. Because renal damage at this stage also usually will be quite advanced, generalized edema and demineralization of bone, with pain in the back, limbs, and joints due to the continuous loss of proteins and minerals, will occur. Finally, in extreme poisoning, bone marrow dysfunction, gastrointestinal symptoms, and mental disturbances will be seen, and death will occur either due to acidosis, anoxia, and cor pulmonale and possibly superimposed pulmonary infection or from severe chronic renal failure.

With early detection and elimination of further exposure, the initial pulmonary and renal stages of chronic cadmium poisoning appear to be reversible. After prolonged inhalation and absorption of cadmium, however, and especially when definite signs of pulmonary emphysema are present, the organic damage will be permanent.

Diagnosis.—The earliest reliable sign of chronic cadmium intoxication is proteinuria. A positive protein reaction, especially when associated with significantly increased cadmium excretion, offers the earliest indication of cadmium nephropathy. Most proteins excreted are of lower molecular weight than albumin and consist of high monomere or dimere γ protein chains.[24] They are difficult to detect by routine screening tests and are best demonstrated quantitatively with sulfosalicylic or trichloroacetic acid. The amount of protein found should be related to the amount of creatinine, osmolarity, or specific gravity. If it appears abnormally high, it should be concentrated and examined electrophoretically.[24] Recent studies have also shown a direct relationship between urinary cadmium concentration and the degree of proteinuria.[17]

The earliest clinical symptoms of chronic cadmium poisoning are yellow rings around the neck of the teeth, persistent watery nasal discharge, marked anosmia, and dyspnea. A high sedimentation rate (due to serum protein imbalance from prolonged proteinuria) and abnormal pulmonary functions may also be significant. Increased urine cadmium concentrations alone indicate exposure only and cannot be taken as evidence of intoxication. However, if combined with low molecular weight proteinuria and the typical symptoms mentioned above, they do justify the diagnosis of chronic cadmium poisoning.

In healthy, nonsmoking individuals, urine concentrations in general should not exceed 2 mg/L but, depending on the cadmium accumulation in their food and environment, may show greater ranges. Age is also an important factor, since the long half-life will lead to a gradual increase of the normal body burden. Tobacco contains 1 to 2 mg cadmium per cigarette, and smokers add constantly to their basic levels. Cadmium concentrations in blood represent recent exposure only and correlate well with neither exposure nor body burden. They should, nevertheless, not exceed 1 mg/100 gm in nonsmokers and 7 mg/100 gm in smokers.[11, 21]

Treatment.—If there is sufficient evidence to suspect chronic cadmium intoxication, immediate removal from exposure and a complete diagnostic workup are mandatory. Once the diagnosis has been confirmed, therapy must be directed at the prevailing kidney or respiratory problems. There is no specific treatment, since chelating agents may cause additional renal damage from cadmium and therefore are contraindicated.

Carcinogenic, Mutagenic and Teratogenic Effects.[11]—The animal literature contains several reports of sarcomata following intramuscular and intravenous injection of rather high concentrations of cadmium oxide, chloride, sulfate, and sulfide in mice and rats. An increase in prostatic cancer has been reported in three epidemiologic surveys, but none of these had statistical significant excesses. Its occurrence in three different groups nevertheless suggests that exposure to certain cadmium compounds may increase the risk of prostatic cancer in man. Mutagenic effects have been observed in yeasts, bacteria, and cells from hamsters and humans. High doses (3 mg/kg) resulted in teratogenic effects in rats, but none have been observed in man.

PREVENTION

Preplacement Examination

The preplacement examination should include laboratory studies for the evaluation of lung, kidney, and liver functions and blood status. Applicants with significant preexisting pathology in any one of these organs should be precluded from exposure to cadmium fumes or dusts.

Health Surveillance[5, 7, 8, 11, 22]

Periodic urine testing, preferably every three months, for proteinuria with sulfosalicylic or trichloroacetic acid will provide the earliest possible indication of harmful cadmium effects. Ventilatory studies (FVC, FEV_1), when conducted regularly and often enough, allow a fairly accurate assessment of lung function changes. Both tests have definite preventive value, since they appear to demonstrate harmful effects early enough to stop their progress by removing the worker from further overexposure. Nevertheless, they are screening tests only, and in case of abnormal results, further detailed assessments of pulmonary and renal function are indicated. Urine cadmium levels should also be determined periodically, since they can be used as an estimate of the body burden. A concentration greater than 10 mg/gm urinary creatinine should be used as an indication for removal from exposure, since above this level kidney disfunction may develop.

Environmental Control[5, 12, 17, 21, 27, 29]

Indoors.—Adequate local exhaust provisions efficient enough to keep cadmium dusts or fumes completely away from the worker's breathing zone are mandatory. In addition, the general air exchanges should be frequent enough to keep the concentration of cadmium below the recommended threshold limit values (TLV). In the United States the TLVs recommended by the American Conference of Governmental Industrial Hygienists are 50 mg/cu m as a time-weighted average for cadmium dusts and salts and 50 mg/cu m for cadmium oxides and fumes. In Finland, the exposure standard requires 10 mg/cu m as a threshold limit for fumes, a level which is also recommended by the International Labor Organization.

In confined spaces, or wherever exhaust systems are not practicable, respirators of the supplied-air or dispensoid-removing type should be supplied and their use made mandatory. The same is required for outdoor and construction work, where crosswinds could blow the fumes right into the worker's breathing zone. Other workers in the vicinity of the hazardous operation should either be removed from the area or afforded the same type of protection.

Outdoors.—In case of torch-burning, welding, or grinding on metal surfaces of unknown composition, on-the-spot tests for cadmium should be conducted either by heating a small area (cadmium will form a gold-yellow, zinc a smoky gray film) or by performing a chemical test, using ammonium nitrate solution, filter paper, and 5% fresh sodium sulfide solution, which, in the presence of cadmium, will reveal a yellowish stain.

Chemical Analysis.[11]—Atomic absorption spectrophotometry (AAS) is today the most common method for the detection of cadmium. The flameless AAS methods allow one to determine accurately 5 mg/kg in foodstuffs and even lower levels in urine.

REFERENCES

1. Axelson B, Piscator M: Renal damage after prolonged exposure to cadmium. *Arch Environ Health* 1966; 12:360.

2. Baader EW: *Berufskrankheiten*. Berlin, Urban & Schwarzenberg, 1960, pp 119–128.
3. Bonnell JA: Cadmium poisoning. *Ann Occup Hyg* 1965; 8:45.
4. Bonnell JA, Ross JH, King E: Renal lesions in experimental cadmium poisoning. *Br J Ind Med* 1960; 17:69.
5. California State Technical Bulletin for Physicians and Industrial Hygienists: *Cadmium Inhalation Poisoning*, ed 2. Sacramento, December 1971.
6. Diechmann WB, Gerarde HW: *Toxicology of Drugs and Chemicals*. New York, Academic Press, 1969.
7. Dunphy B: Acute occupational cadmium poisoning. A critical review of the literature. *J Occup Med* 1967; 9:1.
8. Friberg L: Health hazards of the manufacture of alkaline accumulators with special reference to chronic cadmium poisoning. *Acta Med Scand* 1950; 138 (Suppl 240):1–124.
9. Friberg L: Chronic cadmium poisoning. *AMA Arch Ind Health* 1959; 20:401.
10. Friberg L, et al: *Cadmium in the Environment*, ed 2. Cleveland, CRC Press, 1974.
11. Friberg L, et al: *Handbook on the Toxicology of Metals*. Elsevier North-Holland Biomedical Press, 1979.
12. *ILO Encyclopedia of Occupational Health and Safety*, ed 3. Geneva, International Labour Office, 1983, vol 1, A-K.
13. Holden H: Cadmium fume. *Ann Occup Hyg* 1965; 8:51.
14. Imbus HR, Cholak J, et al: Boron, cadmium, chromium and nickel in blood and urine. *Arch Environ Health* 1963; 6:286.
15. Itokawa Y, et al: Renal and skeletal lesions in experimental cadmium poisoning. *Arch Environ Health* 1974; 28:149.
16. Kazantezis G, et al: Renal tubular malfunction and pulmonary emphysema in cadmium pigment workers. *Q J Med* 1963; 32:32.
17. Lauwerys RR, Buchet JP, et al: Epidemiological survey of workers exposed to cadmium. *Arch Environ Health* 1974; 28:145.
18. Nonjyama K, Sugata Y: Identification of urinary low-molecular weight proteins in renal tubular disorders. *Jap J Hyg* 1972; 27:64.
19. Nordberg QF: Health hazards of environmental cadmium pollution. *Ambio* 1974; 3:55.
20. Patterson JL: The pathology of cadmium smoke poisoning in man and in experimental animals. *J Ind Hyg Toxicol* 1947; 29:294.
21. Patty FA: *Industrial Hygiene and Toxicology*, ed 3. New York, Wiley-Interscience Publication, 1981, vol IIA, pp 1563–1580.
22. Potts CL: Cadmium proteinuria. The health of battery workers exposed to cadmium oxide dust. *Ann Occup Hyg* 1965; 8:55.
23. Piscator M: Proteinuria in chronic cadmium poisoning. I. An electrophoretic and chemical study of urinary and serum proteins from workers with chronic cadmium poisoning. *Arch Environ Health* 1962; 4:607.
24. Piscator M: Proteinuria in chronic cadmium poisoning. III. Electrophoretic and immunoelectrophoretic studies on urinary proteins from cadmium workers. *Arch Environ Health* 1966; 12:335.
25. Princi F: A study of industrial exposures to cadmium. *J Ind Hyg Toxicol* 1947; 29:315.
26. Takase T, et al: On the pathogenesis of so-called "Itai-Itai" disease. *Jap J Clin Med* 1967; 25:200.
27. Threshold Limit Values for Chemical Substances in the Work Environment Adopted by ACGIH for 1986–1987. Cincinnati, Oh, American Conference of Governmental Hygienists, 1985.
28. Tsuchiya K: Proteinuria in chronic cadmium poisoning. *Arch Environ Health* 1962; 4:607.
29. US Dept of Health and Human Services, National Institute for Occupational Safety and Health: *Cadmium*, NIOSH Publ 84–116. Cincinnati, DHHS, NIOSH, *Curr Intell Bull* 42, Sept 27, 1984.
30. Vesa R: Cadmium, occurrence and effects. *Work-Environment-Health* 1972; 9:91.

34

Chromium and Its Compounds

Howard J. Sawyer, M.D.

HISTORY

Chromium was discovered in a relatively rare red-orange mineral, crocoite, by the noted French chemist, Nicholas Vauquelin, in 1797. This mineral, the only natural source of hexavalent chromium, is of minimal commercial importance, but it, and other colored chromates, give the element its name, from the Greek *chromos*, meaning "color." The green of emerald and the red of ruby come from chromium's 1% substitution for aluminum in corundum, Al_2O_3, and beryl, $Be_3Al_2Si_6O_{18}$.[48]

Chromium was first used in chemical production early in the 19th century and "chrome sores" were first noted by Cumin, in 1827, in two dyers who immersed their hands in potassium bichromate solutions.[12] Mackenzie, in 1884, quotes an anecdotal report by a long-time bichromate worker that nasal septal perforations occurred in fellow workers, sometimes within two days after heavy exposures.[41] Early in the 20th century, chromium became widely used in steel production. In Germany, in 1932, Lehman first reported lung cancer among chromate workers.[35]

Today, the main uses for chromium are in alloys, as a principle component of refractories in steel-making furnaces, and in the production of the various chemical forms of chromium. Pigments account for nearly 33% of these chemicals, textiles utilize around 10%, about 25% are used in metal surface treatments and corrosion control, and approximately 25% are used in tanning. Chromium and its compounds protect against rust, provide color, conserve energy as components of catalysts, prevent decay, resist soiling and are used in hundreds of other ways, such as in the manufacturing of foam rubber. In fact, the uses of chromium are so extensive that today's world would be almost unrecognizable without it.

SOURCES, U.S. PRODUCTION, AND NUMBER OF WORKERS EXPOSED

Of the approximately 1,121,000 tons of chromite mined annually, around a quarter (280,000 tons) are consumed in the United States. Chromium has not been mined in the U.S. since 1961, and most of it now comes from South Africa, Russia, and Rhodesia.[46] As its availability becomes potentially less dependable, and primary production costs increase, great amounts are being recycled. The natural, trivalent chromium oxide is always found with iron in the form $FeO.Cr_2O_3$. The ore also contains the oxides of aluminum (around 15%) and magnesium (around 12%) as well as varying amounts of silicates and the oxides of titanium and vanadium.

It is impossible to accurately state how many U.S. workers are exposed to the numerous chromium substances, but the number is conservatively in excess of a million. Although health effects can occur from exposure to trivalent forms, it is in workers exposed to hexavalent compounds that the most serious health problems have been reported. The National Institute for Occupational Safety and Health (NIOSH) lists 104 occupations in which 175,000 workers are so exposed.[45]

THE IMPORTANCE OF VALENCE

Chromium is a very complex and versatile metal whose harmful effects are heavily dependent on valence. In addition to metallic chromium (valence O), other valences are the +2, +3, +4, +5, and +6 combining states.

Divalent chromium is of minor importance in industrial exposures because it readily oxidizes to the trivalent state. Therefore, its harmful effects are mostly those of Cr^{+3}.[43, 11]

The tetravalent and pentavalent forms are essentially unstable. As intermediates in chemical production, they pose no significant human health risks and there are no reports of human illness in workers exposed to them.[30, 37]

Trivalent and hexavalent chromium are the only compounds known to be significantly associated with human disease. Their harmful effects will be easier to understand if the following characteristics are fully appreciated:

1. In nearly all forms likely to exist in the workplace, trivalent chromium is poorly absorbed through the skin. The hexavalent form easily penetrates the skin.[31, 54]

2. Gastric fluids readily reduce hexavalent to trivalent chromium,[15] the valence known to be significantly absorbed intestinally. Reports of the percentage of ingested chromium which is absorbed vary widely from 1%–25%, depending on the particular form and ligand environment.[14, 32, 61] For example, when Cr^{+3} is

in a favorable ligand environment, such as when it is a part of chromium-containing Glucose Tolerance Factor (GTF), absorption is greatly enhanced, up to 25 times that of inorganic chromium.[9, 56] More will be said about this in the section on Nutritional Requirements.

3. In most of the forms likely to be encountered in industry, trivalent chromium's passage through cell membranes is inhibited. Hexavalent chromium is not.[21] Thus, from an *exposure* viewpoint, hexavalent forms are potentially more hazardous.

4. Hexavalent chromium, which readily transits cell membranes, has a short intracellular life, reducing "within minutes to hours" to the potentially carcinogenic trivalent state. An allegory may be helpful. Like the fabled Trojan horse, chromium is thus acceptably disguised as Cr^{+6} to gain cellular entry, only to transform into the *intracellular* carcinogenic form, Cr^{+3}. If the reduction occurs in the cytoplasm, the hazard is low. But if it occurs in the proximity of DNA, the mutagenic potential is significant.

5. Though trivalent chromium is normally inhibited in transiting cell membranes, any that does gain entry can interact, unless trapped in the cytoplasm by appropriate ligands, with nucleic acids, nuclear enzymes, nucleotides and other nuclear substances.[24] It is therefore believed that intracellular trivalent chromium can exert a carcinogenic influence and appears to be the only form of chromiun that is carcinogenic, *but only if it gains access to the nucleus*.

6. Because of the above factors, an understandable confusion occasionally emerges about the carcinogenicity of chromium. Although this led, at one time, to the suspicion that *environmental* trivalent chromium could be a pulmonary carcinogen,[42] no scientific basis has yet developed in support of this hypothesis.[27, 50]

PORTALS OF ENTRY AND LOCAL EFFECTS

Skin Absorption

The importance of valence on skin absorption has already been discussed. Factors favoring skin chromate penetration include increasing pH in the alkaline range, inflammation, open sores, and loss of the skin's normal moisture and oil. Such factors also favor the development of both allergic and irritant skin reactions. Additionally, the solubility, duration of contact, concentration, and pH of the contactant determine the presence and/or degree of both absorption and local reaction. Skin changes have little, if any, relation to air levels.[30] Although skin absorption of trivalent chromium is usually minimal, when certain of the previous factors combine in the right way, especially with the removal of the stratum corneum where Cr^{+3} is normally bound, overwhelming absorption, with severe tissue damage and death, can occur. Such a case was reported by Kelly et al. in a worker accidentally immersed in hot chromium sulfate solution.[29] Examples of skin problems associated with chromium compounds are listed in Table 34–1.

TABLE 34–1.
The Ten Most Important Examples of Skin Problems Associated With Chromium Compounds*

CHROMIUM-CONTAINING MATERIALS OR OBJECTS	JOB OR PLACES OF CONTACT	CHROMIUM COMPOUNDS RESPONSIBLE
Chromium ore	Industrial chromium production	Chromite
Chrome baths	Electro-plating industry	Chromic acid, sodium dichromate
	Graphic trade	Chromates
	Metal industry	Chromates, zinc chromate
Chromate colors and dyes	Painters and decorators, graphic trades, textile, rubber, glass and china industries	Chromic oxide green, chromic hydroxide green, chrome yellow (lead chromate)
Lubricating oils and greases	Metal industry	Chromic oxide
Anticorrosive agents in water system and greases	Diesel locomotive workshops and sheds, central heating and air-conditioning systems	Alkali dichromates
Wood preservation (Wolman salts)	Wood impregnation, furniture industry, carpenters, miners	Alkali dichromates
Cement, cement products, quick-hardening agents for cement (e.g., Sika 1)	Cement production, manufacture of cement products, building trades	Chromates
Cleaning materials (Eau de Javelle), washing and bleaching materials	Homemakers, cleaners, laundry workers	Chromates
Textiles, furs	Textile and fur industries, everyday life	Chromates
Leather and artificial leather tanned with chromium	Leather and footwear industry, everyday life	Chromium sulfate, chromium alum

*Adapted from Polak L: Immunology of chromium, in Burrows D (ed): *Chromium: Metabolism and Toxicity.* Boca Raton, Fla, CRC Press, 1983.

The treatment and prevention of such serious skin absorption formerly included actually removing skin to block toxic chromium absorption.[33] However, newer methods, using ascorbic acid (AA), offer effective means not only of topically reducing Cr^{+6} to Cr^{+3}, but also of doing so in vivo by its intravenous administration. In 1980, Korallus reported treating severe chromate burns with intravenous infusion of 3 gm or more of ascorbic acid. Although chromium excretion was no less than with previous serious burn cases associated with renal failure, none was detected.[31]

A strong skin sensitizer, Cr^{+6} is often found in portland cement, causing cement dermatitis in some workers. Skin application of ascorbic acid and possibly of other reducing agents, such as sodium dithionite, should be considered for use in such susceptible workers.

Ingestion

As stated previously, most chromium is absorbed as Cr^{+3}. Except in deliberate poisonings or unusual accidents, however, ingestion of chromates is of no practical concern in well-controlled industrial environments.

Inhalation

There is no good evidence that inhaled trivalent chromium, at currently allowable concentrations, poses any occupational health risk. The chief concern is with the inhalation of the hexavalent chromates and dichromates, some of which may be carcinogenic in sufficient doses. Additionally, upper airway irritation, with nasal septal perforation, has been reported when workplace concentrations of chromic acid mists were high. Pulmonary sensitization has been reported, although rarely.[52]

Distribution and Elimination

Once absorbed, Cr^{+6} has a short half-life. It can be transported on serum transferrin or may enter erythrocytes or other cells where it is reduced to Cr^{+3}.[25] This chromium is then distributed as shown in Figure 34–1. In the few cases of death due to accidental absorption of high chromium levels, intravascular hemolysis and renal damage predominated.[20, 59] Chromium is eliminated in feces, urine, sweat, skin, and hair. Although it can be found in most tissues, the liver, spleen, muscle, fat, and bone appear to be primary storage sites.[6]

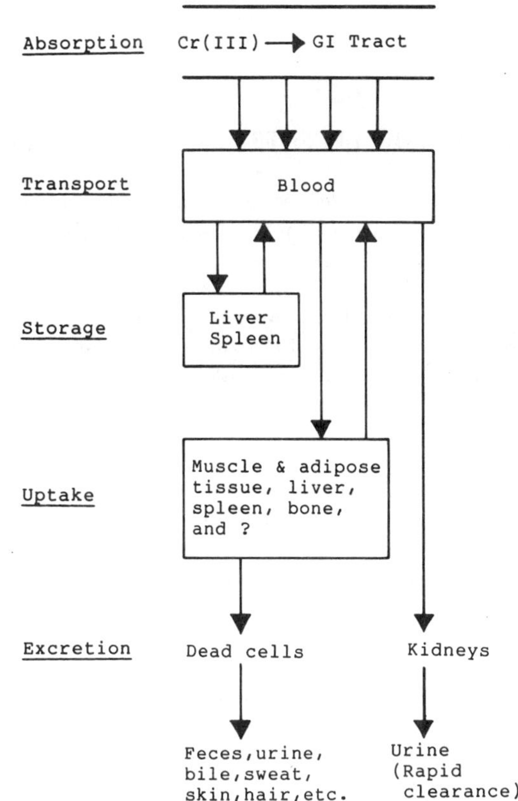

FIG 34–1.
Proposed pathways for chromium (III) in the human body, based on human and animal data. Cr(III) is transported bound mainly to plasma transferrin. (Adapted from Lim TH, Sargent T, Kusubov N: Kinetics of the trace element chromium in the body. *Am J Physiol* 1983; 244(4):R445–454. Used by permission.)

NUTRITIONAL REQUIREMENTS

Although the emphasis of this chapter is on the potential adverse health effects of chromium from occupational exposures, it is very important to realize that chromium is now recognized as an essential trace element. The recommended daily allowance (RDA) is 50–200 μg of inorganic Cr^{+3} but, by taking Cr^{+3} as glucose tolerance factor (GTF), 8–10 μg appear to be equally effective.[56]

Both animal and human experience document that GTF, which has not as yet been isolated and characterized, is an essential cofactor in the binding of insulin to cell receptor sites.[44] Its deficiency can produce a syndrome indistinguishable from diabetes mellitus.[38] Mertz cautions, however, that chromium deficiency should be considered as only one of several nutritional factors associated with impaired glucose tolerance and elevated circulating insulin and cholesterol levels.[44] Other possible nutritional factors include copper, magnesium, and selenium deficiencies.

Chromium differs from most metals in that tissue storage tends to decrease with age, and several studies have indicated that half the adult subjects tested were chromium deficient.[44] Interestingly, injection of insulin, to compensate for reduced endogenous insulin production, may secondarily increase chromium excretion, producing a chromium deficiency that leads to further glucose intolerance. Several human studies have shown that chromium supplementation improved glucose tolerance in diabetics and hyperglycemics.[22, 26, 36, 39]

There are two reported cases of overt chromium deficiency in patients on total parenteral nutrition. They developed severe diabetic-like symptoms, with normal insulin levels. Their symptoms were alleviated by administration of 150 μg of inorganic chromium daily.[18, 28]

Dietary Sources

The richest dietary source of chromium, and the most effective therapeutically, is brewer's yeast. Most meats, fish, fruits, and vegetables are good sources of chromium. Alfalfa, brown sugar, molasses, and dark bread are also high in chromium, as are butter and animal fats.

CARCINOGENIC EFFECTS

As previously indicated, sufficient exposure to specific hexavalent chromium compounds has been associated with an increased risk of lung cancer. The questions are: Which compounds and at what exposures? The answers will never be precisely known, because, during the period when workers were grossly overexposed, industrial hygiene studies and measurements were often meager, inappropriate, inaccurate, or nonexistent. Moreover, only rarely were workers exposed exclusively to one or two specific compounds.

Furthermore, many reported studies are flawed by the lack of information, such as data on individual worker smoking habits, and they are largely based on retrospective studies, and control groups are often inadequate. Still, the following illustrative studies, briefly summarized, provide the best attempt at answering the questions posed above.

In 1932, Lehman first reported the probable relationship between lung cancer and chromium exposure.[35] He was followed by his German countryman, Pfeil, in 1935, who reported on workers exposed to both Cr^{+3} and Cr^{+6}.[53] In 1948, Machle and Gregorius reported an 18–50-fold excess of lung cancer in four of the seven U.S. plants studied, where the main exposures were to calcium chromates and bichromates.[40]

A 1950 study by Anna Baetjer, using Baltimore hospital records, compared occupations among lung cancer cases and those with other diagnoses. Although the study was technically flawed, she found a greater proportion of lung cancer cases among chromate workers.[5]

In 1956, Bidstrup, following up on an earlier negative study, found a nearly fourfold lung cancer increase in workers exposed to bichromates and chromates.[8] In 1953, the U.S. Public Health Service reported that among 897 workers studied, the lung cancer rate was 29 times expected, but the causative compounds were not identified.[23] In 1976, Finklea reported an industry study in which a threefold excess mortality was seen among workers exposed to lead chromate only, and a nearly threefold increase was noted in workers exposed to lead and zinc chromate.[16] Clearly, the above evidence implicates hexavalent chromium compounds as pulmonary carcinogens, suggesting lead, zinc, and perhaps calcium chromates were responsible.

In 1977, Lane and Mass studied chromyl chloride, using tracheal grafts in rats, and found it to cause squamous cell carcinoma and to also act synergistically with benzyprene to cause carcinomas, making this chromate an "inferred carcinogen."[34]

Role of Solubility in Carcinogenesis

From available information, it appears that the ability of hexavalent compounds to produce cancer is a function of their solubility in tissue fluids. In this regard, there are three categories of hexavalent chromium: those which are insoluble, highly soluble, and sparingly or moderately soluble.

Insoluble Compounds.—Inhaled chromates that are insoluble in tissue fluids, such as thallium dichromate, are not known to pose a threat.[2] Although such hexavalent dust particles may stay in the lungs, because they cannot be dissolved from the compounds, they are not available for absorption into cells and are, therefore, harmless.

Highly Soluble Compounds.—Although chromates, such as chromium trioxide (CrO_3), or chromic acid anhydride, as it is also known, can be very corrosive to skin and mucous membranes, and may cause skin ulcers and allergic reactions, there is no clear evidence that they are carcinogenic.[2] One possible explanation is that they are so rapidly absorbed into, and cleared from, the bloodstream and, thus, eliminated quickly from the body, they have less opportunity to enter cells. However, one recent study suggests that these highly soluble compounds may be associated, at sufficiently high concentrations, with lung cancer.[58]

Slightly or Moderately Soluble.—Inhaled chromium compounds that dissolve slowly in tissue fluids, such as calcium chromate, appear to pose the greatest risk of lung cancer.[2, 13] Because they remain in the lung tissue long enough for the slow, steady release of chromate, the likelihood of a steady release of CR^{+6} to pulmonary cells is increased.

Cancer Cell Type Associated With Chromates

Most reports of the association between lung cancer and chromate exposures fail to consider cell type. Generally, they have considered all pulmonary cancers, as a group, in determining an increased incidence. However, a recent Japanese report suggests that small cell carcinomas may be the predominant cell type. The question is far from resolved, however, and possibly a new look at older data, or perhaps new studies, will further elucidate the question.[1]

In summary, there is good reason to suspect zinc, calcium, and lead chromates as human pulmonary carcinogens. Further animal studies may clarify whether other chromates are carcinogenic. Additionally, recent studies involving users, rather than producers, of chromates may further clarify the matter.

OTHER HEALTH EFFECTS

There have been no reports of increased birth defects, impotence, reproductive changes, nonmalignant lung disease, or other medical problems associated with chromium exposures in man.[49] In a properly controlled environment, it is unlikely that such effects will occur.

HAZARDS OF SPECIFIC EXPOSURES

Chromite Ore/Smelter Workers.—Chromite ore, in addition to Cr_2O_3, also contains varying amounts of other minerals, including iron oxide (around 25%), aluminum oxide (around 15%), magnesium oxide (around 12%), and small amounts of other compounds, including silicates and the oxides of titanium and vanadium. Although minor skin irritation is possible, there is no evidence that chromite ore is carcinogenic.[10] The smelting process can, however, produce hazardous substances as seen in Figure 34–2, and appropriate control measures must be taken. However, with regard to metals exposures, control measures that are effective for chromium should be satisfactory for the other potentially less hazardous substances.

Chromium Metal and Alloy Workers.—Chromium metal, stainless steel, and other alloys are not associated with significant medical problems at currently accepted levels of maximum exposure.[19, 55] *Overexposure* has been reported to be associated with nonmalignant lung changes, although other harmful substances were also present in the few cases reported. Workplace air standards are intended primarily to prevent potential lung changes. Metallic forms of chromium are not known to be associated with skin or mucous membrane changes or with lung cancer. Other metals in alloys may, of course, produce their own health changes.

Workers Exposed to Chromyl Chloride and Other Implied Carcinogens.—Very few workers will come into contact with this extremely corrosive, dark-red, fuming liquid which, on contact with water, forms chromic acid anhydride, hydrochloric acid, trivalent chromium chloride, and chlorine gas. Chromyl chloride is a highly soluble form of hexavalent chromium and is not regarded as a significant cause of, or contributor to, human lung

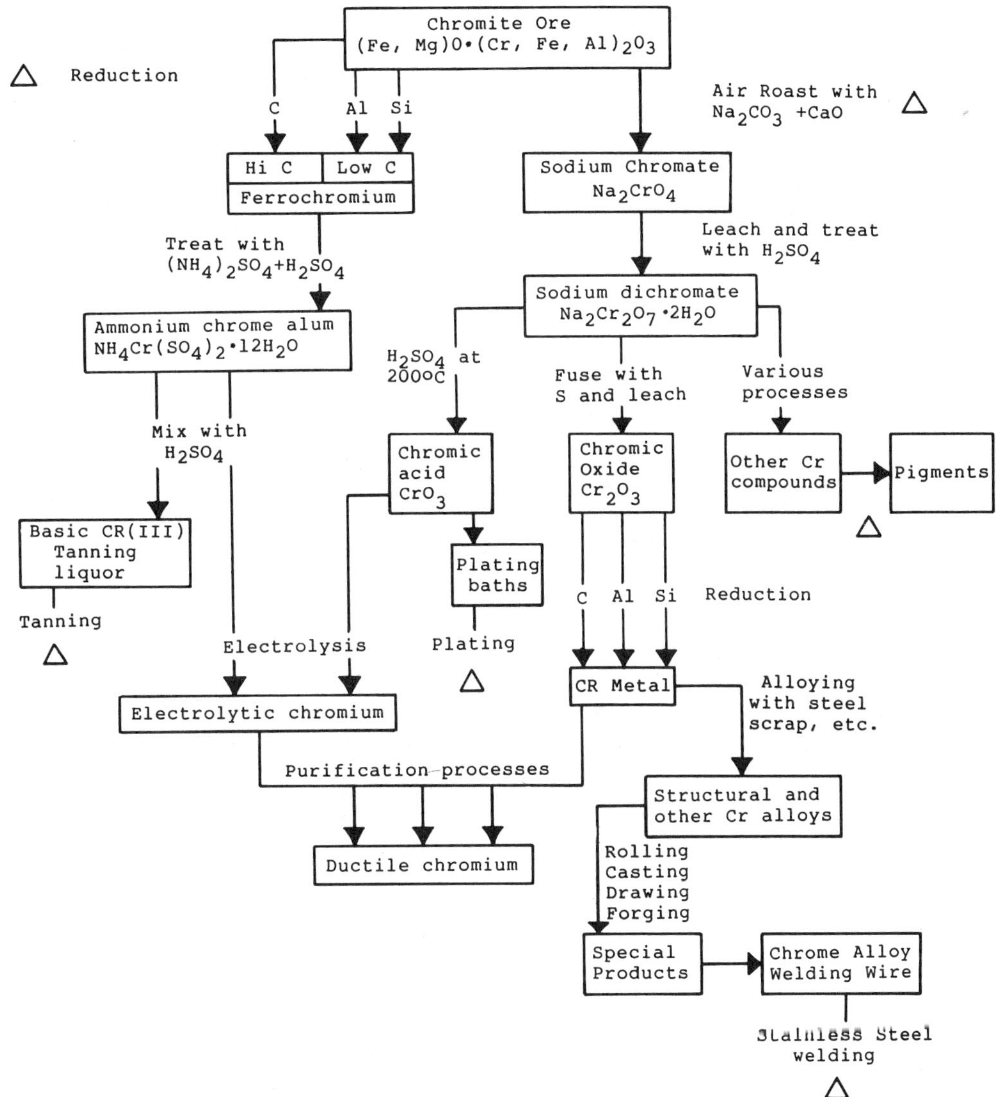

FIG 34–2.
A simplified flow chart summarizing the steps in the production of metallic chromium and some of the important commercial chromium compounds. Processes for which occupational exposure data are available are denoted by the symbol △. (Adapted from Stern RM: Chromium compounds: production and occupational exposure, in Langard S (ed): *Biological and Environmental Aspects of Chromium, Topics in Environmental Health,* Amsterdam, Elsevier North-Holland Biomedical Press, 1982, Vol 5, pp 5–47. Used by permission.)

cancer, although such a possible relationship has been suggested.[3] Based on animal studies, in addition to chromyl chloride, alkaline earth chromates and bichromates and strontium chromates have been suggested as possible lung carcinogens.[47]

Pigment Workers.—As previously indicated, several studies of chromate pigment workers, who have had exposures above currently acceptable standards, report an increased lung cancer risk.[57] The degree of risk appears to depend on the specific pigment, its air concentration, and the nature and duration of exposure. Chromate pigments that appear to have the strongest evidence of lung cancer potential are, as previously indicated, lead and zinc potassium chromates and calcium chromate.

Chromium Plating Workers.—Chrome platers are exposed to chromium trioxide (CrO_3) and its aqueous solution, chromic acid (H_2CrO_4). There is no convincing evidence that these highly corrosive soluble chromates pose a lung cancer risk among chrome platers, although the suggestion of an increased risk has been reported.[17, 58] Today, however, there are additives that reduce the escape of mist by reducing bubbling at electrodes, and newer plating methods, including electroless plating, and other control measures have greatly reduced exposures to these chromates.

Welders of Chromium Alloys.—Several recent reports have focused attention on the possibility that welders of high grade steels may be at increased risk of lung cancer.[7] Soluble and insoluble chromates, chiefly from the welding rod, are present in welding fumes from such steels, but more research is needed to determine whether the suspected cancer originates from the chromium or from other metals, such as nickel. In any case, prudence dictates that, in the welding of high grade steels, the same industrial hygiene precautions should be observed as with known carcinogenic forms, even though the cancer-causing potential of chromium in such alloys is not clearly established.

Ferrochromium Workers.—There are no reports of a significantly increased risk of lung cancer among workers involved in the production of ferrochromium, a metal used in the production of stainless steels and other alloys.[4]

Spray Painters.—Exposures to painters can come from the sandblasting of previously painted surfaces or from spray painting itself. An increased lung cancer risk to spray painters who have been previously overexposed to chromate pigments has been suggested, but there is no indication that painters exposed to currently acceptable levels are at any increased risk of lung cancer.[10]

MONITORING THE HEALTH OF WORKERS EXPOSED TO CHROMIUM COMPOUNDS

Although there is good reason to believe that no increased cancer risk to humans results from hexavalent chromium exposures below present maximum allowable concentrations, medical monitoring of all exposed employees is strongly recommended if for no better reason than to verify a negative correlation.

It is recommended that the monitoring program be the same, regardless of which chromates are involved, at least for the time being. Eventually, some of these recommendations may be modified if continued negative surveillance results indicate the need for change.

Because there is a reported minimal period of ten years before cancer appears in some of those previously overexposed to hexavalent chromium compounds,[8, 51] cancer detection measures such as chest x-ray studies taken sooner than ten years following exposure are not justified. With this in mind, the following is recommended:

1. There is no well-documented value in obtaining urine or other tissue chromium levels for the purpose of removing a worker from exposure.[32] On the other hand, if one is interested in monitoring exposure, biologic monitoring is useful, but only by comparing urine samples at the beginning and at the end of the shift, since chromium levels vary greatly from person to person because of differences in diet and other considerations. If these tests are performed, it is essential that the laboratory be competent and experienced in performing them, because many previously obtained chromium levels were reportedly in error due to sample contamination or poor laboratory technique. The laboratory should be certified by the American Industrial Hygiene Association, or equivalent. Further chromium biologic monitoring information can be obtained from Chapter 13.

2. It is recommended that before work assignments, where hexavalent chromium exposure is likely, the following measures should be taken.

   A. A detailed personal medical and work history should be reviewed by a physician familiar with the potential health risks of exposure to the specific chromium compounds.

   B. A thorough general physical examination by such a physician should be done, with special attention to the skin, mucous membranes, and lungs. Any condition that would potentiate the risk of adverse changes due to chromium exposure (e.g., asthma, dermatitis, prior chromium sensitization) should be noted, and the employee and company should be informed of potential increased risks or special precautions to be taken. If indicated, exclusion from exposure should be advised.

   C. A 14"-x-17" postero/anterior and lateral baseline chest x-ray film should be obtained and retained indefinitely for future comparison.

   D. Spirometry, on equipment and with methods specified by the American Thoracic Society,[60] should be obtained to minimally include Forced Vital Capacity (FVC), forced expiratory volume in one second (FEV_1), and the FEV_1/FVC ratio, chiefly for base-line information. (See chapter 18 for additional details.)

   E. Blood tests to assure normal kidney and liver function and a complete blood count (CBC) should be obtained, initially as a base-line and subsequently to assure that levels toxic to these organs have not been reached.

   F. Urinalysis, to check for protein, glucose, microscopic sediment and specific gravity, should be obtained, for the same reasons given in E above.

3. Once medically approved for chromium VI compound exposure, items A (changes only), B, D, E, and F should be repeated annually. Also, beginning with the tenth year of exposure to any soluble chromium VI compound, anterior and lateral chest x-ray studies and sputum cytology (in those able to produce sputum) may also be useful to verify that lung cancer has not developed. If it is known with absolute certainty that the worker has never been exposed above the maximum allowable concentration, is a nonsmoker, and has meticulous work habits, this precaution may be eliminated.

4. Workers whose potential exposure is to chromium II or III compounds should have their past medical histories reviewed. If there is a history of skin or respiratory problems, medical evaluation and work approval is desirable prior to exposure.

PERSONAL PREVENTIVE MEASURES

In addition to adherence to good personal hygiene and work habits, when considering the risk of lung cancer in persons exposed to chromium compounds, it is important to realize that cigarette smoking, in and of itself, can cause lung cancer. Workers who contact hexavalent chromium compounds should, therefore, be strongly advised not to smoke, to avoid any possible additive carcinogenic effect.

ACCIDENTAL SPILLS

For each specific compound there should be available a Material Safety Data Sheet (MSDS), or equivalent, that discusses the management of potential accidental exposures and first-aid measures. Personnel using a particular substance should be fully aware of the MSDS contents and be proficient in appropriate preventive measures and emergency procedures.

INDUSTRIAL HYGIENE CONSIDERATIONS

The traditional industrial hygiene practices should be followed with chromium compounds, as with any other compound. These measures consist of recognizing the problem, making appropriate measurements of employee exposures, and instituting appropriate exposure control measures. The present Occupational Safety and Health Administration (OSHA) permissible exposure limits (PELs), for eight-hour time-weighted averages, are (1) 0.1 mg/cu m for chromic acid and chromates, as chromium; (2) 0.5 mg/cu m for soluble chromic and chromous salts, as chromium; and (3) 1.0 mg/cu m for chromium metal and "insoluble" salts, as chromium.

The threshold limit values (TLVs) recommended by the American Conference of Governmental Industrial Hygienists (ACGIH) are listed in Table 34–2. (See also Appendix A.) It should be emphasized that in the case of those chromate compounds considered carcinogenic it is always recommended that the concentrations be kept as low as practically achievable.

TABLE 34–2.
ACGIH TLVs for Chromium, 1986–1987

Chromite ore processing (chromate), as Cr	0.05 mg/cu m, (A1a)*
Chromium metal	0.5 mg/cu m
Chromium (II) compounds, as Cr	0.5 mg/cu m
Chromium (III) compounds, as Cr	0.5 mg/cu m
Chromium (VI) compounds, as Cr	
Water-soluble	0.05 mg/cu m
Certain water-insoluble	0.05 mg/cu m, (A1a)*
Chromyl chloride	(0.025 ppm), 0.15 mg/cu m
Lead chromate, as Cr	0.05 mg/cu m (A2a)†

*A1a—*Human Carcinogens:* Substances or substances associated with industrial processes, recognized to have carcinogenic or cocarcinogenic potential, with an assigned TLV.
†A2a—*Industrial Substances Suspect of Carcinogenic Potential for Man:* Chemical substances or substances associated with industrial processes, which are suspected of inducing cancer, based on either (1) limited epidemiologic evidence, exclusive of clinical reports of single cases, or (2) demonstration of carcinogenesis in one or more animal species by appropriate methods.

SUMMARY AND CONCLUSIONS

Chromium is a complex metal, with hundreds of forms, each with a different potential for hazardous health effects. Most, however, pose no greater hazards than many other substances in the workplace, if the potential risks are fully appreciated and appropriate control measures instituted.

ACKNOWLEDGMENTS

I gratefully acknowledge the generous assistance of professors Ralph G. Smith, Ernest Mastromatteo, and Gerald Sattlemeier, for their help in obtaining literature for review, and of Daniel W. Sawyer, for proofreading and preparation of the reference list.

REFERENCES

1. Abe S, Ohsaki Y, Kimura K, et al: Chromate lung cancer with special reference to its cell type and relation to the manufacturing process. *Cancer* 1982; 49:783–87.
2. ACGIH: Documentation of recommendations for TLVs: Chromium, 1986–1987, p 98.
3. ACGIH: Documentation of recommendations for TLVs: Chromyl Chloride, 1986–1987, p 100.
4. Axelsson G, Rylander R, Schmidt A: Mortality and incidence of tumors among ferrochromium workers. *Br J Ind Med* 1980; 37:121–127.
5. Baetjer AM: Pulmonary carcinoma in chromate workers—Incidence on basis of hospital records. *Arch Ind Hyg Occup Med* 1950; 2:505–16.
6. Baetjer AM, Damron C, Budacz V: The distribution and retention of chromium. *Arch Ind Health* 1959; 20:136–150.
7. Becker N, Claude J, Frentzel-Beyme R: Cancer risk of arc welders exposed to fumes containing chromium and nickel. *Scand J Work Environ Health* 1985; 11:2.

8. Bidstrup RL, Case RAM: Carcinoma of the lung in workmen in the bichromate producing industry in Great Britain. *Br J Ind Med* 1956; 13:260–64.
9. Chen NSC, Tsai A, Dyer IA: Effect of chelating agents on chromium absorption in rats. *J Nutr* 1973; 103:1182–86.
10. Chiazze L, Wolfe P: Epidemiology of respiratory cancer and other health effects among workers exposed to chromium: A review of recent literature, in *Proceedings, Chromates Symposium-80*. Pittsburgh, Industrial Hygiene Foundation, 1980.
11. Cotton FA, Wilkinson G: *Advanced Inorganic Chemistry, a Comprehensive Text,* ed 4. New York, John Wiley & Sons, 1980, p 724.
12. Cumin W: Remarks on the medicinal properties of madar, and on the effects of bichromate of potass on the human body. *Edinburgh Med Surg J* 1827; 28:295–312.
13. Dickenson J: Chromate pigments in surface coatings, inks and plastics, in *Proceedings, Chromates Symposium-80*. Pittsburgh, Industrial Hygiene Foundation, 1980.
14. Doisy RJ, Streeten DHP, Levine RA, et al: Effects and metabolism of chromium in normals, elderly subjects and diabetics, in *Trace Substances in Environmental Health II*. Columbia, Mo, University of Missouri Press, 1969, pp 75–82.
15. Donaldson RM, Barreras RF: Intestinal absorption of trace quantities of chromium. *J Lab Clin Med* 1966; 68:484–93.
16. Finklea JF: Lead chromate—An update, written communication, in *The Carcinogenicity of Hexavalent Chromium Compounds: A Literature Review*, a paper prepared by Musch DL. *University of Michigan* EIH 657, 1978.
17. Franchini I, Magnani F, Mutti A: Mortality experience among chrome plating workers. *Scand J Work Environ Health* 1983; 9:247–252.
18. Freund H, Atamian S, Fischer JE: Chromium deficiency during total parenteral nutrition. *JAMA* 1979; 241:496–98.
19. Furst A: Problems in metal carcinogenesis, in Kharasch N (ed): *Trace Metals in Health and Disease*. New York, Raven Press, 1979.
20. Goldman M, Karotkin RH: Acute potassium bichromate poisoning. *Am J Med Sci* 1935; 189:400–403.
21. Gray S, Sterling K: The tagging of red cells and plasma proteins with radioactive chromium. *J Clin Invest* 1950; 29:1604–1613.
22. Gurson CT: The metabolic significance of dietary chromium. *Adv Nutr Res* 1977; I:23–53.
23. *Health of Workers in the Chromate Producing Industry—A Study*, Publ 192. US Public Health Service, Division of Occupational Health, Bureau of State Services, 1953.
24. Herrmann H, Speck LB: Interaction of chromate with nucleic acids in tissues. *Science* 1954; 119:221.
25. Hopkins LL, Schwartz K: Chromium binding to serum proteins, specifically siderophilin. *Biochem Biophys Acta* 1964; 90:484–91.
26. Hopkins LL Jr, Price MG: Effectiveness of chromium (III) in improving the impaired glucose tolerance of middle aged Americans, in *Western Hemisphere Congress*. Puerto Rico, 1968, vol 2, pp 40–41.
27. International Agency for Research on Cancer: Chromium and chromium compounds. *IARC Monog Eval Carcinog Risk Chem Hum* 1980; 23:205–323.
28. Jeejeebhoy KN, Chu RC, Marliss EB, et al: Chromium deficiency, glucose intolerance, and neuropathy reversed by chromium supplementation in a patient receiving long-term total parenteral nutrition. *Am J Clin Nutr* 1977; 30:531–538.
29. Kelly WF, Ackrill P, Day JP, et al: Cutaneous absorption of trivalent chromium: Tissue levels and treatment by exchange transfusion. *Br J Ind Med* 1982; 39:397–400.
30. Koppel W, Hathaway J: The acute chemical effect on chromium compounds in man, in *Proceedings, Chromates Symposium-80*. Pittsburgh, Industrial Hygiene Foundation, 1980, pp 24–31.
31. Korallus U, Harsdorf C, Lewalter J: Experimental bases for ascorbic acid therapy of poisoning by hexavalent chromium compounds. *Int Arch Occup Environ Health* 1984; 53(3):247–256.
32. Kumpulainen J, Lehto J, Koivistoinen P, et al: Determination of chromium in human milk, serum and urine by electrothermal atomic absorption spectrometry without preliminary ashing. *Sci Total Environ* 1983; 31:71–80.
33. Laitung JK, Earley M: The role of surgery in chromic acid burns: Our experience with two patients. *Burns, Incl Thermal Inj* 1984; 10:378–80.
34. Lane BP, Mass MJ: Carcinogenicity and cocarcinogenicity of chromium carbonyl in heterotopic tracheal grafts. *Cancer Res* 1977; 37:1476–1479.
35. Lehman KB: Ist grund zu einer be sonderen beunruhigung wegen auf trepens vun lungen krebs bei chromatarbiteren vorhanden? *Zentralbl Gewerbehyg* 1932; 19:168.
36. Levine RA, Streeten DHP, Doisy RJ: Effects of oral chromium supplementation on the glucose tolerance of elderly human subjects. *Metabolism* 1968; 17:114–25.
37. Lewalter J: Biomonitoring for chrome exposure, in *Proceedings, Chromates Symposium-80*. Pittsburgh, Industrial Hygiene Foundation, 1980, p 276.
38. Lim TH, Sargent T, Kusubov N: Kinetics of trace element chromium (III) in the human body. *Am J Physiol* 1983; 244(4):R445–454.
39. Liu VJK, Morris JS: Relative chromium response as an indicator of chromium status. *Am J Clin Nutr* 1978; 31:972–76.
40. Machle W, Gregorius J: Cancer of the respiratory system in the United States chromate producing industry. *Public Health Rep* 1948; 63:1114–1127.
41. Mackenzie JN: Some observations on the toxic effects of chrome on the nose, throat and ear. *JAMA* 1884; 3:601–603.
42. Mancuso TF, Hueper WC: Occupational cancer and other health hazards in a chromate plant: A medical appraisal, I, Lung cancers in chromate workers. *Ind Med Surg* 1951; 20:358–363.
43. *The Merck Index*, ed 10, Windholz et al (ed). Rahway, NJ, Merck & Co, 1983, pp 315–319.
44. Mertz W: Clinical and public health significance of chromium, in *Clinical, Biochemical and Nutritional Aspects of Trace Elements*. New York, Alan R Liss, Inc, 1982, pp 315–23.
45. Milby TH, Key MM, Gibson RL, et al: Chemical hazards, in Gafafer WM (ed): *Occupational Diseases—A Guide to Their Recognition*, PHS Publ 1097. US Dept of Health, Education and Welfare, Public Health Service, 1964, Sect. VI:120–122.
46. National Research Council: Contingency plans for chromium utilization. Washington, DC, National Academy of Sciences, 1978.
47. National Institute for Occupational Safety and Health: *Occupational Exposure to Chromium VI, Criteria for a Recommended Standard,* 1975.
48. Nelson RD Jr: Chromium chemistry, in *Proceedings, Chromates Symposium-80*. Pittsburgh, Industrial Hygiene Foundation, 1980, p 9.
49. Nieboer E, Yassi A, Haines AT, et al: *Effects of Chromium Compounds on Human Health,* prepared for Ontario Ministry of Labour, ISBN 0-7729-0193-7, 1984, pp 4–39.
50. Norseth T: The carcinogenicity of chromium and its salts. *Br J Ind Med* 1986; 43:649–651.
51. Ohsaki Y, Abe S, Kimura K, et al: Lung cancer in Japanese chromate workers. *Thorax* 1978; 33:372–74.
52. Pepys J: Clinical and therapeutic significance of patterns of allergic reactions of the lungs to extrinsic agents. *Am Rev Respir Dis* 1977; 116:573–88.
53. Pfeil E: Lung tumors as an occupational disease in chromium plants. *Dtsch Med Wochenschr* 1935; 61:1197–1200.

54. Polak L: Immunology of chromium, in Burrows D (ed): *Chromium: Metabolism and Toxicity*. Boca Raton, Fl, CRC Press, 1983, pp 51–136.

55. Rogers G: In vivo production of hexavalent chromium. *Biomaterials* (Guilford, Engl) 1984; 5:4.

56. Saner G: Chromium in nutrition and disease, in *Current Topics in Nutrition and Disease*. New York, Alan R Liss, Inc, 1980, vol 2. Quoted in Jaworski JF: *Chromium Update 1984*. National Research Council Canada, NRCC 23917, p 19, 1984.

57. Satoh K, Fukuda Y, Torii K, et al: Epidemiological study of workers engaged in the manufacture of chromium. *J Occup Med* 23(12):835–38.

58. Silverstein M, Mirer F, et al: Mortality among workers in a die-casting and electroplating plant. *Scand J Work Environ Health* 1981; 7(4):136–165.

59. Sharma BK, Singhal PC, Chugh KS: Intravascular haemolysis and acute renal failure following potassium dichromate poisoning. *Postgrad Med J* 1978; 54:414–15.

60. *Statement of Standardization of Spirometry*. American Thoracic Society, 1987 Update (Approved by ATS Board of Directors March 7, 1987).

61. Underwood EJ: *Trace Elements in Human and Animal Nutrition*, ed 4. New York, Academic Press, 1977, pp 258–270.

62. Waterhouse J: Cancer among chromium platers. *Br J Cancer* 1975; 32:262.

35

Fluorides

Arthur L. Knight, M.D.

Fluorine, the 13th most common element, is one of the most widely distributed of all elements in nature but never found in the elemental state as F_2 which is a yellow gas.[22] It occurs in numerous inorganic and organic compounds with activity of great chemical and physiologic diversity.

Fluorine gas is highly reactive, and with water in air forms hydrofluoric acid (HF), which is corrosive to all common metals and glass. Liquid fluorine is the most powerful chemical oxidizer and the most reactive nonmetal.

Hydrogen fluoride is a colorless liquid with an easily detected odor at a few parts per million, and in water forms hydrofluoric acid. The fluorine ions in hydrofluoric acid readily combine with silica ("glass etching").

Fluorides differ from the other halogens in being more soluble, in resisting formation of higher covalent states, and in bringing about the higher covalency of other elements.

The major source of fluorides comes from the mining of the widespread mineral fluorspar (CaF_2) and the phosphate rock fluoropatite ($Ca_{10}F_2[PO_4]_6$). Large deposits of the latter are found in Florida and are used primarily in the manufacture of fertilizer.[11] Fluorspar heated with sulfuric acid produces hydrofluoric acid. At one time, cryolite (Na_3AlF_6) was mined in Greenland, but now it is mostly manufactured. Elemental fluorine is produced primarily by electrolysis of a fluoride solution.

USES

Fluorine and hydrofluoric acid are used in the manufacture of a tremendous variety of fluoride compounds.

Elemental liquid fluorine is used in producing uranium hexafluoride and as a rocket propellant,[36] as is chlorine trifluoride and bromine pentafluoride.

Industrial fluoride emissions into the atmosphere in the United States total more than 100,000 tons per year, and 88% comes from the manufacture of steel, brick, tile, glass, porcelain, aluminum, fertilizer, and the combustion of coal.[12]

Cryolite is used as an agricultural insecticide and in the manufacture of aluminum.

Fluorine compounds are also important in gold refining, phosphorus extraction, silicate extraction, fluxing agents, coating on welding rods, in metal casting, as insecticides, and in lens coating.

More than 600 million lb of fluorocarbons are manufactured yearly in the United States. They are used as aerosol propellants, foam-blowing agents, solvents, dielectric fluids, degreasers, dry cleaning fluid, ultrasonic cleaners, refrigerants, pharmaceuticals, anesthetics such as methoxyflurane, and in tracheobronchial clearance studies.[4]

The fluorocarbon polymers or fluoroplastics are used in electrical components and insulation, in gaskets and valves and in sealants, in antistick friction-reducing applications and as a nonstick surface on utensils and cookware and bandages, corrosion-resistant linings, long-lasting exterior finishes, and as low-temperature lubricants.

Sodium fluoroacetate, sodium fluoride (NaF) and sodium silicofluoride (Na_2SiF_6) are used as rodenticides, pesticides, and in chemical warfare.

Because of their wide distribution, fluorine compounds are found in nearly all living things, including man, where they play a highly useful[24] and essential role. Nearly all foods contain fluoride. The average United States daily intake in food is 0.2–0.3 mg, with a possible additional 1.0 mg or more in drinking water.[12] Both insufficient and excessive amounts of fluoride are harmful to man's health.[27]

BIOLOGIC EFFECTS

The toxicity of fluorine compounds varies from the most toxic substance, fluoroacetic acid, to several fluorine compounds, such as dichlorodifluoromethane (CCl_2F_2), that have a threshold limit value (TLV) that is exceeded only by carbon dioxide. Ingestion of 1–4 gm of soluble fluoride has been fatal. One percent of the deaths from accidental and suicidal poisoning involve fluorides. Lethal oral doses of fluorides are similar to many other powerful poisons in that they cause nausea, vomiting, diarrhea, central nervous system symptoms, circulatory collapse, respiratory problems, convulsions and death.

Absorption

In general, most fluorides are poorly absorbed from the intact skin but readily absorbed in the lungs and the gastrointestinal tract. The degree and time for absorption vary somewhat with the solubility of the fluoride. However, the fluorides in relatively insoluble rock phosphate dust, when inhaled are rapidly absorbed[8, 9] and give rise in urinary excretion in a fashion similar to that occurring from inhalation of gaseous fluorides.[8]

Metabolism

Fluorides are taken in each day in food and usually in drinking water. Deficiency of fluoride can lead to osteoporosis, calcified abdominal nodes, ligamentous calcification and bone spurs.[27]

Fluoride in trace amounts is found in most body tissues, usually bound to protein and not an active part of the daily intake-excretion process.[45] Fluorine is a normal constituent of the blood and is mostly bound to protein. Only about 10% is ionized.[18] Excessive fluorine intake increases the ionized fluorine in the blood. It is cleared from the blood by either bone deposition, with a biologic half-time of 30 minutes, or by kidney excretion, with a biologic half-time of two to three hours.

Up to 99% of the body burden of fluoride is found in the skeleton.[18] There is an attraction to the skeletal system of a certain level of fluorides. Before this level is reached, a part of the fluorides will be deposited in the bones, and intake of fluoride will exceed excretion. After this level has been reached, the intake of fluoride will approximate the output. If the fluoride intake is excessive, there will be extra fluorides deposited in the bones. If the intake later drops, this bone excess then will be mobilized and excreted. To a degree, this process of excess fluoride buildup in bone is reversible, but if too great or too long, it may become permanent, a condition called fluorosis (chronic fluoride poisoning). In fluorosis, the bone, instead of containing the normal level of fluoride of approximately 0.1%, will contain ten times this amount (1.0%) and may be detectable by x-ray.

Fluoride is deposited on the apatite crystalline lattice of bone by exchange with hydroxyl ions and does not require osteoblasts or osteoclasts. Unlike strontium, it does not replace calcium.

With intake levels up to approximately 3 or 4 mg of fluoride per day, the body likely will excrete the same amount in urine, feces, sweat, tears, and milk. With levels over 4 mg per day, storage in the bones likely will occur.[11]

Fluoride is also selectively taken up by the teeth, especially in the developing stage. Insufficient fluoride can cause an increase in dental caries, optimal amounts are required for maximal dental health, and excess fluoride in the developing stage of the teeth can cause mottling—white or brown spots. With little or no fluoride in the drinking water, most children will have considerable dental caries. One part per million in drinking water protects most teeth from cavity formation and causes very little mottling. At 4 ppm, almost all children will have mottled teeth.

The fluoride content of bile is low.[46]

Increased fluorine is found in the aorta with increasing age. This likely is related to the increasing calcification of the aorta and not to intake.[40] Other ectopic calcifications also store fluoride.

Excretion

The simple fluoride salts are readily excreted in the urine.[26] Urine accounts for more than 90% of the fluoride excretion. If the intake is primarily insoluble fluorides, the level of fecal excretion might reach 30%. If sweating is a major part of the fluid loss, it also could account for one third of the fluoride excretion.[18] It also appears in tears and milk.

When the fluoride level in test animals becomes very high, some kidney damage results.[39]

Prior moderate exposure or no unusual prior exposure does not give a different effect on the excretion of fluoride after a moderate exposure.[9]

When a fluoride-exposed worker no longer is exposed to fluorides, his or her urinary excretion will be in excess of intake for some time—perhaps weeks or longer—until the skeletal load reaches a certain level when the output and intake will become equal.[25]

With the urinary excretion half-life of fluorides as little as two hours, a worker exposed to fluorides will have wide variations of urinary level, depending on the variability and degree of exposure and the time of sampling.

Chloride is 99% reabsorbed by the kidney, resulting in little being excreted. By comparison, however, fluoride is poorly reabsorbed, so that about one third of it filtered by the kidney passes to the bladder to be excreted.

Acute Toxicity

Elemental fluorine and oxygen difluoride are strong oxidizers and are irritating and corrosive to tissue.

Short-term fluorine exposure at 20 mg/cu m for five minutes gives no irreparable respiratory damage, and exposures to 5 mg/cu m for short single exposures should be tolerable from a comfort standpoint.[36] A suggested emergency exposure limit for fluorine is ten minutes at 15 ppm.[18]

Hydrogen Fluoride.—Hydrogen fluoride exposure at 25 mg/cu m gives mild irritation to the eyes and the nose but can be tolerated; short-term exposures to 50 mg/cu m give irritation to the eyes and the nose, and the maximal tolerable exposure to 100 mg/cu m is about one minute.[36] A five-minute emergency exposure limit is said to be 20 ppm.[18]

Hydrogen fluoride at 5–10 ppm causes irritation of the eyes, nose, and throat,[22] possibly with sneezing and lacrimation, whereas at higher concentrations, skin irritation, laryngospasm, tracheal irritation with chest pain, cough, and hemoptysis develop. Its high solubility in water is the reason it is a strong irritant to the upper respiratory tract before pulmonary damage is done.

Inhalation of hydrogen fluoride in concentrations to 4.74 ppm produced no systemic effects. The urine output rose, as did the small amount in the feces. Some stinging of the face and eyes and nasal irritation was noted in concentrations of less than 2 ppm. At 3.39 ppm and higher, redness of the face was noted and, after several days, slight desquamation of the superficial epithelium.[26]

A sour taste in the mouth has been experienced by some workers.

Soluble inorganic salts hydrolyze to form free hydrogen fluoride in contact with tissue; this is very irritating. Less soluble salts are not so irritating but may be harmful on inhalation.

Massive doses of fluoride up to 100 mg per day[17] have been given in the treatment of osteoporosis.[37]

Chlorine trifluoride, a colorless gas used as a rocket propellant is a fire hazard due to its oxidizing ability. It is a primary skin irritant and a strong pulmonary irritant. Boron trifluoride is similar but not quite as irritating.

Sulfur hexafluoride, a colorless, odorless gas used as insulation in electronic tubes, sulfur hexafluoride is physiologically inert.[28] Inhaled as a mixture of 80% with 20% oxygen, it produces tingling, excitement, and altered hearing and is a mild anesthetic.[14] The danger with sulfur hexafluoride is that it can be contaminated with other fluorides of sulfur, such as sulfur pentafluoride[29] and disulfur decafluoride,[38] which are extremely toxic and are respiratory irritants.

Nitrogen trifluoride (NF_3) and tetrafluorohydrazine (N_2F_4) are of a low order of toxicity and act as pulmonary irritants. At high levels of exposure in experimental animals, some hematoxic signs and kidney damage have been noted.[7]

A monofluorinated hydrocarbon, *fluoroacetate*, is very highly toxic. It is found in certain plants in Australia, Brazil, and South Africa, where it was lethal to cattle grazing on them. The fluoroacetate is so toxic because of the very toxic and lethal "protoplasmic poison," fluorocitric acid. The fluoroacetic acid enters the tricarboxylic acid cycle like any two-carbon atom acetate. It is converted by the primary enzymes to fluorocitrate. The enzymes cannot take the fluorocitrate farther and the body then is left with this poison, which blocks the tricarboxylic acid cycle by inhibiting the aconitase enzyme. This disruption of the cell process causes its death. There is no antidote. A couple of drops by any route is likely to be fatal.[7, 33]

Any compound that forms fluoroacetic acid in its biochemical breakdown or metabolism can be predicted to be very toxic. Any fluoroalcohol or w-fluorocarboxylic acid ($F(CH_2)_nCOOH$) with the total carbon atoms in the chain being even is such a product and will be toxic. Those with an odd number of total carbon atoms in the chain will not break down to form fluoroacetic acid and so will not be toxic.[34]

Fluoroacetate poisoning starts with nausea, vomiting, epigastric pain, and excessive salivation, lasting a very few hours. Numbness and a tingling sensation may occur as well as mental apprehension. It affects the central nervous system as well as the cardiovascular system. Muscle twitching, low blood pressure, and blurred vision may develop. Convulsions may be alternated with coma and depression. Death can come from respiratory failure but usually from cardiac irregularity.

The *fluoroalkanes* vary in toxicity. The more chlorine the more toxic they become, but the more fluorine they contain the less toxic they become.[7]

The fluoroalkenes have a double bond that makes them more active and more toxic. The more chlorine or fluorine they contain the more toxic they become.[7]

Fluorocarbons and polyfluorinated compounds.—The outstanding stability of the carbon-fluoride link results in chemical properties very similar to those of the nonfluorinated analogs. Fluorocarbons that appear similar to toxic chlorocarbons are less toxic because of this bond. Carbon tetrachloride (CCl_4) is very toxic, but carbon tetrafluoride (CF_4) is a very inactive, stable, nontoxic gas.

Whereas the unsaturated fluorocarbons are toxic, and the toxicity increases with increased fluorine content, the saturated fluorocarbons become less toxic with additional fluorine atoms.

The polyfluorocarbons offer a wide range of toxicity. Some are mildly irritating to the upper respiratory tract, yet some, such as fluorinated ethylene propylene and Teflon 120 tagged with radioactive fluorine, are used in tracheobronchial clearance studies.[4]

Many halogenated hydrocarbons with chlorine are toxic, and substituting bromine or iodine makes them more toxic, but substituting fluorine usually reduces the toxicity.

Most saturated fluorocarbons are stable, relatively inert, and very slightly toxic. At 2,500 ppm, some adverse effect on the worker's performance and psychomotor skills may occur. A mild central nervous system depression and a mild irritation of the upper respiratory tract may occur also.

The fluoropolymers, when intact, have very low toxicity, but when overheated by an open flame or a hot surface, they will break down. Fluoropolymers such as polytetrafluoroethylene or dichloromonofluoromethane can be safely heated to 200° C. Many fluoropolymers at higher temperatures, particularly about 325° C, yield hydrogen fluoride, hydrochloric acid, and fluorocarbon gases. At higher temperatures,[10] sulfur dioxide, even carbon monoxide, chlorine, phosgene, and perfluoroisobutylene, may be released by heating. The last is very toxic and produces pulmonary edema. Inhalation of these breakdown fumes can produce "polymer fever," similar to metal fume fever, with chills, fever, aches in muscles and joints of one or two days' duration.[7]

Dichlorodifluoromethane (CCl_2F_2).—The most produced fluorocarbon, is another refrigerant and aerosol propellant that, when heated, can break down, producing irritant and toxic products; ordinarily, it is inert physiologically but it can be an asphyxiant. Five percent is said to induce dizziness.

Dichlorotetrafluoroethane is also a refrigerant and aerosol propellant having low toxicity, but 10% causes some irritation and restlessness.

Trichlorotrifluoroethane, a refrigerant and used in dry cleaning, is said to be nontoxic to over 4,000 ppm.[21]

Trifluoroethyl vinyl ether, dibromodichlorotrifluoroethane, and dichlorodifluoroethyl methyl ether are used as anesthetics that produce no liver damage.

Volatile fluorocarbons may produce cardiac arrhythmia when large amounts of epinephrine are secreted endogenously, such as in fear, anger, or exertion.[33]

Effects on the Skin.—Gaseous fluorine causes an instant burn, like fire. Hydrofluoric acid up to a 10% solution may be of no harm if removed shortly after exposure. Concentrations under 20% may have several hours' delay before a burn is detected. Concentrations above 20% are felt quicker and if over 60% are felt immediately.

A case of systemic fluoride poisoning arose from absorption from a hydrofluoric acid burn to 2.5% of body surface. It produced marked stupor, with lack of response to questions for more than a day, severe nausea, hematuria, renal casts, and possible S-T elevation on electrocardiogram (ECG).[3]

The hydrogen fluoride penetrates deeply into the skin also, spreading laterally, causing necrosis even of subcutaneous tissue. In less severe burns, the skin tends to turn white and vesicle formation sometimes is seen with delamination of the skin layers.

Some fluoride compounds are skin irritants and give rise to contact dermatitis, as do the fluorocarbons, by absorbing the skin fat.

Chronic Toxicity

Some cryolite workers have been reported as having a subacute illness, probably due to swallowing cryolite dust.[33] There likely is not any chronic toxicity from fluorine, since an irritant level of 0.1 ppm is not likely to be tolerated.

Small excesses of fluorides in the developing years may lead to mottling of the teeth.

Exposures to levels of 2.4–6.0 mg/cu m of fluoride over many years may give osteosclerotic changes, increased density of the spinal column, some loss of trabecular detail, and some calcification of the intervertebral ligaments, but no physical impairment[11] or overt clinical disease. Some limitation of motion in the dorsolumbar spine can occur. This condition, called fluorosis, can be spontaneous, from diet and water fluorides, or industrial, from fluoride exposure at work. There is no nonskeletal phase to fluorosis.[23] At higher levels, such as was seen in Danish cryolite workers who were crushing and grinding cryolite in a dry state in poor conditions, where intake may have reached 20–80 mg fluoride per day,[17] calcification of the spinal broad ligaments occurred that can give a crippling poker back. Bone and joint disability and bone softening have been seen in cattle, in which chronic effects of fluorides were first described about 100 years ago.

Diagnostic Techniques

There are no pathognomonic signs of acute fluoride poisoning. The great number and variety of compounds with fluorine allow for almost any signs and symptoms to appear and some with great rapidity. Toxicity varies from the most toxic sodium fluoroacetate to primarily asphyxiants, such as sulfur hexafluoride.

Hydrofluoric acid burns sometimes can be suspected by the grayish or whitish skin, the unusual depth for the degree of contact, and failure to respond to usual burn therapy, seen especially if there is involvement of the nail area.

X-Ray.—Radiographic examination of the spine might show the subtle increase in bone density, loss of trabeculation, and calcification of vertebral ligaments found in chronic fluoride poisoning.

Laboratory.—Blood fluoride is mostly protein bound and total fluorides are a poor indication of exposure.[12] The free fluoride ion in the blood[43] is directly related to recent intake, but some fluorides can clear from the blood in a very few hours. Until the 1960s, the blood fluoride that was measured in the laboratory was total fluoride. The custom in laboratories today is to report only the ionized fluoride as the blood fluoride. Most articles on fluorides do not designate what was measured when they mention blood fluorides. Less than 0.05 mg total fluoride per 100 ml is considered a normal blood level by some, whereas others use 0.01 mg/100 ml as a normal limit. In fatal hydrogen fluoride cases, blood levels were 0.3 to 0.4 mg/100 ml.[3]

Urine analysis for fluoride has been more successful in evaluating the degree of fluoride exposure. Fluoride excretion levels of 4 mg of fluoride per liter in urine samples collected at the end of the work shift can be considered the upper limit of normal to serve as a useful reference level for evaluating atmospheric fluoride exposure where industrial environmental concentrations vary widely and in determining the probability of incurring increased bone density.[11] Above 4 mg must be considered suspicious of excessive fluoride exposure.

In evaluating both blood and urine test results for fluorine, the level of fluorine in the drinking water of the employees both at home and at work must be known. Very high water fluorine content can give results above the normal limits.

Treatment

In acute fluorine poisoning, the primary step is to remove the victim from the exposure. Oxygen therapy (100%) has been recommended in such cases. Contaminated clothing should be removed and the patient treated symptomatically.

Swallowed fluoride, such as sodium fluoride, may result in death in two to four hours. If the victim lives longer than four hours, he or she may recover.[17] With swallowed fluoride poisoning, it is advisable to induce vomiting if the person is conscious. Gastric lavage may be effective.

Ingested fluoroacetate is also handled by emptying the stomach contents. Monoacetin (glycerol monoacetate) is a specific antagonist to fluoroacetate and can be given orally, 100 ml diluted with 500 ml of water and repeated in an hour,[34] or intramuscularly, 0.5 ml/kg undiluted each half hour for several hours. Also, it can be given intravenously at the same dose but diluted with 5 parts of isotonic saline.[15] Epileptiform convulsions can be treated with barbiturates. Cardiac irregularities can occur, so monitoring on an ECG when available is advisable.

Patients with fluorohydrocarbon poisoning should not be given epinephrine (Adrenalin) or similar drugs because of the tendency of fluorohydrocarbon to induce cardiac arrhythmia, including ventricular fibrillation.[33]

All acute poisoning cases should be augmented by symptomatic treatment.

A skin burn from hydrofluoric acid always is more severe than its appearance. There is a reaction of the hydrogen ions[5] on the lipids within the cells. Overtreatment is indicated. Knowledge of the concentration of the acid and its length of time on the skin could be valuable in evaluating the condition and the treatment needed. Systemic poisoning has been reported from a fluorine skin burn to 2½% of the body.[3]
Hydrofluoric acid in 20% solution is dangerous, since the burn is not felt soon and hours later is very painful when the skin becomes swollen, turns white or red and gray.

Various therapies have been recommended for hydrofluoric acid burns:

1. Washing with running cool water as soon as possible after the burn for an hour or longer or until other therapy is begun

2. Iced alcohol compresses[3]

3. Magnesium oxide dressings made of 20% magnesium oxide in glycerin

4. Ten percent calcium gluconate injected around and under the burn area.[2] (This is supposed to limit the spread of the acid)

5. Soaking in quaternary ammonium compounds[3]

6. Diethylene triamine (DETA) 1½% solution in a 60% solution of ethyl alcohol used as wet dressings, soaks, or rinsing for an hour or more

Hydrofluoric acid burns that involve the cuticle, sides or bed of a nail should have the nail cut away (under local anesthesia) to allow exposure of the nail bed to treatment. Burned skin or vesicles, if removed, also allow better exposure for treatment of the underlying skin. Large or deep burns may require skin grafting, but it is not done in the acute stage.

Splashes of acid involving the eye should be promptly and copiously rinsed with cool water. If any damage other than conjunctivitis is noted, an ophthalmologist should be consulted immediately.

Small nasal ulcers, usually from chronic exposure to vapor or fumes, demand that the employee be removed from exposure, and the nose should be cleansed and coated with an antibacterial ointment daily until healed.

FLUORINE ANALYSIS

Air Analysis

There is no simple color changing tube or direct meter reading method for determining the amount or type of fluoride in the worker's environment. If the industrial process is releasing both gaseous and particulate fluoride, the problem of analysis is made more difficult and less accurate. Contamination with either silica or aluminum in the collected sample will add complicated steps to the determination.

Standard impingers, bubblers, alkali-treated filter paper, or glass fiber filters and membrane filters can be used. They are efficient collectors of particles above 0.3 μ but vary in reactivity to gaseous fluoride. Choose the collecting system most efficient for the type of fluoride exposure involved. Fumes can be sampled by an electrostatic precipitator.

An automatic hydrogen fluoride recorder was developed for industrial hygiene use.[1] A portable continuous analyzer can be used for gaseous fluorides.[20]

The analysis of the collected sample for fluorides did require separation of contaminants by precipitation, ion exchange,[32] distillation, or diffusion followed by a chemical analysis by gravimetric, enzymatic, titrimetric, colorimetric, or electrochemical method. The sample can be analyzed faster by using the fluorine-specific ion electrode after ashing and buffering.

A qualitative test based on insolubility of thorium fluoride can be used for the determination of fluorine in organic fluorides.[22]

Urine Analysis

Urine containing fluorides has relatively large amounts of other substances that interfere with a fluorine determination by common chemical methods, and the techniques of separation and then of analysis of the fluorides as noted above for air apply to urine. Spectrophotometric analysis can be done; however, it is not specific for fluoride but is based on color development.

The method of choice for urine analysis is the fluorine-specific ion electrode developed in 1966, which made the fluoride determination in urine rapid, simple, and accurate.[41] With this procedure, the pH of the sample being tested must be between 4.5 and 8.[12] If urinary fluoride levels exceed 4–6 mg/L, surveillance of the workers and control of their exposure is advisable.[31]

PRINCIPLES OF CONTROL

Permissible Exposure Limits

Almost two dozen substances containing fluorine are listed in the *Occupational Health Guideline for Chemical Hazards*.[44] The range for these substances varies from 0.02 ppm (tellurium hexafluoride) to 1,000 ppm (trifluoromonobromomethane) and from 0.05 mg/cu m (sodium fluoroacetate) to 7,600 mg/cu m (1,1,2-trichloro-1,2,2-trifluoroethane). The permissible exposure limit (PEL) for dichlorodifluoromethane is 1,000 ppm, but some workers have been affected by a level of 3,000 ppm, and it has been suggested that maybe the PEL should be lowered, especially with its use becoming so widespread.[16]

Controls

Most fluorohydrocarbons are relatively safe and easy to keep within the recommended limits of air exposure. Control of fluorocarbons by ventilation is needed where high concentrations may occur and if used in low areas where the heavy vapor can collect. Caution should be used in entering a confined area or tank where it was used.

Clear and durable labeling when the substances are so diverse as the fluorides are is important, but more important are the knowledge and awareness of the hazards and the instruction in handling given to the employees working with the fluorides.

Personal Protective Equipment

The anhydrous acid should be handled with great care. The face shield should be of plastic, not glass, and apron, boots, and gloves of butyl rubber or neoprene, because natural rubber becomes brittle. Lanolin is of some value as a barrier agent. Cream on the face can protect against hydrogen fluoride in the air that would be irritating to the skin.[26]

Many of the fluorocarbons are good solvents of skin oil, so protective ointment should be used and repeated contact avoided.

Employee Screening

Urinary levels of fluorides can be a rough measure of exposure, as mentioned above under Diagnostic Techniques. It has been suggested that under 4 ppm is safe, that 6 ppm indicates a need for better controls, and over 8 ppm for years will give skeletal changes detectable on x-ray film.[33] X-ray of the spine is not warranted in a screening program for detection of fluoride exposure, since chronic toxicity has been very rare and confined primarily to the cryolite, aluminum, magnesium, and phosphate industries and has not been seen except where environmental conditions were, by today's standards, very poor.

Work Environment

Very small amounts of some inorganic as well as some organic fluorine are toxic on ingestion. Food should not be allowed to be contaminated, and eating should not be allowed in the work area. A strict routine of hand washing before eating should be enforced.

Tobacco and cigarettes should not be carried into the work area nor smoking done where contamination with Teflon dust or other potentially dangerous fluorocarbon is possible.[7]

Eye washer and instant shower facilities should be located near the work areas where spills and splash hazards exist.

Anhydrous acid is shipped in passivated iron cylinders or tanks under pressure. It boils at 20° C. Several of the fluorocarbons boil at low temperatures. They should be opened with caution. Workers should have knowledge of the products with which they are working. Special instruction should be given to those employees involved with dilute hydrofluoric acid so that they realize the dangers from delayed symptoms of burn and the need for quick treatment.

Scrubbing equipment that removes fluorides and ventilation systems need frequent inspections because of the rapid corrosion by hydrofluoric acid. It is advisable to make or coat the system so it is fluoride-resistant. Various calcium hydroxide systems are efficient removers of fluoride.

Many and diverse industrial processes involve fluoride exposure.[19, 43] Most present an easy task of avoiding an acute toxicity hazard by having an awareness of the stability, solubility, and route of entry of the product used, and the nature of the industrial process, and utilizing as simple an environmental control as necessary. It should be remembered that the more complex compounds with fluorides often are toxic because of the chemical nature of the breakdown products.

REFERENCES

1. Adams DF: An automatic hydrogen fluoride recorder proposed for industrial hygiene. *Ann Chem* 1960; 32:1312.
2. Blunt CP: Treatment of hydrofluoric acid burns by injection with calcium gluconate. *Ind Med Surg* 1964; 33:869.
3. Burke WJ, et al: Systemic fluoride poisoning resulting from a fluoride skin burn. *J Occup Med* 1973; 15:39.
4. Camner P, et al: Human tracheobronchial clearance studies. *Arch Environ Health* 1971; 22:444.
5. Cholak J: The occurrence of fluoride in air, food, and water. I. *J Occup Med* 1959; 1:501.
6. Cholak J: Analysis of fluorides. II. *J Occup Med* 1959; 1:648.
7. Clayton JW Jr: The toxicity of fluorocarbons with special reference to chemical constitution. *J Occup Med* 1962; 4:262.
8. Collings GH Jr, et al: Absorption and excretion of inhaled fluorides. *AMA Arch Ind Hyg* 1951; 4:585.
9. Collings GH Jr, et al: Absorption and excretion of inhaled fluorides. *AMA Arch Ind Hyg* 1952; 6:368.
10. Dalhamn T: Freon som orsak till forgiftningsfall. *Nord Hyg Tidskr* 1958; 39:165.
11. Derryberry OM, et al: Fluoride exposure and worker health. *Arch Environ Health* 1963; 6:503.
12. *Fluorides*. Washington, DC, National Academy of Sciences, 1971.
13. Glaser OG, et al: Transplantable malignant cholangiocarcinoma from hamster liver. *Arch Environ Health* 1971; 23:137.
14. Glauser SC, Glauser EC: Sulfur hexafluoride—A gas not certified for human use. *Arch Environ Health* 1966; 13:467.
15. Gosselin RE, Hodge HC, et al: *Clinical Toxicology of Commercial Products*, ed 5. Baltimore, The Williams & Wilkins Co, 1982.
16. Goan MD: Personal communication. Denver, Rocky Mt. Arsenal, 1974.
17. Hodge HC: Highlights of fluoride toxicology. *J Occup Med* 1968; 10:273.
18. Hodge HC, Smith FA: Fluorides, in *Metallic Contaminants and Human Health*. National Institute of Environmental Health, New York, Academic Press, 1972, Ch 7.
19. Hodge HC, Smith FA: Occupational fluoride exposure. *J Occup Med* 1977; 19:12.
20. Howard OH, Weber CW: A portable continuous analyzer for gaseous fluorides in industrial environments. *AMA Arch Ind Health* 1959; 19:355.
21. Imbus HR, Adkins C: Physical examinations of workers exposed to trichlorotrifluoroethane. *Arch Environ Health* 1972; 24:257.
22. Jacobs MB: *The Analytical Toxicology of Industrial Inorganic Poisons*. New York, Interscience Publishers, 1967.
23. Kaltreider NL, et al: Health survey of aluminum workers with special reference to fluoride exposure. *J Occup Med* 1972; 14:531.
24. Kehoe RA: Introduction to symposium: Effects of absorption of fluoride. *Arch Ind Health* 1960; 21:305.
25. Largent EJ: Rates of elimination of fluoride stored in the tissues of man. *Arch Ind Hyg* 1952; 6:37.
26. Largent EJ: The metabolism of fluorides in man. *Arch Ind Health* 1960; 21:318.
27. Leone NC: The effects of the absorption of fluoride I, II, III, VII. *Arch Ind Health* 1960; 21:324.
28. Lester D, Greenberg LA: The toxicity of sulfur hexafluoride. *Arch Ind Hyg* 1950; 2:348.
29. Lester D, Greenberg LA: The toxicity of sulfur pentafluoride. *Arch Ind Hyg* 1950; 2:350.
30. Lutz GA, et al: Environmental hazards of fluorocarbons. Columbus, Oh, Battelle Memorial Institute, July, 1967.
31. Neefus JD, et al: The determination of fluoride in urine, using a fluoride-specific ion electrode. *Am Ind Hyg Assoc J* 1970; 31:96.
32. Nielsen JP, Dangerfield AD: Use of ion exchange resins for determination of atmospheric fluorides. *AMA Arch Ind Health* 1955; 11:61.
33. *Occupational Health and Safety*, vol I, *International Labour Office Encyclopedia of Occupational Health and Safety*, ed 3. Geneva, 1983.
34. Pattison FLM: *Toxic Aliphatic Fluorine Compounds*. Amsterdam, Elsevier Publishing Co, 1959.
35. Princi F: The effects on man of the absorption of fluoride III. *J Occup Med* 1960; 2:92.
36. Ricca PM: Exposure criteria for fluorine rocket propellants. *Arch Environ Health* 1966; 12:399.
37. Rich C, et al: Response to sodium fluoride in severe primary osteoporosis. *Ann Intern Med* 1965; 63:1069.
38. Saunders JP, et al: Some physiological effects of disulfur decafluoride (S_2F_{10}) after intravenous injection in dogs. *AMA Arch Ind Hyg* 1953; 8:436.
39. Smith FA, et al: Investigations on the metabolism of fluoride III. *AMA Arch Ind Health* 1955; 11:2.
40. Smith FA, et al: The effects of the absorption of fluoride V. *Arch Ind Health* 1960; 21:330.
41. Sun MW: Fluorine ion activity electrode for determination of urinary fluoride. *Am Ind Hyg Assoc* 1969; 30:133.
42. Taves DR: Evidence that there are two forms of fluoride in human serum. *Nature* 1968; 217:1050.

43. Ubel FA, Sorenson SD, Roach DE: Health status of plant workers exposed to fluorochemicals—A preliminary report. *Am Ind Hyg Assoc J* 1980; 41:584.
44. US Dept of Health and Human Services: *Occupational Health Guidelines for Chemical Hazards*, DHHS Publ 81-123. Rockville, Md, NIOSH, 1981.
45. Waldbott GL: The physiologic and hygienic aspects of the absorption of inorganic fluorides. *Arch Environ Health* 1961; 2:155.
46. Zipkin I: The effects of the absorption of fluoride IV, VIII. *Arch Ind Health* 1960; 21:329.

36

Lead and Its Compounds*

This chapter is based on the landmark work written by Sven Hernberg, M.D., for the first edition of this book. It has been a privilege to make certain small additions and we are indebted to him. Vernon N. Dodson, M.D., and Carl Zenz, M.D.

Lead is one of the first metals that man learned to use; indeed, there is evidence that it was known as early as 4000 B.C. Both the Egyptians and Hebrews used lead, and the Phoenicians mined lead ores in Spain around 2000 B.C. The Romans were important lead consumers, using metallic lead for piping and for cooking utensils, and lead compounds for pottery glazes. In those days, the mines of Spain and Britain were the main producers. As man developed technically, new uses were invented for lead and its compounds at the onset of the Industrial Revolution, creating a rapid increase in the consumption of lead, and today it is the most widely used nonferrous metal.

Since lead has been used so widely for such a long time, the history of lead poisoning is extensive. Early in ancient times, many of the symptoms of lead poisoning were noted and described, but it was probably Hippocrates (370 B.C.) who was the first to ascribe those symptoms to lead. Nicander, in the second century B.C., was able to relate constipation, colic, pallor, paralysis, and ocular disturbances to lead exposure, and Pliny stated that lead poisoning was common in shipbuilding during the first century A.D.[93] Although those and other early authors were familiar with lead poisoning, this disease became completely forgotten during the Middle Ages. Not before the 16th century did lead again appear in medical literature, when Paracelsus described what he called "the miner's disease." In 1713 Ramazzini noticed that potters who worked with lead showed tremor of the hand followed by paralysis,[93] but in general, very little attention was paid to lead poisoning before the beginning of the 19th century.

The first "modern" description of lead poisoning was the famous study by Tanquerel des Planches, published in 1839 and based upon 1,200 cases of poisoning. It is noteworthy that his study was so complete that only little has later been added to the symptoms and signs of clinical poisoning. Of the isolated manifestations, the hematologic aspects have in particular been subject to a vast amount of study. Attention was drawn to anemia by Laennec in 1831, Andral and Gavarret in 1840, and Malassey in 1873. Garrod, in 1892, was the first to report the increased excretion of porphyrins in the urine, and Behrend, in 1899, to observe erythrocyte stippling. In 1896, Hellström,[81] a practicing physician in Norköping, a highly industrialized city in Sweden, 165 km south of Stockholm, described in great detail various occupations and their comparative risks when working with lead and lead compounds and set forth the hygienic measures to prevent or reduce lead poisoning. The excellent monographs by Aub, Fairhall, Minot, and Reznikoff,[4] Flury,[52] and Cantarow and Trumper,[22] represent the classics of the 20th century.

Despite the extensive knowledge of the cause, clinical knowledge, and prevention of lead poisoning, the disease is still common; although the situation is continuously improving, at least as far as occupational poisoning is concerned. The extremely poor hygienic conditions in industry during the last century and at the beginning of this century are rarely seen nowadays and there is a reduced incidence of poisoning in most industrialized countries. Although there is reason to believe that cases reported nowadays in general are much milder than those some 50 years ago, reported statistics only show the tip of the iceberg and do not usually consider subclinical poisoning. Thus, any favorable trend shown by no means indicates that the problem of occupational lead poisoning is solved yet. The introduction of new uses for lead and lead compounds creates new problems, and although improved, the hygienic conditions are still far from acceptable in a substantial number of workplaces, particularly in small-sized workshops. There is also reason to believe that the industrialization of developing countries will create situations comparable to those in industrialized countries some decades ago. Furthermore, the use of young children as workers throughout the world is a troublesome area of concern (beyond the scope of this book) and only recently publicized by the World Health Organization and others.[8, 127] Thus, lead poisoning still remains one of the most important problems of occupational health.

The restriction of this chapter solely to occupational poisoning would not give a full account of the lead problem. At present, childhood poisoning due to ingestion of flaking lead paint is a public health challenge in the U.S.A. and in many other countries as well, and most physicians in practice will, at least occasionally, come into contact with this problem. Thus, it is necessary for the occupational physician to have at least some insight into pediatric lead poisoning. Another common nonoccupational source of lead poisoning is illicit "moonshine" whiskey. This and other nonoccupational sources of exposure must be known by plant physicians in order to help them evaluate all etiologic possibilities when they are confronted with cases of lead poisoning. Furthermore, a considerable part of our knowledge of the toxicology of lead has been derived from the study of patients with nonoccupational lead poisoning. Lead encephalopathy and lead nephropathy are perhaps the best illustrations of this statement. These are the reasons why it is necessary to include nonoccupational lead poisoning in a review mainly aimed at occupational health practice. And finally, since environmental pollution with lead has become a hot issue in recent years, a short introduction into this controversial area is in order to complete the picture.

PROPERTIES

Lead (atomic weight 207.21, density 11.34) is a bluish or silvery gray, soft, heavy metal with an atomic number of 82. Its melting point is 327.4° C and its boiling point at atmospheric pressure is 1620° C. Molten lead gives off fumes in measurable amounts beginning from 500 to 600° C. Evaporation increases with rising temperature. Lead is malleable but lacks tenacity and contracts considerably on cooling. Elementary lead is poorly soluble in both cold and hot water and in diluted acids. It dissolves in nitric acid, acetic acid, and hot concentrated sulfuric acid. In its compounds, lead occurs in the valence states of +2 and +4. Of them, the former is more common. However, lead also forms red oxide (Pb_3O_4), which is assumed to be a combination of the two valence states. Of the common lead compounds, the acetate and the nitrate are easily soluble in cold water (44.3 and 37.7 gm/100 ml, respectively). Moderately soluble compounds include the chloride (1.0 gm/100 ml), the chromate (0.1 gm/100 ml), and the stearate (0.05 gm/100 ml). The water solubility of other compounds is low (0.012—0.001 gm/100 ml; e.g., the carbonate, the litharge or PbO, the sulfate, and the sulfide) or they are practically insoluble (the basic chromate, the molybdate, the red lead or Pb_3O_4 and the silicate).

Lead also forms organic compounds. Of them, the most important are tetraethyl lead (TEL) and tetramethyl lead (TML). They are practically insoluble in water but dissolve readily in organic solvents, fats, and lipids. They are slightly volatile.

OCCURRENCE

Lead occurs principally as a compound of two isotopes, ^{206}Pb and ^{208}Pb. It is ubiquitously distributed in the earth's crust. The average concentration in the igneous rocks of the earth's continents is 12 ppm down to a depth of about 30 km. The soil film covering the outermost surface of the continents contains an average of about 16 ppm.[34] Uncontaminated natural waters usually contain less than 0.1 ppm of lead, and seawater has been reported to contain from 0.08 to 8 ppm,[161] but in industrial areas where lead is mined, refined, or smelted, or where coal is burned, the lead content in soil may reach several thousand parts per million.[161]

Natural deposits of lead ores occur mainly in Canada, the United States, Mexico, Peru, Ireland, Poland, Sweden, Spain, the Soviet Union, West Germany, Yugoslavia, South-West Africa, China, Japan, North Korea, and Australia.[201] The most abundant lead-containing ore is galena (PbS). Most of the commercial lead is obtained from this mineral. Other important minerals are cerussite (carbonate), anglesite (sulfate), and pryomorphite (chlorophosphate). Lead also occurs as crocoisite (chromate), wulfenite (molybdate), matlockite (chloride) and vanadinite (vanadate).[201]

Because of the ubiquitous distribution of lead, no lead-free environment exists or has ever existed. Thus, man is and always has been submitted to a "background" exposure from ambient air, food and drinking water. This background varies from place to place, and it most probably was lower before the Industrial Revolution than it is today. However, it is always there, and it adds in varying degrees to exposures of other origins.

USES

Total Consumption

Lead probably has the broadest register of application of all nonferrous metals. Exact estimation of the amount produced or consumed annually in the world is difficult because of the lack of reliable statistics and different reporting systems. Expressed as metallic lead, the present annual world production is about 8.9 million metric tons. The consumption is higher than this, however, since more than one third of the lead produced is recycled. For example, production in the United States in 1985 was about 488,000 metric tons and the amount recovered from scrap was nearly 594,000 metric tons. The total U.S. lead consumption in that year was 1,148,000 metric tons.[201]

Uses of Metallic Lead and Alloys

The largest amounts of lead are used in the manufacture of electric storage batteries (grids and oxide). This use accounts for nearly two thirds of the total U.S. consumption. A battery has an average life of 27 months.[201] About 80% of the battery lead is resmelted as scrap (Fig 36–1). Thus, the storage battery industry provides the secondary smelting and refining industry with its most important source of raw material (Fig 36–2). The cable industry uses lead alloys containing small amounts of antimony or arsenic-tin-bismuth alloys for the covering of cables. In the construction industry, lead is used as calking pipe and sheet lead for the prevention of vibration or noise transmission. In industrial construction, sheet lead is also employed in storage tanks, reaction vessels, and other equipment for the manufacture and storage of corrosive chemicals. The ammunition industry uses lead for bullets and shot, and the printing industry uses alloys of lead, antimony, tin, and copper to produce type. Large amounts of lead are also used for soldering—for example, in the tin can industry, in various kinds of repair work, and in the automobile industry, especially in radiator production. Lead as such or in alloys is further used as radiation shielding, as weights and ballast, in collapsible tubes, for terneplate coating, in brass and bronze production, for annealing, galvanizing, and plating, and for numerous other purposes. In several countries, old lead pipes still are in use for interior plumbing and for conveying water to domestic users.

Uses of Compounds

The inorganic lead compounds are used most widely in storage battery production (PbO), as mentioned above, and in the paint

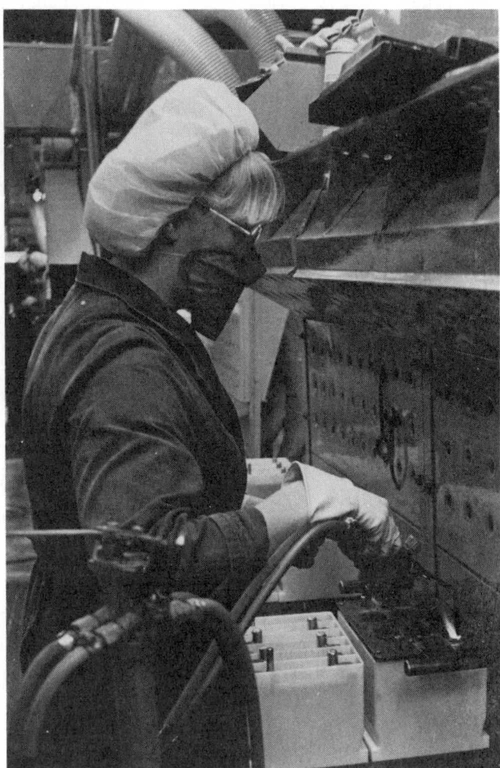

FIG 36–1.
The assembly of electric storage batteries exposes the worker to lead oxide dust. The risk can be reduced substantially by effective local exhaust ventilation.

and pigment industry. Although the use of lead pigments in paints has decreased during the past decades, more than 441,000 metric tons were consumed in 1985 in the United States alone.[201] Basic lead carbonate, basic lead sulfate, leaded zinc oxide, and some lead silicates are used for outdoor paints. Previously, lead paints were used extensively for indoor painting, too, particularly in the United States. Many countries now prohibit by law or regulation indoor paints containing lead. The most important lead pigment for metal coating is red lead (Pb_3O_4) as a primer or rust retardant. Its use is also declining, but other paints used for metal protecting, such as "activated ferrous oxide," contain various amounts of lead. Several pigments, in particular the chromates, are used as colors. The yellow chromate pigments are widely used for traffic marking signs and for the painting of agricultural machines and trucks. Several of the most often seen yellows, greens, and reds are lead chromates, alone or precipitated with other pigments.

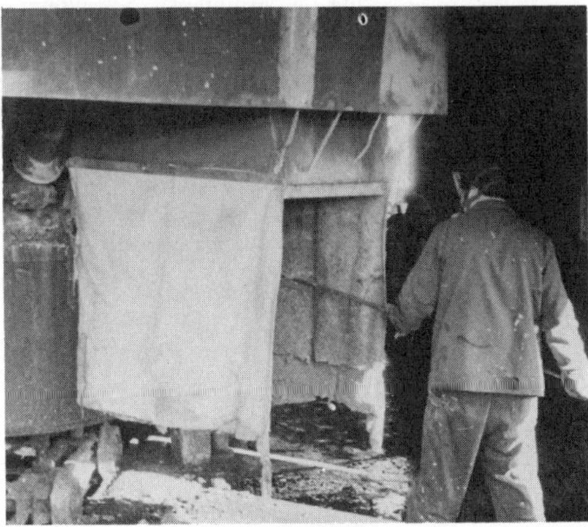

FIG 36–2.
Secondary lead smelting often is performed under primitive conditions in small smelters. The emptying of the furnace gives rise to highly dangerous concentrations of lead fume in the air.

Both inorganic and organic lead compounds have become widely used as stabilizers in the production of polyvinylchloride (PVC) plastics. The ceramics industry uses lead oxides and silicates as glazes for china, porcelain enamels, and glazed tile. Crystal glass, optical glass, and glass for electric purposes contain much lead, too. The picture tube in color television sets is made of lead glass. Other uses include electronic applications, e.g., as for transducers, in ultrasonic cleaners, or as lead telluride in thermoelectric materials. Lead azide has been used for a long time in cartridge primers and primer cord. The use of lead arsenate as an insecticide has greatly declined in recent years, but it represented an important use before World War II.

The petroleum industry has been using lead alkyl since the beginning of the 1920s as an antiknock additive in fuels. In 1923 TEL was introduced and TML in 1959. This consumption has gradually decreased, but it accounted for almost 46,000 metric tons in the United States in 1985, second only to storage battery manufacturing.[201] The recent decisions in a number of countries to gradually reduce the allowable amount of lead additives in gasoline during the 1970s apparently indicates a new trend. Besides the liquid alkyl lead compounds, the petroleum industry also uses litharge (PbO) to remove undesirable sulfur compounds in oil refining.

EXPOSURES

Man's total lead exposure is made up by the background exposure from food, drinking water, and ambient air, which, although neither natural nor desirable, probably has to be considered "normal" in modern society and, in some instances, also by "abnormal" sources, of which occupational exposure is the most common and most important. Of the nonoccupational sources, ingestion of lead-containing objects or of contaminated food and beverages is the most common. The relative importance of the different sources for total exposure shows wide variation. When exposure is abnormally high, there usually is one main cause and the others are less important, although they add up to the total amount absorbed. This is the case, for example, in occupational exposure. However, in polluted areas, such as central districts of big cities, contamination of the general environment has increased the background exposure, at least for certain population groups, to such an extent that it may decrease the tolerance to occupational exposure. In other words, occupations that at one time were considered to be relatively safe may prove risky by reason of the additional burden that environmental exposure may impose; for reasons of clarity, the different exposures will be treated in the following as if they were isolated phenomena. Despite this, the complex nature of exposure should be kept in mind.

Occupational Exposures

The wide use of lead and its compounds has resulted in that quite a substantial part of all industrial workers regularly or occasionally have some contact with them. It must be stressed, however, that the mere presence of lead in a workroom by no means denotes that there is a risk of poisoning. On the contrary, the hazard is determined by the vast number of factors that lead to the occurrence of higher or lower concentrations of respirable (below 5 μ in diameter) lead fumes or lead-containing dust particles in the workroom atmosphere; moreover, these factors show wide variations from one plant to another, even within the same branch of industry. Thus, no simple rule of thumb exists for a general classification of occupations into "dangerous" and "less dangerous" categories. Accordingly, the evaluation of the risk always must be based on scrutiny of the specific working environment. Except for the most extreme cases in which the hazard is either quite obvious or definitely lacking, an evaluation of this kind should include measurements of the concentration of lead in air, sampled from representative sites, and/or determination of the blood or urinary lead concentration of the workers.

In general, factors that determine the magnitude of risk can be divided into three categories. First, the process in itself is important. High processing temperatures, particularly those in excess of 1000° C, extensive fume, dust, or aerosol formation and primitive working methods increase the risk; the more extreme the conditions, the greater the risk. In contrast, low temperatures (below 500° C), low dust formation, and automation promote safety. Second, the adequacy of the elimination technique employed is a determinant. Efficient local and general ventilation and proper prevention of the spreading of lead dust greatly reduce the risk; conversely, a lack of such measures increases the element of danger. Third, the general hygienic level of the workplace should be taken into account. Poor housekeeping, poor personal hygiene, negligence in the use of the elimination methods mentioned above, even if they were available, and general ignorance all raise the risk. This also applies where personal protective equipment is required but not used, or where it is inadequate. For obvious reasons, it is more common to find an accumulation of negatively acting factors in small plants than in large ones. Generally speaking, exposure levels and the risk of poisoning thus are comparatively higher in industries of this type.

Although the importance of local conditions specific to each plant or operation cannot be neglected, general experience has shown some types of work to be more hazardous than others. In each case, the hazard can be attributed to the presence of one or more of the unfavorable factors mentioned above. Since recent systematic measurements of lead in air from the lead-using industry are lacking, it has been necessary to base the evaluation of the average risk in various operations on other criteria, such as the reported occurrence of clinical lead poisoning in various branches of industry.[18, 48, 110, 137, 156, 195, 196, 206]

High-Risk Operations

All operations in which metallic lead or lead-coated materials are burned belong to the category of high-risk operations, since they result in the generation of lead fumes in high concentrations. Welding or cutting of lead constructions or of other metal constructions covered with lead paints always is a hazardous operation, since the temperatures usually reach 1000–3000° C (Figs 36–3 through 36–10). Since analysis of the paint of old construction often is neglected by those responsible for the safety of the welder, the risk may pass unrecognized until the appearance of the first cases of poisoning. Shipbreaking is a well-documented although poorly controlled hazard. Old ships usually are covered with thick layers of lead paint. The cutting of ship frames (often in confined spaces) is done using an oxyacetylene flame, producing a temperature of about 3500° C, which effectively vaporizes both lead and other metals. Also welding or cutting of galvanized or zinc silicate-coated steels gives rise to high concentrations of lead in air. Primary and secondary lead smelting is another procedure in which the risk of poisoning is high. The former produces pig lead predominantly from ores, with a small mixture of scrap. Primary smelters usually are large but few in number. Secondary smelters

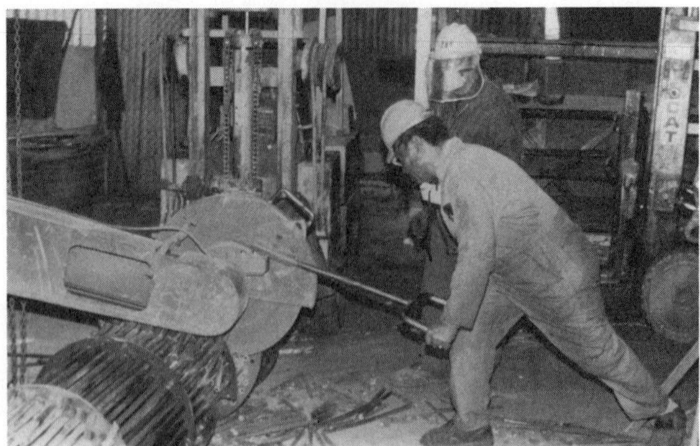

FIG 36–3.
Abrasive cutting of scrap materials and old condenser brass tubes into smaller segments to remelt in bronze production. This cutting can produce dust containing lead and even lead oxide from the heat generated by the cutting action.

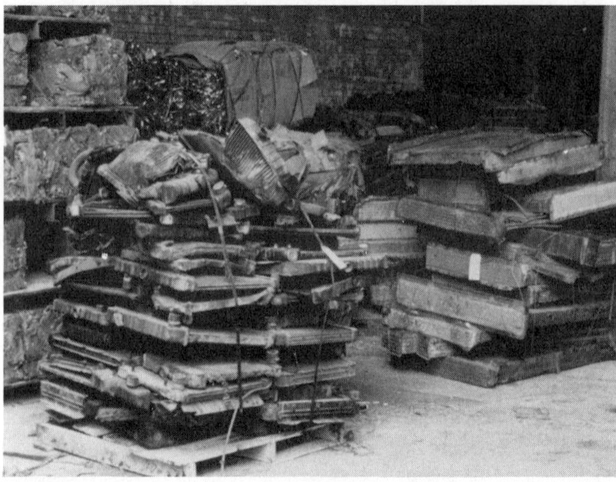

FIG 36–4.
Scrap truck radiators to be recycled into bronze.

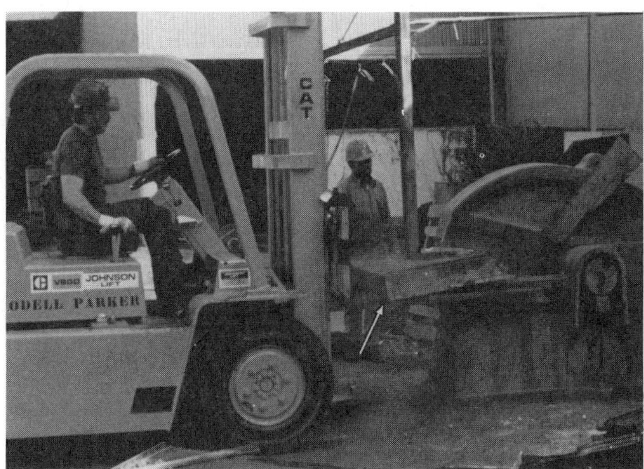

FIG 36–5.
Much scrap reclaiming activity takes place outdoors. In this photograph, scrap truck radiators *(arrow)* are being moved by forklift truck into the cutting shears—generating fine, dust-containing lead, a regular component of brass radiators. Even with outdoor work, these workers had higher blood lead levels than those inside the warehouse.

reclaim lead from scrap, mainly discarded batteries. There are many of these and they can be very small or fairly large enterprises. The risk is partly from the lead fumes generated at the high temperatures required and partly from the lead oxide dust spread around the smelter. Control of the risk has proved to be difficult. Nonferrous foundries often utilize lead alloys. Since many such foundries are small, the working conditions often are uncontrolled, and consequently the risk is high. Storage battery manufacture represents one of the best-known risks.[133] Machine and hand pasting, forming, assembling, and welding of the battery connectors are the jobs in which the risk is highest. Exposure is mainly through lead oxide dust, but the welding operations also generate fumes. Control of the risk has been successful in several large plants, but, especially in small plants, exposure still is high. Spray painting may be hazardous if dust control is ineffective, which often is the case. Mixing of lead salt stabilizers during the production of polyvinylchloride plastic may result in high concentrations of dust containing lead when the operation is done by hand. Automation eliminates the risk.

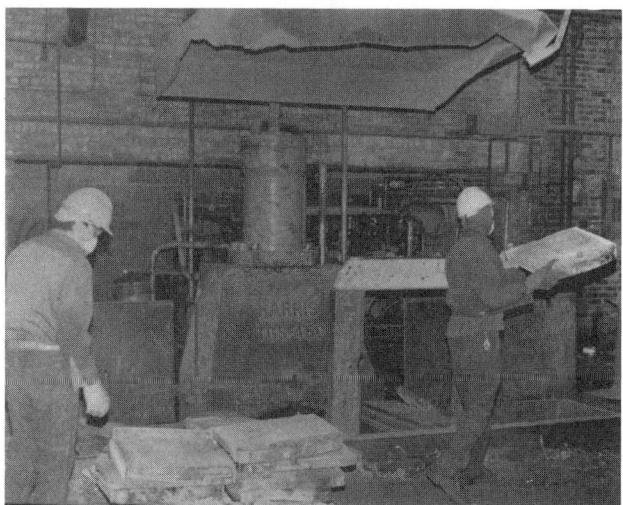

FIG 36–6.
Scrap automotive and truck radiators being thrown into the hydraulic operated compressing machine to make them a suitable size for the melting furnaces. Note working conditions and condition of the old, nonfunctioning hood above.

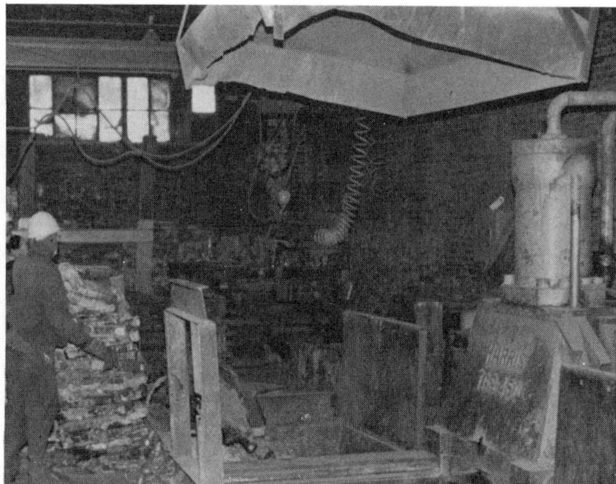

FIG 36–7.
Another view of the scrap compressing area.

In addition, there are several other operations in which the risk may be high. These include mixing of crystal glass mass, sanding or scraping of lead paint, burning of lead in enameling workshops, and repair of automobile radiators.

Moderate-Risk Operations

Exposure to lead further occurs in several other operations in which the risk can be classified as moderate or slight; i.e., the incidence of plumbism usually is low or nil and reported lead con-

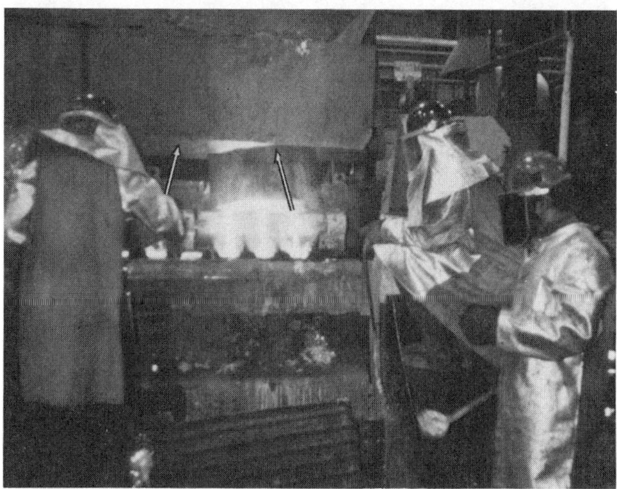

FIG 36–8.
Pouring bronze ingots. Note the exhaust ventilation above the pouring area *(arrows).*

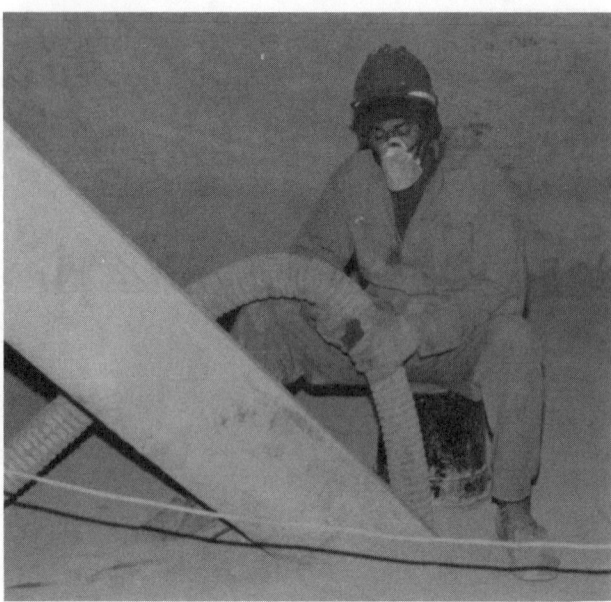

FIG 36–9.
The end product of reclaiming scrap nonferrous materials in the manufacture of fine bronzes. Large quantities of finely divided powder are collected in the "bag house." The powder consists of zinc oxide, which contains 10% to 15% lead oxide (90% of this lead oxide is of fine size and respirable). This scrap must be removed from the factory on a regular basis.

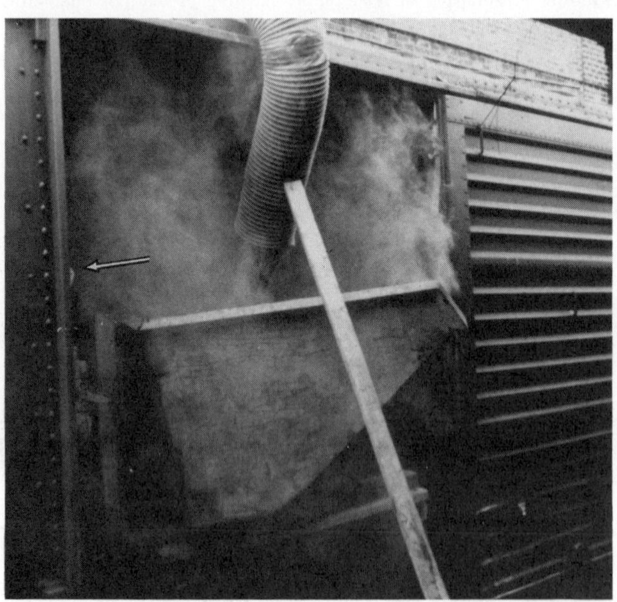

FIG 36–10.
This figure shows the zinc oxide effluent being moved by a forklift truck hopper and being evenly distributed throughout the boxcar. The worker is obscured in this view *(arrow)*. Nearly all of this material is scrap and is delivered to landfill disposal sites. Some of this material may be used as fillers in other industries.

centrations in the air or in the workers' blood or urine have, in general, been around or below the safety norms usually employed.[200] If exposure is intermittent in "high risk" jobs, they may be included in this category. The following categories of workers are exposed to moderate risks: lead miners, solderers, plumbers, cable makers, wire platers, type founders, stereotype setters, certain automobile factory workers, automobile repair mechanics, ship repair workers, including those who add or change lead ballast, lead founders, lead glass blowers, pottery glaze makers, including artists engaged in ceramic glazing (both at home and commercially), enamelers, varnish makers, shot makers, and certain welders. Lead may be added in certain steel casting to improve machinability (Fig 36–11).

Radiation therapists are increasingly using dense, low-melting temperature, heavy metal alloys to shape and block radiation fields. One of the most commonly used of these alloys is Lipowitz's metal, composed of 50% bismuth, 26.7% lead, 13.3% tin, and 10% cadmium.

Low-Exposure Occupations

There are many occupations in which exposure is slight but still in excess of the normal background. The health risk arising from lead exposure can be considered nonexistent in this category of workers. Such groups are traffic police officers, taxi drivers, garage workers, service station attendants, rubber makers, jewelers, linotype setters, pipe fitters and electronic device makers, to mention only a few.

Domestic Exposures

Lead-Glazed Earthenware.—Improperly lead-glazed earthenware has a history of causing lead poisoning.[58] If the temperature used for firing is below 1150° C, the glaze formed is partly soluble because of incomplete fusing of the lead. Large amounts of such pottery are produced under primitive conditions in most Med-

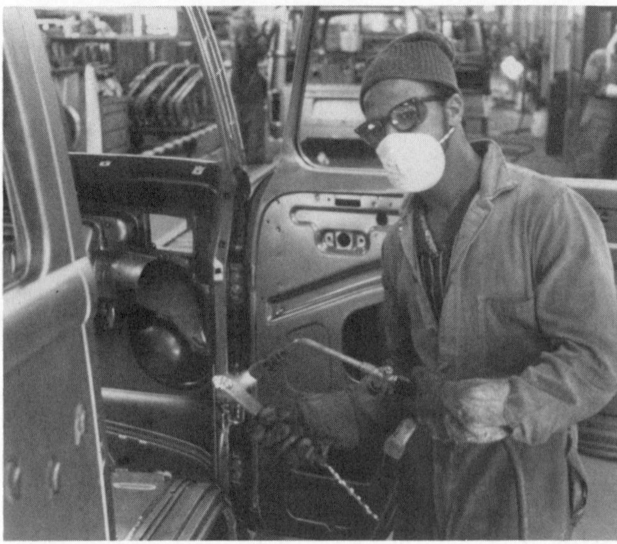

FIG 36–11.
Applying lead-based solder for finishing automotive bodies. A typical van may require up to 3 lb of solder.

iterranean countries, Central America, and several other regions of the world. Since most amateur potters are confined to using comparatively low temperatures, their products may represent a hazard to the public too. It should be noted that stoneware is fired at 1200–1260° C and therefore presents no hazard, but these products are difficult to distinguish from earthenware in the shop. All acidic foods and beverages, such as tomatoes, tomato juice, fruit juices, cola drinks, wine, cider, and pickles and salads stored in vinegar dissolve the lead from the glaze. The amount of dissolved lead increases proportionally with storage time.[36] Lead poisoning from this source is common, even endemic, in countries where such pottery is produced. Poisoning has also occurred in other countries,[80, 106] and a survey of more than 100 imported and domestic earthenware vessels in Canada revealed a lead release considered unsafe (above 7 ppm of lead) in about half of the items.[106]

Illicitly Distilled Whiskey.—Several million gallons of illicit "moonshine" whiskey are produced annually in the United States. The production for 1968 has been estimated to be 36 million (136.26 × 10^6 L) gallons.[141] Production is most widespread in the southeastern parts of the United States. Discarded automobile radiators often are used as condensers and the tubing of the distillation units is smoldered with lead. When hot vapors and alcohol come into contact with lead, some of it dissolves. According to a survey, about 30% of a total of 791 moonshine whiskey samples contained 1 mg/L lead or more.[36] It is self-evident that generous and frequent consumption of such products constitutes a substantial health risk.

Discarded Battery Casings.—Burning of discarded battery casings made of wood or vulcanite in wood-burning stoves has caused severe outbreaks of poisoning.[59] Exposure probably took place by both ingestion and inhalation of lead dust.

Lead in Tap Water.—Lead piping and lead-lined tanks still are important sources of contamination of the tap water in old distribution systems. This problem is not as common in the United States as in some European countries, e.g., in Great Britain. Contamination is worse if the water is artificially softened, naturally soft, humic, or faintly acid. For example, a survey of the Glasgow area has revealed a mean value of 358 μg/L (range 13–1850 μg/L) in overnight water from cold taps.[10] Lead-lined tanks were the heaviest contaminators. Such tap water may cause poisoning in the consumers.[10]

Flaking Lead Paint as a Source of Exposure.—The habit of eating nonfood items (pica) among children makes ingestion of flaking lead paint, crumbling plaster, and putty containing lead an alarming source of poisoning in the United States, and cases have been reported from Great Britain and Australia as well.[29, 36, 54, 69, 97, 138, 140] Paints containing lead were commonly used for indoor painting in the United States before World War II and, to some extent, even after it. An estimate made in 1960 indicated that some 30.6 million dwelling units dated from that period and about 25% were in poor condition.[36] As the buildings decay, the lead paint begins to flake and becomes easily available to the children. Particularly, window sills and frames seem to be attractive.[32] A lead content higher than 1% is considered potentially dangerous, and since the flakes may contain up to 40%, only small amounts are needed to produce poisoning.[36] For obvious reasons, flaking paint is more prevalent in slum districts than elsewhere. Consequently, the lowest socioeconomic group provides five times as many cases as all other groups combined.[138] How severe the problem really is was not realized until some years ago, when the results of case-finding campaigns in a number of major cities became available. According to one estimate, the annual incidence of symptomatic and nonsymptomatic lead poisoning from ingestion of lead paint in the United States might be as high as 250,000 cases.[142]

Exposure From Traffic.—In 1968, the lead emission in the United States from gasoline combustion was 181,000 tons. All other sources combined contributed only some 3,300 tons.[36] Thus, motor traffic is by far the most important cause of today's environmental lead pollution. Downtown areas and other busy districts as well as areas around highways represent locations where such pollution is noted most clearly.[130] Still higher concentrations have been measured around lead smelters. The problems connected with environmental pollution will be dealt with later.

METABOLISM

Absorption

Inorganic lead is absorbed into the human organism by the respiratory and gastrointestinal routes. The former is more important in occupational exposure, whereas the latter predominates in other exposures. Cutaneous absorption of inorganic lead is negligible (Fig 36–12).

Respiratory Absorption

Respiratory absorption of lead depends on three processes—deposition, mucociliary clearance, and alveolar clearance.[189] Deposition occurs in the nasopharyngeal, tracheobronchial, and alveolar compartments and is dependent on particle size and respiratory volume.[138, 151, 160] Deposition in the lungs is maximal (63%) at a particle size of 1 μ and minimal (39%) at 0.1 μ for resting persons (respiratory volume of 10 L/min).[151] Forced respiration diminishes lung deposition. Large particles are deposited more readily in the upper respiratory tract than are small particles.

Mucociliary clearance, which is defined as a combination of mucus flow and ciliary activity, constitutes the process whereby the particles are transported to the pharynx and swallowed. Large particles appear to be transported more quickly than smaller ones.[190] Since the end point of mucociliary clearance is the gastrointestinal tract, particles undergoing this process behave like ingested lead.

Alveolar clearance takes place in three ways:[190] (1) transport to the mucociliary escalator; (2) passage through one of the membranes into the pulmonary tissue; and (3) passage through the pulmonary tissue into the lymph and blood.

Phagocytosis by alveolar macrophages probably is an important mechanism for the transport of lead particles to the mucociliary escalator.[190] The solubility of the lead compounds may to some extent determine the amount absorbed through the lung; however,

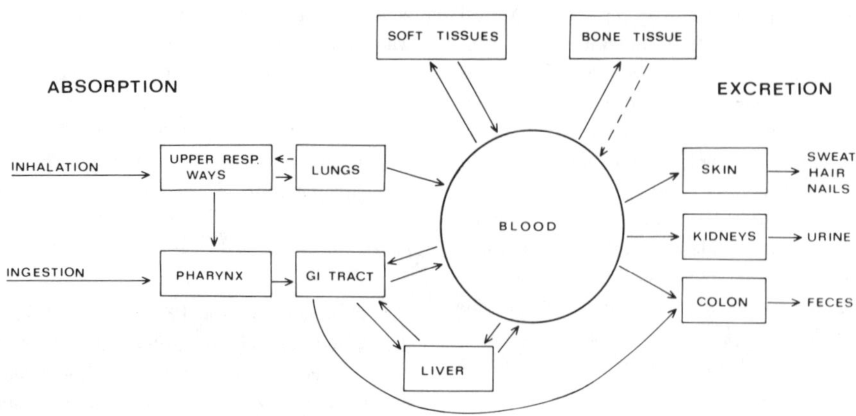

FIG 36–12.
Simplified model of the metabolism of lead in man.

after a long time in the lung, even less-soluble compounds may undergo dissolution.[190]

It is unfortunate that most inhalation studies have paid too little attention to the various factors determining absorption. Consequently, several of the data published are difficult to interpret. A crude estimation of the percentage of inhaled lead reaching the bloodstream would be about 30%–40% (a commonly used figure is 37%), depending on particle size, solubility, respiratory volume, and physiologic interindividual variation. In addition, some pathologic conditions apparently affect pulmonary absorption. Nasal obstruction, resulting in mouth breathing, increases alveolar deposition, whereas bronchial obstruction has the opposite effect. Mucociliary clearance is slower in cigarette smokers than in nonsmokers. Acute upper respiratory tract infections, acute bronchitis, and chronic obstructive bronchitis also impair ciliary activity.[190] The various factors influencing pulmonary absorption of lead not only are of theoretic interest but help us to understand some of the reasons why a given concentration of lead in the air may give rise to quite different blood lead levels in the workers exposed.

Gastrointestinal Absorption

The relative importance of gastrointestinal absorption for total absorption varies depending on the conditions of exposure. As already mentioned, in occupational exposure, it is small compared to respiratory absorption, although the amount that becomes trapped in the upper respiratory tract and is swallowed adds to its importance. Self-evidently, the situation is the reverse when exposure takes place through ingestion. As will be discussed later, ingested lead usually is the main source of exposure for the general population.[103, 175]

Gastrointestinal absorption of lead is not influenced to any great extent by the nature of the compound ingested because of the acid milieu in the stomach.[77] According to Kehoe,[103] absorption measured by determining the difference between lead ingested and lead eliminated in feces and urine is between 5% and 15%. However, according to more recent studies, there may be a wider range of variation. Hursch and Suomela,[95] using ^{212}Pb, found a range of 1.3%–16% in their human studies, and Milev et al.[139] were able to increase absorption in experimental animals from 7% to 49% by increasing the protein content in the food. It is also known that a low content of calcium or iron in the diet increases lead absorption.[183, 184] The same is true for a diet deficient in phosphorus.[65] The explanation may be that absorption of lead through the intestinal mucosa involves a competitive mechanism with regard to calcium.

Circulation, Distribution, and Storage

Lead has a great affinity to erythrocytes and at least 95% of the circulating fraction is bound to these cells. The mechanisms by which lead is bound to the erythrocytes, how it is released from them, and how it is transferred to the tissues are not yet known, although several hypotheses have been advanced. However, it appears that the first site of fixation is the cell membrane.[82] The lead particles probably are first aggregated on the cell surface as a particulate form of lead phosphate,[35] but within a relatively short period, part of the lead becomes associated with a deeper, less accessible structure within the cell.[77]

It is not known how the small fraction remaining in plasma is bound. It is possible that this fraction has more toxicologic importance than erythrocyte lead because of the slow diffusibility of the latter. Plasma lead levels have only rarely been measured because of analytic difficulties, and therefore little is known about their relation to toxic manifestations.

Lead is transported to the organs by the bloodstream and deposited into them as a function of the concentration gradient and the specific affinities of the tissue in question. The total content of lead in the organism is called the *body burden*. Its distribution between different tissues varies. The high affinity of lead to bone is the most remarkable fact. In a steady state, about 90% of the body burden is bound to that tissue.[175] Long bones contain more lead then do flat bones, and even within the former, there are differences in the sense that the ends have higher concentrations than the shafts.[175, 187] Teeth contain more lead than do any of the bones. The concentration of lead in the bones reaches its maximum after the fifth or sixth decade, whereafter a slight decrease occurs.[9, 175, 187]

The manner in which lead is bound to the bones is not completely known. Numerous studies have shown that lead follows the metabolism of calcium. There now is conclusive evidence that the lead deposits in bone consist of at least two compartments. One is firmly bound and partly located in the bone matrix. This fraction probably is made up of "old" lead. Another fraction, apparently "new" lead, is more exchangeable, although it may persist for months and even years after exposure. The exchangeable pool may be bound to the surface of hydroxyapatite, the less exchangeable one being immured in it.[161]

The older literature often stated that acute lead poisoning might occur long after the cessation of exposure. It was thought that a number of factors, among them acute and chronic infections, postoperative acidosis, alcoholism, and fractures, might act as precipitating factors.[22, 177] (A man developed poisoning two years after exposure; multiple fractures may have caused lead mobilization.) Considering the magnitude of the bone pool, only a small percentage of it needs to be mobilized to cause toxic soft tissue concentrations.

Of the soft tissues, the highest concentrations occur in the aorta, the liver, and the kidneys.[9, 175] The concentration in the brain is comparatively low, but inorganic lead does pass the blood-brain barrier. Cortical gray matter and basal ganglia usually show higher concentrations than does cortical white matter.[106] That there are local concentration differences within the brain may be toxicologically more important than the mere fact that lead passes into the brain from the blood.[190]

Lead also passes the placenta.[190] Transplacental passage becomes detectable at 12–14 weeks of gestation, and the fetal whole-body lead content increases from that time on. The distribution of lead in the fetus is similar to that in adults.[6]

Finally, it should be stressed that the lead content of the organism always is in a dynamic state determined by complicated kinetics. The concentration of lead in blood or tissues at any given time thus is a complex multivariate function of absorption, excretion, and other physiologic parameters, such as the dynamics of transfer to and from the tissues.

Excretion

Lead is excreted by several routes, but only renal and gastrointestinal excretion are of practical importance. The feces always contains much lead. Most of it represents unabsorbed lead merely passing through the intestinal tract. The rest is derived from gastrointestinal net excretion (total excretion minus reabsorption). The distinction between unabsorbed and excreted lead has been a serious obstacle for students of true gastrointestinal excretion, and conflicting opinions regarding its importance therefore exist.

Gastrointestinal excretion takes place by (1) active secretion or passive loss of lead with the secretion from various glands, i.e., salivary glands, pancreas, and glands located in the intestinal wall, (2) loss by shedding of epithelial cells, and (3) biliary excretion.[190] An unknown but probably important fraction of lead so excreted is reabsorbed. In animals, biliary excretion appears to be the most important mechanism, but since animal data cannot directly be extrapolated, its role in man remains uncertain. That the total gastrointestinal net excretion is of some importance for the elimination of lead is, however, shown by an experiment in which two human volunteers were given ^{212}Pb intravenously. There was no lead in the feces during the first 24 hours, whereas the urine contained 4.42% of the dose. The figures for the second 24 hours, however, were 1.5% and 1.42%, respectively, which indicates that the fecal route may contribute as much as the urinary one to total excretion.[16]

Renal excretion takes place predominantly, perhaps exclusively, by glomerular filtration.[202] The role of tubular reabsorption is not fully elucidated. Since the concentration of lead in the urine reflects current exposure, measurement of this parameter has gained wide application in occupational health as an exposure test, as will be discussed later.

Other possible routes for lead excretion include sweat, milk, hair, nails, desquamating epithelia, and teeth. From the point of view of clearance from the body, sweat may be of importance in warm climates where sweating is profuse but probably not in temperate climates.[37, 103] Although excretion with milk has little importance from the point of view of clearing lead from the body, it may represent a hazard to the suckling infant. Since there is a relationship between the concentrations of lead in the blood and milk,[78, 146] sucklings of occupationally or otherwise heavily exposed mothers may be exposed to dangerous amounts. Other routes of excretion are mainly of theoretic interest. Lead in hair and teeth has been suggested as a measure of the body burden, but from the point of view of elimination from the organism, these routes are insignificant.

In general, lead is excreted extremely slowly from the body. Its exact biologic half-life is not known, but it may be of the order of ten years for man.[96] Since excreton is slow, accumulation occurs easily. There is no doubt that substantial accumulation always occurs in lead workers, but there has been much dispute about whether or not environmental pollution causes accumulation in the general population. The fact that lead is present in the body in at least four compartments, i.e., (1) a rapid-exchange compartment representing blood and internal organs, (2) the skin and muscles, (3) the exchangeable part of lead in bone, and (4) a very slowly exchangeable part of lead in bone,[159] requires a particularly complex metabolic model to calculate the excretion kinetics. This model has not yet been solved.

GENERAL TOXICOLOGY

In sufficient concentrations, heavy metals can impair any existing biologic activity, and thus there are, theoretically, as many kinds of responses as there are activities. But since there are great variations in the accessibility of biologic components at the organ, tissue, cellular, and molecular level, certain types of responses predominate.[154] For example, all enzyme systems are potentially susceptible to heavy metals, but in the living organism, anatomical structures may limit the accessibility; inert binding sites may compete for the metal ion. For these reasons, there often are considerable differences in sensitivity between different organs and tissues. These considerations also offer explanations for many of the differences in action observed between in vitro and in vivo experiments, for certain interspecies differences, and for why certain responses are typical for clinical poisoning whereas others are not.

In interaction with living matter, lead displays both the general characteristics of heavy metals and some peculiarities.[154] Thus, it is capable of forming complexes with ligands containing sulfur, nitrogen, or oxygen as electron donors. At least the following ligands in living matter may be expected to form more or less stable complexes with lead: $-OH$, $-H_2PO_3$, $-SH$, and $-NH_2$.[165] The biochemical interactions of lead with sulfhydryl groups are thought to be of great toxicologic importance.[166] Lead also has a high affinity to amines and simple amino acids.[70] Chelation is a common phenomenon that often introduces peculiar specificity patterns in the binding of lead ions.[132] Catalytic actions of lead ions may also result in decomposition of organic compounds. In general, the binding of lead ions by biochemical material is strong but rather nonspecific.[154]

Lead may strongly interfere with the activities of enzymes and other proteins of functional significance. As a result of such "poisoning," enzymatic activity will be partially or totally inhibited. The degree of inhibition depends, among other things, on the accessibility of the enzyme, competition from inert ligands in the cell, and the functional significance of the lead-binding ligand of the enzyme. Most important from a functional viewpoint is binding to ligands that participate in the bond formation with the components of the enzyme-substrate complex at the active center of the enzyme.[107] However, binding to other sites may cause changes in the conformation of the enzyme molecule and, in this manner, induce what is called allosteric inhibition.[85]

Both theoretic considerations and experimental evidence have led to the conclusion that the cell membrane is the first and most important site of lead action.[154] The outer surface of the membrane is rich in easily accessible ligands and thus almost all lead is rapidly absorbed on it. For this reason, many important toxic effects of lead are membrane effects. On the other hand, the membrane protects the interior of the cell to some extent, although part of the lead undoubtedly penetrates it. The cell interior, furthermore, has an abundance of inert substances that compete for the lead ions with biologically essential binding sites. Much less is known about the effects of lead on the interior of the cell than of its membrane effects. It has been suggested that impairment of mitochondrial functions, such as cellular respiration, is an important feature of intracellular toxicity.[62] Studies of the effect of lead on various enzymes have revealed almost innumerable isolated functional disturbances. The placing of those findings in perspective is extremely difficult—if not impossible—and, for this reason, no recapitulation of them will be given in this context.

CLINICAL TOXICOLOGY

Hematologic Effects

Anemia is a prominent finding in lead poisoning. It usually is mild to moderate in adults (hemoglobin values ranging from 8 to 12 gm/100 ml), sometimes severe in children. Early in the course of poisoning, and particularly in children, it is microcytic and hypochromic, but in the chronic stage, the anemia often becomes normochromic and normocytic.[82, 203] It is accompanied by pallor of the skin that is out of proportion to the severity of the anemia. Reticulocytosis and basophilic stippling of the erythrocytes are common but nonspecific findings, since both may occur in other diseases as well or they may be absent in lead anemia.

The hematologic abnormalities of lead poisoning can be attributed to the combined effect of (1) the inhibition of hemoglobin synthesis and (2) the shortened life span of circulating erythrocytes, resulting in stimulation of erythropoiesis.

Hemoglobin Synthesis

The inhibitive effect of lead on the formation of hemoglobin has been subject to a vast amount of research; nevertheless, it is not yet completely understood. In order to facilitate the following recapitulation, a simplified schematic outline of heme synthesis is presented in Figure 36–13. Established or suspected sites of lead action are indicated by arrows. The initial step, or formation of δ-aminolevulinic acid (ALA) from activated succinate and glycine, takes place within the mitochondria. The following steps are extramitochondrial whereas the last two steps, again, occur intramitochondrially. The rate of heme synthesis is regulated by negative feedback control. Heme depresses the activity of ALA synthetase, and it is possible that, in addition, both heme and protoporphyrin IX depress ALA dehydratase.[148]

The lead-induced derangement of heme synthesis causes abnormally high excretion of metabolites in the urine. Of these, the levels of ALA and coproporphyrin III always are elevated in lead poisoning,[67, 72, 185] and measurements of these metabolites have gained extensive use as diagnostic tests, as will be discussed later. In severe forms of lead poisoning, the excretion of porphobilinogen, coproporphyrin I and uroporphyrin I increases.[57, 72, 203] Concomitantly, the levels of ALA, coproporphyrin III, porphobilinogen, and protoporphyrin IX in the blood become elevated,[50, 67, 167, 203] All these changes reflect enzyme inhibitions at different steps of heme synthesis. Such inhibition may be caused by direct interaction between lead ions and the enzyme in question, or by the regulative effect of negative feedback from the accumulation of protoporphyrin IX, heme, and other intermediates, or by a combination of both mechanisms.

Of the enzymes involved in heme synthesis, lead inhibits at least ALA dehydratase and ferrochelatase.[45, 60, 128] In addition, it is evident that at least higher concentrations inhibit ALA synthetase and coproporphyrinogen decarboxylase, although the mechanisms of inhibition are not known.[60, 109] Of all known biologic effects of lead, hematologic or otherwise, inhibition of ALA dehydratase is the earliest one. Its activity in circulating erythrocytes always is depressed in lead poisoning,[15, 85, 128] and partial inhibition occurs at lead levels far below those commonly thought to be toxic.[85, 194] The ALA dehydratase assay has been developed into an exposure test for lead[87, 193] (see sections on lead poisoning). However, inhibition of ferrochelatase is the rate-limiting factor for hemoglobin synthesis, since protoporphyrin IX accumulates in the erythrocytes,[167] constituting about 95% of non-iron-bound porphyrins in the red blood cells, commonly termed "free erythrocyte protoporphyrin" (FEP), although it has been shown that this increase from lead toxicity is not "free," but exists as zinc protoporphyrin (ZPP).[113] The FEP increases notably at blood lead levels near 35 μg/100 ml (men) and 25 μg/100 ml (women).[164]

Lead does not interfere with extracellular iron metabolism,

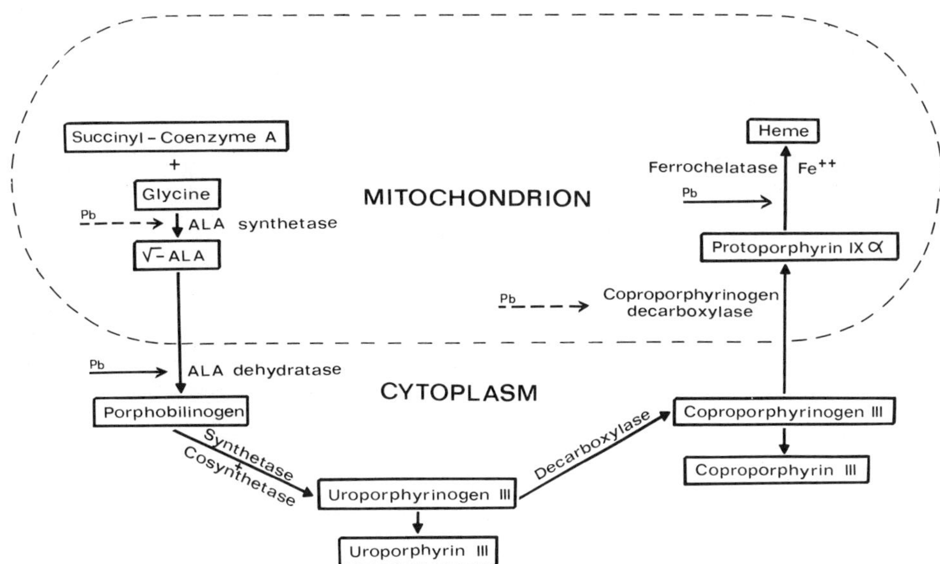

FIG 36–13.
Schematic outline of heme synthesis. The steps where the lead-induced inhibition is strong and well established are indicated by *solid arrows. Dotted arrows* indicate steps where inhibition is less marked.

but the transfer of iron from transferritin into erythrocyte precursors is decreased.[98] As a result, serum iron sometimes becomes elevated. The part of the iron that enters the cell is not completely utilized for hemoglobin formation either, and increase of nonheme iron in the erythrocytes is typical of lead poisoning. Electron microscopic studies have shown so-called ferruginous micelles and aggregations of ferritin in the mitochondria.[14] It now is believed that the basophilic stippling of the immature and mature erythrocytes is made up of fragments of those damaged mitochondria, of microsomal remnants, and of RNA.[14, 100] Since incorporation of glycine into globin is inhibited by lead in vitro, it is possible that the biosynthesis of the protein moiety of the hemoglobin molecule becomes disturbed as well.[101] Production of anomalous hemoglobin (Hb-F) has been reported to occur in lead poisoning, too.[19]

Actions on Circulating Erythrocytes

Shortening of the life span of circulating erythrocytes is the other main mechanism by which lead causes anemia.[67, 77, 203] Present knowledge does not allow quantitative assessment regarding the relative importance of each mechanism; however, it seems that the more acute the poisoning is, the more important is the shortening of erythrocyte life span; conversely, in chronic poisoning, the heme synthesis inhibition is the most prominent feature.[125] In the absence of any inhibition, anemia usually does not develop before the erythrocyte life span is shortened to about 30 days from the normal 128 days. Although the situation is different in lead poisoning where inhibition of heme synthesis hampers the compensating capacity of the bone marrow, some of this capacity apparently is left, and a slight shortening of the erythrocyte life span thus can be tolerated without anemia.[68, 73, 125, 168]

In chronic lead poisoning, the shortening of the erythrocyte life span is moderate and thus slighter than in most hemolytic anemias. Because of the crudeness of the commonly used ^{51}Cr method, it is difficult to give exact data; however, according to several studies, the survival time rarely is reduced below 60 days. Using in vivo labeling with ^{3}H-diisopropyl fluorophosphonate, it has been possible to show slight shortening (to about 100 days) of the erythrocyte life span in a group of heavily exposed lead workers with blood lead levels between 50 and 162 μg/100 ml. The degree of shortening correlated best with that of reticulocytosis but also with anemia, coproporphyrinuria, and PbB.[89] The use of this method also made it possible to state that, at least in chronic exposure, lead shortened the true life span of most or all erythrocytes and that random destruction did not occur.[89] The effect of acute massive doses of lead may be different, however, since random destruction, even leading to intravasal hemolysis, has been reported.[75]

The mechanism by which lead shortens the erythrocyte life span is not well understood.[67, 80, 203] A number of observations show that the osmotic resistance of erythrocytes from patients with lead poisoning is increased.[67, 80, 203]

Increased mechanical fragility has also been reported; however, the studies dealing with this phenomenon are equivocal.[82, 203] It is known that lead interferes with a number of membrane functions.[154] Of them, the cation pump, responsible for maintaining the ionic gradients of sodium and potassium across the cell membrane, is of vital importance for the integrity of the cell. The function of this pump is closely coupled with the activity of membrane Na^{+} and K^{+} activated adenosine triphosphatase. Lead inhibits this enzyme both in vivo and in vitro,[82] which may or may not have a bearing on the shortening of erythrocyte life span. Several other deficiencies in erythrocyte functions have been reported, but the extent to which, if any, they influence erythrocyte viability is completely unclear.

The accelerated removal of erythrocytes from the circulation stimulates erythropoiesis in the bone marrow. Morphologically, the main findings are general hyperplasia and nuclear changes, such as karyorrhexis and mitotic abnormalities. Megaloblasts, polyploid erythroblasts, and sideroblasts often are present. However, the most striking finding is the abundance of stippled erythroblasts. The fact that stippled cells in proportion are more abundant in the bone marrow than in the peripheral blood may be explained by the postulation of two cell populations with different turnover kinetics.[27] Those cells that are morphologically distinguished by basophilic stippling would have a very rapid turnover, perhaps a few days only, whereas the other cells would behave as discussed above.

Dose-Response Considerations

The hematologic effects of lead are the only ones for which dose-response relationships have been established with any satisfactory accuracy, and even this statement presupposes that such an indirect measure as the concentration of PbB (blood lead) stands for dose. The earliest effect is partial inhibition of ALA dehydratase, which becomes measurable at about 20 μg Pb/100 ml blood or even less.[84] Excretion of ALA and oproporphyrins (FEP/ZPP) begins to rise when PbB exceeds 40 μg/100 ml.[178, 194] With increasing PbB values, these changes become more intense. Inhibition of ALA dehydratase displays the best correlation to PbB—coefficients as high as 0.9 have been reported. [84] The correlations for ALA and coproporphyrin are weaker but still of practical significance.[178, 207] Reticulocytosis becomes measurable at PbBs somewhere between 60 and 80 μg/100 ml. In this range, shortening of erythrocyte life span begins to occur as well.[89] For some reason, the degree of anemia correlates poorly, if at all, with PbB. However, a slight drop in the hemoglobin level has been shown at PbB levels of about 50–80 μg/100 ml by following up new lead workers for three to four months.[194] Frank anemia usually does not develop when PbB is below 80 μg/100 ml. At higher PbB levels, all those abnormalities become more and more pronounced, but interindividual variation is large. The dose-response relationship for PbB and protoporphyrin IX (FEP/ZPP) is not known in detail, and the same is true for other, less typical heme synthesis intermediates, such as porphobilinogen. Basophilic stippling of erythrocytes is a poor indicator of lead effect and does not correlate with any other parameter.

Because of the relatively well-established dose-response relationships, several of the hematologic changes described in this chapter serve as diagnostic tests for lead poisoning and as indicators of excessive absorption in the prevention of it. These aspects will be discussed. (See chapter 29 for further discussion on dose-response relationships by R.L. Zielhuis.)

Neurologic Effects

Central Nervous System

Lead encephalopathy formerly was a feared complication of occupational lead poisoning. Nowadays, frank encephalopathy of occupational etiology is rare and the sporadic cases that still occur usually originate in small plants in which industrial hygiene is poor or nonexistent. By far the most serious problem today is encephalopathy as a complication of childhood lead poisoning. Another important etiology is consumption of illicit "moonshine" whiskey or of wine or beverages that have been contaminated by improperly lead-glazed earthenware.[36]

Lead encephalopathy occurs in both acute and chronic forms. In addition, there is a syndrome of permanent brain damage occurring in a large proportion of patients who have survived one or more attacks of acute encephalopathy. Also, subclinical forms of lead-induced brain injury have been described.[46] Those states are not yet well defined, however.

In acute encephalopathy there is swelling of the brain, sometimes in combination with petechial hemorrhages. It is believed that vascular injury is the underlying lesion for the cerebral edema.[36] The most extensive neuronal injury usually is found in the cerebellar cortex, but changes frequently occur in the cerebral cortex as well.[63] Histologically, partial loss of myelin and astrocytic reactions in the white matter are found.[160] The cellular damage may be due to impairment of biochemical metabolic reactions in the brain cells. Since the concentrations of lead in the brains of decreased patients usually have been low compared to most other organs, the central nervous system seems to be particularly vulnerable.[104, 106] In chronic encephalopathy, extensive tissue destruction with cavity formation, as well as thickening of veins with cellular disorganization of their walls, have been described.[168] The latter finding suggests that vascular changes are involved in the development of cerebral injury.

The clinical course of acute lead encephalopathy varies, depending on the age and general condition of the patient, the amount of lead absorbed, the length of exposure, and other concomitant factors, such as chronic alcoholism. Prodromal symptoms may or may not occur. They consist of subtle changes in mental attitude, weakening of memory and of the activity to concentrate, hyperirritability, restlessness, depression, headache, vertigo, and tremor.[36] When the disease progresses, more alarming symptoms indicative of cerebral edema appear. They include vomiting, which may become persistent and forceful, apathy, which develops into drowsiness, stupor, and coma, as well as seizures that may be intractable. Acute encephalopathy may also develop suddenly without warning, often with the onset of seizures. Severe cases progress rapidly to convulsions, coma, and, finally, death from cardiovascular arrest. The onset and course of lead encephalopathy always is unpredictable. Although high blood lead concentrations—usually much above 150 μg/100 ml—are required, other severe symptoms, such as colic, are not always present. Sudden onset of encephalopathy sometimes has occurred in patients whose clinical condition was by no means poor. However, such cases are exceptions. Other manifestations of lead poisoning usually are found, provided that they are looked for and noted.

The prognosis of acute lead encephalopathy is poor. In fatal cases, the patient usually dies within a few days after onset of the first seizure. Before chelation therapy was available, the mortality in childen was about two thirds. Thanks to this treatment, nowadays it is much lower, i.e., about 5%.[30] However, about 25% of those who survive develop permanent brain damage.[185] Although rapid and adequate treatment with chelating agents decreases the risk for permanent brain damage, return to the same hazardous environment increases it to almost 100%.[32] The late encephalopathy may be grave and characterized by severe mental retardation, blindness, and epilepsy with cortical atrophy,[157] or it may be more subtle and characterized by lack of sensory perception and perseverance resulting in poor learning ability and by behavioral disorders such as aggressiveness, destructive behavior, and hostility.[36]

The entity of chronic encephalopathy is complex, since the distinction between the effects of present protracted exposure and those of acute exposure in the past often is impossible. In addition, a number of other factors, such as alcoholism in the adult, influences of the social environment on children, and trauma, infections, and concomitant neurologic diseases in both, often confound the picture. If, despite this, an attempt is made to distinguish between true chronic encephalopathy and late sequelae of acute episodes, it can be said that the former is characterized by a more insidious onset and has a more protracted course. In its mildest forms, it may be detectable by psychologic tests alone. Typical findings in this subclinical state are slow performance of the tests, psychomotor disturbances, impairment of intelligence functions, and personality changes.[74]

The dose-response relationship for the central nervous disorders is not well known. Acute encephalopathy develops only after massive doses, and it seldom is seen when blood lead levels are below 150 μg/100 ml. Also, chronic encephalopathy apparently requires heavy, protracted exposure to develop. The critical dose and duration of exposure, however, have not been determined. The expression of the risk as a function of the concomitant blood lead concentration is not clear, either, since late permanent sequelae of acute encephalopathy often are confused with disorders resulting from current chronic exposure. In the former case, the present blood lead concentration has little connection with the one responsible for the brain damage. Quite naturally, the diffuse and nonspecific character of subclinical disorders renders them still more difficult to relate both to exposure and to the concentration of lead in blood. (See Chapter 50.)

Peripheral Nervous System

Peripheral nervous paralysis, or lead palsy, formerly represented a severe and common complication of occupational lead poisoning. At present, this disorder is seen only sporadically and always under conditions of uncontrolled exposure. The paralysis is characterized by selective involvement of motor neurons, with little or no sensory abnormalities. Another typical feature is that paralysis usually affects extensor muscles, often unilaterally. Since the most heavily used muscle groups are most sensitive, the typical picture is wrist drop of the right hand. However, other muscles of the upper limbs, the extraocular eye muscles, and the extensors of the lower limbs may be involved. Optic neuritis leading to blindness has been reported in children.

According to animal studies, the underlying pathologic lesion is characterized by segmental demyelination and Wallerian degeneration of the peripheral nerves.[55, 173] In man, the nature of lead palsy still remains to be explained. Most data suggest that the lesion is neurogenic and peripheral, usually referred to as neuropathy,[23, 179, 180] but, in some cases, the lesion may be located on the anterior horn cells of the spinal cord.[182]

The clinical picture is characterized by aching and tenderness of the muscles and joints, increased fatigability of the muscles, and fine tremor. Sometimes there may be weakness and lowered tone in the muscles and even atrophy of the extensors of the forearm. The disease then may progress to painless paresis of one or more muscle groups, which, in severe cases, becomes total and ends in typical lead palsy. Recently, subclinical forms, too, have been described. Using electrophysiologic techniques, it has been possible to demonstrate nerve damage in lead workers whose blood lead levels were of the order of 80–120 μg/100 ml and who had varying degrees of clinical or subclinical poisoning but who were completely without any clinical neurologic symptoms.[23, 179, 180] The abnormalities found consisted of slowing of the conduction velocity of the nerves, particularly in the slower fibers and in the distal portions, and electromyographic abnormalities, such as fibrillations and diminished numbers of motor units on maximal contraction.

The prognosis of severe peripheral neuropathy usually is poor. Sometimes milder forms can be healed, but then it is crucial that further exposure is prevented and that effective chelation therapy is started without delay. If chelation is not effective enough, tissue concentrations remain at toxic levels for several months, and this makes the prognosis unfavorable.

The dose-response relationship for peripheral neuropathy is not known in detail. It is generally agreed, however, that frank lead palsy requires severe prolonged exposure to develop, perhaps under conditions in which minor nervous disturbances have been ignored and repeated.[104] At what exposures the first neurophysiologic abnormalities begin to appear is not known, but recent experience from our institute suggests that even lead workers whose blood leads have remained between 40 and 70 μg/100 ml, and never exceeded the latter value, may show slight changes.

Renal Effects

Heavy and prolonged exposure to lead may cause progressive and irreversible renal disease. The older literature contains several reports according to which occupational exposure resulted in chronic interstitial nephritis, often with a fatal outcome.[131] The improvement of industrial hygiene has greatly decreased the number and severity of renal complications from occupational exposure today, but children ingesting lead paint chips and consumers of illicit whiskey still are exposed to a risk.[83, 143]

Lead nephropathy is characterized by a progressive impairment of renal function and often is accompanied by hypertension. The renal damage is chronic interstitial fibrosis, tubular degeneration, and vascular changes in small arteries and arterioles.[56, 143] A peculiar feature is the abundance of intranuclear inclusion bodies in renal tubular lining cells. These bodies are composed of a lead-protein complex in which lead is bound in a nondiffusible form.[64] Goyer and Chisolm[63] have suggested that the inclusion body represents a defense mechanism by which the concentration of lead in cytoplasm will be lowered. Furthermore, since those cells finally are excreted in the urine,[115] this phenomenon would provide the kidneys with a means of getting rid of surplus lead without destroying the viability of the tubular lining cells. The protecting role of the inclusion bodies is also suggested by an animal experiment in which the progression of interstitial fibrosis that developed rapidly after the beginning of exposure stopped concomitantly with the appearance of inclusion bodies.[188]

The functional impairments in lead nephropathy are compatible with damage of the proximal tubuli and are manifested by decreased reabsorption of amino acids, glucose, phosphate, and citric acid.[26, 49] In severe cases, the whole Fanconi triad (hyperaminoaciduria, glucosuria, and hypophosphatemia in combination with hyperphosphaturia) may occur. The functional damage is not necessarily permanent, since even the Fanconi syndrome may be reversible. Its mechanism is not completely understood, but it has been suggested that the decrease in energy production essential for transporting the substances from the tubular lumen across the cell membrane may be responsible.[63]

Saturnine gout is an interesting consequence of decreased tubular function. Lead interferes with the excretion of urates. Consequently, although their formation rate is normal, the uric acid level becomes elevated in the blood, and uric acid crystals are deposited in the joints, quite like in common gout.[49] Saturnine gout differs from the latter in that both sexes are equally involved and in that renal function always is impaired.[49, 143]

Most authors agree that lead nephropathy develops only after heavy, persistent lead exposure, lasting for ten years or more, or after short or repeated episodes of severe acute poisoning. This disorder can, in fact, be regarded as a late sequel of former acute poisoning. The first to draw attention to this was Nye[152] in 1929. He found a high incidence of fatal chronic renal disease in young adults in Queensland who had been poisoned with lead in their childhood. Later, Henderson[83] showed that of 352 adults who had had childhood poisoning 15–40 years earlier, 94 had died of chronic nephritis. The total number of deaths was 165, and nephritis thus accounted for more than half the fatalities. Superficially considered, such findings may suggest that children are more sensitive to lead than are adults. On the other hand, their exposure usually is massive and the poisoning is acute. When adults are similarly exposed, as, for example, heavy consumers of illicit moonshine whiskey, the same syndrome often occurs.[143] Also, heavy industrial exposure may cause renal disease in adults.[129]

Subclinical effects on the kidneys are known to a very little extent only. They appear as slight increases in the excretion of amino acids, glucose, and phosphate in the urine. In experimental animals, the formation of inclusion bodies is one of the earliest effects. They appear even after doses smaller than those required to increase urinary ALA excretion.[64]

Gastrointestinal Effects

The alimentary tract invariably is involved in frank lead poisoning and, as a rule, also milder forms give rise to a variety of gastrointestinal symptoms. The first symptoms begin to appear at PbB concentrations slightly above 80 μg/100 ml. They consist of loss of appetite, digestive disturbances, epigastric discomfort after eating, and either constipation or diarrhea. When the PbB exceeds some 100 μg/100 ml, the likelihood of more severe symptoms increases. These include occasional to frequent colicky abdominal pain and severe constipation. If exposure is not interrupted, classic lead colic develops. The concentration of lead in blood necessary to produce this syndrome usually exceeds 150 μg/100 ml, but wide variations occur. According to Kehoe's[104] excellent description, lead colic is characterized by "sharp onset and recurrent spasms in which the patient writhes in pain, retracts his legs spasmodically to his abdomen, groans, clenches his hands, grits his teeth, with beads of sweat on his brow." This dramatic disorder often results in inappropriate laparotomy, sometimes due to negligence of penetrating the history of the patient, sometimes because the source of exposure is not easily found. If untreated, the colic may persist for several days—even for a week. Intravenous injection of calcium gluconate or other antispasmodic drugs usually results in prompt relief.

The mechanism of colic lies in spasmodic contraction of the smooth muscles of the intestinal wall. The same phenomenon also occurs in the smooth muscles of the arterioles, resulting in pallor of the face, transient elevation of the blood pressure, and decreased glomerular filtration.

Another well-known manifestation of lead exposure is a bluish line on the gums. This so-called Burtonian lead line does not, however, tell anything at all about whether or not the patient has lead *poisoning*. It is formed by precipitated lead sulfide, and it only indicates that the patient has been *exposed* to lead and, in addition, that his dental hygiene is poor.

Cardiovascular Effects

In the acute stages of lead poisoning, and particularly if the patient has colic, the blood pressure often is elevated. Alternatively, hypotonia may occur. The possibility of myocardial damage should not be neglected either.[53] In one study, electrocardiographic changes suggestive of such a disorder were found in 70% of the patients on admission.[181] The main findings were tachycardia, atrial arrhythmia, inverted T waves, and/or an abnormally wide QRS-T angle. Most findings returned to normal after treatment. In another study, there were disturbances in atrioventricular conduction, which returned to normal after treatment but recurred after re-exposure to lead.[147] However, in general, little is known about the acute toxic effects of lead on the cardiovascular system.

The chronic effects have been studied to some extent, but with at least superficially divergent results. Dingwall-Fordyce and Lane[42] found a 2.5-fold excess of cerebrovascular deaths in a population of heavily exposed accumulator factory workers. There was no such excess in less-exposed workers. Since in the United States an earlier epidemiologic study also had failed to reveal any excess mortality from cardiovascular diseases,[44] it may well be that severe, protracted exposure of the type that rarely is seen nowadays is required to produce cardiovascular or cerebrovascular damage. This view is further supported by the fact that there was no effect of moderate lead exposure on the blood pressure in a Swedish study of 364 accumulator factory workers.[38] In view of that and other similar results that have been reported, it appears that work in conditions where exposure is controlled does not give rise to atherosclerosis, hypertension, myocardial infarction, or cerebrovascular disease.

Other Effects

The effect of lead on other systems is not well documented, and also is of less importance from a clinical point of view. However, from the reproductive point of view, the old observations of decreased fertility and increased absorption rate in heavily exposed female workers[75] deserve to be mentioned. Lead also crosses the placenta and may cause fetal injury: for example, neurologic disorders in the child.[75, 153] Recently, also mitotic changes have been found in lymphocytes of lead workers without clinical signs of poisoning.[176]

Lead also impairs thyroid function by preventing the uptake

of iodine, probably by interfering with the pituitary-thyroid axis.[171] Also, the functions of the adrenal and pituitary glands may be impaired.[36]

Some animal experiments have suggested a carcinogenic action of lead. In those studies, adenocarcinoma of the kidneys could be produced by feeding rats lead acetate or by injecting lead phosphate subcutaneously.[36, 42] However, there is no evidence that lead causes cancer in man.[17, 209]

LEAD POISONING

The relevant symptoms and signs of lead effect will be referred to only briefly in the following recapitulation, the purpose of which is to compile the various disorders into clinical syndromes.

Clinical Picture

The first effects of lead exposure occur even in completely symptomless persons. They consist of inhibition of erythrocyte ALA dehydratase activity and, a little later, of increased excretion of ALA and coproporphyrin (FEP/ZPP) in the urine. The earliest subjective symptoms are diffuse and include weariness at the end of the day. The patient is moody and irritable and may fall asleep watching television. Often he loses his interest in leisure-time activities. Such mild symptoms frequently occur with blood lead levels below 80 μg/100 ml. They often begin so insidiously that the patient himself may be unaware of them until he has been away from the exposure for some time. Then, he suddenly realizes that there has been a change for the better in his condition.

With increased absorption, new symptoms develop. They include insomnia, headache and a sweet, metallic taste in the mouth, especially in connection with smoking. Also, symptoms from the gastrointestinal system belong to this stage, and they include loss of appetite, epigastric discomfort, and either constipation or diarrhea. Diffuse muscle pain, tenderness of the joints, and numbness of the legs are common complaints. There may be fine tremor and increased reflexes. At this stage, there often, although not always, is mild anemia, the erythrocyte ALA dehydratase activity is almost completely inhibited, and the urinary ALA and coproporphyrin levels are distinctly elevated (the former usually above 40 or 50 mg/L, the latter above some 1,000–2,000 μg/L). Electrophysiologic examination is likely to reveal slight peripheral neuropathy. These symptoms and signs usually are associated with lead-in-blood levels in the range of 80–120 μg/100 ml or even more and with protracted exposure to lead-in-air levels around 0.3 or 0.5 mg/cu m, but wide variations in sensitivity occur. This type of poisoning still is common in the lead industry, although it is not always reported, because many conservative physicians require more dramatic manifestations to justify a diagnosis of lead poisoning. If no action is taken, attacks of lead colic usually follow. At this stage, all hematologic parameters are pathologic. The hemoglobin value seldom falls below 8 gm/100 ml, but urinary ALA may be as high as 100, even 200 mg/L and the coproporphyrin concentration reaches 5,000–7,000 μg/L (FEP/ZPP often exceeding 500 μg/dl of blood). Corresponding lead-in-blood values usually are above 150 μg/100 ml, and may rise to several hundred micrograms per 100 milliliters in some cases. Particularly when colic is persistent or recurrent, there is risk of peripheral nervous pareses and encephalopathy. These manifestations are rare in occupational poisoning nowadays, but sometimes they occur in consumers of illicit whiskey and are common in children, in whom initial symptoms usually include vomiting, anorexia, apathy, hyperirritability, incoordination, loss of recently acquired skills, and behavioral disorders, such as aggressiveness. Recurrent episodes of colic or protracted exposure at levels producing slighter symptoms are thought to increase the risk of late nephropathy.[117]

If lead compounds are accidentally ingested or if the respiratory exposure has been massive, the onset of poisoning is more acute. Colic and encephalopathy then may develop within weeks or even days. Also, anemia develops quickly, and, in such cases, the hemolytic component dominates. In fact, there may even be intravenous hemolysis and elevation of the serum bilirubin value.

Figure 36–14 is an attempt to relate the onset of different types of symptoms and signs to concomitant blood lead levels. It should be noted that there are wide variations in individual sensitivity and that no definite cutoff points therefore can be defined. The thin portion of the dark area denotes slight effects occurring in part of the exposed population only, whereas the thickening indicates both increasing severity and prevalence of the effect in question. The completely black portion denotes a high intensity of effect in most or all subjects. It should also be stressed that since all dose-response relationships are not known in detail, it has not been possible to avoid a certain degree of arbitrariness. What is important, however, is the continually increasing number and severity of effects with increasing concentrations of PbB, rendering it difficult or impossible to define clear-cut syndromes or to relate the severity of poisoning to given levels of exposure.

Concept of Poisoning

Lead poisoning usually is defined as a clinical disease in which subjective symptoms and objective signs of plumbism occur in combination with typical abnormal laboratory tests. Accordingly, a diagnosis of plumbism should not be made in the absence of overt illness. The acceptance of this definition results in cases that are reported as claims for workers' compensation as being restricted to clinical illness. However, as can be seen from Figure 36–14, before overt clinical symptoms appear there is a "gray" area where functional impairment occurs and where even the subjective well-being may be decreased to some extent. The inclusion of this stage in the concept of poisoning seems justified in today's community, with its increasing demands on "a state of complete physical, mental, and social well-being," as the World Health Organization defines health. Accordingly, subclinical poisoning thus would be defined as a syndrome with slight and vague symptoms but with definite biochemical evidence of functional impairment. Semantically, this stage still can be kept apart from overt poisoning by using different terms such as "plumbism" or "clinical poisoning" for the more severe stages and "mild" or "subclinical" poisoning for the slighter forms (but *not* only "increased absorption," which tells nothing of effects). The crucial point is that the subclinical stage should not be considered acceptable, whatever the term for it, and that preventive and therapeutic action is called for whenever such a disorder is recognized.

However, as has already been pointed out, there are no clear-

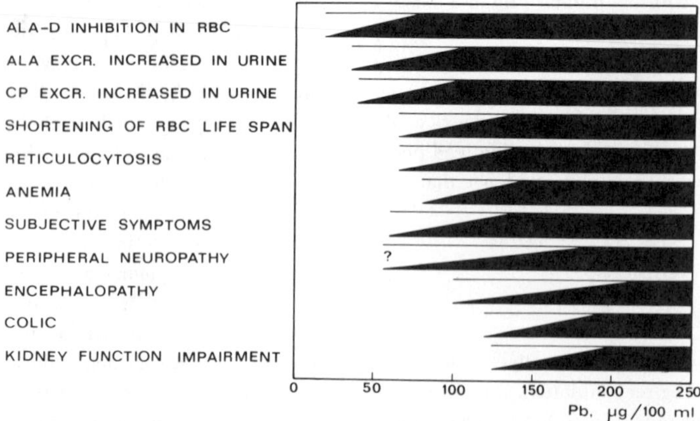

FIG 36–14.
Relationship between blood lead levels and the onset of a number of biologic effects.

cut borders between the different stages of lead effect. All classification systems thus are open to a certain degree of subjectivity. It should also be pointed out that modern techniques have provided us with methods capable of detecting deviations from "normality" so slight as to have no conceivable impact on health at all. Such abnormalities cannot be considered symptoms of poisoning. The problem is to define when a certain deviation from normal becomes unacceptable; this is more a matter of agreement than of facts. As can be expected, there always have been disputes about the definition of the border between acceptable and unacceptable changes. This is not entirely a matter for the medical expert, since the political decision makers, i.e., the governmental bodies, the employers, and the employees, must be given opportunity to express their opinions.

Considering all that, any proposal for classification is doomed to be opposed. If an attempt were made despite this, it would be based on Figure 36–14 and involve the following three categories:

1. No effects or slight effects without any known implication on health. The latter would include partial inhibition of erythrocyte ALA dehydratase and even slight reticulocytosis and a slight increase in the excretion of ALA and coproporphyrin into the urine. This stage would be "acceptable."

2. Mild symptoms, such as weariness, decreased appetite, epigastric discomfort, or loss of initiative, in combination with clearly elevated excretion of ALA and coproporphyrin, slight anemia, and electrophysiologic abnormalities. This stage would be defined as subclinical poisoning and considered to be "unacceptable."

3. Clinical poisoning, which, of course, would also be unacceptable. From Figure 36–14 it can be seen that stage 1 is related to blood lead levels of about 40–80 μg/100 ml or even less, stage 2 with levels between about 60 and 120 μg/100 ml or occasionally more, and stage 3 with levels higher than 100–150 μg/100 ml. There is considerable overlapping due to interindividual differences in sensitivity between the blood lead levels of each category, and no magic border of 80 μg/100 ml or any other value can be distinguished from the dose-response scale. It is quite another matter that some artificial border value can be agreed on and used with more or less wide safety margins to protect workers from having "unacceptable" manifestations of lead.

Diagnosis

The diagnosis of lead poisoning often is said to be difficult, and it is quite true that misdiagnoses are common. The most common mistake is failure to recognize poisoning when it is present, but the reverse may happen as well; i.e., other diseases are mistaken for lead intoxication. No doubt the common denominator for both errors is ignorance, since, generally speaking, the diagnosis of lead poisoning is no more difficult than that of most other diseases.

The first requirement for a correct diagnosis is that the physician remember that lead exists. The second is a good history, detailed enough to allow a quantitative evaluation of the risk. There are certain occupations that are more likely to cause poisoning than others, and nonoccupational sources of exposure should not be forgotten either, as discussed earlier. However, the mere suspicion that lead may be the etiologic factor is crucial, because then one can utilize the special laboratory tests that are available. Of them, the concentration of lead in blood is a key point, since there can be no current poisoning if that level is not elevated. As a general rule, it can be said that the higher the blood lead level is, the greater is the likelihood of lead poisoning. Thinking in terms of probability is important, since there is no well-defined threshold for poisoning. The often-heard statement that poisoning never occurs at a PbB below 80 μg/100 ml does *not* imply that there always is poisoning when that value is exceeded. Furthermore, this statement in itself can be questioned as soon as the subclinical state is included in the concept of poisoning.

However, since all stages of poisoning by definition presuppose functional impairment, the mere demonstration of an elevated blood lead level is not enough for a positive diagnosis. The documentation of functional disturbances using relevant tests must be considered obligatory. Most such tests measure hematologic changes. Of them, the concentration of ALA in serum or urine, the concentration of coproporphyrin in urine, the blood hemoglobin, the reticulocyte count, and the number of stippled red blood cells have been used. The activity of erythrocyte ALA dehydratase always is almost completely inhibited in lead poisoning. Another obligatory finding is elevated FEP/ZPP. The combination of depression of ALA dehydratase activity, increased excretion of

ALA, and increased ZPP levels, is quite specific for lead poisoning. In nonoccupationally exposed workers, ZPP levels are < 2.5 μg/gHb; also the slope of FEP increase is steeper in women. When occupational exposure ceases, the FEP elevation persists out of proportion to current PbB levels. In addition to the tests mentioned above, there are several other examinations that help to complete the picture. Since they are less specific and not necessarily required for the diagnosis, they can be considered descriptive rather than diagnostic. Such examinations are measurement of the erythrocyte survival time, neurophysiologic examinations, kidney function tests, and psychologic testing. The Burtonian lead line on the gums, on the contrary, is no indication of poisoning, merely of exposure. Unfortunately, no numerical border values for "poisoning" or "no poisoning" can be given for any test. Thus, the diagnosis always must be based on the combination of different data, such as a positive history of exposure and typical symptoms and laboratory findings, with a fair amount of sound clinical judgment added.

Differential Diagnosis

Failure to consider the possibility of lead poisoning frequently results in misdiagnosis. Some abdominal disorders bearing a resemblance to lead colic include acute appendicitis, gastric and duodenal ulcer, acute gastroenteritis, acute porphyria, and parasitic infestations. Also, renal colic and poisoning due to other agents may be confused with lead colic. Of the neurologic disorders to be considered, polyneuritis from other causes such as arsenic poisoning, infections (Guillain-Barré syndrome), diabetes, and malnutrition are important. They usually differ from lead palsy by involving sensory nerves and/or by being atypically located. The "Saturday night paralysis" may impose special problems, since it is painless, unilateral, and may involve the radial nerve only. Lead encephalopathy may be confused with other causes of increased intracranial pressure, aseptic meningitis, infections of the meninges, neoplasms, and parasitic infections.

It is quite possible to differentiate all these disorders from lead poisoning, provided that the necessary examinations are performed. The problem with the acute manifestations is that they require quick decisions, leaving no time to wait for blood lead analyses or other time-consuming determinations. This dilemma often has resulted in unnecessary laparotomies, not to mention delay in adequate treatment. A tricky situation occurs when a lead worker develops symptoms that might be due to lead but equally well to some other disease. In such cases, evidence of increased lead absorption is present, perhaps also of functional disturbance. In this situation, it is important to remember that exposure to lead does not protect the worker from incurring other diseases. Consequently, examinations necessary for the exclusion or confirmation of such diseases always should be performed. As mentioned earlier in this chapter, iron deficiency also causes elevated protoporphyrin in the red blood cells.

Occasionally, the failure to find a "natural" diagnosis for a patient displaying bizarre symptoms of various kinds makes the puzzled physician think of lead. If there has been some exposure, the blood lead may be elevated. In this situation, the physician grabs whatever explanation is offered, and such patients then may be diagnosed as cases of lead poisoning on the basis of a slightly elevated PbB only. To prevent such errors, one should remember not to use PbB alone as a diagnostic test, and also keep in mind that lead poisoning is not a vague disorder with all sorts of odd manifestations but a well-defined disease with typical findings.

The most difficult task probably is the establishment (or exclusion) of past lead poisoning as the etiology of some current disease. When several years have passed since the last exposure, the decision is practically impossible to make; especially when there are compensation claims, the history is unreliable. All specific functional tests have returned to normal long ago, and the PbB often is normal too. The only possibility left is the proof of an abnormally high body burden of lead. This is done best by measuring the excretion of lead in urine on provocation with CaEDTA (calcium disodium edetate) or some other chelating agent. This test now is considered to be the most reliable way short of bone biopsy to demonstrate an increased body burden when high-level exposure took place in the past.[36] In addition, the level of ZPP may remain elevated for a long time after termination of exposure.[92, 167] However, the snag is that these tests reveal past *exposure* only, not past *poisoning*. Consequently, they fail to provide the information looked for.

Treatment

The treatment of lead poisoning is based on the prompt termination of exposure and on the use of chelating agents. The first requirement is categoric. The second is determined by the severity of poisoning; at present, the greatest issue is whether asymptomatic patients should be treated or not.

The most commonly used therapeutic chelating agents are CaEDTA, BAL, and D-penicillamine. Of them, the first two mentioned should be administered parenterally to be effective, whereas D-penicillamine can be given perorally. As always when therapy is concerned, there are innumerable regimens in use; unfortunately, there are few systematic trials done where the different methods of treatment have been scientifically compared. For this reason, it is not easy to judge which method is superior.

The general rule is that the more severe the symptoms are, the more active the treatment should be. According to my personal experience, intravenous infusions of 2 gm of CaEDTA diluted in 500 ml of physiologic saline in two to three five-day courses with a two- to five-day rest period are effective in cases without encephalopathy. Chisolm,[30] who has compared the effects of different treatments, recommends the following regimen: In acute encephalopathy, intramuscular injections of BAL-CaEDTA (BAL = 2.5 mg/kg/dose, CaEDTA = 8.0 mg/kg/dose) should be given for five to seven days, followed by a second five-day course if PbB is above 80 μg/100 ml two to three weeks after the first course. The therapy then should be continued with a three- to six-month course of oral D-penicillamine (500–750 mg/24 hr). When colic and other abdominal symptoms dominate, a three- to five-day course of intramuscular BAL-CaEDTA should be given, followed by oral D-penicillamine for about two months or until the urinary excretion of lead is less than 500 μg/24 hr. In painless peripheral neuropathy, the basic treatment is oral D-penicillamine for one to two months except when the blood lead is above 100 μg/100 ml. In that case, the treatment should be started with a three- to five-day course of BAL-CaEDTA. Sometimes symptomatic treatment may be necessary too. Colic is rapidly relieved by intravenous injection of calcium gluconate or other antispasmodic agents. Encephalopathic symptoms are treated according to the same principles as in children.

Chisolm also recommends a three- to five-day course of BAL-CaEDTA followed by oral penicillamine for one to two months in asymptomatic patients with the PbB above 100 μg/100 ml, and a brief course of oral D-penicillamine when it is 80–100 μg/100 ml. The idea of treating asymptomatic patients with chelating agents is not generally accepted, however. In occupational exposure, the step from this practice to the prophylactic use of these agents is a small one. Since the only acceptable prophylaxis is control of exposure, it may be prudent to withhold chelating agents when treating asymptomatic patients. Of course, such a restrictive attitude prolongs the time the worker has to stay unexposed and therefore may seem uneconomic. But once the employer notices that prophylactic chelation therapy is an inexpensive substitute for hygienic improvements, there is the risk of the management neglecting to control exposure.

All chelating agents may have side effects. First, they mobilize iron and essential trace metals, such as zinc and copper. Second, CaEDTA may produce reversible nephrosis, hypokalemia, hypercalcemia, and fever.[30] Safe treatment requires regular and frequent determinations of serum electrolytes, serum creatinine, calcium, and phosphorus, as well as examination of the urinary sediment. Also, D-penicillamine has adverse side effects, such as eosinophilia, skin rashes, fever, coagulation disturbances, leukopenia, and nephrotic syndrome. Since this drug is related to penicillin, those who are allergic to the latter should not receive D-penicillamine. For these reasons, long therapeutic courses in particular should be prescribed with caution.

After termination of the chelation therapy, the patient should be observed regularly for a long period. Return to the toxic environment is not advisable, although often it is unavoidable. Under no circumstances should it be permitted until the PbB is well below 50 μg/100 ml.

Treatment of childhood poisoning always belongs to a special hospital. Because of the frequent involvement of the central nervous system, one of the main aims is to control encephalopathic symptoms. The first task is to establish adequate urine flow by intravenous infusions of 10% dextrose or mannitol. Seizures are controlled by diazepam, paraldehyde, or, in long-term therapy, by barbiturates and diphenylhydantoin.[30] Chelation therapy is based on the combination of CaEDTA and BAL. The addition of the latter drug accelerates urinary lead excretion and prevents the accentuation of the toxic lead effects that sometimes occur after therapy with CaEDTA.[30] The therapy then may be continued with a long-term course of D-penicillamine. The most important matter, however, is prevention of recurrent exposure and treatment of the underlying social situation.

Hryhorczuk et al.[92] observed a temporal fall of zinc protoporphyrin (ZPP) levels in whole blood in 51 workers with chronic lead intoxication who were removed from exposure, treated with intravenous CaEDTA, and followed for a period of 2,273 days. Levels of ZPP fell, with a mean half-life of 68 days, to a mean base level of 36 μg/dl of whole blood. The base-line ZZP level was positively associated with the length of exposure ($P < .01$) and the blood lead half-life ($P < .001$). The amount of EDTA received had no apparent effect on ZPP levels, suggesting that the fall of ZPP levels is largely a function of red blood cell turnover. The base-line ZPP level appears to be a useful biologic index of the biologically active pool of lead for at least two years after removal from exposure.

EPIDEMIOLOGIC ASPECTS—A SHORT RECAPITULATION

Epidemiologic methods have not been applied to any great extent in the study of disorders related to lead exposure. This is unfortunate, since the result is that many important questions still are without answers. There are in particular three problem complexes in which an epidemiologic approach would be rewarding. The first comprises the prevalence of exposure to given intensities of lead in various branches, i.e., how many workers are exposed to how much in different types of factories in a geographic area. Such information is valuable for the planning of prevention programs and for the estimation of what resources (such as manpower, laboratory capacity, sampling capacity) are needed.

The second problem comprises the prevalence and incidence of specific lead-induced disease, including the whole range from clinical poisoning to slight biologic disturbances. The information gained from such studies completes that from exposure studies and shows the severity of the problem. Self-evidently, the study of dose-response relationships belongs to this complex.

The third problem is, perhaps, the most thrilling one. It consists of the study of the relationship between exposure to lead and nonspecific disease. We know little of this. If more such studies had been performed in industry, the present confusion regarding the health effects of environmental lead pollution would have been less complex, since at least part of the data so collected could have been extrapolated. At least a noneffect level for several potential disorders might have been detected.

Since systematic data regarding all three problem complexes are scanty indeed, it seemed more appropriate to combine them with the corresponding clinical findings or descriptions of exposures. In this context only, some complementary and summarizing remarks will be made. (See Chapter 71 on occupational epidemiology by S. Hernberg.)

Prevalence of Exposure

As already discussed, accumulated knowledge has made it possible to crudely classify high-, moderate- and low-exposure jobs. However, since there is almost complete lack of extensive systematic studies aiming at the estimation of the number of workers exposed to given intensities in different branches, it is quite impossible to give any national or other figures of the size of the populations concerned. Holmqvist reported a study in which about 2,000 PbBs were measured in a large Swedish lead smelter.[91] He found values ranging from 15 to 110 μg/100 ml and the means for the subgroups were between 43 and 54 μg/100 ml. Thus, he was able to accurately establish the level of exposure in different jobs in that smelter. Attempts have been made on a nationwide scale to estimate the magnitude of exposure in different branches of the lead-producing and lead-using industry and thus provide data for the planning of a preventive program.[90] However, since great variations between different countries may be expected, studies must be interpreted with great caution from the point of view of generalization with other countries. Thus, each country should collect its own systematic exposure data from different branches in order to be able to plan preventive programs.

Data on nonoccupational lead exposure are sporadic as well. Exposures from flaking lead paint, illicit whiskey, and improperly glazed earthenware have been touched on and therefore will not be repeated here.

Prevalence and Incidence of Specific Lead-Induced Disease

The incidence of occupational lead poisoning is best reflected in official national statistics in countries where such records are kept. In general, these statistics show declining trends over the years. Such statistics also show, as already mentioned, that smelting or burning of lead, shipbreaking, manufacture of storage batteries, and certain other occupations cause by far the largest number of cases of clinical poisoning. However, such statistics only show the tip of the iceberg and, therefore, tell nothing of subclinical poisoning. There is, furthermore, reason to believe that the ignorance of many physicians results in underreporting; sometimes, perhaps, also in overreporting. From an epidemiologic viewpoint, the most serious deficiency of official statistics is that they do not give information concerning the population at risk, i.e., the number of workers exposed to different intensities in different branches. For this reason, it is impossible from this source alone to compare the incidence of poisoning in different branches or even to gain meaningful comparative information concerning the national incidences in different countries.

Systematic surveys of the incidence or prevalence of poisoning in different countries or even in single branches are extremely scanty. In a survey of nine shipyards in Scotland and northeast England, anemia was found in 36% of 225 burners.[137] In Finland, the yearly incidence of lead poisoning in the accumulator industry was about 10% in 1970. Of all workers, 44% had PbBs in excess of 70 μg/100 ml.[196] According to an earlier Swiss study, about half of the workers in accumulator (battery) manufacture had objective manifestations of lead poisoning.[47] In Holland, a total decline to about one third had occurred in the number of cases of lead poisoning in the period 1953–1954 to 1963–1964. This was due mostly to the sharp decrease of reported cases in the accumulator and lead pigment industries.[186] These are just a few examples of the types of studies needed to collect the data necessary for an overview of the epidemiology of lead poisoning. Needless to say, such studies should not concentrate on clinical poisoning only but on all manifestations of lead-induced biologic impairment. Because of the almost complete lack of such studies, the conclusion is that very few, if any, reliable data are available on the epidemiology of occupational lead poisoning.

The situation for childhood poisoning is somewhat better. Thanks to recent intensive activities in the United States, the magnitude of the problem has been realized. The data available suggest that 5%–10% of preschool children residing in slum districts consume enough lead paint to have "increased absorption" and that approximately 1% have clinical lead poisoning.[36] The incidence is higher in the summer than during the winter.[36] Similar data from other countries are missing.

Dose-response considerations were discussed in preceding sections and will not be repeated here.

Relationship With Nonspecific Disease

For the study of cause-effect relationships between exposure to lead and a given disorder, epidemiology offers its classic study designs: cross-sectional studies, cohort studies (retrospective or prospective), and case-control studies.

An example of the cross-sectional design is the comparison of the present health state of occupational groups with documented exposure with that of control groups. This type of study is the one used most often, but the information usually is confused by selection and other uncontrollable errors. The Swedish study of blood pressures in the accumulator industry mentioned before is an example of this design.[38] Cohort studies, in general, are more informative but also more time-consuming and more expensive. To my knowledge, not a single prospective cohort study aiming at the elucidation of a cause-effect relationship between lead exposure and nonspecific disease has been published. Retrospective cohort studies are not frequent, either, as far as occupational exposure is concerned. The most well-known one probably is Dingwall-Fordyce and Lane's mortality study showing an excess of deaths from cerebrovascular disease among heavily exposed battery workers.[42] The authors originally had planned their study to answer whether or not lead exposure caused cancer; no indication of this was found, however. This study is mentioned here only to illustrate the use of the retrospective cohort design; the relationship between lead on the one hand and cardiovascular disease or cancer on the other has been discussed. Earlier retrospective designs have further been used in connection with pediatric poisoning to show the relationship between lead exposure and renal disease.[83]

The application of the case-control design is best made by comparing the tissue concentrations of lead in persons who have died from a given disease with those of persons who did not suffer from the disease but who were otherwise similar. This is not a common approach in lead toxicity research, either. So far, only renal disease and multiple sclerosis have been studied using this design. In Queensland, Henderson and Inglis[83] found higher bone lead concentrations in patients with no known etiology to their renal disease as compared to those with known etiology. The findings were interpreted as confirming the role of childhood lead poisoning as a causative agent for renal disease. As to multiple sclerosis, one study showed that the lead content of teeth was higher than normal in patients with that disease,[21] but, in another study, no relationship between the lead content of other tissues could be found between patients and controls.[20] The interpretation of such data is difficult without any knowledge of the mechanism(s) involved. The examples cited illustrate that epidemiology is just one of the tools for the study of causal connections.

In conclusion, much remains to be done in the field of epidemiology of potentially lead-related disorders. In some instances, it seems as if epidemiologic methods wold be best suited for the study of them, whereas, in others, the problem appears to be insoluble using these methods because of too many uncontrollable disconcerting factors.

PREVENTION OF POISONING

Technical Control of Occupational Exposures

Exposure to lead or its compounds can be made safe, provided that the average concentration in the air is kept below a given level, the TLV (threshold limit value). At present, it is proposed that this level should be 0.15 mg/cu m (ACGIH) for lead and its compounds and 0.1 mg/cu m (NIOSH) (except for tetraethyl lead) in the United States.[2, 200] This standard is a time-weighted average exposure for eight hours a day, 40 hours a week, for a working lifetime. It has already been adopted in several western European countries. In Sweden, the TLV was lowered to 0.1 mg/cu m in 1974. Socialistic countries in general recommend lower values, since they base their standards on other norms. Thus, the maximum acceptable concentration (MAC) for the Soviet Union is 0.01 mg/cu m, that for Hungary 0.02 mg/cu m, and that for Poland and Czechoslovakia 0.05 mg/cu m. Great efforts, calling for a combination of different methods and procedures of technical, hygienic, and medical character, often are needed for compliance with the hygienic standards. A short recapitulation of the main principles follows.

Substitution by Less-Toxic Substances.—The ideal method of prevention is the substitution for a toxic agent of one less toxic in nature. In the case of lead, this has been achieved by the substitution for lead carbonate paint (white lead) of other pigments that now are so readily available that some countries have completely prohibited the use of white lead for indoor painting. Such regulations not only protect painters and paint manufacturers but also the general public by the prevention of disastrous epidemics of childhood lead poisoning from the ingestion of flaking paint. Moreover, red lead (Pb_3O_4) is increasingly being substituted for by less-toxic paints. In the pottery industry, the introduction of insoluble, fritted lead polysilicates as glazes has somewhat diminished the exposure, although not to the extent of completely eliminating the risk of poisoning. However, in the vast majority of operations, no possibility exists for the substitution for lead and its compounds; consequently, other methods of prevention must be applied.

Planning of New Plants or Operations.—The technical control of lead exposure follows the principles applied in technical hygiene in general. This entails that, as a rule, old plants are more difficult to control than are new ones. Obviously, the best results are achieved by consideration of the safety aspects at the planning stage. If possible, when the plant is being planned, all the hazardous types of exposure should be concentrated in a single area in which special control processes can be utilized, and not dispersed around the plant. Encapsulation and other methods of isolation of the dangerous process prevent dust and fumes from spreading around, especially when maintained at slight underpressure; thus, procedures of this type should be applied whenever practicable. Mechanization and automation reduce the number of workers exposed and often also prevent the escape of lead into the atmosphere. Plain, smooth surfaces should be designed for all departments with risk of exposure, and dust control is greatly facilitated by the avoidance of nooks and corners (Fig 36–15).

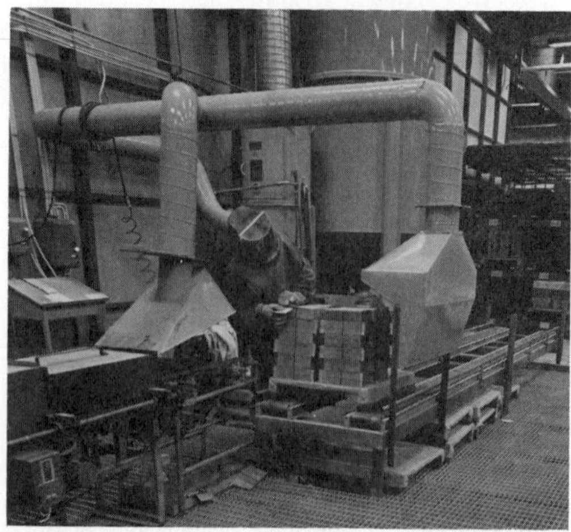

FIG 36–15.
The concentration of lead dust in air can be highly reduced by effective combination of different methods. In this storage battery factory, the floor is constructed of a metal grid, under which water is flowing. Powerful local exhaust ventilation, both from the side and from above, eliminates the dust at the source.

Ventilation.—Effective local exhaust ventilation is one of the best methods for the control of atmospheric contamination, but the air must not be recirculated or discarded in a way that would cause environmental pollution. Self-evidently, good general ventilation is of paramount importance also. Although lead dust is heavy, respirable lead is made up of small particles capable of staying in the air for long periods. For this reason, it is more effective to place the exhaust hood above the process than below it. It should be stressed that open windows and doors may spoil an otherwise effective ventilation system, that changes in the working procedure may have the same effect, and that the ventilation, filtration, and precipitation equipment may undergo deterioration. All of these are circumstances that augment the risk (Figs 36–16 through 36–19).

Prevention of the Spreading of Dust and Fumes.—The spreading of dust can be controlled further by keeping the floor permanently moistened and by frequent vacuum cleaning. However, it should be noted that splashing water on molten lead results in violent explosions. The practice of vigorously sweeping up floors in departments where lead or its compounds are used is dangerous. If, of necessity, sweeping must be done, liberal quantities of oiled sawdust should first be applied to the floor. The use of compressed air to blow lead dust from floors, walls, and ledges should be strictly prohibited, and all other activities that whirl up dust, such as cleaning of walls and constructions as well as maintenance and repair, should be performed outside the working shift by well-protected, special workers. Operations involving burning of metals coated with paint of unknown composition should not be allowed before samples of the paint have been analyzed for lead.

Housekeeping.—Even the best technical control system fails if housekeeping is poor. Constant supervision is needed to ensure proper use of the control methods mentioned above. Edu-

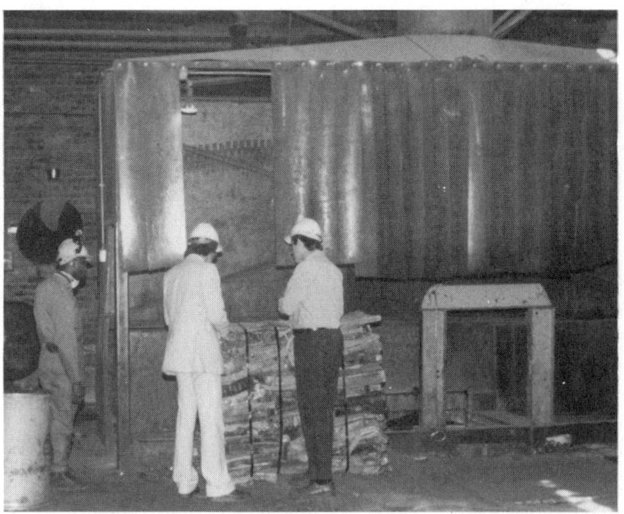

FIG 36–16.
A new, specially designed exhaust for control of the lead dust created by the compressing of the scrap radiators. Compare work area with that shown in Figures 36–6 and 36–7. (This design and installation cost $70,000 in 1983.)

cation of the management and the supervisors is imperative. Besides this, all workers should be apprised of the hazards entailed, the relevant symptoms, and proper precautions, and supervision should be exercised to ensure that the rules are obeyed.

Smoking cannot be allowed in a workroom where a lead hazard exists. Washing facilities, including showers, must be available and used, and each employee should be provided with full-body work clothing and a hat. Work clothing should be vacuumed before being removed and changed at least twice a week. Work and street clothing should not be stored in the same lockers. Food preparation, dispensing, and eating should be prohibited in lead work areas. Whenever the average concentration of lead in air exceeds the TLV, working overtime is not recommended.

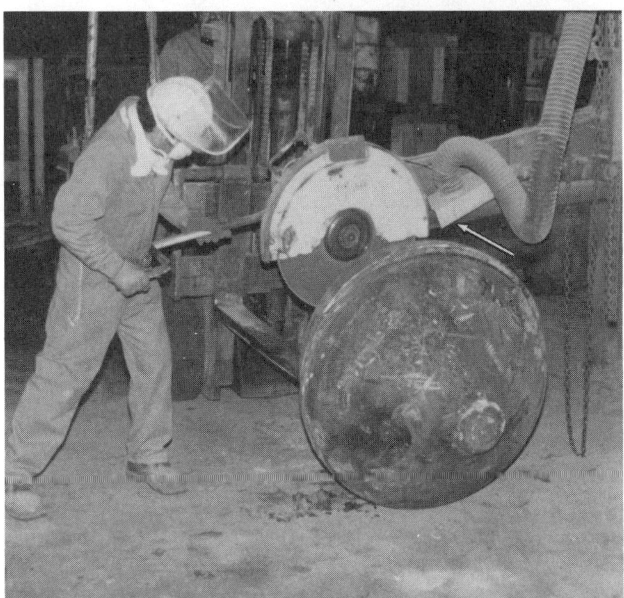

FIG 36–17
Abrasive wheel used to cut large bronze scrap object; note exhaust ventilation attached to collect effluents produced by the abrasive cutting action *(arrow)*.

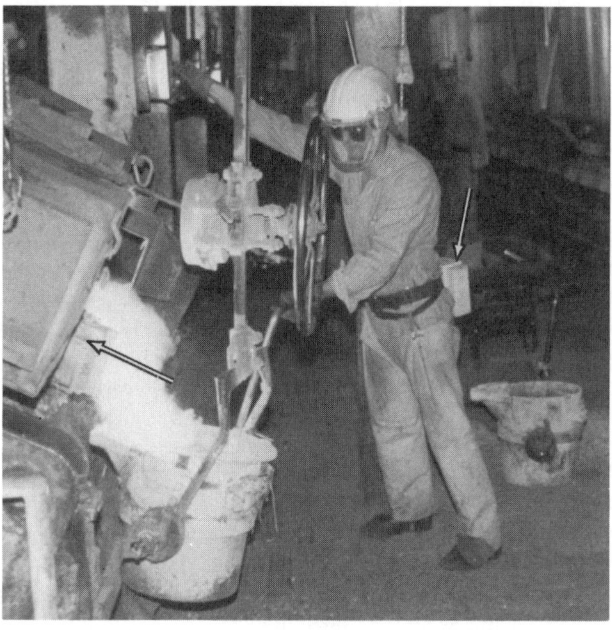

FIG 36–18.
A view of the pouring area of a modern brass foundry. Note the protective equipment worn by the worker—a helmet supplied with filtered air from a portable battery powered device. Also note the exhaust ventilation system *(arrow)*. After extensive design and engineering of an entirely new exhaust ventilating system for this pouring area, the environmental levels of lead were found to be well within acceptable standards, but the workers persisted in wearing their helmets for personal reasons and for cooling comfort, although the filters in the portable system were no longer needed.

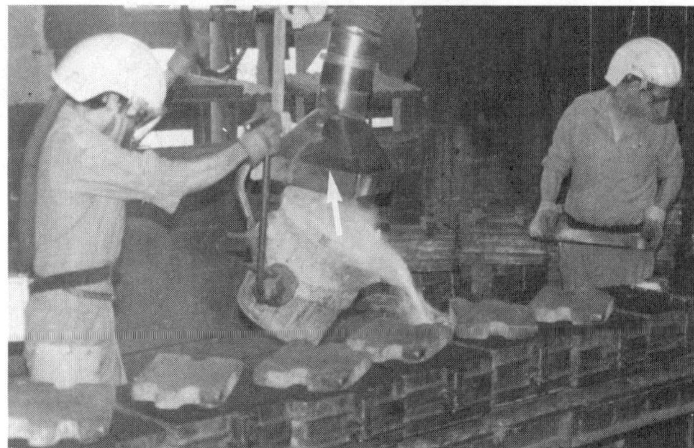

FIG 36–19.
In the molding area, a central exhaust ventilation was an engineering impossibility, and portable exhaust *(arrow)* was required. With a properly functioning overhead movable exhaust system, the employee helmets were redundant.

The worker should also be taught to avoid, whenever possible, areas in which the lead concentrations are particularly high. When engaged in burning or welding outdoors, the worker always should place himself upwind. It is obvious that, along with improving standards of technical prevention measures, the relative importance of good housekeeping increases.

Monitoring of the Lead in Air.—According to the recommendations endorsed by the National Institute for Occupational Safety and Health (NIOSH), the concentration of lead in air should be measured using adequate methods at least once every six months. If the concentrations exceed the standards given, measurements should be made every three months until two consecutive samplings have indicated safe conditions. Moreover, a sufficient number of breathing zone samples for calculations of the time-weighted average for every operation always should be collected.[200] When concentrations that exceed half the standard level are found, warning signs should be affixed in the workroom. The average lead level determines how often and by which methods biologic monitoring should be effected.[11]

Personal Protective Equipment.—Personal protective equipment should be used when the engineering control measures adopted fail to ensure a safe working environment or for occasional brief exposures above the TLV or for emergencies. It should be stressed that respirators merely represent a substitute for technical control measures and should never be regarded as the primary method of protection. There are many types of respirators on the market, but not all of them are adequate. To be effective, the respirator should meet certain requirements, such as those outlined in the American National Standard for Respiratory Protection Z88.2-1969.[3] Fumes and dust require different types of respirators and, if both are present, the recommended usage is that for fumes.

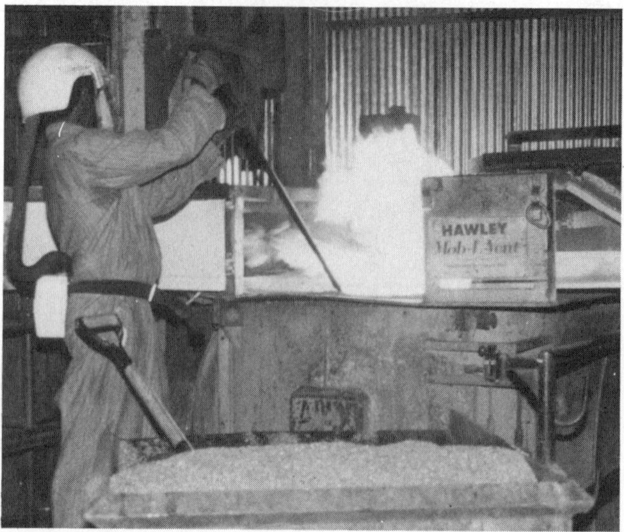

FIG 36–20.
Scrap brass being reclaimed in the melting area. Local exhaust ventilation was later provided.

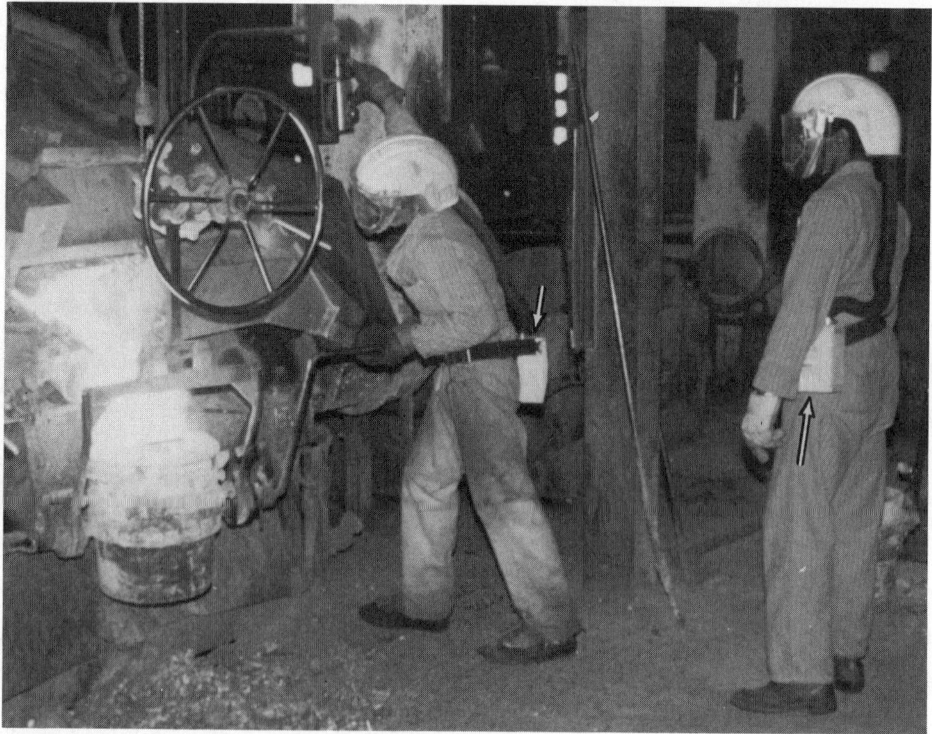

FIG 36–21.
Filling a ladle with molten brass. Tests of air in the breathing zone of each worker revealed no detectable lead with use of the filtered air supplied through the battery powered devices *(arrows).*

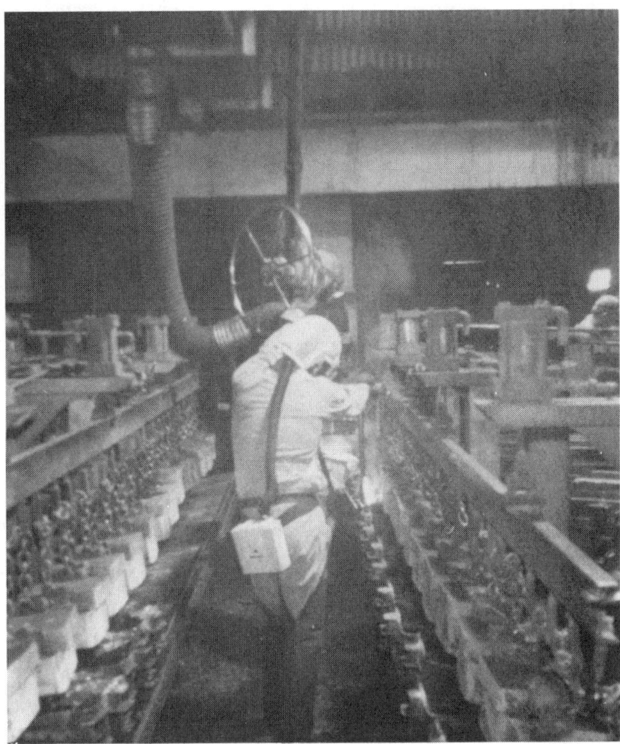

FIG 36–22.
Another view of the large pouring area in the brass foundry.

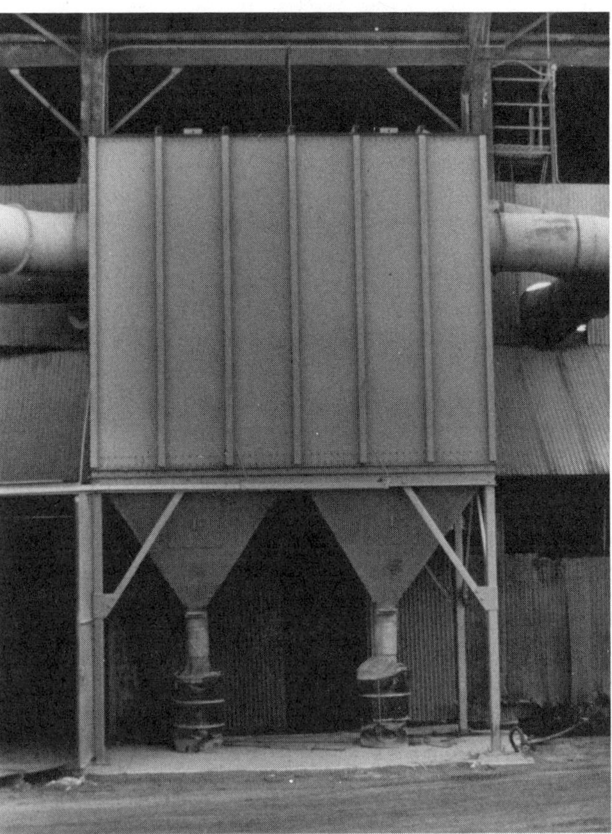

FIG 36–23.
Dust collecting system after plant modernization. Compare with conditions shown in Figures 36–9 and 36–10 (from the same company producing high-grade bronze).

At high concentrations (above 15 mg/cu m), only air-purifying positive-pressure respirators are to be recommended[200] (Figs 36–20 through 36–22).

Impact of Technical Prevention.—Effective combination of the measures described above renders it technically possible to control most exposures, although the financial requirements may be substantial. The most important exceptions are the burning and welding of old lead or lead-painted constructions, for which no effective methods exist. Moreover, primary and secondary lead smelting, particularly in old smelters, is hard to control (Fig 36–23).

Medical Control of Occupational Exposure

No prevention program is satisfactory without regular medical surveillance. The essential part of this surveillance is frequent biologic monitoring of the workers by means of one or more of the comparatively reliable exposure tests developed for lead. Biologic monitoring is at least as important as technical monitoring and is superior to it in the provision of information on personal exposure and the degree of hazard, which depends on a number of factors other than the current concentration of lead in air. These factors include exposure from sources other than occupational ones, the magnitude of the body burden, variations in the level of personal hygiene, the use of respirators, differences in working habits, and intercurrent disease.

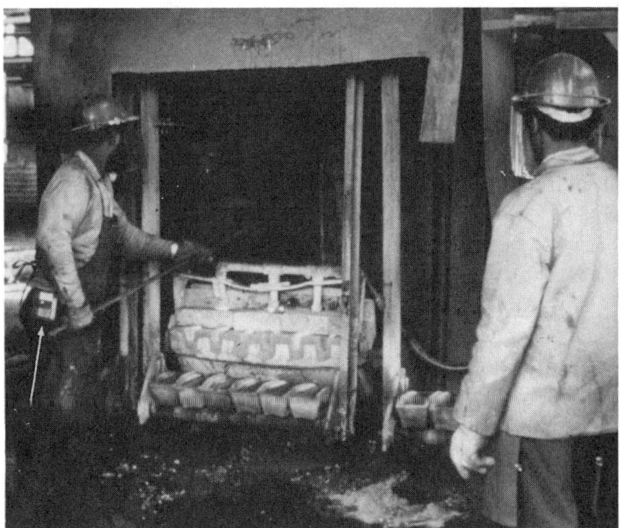

FIG 36–24.
Pouring bronze ingots. (Note the portable battery powered pump [*arrow*] to collect breathing zone workroom air samples for analysis.)

Preemployment Examination

All workers to be exposed to lead should be submitted to preemployment examination. In several countries, such preemployment examinations are required by law. The aim of the examination is that of preventing workers with dispositions suggestive of higher than normal sensitivity to lead from being exposed. Such dispositions are nail biting, anemia, porphyria, cardiovascular disease, recurrent peptic ulcer or gastritis, psychiatric and neurologic disease, neurasthenic disorders, renal and hepatic disease, and all other conditions that significantly impair health. In many countries, the employment of workers below 18 years of age is prohibited. The preemployment examination thus should include a carefully compiled history, a physical examination, a chest x-ray, complete blood count (CBC), blood lead and ZPP determinations, routine urinalysis, and other tests necessary to ensure that the worker is free from significant disorders. Medical records should be kept and should contain all relevant data.

A very difficult question is whether women in the reproductive age should be employed at all in lead works because of the risk for the embryo in case of pregnancy. There is sufficient evidence to prove that lead passes the placenta, so the levels in the embryo will reflect those of the mother. On the other hand, there is not yet conclusive evidence of any particular sensitivity of the embryo, although common sense makes one likely to suspect such a hypersensitivity. In the book *Lead: Airborne Lead in Perspective,*[36] the National Academy of Sciences concludes its review in the following way: "Clinical responses to moderate increases in soft-tissue lead are still ill defined, particularly in very young children. Nevertheless, a rapidly growing child's response to moderately increased lead content may well differ from that of an adult, despite the current inability to perceive the response." Thus, it seems prudent to regard developing embryos as a risk group.

Many experts now believe that 40 μg/100 ml is the upper tolerance limit for the general adult population, but only 25 μg/100 ml should be acceptable for an embryo.[25] Under no circumstances can commonly employed occupational norms be applied. Accordingly, any exposure resulting in 35–40 μg/100 ml in the mother's blood should be regarded as unacceptable, and pregnant women should not be allowed to be exposed to such intensities. In this situation, the decision is simple.

But most women enter their employment without being pregnant and the problem does not arise until the pregnancy starts. Should the use of female workers in the reproductive age in lead works be completely prohibited only because of the "risk" of later pregnancy? It is hard to believe that such a prohibition would work in practice; analogously, all other toxic exposures then should be forbidden also. Thus, the prevention of an embryo from becoming overexposed must rely, rather, on intensive health education, stressing the possible dangers should the woman become pregnant, and the demand of immediate report to the health service when this happens. It should also be assured that another job with the same economic and social conditions will be arranged in case of pregnancy to ensure reporting.

Biologic Monitoring.

Several exposure tests are available for the biologic monitoring of exposed workers. The system to be preferred is determined principally by the reliability of the tests, but economic factors and the availability of well-equipped laboratories also play their parts. The best parameter to use is the measurement of lead in the blood (PbB).[1] (See Chapter 13 on biologic monitoring.)

The National Institute for Safety and Health[200] recently has given recommendations for the medical monitoring of workers exposed to more than half the TLV, or for working conditions that give rise to the belief that operations produce unusual exposure excursions, or that experimental samples do not adequately indicate worker exposure. According to these recommendations, biologic monitoring, preferably PbB measurement, should be performed regularly every six months for half the workers; this means a check for everyone at least once a year. Whenever environmental sampling and analysis shows that the concentration of lead in air reaches or exceeds the TLV, blood analysis shall be conducted quarterly, with each worker sampled semiannually. A PbB of 60 μg/100 gm or more is considered indicative of unacceptable absorption. Such values urge more frequent monitoring, removal of the worker from the toxic environment, and improvement of the environmental controls. The National Institute for Safety and Health also recommends annual medical examinations when unacceptable absorption of lead occurs or when the environmental levels attain or exceed the TLV (Fig 36–24).

The NIOSH system relies heavily on regular environmental monitoring. In countries lacking such resources—and they form the majority—control has by tradition been based on medical monitoring. The fact that there are several biologic tests besides lead in blood or urine has created a variety of different monitoring systems.

It is obvious that the more complete the test battery is and the more frequent the intervals are, the more perfect will be the result from the aspect of safety. However, as already mentioned, economic considerations and limitations of the analytic capacity call for compromises with regard to both aspects.

It is advantageous to combine measurements of PbB, ZPP in urine, and the blood hemoglobin. The PbB monitors exposure, and the last two indicate response. Inclusion of ZPP in the test battery has the advantage both of revealing those individuals who react most sensitively and also of allowing a narrowing of the safety margin for PbB by providing additional information. The number of false positives thus declines.

Lerner et al.[126] measured zinc protoporphyrin (ZPP), free erythrocyte protoporphyrin (FEP), and blood lead (PbB) on 101 workers in a primary lead smelter immediately as they reported for work upon return from a ten-week strike, during which there was no known extraordinary exposure to lead. These measurements were repeated at 2, 6, 10, 35, and 50 weeks following reexposure. The results of this study indicate that FEP or ZPP may be a poor predictor of blood lead in occupationally exposed workers, according to Lerner et al. This is particularly true during more rapid changes in blood lead, such as when a worker is newly introduced to or removed from the lead environment. Monitoring lead workers with FEP or ZPP could give misleading information relative to blood lead if the normal lag in the rise and fall of protoporphyrin IX (PP) in the peripheral blood relative to blood lead is not considered. Blood lead responds more rapidly and remains a better indicator of lead exposure than FEP or ZPP. Also, Lerner and coauthors stated, slight quantitative differences between FEP and

ZPP are clinically inconsequential and their comparable quantitative values may be used interchangeably.

On the basis of experience and studies of the intercorrelation of parameters, the following recommendations were given for the interpretation of the most frequently used biochemical monitors:[88, 121, 204, 205, 208] blood lead (men)—40 μg/100 ml, and blood lead (women)—30 μg/100 ml. When the tests exceed these values, action must be taken to remove the worker from the toxic environment. However, it should be noted that even in the best laboratories there may be a 10% error in a specific lead determination. Thus, a measured value of 40 μg/100 ml actually may have a true value of almost 45 μg/100 ml. In order to ensure better safety, 50 μg/100 ml consequently is more appropriate as an upper limit.[200] In fact, that standard is applied in many countries.

The intervals between the biologic monitoring depend on the degree of risk, but to some extent also on what can be considered reasonable from the economic viewpoint. In high-risk jobs where a significant proportion, say about 50% or more, of the test results of the group is above the standards, frequent monitoring is necessary. This means intervals as short as one month or even less. (It is self-evident that such conditions are not acceptable at all and that all efforts must be devoted to the improvement of the hygienic level.) Bimonthly monitoring is advisable when about 20%–50% of the tests are above the standards, and about 10% of such values require monitoring every third month. In view of the foregoing discussion, the following general rules for biologic monitoring may be given.

1. The higher the risk, the more frequent the monitoring should be.
2. Measurement of PbB always should be included in the test battery.
3. When the PbB exceeds an agreed-on level, or whenever exposure is known to be hazardous, supplementary tests such as ZPP or FEP should be included.[158, 197, 198]
4. Medical examination is required on indications of unsafe absorption.
5. Competent laboratories under regular control should be used for the analyses, and the medical evaluation should be in the hands of a physician familiar with the toxicology of lead.

When the PbB, FEP, or ZPP exceeds the specified upper limits, the worker should be removed from exposure until his or her values have returned to safe levels. It is prudent to apply a safety margin in this situation to avoid rapid recurrence. If 60 μg/100 ml is considered the safe upper limit, the PbB should be below 40 μg/100 ml before the worker can be allowed to return to the exposed (but supposedly hygienically improved) work situation. Usually, several months, even years, are required before this is achieved. The general rule is, the higher the body burden, the longer is the time required; this fact is not generally known or appreciated. Workers with high body burdens are more than normally sensitive to recurrent exposure. Quite often, it proves necessary to remove such workers from exposed jobs permanently.

Finally, it should be stressed that no diet, milk, vitamin, or medicinal preparation can be recommended for the prevention of lead poisoning. The only approved means is that of technical and hygienic control. At times, the prophylactic use of chelating agents may seem tempting, but this practice must be strictly condemned, since it will result in negligence of technical control (of course, therapeutic use of those agents is quite another matter). Moreover, the chelation of essential trace metals and other side effects may in itself represent a risk. It is extremely strange indeed that this method of "prevention" finds widespread use in such a large number of European countries.

Childhood Poisoning

The principles for the prevention of childhood poisoning are (1) prohibition of the use of lead paints in indoor painting, (2) sanitation of decaying buildings, (3) case-finding campaigns and other screening programs, (4) education, and (5) treatment of the medical, psychologic, and social conditions that are the underlying reasons for pica. In many European countries, indoor use of lead paints has been prohibited for decades. In 1970, only four states and ten municipalities in the United States had laws or ordinances prohibiting indoor painting with lead paint.[36] Some of them also require the removal or covering of lead paints for dwellings where PbBs in excess of 60 μg/100 ml have been measured from the children. In January of 1971, the Lead Based Paint Poisoning Prevention Act was signed into law, and this probably will help local governments in the battle against lead poisoning.

In recent years, a new element of concern has been added to occupational hazards of lead exposures with reports of increased lead absorption in the children of lead workers.[5, 24, 25] Home contamination lead dust brought home on workers' clothing was found responsible for certain observed effects in children, which included elevated blood lead values and erythrocyte protoporphyrin levels. (In some of the lead-intoxicated children, hospitalization and chelation therapy were required.)

ALKYL LEAD COMPOUNDS

The only alkyl lead compounds of practical significance are tetraethyl lead (TEL) and tetramethyl lead (TML), which are used as antiknock agents in gasoline. The former was introduced in 1923 and the latter in 1959. Both compounds are lipid-soluble liquids. TML is more volatile than TEL; the boiling point for the former is 110° C and for the latter is 199° C. Although the alkyl leads are used exclusively as antiknock agents, they represented about 46,000 metric tons of the total lead consumption in the United States in 1985, second only to what was consumed in storage battery manufacturing.[201]

Exposures

All forms of exposure are connected with the production, distribution, and handling of alkyl leads. In the manufacturing plant, the risk usually is low because of the strict precautions employed. However, the manufacture of TEL sometimes has been attempted under improvised conditions without any hygienic or medical supervision. Under such circumstances, the risk, of course, is high; consequently, cases of poisoning have occurred.[170] The transportation of alkyl lead compounds from the manufacturing plant to the petroleum refinery has a good record, and poisoning in general does not result from this activity. Generally speaking, the same can be said about the handling of TEL and TML in gasoline refineries. The procedures involve transfer of the antiknock compounds from shipping containers into storage tanks and mixing of them into gasoline. Since the potential danger involved in these procedures is so obvious, early anticipation of it has resulted in preventive measures effective enough to avoid serious health effects. Accidents and failure of equipment represent great hazards.

The most important exposure from the toxicologic point of view occurs in the cleaning and repairing of tanks for the storage of leaded gasoline. These tanks often contain a bottom sludge with a high content of TEL or TML. Cleaning usually is performed by special working teams of 2–20 men who use some hours to some days for the procedure. Exposure occurs by both the cutaneous and the respiratory routes; both exposure routes can be protected effectively by appropriate clothing. It should be noted that not all tanks present hazardous conditions; however, it is impossible to predict in advance which tank is dangerous and which one is not.[170] In other words, the mere entering of a tank does not necessarily expose the worker to dangerous conditions. On the other hand, there are indeed dangerous tanks. Consequently, the cleaning and repair of storage tanks is by far the most important cause of TEL poisoning and therefore always calls for strict precautions.[170]

Finally, there may be a theoretic possibility of overexposure when leaded gasoline is used for cleaning or degreasing (for which it is not intended) in poorly ventilated workrooms. However, since the gasoline itself is highly volatile, its smell and the symptoms provoked by the high concentrations formed usually limit exposure to TEL. Another possibility is cutaneous absorption through repeated skin contact with leaded gasoline; this possibility is hypothetic, however.

Toxicology

Because of their lipid solubility, the alkyl leads are readily absorbed through the intact skin and the mucous membranes. For the same reason, they readily penetrate the blood-brain barrier. In the blood, a high proportion of the alkyl leads is located in the lipid fraction—about three times more than is the case with inorganic lead.[10] In general, the alkyl lead compounds find their way to organs with high lipid content, such as the central nervous system. In the organism, TEL becomes metabolized by the liver to trialkyl lead, which is water-soluble, and to inorganic lead.[39] It is believed that triethyl lead is responsible for the toxic manifestations of TEL poisoning. The lethal dose for rats is about 11 mg/kg for TEL and about 83 mg/kg for TML.[172] Thus, there is at least a sevenfold difference in acute toxicity between these compounds. This difference eliminates the hazards caused by the higher volatility of TML.

Obviously, the development of poisoning in man requires sufficient exposure. More specifically, there must be a history of prolonged skin contact with undiluted TEL, or of the spending of several hours to several days in an atmosphere containing high concentrations of this compound. (Since the literature on TML poisoning is scanty, the following passages deal with TEL unless otherwise stated.) When the exposure time is a matter of hours, concentrations above 10 mg/cu m usually are required to produce TEL poisoning. The longer the exposure time is, the lower is the dangerous concentration. The TLV for TEL[2] now is 1.0 μg/cu m, and the concentration in air that is safe for shorter occasions may be expressed as a curve indicating that 1 mg, 0.6 mg, 0.4 mg and 0.28 mg/cu m are safe for one, two, three, and four hours, respectively.[170]

Clinical Picture of TEL Poisoning

Poisoning usually starts with nonspecific symptoms. In mild cases, there is no further progress, and the symptoms subside in some days, but sometimes these symptoms are prodromes of a more severe disease. After massive exposure, TEL intoxication may also have a sudden, dramatic onset. The general rule is that the length of the time intervening between exposure and the onset of the earliest symptoms relates to the severity of the illness; i.e., the shorter the time, the more severe is the intoxication.

The mild intoxication, or the prodromal stage of a more severe illness, is characterized by nervous instability. Common symptoms include insomnia, troubled dreams, emotional instability, and heightened and erratic physical activity. Gastrointestinal symptoms include anorexia, vomiting, and minor diarrhea. On examination, the patient often shows marked tremor, increased tendon reflexes, pallor, and lowering of the blood pressure. A remarkable feature is the absence of changes in the blood count or of any increase in heme synthesis metabolites, i.e., ALA, coproporphyrin, or porphobilinogen in the urine. This is one of the most important differences between poisoning with inorganic lead and TEL; consequently, disturbances of heme synthesis are of no diagnostic or preventive value in TEL poisoning. The only exception is inhibition of erythrocyte ALA dehydratase, which, according to a recent study, occurs in TEL poisoning without concomitant increase in ALA excretion.[10]

In severe cases, the prodromal stage develops into violent symptoms, sometimes gradually but most often suddenly. These consist of delusions, hallucinations, and hyperactivity, with constant moving, loud shouting, and laughing. The hyperactivity may go on continually for several days before it ends up in coma and death or, alternatively, in recovery. Once coma has developed, the prognosis is severe. During recovery, which may take some weeks or even months, mild nervous symptoms often persist for some time. The treatment is symptomatic only, since no specific therapy is known. Heavy and prolonged sedation with barbiturates or diazepam often is necessary. Water and electrolyte balance must be cared for. Chelating agents cause a slight increase in the excretion of lead but they have no certified effect on recovery.[10]

Prevention

Any prevention program must be based on the availability of proper technical facilities, strict regulations, effective protective clothing, and regular hygienic and biologic monitoring. The mixing of TEL or TML with gasoline always should be performed using proper equipment and under strict surveillance. The most difficult operation to control is the cleaning of tanks that have been used for storage of leaded gasoline. It should be strictly forbidden to enter any tank without proper full-body protective clothing and an airline mask. The biologic monitoring usually has been based on regular measurements of lead in urine, the level of which should be kept below 150 μg/L.

There are not data enough to allow definite statements concerning the upper limit for safe levels in blood.

ANALYTIC ASPECTS

Air Sampling

Sampling for atmospheric lead dust and/or fumes can be done either from fixed sites or by personal samplers. Both methods have their own indications. For the collection of the sample, either 0.45 or 0.8 μ pore cellulose membrane filters or electrostatic precipitators may be used. The National Institute for Safety and Health recommends the first-mentioned procedure.[200] The air is drawn through the filter mounted in a filter holder at a flow rate of 1–4 L per minute.[200] The Millipore HA filter recommended by the American Society for Testing and Materials is reported to have a 99.9% efficiency for collecting particles above 0.03 μ.[200] A minimal sample of 100 L is necessary to provide accurate results, but larger sample volumes are encouraged.[200]

Sampling of Biologic Materials

The most common materials are blood and urine, but, recently, hair samples also have been suggested for the estimation of exposure to lead.[76] A common feature for all biologic samples is that lead is present in minute amounts. This requires meticulous care and avoidance of contamination at all steps of sampling and analyzing. Some recent interlaboratory comparisons have shown that these requirements often definitely are not achieved.[13, 105] To avoid contamination, lead-free materials should be used. Of the plastics, polypropylene and Teflon are best suited. All plastic and glassware used should be washed with mineral acids, e.g., 10% nitric acid, or with the newer commercial washing materials, e.g., Newamat or Deconex, and then rinsed in copious amounts of double-distilled, ion-free water. Anticoagulants as well as all reagents used in the analysis should be "lead free." A lead-free tube is manufactured by Becton, Dickinson and Company (B-D). It is easily identified by its royal (dark) blue-colored stopper. B-D certifies that these tubes have been analyzed for trace element content and have been found free of these at the concentrations specified below. The tube is particularly suitable for blood lead determinations since it introduces no detectable lead into the sample. A sample copy of the certificate enclosed by B-D in each box of these vacutainers is shown in Table 36–1.

Needles should be of stainless steel with a polypropylene hub. Glassware that may have come into contact with samples containing much lead must be isolated and carefully deleaded before being used again. As pointed out earlier, blood samples are preferred to urine samples. If, for some reason, the latter are used, there always is a conflict between the optimal requirement of 24-hour samples and the practical difficulties in collecting them from actively working people. The latter aspect usually weighs more, and "spot samples" thus are chosen. However, the basic requirements for using such samples are that they be collected during the work shift at the same time of the day each time, that they have a volume of at least 100 ml, and that their specific gravity is 1.010 or more.

TABLE 36–1.

Product Information Notice
This product is suitable for usual laboratory use and is especially useful for collection of specimens for trace element determinations.

TRACE ELEMENT† LEVELS OF THE TUBES ARE:

TEST	VALUE PPM	TEST	VALUE PPM
Zinc	0.20	Manganese	< .01*
Lead	< .01*	Cadmium	< .01*
Iron	0.12	Arsenic	< .02*
Copper	< .09	Antimony	< .04*
Calcium	0.60	Magnesium	0.10

*Flameless technique
†Determined by acid extraction of the stoppered tube utilizing Atomic Absorption Spectroscopy (AAS).

The experiences with hair samples still are too preliminary to allow any recommendations; however, the greatest problems are connected with external contamination and how vigorously this can be removed.

Analytic Methods for Lead

There are several analytic methods that yield reliable results, provided that care is taken to avoid contamination or loss of lead during the pretreatment of the sample and provided that the analysis is in the hands of well-trained technicians. Lead can be measured from biologic or atmospheric samples, e.g., by mass spectrography, colorimetric dithizone methods, atomic absorption spectrophotometry, polarography, and anodic stripping voltammetry. Each method, of course, requires appropriate sample pretreatment. Of the techniques mentioned, atomic absorption spectrophotometry is becoming the method of choice because of its sensitivity, accuracy, and speed. Mass spectrography is considered to be the most accurate method, but its expensiveness limits its use. Polarography still is used in several European countries, but it is a slow method, and it has yielded poor comparability in interlaboratory studies.[105] Of the newer methods, anodic stripping voltammetry is extremely sensitive and seems to be promising,[7] but enough experience still is lacking. Micromethods based on some of the techniques mentioned are also being introduced. Their advantage is that they require such small amounts of samples as to render venipuncture unnecessary, but their disadvantage is that the risk of contamination from the skin increases in proportion to the decreasing size of the blood sample.

Quality Control

It is a well-known fact that lead analyses, irrespective of the method used, are subject to extremely severe methodologic errors unless meticulous care is taken to avoid them. A comparative interlaboratory study made in the United States showed quite alarming results,[105] and a more recent one in Europe[13] was at least equally depressing. For example, in the latter study, there was a ninefold range in the results obtained from the same blood sample. Even in the hands of the best analyst, there may be a 10% error in a specific lead determination. Thus, in order to ensure satisfactory reliability, continuous and efficient quality control is needed. Such control should include regular checking of standards and reagents, routine use of duplicate determinations, regular inclusion of samples in the test series to which known amounts of lead have been added, and, finally, regular interlaboratory comparison programs.

Sample Collection and Analytic Methods for Other Exposure Tests

The tests that will be considered in this context are urinary ALA and erythrocyte ALA dehydratase. The crucial matter here is not contamination but the instability of ALA or of the activity of ALA dehydratase. Since light may degrade ALA, urine samples should be collected in nontransparent flasks and stored in the dark at 4° C until analysis. Freezing should be avoided, since there may be serious losses. δ-aminolevulinic acid is stable in acid solutions; thus, enough hydrochloric acid or glacial acetic acid should be added to keep the pH below 5. Provided that these requirements are met, samples can be stored for months. The use of lead-free equipment is recommended, since analysis of urinary lead then becomes possible from the same samples, if desired.

There are three common methods for the determination of ALA. The original method described by Mauzerall and Granick[135] is the most exact but the most cumbersome one. The simpler and speedier modifications developed by Davies[41] and by Grabecki et al.[66] are not so specific and give slightly higher values. However, for routine use, both methods are quite satisfactory and therefore can be recommended for practical reasons. Recently, also, an automatic method for ALA that appears to be quite satisfactory has been developed.[119]

δ-aminolevulinic acid dehydratase is unstable in blood samples, but no significant loss of activity has been shown to occur when samples have been stored for periods up to five hours at 3°, 25°, and 30° C. Analyses, therefore, should be done as soon as possible, and at least within five hours from sampling.[84, 149] The assay that has achieved widest use was developed originally by Bonsignore et al.[15] However, newer modifications have improved it considerably.[149] It is important to use stable buffers such as phosphate buffers and to avoid exposure of the sample to light during incubation. By adjusting the incubation pH from the commonly used 6.8 to 6.4 or even less, the sensitivity of the test can be decreased without loss of accuracy, thereby rendering it more suitable for the monitoring of occupationally exposed workers.[149]

The FEP concentrations are readily ascertained by means of fluorometry; FEP is usually found below 80 μg/dl in men (mean about 50) and is essentially similar for women.[163]

LEAD AS A POLLUTANT OF THE GENERAL ENVIRONMENT

So far, this treatise has focused on occupational lead poisoning, and the problems caused by the dispersion of lead in the general environment have been mentioned only in passing. However, it has already been stressed that a person's total exposure is made up of the sum of several contributing sources. One of them is the "background" from food, drinking water, and ambient air. For this reason, a brief review of the factors determining this background exposure and its impact on health seems indicated. Connected to this problem are several crucial questions, and the most critical ones seem to be the following.

1. What are the patterns of pollution?
2. Is exposure from food, drinking water, and inhaled air increasing?
3. Are human beings presently accumulating lead from environmental exposure?
4. If so, have there occurred any health effects resulting from such accumulation?
5. What are the prospects if the present trend of pollution continues?

The answers to these questions are by no means simple and straightforward, and there are few fields at the moment in which the opinions are so inflamed. The following attempts to summarize the controversial topic of environmental pollution with lead should be regarded with this fact in mind.

Patterns of Pollution

As already stated, lead is a ubiquitous element, and there has never existed a completely lead-free environment. Natural sources that contribute to the emission of lead into the atmosphere include silicate dust, volcanic halogen aerosols, forest fire smoke, aerosolic sea salts, and meteoritic and meteoric smoke.[155] However, man's activities have by far outstripped this "natural pollution," which has been estimated to equal about 0.0005 μg/cu m air only.[155] The first significant step was the Industrial Revolution, which increased the need for lead and its compounds; consequently, the smelting of lead ores expanded. The primitive methods used in the 18th century caused heavy local pollution because of great loss of lead in the air. During the 19th century, the smelting procedures improved somewhat, and in the 20th century, it became really economic to recover lead from smelter fumes. Thus, pollution from lead smelting has decreased in general, although there are several exceptions.[43, 150] Another source of pollution that emerged from the Industrial Revolution was the increase of coal burning in industry. Coal contains about 7 ppm of lead and the silicate material of fly ash may contain as much as 100 ppm.[155]

The most drastic change in the pollution pattern took place in the 1920s, however, when the use of alkyl lead compounds as antiknock agents in gasoline was introduced. The rising trend has been sharp. In 1933, only 10,000 tons of lead alkyls were burned in the Northern Hemisphere as compared to 300,000 tons in 1966.[145] Today, combustion of leaded gasoline is responsible for about 98% of the total lead emission in the United States. It has been estimated that this source accounted for 181,000 tons in 1948 as compared to 920 tons from coal combustion and 958 tons from primary and secondary lead smelting.[36] Thus, not only the amount of lead emitted but also the pattern of emission have changed substantially during this century.

The increased emission into the atmosphere due to the Industrial Revolution and, in particular, due to the use of alkyl leads has been studied from the ice caps of the Northern Hemisphere. The lead content in annual layers of the ice cap of Greenland increased by about 400% between 1750 and 1935, which reflects the industrial revolution. But, between 1935 and 1965, the concentrations tripled; this clearly shows the effect of leaded gasoline. In the Antarctic, such an effect is not evident, however.[145] Old moss materials preserved in botanic herbaria have also been used to prove that the lead pollution has increased. In a Swedish study, there was a fourfold increase from 1850 to the present.[169]

Cycling of Lead

Lead is not evenly distributed in the environment. There is a logarithmic increase in atmospheric lead concentration from mid-ocean to remote high mountains, to seashore, to suburban, and to urban environments.[36] However, the lead does not remain in the atmosphere forever. Approximately half of the amount emitted by cars is removed by gravity within about 100 m from the source. The rest stays airborne for about 7–30 days and is gradually removed by aggregation or precipitation, rain being the main cleaner.[36] The lead content of soils probably becomes slowly increased by precipitation. Part of the lead also reaches the seas, either directly or through the draining of streets in urban areas, but in rural areas, the atmospheric washout is to a great extent held in the clay fraction of the soil, which means that it contributes only little to surface water pollution.[112] Much of the lead entering aquatic systems is removed by sedimentation because its solubility is low. This means that both air and aquatic systems possess a cleaning mechanism.

Precipitation tends gradually to increase the lead content of soils, but, from this, it does not automatically follow that plants take up that lead, because its solubility is low. Although to some extent plants can absorb lead through their roots, even wide variations of the lead concentrations in the soil are not reflected by similar variations in the plants.[36] Within a plant there is a natural accumulation of lead in the leafy portions in both polluted and unpolluted conditions.[191] This is explained both by translocation within the plant and by deposition on the surface from fallout. Usually, the lead concentrations on the surface of foliage are proportional to those in the air, and roughly half of the lead can be removed by washing with water. Parts that are less exposed to fallout, to which category most edible plant materials belong, show little effect of contamination.[36] From the point of view of cycling of lead, these facts indicate that such leafy vegetables as lettuce and cabbage and, of course, grass are the most important sources for the transfer of lead to herbivorous animals and to man. Considering that most of the lead emitted is deposited near the source (along highways, in downtown areas, and around industry), vegetables containing much lead are confined to restricted areas. This fact naturally creates local problems but, as a whole, it acts to limit the amount of emitted lead entering food chains. Another important barrier for the cycling of lead is its tendency to become deposited in the bones. Thus, only a small fraction remains available in meat for carnivorous animals and man. In other words, lead behaves quite unlike mercury in ecosystems in the sense that it does not enrich in ecologic chains, rather the opposite.

Sources of Exposure

When no "abnormal" sources are present, man's total exposure to lead is made up by that from drinking water, food, and inhaled air. Drinking water usually originates from rivers and lakes. Most values reported from water supplies have been withinn the limits recommended by both the U.S. Public Health Service and the World Health Organization (i.e., 0.05 mg/L). According to a nationwide community water supply survey in nine different areas of the United States in 1969, only 41 of the 2,595 samples studied contained more than 0.05 mg/L.[142] However, where lead plumbing systems still are in use, the situation may be quite different for tap water; but, on the average, drinking water contributes a small amount only to man's total lead exposure. Assuming 20 μg/liter and a daily consumption of 1 L, the lead absorbed from water would equal 2 μg/day only. However, since children drink more in proportion to their body weight, the importance of lead in drinking water is greater for them.

Man's exposure from foods depends on their natural lead content, factors that may increase it, and the amount of food ingested. The "natural" lead content of food probably is not more than about 0.01 μg/gm wet weight.[155] However, all food studies performed show higher values.[93, 103, 124, 174] There are both national differences and extremely broad variations within a country for the same foodstuff, not to mention different foodstuffs. This renders the calculation of an average daily intake from such data difficult. No food or group of foods is either a large or a constant contributor of lead in man because the traditional diet, at least in the United States and Europe, is composed of a wide variety of items. For this reason, calculations of the daily intake should be based on a "double portion" technique or some other adequate method rather than on extrapolations from concentrations in separate foodstuffs. Furthermore, the population studied should be representative and large enough. Unfortunately, sufficient data from such studies are lacking. With these reservations and considering that there is a wide range of variation (100–500 μg/day),[174] the average daily intake from food for Americans is about 300 μg/day.[79, 103] The daily dietary intake for 1–3-year-old children averages 130 μg/day,[7, 32] which is proportionally greater than for adults. Assuming an average 10% net absorption rate in the intestine, the contribution of lead in food to total intake thus would be about 30 μg/day.

The literature on lead in air is extensive indeed. The most important emission products from gasoline are in particles of equivalent diameters between 2 and 10 μ—lead bromochloride (PbClBr)—and in particles smaller than 1μ—α and β ammonium chloride and lead bromochloride ($NH_4Cl \cdot 2\,PbCl \cdot Br$, $2NH_4Cl \cdot PbCl \cdot Br$), minor quantities of lead sulfate, and the mixed oxide and halide ($PbO \cdot PbCl \cdot Br \cdot H_2O$). Very small amounts of TEL and TML may escape into the atmosphere during evaporation of gasoline.[36] Most particles are below 1 μ in diameter. Their mass median equivalent diameter has been thought to range from 0.18 to 0.42 μ,[123, 162] but, according to recent research, also heavy deposits of particles ranging from 300 to 3000 μ in diameter are formed.[71, 100] The general pattern is that urban air contains more lead than does rural air and that there is a correlation with traffic density. Thus, downtown areas of big metropolises, busy streets, and the vicinity of freeways regularly show the highest concentrations.[36, 161] Locally, still higher concentrations have been found around lead smelters.[43] The concentration of lead in air in nonurban areas in the United States[199] ranges from undetectable to 0.17 μg/cu m. By contrast, urban areas usually have averages ranging from 1 to 3 μg/cu m, with peaks of 14–25 μg/cu m during rush hours.[130] The variation between suburban and urban areas usually is at least fivefold.

Man's exposure from airborne lead thus varies substantially, depending on where he lives and where he spends his days. The variability is increased further by the amount of air inhaled, which, in turn, depends on the degree of physical activity. At rest, man inhales about 11 cu m/24 hr, but if he performs light work for eight hours and has light leisure-time activity for another eight hours, the amount rises to 23 L. Thus, depending on the site of dwelling and the degree of activity, the amount of lead taken in by respiration may vary between 1.1 μg for a rural man at rest and 57.0 μg for a man engaged in light work and residing in a downtown area with an average concentration of 2.5 μg/cu m. Supposing an average retention of 37%, this would correspond to 0.4 and 21 μg/day, respectively. Table 36–2 shows the relative importance of airborne lead for total intake under various conditions. However, when considering these figures, it also must be remembered that excretion increases with increasing intake, and that only a fraction of the latter will be retained. It thus can be concluded that intake from food usually is the principal source for the general population, that drinking water contributes little, and that intake from inhaled air becomes important only in areas with dense traffic.

Does Man Accumulate More Lead Than Before?

Although the concentration of airborne lead in urban areas no doubt has increased during the past decades, it is difficult to estimate whether man's total intake of lead has increased or not. This may sound like a paradox, but the explanation is that other sources of exposure may have decreased. These include contamination of drinking water from lead plumbing systems or of foodstuffs from lead arsenate insecticides, leaded kitchenware and earthenware, or improperly soldered conserve cans. Since no systematic studies were performed in the beginning of this century and since the analytic methods for lead some decades ago were unreliable, it probably is impossible to find an answer to this problem. It may be suggested that the total exposure has decreased in rural environments but increased somewhat in urban areas; but of course, this is speculation.

Furthermore, two other difficult problems are connected to this question. One is whether man accumulates lead with age or not, under present conditions, and the other is whether the body burden today in general is higher than before the introduction of alkyl leads in gasoline. According to the scanty information available from tissue analyses, there seems to occur a slight accumulation of lead up to the age of 50. Schroeder and Tipton[175] have estimated the mean body burden of "The Standard American" to be 121 mg. It is quite obvious that children do not contain such quantities. Accumulation probably starts at an early age and reaches its maximum at the age of 50. The reasons for the slight decline after this age are not known for certain. However, since most of the lead is bound to bones, the biologic importance of such an accumulation is not clear and probably is insignificant. It should be stressed that increased absorption of lead results in increased excretion as well.[103] This means that only part of the surplus lead becomes incorporated in the body, the rest being excreted. Exactly at what magnitude of absorption accumulation begins is not known.

Lack of reliable analytic data from the past makes it impossible to judge whether the body burden currently is higher than before. It has been claimed that the prevailing total body burden today is about 100 times the "natural" level.[155] Some studies on fossil bones have shown lead concentrations close to 1% or less of today's concentrations, but studies of this type are vulnerable to several errors, such as depletion of lead in acid soils.[99] Obviously, the accumulation problem cannot be solved for certain by this approach. In order to find out the effect of different conditions on the magnitude of lead absorption, it probably is more fruitful to compare different population groups with respect to their PbBs. To what extent that parameter reflects the body burden remains to be determined, but at least it is the best indicator available for the present exposure, all routes considered together.

TABLE 36–2.
Absorption of Lead Under Various Tentative Conditions of Lead in Air and Physical Activity

	ABSORPTION OF LEAD, μG/24 HOURS				
LOCATION	DRINKING WATER (AMOUNT ABSORBED)	FOOD (AMOUNT ABSORBED 10%)	INHALED AIR (AMOUNT ABSORBED 10%)	TOTAL	PERCENT FROM THE AIR
Rural	2	30 (10–50)	1	33 (13–53)	3 (8–2)
Suburban Pb in air 1 μg/cu m Respiration 15/24 hr	2	30 (10–50)	6	38 (18–58)	16 (33–10)
Suburban Pb in air 1 μg/cu m Respiration 23 cu m/24 hr	2	30 (10–50)	8	40 (20–50)	20 (40–16)
Urban Pb in air 2.0 μg/cu m Respiration 15 cu m/24 hr	2	30 (10–50	10	42 (22–62)	24 (45–16)
Urban Ph in air 2.0 μg/cu m Respiration 23 cu m/24 hr	2	30 (10–50)	17	49 (26–69)	35 (59–25)

Most available data show that populations residing in areas where pollution with airborne lead is intensive have higher blood lead concentrations than those living in low-pollution areas.[40, 61, 90, 108, 130, 150, 192] To what extent this applies to concentrations below 2 μg/cu m is at present subject to dispute. One reason for this is that unless dietary lead is kept constant (which is extremely difficult), it is impossible to observe any effect on PbB of air lead concentrations in that range, since even small variations in the former tend to mask those of the latter.

Potential Health Impact of Environmental Lead

Does environmental pollution with lead constitute a health hazard to the general population? This perhaps is the most controversial question today. Many reasons explain why there are more opinions than facts. First, pertinent epidemiologic studies are scant so there are no data available. Second, such studies would be extremely difficult, if at all possible, because of the abundance of confusing factors. Third, one should consider not only specific manifestations of lead toxicity but also quite nonspecific diseases. That would mean the entering of such vague areas as psychologic disturbances and premature aging, to mention two examples only. Fourth, one should be able to foresee the future effects of an ever-increasing world consumption of lead additives, at least for some decades ahead, which means extrapolating from something one does not even know. Finally, the enormous economic interests involved introduces the question of what costs are reasonable for the elimination or avoidance in the future of a given degree of health effect (in other words, could these monies be spent more effectively in another way from the point of view of health promotion?).

When one tries to evaluate the health impacts of environmental pollution with lead, one must at least consider the risk of (1) acute poisoning, (2) chronic poisoning from a lifetime's exposure, including nonspecific disease, (3) genetic damage, and (4) fetal damage.

Acute poisoning is common in slum district children, but the overwhelming cause for this is ingestion of flaking lead paint. No cases of acute poisoning from airborne lead in the general population are known; therefore, this aspect will not be treated further here.

When considering the possibility of chronic poisoning, one should also pay attention to atypical or nonspecific forms, such as increased load on adaptive functions, resulting in decreased resistance to chemical or microbiologic stresses, diffuse neuropsychiatric disorders, or accelerated aging. In short, it can be said that, with regard to the general population, more needs to be known about such effects arising from environmental contamination with lead and that experience from occupational exposure has not been systematically collected so as to provide guidelines.

The same can be said about genetic damage. There are some studies showing chromosome aberrations at exposure levels (in industry) considered to be toxic,[176] but the interpretation of those findings is not possible at present (see Chapter 51).

Fetal damage, on the other hand, is a potential hazard deserving close attention. First, it is conceivable that the fetus is more sensitive to toxic effects than are adults. Second, lead passes readily through the placenta.[6, 47, 120] There apparently is a relationship between the blood lead of the mother and that of the fetus, which is discussed by Messite and Bond in Chapter 54.

It is unfortunate that one must conclude that there is more speculation than there are facts about the hazards of present environmental pollution, not to mention the future trend. Everybody who tries to make a synthesis of the vast and conflicting literature should consider (1) that other sources of exposure (occupational, domestic, etc.) may confound the situation, (2) that the upper range of a distribution of PbBs in a population is more relevant than the average for enforcing standards, (3) that even the most vulnerable part of the population should be defined and protected, and (4) that possible adverse effects in the population must be well defined. The last requirement often is neglected; to fill this gap, experience from occupational health should be systematized and utilized.

CONCLUSION

If all potential hazards or toxic work exposures were properly controlled to minimize or eliminate exposure of employees, and if, for example, the high-volume exhaust system is functioning adequately, there would be less concern about lead absorption by employees on the job, and the setting up and maintenance of "lead screening" programs would be unnecessary. But factory conditions are rarely ideal; thus, exposure to, absorption of, and intoxication from lead and its compounds pose a never-ending problem in industry.

Common expressions "control" and "supervision" of the worker exposed to various toxic materials ought to give way to redirection to and emphasis on designing, installing, and maintaining clean working areas. If hygienic studies of workplaces reveal lead levels ranging from 40 μ to 60 μ/cu m or more during an eight-hour shift and engineering controls that are less than desirable, with dirty work areas and poor personal hygiene, then appropriate action is necessary.

First, respirable lead levels must be reduced. Other clean-up measures, including restrictions on eating, smoking, and drinking in the work areas should be enforced. To make all this workable, *decent* eating areas must be designated; kept clean with equipment to store food and liquids—the air must be of known cleanliness! Also, the employer must provide suitable wash-up facilities (including showers); separate lockers for each employee, one for street clothes and personal shoes; a separate locker for work clothing and work shoes. Work clothes should be provided by the employer along with appropriate laundry arrangements. No work clothes and shoes permitted to be taken home. Medical screening to include occupational and medical history, physical examination, and a venous blood sample for lead analysis should be instituted.

The 1978 criteria document on lead by the National Institute for Occupational Safety and Health (NIOSH) states that "unacceptable absorption of lead posing a risk of lead poisoning (in adults) is demonstrated at lead levels of 60 μg/100 ml of whole blood or greater. Excellent as they are, "criteria documents" are not substitutes for good clinical judgment. Furthermore, laboratories that perform blood and urine analyses for lead must demonstrate competence and provide the limits of variation and error of their results; this variation in current laboratory techniques can be large (±20 μg). If the blood level of lead is found to be elevated by a few micrograms above the established "upper level" and the worker is asymptomatic, it is advisable to take additional blood samples and use different laboratories. A worker should not be removed from the job without good clinical cause, and since laboratory results vary widely, this decision must not be based on a single test. Repeated blood lead determinations after one to two weeks will be useful for confirming absorption and following the course of possible toxicity.

Again, it must be emphasized that treatment with chelating agents should not be instituted in the absence of strong clinical findings. Chelating agents must be used with caution, for side effects such as kidney damage can occur. "Deleading" of a worker must not be undertaken while the worker remains exposed to lead. Sound occupational health practice is based on two major fundamentals, control of contaminants at the worksite by engineering and hygienic measures (including environmental monitoring) and good medical surveillance. Neither of these should be substituted as a replacement for the other!

REFERENCES

1. Aitio A, Riihimäki V, Vaino H (eds): *Biological Monitoring and Surveillance of Workers Exposed to Chemicals*. Washington, DC, Hemisphere Publishing, 1984.
2. American Conference of Governmental Industrial Hygienists: *Threshold Limit Values for Substances in Workroom Air*, 1986–87. Cincinnati, Oh, ACGIH, Ohio, 1986.
3. *American National Standard for Respiratory Protection* Z88.2-1969. New York, United States of America Standards Institute, Inc, 1969.
4. Aub JC, et al: *Lead Poisoning*. Baltimore, Williams & Wilkins Co, 1962.
5. Baker E Jr, Folland D, Taylor T, et al: Lead poisoning in children of lead workers—Home contamination with industrial dust. *New Engl J Med* 1977; 296(5):260–261.
6. Barltrop D: Transfer of lead to the human foetus, in Barltrop D, Burland WL (eds): *Mineral Metabolism in Pediatrics*. Philadelphia, FA Davis Co, 1969.
7. Barltrop D, Killala JP: Faecal excretion of lead by children. *Lancet* 1967; 2:1017.
8. Barn Arbete: *Arbetsmiljö*: 7, Föreningen för Arbetarskyyd, Stockholm, 1984, pp 14–25.
9. Barry PSI, Mossman DB: Lead concentrations in human tissues. *Br J Ind Med* 1970; 27:339.
10. Beattie AD, et al: Environmental lead pollution in an urban softwater area. *Br Med J* 1972; 2:491.
11. Berg BA, Zenz C: Environmental and clinical control of lead exposure in a non-ferrous foundry. *Am Ind Hyg Assoc J* 1967; 28:175.
12. Berk PD, et al: Hematologic and biochemical studies in a case of lead poisoning. *Am J Med* 1970; 48:137.
13. Berlin A, Del Castilho P, Smeets J: European Intercomparison Programmes: a) Lead in Air, b) Lead in Blood, c) ALA in Urine, d) ALAD in Blood. *Proceedings, International Symposium on the Environmental Health Aspects of Lead*, Amsterdam, Oct 2–6, 1972. Luxembourg, Commission of the European Communities, 1973.
14. Bessis MC, Jensen WN: Sideroblastic anemia, mitochondria and erythroblastic iron. *Br J Haematol* 1965; 11:49.
15. Bonsignore D, Calissano P, Cartasegna C: Un semplice metode per la determinazione della δ-amino-levulinico-deitratase nel sangue. Comportamento dell 'enzima nell'intossicazione saturnina. *Med Lav* 1965; 56:199.
16. Booker DV, et al: Uptake of radioactive lead following inhalation and injection. *Br J Radiol* 1969; 42:457.
17. Boyland E, et al: The induction of renal tumours by feeding lead acetate to rats. *Br J Cancer* 1962; 16:283.
18. Brandt AD, Reichenbach GS: Lead exposures at the government printing office. *J Ind Hyg Toxicol* 1943; 25:445.
19. Buczkowski M: Der Einfluss der Bleivergiftung auf die Bildung von fetalem Hämoglobin. *Arch Gewerbepathol Gewerbehyg* 1964; 20:537.
20. Butler EJ: Chronic neurological disease as a possible form of lead poisoning. *J Neurol Neurosurg Psychiatry* 1952; 15:119.
21. Cambell AMG, et al: Lead in relation to disseminated sclerosis. *Brain* 1950; 73:52.
22. Cantarow A, Trumper M: *Lead Poisoning*. Baltimore, Williams & Wilkins Co, 1944.
23. Catton MJ, et al: Subclinical neuropathy in lead workers. *Br Med J* 1970; 2:80.
24. Centers for Disease Control, US Dept of Health and Human Services: Lead poisoning in children of battery plant employees—North Carolina. *Epidemiologic Notes and Reports* Sept 30, 1977; vol 26, no 29.
25. Centers for Disease Control, US Dept of Health and Human Services: *Preventing Lead Poisoning in Young Children*. Atlanta, Ga, CDC, Public Health Service September, 1984.
26. Chisolm JJ Jr: Aminoaciduria as a manifestation of renal tubular injury in lead intoxication and a comparison with patterns of aminoaciduria seen in other diseases. *J Pediatr* 1962; 60:1.
27. Chisolm JJ Jr: Disturbances in the biosyntheses of heme in lead intoxication. *J Pediatr* 1964; 64:174.
28. Chisolm JJ Jr: Childhood lead intoxication. Diagnosis, management and prevention. *Med Times* 1970; 98:92.
29. Chisolm JJ Jr: Lead poisoning. *Sci Am* 1971; 224:15.
30. Chisolm JJ Jr: Treatment of lead poisoning. *Mod Treat* 1971; 8:593.
31. Chisolm JJ Jr, Harrison HE: Quantitative urinary coproporphyrin excretion and its relation to edathamil calcium disodium administration in children with acute lead intoxication. *J Clin Invest* 1956; 35:1131.
32. Chisolm JJ Jr, Harrison HE: The exposure of children to lead. *Pediatrics* 1956; 18:943.
33. Chisolm JJ Jr, Kaplan E: Lead poisoning in childhood—Comprehensive management and prevention. *J Pediatr* 1968; 73:942.
34. Chow TJ, Patterson CC: The occurrence and significance of lead isotopes in pelagic sediments. *Geochim Cosmochim Acta* 1962; 26:263.
35. Clarkson TW, Kench JE: Uptake of load by human erythrocytes in vitro. *Biochem J* 1958; 69:432.
36. Committee on Biologic Effects of Atmospheric Pollutants Division of Medical Sciences National Research Council: *Lead: Airborne Lead in Perspective*. Washington, DC, National Academy of Sciences, 1972.
37. Consolazio CF, et al: *The Trace Mineral Losses in Sweat*, Rep 284. Natick, Mass, US Army Medical Research and Nutrition Laboratory, 1964.
38. Cramér K, Dahlberg L: Incidence of hypertension among lead workers. A follow-up study based on regular control over 20 years. *Br J Ind Med* 1966; 23:101.
39. Cremer JE: Toxicology and biochemistry of alkyl lead compounds. *Occup Health Rev* 1965; 17:14.
40. Daines RH, et al: Air levels of lead inside and outside of homes. *Ind Med Surg* 1972; 41:26.
41. Davies TAL: The early detection of absorption of toxic materials (abridged). *Proc R Soc Med* 1968; 61:911.

42. Dingwall-Fordyce I, Lane RE: A follow-up study of lead workers. *Br J Ind Med* 1963; 20:313.
43. Djurić D, et al: Environmental contamination by lead from a mine and smelter. *Arch Environ Health* 1971; 23:275.
44. Dreesen WC, et al: The control of the lead hazard in the storage battery industry. *Public Health Service Bull* 1941; no 262.
45. Dresel EIB, Falk JE: Studies on the biosynthesis of blood pigments: 3. Haem and porphyrin formation from δ-aminolaevulinic acid and from porphobilinogen in haemolysed chicken erythrocytes. *Biochem J* 1956; 63:80.
46. Editorial, Subclinical lead poisoning. *Lancet* 1973; 1:87.
47. Egli VR, et al: Die Verbreitung der chronischen Bleivergiftung in Akkumulatoren-und Bleifarbenfabriken. *Schweiz Med Wochenschr* 1957; 87:1171.
48. Elkins HB: *The Chemistry of Industrial Toxicology*, ed 2. New York, John Wiley & Sons, 1959.
49. Emmerson BT: The clinical differentiation of lead gout from primary gout. *Arthritis Rheum* 1968; 11:623.
50. Feldman F, et al: Serum δ-aminolaevulinic acid in plumbism. *J Pediatr* 1969; 74:917.
51. Finklea JF, et al: Transplacental transfer of toxic metals. Working Paper for the Task Group of Metal Accumulation, Buenos Aires, 1972.
52. Flury F: Blei, Heffter-Heubner: Handbuch der experimentellen Pharmakologie. Berlin, Springer-Verlag, 1934, vol 3.
53. Freeman R: Reversible myocarditis due to chronic lead poisoning in childhood. *Arch Dis Child* 1965; 40:389.
54. Freeman R: Chronic lead poisoning in children. A review of 90 children diagnosed in Sydney, 1948–1967. 1. Epidemiological aspects. *Med J Aust* 1970; 1:640.
55. Fullerton PM: Chronic peripheral neuropathy produced by lead poisoning in guinea-pigs. *J Neuropathol Exp Neurol* 1966; 25:214.
56. Galle P, Morel-Maroger L: Les lésions rénales du saturnisme humain et expérimental. *Nephron* 1965; 2:273.
57. Gibson SLM, Mackenzie JC, Goldberg A: The diagnosis of industrial lead poisoning. *Br J Ind Med* 1968; 25:40.
58. Gilfillan SC: Lead poisoning and the fall of Rome. *J Occup Med* 1965; 7:53.
59. Gillet JA: An outbreak of lead poisoning (In the Canklow district of Rotherdam). *Public Health* 1955; 1:1118.
60. Goldberg A, et al: Studies on the biosyntheses of heme in vitro by avian erythrocytes. *Blood* 1956; 11:821.
61. Goldsmith JR, Hexter AC: Respiratory exposure to lead: Epidemiological and experimental dose-response relationships. *Science* 1967; 158:132.
62. Goyer RA: Lead toxicity: A problem in environmental pathology. *Am J Pathol* 1971; 64:167.
63. Goyer RA, Chisolm JJ: Lead, in Lee Douglas HK (ed): *Metallic Contaminants and Human Health*. New York: Academic Press, 1972.
64. Goyer RA, et al: Lead dosage and the role of the intranuclear inclusion body. *Arch Environ Health* 1970; 20:705.
65. Goyer RA, Mahaffey KR: Susceptibility to lead toxicity. *Environ Health Perspect* 1972; 1:73.
66. Grabecki J, Daduch T, Urbanowicz H: Die einfachen Bestimmungsmetoden der δ-Aminolävulinsäure im Harn. *Int Arch Gewerbepathol Gewerbehyg* 1967; 23:226.
67. Griggs RC: Lead Poisoning: Hematologic aspects. *Prog Hematol* 1964; 4:117.
68. Griggs RC, Harris JW: Erythrocyte survival and heme synthesis in lead poisoning. *Clin Res* 1958; 6:188.
69. Griggs RC, et al: Environmental factors in childhood lead poisoning. JAMA 1964; 187:703.
70. Gurd FRN, Wilcox PE: Complex formation between metallic cations and proteins, peptides, and amino acids. *Adv Protein Chem* 1956; 11:311.
71. Habibi K: Characterization of particulate lead in vehicle exhaust experimental techniques. *Environ Sci Tech* 1970; 4:239.
72. Haeger-Aronsen B: Studies on urinary excretion of δ-aminolaevulinic acid and other haem precursors in lead workers and lead-intoxicated rabbits. *Scand J Clin Lab Invest* 1960; 12:12.
73. Hänninen H: Personal communication.
74. Hamilton A, Hardy HL: *Industrial Toxicology*, ed 2. New York, Hoeber, 1949.
75. Hammer DI, et al: Trace metals in human hair as a simple epidemiologic monitor of environmental exposure. *Am J Epidemiol* 1971; 93:84.
76. Hammond PB: Lead poisoning. An old problem with a new dimension. *Esssays Toxicol* 1969; 1:115.
77. Hammond PB, Aronsen AL: Lead poisoning in cattle and horses in the vicinity of a smelter. *Ann NY Acad Sci* 1964; 111:595.
78. Harris RW, Elsea WR: Ceramic glaze as a source of lead poisoning. *JAMA* 1967; 202:644.
79. Harley JH: Discussion. Sources of lead in perennial ryegrass and radishes. *Environ Sci Tech* 1970; 4:225.
80. Hasan J, Hernberg S: Interactions of inorganic lead with human red blood cells. *Work Environ Health* 1966; 2:26.
81. Hellström J: *Om Yrkessjukdomar Och Industriell Hygien:* Hälsovännens Flygskrifter, Ne. 26, Hälsovännens Förlagsexpedition, Stockholm, 1896.
82. Henderson DA: A follow-up of cases of plumbism in children. *Australas Ann Med* 1954; 3:219.
83. Henderson DA, Inglis JA: The lead content of bone in chronic Bright's Disease. *Australas Ann Med* 1957; 6:145.
84. Hernberg S, Nikkanen J: Effect of lead on δ-aminolaevulinic acid dehydratase. A selective review. *Pracov Lék* 1972; 24:77.
85. Hernberg S, et al: δ-aminolevulinic acid dehydratase as a measure of lead exposure. *Arch Environ Health* 1970; 21:140.
86. Hernberg S: Lead, in Zenz C (ed): *Occupational Medicine: Principles and Practical Applications*. Chicago, Year Book Medical Publishers, 1975.
87. Hernberg S, Nurminen M, Hasan J: Non-random shortening of red cell survival times in men exposed to lead. *Environ Res* 1967; 1:247.
88. Hernberg S: Lead, in Aitio A, Riihimäki V, Vainio H (eds): *Biological Monitoring and Surveillance of Workers Exposed to Chemicals*. Washington, DC, Hemisphere, 1984, pp 19–27.
89. Hofreuter DH, et al: The public health significance of atmospheric lead. *Arch Environ Health* 1961; 3:568.
90. Holmqvist I: Blood lead determinations in control of exposed workers. *Arch Hig Rada Toksikol* 1969; 20(Suppl 4):43.
91. Horiuchi K: Lead in the environment and its effect on man in Japan. *Osaka City Med J* 1970; 16:1.
92. Hryhorczuk DO, et al: The fall of zinc protoporphyrin levels in workers treated for chronic lead intoxication. *J Occup Med* 1985; 27:816.
93. Hunter D: *The Disease of Occupations*, ed 4. Aulesbury, The English Universities Press, Ltd, by Hazell Watson and Viney Ltd, 1969.
94. Hursch JB, Suomela J: Absorption of ^{212}Pb from the gastrointestinal tract of man. *Acta Radiol* 1968; 7:108.
95. Hutchison HE, Stark JM: The anemia of lead poisoning. *J Clin Pathol* 1961; 14:548.
96. International Commission on radiological protection: *Recommendations of the International Commission on Radiological Protection*.

Report on Committee II on Permissible Dose for Internal Radiation, ICRP Publ 2. London, Pergamon Press, 1959.

97. Jacobziner H: Lead poisoning in childhood: Epidemiology, manifestations and prevention. *Clin Pediatr (Phila)* 1966; 5:277.
98. Jandl JH, et al: Transfer of iron from serum iron-binding protein to human reticulocytes. *J Clin Invest* 1959; 38:161.
99. Jawrowski Z: Stable lead in fossil ice and bones. *Nature* 1968; 217:152.
100. Jensen WN, Moreno GD, Bessis MC: An electron microscopic description of basophilic stippling in red cells. *Blood* 1965; 25:933.
101. Kassenaar A, Morell H, London IM: Incorporation of glycine into globin and the synthesis of heme in vitro in duck erythrocytes. *J Biol Chem* 1957; 229:424.
102. Keenan RG, et al: "USPHS" method for determining lead in air and in biological materials. *Am Ind Hyg Assoc J* 1963; 24:481.
103. Kehoe RA: The Harben Lectures, 1960. The metabolism of lead in man in health and disease. London, McCorquodale and Company, Ltd, 1961.
104. Kehoe RA: Occupational lead poisoning. 2. Chemical signs of the absorption of lead. *J Occup Med* 1972; 14:390.
105. Keppler JF, et al: Interlaboratory evaluation of the reliability of blood lead analysis. *Am Ind Hyg Assoc J* 1970; 31:412.
106. Klein M, et al: Earthenware containers as a source of fatal lead poisoning. Case study and public health consideration. *N Engl J Med* 1970; 283:283.
107. Klotz IM: Thermodynamic and molecular properties of some metal protein complexes, in McElroy SD, Glass B (eds): *A Symposium on the Mechanism of Enzyme Action*. Baltimore, Johns Hopkins Press, 1954.
108. Knelson JH, et al: Kinetics of respiratory lead uptake in humans, in *Proceedings of International Symposium on the Environmental Health Aspects of Lead,* Amsterdam, Oct 2–6, 1972. Luxembourg, Commission of the European Communities, 1973.
109. Kreimer-Birnbaum M, Grinstein M: Porphyrin biosynthesis. III. Porphyrin metabolism in experimental lead poisoning. *Biochem Biophys Acta* 1965; 111:110.
110. Kunhenn H: In Deutsche Gesellschaft für Arbeitsschutz: Blei—Neuere Erkenntnisse aus arbeitsmedizinischer und arbeitsschutztechnischer Sicht. *Arbeitsschutz und Arbeitsmedizin* (suppl) 1967; 2:103.
111. Laabe RF: History and Background of Protoporphyrin Testing. *Clin Chem* 1977; 23(2):256–259.
112. Lagerwerff JV, Specht AW: Contamination of roadside soil and vegetation with cadmium, nickel, lead and zinc. *Environ Sci Tech* 1970; 4:583.
113. Lamola AA, Yamane T: Zinc protoporphyrin, in the patients with lead intoxication and iron deficiency anemia. *Science* 1974; 186:936.
114. Lamola A, Joselow M, Yamane T: Zinc protoporphyrin (ZPP), a simple sensitive, fluorometric screening test for lead poisoning. *Clin Chem* 1975; 21:93.
115. Landing B, Nakai H: Histochemical properties of renal lead-inclusions and their demonstration in urinary sediment. *Am J Clin Pathol* 1959; 32:499.
116. Lane RE: The care of the lead worker. *Br J Ind Med* 1949; 6:125.
117. Lane RE: The clinical aspects of poisoning by inorganic lead compounds. *Ann Occup Hyg* 1965; 8:31.
118. Lane RE, et al: Diagnosis of inorganic lead poisoning: A statement. *Br Med J* 1968; 4:501.
119. Lauwerys R: Le diagnostic biologique d'exposition excessive au plomb. *Louvain Méd* 1972; 91:19.
120. Lauwerys R, Buchet JP, Roels HA, et al: Placental transfer of lead, mercury, cadmium and carbon monoxide in women. 1. Comparison of the frequency distributions of the biological indices in maternal and umbilical cord blood. *Environ Res* 1978; 15:278.
121. Lauwerys RR: *Industrial Chemical Exposure: Guidelines for Biological Monitoring*. Davis, Cal, Biomedical Publications, 1983.
122. Lawther PJ, et al: More observations of airborne lead, in *Proceedings of International Symposium on the Environmental Health Aspects of Lead,* Amsterdam, Oct 2–6, 1972. Luxembourg, Commission of the European Communities, 1973.
123. Lee RE, Patterson RK, Wagman J: Particle-size distribution of metal components in urban air. *Environ Sci Tech* 1968; 2:288.
124. Lehnert G, et al: Usuelle Bleibelastung durch Nahrungsmittel und Getränke. *Arch Hyg* 1969; 153:403.
125. Leikin S, Eng G: Erythrokinetic studies of the anemia of lead poisoning. *Pediatrics* 1963; 31:996.
126. Lerner S, Gartside P, Bernard R: Free erythrocyte protoporphyrin, zinc protoporphyrin and blood lead in newly re-exposed smelter workers: A prospective study. *Am Ind Hyg Assoc J* 1982; 43:516–519.
127. Levin L: Too young to work. *World Health* 1984; Jan–Feb.
128. Lichtman HC, Feldman F: In vitro pyrrole and porphyrin synthesis in lead poisoning and iron deficiency. *J Clin Invest* 1963; 42:830.
129. Lilis R, et al: Nephropathy in chronic lead poisoning. *Br J Ind Med* 1968; 25:196.
130. Ludwig JH, et al: Survey of lead in the atmosphere of three urban communities: A summary. *Am Ind Hyg Assoc J* 1965; 26:270.
131. Malcolm D: The effect of lead on the kidney. *Trans Soc Occup Med* 1970; 20:50.
132. Martell AE, Calvin M: The chemistry of the metal chelate compounds. New York, Prentice-Hall, 1952.
133. Martinez EG, Junco Muñoz PR, Ballesteros MG, et al: Toxic effects of lead impurities found in aluminum factories. *Am J Ind Med* 1981; 2:161–165.
134. Marvert HS, Schmid R: The porphyrias, in Stanbury JB, et al (eds): *The Metabolic Basis of Inherited Disease*. New York, McGraw-Hill Book Co, 1972.
135. Mauzerall D, Granick S: The occurrence and determination of δ-aminolevulinic acid and porphobilinogen in urine. *J Biol Chem* 1956; 219:435.
136. McCabe LJ: Metal levels found in distribution samples. Presented at American Water Works Association Seminar on Corrosion by Soft Water, Washington, DC, June 21, 1970.
137. McCallum RI, Sanderson JT, Richards AE: The lead hazard in shipbreaking: The prevalence of anemia in burners. *Ann Occup Hyg* 1968; 11:101.
138. Miano S: The problem of lead poisoning in children. *J Environ Health* 1964; 27:510.
139. Milev N, Sattler EL, Menden E: Aufnahme und Einlagerung von Blei im Körper unter verschidenen Ernährungsbedingungen. *Med Ernähr* 1970; 11:29.
140. Moncrieff AA, et al: Lead poisoning in children. *Arch Dis Child* 1964; 39:1.
141. *Moonshine: The Rotgut Racket*. New York, Licensed Beverage Industry, Inc, 1969.
142. Moore JE: Community aspects of childhood lead poisoning. *Am J Public Health* 1970; 60:1430.
143. Morgan JM, Hartley MW, Miller RE: Nephropathy in chronic lead poisoning. *Arch Intern Med* 1966; 118:17.
144. Muir DCF, Davies CN: The deposition of 0.5 μ diameter aerosols in the lungs of man. *Ann Occup Hyg* 1967; 10:161.
145. Murozumi M, Chow TJ, Patterson C: Chemical concentrations of pollutant lead aerosols, terrestrial dusts, and sea salts in Greenland and Antarctic snow strata. *Geochem Cosmochim Acta* 1969; 33:1247.

146. Murthy GK, Rhea US: Cadmium, copper, iron, lead, manganese and zinc in evaporated milk, infant milk products and human milk. *J Dairy Sci* 1971; 54:1001.
147. Myerson RM, Eisenhauer JH: Atrioventricular conduction defects in lead poisoning. *Am J Cardiol* 1963; 11:409.
148. Nandi DL, Baker-Cohen KF, Shemin D: δ-aminolevulinic acid dehydratase of rhodopseudomonas spheroides. I. Isolation and properties. *J Biol Chem* 1968; 243:1224.
149. Nikkanen J, Hernberg S, Tola S: Modifications of the δ-aminolevulinic acid dehydratase test and their significance for assessing different intensities of lead exposure. *Work Environ Health* 1972; 9:46.
150. Nordman CH, et al: Blood lead levels and erythrocyte δ-aminolevulinic acid dehydratase activity in people living around a secondary lead smelter. *Work Environ Health* 1973; 10:19.
151. Nozaki K: Method for studies on inhaled particles in human respiratory system and retention of lead fume. *Ind Health* 1966; 4:118.
152. Nye LJJ: An investigation of the extraordinary incidence of chronic nephritis in young people in Queensland. *Med J Aust* 1929; 2:145.
153. Palmisalo PA, Sneed RC, Cassady G: Untaxed whiskey and fetal lead exposure. *J Pediatr* 1969; 75:869.
154. Passow H, Rothstein A, Clarkson TW: The general pharmacology of the heavy metals. *Pharmacol Rev* 1961; 13:185.
155. Patterson CC: Contaminated and natural lead environments of man. *Arch Environ Health* 1965; 11:344.
156. Pegues WL: Lead fume from welding on galvanized and zinc-silicate coated steels. *Am Ind Hyg Assoc J* 1960; 21:252.
157. Perlstein MA, Attala R: Neurologic sequelae of plumbism in children. *Clin Pediatr* 1966; 5:292.
158. Piomelli S: Free erythrocyte porphyrins in the detection of undue absorption of Pb and of Fe deficiency. *Clin Chem* 1977; 2:264–269.
159. Piotrovski J: *The Application of Metabolic and Excretion Criteria Problems of Medical Toxicology*. Bethesda, Md, US Dept of Health, Education and Welfare, Public Health Service, National Institutes of Health, 1971.
160. Popoff N, Weinberg S, Feigin I: Pathologic observations in lead encephalopathy. (With special reference to the vascular changes). *Neurology (Minneapolis)* 1963; 13:101.
161. *Proceedings of a Working Group on the Hazards to Health of Persistent Substances in Water*. Convened by the Regional Office for Europe of the World Health Organization, Helsinki, 1972. Working paper on lead prepared by Hernberg S, Nordman CH.
162. Robinson E, Ludwig FL: Particle size distribution of urban lead aerosols. *J Air Pollut Control Assoc* 1967; 17:664.
163. Roels HA, Balis-Jacques MN, Buchet JP, et al: The influence of sex and chelation therapy on erythrocyte protoporphyrin and urinary δ-aminolevulinic acid in lead exposed workers. *J Occup Med* 1979; 21:527.
164. Roels HA, Lauwerys R, Buchet JP, et al: Response of free erythrocyte porphyrin and urinary δ-aminolevulinic acid in men and women moderately exposed to lead. *Int Arch Arbeitsmed* 1975; 34:97.
165. Rothstein A: Ion Exchange Properties of Cells and Tissues, AEP Rep UR-404. Rochester, NY, University of Rochester, 1955.
166. Rothstein A, Weed RJ: *The Functional Significance of Sulfhydryl Groups in the Cell Membrane*, AEP Rep UR-633. Rochester, NY, University of Rochester, 1963.
167. Rubino GF, et al: Erythrocyte copper and porphyrins in lead poisoning. *Br J Haematol* 1958; 4:103.
168. Rubino GF, Prato V, Fiorina L: L'Anemia da piombo: Sua natura e patogenesi. *Folia Med (Napoli)* 1959; 42:1.
169. Rühling Å, Tyler G: An ecological approach to the lead problem. *Nature* 1968; 121:321.
170. Sanders LW: Tetraethyllead intoxication. *Arch Environ Health* 1964;
171. Sandstead HH, et al: Lead intoxication and the thyroid. *Arch Intern Med* 1969; 123:623.
172. Schepers GWH: Tetraethyllead and tetramethyllead. *Arch Environ Health* 1964; 8:277.
173. Schlaepfer WW: Experimental lead neuropathy: A disease of the supporting cells in the peripheral nervous system. *J Neuropathol Exp Neurol* 1969; 28:401.
174. Schroeder HA, et al: Abnormal trace metals in man: Lead. *J Chronic Dis* 1961; 14:408.
175. Schroeder HA, Tipton IH: The human body burden of lead. *Arch Environ Health* 1968; 17:965.
176. Schwanitz G, Lehnert G, Gebhart E: Chromosomenschäden bei beruflicher Bleibelastung. *Dtsch Med Wochenschr* 1970; 95:1636.
177. Schwartz S: Studies of porphyrin metabolism. The effect of metals on coproporphyrin excretion, in Tannebaum A (ed): *Toxicology of Uranium*. New York, McGraw-Hill Book Co, 1951.
178. Selander S, Cramér K: Interrelationships between lead in blood, lead in urine, and ALA in urine during lead work. *Br J Ind Med* 1970; 27:28.
179. Seppäläinen AM, Hernberg S: Sensitive technique for detecting subclinical lead neuropathy. *Br J Ind Med* 1972; 29:443.
180. Sessa T, Ferrari E, Colucci d'Amato C: Velocita di conduzione nervosa nei saturnini. *Folia Med (Napoli)* 1965; 48:658.
181. Silver W, Rodriquez-Torres R: Electrocardiographic studies in children with lead poisoning. *Pediatrics* 1968; 41:1124.
182. Simpson JA, Seaten DA, Adams JF: Response to treatment with chelating agents of anemia, chronic encephalopathy, and myelopathy due to lead poisoning, *J Neurol Neurosurg Psychiatry* 1964; 27:536.
183. Six KM, Goyer RA: Experimental enhancement of lead toxicity by low dietary calcium. *J Lab Clin Med* 1970; 76:933.
184. Six KM, Goyer RA: The influence of iron deficiency on tissue content and toxicity of ingested lead in the rat. *J Lab Clin Med* 1972; 79:128.
185. Smith HD, et al: Sequela of pica with and without lead poisoning. *Am J Dis Child* 1963; 105:609.
186. Staverman HJ, Zielhuis RL: Industriële loodvergiftiging in Nederland. Een vergelijkend onderzoek over 1953 t/m 1964. *Tÿdschr Soc Geneeskd* 1967; 45:2.
187. Strehlow CD, Kneip TJ: The distribution of lead and zinc in the human skeleton, AIHA refresher course. *Am Ind Hyg Assoc J* 1968; 29:114.
188. Tange JD, Hayward NJ, Bremner DA: Renal lesions in experimental plumbism and their clinical implications. *Australas Ann Med* 1965; 14:49.
189. Task Group on Lung Dynamics: Deposition and retention models for internal dosimetry of the human respiratory tract. *Health Phys* 1966; 12:173.
190. Task Group on Metal Accumulation: Accumulation of toxic metals in total body and critical organs with special reference to absorption, excretion and biological half-times. *Arch Environ Health* 1973; 27:53.
191. Ter Haar GL: Air as a source of lead in edible crops. *Environ Sci Tech* 1970; 4:226.
192. Thomas HV, et al: Blood lead of persons living near freeways. *Arch Environ Health* 1967; 15:695.
193. Tola S: The effect of blood lead concentration, age, sex and time of exposure upon erythrocyte δ-aminolevulinic acid dehydratase activity. *Work Environ Health* 1973; 10:26.
194. Tola S, et al: Parameters indicative of absorption and biological effect in new lead exposure: A prospective study. *Br J Ind Med* 1973; 30:134.
195. Tola S, Hernberg S, Nikkanen J: *Detection of Lead Exposure in*

Shipyards, in Safety and Health in Ship Building and Ship Repairing, Occupational Safety and Health Series, 27. Geneva, International Labour Office, 1972.

196. Tola S, et al: Occupational lead exposure in Finland: I. Electric storage battery manufacturing and repair. *Work Environ Health* 1971; 8:81.
197. Tomokuni K, Osaka I, Ogata M: Erythrocyte protoporphyrin test for occupational lead exposure. *Arch Environ Health* 1975; 30:588.
198. Tsuchija K: Lead, in Friberg L, Nordberg GF, Vouk VB (eds): *Handbook of Toxicology of Metals*, Amsterdam, Elsevier, 1979.
199. US Dept of Health, Education and Welfare, Public Health Service, Division of Air Pollution: *Survey of Lead in the Atmosphere of Three Urban Communities*, PHS Publ 999-AP-12. Cincinnati, Oh, Public Health Service, 1965.
200. US Dept of Health, Education and Welfare: Criteria for a Recommended Standard . . . Occupational Exposure to Inorganic Lead. Public Health Service, Health Services and Mental Health Administration, National Institute for Occupational Safety and Health, 1978.
201. US Dept of the Interior: *Minerals Yearbook for 1985*. Washington, DC, Government Printing Office, 1985, vol 1.
202. Vostal J: Mechanisms of lead excretion. *Biochem Pharmacol* 1963; 2:207.
203. Waldron HA: The anemia of lead poisoning: A review. *Br J Ind Med* 1966; 23:83.
204. World Health Organization: *Environmental health criteria 3, Lead*. Geneva, WHO, 1977.
205. World Health Organization: *Report of a study group: Recommended Health-Based Limits in Occupational Exposure to Heavy Metals*, Tech Rep 647. Geneva, WHO, 1980.
206. Zielhuis RL: De industriële loodintoxicatie in Nederland. Beschouwingen en onderzoekingen, Verhandeling van het Nederlands Instituut voor praeventieve geneeskunde XLVI, 1959.
207. Zielhuis RL: Interrelationship of biochemical responses to the absorption of inorganic lead. *Arch Environ Health* 1971; 23:299.
208. Zielhuis RL: Lead, in Parmeggiani L (ed): *Encyclopedia of Occupational Health and Safety*, ed 3. Geneva, International Labor Office, 1983, pp 1200–1205.
209. Zollinger HU: Durch chronische Bleivergiftung erzeuge Nierenadenome und -carcinome bei Ratten und ihre Beziehungen zu den entsprechenden Neubildungen des Menschen. *Virchows Arch* 1953; 323:694.

37

Manganese and Its Compounds

Shiro Tanaka, M.D., M.S.

NATURAL OCCURRENCES AND CHEMICAL PROPERTIES

Manganese is widely distributed in the earth's crust and is calculated to be the 12th most abundant element. Deposits of manganese ore of high concentration are found in African countries (Gabon, Ghana, Morocco, The Republic of South Africa, and Zaire), Australia, Brazil, China, India, and the U.S.S.R. Deposits of lower-grade ore are found in various parts of the United States.[46] It is known that there are vast deposits of manganese oxide nodules on the ocean floor which may be commercially exploited in the future.[46]

The chemical symbol for manganese is Mn; it has an atomic weight of 54.94, the specific gravity is 7.2, and the melting point is 1,260° C.[57] In its chemical behavior, manganese is similar to iron and often is associated with iron in its natural occurrence. Manganese can have valences of 1, 2, 3, 4, 6, or 7 in its compounds and is divalent in the most stable salts. Manganese does not occur naturally as the metal. Pyrolusite, a mineral form of manganese dioxide (MnO_2), is one of the more common and commercially important ores.[46] Other manganese ores include braunite (Mn_2O_3 + $xMnSiO_3$), hausmannite (Mn_3O_4), manganite ($MnO[OH]$), and psilomelane (MnO_2 + x[MnO, BaO, K_2O, H_2O]).[54]

INDUSTRIAL USES AND EXPOSURES

Manganese ores are mined by both open-pit and underground mining, and methods vary from primitive to modern. In particular, the job of drilling with pneumatic drills has been reported to be one of the most significant sources of manganese exposure and poisoning.[48, 50, 54, 63] The ores are washed, separated from rocks, crushed, and, in some cases, roasted, sintered, and nodulized before shipment.[46] After shipment, manganese ores are crushed to a smaller size, ground, and bagged for further industrial uses. This grinding process has also been responsible for a great number of caes of manganese poisoning.[10, 17, 18, 24]

Manganese is essential to the production of steel and is used for the production of important alloys with copper, aluminum, magnesium, and cast iron. More than 80% of manganese used in the United States is consumed in the production of alloys, steel and iron.[31] Manganese serves in steelmaking to nullify the undesirable effects of sulfur (such as reduced ductility), as a deoxidizer and alloying agent to provide strength and hardness.[46] Standard high-carbon ferromanganese contains 78%–82% manganese and silicon-manganese contains 65%–68% manganese. Poisoning has occurred among workers making such alloys,[30, 56] among workers crushing and screening ferromanganese,[56] and among workers performing arc welding or arc burning of steel that contained as low as 11%–14% manganese.[58, 61] A crane operator who worked over the furnaces which melted steel and manganese ore was also affected.[51]

In the chemical industries, manganese dioxide ores are used in the production of hydroquinone, potassium permanganate, and manganese sulfate. Manganese sulfate is added to fertilizers to provide this trace element to soil. Manganous oxide (MnO) is added to animal and poultry feed.[46] The common dry cell battery uses manganese dioxide as a depolarizer. Cases of manganese poisoning have also been reported from the process of battery manufacturing.[19]

Chemicals containing manganese are used in the ceramics industries to color glass, face brick, and to make other ceramic products. Welding rods and fluxes contain manganese. In other applications, manganese dioxides and other compounds are used in the manufacture of dyes, paint, varnish, dryers, fungicides, and pharmaceuticals.[46] Manganese tricarbonyl compounds, which will be discussed later in this chapter, are used as smoke-inhibitor additives to fuel oil and as antiknock additives to gasoline.

In 1984, a total of 1,076,631 short tons of manganese were consumed in the United States; 744,832 short tons (69%) were used for making manganese alloys and metals, and the rest for the manufacture of pig iron and steel (14%) and dry cells, chemicals, and other items (17%).[31] Estimates of number of U.S. workers potentially exposed to manganese and its compounds range from 68,000 to 185,000.[45]

BIOLOGIC EFFECTS

Several extensive reviews on the biologic effects of manganese have appeared in the literature during the past several decades.[13, 22, 46, 57, 59, 62]

Physiologic Role

Manganese is considered an essential mineral for human beings and animals. It has been shown to be necessary for normal bone formation and for synthesis of chondroitin sulfate. Although manganese deficiency has been reported to cause skeletal deformities, sterility, and neonatal deaths in various animal species, similar effects of manganese deficiency have not been found in man.[46] Cotzias and his co-workers reported that normal manganese concentration is required for optimal melanocyte function and for the metabolism of catecholamines in the brain.[14]

The daily intake of manganese in human diets varies considerably with the nature of the diet, but averages from 3 to 7 mg. It has been estimated that a normal 70-kg man has a total of 12–20 mg of manganese in his body. Manganese is widely distributed throughout the body and tends to concentrate in the mitochondria.[38]

In animal feeding studies,[46] rats tolerated high concentrations of dietary manganese, their growth rate being unaffected by concentrations as high as 2,000 ppm. Dietary supplements of 820 ppm had no detectable effect on the growth or appetite of calves, but at 2,460 ppm they showed decreased food intake and decreased body weight gains.

Route of Entry and Absorption

Inhalation is the major route of entry in occupational manganese poisoning, although excessive gastrointestinal absorption may also occur in settings of poor industrial or personal hygiene.[17] Tricarbonyls of manganese can be absorbed through the skin.[4] Intoxication from contaminated drinking water has also been documented.[32]

In a study by Greenberg, et al.[25] only about 4% of orally administered radioactive manganese (as $MnCl_2$) was absorbed by rats. Injected radioactive manganese (as $MnCl_2$) disappeared rapidly from the bloodstream, and 10%–30% of the dose was accumulated in the liver.[25]

Manganese is excreted almost totally via the gastrointestinal tract, being secreted through the intestinal wall and eliminated in the bile. Very little manganese is excreted in the urine.[25] Seventy percent of injected radioactive manganese is eliminated via a moderately slow pathway with an average half-life of 39 days, while the rest takes a more rapid pathway with a half-life of four days.[36]

The usual range of manganese concentrations in biologic samples of nonexposed adults is 0.8–1.6 μg/100 ml for blood,[8] and 0.11–2.67 μg/L (geometric mean: 0.56 μg/L) for urine.[60] These values are about ten times as low as the values reported in previous years.[11] This downward shift is probably due to the improved sensitivity of analytical methodology available in recent years, rather than to decreased intake of manganese.

INDUSTRIAL MANGANESE POISONING

The industrial toxicity of manganese may be grouped into two major categories: a chronic disorder of the central nervous system resembling parkinsonism, and a form of lobar pneumonia called manganic pneumonia. It is customary that the term *manganism* or *manganese poisoning* refers to the chronic neurologic disorder caused by manganese.

Manganism

The first report of manganism was made in 1837 by Couper,[17] who had observed the development of neurologic abnormalities among men employed in grinding the black oxide of manganese. Since that time, numerous cases have been reported from many countries, with 353 reported cases in the literature at the time of Fairhall and Neal's review in 1940.[22] Cases continue to be reported in the more recent literature.[12, 19, 26, 30, 51, 56, 62] It is suspected that many more cases occur but go unrecognized, undiagnosed, or unreported.[58]

Signs and Symptoms

The symptoms of manganism resemble Parkinson's disease and are accompanied by lesions in the extrapyramidal tract of the brain. Marked morphologic changes and degeneration of neurons occur in the gray matter of the midbrain and in the basal ganglia in affected individuals.[5, 9] It is believed that manganese injures the dopaminergic components of the extrapyramidal system in a manner paralleling parkinsonism.[41]

The onset of the disease is insidious and appears after months or years of exposure to manganese. In one reported case series, latency ranged from 1 month to ten years.[50] The median was one to two years (24%); six patients had a latency of one to three months, and two patients more than ten years. There are reports that patients developed major symptoms several years after exposure to manganese had ceased.[12, 52]

The disease is roughly divided into two stages. The first, or early, stage is characterized by subjective symptoms reflecting emotional instability and irritability. The second stage is characterized by the manifestation of neurologic signs. (Some investigators divide the disease into prodromal, intermediate, and established phases.[50]) Lists of clinical features have been provided by previous investigators,[10, 12, 18, 24, 39, 48, 50, 54] and are summarized in Table 37–1.

In the early stage, the patient develops or complains of apathy, asthenia, anorexia, lassitude, insomnia, or somnolence, and slowed or clumsy movements. He may show a form of aggressiveness and mental excitement, termed manganese psychosis. At this stage, many patients complain of decreased libido or sexual impotence,[24, 50] which, in some instances, may be preceded by a short period of increased libido.[50] Other reported symptoms are muscle pains and cramps, lumbar pain, headache, giddiness, clumsiness in movements, difficulty in speech and gait, increased salivation, profuse sweating, and paresthesias. The duration of this stage is variable and difficult to determine, and it appears to depend on the degree of exposure. However, it is estimated to last from one to several months. Thereafter, the condition slowly progresses to the next stage unless the worker is removed from exposure.

The second, or advanced, stage is characterized by various neurologic abnormalities similar to those of parkinsonism. Difficulties in coordinating movements, which had been felt only by the

TABLE 37–1.

Reported Prevalence Rates of Symptoms and Signs Among Manganism Patients*

SYMPTOMS AND SIGNS	PERCENTAGE†
Symptoms:	
1. General malaise, weakness or fatigability	77–100
2. Clumsy movement, including difficulty in walking	77–100
3. Somnolence, and/or insomnia	46–100
4. Speech disturbance, including slurred speech	33–100
5. Tremor	62–91
6. Muscle aches, cramps, weakness, or stiffness	50–82
7. Loss of libido or impotence	27–83
8. Headache	38–80
9. Loss of memory or forgetfulness	31–75
10. Irritability, excitability, or nervousness	40–69
11. Nightmare and/or hallucination	25–40
12. Excessive salivation and/or sweating	5–87
13. Other symptoms reported: Anorexia, dysphagia, dysuria, lumbago, vertigo, paresthesia	
Signs:	
1. Gait disturbance including propulsion, retropulsion, difficulty in turning	67–100
2. Speech disorder, including slurring	62–83
3. Muscle rigidity (all types)	8–87
Expressionless face	62–83
Monotonous speech	20–47
Micrographia	8–67
Cogwheel resistance	8–23
4. Adiadochokinesis	30–80
5. Sudden laughter or weeping	46–67
6. Tremor of extremities and/or body	38–67
7. Reduced muscle strength	31–55
8. Other signs reported: Convergence disorder, diplopia, nystagmus, torticollis, hyperreflexia, sensory defects.	

*Data from Cook et al.,[12] Edsall et al.,[18] Flinn et al.,[24] Mena et al.,[39] Radier,[50] and Schuler et al.[54]

†Percentage figures are listed only to provide readers with a general idea about relative frequency of these symptoms and signs, since there is considerable variation in reported patient populations, definition of abnormal conditions, and method of medical evaluation.

patient, now may become manifest to observers. This may be the first time that the patient is brought to a physician's attention, and particular questions may have to be asked to elicit symptoms of the previous stage. The patient's speech becomes monotonous with economized tongue and lip movement to produce slurring. The facial movements are diminished, presenting a "mask-like" face. The gait is troubled by propulsion; on walking down a hill, the patient must go faster and faster because he cannot control the pace of his walk. Walking backward or turning quickly on the level becomes almost impossible. When pushed from the front, a patient loses balance and falls backward.

As the disease advances, the gait becomes slower, more labored, and spastic. A peculiar, high-stepped gait termed *Hehnetritt* (cock-walk) may be observed.[18] On passive flexion of the extremities, muscle rigidity may give a cogwheel resistance to the examiner's hand. Impulsive laughter, or spasmodic weeping, which occurs without reason, is seen frequently. Standing up from a chair without using the hands or lifting a weight from the floor becomes very difficult.

Handwriting becomes shaky, and micrographia is noted. Fine tremors of the fingers and extended tongue, as well as gross rhythmic movements of arms and legs, are observed. Adiadochokinesis is evident in many cases. This is thought to be due to poor muscle control rather than to loss of proprioceptive sense.[24] When the pyramidal tracts are affected, pyramidal signs such as the Babinski sign or increased tendon reflexes may be elicited with ankle and patellar clonus.

Other less frequently reported symptoms and signs are dysphagia, nystagmus, convergence disturbance, and torticollis. Schuler et al.[54] reported changes in superficial and deep sensation in four of their 15 cases. Although they also reported three cases of hearing impairment, industrial noise as the cause of that finding was not ruled out. Visual sense is in general well preserved. However, two of Schuler's cases complained of diplopia. Dysuria and urinary incontinence have also been reported.[58] Mental capacity may be diminished in some cases.[12]

It is noted here that some investigators object to grouping manganism together with parkinsonism. For example, Barbeau et al. maintain that manganism is predominantly a dystonic disease.[7] (Dystonia is defined as a "postural instability of complementary muscle groups.") Pathologically, the pallidum, putamen, and caudate nucleus are affected in manganism,[5, 9] while the substantia nigra, locus ceruleus, and dorsal nucleus of the vagus are damaged in parkinsonism.[2] Klawans et al.[33] note on the basis of their review that the tremor in manganism is frequently an intention tremor, while in parkinsonism it is the classical resting tremor. For the purpose of screening, however, these distinctions are not considered critical.

Diagnosis of Manganism

Careful review of the occupational history is most important. Diagnostic problems arise when the physician does not suspect an occupational origin for a worker's complaints or is not familiar with the toxic effects of manganese. Many worker-patients may not necessarily be aware of the toxicity of materials with which they are working, or to which they are occupationally exposed. Sometimes the word *manganese* is confused with the word *magnesium*.[58] Early diagnosis is often made difficult due to the insidious onset and progress of the disease. Because of manganese-induced apathy, the patient may not voluntarily seek medical help. Symptoms may be mistaken by a worker's family, fellow workers, or even by the medical staff as unrelated to his job. If an occupational cause is suspected, the physician should not hesitate to obtain exact information by contacting the patient's employer or the appropriate federal or state occupational safety and health agency.

If a worker known to be exposed to manganese is found to have symptoms and signs similar to those described in the previous sections, there is a strong suspicion of manganism, and the worker should be more closely examined, preferably by a neurologist.

At a workplace with known manganese exposures, a periodic

screening program should be conducted to detect the earliest indication of overexposure, including blood and/or urine analysis for manganese and review of symptoms and signs (see Prevention section).

The usefulness of manganese analysis in blood or urine for diagnosis of manganism has been controversial.[19, 30] The main reason for this controversy may be that there has been no definitive relationship established between biologic manganese levels and the severity of clinical signs and symptoms.[12, 15, 58] This uncertainty is probably the result of the very chronic and insidious nature of the poisoning, a fairly rapid turnover of body manganese, the cross-sectional nature of the past investigations, and the rather insensitive analytic methodology of the past. If a biologic monitoring program is established with a preemployment level as a baseline, and worker's levels of manganese are followed with concurrent medical and environmental monitoring, a better correlation may be elicited.

In view of the recently revealed lower levels of manganese among nonexposed population (see Route of Entry and Absorption), levels above the range of 5–10 μg/100 ml for blood and above 5–10 μg/L for urine may be indicative of increased manganese exposure and absorption. Such determinations are made by means of flameless atomic absorption spectrophotometry.[8, 60] Elevated levels may not by themselves necessarily establish a diagnosis of manganism, but they should call for a closer examination of the worker's health status and the exposure conditions. A good correlation of atmospheric and urinary manganese levels in exposed workers was observed on a group basis.[58]

Differential diagnosis of manganism should rule out parkinsonism of nonoccupational origin (absence of occupational exposure and higher age—idiopathic parkinsonism is very rare in persons under age 45), Wilson's disease (presence of hepatic involvement and Kayser-Fleischer ring), multiple sclerosis (presence of visual and other sensory disturbances, nystagmus, and history of temporary remissions), and neurosyphilis. Comparison of manganese excretion in the urine samples of pre- and postchelation therapy may be of diagnostic value.[52, 61]

Prognosis and Treatment of Manganism

If manganese poisoning is detected in its early stage and the worker removed from exposure promptly, the neurologic abnormalities will disappear without specific treatment.[18] Spontaneous recovery may take one to three months. It is believed that in such cases the brain cells were only functionally impaired. The body's natural clearance mechanism is considered sufficient in removing excess manganese. However, chelation therapy using calcium disodium ethylenediaminetetraacetic acid (CaEDTA) may be attempted to accelerate the elimination process.[34, 49]

For patients in the second stage of the poisoning, the effectiveness of removal from exposure and CaEDTA therapy has been variable,[49, 61] apparently depending on the presence or absence of irreversible cell damage in the brain.[50, 61] It is likely that in those who do not improve on removal and chelation therapy, permanent neuronal damage has occurred. On the other hand, Cook et al.[12] reported that temporary improvements after chelation therapy were observed in four of six patients with well-established manganism.

Once established, manganism is an intractable and permanently disabling occupational disease for which there is no cure. Although there is no immediate threat to life, patients suffer a miserable condition for the rest of their lives. Progress in research on the pathogenesis and therapy of parkinsonism and manganism, however, has occurred in recent years.[16]

In both parkinsonism and manganism, brain cells are depleted of the catecholamine neurotransmitters and of melanin. Based on this information, investigators administered the biochemical precursor of the catecholamine neurotransmitters, L-dopa (levodopa; 3,4-dihydroxyphenylalanine) to parkinsonism patients and observed clinical improvement. Because of the clinical similarities of idiopathic parkinsonism and manganism, L-dopa has also been utilized in manganism patients with some success.

Mena et al.[41] administered slowly increasing oral doses of L-dopa up to 8 gm per day to eight patients with manganism. Five of the six patients with hypokinetic features and both of those two with dystonic features showed improvement. One of the hypokinetic patients experienced aggravation of his symptoms on this treatment but subsequently was improved by a 3-gm daily dose of D,L-5-hydroxytryptophane. Rosenstock et al.[51] reported on a patient who showed improvements of abnormal reflexes, disturbed mentation and speech, adiadochokinesis, and bradykinesia when treated with 6–12 gm daily of levodopa for four months. There was, however, no improvement in dystonia.

Greenhouse[26] reported on four cases of manganism that were not improved by levodopa and suggested that there might be a difference in pathophysiology among the patients. In a study of six patients who did not respond well to the levodopa therapy, Cook et al.[12] suggested a correlation between muscle tone and response to levodopa by stating that, in the absence of rigidity or dystonia, or both, levodopa is ineffective for treatment of chronic manganism.

In a study of parkinsonism cases, a low-protein diet was found to be effective in stabilizing symptoms and reducing the required dose of levodopa. It is postulated that this effect occurs because the amino acid levodopa is competitively intercepted in peripheral tissues by dietary amino acid. In addition to reducing protein intake, α-methyldopa hydrazine (MK-486) has been used successfully to prevent the rapid metabolism of levodopa to dopamine. This was effective in preventing the "off-on" phenomenon (episodic loss of symptomatic control) during the course of long-term use of levodopa for parkinsonism.[43]

It is expected that future progress in the therapeutic strategy will bring further improvement in treatment of manganism. However, it should be emphasized here that the best treatment still lies in the prevention of the poisoning.

Prevention of Manganism

The preventive program must consist of industrial hygiene control, education, and a medical program.

Industrial Hygiene Control.—The type and magnitude of the exposure must be evaluated by a qualified person, and adequate control measures should be established to keep the exposure levels below current standards.[63] Engineering controls include process enclosures, general ventilation, local exhaust ventilation, wetting of dust, and remote handling. When necessary, personal protective equipment, such as certified respirators or airline respirators, should be used.[58] Such equipment must be checked periodically and maintained properly. The fact that manganese metal dust cloud is explosive must be kept in mind.[57]

Education.—Supervisors as well as workers must be properly informed of the hazard of manganese exposure. Employees should be educated concerning proper methods of handling toxic materials, using personal protective equipment and recognizing and reporting abnormal symptoms. Ignorance of these fundamentals has resulted in many irreversible disabilities.[58] There is the need for proper labeling of chemical materials containing manganese or other toxic substances.

Medical Program.—The baseline health status of manganese workers must be established by the preplacement medical examination, and their subsequent health status be monitored at periodic intervals.[50, 53, 58, 62] These intervals may vary from 1 to 12 months, depending on the type and degree of exposure. The program should include review of symptoms and signs, and blood and/or urine manganese analysis conducted by a dependable laboratory. If a worker is found to have some of the symptoms and signs listed in Table 37–1, or if the blood or urine manganese level is above the reported normal range (see Diagnosis of Manganism), he or she must be evaluated further and, if indicated, removed from the exposure and followed up with neurologic examinations.

A variety of neurobehavioral tests have been proposed for the evaluation of neurotoxicity resulting from occupational exposure.[6, 29] Of these tests, it is expected that a battery consisting of a personality test, a mood test (e.g., The Profile of Mood Status [POMS]), and a motor test (e.g., dexterity test) may prove to be valuable for detection of early manganese poisoning. Unfortunately, however, these tests have not yet been systematically applied to or validated on manganese workers, with the exception that in the grip strength test grip strength has been found to be reduced in manganism patients.[52] Therefore, the establishment of their usefulness for detection of manganism must await further investigation.

Some investigators reported that there was a remarkable variation in individual susceptibility to manganese under similar exposure conditions.[10, 19, 48] Although the exact nature of this phenomenon is not fully understood, nutritional deficiency, in particular iron deficiency anemia, has been advanced as an important factor in worker susceptibility to manganism.[40, 55] Since there are atomic similarities between iron and manganese, an iron-deficient body may absorb manganese more readily than one with adequate iron supply.[42] Although this hypothesis has not been confirmed epidemiologically among exposed workers, it would be prudent to add a hemoglobin determination to preplacement and periodic medical examination of manganese workers. If anemia is detected, its cause should be investigated and treated before the worker is placed on or returned to work with manganese exposure.[53]

The medical program should include screening of workers for pulmonary insufficiency in view of the exposure to dust and also provide counseling for cessation of smoking.[53]

Manganic Pneumonia

In 1921, Brezina first reported five pneumonia deaths among ten manganese workers in an Italian pyrolusite industry.[46] In 1939, Elstad reported an epidemic of lobar pneumonia in the town of Sauda, Norway.[46] A plant near the town smelted ferromanganese that contained 80% manganese and silicon manganese. Smoke from the furnace containing silica and manganese oxides polluted the town, which is located on the shore of a fjord. During the years with heavy pollution, lobar pneumonia accounted for 32.3% of all deaths in Sauda, affecting not only plant workers but other inhabitants of the community. The corresponding figure for all of Norway was 3.65%. Lloyd Davies[35] reported that the incidence of pneumonia among the men exposed to the dust of oxides of manganese in the manufacture of potassium permanganate was 36 times as high as that in an unexposed but otherwise similar group.

Other cases of manganic pneumonia have been reported from many different countries. However, there has been a lack of similar reports in the United States. Whether this is due to the genuine absence of manganic pneumonia or to the lack of epidemiologic investigations remains unknown.

From the results of animal experiments in which groups of animals were exposed to pathogens with or without manganese oxide, it has been postulated that manganese may potentiate infectious processes.[1, 37] The exact mechanism of such potentiation, however, has not been elucidated.

ORGANIC MANGANESE COMPOUNDS

In this group of compounds, cyclopentadienyl manganese tricarbonyl (CMT) and methylcyclopentadienyl manganese tricarbonyl (MMT) have been studied for their toxicity. The following information pertains mainly to MMT (Fig 37–1).

MMT is a dark orange liquid characterized by a herbaceous odor, low volatility (vapor pressure 9.3 mm Hg at 100° C), and high thermal stability (a boiling point of 232° C at 760 mm Hg and a closed-cup flash point of 96° C) but is subject to rapid photochemical decomposition.[20]

In the molecular structure, the manganese tricarbonyl moiety is not attached to a specific carbon atom, but instead the manganese atom is in a different plane and is bound to all of the carbon atoms in the ring, as depicted by a term "sandwiched." Manganese comprises about 25% of the compound's molecular weight.

MMT has been added to fuel oil as a smoke inhibitor or a combustion improver and also has been suggested as an antiknock additive to gasoline, supplementing or substituting tetraethyl lead. However, the latter use in unleaded gasoline has not been ap-

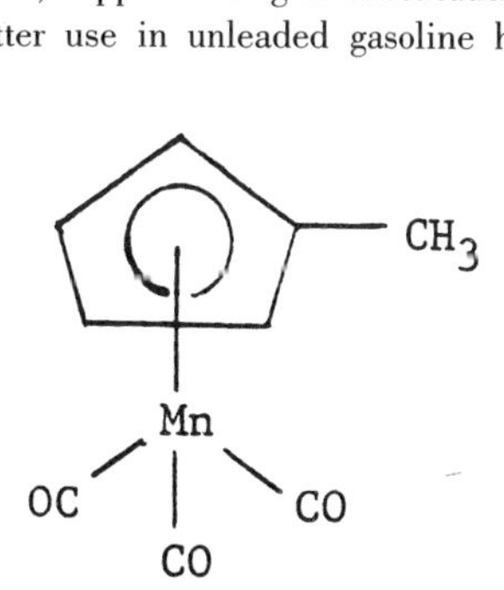

CH_3 Mn OC CO CO

FIG 37–1.
MMT—methylcyclopentadienyl manganese tricarbonyl.

proved in the United States by the Environmental Protection Agency.[23] As of 1983, MMT was used in about 25% of all regular leaded gasoline in the U.S. and in all unleaded gasoline in Canada, at a rate of 0.03–0.04 gm (as manganese) per U.S. gallon.

Moore et al. studied the metabolism of MMT using radioactive manganese in rats.[44] Following oral or intravenous administration of ^{54}Mn-tagged MMT, most of the radioactivity was excreted into the urine and feces in the first few days of administration. This route of excretion is contrasted to that of inorganic manganese (e.g., $MnCl_2$) which is excreted very little by way of the urine.

Toxicity of a Manganese Tricarbonyl

The data from animal studies on the toxicity of MMT indicate that the toxicity depended on the species of animal, rats being more susceptible than others. Hinderer[27] reported that the LD_{50} of MMT was 58 mg/kg in the rat and 230 mg/kg in the mouse. By inhalation, the LC_{50} in the rat was 247 mg/cu m air for a one-hour exposure and 76 mg/cu m for a four-hour exposure. The LD_{50} of MMT applied to the skin of the rabbit ranged from 140 to 795 mg/kg, depending on the testing laboratory. Reactions of animals varied from none to excitation, tremors, convulsions, and bloody diarrhea. Gross pathologic changes were observed in the lungs, liver, kidneys, and spleen.

Although manganese carbonyls can be absorbed through the skin,[4] MMT is not strongly irritating to the skin or eye. Therefore, exposed workers should be cautioned not to depend on irritation as a warning sign of exposure. They should be instructed to wash the skin and change their clothing as soon as contamination with MMT occurs.

While no epidemiologic or other systematic studies of workers exposed to organic manganese compounds have been reported, a few episodes of inadvertent worker exposure have been documented by the manufacturer of MMT.[21] It appears that transfer of the liquid provides opportunities for contamination of clothes and dermal exposure. In one incident two men wearing rubber gloves and air masks got their clothing (shoes and socks, in particular) wet with MMT. They kept working for about 1.5 hours before they changed clothes and reported to the medical department. They had no symptoms other than a slight burning sensation on the skin. No abnormalities were found on physical examination. Urinary manganese levels on the same day were 46 and 137 µg/L, and dropped to 2.9 and 3.4 µg/L, respectively, a few weeks later. In another incident in which six workers were dermally exposed for up to 30 minutes, headache was reported by four, nausea by four, dyspnea by three, chest tightness by one, and paresthesia by one. These symptoms appeared five minutes to an hour after exposure and subsided in two hours in four cases; the remaining two reported abdominal distress for two days.

RECOMMENDED EXPOSURE LIMITS

There is a wide range (from 0.3 to 6 mg/cu m) in the levels of manganese to which workers in various countries are permitted to be exposed.[28] This wide range is probably due to different concepts, interpretations, and legal applications of these limits by the different countries.

In the United States, the permissible exposure limit[47] for manganese dust and compounds (as Mn) is a ceiling value of 5 mg/cu m. Some investigators question the adequacy of protection afforded by this level and favor more strict exposure control.[1] The American Conference of Governmental Industrial Hygienists (ACGIH) prescribes that the threshold limit value (TLV) for manganese fumes be 1 mg/cu m TWA (time-weighted average) and 3 mg/cu m STEL (short-term exposure limit).[3] Cyclopentadienyl manganese tricarbonyl (CMT) has a TLV (as Mn) of 0.1 mg/cu m TWA and 0.3 mg/cu m STEL. The TLV (as Mn) for methylcyclopentadienyl manganese tricarbonyl (MMT) is 0.2 mg/cu m and 0.6 mg/cu m STEL. Both CMT and MMT have a notation for skin absorption.[3]

REFERENCES

1. Adkins B, et al: Increased pulmonary susceptibility to streptococcal infection following inhalation of manganese oxide. *Environ Res* 1980; 23:110.
2. Alvord EC, et al: The pathology of Parkinsonism: A comparison of degenerations in cerebral cortex and brain stem, in McDowell F, Barbeau A (eds): *Advances in Neurology*. Raven Press, New York, 1974, vol 5, p 175.
3. American Conference of Governmental Industrial Hygienists: *Threshold Limit Values for Chemical Substances and Physical Agents in the Work Environment with Intended Changes for 1986–87*. Cincinnati, ACGIH, 1986.
4. Arkhipova OB, et al: Toxicity within a factory of the vapor of new antiknock compound, manganese cyclopentadienyltricarbonyl. *Hyg Sanit* 1965; 30:40.
5. Ashizawa R: Uber einem Sektionsfall von chronischer Manganvergiftung. *Jap J Med Sci* 1927; 1:173.
6. Baker EL, et al: Monitoring neurotoxins in industry—Development of a neurobehavioral test battery. *J Occup Med* 1983; 25:125.
7. Barbeau A, et al: Role of manganese in dystonia, in Eldridge R, Fahn S (eds): *Advances in Neurology*. Raven Press, New York, 1976, vol 14, p 339.
8. Buchet JP, et al: Determination of manganese in blood and urine by flameless atomic absorption spectrophotometry. *Clin Chim Acta* 1976; 73:481.
9. Canavan MM, et al: Chronic manganese poisoning. *Arch Neurol Psychiat* 1934; 32:501.
10. Casamajor L: An unusual form of mineral poisoning affecting the nervous system: Manganese? *JAMA* 1913; 60:646.
11. Cholak J, Hubbard DM: Determination of manganese in air and biological material. *Am Ind Hyg Assoc J* 1960; 21:356.
12. Cook DG, et al: Chronic manganese intoxication. *Arch Neurol* 1974; 30:59.
13. Cotzias GC: Manganese in health and disease. *Physiol Rev* 1958; 38:503.
14. Cotzias GC, et al: Manganese in melanin. *Nature* 1964; 201:1228.
15. Cotzias GC, et al: Chronic manganese poisoning: Clearance of tissue manganese concentrations with persistence of the neurological picture. *Neurology* 1968; 18:376.
16. Cotzias GC, et al: Metabolic modification of Parkinson's disease and of chronic manganese poisoning. *Ann Rev Med* 1971; 22:305.
17. Couper J: On the effects of black oxide of manganese when inhaled into the lungs. *Br Ann Med Pharm* 1837; 1:41.
18. Edsall DL, et al: The occurrence, course and prevention of chronic manganese poisoning. *J Ind Hyg* 1919; 1:183.
19. Emara AM, et al: Chronic manganese poisoning in the dry battery industry. *Br J Ind Med* 1971; 28:78.

20. Ethyl Corporation: *"Ethyl" Antiknock compound—Manganese,* Rep TS-213. Ferndale, Mich, Ethyl Corporation, 1971.
21. Ethyl Corporation: *A Medical Guide-"Ethyl MMT."* Baton Rouge, La, Ethyl Corporation, 1977.
22. Fairhall LT, Neal PA: *Industrial Manganese Poisoning,* National Institute of Health Bull 182. Washington, DC, US Government Printing Office, 1943.
23. Ethyl Corp: Denial of Application for Fuel Waiver; Summary of Decision. *Federal Register* 46:58360 (Dec 1) 1981.
24. Flinn RH, et al: *Chronic Manganese Poisoning in an Ore-Crushing Mill,* Public Health Bull 247. Washington, DC, US Government Printing Office, 1940.
25. Greenberg DM, et al: Studies in mineral metabolism with the aid of artificial radioactive isotopes. VII. The distribution and excretion, particularly by way of the bile, of iron, cobalt, and manganese. *J Biol Chem* 1943; 147:749.
26. Greenhouse AH: Manganese intoxication in the United States. *Trans Am Neurol Assoc* 1971; 96:248.
27. Hinderer RK: Toxicity studies of methylcyclopentadienyl manganese tricarbonyl (MMT). *Am Ind Hyg Assoc J* 1979; 40:164.
28. International Labour Office: *Occupational Exposure Limits for Airborne Toxic Substances,* ed 2. *A Tabular Compilation of Values from Selected Countries,* Occupational Safety & Health Series 37. Geneva, ILO, 1983.
29. Johnson BL, Anger WK: *Behavioral Toxicology,* in Rom WR (ed): *Environmental and Occupational Medicine.* Boston, Little, Brown & Co, 1983, p 329.
30. Jonderko G, et al: Problems of chronic manganese poisoning on the basis of investigations of workers at a manganese alloy foundry. *Int Arch Arbeitsmed* 1971; 28:250.
31. Jones TS: *Manganese,* in *Minerals Yearbook,* vol I, *Metals and Minerals.* Washington, DC, Bureau of Mines, US Dept. of the Interior. US Government Printing Office, 1985, p 573.
32. Kawamura R, et al: Intoxication by manganese in well water. *Kitasato Arch Exp Med* 1941; 18:145.
33. Klawans H, et al: Theoretical implications of the use of L-DOPA in Parkinsonism—A review. *Acta Neurol Scand* 1970; 46:409.
34. Kosai MF, Boyle AJ: Ethylenediaminetetraacetic acid in manganese poisoning of rats. *Ind Med Surg* 1956; 25:1.
35. Lloyd Davies TA: Manganese pneumonitis. *Br J Ind Med* 1946; 3:111.
36. Mahoney JP, Small WJ: Studies on manganese-III. The biological half-life of radiomanganese in man and factors which affect this half-life. *J Clin Invest* 1968; 47:643.
37. Maigetter RZ, et al: Potentiating effects of manganese dioxide on experimental respiratory infections. *Environ Res* 1976; 11:386.
38. Maynard LS, Cotzias GC: The partition of manganese among organs and intracellular organelles of the rat. *J Biol Chem* 1955; 214:489.
39. Mena I, et al: Chronic manganese poisoning: Clinical picture and manganese turnover. *Neurology* 1967; 17:128.
40. Mena I, et al: Chronic manganese poisoning—Individual susceptibility and absorption of iron. *Neurology* 1969; 19:1000.
41. Mena I, et al: Modification of chronic manganese poisoning. *New Engl J Med* 1970; 282:5.
42. Mena I: The role of manganese in human disease. *Ann Clin Lab Sci* 1974; 4:487.
43. Mena I, Cotzias GC: Protein intake and treatment of Parkinson's disease with levodopa. *New Engl J Med* 1975; 292:181.
44. Moore W, et al: Metabolic aspects of methylcyclopentadienyl manganese tricarbonyl in rats. *Environ Res* 1974; 8:171.
45. National Institute for Occupational Safety and Health: A computer printout on manganese from the National Occupational Hazard Survey (NOHS) data base collected during the period 1972–74. Cincinnati, Oh, NIOSH, Hazard Section, Surveillance Branch, 1976.
46. National Research Council: *Manganese—Publication of the Panel on Manganese, Committee on Medical & Biologic Effects of Environmental Pollutants.* Washington, DC, National Academy of Sciences, 1973.
47. Occupational Safety and Health Administration: *General Industry Occupational Safety and Health Standard,* Section 29, CFR 1910.1000.
48. Penalver R: Manganese poisoning. *Ind Med Surg* 1955; 24:1.
49. Penalver R: Diagnosis and treatment of manganese intoxication. *AMA Arch Ind Health* 1957; 16:64.
50. Rodier J: Manganese poisoning in Moroccan miners. *Br J Ind Med* 1955; 12:21.
51. Rosenstock HA, et al: Chronic manganism. Neurologic and laboratory studies during treatment with levodopa. *JAMA* 1971; 217:1354.
52. Sano S, et al: An epidemiological survey and clinical investigations on retired workers from manganese mines and ore grinders in Kyoto Prefecture. *Nippon Eiseigaku Zasshi (Japan J Hyg)* 1982; 37:566.
53. Šărić M: Manganese, alloys and compounds, in Parmeggiani L (ed): *Encyclopaedia of Occupational Health and Safety,* ed 3 rev. Geneva, International Labour Office, 1983, vol 2.
54. Schuler P, et al: Manganese poisoning—Environmental and medical study at a Chilean mine. *Ind Med Surg* 1957; 26:167.
55. Shukla GS, Chandra SV: Manganese induced morphological and biochemical changes in the brain of iron deficient rats. *Ind Health* 1976; 14:87.
56. Smyth LT, et al: Clinical manganism and exposure to manganese in the production and processing of ferromanganese alloy. *J Occup Med* 1973; 15:101.
57. Stokinger HE: Manganese, in Clayton GD, Clayton FE (eds): *Patty's Industrial Hygiene and Toxicology,* ed 3 rev. Vol 2A *Toxicology.* New York, John Wiley & Sons, 1981, p 1749.
58. Tanaka S, Lieben J: Manganese poisoning, and exposure in Pennsylvania. *Arch Environ Health* 1969; 19:674.
59. von Oettingen WF: Manganese: Its distribution, pharmacology, and health hazards. *Physiol Rev* 1935; 15:175.
60. Watanabe T, et al: Determination of urinary manganese by the direct chelation method and flameless atomic absorption spectrophotometry. *Br J Ind Med* 1978; 35:73.
61. Whitlock CM, et al: Chronic neurological disease in two manganese steel workers. *Am Ind Hyg Assoc J* 1966; 27:454.
62. World Health Organization: *Manganese, Environmental Health Criteria* 17. Geneva, WHO, 1981.
63. Wynter JE: The prevention of manganese poisoning. *Ind Med Surg* 1962; 31:308.

38

Mercury and Its Compounds

Arthur L. Knight, M.D.

Prehistoric man used a red stone of mercury ore (cinnabar, mercury sulfide, HgS) to color the drawings on his cave walls, and metallic mercury was known to the ancient Egyptians. Man soon determined mercury mining to be hazardous to health and life; consequently, mines were primarily worked by slaves and convicts.

In 1557, a Frenchman, Jean Fernel, was the first to describe the symptoms and signs of poisoning by mercury during the period that a mercury compound, mercurous chloride (calomel, HgCl), was beginning to be used in medicine as a diuretic.

Mercury was the first substance to be the cause of legislation to control the occupational disease it caused. In 1665, the workday in Idrija, Yugoslavia, was reduced to six hours in the mercury mines instead of the 14 hours prevalent in the workplaces at that time.

Ramazzini described the plight of the mercury miners; a century later, several investigators described the problems of the workers in the felt hat industry.[42] In 1865, C. L. Dodgson (Lewis Carroll) wrote *Alice's Adventures in Wonderland*, in which the character of the Mad Hatter apparently was a good example of mercury poisoning.[24]

Although mercury is rarer than uranium or platinum, it is more available, because it exists in high concentrated ores that are readily available and easily refined. As world production and usage of mercury rapidly advanced in the 20th century, it became apparent that it would be a widespread hazard that would present itself to man, not only in the mine[27] and industry but at home, in the school, in his food,[10] and in plant life. In 1971, the world production of mercury was estimated at 11,600 tons. The United States uses about one sixth of this production; half is imported from Canada, Spain, Italy, and Mexico, the remainder coming from domestic production, primarily in California, Alaska, Idaho, and Nevada.

SOURCES

Mercury is obtained primarily from the ore cinnabar. One method involves heating of the ore to 500° C in the presence of oxygen (air), permitting the sulfur to combine with oxygen, leaving the metallic mercury as a vapor that is easily condensed. Cinnabar can also be heated with lime, and the sulfur will combine with the calcium, leaving metallic mercury vapor. There are other methods, but mercury nearly always is purified by distillation.[11]

PHYSICAL PROPERTIES

Mercury has the symbol Hg, derived from the Greek word hydrargyros, meaning "water silver" because it is a silvery liquid at ordinary room temperatures. It has a melting point of −38.87° C and a boiling point of 357.0° C. Mercury has an atomic number of 80 and an atomic weight of 200.61. With a specific gravity of 13.55, mercury will allow lead to float on its surface. The mercury atom has five shells of electrons complete (2, 8, 18, 32, 18), an incomplete shell of two electrons, and a valence of +2. This gives the usual mercuric compounds. Two mercury atoms can combine and form the ion Hg_2^{++} with an apparent valence of +1, giving us the mercurous compounds. Mercury readily forms complex ions with shared electrons, coordinate covalent bonds, which give us the important organomercurial compounds.

Mercury vaporizes readily at ordinary temperatures, is a good conductor of electricity, has a linear expansion, does not wet glass, absorbs ultraviolet resonance light at 2,537 Å, and is insoluble in water and soluble in dilute nitric acid. Most metals other than iron and platinum dissolve in or amalgamate with mercury. The mercury vapor-holding capability of air is increased by increased temperature. At 40° C, air can hold more than four times what it can hold of mercury vapor at 20° C. The amount of mercury vapor in the air is also affected by pressure, rate of air exchange, and the amount of mercury surface exposed.

USES OF MERCURY

Mercury is used in the manufacture of many medical instruments, including blood pressure apparatus, thermometers, and pacemakers. The pharmaceutical industry produces many products that contain mercury that are used as antiseptics, diuretics, cathartics, and the once popular inorganic and organic mercury compounds used in the treatment of syphilis.

Metallic mercury is used in the manufacture of scientific instruments, such as barometers, mercury-arc rectifers that produce

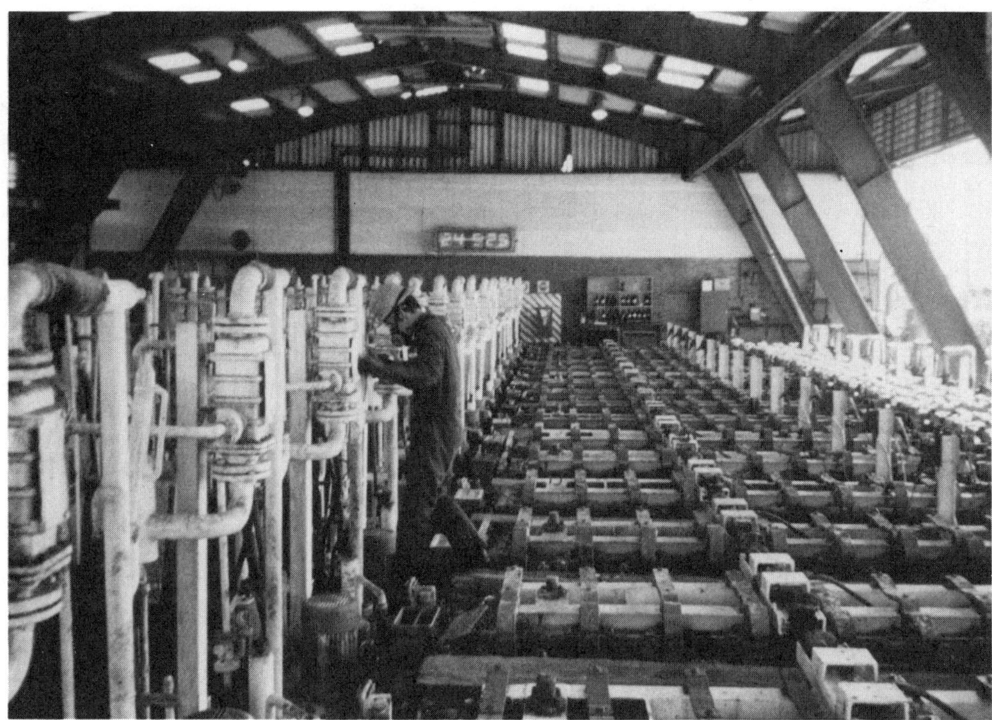

FIG 38–1.
A view of a chlorine production facility where large quantities of metallic mercury are used. Leaks from pumps and fittings are a constant concern and there is regular inspection and maintenance by the workers who are tested regularly for urinary mercury excretion. In addition, the air is monitored.

ultraviolet light, and automatic thermostats. The electrical industry further uses metallic mercury in the silent light switch, in fluorescent lamps, which often are activated by mercury vapor, and in many of the more powerful street lamps. Mercury is also used in some gold mining to amalgamate the gold. It was also used in the separation of lithium 6 in the hydrogen bomb.

The manufacture, repair, and maintenance of electrical meters and the manufacture of amalgams with copper, tin, silver, or gold consume large amounts of mercury (Fig 38–1). It is widely used in the chemical industry for the production of many mercury compounds, caustic soda, and glacial acetic acid. Dentists use mercury as a component in the "silver" filling. Mercury is used as a catalyst in some chemical processes, one of its main uses being in the manufacture of chlorine. Mercury is used in the manufacture of some aluminum alloys and, unfortunately, still is found in some children's electrical and chemistry kits and toys. Some precision machines are floated in mercury in order to avoid earth-transmitted vibrations.

Inorganic mercury compounds are used in the felt hat industry;[3] where the nitrate is used in the "carrotting" of rabbit fur to cause it to form a tenacious felt; a mercuric nitrate solution is used in the treatment of fur to make it pliable for shaping. Inorganic mercury compounds are also found in pigments, paints, dyes, tattooing materials, embalming preparations, wood preservatives, fingerprinting compounds, herbicides, insecticides, spermicidal jellies, pesticides, germicides in soap, fireworks, percussion caps, long-life mercury batteries, and fungicides. Both mercurous chloride and mercuric chloride are used in treating and protecting seeds and seedlings, and in earthworm control.

Mercury compounds are found in paint additives to inhibit the growth of bacteria and mildew, and mercury often is an ingredient in floor wax, furniture polish, and fabric softeners. Organic mercury compounds are used in the manufacture of seed dressings, as a fungicide for treating seed, and for preventing mold on turf. Some organic mercury compounds are used for local external antiseptic products; they are also used in laundry and diaper services. These alkyl compounds are used in the machinery of paper mills to prevent the formation of "slime." These fungicides in mechanical pulp and paper mills (such as phenyl-mercury-acetate to improve storage) as well as other industrial mercury discharges (e.g., those from the chlor-alkali industry and various plastics manufacturers) have been reported as great sources of environmental mercury contamination. Mercuric fulminate is used as an explosive primer. An interesting process, frozen-mercury investment casting, was pointed out by Kramer and Goldwater in 1956.[26]

BIOLOGIC EFFECTS OF MERCURY

Mercury, as the metal or in most of its many inorganic and organic forms, is a protoplasmic poison hazardous to all forms of life. Some of the confusion that arose from the various medical reports regarding mercury was generated because it has different properties, modes of action, and effects, depending on many factors, including the form it presents as well as the concentration, route of entry, and duration of exposure.[12, 17, 19, 28]

It was known for centuries that the mining of mercury caused disease, but in the early 19th century it became apparent that mercury was a greater hazard than had been realized. In 1803, a fire in a mercury mine produced 900 neighborhood cases in Idrija, Yugoslavia. The inhabitants developed muscle tremors and the domestic animals were affected also. In 1810, broken mercury containers on a British ship resulted in the death of all birds and cattle aboard; 200 persons developed symptoms of mercury poisoning, with three deaths.

Today, mercury is a greater hazard in our schools, laboratories, hospitals, museums, dental and medical offices, and homes than it need be, because most people do not realize that mercury is an airborne poison and they have never considered that it vaporizes at room temperature. For example, to avoid mercury exposure, dentists should not use carpeting in treatment rooms or leave old amalgams or mercury in open containers.

Mercury is more toxic than lead. Its toxicity, in general, depends on the release of the mercuric ion. However, mercury should be thought of in terms of four different categories—the metal, the inorganic compounds, the organic alkyl mercury, and the other organic mercury compounds.

The toxicology of mercury is well documented in the medical literature. Notable are the numerous research papers by Goldwater et al.,[21–24] the chapter written by Stokinger[40] in the textbook *Industrial Hygiene and Toxicology*, the book *Toxicology of Mercury and Its Compounds* by Bidstrup,[9] a critical review of the literature on mercury toxicity by Battigelli,[4, 5] and the papers on body retention of mercury by Berlin et al.[8]

Skin contact with metallic mercury results in no significant absorption. Some people have developed a sensitivity to mercury that resulted in a dermatitis.[35]

Some inorganic mercury compounds, such as mercuric chloride and potassium mercuric iodide, can have 3% or 4% absorbed from the skin in a five-hour period.[44]

Organic mercury compounds may be toxic on skin contact, as is methylmercuric dicyanamide.

Taken orally, metallic mercury apparently is affected very little and is relatively harmless, depending on the surface exposed. Some sulfide forms on the surface and is absorbed. Ingested inorganic mercury compounds vary widely in their absorption and toxic effect. Mercurous chloride has a low toxicity, is not metabolized, with approximately 15% absorption from the gastrointestinal tract, and has been used as a medicine for centuries. Mercuric chloride is very toxic and corrosive and earlier in this century was one of the common methods of suicide.

Some organic mercury compounds, such as methylmercury chloride, are almost completely absorbed. Environmental methylmercury contamination combining with protein in fish was the cause of mercury poisoning in the Minamata area of Japan in 1953.[39] That was the first major publicity that began the environmental mercury scare and initiated studies elsewhere in the world.[25]

Inhalation of mercury vapor and dust of mercury compounds has been the major cause of occupational mercury poisoning.

Acute and Chronic Mercury Poisoning

Acute mercury poisoning can occur from inhalation of high concentrations of mercury vapor or dust. If the concentration of mercury vapor is high enough, the exposure will result in tightness and pain in the chest, difficulty in breathing, coughing, and, shortly thereafter, a metallic taste, nausea, abdominal pain, vomiting, diarrhea, headache, and occasionally albuminuria. Death may occur at any point. In three or four days, the salivary glands swell, gingivitis develops, and gastroenteritis symptoms and nephritis appear. In most cases, the patient will recover in one to two weeks. The more severe cases will develop psychopathologic symptoms and muscle tremors. These have, in fact, become chronic types and the symptoms based on neurologic damage may be permanent.

Chronic mercury poisoning usually is what is meant when the term *mercurialism* is used. It can occur from inhalation or ingestion and be aggravated by skin absorption. It is the mercurial poisoning found most commonly in the occupational setting.[30, 45] The symptoms may first occur after a very few weeks of exposure, or they may not become apparent for several years. The more intense the exposure has been, the more the symptoms will relate to the mouth, the kidney, and the respiratory and gastrointestinal systems. The more prolonged and the lower the level of exposure, the more likely the symptoms and signs will be pathoneurologic in nature. Most cases have a blending of both.

The chronic poisoning effect is also related to the physiochemical properties of the material inhaled or ingested.

Signs and Symptoms of Chronic Poisoning

Chronic poisoning has been reported frequently and with a great variety of *signs and symptoms* observed. In the mouth area, a generalized inflammation may occur. The gums become tender; a gingivitis and discolored gums, sometimes with bluish black dots along the gum line, may occur. The teeth become loosened and alveolar destruction can be seen on x-ray. The salivary glands may swell and mercury is excreted in the saliva. Some report increased salivation and others complain of dryness in the mouth. A stomatitis can occur as well as a tremor of the tongue. A speech defect is common in severe cases. There may be nasal irritation, epistaxis, disturbances of taste and smell, loss of appetite, facial pallor, and anemia.

The most common but usually not the first sign of chronic mercurial poisoning is *tremor*.[47] This may occur in the eyelids but is observed most frequently in the fingers and later in the arms and legs. Severe cases can develop rigidity. An effect on handwriting because of the intention tremor has been a frequent observation. Neuralgia, paresthesias, ataxia, exaggerated knee jerks, and altered plantar reflexes have been reported.[29]

Vasomotor disturbances can cause excessive perspiration and uncontrolled blushing. Ocular lesions, including coloring of the anterior capsule of the crystalline lens, can occur. Decreased peripheral vision may be present and blindness can result.

Personality changes are the most common findings in chronic mercurial poisoning. In mild cases, these may occur with no other signs or symptoms apparent. The psychopathologic effects have been described as erethism, irritability, irascibility, criticalness, excitability, fearfulness, restlessness, insomnia, inability to concentrate, melancholy, depression, shyness, timidity, moroseness, fatigue, weakness, and drowsiness. The person may appear indecisive or have a memory defect. Headache and digestive disturbances often are present.

The toxic biologic effects of mercury are, like the symptoms of mercurialism, variable with the level of exposure, mode of attack, and disposition. Some changes occur in the enzyme systems of workers whose exposure to mercury is well below the NIOSH recommended permissible exposure limit (PEL) of 0.05 mg/cu m. At an average airborne mercury level of 0.028 mg/cu m, lab technicians exhibited a significant decrease in red blood cell cholinesterase activity and an increase in plasma galactosidase and catalase activities.

Absorption and Excretion

Elemental mercury and mercurous compounds appear to be readily absorbed from the alveoli of the lungs and presumably are oxidized to mercuric salts.[2] Metallic mercury may, however, because of its solubility in liquids, be easily diffused through the lipid-containing cell membrane of the alveolar wall and later transported, attached to blood lipid, to other tissues to be oxidized and bond itself to a protein, making further release difficult. Mercury has a cumulative effect and has a tendency to deposit in certain organs, most notably the brain, liver, and kidney, although it can be found in nearly all tissues. The hair has been used as a method of assessing mercury intake and so has the saliva.

Excretion of mercury occurs in internal systems such as the biliary and salivary. The main route of excretion is via the urine, although some mercury is excreted in feces and sweat.[20, 36] Some observers have noted that victims of mercury poisoning had an abnormal breath smell. Mercury is transferred to the infant through the mother's milk. Excretion of mercury may continue for months after the exposure to mercury has stopped.

In general, the unstable organic mercury compounds degenerate into inorganic mercury and give toxic patterns similar to the inorganic salts. The more stable organic mercury compounds, such as the alkylmercury compounds, may not produce effects as quickly but they do act on the nervous system and may result in permanent changes.[16]

The excretion of mercury in the urine bears a relation to the mercury exposure but varies widely in individual cases because of many variable factors.[31] Excretion becomes more significant of the amount of exposure when studying group exposures. After an injection of methylmercuric salts, inorganic mercury was found in the blood, brain, bile, liver, kidney, and spleen, and preferentially excreted in the feces. Oyanguran[38] found a relationship between urinary concentration of mercury and the working conditions and a direct relationship between clinical symptoms and the length of exposure, especially if the exposure had been a long one. Mastromatteo[32] reported on eight cases of mercury poisoning with very different urinary levels but with similar symptoms.

Diagnosis of Mercury Poisoning

The *diagnosis* of mercury poisoning will depend primarily on the *history*. Considering the many uses and widespread distribution of mercury in products and in the environment, it should be borne in mind when a patient presents any of the symptoms.

The basic *symptom group* of chronic mercury poisoning consists of (1) psychic changes, (2) gum abnormality, and (3) tremor.

Psychic changes usually reflect hostility, withdrawal, neglect of family, and work deterioration.

Gums may show tenderness and swelling, bleed easily, and have a dark line or spots. Some patients complain of a bad taste.

Tremor is the most commonly mentioned symptom of mercurialism and often is noted by the patient as a difficulty in writing. Other parts of the body can be involved. The intention tremor is fine and fairly rhythmic at about six movements per second, which increases with effort and is bilateral.

Other symptoms that may induce the patient to see the physician are headache, loss of appetite, loss of weight, uncontrollable blushing, and weakness.

The signs on examination would also include the gum problems, psychic abnormality and tremors. The tremors can be exaggerated by line tracing, point tests, and having the subject eager to comply. In advanced cases, the tremor may be widespread and coarse or rigidity can have developed (clonic spasm). The knee jerks may be exaggerated. Rarely, a brownish discoloration may be seen on the anterior capsule of the lens. Dermatographia also may be a sign.

The *laboratory* may be of help in the diagnosis. The standard blood tests offer no help except for an anemia and erythropenia in severe, chronically exposed cases. Lymphocytosis has been reported. Mercury levels in the blood, hair,[37] and saliva have been investigated. Blood mercury may run as high as 9 μg/100 ml in the normal population.[23] Urine analysis for mercury often has shown poor correlation between signs and symptoms on the one hand and urinary mercury on the other. Nonetheless, in suspected mercury poisoning, a determination of mercury in the urine should be made. A 24-hour specimen is preferable. Special mercury-free bottles and stoppers must be used for collecting the blood or urine specimen. Of great importance is that blood and urine analysis for mercury at many laboratories will not be reliable. The variety of opinions concerning normal urinary levels of mercury is summarized by Danziger and Possick.[14] The *Technical Bulletin for Physicians* issued in 1967 by the state of California contains a table to be used as a tentative guideline for interpretation of urine mercury levels (Table 38–1). Surface electromyography might help to identify individuals with minimal mercury body burdens.[18]

TREATMENT

Treatment of acute poisoning by ingestion consists of gastric lavage with 5%–10% sodium formaldehyde sulfoxylate solution,[40] leaving 100–200 ml of the solution in the stomach. BAL (dimercaprol), 5 mg/kg of body weight, must be given early to be effective. It is more effective in an alkaline urine. Deichmann and Gerarde[15] state that oral therapy (including 1 teaspoonful of potas-

TABLE 38–1.
Guide for Workers Exposed to Inorganic Mercury*

INDICATION	LEVEL OF MERCURY IN URINE (μg/L)
Normal	Below 10
Increased absorption	Above 50
Warning level	Above 100
Hazardous level—remove from further exposure	Above 200
Symptoms of poisoning may appear	Above 300

*Do not use these standards for workers using organic mercury compounds where excretion over 50 μg/L is the hazardous level. Exposures in California mines and mills are limited to inorganic mercury. Organic mercury is used commonly as a fungicide. (From State of California, Department of Health.)

sium bitartrate and 1 teaspoonful of sodium citrate in water or orange juice) promotes the excretion of mercury.

Acute poisoning by inhalation is also treated early with BAL. Signs of acute distress, such as shock or respiratory distress, are treated in the usual manner. Alkylmercury skin burns should be treated by prompt removal of the blister fluid and the overlying skin.[7] Acute and chronic mercury poisoning treatment with glutamic acid was investigated by Winter et al.[46]

Treatment of chronic mercury poisoning must begin by removing the patient from the exposure. A check of the other workers and testing of the environment, both inside and outside, for mercury concentrations should be done. Mild sedation or psychotherapy may be needed for the mentally perturbed. Clarkson et al.[13] report that polythiol resin added to the diet of mice doubles the excretion rate of mercury in the feces. The inducing of sweating by exercise and heat removes significant amounts of mercury with the sweat.[31] BAL is not as effective in chronic poisoning as it is in acute poisoning, but it does increase the urinary output of mercury. Aposhian et al.[1] have reported on the sulfhydryl compounds in the treatment of mercury poisoning and found oral *N*-acetyl-*dl* penicillamine and *d*-penicillamine to be the more effective and least toxic. Woodcock[48] found that calcium disodium versenate ($CaNa_2EDTA$) increased urinary excretion.

ENVIRONMENTAL TESTING

Mercury analysis at the workplace can be done in several ways. Careful technique and selection of place and time for sampling to give results representative of the work environment are needed.

Indicator tubes based on color changes with mercury are fast, simple, sensitive, and accurate if used properly under the appropriate conditions. An instrument with a precision pump should be used, avoiding use of the "squeeze bulb" type. Avoid using old tubes, taking samples in cold or heat extremes, and storing tubes in the heat. Care should be taken in interpreting results when other air contaminants may be present.

Goldwater et al.[23] suggest that atmospheric tests be run on Monday morning after there may have been minimal ventilation for two days. In laboratories where air temperature and humidity are precisely controlled, be sure in weather extremes that enough make-up air is added to control the mercury vapor accumulation.

When the air to be sampled contains a considerable amount of mercury as dust, it is best to use a collecting system that will also capture the dust.

If the exposure is to mercury vapor alone and there is no dust or smoke in the air to interfere with a light beam, a mercury vapor meter can be used. This direct-reading instrument is based on the principle that mercury absorbs ultraviolet light of 2537 Å. Carbon dioxide and ozone also absorb this light and could give inaccurate mercury readings if either is in significant quantity in the air being tested.

A personnel monitoring apparatus using metallic silver wool to pick up the mercury vapor was developed by Bell in 1973,[6] and a passive monitor using gold foil by 3M Company in 1977.[34]

LIMITING EXPOSURE

Environmental Mercury Exposure

Mercury as an environmental hazard has been reviewed extensively by Vostal and Clarkson.[43] Major sources of mercury pollution in the United States have been such industrial manufacturers as the pulp and paper industry and the users of mercury compounds, e.g., the use of pesticides in agriculture. Both of these sources of pollution have been greatly reduced in the past few years. The major sources of air contamination with mercury have been the refining of ore, electrical manufacturing, and chlorine and caustic soda processing. It is estimated that a stack loss of only 1% when refining mercury ore in the United States would put 9 tons of mercury into the atmosphere each year. A 5% stack loss can occur. Goldwater et al.[23] sampled office air in New York City in an area that did not use mercury and found that the mercury vapor was as high as 0.05 mg/cu m. Since 1970, the amount of mercury imported, produced, and used has been reduced, with resulting reduction in mercury pollution, an anticipated continuing trend.

Occupational Mercury Exposure

The recommendation of the National Institute for Occupational Safety and Health for mercury exposure is 0.05 mg/cu m as an eight-hour time-weighted average. The Occupational Safety and Health Administration standard is 0.1 mg/cu m as a ceiling value.[41]

Control of mercury exposure in industry can be accomplished most readily by engineering methods. Where mercury is used at normal temperatures, good ventilation should be maintained, but filtration of the ventilated air before release may be required. In processes in which mercury is heated, better control of the effluent is required, and a condensation and collection system to contain the mercury is a strict requirement.

It must be remembered that mercury sometimes is a contaminant in other ores, especially gold and zinc, and should not be allowed to be discharged into the environment with the waste. On occasion, the reclaimed mercury has proved to be a valuable byproduct.

A substitution for mercury eliminates the problem at the manufacturing source. We do not need to manufacture mercury blood pressure apparatus, thermometers, barometers, and other equipment for regular use when satisfactory substitutes are available.

The work area where mercury is used should be easily cleanable and have a nonporous surface on the floor and the bench. Where metallic mercury may spill, the floor should slope to a collection cup.

Protective clothing for mercury workers should have a nonporous surface and be without cuffs or pockets. When working with dusty mercury compounds, the worker should have a locker for street clothes and a locker for clean work clothes, which are supplied daily. There should be a shower facility located between the two lockers. Workers should be advised about washing their hands before eating, smoking, or drinking, and they might be advised to rinse their mouths before eating or drinking.

If adequate exhaust ventilation is not present, respirators must be provided where the threshold limit value (TLV) is approached or exceeded regardless of the length of exposure. Employees should have their personal respirator, be instructed in its use, and have replaceable filters available. There should be a regular cleaning and inspection program for the respirators, and the use of respirators should be on a short-term basis only.

In areas in which there is a potential mercury exposure, warning signs should be posted.

Eating and smoking in the workplace are not permitted, and an uncontaminated and easily cleanable area should be available for storage and eating of food and for personal hygiene.

Metallic *mercury spills* must receive prompt attention. The larger particles can be recovered easily; small particles in cracks are not removed by the high-powered vacuum with its mercury trap. Washing the area likely will remove most of the particles. Several commercial mercury decontaminating powders or solutions are available and may be of some value. The area of the spill should have air tests for mercury after the cleaning has been completed.

Before starting work, each employee should be made familiar with the hazards, methods of control, medical aspects, safe methods of working, and emergency procedures in an area in which there is potential exposure.

Preemployment Examination.—*Preemployment evaluation* of any worker to be assigned to work with mercury should include a history of previous mercury exposure, central nervous system disorders and renal disease. An appraisal of the gums and the number of silver fillings might be done. Workers with extensive or chronic dermatitis should not be assigned to work with possible mercury exposure. A routine urine analysis should be done, including the microscopic examination. Some might advocate a urine mercury determination as a base figure against which to compare future urine mercury findings, but a single test may prove inadequate. Lovejoy et al.[31] suggest that any individual with mercurialentis on preemployment not be put at work with potential exposure to mercury. It once was popular to give milk to lead workers, a practice still seen in many countries today. Should we be adding polythiol resin[13] to the food of workers exposed to mercury? Certainly not, since proper occupational hygienic and engineering measures can reduce contamination and control worker exposures to levels beneath those set forth in the TLV guide.[41]

Biologic Monitoring.—*Periodic evaluation* of employees and their environment should be based on the amount of exposure. Where workplace air tests reveal no appreciable mercury, repeating the tests every six months or year should be sufficient. Atmospheric tests should be done whenever the method of mercury usage changes or the employees working with the processes change. If air tests show mercury within the upper half of the TLV, air sampling should be done on a monthly to three-month schedule and employees given a repeat of their preemployment evaluations, including a urine mercury determination at six-month to one-year intervals. If air concentrations reveal mercury to be above the TLV, corrective measures must be taken to reduce the hazard. In this case, the worker should have an immediate medical evaluation, including urine mercury determinations.

REFERENCES

1. Aposhian HV, et al: *N*-acetyl-*dl*-penicillamine, a new oral protective agent against the lethal effects of mercuric chloride. *J Pharmacol Toxicol* 1959; 126:131.
2. Ashe WF, et al: Behavior of mercury in the animal organism following inhalation. *AMA Arch Ind Hyg* 1953; 7:19.
3. Baldi G, et al: Chronic mercurialism in felt hat industries, abstract. *AMA Arch Ind Hyg* 1953; 8:487.
4. Battigelli MC: Mercury toxicity from industrial exposure. Pt I. *J Occup Med* 1960; 2:337.
5. Battigelli MC: Mercury toxicity from industrial exposure. Pt II. *J Occup Med* 1960; 2:394.
6. Bell ZG, et al: A method to determine mercury time-weighted average (TWA) exposures. *J Occup Med* 1973; 15:340 and 420.
7. Berkhout PG, Ladd PG, Goldwater LJ: Treatment of skin burns due to alkyl mercury. *Arch Environ Health* 1961; 3:106.
8. Berlin M, et al: 8 papers on accumulation, retention and excretion of mercury. *Arch Environ Health* 1963; 18:42–50, 719–729.
9. Bidstrup PL: *Toxicology of Mercury and Its Compounds*. New York, Elsevier North-Holland, Inc, 1964.
10. Birke G, et al: Studies on humans exposed to methyl mercury through fish consumption. *Arch Environ Health* 1972; 25:77.
11. Browning E: *Toxicity of Industrial Metals*. London, Butterworths, 1961.
12. Clarkson TW: Biochemical aspects of mercury poisoning. *J Occup Med* 1968; 10:351.
13. Clarkson TW, et al: Excretion and absorption of methyl mercury after polythiol resin treatment. *Arch Environ Health* 1973; 26:176.
14. Danziger SJ, Possick PA: Metallic mercury exposure in scientific glassware manufacturing plants. *J Occup Med* 1973; 15:15.
15. Deichmann WB, Gerarde HW: *Toxicology of Drugs and Chemicals*. New York, Academic Press, 1969.
16. Derban LKA: Poisoning due to alkylmercury fungicide. *Arch Environ Health* 1974; 28:49.
17. Dinman BD: Organic mercury, *AMA Arch Ind Health* 1958; 18:248.
18. Dinman BD: in Horvath M: *Adverse Effects of Environmental Chemicals*, vol 1, *Functional Tests*. New York, Elsevier North-Holland Inc, 1973, p 165.

19. Friberg L: Kidney injury after chronic exposure to inorganic mercury. *AMA Arch Ind Hyg* 1953; 8:149.
20. Gage JC: The distribution and excretion of inhaled mercury vapor. *Br J Ind Med* 1961; 18:287.
21. Goldwater L, et al: Mercury exposure in a university laboratory. *AMA Arch Ind Health* 1956; 13:245.
22. Goldwater LJ, et al: Acute exposure to phenylmercuric acetate. *J Occup Med* 1964; 6:227.
23. Goldwater LJ, et al: Absorption and excretion of mercury in man, I-XIV. *Arch Environ Health* 1962; 17:39–43.
24. Goldwater LJ: Facts about mercury. *Arch Environ Health* 1971; 22:513.
25. Kershaw TG, et al: The relationship between blood levels and dose of methylmercury in man. *Arch Environ Health* 1980; 35:28.
26. Kramer I, Goldwater LJ: Investment casting by the frozen-mercury process. *AMA Arch Ind Health* 1956; 13:29.
27. Ladd AC, et al: Absorption and excretion of mercury in miners. *J Occup Med* 1966; 8:127.
28. Lauwerys RR, Bucket JP: Occupational exposure to mercury vapors and biological action. *Arch Environ Health* 1973; 27:65.
29. Levine SP, et al: Elemental mercury exposure: Peripheral neurotoxicity. *Br J Ind Med* 1982; 39:136.
30. Lewis L: Mercury poisoning in tungsten-molybdenum rod and wire manufacturing industry. *JAMA* 1945; 129:123.
31. Lovejoy HB, et al: Mercury, recommendations for medical evaluation of mercury exposed workers in the chlor-alkali industry. *J Occup Med* 1973; 15:340, 420, 501, 590, 647, 964.
32. Mastromatteo E: Recent occupational health experiences in Ontario. *J Occup Med* 1965; 7:502.
33. McCammon CS, et al: A comparison of four personal sampling methods for the determination of mercury vapor. *Am Ind Hyg Assoc J* 1980; 41:528.
34. McCammon CS, et al: An Evaluation of a passive monitor for mercury vapor. *Am Ind Hyg Assoc J* 1977; 38:378.
35. Miedler J, Forbers JD: Allergic contact dermatitis due to metallic mercury. *Arch Environ Health* 1968; 17:960.
36. Noe FE: Chronic mercurial intoxication. *Ind Med Surg* 1960; 29:559.
37. Nord PJ, et al: Mercury in human hair. *Arch Environ Health* 1973; 27:40.
38. Oyanguran H: Mercury poisoning among personnel of hospital laboratories. *Ind Med Surg* 1964; 33:468.
39. Putman JJ: Quicksilver and slow death. *Natl Geogr Mag* 1972; 144:507.
40. Stokinger HE: Mercury, in *Pattys' Industrial Hygiene and Toxicology*, ed 3. New York, Wiley-Interscience Publishing, 1981, vol 11A, p 1969.
41. US Dept. of Health and Human Services: NIOSH Recommendations for Occupational Safety and Health Standards. *MMWR* 1986; 35 (suppl 1).
42. Vigliani EC, Baldi G: Una insolita epidemia di mercurialismo in una fabbrica di cappelli di feltro. *Med Lav* 1949; 40:65.
43. Vostal JJ, Clarkson TW: Mercury as an environmental hazard. *J Occup Med* 1973; 15:649.
44. Wahlberg J: Absorption and excretion of toxic materials. Report of subcommittee on toxicology at meeting of Perma Comm Int Assoc Occup Health in Bulgaria, Sept 1971. *Nord Hyg Tidskr* 1971; 53:80.
45. West I, Lim J: Mercury poisoning among workers in California's mercury mills. *J Occup Med* 1968; 10:697.
46. Winter D, et al: The protective action of glutamic acid. *Arch Environ Health* 1968; 16:626.
47. Wood RW, et al: Hand tremor induced by industrial exposure to inorganic mercury. *Arch Environ Health* 1973; 26:249.
48. Woodcock SM: Case illustrating the effect of calcium disodium versenate on chronic mercury poisoning. *Br J Ind Med* 1958; 15:207.
49. Yamaguchi S, et al: Alkylmercury in caustic soda factory. *Arch Environ Health* 1971; 23:196.

39

Nickel and Its Compounds

Ernest Mastromatteo, M.D.

Nickel was first isolated in impure form in 1751 by Cronstedt from an ore containing niccolite (NiAs).[1] An ore of this type had earlier caused trouble in the smelting of copper and silver in Saxony, yielding an unusually brittle product. This interfering substance was referred to as "kupfernick" after "Old Nick" and his mischievous gnomes, and Cronstedt applied the name "nickel" to this new element. The pure metal was first prepared by Richter in 1804 and he described some of the useful properties of nickel.

Nickel is widely distributed in nature, forming about 0.008% of the earth's crust (0.01% in igneous rocks). Nickel ranks 24th among the elements in order of abundance on the earth; nickel is more abundant than copper, lead, and zinc. The core of the earth contains about 8.5% nickel. Meteorites have been found to contain 5%–50% nickel. Nickel is also an important constituent of deep-sea nodules, comprising about 1.5%. Nickel ores are of two main types: oxide ores (laterites) and sulfide ores.

Laterites are formed by the long-term weathering of igneous rocks which are rich in magnesia and iron and contain about 0.25% nickel. Water leaching over a long period of time removes the iron and magnesia, leaving a nickel-enriched residue. Some nickel is found as nickel magnesium silicate (garnierite).

Sulfide ores contain a mixture of metal sulfides, principally pentlandite ($(FeNi)_9S_8$), chalcopyrite ($CuFeS_2$), and pyrrhotite (Fe_7S_8) in varying proportions. Canada's sulfide ores in the Sudbury region of Ontario, Canada still provide a major share of the nickel used in the Western World. Other elements present in the Sudbury sulfide ores are also recovered, including copper, iron, cobalt, sulfur, selenium, tellurium, silver, gold, and metals of the platinum group.

Laterite deposits have been mined in many regions of the world, including New Caledonia, Cuba, the Dominican Republic, Indonesia, the Soviet Union, Greece, Colombia, the Philippines, and Guatemala. Laterite deposits in Oregon have been mined. The New Caledonia laterite deposits have been mined since 1873.

In addition to the major nickel sulfide ore body in the Sudbury area, sulfide ores are also mined in Manitoba, the Soviet Union, Australia, South Africa, Zimbabwe, and Finland.

Other nickel ores include the nickel-arsenicals and the nickel-antimonials, including NiAs, NiAsS, and NiSb, but these are of much less commercial importance.

MINING, SMELTING AND REFINING OF NICKEL

The main steps in the production of nickel metal and other nickel products from the sulfide and laterite deposits are shown in Figure 39–1 and Figure 39–2 respectively.

In earlier refining operations of the sulfide ores, high-temperature roasting by calcining and sintering operations were carried out on the impure nickel sulfide matte (now principally nickel subsulfide [Ni_3S_2]) to produce nickel oxide. These earlier operations—particularly open sintering—were very dusty. Later studies demonstrated that workers employed at calcining and sintering of nickel matte were at much higher risk of having cancer of the lung and nasal sinus develop. These operations were eliminated from nickel refinery operations by 1963, and now nickel matte roasting, where it is done, is done in enclosed fluid bed roasters.

Another early process used in nickel refining is the Mond process, named after the chemist who first discovered it. In this process, carbon monoxide gas is passed over finely divided nickel at 50° C, forming nickel tetracarbonyl ($Ni(Co)_4$), which is in turn decomposed above 60° C to yield high-purity nickel. This process has been in use in nickel refining since 1902. Nickel carbonyl is a very toxic gas and presumed by many early authors to be the carcinogen responsible for the increase in respiratory cancer among nickel refinery workers. The toxicity of nickel carbonyl will be dealt with in more detail later in this chapter.

Detailed information on the geology and worldwide distribution of nickel ores and on the mining, smelting and refining of nickel is provided in the definitive textbook on this subject, entitled *The Winning of Nickel*.[8]

PROPERTIES OF NICKEL

Nickel is a very silvery metal with an atomic weight of 58.7. It has a specific gravity of 8.9, a melting point of 1455° C and a boiling point of 2900° C. The metal is insoluble in hot or cold water. It is soluble in dilute nitric acid and only slightly soluble in hydrochloric and sulfuric acids. Nickel occurs in nature in the

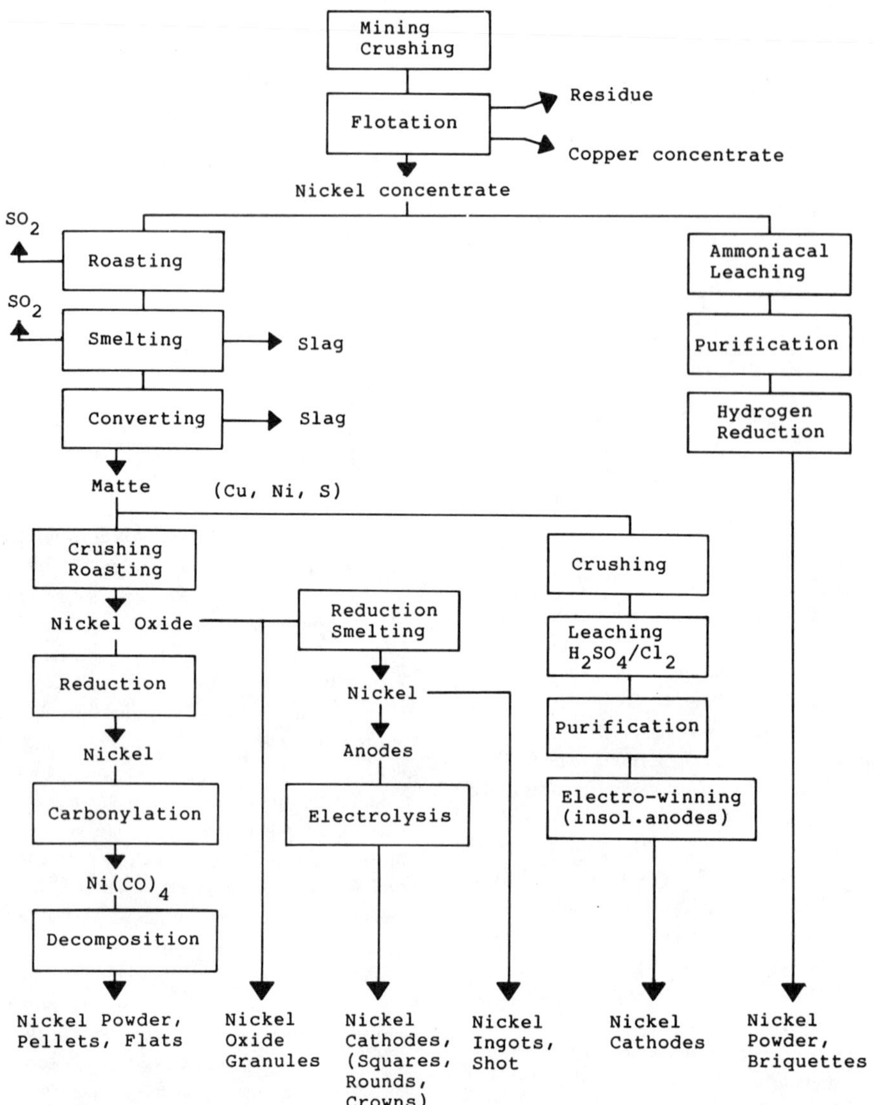

FIG 39–1.
Extraction and refining of nickel and compounds from sulfide ores.

zero-valent and divalent states. Other valence states are possible (−1, +1, +3, and +4), but these occur very infrequently.[3]

Nickel and its alloys are important because of their properties of hardness, toughness, and resistance to oxidation and corrosion. Nickel also has important magnetic properties.

USES OF NICKEL

When combined with other metals, nickel provides strength, corrosion resistance, and useful magnetic properties over a wide range of temperatures. The major uses of nickel include:

1. Production of stainless steels. There are many varieties of stainless steel. A common variety contains 8% nickel and 18% chromium.

2. Production of nickel alloys. The major nickel alloys include (a) nickel-copper (66.5% nickel; 30% copper), used for marine components, ship propellors, and desalination plants; (b) nickel-chromium (41.5%–73.0% nickel; 15.5%–30% chromium), used in jet engine parts, high temperature reaction vessels, furnaces, and heating elements for stoves; (c) nickel-iron-chromium (25.5%–42% nickel; 30%–46% iron; 18.5%–21.5% chromium), used for cryogenic purposes and storage of liquified gases; and (d) nickel-aluminum, used for permanent magnets.

3. Production of nickel cast iron.

4. Electroplating and electroforming. Nickel metal, nickel sulfate, nickel chloride, and nickel sulfamate are the main nickel products used in electroplating.

5. Manufacture of alkaline (nickel-cadmium) batteries.

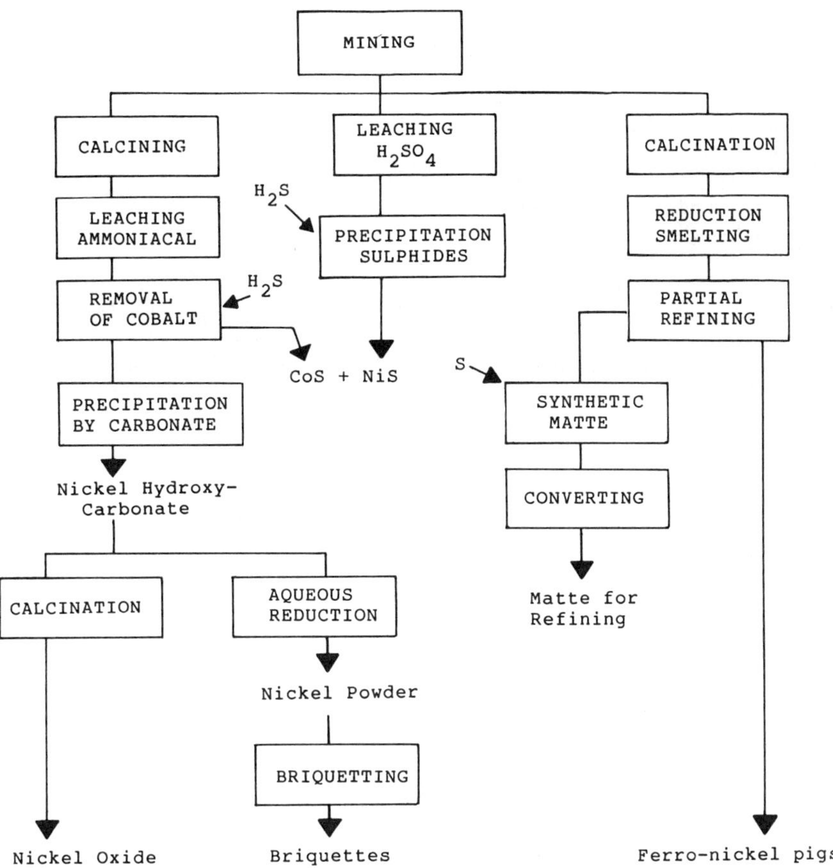

FIG 39–2.
Extraction and refining of nickel and compounds from oxide and silicate ores.

6. Catalyst uses. Raney metal is derived from an aluminum-nickel alloy (50% nickel; 50% aluminum). The alloy is ground and the aluminum removed by controlled leaching with caustic soda. The resulting product, now called Raney metal, is used as a catalyst for the hydrogenation of fats and oils. Nickel oxide and other compounds of nickel are used as catalysts. Other catalyst uses for nickel include desulfurization of oils, production of hydrocarbons by polymerization, and the production of ammonia.

7. Manufacture of coins. Nickel and nickel-copper alloys are mainly used.

8. Production of welding products including coated electrodes and filler wire for welding of nickel and high nickel alloys.

9. Production of sintered components. Nickel-containing ferrous alloys are widely used in the automotive industry. Nickel powders are used in some hard metal tools.

10. Inorganic pigments. Nickel has some use as an inorganic pigment for enamels and ceramics where resistance to high temperature and corrosion are important. An example of a typical pigment of this type is $(Ti,Ni,Sb)O_2$.

11. Electronic uses. Nickel containing compounds (ferrites) are used in electronic and computer equipment.

NICKEL IN THE GENERAL ENVIRONMENT

The general atmosphere in United States cities contains 0.02 μg Ni/cu m on average; rural areas average 0.006 μg Ni/cu m.[14] Small amounts of nickel are found in coal and petroleum. The combustion of these fossil fuels provides the major contribution to ambient nickel levels.

Public water supplies contain an average of 5 μg Ni/L. Seawater contains 0.1 to 0.5 μg/L.

Local airborne, soil, and surface concentrations of nickel are higher around those locations where nickel is mined, smelted, or refined or where high nickel alloys are produced or used. No adverse health effects among community residents, however, have been linked to these operations or to the low ambient levels of nickel present in air or water.

Nickel is also found in many foodstuffs, including tea, cocoa, baking soda, and some ground nuts. Dietary intake of nickel also results from the use of stainless steel cooking utensils. The use of nickel catalysts in hydrogenation may give rise to food residues containing nickel. Schroeder et al. in 1962[64] estimated that the average dietary intake of nickel in the United States was from 300 to 600 μg per day. This daily dietary intake is not associated with any known adverse health effect, except perhaps in some individ-

TABLE 39–1.
Occupational Exposure to Airborne Nickel*

OCCUPATIONAL GROUP	AIRBORNE NICKEL EXPOSURE (MG CU M)
1. Primary Production of Nickel	
Underground miners, sulfide mines	0.025
Open pit miners, laterite mines	0.05
Grinders and concentrating nickel	<0.05
Smelter workers	0.05–1.0
Nickel refinery workers	<1.0
Packaging nickel powders	<1.0
Discontinued calcining and sintering operations	25–30
Electrolytic tank house worker	0.02–0.3 (soluble forms)
Carbonyl refinery worker	<0.35 (gaseous form)
2. Uses of Nickel	
High nickel alloys	0.06–0.1
Manufacture and welding stainless steel	0.01–0.1
Nickel foundry workers	0.01–0.3
Electroplating of nickel	0.004–0.01 (soluble forms)
Nickel cadmium battery workers	0.4
Production wrought nickel	1.5

*Modified from Warner JS: Occupational exposure to airborne nickel in producing and using primary nickel products, in *Nickel in the Human Environment,* IARC Sci Publ 53. Lyon, France, International Agency for Research on Cancer, 1984, pp 419–437.

uals who have a marked skin or respiratory sensitivity to nickel. More study is needed on this. The United States Food and Drug Administration concluded, however, that the present levels of nickel residues in food should be categorized as a GRAS substance (generally recognized as safe).[28]

Dermatitis from exposure to nickel is fairly widespread among the general population. Up to 10% of persons seen in dermatologic practice, not occupationally exposed to nickel, show a positive reaction on skin patch testing with nickel sulfate. Most of these are women in whom the use of jewelry containing nickel, particularly pierced earrings, is believed to play the major part.

There are other aspects concerning exposure to nickel by the general public which are outside the scope of this chapter. For example, questions have been raised about the use of nickel in dental alloys and in surgical implants and the nickel content of dialysate fluids.

NICKEL IN THE OCCUPATIONAL ENVIRONMENT

The United States National Institute of Occupational Safety and Health (NIOSH) estimated that 250,000 workers in the United States were exposed to nickel and its inorganic compounds.[47] Exposures may occur at any stage in the production or use of nickel.

Warner[85] has documented the available information on occupational exposure to airborne nickel in its production and use. Some of this information is summarized in Table 39–1 for different nickel-exposed occupation groups.

These values should be compared with the current permissible exposure level of the Occupational Safety and Health Administration in the United States which is 1 mg/cu m for nickel metal and its inorganic compounds and 0.007 mg/cu m for nickel carbonyl.[84] The current threshold limit value[81] of the American Conference of Governmental Industrial Hygienists is as follows:

Nickel metal	1 mg/cu m
Nickel, soluble compounds as Ni	0.1 mg/cu m
Nickel carbonyl	0.35 mg/cu m
Nickel sulfide roasting, as Ni	1 mg/cu m A1a*

Because of the diversity of these exposures, the variety of nickel forms encountered, and the presence of other agents, the documentation of occupation exposure to nickel should include: (1) the concentration of the airborne dust and its nickel content; (2) the specific form or forms of nickel present; (3) the size range of the airborne particulates; (4) the presence of other contaminants, e.g., sulfur dioxide, polynuclear hydrocarbons, or asbestos fibers; and (5) the relationship of nickel and other airborne contaminants to their appropriate occupational exposure limits.

Reported Health Effects From Occupational Exposure to Nickel and Nickel Compounds

Reported and potential health effects as a result of occupational exposure to nickel metal and to inorganic compounds of nickel include: (1) increased risk of nasal sinus, lung, and possibly laryngeal cancer among nickel refinery workers; (2) increased risk of gastric cancer; (3) increased risk of sarcoma; (4) chronic irritation of the upper respiratory tract manifested by rhinitis, sinusitis, perforation of the nasal septum, and loss of the sense of smell; (5) pulmonary irritation and pulmonary fibrosis; (6) pneumoconiosis;

*The designation A1a denotes a human carcinogen.

(7) bronchial asthma; (8) increased susceptibility to respiratory infections; and (9) dermatitis.

Occasional accidental ingestion of nickel compounds, especially with relatively large amounts of the water-soluble forms, have given rise to acute effects. Nickel carbonyl gas, which is used in some refining operations, is highly toxic, producing pneumonitis.

Each of these repeated health effects is reviewed in this chapter with a distinction between occupational exposures in primary production, including refining of nickel, and those in the use of nickel and its compounds.

Acute Toxicity

The published information on the acute toxicity of nickel and nickel compounds is well documented and summarized in the United States National Academy of Sciences publication on nickel.[14]

Metallic nickel is relatively non-toxic on oral ingestion. Stokinger noted that dogs given 1–3 gm/kg body weight/day by mouth showed no apparent adverse effects.[69] Inorganic nickel compounds are well tolerated when given orally in rodents and other experimental animals in doses of about 500 mg/kg, although soluble salts give rise to gastric irritation. The acute oral LD_{50} was recently determined for a number of nickel compounds in Sprague-Dawley rats.[29] The results are shown in Table 39–2.

Soluble salts when administered intravenously, subcutaneously, intraperitoneally, or by any other parenteral route, are highly toxic. For example, the LD_{50} of nickel chloride in the rat is 11 mg/kg on intraperitoneal injection.

In the late 19th century nickel salts were used as oral therapeutic agents for rheumatism and epilepsy. Daily doses of nickel sulfate and nickel bromide of up to 500 mg daily were well tolerated in patients.[21]

TABLE 39–2.
Lethal Dose of Nickel Compounds Given Orally to Sprague-Dawley Rats*

FORM OF NICKEL	ORAL LD_{50} (MG/KG)
Ni metal powder	>9,000
Ferronickel (30% Ni)	>5,000
NiO, black	>5,000
NiO, green	>5,000
NiS, amorphous	>5,000
Ni_3S_2	>5,000
$Ni(OH)_2$	1,600
$NiCO_3 \cdot xH_2O$	1,044
$Ni(NH)_4(SO_4)_2$	420
$NiSO_4 \cdot 6H_2O$	300
$NiCl_2 \cdot 6H_2O$	200

*From Food and Drug Research Laboratory, Inc: Acute oral toxicity of seventeen nickel/cobalt samples in Sprague-Dawley rats. Report submitted to Nickel Producers Environmental Research Association, 1984.

NICKEL CARBONYL

Nickel carbonyl is a volatile liquid which is highly toxic. Exposure to airborne concentrations of about 30 parts per million (ppm) for 30 minutes may be lethal to humans. Initially, headache, discomfort, fatigue, weakness, nausea, vomiting, and influenza-type symptoms appear. These initial symptoms usually clear but may be followed in 12–36 hours by more severe symptoms similar to pneumonia, such as shortness of breath, pallor, chest pain, and difficulty in breathing. Nickel carbonyl causes a severe pneumonitis which may result in death, depending on the severity of exposure. The potentially high acute toxicity of nickel carbonyl is well recognized and appropriate precautions are necessary where nickel carbonyl is used.

The determination of nickel in urine provides a useful indication of the severity of exposure to nickel carbonyl and also serves as a guide to the treatment which should be given. Sunderman and Sunderman[75] have classified human exposure to nickel carbonyl based on the initial nickel determination in urine, as shown in Table 39–3.

Diethyldithiocarbamate (dithiocarb) is the chelating agent of choice to use in nickel carbonyl poisoning. Sunderman[72] developed a therapeutic regimen for the administration of dithiocarb in nickel carbonyl cases.

Sunderman et al. have reported that nickel carbonyl is a carcinogen in experimental exposure to rats.[71, 73, 74] The International Agency for Research on Cancer, however, did not consider that the evidence for carcinogenicity of nickel carbonyl in experimental animals was conclusive.[34] The American Conference of Governmental Industrial Hygienists Threshold Limit Value (TLV) Committee in 1975 raised the TLV of nickel carbonyl from 1 to 50 parts per billion (ppb) because the committee felt that nickel carbonyl had not been demonstrated to be a human carcinogen.[80] A recent unpublished study of nickel refinery workers "gassed" by nickel carbonyl showed no statistically significant increase in lung cancer incidence as a consequence of the gassing by nickel carbonyl.[45] The study cohort, however, is small.

TABLE 39–3.
Classification of Human Exposure to Nickel Carbonyl*

CLASSIFICATION	LEVEL OF NICKEL IN URINE
Mild	<10 μg/100 ml
Moderate	10–50 μg/100 ml
Severe	>50 μg/100 ml

*Modified from Sunderman FW, Sunderman FW Jr: Nickel poisoning. VII. Dithiocarb: A new therapeutic agent for persons exposed to nickel carbonyl. *Am J Med Sci* 1958; 236:26–31.

Dermatitis

Dermatitis in workers engaged in nickel-plating was first reported in 1889.[6] Samitz, writing the National Academy of Sciences document on nickel,[14] described two forms of nickel dermatitis—an eczematous contact dermatitis ("nickel itch") and atopic dermatitis. Nickel itch in platers is increased in the summer months when the temperature and humidity in the shops are high and there is increased sweating. Samitz noted that nickel dermatitis was seen infrequently as an occupational disease. Marcussen[42] studied 621 Danes with nickel dermatitis. Of these, 4% were nickel-platers, 9.5% had other occupational exposure to nickel, and 86.5% had nonoccupational exposures. Marcussen concluded that the risk of skin sensitization was greater from off-the-job exposure to nickel than from the workplace exposure. Other studies of patients with dermatitis show that about 7% reacted positively to patch testing with nickel sulfate.[67, 41] Raithel et al.[54] reported that 7.7% of occupational skin diseases noted in the Federal Republic of Germany in 1978 to 1981 were caused by exposure to nickel.

Cancer in Nickel Refinery Workers

Increased risk of occupational cancer has been reported among nickel refinery workers from Great Britain, Canada, Norway, Germany, New Caledonia, and the Soviet Union.

Great Britain.—The first reports of increased risk of nasal sinus cancer were noted in 1932 in workers from a nickel refinery in Clydach, Wales. This refinery began operations in 1902 using the Mond carbonyl process for refining nickel. Processes at Clydach involved crushing and grinding of nickel-copper matte received from Canada, calcining crushed matte to produce nickel and copper oxides, extracting copper by sulfuric acid, reduction of nickel oxide, and refining with nickel carbonyl. The matte received in Clydach varied. Before 1933 it contained 40%–45% nickel; after 1933 it contained 74% nickel. Since 1961, nickel oxide from fluid bed roasters has been directly refined by the carbonyl process.

The earliest epidemiologic study was carried out by Hill in 1939.[33] Hill found a relative risk of 22 for nasal cancer and 16 for lung cancer among the nickel refinery workers.

By 1949, 47 sinus and 82 lung cancer cases were known. In this year, cancer of the nasal cavities and cancer of the lung were designated as industrial diseases in Great Britain among nickel refinery workers "in any occupation in a factory where nickel is produced by decomposition of a gaseous nickel compound involving work in or about a building or buildings in which the process is carried out."[12]

Two epidemiologic studies were reported by Morgan[44] and Doll[22] in 1958. By this time 61 nasal and 131 lung cancer deaths in workers from this refinery were known. Morgan noted that there were no nasal cancer cases among workers entering employment after 1924. It is evident that the increased risk was sharply decreased, but not completely eliminated for lung cancer after 1924, as shown by later studies. Morgan suggested in his article that exposure to hot furnace dusts and not to nickel carbonyl was responsible for the increase in respiratory cancer. The reduction was attributed in part to the wearing of cotton gauze masks by furnace workers, the use of arsenic-free acid in refining, and improvements in ventilation. All of these changes began in the early 1920s.

Airborne concentrations of dust were very high in the early years. Air sampling in the early years was not complete but dust counts were done. These have been used to estimate average mass concentrations of dust, as shown in Table 39–4.

Follow-up studies were carried out by Doll and his associates on the men employed in the Clydach Nickel Refinery.[23, 24] Mortality from lung and sinus cancer and from all causes was analyzed by year of first employment. These authors concluded that the increased risk of respiratory cancer persisted until at least 1930, which accorded better with the process changes.

Morgan[45] carried out a study of 84 workers who had been gassed with nickel carbonyl and required medical treatment. Although the numbers involved are small, he found no significant difference in cancer incidence in this group with that expected on the basis of age and sex-specific national mortality rates. Cuckle and his colleagues[20] studied the causes of death in a small cohort of refinery workers exposed entirely or primarily to soluble salts of nickel. They found no sinus cancers. There was an increase in the lung cancer deaths, but the small size of the group limited this study.

Norway.—A nickel refinery began operations in Kristiansand, Norway, in 1910 and used Norwegian ore. In 1928 the refinery began processing nickel matte sent from Canada. The refinery was closed from 1940 to 1945. After the war, nickel sulfide matte was again sent from Canada for refining by the electrolytic process. Nickel carbonyl was not used at this Norwegian refinery.

In 1950 Løken[40] reported three cases of lung cancer among workers from this refinery. In 1973 Pedersen et al.[51] carried out an epidemiologic study. Workers employed in more than one department were classified by the department in which the longest time was spent. Norwegian Cancer Registry data were used to determine the expected number of cases, and mortality rates for Norway were used to determine the expected number of deaths. This study showed that workers in all the occupational groups had increased risk of developing cancers of the respiratory tract. The risk was greatest in workers in the roasting and smelting group and in the electrolysis group. In addition to lung and sinus cancer, the incidence of laryngeal cancer was increased in the roasting and smelting group.

Canada.—Calcining and, later, sintering of nickel sulfide matte and electrolytic refining operations were carried out in a nickel refinery in Port Colborne, Ontario, which commenced op-

TABLE 39–4.
Average Airborne Concentrations of Nickel Dust in Nickel Refining

NICKEL REFINERY OPERATION	DUST CONCENTRATION (AS Ni) (MG/CU M)
Grinding plant	25 (range 7 to 95.5)
Calciner	31.5
Carbonyl process dusts	6

erations in 1918. The nickel carbonyl process was not used. In 1959 Sutherland[77] on the Ontario Health Department studied a cohort of 2,355 refinery workers followed from 1930 to 1957. He found seven deaths from sinus cancer and 19 from lung cancer, giving relative risk ratios of 37:1 and 2:1, respectively, when compared to Ontario men. Sutherland analyzed the occupational exposures in his cohort and concluded that nearly all the excess deaths from sinus and lung cancer occurred in workers exposed to furnace dusts in calcining and sintering. Sintering was done on down-draft traveling grate sinter machines which operated at a temperature of 1,650° C. Sinter feed comprised nickel sulfide matte, recirculated sinter, and coke. The sintering operation was very dusty. Air sampling by the Ontario Department of Health on one occasion in 1953 showed an average concentration of 340 mg/cu m of total airborne dust. The Sutherland study was updated to cover the period 1930 to 1970.[49] By this time there were 24 sinus cancer and 76 lung cancer deaths.

At Copper Cliff, Ontario, sulfide ore has been smelted since 1888. In 1948 a sintering plant was installed at Copper Cliff. This sinter plant operated until April 1963 when the conversion to fluid bed roasters was completed.[48] The sintering operation was similar to that carried out in Port Colborne, with an average plant population of 500 workers over the years 1948–1963. The exposure was to hot dust from the conversion of impure nickel sulfide matte to nickel oxide. Dust sampling data are not available, but one sample from the sinter plant taken in 1960 showed a total airborne dust concentration of 46 mg/cu m. Sutherland carried out an epidemiologic study of 483 sinter plant workers.[76] Workers exposed five years or more showed a relative risk of 10.9 for lung cancer.

In 1971 Sutherland[78] carried out a study of 831 workers from the Copper Cliff complex, classified into five occupational groups—converter, mill and separation, copper refinery, underground mining, and mixed exposure. The study covered the period 1950–1967. It was carried out primarily to examine chronic respiratory disease in converter workers. The number of deaths from lung cancer was increased in all groups except the mixed exposure group, but the increase was not statistically significant.

Other sinter plants were also operated at Coniston and Falconbridge in Ontario. These plants were also very dusty but the operating temperatures were lower (1,000° to 1,100° C) and the product was nickel sulfide, not nickel oxide. Dust concentrations at Coniston varied from 5 to 125 mg/cu m of total airborne dust. There has been no evidence of any increased risk of respiratory cancer among these sinter workers.

In 1977, the NIOSH criteria document on nickel[47] concluded, ". . . in the absence of evidence to the contrary, nickel metal and all inorganic nickel compounds, when airborne, should be considered carcinogens." Should evidence show that this conclusion was invalid, NIOSH would reevaluate its conclusion.

The International Agency for Research on Cancer (IARC) has undertaken the evaluation of the carcinogenic risk of chemicals and chemical processes to humans. In 1973 IARC concluded, "In the past, there has been an excessive risk of cancers of the nasal sinus and lung among nickel refinery workers who inhaled nickel-containing dusts from crude ores. It is probable that nickel in some form is carcinogenic."[34] In the 1976 update,[35] IARC took note of the report by Ottolenghi et al.,[50] which showed pulmonary tumors in rats from inhalation of nickel subsulfide (Ni_3S_2). In 1979 IARC published a further reevaluation.[36] Chemicals and processes were divided into different categories depending on the quality of the evidence. Nickel refining was assigned to group 1 (sufficient evidence of carcinogenicity to men) and nickel metal and certain nickel compounds were assigned to group 2A (evidence "almost" sufficient).

In view of the NIOSH and IARC conclusions and recommendations, there was great need for additional epidemiologic and other studies to review the risks of occupational exposure to nickel in both the primary production and use of nickel. Since these reports, additional studies on Canadian refinery workers have been completed and these are briefly reviewed below.

Roberts and his colleagues[58–60] carried out a study of a large cohort of Inco workers with six months or more of employment history. Their cohort numbered 54,724 workers. The cohort was followed from 1950 to 1976. Mortality was ascertained and compared to that expected for Ontario men. The workers were divided into 14 occupational groups for analytic purposes. The study showed that the respiratory cancer exam was restricted to the sintering, calcining, and leaching occupational group. There was no excess among miners, concentrators, smelters, or other groups. These studies confirmed the original conclusions that the excess respiratory cancer risk was restricted to specific operations.

A similar study was carried out in a cohort in 11,594 Ontario Falconbridge workers.[65] High temperature sintering and calcining were never carried out in the Ontario operations of this company. This study showed no excess of sinus or lung cancer. The matte produced in Ontario was shipped to Norway for refining and it was in Norway that the increased risk of sinus and lung cancer were noted.

A major study of mortality of hard rock miners in Ontario[46] showed no excess of respiratory cancer among nickel-copper miners, whereas uranium and gold miners showed an excess of lung cancer.

Other recent studies of nickel refinery workers have been reported. Egedahl and Rice[25] found no excess of respiratory cancer among a cohort of 720 workers employed in a nonpyrometallurgical nickel refinery. Cooper and Wong[17] studied a cohort of 1,307 workers employed in a U.S. laterite operation in Oregon. No excess of respiratory cancer was found.

Soviet Union.—Saknyn and Shabynina in 1970[63] reported an increase in lung and gastric cancer in nickel refinery workers in a U.S.S.R. plant in the Urals. The refinery was engaged in the preparation of nickel oxide ore, roasting, and smelting. The authors found that the relative risk ratio of lung cancer was 1.8:1 compared to residents of a nearby city. They also found that the death rate from sarcomas was increased eightfold. Tatarskaya[79] reported two cases of sinus cancer among workers engaged in electrolytic refining of nickel. He reported development of nasal irritation and anosmia in workers exposed to aerosols containing nickel from the electrolytic refining operations. Znamenskii[88] noted "many" cases of lung cancer and "several" cases of sinus cancer among workers employed in extracting and processing nickel ore.

The reports from the Soviet Union, unfortunately, lack sufficient details for critical analysis.

German Democratic Republic.—Rockstroh[61] reported that there was an increase in lung cancer in a nickel smelting plant. Forty-five cases of lung cancer were reported between 1928 and

1956. The workers, however, were also exposed to arsenic, cobalt, copper, bismuth, benzopyrene, and other chemicals.

France.—A nickel refinery has been located at Le Havre for about 100 years. There have been no reports of increase in sinus or lung cancer from workers of this refinery, but no formal epidemiologic study has been done. This refinery treated a nickel sulfide matte made from laterite ore.

New Caledonia.—Laterite ores have been mined and smelted in New Caledonia for a long time. Lessard et al.[39] carried out a case control study of lung cancer cases. They concluded that increased risk of lung cancer was associated with cigarette smoking, proximity of residence of a nickel smelter, and employment in the nickel smelter. Goldberg and colleagues[31, 32] carried out a major and more detailed study of the New Caledonia workers and reported no excess of respiratory cancer.

Cancer in Workers Using Nickel

Reference has been made earlier to occupational exposure to nickel in other operations such as the production and use of high-nickel alloys, manufacture of stainless steels, nickel plating, and welding, grinding, and pickling of nickel alloys and stainless steels. Epidemiologic studies in such groups of workers have been few. There is also some difficulty in assessing these exposures, because they commonly involve exposure to other substances, e.g., to hexavalent chromium in electroplating and in welding stainless steel.

Because of the NIOSH conclusion and the 1979 IARC reevaluation cited above, the need for studies among nickel users was apparent. These studies are reviewed below.

Nickel Powder.—Godbold and Tompkins[30] carried out a long-term study of 814 workers exposed to finely divided nickel powder of respirable size. This cohort was followed from 1948 to 1972. There was no evidence of increased risk of respiratory cancer in this cohort. Cragle et al.[19] extended the study period from 1948 to 1977 and again found no evidence of any increase in respiratory cancer.

High Nickel Alloy Manufacture.—Nickel alloys are produced in a plant in Huntington, West Virginia, since operations began in 1922. Enterline carried out a study of 815 retired workers.[26] He found two deaths from sinus cancer. There was an increased relative risk from lung cancer shown, but this was not statistically significant. Enterline and Marsh[27] studied a cohort of 1,852 workers who worked at least one year at this plant prior to January 1, 1948. There was no significant increase in deaths from lung cancer in any of the five occupational groups studied. Three deaths from sinus cancer were found, including the two reported earlier by Enterline. The three workers who died of sinus cancer worked during the period 1922–1948, when calcining of impure nickel sulfide matte was done at Huntington—the same calcining operation as carried out at Clydach, Wales, and at Port Colborne and Copper Cliff, Ontario. There was no excess of lung cancer among the high-nickel alloy plant workers; there was an excess of sinus cancers that was related to the earlier sintering operations.

Redmond[55] reported on a cohort mortality study of over 28,000 workers in 12 U.S. plants producing high-nickel alloys. No excess of nasal or lung cancer was found.

Cox et al.[18] studied a cohort of 1,925 men engaged in high-nickel alloy production. He found no sinus cancer or increase in lung cancer.

Nickel Plating.—The Registrar-General in the U.K.[57] has reported a significant increase in the proportion of deaths due to cancer of the lung and intestine, which could not be explained by social class differences, in "electroplaters, dip platers and related workers." No specific exposure information is available.

A proportionate mortality study was carried out in U.S. platers, polishers, and buffers. Deaths were identified by union obituary notices and death certificates obtained. Proportionate mortality for esophageal and liver cancer was increased but not for lung or sinus cancer.[7]

The principal difficulty with the studies reported above is the assessment of health effects due to nickel where there is concomitant exposure to other substances such as chromium, acid mist, alkali mist, and other chemicals used in the plating industry. Plating baths may give rise to aerosols of soluble nickel. Workers engaged in buffing and polishing in electroplating shops would be exposed to metallic nickel, nickel oxide, and abrasive dusts.

Burges of the U.K. Employment Advisory Service studied 900 nickel platers. He found no cases of sinus cancer, but he identified a statistically significant excess in stomach cancer.[11] He cautioned that the study was limited because of its size.

Welding on Nickel and Nickel-Alloys.—The Registrar General in the U.K.[57] reported an increase in the proportion of deaths due to lung cancer in gas and electric welders and cutters. This increase was, however, not statistically significant.

Stern in Denmark[68] collected fume from arc welding of stainless steel. This fume was tested by the Ames microbiologic assay system and found to be positive. Stern felt that hexavalent chromium, present in the fume, was likely responsible, but nickel has not been ruled out.

Sjögren[66] and Polednak[53] studied mortality in nickel-exposed welders and did not find increases in sinus or lung cancer. Both these studies have marked limitation because of sample size and methodology. At present, there is no evidence of increased risk of lung cancer in welders exposed to nickel. Peto[52] noted that lung cancer studies in welders are confounded by differences in cigarette smoking and by exposure to asbestos in shipyard welding.

Stainless Steel Manufacture.—Redmond[56] analyzed the existing computerized records for the Allegheny County Steelworkers Study. She found no cases of sinus cancers among those members of the cohort engaged in stainless steel manufacture. Lung cancer was not increased in this group, but the data were not considered too reliable.

Cornell[15] studied proportional mortality in 4,487 deaths in workers from seven U.S. plants engaged in the production of stainless steel and low-nickel alloy steels. There were no cases of sinus cancer nor any excess of lung cancer.

Nickel/Chromium Foundry Work.—Cornell and Landis[16] carried out a proportional mortality study of all deaths occurring in 26 U.S. foundries from 1968 to 1979. The mortality experience of 851 foundry workers exposed to nickel/chromium was compared to that of 141 not so exposed. No excess of respiratory cancer was found in the nickel-chromium exposed group.

Exposure to Soluble Nickel Salts.—Mention has already been made of the study of Clydach refinery workers engaged in the manufacture of soluble nickel salts.[42] Workers from this plant showed no deaths from sinus cancer. The deaths from lung cancer were not significantly different from that of United Kingdom men.

Workers producing soluble nickel salts also have exposure to insoluble forms of nickel, principally the metal and oxide, and some had previous exposure to nickel refinery operations.

Other Nickel Exposures.—Tsuchiya[83] carried out a proportionate mortality study by occupational groups, and he reported a significant increase in lung cancer among nickel-exposed workers. The nickel exposures were described only in general terms. It is difficult to draw conclusions about nickel from this study.

Bernacki et al.[4] carried out a retrospective case control mortality study of all known lung cancers occurring in workers in a large aircraft factory using high-nickel alloys. The workers were exposed to nickel in welding, plating, grinding, buffing, and melting of nickel and its alloys. Bernacki found that nickel exposure was not associated with any increase in the risk of developing lung cancer in workers.

Rousch et al.,[62] using data from the Connecticut Tumor Registry and from city directories, determined the occupational exposures of individuals reported to have cancer of the nasal sinuses for the years 1950 to 1975. The author found no increase in nasal sinus cancer in occupations classified as having nickel exposure, whereas there was a significant increase in those occupations with exposure to wood dust and to oil mist.

As noted earlier, Blair[7] did a proportional mortality study of union members engaged in metal polishing and nickel finishing. No excess of lung or sinus cancer was found.

Burch et al.[10] carried out a case control study of 204 patients with laryngeal cancer and 204 neighborhood controls. Exposure to nickel was examined and no association was found between nickel exposure and laryngeal cancer. An association was found with smoking and with exposure to asbestos.

Individual Case Reports.—Sinus cancer has been reported in individual case history reports. One case occurred in a worker engaged in buffing and grinding stainless steel knives and forks.[9] Another occurred in a worker involved in nickel electroplating operations.[70] It is impossible to determine whether these cases occurred as isolated episodes or as a result of exposure to nickel.

Nasal Effects

Tatarskaya[79] and Kicharin[38] have reported nasal irritation, damage to the nasal mucosa, perforation of the nasal septum, and loss of smell in workers exposed to nickel aerosols. Such reports are not common. Often it is difficult to rule out the effects of other contaminants.

Asthma

Asthmatic illness has been attributed to exposure to nickel[13, 43, 82] in the form of individual case reports. Despite the widespread use of nickel throughout the industry, respiratory allergy to nickel is uncommon. In the report by Tolot et al.[82] there was mixed exposure to chromium and aniline as well. It is likely, however, that specific episodes of asthma from exposure to nickel have occurred.

Pulmonary Fibrosis (Pneumoconiosis)

A few authors have reported that workers inhaling nickel dusts develop pulmonary changes with fibrosis.[87, 37] In view of the widespread use of nickel in industry, it does not appear that the inhalation of nickel-containing dusts gives rise to a specific pneumoconiosis or to chronic respiratory disease. There have been no specific epidemiologic studies on chronic pulmonary disease in nickel workers, apart from lung cancer. A number of mortality studies in nickel refinery workers, however, do not indicate any increase in the relative risk ratio for nonmalignant respiratory disease,[22, 44, 48, 77] except for those exposed to sulfur dioxide in smelting sulfide ores.[78]

WORKER HEALTH SURVEILLANCE

The purpose of health surveillance of workers is to identify at as early a stage as possible any variation in the health of employees which may be related to their working conditions, including their exposure to nickel and nickel compounds. The individual worker or groups of workers should benefit from the health surveillance procedures included in the program by showing reduced morbidity or mortality. Health surveillance procedures should not be offered or used as a substitute for proper environmental control measures. Only those procedures that are relevant to the industry or processes should be adopted. Continuing assessment should be made of the validity of the current health surveillance procedures and the applicability of new surveillance procedures as they become available.

Health surveillance programs include initial and periodic examinations supplemented by additional tests and procedures as appropriate, including biologic monitoring, chest radiography, sputum cytology, patch testing, and pulmonary function testing.

Good records are vital to all systems of health surveillance. These records should be accurate, readily retrievable, and maintained in a confidential fashion.

For any health surveillance program it is necessary to know what adverse health effects may be expected in exposed workers, whether these changes can be reliably detected and measured, whether there are remedial actions available to reverse or arrest these changes, and whether there are available resources for the program.

For the purpose of inclusion in any surveillance program, a "nickel worker" should be defined; all workers exposed to nickel and nickel compounds at 50% or more of the applicable exposure limits may be defined as "nickel workers."

The following are suggested for consideration in the health surveillance of nickel workers:

Initial Health Assessment

The initial health assessment should include:

1. A detailed occupational history
2. Specific reference to skin and respiratory system conditions
3. Smoking history
4. Family history
5. Assessment of the individual's ability to wear respiratory protection where necessary
6. A base-line chest x-ray

Routine initial skin testing for nickel sensitivity is not recommended. The routine use of a validated respiratory disease questionnaire and pulmonary function testing is not recommended. The latter procedures may be used if desired for base-line information. The determination of nickel in plasma and serum is feasible, but the significance of such measurements to possible long-term health effects has not been established. If it is decided to include biologic monitoring for nickel, it should be clearly indicated to individuals in the work force that, at present, biologic measurements cannot be related to health effects.[88] As noted above, however, urinary nickel levels are useful in assessing the severity of exposure to nickel carbonyl and the treatment regimen for overexposure to this nickel compound.

Periodic and Special Health Assessments

Periodic and special health assessments should include:

1. The reporting of skin and respiratory complaints, plus any other condition the worker feels may be associated with nickel exposure

2. Periodic assessment of sickness absence records, with special note of skin and respiratory tract conditions

3. Review of workers on return to work after prolonged or repeated sickness absence and assessment of fitness to return to work in exposure to nickel or nickel compounds

4. Skin tests for workers who develop dermatitis (usually 0.5% nickel sulfate) and, if positive for nickel, alternative employment provided, where available

5. A validated respiratory disease questionnaire and pulmonary function testing for workers who develop allergic asthma or who are suspected to be at increased risk of developing allergic asthma

With regard to the health surveillance of workers believed to be at greater risk of developing nasal sinus and lung cancer (e.g., former sinter plant workers), chest radiography, sputum cytology and nasal biopsy have not been found to satisfy the criteria for routine screening procedures.[86] Aitio[2] also noted that cytogenic methods do not seem appropriate for assessing risk or exposure in nickel workers. Cytogenic methods including chromosome gaps requires further research as surveillance procedures.

REFERENCES

1. Adamec JB, Kihlgren TE: Nickel and nickel alloys, in *Kirk-Othmer Encyclopedia of Chemical Technology*, ed 2. New York, Interscience Publishers, 1967, vol 13, pp 735–753.
2. Aitio A: Biological monitoring of occupational exposure to nickel, in *Nickel in the Human Environment, IARC Sci Publ* 53. Lyon France, International Agency for Research on Cancer, 1984, pp 497–505.
3. Antonsen DH, Springer DB: Nickel compounds, in *Kirk-Othmer Encyclopedia of Chemical Technology*, ed 2. New York, Interscience Publishers, 1967, vol 13, pp 753–765.
4. Bernacki EJ, Parsons GE, Sunderman FW Jr: Investigation of exposure to nickel and lung cancer mortality: Case control study at an aircraft engine factory. *Ann Clin Lab Sci* 1978; 8:190–194.
5. Bishop CM: Health surveillance of workers exposed to nickel and its compounds, in Brown SS, Sunderman FW Jr (eds): *Progress in Nickel Toxicology*. Cambridge, University Press, 1985, pp 227–230.
6. Blaschko A: Occupational dermatosis—Contribution to industrial hygiene. *Dtsch Med Wochenschr* 1889; 15:925–927 (German).
7. Blair A: Mortality among workers in metal polishing and plating industry. *J Occup Med* 1980; 22:158–162.
8. Boldt JR Jr, Queneau P: *The Winning of Nickel*. Toronto, Longmans Canada Limited, 1967.
9. Bourasset A, Galland G: Carcinoma of the respiratory tract and exposure to nickel salts. *Arch Mal Prof Med Trav Secur Soc* 1966; 27:227–229.
10. Burch JO, Howe GR, Miller AB: Tobacco, alcohol, asbestos and nickel in the etiology of cancer of the larynx: A case control study. *J Natl Cancer Inst* 1981; 67:1219–1224.
11. Burges DCL: Mortality study of nickel platers, in Brown SS, Sunderman FW Jr (eds): *Nickel Toxicology*. London, Academic Press, 1980, pp 15–18.
12. Cancer of the nasal cavities and lung in nickel refinery workers. Great Britain, Industrial Injuries Act, 1949.
13. Cirla AM, Bernabeo F, Ottoboni F, et al: Nickel induced occupational asthma: Immunological and clinical aspects, in Brown SS, Sunderman FW Jr (eds): *Progress in Nickel Toxicology*. Cambridge, University Press, 1985, pp 165–168.
14. Committee on Medical and Biologic Effects of Environmental Pollutants: *Nickel*. Washington, DC, National Academy of Sciences, National Research Council, Division of Medical Sciences, 1975.
15. Cornell RG: Mortality patterns among stainless steel workers, in *Nickel in the Human Environment, IARC Sci Publ* 53. Lyon, France, International Agency for Research on Cancer, 1984, pp 65–71.
16. Cornell RG, Landis JR: Mortality patterns among nickel/chromium alloy foundry workers, in *Nickel in the Human Environment, IARC Sci Publ* 53. Lyon, France, International Agency for Research on Cancer, 1984, pp 87–93.
17. Cooper WC, Wong O: *A Study of Mortality in a Population of Nickel Miners and Smelter Workers*. Riddle, Ore, a report to the Hanna Nickel Smelting Company, 1981.
18. Cox JE, Doll R, Scott WA, et al: Mortality of nickel workers: Experience with men working with metallic nickel. *Br J Ind Med* 1981; 38:235–239.
19. Cragle DL, Hollis DR, Newport TH: A retrospective cohort mortality study among workers occupationally exposed to metallic nickel powder at the Oak Ridge Gaseous Diffusion Plant, in *Nickel in the Human Environment, IARC Sci Publ* 53. Lyon, France, International Agency for Research on Cancer, 1985, pp 57–63.

20. Cuckle H, Doll R, Morgan LG: Mortality study of men working with soluble nickel compounds, in Brown SS, Sunderman FW Jr (eds): *Nickel Toxicology*. London, Academic Press, 1980, pp 11–14.
21. DaCosta JM: Observations on the salts of nickel especially the bromide of nickel. *Med News* 1883; 43:337–338.
22. Doll R: Cancer of the lung and nose in nickel workers. *Br J Ind Med* 1958; 15:217–223.
23. Doll R, Mathews JD, Morgan LG: Cancers of the lung and nasal sinuses in nickel workers: A reassessment of the period of risk. *Br J Ind Med* 1977; 34:102–105.
24. Doll R, Morgan LG, Speizer FE: Cancer of the lung and nasal sinuses in nickel workers. *Br J Ind Med* 1970; 24:623–632.
25. Egedahl R, Rice E: Cancer incidence at a hydrometallurgical nickel refinery, in *Nickel in the Human Environment, IARC, Sci Publ* 53. Lyon, France, International Agency for Research on Cancer, 1984, pp 47–55.
26. Enterline PE: A study of the mortality and disability experience of workers from a nickel plant. Unpublished report submitted to the National Institute for Occupational Safety and Health by PE Enterline, November, 1976.
27. Enterline PE, Marsh GM: Mortality among workers in a nickel refinery and alloy manufacturing plant in West Virginia. *J Natl Cancer Inst* 1982; 68:925–933.
28. *Evaluation of the Health Aspects of Nickel as a Food Ingredient*, Contract FDA 223-75-2004. Bethesda, Md, Life Sciences Research Office, Federation of American Societies for Experimental Biology, 1979.
29. Food & Drug Research Laboratory, Inc: Acute oral toxicity of seventeen nickel/cobalt samples in Sprague-Dawley rats. Report submitted to Nickel Producers Environmental Research Association, 1984.
30. Godbold JH, Tompkins EA: A long-term mortality study of workers occupationally exposed to metallic nickel in the Oak Ridge Gaseous Diffusion Plant. *J Occup Med* 1979; 21:799–806.
31. Goldberg P, Blanc M, Fuhrer R, et al: Incidence of respiratory cancers among workers in a factory extracting and refining nickel and in the general population in New Caledonia, in Brown SS, Sunderman FW Jr (eds): *Progress in Nickel Toxicology*. Cambridge, University Press, 1985, pp 211–214.
32. Goldberg M, Fuhrer R, Brodeur J-M, et al: Cancer of the respiratory passages among workers of a factory extracting and refining nickel in New Caledonia: A case control study within a cohort, in Brown SS, Sunderman FW Jr (eds): *Progress in Nickel Toxicology*. Cambridge, University Press, 1985, pp 215–218.
33. Hill AB: Unpublished 1939 report to the Mond Nickel Company submitted to NIOSH by the International Nickel Company Limited, Toronto, 1976.
34. International Agency for Research on Cancer: Nickel and inorganic nickel compounds. *IARC Monogr Eval Carcinog Risk Chemi Man* 1973; 2:126–149.
35. International Agency for Research on Cancer: Nickel and nickel compounds. *IARC Monogr Eval Carcinog Risk Chemi Man* 1976; 2:75–112.
36. International Agency for Research on Cancer: *IARC Monographs*, Vol 1–20. *Chemicals and Industrial Processes Associated with Cancer in Humans*, IARC Monograph Suppl 1. Lyon, France, IARC, 1979.
37. Jones JG, Warner CG: Chronic exposure to iron oxide, chromium oxide, and nickel oxide fumes in metal dressers in a steelworks. *Br J Ind Med* 1972; 29:168–177.
38. Kicharin GM: Occupational disorders of the nose and nasal sinuses in workers of an electrolytic nickel refining plant. *Gig Tr Prof Zabol* 1970; 14:38–40 (Russian).
39. Lessard R, Reed D, Maheux B: Lung cancer in New Caledonia, a nickel smelting island. *J Occup Med* 1978; 20:815–817.
40. Løken AC: Lung cancer in nickel workers. *Tidsski Nor Laegeforen* 1950; 70:376–378 (Norwegian).
41. Malten KE, Fregert S, Bandmann HJ, et al: Occupational dermatitis in five European dermatological departments. *Berufs-Dermatosen* 1971; 19:1–14.
42. Marcussen PV: Ecological considerations on nickel dermatitis. *Br J Ind Med* 1960: 17:65–68.
43. McConnell LH, Fink JN, Schleuter DP, et al: Asthma caused by nickel sensitivity. *Ann Intern Med* 1973; 78:888–890.
44. Morgan JG: Some observations on the incidence of respiratory cancer in nickel workers. *Br J Ind Med* 1958; 15:224–234.
45. Morgan LG: Personal communication, 1979.
46. Muller J, Kusiak R, Suranuyi G: Ontario Miners Mortality Study Report to the Governments of Ontario and Canada. Ontario, Canadian Government Department of Mines, 1983.
47. National Institute for Occupational Safety and Health: *Criteria for a Recommended Standard for Occupational Exposure to Inorganic Nickel*. Washington, DC, NIOSH, Dept of Health, Education and Welfare, 1977.
48. *Nickel and Its Inorganic Compounds (Including Nickel Carbonyl)*. Unpublished report submitted to NIOSH by the International Nickel Company of Canada Limited and International Nickel (US) Incorporated, 1976.
49. *Nickel and Its Inorganic Compounds (Including Nickel Carbonyl)*. Unpublished supplementary report submitted to NIOSH by International Nickel Company of Canada Limited and International Nickel (US) Incorporated, 1976.
50. Ottolenghi AD, Haseman JK, Payne WW, et al: Inhalation studies of nickel sulfide in pulmonary carcinogenesis of rats. *J Natl Cancer Inst* 1974; 54:1165–1172.
51. Pedersen E, Hogetveit AC, Andersen A: Cancer of the respiratory organs among workers at a nickel refinery in Norway. *Int J Cancer* 1973; 12:32–41.
52. Peto J: Lung cancers in welders. Paper presented to International Conference on Health Hazards in Welding, Copenhagen, Denmark, 1985.
53. Polednak AP: Mortality among welders, including a group exposed to nickel oxide. *Arch Environ Health* 1981; 36:235–242.
54. Raithel HJ, Schaller KH, Valentin H: Medical and toxicological aspects of occupational nickel exposure in the Federal Republic of Germany—Clinical results (carcinogenicity, sensitization) and preventive measures (biological monitoring), in *Nickel in the Human Environment, IARC Sci Publ* 53. Lyon, France, International Agency for Research on Cancer, 1984.
55. Redmond CK: Site-specific cancer mortality among workers involved in the production of high nickel alloys, in *Nickel in the Human Environment, IARC Scientific Publ* 53. Lyon, France, International Agency for Research on Cancer, 1984, pp 73–86.
56. Redmond CK: Respiratory disease in stainless steel workers. Unpublished report submitted to Inco Limited, 1978.
57. Registrar-General: *The Registrar-General's Decennial Supplement for England and Wales 1970–1972*. *Occupational Mortality Tables*. London, Register General, 1978.
58. Roberts RS, Julian JA: Mortality studies in Ontario nickel workers, in Brown SS, Sunderman FW Jr (eds): *Nickel Toxicology*. London, Academic Press, 1980, pp 27–30.
59. Roberts RS, Julian JA: Mortality study of Canadian nickel miners, in Wagner WL, Rom WN, Merchant JA (eds): *Health Issues Related to Metal and Nonmetallic Mining*. Woburn, Mass, Butterworth Publishers, 1983, pp 241–260.
60. Roberts RS, Julian JA, Muir DCF, et al: Cancer mortality associated with the high-temperature oxidation of nickel subsulfide, in *Nickel in the Human Environment, IARC Sci Publ* 53. Lyon, France, International Agency for Research on Cancer, 1984, pp 23–35.

61. Rockstroh H: On the etiology of bronchial cancer in arsenic processing nickel smelting plants. *Arch Gesch wulstforsch* 1959; 14:151–162 (German).
62. Rousch GL, Meigs JW, Kelly J, et al: Sinonasal cancer and occupation: A case control study. *Am J Epidemiol* 1980; 111:183–193.
63. Saknyn AC, Shabynina NK: Some statistical materials on carcinogenic hazards in the production of nickel on an ore oxide base. *Gig Tr Prof Zabol* 1970; 14:10–13 (Russian).
64. Schroeder HA, Balassa JJ, Tipton IH: Abnormal trace elements in man—Nickel. *J Chron Dis* 1962; 15:51–65.
65. Shannon HS, Julian JA, Muir DCF, et al: A mortality study of Falconbridge workers, in *Nickel in the Human Environment, IARC Sci Publ* 53. Lyon, France, International Agency for Research on Cancer, 1984, pp 117–124.
66. Sjögren B: A retrospective cohort study of mortality among stainless steel welders. *Scand J Work Environ Health* 1980; 6:197–200.
67. Skog E, Thyresson N: The occupational significance of some common contact allergens. *Acta Derm Venereol* 1953; 33:65–74.
68. Stern RM: A chemical, physical and biological assay of welding fumes. Report of the Danish Welding Institute, Copenhagen, 1977.
69. Stokinger HE: Nickel in Clayton GD, Clayton F (eds): *Patty's Industrial Hygiene and Toxicology*. New York, John Wiley & Sons, New York, pp 1820–1841.
70. Sunderman FW Jr: The current status of nickel carcinogenesis. *Ann Clin Lab Sci* 1973; 3:156–180.
71. Sunderman FW: Metastasizing pulmonary tumors in rats induced by the inhalation of nickel carbonyl, in Seviri L (ed): *Lung Tumors in Animals*, 1985. Proceedings of the third quadrenial conference on cancer, University of Perugia, June 24–29, 1965, Perugia, Italy.
72. Sunderman FW Jr: The treatment of acute nickel carbonyl poisoning with sodium diethyldithiocarbonate. *Ann Clin Res* 1971; 3:182–185.
73. Sunderman FW, Donnelly AJ: Studies of nickel carcinogenesis. Metastasizing pulmonary tumors in rats induced by the inhalation of nickel carbonyl. *Am J Path* 1965; 46:1027–1041.
74. Sunderman FW, Donnelly AJ, West B, et al: Nickel poisoning IX. Carcinogenesis in rats exposed to nickel carbonyl. *AMA Arch Ind Health* 1959; 20:36–41.
75. Sunderman FW, Sunderman FW Jr: Nickel poisoning VIII. Dithiocarb: A new therapeutic agent for persons exposed to nickel carbonyl. *Am J Med Sci* 1958; 236:26–31.
76. Sutherland RB: *Mortality Among Sinter Workers—International Nickel Company of Canada, Copper Cliff Smelter*. Toronto, Ontario Department of Health, 1969.
77. Sutherland RB: *Mortality Among Sinter Workers—International Nickel Company of Canada, Limited, Port Colborne Nickel Refinery*. Toronto, Ontario Department of Health, 1969.
78. Sutherland RB: *Morbidity and Mortality in Selected Occupations at the International Nickel Company of Canada Limited; Copper Cliff, Ontario 1950–1967*. Toronto, Ontario Department of Health, 1969.
79. Tartarskaya AD: Occupational diseases of upper respiratory tracts in persons employed in electrolytic refining departments. *Gig Tr Prof Zabol* 1960; 6:35–38 (Russian).
80. *Threshold Limit Values for Chemical Substances and Physical Agents in the Workroom Environment With Intended Changes for 1975*. Cincinnati, Oh, American Conference of Governmental Industrial Hygienist, 1975.
81. *Threshold Limit Values for Chemical Substances in the Work Environment Adopted by ACGIH with Intended Changes for 1986–1987*. Cincinnati, Oh, American Conference of Governmental Industrial Hygienists, 1986.
82. Tolot F, Brodeur P, Neulat G: Asthmatic forms of lung disease in workers exposed to chromium, nickel and aniline inhalation. *Arch Mal Prof Trav Secur Soc* 1956; 18:291–293
83. Tsuchiya K: The relationship of occupation to cancer, especially cancer of the lung. *Cancer* 1965; 18:136–144.
84. United States (1979) CFR Title 29, Chap 17, Pt 1910, Subpart Z.
85. Warner JS: Occupational exposure to airborne nickel in producing and using primary nickel products, in *Nickel in the Human Environment, IARC Sci Publ* 53. Lyon, France, International Agency for Research on Cancer, 1984, pp 419–437.
86. World Health Organization: Lung cancer: Epidemiology, treatment, prevention. Reappraisal of the present situation in prevention and control of lung cancer. *Bull WHO* 1982; 60:809–819.
87. Zislin DM, Ganjuskina SM, Dubilina ES, et al: Residual pulmonary volume in the complex assessment of the functional state of the respiratory system in the initial stage of pneumoconiosis and suspected pneumoconiosis. *Gig Tr Prof Zabol* 1969; 13:26–29 (Russian).
88. Znamenskii SV: Occupational bronchogenic cancers in workers extracting, isolating and reprocessing nickel ore. *Vop Onkol* 1963; 9:130 (Russian).

40

The Rare Earths

Arthur L. Knight, M.D.

OCCURRENCE AND CHEMICAL PROPERTIES

The term *rare earths* usually refers to the lanthanum series (atomic numbers 57–71) with yttrium (39), also called the lanthanons (39, 57–71). They are found together in various combinations in many ores, such as monazite (65% or more rare earth metal oxides), xenotime, gadolinite, samarskite, fergusonite, apatite, euxenite, bastnaesite (90% rare earth metal oxides), mainly in Norway, Sweden, the United States (Idaho, California, and South Carolina), Canada (Ontario), and Brazil. Other terms, often used loosely, are also in use, such as lantanide elements (58–71), 4 f transition elements (58–70) and rare earth metals (21, 39, 57–71).

The rare earths are part of the transition metals, group III of the first series of the periodic table. They have similar molecular structures. In the lanthanum series (57–71), each metal has two outer electrons and eight or nine in the next inner shell. They vary in the third shell from outside. In general, each element above lanthanum (57) has one electron more in that third layer than the element below it. This makes the mass greater and the atomic weights increase, but the addition of electrons to the inner shells makes little change in the physical and chemical properties. Thus, the rare earths are very similar. This makes separation of them difficult.[18] All are relatively soft metals, malleable, with a bright silver luster, although some oxidize readily in air. Table 40–1 illustrates that in some qualities the rare earth metals show marked differences.[15]

Although most were discovered in the 19th century, it was not until the middle of the 20th century that most rare earth metals were available commercially in relatively pure form. The most common, cerium, is more abundant than lead or copper. In the hydrate form with a purity of about 90%, contaminated with 8% of other rare earths and a total of 2% of thorium oxide, iron, sodium potassium, calcium, sulfate and chloride, it is the cheapest at a few dollars per pound. Promethium does not exist in the natural state but is produced as a fission product, usually from neodymium. Thulium, the rarest in very pure form, costs several thousand dollars per pound. The great purity is achieved by the ion exchange process. The rare earth metals, as well as the chloride, nitrate, sulfate and oxalate salts, are available commercially.

INDUSTRIAL PROCESSES AND USES

The rare earths are the subject of much research and new uses will be found. The complexity of the subject can be illustrated by the use of cerium in optical glass. Cerium can be used in coloring glass yellow, yet is used in a smaller quantity to enhance the clarity of white glass. It can be used to give a blue fluorescent quality to glass if made in reducing conditions, but if made in an oxidizing process it produces no fluorescence. It is also used to prevent color change in glass on exposure to ultraviolet light. It also can make stable visible color in glass.

Cerium has replaced rouge in polishing glass. It is also used in dyeing and in the textile industry for mildew-proofing. It is used to manufacture lighter flints and tracer bullets. Cerium constitutes about 50% of the make-up of misch metal used in magnesium and ferrous alloys.

Praseodymium is used to color glass, to make carbon arc cores for lights in theater projection machines, searchlights, and other intense lighting situations. Like most of the rare earth metals, it is used in alloys.

Neodymium makes a purple glass. It is used to make glass-blower's glass because it absorbs yellow. It is used in doping glass lasers. It is a source of promethium.

Promethium provides an important radioactive source, as do the radioactive isotopes of the other rare earth metals. Promethium is used on luminescent dials.

Samarium is used in making infrared-absorbing glass. Like europium, it is also used as a dopant for lasers and as a neutron absorber (see Table 40–1) in nuclear reactors as well as a constituent of color television phosphors.

Gadolinium has a high neutron absorption factor (see Table 40–1) and is used in control rods in reactors. As an alloy, it improves the high-temperature character of iron and chromium.

Terbium is used as a solid-state and laser dopant.

Erbium is used in metallurgy and nuclear research and to color glass and porcelain.

Thulium has 16 important isotopes. Isotope 170 is used in small portable radiation units.

Ytterbium is another rare earth that is used in lasers, in alloys, and as an x-ray source for portable irradiation devices.

Yttrium is used in some optical glasses, in ceramics, and in

TABLE 40–1.
Qualities of the Rare Earth Metals

Element	Symbol	Atomic Number	Atomic Weight	PPM in Earth Crust*	Valence†	Corrodes or Resists‡	Hardness DPH kg/sq mm	Neutron Absorption Barns/Atom	Intraperitoneal‖ Toxicity Chloride	Fluorescence in Glass (Oxidizing)	Fluorescence in Glass (Reducing)	
Lanthanum	La	57	139	18		C	40	8.9	372			
Cerium	Ce	58	140	46	4	C	25	0.7	352	None	Blue	CERIUM GROUP
Praseodymium	Pr	59	141	10	4	C	40	11	358		Brown	
Neodymium	Nd	60	144	24		C	35	48	600	None		
Promethium	Pm	61	147	0								
Samarium	Sm	62	150	10	2	CR	45	5,600	585	Orange	Orange	
Europium	Eu	63	152	10	2	C§	20	4,300	550	Red	Purple	
Gadolinium	Gd	64	157	10		R	55	46,000	550	None	None	TERBIUM GROUP
Terbium	Tb	65	159	10	4	R	60	45	550	Green	Greenish white	
Dysprosium	Dy	66	163	10		R	55	1,100	585	Yellowish white	Yellowish white	
Holmium	Ho	67	165	10		R	60	64	560	None		
Erbium	Er	68	167	10		R	70	166	535	Yellow	Orange	
Thulium	Tm	69	169	10		R	65	125	485	Blue	Blue	YTTRIUM GROUP
Ytterbium	Yb	70	173	10	2	R	25	37	395	None	Orange	
Lutetium	Lu	71	175	10		R	85	111	315	None		
Yttrium	Y	39	89	40		R		1.31	88			
Scandium	Sc	21	45						755			

*Copper 45. Cerium more abundant than lead.
†In addition to the normal valence of 3 that all have, the divalent is stable with relatively high vapor pressure.
‡Metal corrodes easily, oxidizes in air and is flammable—C. Metal is fairly resistant to oxidation in air—R.
§Europium can burn spontaneously in air.
‖LD_{50} mice, intraperitoneal injection chloride salt. (Haley et al.[14])

color TV tubes, and to increase the strength of magnesium and aluminum alloys. Levels of needed respiratory protection are outlined in the National Institute for Occupational Safety and Health (NIOSH) Health Guidelines for Yttrium.[25]

BIOLOGIC EFFECTS

Most of the toxicologic data are derived from animal investigations.

Sex Difference

The acute toxicity studies to establish LD_{50} data with IV cerium show that female rats are 11 times more susceptible than the males. With other rare earths, this sex difference becomes less as the atomic number increases.[4] With several of the rare earth chlorides, liver damage is more common in the male. Ytterbium chloride can cause gastric hemorrhage but has been detected only in the female.

Absorption

The rare earth metals are not absorbed from the skin, are poorly absorbed from the gastrointestinal tract, and are slowly absorbed from the lung or on injection. On absorption, scandium and the rare earth metals tend to collect in the liver and the skeleton. There is a transition to more bone storage with the rare earths of higher atomic number.

The absorption on injection is more dependent on the type of salt, such as oxide, chloride, nitrate, acetate, sulfate, or fluoride, than on which rare earth is involved.

Complexing the rare earth with citrate may increase the absorption 95% by reducing the precipitation and inflammation. However, this does increase the toxicity.

A rare earth chloride intraperitoneally has a toxic reaction of progressive local inflammatory changes resulting in peritonitis and hemorrhagic ascites. The toxic effect or reaction with the citrate complex and its faster absorption has a stage of dyspnea and pulmonary edema followed by liver edema and portal congestion as well as pleural effusion and pulmonary hyperemia.[9]

The rare earth salts precipitate very rapidly in the physiologic pH ranges, since the isoelectric point of these compounds is below pH 7.[9] The hydrolyzed portion remains at the site, but the complexes formed with the nucleic acids and proteins are absorbed by blood as colloids and are deposited in the liver, spleen and bone marrow. They are slowly ionized and return to the blood as bound proteins that are removed by the hepatic cells. The rare earth then is excreted in the bile.[17]

Lanthanum may be 15% unabsorbed from the injection site after four days and holmium 95% unabsorbed in this time.

Inhalation

Inhaled cerium citrate, chloride, and cerium entrapped in fused-clay particles[21] cleared the body rapidly, with 10% clay, 20% chloride, and less than 30% of the citrate remaining by the end of 20 days. At 120 days, 25% citrate, 10% chloride, and 2% clay still were present. Ninety percent of the cerium clay that remained was in the lungs. The more soluble cerium citrate and chloride appear more readily in the liver and bones, where they apparently are not released so easily. All three are excreted primarily by the feces (90% or more) but also by the urine (10%). The amounts of cerium citrate and chloride in the liver slowly decreased after the first 20 days, but the amounts of these in the bone slowly increased after the first 20 days. The cerium chloride had a more rapid early urinary excretion than did the cerium citrate.

Inhalation of gadolinium oxide was injurious to the lungs and resulted in an increase in pneumonia cases. Some calcification of the lungs was noted. Granulomatous inflammation occurred with gadolinium chloride. No increase in lung tumors was found.[1]

Excretion

Elimination of rare earths is primarily fecal, and after deposition in the skeleton it may take years before removal is completed. Starvation lessened the excretion.[17]

Metabolism

Lanthanum, like some other of the lower atomic number rare earth metals such as yttrium, has a lot of similarity chemically and biologically to aluminum. It can replace aluminum as the needed metal in the liver succinic dehydrogenase enzyme system. It inhibits adenosine phosphate activity, as does yttrium.[6]

Several of the rare earth metal compounds have been used in medicine. Cerous nitrate was used in a solution of 1:1000 as an antiseptic, and as an astringent.[3] Cerium iodide was effective in treating puerperal infection.[3] In relieving vomiting of pregnancy, cerium oxalate was useful. Ceric nitrate served as a nerve tonic and cerium carbonate as a sedative.

Lanthanum, neodymium, and cerium were all used to prevent blood clotting through an antiprothrombin action.[2] It was found that they could induce hemorrhages.[20] Hemoglobinuria has been noted in patients who received neodymium compound as an anticoagulant.

Toxicity

The lanthanons are relatively nontoxic. Only terbium chloride has been noted to be an irritant to the intact skin. Gadolinium and samarium chlorides produced ulcers on abraded skin. Lutetium and europium chlorides caused extensive scarring on abraded skin and, along with dysprosium, holmium, and erbium, produced nodules from intradermal injection.[14]

The chloride of each of the rare earths caused ocular irritation in the form of a transient conjunctivitis. In addition, terbium chloride produced corneal damage. The lanthanons can produce opacity to the abraded cornea.[22]

The large amounts of rare earth chloride injected intraperitoneally to produce LD_{50} data are shown in Table 40–1.

Like gadolinium chloride, intratracheal administration of oxides of yttrium, neodymium, and cerium in rats produced granulomas of the lung.[14]

There can be synergistic toxicity with simultaneous exposure to *some* rare earth compounds and ionizing radiation as might occur in an explosive nuclear reactor accident.[7]

Acute Toxicity.—If in great enough quantity, the rare earth compounds can produce, on inhalation, acute chemical irritation pneumonitis, and bronchitis.

The acute toxicity with injection was investigated by Graca et al.[10] Rare earth compounds have, in general, a mild depressant physiologic effect. The blood pressure and respiratory rate, if affected, are lowered. The heart rate is reduced. A leukopenia has been observed in dogs. The blood coagulation time increases, except with samarium. The blood prothrombin time increased but there is a decreasing effect with increase in atomic number, except for ytterbium.

Headache and nausea from dust and fumes from using cored arc light carbons containing lanthanum has been reported.[8] In some experimental studies with rare earths, weight loss was noted.[19]

DIAGNOSTIC METHODS

There are no signs or symptoms pathognomonic of toxicity from lanthanons. A history of exposure would be necessary in making the diagnosis. A chest x-ray after massive acute inhalation might show signs of edema or pneumonitis. Fibrous nodules have been found in the lung in experimental animals after lanthanon exposure, but the same has never been noted in exposed workers. Blood levels have never been established. Excretion of the rare earth metals in the urine is a small part of the total excretion by the body but could be measured accurately. No standards of urinary level have been established, because it is not yet known if there is a correlation between the urinary level and either the exposure or the fecal excretion.

Fecal excretion of lanthanons is measurable. The level of excretion varies greatly with the route of exposure and the solubility of the lanthanon. No indices of toxicity based on fecal excretion have been established, but fecal levels do afford an inconvenient method of monitoring exposure.

TREATMENT

As noted before, some lanthanons delay healing, cause irritation and ulcers on abraded skin and form nodules intradermally. Extra care should be used in treating wounds contaminated with a lanthanon.[16]

If lanthanon toxicity is suspected, the patient should be removed from further exposure. There is no specific therapy, and treatment of any findings that are believed to be related to the lanthanon exposure, such as acute chemical pneumonitis, hematuria or leukopenia, are treated in the usual manner. Is there any therapeutic implication in the fact that Herman and Clark[17] found that starvation lessened excretion of lanthanons?

RARE EARTH ANALYSIS

Analysis of rare earths by quick or inexpensive means does not exist. Because of the similar physical and chemical natures of the rare earths to one another and the variety of common contaminants, there are many methods of qualitative and quantitative analysis.

Most rare earths are a mixture, although highly purified products are becoming more plentiful.

Analysis becomes more complex if you wish to determine the total rare earth content and also which rare earths are involved.

Total content can be found by a chemical method, usually precipitation as the hydroxide or oxalate, or a volumetric titration with a complexing agent.

The individual elements, except for cerium and possibly europium, which is best determined chemically by volumetric methods with persulfate oxidation titration, are determined by physical measurements. Absorption and x-ray fluorescence spectra can be used for macro amounts and emission spectra for low levels.

Flame photometry is not suitable for most rare earths because of interferences. It is applicable for use with lanthanon, neodymium, and ytterbium.[18]

Spectrographic analysis requires an instrument with good dispersion, preferably with a controlled atmosphere. It is fairly accurate in identifying each rare earth, especially in trace amounts.

With the exception of cerium, atomic absorption spectrophotometry is the method of choice for rare earth quantitative determination.

PRINCIPLES OF CONTROL

The Occupational Safety and Health Administration (OSHA) permissible exposure limit (PEL) for yttrium is 1 mg/cu m as an eight-hour time weighted average (TWA). The rare earths have such a low level of toxicity that the PEL for yttrium is more than adequate for the other rare earths.

Very often the rare earth used in industry is only a small part of the total contents of that industrial process. In such cases, the other substances are the determinants of the degree of control. Europium and vanadium in the TV industry are examples of this.[23]

Environmental Control

Environmental control is concerned only with inhalation. Incidental ingestion is harmless.

Heated rare earths may give off toxic fumes that should be controlled. Dusts should be vented adequately. The yttrium PEL should be applied to all rare earth operations. Levels of needed respiratory protection are outlined in NIOSH Health Guidelines for yttrium.[25]

Gloves, protective eyewear, and such other protective equipment as may be necessary should be used to prevent terbium from coming into contact with the skin until patch testing has shown no irritation response in the worker.

Preemployment Examination

Applicants with corneal injuries, keratoconus, or conjunctivitis should not be exposed to rare earth dusts.

Applicants with skin cuts, abrasions, or dermatitis should not be employed where contact with the rare earths of the terbium and yttrium groups would occur (see Table 40–1). Exclude from work with significant rare earth exposures applicants with chronic lung disease, x-ray evidence of fine lung opacities, increased blood coagulation time, or leukopenia.[10]

ISOTOPES

Isotopes of rare earths are numerous and are used in industry and medicine. The uses and precautions are primarily based on the radioactivity.

Ytterbium 169 emits γ-rays and is used in radiography of small castings and other small materials.[11] It has an advantage over x-ray in that no hazard from electrical shock or explosion can occur and it is lighter.

To reduce the radioactive hazard from luminous paint on clocks and instrument dials, promethium 147, a β emitter, is used. This poses a problem in control of exposure, as lung and gastrointestinal tract exposure can be estimated only by feces examinations.[25]

Several rare earth isotopes are used in needles and pellets to treat cancer. Because of the tendency of some rare earths to stay at the site of injection, some are used by injection to treat cancer. However, cerium fluoride on inhalation can produce bronchogenic cancer.[5]

REFERENCES

1. Ball RA: Chronic toxicity of gadolinium oxide for mice following exposure by inhalation. *Arch Environ Health* 1966; 13:601.
2. Beaser SB, et al: The anticoagulant effects in rabbits and man of the intravenous injection of salts of the rare earth metals. *J Clin Invest* 1942; 21:447.
3. Browning E: *Toxicity of Industrial Metals*. London, Butterworths, 1961.
4. Bruce DW, et al: The acute mammalian toxicity of rare earth nitrates and oxides. *Toxicol Appl Pharmacol* 1963; 5:750.

5. Cember H, et al: Bronchogenic carcinoma from rdioactive cerium fluoride, *AMA Arch Ind Health* 1959; 19:14.
6. Cochran KW, et al: Acute toxicity of zirconium, columbium, strontium, lanthanum, cesium, tantalum, and yttrium. *Arch Ind Hyg* 1950; 1:637.
7. DuBois KP, Hietbrink E: Studies on the toxicity of rare earth compounds and their influence on radiation lethality. *USAF Radiation Laboratory Progress Reports* 1960; 34–36.
8. Fairhall LT: *Industrial Toxicology*, ed 2. Baltimore, Williams & Wilkins Co, 1957, pp 67–68.
9. Graca JG, et al: Comparative toxicity of stable rare earth compounds. I. *AMA Arch Ind Health* 1957; 15:9.
10. Graca JG, et al: Comparative toxicity of stable rare earth compounds. II and III. *Arch Environ Health* 1962; 5:437, and 1964; 8:555.
11. Green FL: Uses and safety aspects of the low-energy source ytterbium 169. *Am Ind Hyg Assoc* 1966; 27:444.
12. Haley TJ, et al: Toxicological and pharmacological effects of gadolinium and samarium chlorides. *Br J Pharmacol* 1961; 17:526.
13. Haley TJ, et al: Pharmacology and toxicology of terbium, thulium, and ytterbium chlorides, and pharmacology and toxicology of dysprosium, holmium, and erbium chlorides. *Toxicol Appl Pharmacol* 1963; 5:427, and 1966; 8:37.
14. Haley TJ, et al: Pharmacology and toxicology of lutetium chloride, pharmacology and toxicology of europium chloride and pharmacology and toxicology of the rare earth elements. *J Pharmacol Sci* 1964; 53:1186, 1965; 54:643, and 54:663.
15. Hampel CA (ed): *Rare Metals Handbook*, ed 2. London, Reinhold Publishing Corp, 1961, pp 393–417 and 653–666.
16. Hartwig QL, et al: Some toxic effects of yttrium and lanthanum and other rare earths. *AMA Arch Ind Health* 1958; 18:505.
17. Herman MW, Clark AJ: Excretion and body distribution of promethium 147. *Arch Environ Health* 1973; 26:200.
18. Kolthoff IM, Elving PJ: *Treatise on Analytical Chemistry*, Part II, vol 8, *The Rare Earths*. New York, Interscience Publishers, 1963.
19. Kryker GC, Cress EA: Acute toxicity of yttrium, lanthanum and other rare earths. *AMA Arch Ind Health* 1957; 16:475.
20. Machlin LJ, et al: Relative toxicity of lanthanum, tantalum, and thorium compounds in the developing chick embryo. *AMA Arch Ind Hyg* 1952; 6:441.
21. Morgan BN, et al: Influence of the chemical state of cerium 144 on its metabolism following inhalation by mice. *Am Ind Hyg Assoc J* 1970; 31:479.
22. Patty FA, (ed): *Industrial Hygiene and Toxicology*, ed 2. New York; Interscience Publishers, 1962, vol II, pp 1058–1067.
22a. Sabbioni E, Pietra R, Gaglione P, et al: Long-term occupational risk of rare-earth pneumoconiosis—A case report as investigated by neutron activation analysis, in *The Science of the Total Environment*, vol 26. Amsterdam, Elsevier, 1982, pp 19–32.
23. Tebrock HE, Mackle W: Exposure to europium-activated yttrium orthovanadate: A cathodoluminescent phosphor. *J Occup Med* 1968; 10:692.
24. US Dept of Health and Human Services: *Occupational Health Guideline for Yttrium*. Occupational Health Guides for Chemical Hazards, DHHS Publ 81–123, Rockville, Md, NIOSH, 1981.
25. Vennart J: The usage of radioactive luminous compound and the need for biological monitoring of workers. *Health Phys* 1967; 13:959.

41

Selenium, Tellurium, and Osmium

Thomas H. F. Smith, Ph.D.

SELENIUM

History

Selenium is a paradoxical element. It is toxic to animals at concentrations which occur in the environment and is at the same time essential to human beings in varying amounts from traces to parts per million.

Although Arnold De Villanova spoke of a *Sulphur Rubeum* as early as the 14th Century, the credit for the isolation and identification of selenium is given to Berzelius,[2] who published his definitive work in 1818. Since it resembled tellurium, he chose to call it after the Greek word for the moon—*selene*, since tellurium was named for the earth—*tellus* (Latin, poetic). In deference to Berzelius, one of the sellentine ores was later called Berzelianite (Cu_2Se).

Chemical and Physical Properties

Selenium has an atomic number of 34 and atomic weight of 78.96. It lies between sulfur and tellurium in group VIa and between arsenic and bromine in period 4 of the periodic table.

It is strikingly similar to sulfur in most of its chemistry. Its important oxidation states are −2, 0, +2, +4, and +6. As far as it is known, the +2 state does not occur in nature. There are six stable isotopes and a number of artificially produced radioisotopes. It exists in six allotropic modifications including in amorphous, vitreous, and crystalline form and a colloidal form, which at 1 part per 10,000 in water imparts a distinct reddish tinge.

Hexagonal grey crystalline selenium is a stable metal and a good conductor of electricity and is a photo conductor allotrope. This electroconductivity is low in the dark but increases several hundredfold on exposure to light.

In many reactions selenium acts as an oxidant as well as a reductant, making it a very versatile substance. Binary compounds of selenium with 58 metals, eight nonmetals, and alloys with three other elements have been described.

The only important hydride of selenium is hydrogen selenide (H_2Se), a colorless, flammable gas with a distinctly unpleasant odor which is more toxic than hydrogen sulfide but less stable. It also reacts readily with halogens and nitrogen.

Occurrence and Use

At a concentration of 0.68 atoms per 10,000 atoms of silicon, selenium is the 30th element of cosmic abundance. It ranks about 70th in the order of crustal abundance, the average amount in rocks being 0.05 ppm.[12]

It occurs mostly in conjunction with sulphur where it is isomorphous. In hydrothermal deposits it is associated isothermally with silver, gold, antimony and mercury.

Since it forms natural compounds with 16 other elements and is a main constituent in 39 mineral species and a minor component in 17 more, it might well be considered as one of the more ubiquitous elements.

In seawater it occurs at about 0.090 μg/L, mostly as $(SeO_4)^{-2}$. It is absorbed by marine organisms and is concentrated in soils.[4]

In the air selenium has been detected at 0.001 μg/cu m. This can be reasonably and accurately determined by measuring sulfur, since the ratio is usually 1×10^{-4} (Se:S).

It occurs in alkaline soils as water-soluble selenates readily available to plants, where accumulation in sufficient quantities has led to livestock poisoning.

Data on selenium in drinking water is limited, but it is usually present at less than 1 μg/L. It has been found in wells in certain regions at levels as high as 2,680 μg/L. The permissible criterion for selenium is 10 ppb.

Selenium has nearly as many diverse applications as it has appearances in nature. It is used in hardening and toughening metals and to increase resistance to abrasion in rubber hose and cable coverings. Glass and ceramic industries use it, as well as the cosmetics industry in antidandruff shampoos. It is especially useful as pesticide specific for aphids in carnation cultivation.

Since it has the remarkable property of increased electrical conductivity in the presence of light, it is widely used in photo electric cells and rectifiers.

Metabolism

The metabolic features of selenium have been studied chiefly from the point of view of animal toxicology; although there are an abundance of comprehensive reviews on this element.[4, 6, 7, 13–15]

Elemental forms of selenium are probably not absorbed from the gastrointestinal tract. The average body burden is estimated to be 14.6 mg, with the greatest concentrations being found in the kidney, with the liver having about 50% of the amount found in the kidney. Human blood contains selenium with an erythrocyte plasma ratio of approximately 3:1. It is excreted in urine at about twice the amount present in feces. Normal levels range from 0 to 15 μg/100 ml, so this can be an indicator or index of excessive exposure or intake.

Similar to tellurium, it provides "garlic breath," due to dimethyl selenide. It also transgresses the placental barrier and is found in newborns.

Two major metabolic pathways exist in the body. The first is methylation, dimethylation, and trimethylation, and the other is direct incorporation or binding in proteins. In this case, it substitutes itself for sulfur in methionine or as a selenotrisulfide. There is no direct proof of homeostasis of this substance, but there are good indications that it exists.

Toxic Effects

Selenium compounds are the most toxic of the Group VIa elements. Selenosis is produced by both inorganic and organic forms. This subject has been reviewed extensively.[6, 11, 14, 15] Toxicity varies with the chemical form and the species involved.

In humans, it is initially a severe irritant to skin, mucous membranes, and the respiratory tract. The chief occupational exposure complaint is dermatitis, probably one to dusts or the oxides. Selenium oxychloride destroys skin on contact. In the eye, a condition known as "rose eye," a pinkish allergic condition of the eyelids is obvious. This is often accompanied by a conjuctivitis or the palpebral conjunctiva. Possible liver damage is a risk with high exposures to selenium compounds.

The earliest reference to industrial selenium poisoning was a report by Hamilton[8] in 1925, in which she described a condition she called "rose cold." She first recognized this condition in 1917, but did not publish her findings until eight years later for reasons not explained. The symptoms noted included coryza-like symptoms, acute sore throat, lacrimation, a metallic taste, garlic breath, and a gastrointestinal disturbance.

Marco Polo reported in 1295 a disease called "hoof rot" in horses in the Nan Shan and Tien Shan mountains of Turkestan, which was obviously a form of selenosis from ingesting grass from the selenium rich soil in this area.

Buchan[5] reported a case of sore throat attributed to the use of a selenium red ("Cadmium red" or cadmium sulfoselenide) lipstick. This colorant was banned for cosmetic use in 1938, but serves to demonstrate another case of exposure by an unsuspecting user.

Interestingly, selenium has been accused of being both a carcinogen and an anticarcinogen. The weight of the evidence is inconclusive in either direction and will require further examination before a conclusive decision can be reached.[10]

Mutagenic data is similarly contradictory. Teratogenic and antiteratogenic effects have likewise been reported. However, it has been documented that Indians in an area of Colombia, South America, where the black "peladero" soil contains extremely high concentrations of selenium, have had malformed infants by parents with symptoms of selenium intoxication. Loss of hair and nails was also observed. The accidental exposure of several female laboratory workers resulted in the termination of several pregnancies by miscarriages and the birth of one bilateral clubfoot infant.[9]

Medical Surveillance

Preemployment and periodic examinations should consider the skin, eyes, liver, respiratory tract, kidney, and liver functions and preexisting disorders or diseases. The fingernails should be carefully examined as an indicator of exposure. Measurement of urinary excretion of selenium is useful if comparison data is available. Levels should be maintained below 0.1 mg/L. The threshold limit value time-weighted average for selenium is currently 0.02 mg/m^3. The short-term exposure limit (STEL) is the same.

Treatment

First aid should consist of irrigating the affected area immediately and thoroughly with water. If selenium is inhaled, remove the patient to fresh air and give artificial respiration, if required. If selenium is swallowed, give the patient copious amounts of water.

Suitable methods for treating systemic poisoning are singularly lacking. Various substances have been examined and discarded. Amdur[1] indicates the use of BAL (dimercaprol) is contraindicated.

A 10% sodium thiosulfate ointment is recommended for the treatment of burns.

REFERENCES

SELENIUM

1. Amdur ML: Selenium. *Arch Ind Health* 1958; 17:665.
2. Berzelius JJ: Selenium. *Acad. Handl. (Stockh)* 1818; 39:13.
3. Brown SS, Savoy J: *Chemical Toxicity and Clinical Chemistry of Metals*. New York, Academic Press, 1983.
4. Browning E: *Toxicity or Industrial Metals*, ed 2. London, Butterworths, 1969.
5. Buchan RF: Industrial selenosis. *J Occup Med* 1947; 3:439.
6. Dudley HC: Toxicology of selenium. Am J Hyg 1936; 24:227.
7. Glover JR: Selenium and its industrial toxicology. *Ind Med Surg* 1970; 39:50.
8. Hamilton A: *Industrial Poisons in the US*. New York, MacMillan Publishing Co, 1925.
9. Hansson E, Jacobson SO: *Biochem Biophys Acta* 1966; 115:285–293.
10. Lewis A: *Selenium: The Facts About This Essential Element*. New York, Cancer Control Society, 1983.
11. National Academy of Sciences: *Selenium*. Washington, DC, US Government Printing Office, 1976.
12. Rosenfeld I, Beath OA: Chemistry of selenium, in *Selenium, Geobotany, Biochemistry, Toxicity and Nutrition*. New York, Academic Press, 1964.
13. Schamberger RJ: *Biochemistry of Selenium*, vol 2, *Biochemistry of the Elements*. New York, Plenum Press, 1983.
14. Wilbur CG: Toxicology or selenium: A review. *Clin Toxicol* 1980; 17:171–230.
15. Wilbur CG: *Selenium: A Potential Environmental Poison and a Necessary Food Constituent*. Springfield, Ill, Charles C Thomas, Publisher, 1983.

TELLURIUM

History

Up until the end of the 18th century, tellurium was considered to be a "white gold," possibly an alloy of antimony and bismuth, found in sandstone near Zalantha, Transylvania. About 1792, Muller von Reichenstein[10] showed that it contained neither of these metals. He suspected it was a new metal, but didn't know what. He temporarily called it *metalium problematicum* or *aurum paradoxium*. How it ultimately became known as tellurium, from the Latin (poetic) *tellus,* meaning *the earth,* is not clearly evident.

In spite of its industrial uses to varying degrees from the early 1800s, the First International Symposium on Industrial Uses of Selenium and Tellurium was not held until 1965 in New York City. Interestingly, the Selenium-Tellurium Development Association, Inc., is composed of only eight members—four of them are American, two Canadian, one Swedish, and one Japanese. At the Second Annual Symposium in 1980, 140 producers and dealers were in attendance. This information is provided as an indication of the growing number of individuals likely to be encountering or to be exposed to this substance and its increasing importance to the occupational physician.

Occurrence and Use

Tellurium is found to some extent in the free state, but chiefly associated with ores such as slyvanite, $(AgAu)Te_2$. Also called krennerite, black tellurium, or nagyagite $(AgPb)_2TeS(Sb_2)$,[4] Kessite (AG_2Te), and tetradymite (Bi_2Te_2S).

Tellurium is about the 40th element in cosmic abundance and 71st in the earth's crust. It composes about 10^{-9}% of the earth's crust. It is found as a free element in Central Europe, Colorado, and Bolivia, and with selenium in sulfur deposits in Japan.

It occurs as a main component of 40 mineral species and a minor constituent of an undetermined number of others.

No spectrographically detectable amounts have been found in U.S. rivers.[7] An estimate has been made that coal combustion in the U.S. releases about 40 tons of tellurium in fly ash per year.

Schroeder et al.[11] reported that the garlic plant is high in tellurium compound derived from the soil and draws an analogy to the garlic breath odor of workers exposed to this metal.

The estimated tellurium consumption in metallurgy is 79%, in chemical, rubber, plastics, and glass, 18%, and in the electronic and electrical industry, 3%. In metallurgy, it improves the properties of steel and cast iron and copper- and lead-based alloys.

Tellurium rectifiers have been developed, but their manufacture and use is undocumented. Some tellurium is used in semiconductor lasers and as a dopant in alloys. Tellurium also has been used in amorphous memory devices and in electrophotographic materials and photoreceptors. A zinc, cadmium, and indium-tellurium combination is useful in solid state image conversion devices.

Chemistry and Physical Properties

Tellurium has an atomic number of 52 and an atomic weight of 127.6. It is the most electropositive element in subgroup VIA and has multiple electron states of -2, 0, $+2$, $+4$, and $+6$. In the elemental state it is a coarse, crystalline, silver-white solid with a metallic luster. It is insoluble in water and does not easily form an oxide when heated in air. It will form di- and trivalent oxides and water-soluble tellurite and teleurate anions. Cationic salts are unstable and hydrolyze to oxides and oxyacids. Telluric acid forms stable polymeric chains in aqueous solutions. It burns with a blue flame to form tellurium dioxide.

Tellurium is positioned between selenium and polonium in group VIA and between antimony and iodine in period 4. It is more metallic than oxygen, sulfur, and selenium, but resembles them in its chemical properties. While oxygen and sulfur are nonmetals and electrical insulators, tellurium is a semiconductor.

At least 21 isotopes are known, with mass numbers from 114 to 134. Eight of these are stable. Tellurium illustrates the rule that elements with even atomic numbers have more isotopes than those with odd numbers.

Tellurium forms a continuous range of isomorphous solid solutions with gray selenium. These contain chains of more or less random selenium and tellurium atoms.

It exists in two allotropic modifications, a crystalline and amorphous form. The crystalline form has extremely low electrical conductivity. It melts at 449.8° C and boils at 1,390° C. On the Moh scale it has a hardness of 2.5 and is insoluble in all solvents. A red colloidal sol of tellurium can be produced by reducing telluric acid with hydrazine.

The only known hydride is hydrogen telluride (H_2Te). This is a colorless gas with an offensive odor and is about equally toxic with hydrogen selenide. It will also react with halogens, the most important compound being tellurium hexafluoride.

The electrical resistance of tellurium varies greatly with the amount of impurities and decreases markedly as temperature or compression increase.

Metabolism

The metabolism of tellurium in mammals has not been studied extensively. The biochemistry was reviewed by Amdur[1, 2] and the toxicology by Cooper[5] and Cerwenka and Cooper.[6] There is no quantitative information on respiratory absorption, but evidence exists for expiratory excretion of tellurite compounds, producing the characteristic "garlic breath" of exposed individuals. This is due to the methylation to volatile dimethyltelluride. It is apparently absorbed through the intact skin and from the gastrointestinal tract. In the blood it complexes with plasma proteins and very little enters the erythrocytes. Bone and kidneys retain it longer than soft tissues. Excretion is mostly in urine and feces. If the administration is parenteral, urinary excretion will predominate. If oral, the greater amount will appear in the feces. At least in rats, tellurium crosses the blood-brain barrier and affects the nervous system. Demyelination of the sciatic nerve and spinal roots have been observed in animal studies.

There does not appear to be any specific metabolic detoxification mechanism for tellurium.

No reliable data exists on normal values for tellurium in humans and it is not considered to be an important micronutrient. Of the 600-mg (average) body burden in the human, 90% is found in the bones.

Toxic Effects

Exposure to tellurium vapor or hydrogen telluride has been reported to cause respiratory irritation. Several cases, two of which were fatal, resulted from the accidental use by mistake of sodium tellurite in a retrograde pyelography. Stupor, cyanosis, vomiting, and unconciousness preceded death.[8] Blackadder and Manderson[3] reported on two cases of occupational absorption.

Experimentally, tellurium was found to produce hydrocephalus in newborn rats when the mothers were fed high concentrations. From a teratogenic aspect, it would appear this is a direct embrotoxic action. There is no evidence for carcinogenicity, although some chromosome breakage was observed in human leukocytes treated in vitro with sodium and ammonium salts.

> **Case Report.**—Man, 18 years, who was packaging tellurium oxide powder for less than three weeks in very dusty, uncontrolled working conditions, sought medical advice, mainly because of family complaints about his offensive body odors. The physical examination and routine blood and urine studies were normal, and tellurium was detected in his blood. (Unfortunately, no workroom air level measurements could be taken, as the plant was small—one owner, few employees. Local and federal regulations are unresponsive to such situations.) His body odor persisted for two months. No follow-up was possible.[9]

The acute toxic effects of tellurium are similar to those of arsenic in many respects.

Medical Surveillance

The ACGIH-recommended TLV for tellurium is 0.1 mg/cu m. However, experience has shown that the concentration should be controlled to 0.01 mg/cu m to prevent the characteristic and offensive "garlic breath" symptoms. This, fortunately, is a very significant early warning sign of potential intoxication.

There are no known medical conditions that would be a specific contraindication for exclusion from working with tellurium or its compounds.

There is no specific antidote for poisoning by tellurium compounds, and in spite of previous suggestions, the use of BAL or ascorbic acid is not currently recommended. Actually, there are indications that BAL might potentiate the toxicity of tellurium.[1, 2]

REFERENCES

TELLURIUM

1. Amdur ML: Tellurium. *Occup Med* 1947; 3:386.
2. Amdur ML: Tellurium oxide. *Arch Ind Health* 1958; 17:665.
3. Blackadder FS, Manderson WG: Occupational absorption of tellurium: A report of two cases. *Br J Ind Med* 1975; 32:59 61.
4. Browning: The toxicity of industrial metals, ed 2. London, Butterworths, 1969, pp 310–316.
5. Cooper WC (ed): *Tellurium*. New York, Van Nostrand-Reinhold, 1971.
6. Cerwenka EA Jr, Cooper WC: Toxicology of selenium and tellurium and their compounds. *Arch Environ Health* 1961; 3:189–200.
7. Durum WH: Trace metals, in *Proceedings, Conference on Physiological Aspects of Water Quality*. Washington, DC, US Public Health Service, 1960, p. 51.
8. Keall JHH, Martin NH, Tunbridge RE: Three cases of accidental poisoning by sodium tellurite. *Br J Ind Med* 1946; 3:175.
9. Mayer J: Personal communication to C Zenz, August, 1984.
10. Mellor JW: *Comprehensive Treatise on Inorganic and Theoretical Chemistry*. New York, Longmans Green and Co, 1930.
11. Schroder HA, et al: Abnormal trace elements in man. Tellurium. *J Chronic Dis* 1967; 20:147.

OSMIUM

History

Osmium is the heaviest inorganic substance known (density 27.59). It was isolated in 1804 by Tennant from the aqua regia insoluble residues of platinum. Its associate is iridium, named for *iris* (the *rainbow*), due to the color of the salts. Osmium was less dignified in its christening, and derived its name from *osmos* (Greek, meaning a *smell* or *odor*), due to the pungent, chlorine-like smell of its volatile oxide. (At first, Tennant considered calling it *petenium*—from *winged* (volatile), but that idea was discarded.)

Occurrence and Use

Osmium is present in the earth's crust at very low concentrations (6.0×10^{-12}). It is usually found in association with platinum ores from Colombia, Chile, Brazil, Russia and Alaska, Oregon, and California, in the U.S.A. In many of the Russian deposits it occurs as osmiridium or syserkite (more than 40% osmium) or as iridiosmium or nevyanskite (less than 40% osmium). Actually, the line of demarcation is ill-defined.

It is readily separated and isolated to a high degree of purity because it readily forms a volatile tetroxide, or in solution, osmic acid. It can be either distilled off or recovered by neutralizing and evaporating to dryness.

Osmium is used as a catalyst in the synthesis of ammonia and in the hydrogenation of organic compounds. It forms solid-solutions alloys with other metals in the platinum family and also with iron, cobalt, nickel, tin, and zinc. With the latter two, it forms brittle, intermetallic compounds. It imparts excellent corrosion resistance and hardness when combined with other metals.

Chemical and Physical Properties

Osmium resides in group VIII of the periodic table and appears horizontally in the sixth row, which relates it to few substances of great physiologic importance other than remotely to platinum, gold, mercury, and lead, with which it shares few similarities in behavior.

It has an atomic number of 76 and an atomic weight of 190.2° C, with a high melting point of 3,045° C and a boiling point of 5,020° C.

Physically, it is a blue-white, hard metal in the pure state. It is lustrous and brittle, with a close-packed hexagonal crystalline structure. It is insoluble in water and only slightly soluble in aqua regia or nitric acid. A blue oxide (OsO_2) forms at room temperature in air, but prior to this, OsO_4 and OsO_3 volatilize off. These are very toxic substances, and because of their ready formation, they complicate both the analysis and refining of osmium.

Because of its hardness (7.0 on the Moh scale) it is virtually impossible to machine or process solid, pure osmium or its alloys. It must be cast molten or fabricated by powder metallurgy techniques. The latter provides the potential for dust inhalation, the former for fumes of the oxides.

Chemically, osmium combines irreversibly with hydrogen. It does not oxidize in air or oxygen at 100° C, but it will do so at elevated temperatures or in the presence of water vapors. It will form stable tri, tetra, and octavalent compounds, and coordinates readily with atoms and molecules to form hexahalo, cyano, nitro, and carbonyl coordination complexes with tetrahedral configurations. Most of these are unstable.

Because of the rapid electron exchange between coordinately saturated Os^{+4} and Os^{+3} complexes, they may be involved in oxidation and reduction reactions in living organisms.

The most widely recognized osmium derivative is the tetroxide, also known as osmic acid (OsO_4). This is a black crystalline material with a burning taste and halogen (chlorine) odor. It is volatile at room temperatures and rapidly reduces in the presence of organic matter. It is used as a fixative in electron microscopy and as the acid form for staining fat selectively in ordinary histologic techniques.

Metabolism

There is no evidence to support the suggestion that osmium is an essential micronutrient.[2] Reports regarding its absorption, distribution, retention, and excretion are scant. Some data indicate that ingested insoluble salts are excreted in the feces. Parentally injected salts remain at the sites of introduction, usually reduced to the metal. Minute intravenous doses distribute into soft tissues, but about 80% is excreted within a week. By inhalation, osmic acid vapors are retained in the lungs and respiratory tract, causing severe irritation and black discoloration, due to the reduction of the osmic acid to the metallic form.

Toxic Effects

The toxic effects of osmium have not been studied in animals.[5] The sparse data available have been recorded from isolated instances of accidental human exposures. Osmium tetroxide has received some, but not a great amount, of attention in this respect.

In 1927, Gmelin[1] conducted animal studies with osmium salts, from which he reported that they acted upon the stomach, quickly causing vomiting, and in the respiratory system, causing the copious discharge of a serous fluid and a stoppage of respiration. A subsequent injection (dose not specified) resulted in paralysis of the extremities and death.

Human deaths have been reported from poisoning with osmium metal.[7] The limited reports available indicate it behaves similarly to platinum in attacking mucous membranes, the respiratory tract, and ocular tissue.

The data are most confusing to analyze, since osmium tetroxide is discussed interchangeably with osmium, as if they were one and the same substance. Since the tetroxide is more likely to be the encountered industrial poison, it is to this that most reference texts address themselves.

The NIOSH *Occupational Health Guideline for Osmium Tetroxide*[6] is the best reference work for the occupational physician. It indicates that the current TWA is 0.002 mg/cu m, and the ACGIH TLV is 0.0002 mg/cu m. Warnings are issued that it will produce severe eye damage, with tearing and irritation. Subsequent keratitis epithelia with corneal edema and browning of the sclera and cornea has been reported. Chronic, impaired pulmonary function is exacerbated, and based upon animal studies, preexisting kidney damage could be worsened. It is also a skin irritant.

Medical Surveillance

It is advisable to screen employees for preexisting eye, kidney, respiratory or dermatologic conditions, as all of these will predispose their susceptibility to osmium tetroxide. Periodic medical examinations are advisable in all cases.

In emergencies, remove the material by washing the exposed area thoroughly or administering large amounts of water (for oral ingestions). First aid for inhalation would be immediate removal from the area and artificial respiration if breathing has stopped.

No information on chronic effects was discovered in a literature search on this substance. An interesting volume on osmium[4] was published by Ann Arbor Press, but it is now out of print and difficult to obtain. The seriously interested may want to pursue a search for this comprehensive tome.

REFERENCES

OSMIUM

1. Browning E: *Toxicity of Industrial Metals*, ed 2. London, Butterworths, 1969.
2. Luckey TD, Venugopal B, Hutcheson D: *Heavy Metal Toxicity, Safety and Hormonology*. New York, Academic Press, 1975.
3. Mellor JW: *Comprehensive Treatise on Inorganic and Theoretical Chemistry*. New York, Longmans Green and Co, 1930.
4. Smith Ivan C, Carson BL, Ferguson TL (eds): *Palladium/Osmium*, vol IV, *Chemicals in the Environment*. Ann Arbor, Ann Arbor Press, 1977.
5. Stockinger H: in Patty FA, Irish DD (eds): *Industrial Hygiene and Toxicology*, ed 3. New York, Wiley-Interscience, 1981, vol 2A, pp 1505–1517.
6. US Department of Health and Human Services: *Occupational Health Guideline for Osmium Tetroxide*. Occupational Health Guide for Chemical Hazards, DHHS Publ 81-123, Rockville, Md, NIOSH, 1981.
7. Viotti G, Valbonesi M, Ardino V: Su tre casi di intosicazione da osmio (three cases of osmium intoxication). *Lav Med* (Genoa) 1969; 23:77–82.

42

Gallium, Germanium, and Indium

Thomas H. F. Smith, Ph.D

At first it may appear strange to the reader that gallium, germanium, and indium should be grouped together, but as this chapter unfolds, it will become apparent why this combination was chosen. The close similarities and applications of these materials makes this combined discourse a most rational approach to the consideration of the occupational aspects of these substances.

Gallium and indium are associated vertically in the group IIIA elements of the periodic table. Gallium, germanium, and arsenic are members of the same fourth horizontal period, and indium and antimony are related in the fifth period.

These relationships are of interest for a number of reasons. A review of the intrinsic toxicity of metals, relevant to their position in the vertical groups of the periodic table, reveals interesting sequences between toxicity, electropositivity, and solubility.[30] Toxicity increases proportionately with the electropositivity and solubility of metal cations in lipids and water. Toxicity increases further with the formation of covalent and coordinate valent compounds, more so than with electrovalent combinations. Within the vertical group, greater toxicity is associated with an increase in the atomic weight or a higher atomic number. Heavy metals form irreversible stable complexes with biologic macromolecules, thus changing their configuration and biologic function and activity.

An examination of the horizontal period relationships reveals, again, a pattern of toxicity that increases with successive periods. Usually there is a decrease in toxicity of metal cations from groups I to IV, and an increase with metal anion (oxyacids exhibiting the maximum valence state) from groups V to VII. This greater electropositivity of the metals of the fifth horizontal period, renders them more toxic than the elements of the fourth series. Some of the intrinsic toxicity of the group IV metals (gallium, germanium, arsenic) is masked by the hydrolysis of their soluble salts at tissue pH levels and subsequent olation. These metals exhibit electroneutral and amphoteric characteristics with variable valences. Tetravalence is common with the anions of the lighter metals, e.g., germanium. Usually, the higher the valence, the lower the toxicity.

Another reason for the examination of these elements as a trilogy is the fact that, while relatively small amounts are used industrially, they are becoming increasingly important in the semiconductor and communication industries. More and more instances will be seen of the combination of gallium, germanium, and indium with arsenic, antimony, and phosphorus, as well as in alloys with each other. The gaseous reactive forms of these metalloids, hydrides, arsenides, antimonides, and phosphides also share with arsine and stibine potentially toxic properties, and these are the main forms in which they are used.

HISTORY

Gallium was predicted to exist by Mendeleef in 1871, but was not isolated until four years later by DeBouisbaudran,[2] who named it after his native land (*Gallia*, Latin for France). The work of DeBouisbaudran was not published until 1877, when he explained how he had noted a gap between the regularity of the spectral lines of aluminum and indium in group III of the elements. After examining hundreds of samples of ores, he discovered the missing element in a sample of zincblende from the Pyrenees. This represented a significant achievement, since gallium does not exist in the free state in nature, nor are there any specific gallium ores.

Germanium was isolated by Winkler[32] in Germany in 1886. In a surge of patriotism, he named this element in honor of his native land (*Germania* in Latin). Germanium is also always found in combination with other elements and never in the free state, and extensive deposits of germanium ores are rare.

Indium was discovered in 1863 spectroscopically by Reich and Richter[21] in Freiburg pitchblende, in Germany. The spectrum showed an intense blue line and a second fainter blue line, and from this indigo color they conceived the name *Indium*. Indium is found widely distributed in ores of zinc, tin, manganese, and antimony, but only in very low concentrations. Dark sphalerite (ZnS), narmatite, christophite (FeS:ZnS), and siderite are the most common ores.

In spite of their identification well before the turn of the century, these substances were not isolated in sufficient quantities to be of any commercial interest or importance for over 50 years. Gallium was only an experimental curiosity until well into the 1970s. Germanium came into prominence in World War II for the preparation of diodes and was largely responsible for the "revolution in electronics." Indium likewise was not produced in appreciable quantities for industrial purposes until about 1940, with the development of improved electrolytic processes.[13] Geckler and Marchi[9] reported that in 1934, indium was first employed in dental gold amalgam. It was estimated that 90% of gold crowns with porcelain veneers contained 1% indium. During World War II, it was used in aircraft bearings to withstand high temperatures and acidic oils.

Precise figures of the worldwide production of these metals is quite difficult to obtain. Ten years ago, it was estimated that the world production of gallium was about 10,000 kg and sold at a price of $750 per kilogram. This amount has unquestionably increased since that time. Germanium worldwide, in the same year, totalled 369,000 kg. U.S. production, however, had fallen to 61,000 kg from a 1954 high of 90,000 kg, owing to a decline in the demand for germanium in semiconductors. Because of the limited nature of the indium market, U.S. production figures for 1984 are not known. It has been estimated that 2,100 kg were imported in 1984.

GEOCHEMISTRY AND OCCURRENCE

Gallium is widely distributed in the earth's lithosphere, but never in a free state. The earth's crust contains about 5 ppm or 15 gm/ton.[10] This is about equal to lead and 30 times more than mercury. The richest source is the mineral germanite (7 $CuSFeSGeS_2$), a copper sulfate ore found mostly in South West Africa. It contains about 0.5%–0.7% gallium. Bauxite, an aluminum ore, contains 0.01%–0.05%, and lesser concentrations are found in Sphalerite (ZnS). Gallium is also found in varying amounts in coal, and can be recovered from fluegas.

No information is available about the presence of gallium in seawater or human body tissue, although traces (1 ppm) have been detected in the human skeleton. It is not considered to be an essential element in human nutrition.

Germanium is likewise never found in the pure state but usually in ores such as argyrodite (Ag_8GeS_6), which contains 5.7%, or germanite, which contains up to 10%. These also are found mostly in South West Africa and Zaire. It is present in many coals and as much as 3% can be recovered from the burning fluegas. Enargenite, a copper-arsenic sulfide, is found in the U.S. but only yields about 0.03%, which is not of commercial importance.

Indium is also present in the earth's surface in minute quantities of 0.1% or less. It is found in the hydrosphere, in both fresh and salt water, at concentrations up to 500 ppb near mining, milling, and smelting plants, and in freshwater mud in these locations up to 45 ppm. Much less indium is found in seawater (0.00002–0.007 ppb). It is an ambiguous component of the atmosphere, being found at levels of 0.00053 μg/cu m at the south pole. Maximum concentrations are measured near refining operations. In Idaho, 43 μg/cu m; in California, 8.6 μg/cu m; with 5.3 μg/cu m in Cleveland, Ohio, and 4 μg/cu m in Tucson, Arizona; near a nuclear power plant in Budapest, Hungary, 39 μg/cu m was measured.

CHEMICAL AND PHYSICAL PROPERTIES

Gallium has an atomic number of 31 and an atomic weight of 69.72. It is a member of group III of the periodic table, with a density of 5.91. It is liquid at slightly above room temperatures (29.75° C) and the molten metal is silver white. It boils at 1,700° C. Like water, it expands on freezing but can be supercooled and remain liquid at 0° C. Its freezing point is lower than any metal except mercury, which is −39° C.

Gallium is chemically similar to aluminum, being amphoteric, but slightly more acidic. It has a normal valence of +3, but is trivalent and can exist as +1 or +2. Cationic salts undergo hydrolysis to hydroxides in dilute aqueous solutions. Anionic gallates are stable and water-soluble. Halides tend to be bimolecular in the gaseous state. Complexes are tetrahedral in geometry. Gallium binds to the microbial protein, transferrin, with the same stochiometry as iron. Chlorides are not stable at physiologic pH and tend to hydrolyze to colloidal hydroxides ($GaOH_3$). It has an electrode potential of −0.56, placing it between zinc and indium.

It has been postulated that gallium forms a dimeric molecule with hydrogen to form digallane or gallium hydride (GaH_3) or perhaps Ga_2H_6, in a bridged structure similar to diborane. This is a volatile liquid and it decomposes at 130° C. Unfortunately, there is no direct experimental evidence to support this premise.

Since much of the impetus for preparing this section was due to an interest in gallium arsenide (GaAs), mention should be made of that compound and its peculiar properties. Gallium arsenide can be used for translating mechanical motion into electrical impulses. A moveable grating is imposed between a light-emitting source (a gallium arsenide diode) and a photosensitive gallium arsenide reversed biased diode (the former is forward biased). When the grating is attached to a diaphragm or other mechanical system, its motion can modulate light as it impinges on the junction of the reversed biased diode. This cationic form of gallium has given excellent results in various semiconductor applications at higher temperatures and both lower and higher frequencies than are useable with either germanium or silicon.

The continuing and intensifying interest in gallium increases the real potential for occupational exposure hazards, since research scientists tend to be more cavalier in their attitudes and concerns than manufacturing employees. An extensive review on gallium has been published by De La Breteque[3] and those interested are encouraged to examine it.

Germanium has an atomic number of 32 and an atomic weight of 72.6. It is a member of group IVB, along with carbon, silicon, tin, and lead. Germanium, like its associates, has both metallic and nonmetallic properties. From the viewpoint of the biologist, these can be considered to be chemical hemaphrodites, in that they can either be the donor or receiver in the formation of new chemical entities, acting in a positive or a negative fashion. Normally germanium has a valence of +2 or +4. The bicovalent compounds of germanium are few, and there is no evidence that the atom ever exerts two covalent bonds in a discrete molecule. It is less electronegative and more metallic than carbon or silicon.

The majority of the time the atom is quadrivalent. It is almost never diagonally or triagonally hybridized, but it can be tetrahedrally hybridized to form hybrides, halides, and alkyl or aryl organometallic compounds. The hydrides can take the form of GeH_4, Ge_2H_6, or GeH_8. Monogermane (GeH_4) is a gas, liquifying at low temperatures and only reasonably stable at room temperature. Fortunately, it is not explosive below 130° C.

In a pure state, germanium is a greyish white, lustrous, brittle metalloid. It melts at 937.4° C and boils at 2,830° C.

Germanium possesses the unique property of semidirectional transmission of electricity. It is also unusual in being highly transparent to infrared light. This, coupled with its high index of refraction, makes it particularly desirable in specialized optical instruments. Crystalline germanium is a true semiconductor. Depending upon the type and amounts of impurities present, it will be an "n" or a "p" type. In semiconductor applications it is frequently alloyed with arsenic, antimony, gallium, or indium.

Indium has an atomic number of 49 and an atomic weight of 114.76. It is a silvery white, soft, malleable metal, unaffected by air or alkalis. It melts at 156° C and boils at 2,075° C.

The indic ion is colorless and has a valence of +3. Indium is a member of group IIIA. Electromotively, it falls between iron and tin. It is slightly less amphoteric than gallium but more electropositive. It also binds to transferrin, but to a lesser degree. Indium ions do bind to free and bound phosphate groups in biologic fluids and tissue. It will form alloys in four systems: binary, ternary, quaternary, and quinary. With the elements of group III and V (arsenic, antimony, phosphorus) it forms an intermetallic semiconductor, with promising properties.

Combined with gallium (24% indium and 76% gallium), it forms a eutectic which melts at 16° C, is liquid at room temperature, and has the unique property of wetting glass for metal-to-glass or glass-to-glass seals, where high temperatures cannot be used.

Indium exhibits mono-, di-, and trivalent states, but is most commonly found as +3. It forms arsenides, antimonides, phosphides, and hydrides. Indium hydride or indane (InH_3) is an unstable gas except in ether solutions at subzero temperatures. It complexes with gallium and other metalloids and also forms alloys with higher metals. With halogens it forms complexes such as indium hexafluoride $(InF_6)^{-3}$. Covalent complexes are tetrahedral.

For the most part, indium chemistry is not closely analogous to gallium and thallium. Indium +3 salts begin to precipitate as $In(OH)_3$ and basic salts at a pH of 3.4. The hydroxide is probably the major form assumed by industrial discharges of ionic indium in freshwater. In seawater it is more likely to be present as $(InOH)^{+2}$ or $(InOH_4)^-$. At pH 10, soluble indates form.

Indium is not considered to be an essential nutrient for mammals, in spite of its widespread traces in foods of plant origin.

Extensive reviews on indium have been published by Smith, Carson, and Hoffmeister[24] and Lutwick.[14] Again, the interested reader is directed to these for more details.

ABSORPTION, METABOLISM, EXCRETION, AND TOXIC EFFECTS

Gallium, germanium and indium have not been extensively examined toxicologically. Overall, there is a dirth of information regarding occupational exposures or health effects. For the most part, only animal investigations on the toxicity of these elements appear in the literature, and many of these are studies on compounds, salts, or derivatives, rather than on the pure substance.

However, since occupational exposures may be the basis for future knowledge about the toxic effects of these materials, it appears prudent to examine the facts that are available as a guideline to future understanding and investigations. Each of the elements will be explored individually from the aspects of absorption, metabolism, distribution, and excretion, with comments about the toxic effects reported in animal species.

Gallium

Gallium is not readily absorbed from the gastrointestinal tract, owing to the hydrolysis of GA^{+3} salts to the insoluble and unabsorbable hydroxide, $Ga(OH)_3$. When injected subcutaneously or intravenously as citrate or lactate salt, it will disappear in a short period after administration (four hours), and in the case of the citrate, 30%–48% is deposited in bone, 1%–2% is excreted in the feces, and 30%–55% leaves through the kidneys and urine. The lactate follows a similar pattern, but appreciable amounts of this salt are retained by the liver and kidneys for almost a month. Osteolysis from the bones does not start until almost three months after the initial administration. Subcutaneously, gallium as a metal or alloy produces in situ necrosis with subcutaneous inflammation. Renal tubular damage results from parenteral doses. This leads to decreased blood pH, lowering of sodium and potassium in serum, uncompensated acidosis, and elevated blood urea nitrogen and blood sugar, followed by albuminuria and glycosuria. Gallium can be a neuromuscular toxin, producing hyperexcitability, blindness, and terminal paralysis. Symptoms following intravenous dosing are often anorexia, nausea, itching, edema, dermatitis, and lymphopenia.

The hydroxide, mentioned earlier, is immediately lethal when introduced intravenously. There does not appear to be any biodetoxification mechanism for gallium in the human. The lack of this homeostatic mechanism and the retention of gallium in bone would preclude a gradual accumulation with age and exposure. This remains to be confirmed.

Brucer, Andrews, and Bruner[1] presented a comprehensive study in 1960 on the physiologic and pharmacologic effects of gallium in animals. Dudley et al.[4–7] studied gallium extensively in laboratory animals. The most significant and possibly clinically related effects observed were swollen lymph nodes, nuclear fragmentation and necrosis of lymphoid tissue, renal damage similar to that caused by mercury, aplastic bone marrow changes, photophobia, and blindness (in rats). No inhalation studies above have been reported to date. Ferm and Carpenter[8] found no teratogenic or embryopathic effects in hamsters from the intravenous administration of 40 mg/kg.

A single case of occupational poisoning[8] is the only known incident of human intoxication with gallium. This was a 43-year-old woman who was exposed to gallium fluoride fumes. She experienced a petechial rash on the forearm and hand, with neurologic symptoms after a few days. The rash cleared in two weeks, but muscular weakness and pain persisted for three months. This of course does not represent a pure gallium toxicity case but is mentioned since it was the only one uncovered in the literature.

Gallium as a metallic crystal was patch tested on humans by Meek et al.[16] and no positive reaction resulted. No information was uncovered regarding the toxicity of gallium hydride (digallane, Ga_2H_6). One suggestion was found that it may resemble diborane, but this was not confirmed.

Gallium arsenide was only recently subjected to a preliminary inhalation study by Webb, Sipes, and Carter.[31] This is the first serious approach to any toxicologic examination of what will soon be the most important industrial form of this element. Two papers did appear in the literature which purport lung fibrosis due to gallium arsenide particles by inhalation,[23, 26] but neither is well-documented and they are included solely for comprehensive coverage of the subject since they refer to human health effects.

Germanium

Germanium has not enjoyed an abundance of attention in the recent scientific literature on toxicology. No sophisticated modern biochemical techniques have been applied to studying the metabolic pathways of this element in the body. Short reviews on the toxicology of germanium appears in more publications covering a variety of metals and metalloids by Mogilevskaja[18] and Underwood.[28]

The inhalation of germanium particles was examined and the rate of clearance was exponential. Fifty-two percent was excreted in 24 hours while 18% remained for seven days postexposure. It enters the circulation and appears in the kidneys and liver one hour after exposure. Germanium in various forms is absorbed from the gastrointestinal tract and excreted in the urine (68%) and the feces (9.7%) within 24 hours of administration. It is fairly equally distributed between plasma and red blood cells but is not bound to plasma proteins. Germanium may be transported in the blood, unbound to protein, since it leaves the bloodstream in a few hours. It is widely distributed in body tissue and not selectively retained by any single tissue. Often, within a week it has even disappeared from the tissues in which it was detected. Generally speaking, it has a fairly low systemic toxicity to mammals. Degenerative effects were observed in the liver and kidneys in some investigations. Early work suggested it may have a stimulatory effect on the erythropoietic system, but this was never confirmed. Animal studies to detect mutagenicity, teratogenicity, and carcinogenicity did not produce any positive evidence. No data were found regarding human exposures or effects. One effect which may have human relevance is the profound ability of germanium to disturb water balance when high exposure levels are expected. This leads to hemoconcentration, a fall in blood pressure, and hypothermia.[22]

Germane or germanium hydride (GeH_4) was closely examined by Paneth in 1928.[20] Like arsine and stibine, it is a hemolytic gas, but less toxic than arsine. No human fatalities have been reported. A possibility for neurologic signs (excitation, impaired locomotor activity, listlessness, hypothermia, and convulsions) has been suggested by Gus'kova.[11, 12] Germane is a strong irritant, with an irritation threshold of 13 mg/cu m. At this concentration it depresses pulmonary cell reactions. As the level increases, the respiratory rhythm and rate changes, and catarrh-desquamative bronchitis often results.

Indium

Indium compounds are often toxic, depending on the route of administration and the substance that contains them. Soluble salts are more toxic than other forms. Intravenously in rats, fractions of 1 mg/kg of certain salts are rapidly lethal. The colloidal, hydrated oxide is 40 times as toxic intravenously as a corresponding dose of indium chloride. Inhalation of insoluble dust (indium oxide, In_2O_3) produces atypical pulmonary inflammatory reactions, with a paucity of cellular exudate. No fibrosis results from the healing process, but the dust produces a widespread alveolar stasis resembling alveolar proteinosis, in which alveolar clearance is reduced. McCord et al.[15] provide a brief review of the literature on indium. Interestingly it is noted that ingested indium oxide produces no harmful effects. However, in a hydrate or colloidal form, there appears to be an unusual activation or biotransformation of this compound in macrophages or hepatic lysosomes, following its phagocytosis. The hepatic phagocytes accumulate and concentrate the indium in the reticuloendothelial cells from which it leaks out and damages hepatic parenchymal cells. This is unusual, since these cells are generally associated with detoxifying or inactivating toxic agents.

Indium is also a powerful "direct calcifier," producing this effect in connective tissue, when introduced.

The metabolism of indium, similar to its toxicity, is form dependent. Indium chloride binds in the blood plasma to transferrin, with small amounts binding to the α-globulin and albumin. Colloidal aggregates are, on the other hand, phagocytized.

Distribution is generally uniform, with skin, muscle, and bone accumulating much of the dose. About 60% leaves the lungs in a two-week period, but in nine weeks only 82% is gone. Fecal excretion accounts for 50% and urinary excretion for 8% of an administered dose.

There are no specific detoxification mechanisms reported for indium. (Interestingly, it accumulates in solid tumors in man, but does not inhibit their growth.)

Intravenous administration of ionic indium to hamsters was reported to produce teratogenic effects[8] below 1 mg/kg and embryo-lethality at 9–20 mg/kg. No mutagenicity or carcinogenicity information was discovered.

It is known that indium produces a hydride, indane (InH_3). This is an unstable gas, and since it exists only at subzero temperatures, it is not surprising that it has not been studied or reported on.

McCord[15] did not produce skin sensitization in human beings from the metallic form. However, others have reported it to be a local irritant on skin contact.[19]

Data involving humans is very limited. Stockinger[25] comments that no occupational exposure has been reported. Utidjian[29] has reported on a single isolated case of gallium fluoride exposure.

PERMISSIBLE EXPOSURES

The American Conference of Governmental Hygienists[27] has not set any values for gallium, and this is a situation which will require remedy in the near future. Germanium as a metal has no threshold limit value (TLV), but germane (germanium tetrahydride) is currently set at 0.2 ppm (0.6 mg/cu m) with a short-term exposure limit (STEL) of 0.6 ppm (1.8/cu m). In the U.S.S.R., the maximum allowable concentration (MAC) is 5 mg/cu m.

Indium has a TLV of 10 ppm (0.1 mg/cu m) with a proposed STEL of 3 ppm (0.3 mg/cu m) for 1985, lowered from the 1980 value of 15 ppm (70 mg/cu m).

SUMMARY

It is not possible to offer firm conclusions in this section, because knowledge of the toxicity of these critical elements is still scanty. Much remains to be explored, and the toxic symptoms, manifestations, diagnosis, and treatment of occupational exposures to this chemical trinity challenge the efforts of toxicologists to respond. It is hoped that by the time this textbook is again revised and updated, it will be possible to elaborate more completely on the health effects of these elements on human beings.

REFERENCES

1. Brucer M, Andrews GA, Bruner HD: Study on gallium. *Radiology* 1953; 61:534–512.
2. De Boisbaudran ML: Sur un nouveau metal, le gallium (On a new metal, gallium). *Ann Chim Phys* 1877; 10:100.
3. De La Breteque P: Gallium (in French). *Information Bull* 12. Alusuissee-France SA, 1974.
4. Dudley HC, Henry KE, Lindsley BF: Studies on the toxic action of gallium (I). *J Pharmacol Exp Therap* 1950; 98:409–417.
5. Dudley HC, Levine MD: Gallium toxicity. *J Pharmacol* 1949; 95:487–493.
6. Dudley JC, Marrer HH: Gallium metabolism—Deposition and clearance from bone. *J Pharmacol Exp Therap* 1952; 106:129–134.
7. Dudley HC, Munn JI, Henry KE: Studies on the metabolism of gallium (II). *J Pharmacol Exp Therap* 1950; 98:105–110.
8. Ferm VH, Carpenter SJ: Teratogenic and embryopathic effects of indium, gallium and germanium. *Toxicol Appl Pharmacol* 1970; 16:166–170.
9. Geckler RP, Marchi LE: Indium. *J Chem Ed* 1944; X:407–411.
10. Goldschmidt VM: The principles of distribution of chemical elements in minerals and rocks. *J Chem Soc* 1937; 1:655–662
11. Gus'kova EJ, Barina MD: O bezopasnoti rabotys gidridom germanija. (Occupation Safety and Germanium Hydride) Bezopasnost-truda. *v Promylslennosti* 1974; 1:40–41 (Moscow).
12. Gus'kova EI: K Toksikologii gidrida germaija. (Toxicology of germanium hydride). *Gig Tr i Prof Zabol* 1974; 2:56–57 (Moscow).
13. Linford HB: Indium. *Chem Eng News* 1940; 18:624–628.
14. Lutwick MT: Indium, ed 2. Utica, NY, The Indium Corporation of America, 1959.
15. McCord CP, Meek SF, Harrold GC, et al: The physiological properties of indium and its compounds. *J Ind Hyg Toxicol* 1942; 24:243–254.
16. Meek SF, Harrold GC, McCord CP: Toxicity of gallium. *Ind Med Surg* 1943; 12:9–14.
17. Meigs JW: Gallium fluoride poisoning: A problem case with skin effects and neurological sequence. *J Occup Med* 1972; 14:925.
18. Mogilevskaja O Ja: Gallium toxicity, in Mogilevskaja O Ja, Izreal' son ZI, Suvorov SV (eds): *Problems of Industrial Hygiene and Occupational Pathology in Work with Rare Metals*. Moscow, Medicina, 1973, pp 227–239.
19. Muroma A: Skin reactions produced by certain metallic salts. *An Tev Exp Biol Fenn* 1961; 39(3):277–279.
20. Paneth F: Radioelements as indicators and other selected topics in inorganic chemistry. New York, McGraw-Hill Book Co, 1928.
21. Reich F, Richter Th: Vorlaufige notiz uber ein neues metall (Preliminary notice concerning a new metal). *J Prakt Chem* 1863; 89:441–442.
22. Rosenfeld G, Wallace EJ: Studies of the acute and chronic toxicity of germanium. *Naval Med Res Inst Rep* 46, 1952.
23. Rosenina TA: Toksikologicheskaya kharakteristika antimonida. Indiyai arsenida galliya - Novykh poluprovodinikovykh materialov. (Toxicological features of antimony, indium, and gallium arsenide. A new group of semi-conductors.) *Gig Tr Prof Zabol ISS* 1966; 10(5):30–33 (Russian).
24. Smith IC, Carson BL, Hoffmeister F: *Trace Metals in the Environment*, vol 5, *Indium*. Ann Arbor, Ann Arbor Science Publishers, 1978.
25. Stockinger H: The metals, in Clayton GD, Clayton FE (eds): *Patty's Industrial Hygiene and Toxicology*, ed 3. New York, Wiley Interscience, 1982, pp 1632–1636.
26. Tarasenko NY, Fadeev AI: Problemy gigieny trude v svyazis primeneniem v naroonom chozyaistve soedinenii galliya i indiya (Problems of industrial hygiene related to the use of gallium and indium combinations in the national economy). *Gig Sanit ISS* 1980; 10:13–16.
27. TLVs for Chemical Substances in the Environment Adopted by ACGIH 1986–1987. Cincinnati, Oh, American Conference of Governmental Hygienists, 1986.
28. Underwood EJ: Gallium, in *Trace Metal in Human and Animal Nutrition*, ed 2. New York, Academic Press, 1977.
29. Utidjian H: Gallium fluoride poisoning. *J Occup Med* 1973; 15(2):134.
30. Venugopal B, Luckey TD: *Metal Toxicity in Mammals*, vol 1, *Physiological and Chemical Basis for Metal Toxicity*. New York, Plenum Press, 1978. (See also vol 2, *Chemical Toxicity of Metals and Metaloids*.)
31. Webb DR, Sipes IG, Carter DE: In-vitro solubility and in-vivo toxicity of gallium arsenide. *Toxicol Appl Pharmacol* 1984; 76:96–104.
32. Winkler C: Mitheilugen uber das germanium (Discussion of germanium). *J Prakt Chem* 1886; 105:343.

43

Tungsten, Cobalt, and Their Compounds

Rolf Alexandersson, M.D.

TUNGSTEN AND ITS COMPOUNDS

Tungsten (W) is a steel-gray to tin-white metal which occurs in nature together with other minerals such as tungstate of calcium, iron, and manganese. The commercial tungstate minerals are wolframite ($[FeMn]WO_4$), scheelite ($CaWO_4$), feberite ($FeWO_4$), and hubnerite ($MnWO_4$). Worldwide, wolframite is the most important ore containing tungsten, whereas scheelite is the principal domestic ore in the U.S. Most tungsten deposits are low grade and are upgraded by concentration techniques. The tungsten concentrates produced contain at least 60% tungsten oxide. Worldwide production of tungsten concentrates in 1984 was 49,800 tons.

Uses and Exposures

Tungsten is a very hard metal with extreme resistance to heat. It is therefore used to increase hardness, toughness, elasticity, and tensile strength of steel. Because of its extreme hardness, tungsten cement carbide has replaced diamond (hard metal has 90% of the hardness of diamond) in, for example, rock drills. The majority of tungsten is made into cemented tungsten carbide, i.e., hard metal. It is an alloy consisting of mainly wolfram (tungsten) carbide (70%–95%) and cobalt as a binder (5%–25%).[2] Depending on the quality desired, various amounts of other metals, such as titanium, tantalum and molybdenum can be added. Wolfram carbide, after being milled to a fine powder, is mixed with finely milled metallic cobalt. The mixed powder is pressed into roughly desired shapes and heated under pressure to about 1,000° C. This gives the material enough hardness to be ground more finely. This is done by dry grinding. Then the product is heated to about 1,500° C (above the melting point of cobalt). Finally, the pieces are ground to very exact shapes by diamond grinding.[2]

Potential occupational exposures to sodium tungstate are found in the textile industry, where the compound is used as a mordant and fireproofing agent, and in the production of tungsten from some of its ores, where sodium tungstate is an intermediate product. Potential exposures to tungsten and its compounds are also found in the ceramics, lubricants, plastics, printing inks, paint, and photographic industries.

Occupations with potential exposure to tungsten and its compounds are: cemented tungsten carbide workers, alloy makers, carbonyl workers, ceramic workers, cement makers, dye makers dyers, flameproofers, high-speed tool steelworkers, incandescent-lamp makers, industrial chemical synthesizers, ink makers, melting-pouring-casting workers, metal sprayers, ore-refining and foundry workers, pigment makers, paper makers, penpoint makers, petroleum refinery workers, photographic developers, spark plug makers, textile dryers, tool grinders, tungsten and molybdenum miners, waterproofing makers, and welders. The National Institute for Occupational Safety and Health (NIOSH) estimates that at least 30,000 employees in the United States are potentially exposed to tungsten and its compounds, based on actual observations in the National Occupational Hazards Survey.

Hazards

The major problem associated with occupational exposures to tungsten and its compounds is the respiratory disease caused by cemented tungsten dust. In the cemented tungsten carbide (hard-metal) industry, exposure to a combination of cobalt and tungsten sometimes has resulted in a "hard-metal disease," a disabling, progressive, interstitial pneumonitis, fibrosis, or pneumoconiosis.[3, 7, 14, 16] Other manifestations can be bronchial asthma or obstructive symptoms.[1, 4, 18, 20]

Animal Studies.—Animal experiments by Harding,[10] Lundgren and Swensson,[13] Delahant[6] and Schepers[19] indicate that cobalt and not tungsten itself is the hazardous material.

Kerfoot et al.[11] exposed miniature swine to pure cobalt metal powder at air concentrations of 0.1 and 1.0 mg/cu m, six hours a day, five days a week for several months. After three months, they demonstrated by electron microscopy thickening and collagenization of lung septa and a decrease in lung function, i.e., lung compliance, compared to control animals. Kerfoot concluded from this study that the present threshold limit value (TLV) of 0.1 mg/cu m (adopted in 1979, dust and fumes as cobalt) for cobalt seems to be inadequate.

These animal results of exposure to tungsten metal dust and

dust of wolfram carbide compared to those of cobalt metal dust would suggest that the toxic effect of tungsten cemented carbide dust on the lungs is due more to cobalt than to tungsten itself.

Human Beings.—Most information on human toxicity is chronic in nature and originates from case reports and studies from the hard-metal industries.

Rare cases of hard-metal pneumoconiosis have been reported by hard-metal workers. The exposure periods for the development of the disease have ranged from one month to 28 years, but the most common exposure time exceeds ten years.[17] The hard-metal disease is characterized by a fibrotic reaction in the lung parenchyma. Chest x-rays of affected workers may show diffuse bilateral, linear, patchy shadows and various types of nodular opacities in the middle or lower lobe.[17, 20] In rare cases the interstitial infiltration and fibrosis have been fatal,[5] but mostly the subjective reactions seem to be relieved after the workers have been removed from the work environment.[20]

The hard-metal disease usually develops in tungsten tool industries where the exposure to total dust has ranged between 2 mg/cu m and 10.5 mg/cu m[20] with a cobalt concentration between 0.1 and 2.0 mg/cu m.

Obstructive lung disease may also develop in workroom concentrations of tungsten cemented dust lower than those necessary to cause fibrosis. A few studies have shown an overfrequency of bronchial asthma among hard-metal workers. The workers have fewer symptoms during holidays.[1, 20] Further evidence that a comparably low concentration of wolfram carbide and cobalt in the air also significantly impairs the lung function of workers has been provided by Alexandersson in 1979.[1] In a cross-sectional study, he examined hard-metal exposed workers in different plants in Sweden. Pulmonary function was measured by spirometry and single-breath nitrogen washout. Unexposed control groups were matched with regard to sex, height, and smoking habits. Irritation of the respiratory system was a common complaint of exposed persons. An average exposure level of 1.2 mg total dust/cu m, 0.6 mg/cu m tungsten, and 0.06 mg/cu m cobalt[2] caused symptoms that were mainly obstructive. These reactions occurred during a single eight-hour day and decreased overnight or over the weekend. However, a difference between the exposed workers and the matched controls persisted on Monday morning or after four weeks of holiday. A chronic effect can thus not be excluded. Because there appeared to be a dose-related effect to cobalt, it seems reasonable to suspect cobalt as the hazard metal.

In accordance with the Swedish data, Roto[18] in a case-controlled study, showed that workers who had been exposed to cobalt sulphate dust developed occupational asthma more often than control workers. The relative risk for asthma was about five times higher for cobalt in the air, which varied between 0.05 and 0.1 mg/cu m.

Other Effects

According to Schepers[19] neither tungsten, wolfram carbide, nor hubnerite induced tumors in guinea pigs when they were intratracheally introduced. Exposure to cemented tungsten carbide has been reported to be associated with dermatitis, but mostly with other components in the metal, such as cobalt, nickel, or chromium.[8, 9, 15] Soluble tungsten compounds, such as sodium salts and tungsten acid, have the potential for causing central nervous system and gastrointestinal effects, but there are no reported cases.

Threshold Level Values

The American Conference of Governmental Hygienists (ACGIH) has two limits for exposure. Insoluble tungsten compounds, have an eight-hour time-weighted average (TWA) threshold limit value (TLV) of 5 mg/cu m and soluble compounds have a TWA TLV of 1 mg/cu m. However, it is important to combine the TLV with other components in the cemented tungsten carbide, especially cobalt. From experimental animal studies and group studies on humans, it seems reasonable to lower the TWA TLV on cobalt to less than 0.06 mg/cu m (see Cobalt and Its Compounds).

REFERENCES

TUNGSTEN

1. Alexandersson R: Studies on effects of exposure to cobalt. VI. Exposure, uptake and pulmonary effects of cobalt in the hardmetal industry (in Swedish with English summary). *Arbete och Hälsa* 1979; 10:1–24.
2. Alexandersson R, Bergmann K: Studies on effects of exposure to cobalt: I. Investigation of exposure conditions in the hardmetal industry (in Swedish with English summary). *Arbete och Hälsa* 1978; 20:1–25.
3. Bech AO: Hard metal disease and tool room grinding. *J Soc Occup Med* 1974; 24:11–16.
4. Bruckner HC: Extrinsic asthma in a tungsten carbide worker. *J Occup Med* 1967; 9:518–519.
5. Coates EO, Watson JHL: Diffuse interstitial lung disease in tungsten carbide workers. *Ann Intern Med* 1971; 75:709–716.
6. Delahant AB: An experimental study of the effects of rare metal on animal lungs. *AMA Arch Ind Health* 1955; 12:116–120.
7. Fairhall LT, Castberg HT, Carosso NJ, Brinton HP: Industrial hygiene aspects of the cemented tungsten carbide industry. *Occup Med* 1947; 4:371–378.
8. Fisher AA: *Contact Dermatitis*, ed 2. Philadelphia, Lea & Febiger, 1973.
9. Fregert S: *Manual of Contact Dermatitis*. Copenhagen, Munsgaard, 1974.
10. Harding HE: Notes on the toxicology of metal cobalt. *Br J Ind Med* 1950; 7:76–78.
11. Kerfoot E, Fredrick W, Domeier E: Cobalt metal inhalation studies on miniature swine. *Am Ind Hyg Assoc J* 1975; 36(1):17–25.
12. Lictenstein ME, Bartl F, Pierce RT: Control of cobalt exposure during wet process tungsten carbide grinding. *Am Ind Hyg Assoc J* 1975; 36(12):879.
13. Lundgren KD, Swensson A: Experimental investigations using the method of Miller and Sayers on the effects upon animals of cemented tungsten carbides and the powders used as raw material. *Arch Med Scand* 1953; 145:20–27
14. Lundgren KD, Öhman H: Pneumokoniose in der hardmetallindustrie. *Virchows Arch Pathol Anat Physiol* 1954; 325:259–284.
15. Menne T: Relationship between cobalt and nickel sensitization in females. *Contact Dermatitis* 1980; 6:337–340.
16. Miller CW, Davis MW, Goldman A, et al: Pneumoconiosis in the tungsten-carbide tool industry. *Arch Ind Hyg Occup Med* 1953; 8:443–465.
17. Parkes WR: Occupational lung disorders, ed 2. London, Butterworth & Co, 1982, pp 464–467.

18. Roto P: Asthma, symptoms of chronic bronchitis and ventilatory capacity among cobalt and zinc production workers. *Scand J Work Environ Health* 1980; 6(Suppl 1):1–49.
19. Schepers GWH: The biological action of cobaltic oxide. *Arch Ind Health* 1955; 12(2):124–126.
20. Tolot F, Girard R, Dortit G, et al: Manifestations pulmonaires des "métaux durs": Troubles irritatifs et fibrose (euquête et observations cliniques). *Arch Mal Prof* 1970; 31:453–470.

COBALT AND ITS COMPOUNDS

Cobalt (Co) is a silvery bluish-white metal with magnetic properties but passes at 1,115° C into a nonmagnetic form. Cobalt has an atomic weight of 58.9, a specific gravity of 8.9, and a melting point of 1,493° C. Ambient concentrations of cobalt are usually low. In soil, the cobalt concentration ranges from 1 mg/kg to 40 mg/kg. The world consumption of cobalt ranges between 25,000 and 35,000 tons.[7]

Industrial Uses and Exposures

Potential occupational exposures and uses of cobalt metal are in alloying processes such as steel cutting, grinding, welding, and melting. Pure cobalt metal, as a fine powder, is used as a catalyst and also an additive to certain paints, coatings and resins, and in magnet alloys, and various compounds are added to feed-stock and other animal nutritives. For centuries, it has been used by humans for the coloring of pottery and glass. Since 1927, it has been used as a component in alloys as a binder. Alloys containing cobalt are more resistant to oxidation and high temperature and are of high strength. These physical characteristics make the use of cobalt increasingly important in the tungsten carbide tool industries. It is also used as high strength alloy in the electrical, aircraft, and automobile industry; the estimated potential worker exposure to cobalt is high (Table 43–1).

TABLE 43–1.
Estimated Potential Worker Exposure to Cobalt*

SUBSTANCE	NUMBER OF WORKERS
Cobalt metal	235,000
Cobalt oxides	867,000
Cobalt drier†	301,000
Cobalt paste drier‡	8,300
Cobalt naphthenate	79,000
Cobalt neodecanoate	1,300
Cobalt octanoate	8,100
Cobalt tallate	19,000
Cobalt titanate	900
Cobaltous acetate	21,000
Cobaltous carbonate	5,100
Cobaltous chloride	10,000
Cobaltous nitrate	8,600
Cobaltous oxalate	1,700
Cobaltous sulfate	8,300
Cobalt cyanide	7,200
Cobalt hydroxide	2,500
Cobalt 2-ethylhexoate	3,900

*From the NIOSH National Occupational Hazard Survey, 1972–74.
†Many of these workers would be potentially exposed to only small amounts of cobalt through inhalation, ingestion, or dermal contact. The exposure estimates are not additive, since some workers would be exposed to more than one compound.
‡Substance(s) comprising the drier were not identified.

Production of alloys and "hard metal" accounts for 70% of cobalt use. Work exposures in eight cemented tungsten carbide plants in Sweden have been evaluated by Alexandersson and Bergman.[5] Their findings revealed that exposure to cobalt varies a great deal from one category of production personnel to another. Some particles are small enough to penetrate to the alveolar level. Typical concentrations in the working environment range from 0.001 mg/cu m to 1.7 mg/cu m. The highest levels of exposure to cobalt occur among groups handling presintered materials, as powder handling, with declining levels among press operators and shapers (the mean value for these categories is 0.06–0.01 mg/cu m), dry-grinders (0.012 mg/cu m), wet-grinders (0.008 mg/cu m), flat-grinders (0.003 mg/cu m), and inspection personnel (0.002 mg/cu m).

Metabolism

Cobalt is essential to humans as a necessary component of cyanocobolamin or vitamin B_{12}. No other function for cobalt has been established.[38]

Absorption.—The most important occupational exposure to cobalt is through inhalation.[6, 40] The gastrointestinal absorption of soluble cobalt compounds, such as cobalt chloride ($CoCl_2$), has been reported to be between 5% and 44%[33, 34, 39] with a mean absorption around 18%. Nothing is reported about skin absorption.

Distribution and Excretion.—The absorption of cobalt in the lungs is very rapid. Excretion takes place predominantly in the urine.[6] After absorption, cobalt is distributed mainly to the liver, but it has also been found in heart muscle tissue.[1, 37] Alexandersson and Lidums[6] followed the concentration in urine from Friday after the work shift to Monday morning before the work shift. The results showed a rapid decrease of the urinary concentration of cobalt during the first 20–30 hours after exposure when the exposure was relatively high (Fig 43–1). The decrease was less pronounced when the exposure was lower. Then a period with prolonged excretion followed, with some persons not reaching the "normal zone" even after four weeks of vacation. In the same studies, the normal values of cobalt was 8.5 nmol/L in the blood and 6.8 nmol/L in the urine of a nonoccupationally exposed group. Another group of exposed persons was followed for a whole work week. The exposure of each person was determined by means of personal air samples and the concentration in urine was checked every morning and afternoon (Fig 43–2). Each shift was found to increase urinary cobalt concentration, with a consistent decrease the following morning. When the average exposure in the air for the whole week was compared with the cobalt concentration in urine, the correlation coefficient on Friday afternoon was 0.79 and

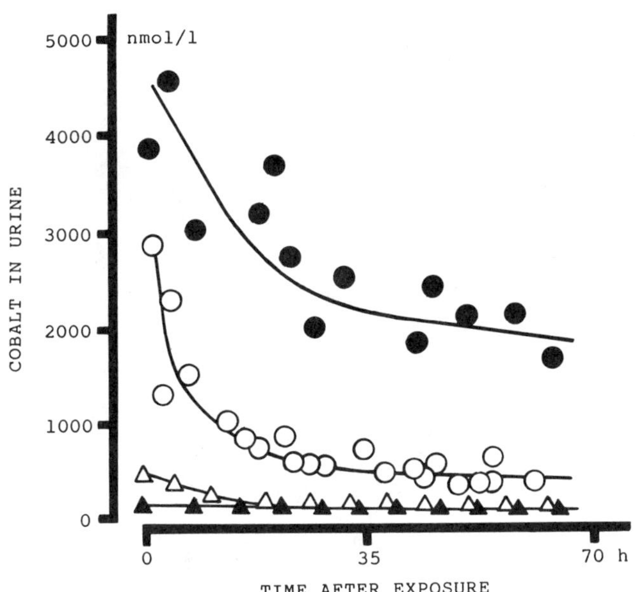

FIG 43–1.
Urinary concentration of cobalt at different times after exposure to cobalt dust. Four persons with different degrees of exposure.

on Monday morning was 0.81. For blood, the correlation coefficient was 0.87 and 0.76, respectively.

Biologic Effects

Respiratory Effects.—Rare cases of pneumoconiosis have been observed in the carbide producing industry, especially during earlier years.[26] The disease developed after one month to 28 years of exposure to cobalt at workroom concentrations in the order of, or exceeding, 0.2 mg/cu m.[10] Occupational medical analyses and experiments on animals pointed to cobalt as the substance probably causing the condition.[11, 16, 22, 32] Kerfoot et al.[20] designed an animal inhalation study simulating the conditions under which workers in the tungsten carbide industry are exposed to cobalt metal powder. Miniature swine were exposed to cobalt at both 1.0 mg/cu m and 0.1 mg/cu m (which is the present TLV for workers adopted by the ACGIH in 1984) for three months daily, six hours per day, five days a week. The study resulted in the appearance of pulmonary disease evidenced by a marked decrease in lung compliance and an increase in the amount of collagen in the central areas of the pulmonary alveolar septa.

Toward the end of 1960, the persons exposed to cemented carbide once more complained of diffuse respiratory troubles in the form of coughing and dyspnea.[28]

Six groups of workers from the tungsten carbide industry with different degrees of exposure to cobalt have been studied by Alexandersson.[2] Pulmonary function was measured by spirometry and with a single-breath nitrogen washout. Unexposed control groups were matched with regard to sex, height, and smoking habits. Irritation of the respiratory passages was a common complaint of exposed persons. An average cobalt exposure level of 0.06 mg/cu m causes symptoms that are mainly obstructive. These reactions can occur during a single eight-hour day and decrease overnight or over the weekend. However, a difference between the exposed workers and the matched controls persists on Monday morning or after four weeks of holiday. A chronic reduction in the pulmonary function can thus not be excluded. There also appears to be a dose-related effect. The responses to cobalt were more marked in smokers than nonsmokers. In conclusion, exposure to cobalt below the TLV (0.1 mg/cu m) at the time of the investigation (1978) resulted in acute but, in general, subsiding pulmonary effects, interpreted as airway obstruction. For the most exposed subjects, a chronic reduction in lung function could not be excluded.

Skin Effects.—Cases of cobalt skin allergy are well-documented.[12, 13, 31, 35] Isolated skin allergy is, however, uncommon and mostly associated with other types of contact allergies, i.e., nickel.[24]

Myocardial Effects.—Cases of myocardial disorders have been observed in patients with a high consumption of beer after breweries had added cobalt compounds to stabilize the froth.[9, 21, 23, 36] The clinical picture of myocardial disorders observed in cobalt or production workers is similar to that of beer drinkers' disease.[8] In one case, a hard-metal worker with four years of occupational exposure to cobalt died of cardiac insufficiency.[19]

In two Swedish cross-sectional studies of workers in the hard metal industry, Alexandersson and Atterhög[3, 4] have studied the heart effects of exposure to cobalt in three groups with different exposure to cobalt. One of the groups, wet-grinders, had an overfrequency of the symptoms "dyspnea and shortness of breath" and "tightness in the chest," but without pulmonary dysfunction, compared to matched controls. They also had an overfrequency of electrocardiogram (ECG) ST- and T-depressions and an overfrequency of ectopic beats. The changes were small, and after four weeks of holiday, the ECG changes decreased significantly to the level of the unexposed controls, indicating that the ECG changes recorded at work among wet-grinders are reversible and not chronic.

Carcinogenic Effects.—Cobalt powder, cobalt oxide, and cobalt sulfide have been reported to induce sarcomata in rats.[15] However, no data have been published so far about cancer mortality or morbidity among workers occupationally exposed to only cobalt without other suspected carcinogenic substances in the air.

Other Effects.—Polycythemia[41] and subsequent development of thyroid hyperplasia[14, 29] have occurred following ingestion of cobalt salts. However, there is no evidence of these effects in occupationally exposed workers. Cobalt does not appear to have a strong mutagenic[18, 25, 27] or teratogenic effect.[14] Alexandersson and Hogstedt[6a] investigated the mortality pattern of 1,876 male hard metal workers with at least five years of occupational exposure to cobalt in four Swedish hard metal factories. The number of deceased men with different causes of death during 1951–1982 has been compared with expected numbers based on national statistics. Individual exposures had been assessed during different time periods and thereafter the study population has been divided into two exposure categories. The lower of these categories had been exposed to 0.001–0.01 mg cobalt/cu m and the higher category had

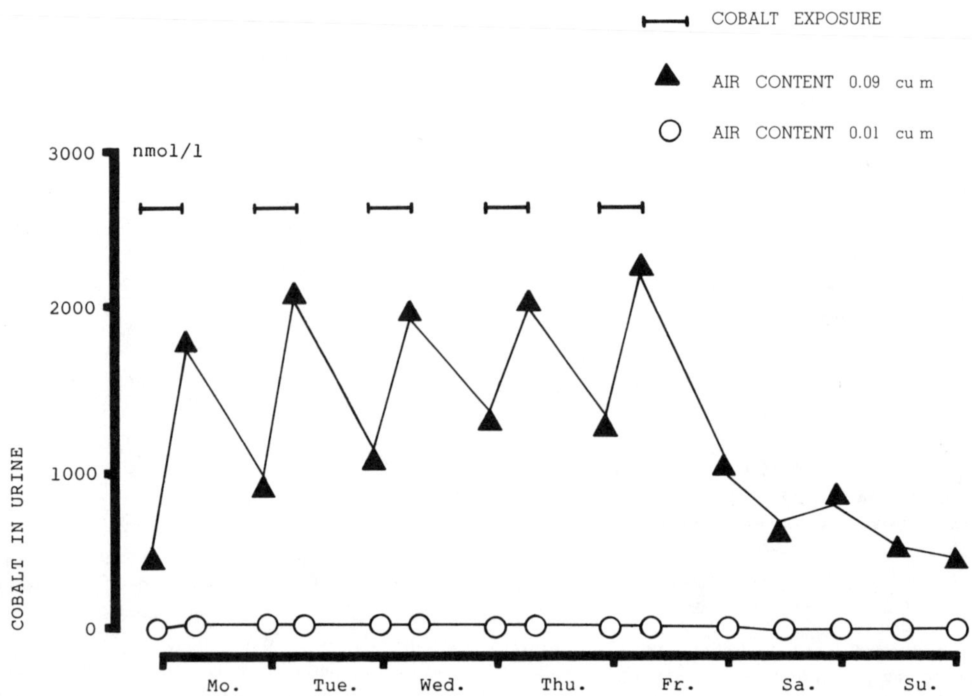

FIG 43–2.
The mean value for cobalt concentration in urine before and at the end of every workday during one week and during the subsequent weekend. One high-exposure and one low-exposure group.

been exposed to 0.01–1.0 mg cobalt/cu m. The cobalt exposure has only been reduced moderately since 1940–1950 in the low exposure subcohort while a substantial reduction has been achieved in the higher exposure subcohort. 172 deaths prior to the age of 80 were recorded compared with 202 expected according to the national statistics. However, an increased risk of pulmonary fibrosis and lung cancer was found although without a definite exposure response pattern. A nonsignificant increase in deaths from ischemic heart disease was also noticed in the high exposure subgroup 20 years after first time of exposure. Further follow-up is needed in order to assess the risks with greater certainty but the results indicate that the cobalt exposure should be kept as low as possible.

Threshold Level Values

Present TLV values in different countries throughout the world range from 0.05 to 0.5 mg/cu m with the Nordic countries having the lowest values and Poland and U.S.S.R. the highest.[30] In view of the findings obtained after a relatively short period of cobalt exposure at 0.1 mg/cu m, as in the miniature swine studies, and the fact that workers in group studies have obstructive findings in their lungs after a mean exposure of 0.06 mg/cu m it seems reasonable that the TLV should be less than 0.1 mg/cu m and also 0.06 mg/cu m. In the U.S.A., the TLV is 0.1 mg/cu m, but with a recommendation to lower the value to 0.05 mg/cu m (ACGIH, 1985).

REFERENCES

COBALT AND ITS COMPOUNDS

1. Alexander CS: Cobalt-beer cardiomyopathy (including a general review on toxicology). *Am J Med* 1972; 53:395–417.
2. Alexandersson R: Studies on effects of exposure to cobalt. VI. Exposure, uptake and pulmonary effects of cobalt in the hardmetal industry (in Swedish with English summary). *Arbete och Hälsa* 1979; 10:1–24.
3. Alexandersson R, Atterhög J-H: Studies on effects of exposure to cobalt. VII. Heart effects of exposure to cobalt in Swedish hardmetal industry (in Swedish with English summary). *Arbete och Hälsa* 1980; 9:1–21.
4. Alexandersson, RS, Atterhög J-H: Comparision of electrocardiograms among wetgrinders in Swedish hardmetal industry before and after four weeks holiday (in Swedish with English summary). *Arbete och Hälsa* 1983; 18:1–15.
5. Alexandersson R, Bergman K: Studies on effects of exposure to cobalt. I. Investigation of exposure conditions in the hardmetal industry (in Swedish with English summary). *Arbete och Hälsa* 1978; 20:1–25.
6. Alexandersson R, Lidums V: Studies on effects of exposure to cobalt. IV. Cobalt concentrations in blood and urine as indicators of exposure (in Swedish with English summary). *Arbete och Hälsa* 1979; 8:1–23.

6a. Alexandersson R, Hogstedt C. Mortality among hardmetal workers in Sweden (in Swedish with English summary). *Arbete och Hälsa* 1987; in press.

7. American Metal Market: *Metal Statistics*. New York, American Metal Market, 1985, pp 57–58.
8. Bech AO, Kipling MD, Heather JC: Hard metal disease. *Br J Ind Med* 1962; 19:239–252.

9. Bonenfant JL, Miller LW, Roy PE: Quebec beer drinkers cardiomyopathy: Pathological studies. *Can Med Assoc J* 1967; 97:910.
10. Coates EO, Watson JHL: Diffuse interstitial lung disease in tungsten carbide workers. *Ann Intern Med* 1971; 75:709–716.
11. Delahant AB: An experimental study of the effects of rare metal on animal lungs. *AMA Arch Ind Health* 1955; 12:116–120.
12. Fisher AA: *Contact Dermatitis*, ed 2. Philadelphia, Lea & Febiger, 1973.
13. Fregerts S: *Manual of Contact Dermatitis*. Copenhagen, Munksgaard, 1974.
14. Friberg L, Nordberg G, Vouk V: *Cobalt in Handbook on the Toxicology of Metals*. New York, Elsevier North-Holland, 1979, pp 403–407.
15. Gilman JP, Ruckerbauer GM: Metal carcinogenesis. I. Observations on the carcinogenicity of a refinery dust, cobalt oxide, and colloidal thorium dioxide. *Cancer Res* 1962; 22:152–157.
16. Harding HE: Notes on the toxicology of metal cobalt. *Br J Ind Med* 1950; 7:76–78.
17. Hewitt PJ, Hichs R: Neutron activation analysis of blood and body tissues from rats exposed to welding fumes in nuclear activation techniques in the life sciences. Proceedings of a symposium April 10–14, 1972. Vienna, International Atomic Energy Agency, 1972.
18. Kanematsu N, Hara M, Kada T: Rec. assay and mutagenicity studies on metal compounds. *Mutat Res* 1980; 77(2):109–116.
19. Kennedy AJ, Dornan JD, King R: Fatal myocardial disease associated with industrial exposure to cobalt. *Lancet* Feb 1981; 21:412–413.
20. Kerfoot E, Fredrick W, Domeier E: Cobalt metal inhalation studies on miniature swine. *Am Ind Hyg Assoc J* 1975; 36:(1)17–25.
21. Kesteloot H, Roelandt J, Claes JH, et al: An enquiry into the role of cobalt in the heart disease of chronic beer drinkers. *Circulation* 1968; 37:854–864.
22. Lundgren KD, Swensson Å: Experimental investigations using the method of Miller and Sayers on the effects upon animals of cemented tungsten carbides and the powders used as raw material. *Arch Med Scand* 1953; 145:20–27.
23. McDermott PH, Delaney RL, Eagan JD, et al: Myocardosis and cardiac failure in men. *JAMA* 1966; 198:(3)253–256.
24. Menne T: Relationship between cobalt and nickel sensitization in females. *Contact Dermatitis* 1980; 6:337–340.
25. Miyaki M, Akamatsu N, Ono T, et al: Mutagenicity of metal cations in cultured cells from chinese hamster. *Mutat Res* 1979; 68:259–263.
26. Parkes WR: *Occupational Lung Disorders*, ed 2. London, Butterworth & Co, 1983, pp 464–467.
27. Paton GR, Allison AC: Chromosome damage in human cell cultures induced by metal salts. *Mutat Res* 1972; 16:332–336.
28. Resare D, Swensson Å: Enkätundersökning av hälsotillståandet hos anställda i hårdmetallindustri. *Arbete och Hälsa* 1977; 6:1–19.
29. Roy PE, Bonenfant JL, Turcot L: Thyroid changes in cases of Quebec beer drinkers' myocardosis. *Am J Clin Pathol* 1968; 50:234–239.
30. Roto P: Cobalt: Nordic expert group for documentation of occupational exposure limits (in Swedish with English summary). *Arbete och Hälsa*. 1982; 16:1–32.
31. Rudzki E, Kohutnicki Z: Occupational allergens in bricklayers. *Med Pracy* 1971; 22:515–519.
32. Schepers GWH: The biological action of cobaltic oxide. *Arch Ind Health* 1955; 12(2):124–146.
33. Smith T, Edmonds CJ, Barnaby CF: Absorption and retention of cobalt in man by whole body counting. *Health Phys* 1972; 22:359–367.
34. Sorbie J, Olatunbosun D, Corbett WEN, et al: Cobalt excretion test for the assessment of body iron stones. *Can Med Assoc J* 1971; 104:777–782.
35. Spruit D, Malten KE: Occupational cobalt and chromium dermatitis in offset printing factory. *Dermatologica* 1975; 151:34–42.
36. Sullivan JF, George R, Bluvas R, et al: Myocardiopathy of beer drinkers: Subsequent course. *Ann Intern Med* 1969; 70:277–282.
37. Sumino K, Hayakawa K, Shibata T, et al: Heavy metals in normal Japanese tissues. *Arch Environ Health* 1975; 30:487–494.
38. Underwood: Cobalt and manganese. World Health Organization Expert Committee on Trace Elements in Human Nutrition. *WHO Tech Rep Ser* 1973; 532 (Geneva).
39. Valberg LS, Ludwig J, Olatunbosun D: Alteration in cobalt absorption in patients with disorders of iron metabolism. *Gastroenterology* 1969; 56:241–251.
40. Wienzierl SM, Webb M: Interaction of carcinogenic metals with tissue and body fluids. *Br J Cancer* 1972; 26:279–291.
41. Wolters H-G: Zur wirkung von kobalt auf die erythropoese. *Blut* 1970; 21:105–117.

44

Vanadium and Its Compounds

Carl Zenz, M.D.

OCCURRENCE AND DISTRIBUTION

Vanadium (V) was discovered by Nils Gabriel Sefström, at the mining school in Falun, Sweden, in 1831. He noted an unusual component present in certain iron ore and slags from Taberg (in the Småland province of Sweden) and isolated an oxide that produced brilliant multicolors, which he believed to be an element, naming it after Vanadis, the Nordic goddess of beauty. However, it was not until 1927 that pure vanadium metal was prepared. With an atomic number of 23 and atomic weight of 50.95, vanadium is a metallic element of group V of the periodic system, related to niobium, phosphorus, and tantalum.

Vanadium does not occur in the earth's crust as a free metal but rather as relatively insoluble salts in which vanadium most commonly is in the trivalent state. Vanadium can be extracted from the following mineral resources: carnotite, a uranium-vanadium mineral; phosphate rock deposits; titaniferous magnetite; and vanadiferous clays. Vanadium also occurs in small amounts in fossil fuels. Vanadium ranks 22nd among the elements in the earth's crust, averaging about 150 mg/kg, and is found in minute quantities in many foods. Shellfish contain high concentrations of vanadium, which probably accounts for the vanadium in fuel oils. (A review of vanadium in the general environment may be found in references 21 and 40.)

In 1984, world production from ores and concentrates was 38,500 short tons. In the United States, vanadium and vanadium compound production was drastically reduced in 1984, primarily because of the slump in steel production. For 1984, production figures from ores and concentrates were: Australia, 110 tons; China, 5,000 tons; Finland (in vanadium pentoxide [V_2O_5]), 3,470 tons (from one underground mine and one open pit mine); Norway, 120 tons; South Africa, 13,200 tons; U.S.S.R., 10,500 tons; United States (in recoverable vanadium), 4,100 tons. Production from petroleum residues, ashes, and spent catalyts: Japan (in vanadium pentoxide product), 550 tons; United States (in vanadium pentoxide and ferrovanadium product), 1,500 tons. The Finnish company, Rautaruukki, with the United Nations Development program, have evaluated high-grade vanadium deposits recently discovered in Burundi, with early drilling indicating over 6 million tons of ore with up to 1.5% vanadium pentoxide.[18]

EXTRACTION AND PRODUCTION

Ores, slags, and boiler residues containing vanadium in a low state of oxidation must be roasted with salt, soda ash, or sodium sulphate to convert the vanadium to water-soluble sodium vanadate ($NaVO_3$). The roasted product is then leached in water or soda ash solution and then sometimes leached with dilute acid. Oxidized ores such as carnotite can be leached with sulfuric acid without roasting. Vanadium is precipitated from water-leach or soda-leach solutions by adding sulfuric acid to a pH of about 2.5. The precipitate is sodium polyvanadate (approximately $[H_2Na]_4V_6O_{17}$ or $[H_2Na]_6V_{10}O_{28}$). Acid-leach liquors containing vanadium are treated by solvent extraction or ion exchange to separate uranium and any impurities present.

The roasting and leaching procedure is sometimes used to extract vanadium from titaniferous magnetite, but a more common procedure, used in the U.S.S.R. and South Africa, is to smelt the magnetite and produce vanadium-bearing pig iron. The pig iron is blown with oxygen and the vanadium is recovered in a slag containing 15%–25% vanadium pentoxide. The slag is roasted and leached to extract vanadium or is used to produce ferrovanadium by a direct reduction process. Reduction of the fused oxide with aluminum produces a commercial grade of metal containing 90% vanadium. Metal containing over 99% vanadium is produced by calcium reduction of vanadium pentoxide in a steel bomb or by reduction of vanadium trichloride (VCl_3) with magnesium or sodium in an argon atmosphere. Carbon reduction of vanadium trioxide (V_2O_3) at 1,700° C in a vacuum has also been used to produce high-purity vanadium. The purest metal, 99.95%, is produced by electrolytic refining of impure grades in a fused salt bath.

Ferrovanadium containing 50%–55% or 70%–80% vanadium is produced by aluminum reduction of a mixture of fused oxide and either iron scale or punchings. Although external heat is not needed if iron scale is used, better vanadium recovery is achieved by using an electric furnace. Silicon metal or ferrosilicon can be used instead of aluminum to reduce the fused oxide, but this requires a two-step process for high vanadium recovery. Ferrosilicon is also used for producing ferrovanadium from vanadium-bearing slags; some of the iron in the slag can be removed by a preliminary ferrosilicon reduction step. Carbon reduction in an electric furnace to produce ferrovanadium has been discontinued. Commercial vanadium carbide (V_2C) for use as an additive to steel is made by carbon reduction of vanadium tetroxide (V_2O_4) in a vacuum. Aluminum-vanadium alloys for the titanium industry are made by aluminum reduction of fused oxide.

CHEMISTRY

Vanadium forms compounds in four valency states. Pentavalent vanadium is nominally acidic with well-defined amphoteric properties. The oxide, V_2O_5, dissolves in alkalis to form a series of meta-, ortho-, pyro-, and polyvanadates, depending upon the pH. Vanadium pentoxide reacts with halides to form $VOCl_3$, VOF_3, and $VOBr_3$. Reaction of metallic vanadium with fluorine yields VF_5.

The tetravalent oxide, VO_2, is formed by reduction of vanadium pentoxide with ammonia or other reductants. It is amphoteric and dissolves in acids to give $(VO)^{2+}$ salts such as $VOSO_4$ and $VOCl_2$. These salts form deep-blue solutions. Chlorination of vanadium at 300° C produces vanadium tetrachloride (VCl_4).

The basic trivalent oxide, V_2O_3, is formed by reduction of V_2O_5 with hydrogen or ammonia at 650° C. It is insoluble in water or alkalis and does not react readily with acids. The chloride, VCl_3, is made by reduction of VCl_4.

The divalent oxide, VO, is best prepared by reduction of V_2O_5 with hydrogen at 1,700° C. It has a metallic luster and good electrical conductivity, and possibly was mistaken for metal by early experimenters. It is insoluble in water or alkalis, but dissolves in acid to form divalent salts.

As noted above, vanadium residues from fly ash, slags, and spent vanadium catalysts apparently are being used in the production of vanadium products in the United States and elsewhere. These sources generally have a considerably higher vanadium concentration than naturally occurring ores and, therefore, account for a greater concern in handling and preventing general contamination. Ash from petroleum-fired facilities, for example, may contain up to 70% vanadium pentoxide, although the concentration varies significantly, depending on the vanadium content of the fuel oil. Vanadium pentoxide concentrations of 5%–18% have been reported for fly ash residues commonly processed. Although reported as vanadium pentoxide, the vanadium present in fly ash rarely is in this form, and most probably exists in one of several reduced forms—as vanadium tetroxide, trioxide, and dioxide—but not necessarily in the form of simple vanadium oxides. Vanadium-rich slags also represent a potential source of vanadium. Processing of a vanadiferous magnetite ore reportedly provides a vanadium pentoxide concentration of 20%–25% in the slag.

Almost all the coal consumed in the United States contains some vanadium. From the Bureau of Mines data, the weighted average vanadium content of coal mined in the United States is about 30 ppm. The estimate indicates that about 1,750 tons of vanadium were emitted in 1969 as a result of burning bituminous coal and perhaps an additional 375 tons as a result of burning anthracite coal.[1]

Nearly all crude oils of petroleum origin contain vanadium as an impurity; the concentration can vary from less than 1 to as high as 1,400 ppm, depending on the source of the crude oil. In a report prepared for the Environmental Protection Agency,[4] it was estimated that the residual fuel oils burned in the United States in 1968 contained a total of slightly under 19,000 tons of vanadium and that 90% of this total (some 17,000 tons) was emitted into the air.

During the early 1960s, large numbers of U.S. military personnel and their families stationed in Japan developed a high incidence of upper respiratory symptoms—a condition referred to as "Yokohama asthma." Many factors were investigated in the search for the etiologic agent, and vanadium oxides were among the agents studied. Vanadium oxides were suspected because of the new sources of Japan's oil supply after World War II. Before the war, fuel oil low in vanadium had been obtained from Indonesia. This source dwindled, and postwar arrangements were made with Middle East suppliers whose oil contained considerably more vanadium. Vanadium was never proved to be the etiologic agent accountable for Yokohama asthma, but it might have been a contributing factor.

USE IN METALLURGIC AND CHEMICAL INDUSTRIES

Ferrovanadium, mainly an alloy of iron and vanadium containing 50%–80% vanadium, is one of the most common commercial forms in which vanadium is added in steelmaking. Aluminothermic vanadium, an alloy of aluminum and vanadium, is used in titanium alloy production. Vanadium carbide is used in the iron and steel industry and is added either as ferrovanadium or as vanadium carbides (VC and V_2C). Apart from its use in steels, vanadium is a major alloying element in high-strength titanium alloys. The alloy of greatest production for many years has contained 4% vanadium. Metallurgic products containing vanadium, particularly steel and titanium alloys, are themselves often processed, e.g., by flame cutting, welding, and brazing for joining. Processing operations involving high temperatures are of particular interest, because they may involve considerable smoke and fume.

The principal uses of vanadium in the production of chemicals are as catalysts in the synthesis of sulfuric acid and in the oxidation of numerous organic compounds to commercial products. The oxidation of sulfur dioxide to sulfur trioxide in the production of acid consumes by far the largest amount of vanadium (estimated at 80 tons of vanadium pentoxide in 1982). Vanadium pentoxide on asbestos as a carrier is reported to be the preferred catalyst for the reaction.

In dye manufacture and dyeing, vanadium compounds are widely used in the production of aniline black. Vanadium salts are added as catalysts to a mixture of aniline hydrochloride and potassium or sodium chlorate. Vanadium compounds are used as mordants in the dyeing and printing of cotton, and particularly for fixing aniline black on silk. Ammonium metavanadate has been used as a catalyst in the dyeing of leather and fur. Some modern quick-drying inks depend on the addition of ammonium metavanadate for their performance. Closely allied to the chemical industry is polymer synthesis and processing. Ammonium metavanadate continues to play a primary role in various ceramic glazes, particularly the zircon vanadium blues. These glazes are not used in dinnerware but in such applications as wall tile.

Vanadium compounds such as vanadium oxychloride, vanadium tetrachloride, and vanadium triacetylacetonate are used as catalysts in polymerization processes to produce soluble copolymers derived from ethylene and propylene. There is also substantial use in the manufacture of synthetic rubber of the ethylene-propylene-diene types.[21]

Other processes using vanadium catalysts are: manufacture of phthalic anhydride, maleic anhydride, production of aniline black, oxidation of cyclohexane to adipic acid, oxidation of ethylene to acetaldehyde, oxidation of anthracene to anthroaquinone, oxidation of toluene or xylene to aromatic acids, oxidation of furfural to fumaric acid, oxidation of hydroquinone to quinone, oxidation of butene-2 and 1,3-butadiene to maleic anhydride, ammonolysis oxidation toluene, m-xylene, p-xylene, and propylene, preparation of vinyl acetate from ethylene, manufacture of cyclohexylamine from cyclohexanol and ammonia, and catalytic combustion of exhaust gases. Vanadium pentoxide is used in gram quantities to make miniature batteries for pacemakers, etc.

EFFECTS ON MAN

Occupational Exposures

The route of entry most common in occupational exposures is through the respiratory system, although entry can also be via the gastrointestinal system as part of the overall airborne exposure. Uptake in human beings through ingestion or by direct injection into the circulatory system is uncommon, being encountered only in experimental situations.

Studies based on 19 workers exposed to vanadium pentoxide for periods of a few months to several years were reported by Symanski.[33] He concluded that there is a characteristic picture and that the symptoms are due entirely to the irritating effects of vanadium on the mucous membranes of the respiratory tract and on the conjunctiva. In all his cases, he observed conjunctivitis, rhinitis with watery discharge, "sore throat," and persistent cough with pressure over the chest and many rhonchi. He pointed out that severe chronic bronchitis might occur, possibly with bronchiectasis, and he emphasized that he had observed no gastrointestinal symptoms, no signs of lowered activity of the blood-forming organs or any symptoms or organic injuries of the kidneys or the nervous system. Symanski believed that there was no reason to suspect an absorptive poisoning effect, but he did not present any tissue or body fluid analyses or histologic data to support this contention.

Sjöberg published a classic presentation[28] of his clinical and experimental investigation on the effect on man and animals of the inhalation of vanadium pentoxide dust. His series of workers had been exposed to dust during the manufacture of vanadium pentoxide and observed over a two-year period. Symptoms consisted chiefly of slight conjunctivitis and irritation of the nasal mucosa—in most cases with nasal catarrh and moderate pathologic changes in the mucous membrane. Acute and chronic hyperplastic changes in the mucous membrane—in many cases of "allergic type"—predominated at the final examinations. The most characteristic symptoms were coughing (in most cases violent, in some merely irritation of the throat) with or without expectoration, wheezing sounds in the chest (also heard on auscultation), and dyspnea. No chronic changes in the lungs (pneumoconiosis, fibrosis, emphysema) were demonstrated. There was no discoloration of the tongue, and urine vanadium was demonstrated by spectral analysis. Eczema was present in some, probably attributable to "hypersensitivity."

Williams[37] reported an incident in which boiler cleaners sustained vanadium intoxication. Primary symptoms occurred a half hour to 12 hours after starting work and consisted of rhinorrhea, sneezing, watering of the eyes, sore throat, and substernal soreness; the secondary symptoms appeared after 6–24 hours and consisted of a dry cough, wheezing, severe dyspnea, lassitude, and depression, with a disinclination to follow the usual evening activities. A greenish black coating developed on the tongue; this faded two to three days after removal from contact with the petroleum soot. In some cases, the cough became paroxysmal and productive. The symptoms continued while the subjects were at work and did not become less severe until three days after removal from the exposure. In one man, the wheezing and dyspnea persisted for more than a week, but no permanent effects were noted.

Browne[2] studied vanadium poisoning in 12 men exposed to exhausts from gas turbines using heavy residual fuels. The symptoms noted occurred between the first and 14th days of exposure and were generally similar to those described by Williams except that there was some bleeding rather than running of the nose. Browne reported skin effects but did not observe mental depression. Browne and Steele[3] surveyed three catalytic oil-gas plants in which the nickel-impregnated catalyst became coated with fuel oil ash containing vanadium. These coatings had to be manually cleaned periodically by removing and sieving and adding new catalyst to replace losses, all resulting in high concentrations of pentoxide dust. The men employed in the changing process wore goggles, respirators, and protective clothing.

Lewis[17] reported a study of 24 men who had worked with vanadium without exposure to other metals for more than six months. He was one of the first investigators to describe bronchospasm, which persisted in some cases for two to three days after cessation of exposure. He found significant differences in symptoms and physical findings between controls and exposed workers. Eye, nose, and throat irritations, cough, wheezing, and productive sputum were among the most significant symptoms; infected pharynx, green tongue, and wheezes, rales, or rhonchi were among the most significant of the physical findings. The effects of irritation of mucosal surfaces by vanadium were evident and consistent with the symptoms elicited. Wheezes, fine rales, and rhonchi were heard often on auscultation of the chest, and infection of the pharynx and nasal mucosa was common in the exposed group. Lewis also noted a green coloration of the tongue, a harmless pigmentation that is a result of the deposition of vanadium salts of reduced valency forms; it varied from a pale green to a dark greenish black and was described first by Wyers[38] in 1946. In Lewis's study,[17] it was observed in 9 of 24 workers. The average concentration of vanadium found in the urine of the control group was 11.6 μg/L; the mean of the exposed group was 46.7 μg/L.

Zenz, Bartlett, and Thiede[43] reported responses from 18 men engaged in pelletizing pure vanadium pentoxide. The clinical picture of acute illness appeared remarkably uniform among these workers. The syndrome consisted of a rapidly developing mild conjunctivitis, severe pharyngeal irritation, and nonproductive persistent cough, followed by diffuse rales and bronchospasm. After severe exposure, four men complained of skin "itch" and a sensation of "heat" in the face and forearms, but no objective evidence of skin irritation was found. A striking feature among the acute intoxications was the increased severity of symptoms with repeated exposures of lesser time and intensity. The severity of the symptoms developing after second and third or subsequent exposures was so dramatic as to suggest a sensitivity reaction rather than an effect of cumulative dosage. Although these recurrent symptoms appeared more severe than the original illness, there was no clinical evidence that these exacerbations were of longer duration.

Milby (in a personal communication) described an incident in which 21 workers were assigned to a job at a refinery where they were called on to install new catalytic converter tubes. Each tube contained a large number of pipes about 7/8 in. in diameter and 10 ft long, which were to be filled with small pellets of vanadium pentoxide. The workers used a small measuring cup to drop the pellets into the tubes in such a fashion as to prevent their clogging the channels near the top. "Dust masks" and goggles were supplied. The principal dust exposure occurred when the pellets were dumped into a bin before the men dropped them into the converter pipes, work carried on during all three shifts. After about 72 hours, or three working days of exposure, the workers began to complain of nasal, ocular, and bronchial irritation and, by the fourth day, most were very ill. Common symptoms were upper respiratory irritation, eye irritation, chest pain, cough, and increasing shortness of breath, which became severe enough to be disabling to all. Other reported symptoms were blurred vision, ringing in the ears, dizziness, palpitations, nausea, vomiting, deep bone pain, headache, and loss of appetite. No permanent sequelae occurred. The pellets contained 11.7% vanadium pentoxide with a trace of cobalt. Dust samples taken during the shaking of these pellets indicated that the average particle diameter was 1.1–1.5 mμ. Unfortunately, dust concentration during exposure was not given.

Tebrock and Machle[34] described "exposure of a plant population to a vanadium-bearing phosphor (europium yttrium orthovanadate) at a mean level of 0.84 mg/cu m of air for five years that resulted in an increase of 30% in the annual rate of minimal injury by vanadium." They concluded that no chronic or systemic effects were found, no significant chest x-ray changes were seen in the 1960–1967 period, and the incorporation of vanadium as the orthovanadate into the crystalline lattice of the phosphor apparently results in the formation of a compound of much lower toxicity than that of vanadium pentoxide alone.

Kiviluoto et al.[11] reported on their studies of effects of vanadium (pentoxide) on 63 men—18 aged 19–29, 14 aged 30–39, and 31 aged 40–56 years. Four men had been exposed for 8.8 years, 23 for 14 years, and 20 for 20 years. (The average length of employment was 11 years.) Concentration of levels of vanadium dust were determined by standard industrial hygiene procedures with analysis by atomic absorption spectrophotometry (graphite furnace method); these procedures were conducted since 1970, with average amounts of vanadium between 0.2 and 0.5 mg/cu m, and a total of 64 samples taken between 1970 and 1975. Early in 1976, steps were taken to reduce dust by flushing the factory floors, thereafter the levels were about 0.01–0.04 mg/cu m. In the spring of 1976, 194 air samples were collected—114 from workers' breathing zones and the remainder at various stationary locations. The authors noted, "in addition to vanadium, the air contained inert magnetite dust" (amounts not stated), and near sintering furnaces, sulfur dioxide levels were determined, these never exceeding 0.5 mg/cu m. Their investigation focused on macroscopic and microscopic studies of the upper respiratory tract and a reference group of workers was selected and similarly studied. Ten workers with the least employment service were eliminated. Smears from the nasal mucosa were taken, as were biopsies from the middle part of the nasal inferior turbinates. Nasal smears and sputum cells were studied. The biopsies from the vanadium workers showed a statistically significant increase in numbers of plasma and round cells, with a nearly characteristic histologic picture. Since there were no significant changes in numbers of eosinophils, the authors stated that the cellular changes found were not of allergic origin. Of special note is that this is the first study of workers exposed to vanadium which included a macroscopic, cytologic, and histologic study of the respiratory tract. Also noteworthy is that the subepithelial inflammatory cell localization and hyperemia in the nasal mucosa of rabbits was described by Sjöberg in his classic report in 1950.

Gylseth et al.[8] conducted an investigation of 17 workers in a ferroalloy plant in order to correlate urinary and blood vanadium levels with their working conditions. This factory began production of pig iron in 1927, initiating a new process in 1956 which permitted vanadium contaminants in the iron to form stable oxides, removed as slag, by blowing oxygen through the liquid iron. This slag contains 12%–13% vanadium. The iron is removed by conventional magnetic separation, the vanadium slag is melted in an electrofurnace with the addition of calcium carbonate and ferrosilicon, and the reduced product contains 50% vanadium, 38% iron, 7% silicon, and 2% manganese. The workers were exposed to the slag dust which contained mainly vanadium pentoxide—the authors reported that other oxides may have been present (VO_2 and V_2O_3). During the reduction phase, pot men are exposed to a mixture of metal and oxide fumes of iron and vanadium. During crushing and packing, workers are exposed to ferrovanadium dust. In order to look for differences between those with "little or no exposure" and those with "moderate to high exposure," they were divided into two groups: group A consisted of six persons working at the pig iron furnace who had none to low exposure, group B was 11 persons working in slag production, on the ferrovanadium furnace, and in the crushing and packing area who had moderate to high exposure. Daily vanadium exposure of those in group B were determined utilizing personal (breathing zone) sampling devices on four successive days (Monday–Thursday). Blood and urine samples were collected from both groups before and after the work shift on the first day and after the shift on the fourth day. The usual industrial hygiene techniques were employed in monitoring and were analyzed by means of electrothermal atomic absorption spectrophotometry. Urine and blood vanadium concentrations were measured by means of neutron activation analysis. The worksite air vanadium levels apparently ranged between 0.02 mg/cu m to more than 1.0 mg/cu m, with most below 0.1 mg/cu m. Gylseth and co-workers stated that a comparison of the exposure and concentration of vanadium in the blood and urine demonstrates that the urinary concentration adjusted for creatinine concentration is the mos reliable exposure indicator. They noted that at the exposure levels encountered, the blood vanadium and urine vanadium values for a single worker can give no clear information about exposure level, but on a group basis, blood vanadium and urine vanadium analysis can be used to reveal exposure, and under certain conditions, the urine vanadium level may give an indication of the exposure level. They clearly noted that "the differences are small and the method difficult and expensive, so for routine control, other criteria should be sought for the control of vanadium dust exposure." According to Gylseth et al., the normal values for vanadium in blood are less than 20 nmol/L and the corresponding urine values are less than 3.5 nmol/mmol of creatinine.

Changes in lung function after exposure to vanadium compounds in fuel oil ash were reported by Lees,[15] who observed and studied 17 workers at a large oil-fired electricity-generating station which used Arabian oil with 200 ppm vanadium content. Because of Lees' thoroughness and clear description of the working conditions (and following, striking findings), his observations are set forth:

> "The products of combustion are recirculated through the boiler before being exhausted via precipitators to a 200-m stack. The combustible components of ash are thus burnt off, leaving a high concentration of vanadium in the final waste product. Some of the final ash falls to the bottom of the boiler, the remainder being caught in the precipitators. The design of the boilers is such that much of the ash forms clinker on the sloping collection sides of the bottom hopper. Periodic removal of the ash and clinker necessitates the entry of men into the hopper to shovel out ash and break clinker with crowbars. This is a dusty operation, and the men engaged in it wear complete disposable coveralls and face masks fitted with cannister filters. Despite this, many symptoms were reported by the men doing this job. On two separate occasions I was able to observe 17 men exposed to bottom ash during cleaning operations. While the men work in crews of six to eight, with one supervisor, only two or three men work in the hopper at a time. They work in rotation so that during an eight-hour shift each man has about two hours of exposure to the dust."

The bottom ash at this generating station had an average vanadium content of 15.3%, while the vanadium content of the crusted deposits, or clinker, had been measured at 24.2%–35%. Breathing zone air monitoring for respirable dust (under 10 μ) was taken from four men, yielding a mean time-weighted average of 523 μg/cu m, suggesting a total dust concentration exceeding 26 mg/cu m. Furthermore, 2% of the dust particles were less than 10 μ in size. Although the workers wore cartridge filter respirators, subsequent testing revealed *peak leakages of up to 9%* of the respirators due to imperfect facial sealing. (With this type of labor intensive cleaning, the average worker's respiratory minute volume must have been greater than 20 L/min, perhaps 30 L/min or more.[42] This represents a marked potential for intake of dust, nearly 2–3 L/min of unfiltered air.)

Serial spirometry was performed on each subject at 24-hour intervals, starting on the day work began and for three days thereafter; a final spirometric record was obtained on the eighth day after initial exposure.

On the day after completing the cleaning operation, the men were clinically examined and their symptoms were recorded. None of the 17 men gave a preexposure history of eye, skin, or respiratory symptoms, but a total of 44 symptoms were reported during the study. There were no positive patch skin tests.

Spirometry was repeated four weeks after exposure and was found to have returned to preexposure levels in all cases. Clinical examination after dust exposure provided no surprises in the light of the reported symptoms. Coarse rhonchi were audible in all who complained of wheezing, while widespread rales were found in two others. No areas of consolidation were noted. Urine samples were obtained on the morning after first exposure. One man who was a study volunteer worked one hour in the hopper with only a simple paper face mask. This person's urinary vanadium level was 280 μg/L (5.488 μmol/L), exceeding the threshold of 40 μg/L (0.784 μmol/L) for this specific test. The volunteer sustained severe discomfort 18 hours after exposure. Pronounced reductions in forced vital capacity (mean 0.5 L), forced expiratory volume (mean 0.5 L), and forced midexpiratory flow (mean 1.16 L/sec) occurred within 24 hours of first exposure and did not return to preexposure levels, but four weeks after exposure no residual defects were noted. Lees suggested that, because of the timing, duration, and quality of changes in lung function, these responses could not be attributed solely to reflex bronchial reaction to irritation by an inert dust.

All the symptoms encountered have been reported previously by other authors. Only one observation of greenish-black tongue discoloration was made. That sign is thought to be evidence of exposure only and not a manifestation of toxicity. Lees noted this color change after applying some dust to the moist tongue without having had any other exposure to vanadium.

Generally, symptoms disappeared within four days of the end of exposure, but half of the men who complained of cough continued to have it until the sixth day. All abnormalities noted on auscultation had disappeared within five days. Thus, symptoms and signs associated with exposure had resolved several days before lung function tests had returned to preexposure levels.

Absorption, Metabolism, Storage, and Excretion

As mentioned earlier, entry is mainly through the respiratory route. Human tissues generally accumulate less vanadium than do those of wild animals. Vanadium was found, however, in more than half the lung samples studied, and an increase in vanadium was noted with increased age, especially in people over age 60.[35] Next in frequency of occurrence of vanadium were the lower small and large intestines, as well as the omentum. No other tissue seemed to retain vanadium to any great extent, and no vanadium was detected in the human aorta, brain, muscle, ovary, or testis.

There is significantly more vanadium in the lungs of people living in the Middle East than in those of people from the United States, Africa, and the Far East. Vanadium was found in 12 of 101 aortas and in 21 of 152 kidneys taken from subjects in the Middle East, whereas no vanadium was found in these tissues from American subjects.

Data concerning vanadium content of foods are sparse, but from these data, the following observations can be made: Vanadium is incorporated into foods from both plant and animal sources. The amount that a particular plant species takes up is variable and probably reflects to some extent the vanadium available in the soil. The amount in animal foods probably reflects the diet. Seafoods are higher in vanadium, as are animal tissues in cases in which dietary vanadium has been increased. Vanadium in foods probably is around a few parts per billion.

Vanadium salts are poorly absorbed in the intestine. Even when they are ingested in a soluble form, only about 1% of a given quantity is absorbed. Vanadium that is absorbed is excreted rapidly, with about 60% of a given absorbed quantity being excreted in the urine in 24 hours. Only small amounts of vanadium are stored, and vanadium that enters bone is mobilized more slowly than from other tissues. Because of the low absorption of vanadium and its relatively rapid excretion, it is less toxic than other metals that do not have these characteristics.

Stokinger[32] pointed out that vanadium at extremely low tissue concentrations (1 μg/gm of tissue) can induce derangements of basic metabolic processes that are not manifest clinically or felt by the subject. Stockinger found that the cystine content of fingernails decreased after chronic, low-grade exposure to vanadium. Later, however, Kiviluoto, et al.[13] studied workers with an average of 14 years exposure (at levels 0.1–0.6 mg/m^3) who did not have fingernail cystine levels different from unexposed controls.

Other metabolic effects appear to include lowering of cholesterol synthesis (particularly in younger animals and man), a reduction in coenzyme A and coenzyme Q production, and activation of monoamine oxidase. These are noted in greater detail in the Vanadium report prepared by the Panel on Vanadium, Committee on Biologic Effects of Atmospheric Pollutants, National Research Council, National Academy of Sciences–National Academy of Engineering.[20]

Although no evidence of nutritional essentiality for man was found, vanadium is known to be essential for laboratory animals and probably will be shown to be essential for man also. There is no evidence in the literature for any indication of mutagenicity, carcinogenicity, or alterations of the immune systems in man or animals.

EXPERIMENTAL STUDIES

Few experimental studies in which humans have been exposed to vanadium oxide dusts have been made. Zenz and Berg[41] conducted such a study on nine healthy volunteer subjects, 27–44 years of age. Vanadium, 0.013 mg/100 ml, was found in the urine three days after exposure; none was detectable a week after exposure. Maximal fecal vanadium was 0.003 mg/gm, and none detected after two weeks. Acute manifestations of marked pulmonary irritation were observed in all subjects.

Sjöberg[28] conducted long-term inhalation studies exposing rabbits for one hour a day to vanadium pentoxide at 20–40 mg/cu m for several months. Pathologic changes found included chronic rhinitis and tracheitis, emphysema, and patches of lung atelectasis with bronchopneumonia; in some cases, pyelonephritis was seen. Vanadium could again be detected in the lung, liver, and kidney, but not in the intestine, as in the heavily exposed group. Continuous exposure to a concentration of 10–30 mg/cu m was distinctly toxic to rabbits, causing bronchitis and pneumonia, loss of weight, and bloody diarrhea. With rats, 10 mg/cu m was toxic, and a small exposure of 3–5 mg/cu m caused symptoms after two months; a lethal exposure was considered to be 70 mg/cu m if prolonged for more than 20 hours.

In a series of experiments, Roschin[26] and Roschin et al.[25] exposed rabbits to vanadium trioxide aerosol at 40–75 mg/cu m for two hours a day over a period of 9–12 months. The animals showed signs of a general toxic effect, such as profuse nasal discharge of mucus and sneezing, and attacks of bronchial asthma were noted in some animals.

Rats exposed to vanadium trioxide showed changes in the respiratory system that included suppurative bronchitis, septic bronchopneumonia, pulmonary emphysema, formation of cellular-dust foci with signs of necrobiosis in the phagocytes, and moderate interstitial pulmonary sclerosis.

Rabbits and rats exposed to vanadium chloride (VCl_3) showed more marked histopathologic changes in internal organs than those exposed to vanadium trioxide. They were characterized by protein and fatty dystrophies of the cells of the liver, kidney, and myocardium, arterial necrosis of the tissues of some organs, and reduction in the ribonucleic acid and deoxyribonucleic acid content of the cells of the liver, kidney, myocardium, stomach, intestine and lung. Thus, vanadium chloride proved to be more toxic than vanadium trioxide under the same experimental conditions.

The aerosols of vanadium, vanadium carbide and ferrovanadium were not considered highly toxic. Exposure to vanadium carbide and vanadium dust was found to produce a slight, unstable, statistically insignificant biochemical change in the blood.

In all cases, the chief damage was to the respiratory tract, but no fibrotic changes or specific chronic lesions were observed in the lungs. The presence of vanadium in several organs was evidence of its absorption; this absorption probably was rapid, inasmuch as the lungs in the long-term experiments contained no more particles than did those of animals exposed for a short period. Symptoms of vanadium toxicity consisted of depression of the respiratory center, constriction of the peripheral arteries of the viscera, hyperperistalsis and enteritis. Other effects included congestion, with focal hemorrhages in the lungs, fatty degeneration of the liver and damage to the convoluted tubules of the kidneys.

Roschin[25, 26] pointed out that the degree of vanadium toxicity depends on the dispersion and solubility of vanadium aerosols in biologic media. He also noted that the toxicity depends on valence, i.e., it increases with increasing valence, with pentavalent vanadium being most toxic. In addition, it is toxic both as a cation and as an anion. For additional details from numerous other animal studies refer to the NIOSH Criteria Document on Vanadium.[21]

DIAGNOSIS

It is not always easy to distinguish the disease picture from acute infection of the respiratory tract. The history of exposure to vanadium and its compounds must be ascertained. If dust exposure is suspected, an analysis of the material(s) producing the dust should be made to include the mean particle size distribution. Determination of concentration of the vanadium compound in the worker's breathing zone must be made, or reconstructed with another worker. Determination of the vanadium concentration in the urine may be helpful, if the exposure was recent (less than two weeks). (Not all excessively dusty exposures, i.e., to V_2O_5, involve small particles; many production processes use vanadium compounds that appear to be extremely fine, but on analysis, reveal particle sizes above 50 μ or 100 μ.) As described earlier, vanadium is rapidly excreted in the urine and in vanadium-exposed workers, higher levels are seen than in those nonexposed. The urine V concentrations may be measured daily, but 5 to 7 days is sufficient to note the decrease in the V levels, assuming work exposure has stopped, or otherwise has been controlled. There are no other useful clinical or laboratory tests to determine or verify exposure; workroom air sampling is required. Nose bleeds are rarely seen; skin allergy is rare and occupational exposures causing allergies have not been reported. Skin patch tests are of no diagnostic value; two cases reported to have "positive skin patch tests" were patients who had prosthetic (metallic) hip joints and they also had allergies to other metals.[5, 23] Expectations for observing discoloration of the gums, teeth, and tongue ("green tongue") are uncommon, even with heavy exposures, and may be related to poor personal hygiene.[15, 43]

Nearly always, pulmonary function tests are normal. Only Lees[15] reported some decreases in ventilatory function, but these workers were heavily exposed to (boiler) flue dust containing up to 20% V_2O_5, but other dust components were not stated.

The history of exposure, i.e., a detailed description of the job, is most important: "We were changing the catalyst," or, "I was running a pelletizing mill." Commonly noted is the lack of respiratory protective equipment, or improper fit or failure to use the mask issued. The rapid (or marked) reduction in the repeated urinalyses will confirm that excess exposure and intake has occurred and symptoms and signs resulted from the job. Many studies have shown that V concentrations in the urine of nonexposed workers have very low levels, below 50 nmol/L (2.5 μg/L) (see Chapter 13).

Treatment of responses to over-exposure is symptomatic and assurances given the worker that no permanent damage will develop. There is no evidence that vanadium and its compounds are mutagenic or carcinogenic in man.

Environmental and "Medical" Controls

Several methods have been used to sample airborne vanadium. Ideally, all particles, regardless of particle size, should be collected in order to be representative of the worker's actual exposure and air sampling should be performed by personal sampling whenever possible. Vanadium is readily determined by a number of analytic techniques with very accurate determinations of vanadium made possible using neutron activation analysis. Of all the analytical procedures discussed in the literature, and in use, atomic absorption spectrophotometry is the most commonly used for trace metal analysis because it is simple, rapid, sensitive, selective, and widely available. For credible interpretations of analytic results, the laboratories used should be accredited by regulatory agencies or by professional standards associations.

Engineering Controls

Engineering design for operations and processes involving vanadium and vanadium compounds should be directed toward controlling inhalation exposures and minimizing skin and eye contact with the dust. Properly designed and maintained ventilation systems can prevent dispersal of vanadium compounds into the workroom atmosphere and reduce or eliminate surface accumulation, reducing the chances of resuspension. Where closed systems cannot be adequately designed or effectively used, local exhaust systems with collection hoods at potential contamination sources should be provided.

Warning labels indicating skin, eye, and respiratory irritation hazards and requiring the use of adequate ventilation should be on containers used to transport various vanadium compounds, particularly fused flakes and fine granular ammonium metavanadate, vanadium pentoxide, trichloride, oxytrichloride, and tetrachloride. Maintenance and repair workers pose special problems with regard to potential exposure; there must be careful supervision, and these workers must wear the appropriate protective equipment and clothing.

Respiratory Protection

Some industrial processes produce simultaneous exposure to particulate vanadium compounds and to vapors of volatile com-

TABLE 44–1.
Major Responses in Man to Short-Term Inhalation of Vanadium and Certain Compounds*

SUBSTANCE	MG/V/CU M	TIME	EFFECTS	REF
V_2O_5	10–32	2–5 d	Bronchial irritation, discolored tongue	37
V_2O_5	0.6	8 h	Bronchial irritation, cough	41
V_2O_5	0.6	5 min	Cough	41
V_2O_5	0.3	8 h	Bronchial irritation, cough	43
V_2O_5 (in soot)	0.3	—	Bronchial irritation, cough Reduced lung function, conjunctivitis	15
V_2O_5	0.1	8 h	Cough	41
V_2O_5	0.06	8 h	Cough, mucus production	41
V_2O_5 and NH_4VO_3	0.04 to 0.4	—	Bronchial irritation Discolored tongue	6
V-A1 alloy	—	—	Bronchial irritation Discolored tongue	24
Ferro-vanadium	—	—	Bronchial irritation Irritation of eyes	17
Metallic V	—	—	Bronchial irritation	17

*Modified from Scientific Basis for Swedish Occupational Standards IV, Criteria Group for Occupational Standards, Arbete och Hälsa. 1983; 36:115. Solna, Sweden, National Board of Occupational Safety and Health. (This report is based mainly on two criteria documents.[8, 22])

TABLE 44–2.
Some Epidemiologic Reports*

SUBSTANCE	MG/V/CU M	TIME	EFFECTS	REF
Vanadium ore	0.01–2.12	<3 yrs	Bronchial irritation Eye irritation	36
V_2O_5	0.01–0.52	2.5 yrs	Bronchial irritation	17
V_2O_5	0.1–0.3	11 yrs	Bronchial irritation	12
V_2O_5	—	6 yrs	Cough, chest pains	38

*Modified from Scientific Basis for Swedish Occupational Standards IV, Criteria Group for Occupational Standards, Arbete och Hälsa. 1983; 36:115. Solna, Sweden, National Board of Occupational Safety and Health. Sweden. (This report is based mainly on two criteria documents.[8, 22])

pounds, as vanadium halides. In these areas, the employee must be given the recommended type of respirator that will provide protection against both particulate form and vapor.

Workers in confined spaces, such as boiler cleaners, should wear acid-resistant suits that fit snugly over wrists and ankles, suitable gauntlet gloves, and rubber boots. A suitable respirator should be worn, preferably an air-fed hood to cover the head and shoulders (see Chapter 2).

Good sanitation and personal hygiene is necessary. The employer should provide facilities and separate lockers for work (including shoes) and for street clothes and showers.

Medical Surveillance

Preplacement medical examinations are not useful, even if the potential for exposure to vanadium compounds exists. Certainly, any evidence of active, chronic eye or skin disorders, respiratory problems, or troublesome allergies are present, then over-exposure to vanadium compounds might cause aggravation. Because symptoms of bronchial asthma and bronchitis may be found in ("normal") worker populations potentially exposed when working with vanadium compounds, "pulmonary function tests" may be considered, if only to assure workers that no permanent pulmonary damage has occurred. There is no need for annual pulmonary function tests if work exposures are properly controlled. As clearly described by Lees, the pulmonary spirometric findings in a single worker may not prove as meaningful as the results found in several workers from the same contaminated work area. If workers have not had recent excess exposure, then routine spirometry is not recommended. Chest x-rays need not be performed routinely, but at the discretion of the responsible physician based on his knowledge of work exposure and clinical findings. There is no evidence that vanadium causes emphysema in man.

Occupational Exposure Limits and Threshold Limit Values

As described in this chapter, vanadium compounds such as the oxides and vanadates are known to cause respiratory tract irritation, with eye and skin irritation under certain heavily contaminated work conditions. While there is little information on the halides, it is reasonable to assume, because they decompose to halide acids and vanadium oxides, that they will cause similar acute effects. Other forms of vanadium, for example, ferrovanadium, other alloys of vanadium, vanadium metal, and vanadium carbide are much less active and cause lesser irritant or toxic effects, if any. Critical effects to vanadium and vanadium compound dusts have been noted at exposures of 0.06 mg/V/cu m during one workshift, with symptoms disappearing a few weeks after exposure ceased. There is some evidence of pulmonary "sensitization" on repeated heavier exposures. See Tables 44–1 and 44–2. The ACGIH TLV is 0.05 mg/cu m respirable dust and fumes as V_2O_5; the OSHA TLV is 0.5 mg/cu m (dust ceiling); 0.1 mg/cu m (fume); and NIOSH: 0.05 mg/cu m (15 minute-ceiling).

REFERENCES

1. Abernathy RF, Peterson MJ, Gibson FH: Spectrochemical Analyses of Coal Ash for Trace Elements. Bureau of Mines Report of Investigations #7281, Pittsburgh, US Dept of Interior, 1969.
2. Browne RC: Vanadium poisoning from gas turbines. *Br J Ind Med* 1955; 12:57.
3. Browne RC, Steele J: The control of the vanadium hazard in catalytic oil-gas plants. *Ann Occup Hyg* 1963; 6:75.
4. Davis WE, et al: National Inventory of Sources and Emissions—Arsenic, Beryllium, Manganese, Mercury and Vanadium. Vanadium, Section V, 1968, Report for Environmental Protection Agency, Leawood, Kansas, WE Davis & Assoc, 1971.
5. Elves MW, Wilson JN, Scales JT, et al: Incidence of metal sensitivity in patients with total joint replacements. *Br Med J* 1975; 4:376.
6. Faulkner Hudson TG: *Vanadium—Toxicology and Biological Significance*. New York, Elsevier North-Holland, Inc, 1964.
7. Gylseth B, Leira H, Stennes E, et al: Vanadium in the blood and urine of workers in a ferroalloy plant. *Scand J Work Environ Health* 1979; 5:188.
8. Gylseth B, Hansen TV: Nordiska expertgruppen for gränsvärdesdokumentation. 33. Vanadin. Arbete och Hälsa. (In Norwegian, with English summary.) 1982; vol 18.
9. Hopkins LL, Jr, Mohr HE: The biological essentiality of vanadium, in Mertz W, Cornatzer, WE (eds): *Newer Trace Elements in Nutrition*. New York, Marcel Dekker, Inc, 1971, pp 195–213.
10. Kanematsu N, Hara M, Kada T: Assay and mutagenicity studies on metal compounds. *Mut Res* 1980; 77:109.
11. Kiviluoto M, Räsänen O, Rinne A, et al: Effects of vanadium on the upper respiratory tract of workers in a vanadium factory. A macroscopic and microscopic study. *Scand J Work Environ Health* 1979; 5:50.
12. Kiviluoto M: Observations on the lungs of vanadium workers. *Br J Ind Med* 1980; 37:363.
13. Kiviluoto M, Pyy L, Pakarinen A: Fingernail cystine of vanadium workers. *Int Arch Occup Environ Health* 1980; 46:179.
14. Kiviluoto M, Pakarinen A, Pyy L: Serum and urinary vanadium of workers processing vanadium pentoxide. *Int Arch Occup Environ Health* 1981; 48:251.
15. Lees REM: Changes in lung function after exposure to vanadium compounds in fuel oil ash. *Br J Ind Med* 1980; 37:253.
16. Lees R: Vanadium, in *Occupational Health in Ontario*, vol 6, 4:177, 1985, Toronto, Ontario.
17. Lewis CE: The biological effects of vanadium. II. The signs and symptoms of occupational vanadium exposure. *Arch Ind Health* 1959; 19:497.
18. Minerals Yearbook, Metals and Minerals, Vol I. Washington DC, US Government Printing Office, 1985.
19. Mountain JT, Stockell FR, Stockinger HE: Fingernail cystine as an early indicator of metabolic changes in vanadium workers. *Arch Ind Health* 1955; 12:494.
20. National Academy of Sciences, National Research Council, Division of Engineering: Trends in the Use of Vanadium. A Report of the Na-

tional Materials Advisory Board, No. NMAB-267. Springfield, Virginia, Clearinghouse for Federal Scientific & Technical Information, 1970.

21. National Academy of Sciences, National Research Council, National Academy of Engineering: Vanadium, Committee on Biological Effects of Atmospheric Pollutants. Washington, DC, 1974.
22. Occupational Exposure to Vanadium, Criteria for a Recommended Standard. NIOSH, U.S. Department of Health and Human Services, PHS, Centers for Disease Control, Cincinnati, Ohio, 1977.
23. Oleffer J, Wilmet J: Generalized dermatitis from an osteosynthesis screw. *Cont Derm* 1980; 6:365.
24. Roberts WC: The ferroalloy industry. Hazards of the alloys and semimetallics. Part II. *J Occup Med* 1965; 7:71–77.
25. Roschin IV, et al: Effect on organism of vanadium trioxide. *Fed Proc* 1965; 24:611.
26. Roschin IV: Toxicology of vanadium compounds used in modern industry. *Gig Sanit* 1967; 32:26.
27. Schroeder HA, Malassa JJ, Tipton IH: Abnormal trace of metals in man—Vanadium. *J Chron Dis* 1963; 16:1047.
28. Sjöberg SG: Vanadium pentoxide dust: A clinical and experimental investigation on its effect after inhalation. *Acta Med Scand* 1950; 138(Suppl 238).
29. Sjöberg SG: Vanadium bronchitis after cleaning oil burning steam boilers. (In Swedish, summary in English.) *Nord Hyg Tidskr* 1954; 35:45.
30. Sjöberg SG: Vanadium bronchitis from cleaning oil-fired boilers. *Arch Ind Health* 1955; 11:505.
31. Sjöberg SG: Vanadium dust, chronic bronchitis and possible risk of emphysema. *Acta Med Scand* 1956; 154:381.
32. Stokinger HE: Vanadium, in Patty FA (ed): *Industrial Hygiene and Toxicology* (ed 2). New York, Interscience Publishers, Inc, 1962, pp 1171–1181.
33. Symanski J: Gewerbliche Vanadin-schadigungen, ihr Enstehung and Symptomatologie. *Arch Gewerbepath Gewerbehyg* 1939; 9:295.
34. Tebrock HE, Machle W: Exposure to europium-activated yttrium orthovanadate: A cathodoluminescent phosphor. *J Occup Med* 1968; 10:692.
35. Tipton IH, Shafer JJ: Statistical analysis of lung trace elements levels. *Arch Environ Health* 1964; 8:58.
36. Vintinner FJ, Vallenas R, Carlin CE, et al: Study of the health of workers employed in mining and processing of vanadium ore. *Arch Ind Health* 1955; 12:635.
37. Williams N: Vanadium poisoning from cleaning oil-fired boilers. *Br J Ind Med* 1952; 9:50.
38. Wyers H: Some toxic effects of vanadium pentoxide. *Br J Ind Med* 1946; 3:177.
39. Yakawa M, Amano K, Suzuku-Yasumoto M, et al: Distribution of trace elements in the human body determined by neutron activation analysis. *Arch Environ Health* 1980; 35:36.
40. Zenz C: Vanadium, in Waldron HA (ed): *Metals in the Environment*. London, Academic Press, 1980, pp 293–327.
41. Zenz C, Berg BA: Human responses to controlled vanadium pentoxide exposure. *Arch Environ Health* 1967; 14:709.
42. Zenz C, Staples G: An ergonomic study of body positions related to energy expenditure during foundry chipping. *J Occup Med* 1967; 9:449.
43. Zenz C, Bartlett JP, Thiede WH: Acute vanadium pentoxide intoxication. *Arch Environ Health* 1962; 5:542.

45

Other Metals

Donald M. Rowe, M.D.

Joseph A. Solomayer, M.D., Sc.D.

Carl Zenz, M.D.

In this chapter, pertinent occupational health aspects of the following metals and their commonly used compounds are described:

Aluminum
Barium
Bismuth
Boron
Copper
Hafnium
Iron
Lithium
Magnesium
Molybdenum
Palladium
Platinum
Rhenium
Rhodium
Silver
Strontium
Tantalum
Thallium
Tin
Titanium
Zinc
Zirconium

Throughout the world, millions are working in mines (underground, open-pit), quarries, tunnels, drilling rigs (on land and water), exposed to the entire spectrum of potential work hazards (Fig 45–1). Not uncommonly, working conditions can be exceedingly harsh. Even with modern transport, seeking new locations by exploration for the expanding needs of industry and growing demands of societies can be dangerous, time-consuming and costly. Occupational stresses range from psychologic (distant travel may be involved with time zone changes, long working hours and shift changes, darkness, loneliness, other languages, new diseases, risks from trauma, etc.) to severe extremes and variations of physical stress, often combined. There may be climatic extremes—high altitudes, bitter cold or heat, high humidity or ever-present rain, to extreme desert dryness with intense radiant heat; at times high wind velocities and wind chill; poor illumination or marked glare, heavy physical work loads, demanding high energy expenditure. Noise and vibration may be present to varying degrees. In addition to the previously mentioned potential psychologic stresses, many subtle factors may be present. These can include unknown, but present, background radiation levels (in certain mines and factories), breakdown products from lubricating oils and greases from equipment (engines, motors, pumps, electrical wiring, etc.), byproducts of explosive blasting. Even nutrition can be influencing: there may be a limited supply of foods, with deficiencies of minerals, proteins and vitamins. Other subtle agents with far-reaching and potentially debilitating effects are various dusts; prominent are the asbestos fibers and silica particles encountered in many mining and quarrying operations. Hazards exist in transport of materials and minerals for crushing and grinding for smelting, refining, finishing, and packaging; interwoven is maintenance of equipment. Products move to warehouses, petrochemical plants, foundries, machine shops, and laboratories, to farms; some to schools and homes for crafts, artwork, and hobbies. Broadly then, men, women (and children) are working in "high-tech" industries, i.e., from Japan and California, but in sharp contrast, also, in open gem mines in Brazil to underground activities for construction of subways, storage facilities, manufacturing, military needs, living quarters, often beneath large cities. Work exposures often include many substances and materials; single exposures are uncommon. For certain metals, their oxides and their compounds, there is little or no animal or human exposure data reported in the literature. The following general references will prove useful.

REFERENCES

1. Aitio A, Riihimaki V, Vainio H, (eds): *Biological Monitoring and Surveillance of Workers Exposed to Chemicals.* New York, Hemisphere, 1984.
2. American Conference of Governmental Industrial Hygienists: *Documentation of the Threshold Limit Values for Substances in Workroom Air*, ed 5. Cincinnati, 1986.
3. Friberg L, Nordberg GF, Vouk VB (eds): *Handbook of Toxicology of Metals.* Amsterdam, Elsevier-North Holland, 1979.
4. Waldron HA (ed): *Metals in the Environment.* London, Academic Press, 1980.
5. *Minerals Yearbook 1985, Volume I, Metals and Minerals.* Bureau of Mines, United States Department of the Interior, US Government Printing Office, Washington, DC, 1985.
6. NIOSH Recommendations for Occupational Health Standards, Morbidity and Mortality Weekly Report, Supplement September 26, 1986, Vol 35, No 1S, US Department of Health and Human Ser-

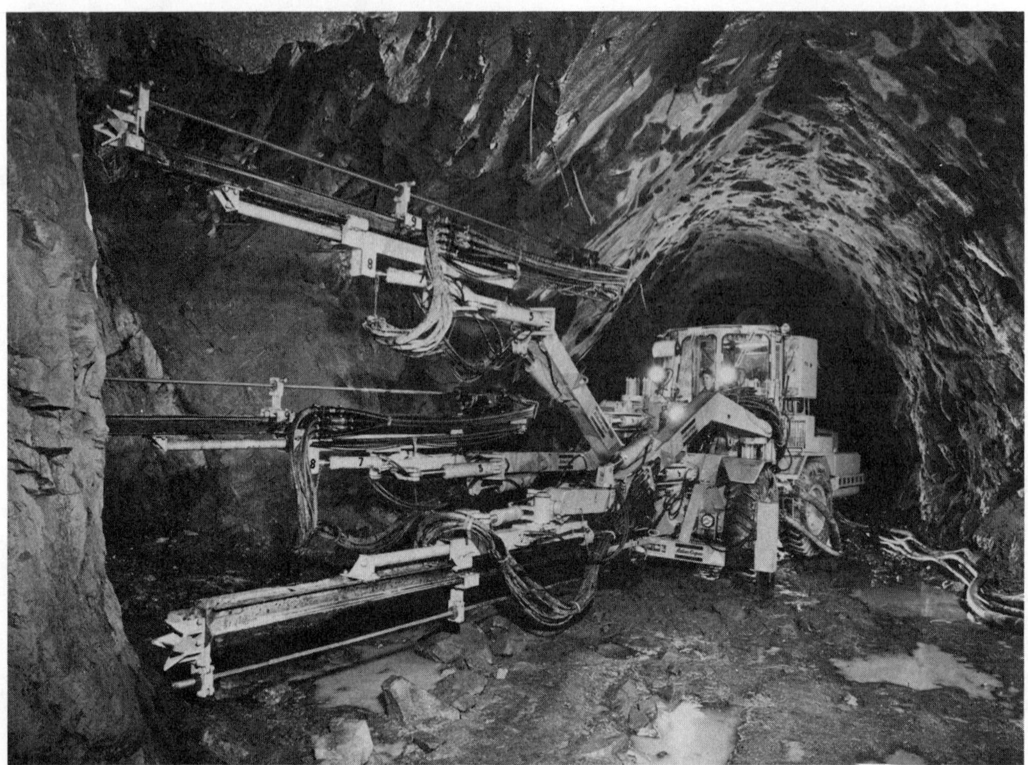

FIG 45–1.
Photograph shows an example of ideal worker protection for a hostile mining environment—a drilling rig of advanced design with emphasis on the operator as well as the working environment. One worker can use three rock drills from an ergonomically-planned position with maximum visibility. The rig is sound and vibration-damped, air conditioned with clean air and special exhaust purification system, including catalyzer-scrubber. The worker is safely enveloped in a "micro-climate" representing a most effective barrier against hazardous working conditions, commonly encountered in tunneling for sewage systems, water, power stations, storage, underground transport, and mining. Compare with the typical mine drilling rig seen in figure 2–14. (Courtesy of Atlas Copco AB, Stockholm, Sweden.)

vices, Public Health Service, National Institute for Occupational Safety and Health, Centers for Disease Control, Atlanta, Georgia.

7. Considine D, Considine G (eds): *The Encyclopedia of Chemistry*, ed 4. New York, Van Nostrand Reinhold Co., 1984.
8. Parmeggiani L (ed): *The Encyclopedia of Occupational Health and Safety*, ed 3. Geneva, International Labor Office, 1983.
9. *The Merck Index*, ed 10. Rahway, NJ, Merck & Co, Inc, 1983.
10. LaDou J (ed): *The Microelectronics Industry*. State of the Art Reviews, Occupational Medicine, 1:1, January-March, Philadelphia, Hanley & Belfus, Inc, 1986.
11. World Health Organization: *Health Effects of Combined Exposures in the Work Environment*. Geneva, 1980.
12. World Health Organization: *Occupational Health Aspects of Cosntruction Work*. Geneva, 1983.
13. World Health Organization: *Early Detection of Occupational Diseases*. Geneva, 1986.

ALUMINUM AND ITS COMPOUNDS

By weight (8.13%), aluminum (Al) is the third most common element in the earth's crust, after oxygen and nitrogen, making it the most abundant metal. Bauxite (hydrated aluminum oxide and iron oxides) is the main ore, followed by cryolite (Na_3AlF_6).

Although aluminum metal was first made in 1824, the discovery of the electrolytic reduction process in 1886 (Hall, United States, and Heroult, France) led to practical production. The aluminum oxide is dissolved in molten cryolite, decomposed by a low-voltage, high-amperage current with consumable carbon-mixture anodes and the metal deposited on the cathode in the furnace. This method is in use today, with worldwide production in 1982 of 14,600,000 short tons.[4] Ninety-three percent of bauxite is refined to produce alumina; about 2.07 tons of bauxite are needed to make 1 ton of (dry) calcined alumina. To produce 3 lb of aluminum requires one *kilowatt-day* of energy, consuming 1½ lb of anode and 6 lb of alumina, which is in turn purified from 12 lb of bauxite.[2, 7]

Uses

Aluminum enjoys a vast use: it is used in construction and in the manufacture of beverage and food containers, autos, trucks, electrical products, various machines and parts, and cooking utensils. In wire form, it is used in welding. As a fine powder, it is used in explosives, solid rocket propellants, and paints. Another major use is found in making various alloys. Alumina is used as a starting compound to make refractories (furnace and other), abrasives, and synthetic rubies and sapphires (for small bearings). Alumina is also used in ceramics, as a dessicant, for antacids, in antiperspirants, and as a catalyst for organic synthesis.

Occupational Exposures.—Several authors have described the varied (and concomitant) potential hazards associated with the manufacturing processes.[1, 3, 4] Occupational exposures are mainly through inhalation, and a considerable body of literature provides documentation of acute and chronic pulmonary effects in workers in several industries.[7] (For clinical details, refer to Levy, Chapter 14.) Other effects on workers are less well defined, with little supporting documentation of the systemic effects of aluminum compounds. For example, aluminum chloride ($AlCl_3$), a fine powder used extensively in petroleum cracking and in making synthetic polyisoprene, is capable of forming at room temperature and is a severe irritant to skin and mucus membranes. Other aluminum compounds, notably alkyl types, are very reactive and are used as catalysts in polyethylene manufacturing.

Absorption, Metabolism, and Toxic Responses.—Although aluminum is known to be a nonessential trace element in man, its rate of absorption via the pulmonary system and its metabolism is not clear. Aluminum is detected in the blood and urine of exposed workers, but there are many variables, and reports in the literature have not pin-pointed concentrations which might indicate levels leading to toxic responses.

Mussi et al.[5] studied seven workers. Four of them worked on electric aluminum wire welding and were exposed to fumes, and three polished and cut aluminum wire and were exposed to aluminum dust. Workroom air sampling for fumes ranged from 1.0 mg/cu m to 6.2 mg/cu m; and for dusts, 1.0 mg/ cu m to 4.5 mg/ cu m. It is of interest that plasma aluminum levels in the workers were essentially within the same range as that found in a nonoccupationally exposed group. However, urinary levels were much higher for the men exposed to fumes, as expected. Two weeks after exposure, urinary levels had decreased to levels close to those of the nonexposed. Despite the small worker sample, this study demonstrated that an evaluation of the difference between urinary aluminium levels at the beginning and end of the working day could provide information on the degree of exposure on that day; and evaluation of the difference between urinary aluminium levels on Friday morning and Monday morning may reflect the degree of total exposure over the four previous days.

Aluminum and aluminum oxide have a low resorption rate. Aluminum concentration in serum appears to be an indicator of body burden, and the aluminum urine concentration seems to be an indicator of current exposure.[6] Sjögren et al.[8] measured urinary excretion in 23 welders before and after an exposure free interval of 16 to 37 days. Air concentrations were determined on these men on the same work day as the first urinary sampling. They reported that the biologic half-time of aluminum excreted in the urine of welders exposed less than 1 year was about 9 days; welders exposed for more than 10 years reflected a biologic half-time of 6 months or longer.

For discussion of the many factors involved in assessing the validity of biologic monitoring, refer to Aitio and co-authors, Chapter 13.

REFERENCES

1. Dinman BD: Aluminum, alloys and compounds, in *Encyclopedia of Health and Safety*, ed 3. Geneva, International Labor Organization, 1983.
2. Considine D, Considine G (eds): *The Encyclopedia of Chemistry*, ed 4. New York, Van Nostrand Reinhold Co, 1984.
3. Hughes JP (ed): *Health Protection in Primary Aluminium Production.* Proceedings of a Seminar. Copenhagen, June 28–30, 1977. London, 1978.
4. Martinez EG, Munoz PRJ, Ballesteros GM, et al: Toxic effects of lead impurities found in aluminum factories. *Am J Ind Med* 1981; 2:161–165.
5. Mussi I, et al: Behaviour of plasma and urinary aluminium levels in occupationally exposed subjects. *Int Arch Occup Environ Health* 1984; 54:155–161.
6. Schaller KH, Valentin H: Aluminium, Alessio L, Berlin A, Boni M, et al (eds): in *Biological Indicators For The Assessment of Human Exposure to Industrial Chemicals.* Varese, Italy, Joint Research Centre Ispra Establishment, 1984.
7. Sjögren B: Respiratory disorders and biological monitoring among electric-arc welders and brazers (Doctoral dissertation). *Arbete och Hälsa* 1985; 9.
8. Sjögren B, Elinder C-G, Lidums V, et al: Uptake and urinary excretion of aluminum by welders. *Arbete och Hälsa* 1986; 16.
9. Taylor W: Manufacturing processes—Aluminium manufacture. *J Soc Occup Med* 1978; 28:25–26.

BARIUM AND ITS COMPOUNDS

Barium (Ba) is a silver-white metal, slightly harder than lead. It is malleable, machinable, and extrudable. It is the densest of the alkaline earth metals, hence its name, from the Greek, *barys* (heavy). Barium makes up about 0.4%–0.5% of the earth's crust. Barite or barytes ($BaSO_4$) and witherite ($BaCO_3$) are the most common mineral forms. The estimated annual world production of barite is 6,600,000 short tons, and 1,650,000 short tons are produced in the United States.[3]

Uses

Natural barite is mainly used for well drilling "mud," and alloys with aluminum magnesium and other metals are readily made. Most compounds are made from barite. Barium carbonate is used in water treatment, as flux in ceramics, as a component of welding rod fluxes, in optical glass and fine glassware, and in making barium ferrite ceramic magnets (with iron oxide), which are used in speakers, small motors, and various electronic devices. Barium chloride and nitrate are used in flares, fireworks, and tracer bullets. Barium oxide is used in making lubricating oil detergents. Insoluble barium sulfate is used extensively as a radiopaque contrast medium in radiology departments and is not absorbed by the gut. It is used as an extender or filler in cement, paint, paper, soap, rubber, linoleum, and plastics. Potential primary occupational exposures occur in refining barite (barytes) ores and in lithopone manufacture. Lithopone is used extensively as a white pigment in paints and consists of 20% barium sulfate, 30% zinc sulfide, and up to 8% zinc oxide. Compounds containing barium salts come into the home as hair removers (barium sulfide), insecticides, rodenticides, matches, and art paint pigments.

It is important to recognize soluble barium salts ($BaCO_3$, $BaCl_2$, BaNO, BaS) as potentially dangerous materials when ingested, since they are rapidly absorbed from the gastrointestinal system and are fatal to man in amounts less than 1 gm. Therefore, small or bulk amounts should be handled with care.

Toxicology

Ingestion of soluble barium compounds in man causes gastroenteritis, muscular paralysis, slow pulse rate, extrasystoles, and marked hypokalemia. This hypokalemia is believed to be the cause for skeletal muscle paralysis, which can progress to involve respiratory muscles.[12] The barium ion causes stimulation of smooth, striated, and cardiac muscle.[2, 7] Cardiotoxic effects have been shown to be reversible by potassium administration.[9] Muscle cramping and twitching may occur, and small amounts of barium in cerebrospinal fluid lead to convulsions. Marked hypertension due to smooth muscle spasms in arterioles occurs. These effects have been demonstrated in several animal studies.[8] Aqueous solutions of barium hydroxide and barium oxide are strongly alkaline and can cause severe burns to the eye and skin irritation. Pneumoconiosis (baritosis) has been identified with heavy exposures to finely divided particles of barium sulfate and barium oxide and lithopone. This benign pneumoconiosis does not result in impairment of ventilatory function, although signs of mild bronchial irritation may occur. Characteristic x-ray changes are those of small, dense, circumscribed nodules evenly distributed throughout the lung fields, reflecting the radio-opacity of the barium dust.[5]

There is little information on barium metabolism, but it is an essential trace element; the average daily intake in man is estimated to be 1.2 mg. Schroeder et al.[10] found that the average barium level in human plasma is 79 μg/L. Since barium and calcium are closely related in the elemental periodic order, up to 93% of the body burden is concentrated in the skeletal system.

In addition to inhalation, there is rapid skin absorption with burns. Dare et al.[4] studied various commonly used welding electrodes using barium compounds as fluxes in ore welding. They studied five welders working in a 12 × 4 × 3-m tent with natural ventilation for a three-hour period, with actual fume generation taking 30% of this time. Analyses revealed that fumes from a cored-wire electrode with barium fluoride flux contain more than 16% barium (soluble in water). Stick electrodes with barium carbonate flux produced fumes with 15%–30% barium in readily soluble form. Urine samples for barium analysis taken at the end of the three-hour exposure and the next morning resulted in elevated barium levels; averaging 120 μ/L and 48 μg/L, respectively.

Stewart and Hummel[11] described a case report with barium poisoning secondary to a barium chloride burn.

> Case Report.—Man, 62, in previously good health, was burned over his face, arms and legs with molten barium chloride while at work. While the man was cleaning out a furnace used to heat barium chloride-treated steel, an explosion occurred when the patient's jackhammer hit a pocket of molten barium chloride, resulting in spattering of molten barium chloride over the patient. The admitting chest x-ray film revealed multiple radio-opaque foreign bodies scattered over the left chest, corresponding to the burned areas. The patient was immediately transferred from the emergency room to the burn special care unit. His burns were debrided, washed, and covered with silver sulfadiazine (Silvadene, Marion). Further cleaning and debridement were followed by repeat chest, skull, and extremity x-ray films, which showed no evidence of residual barium on the skin. The patient vomited, and cardiac monitoring revealed that the bigeminy that had been found on the admitting ECG and had persisted for nine hours postburn, had spontaneously converted to normal sinus rhythm. His potassium level dropped and plasma barium levels were measured. Approximately two hours postburn, the plasma barium level was 12.4 mg/L. At 4, 8, 12, and 18 hours postburn, the plasma barium levels were 10.3, 8.2, 8.9, and 4.0 mg/L, respectively. His initial blood pressure of 180/114 mm Hg fell. There was an uneventful recovery (with successful skin grafts) within 38 hospital days. There were close clinical and laboratory observation and appropriate intravenous potassium therapy.

Stewart and Hummel emphasized the need for frequent checks of serum potassium and aggressive intravenous replacement of potassium in this first report in the literature describing toxic barium levels.

Exposure Limit Recommendations

Work exposure levels of soluble barium compounds must be kept under the threshold limit value (TLV) of 0.5 mg/cu m. Good ventilation and housekeeping are imperative, as is proper personal hygiene and safe work practices.

Further, Dare et al. stated:

> The minimum requirements for control of hazards from barium in welding processes may be summarized as follows:
>
> 1. Improved labelling of wire and stick electrodes, including provision of easily available and explicit hazard data sheets provided by the manufacturers for worker education.
> 2. Understanding by the users and occupational hygienists of the various processes involved whereby barium constituents of the flux can present occupational hazards.
> 3. Assessment of surface and air contaminants, noting that, for the electrodes examined, specific analysis for barium (and possibly other constituents) in the fume would be necessary for comparison with the appropriate limit—in the case of soluble barium, a 0.5 mg/cu m limit for total welding fume, not otherwise classified, would not provide an adequate control of fume exposures from the barium-containing electrodes examined here.
> 4. Adoption of ventilation or other measures to control inhalation risks.
> 5. Segregation of working area and waste produced to control ingestion risks from surfaces. Improved work practice and waste disposal may be necessary.

REFERENCES

1. American Conference of Governmental Industrial Hygienists: *Documentation of the Threshold Limit Values for Substances in Workroom Air*, ed 5. Cincinnati, Oh, ACGIH, 1986.
2. Bernine J: Hypokalemia of barium poisoning, letter. *Lancet* 1975; 1:110.

3. Bureau of Mines, US Dept of the Interior: *Minerals Yearbook*. Washington, DC, US Government Printing Office, 1985.
4. Dare P, Hewitt P, Hicks R, et al: Short communication: Barium in welding fume. *Ann Occup Hyg* 1984; 28:445–448.
5. Doig A: Baritosis: A benign pneumoconiosis. *Thorax* 1976; 31:1.
6. Goodman L, Gilman, A: *The Pharmacological Basis of Therapeutics*, ed 7. New York, Macmillan Publishing Co, 1985.
7. Gould D, et al: Barium sulfide poisoning. *Arch Intern Med* 1973; 132:891–894.
8. Jaklinske A, Jerzy M, Przegalinski E: Experimental studies on barium poisoning. *J Forensic Med* 1967; 14:13.
9. Roza O, Berman L: The pathophysiology of barium hypokalemic and cardiovascular effects. *J Pharmacol Exp Ther* 1971; 177:433–439.
10. Schroeder H, Tipton I, Nason A: Trace metals in man: Strontium and barium. *J Chronic Dis* 1972; 25:491–517.
11. Stewart D, Hummel R: Acute poisoning by a barium chloride burn. *J Trauma*, 1984; 24:768–770.
12. Wetherill S, et al: Acute renal failure associated with barium chloride poisoning. *Ann Intern Med* 1981; 95:187–188.

BISMUTH AND ITS COMPOUNDS

Worldwide, more than 7 million lb of bismuth are produced annually. About 40% is refined in the United States. Most bismuth is obtained as a by-product of copper and lead refining and smelting.

Bismuth is used in malleable iron; it is added to aluminum and steel for better machinability and has great use in alloys of low melting points, "fusible alloys," and in safety devices such as automatic fire sprinkler valves. Many compounds are readily formed. Bismuth telluride is used for semiconductors. Bismuth oxide, hydroxide, nitrate, and oxychloride are used in cosmetics (the oxychloride is a pearlescent ingredient). Bismuth phosphomolybdate is used as a catalyst in acrylonitrile fiber manufacture. The subcarbonate and subnitrate are well known as medicinals.

Bismuth and its compounds are considered the least toxic of the heavy metals. If occupational exposures have occurred, reports are not found in the literature. However, animal inhalation studies of bismuth telluride "doped" with selenium sulfide (see Chapter 41) have produced a "mild" granulomatous pulmonary response, apparently reversible. Because of this, the TLV of the American Conference of Governmental Industrial Hygienists (ACGIH) is 5 mg/cu m.

REFERENCE

1. Galland MC, Rodor F, Jougland J: Bismuth et encephalopathie. (Bismuth and encephalopathy). *Medecine et Hygiene* (Geneva) 1979; Aug 15.

BORON AND ITS COMPOUNDS

Boron

Boron (B) is considered a metalloidal element, occurring mainly as sodium borate ($Na_2B_4O_7$), but also as calcium borate. As borax ($Na_2B_4O_7{\cdot}10H_2O$), it has been used commercially for hundreds of years. The world production of boron minerals was 2,700,000 short tons in 1985.[2] Boron is used in degassing and deoxidizing metals, it is alloyed with aluminum, and to harden steel, it is added as ferroboron or manganese-boron. It has important use in atomic reactors as a neutron absorber.

Borates are used to make glass fibers for insulation and for the glass-fiber-reinforcing of plastics, the two main areas of demand. Another major use is to make textile-grade glass fibers. U.S.-produced colemanite, orthoboric acid, ulexite-probertite, borax pentahydrate, and Turkish colemanite are essential raw materials for manufacturing high-tensile-strength glass-fiber composites for use in a range of products that include aircraft, automobiles, and sports equipment. Consumption of borates (colemanite, anhydrous borax, borax decahydrate and pentahydrate, orthoboric acid, and anhydrous boric acid) in the manufacture of special borosilicate glasses is a major end use.

Boron compounds in cleaning and bleaching have been important but are declining. Boron compounds find application in the manufacture of biologic growth control chemicals for use in water treatment, algicides, fertilizers, herbicides, and insecticides. Boron compounds are used in metallurgic processes as fluxes, as shielding slag in the nonferrous metallurgical industry, and as components in plating baths in the electroplating industry.[2]

It is known that boron is a trace element in animal tissues and in plants; its role is unclear. "Normal" boron concentration in the blood of man is 9.8 μg/100 gm, ranging from 3.9 to 36.5 μg/100 gm. In urine, the concentration is 715 μg/L, ranging from 40 to 6,600 μg/L.[1] Trace amounts of boron in coal ash are of concern for environmental effects. Boron concentrations exceeding 2 mg/L can cause plant toxication. Boron concentrations in coal range between 5 and 200 mg/kg, of which up to 71% could become airborne on combustion.[3] In general, most boron compounds are irritants to the skin and mucus membranes; some are corrosive.

REFERENCES

1. *Criteria for a Recommended Standard—Occupational Exposure to Boron Trifluoride*, DHEW (NIOSH) Publ. 77–122. Cincinnati, Oh, National Institute for Occupational Safety and Health, 1976.
2. Lyday PA: Boron, in *Minerals Yearbook 1985, Vol I. Metals and Minerals*. Washington, DC, US Dept of the Interior, Bureau of Mines, US Government Printing Office, 1985.
3. Pagenkopf GK, Connolly JM: Retention of boron by coal ash. *Environ Sci Technol* 1982; 16:9.

Boron Oxide

Boron oxide (B_2O_3), also known as anhydrous boric acid or boric anhydride, appears as colorless, glassy granules or flakes with no odor. It is used in the manufacture of metal borates and in the preparation of fluxes. Boron oxide is also used in the manufacture of glass to produce heat-resistance. It is used as a herbicide and as a fire-resistant additive in enamel and paints.

Toxicology.—Boron oxide aerosol is of low toxicity. At high levels, it is mildly irritating to the mucous membranes of animals. Repeated exposure of rats to an aerosol at a concentration of 470 mg/cu m for ten weeks caused only mild nasal irritation; repeated exposure of rats to 77 mg/cu m for 23 weeks resulted in elevated creatinine and boron content of the urine, in addition to increased urinary volume. Grant states that boron oxide "tested on rabbit eyes in the form of a dust has been found to cause almost immediate irritation of the conjunctiva."[3] Conjunctivitis was probably the result of the exothermic reaction of boron oxide with water to form boric acid. Topical application of boron oxide dust to the clipped backs of rabbits produced erythema that persisted for two to three days.

Permissible Exposure Limit.—The current Occupational Safety and Health Administration (OSHA) standard for boron oxide is 15 mg/cu m averaged over an eight-hour work shift. The ACGIH has recommended for boron oxide a TLV of 10 mg/cu m.[1]

REFERENCES

1. American Conference of Governmental Industrial Hygienists: Boron Oxide, in *Documentation of the Threshold Limit Values for Substances in Workroom Air,* ed 5. Cincinnati, Oh, ACGIH, 1986.
2. Deichmann WB, Gerarde HW: *Toxicology of Drugs and Chemicals*. New York, Academic Press, 1969.
3. Grant WM: *Toxicology of the Eye,* ed 4. Springfield, Ill, Charles C Thomas, 1974.
4. International Labour Office: *Encyclopedia of Occupational Health and Safety,* ed 3. Geneva, International Labor Office, 1983.
5. Wilding JL, et al: The toxicity of boron oxide. *Am Ind Hyg Assoc J* 1959; 20:284–289.

Boron Trifluoride

Boron trifluoride (BF_3) is a colorless gas that is stable in dry atmospheres. At present, boron trifluoride is known to be produced as a specialty chemical by only one U.S. company, whose production figures are not available. Although the predominant use of boron trifluoride is as a catalyst, that is not its only use *(synthesis of:* saturated hydrocarbons, alcohols, olefins, ketones, ethers and sulfur compounds; *condensation of:* acid with olefin, acid with acetylene, acid with alcohol, nitrite with alcohol, amide with alcohol and aldols; *dehydration of:* alcohols, acids, and ketones; *alkylation of:* paraffinic hydrocarbons, alkyl esters, and aromatic hydrocarbons; *polymerization of:* ethylene, propylene, butylene, isobutylene, vinyl compounds, dienes, and cyclic oxides; and for some epoxy resin curing).

The magnesium industry utilizes the fire-retardant and antioxidant properties of boron trifluoride in casting and heat treating. Nuclear applications of boron trifluoride include neutron detector instruments, boron-10 enrichment, and the production of neutron-absorbing salts for molten-salt breeder reactors. Boron trifluoride has also been identified as having insecticidal properties. Employees with potential exposure to boron trifluoride include the initial manufacturers, magnesium founders, organic synthesizers, neutron detector instrument manufacturers and fumigant producers. The NIOSH estimates that 50,000 employees are potentially exposed to boron trifluoride in the United States.

On contact with air, boron trifluoride gas immediately reacts with water vapor to form a mist that, at a high enough concentration, may provide a visible warning of its presence. Boron trifluoride gas is a severe irritant of the lungs, eyes, and skin. Exposure of six animal species to 100 ppm for 30 days resulted in a high mortality rate. Exposure of animals to a concentration of 42 mg/cu m (approximately 15 ppm) for an unspecified period was fatal in some cases; autopsy findings were pneumonitis and degenerative changes in the renal tubules. Repeated exposure of mice to 15 ppm for 30 days resulted in mortality of 19% due to pulmonary irritation; rats similarly exposed for two weeks developed hypoplasia of the teeth and deposition of fluoride up to 25 times normal levels, both in the incisors and in femoral epiphyses. Three species of animals repeatedly exposed to levels of 12.8, 7.7, or 3 ppm for periods up to six months developed pneumonitis and evidence of dental fluorosis; the higher concentrations caused deaths in guinea pigs. In man, the gas in high concentration produces burns of the eyes and skin similar to those caused by hydrogen fluoride but less severe. Workers exposed to concentrations of up to 90 mg/cu m (approximately 32 ppm) for 10–15 years developed dryness of the nasal mucous membranes and epistaxis. No chronic effects have been observed in workers who were exposed to low concentrations at frequent intervals over a period of years.[2, 4]

The present federal standard is a ceiling value of 1 ppm (3 mg/cu m), which was based on the 1-ppm ceiling ACGIH TLV for boron trifluoride.

In the absence of a suitable monitoring method, the NIOSH recommends that medical surveillance, including comprehensive preplacement and annual periodic examinations, be made available to all workers employed in areas where boron trifluoride is manufactured, used, handled or is evolved as a result of chemical processes. Engineering controls should be used to maintain boron trifluoride concentrations at the lowest feasible level. Air-supplied respirators should be used only in certain nonroutine situations or in emergency situations when air concentrations of boron trifluoride are sufficient to form a visible mist.

REFERENCES

1. Allied Chemical Corporation: *Material Safety Data Sheet, Boron Trifluoride*. Morristown, NJ, 1980.
2. American Conference of Governmental Industrial Hygienists: Boron trifluoride, in *Documentation of the Threshold Limit Values for Substances in Workroom Air,* ed 5. Cincinnati, Oh, ACGIH, 1986.
3. Levinskas GJ: *Boron, Metallo-Boron Compounds and Boranes,* Adams RM (ed). New York, Interscience, 1964, p 726.
4. National Institute for Occupational Safety and Health, US Dept of Health, Education, and Welfare: *Criteria for a Recommended Standard: Occupational Exposure to Boron Trifluoride*. Cincinnati, Oh, NIOSH, 1978.
5. Torkelson TR, et al: The toxicity of boron trifluoride when inhaled by laboratory animals. *Am Ind Hyg Assoc J* 1961; 22:263.

Diborane

Diborane (B_2H_6), also known as boroethane, is a colorless gas with a repulsive, sweet odor. It is used as a reducing agent in the synthesis of organic chemical intermediates. It is a component or additive for high-energy fuels and a catalyst in olefin polymerization. In the electronics industry, diborane is used to improve crystal growth or to impart electrical properties in pure crystals.

Toxicology.—Diborane gas is a pulmonary irritant. The LC_{50} for rats was 50 ppm for four hours. In other animal experiments, acute exposure caused pulmonary edema and hemorrhage and temporary damage to the liver and kidneys.[5, 9, 10] In human beings, overexposure results in a sensation of tightness in the chest, leading to precordial pain, shortness of breath, nonproductive cough, and sometimes nausea. Prolonged exposure to low concentrations causes headache, light-headedness, vertigo, chills, and, less frequently, fever. Fatigue or weakness occurs and may persist for several hours. Tremor or muscular fasciculations occur infrequently and are usually localized and of short duration. Diborane gas has not been found to have significant effects upon contact with skin or mucous membranes, although high concentrations may cause eye irritation.[1, 4, 6]

Permissible Exposure Limit.—The current OSHA standard for diborane is 0.1 ppm averaged over an eight-hour work shift. This may also be expressed as 0.1 mg/cu m.

REFERENCES

1. Cordasco EM, et al: Pulmonary aspects of some toxic experimental space fuels. *Dis Chest* 1962; 41:68–74.
2. Holzmann RT (ed): *Production of the Boranes and Related Research.* New York, Academic Press, 1967.
3. International Labour Office: *Encyclopedia of Occupational Health and Safety*, ed 3. Geneva, International Labor Office, 1983.
4. Krackow EH: Toxicity and health hazards of boron hydrides. *AMA Arch Ind Hyg Occup Med* 1953; 8:335–339.
5. Kunkel AM, et al: Some pharmacological effects of diborane. *AMA Arch Ind Health* 1956; 3:346–351.
6. Lowe HJ, Freeman G: Boron hydride (borane) intoxication in man. *AMA Arch Ind Health* 1957; 16:523–533.
7. Manufacturing Chemists Association, Inc: *Chemical Safety Data Sheet SD-84, Boron Hydrides.* Washington DC, MCA, Inc, 1967.
8. Roush G Jr: The toxicology of the boranes. *J Occup Med* 1959; 1:46–52.
9. Rozendaal HM: Clinical observations on the toxicology of boron hydrides. *AMA Arch Ind Hyg Occup Med* 1951; 4:257–260.
10. Stumpe AR: Toxicity of diborane in high concentrations. *AMA Arch Ind Health* 1960; 21:519–524.

Pentaborane

Pentaborane (B_5H_9), also known as stable pentaborane or pentaboron anhydride, is a colorless liquid with a strong, pungent odor. It is used in chemical research, as jet and rocket fuels, catalysts, corrosion inhibitor-fluxing agents, and oxygen scavengers. The higher boranes and alkyl boranes—ethyl pentaborane and various hydrides—are chemical intermediates; these are not industrial chemicals.

Toxicology.—Pentaborane vapor affects the nervous system and causes signs of both hyperexcitability and narcosis. Exposure of rats to 10 ppm for two hours was fatal. Effects included weakness, incoordination, corneal opacities, tremors, and convulsions. Other animal studies have indicated that kidney and liver damage may occur.[3]

In human beings, the onset of symptoms may be delayed up to 48 hours after exposure. Dizziness, headache, and drowsiness are common. Other symptoms include fatigue, incoordination, and tremor. After exposure to higher concentrations, the onset of symptoms may be prompt and include tonic spasms of the muscles of the face, neck, abdomen, and extremities. After severe exposures, convulsive seizures may occur.[4, 7]

The results of animal exposure to pentaborane for 60 minutes are: 8 ppm, some decrement in performance of learned tasks and slight signs of toxicity; 15 ppm, convulsions; 30 ppm, convulsions and death. Severe irritation and corneal opacity of the eyes of test animals occurred from exposure to the vapor. The liquid on the skin of animals caused acute inflammation.[6]

Permissible exposure limit.—The current OSHA standard for pentaborane is 0.005 ppm, or 0.01 mg/cu m, over an eight-hour work shift.

REFERENCES

1. Holzmann RT (ed): *Production of the Boranes and Related Research*, Academic Press, New York, 1967.
2. International Labour Office: *Encyclopedia of Occupational Health and Safety*, ed 3. Geneva, International Labor Office, 1983.
3. Krackow EH: Toxicity and health hazards of boron hydrides. *AMA Arch Ind Hyg Occup Med* 1953; 8:335–339.
4. Lowe HJ, Freeman G: Boron hydride (borane) intoxication in man. *AMA Arch Ind Health* 1957; 16:523–533.
5. Manufacturing Chemists Association, Inc: *Chemical Safety Data Sheet SD-84, Boron Hydrides.* Washington, DC, MCA, Inc, 1967.
6. Roush G Jr: The toxicology of the boranes. *J Occup Med* 1959; 1:46–52.
7. Rozendaal HM: Clinical observations on the toxicology of boron hydrides. *AMA Arch Ind Hyg Occup Med* 1951; 4:257–260.

COPPER AND COPPER COMPOUNDS

Copper is the 26th most abundant element in the earth's crust at about 0.01%. It is often found in pure form, but is usually mined (both underground and in open pits) as sulphide ores: copper sulfide (CuS), chalcocite (Cu_2S), chalcopyrite ($CuFeS_2$), bornite (Cu_3FS_3), malachite (the well-known "malachite green,") ($Cu_2CO_3[OH]_2$), and various other oxides. Copper has been used by man since very early times, antedating the bronze age. World production in 1985 was 8.1 million tons. From an occupational health view, there must be awareness that exposure to copper or copper compounds often is accompanied by other substances, such as oxides of arsenic, cadmium, iron, sulfur, zinc, and others. The chief hazards are inhalation of copper (oxide) fumes or dusts in smelters and in grinding, cutting, welding, and packaging of various compounds (Fig 45–2).

Toxicology

Although copper is an essential trace element in man, exposure to fumes or dust can cause acute upper respiratory tract irritation. Occasionally, metal fume fever can occur (see section on Zinc, this chapter). Poisoning by ingestion is rare in industry.

Inhalation of copper fume results in irritation of the upper respiratory tract and an influenza-like illness called "metal fume fever." Signs and symptoms of metal fume fever include chills, muscle aches, nausea, fever, dry throat, cough, weakness, and

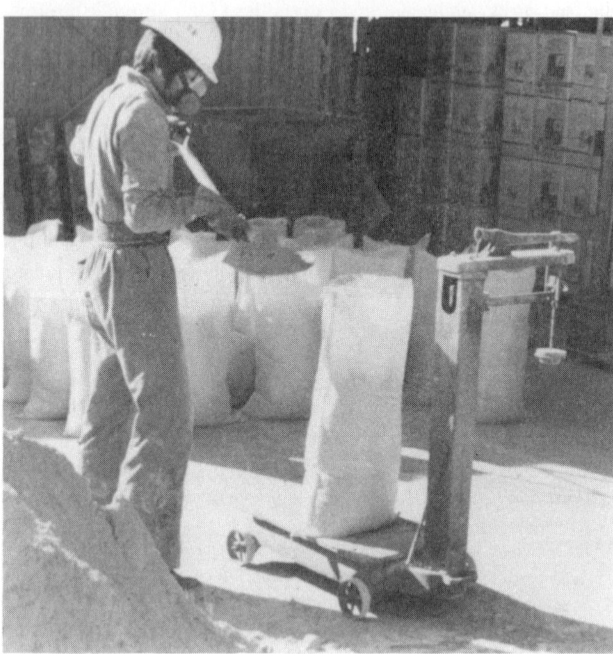

FIG 45–2.
Packaging copper sulfate.

lassitude. Leucocytosis occurs, up to 12,000 to 16,000/cu m. Recovery is usually rapid, and there are no sequelae. Most workers develop an "immunity," but it is quickly lost. Attacks tend to be more severe on the first day of the workweek.

Other effects from copper fume are irritation of the upper respiratory tract, ulceration and perforation of the nasal septum, metallic or sweet taste, and in some instances, discoloration of the skin and hair. Exposure of workers to concentrations of 1–3 mg/cu m for short periods resulted in altered taste responses, but no nausea; levels of 0.02–0.4 mg/cu m produced no complaints. There may be transient irritation of the eyes following exposure to the fine dust of oxidation products of copper. Armstrong et al.[1] reported an outbreak of metal fume fever among workers involved in cutting brass pipes with electric cutting torches in an enclosed, poorly ventilated steam condenser. Twenty-six workers were affected; the most commonly reported symptoms were fever (21), dyspnea (23), chills (21), headache (21), and nausea (19). Fourteen of the workers experienced the symptom of an unusual sweet or metallic taste in the mouth. Clinical signs were limited to wheezing or rales in eight patients. Leukocytosis and an increase in band cell forms were noted in 21 and 20 of 24 workers, respectively. (The white blood cell count ranged from 12,300 to 24,600/cu mm.) The median time interval between exposure and onset of symptoms was five hours. None of three workers who spent less than one hour in the condenser became ill, whereas 25 of 26 of those who spent more than one hour became ill. Five of 12 workers had urine copper levels in excess of 0.05 mg/L. Chronic, heavy exposures may produce various health effects, such as the respiratory symptoms mentioned, dermatitis, and gastrointestinal distress.

Complaints of metallic taste and irritation of nasal and oral mucosa from sheet-metal workers resulted in a study of 11 workers and their working conditions by Askergren and Mellgren.[2] Copper that is used for roofing and other exterior fittings, such as flashing and guttering, is treated to give a "patina" appearance—the typical "green" found on old statues and other bronze items. When this sheeting must be worked, i.e., cut and ground, dust from the patina is produced. An analysis of the dust revealed the following components and their percentages: Copper hydroxide nitrate ($Cu[NO_3]_2 \cdot 3Cu[OH]_2$), 26%; copper hydroxide sulfate ($CuSO_4 \cdot 3Cu[OH]_2$), 25%; copper hydroxide chloride ($CuCl_2 \cdot 3Cu[OH]_2$), 1%; copper hydroxide carbonate ($CuCO_3 \cdot Cu[OH]_2$), 1%; copper silicate ($CuSiO_3$), 22%; cupric oxide (CuO), 17%; ferric oxide (Fe_2O_3), 4%; and water (H_2O), 4%. Duration of work on this sheeting ranged from one month (five years earlier) to 60 months. Nine of the ten workers complained about a sweet taste with work, seven complained of a runny nose, and six a feeling of mucosal irritation in the mouth or eyes. Eight reported that their distress began almost immediately after work began; the other two experienced no discomfort until after one to two hours. However, ventilation was reported to have had great importance. Half of the subjects were free from complaints two to three hours after work, while distress disappeared in the remaining subjects after an hour or so. Two complained of residual discomfort, one of irritation of the conjunctiva with lacrimation, and the other of lesions in his nose on a few occasions. Four of the ten sheet-metal workers displayed atrophic mucosal changes. These four were also the ones with the longest exposure time. It is notable that one of the examined subjects had not been exposed to the substances for at least six months prior to the examination. One even reported a previous exposure occasion five years earlier. Previously, workers did not use respiratory protective devices, but the authors recommended that respirators be used and wetting of the materials be done.

Pimentel et al.[8, 9] and Villar[13] have reported granulomatous and fibrotic lung changes in vineyard sprayers in Portugal who used "Bordeaux" mixture (1%–2% aqueous copper sulfate and hydrated lime, a pesticide no longer used in the U.S.). Experimental studies in mice by Eckert and Jerochin[6] supported these findings that copper was the etiologic agent. One hundred workers grinding copper and sieving high purity copper dust for four years with exposure concentrations up to 464 mg/cu m were reported by Suciu et al.[11] (India). The serum copper concentrations in these workers ranged from 0.8 to over 2 mg/L, compared to concentrations of 0.8–1.2 mg/L in nonexposed subjects. In contrast to these high levels, Clausen and Rastogi,[4] studied auto workers with exposure levels from 0.03 to 0.84 μg/cu m, with blood copper levels comparable to a nonoccupational group. Biologic tests for occupationally exposed workers are of uncertain value,[4, 12] especially at air concentrations near current ACGIH TLV levels (1 mg/cu m).

REFERENCES

1. Armstrong C, Moore L, Hackler R, et al: An outbreak of metal fume fever, diagnostic use of urinary copper and zinc determinations. *J Med* 1983; 25:886–888.
2. Askergren A, Mellgren M: Changes in the nasal mucosa after exposure to copper salt dust. A preliminary report. *Scand J Work Environ Health* 1975; 1:45–49.
3. Baselt R: Biological monitoring methods for industrial chemicals. Davis, Cal, Biomedical Publications, 1980, pp 88–91.

4. Clausen J, Rastogi S: Heavy metal pollution among autoworkers. II. Cadmium, chromium, copper, manganese and nickel. *Br J Ind Med* 1977; 34:216–220.
5. Cohen S: A review of the health hazards from copper exposure. *J Occup Med* 1974; 16:621.
6. Eckert H, Jerochin S: Lungenveranderungen durch Kupfersulfat. *Z Erkrank Atm -Org* 1982; 158:270–276.
7. Enterline Ph, Marsh G: Cancer among workers exposed to arsenic and other substances in a copper smelter. *Am J Epidemiol* 1982; 116:895–911.
8. Pimentel C, Marques F: Vineyard sprayer's lung: A new occupational disease. *Thorax* 1969; 24:678–688.
9. Pimentel C, Menezes A: Liver granulomas containing copper in vineyard sprayer's lung. *Am Rev Respir Dis* 1975; 111:189.
10. Roi R, Twon W, Hunter W, et al: *Occupational Health Guidelines for Chemical Risk.* Luxembourg, Commission of the European Communities, Directorate General Information Market and Innovation EUR 8513, 1983.
11. Suciu I, Lazar V, Ilea E: Copper poisoning in workers from copper electrolysis, in Zaidu SG (ed): *Environmental Pollution and Human Health.* Lucknow, India, Indian Toxicology Research Centre, 1977, pp 211.
12. Triebig G, Schaller K: Copper, Alessio L, Berlin A, Boni M (eds): in *Biological Indicators For The Assessment of Human Exposure to Industrial Chemicals.* Varese, Italy, Joint Research Centre Ispra Establishment, 1984.
13. Villar T: Vineyard sprayer's lung. *Am Rev Respir Dis* 1974; 110:545.
14. Wagner W: Environmental conditions in U.S. copper smelters. Washington DC, US Government Printing Office, 1975.

IRON OXIDE AND HEMATITE

Hematite, a major source of iron, is found in two forms–red hematite (red iron ore), consisting of about 70% iron (Fe_2O_3), and brown hematite, a hydrated sesquioxide of iron, with 42% iron content. Of importance is that most ores mined may contain between 10% and 12% free silica.

Occupational exposures may occur to dust and fumes of iron oxide in mining, both underground or open-pit, to chippers and grinders, arc welders, in various metal processing in foundries, and in silver polishing (using fine iron oxide as a polishing rouge).

Inhalation of iron oxide fume or dust may cause a clinical entity known as "benign pneumoconiosis," often labeled "siderosis," based on x-ray findings and work history. Iron oxide alone does not cause fibrosis in the lungs of animals, and it is probable that the same applies in humans.[6] Heavy exposures of six to ten years usually are required before changes recognizable by x-ray can occur; the retained dust gives x-ray shadows that may be indistinguishable from fibrotic pneumoconiosis.[4, 10]

Eight of 25 welders exposed chiefly to iron oxide for an average of 18.7 (range 3–32) years had reticulonodular shadows on chest x-ray films consistent with siderosis but no reduction in pulmonary function; exposure levels[4, 9] ranged from 0.65 to 47 mg/cu m. In another study, 16 welders with an average exposure of 17.1 (range 7–30) years also had x-ray studies that suggested siderosis and spirograms that were normal; however, the static and functional compliance of the lungs was reduced. Some of the welders were smokers.[11] The welders with the lowest compliance complained of dyspnea. Signs of "benign pneumoconiosis" with x-ray shadows that may be indistinguishable from fibrotic pneumoconiosis are found. It should be noted that in industrial situations, iron oxide fumes usually exist with other metallic fumes, and the effects of the combined substances should be considered.

Axelson and Sjöberg[1] studied a working population with high exposure to iron oxides who were engaged in sulfuric acid production from pyrite ore (FeS_2). Some 500 workers had been annually occupied in a factory founded in 1905 with particularly heavy iron oxide exposure throughout the years up to the mid-1950s. The production process used was based on oxidation of pyrite ore to produce sulfur dioxide, which was further oxidized to sulfur trioxide. The remaining content of the pyrite is iron oxides, almost exclusively hematite (Fe_2O_3), with 1%–2% of copper and small amounts of arsenic, nickel, and cobalt metals found as impurities along with the iron oxides. The arsenic content (as iron arsenate, $FeAsO_4$) was estimated at about 0.01%–0.1% (based on arsenic weight), whereas most of the copper was extracted. It was estimated that the iron oxide content of the factory air might have been in the order of 50–100 mg/cu m for many of the workers through a considerable time of the shift. It was well known that a heavy, dark "mist" of iron oxide was characteristic in several workplaces in this factory. The particle size was estimated to have been less than 10 μ for 25% of the dust, with 5%–10% less than 5 μ. Axelson and Sjöberg added that, despite the very heavy exposures, no cases of siderosis were found in this plant. In this case-reference study, Axelson and Sjöberg found no excess cancer in the respiratory system or other sites. It was suggested that earlier reports of respiratory cancers thought to be associated with iron oxides might be due to other, concomitant risk factors.

Judging from experiences in Sweden,[2] the increased lung cancer mortality among various mining populations was explained to be most likely due to exposure to radon and radon daughters rather than to iron oxides, along with a possible relationship to diesel exhaust gases.[7] Hernberg[5] summarized the evidences for and against the carcinogenic properties of iron ore dust and concluded that the carcinogenic effect for humans still is an open question.

An epidemiologic survey of welders was conducted in the Caterpillar Tractor Company plants in Peoria, Illinois, by Emmett et al.[3] in 1976 (Figs 45–3 and 45–4). Comparison groups consisted of 77 white men who had been welders at this plant for a total of longer than 10 years, 75 white men who were not welders but had been employed in other crafts in the vicinity of welding operations at this plant for more than eight years and 58 white male parts and tool employees who had neither worked as welders nor in the vicinity of welding operations but had been employed at this plant for more than 10 years. The investigators reported a statistically significant increase in the prevalence of cough in the morning and at other times during the day in the welders. Those in the welding and exposed groups reported significantly more phlegm at times other than the morning compared with the control group. There was no significant difference in the prevalence of other chest symptoms, of major respiratory illness, of abnormalities on physical examination of the respiratory system, or of abnormalities detectable on posteroanterior chest x-ray among the groups. The observed/expected forced expiratory volume (FEV_1) and observed/expected maximal midexpiratory flow (MMF) were significantly reduced in smokers contrasted with nonsmokers. There was a significant reduction in the observed/expected FEV_1 and observed/expected

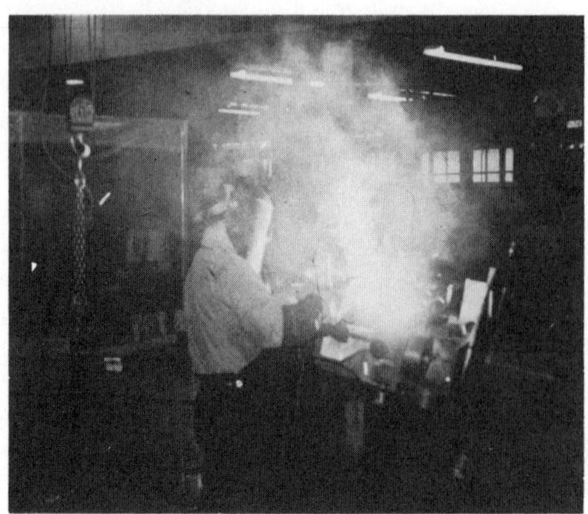

FIG 45–3.
Production welding before exhaust system was installed. Note dense fumes, which are mainly iron oxide.

forced vital capacity (FVC) in both the welding and exposed groups compared with the controls. There were indications that smoking and occupation might interact in producing decrements in observed/expected FVC, observed/expected FEV_1, and observed/expected MMF. The decrements in pulmonary function compared to the control group were similar in both the welding and exposed groups, suggesting that other factors rather than the ambient workplace atmospheres might be responsible, concomitant factors studied and reported by Jörgensen.[8]

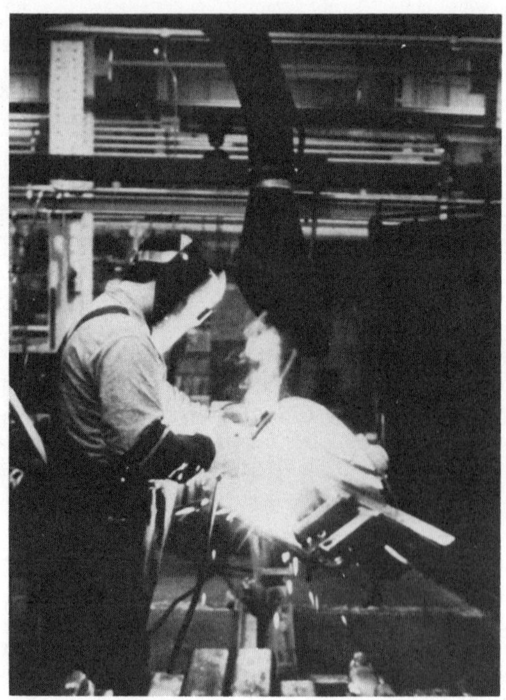

FIG 45–4.
Welding fumes effectively captured by local exhaust. The materials in the air are collected on a special filter, similar to that of a vacuum cleaner.

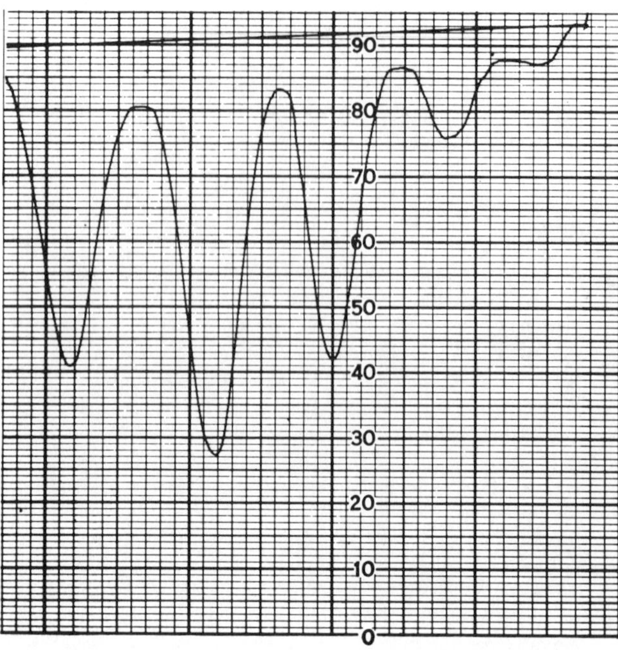

FIG 45–5.
Lactic dehydrogenase zymogram. Impression: normal total but there is an elevation in factor III. Pulmonary parenchyma is especially rich in isoenzyme factor III.

The 1985 TLV for iron oxide fumes is 5 mg/cu m. Methods of control are seen in Figure 45–4. (See Sjögren, Chapter 65, Effects of Gases and Particles in Welding and Soldering.)

REFERENCES

1. Axelson O, Sjöberg A: A case-referent study on cancer incidence and exposure to iron oxide dust. *J Occup Med* 1979; 21:419.
2. Axelson O, Sundell L: Mining, lung cancer and smoking. *Scand J Work Environ Health* 1978; 4:46.
3. Emmett E, Buncher C, Suskind R: An epidemiologic survey of welders. Cincinnati, Oh, University of Cincinnati, Dept of Environmental Health, 1976.
4. Harding HE, et al: Clinical, radiographic, and pathological studies of the lungs of electric-arc and oxyacetylene welders. *Lancet* 1958; 2:394.
5. Hernberg S: Incidence of cancer in populations with exceptional exposure to metals, in *Origins of Human Cancer*. Cold Spring Harbor Laboratory, 1977.
6. Jones G, Warner C: Chronic exposure to iron oxide, chromium oxide, and nickel oxide fumes of metal dressers in a steelworks. *Br J Ind Med* 1972; 29:169.
7. Jörgensen H: A study of mortality from lung cancer among miners in Kiruna, 1950–1970. *Work Environ Health* 1973; 10:127.
8. Jörgensen HS: Medical and hygenic health problems in an iron ore mine with special reference to repiratory illness. Arbete och Hälsa 1986;22.
9. Kleinfeld M, et al: Welders' siderosis. *Arch Environ Health* 1969; 19:70.
10. Sentz F, Rakow A: Exposure to iron oxide fume at arcair and powder-burning operations. *Am Ind Hyg Assoc J* 1969; 30:143.
11. Stanexcu D, et al: Aspects of pulmonary mechanics in arc welders' siderosis. *Br J Ind Med* 1967; 24:143.

LITHIUM AND ITS COMPOUNDS

Lithium (Li), with an atomic number of 3, is the lightest metallic element. It has enormous usage throughout the world. The United States is the largest producing country: nearly 11 million lb of lithium carbonate (Li_2CO_3) and 800,000 lb of lithium hydroxide ($LiOH\text{-}H_2O$) were exported to other countries in 1985. Ferrell reported:

> . . . most of the mineral concentrate is converted to lithium compounds and metal. The most widely used compound, lithium carbonate, can be added to aluminum potlines to reduce electricity consumption and fluorine emissions. It is also used to produce both ground-coat and cover-coat frits for vitreous enameling of steel. For this use, lithium functions as a flux to lower firing temperatures and reduces thermal expansion to extend the life of the enamel coating.
>
> The second most widely used lithium compound, lithium hydroxide, is used to manufacture lithium grease, which withstands temperature extremes better than most other greases. Less widely consumed lithium compounds include lithium bromide, which is used in absorption-refrigeration air-conditioning systems; lithium chloride, which is valued as a dehumidifying agent; and lithium hypochlorite, which serves as a sanitizer for swimming pools. Alkyllithium compounds, principally n-butyllithium, are used in synthetic rubber manufacturing.
>
> Lithium metal for lithium batteries give twice the service life of typical alkaline cells and, according to some sources, higher energy density and greater resistance to extremes of heat and cold. Disposable lithium batteries offer high-energy density and long life and find application in calculators, flashlights, pacemakers, and memory circuits. Secondary, or rechargeable, lithium batteries have potential for use in electric vehicles and power plant systems requiring peak load reserve energy.
>
> Some mineral (lithium) concentrates, possibly as much as 10% of total production, are used directly by the glass and ceramics industry as a powerful fluxing agent. In addition, use of lithium instead of soda or potash imparts a greater chemical durability and thermal shock resistance to the finished material.[3] Because of these intrinsic qualities, lithium mineral concentrate is preferred as a glass material in the manufacture of cathode ray tubes and sealed-beam headlights and as a ceramic material in heat-resistant cookware.

Lithium has great use in the preparation of numerous organic compounds. Despite this widespread use of lithium and its compounds, reports of toxic responses in man are rare. (Lithium carbonate is used in treating manic-depressive disease. The lithium ion is believed to exert its effect on monoamine metabolism in the brain.) The only compound that is reported as a severe hazard is lithium hydride (LiH), which is used as a condensing agent in chemical synthesis with acid esters and ketones, as a dessicant, a reducing agent and as a hydrogen source. Exposure is by inhalation. Ingestion of lithium in industry is rare.

Toxicology

Lithium hydride is a severe irritant of the eyes, mucous membranes, and skin due to the formation of lithium hydroxide on moist surfaces and its caustic action.[1]

The inherent toxicity of the lithium ion is high; a few milliequivalents in the plasma evokes serious symptoms and signs of nervous system effects: anorexia, nausea, muscle twitches, apathy, mental confusion, tremor, blurring of vision, coma, and death.[1]

An explosion of a cylinder of lithium hydride with eye contact and swallowing of a small amount by a technician caused burns which resulted in scarring of both corneas and produced strictures of larynx, trachea, bronchi, and esophagus; delayed death ensued.[2]

In man, brief exposure to 0.5 mg/cu m caused sneezing, to which some degree of tolerance was acquired.[2]

Exposure of animals to concentrations of 5–55 mg/cu m of lithium hydride caused sneezing and coughing; levels of 10 mg/cu m corroded the body fur and skin of the legs, and there was occasionally severe inflammation of the eyes and nasal septum.[4] Lesions of the nose and legs were similar to thermal burns and were attributed to the alkalinity of the hydrolysis product of lithium hydride.[2]

The TLV was set at a level to prevent nasal irritation—0.25 mg/cu m.

REFERENCES

1. American Conference of Governmental Hygienists: Lithium hydride, in *Documentation of the TLVs for Substances in Workroom Air*, ed 5. Cincinnati, Oh, ACGIH, 1986.
2. Cracovaner AJ: Stenosis after explosion of lithium hydride. *Arch Otolaryngol* 1964; 80:87.
3. Searles JP: Lithium, in *Minerals Yearbook, 1985. Vol I. Metals and Minerals*. Washington, DC, US Dept of the Interior, Bureau of Mines, US Government Printing Office, 1985.
4. Spiegl CJ et al: Acute inhalation toxicity of lithium hydride. *AMA Arch Ind Health* 1956, 14:468.

MAGNESIUM AND ITS COMPOUNDS

Magnesium is the lightest structural metal. Aluminum is 1½ times heavier and steel is 4½ times heavier. It is widely present as it is the eighth most abundant element and sixth most common metal, exceeded only by aluminum and iron. Magnesium is obtained from seawater, and there are ores rich in magnesium, such as dolomite and magnesite.

Uses

There is an enormous use in structural applications, especially aircraft. Further, magnesium is used to make portable tools, parts for machines, engines, sporting goods, office equipment—it has nearly endless uses in casting, forging, and extruding processes. It is alloyed with aluminum, lead, zinc, and other metals. It is used as an additive in iron foundries making ductile cast iron. (See Fig 45–2—the brilliant "flash" is magnesium metal being shoveled in or thrown in bags, into molten iron.)

Magnesium has a role in organic chemistry reactions. It is used in certain batteries and as a corrosion preventive in tanks, ship bottoms, and pipelines by cathodic action. Magnesium is a reducing agent in making metallic beryllium, titanium, uranium, and zirconium. There is heavy use in fireworks and flares for military applications.

There are numerous magnesium compounds in use. The most common are: magnesium carbonate (used in ceramics, glass making, inks, fertilizers, insulation, chemicals, and rubber products), magnesium chloride (used as a flocculating agent, treatment for fire resistance, and prevention of drying, in ceramics and paper, and for production of metallic magnesium), magnesium hydroxide (used in sulfite pulp, uranium processing, in medicines, and sugar refining), magnesium oxide (magnesia) (for refractories, in cement, insulation, in rubber, fertilizers, rayon processing and paper manufacture); magnesium sulfate (epsom salt) (in leather tanning, mordant assist in textile dyeing, paper sizing, in cement, ceramics, explosives, in matches, and for medicines).

Toxicology

Probably, the main occupational hazard that magnesium presents is a fire hazard, since it ignites readily. Magnesium and its alloys are considered to be of low toxicity. Experience with magnesium oxide and magnesium oxide fumes has been shown to be a mild irritant to the eyes and nasal mucosa. Examination of 95 workers exposed to an unspecified concentration of magnesium oxide dust revealed slight irritation of the eyes and nose. The magnesium level in the serum of 60% of those examined was above the normal upper limit of 3.5 mg%. Experimental subjects exposed to fresh magnesium oxide fume developed metal fume fever. Symptoms included fever, cough, oppression in the chest, and leukocytosis. There are no reports of metal fume fever resulting from occupational exposure. Metal magnesium slivers produce a gaseous reaction and cause a slow-healing burn with ulceration, but this has not been reported for magnesium oxide.

Permissible Exposure Limit

The current OSHA standard for magnesium oxide fume is 15 mg/cu m averaged over an eight-hour work shift. The ACGIH has recommended for magnesium oxide fume a TLV of 10 mg/cu m.

REFERENCES

1. American Conference Governmental Hygienists: Magnesium oxide fume, in *Documentation of the TLVs for Substances in Workroom Air*, ed 5. Cincinnati, Oh, ACGIH, 1986.
2. Drinker KR, Thomson RM, Finn JL: Metal fume fever. The effects of inhaled magnesium oxide fume. *J Ind Hyg* 1927; 9:187.
3. *Magnesium*, Data Sheet 426, Revision A. Chicago, National Safety Council, 1975.

MOLYBDENUM AND ITS COMPOUNDS

Molybdenum (Mo) was discovered by Scheele in 1778, but metallic molybdenum was not isolated until 1782.

The largest molybdenum deposits are found in the western hemisphere, the United States providing almost one third of world supply (world production in 1984 was 215,000,000 lb). Molybdenum is obtained both from primary mining operations and as a by-product in some copper mining operations.

The most abundant mineral in both primary and by-product mining is molybdenite (MoS_2). Less important minerals are wulfenite ($PbMoO_4$) and powellite ($Ca[MoW]O_4$).

Uses

Most molybdenite concentrate is roasted to molybdic oxide (MoO_3), a product directly usable in some iron and steel-making processes. Molybdic oxide can be converted to ammonium molybdate ($[NH_2]\ Mo_2O_7$), a high-purity material used in the manufacture of chemicals.

Pure molybdic oxide or ammonium molybdate is used in preparing powder metallurgy or vacuum-arc-cast molybdenum metal. Molybdenum powder is also used in the manufacture of catalysts and as feedstock for molybdenum metal spraying.

Some molybdenite concentrate is purified to a grade of molybdenum sulfide used in the manufacture of a dry lubricant.

Molybdenum forms compounds with valence states of 0, +2, +3, +4, +5, and +6.

The most common oxides are molybdenum dioxide and molybdem trioxide. At least seven intermediate oxides have been identified. The dioxide is readily converted to the trioxide by heating in an oxidizing atmosphere.

The trioxide is an acid anhydride forming molybdic acid (H_2MoO_4). The salts of molybdic acid form an important family of compounds called molybdates.

Molybdenum pentachloride ($MoCl_5$) has been used in the vapor phase deposition of molybdenum coatings.

Molybdenum hexacarbonyl ($Mo[CO]_4$) reacts with a variety of organic compounds to yield organomolybdenum compounds.

Molybdenum forms a series of homologous compounds with sulfur, selenium, and tellurium.

Molybdenum forms many organometallic compounds because of its many valence states and great complexing power. Molybdenum forms chelates with nitrogen, sulfur, and oxygen and a series of esters with alcohols, phenols, and hydroxy acids. Molybdenum forms alkyl and aryl derivatives as well as complexes with cyanides, olefins, and acetylenes.

Examples of organic compound applications include molybdenum acetylacetonate as a catalyst for the polymerization of ethylene and for the formation of polyurethane foam, molybdenum oxalate in certain photochemical systems, and molybdenum dithiocarbamate as a lubricant additive.

Approximately 85% of molybdenum production now goes into the manufacture of alloy steels, tool and high-speed steels, stainless steel, and alloy cast irons.

Superalloys, the materials used in the turbine wheels and blades of jet engines, usually contain molybdenum. The molybdenum content of superalloys varies over a wide range and can go as high as 30%.

Molybdenum-containing catalysts are now used in many petroleum and chemical processes. Molybdenum compounds may serve as principal catalysts or as activators and promotors of other catalysts.

Hydrocracking, alkylation, and reforming are important processes utilizing molybdenum catalysts.

Pigments containing zinc molybdate have been developed that have shown exceptional stability and anticorrosion properties and have a very low toxicity level. A pigment of long-standing use is molybdenum orange. This pigment is formed by coprecipitation of lead chromate and lead molybdate.

Potential occupational exposures may occur during liberation from mining and processing ore, from grinding and other abrasive action on metal or alloys, in oxyacetylene cutting, and from dusts of compounds, and upon skin contact. As with other metals, i.e., platinum, the more readily soluble compounds appear to be more toxic.

Toxicology

There are few reports of toxic effects in man, with elevated levels found in plasma and urine after inhalation of molybdenum dust.[11] Following exposure to average air concentrations of molybdenum (9.4 mg/cu m) during a work shift, worker plasma concentrations ranged from 9 ng/ml to 365 ng/ml (average, 122 ng/ml), a control group showing less than 34 ng/ml. In this plant producing molybdenum oxide from molybdenum sulfide, the 25 workers (with average employment time of four years) complained of headaches and aching joints more than the control group did and they experienced an increase of serum uric acid and ceruloplasmin. A Russian study[3] reported increased serum uric acid levels and joint aches in 34 of 37 workers. Goutlike symptoms have been reported in some areas in Armenia where there is a high food intake of molybdenum.[3] X-ray appearance of pneumoconiosis was reported in 3 of 19 Russian workers exposed to metallic molybdenum or molybdenum trioxide, exposure periods from four to seven years, with molybdenum concentrations between 1 and 19 mg/cu m.[3]

Molybdenum is an essential trace element for animals and plants.[3, 10] Molybdenum compounds inhaled in high concentrations caused respiratory mucous membrane changes in animals.[3] In small animals, gastrointestinal absorption is between 40% and 85% (in man, it is about 50%).[3, 6, 10] Livestock have been shown to be sensitive to high levels of molybdenum in food, with molybdenum poisoning in ruminates presenting findings similar to copper deficiency: loss of appetite, diarrhea, hair discoloration, joint abnormalities, and in severe cases, death.[4] Molybdenum impedes intake of copper, if sulfate intake is inadequate. Molybdenum deficiency can produce chronic copper poisoning in livestock.[10] Molybdenum is excreted mainly through the kidney.[1, 7]

Permissible Exposure Limit

The ACGIH TLV for molybdenum is 5 mg/cu m (soluble compounds) and 10 mg/cu m (insoluble).

REFERENCES

1. Bell MC, Diggs BG, Lowrey RS, et al: Comparison of Mo^{99} metabolism in swine and cattle as affected by stable molybdenum. *J Nutr* 1964; 84:367–372.
2. Considine D, Considine G (eds): *The Encyclopedia of Chemistry*, ed 4. New York, Van Nostrand Reinhold Co, 1984.
3. Friberg L: Molybdenum, in Friberg L, Nordberg GF, Vouk VB (eds): *Handbook of the Toxicology of Metals*. Amsterdam, Elsevier, 1980, pp 531–539.
4. Jarrell WM, Page AL, Elseewi AA: Molybdenum in the environment. *Residue Rev* 1980; 74:1–43.
5. *Minerals Yearbook, vol 1. Metals and Minerals*. Washington, DC, US Dept of the Interior, Bureau of Mines, US Government Printing Office, 1985.
6. Neilands JB, Strong FM, Elvehjem CA: Molybdenum in the nutrition of the rat. *J Biol Chem* 1948; 172:431–439.
7. Robinson GA, McCarter A, Rowsell MC, et al: The biological half-life of molybdenum-99 in normal and nutritionally deficient cows. *Am J Vet Res* 1964; 25:1040–1043.
8. Tipton IH, Stewart PL, Bickson J: Patterns of elemental excretion in long-term balance studies. *Health Phys* 1969; 16:455–462.
9. Underwood EJ: Trace metals in human and animal health. *J Hum Nutr* 1981; 35:37–48.
10. Van Campen DR, Mitchell EA: Absorption of Cu^{64}, Zn^{65}, Mo^{99} and Fe^{59} from ligated segments of the rat gastrointestinal tract. *J Nutr* 1965; 86:120–124.
11. Walravens PA, Moure-Eraso R, Solomons CC, et al: Biochemical abnormalities in workers exposed to molybdenum dust. *Arch Environ Health* 1979; 34:302–308.
12. Wester PO: Trace element balances in relation to variations in calcium intake. *Atherosclerosis* 1974; 20:207–215.

PLATINUM AND PLATINUM-GROUP METALS

The platinum group consists of platinum, palladium, indium, osmium, rhodium and ruthenium. Excluding the United States, world production of these metals in 1985 was estimated at 7.9 million troy ounces. These metals occur together in many areas throughout the world, with the main sources located where copper and nickel are mined: at Sudbury, Canada; in the Transvaal, South Africa; and in Siberia and in the Kola Peninsula, U.S.S.R. Approximately 95% of all platinum is mined in South Africa and the U.S.S.R., with Canada and Colombia producing most of the balance.

Uses

Platinum is extensively alloyed with other metals: copper, gold, iridium, rhodium, ruthenium, and cobalt (the cobalt-platinum alloy has strong magnetic properties). Most applications using platinum depend on its catalytic powers. In the petroleum industry, platinum catalyzes the isomerization of hydrocarbons in gasolines to improve octane rating; platinum is also used for other synthesis of hydrocarbons in petrochemical production. The chemical industry employs platinum-rhodium gauze catalysts in the production of nitric acid from ammonia or of hydrogen cyanide. Finally, dispersed platinum catalysts are used in the production of pharmaceuticals such as vitamins and especially in hydrogenation.

In addition to these catalytic applications in the petrochemical industries, the greatest use of platinum is its role in automotive exhaust systems as "catalytic converters." In 1984, the European Commission recommended that member countries enforce the introduction of lead-free fuel and antipollution measures for vehicles, so it is estimated that the European automobile industry will be using about 400,000 oz of platinum by the 1990s, which is about 80% of present U.S. auto industry consumption.

In 1984, there were 46 small fuel cells, each with 40-kW power, constructed in the U.S. and Japan for restaurants, hospitals, and swimming baths. A few 5–10-kW cells are being built for forklift trucks, military generators, milk trucks, and urban buses. These fuel cells are reported to have electrical efficiency 50%–100% more than present power units.

New consumption areas are coins and small bars. The 1-oz platinum Noble, marketed toward the end of 1983, sells at 5,000 oz· a month.

Platinum is used for resistance thermometers and in thermal couples, often alloyed with rhodium. The rhodium-platinum alloy has been used for high temperature furnaces and in the manufacture of spinnerettes used in synthetic and glass fiber production. The chemical industry has great use for platinum in lining vessels.

Platinum is often alloyed with iridium for jewelry, in electrodes for electrolytic oxidations, electrical contacts, for razor blades, industrial rubies for lasers, and spark plugs.

Some platinum compounds are: ammonium hexachloroplatinate ($[NH_4]_2PtCl_6$), chloroplatinic acid (H_2PtCl_6), platinic chloride ($PtCl_4$), platinic oxide (PtO_2), platinum hexafluoride (PtF_6), potassium hexachloroplatinate (K_2PtCl_6). Some of these compounds have been used in photographic work.

At the mines, ores are concentrated by floatation yielding a rich concentrate of the platinum-group metals. Final refining may take place in different countries. The concentrate is dissolved in hydrochloric acid and chlorine; after gold is precipitated, other metals present are precipitated or their volatile tetroxides are distilled. This solution of platinum and palladium is treated with ammonium chloride to precipitate platinum as ammonium hexachloroplatinate, known as "yellow salt." Further refining produces platinum 99.99% pure. In these refining workshops, exposures can occur during the handling of the halogenated compounds of platinum.

Toxicology

One of the first occupational studies of platinum refinery workers was undertaken by Hunter et al.[9] (reported in 1945) who studied all workers in four refineries of 91 men examined, 52 had symptoms including repeated sneezing with running nose, tightness of the chest, shortness of breath, and wheezing, which persisted as long as the workers were in the factory and for about one hour after they left. Also, many stated they would wake in the early hours of the morning with a bout of dry coughing lasting between a half and one hour. Hunter and co-workers estimated workplace atmospheric air to contain platinum levels ranging from 1.0 μg/cu m to 1,700 μg/cu m; at different locations and with various work stages. In 1951, Roberts[17] reported a five-year study of 21 workers in a platinum refinery, noting that all had some form of platinum allergy, with 50% reporting symptoms. Unfortunately, Roberts described these conditions as "platinosis," suggesting to future readers that a chronic fibrogenic lung disease developed from the exposures, while the correct term should have been "allergy to platinum compounds."

Hughes[8] undertook an investigation of environmental and clinical factors in the largest refinery in Western Europe, producing all platinum group metals from primary and secondary materials. Approximately 150 workers were studied (regular medical surveillance had been ongoing since 1967). All potential employees are given a questionnaire for previous occupational and medical history, with attention being paid to previous asthma, allergy, lung disease, family history of allergies and smoking habits. All potential employees were given a skin prick test for atopic status using house dust, house dust mite, and mixed grass pollens. They were also given a skin prick test with three platinum salts—ammonium hexachloroplatinate, sodium tetrachloroplatinite, and sodium hexachloroplatinate at 10^{-3} gm/ml—to determine whether sensitization had occurred in previous employment, e.g., previous employment in a platinum refinery, university department, catalyst production, or laboratory work. In addition, a lung function assessment and a medical examination were performed. Thirty-five percent of persons examined before employment were found to be atopic. (See Mathias, Chapter 10, for a discussion of the specificity of some metal salts for inducing type I IgE-mediated allergic reaction by skin testing.[4, 6, 15])

Hughes described details of the skin prick tests performed on all potentially exposed workers, done at three-month intervals, to detect any sensitization before symptoms appeared. The dosage of platinum salts used in the tests was small (10^{-3} gm/ml of solution, in absolute terms, is 3×10^{-9} gm of platinum salt—work exposures can be many times greater than this). No adverse reactions were observed, in contrast to previous reports of adverse reactions following scratch and intracutaneous tests. In most, symptoms preceded positive skin tests, but in a minority, the prick test remained negative despite clinical findings that sensitization had occurred. The possibility of sensitizing workers by repeated skin testing is questioned, but in practice, this did not occur.[3]

All workers in whom a diagnosis of platinum allergy was made along with symptoms or an indication of decreasing lung function were recommended to leave the factory site. Previously, efforts were made to move these workers to other areas where exposure was thought to be nil, but many were so exquisitely sensitive to small amounts of platinum salts that work-related symptoms persisted. All who left the factory rapidly lost all symptoms and recovered completely, but some with a positive skin prick test to platinum salts have been seen to revert to a negative test after cessation of exposure.

The literature shows many dermatitis cases attributed to platinum in refinery workers and other occupations, with suggestions this is due to a type IV allergic response. However, Hughes stated that, after 12 years' surveillance of this platinum refinery, a true contact dermatitis is extremely rare and that the dermatitis seen is of a primary irritant nature following exposure to strong acids and alkalis. Urticaria follows splashing with solutions containing platinum salts and in some instances it is the first indication of sensitization. Dermatitis in the refinery workers can be high and can develop rapidly. Sensitization has been seen ten days after starting work in the refinery.

Preventive measures similar to that for control of lead, isocyanates, and similarly potentially irritative and toxic substances is imperative for workers with potential exposure to the soluble platinum compounds. Excluding atopic persons has proven to be important, and when the diagnosis of platinum allergy is made, the affected person should be moved from the workplace and away from any possible further contact. (See Levy, Chapter 14, for a description of platinum respiratory reactions.)

Permissible Exposure Limits

The current OSHA standard for soluble platinum salts (as platinum) is 0.002 mg/cu m averaged over an eight-hour work shift. The TLV for platinum metal is 1 mg/cu m.

REFERENCES

1. American Conference of Governmental Industrial Hygienists: Platinum (Soluble Salts as Pt), in *Documentation of the Threshold Limit Values for Substances in Workroom Air*, ed 5. Cincinnati, ACGIH, 1986.
2. Campbell F, et al: Dermal irritancy of metal compounds. *Arch Environ Health* 1975; 30:168–170.
3. Clarke CW, Pepys J: Platinum group metals, in *Medical and Biological Effects of Environmental Pollutants*. Washington DC, National Academy of Sciences, 1977, p 109.
4. Cleare MJ, Hughes EG, Jacoby B, et al: Immediate (type I) allergic responses to platinum compounds. *Clin Allergy* 1976; 6:183.
5. Considene D, Considene G (eds): *The Encyclopedia of Chemistry*, ed 4. New York, Van Nostrand Reinhold Co, 1984.
6. Cromwell O, Pepys J, Parish WE, et al: Specific IgE antibodies to platinum salts in sensitized workers. *Clin Allergy* 1979; 9:109.
7. Freedman SO, Krupey J: Respiratory allergy caused by platinum salts. *J Allergy* 1968; 42:233.
8. Hughes EG: Medical surveillance of platinum refinery workers. *J Soc Occup Med* 1980; 30:27–30.
9. Hunter D, Milton R, Perry KMA: Asthma caused by complex salts of platinum. *Br J Ind Med* 1945; 2:92.
10. Levene GM: Platinum sensitivity. *Br J Dermatol* 1971; 85:590.
11. Mastromatteo E: Platinum, alloys and compounds, in *The Encyclopedia of Health and Safety*. Geneva, International Labour Office, 1983.
12. Milne JEA: A case of platinosis. *Med J Aust* 1970; 25:1194.
13. *Minerals Yearbook 1985*, vol 1, *Metals and Minerals*. Washington, DC, US Dept of the Interior, Bureau of Mines, Superintendent of Documents, US Government Printing Office, 1985.
14. Parrot JL, Hebert R, Saindelle A, et al: Platinum and platinosis. Allergy and histamine release due to some platinum salts. *Arch Environ Health* 1969; 19:685.
15. Pepys J, Paris WE, Cromwell O, et al: Passive transfer in man and the monkey of type I allergy due to heat labile and heat stable antibody to complex salts of platinum. *Clin Allergy* 1979; 9:99.
16. Pepys J, Pickering CAC, Hughes EG: Asthma due to inhaled chemical agents-complex salts of platinum. *Clin Allergy* 1972; 2:391.
17. Roberts FA: Platinosis. A five year study of the effects of soluble platinum salts on employees in a platinum laboratory and refinery. *Arch Ind Hyg* 1951; 4:549.
18. Roshchin AV, Veselov VG, Panova AI: Industrial toxicology of metals of the platinum group. *J Hyg Epidemiol Microbiol Immunol* 1984; 28:17–24.

SILVER AND ITS COMPOUNDS

World production of silver in 1985 was 412 million troy ounces. Peru is the greatest producing country, followed by Mexico, the U.S.S.R., the United States, and Canada. Natural occurrence is mainly its sulfide form (Ag_2S), but more than half of that produced is a by-product of lead and copper production. Native gold is also a large source. There is much reclaiming from scrap and from x-ray and photographic films (see Chapter 47, Cyanides). Its main uses are for electrical conducting components, electrical contacts, for silverware, in photography and plating, in photochromic glass, for corrosion-resistant parts in chemical making, as a catalyst in certain hydrogenation or oxidation processes, in jewelry, in dental amalgams, and in coins. (Formerly, U.S. coins were 90% silver and 10% copper; now there is no silver in dimes and quarters and only 40% in half dollars.) Some important alloys are: sterling silver, which is 92.5% silver and 7.5% copper; silver-copper-zinc, as "silver solders"; silver-lead, which is used in special batteries; and silver-cadmium alloys for bearings, which are made of 97% cadmium, 2% silver, and 1% copper or nickel. There are numerous compounds; the *Merck Index* lists 32. Probably the most important compound is silver nitrate ($AgNO_3$), long used as a topical antiseptic and for the prevention of ophthalmia neonatorum. The halides are the basis for the light sensitivity of photographic emulsions.

Toxicology

Skin disfiguration can occur when pieces or particles of metallic silver penetrate the skin, producing pigmented lesions similar to tattooing, a permanent pigmentation. This localized argyria may be localized in the skin, eyes, or mucous membranes, appearing as grey-blue patches, without evidence of tissue reaction.[1, 3] With chronic inhalation (above respirable limits of 0.01 mg/cu m or oral accumulative doses from 1 to 5 gm of silver[1]), there is a generalized argyria recognized by widespread pigmentation of the skin and first seen in the conjunctiva, with some localization in the inner canthus. Argyrosis of the respiratory tract has been described in two workers involved in the manufacture of silver nitrate; their only symptom was mild chronic bronchitis. Bronchoscopy revealed tracheobronchial pigmentation; biopsy of the nasal mucous membrane showed silver deposition in the subepithelial area.[1] Nearly all the silver salts are irritating to the mucous membranes and to the skin (depending on concentration, if liquid, the duration of contact of the liquid or solid, and the temperature). Silver nitrate is a powerful oxidizer, caustic and corrosive. As a dust, silver nitrate can cause conjunctivitis, argyria, and even blindness. Silver oxide (Ag_2O) is also a strong oxidizer, used in special battery making, for glass (polishing and giving a yellow color), as a catalyst, for purifying water for drinking, and as an ointment or in a solution for germicidal use. Contact and inhalation must be prevented.

Permissible Exposure Limit

The current OSHA standard for silver metal and soluble silver compounds is 0.01 mg/cu m averaged over an eight-hour work shift. The ACGIH (1985–86) TWA for silver metal is 0.1 mg/cu m, and for soluble compounds (as Ag), 0.01 mg/cu m.

REFERENCES

1. Browning E: *Toxicity of Industrial Metals*, ed 2. London, Butterworth & Co, 1969.
2. American Conference Governmental Industrial Hygienists: Silver, in

Documentation of the TLVs for Substances in Workroom Air, ed 5. Cincinnati, ACGIH, 1986.

3. Rosenman KD, Moss A, Kon S: Argyria: Clinical implications of exposure to silver nitrate and silver oxide. *J Occup Med* 1979; 21:430–435.

Strontium (Sr)

Strontium is one of the alkaline earth elements, located between calcium and barium on the periodic table; its chemical and physical properties resemble barium and calcium. Metallic or elemental strontium is produced by electrolysis, but commercial quantities are small, since barium and calcium are more common and readily usable. World production is estimated to be about 130,000 short tons. Strontium compound consumption is estimated about 80% as carbonate, 15% as nitrate, and 5% for chloride, chromate, phosphate, oxide, peroxide, sulfide, and many others.

Strontium compounds have had long use in military and civil applications for flares, in tracer bullets, and in fireworks for entertainment because of the intense and brilliant red colors imparted, especially from the nitrate, but also carbonate, chlorate chloride, oxalate, or sulfate compounds. Other applications are found in the manufacture of ferrite-ceramic magnets (with strontium carbonate) for many small motors, (audio) speakers; in the front end of television tubes to reduce x-ray emissions; to increase iridescence in some glass; the chromate as a yellow pigment; the sulfide for luminous paints; the bromide for diagnostic x-ray film screens. Other uses are found in fluorescent lights, in certain plastics polymerization, special electronic devices, various coatings and paints, and in welding fluxes.

The main hazard of metallic strontium is that of fire or explosion; contact with moisture or water causes a rapid reaction with production of hydrogen, creating a potential explosive threat. Major hazards of the compounds, especially the nitrate, chlorate, and peroxide are fire and explosivity, as these substances are powerful oxidizing agents (as attested by their widespread usage in pyrotechnic applications mentioned above. Under occupational conditions, oral exposures are rare and the few animal studies made have revealed an LD_{50} of 400–500 mg/kg for the salts.

The greatest danger to humans is that from the artificial isotopes ^{89}Sr and ^{90}Sr produced in nuclear reactions; fallout of ^{90}Sr, mainly from atmospheric nuclear explosions (and power-plant reactor accidents) has caused great concern. These isotopes are deposited in bones acting as a source of internal radiation. The ^{90}Sr has a half-life of 28 years, and emits beta particles that damage marrow. (See Chapter 26 for full discussion of these important aspects.)

REFERENCES

1. Kroes R, Den Tonkelaar EM, Minderhoud A, et al: Short term toxicity of strontium chloride in rats. *Toxicology (Amsterdam)* 1977; 7:11–21.
2. Considine D, Considine G (eds): *The Encyclopedia of Chemistry*, ed 4. New York, Van Nostrand Reinhold Co, 1984.
3. *Minerals Yearbook 1985*, vol 1, *Metals and Minerals*. Bureau of Mines, US Department of the Interior, US Government Printing Office, Washington, DC.
4. US Department of Health and Human Services: *Occupational Health Guidelines for Strontium*. Occupational Health Guides for Chemical Hazards, DHHS Publ 81-123, Rockville, Md, NIOSH, 1981.

THALLIUM AND THALLIUM COMPOUNDS

Thallium (Tl), named after its bright green spectroscopic line, is estimated to be present in the earth's crust in amounts equal to that of mercury and is recovered mainly from sulfide minerals during lead and zinc smelting. Thallium is also recovered from cadmium-containing flue dusts. The first main use was in the 1920s, when thallium sulfate was the main component of rat poison. This compound was widely used as a rodenticide until recently, when anticoagulants replaced it as a general rodenticide. The marked toxicity of thallium compounds has long been recognized, mainly because of poisoning arising from accidental ingestion of the rodenticide, from therapeutic uses (as a depilatory) and in suicidal attempts. Occupational exposures may occur in production and ore processing, during certain alloying manufacture, or when using compounds for pharmaceuticals or for glass for special lenses and prisms. (Thallium in combination with arsenic and sulfur forms low melting-point glass.) Thallium is also used in detecting radiation in the infrared range (thallium, oxysulfide, and mixed thallium bromide codide crystals are used). Additionally, thallium is used in some semiconductors. In 1979, Schaller et al.[8] studied worker exposures from cement factories that produced a special resistant cement using additives of thallium containing iron pyrites.

Toxicology

Entry into the body can result from inhalation of dust or fumes and absorption through the skin. Ingestion is rare in the industrial setting. It appears that thallium is a general cytotoxic agent, the thallium-I-ions being treated by the organism as potassium ions, with rapid systemic transport, nearly all into the cells. The elimination half-life is about four days.[6] Thallium concentration is higher in the kidneys than in other tissues, although a marked concentration is also found in the central nervous system, based on animal studies.[2]

Many deaths have resulted from ingestion of the lethal oral dose of thallium acetate, which in man is estimated to be about 12 mg/kg body weight. Ingestion causes nausea, vomiting, diarrhea, abdominal pain, and gastrointestinal hemorrhage, usually occurring within one to three days. These are followed or accompanied by ptosis, strabismus, peripheral neuritis, pain, weakness, paresthesias in the legs, tremor, retrosternal tightness, and chest pain. Severe alopecia usually occurs after two to three weeks and is thought to be pathognomonic, but may not always occur, even with severe poisoning. Severe intoxication may result in prostration, tachycardia, blood pressure fluctuations, convulsive seizures, choreaform movements, and psychosis. Recovery may be complete, but permanent residual effects, such as ataxia, optic atrophy, tremor, mental abnormalities, and foot-drop, have been reported.

In cases of fatal intoxication, typical autopsy findings include pulmonary edema, necrosis of the liver, nephritis, and degenerative changes in peripheral axons.

In a study of 15 workers who had handled solutions of organic thallium salts over a 7.5-year period, six workers suffered thallium intoxication. The chief complaints were abdominal pain, fatigue, weight loss, pain in the legs, and nervous irritability. Three of the workers had albuminuria and one had hematuria.

In 1979, plant and animal damage from environmental contamination of thallium-containing emissions from a cement factory resulted in a new look at the levels of occupational thallium exposures which previously had been considered low. Schaller et al.[8] conducted detailed studies of workers in three cement factories where thallium-containing additives were used. They examined 128 men from all production areas, who had a mean exposure of 19.5 years (range, 1–42 years). Schaller and co-workers determined that the roasted pyrites contained 300 ppm thallium and that the collected dusts from the electrofilters (which must be maintained) contained thallium oxides (Tl_2O and Tl_2O_3) and thallium hydroxide (TlOH). The chief findings were worker urinary thallium concentrations significantly higher (up to 30 μg/L) than those found in "normal" persons. Relatively high excretions were associated with the furnace workers, since the roasting process causes enrichment of thallium. (The thallium escapes at the high temperatures, cools, and is found in the filter dust.)

The usefulness of urinary thallium measurement as a rapid biologic screening method was described with detailed clarity by Marcus,[4] who studied and reported his findings of workers engaged in manufacturing special alloy anode plates for use in seawater batteries, which are used for powering sonobuoys, torpedo propulsion, various marine emergency devices, and in radiosonde balloons. One of the magnesium alloys used is composed of 7% magnesium, 88% aluminum, and 5% thallium. Marcus provided an excellent process flow diagram which is most suitable and adaptable for use in other occupational health exposure investigations. Using personal monitors, random workroom air samples that were taken revealed a maximum thallium of 0.022 mg/cu m. Samples in the rolling mill scratchbrushing area were 0.014 mg/cu m (maximum). These levels were attained after a strict code of practice was developed and followed. Previously, results in September 1976 showed that out of a population of 39, seven workers had urinary thallium levels between 50 μg/L and 100 μg/L, three had values up to 236 μg/L, while the remaining 29 had levels below 50 μg/L. Following the introduction of a code of practice, urine screening has shown that the safeguards introduced have reduced absorption. Typical results were obtained in September 1981, with the highest individual level being 5.2 μg/L.

In human beings, thallium is present as a naturally occurring trace element.[9] A urine thallium level of 300 μg/L is suggested as the threshold for poisoning, according to Glomme.[3] Marcus considers this too high, suggesting an action level of 50 μg/L. There is no evidence to support the possibility of thallium presenting a carcinogenic, mutagenic, or teratogenic risk in humans

Permissible Exposure Limit

The current OSHA standard for soluble thallium compounds is 0.1 mg/cu m averaged over an eight-hour work shift.

REFERENCES

1. American Conference of Governmental Industrial Hygienists: Thallium, *Documentation of the Threshold Limit Values for Substances in Workroom Air*, ed 4. Cincinnati, Oh, ACGIH, 1980.
2. Banks W, Pleasure D, Suzuki J, et al: Thallium poisoning. *Arch Neurol* 1972; 26:456.
3. Glomme J: Thallium and compounds, in *Encyclopaedia of Occupational Health and Safety*, ed 3. Geneva, International Labour office, 1983.
4. Marcus R: Investigation of a working population exposed to thallium. *J Soc Occup Med* 1985, 35:4–9.
5. Paulson G, et al: Thallium intoxication treated with dithizone and hemodialysis. *Arch Intern Med* 1972; 129:100–103.
6. Rauws A: Thallium pharmacokinetics and its modification by Prussian blue. *Chem Abstr* 1975; 82:16780X.
7. Richeson E: Industrial thallium intoxication. *Ind Med Surg* 1958; 27:607–619.
8. Schaller K, Manke G, Raithel H, et al: Investigations of thallium-exposed workers in cement factories. *Int Arch Occup Environ Health* 1980; 47:223–231.
9. Smith I, Carson B: *Trace Metals in the Environment, Vol 1. Thallium*. Ann Arbor, Ann Arbor Science, 1977.

TIN AND ITS COMPOUNDS

The primary source of tin (Sn) is cassiterite (SnO_2). World mine production of tin in 1985 was 191,000 metric tons. The main sources of tin are Malaysia, Thailand, Indonesia, Bolivia, and China, with the U.S.S.R. now ranking second. No ores of commercial value are found in the United States.[11]

Uses

Tin is easily melted (its melting point is 232° C) and readily alloys with other metals and in liquid form. Tin "coats" and joins other metals, a property long known and widely used to make solders and "tinplate," which is low-carbon steel, thinly tin-plated. Formerly, tinplate was the largest use of primary tin, but aluminum containers now exceed the traditional "tin cans" in production. In the United States (1982), out of 90 billion metal cans shipped, tinplate accounted for 41% and aluminum for 59%. Solders now are tin's largest applications. "Soft solders" are tin and lead alloys.

Copper-tin alloys are called "bronzes," but may contain small amounts of other metals, e.g., silicon, lead, or zinc. High tin-antimony-copper alloys are used as babbit (bearings), in die castings, and in pewter. (Pewter is composed of 91% tin, 7% antimony, and 2% copper; softer pewter has 95% tin.) Lead alloys containing antimony and tin are common materials for bearings and also for printing type.

Because of tin's low melting point and high boiling point (2,270° C), it has provided the ideal method to produce "float glass," (molten glass on molten tin) to fabricate high quality window glass. Its long use as a plating for household utensils and for food storage attests to its nontoxicity.

Stannous sulfate, chloride, fluoride, and fluoborate salts and the potassium or sodium stannates are used for the electroplating of tin and tin alloys. Stannous fluoride is well-known as a toothpaste additive. Stannous oxide (SnO) and stannic chloride ($SnCl_4$) are used in preparation of other tin compounds.

Toxicology

Although no systemic toxic effects have been reported with inorganic tin compounds, some can cause skin or eye irritation from acid or alkaline reactions with water: stannous chloride and stannous sulfate are strongly acid, and potassium and sodium stannate are strongly alkaline.[1] Prolonged inhalation of fine tin oxide dust (silica-free) in heavy amounts can lead to a benign penumoconiosis ("stannosis") without pulmonary function impairment: the radiologic findings are similar to baritosis.[4, 8] The TLV for tin oxide is 2 mg/cu m (except SnH_4 and SnO_2).

In contrast to the above mentioned inorganic tin compounds, organic tin compounds are highly toxic. Some organic tin compounds are used in polyvinyl chloride plastics as stabilizers to prevent darkening and breakdown. The chief tin compounds are dibutyltin, dioctyltin, dimethyltin chloride, and trimethyltin chloride. When compounded into the final plastic product, they are nontoxic. The alkyl and aryl series of organic tin compounds were found to have biocidal and fungicidal properties in the early 1950s and are now widely used in wood preservatives (consumer and industrial), in paper and textile making (dyeing and printing), in paints, in agricultural fungicides and insecticides, and in hospital disinfectants.[5]

Organotin compounds cause irritation of the eyes, mucous membranes, and skin; some produce cerebral edema and others cause hepatic necrosis.[7]

The most toxic are the trialkyltins, followed by the dialkyltins and monoalkyltins. The tetraalkyltins are metabolized to their trialkyltin homologs; their effects are those of the trialkyltins. The severity of effects is dependent upon the rate of the metabolic conversion and the amount and duration of work exposures. In each organotin group, the ethyl derivative is the most toxic.[2, 3, 6, 14]

Tributyltin ($[C_4H_9]SnCl_3$).—Workers exposed to the vapor or fume of tributyltin compounds developed sore throat and cough several hours after exposure. When a worker was splashed in the face with a tributyltin compound, lacrimation and severe conjunctivitis appeared within minutes and persisted for four days, despite immediate lavage. After seven days the eyes appeared normal. Chemical burns may result after only brief contact with the skin. Pain is moderate, and itching is the chief symptom. Healing is usually complete within seven to ten days.[2, 10]

Triphenyltin Acetate ($[C_6H_5]SnCl_3$).—Liver damage has been reported from occupational exposure to triphenyltin acetate. In two cases, both developed hepatomegaly and one had slightly elevated SGPT and SGOT activity. Exposure to a 20% solution produced skin irritation two days after prolonged contact with contaminated clothing. Other nonspecific effects of exposure have included headache, nausea, vomiting, diarrhea, and blurred vision.[2, 13, 14]

Bis (Tributyltin) Oxide (TBTO).—This is an irritant to the eyes and respiratory tract.

Dimethyl and Trimethyltin Chloride ($[CH_3]_2SnCl$ and $[CH_3]_3Sn$ Cl).—Rey et al.[12] observed and treated six workers from a chemical plant who were exposed to dimethyl and trimethyltin chloride while cleaning a vessel. The liquid phase contained a solution of 75% dimethyltin chloride and 25% trimethyltin chloride, while the gas phase had concentrations of the two substances at approximately 50% each. Duration of exposure varied among the six workers, with maximal exposure being nine ten-minute exposures in three working days. All workers allegedly wore the prescribed protective clothing and gas masks.

The first symptoms arose following a latent period of one to three days. These included headache, tinnitus, deafness, impaired memory, disorientation, aggressiveness, psychotic behavior, syncope, loss of consciousness, and, in the most severe cases, respiratory depression, requiring ventilatory assistance. Significantly increased tin excretion was detected in the urine of all patients. Those who were most ill had the highest urinary tin concentrations. Urinary tin levels were from 625 ppb to 1,600 ppb. There were epileptic activity demonstrated by electroencephalogram (EEG) and leukocytosis in all six patients and the need for artificial ventilation in three of them. Pronounced EEG alterations were present, similar to that seen in temporal lobe seizures.

Therapeutically, dexamethasone was administered to treat cerebral edema in all. Plasma separation was chosen because of the recognized high protein-binding of tin, and it was carried out in four patients. However, it did not lead to the expected decline in tin excretion via the urine, and plasma-tin levels could not be found. The patient with the highest tin levels died 12 days after initial exposure and had suffered coma, respiratory depression, acute respiratory distress syndrome, shock, anuria, and liver cell damage. The postmortem studies confirmed clinical impressions: microscopic sections revealed massive fatty degeneration of liver cells and necrosis, shock kidneys, and cerebral edema with irreversible cell damage in the area of the nucleus amygdaloideus, typical for trimethyltin chloride intoxication. These findings correlate with observed epileptic activity and the dream attacks.

The patient with the second highest urinary tin levels developed a severe and permanent neurologic defect syndrome, characterized by extrapyramidal hyperkinesis and severe cerebral defects. The third most severely intoxicated patient sustained severe deficits with memory dysfunction and aggressiveness. The remaining three patients appeared clinically healthy and returned to work, although they complained of memory loss for some six months. This striking report by Rey and co-authors strongly demonstrates the need for mandatory and strict engineering, hygienic control measures, and close supervision. The TLV of 0.1 mg/cu m for dimethyltin and trimethyltin chloride appears appropriate.

REFERENCES

1. American Conference of Governmental Industrial Hygienists: *Documentation of the Threshold Limit Values for Substances in Workroom Air,* ed 5. Cincinnati, Oh, ACGIH, 1986.
2. Barnes J, Stoner H: The toxicology of tin compounds. *Pharmacol Rev* 1959; 11:211.
3. Brown A, Aldridge W, Street B, et al: The behavioral and neuropathologic sequelae of intoxication by trimethyltin compounds in the rat. *Am J Pathol* 1979; 97:59.

4. Cole C, Davies JVSA, Kipling M, et al: Stannosis in hearth tinners. *Br J Ind Med* 1964; 21:235–241.
5. Considine D, Considine G (eds): *The Encyclopedia of Chemistry*, ed 4. New York, Van Nostrand Reinhold Co, 1984.
6. Criteria for a recommended standard: Occupational exposure to organotin compounds, DHEW (NIOSH) Publ. 77–115. Cincinnati, Oh, National Institute for Occupational Safety and Health, 1976.
7. Fortemps E, Amand G, Bomboir A, et al: Trimethyltin poisoning—Report of two cases. *Int Arch Occup Environ Health* 1978; 41:1.
8. Fox A, Goldblatt P, Kinlen L: A study of the mortality of Cornish tin miners. *Br J Ind Med* 1981; 38:378–380.
9. Louria D, Joselow M, Browder A: The human toxicity of certain trace elements. *Ann Intern Med* 1972; 76:307.
10. Lyle W: Lesions of the skin in process workers caused by contact with butyl tin compounds. *Br J Ind Med* 1958; 15:193.
11. *Minerals Yearbook*, vol 1. *Metals and Minerals*. Washington, DC, US Dept of the Interior, Bureau of Mines, US Government Printing Office, 1985.
12. Rey C, Reinecke H, Besser R: Methyltin intoxication in six men: Toxicologic and clinical aspects. *Vet Hum Toxicol* 1984; 26:2.
13. Shanor S, Davis E: Acute and subacute toxicology and safety evaluation of triphenyl tin hydroxide (Vancide WS). *Clin Toxicol* 1978; 13:281–296.
14. Tin and organotin compounds—A preliminary review. *Environmental Health Criteria* 15. Geneva, World Health Organization, 1980.

TITANIUM AND COMPOUNDS

Titanium is ninth in abundance of the elements making up the crust of the earth, accounting for 0.63% of the total. It is exceeded in amount only by aluminum, iron, and magnesium.

Most common titanium minerals are ilmenite (iron titanate), and rutile (titanium dioxide). The largest deposits of rutile are in Australia. World production of ilmenite concentrate in 1985 was 3.6 million short tons; of titaniferous slag, 1,170,000 short tons; and of natural rutile concentrate, 401,000 short tons.

Titanium metal is very resistant to corrosion. Most titanium goes into military hardware, largely for airplane parts. Smaller amounts go into guided-missile parts, airborne equipment, and space vehicles. The largest industrial uses are in the construction of parts of commercial airplanes and of chemical plant equipment.

The titanium that is used as a construction material is usually in the form of alloys. Alloying elements are aluminum, iron, manganese, chromium, molybdenum, and vanadium.

Titanium forms four well-defined oxides: titanium monoxide (TiO), dititanium trioxide (Ti_2O_3), titanium dioxide (TiO_2), and titanium trioxide (TiO_3).

Titanium dioxide, because of its extreme whiteness and brightness, is widely used as a white pigment in paints, lacquers, and enamels, paper, floor coverings, rubber, coated fabrics and textiles, printing ink, plastics, roofing granules, welding rods, synthetic fabrics, ceramics, and cosmetics.

Anhydrous titanium tetrachloride liquid is employed in producing smoke screens and as a catalyst in many organic reactions.

Many organic compounds of titanium, such as esters, alcoholates, phenylates, and complexes, have been prepared. Titanium is a constituent of a number of permanent metallized azo dyes. A very large number of complex compounds of titanium have been prepared.

There is scant human health data in the literature about titanium compounds. Of the many compounds in use, the greatest experience is that with titanium dioxide (TiO_2), also called "rutile," "anatase," or "brookite," a white, odorless powder that is usually considered a nuisance dust.

Toxicology

Titanium dioxide dust is a mild pulmonary irritant. Rats repeatedly exposed to concentrations of 10 to 328 million particles per cubic foot of air (mppcf) for as long as 13 months showed small focal areas of emphysema, which were attributed to large deposits of dust; there was no evidence of any specific lesion being produced by titanium dioxide.[2]

Three of 15 workers who had been exposed to titanium dioxide dust showed radiographic signs in the lungs resembling "slight fibrosis," but disabling disease did not occur; the magnitude and duration of exposure were not specified.

In the lungs of three workers involved in processing titanium dioxide pigments, deposits of the dust in the pulmonary interstitium were associated with cell destruction and slight fibrosis; the findings indicated that titanium dioxide is a mild pulmonary irritant.[1, 5]

Reline et al.[6] reported granulomatous pulmonary disease in a 45-year-old man who worked for 13 years as a furnace feeder in an aluminum smelter. Lung biopsy revealed aluminum in combination with other metals, including titanium, zinc, and nickel (61%), various aluminum silicates (35%), and silica (2%). Immunologic testing demonstrated a lymphocytic proliferative response to titanium chloride. Concentrations of workroom air contaminants were unknown and the authors stated that a causal relationship between titanium and the observed changes could not be proved.

Permissible Exposure Limit

The current OSHA standard for titanium dioxide is 15 mg/cu m (total dust) averaged over an eight-hour work shift. ACGIH has recommended for titanium dioxide a TLV of 10 mg/cu m.

REFERENCES

1. American Conference of Governmental Industrial Hygienists: Titanium dioxide, in *Documentation of the Threshold Limit Values for Substances in Workroom Air*, ed 5. Cincinnati, Oh, ACGIH, 1986.
2. Christie H, et al: Pulmonary effects of inhalation of titanium dioxide by rats. *Am Ind Hyg Assoc J* 1963; 24:42–46.
3. Grant WM: *Toxicology of the Eye*, ed. 2. Springfield, Ill, Charles C Thomas, 1974.
4. *Minerals Yearbook*, vol 1. *Metals and Minerals*. Washington, DC, US Dept of the Interior, Bureau of Mines, US Government Printing Office, 1985.
5. Titanium. *Environmental Health Criteria* 24. Geneva, World Health Organization, 1982.
6. Reline S, et al: Granulomatous disease associated with pulmonary deposition of titanium. *Br J Ind Med* 1986; 10:652.

ZINC AND ITS COMPOUNDS

In order of abundance, zinc ore occurs as zinc sulfide (zinc blend) (ZnS) and the carbonate (calamine). Zinc sulfide ore occurs in complex ore deposits of galena (lead sulfide) and pyrite (iron disulfide). Complex zinc mineral deposits may also contain varying amounts of cadmium, arsenic, and manganese.[5, 6] The use of zinc products may expose workers to more serious toxic fumes than zinc alone.

Refined metallic slab zinc has a silvery white appearance in the nonoxidized form. Zinc is not malleable at room temperature but becomes workable into plates, sheets, or wire at 110–150° C. Zinc melts at 419.47° C and boils at 907° C.[14] Exposure of metallic zinc or zinc fumes to an oxidizing atmosphere converts zinc to the oxidized form, zinc oxide (ZnO).

Uses

Zinc is an essential element metal in enzymes and metabolism in biologic systems. It was first reported by Keilin and Mann[13] as a constituent of carbonic anhydrase, essential to respiration. Since 1950, the literature has become voluminous with the subject of zinc-metallo enzymes.

One of the principal uses of metallic zinc, slab zinc, is to galvanize iron or steel to prevent oxidation. Slab zinc is used in alloys and zinc die castings, which accounts for approximately 80% of slab zinc used in U.S. industry.[7] The zinc alloy in die castings is used in the automobile, electrical appliances, hardware, toy, and light machine industries. In the foundry industry, it is used in brass and in alloying with nickel, aluminum, and magnesium.

Zinc oxide and the salts of zinc, zinc chloride ($ZnCl_2$) and zinc sulfate ($ZnSO_4$), are used in the rubber, ceramic, chemical (including pharmaceutical), agriculture, and paint industries.

One important occupational use of zinc chloride is in soldering fluxes.

The most common occupational exposure is to zinc oxide fumes secondary to torch welding and cutting operations.[2, 8, 12] Less common exposure is to fumes from foundry operations in which brass or alloys of zinc are melted. Foundry operations involving zinc usually are controlled well enough to avoid excessive exposure to zinc fumes. The unusual pour in a brass foundry of a high-zinc alloy may produce excessive exposure.

Repairing of castings, welding, and scraping operations of various alloys containing zinc in the average shop are, at best, haphazardly ventilated in present-day operations.

Except for the inexperienced worker, welders are aware of the discomfort associated with zinc fumes. The usual story in repairing operations is that the hazard is not considered serious and attempts at securing good ventilation are not important because "the job will not take too much time."[11]

In soldering or brazing operations involving zinc chloride as a flux, the caustic hazard to skin and lungs might be overlooked.

Toxicology

Metal fume fever may be caused by many metallic oxides.[2, 6, 8, 14, 16] The onset of symptoms of metal fume fever associated with fresh zinc oxide fume exposure is primarily respiratory. The patient may complain of upper respiratory irritation, chest pain, and coughing shortly after excessive exposure to zinc oxide fumes. Experienced metal workers who are familiar with zinc or brass chills may report this to their family physician as a "cold that is settling in my chest."[8] A slanted history is misleading, since the worker believes that some treatment with an antibiotic will help but is afraid to relate the real story of his negligence. He is concerned that he may be removed from his job. A good history may reveal marked thirst and a metallic taste in the mouth. Malaise, chills, and fever (101–102° F) may occur four to six hours after exposure and last one to three hours.[11]

Physically, the patient appears distressed, his pulse is elevated (100–120 beats per minute), and he has fine crepitant rales in the lower lung fields. Laboratory data may include elevated sedimentation rate and white blood cell count in the range of 11,000–16,000/cu mm, with a marked shift to early band forms of neutrophils. Lactic dehydrogenase enzyme and pulmonary factor III may be elevated[2, 8] (Fig 45–5). McCord[14] has postulated that metal fume fever is an immunologic disease. As yet, this postulate remains unconfirmed.

Handling zinc chloride or working with soldering fluxes containing zinc chloride may produce irritation of the mucous membranes and ulceration of the exposed skin of the hands and arms from its caustic action. Severe forms of zinc chloride dermatitis are

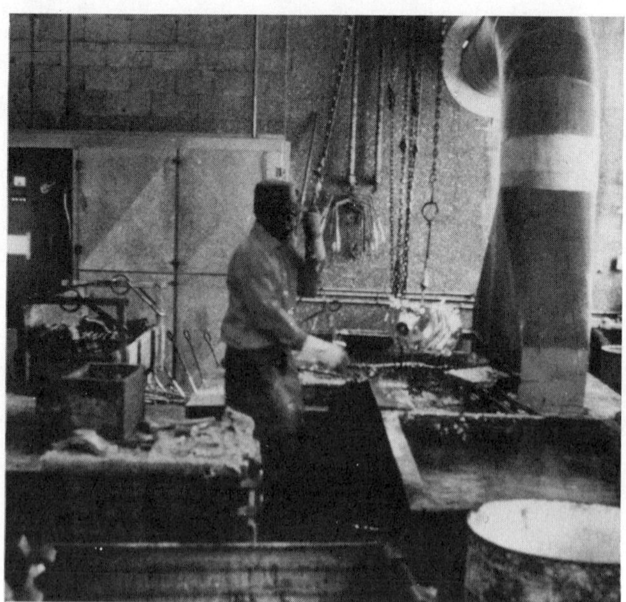

FIG 45–6.
Note ventilation present in zinc galvanizing. Zinc has a fairly low melting point (419°C); a fairly high boiling point (907°C) makes it ideal as a hot dip operation (zinc oxide fumes are not formed until the boiling point is reached). Respiratory protection is not needed because of the low temperatures involved.

associated with wood preserving.[14] The most severe reaction to zinc chloride is to its fume, which is experienced rarely in industry, except in accidents, and leads to death from pulmonary edema and respiratory collapse.[10]

Chronic exposures to high zinc concentrations may cause symptoms of irritative gastritis.[9] The gastric effect is assumed to be due to high secretion of zinc salts into the stomach.

Zinc Stearate.—The inhalation of zinc stearate has been reported to cause bronchopneumonia in infants, with fatal results.[1] A case of fibrous pneumonia due to inhalation of zinc stearate and death due to pneumoconiosis with probable heart failure has been reported in a 29-year-old rubber worker.[5]

According to the 1986 ACGIH TLV recommendation, zinc stearate is considered a nuisance particulate with levels of 30 mppcf or 10 mg/cu m.

A study carried out by Bourne and co-workers[5] of 18 employees in a small rubber manufacturing plant exposed to concentrations of 4.4–7.8 mg/cu m of zinc stearate for three months to five years revealed their health to be essentially normal on the basis of laboratory study and health histories. All but two had had chest x-rays within the preceding two years of study. These x-rays and three others taken at the time of the study showed no pathologic changes. All the workers were found to have redness of nasal mucous membrane and three had excoriation of the membrane. Reexamination of these employees nine months later showed this redness and excoriation to have persisted.

Zinc Sulfate.—Zinc sulfate is used therapeutically to enhance wound healing in doses to 600 mg daily. A case of metallic zinc poisoning by self administration of 12 gm of elemental zinc for wound healing was reported by Murphy.[15]

Treatment

Fortunately, in the majority of cases, intoxication by ingested zinc salts or inhaled zinc fumes is a self-limiting disease. Symptomatic relief from pain and supportive therapy is all that is medically indicated in the common case. Chelating agents such as calcium disodium EDTA (ethylenediaminetetraacetic acid), which are used in chelating zinc from the bloodstream, rarely is indicated.[15]

Recommendations

All cases of zinc fume intoxication will be prevented with the proper control of fumes below 5 mg/cu m by engineering controls.[8] Exhaust ventilation is the most effective control of freshly generated zinc oxide fumes. Education of metal repairpersons as to the hazards and proper use of temporary ventilation for large repair jobs is essential. A properly fitting respirator with a filter cartridge suitable for fumes is effective in unusual jobs requiring respirators for short exposures.

REFERENCES

1. American Conference of Governmental Industrial Hygienists: *Documentation of the Threshold Limit Values for Substances in Workroom Air*, ed 4. Cincinnati, Oh, ACGIH, 1980.
2. Anseline P: Zinc fume fever. *Med J Aust* 1972; 2:316.
3. Argus MF, Hoch-Ligeti C: Comparative study of the carcinogenic activity of nitrosamines. *J Natl Cancer Inst* 1961; 27:695.
4. Bertelli G., Cortona G, Odone P, et al: Zinc, in Alessio L, Berlin A, Boni M, et al: *Biological Indicators for the Assessment of Human Exposure to Industrial Chemicals*. Varese, Italy, Joint Research Centre Ispra Establishment, 1984.
5. Bourne HG, Yee HT, Seferian S: The toxicity of rubber additives. Arch Environ Health 1968; 16:700.
6. Browning E: *Toxicity of Industrial Metals*. London, Butterworth, 1961.
7. Bureau of Mines: *Minerals Yearbook 1971*, vol 1. Washington, DC, 1985.
8. Criteria for a recommended standard: Occupational exposure to zinc oxide, HEW (NIOSH) Publ 76–104. Rockville, Md, National Institute for Occupational Safety and Health, 1975.
9. Dalager NA, Mason TJ, Fraumeni JF, et al: Cancer mortality among workers exposed to zinc chromate paints. *J Occup Med* 1980; 22:25–29.
10. Evans EH: Casualties following exposure to zinc chloride smoke. *Lancet* 1945; 2:368.
11. Fishburn C, and Zenz C: Metal fume fever. *J Occup Med* 1969; 11:142.
12. Hamdi E: Chronic exposure to zinc of furnace operators in a brass foundry. *Br J Ind Med* 1969; 26:126.
13. Keilin D, Mann T: Carbonic anhydrase purification and the nature of the enzyme. *J Biochem* 1940; 39:1163.
14. McCord CP: Metal fume fever as an immunological disease. *Ind Med Surg* 1960; 29:101.
15. Murphy J: Intoxication following ingestion of elemental zinc. *JAMA* 1970; 212:2119.
16. Papp JP: Metal fume fever. Case report. *Postgrad Med* 1968; 43:160.
17. Patty FA (ed): *Industrial Hygiene and Toxicology*, ed 3. New York, Interscience Publishers, Inc, 1978.
18. Soffer A: *Chelation Therapy*. Springfield, Ill, Charles C Thomas, Publisher, 1964.
19. Uotila U, Noro L: Lo stearato di zinco come causa di pneumonoconiosi. *Folia Med (Naples)* 1957; 40:245.

ZIRCONIUM AND ZIRCONIUM COMPOUNDS

Typical compounds are: zirconium oxide (ZrO_2), zirconium oxychloride ($ZrOCl_2 \cdot 8H_2O$), zirconium tetrachloride ($ZrCl_4$), zirconium hydride (ZrH_2), and zirconyl acetate ($H_2ZrO_2[C_2H_3O_2]_2$).

Potential occupational exposures to zirconium may be encountered during liberation from refining and casting operations, during preparation of alloys, and in the manufacture of metal or alloys in nuclear power, aerospace, and various chemical industries. Zirconium is also used in the manufacture of ceramics, glass, and porcelains, in the synthesis of pigments, dyes, and water repellants, in tanning operations, and for abrasive and polishing materials. Zirconium is used as igniters in the manufacture of munitions and other items such as detonators, and in lighter flints. Zirconium is used to make skin ointments and antiperspirants. Zirconium is a "gas getter" in the manufacture of high-vacuum tubes. It is used as a deoxidizer, denitrifier, and desulfurizer in iron and steel manufacture and may be liberated from chemical synthesis. Inhalation and contact with eyes or skin may be damaging, depending on the concentration, temperature, and compound (or presence of other substances).

Toxicology

Zirconium compounds are generally of low toxicity, although granulomata have been produced by repeated topical applications of zirconium salts to human skin. In rats, the oral LD_{50} of several zirconium compounds ranged from 2.5 to 10 gm/kg. Repeated inhalation of zirconium tetrachloride mist by dogs for two months at 6 mg/cu m as zirconium caused slight decreases in hemoglobin and in erythrocyte counts, with some increases in mortality over that of controls; these effects may have been due to the liberation of hydrogen chloride.[1] However, animals exposed to zirconium dioxide dust for one month at 75 mg/cu m as zirconium showed no detectable effects. Rats exposed to high concentrations of zirconium silicate dust for seven months developed radiographic shadows in the lungs; these were attributed solely to the deposition of the radiopaque particles, since histologic examination showed no cellular reaction.[6]

A study of 22 workers exposed to fumes from a zirconium reduction process for one to five years revealed no abnormalities referable to the exposure. Hadjimichael and Brubaker[2] studied 32 men who worked as handfinishers of zirconium fabricated nuclear fuel components from one to 17 years (an average of 4.9 years). A control group was also studied in this plant. The finishing process was done with small hand-held sanders using silicon carbide abrasives as well as cloth strips with aluminum oxide and silicon carbide abrasives, small amounts of phenolic resins, and rubber cement as bonding agents. The dust produced was analyzed; breathing zone samples revealed quantities ranging from 5.75 to 14.7 mg/cu m. Atomic absorption analysis showed that 25% of the dust was zirconium; the remainder was silicon carbide, binding agent, and general shop dust. Particle size analysis indicated that 64% of the particles were less than 5 μ in diameter, 21% between 5 and 10 μ, and 14% greater than 10 μ. Multiple breathing zone samples varied between 0.67 and 3.2 mg/cu m of zirconium, with 60% of the particles being less than 2 μ and 95% less than 10 μ in diameter. In the addition to the worker air monitoring, all workers and control groups completed a standardized respiratory questionnaire, posteroanterior chest radiographs were taken and submitted to a "B" reader, and expiratory lung function tests performed. The authors were unable to demonstrate adverse effects in these workers.

There are no other well-documented cases of toxic effects from industrial exposure. Granulomata of the human axillary skin have occurred from use of deodorants containing zirconium, although the metal is not regarded as a skin sensitizer in other types of exposure.[5]

Permissible Exposure Limit

The current OSHA standard for zirconium compounds is 5 mg/cu m averaged over an eight-hour work shift.

REFERENCES

1. Cochran KW, et al: Acute toxicity of zirconium, strontium, lanthanum, cesium, tantalum and yttrium. *AMA Arch Ind Hyg Occup Med* 1950; I:537–50.
2. Hadjimichael O, Brubaker R: Evaluation of an occupational respiratory exposure to a zirconium-containing dust. *J Occup Med* 1981; 23:
3. International Labour Office: *Encyclopedia of Occupational Health and Safety*, ed 3. New York, McGraw-Hill Book Co, 1982.
4. Shelley WB, Hurley HJ: The allergic origin of zirconium deodorant granulomas. *Br J Dermatol* 1958; 70:75–101.
5. Williams RM, Skipworth GB: Zirconium granulomas of the glabrous skin following treatment of rhus dermatitis. *Arch Dermatol* 1959; 80:63–66/273–276.
6. Zhilova NA, Kasparov AA: Toxicological studies of niobium and zirconium chlorides, in *Hygiene and Sanitation*. Washington, DC, Environmental Protection Agency and National Science Foundation, 1966, vol 31, pp 328–330.

HAFNIUM AND COMPOUNDS

Hafnium (Hf) is found in association with zirconium ores, production based on zircon ($ZrSiO_4$) concentrates which contain 0.5 to 2% hafnium. It has outstanding corrosion resistance, accounting for some of its major applications: control rods in atomic reactors in nuclear-powered submarines and other reactors for power; for alloying with other metals (niobium, tantalum, tungsten); in electronic components; in certain optical glasses (HfO_2); and to produce corrosion-proof films on base metals, i.e., some rocket engine components.

Hafnium dust has very low toxicity. Other than fire or explosion hazards no health hazards have been reported, but hafnium salts can irritate the eyes and skin. Liver damage has been produced in experimental animals. In mice, the LD_{50} of hafnyl chloride by intraperitoneal injection was 112 mg/kg.[2] In cats, intravenous administration of hafnyl chloride at 10 mg/kg was fatal.[2] Rats fed a diet containing 1% for 12 weeks showed slight changes in the liver, consisting of perinuclear vacuolization of the parenchymal cells and coarse granularity of the cytoplasm.[1] Application of 1 mg of hafnium chloride to the eyes of rabbits produced transient irritation. Topical application of hafnium chloride crystals to unabraded rabbit skin produced transient edema and erythema; application to abraded skin caused ulceration.[2]

The TLV was set at a level to prevent systemic injury (0.5 mg/cu m).

REFERENCES

1. Manufacturing Chemists Association, Inc: Chemical Safety Data Sheet SD-92, Zirconium and Hafnium Powder. Washington, DC, 1966.
2. Haley TJ, Raymond K, Komesu N, et al: The toxicologic and pharmacologic effects of hafnium salts. *Toxicol Appl Pharmacol* 1962; 4:238.
3. American Conference of Industrial Hygienists: *Hafnium: Documentation of the TLVs for Substances in Workroom Air*, ed 5. Cincinnati, 1986.

PALLADIUM AND COMPOUNDS

Palladium (Pd) is found with platinum gold and nickel ores. Its main use is for electrical components, usually alloyed with copper and silver, i.e. contacts. Other major uses are as the catalyst to produce sulfuric acid, and for hydrogenation reactions, particularly that of acetylene to ethylene. Smaller amounts are used in jewelry and a gold alloy, decolorized with palladium, "white gold." Compounds in use are palladium oxide (PdO), used as a catalyst in certain organic synthesis; palladium chloride ($PdCl_2$) which has enjoyed long use in photography for special toning effects; palladium iodide (PdI_2); and palladium nitrate and palladium trifbionide which are used in specific reactions such as "detector tubes." Despite the wide use, especially the handling of materials in laboratories and in photography, no occupational poisoning has been shown. Palladium and compounds are not listed in the ACGIH TLV guide for 1986–87.

REFERENCES

1. Platinum-group metals: Committee on Medical and Biologic Effects of Environmental Pollutants, Washington, DC, National Academy of Sciences, 1977.
2. Campbell KI, Hall LL, et al: Dermal irritancy of metal compounds. Studies with palladium, platinum, lead and manganese compounds. *Arch Environ Health* (Chicago) 1975; April, p 168.
3. Mastromatteo E: in Parmeggiani L (ed): *The International Encyclopedia of Health and Safety*, ed 3. Geneva, International Labour Office, 1983.
4. Moore W, et al: Biological fate of ^{103}Pd in rats following different routes of exposure. *Environmental Research*, New York, Academic Press, October, 1974.

RHENIUM AND ITS COMPOUNDS

Rhenium (Re) is found in minute amounts in various ores, worldwide, including platinum, copper sulfides, manganese oxides, but is extracted from molybdenite ore (MoS_2). There are many rhenium compounds: rhenium heptoxide (Re_2O_7); rhenium hexafluoride (ReF_6); rhenium oxychloride (ReO_3Cl); and rhenium trioxide (ReO_3). The main uses are as catalysts; either alone or with some compounds, in alloys with platinum, silver, tungsten, in the dehydrogenation of alcohols, synthesis of ammonia, hydrogenation of coal, coal tar and mineral oil, oxidation of ammonia and the oxidation of sulfur dioxide to sulfur trioxide. Rhenium-platinum catalysts are used in petroleum refineries for production of high-octane gasoline accounting for a major portion of use of rhenium. Reforming platinum-rhenium catalysts are used to produce benzene, toluene, and xylenes. Smaller amounts are used in plating jewelry, instruments, electrical contacts, and thermocouples. Although some compounds are irritating to the eyes and skin, no toxic effects in animals or man have been reported.

REFERENCES

1. Mastromatteo E, in Parmeggiani L (ed): *The International Encyclopedia of Health and Safety*, ed 3. Geneva, International Labour Office, 1983.

RHODIUM AND COMPOUNDS

Rhodium (Rh) is a member of the platinum group, occurring with the other platinum metals. The metal has high reflectance and corrosion resistance, making it useful for electrodeposition on mirrors and other optical surfaces. Its main use is in alloying with platinum for thermocouples, (high temperature) furnace windings, bushings and fine nozzles for glass fiber spinning, and as catalysts for making ammonia and for synthesis of hydrogen cyanide. For plating, rhodium phosphates or sulfates are used. Rhodium alone as a catalyst is used in the hydrogenation of benzene to cyclohexane and in the oxidation of primary alcohols to aldehydes. No toxic effects from rhodium metal dust or fumes has been reported in animals or man. Although there is no evidence that sensitization occurs from exposure, because of rhodium's similarity to platinum in the periodic table, a TLV of 1 mg/cu m is recommended. Similarly, based on analogy with platinum, the TLV for soluble rhodium compounds is 0.01 mg/cu m, although no allergic manifestations in humans have been reported.

REFERENCES

1. ACGIH: Rhodium as Rh. *Documentation of the TLVs for Substances in Workroom Air*, ed 5. Cincinnati, 1986, p 222.
2. Grant WM: Toxicology of the eye, ed 2. Springfield, Charles C Thomas, 1974, p 887.
3. Mastromatteo E, in Parmeggiani L (ed): *The International Encyclopedia of Health and Safety*, ed 3. Geneva, International Labour Office, 1983.
4. Platinum-group metals: Committee on Medical and Biological Effects of Environmental Pollutants. Washington, DC, National Academy of Sciences, 1977, p 232.

TANTALUM AND COMPOUNDS

Tantalum (Ta) was used as the first workable metallic lamp filament in 1906. Its special properties have had application for the manufacture of corrosion resistant equipment since the early 1930s. One of the main uses for tantalum is in the production of high quality capacitors. As a metal, it is inert to human body fluids and tissues, making it useful for surgical implantations. Fine Ta powder has been used as a pulmonary x-ray contrast medium. Despite this inertness, earlier studies, using tantalum oxide in guinea pigs by the intratracheal route, produced a transient bronchitis, interstitial pneumonitis, and hyperemia with some slight residual sequelae in the form of focal hypertrophic emphysema and organizing pneumonitis around metallic deposits. There was slight epithelial hyperplasia in the bronchi and bronchioles.[3] Because of this, the TLV was recommended at 5 mg/cu m, even though no systemic effects have been reported in man.

REFERENCES

1. ACGIH: Tantalum (metal and oxide dusts). *Documentation of the TLVs for Substances in Workroom Air*, ed 5. Cincinnati, 1986.
2. Delahant AB: An experimental study of the effects of rare metals on animal lungs. *Arch Ind Health* 1955; 12:116.
3. Schepers GWH: The biologic action of tantalum oxide. *Arch Ind Health* 1955; 12:121.

46

Occupational Health Aspects of Pesticides: Clinical and Hygienic Principles

Florence Ebert, R.N., C.O.H.N.

Raymond D. Harbison, Ph.D.

Carl Zenz, M.D.

With worldwide, ceaseless demand for foodstuffs, control of vegetation, crop preparation, storage (of seeds and edibles), shipment, and distribution from the field into the home, there are parallel research, production, formulating and packaging, storage, shipping and distributing, supplying and application of an array of pesticides, creating a chain of events with potential occupational health impact. A general overview is presented here, emphasizing occupational medical and hygienic principles applicable to selected substances and major groups of compounds in common use. Frequently overlooked are chemical measures applied worldwide for disease control in fish, fowl, wild game, and livestock of all varieties. Occupational exposures may occur inadvertently with those who work with animal disease control as well as with growers, harvesters, packagers, handlers, and sellers of flowers. The environmental impact of pesticides is beyond the scope of this chapter, and the reader is referred to the references.

The continuing need for crop protection and the control of disease-spreading rodents and pests is clear. In areas where mechanization and an integrated scientific approach to agriculture are well established, the farmer wants more crops of better quality, based largely on consumer ("societal") demands. In other areas, where populations expand faster than agriculture, the question becomes not only one of the quality of foods and fibers produced but of life itself. For this reason, the regulatory restraints imposed on the use of agricultural crop protection agents in one country may be inappropriate for the same product's use in another part of the world.

Currently, each government sets its own policies for use, based on each country's own needs and priorities. Regulatory uniformity is being discussed by agricultural experts and government officials as the worldwide agricultural community attempts to establish common standards of safety in handling, safety in use, and environmental considerations.

The use of chemical compounds for protecting crops is not a 20th-century innovation. Actually, chemical crop protection predates Biblical times, when farmers used sulfur to control mildew. Nicotine was widely used in France as early as 1690 to kill lace bugs, and in the United States in the 1860s arsenic-based compounds were used to control the potato beetle.

Since the early 1940s, when organic insecticides were first introduced, thousands of new compounds have been developed to help farmers control the pests that destroy their crops.

The United States Federal Insecticide Fungicide and Rodenticide Act (FIFRA) defines a pesticide as:

> 1. Any substance or mixture of substances intended for preventing, destroying, repelling or mitigating any pest (insect, rodent, nematode, fungus, weed, other forms of terrestrial or aquatic plant or animal life or viruses, bacteria or other microorganisms, except microorganisms on or in man or other living animals), which the administrator of the Environmental Protection Agency (EPA) declares to be a pest, and
> 2. Any substance or mixture of substances intended for use as a plant regulator, defoliant or desiccant.[30]

There are approximately 1,500 active ingredients in common use registered by the EPA. In addition, there are numerous pesticide active ingredients that are registered on an experimental basis only or that are produced in the United States for export only. Pesticides are an extremely diverse group of substances with a wide potential for a variety of toxic effects. These substances range in acute toxicity from the lethal at low doses, such as strychnine, to the edible in relatively large quantities, such as sodium chloride.

With many pesticides, the possibility of dermal exposure with subsequent absorption through the skin may present a greater problem to workers than does exposure through inhalation. However, it must be emphasized that both routes of absorption may occur concomitantly. Some of the compounds have been known to produce carcinogenic, teratogenic, mutagenic, and neurotoxic effects, as well as alterations of reproductive processes or functions in experimental animals and in man.

Early-used pesticides were materials of natural origin, such as the salts of arsenic, copper, lead, mercury, and zinc, leading into the era of the synthetic organic pesticides, which began with the discovery of the insecticidal activity of DDT in 1939. Research continued to develop a wide variety of other synthetic pesticides, and there are now more than 40,000 registered pesticide compounds in the United States.[97]

More than 4 billion kg of pesticide-active ingredients were produced in 1984 in this country. Of this vast total, about 1.6 billion kg were herbicides, 1.5 billion kg were insecticides, and the remainder fungicides. Domestic industrial capacity increased by 12% in 1976 and 5% in 1982, and this trend is expected to continue. Approximately 90% of present-day pesticides are organic compounds, with insecticides consisting primarily of the organochlorine compounds, the organophosphate compounds, and the carbamate compounds. Fumigants include the halogenated hydrocarbons and certain inorganic gases. The herbicides include the amides, arsenicals, carbamates and thiocarbamates, and substituted ureas. Fungicides include thiocarbamates, phthalimides, and organotin compounds. A listing of significant pesticides with corresponding chemical identities and main uses is found in the Glossary at the end of the chapter.

Often overlooked is the well-known compound called "creosote," a preservative long known for its ability to kill both fungi and boring insects likely to infest wood. Creosote is a mixture of phenols derived from wood or bituminous coal by distillation and used principally as a wood preservative. In the United States, more than 0.5 billion kg of creosote are produced annually, an amount nearly equaling that of the synthetic organic pesticides produced.

The inorganic pesticides, which account for the remaining 10% of production, include calcium arsenate, lead arsenate, arsenic acid, borate sulfur, and sodium chloride.

Most insecticides are synthesized from other chemicals, and it is during these beginning stages that occupational exposure can occur. These materials have been classified according to the chemical vernacular as the "chlorinated hydrocarbons" (DDT being the most well known of this group) and "organophosphate compounds" (parathion, as a chief example) and marketed under a host of trade and generic names—Abate, azinphosmethyl (Guthion), carbophenothion (Trithion), chloropyrifos (Dursban), demeton (Systax), Diazinon, dicapthon (DiCaptan), etc. A special class is termed "carbamates." Among these are the well-known carbaryl (Sevin), aldicarb (Temik), carbofuran (Furadan), fometanate HCl (Carzol), metalkamate (Bux), and methomyl (Lannate).

As mentioned earlier, the inorganic arsenicals were among the earliest insecticides used throughout the world: lead arsenate, "Paris green," and sodium arsenite (these will be discussed briefly).

Certain other well-known chemicals, because of their inherent toxic nature, have been used as "fumigants," usually in areas that can be safely sealed off and any human contact scrupulously restricted. Typical fumigants are:

1. Cyanides: Acrylonitrile, calcium cyanide (Cyanogas), hydrogen cyanide, etc. (see Chapter 47)
2. Halogens: Methyl bromide and sulfuryl fluoride (Vikane)
3. Phosphines: Aluminum phosphide (Celphos, Phostoxin)

Herbicides, commonly called "weed-killers," are produced in large quantities to control growth of weeds and other undesirable plants in lawns, along highways, railroads, and airports. Factory occupational exposures are overshadowed by exposures during private use. Prominent herbicides are endothal (dicarboxylic acid derivative) and diquat and paraquat (quaternary ammonia derivatives).

The organic acids and some of their common derivatives are cacodylic acid, dichlorophenoxyacetic acid (2,4-D), DSMA, MSMA (sodium methanearsonate), Silvex (2,4,5-TP), fenuron TCA (Urab), and monuron (Telvar).

Rodenticides constitute another major class: Diphacinone (Diphacin), Fumarin, Pival (Pivalyn), PMP (Valane), and warfarin.

Manufacturers usually operate integrated chemical synthesis plants and may produce many other chemical products in addition to pesticides. The work force normally includes chemists, engineers, managers, skilled chemical operators, pipe-fitters, electricians, laborers, truck drivers, and warehouse workers.

Manufacturing includes pretreatment of reactants (change of size, temperature, and state), reaction, purification, and posttreatment of products (change of size, and state). Raw materials for manufacture are delivered in bulk by pipeline, railroad car, barge, or tank trucks, or may be produced in-plant, often as by-products of other reactions. Manufacturers may produce several pesticide active ingredients at a single plant, which usually consists of several separate but interconnectable production areas or subplants. A subplant contains the equipment necessary for carrying out all the unit processes and operations, such as reaction, distillation, filtration, and mixing, which are necessary to synthesize a product from raw materials. Subplant equipment may include mills, screens, hoppers, tanks, reactors, absorption columns, cooling towers, stills, filters, centrifuges, and dryers. Process monitoring, sampling and analyses are performed to determine temperatures, pressures, flow rates, densities and composition changes in order to control the chemical reactions. The production of pesticides involves complex chemical processes, including chlorination, alkylation, nitration, phosphorylation, sulfonation, and bromination.

Pesticide-formulating establishments generally are smaller than manufacturing establishments. Employees may include engineers, chemists, operators, and laborers. There are major variations among formulators both in size and in operating practices. Seventy-one percent of all formulating establishments employ less than 20 employees. Only 6% of all establishments employ more than 100 employees, but these larger plants dominate total production. Formulators with 100 or more employees account for 56% of production, whereas formulators with fewer than 20 employees account for only 12.5% of all production.[96, 97]

A formulating operation generally is less complex than a manufacturing operation (Fig 46–1). Usually, a formulator receives concentrated active ingredients from a manufacturer and dilutes them with various nonpesticidal materials known as "inerts." The term "inert" refers to the effect of the substance on the target organism relative to the effect of the pesticide on that organism. However, as with any chemical, a toxic effect can be obtained with

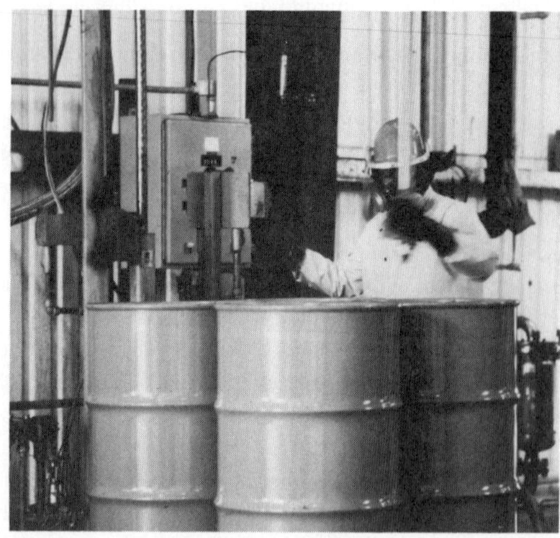

FIG 46–1.
Filling drums—the end stage of the manufacturing process.

any inert at some dose, and many so-called inerts are more toxic to man than the term would lead one to believe. The formulating process may also include physical or chemical treatment to yield particular product forms: dust, powder, wettable powder, granule, pellet, emulsifiable concentrate, capsule, or aerosol. Further processing may be done by wholesalers, retailers, repackagers, or end users. With a few exceptions, formulating is a simple process varying in type according to the desired end product.

The preparation of dust and powder pesticide formulations entails dispensing from hoppers, screening for size, and mixing with flour, silica, sulfur, lime, gypsum, talc, or clay in a hammer mill, roller mill, or other type of mill. Granule formulating consists of dispensing and sizing the inert (e.g., clay, vermiculite, ground corncobs, diatomaceous earth), dissolving or melting the pesticide in a tank, and then spraying the pesticide onto the inert in a mixer.

Frequently overlooked when evaluating exposure is the potential role of the vehicle. In the laboratory, new products can be dissolved in a variety of solvents. In the field, however, the delivery medium is mainly water, so one of four basic formulations is used: emulsifiable concentrates, wettable powders, dusts, or granular materials. However, solvents or mixtures of solvents can be used to a limited degree. Primarily, these are hydrocarbons such as diesel oil, gasoline, kerosene, or xylene, with or without water, and "wetting" or "dispersing" agents.

Occupational exposures are not limited to the pesticide manufacture and formulation operations already described. The American Public Health Association (1979) estimates that, almost daily, nearly 1,275,000 U.S. farm workers are exposed to pesticides. This estimate does not take into account children (preschool and older) who work part or full time, nor does it consider wives of "migrant workers" who join their husbands in field work, often while pregnant and continuing work as long as possible before delivery.

Various physical and chemical properties of materials present during the manufacture and formulation of pesticides significantly affect the magnitude and/or subsequent effects of exposure. The following sections describe possible routes of exposure and certain physical, chemical, and toxicologic properties.

AERIAL SPRAYING (Fig 46–2)

Gribetz et al.[43] determined the physiologic and subjective effects of heat stress in the cockpits of agricultural spray pilots. Nine pilots flying for a large Israeli aerial spray company were studied. The pilots' daily workload was demanding (early work hours, four to five hours' flight time, 10–15 takeoffs and landings, several hundred 180° turns, and frequent passes under telephone and power lines) and included exposures to noise, vibrations, gravitation forces, and various pesticides in addition to heat. The heat stress produced in the cockpits exceeded the heat exposure threshold limit value (TLV) for continual heavy work (25° C) ten out of ten times and was sustained for periods of up to 3½ hours. The heat stress exceeded TLVs for continual moderate work (26.7° C) seven out of ten times.

Cockpit air cooling was suggested as a necessary measure for preventing heat stress in hot climates. The need for appropriate filter technologies to prevent pesticide exposure during flight was noted as well as precautionary cockpit monitoring for pesticides and carbon monoxide. An unresolved question was whether conventional threshold standards for heat exposure are appropriate for spray pilots. (Standards are based on the prevention of symptoms more gross than the subtle psychomotor changes in pilot performance.) Heat and dehydration, together with other hazards (g-forces, organophosphates), are hypothesized to produce fluid loss, peripheral vasodilatation, and blood pressure drops, and decreased threshold exposures to all these hazards may pose an insidious danger. Therefore, engineering and other measures to prevent heat stress and dehydration should rank high as part of a comprehensive program to protect the health and performance levels of agricultural spray pilots.[38]

Workers assigned as "flagmen" during aerial application are especially vulnerable to overspray and contamination. Suitable respiratory protective equipment and clothing are required. (Preferably, other means for directing aerial applications should be used.)

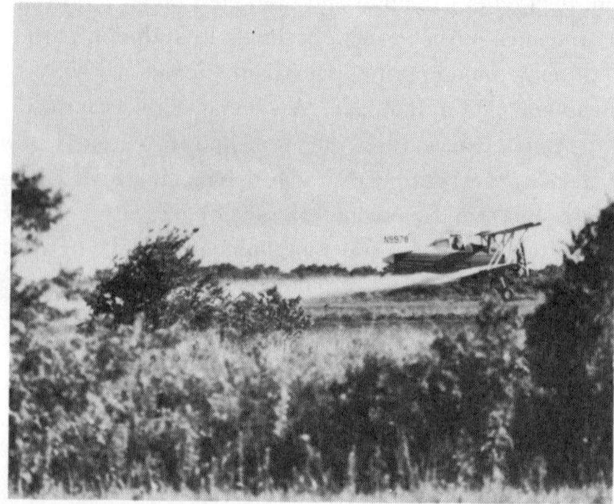

FIG 46–2.
Aerial application. Hazards involved include mixing and loading of the chemicals, fatigue and heat stress—frequently overlooked in assessing work exposures.

INHALATION EXPOSURES

The inhalation of pesticide dusts, vapors, mists, and gases may represent a significant occupational hazard.

In pesticide operations, dusts are generated by the mechanical agitation of solid material, such as milling or grinding. Note that fine dusts can be generated as a result of dry sweeping or vehicle traffic over an area contaminated with "coarser" material.

Dust hazards may involve the formulation of wettable powders, granules, or baits. The "finer" the solid material, the greater is the potential problem of workplace emissions and subsequent contamination of the general work area (Fig 46–3).

Retention of particles within the lungs depends on many factors: size, shape hydroscopicity, density, reactivity, and inhalation process (nasal or oral). Hayes[49] speculated that, in the absence of specific information on a particulate, it can be assumed that about 25% of inhaled material would be exhaled, about 50% would be deposited in the upper respiratory passages and subsequently swallowed, and about 25% would be deposited in the lower respiratory passages. Even dusts too large to be considered "respirable" may present a potential hazard due to deposition in the throat, with subsequent ingestion.

The volatility of the material affects the environmental concentration and thus is a significant factor in respiratory exposure. Vapor pressures of pesticides vary from nonvolatile materials such as DDT and dieldrin to compounds with extremely high vapor pressures such as methylbromide and dichlorvos. Some fumigants such as phosgene and ethylene oxide are gases at standard temperature and pressure.

For all pesticides, both the aerosol (dust or mist) and vapor/gas component of the total potential inhalation exposure must be considered.

DERMAL EXPOSURE

Employees frequently experience dermal exposure to pesticides, with subsequent absorption through the skin. The rate at which a pesticide is absorbed through the skin is determined by the nature of the compound, the condition of the skin, and external factors, such as temperature. The most rapid and complete absorption occurs with pesticides that have some solubility in both water and lipid.[138]

Skin absorption for a specific pesticide is also related to the area of skin exposed, duration of exposure and the region exposed (Fig 46–4). Different areas of the human skin absorb chemicals at different rates. Maibach and co-workers[78] determined that the parathion absorption rate was significantly higher for the scrotal skin, axilla, head, and neck areas than for the hands or arms.

The degree and rate of skin absorption may be increased if the skin barrier is injured due to washing with solvents, irradiation, and thermal/chemical burns.[50] Other factors include increased circulation of blood through the dermis of the skin and sweat rate.

Fine powders tend to be absorbed more readily than coarse powders for equivalent contact. Hayes[50] found that very finely ground technical dieldrin was absorbed as readily as dieldrin applied to the skin in solutions. In contrast, coarsely ground dieldrin powder was not as well absorbed (See Chapter 10 for additional clinical details.)

INGESTION EXPOSURE

Oral exposures may occur through accidental splashing of liquid pesticide into the mouth, by smoking/eating with pesticide-contaminated hands or with accidentally contaminated food or smoking materials, by rubbing the mouth area with contaminated hands, and by swallowing inhaled material that either entered the upper respiratory tract or was swept up by ciliary action into the trachea.

The degree of hazard is related to the extent of absorption of the specific pesticide for the specific portion of the gastrointestinal system involved.

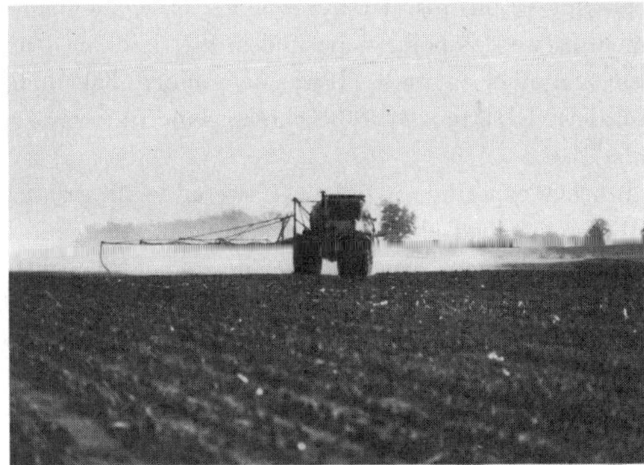

FIG 46–3.
Large-scale agricultural pesticide application using pressurized spraying.

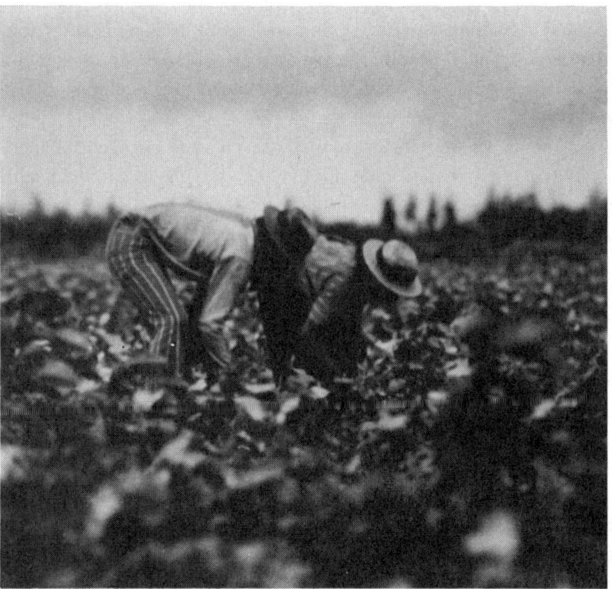

FIG 46–4.
Workers picking crops in fields which have had applications of pesticides—a very common scene throughout the world.

OCULAR EXPOSURE

Ocular exposure usually is a result of accidental spills/splashes. Acute local effects may be produced on the eye or associated structure (eyelids, conjunctiva) in the absence of systemic effects.

During the past decade, the possibility of visual impairment following chronic pesticide exposure has gained importance. Ishikawa et al.[57, 58] reported ocular disease attributed to chronic organophosphate pesticide exposure. In 1977, the Japanese government restricted the use of parathion, EPN, and TEPP[59] and the Japanese Ministry of Public Welfare set forth standards for ocular conditions stemming from these pesticides.

Plestina and Piukovic-Plestina[109] noted the lack of published information on ocular effects and conducted a study of workers engaged in pesticide formulation for five years or longer. Sixty-three workers were divided into three groups according to pesticide exposure. The ophthalmologic data sought included measurement of corneal curvature, visual acuity, accommodation and focusing, intraocular pressure, visual fields, dark adaptation, color vision, and retinal fields. Pupillary size and reaction were not recorded. Group A consisted of 31 workers selected according to the length of time each worker had been engaged in pesticide production. All of them were well-trained permanent staff, mostly involved in the production of pesticide emulsions.

Initially, working conditions ot those occupationally exposed to pesticides were rather poor, but they improved gradually. The active ingredients produced were predominantly, but not exclusively, anticholinesterase compounds, consisting mainly of different types of dimethoxy- and diethoxyphosphates, thiophosphates, and carbamates. A few compounds were chlorinated hydrocarbons or herbicides. Workers had no fixed working place, and a system of irregular rotation was introduced to equalize exposure. Usual working time was eight hours a day, five days a week for nine to ten months a year. However, overtime work was quite common, particularly when seasonal production had to be increased. A regular monitoring of cholinesterase activity showed an association between overtime work and decreased blood cholinesterase activity.

Among 12 workers in group B, seven were engaged for more than five years in pesticide application, largely in public health programs, but also in disinfestation of food stores. Two workers were pilots who applied pesticides in agriculture, and those remaining supervised pesticide production. Common factors for all workers in this group were irregular exposure, good protective measures, and good working conditions. All this accounted for a considerably milder exposure than for workers in group A. Again, the active materials were predominantly anticholinesterase compounds, except for the pilots, who were equally exposed to different fertilizers and herbicides. Blood cholinesterase activity data, monitored over a long period, did not reveal any toxicologically meaningful pattern of enzyme inhibition. Similarly, other routine biochemical and hematologic tests required by clinicians at their periodic medical checkups were normal.

Group C, a group of 20 subjects, was formed to serve as control. The workers were recruited from among those of similar socioeconomic status as were the two preceding groups. They were matched by age and habits, but had no closer contact with pesticides than the general population. They worked either in internal transport or in the storage of end products that were not insecticides. Thus, except by sex, the three groups were matched as closely as possible.

Plestina's and Piukovic-Plestiņa's main findings in these workers were a decreased dark adaptation, a mild constriction of peripheral visual fields (3%–4%), and slightly more conjunctival injection. In this report, as noted in others, "highly" exposed and "heavily" exposed terms are not defined. In the United States, optic atrophy or other visual sequelae from work exposures to organophosphate pesticides has not been observed.[86]

CHLORINATED HYDROCARBON COMPOUNDS

Summaries of the salient toxicologic aspects of the most representative chlorinated hydrocarbon compounds are set forth.

DDT

DDT (1,1-bis [*p*-chloropheny]2,2,2-trichloroethane) was first used in 1947 and gained worldwide acceptance in malaria eradication programs but now is banned in most countries. A brief background description can serve as reference to other related "chlorinated hydrocarbon" insecticides with somewhat similar chemical structures.

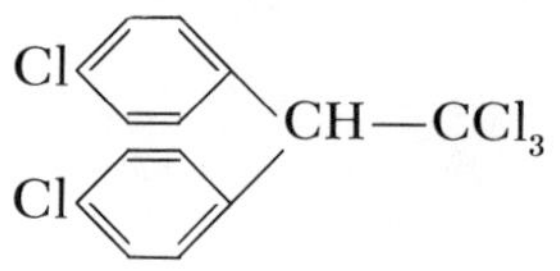

Cl
CH—CCl_3
Cl

The American Conference of Governmental Industrial Hygienists (ACGIH) threshold limit value (TLV) for DDT is 1 mg/cu m of air for an eight-hour time-weighted average (TWA).

As an insecticide, DDT proved to be cheaper and much more effective against many insect species than the previously used natural insecticides. Although its acute toxicity to mammals and man was low (because of its low water solubility, its low vapor pressure, and lack of reactivity with oxygen), it had a long persistence following spraying or dusting. DDT was found to accumulate in the environment as well as being deposited in the lipids of mammals, birds, fish, and other creatures. It was determined that, under certain conditions, DDT proved to be carcinogenic in several strains of animals.[93]

With heavy exposure to DDT dust, eye and skin irritation can result. At chronic high absorbed doses for man, the central nervous system is affected, causing paresthesias and tremors. With sufficient exposure (usually occurring with accidental ingestion of 10 mg/kg or greater), convulsions have occurred in some persons within two to three hours after ingestion. Clinically, excessive and chronic exposure is characterized by malaise, headache, dizziness, paresthesias of the tongue, face, and lips, a feeling of apprehension, tremors, and sometimes confusion. Severe intoxication may result in convulsions, and ingestion of very large doses induces vomiting. Fortunately, recovery occurs in most cases within 24 hours, with few residual effects. Chronic poisoning in man has not been reported.

Laws et al.[74] reported on the clinical evaluation and laboratory findings of 31 workers exposed to an equivalent of 3.6–18 mg daily over a period of 21 years without evidence of hepatotoxicity. An increased activity of hepatic microsomal enzymes was noted, but no apparent evidence of reduction of general health. Earlier investigations by Laws et al.[75] involving a study of 20 workers exposed to DDT for a period of 11–19 years, with a daily intake of 18 mg per person, demonstrated that the isomers and metabolites of DDT in fat range from 38 to 647 ppm (compared with an average of 8 ppm for the general population). DDE (1,1-bis[p-chlorophenyl]-2,2-dichloroethylene) is the major excretory product in workers exposed to DDT.[25]

The hepatocarcinogenicity of DDE has been shown and confirmed in various strains of mice by chronic oral feeding studies, and liver cell tumors were found in both sexes of the experimental animals (mice), with metastases to the lung.[55]

Methoxychlor

Methoxychlor, another much-used insecticide that is closely related to DDT, is a solid, with main exposure through inhalation. It is a substance of low toxicity with no reported effects in humans. The substitution of the methoxy groups for chlorine, as noted in the formula below, decreases considerably the toxicity of methoxychlor. Thus, whereas the oral LD_{50} for DDT in male rats is about 200 mg/kg, the oral LD_{50} for methoxychlor in rats is about 5,000 mg/kg.

The TLV for methoxychlor is 10 mg/cu m.

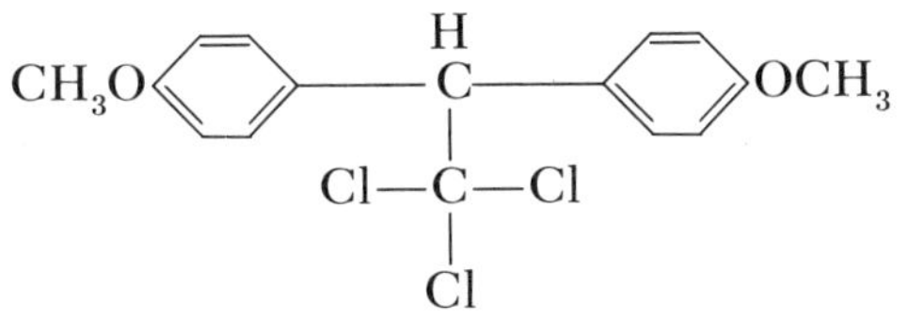

H
CH_3O–⟨benzene⟩–C–⟨benzene⟩–OCH_3
Cl—C—Cl
Cl

Benzene Hexachloride (Lindane)

The TLV is 0.5 mg/cu m.

Benzene hexachloride is an insecticide for agricultural and residential use effective against lice, fleas, ticks, flies, mosquitoes, carpet beetles, and clothes moths and is used in Kwell shampoo and spray for body lice.

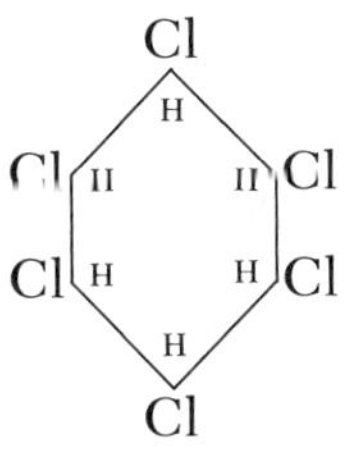

Cl
H
Cl H H Cl
Cl H H Cl
H
Cl

Benzene hexachloride (BHC), 1, 2, 3, 4, 5, 6-hexachlorcyclohexane, has six isomers, with the γ-isomer noted to have insecticidal properties (since 1942) and named "lindane" in honor of Van der Linden, discoverer of four isomers. Lindane has a fumigant action, as it is about 100 times more volatile than DDT. The insecticidal toxicity of BHC is based chiefly on the content of its most toxic component, the γ-isomer, which is about 50–10,000 times more potent than the other isomers. The isomers have different toxic actions, with the γ- and α-isomers acting as central nervous system stimulants and the β- and δ-isomers being CNS depressants. Occupational exposures may occur by inhalation and skin absorption, rarely by ingestion. Exposure to the vapor causes eye, nose, and throat irritation, and continued exposure can cause nausea and headache.

In Sweden, Kolmodin-Hedman and her co-workers[70] studied groups of workers who used lindane and DDT in various concentrations during several types of agricultural activities between 1974 and 1977. Different methods of treatment were observed: dipping, spraying in a spray tunnel, and spraying on fields. Also, exposure in connection with handling of the treated plants was studied and the concentration of the substances in the air above treated plants was measured. Exposures were determined as concentrations in the air, as a result of both personal and stationary air sampling. The uptake was measured as the plasma concentration of the substances. Exposures varied a great deal, but the concentration of lindane or DDT in air never was higher than one half of the TLV value. On the whole, no uptake of DDT (increased DDT in plasma) could be demonstrated. Working with lindane gave a small and variable but significant increase of the lindane concentration in plasma, which disappeared very rapidly when exposure was stopped. The concentration of lindane in plasma never was so high as to cause alteration of liver enzyme function. No symptoms related to exposure were found.

Further studies by Kolmodin-Hedman et al.[72] involved workers who treated pine and fir trees with an emulsion containing 1% lindane. Ten persons packed these plants for two days indoors. After packing for two days, their plasma levels of lindane were 1.2–25.7 ng/ml. Plasma levels decreased to half the initial value in three to five days. Planting resulted in plasma levels of lindane of 0.2–22.3 ng/ml at the end of the first week. Despite continued planting, the lindane levels decreased to 0.2–3.5 ng/ml at the end of the second week. Symptoms were not noted with higher frequency in a group of planters exposed to lindane compared to a group of planters who worked with unprepared plants, and symptoms did not correlate with higher plasma levels of lindane.

In another investigation, Kolmodin-Hedman et al.[73] studied 11 workers who treated pine and fir trees with a solution containing 1% lindane. Eight workers packed plants for one week and 60 persons thereafter planted them for one to two weeks. Exposure to dry lindane powder resulted in a plasma lindane level of 44.0 and 28.0 ng/ml, respectively. The packing personnel had plasma levels of 10.5 ± 6.8 ng/ml. After one month, the high values had declined and were about 1 ng/ml. The investigators thought that plasma levels exceeding 10 ng/ml might induce liver microsomal enzyme changes.

Lindane has been suspected to cause aplastic anemia, but reports have not been conclusive in humans. Fatalities have occurred following accidental ingestion (estimated fatal oral dose 150 mg/kg), with severe convulsions, respiratory distress, and cyanosis.[48]

Dieldrin

The TLV is 0.25 mg/cu m.

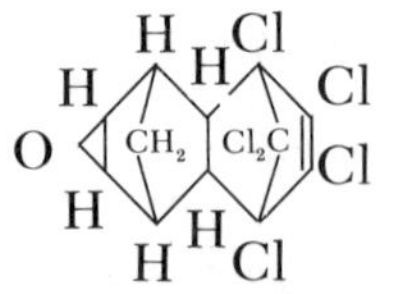

Among the chlorinated cyclodienes, dieldrin is the most frequently used pesticide. Main occupational exposure may occur through inhalation, skin absorption, and ingestion. Dieldrin is considered a convulsant and has been known to cause liver cancer in mice.[56, 105] Early symptoms of overexposure include malaise, increased sweating, headache, dizziness, nausea, vomiting, and, with high exposures, myoclonic jerking of the extremities. Clonic and tonic convulsions, which may be followed by coma, have occurred. Brown et al.[15] reported case studies of five workers who had been exposed to aldrin-dieldrin and were found to have suffered one or more convulsive seizures and/or myoclonic limb movements. They noted that the blood concentration of dieldrin during the acute phase ranged from 16 to 62 μg/100 gm of blood. The analysis of blood for dieldrin concentration may assist in estimating the extent of absorption following exposure.

Aldrin

The TLV is 0.25 mg/cu m.

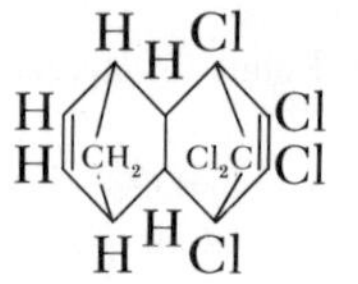

This insecticide is an odorless, white, crystalline solid readily absorbed through the skin and by inhalation. It is rapidly metabolized into dieldrin, and, in cases of acute poisoning, these compounds can produce generalized convulsions. In the same report by Brown et al.,[15] the five workers were exposed to aldrin concentrations up to 8.5 mg/cu m. Other early symptoms of aldrin intoxication resemble those of dieldrin.[60]

Endrin

The TLV is 0.1 mg/cu m.

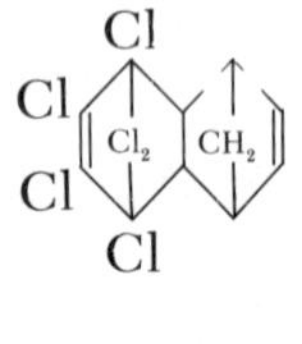

In addition to use as an insecticide, endrin is also utilized as an aviacide and rodenticide and is readily absorbed through the skin and by inhalation and ingestion. Its chief toxic effect is as a convulsant; in human beings, the early effects of acute intoxication are sudden epileptiform convulsions, lasting for several minutes, which can occur from 30 minutes up to 10 hours following overexposure. Coble et al.[21] described dysrhythmic changes, often preceding convulsions, and showed that removal from exposure generally results in a normal electroencephalogram within one to six months. In most cases, recovery is rapid, but anorexia, lethargy, weakness, headache, and dizziness may persist for two to four weeks. Jager[60] reported that in less severe cases of endrin intoxication, the main complaints were headache, dizziness, abdominal distress, nausea, vomiting, insomnia, and occasionally slight mental confusion. Many fatalities have occurred from ingestion of endrin, usually from accidental intake of bread made with contaminated flour. Such cases result in sudden onset of convulsions, with serum endrin levels of 0.053 ppm 30 minutes after the convulsion and 0.083 ppm after 20 hours. A high incidence of fetal organogenesis was reported in golden hamsters fed single doses of 2.5 mg/kg of endrin. Ottolenghi et al.[105] reported congenital anomalies and growth retardation in offspring, and rats fed a diet of 100 ppm of endrin for two years developed degenerative changes.[60]

Chlordane

The TLV is 0.5 mg/cu m (1985).

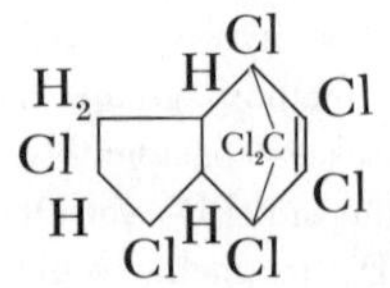

Technical chlordane is an insecticide with a physical appearance of an amber-colored viscous liquid having a low vapor pressure. It is a member of the cyclodiene group of chlorinated insecticides, which includes aldrin, dieldrin, endrin, and DDT, and exhibits a similar chemical structure. Introduced in 1945, chlordane was widely used for household and garden pesticide applications but currently, in the United States, 100% of the production of chlordane is used exclusively for subterranean termite control, and no longer used for agricultural applications.

Since chlordane is relatively persistent in the environment, having a half-life of one year, the known probability for human exposure has resulted in action by the Enviromental Protection Agency to suspend its agricultural use in 1975, effective August, 1976. Current use of chlordane for termite control is exempted from the EPA order. Termiticide applications (1% in water solution) of chlordane are strictly regulated as to usage, primarily by licensed pest control operators and in accordance with the existing state regulations where the application is to be performed. This exclusive non-crop usage has resulted in the reduction of the quantity of chlordane produced. There is one plant in the United States producing nearly 5 million kg annually, with about 70 workers, average 29 years of service and an average age of 53 (1985). Before the imposition of strict control measures in this facility, initiated in 1979, industrial hygiene studies revealed work room air levels between 200 to 750 μg/cu m of chlordane. Based on studies of employee records, comprehensive clinical and laboratory examinations between 1979 through 1985, no evidence of health problems attributable to chlordane could be found.[144]

Occupational exposures may occur most commonly through inhalation or skin absorption when carelessly used, i.e., by termite control applicators, or with other use in the field. Chlordane is a persistent, non-systemic stomach and contact insecticide and is non-phytocidal at insecticidal concentrations. It is readily absorbed from the gastrointestinal tract, the respiratory tract and percutaneously and is considered moderately toxic on ingestion. It is stored in the fat, maximum levels being attained about five days after the beginning of daily doses. There is also some accumulation in glandular tissue. Chlordane is removed fairly rapidly from the fat with very little detectable 20 days after cessation of exposure. Excess inhalation and absorption by humans have produced symptoms indicative of dysfunction of the nervous system, principally that of the brain. Major manifestations of overexposures have included apprehension, excitability, dizziness, headache, disorientation, weakness, paresthesias, muscle twitching, tonic and clonic convulsions (often epileptiform), and unconsciousness. When absorbed dermally, apprehension, twitching, tremors, and confusion may be the first symptoms. Respiratory depression may occur. Pallor occurs in moderate to severe poisoning. Cyanosis may result as convulsive activity interferes with respiration.[88] Although convulsive activity may be severe, the prognosis is not hopeless. Fatalities have occurred following heavy absorption, but there is complete recovery if prompt medical attention is given and convulsions controlled with vital functions sustained.[22] Nausea and vomiting have been noted soon after ingestion either through accident or suicidal intent. The ingestion of 6 gm (100 mg/kg) in a suicide attempt resulted in severe burns of the mouth, severe gastritis, diffuse pneumonia, anuria, convulsions, and mania, with death occurring after 9½ days.[50] Derbes et al.[26] describe the case of a female worker who had spilled a solution of 25% chlordane and DDT on her clothing, with convulsions occurring 40 minutes later and death shortly thereafter (the contaminated clothing was not immediately removed). However, there is scant published data with primate experimental studies designed to observe acute or chronic effects on the embryo, fetus, pregnant or lactating females. An analysis carried out by the Carcinogenesis Program of the National Cancer Institute found that chlordane fed in the diets of test mice produced hepatocellular carcinoma but these hepatocellular carcinomas did not appear in rats fed chlordane.[91] Although these results are definitive for animals, human risk has not been predictable.

A 90-day inhalation study using rats and monkeys exposed to technical chlordane at concentrations of 0.1, 0.98 and 9.23 μ/L for 8 hr/day, 5 days/week was made. An increased enlargement of the liver and thyroid was found in the high exposed rats after 90 days' exposure; 13 weeks after exposure there were no macroscopic alterations. Increased liver and kidney weight was noted for the high exposed male and female rats after 90 days' exposure, but not after 13 weeks following cessation of exposure. With the monkeys, no abnormalities with respect to clinical signs, respiratory/pulmonary tests, hematology, blood chemistries, urinalyses, and macroscopic and microscopic studies were discerned. Only mean thyroid and liver weights for the high exposed monkeys were greater than controls. The no-effect level established in this study in the rat was 0.1 μ/L; for the monkey, in excess of 9.23 μ/L.[145] At the present, there are no accepted standards or limits for airborne and/or contact exposures in human habitations; however, for working conditions, a TLV of 0.5 mg/cu m and a STEL of 20 mg/cu m are believed to be sufficiently low to prevent systemic injury.[1] The Committee on Toxicology (NRC, 1979) suggested an interim guideline for airborne chlordane in military housing of 10 μg/cu m.[91]

Heptachlor

The TLV is 0.5 mg/cu m.

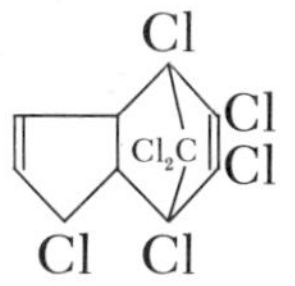

Cl
Cl_2C Cl Cl
Cl Cl

Heptachlor is chemically related to chlordane, and symptoms of excessive exposure to heptachlor would closely parallel those previously described for chlordane. Its effects would be principally on the nervous system, with headache, dizziness, weakness, and, in severe cases, convulsions being the most commonly reported symptoms. In an occupational environment, exposure may occur through inhalation, dermal contact, and possibly the oral route. Heptachlor may be absorbed through the skin and this action may be enhanced by organic solvents mixed with heptachlor. Heptachlor is acutely more toxic than chlordane. Following feeding of 90 mg/kg in rats, convulsions have been noted with effects occurring within 30–60 minutes. Necropsy revealed liver necrosis in the rats, and repeated applications of a 20 mg/kg solution to the skin of rats revealed a toxic cumulative action. Heptachlor has been tested under the carcinogenesis program of the National Cancer Institute (NCI), selected by the NCI for bioassay because of known biologic effects of low doses over extended periods of time and because of its persistence in the environment and the probability of continued human exposure. Under test conditions, heptachlor was found to be carcinogenic for liver in mice.[124] A study of workers engaged in the manufacture of heptachlor concluded that there was no overall excess of deaths from cancer, even among workers followed 20 or more years after entry into the occupation.[136] The World Health Organization in 1967 established a maximal daily intake for heptachlor and its epoxide of 0.005 mg/kg of body weight. Measurement of average U.S. intake in 1970 indicated levels well below the "acceptable" level.[112]

Toxaphene

The TLV is 0.5 mg/cu m.

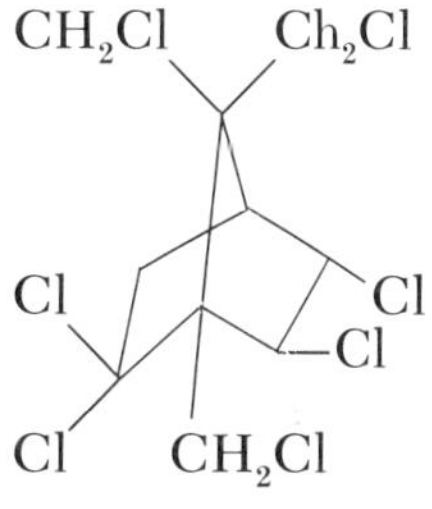

CH_2Cl Ch_2Cl
Cl Cl
Cl
Cl CH_2Cl

This yellow, waxlike compound is prepared by chlorinating bicyclic terpene-camphene to contain up to 69% chlorine. In

1976, toxaphene production in the United States amounted to more than 50 million kg, with about 85% for use on cotton crops. Other major uses are on cattle and swine, and on soybeans, corn, wheat and peanuts. Substantial amounts also are used for lettuce, tomatoes, and other food crops. Standard commercial formulation is a dust containing 20% toxaphene, and emulsifiable concentrates contain up to 1 kg toxaphene per liter; oil solutions are 90% toxaphene, and wettable powders are 40% toxaphene. Toxaphene also is mixed with other insecticide chemicals for a variety of uses. Toxaphene is highly toxic to most fish species and was added to open waters at levels between 0.5 and 0.2 ppm to destroy unwanted fish.

Strobane is a substance similar to toxaphene, prepared by chlorinating camphene and pinene to contain 65% chlorine, and is also widely used, since it is inexpensive, with a residue effect. Exposure may occur through inhalation, skin absorption, and, rarely, by accidental ingestion. Moderate skin irritation has been reported, but there have been few occupational exposures. Warraki[137] described two cases of pneumonitis in sprayers. Nonfatal poisonings by ingestion have shown symptoms of nausea, mental confusion, "jerking" of arms and legs, and convulsions. The estimated accidental fatal oral dose in man is 2–7 gm, with severe effects within a half hour after ingestion and frequent, violent convulsions and a rapid cyanosis.

There are no specific tests for toxaphene poisoning. Prompt application of soap and water for skin decontamination is recommended. If severe toxaphene poisoning is recognized, convulsions must be controlled by administration of intramuscular or intravenous sodium phenobarbital or diazepam.

Analysis and evaluation of data from bioassay studies by the National Cancer Institute revealed that, under test conditions, toxaphene was carcinogenic to male and female mice, causing cancers of the liver. Development of cancerous and noncancerous tumors in the thyroid glands of male and female rats suggested, but did not establish conclusively, that toxaphene was carcinogenic in rats as well.[130] (It is to be noted that this substance has been used for more than 32 years.)

As discussed for lindane and extensively studied and reported by Kolmodin-Hedman et al., organochlorine pesticides can be determined in blood by gas chromatography, with plasma levels providing a satisfactory measurement of total body burden. This has been demonstrated in man and in laboratory animals for *p,p'*DDT, lindane, dieldrin, and endrin. Jager[60] states that the threshold level in the blood below which no signs or symptoms of intoxication occur is at 0.20 μg/ml for dieldrin. Brown et al.[15] placed the threshold level for dieldrin in the blood at 0.15 μg/ml.

ORGANOPHOSPHATES

This group of insecticides is classified according to a common mode of toxic action, related to the inhibition of the enzyme cholinesterase, so that, as a group, these substances are called "cholinesterase inhibitors." However, the toxicity of the various organophosphate compounds can vary widely, ranging from the highly toxic, such as TEPP (tetraethylpyrophosphate) with an LD_{50} of 1 mg/kg, to compounds with a low order of acute toxicity, such as Abate with an LD_{50} of more than 8 gm/kg. Nearly all of the organophosphate insecticides are readily absorbed by inhalation, ingestion, and through intact skin.

Occupationally, the most common exposures occur during manufacture, packaging, handling during shipping, storage, and formulating for actual use in homes and agricultural settings. There is a great similarity of symptoms and signs of overexposure to the organophosphate insecticides that are caused by the inactivation or inhibition of the enzyme cholinesterase, resulting in an accumulation of acetylcholine at synapses in the peripheral nervous system. The developmental sequence of systemic effects can vary with the route of entry. Although acute toxicity usually is rapid in onset, symptoms may be delayed up to 12 hours. With inhalation overexposure, respiratory and ocular effects appear, initially usually within minutes. It has been noted that skin absorption is more frequent with increased workplace temperatures.

For simplification of the discussion of the toxic responses, the organophosphate compounds may be considered as a group, the first or mild symptoms and signs developing as anorexia, headache, dizziness, weakness, anxiety, tremors of tongue and eyelids, miosis, and impairment of visual acuity. With moderate exposure, symptoms and signs are increased sweating, nausea, excess salivation, lacrimation, abdominal cramps, vomiting, a slow pulse, and muscle tremors. With severe overexposure, pinpoint and nonreactive pupils develop, along with respiratory difficulty, diarrhea, pulmonary edema, cyanosis, loss of sphincter control, convulsions, coma, and heart block. Following severe intoxication by any route, the excess acetylcholine at the neuromuscular junctions of skeletal muscles is the cause of the weakness, easily aggravated by exertion, along with muscle fasciculations leading to eventual paralysis with the most serious consequence being that of respiratory muscle paralysis. Central nervous system effects include dizziness, slurred speech, ataxia, confusion, Cheyne-Stokes respiration, convulsions, coma, and loss of reflexes. There are multiple cardiovascular responses, including fall in blood pressure and cardiac irregularities, and a complete heart block may occur. Fortunately, complete recovery usually occurs within a week, but there is an increased susceptibility to the effects of the anticholinesterase chemicals, in some persons persisting up to several weeks following exposure.

Occupational exposure concentrations insufficient to produce symptoms following single exposures can readily result in the onset of symptoms with continued daily exposures. It is emphasized that *a worker who has recovered from the acute phase of intoxication remains hypersusceptible for up to several weeks.* Any of the anticholinesterase compounds inactivate cholinesterase by phosphorylation of the active site of the enzyme to form dimethylphosphoryl enzyme. In the subsequent 24–48 hours after exposure there is a process termed "aging" of conversion to the monomethylphosphoryl enzyme. This so-called aging is of clinical importance, since during the treatment of organophosphate intoxication the cholinesterase reactivators, such as pralidoxime (2-PAM, Protopam) chloride, are ineffective after "aging" has occurred.[62, 96]

Diagnostic Test Procedures

Two types of cholinesterase are clinically significant: true acetylcholinesterase, found principally in the nervous system and the red blod cells, and the pseudo- or butyrylcholinesterase, found in the plasma, the liver and the nervous system. Both types are inhibited by the organophosphate compounds, *but the level of depression of the red blood cholinesterase is a more reliable indicator of clinically significant reduction of cholinesterase activity.* Verification of organophosphate intoxication may be determined from laboratory evidence of the amount of depression of red blood cell cholinesterase activity to a level considerably below preexposure levels—that is, a reduction of at least 50%, or much lower. The measurement of the enzyme cholinesterase is very difficult and usually not done. The activity (hydrolytic capacity) of the enzyme is usually measured. With each method for estimating cholinesterase activity of blood there can be an associated difference of normal values and reporting units. The laboratory report of cholinesterase determinations must state the units involved along with the appropriate normal range for that laboratory. The clinically usually acceptable normal range of red blood cell cholinesterase activity (by the Michel method) in Δ pH per hour is 0.39–1.02 for men and 0.34–1.10 for women. The normal range of the enzyme activity in Δ pH per hour of plasma is 0.04–1.63 for men and 0.24–1.54 for women. There is regeneration of cholinesterase primarily by the synthesis of new enzyme, which takes place at the rate of approximately 1% per day.

Average baseline values of erythrocyte and plasma ChE (cholinesterase) activity determined for healthy nonexposed men and women are given in Table 46–1. The value for average red blood cell (RBC) ChE activity for men is drawn from Wolfsie and Winter.[140] The value for women is obtained by multiplying the average RBC ChE activity figure for men by the ratio of mean ΔpH/hr for women to mean ΔpH/hr for men derived from the data of Rider et al.[114] The use of the data of Wolfsie and Winter allows for the increased packing and possible contamination of RBCs by plasma ChE. Plasma ChE values were selected from Rider et al., since their larger data base probably provides a closer approximation of the true population mean of normal values for plasma ChE activity. For the same reason, their data provide the most reliable women/men ratio for RBC ChE activities. The data of Wolfsie and Winter and Rider et al. are presented in Table 46–2.

TABLE 46–1.
Mean Baseline Values of Erythrocyte and Plasma Cholinesterase in Men and Women (ΔpH/Hr)

	Erythrocyte Cholinesterase	
	Men	*Women*
Mean	0.861	0.843
	Plasma Cholinesterase	
Mean	0.953	0.817

Treatment

Depending on the compounds involved and the occupational factors occurring at the time of exposure, treatment may be directed to simple removal from exposure in mild or suspected cases or to the most severe clinical intoxication requiring hospitalization and intensive care with special antidotal measures.

Initially, it is of utmost importance to decontaminate the exposed worker rapidly. It is an important reminder that persons undertaking decontamination must be protected with proper work clothes and gloves to avoid contaminating themselves, as well as having had prior education as to how to respond to such events. Contaminated work clothing, including shoes and socks, must be removed quickly, followed by thorough washing with soap and water or detergent and generous amounts of water, preferably under a shower or even submersion, if available, in the field.[97] The hair should be shampooed, and fingernails and toenails should be cleaned as well. Contaminated articles of clothing must be placed in plastic bags, marked as contaminated and diposed of properly.

It is wise and preferable to transport the sick worker to the nearest facility, making note of the substances that may have caused the illness. Because of the danger of pulmonary complications and the possible need for artificial respiration, care must be given to the removal of excess secretions and provision made for a patent airway. Anticonvulsant medication may be necessary, and, if cyanosis has been overcome, atropine should be given intravenously in doses of 2–4 mg. (This amount of atropine is about ten times the amount ordinarily administered for other medical conditions in which atropine is used.) This dose may be repeated at five- to ten-minute intervals until signs of atropinization appear—a dry, flushed skin, a tachycardia as high as 140 beats per minute, and pupillary dilation. A mild degree of such atropinization should be maintained for at least 48 hours. Doses of pralidoxime (2-PAM, Protopam) chloride as a cholinesterase reactivator can be given in doses of 1 gm intravenously at a rate not in excess of 500 mg/min to complement the action of the atropine. (After an hour, a second dose, 1 gm, may be given if muscle weakness has not improved.) Treatment with 2-PAM is effective if given within 24 hours after intoxication. *Avoid morphine, theophylline, aminophylline, barbiturates, and phenothiazines!* Blood samples for cholinesterase tests should be drawn in 10-ml quantities in heparinized tubes, prefer-

TABLE 46–2.
Normal Values for Circulating Cholinesterases in Healthy Nonexposed Persons*

	ERYTHROCYTE CHOLINESTERASE ACTIVITY (ΔpH/Hr)			PLASMA CHOLINESTERASE ACTIVITY (ΔpH/Hr)			
SUBJECTS	RANGE	MEAN	SD	RANGE	MEAN	SD	REFERENCE
400 men	0.58–0.95	0.766	0.081	0.52–1.39	0.953	0.187	109†
400 women	0.56–0.94	0.750	0.082	0.38–1.25	0.817	0.187	109†
255 men	0.554–1.252	0.861	0.091	0.408–1.652	0.912	0.112	133‡

*Method of Michel.[85]
†Ranges, means, and standard deviations in this study are estimates based on data extrapolated to age 40; ranges reflect elimination of highest 1% and lowest 1% of values.
‡Analytic method modified for smaller blood sample.

ably before the 2-PAM is given. In addition, urine *p*-nitrophenol may verify or indicate exposure.

To reiterate: speed in initiating therapy is essential; *no* atropine is to be given to a cyanotic person; oral atropine never is used, and atropine prophylaxis *is not condoned!*

Cholinesterase levels of 30%–50% of normal indicate exposure, although symptoms in some individuals may not appear until the level falls to 20% or less. The worker whose cholinesterase falls to or below 40% of the preexposure baseline must be removed from further exposure until the activity returns to within 80% of the preexposure baseline.

Hayes[48–50] noted that measurement of cholinesterase activity and pesticide metabolite determination in urine yield complementary findings, since metabolite excretion occurs rapidly whereas enzyme activity recovers slowly. Cholinesterase activity determination integrates the effects of exposure during a long interval (several weeks) whereas metabolite measurement gives information on very recent exposure.[77]

Some selected and widely used organophosphate compounds follow (see Glossary for a more comprehensive listing).

Parathion (0, 0-diethyl-0-*p*-nitrophenyl thiophosphate)

This is a widely used acaricide/insecticide. In its liquid form, it has a high boiling point and low vapor pressure. It is supplied as a dust or as a liquid for further dilution before spraying. Overexposure in the factory or in the field may result from inhalation or skin contact.

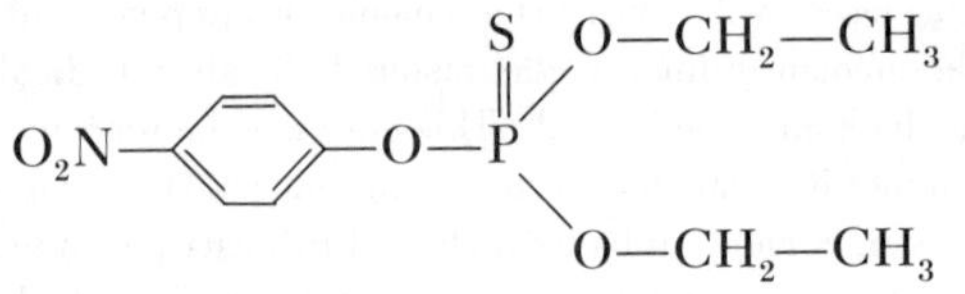

$$O_2N\text{—}C_6H_4\text{—}O\text{—}P(=S)(O\text{—}CH_2\text{—}CH_3)(O\text{—}CH_2\text{—}CH_3)$$

The minimal lethal oral dose of parathion for man has been estimated to range from less than 10 mg up to 125 mg. Arterberry et al.[5] observed and reported findings in 115 workers exposed to parathion under various conditions, the majority excreting significant amounts of *p*-nitrophenol in the urine, whereas those with heavier exposures had a measurable decrease in blood cholinesterase. One of its metabolites, paraoxon, is the active inhibitor of cholinesterase.

Measurement of urinary *p*-nitrophenol excretion has been found to be a reliable index of parathion exposure, even more sensitive as an absorption index than a decrease in blood cholinesterase activity. A biologic threshold of 100 μg/L in urine has been proposed. This may provide a high margin of safety, since excretion rates of more than 100 μg/L have been found in sprayers exposed to parathion without symptoms of intoxication, according to Wolfe et al.[139]

Some clinicians have thought that absorption of parathion can be tolerated without illness and with little or no reduction in cholinesterase activity as long as the concentration of *p*-nitrophenol in urine does not rise much above 2 mg/L. However, poisoning has been reported by Arterberry et al.[5] in which the *p*-nitrophenol excretion was lower than 2 mg/L (0.9, 0.57, and 1.6 mg/L[49, 100]).

Methyl Parathion

The TLV is 0.2 mg/cu m.

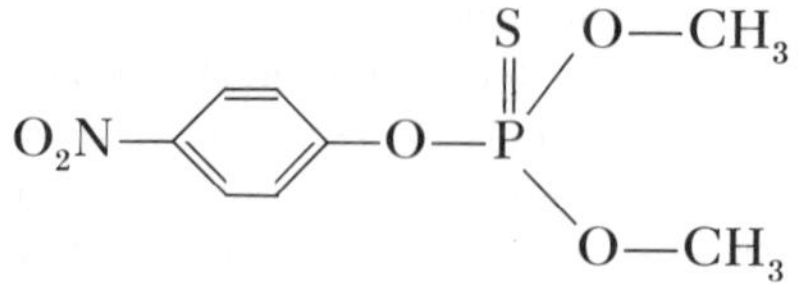

$$O_2N\text{—}C_6H_4\text{—}O\text{—}P(=S)(O\text{—}CH_3)(O\text{—}CH_3)$$

Methyl parathion itself is not a strong cholinesterase inhibitor, but one of its metabolites, methyl paraoxon, is an active cholinesterase inhibitor and inactivates cholinesterase to those compounds mentioned earlier. The minimal lethal oral dose for adults appears to be less than 1.84 gm, and data from human intoxication from this compound are not detailed enough to identify the range between the doses producing initial symptoms and those severe or fatal.[99]

Roan et al.[115] found the determination of ethyl or methyl parathion in serum samples by gas chromatography to be more sensitive than urine *p*-nitrophenol measurements. Several other anticholinesterase pesticides are amenable to analysis by unsophisticated techniques. Measurement of these metabolites may indicate a biochemical test of exposure, but insufficient human data exist for the proposal of credible biologic threshold limit values for most of these metabolites, and additional studies are needed for exposed worker evaluation.

Malathion

The TLV is 10 mg/ cu m.

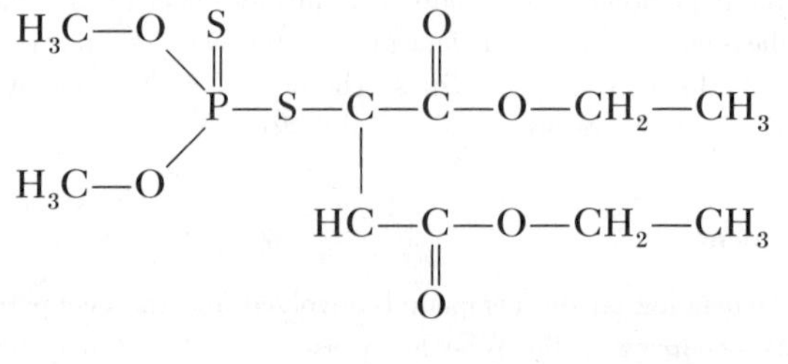

$$(H_3C\text{—}O)_2P(=S)\text{—}S\text{—}CH(C(=O)\text{—}O\text{—}CH_2\text{—}CH_3)\text{—}CH_2\text{—}C(=O)\text{—}O\text{—}CH_2\text{—}CH_3$$

This colorless to light amber liquid insecticide is of a relatively low order of toxicity when compared to the other organophosphates. Although malathion has only a mild direct inhibitory action on cholinesterase, one of its metabolites, malaoxon, is an active inhibitor, and both malathion and malaoxon are rapidly detoxified by the liver esterases and other organs. This apparent rapid metabolism is the main reason for the lower toxicity of this compound. Malaoxon otherwise inactivates cholinesterase in the toxic sequence similar to the other organophosphates described. The relative safety of malathion to man has been demonstrated repeatedly. Culver et al.[23] studied a group of workers with average exposure of 3.3 mg/cu m for five hours (maximum of 56 mg/cu m), finding that the cholinesterase levels in the blood were not significantly lowered, and no worker exhibited signs of cholinesterase inhibition. Golz,[36] using a controlled human exposure to malathion in which four men were exposed one hour daily for 42 days to 85 mg/cu m, found moderate nasal irritation and conjunctivitis but no cholinergic symptoms and signs. Nonlethal intoxication occurring in agricultural workers usually has been the result of gross exposures with concomitant skin absorption.[98] Nearly all reported fatalities from malathion have been through ingestion. Milby[87] reported that malathion has caused skin sensitization, and dermatitis may occur under conditions of heavy field use.

Baker et al.[8] described an epidemic of malathion intoxication, estimated to have affected 2,800 workers in the Pakistan malaria-control program, that was attributed to a combination of poor pesticide-handling techniques among spray team workers and to increased concentrations of toxic by-products in two of the three pesticide formulations used (isomalathion and *o,o,s*-trimethyl phosphorodithioate). Cholinesterase depression in field personnel was greatest in those using the pesticide brands with the highest concentrations of isomalathion and other malathion degradation products. Workers with greatest dermal exposure to malathion (sprayers and mixers) were more severely affected than supervisors. Cholinesterase activities were highest on Monday and fell during the week, reflecting cumulative effects of repeated exposures. The proscription of the use of the contaminated pesticide and special instructions in pesticide-handling techniques halted the epidemic.

Dermal absorption from excessive skin contact during spraying and mixing operations was the primary route of pesticide uptake; respiratory exposure was relatively unimportant, according to the authors, who estimated the average daily dermal exposure for sprayers to have been 330 mg of malathion (applying measured exposure rates to a body surface area of 1.75 cu m) and the percutaneously absorbed dose to have been 26 mg/day (based on 8% absorption of the pesticide). Baker et al. observed the cholinesterase depression and illness at this exposure level to be consistent with controlled studies, which found the minimal effective dose of malathion to range from 24 to 48 mg/day. Carriers and surfactants used in the manufacture of malathion water-dispersible powders were believed to be important in the formation of isomalathion and other toxic components in powders held under tropical storage conditions. A comprehensive training and medical surveillance program was developed to prevent recurrence of pesticide toxicity during the next spray season.

Mevinphos (Phosdrin) $(CH_3O)_2PO_2(CH_3)C = CHC(O)OCH_3$

The TLV is 0.01 ppm.

$$CH_3O{-}\overset{\overset{\displaystyle O}{\uparrow}}{P}{-}O\overset{\overset{\displaystyle CH_3}{|}}{C}{-}CHCOOH_3 \quad (P{-}OCH_3)$$

Holmes et al.[53] described two cases of moderate intoxication to this insecticide, with urinary excretion of dimethylphosphate, a metabolite of mevinphos, as late as 50 hours after exposure. Therefore, this metabolite present in urine may be useful in estimating absorption.

EPN (0-ethyl-0-*p*-nitrophenyl phenylphosphonothioate)

The TLV is 0.5 mg/cu m.

$$(C_2H_5O)(C_6H_5)P(=S){-}O{-}C_6H_4{-}NO_2$$

This parathion analogue differs somewhat, as it has a direct carbon-phosphorus link and is less volatile than parathion. EPN is used as an acaricide and insecticide for orchard pests and some soil insects and is relatively toxic to mammals, with an acute oral LD_{50} in rats of 8–36 mg/kg.[50, 62] EPN is suspected of delayed neurotoxicity, based on experimental evidence in chickens.[96]

Demeton

Demeton is known commercially as Systox and is a mixture of two isomers having a strong mercaptan odor. This systemic insecticide is highly toxic to mammals (oral LD_{50} in rats of 2–12 mg/kg) and has a long residual life within plants.

$$(C_2H_5O)_2\overset{\overset{\displaystyle O}{\|}}{P}{-}S{-}CH_2CH_2{-}S{-}CH_2CH_3 \quad \leftarrow \text{Thiol isomer}$$

$$(C_2H_5O)_2\overset{\overset{\displaystyle S}{\|}}{P}{-}O{-}CH_2CH_2{-}S{-}CH_2CH_3 \quad \leftarrow \text{Thiono isomer}$$

The used mixture consists of 65 parts thiono and 35 parts thiol isomers. At least four fatal, several severe, nonfatal, and several mild cases of demeton poisoning have been reported.[48]

Dichlorvos

The TLV is 1 mg/cu m.

$$(H_3C{-}O)_2P(=O){-}O{-}CH{=}CCl_2$$

This substance has a much higher vapor pressure than most other similar chemicals, with an extremely high toxicity for many insects but presenting little hazard to man from inhalation. Dichlorvos is applied as a film to plastic strips that may be suspended in the room or areas to be cleared of flying insects as a space fumigant. These are commonly known as "s-strips" and are very effective against flies and mosquitoes, the insects being killed by exposure to the substance.[8]

Naled (1,2-dibromo-2,2-dichloroethyl dimethyl phosphate)

The TLV is 3 mg/cu m.

$$(CH_3O)_2P(=O)—O—CH(Br)CBrCl_2$$

This compound is essentially a dibrominated dichlorvos, acting as a contact insecticide. The acute oral lethal dose (LD_{50}) to rats is about 430 mg/kg, relatively low compared to parathion but greater than malathion. Edmundson and Davies[29] described dermatitis in 9 of 12 women who were cutting tops of unflowered chrysanthemum plants which had been sprayed with naled. The dermatitis involved the exposed skin of the face, neck, and hands, apparently from exposure within two hours after plant spraying. It is known that naled hydrolyzes within two hours, simplifying control of contact exposures by allowing time before cutting plants.

Ronnel

The TLV is 10 mg/cu m.

$$Cl_3C_6H_2—O—P(=S)(O—CH_3)_2$$

This white crystalline powder is a weak cholinesterase inhibitor used in animal feed to kill external as well as internal parasites and actually is used as a systemic insecticide in livestock care. Occupational exposure occurs mainly by inhalation, not by skin absorption and rarely by ingestion. It is a weak cholinesterase inhibitor, affecting primarily the pseudocholinesterases of the blood plasma rather than the erythrocyte acetylcholinesterase. McCollister et al.,[81] using humans as subjects, evaluated the primary skin-irritating and skin-sensitizing potential of ronnel. Fifty subjects received three applications per week for three weeks of gauze saturated with a 10% suspension of ronnel in sesame oil without significant effects on the skin. Application of small amounts of powder into the eyes of rabbits produced slight discomfort and transient conjunctival irritation, subsiding in 48 hours. The LD_{50} for the rat is about 3,000 mg/kg and presumably, therefore, ronnel is one of the least toxic insecticides to man.

Tetraethylpyrophosphate $(C_2H_5)_4P_2O_7$

The TLV is 0.004 ppm.

$$(C_2H_5O)_2P(\rightarrow O)—O—P(\rightarrow O)(OC_2H^5)(OC_2H_5)$$

Commonly known as TEPP, this colorless, odorless liquid is a widely used insecticide and may be systemically absorbed via inhalation, skin, or ingestion. Quinby and Doornink[110] reported mild intoxication in 15 people exposed to a dust of 1% TEPP, the predominant symptoms being shortness of breath occurring after breathing dust-laden air for 30 minutes. Symptoms subsided rapidly when exposure was terminated.

Ten cases of possible organophosphate pesticide poisoning in florists exposed to pesticide residues on cut flowers were reported by Morse et al.,[89] who conducted a prospective random-sample survey to determine residual pesticide levels on flowers imported into Miami, Florida. Sampling of flowers imported into Miami on three days in January, 1977 showed that 18 (17.7%) of 105 lots contained pesticide residue levels up to 5 ppm and that three lots had levels up to 400 ppm. Twenty quarantine workers in Miami and 12 commercial florists exposed to contaminated flowers were clinically examined. Occasional nonspecific symptoms compatible with possible organophosphate exposure were noted, but no abnormalities in plasma or red blood cell cholinesterase levels were found. This study documents a previously unrecognized potential source of occupational pesticide exposure, and the authors suggest that safety standards should be set for residue levels on cut flowers.

CARBAMATES

Carbamates are derivatives of carbamic acid (CO_2NH_3), differing from the chlorinated hydrocarbon and organophosphate insecticides by the absence of chlorine and phosphorus. Work exposures may occur from inhalation, skin absorption and, rarely, ingestion. Clinically, toxic responses are similar to those of the organophosphates, as carbamates are anticholinesterase agents with the characteristic of having rapid reversibility of inhibition of the enzyme. Typical of this class of insecticides is carbaryl, commonly sold under the trade name Sevin. It has a low mammalian toxicity with a wide spectrum against nearly 150 insect species. Carbaryl dusts at 2%–5% concentrations are used to kill fleas on dogs and cats (except puppies and kittens under 4 weeks old). With DDT restricted in the United States, carbaryl dust is one of the insecticides useful to control the rat flea in murine typhus control programs and also wild rodent fleas in rural plague control. Sprays and dusts have been applied in adult mosquito control.

The TLV is 5 mg/cu m.

$$H_3C—NH—C(=O)—O—C_{10}H_7$$

Because carbaryl is metabolized rapidly, monitoring of exposure and measurements of the cholinesterase levels may not indicate the true magnitude of occupational exposure, which can be clinically misleading. Best and Murray[12] studied 59 workers exposed to concentrations ranging from 0.23 to 31 mg/cu m during a 19-month period, noting that there were no symptoms or signs of anticholinesterase activity. In the most heavily exposed workers, relatively large amounts of l-naphthol, a metabolite of carbaryl, were excreted in the urine, and the blood cholinesterase activity was only slightly depressed. They concluded that an excretion level of total l-naphthol significantly above 500 μg/100 ml of urine indicated absorption and metabolism of carbaryl. Concentrated solutions may produce skin irritation and systemic intoxication. Oral administration of carbaryl to guinea pigs during organogenesis was teratogenic at dose levels of 300 mg/kg and in beagle dogs in doses of 25 mg/kg (see Chapter 2 for details). Because of the rapidly reversible inhibition of cholinesterase, 2-PAM and other oxine reactivators are not used in treatment of carbaryl intoxication.[95]

Other carbamates are methomyl (Lannate), propoxur (Baygon), and carbofuran (Furadan); the mode of action is identical to carbaryl. The TLVs for methomyl, propoxur, and carbofuran are 2.5 mg/cu m, 0.5 mg/cu m, and 0.1 mg/cu m, respectively.

NONANTICHOLINESTERASE EFFECTS

There is evidence that many organophosphate compounds can inhibit enzyme systems other than cholinesterase. Tri-orthocresyl phosphate (TOCP), for example, inhibits an enzyme contained in nerve cells, and this inhibition can initiate a sequence of events that may end with loss of function and structural changes in affected nerve fibers. The physiologic function of this enzyme is not known, but, because of the delayed neurotoxicity that follows its inhibition, it has become known as neurotoxic esterase.[66]

Roberts[119] reported evidence for other nonanticholinesterase actions of organophosphate compounds from the observation that mipafox and leptophos, when given to rats for 35 days at dose levels of 5 mg/kg and 10 mg/kg, respectively, reduced the dopamine level in the corpus striatum. The functional changes associated with a reduction in striatal dopamine include akinesia, rigidity, and tremor in man and in experimental animals, and this action may contribute to the ataxia found in experimental and occupational exposures to certain organophosphate compounds such as mipafox and leptophos.

Another region of the brain with both cholinergic and adrenergic synapses is the optic tectum, where a change in the balance between acetylcholine and dopamine could lead to various visual and perceptual defects. Neurophysiologic evidence for this has been found in pigeons experimentally exposed to a single dose of mevinphos of 0.1 mg/kg. These effects assume importance for *spray pilots* and others whose work requires coordination of visual and motor skills. When atropine is used to suppress the acute anticholinesterase effects of organophosphate exposure, it may also cause central neurologic disturbances, particularly when given in large doses.[119]

Axonal degeneration followed by degeneration of myelin sheath cells in peripheral nerves and, in some cases, degeneration of tracts within the spinal cord have been observed as a result of prolonged exposure to such organophosphate compounds as tri-o-cresyl phosphate, mipafox,[13] and leptophos.[141] Demyelination was the probable explanation seen in poisoning caused by tri-o-cresyl phosphate.[65]

It is known that some fluoro-organophosphate compounds cause delayed neurotoxicity.[2, 3, 61, 118] Hexane[141] and other hydrocarbon solvents have caused polyneuropathy.[19, 142] Simplified methods of electromyography (EMG) have been developed, using surface electrodes to stimulate the ulnar nerve and to record action potentials from the adductor muscle of the thumb.[17] These methods are not specific for organophosphorus compounds or for anticholinesterase effects but may detect subtle and early changes in nerve and muscle function. Electromyography (EMG) has been used to evaluate exposure of workers to several organophosphate pesticides.[61, 126]

Mevinphos, an organophosphate, was administered to male volunteers by Verberk and Salle[135] with a dose of 25 μg/kg daily for 28 days, comparing findings with a control group. A 7% decrease in slow fiber motor nerve conduction velocity and a 38% increase in Achilles tendon reflex force were found after exposure. No effect on neuromuscular transmission was observed, and the red blood cell cholinesterase depression was 19%.

To determine if cholinesterase inhibition might affect neuromuscular transmission in exposed workers, Stålberg et al.[126] utilized electromyography to study 11 men commercially applying insecticides. All were sprayers, working daily with solutions of 4% lindane, 0.2% pyrethrum, 0.125% piperonylbutoxide, 2.5% malathion or 2% bromophos in kerosene, with intermittent exposure to 0.5% diazinon and dursbane. The workers' employment periods varied between 1 and 24 years. All were equipped with routine protective devices such as respirators, boots, overalls, and gloves, and all were examined clinically and neurophysiologically, along with measurements of blood cholinesterase activity. They formed their own reference group, since measurements were also made after one to four weeks of nonexposure (preexposure values). Measurements following exposure generally were made within 1–24 hours after a period of spray work, with exposure values taken during spring and preexposure values after summer vacation. Blood samples for cholinesterase activity and analysis were taken immediately before each EMG investigation. Cholinesterase activity of plasma and erythrocytes was determined with a gasometric technique, using whole blood samples with activity expressed in microliters of carbon dioxide evolved in 30 min/50 μl blood or simply b_{30}.

Slight changes in plasma cholinesterase activity were not correlated with disturbed neuromuscular transmission in the subjects.

Lower sensory nerve conduction velocities after work in seven subjects was found, with average reduction for the group small (3%) but statistically significant ($P = .05$). Reduced conduction velocity usually is a sign of neuropathy, which was thought might be present in some of the workers. The increased jitter values seen in some recordings were thought to indicate an uncertain impulse transmission in reinnervation structures (nerve sprouts, immature motor endplates[64]) but did not relate to acute exposure and preceding denervation due to neuropathy, as suggested by Stålberg et al.

Stålberg and his co-investigators indicated that a peripheral neuropathy could cause a reduced surface action potential, for example, due to reduced excitability (demyelination) or axonal degeneration, and concluded that the slight neurophysiologic abnormalities found in this investigation were unrelated to a lowered cholinesterase activity.

Persisting electroencephalogram (EEG) changes in men following exposure to the organophosphate ester Sarin were reported by Duffy,[28] who recorded the brain wave activity of 67 workers exposed at least once, but not in the preceding year, and described a significant difference from that of 26 workers who had no prior exposure to Sarin. The brain waves of the unexposed workers also differed significantly from those of 38 exposed workers who had three or more exposures within the preceding six years, but excluding the most recent years, according to Duffy. Worker exposure levels were not given. Activity in the β range was greater in the exposed workers than in the nonexposed, being the chief difference between the observed groups. However, Duffy stated that the exposed group revealed a greater number of EEGs with decreased α activity, increased epochs of slow activity, and deviation of background activity with faster or slower rhythms, which did not have clear diagnostic value, since the electroencephalographer's interpretations were at a level of chance, only 49.5%.

Sarin (Isopropyl Methylphosphonofluoride)

```
                  O
                  |
(CH3)2CHO—P—F
                  |
                 CH3
```

Tabun (not in use)

```
            O
            |
(CH3)2N—P—CN
            |
           OC2H
```

Sarin is the most toxic of the "nerve gases." It is related to tabun, and both are extremely active cholinesterase inhibitors, much more severe in activity than parathion. The lethal dose for man is estimated to be 0.01 mg/kg.

OTHER CLINICAL ASPECTS OF ORGANOPHOSPHATE AND CARBAMATE INSECTICIDES—A REITERATION

Depression of plasma and/or erythrocyte cholinesterase is considered a good index of the absorption of cholinesterase-inhibiting pesticides (organophosphate esters, *N*-methyl or *N*-dimethyl carbamate esters). The selection of the enzyme activity to be determined (red blood cell or plasma) depends on the relative affinity of the pesticide for both enzymes; there is interindividual variability in blood cholinesterase activity, and it is important to compare exposure values with preexposure levels, with a 50% reduction in activity dictating removal of the worker from continued exposure. Cholinesterase enzyme determinations are sufficiently sensitive and specific for monitoring programs (if preexposure activities are known); problems can occur with inadequate sample preservation before analyses, and urinary metabolites may be sought. Various techniques available for measuring these enzymes have been reported, but it must be pointed out that the *inhibition* of the *enzymes by free active pesticides can occur during blood storage;* the cholinesterase activity may not indicate the true activity in vivo. Carbamylated cholinesterases and some phosphorylated cholinesterases can be reactivated during storage, and *further inhibition or partial recovery after sampling* must be recognized in determining conditions of assay.[88]

Serum activity is within normal ranges in patients manifesting myasthenia gravis, bronchial asthma, epilepsy, hyperthyroidism, hypertension, and diabetes mellitus.

In addition to the organophosphate and carbamate compounds, depression of serum cholinesterase activity is produced by suxamethonium and certain other substances. Short-term depression is caused by adrenaline, antipyrine and antipyrine derivatives, amidone and isoamidone, antimalarial drugs, atropine, barbiturates, caffeine, chloroform, codeine, Dilaudid, ether, folic acid, morphine, para-aminobenzoic acid, phenothiazine derivatives, physostigmine, procaine hydrochloride, Prostigmin, quaternary ammonium compounds, quinine, sulfanilamides, tetraethylammonium chloride, theobromine, theophylline, thiamine, and vitamin K. Long-term depression is caused by alkyl fluorophosphates.

Other factors affecting these levels may be impairment of liver function, certain anemias, malnutrition, and pregnancy. Howard et al.[54] observed six healthy young women before and during pregnancy, noting a significant fall in plasma cholinesterase activity in the first three months of normal pregnancy. There was some evidence of return to normal prepregnancy levels in later pregnancy. No hypothesis was suggested to account for this phenomenon, although it seems possible that it may be the result of altered liver enzyme synthesis. None was exposed to organophosphates or other cholinesterase depressants. The percentage fall ranged from 17.7 to 46.4, but values returned to normal later in pregnancy. These findings introduce another important variable into the routine biologic monitoring of female workers exposed to anticholinesterase compounds, complicating assessment of the significance of depressions of cholinesterase activity in relation to exposure to organophosphates and similar compounds.

To reemphasize: The important difference in the toxicology between *organophosphate* and *carbamate* insecticides is that the organophosphate compounds almost *irreversibly* phosphorylate the acetylcholinesterase, whereas the *carbamates cause reversible* carbamylation of the enzyme. In man, organophosphate exposure can cause depression of plasma cholinesterase to persist for one to three weeks; red blood cell depression can persist up to 12 weeks. With carbamate poisoning, plasma and red blood cell cholinesterase may be depressed, but usually return to normal within a few hours after exposure.[88]

A summary of emergency medical treatment for acute insecticide poisoning is given in Table 46–3.

TABLE 46–3.

A Summary of Emergency Medical Treatment for Acute Insecticide Poisoning (Some Typical Compounds)

ORGANOPHOSPHATES (Irreversible Cholinesterase Inhibitors)	CARBAMATES (Reversible Cholinesterase Inhibitors)	CHLORINATED HYDROCARBONS
Chlorpyrifos (Dursban) Diazinon Dichlorvos (Vapona, DDVP) Dimethoate (Cygon) Fenthion (Baytex, Entex) Rabon (Gardona) Malathion Methyl parathion Parathion Naled (Dibrom) Ronnel (Korian) Trichlorfon (Dipterex)	Carbaryl (Sevin) Dimetilan Landrin Propoxur (Baygon	CNS depressant/stimulant aldrin—BHC chlordane—DDT dieldrin heptachlor—lindane mirex toxaphene In general, these act on the central nervous system to stimulate or depress, varying by compound
Symptoms and Signs		
1. MILD—headache, dizziness, weakness, anxiety, miosis, impairment of visual acuity 2. MODERATE—nausea, salivation, lacrimation, abdominal cramps, vomiting, sweating, slow pulse, muscle tremors 3. SEVERE—diarrhea, pinpoint and nonreactive pupils, respiratory difficulty, pulmonary edema, cyanosis, loss of sphincter control, convulsions, coma and death	Constriction of pupils Salivation Profuse sweating Lassitude Muscle incoordination Nausea Vomiting Diarrhea Epigastric pain Tightness in chest	Typical onset—20 min to 4 hr Nausea Vomiting Restlessness Tremor Apprehension Convulsions Coma Respiratory failure Death DO NOT INDUCE EMESIS IF THE INGESTED POISON IS PRINCIPALLY A HYDROCARBON SOLVENT (e.g., kerosene)
Therapy		
1. Support respiration. Keep airways clear. Use artificial respiration with oxygen if cyanosis is indicated. Death from pesticide poisoning usually is due to respiratory failure. 2. Decontamination as indicated. Remove contaminated clothing. Wash skin, hair, and fingernails with soap and water. Sponge with alcohol. Cleanse eyes. If ingested, lavage stomach with 5% sodium bicarbonate if person is not vomiting. Protect first-aid and medical personnel!! 3. Draw 5 ml heparinized blood for cholinesterase determination. Save samples of first urine and first/early vomitus for possible laboratory analysis. 4. Consult insecticide label under "ACTIVE INGREDIENTS" for specific chemicals involved. 5. When mixtures of organophosphates and chlorinated hydrocarbons are involved (e.g., endrin and methyl parathion), give specific treatment for organophosphates first and indicated support therapy and decontamination.		
ANTIDOTE	ANTIDOTE	TREATMENT
1. Adults: After cyanosis is overcome, use atropine sulfate, 2–4 mg intravenously. Repeat doses at 5–10-minute intervals until signs of atropinization appear. Maintain for 24 hours or longer if necessary. 2. Children: Atropine sulfate in proportion to body weight: approx. 0.05 mg/kg. 3. Support atropine treatment with 2-PAM (pralidoxime chloride) (Protopam Chloride, Ayerst). a. Adult dose: 1 gm, slowly, intravenously b. Infants: 0.25 gm, slowly, intravenously NOTE: Contraindicated are morphine, aminophylline, theophylline, phenothiazine tranquilizers, and barbiturates.	1. Adults: After cyanosis is overcome, use atropine sulfate, 2–4 mg intravenously. Repeat dose at 5–10-minute intervals until signs of atropinization appear. Maintain for 24 hr or longer if necessary. 2. Children: Atropine sulfate in proportion to body weight: approx. 0.05 mg/kg. NOTE: 2-PAM is contraindicated in carbamate insecticide poisoning. Also avoid morphine, aminophylline, theophylline, phenothiazine tranquilizers, and barbiturates.	1. Gastric lavage with 2–4 L tap water. Catharsis with 30 gm (10 oz) sodium sulfate in 1 cup of water 2. Barbiturates in appropriate dosages repeated as necessary for restlessness or convulsions 3. Avoid oils, oil laxatives, and epinephrine (adrenalin). Do not give stimulants. 4. Give calcium gluconate (10% in 10-ml ampules) intravenously every 4 hr.

FOR SPECIFIC INFORMATION: CALL NEAREST POISON CONTROL CENTER.

HERBICIDES

Herbicides are compounds intended for killing plants or interrupting their normal growth—for example, the elimination of dandelions in lawn grasses.

The chlorophenoxy herbicides are one well-known class of herbicides, including 2,4,5-T(2,4,5-trichlorophenoxyacetic acid) and 2,4-D(2,4-dichlorophenoxyacetic acid).

$$\text{Cl}(\text{Cl})\text{C}_6\text{H}_3\text{—O—CH}_2\text{—C(=O)—OH} \qquad \text{Cl}(\text{Cl})(\text{Cl})\text{C}_6\text{H}_2\text{—O—CH}_2\text{—C(=O)—OH}$$

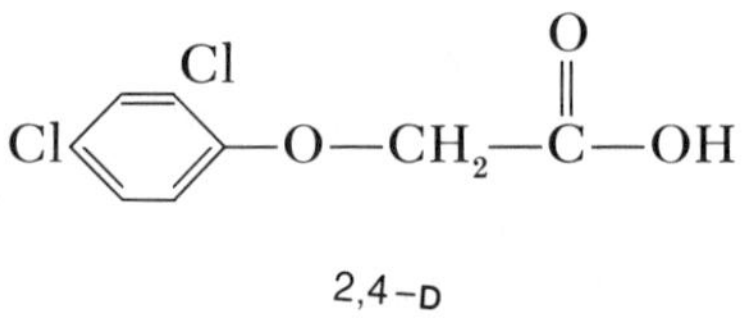

2,4-D 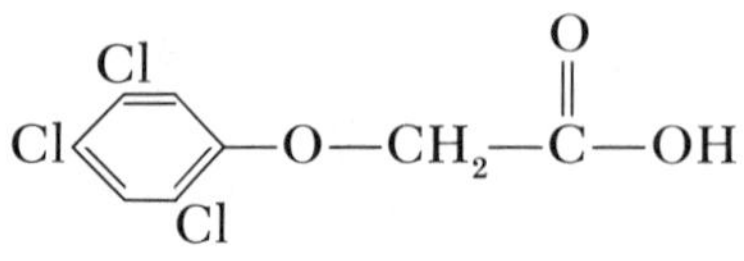 2,4,5-T

Enormous quantities of 2,4,5-T and 2,4-D (in excess of 6,000,000 kg annually) are produced and used throughout the world. The materials are formulated as emulsifiable concentrates for air or ground spray applications.

During the manufacture of 2,4,5-T, the 2,4,5-trichlorophenol intermediate can react with itself to produce TCDD (2,3,7,8-tetrachlorodibenzopara-dioxin). Although 2,4,5-T and 2,4-D have essentially low toxicity for animals and man, TCDD is one of the most toxic compounds known.

$$\text{Cl}_3\text{C}_6\text{H}_2\text{OH} + \text{HOC}_6\text{H}_2\text{Cl}_3 \rightarrow \text{TCDD} + 2\ \text{HCl}$$

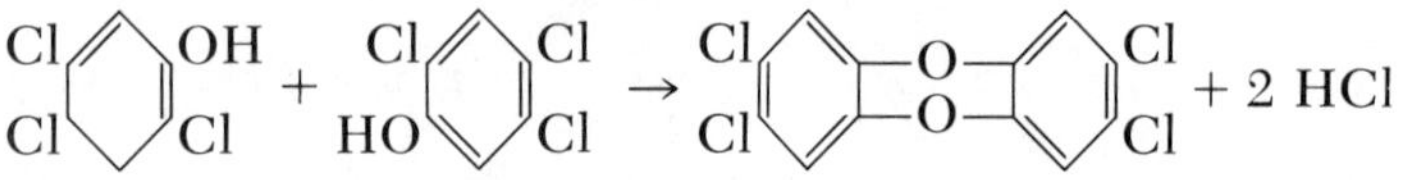

TCDD

The intense toxicity of TCDD, called "dioxin," was underscored in 1976 in an accident in the ICMESA factory producing 2,4,5-trichlorophenol (used to make the bactericide hexachlorophene as well as the herbicide 2,4,5-T). The reactor vessel heat-regulating valves failed, with safety valve blowout, exhausting an estimated 10% of the contents into the external plant atmosphere, forming a huge cloud reported to contain some 500 kg 2,4,5-T and 2 (or more) kg of TCDD. An area about 5 km long and 700 m wide was contaminated in the nearby town of Seveso (population 17,000) 20 km north of Milan, Italy. Of the 14 workers in the plant, or who entered the area shortly thereafter, 13 had abnormal liver function tests, but normal ones within two weeks. Some workers developed mild chloracne. The entire plant was contaminated by TCDD, and, inadvertently, production was resumed in some areas. Within six months, 79 chloracne cases were noted, especially in maintenance workers. Evacuation of a large segment of the community was ordered, involving hundreds of people of all ages. About 2,000 persons were exposed to TCDD, 300 of whom were treated for skin disorders. More than 1,100 animals were killed by direct exposure (up to 225 ng TCDD per gm of tissue were found in dead rabbit livers). Occupational health services were initiated to observe the 60 plant workers and a large-scale epidemiologic program was enacted involving the 200,000 people in the area to investigate long-term effects.

Because of the potential for contamination of the herbicide 2,4,5-T and Silvex, the EPA in April, 1979, suspended use for crops used for human food, around aquatic areas and recreational areas, and around homes. In the United States, current allowed use is only on pastures, rangelands, rights of way, and for rice crops. In the late 1970s, more than 2 million kg were used in the United States for commercial weed control and more than 1 million kg on pastures and rangelands.

2,4-D is a systemic herbicide widely used for control of broadleaf weeds in cereal crops and sugar cane and on turf, pastures, and non-croplands. It is also used to control the ripening of bananas and citrus fruits and to delay preharvest dropping of some fruits and is used in some countries as a fungicide for the control of Alternaria rots when lemons are to be held for storage.

2,4-D was used to defoliate jungle areas in South Viet Nam, where it was a component of "Agent Orange" (a 50:50 mixture of the *n*-butyl esters of 2,4-D and 2,4,5-T, containing up to 30 mg/kg TCDD). About 40 million L of "Agent Orange" were sprayed in South Viet Nam between 1965 and 1971 for defoliation or crop destruction.

2,4,5-T was banned in Italy in 1970 and also banned in the Netherlands and Sweden. The 1979 ACGIH TLV for 2,4,5-T is 10 mg/cu m for an eight-hour TWA.

The 1979 ACGIH TLV for 2,4-D is 10 mg/cu m for an eight-hour TWA. The corresponding standard in West Germany is also 10 mg/cu m, and the acceptable ceiling concentration in the USSR[111] is 1 mg/cu m.

Occupational Exposure

2,4,5-T dust is a slight skin irritant, but it and 2,4-D may cause dermatitis on prolonged skin contact. Occupational exposure to phenoxy acids (2,4-D and 2,4,5-T) has been studied in forestry work with four tractor sprayers spraying a 2% emulsion in water and the phenoxy acid levels in the breathing zone of the subjects determined by Kolmodin-Hedman et al.[71] The phenoxy acid levels in plasma and urine were determined by electron capture gas chromatography and the air samples analyzed by UV-spectrophotometry and thin-layer chromatography. The air levels of phenoxy acids ranged between 0.1 and 0.2 mg/cu m, with occasional higher levels (about 1 mg/cu m) obviously due to contamination of the impinger flash by larger droplets. Plasma and urine levels were followed during a week of exposed work and for 36 hours after exposure. Plasma levels ranged from the detection limit up to 0.1–0.2 μg/ml. The levels varied due to intermittent exposure. After exposure, these levels declined to near the detection limit overnight. Mean urinary levels of phenoxy acids were (2,4-D and 2,4,5-T, respectively) 8 and 4.5 μg/ml, ranging from 3 to 14 μg/ml for 2,4-D and 1 to 11 μg/ml for 2,4,5-T in the afternoon of the day of exposure. In a second investigation, the mean 24-hour excretion in urine was 9 mg of 2,4-D and around 1 mg of 2,4,5-T. Urinary elimination was rapid. Absorption seemed to be caused by inhalation and dermal exposure, but the conditions did not allow an assessment of the relative importance of these channels of uptake. Improved hygienic conditions are suggested to decrease exposure. None of the subjects reported clinical symptoms except one, who had slight irritation of the eyes after direct contact with the spray liquid. In control subjects with a low and indirect exposure, no 2,4-D and 2,4,5-T could be detected in plasma or urine. The authors concluded that exposure to 2,4-D and 2,4,5-T could best be followed by measurement of the phenoxy acid levels in the urine, with sampling preferably made in the afternoon of an exposed working day or within a day following exposure. The lowest detectable concentration in urine of 2,4-D and 2,4,5-T is 0.05 μg/ml. A variety of toxicologic effects have been reported in workers engaged in manufacturing 2,4,5-T and 2,4-D. Chloracne, liver disorders, neurologic and behavioral changes, and signs of porphyria cutanea tarda are among the more frequently reported clinical findings.

Chloracne, one of the common and prominent features of TCDD exposure, is characterized by inclusion cysts, comedones and pustules, with scarring of the skin, more often on the face, but on other areas of the body as well. Blepharoconjunctivitis and irritation of other mucous membranes have been noted. The chloracne may be preceded by erythematous and edematous skin. Latency between exposure and the appearance of signs of chloracne ranges from a few weeks to several months, according to May.[79]

Chloracne and liver impairment, formerly thought to be caused by the chlorophenols, were shown to be due to TCDD, but the actual cause of certain other findings, particularly the neurologic ones, may also be from other substances, such as 2,4-D or chlorophenols. Chloracne affected 60 workers at the 2,4,5-T factory of the Dow Chemical Company in Midland, Michigan, in 1964.[31]

Eleven of 29 subjects with features of chloracne working in a 2,4-D and 2,4,5-T-producing factory of the Diamond Alkali Company, Newark, New Jersey, also showed increased uroporphyrin excretion. In three cases, a diagnosis of porphyria cutanea tarda was unquestionable; two of these had raised serum glutamic oxaloacetic transaminase levels. Many of the workers, regardless of uroporphyrinuria, had hirsutism, hyperpigmentation, increased skin fragility, and vesiculobullous eruptions on exposed areas of skin.[14, 31]

Similar findings were described by Jirásek et al.,[63] who reported 76 cases of chloracne between 1965 and 1968 in a factory in Czechoslovakia producing 2,4,5-T and pentachlorophenol. These effects were attributed to TCDD. Fifty-five patients were submitted to medical follow-ups for more than five years. Four deaths were observed, two of which were from bronchogenic carcinomas. Some of the workers had symptoms of porphyria cutanea tarda, uroporphyrinuria, abnormal liver tests (bilirubin, serum glutamic oxaloacetic transaminase, serous glutamic pyruvic transaminase, and bromosulphthalein), and liver enlargement. The majority of workers were reported to have "severe neurasthenia" and "depressive syndrome." In 17, signs of peripheral neuropathy, notably in the lower extremities, were confirmed by electromyographic studies. More than half showed increased blood cholesterol and total lipids. In 1949, an accident occurred at the 2,4,5-T-producing factory of the Monsanto Chemical Company in Nitro, West Virginia; 228 people were affected. Symptoms included chloracne, melanosis, muscle aches and pain, fatigue, nervousness, and intolerance to cold.[31]

Czeizel and Király[24] studied the frequency of chromosome aberrations in the peripheral blood lymphocytes of 76 workers at a Budapest chemical factory producing herbicides and in 33 controls. Thirty-six workers had been exposed to 2,4,5-trichlorophenoxyethanol (TCPE) and 26 to Buvinol, a combination herbicide containing TCPE and 2-chloro-6-ethylamino-4-isopropylamino-1,3,5-triazine (atrazine); 14 had never been engaged in herbicide production or use. The TCDD contamination of the final products was said to be less than 0.1 mg/kg and generally not more than 0.05 mg/kg. The frequency of chromatid-type and unstable chromosome aberrations was found to be statistically significantly higher in the factory workers, whether they had been directly exposed in herbicide production or not. The aberrations were more frequent among workers preparing Buvinol and TCPE than in other factory workers, but the difference was significant only for the chromatid-type effect.

Hardell and Sandström[44] investigated workers engaged as herbicide applicators in northern Sweden and found a number of patients with soft-tissue sarcomas and previous exposure to phenoxyacetic acids. Due to this observation, a matched case-control study was performed with consideration for exposure to chlorophenols included. The results showed that exposure to phenoxyacetic acids or chlorophenols gave an approximately sixfold increase of the risk for this type of tumor. They considered it most unlikely that the results were influenced by uncontrolled confounding factors or other defects in the validity of the study. A specific evaluation of the effect of separate chemical substances was not possible, since nearly all exposed persons were also exposed to chlorinated dioxins, including their most potent form, 2,3,7,8-tetrachlorodibenzo-*p*-dioxin (TCDD). They were not able to determine if the carcinogenic effect was exerted by these compounds or by impurities such as chlorinated dibenzodioxins and dibenzofurans that in almost all cases were part of the commercial preparations used. The authors suggested that the increased risk for this type of tumor after exposure to phenoxyacetic acids or chlorophenols may be caused by the pure chemical substances, impurities in the commercial preparations, or a combination of both.

Axelson and Sundell[6] studied a cohort of Swedish railway workers exposed to a variety of herbicides, finding a significant twofold excess of all cancers observed in exposed workers, as compared to the Swedish national average. The situation was difficult to evaluate because of the combined exposure of many workers to more than one herbicide. Most of the excess, however, seemed to be due to exposure to 3-amino-1,2,4-triazole (amitrole); within the subgroups that had been exposed to phenoxy acids (2,4-D and/or 2,4,5-T), only a small difference was detected: 5 cancers at all sites observed versus 2.8 expected. The authors state that the use of 2,4-D and 2,4,5-T probably had been higher than what they could trace.

Thiess and Goldmann[131] traced four cancer deaths (one lung carcinoma at 54 years, two gastric carcinomas at 64 and 77 years, and one colonic carcinoma at 70 years) out of 15 deaths occurring in a cohort of 53 workers exposed accidentally to TCDD at the BASF factory in Ludwigshafen, West Germany, in 1953.

There are reports describing the occurrence of cancer in workers exposed to TCDD. Jirásek et al.[63] followed 55 subjects of a cohort of 78 exposed workers for five to six years: four deaths were observed, two of which were from bronchogenic carcinoma at 47 and 59 years. Smoking history was not reported and no causal conclusion was drawn. However, if 1965 WHO lung cancer mortality rates for Czechoslovakia were applied to the age structure of the whole cohort of 78 workers, the expected number of lung cancer deaths in five years would be only 0.12.

Recently, chemical processes for 2,4,5-trichlorophenol production that do not cause TCDD to be formed have been inaugurated so that production of these herbicides is free from the TCDD hazard. The herbicide Dalapan (2,4-dichloropropionic acid) is a substitute herbicide having a low toxicity for animals and man.

In addition, TCDD-contaminated pesticides, several other types of pesticides, and their intermediates have been associated with chloracne. Chlorinated naphthalenes, diphenyls, diphenyl oxides, azoxybenzenes, and chlorinated dibenzofurans have been implicated in producing chloracne and hyperpigmentation of the skin. Further discussion on dioxin and phenoxy acids is presented in Chapter 47.

Paraquat (1,1′-dimethyl-4,4′-bipyridilium dichloride)

The TLV is 0.1 mg/cu m.

$$H_3C—{}^{+}N\langle\;\rangle—\langle\;\rangle N^{+}—CH_3 \cdot Cl_2$$

Paraquat has worldwide use in killing leafy plants and in harvesting cotton (by spray) in order to desiccate the leaves to defoliate the plants, making the cotton bolls easier to be picked mechanically. In use in field applications, paraquat is rapidly decomposed and inactivated by the action of sunlight. The sale and use of paraquat is carefully regulated in most countries and generally is formulated as a 20% solution that is sprayed on the desired areas. The solutions often contain surfactants as wetting agents and ordinarily are mixed or added to the spray shortly before use. Paraquat is applied on large areas by aerial spraying. It gained prominence in 1978 when used to destroy marijuana crops in Mexico, causing much concern to users of marijuana, but actual paraquat toxicity was ruled out by a CDC investigation.[108, 127]

Although paraquat had been studied mainly in laboratories since 1933, reports on occupational intoxication had not been made until the 1960s, when this compound was introduced for agricultural use. The first report of intoxication to paraquat was due to accidental ingestion in two young men who consumed a small quantity of paraquat concentrate mistakenly thought to contain an alcoholic beverage. Death occurred within several days from a rapidly developing and progressive fibrosis of the lungs.[108] These examples, along with laboratory animal studies, revealed that paraquat by ingestion was extremely toxic and rapid in action, producing irreversible lung damage even though elimination in the urine was quite rapid.

Vaziri et al.[133] studied three patients with paraquat poisoning, two due to suicidal ingestion (a 56-year-old woman ingested a "large cup" of paraquat, a 16-year-old boy a "mouthful," and a 17-year-old boy a "mouthful" by accident). Renal function studies revealed acute renal failure observed in all three cases. The glomerular filtration rate improved for two patients who survived three weeks, illustrating the reversible nature of paraquat-induced acute renal failure. A mild-to-moderate transient proteinuria was observed during the first and second weeks following paraquat ingestion. Renal glucosuria, marked amino aciduria and increased fractional excretion of phosphorus, sodium, and uric acid were observed. These findings, which have not been described previously in man, are indicative of proximal tubular dysfunction and parallel observations previously made in experimental animals.

Symptoms that have been displayed by agricultural workers subjected to excessive periods of paraquat spray exposure are related to local irritation and include nosebleed, upper respiratory and buccal mucous membrane inflammation, cough, headache, eye irritation, skin irritation, and damaged fingernails with transverse bands of nail discoloration; other lesions were loss of nail surface, ridging, gross nail deformities, and, in some, loss of the nail.[128] These signs of overexposure should be sufficient indicators for removal of the worker from the area and prevention of further overexposure. Although absorption via healthy skin is thought to be minimal, injured skin, i.e., abraded or having small lacerations, can enhance absorption, and contamination of scrotal skin must be avoided.

Experimental Toxicology.—Ingestion of paraquat by laboratory animals produces signs of poisoning similar to those described for man, which include oral and pharyngeal irritation in addition to pulmonary and possible renal complications.

Carefully controlled skin exposure studies, which eliminate the possibility of ingestion, failed to demonstrate any signs of lung toxicity. However, a 20% decrease in body weight was reported in the paraquat-treated animals. Acute dermal exposure to paraquat concentrate has produced mild erythema, hyperkeratoses, and desquamation in rats and rabbits. The effects were diminished when typical field spray concentrations were used.[20]

Prolonged exposure to respirable paraquat spray has been demonstrated to produce pulmonary congestion and edema in rats.[20] The reaction is immediate, resulting in the development of chemical pneumonitis in the form of congestion and edema. This does not resemble the syndrome seen following ingestion. Discoloration, swelling, and clouding of renal tissue in rats subjected to paraquat aerosol inhalation indicated that the herbicide may be partially absorbed by this route. It must be noted that agricultural sprays have much larger particles and, therefore, do not reach the alveoli.

Investigations have been conducted on the possible hazard from dust from paraquat-treated soils. Rats, mice, guinea pigs, and rabbits were exposed to a dust cloud containing 500 ppm paraquat at a level of 10 gm/cu m, of which 0.25 gm/cu m was respirable. No effects were noted.

Two-year feeding studies were conducted in mice using 9, 25, 50, and 75 ppm paraquat cation in the diet without evidence of carcinogenic activity. Paraquat was tested to determine if dominant lethal gene formation occurred in mice. No mutagenic properties were demonstrated. However, certain antifertility effects were noted in mice administered 17.3 mg paraquat cation/kg orally. There was a decreased percentage of pregnancies in treated mice. No differences were found between control and treated animals regarding the number of fetal deaths.[20]

No teratologic effects have been reported from dietary intake of paraquat in experimental animals.[107] A three-generation, two-litter reproduction study on rats sustained on diets containing 30 and 100 ppm paraquat cation demonstrated that the compound did not influence the growth or fertility of the treated animals or their offspring, nor were any teratogenic effects noted.

An extensive report on the toxicology of paraquat, diquat, and morfamquat was published by Pasi[107] in 1978.

Clinical.—Paraquat can be determined in urine and dialysate. However, the technique is lengthy and requires ion-exchange resins not generally available. In emergencies, paraquat levels should be determined, but treatment should not be delayed. Obtain a 100-ml urine sample and/or a dialysate sample and store under refrigeration until arrangements for analysis are made.* The Chevron Chemical Company's Environmental Health Group has prepared a valuable document describing paraquat poisoning, signs and symptoms, along with treatment.[106]

Urea Derivatives

Certain urea derivatives are commonly used as herbicides. Some of these are monuron (Monurex, Telvar), diuron (Di-on, diurex, Karmex) and others.

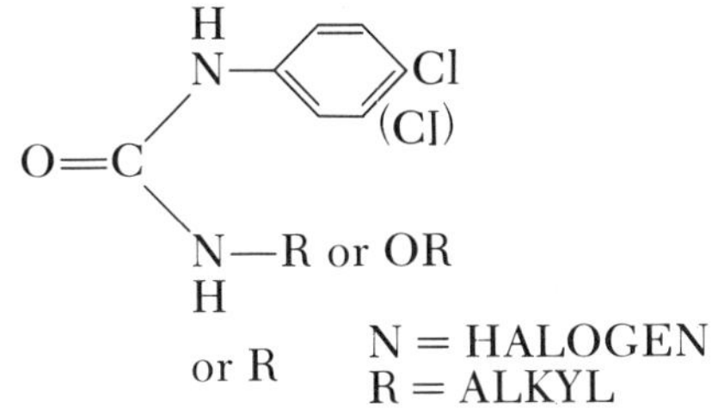

```
        H
        N—⟨phenyl⟩—Cl
       /          (Cl)
  O=C
       \
        N—R or OR
        H
        or R        N = HALOGEN
                    R = ALKYL
```

Some uracil compounds are bromacil (Borea, Hyvar X, Hyvar X-2), terbacil (Sinbar) and others. Triazines: atrazine (Atarex, Atranex, Primatol A, etc.) and a host of other trade names. Occupational exposures to these compounds rarely have produced adverse effects, and most of these effects have been skin irritation following prolonged contact.

*The Chevron Chemical Company will perform urine and dialysate analysis for paraquat at no cost. Arrangements for this service can be made by telephoning the Chevron Poison Information Center—(415) 233–3737.

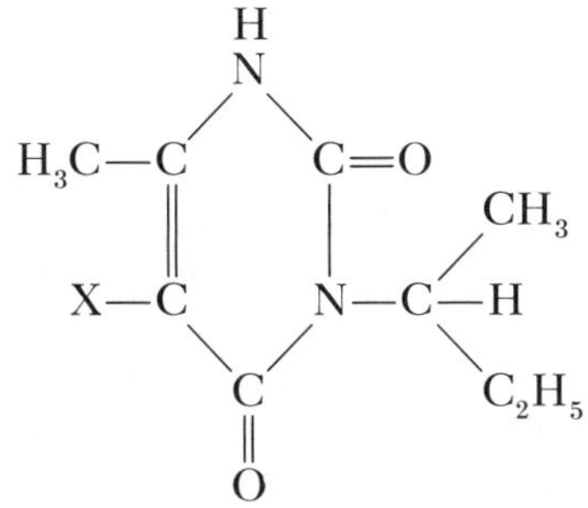

```
            H
            N
          /   \
  H3C—C         C=O
      ||        |        CH3
                        /
   X—C          N—C—H
      \        /     \
         C              C2H5
         ||
         O
```

Although certain newer herbicides show low systemic toxicity in laboratory animals, most are irritating to the skin, eyes, and the upper respiratory system. The acetanilids and acetamides have demonstrated severe skin sensitization reactions. Application formulations include petroleum distillates. Selected products are alachlor (Lasso), allidochlor (Randox), chloropropham, propachlor (Ramrod), and propanil (Stam, Propanex).

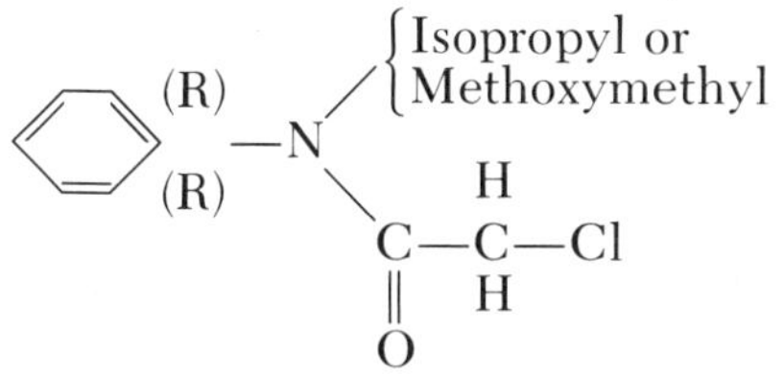

```
                          {Isopropyl or
              (R)        / {Methoxymethyl
  ⟨phenyl⟩       —N
              (R)        \       H
                          C—C—Cl
                          ||   H
                          O
```

FUNGICIDES

Fruit trees, vegetable crops, and ornamentals, as well as germinating seeds, are subject to fungal attack unless protected. There are several classes of fungicides in common use. Sulfur, the earliest chemical used, still is available in a wettable powder or sold as "lime-sulfur" and is relatively nontoxic to man.

Fungicides include forms of copper and sulfur, mercury, complexes of cadmium, iron, manganese and zinc, along with a variety of organic compounds (common examples are disulfiram, ferbam, nabam, ziram, and zineb). Use of certain metallic compounds, especially mercurials, now is forbidden in many countries because of their toxicity.

Wood preservatives include three classes: creosote (evaporates slowly, insoluble in water), certain metallic salts (injected as water solution into wood), and other chemicals (inorganic solvents).

Creosote

Creosote is an oily distillate obtained from either coal or wood tar and is a mixture of more than 150 compounds. Coal-tar creosote or creosote oil is used mainly as a wood preservative to protect against fungi, shipworms, and termites. About 100 million kg are used in the United States to pressure-impregnate building lumber, factory floor blocks, pilings, and telephone poles.

Creosote is highly toxic to wood-destroying organisms and has a low rate of evaporation. The National Institute for Safety and Health has recommended a 0.1 mg/cu m permissible limit for an eight-hour TWA exposure.

Creosote can be absorbed through the skin and is extremely irritating to human skin. Vapors can produce an intense burning sensation of the mucous membranes of the eyes and upper respiratory system. Eye injuries include conjunctivitis, keratitis, and corneal scarring. To be noted is that treated wood retains creosote for more than 25 years; therefore, caution is advised in handling and sawing old creosoted lumber (much heat is generated from the saw cutting teeth, increasing vapor production as well as throwing off much dust and particles of wood, easily lodging on skin and in clothing and creating inhalation exposure hazards and danger to the eyes). Suitable clothing and eye protection are necessary as well as wash-up facilities for workers. Other than conservative therapy and prevention of secondary skin infection, there is no satisfactory treatment for creosote irritation.

Pentachlorophenol

The TLV is 0.5 mg/cu m.

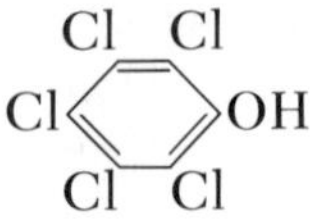

This compound is used as a fungicide and for slime control in the manufacture of paper pulp. It is also used in the United States for agricultural seed treatment and as a wood preservative against termites, molds, and wood-boring insects. Pentachlorophenol is used as a preharvest defoliant and a general herbicide. It is readily absorbed through the skin and by inhalation. Other nonpesticide uses include processing of glues, oils, leather, paints, and textiles, and it has been incorporated into certain shampoos.

Exposure can cause irritation to the eyes and upper respiratory system, and prolonged skin exposure causes an acneiform dermatitis. Hyperpyrexia and an increase in metabolic rate have been shown in humans following systemic absorption. Human exposure to dust or mist concentrations of 1 mg/cu m or more causes discomfort in the nose and throat, along with violent sneezing and coughing. As little as 0.3 mg/cu m has caused nose irritation, but workers have become inured to concentrations up to 2.4 mg/cu m. Because this substance easily penetrates intact skin and the systemic concentration is cumulative, fatalities have been reported. Symptoms of intoxication are anorexia, sweating, weight loss and weakness, as well as headache, dizziness, nausea, vomiting, dyspnea, and chest pain. Body temperature has been observed as extremely high, and death has occurred as early as three hours after onset of symptoms, with risk of serious intoxication increased during hot weather, according to Bergner et al.[10] Acneiform dermatitis has been reported with chronic low-level dermal exposures in ten workers engaged in production of this compound for five to ten months. Also, widely disseminated skin eruptions were noted by Baader and Bauer[7] in their case reports describing small and large furuncles and brown pigmentation. Some workers were reported to develop severe bronchitis. More than a year following cessation of exposure, all but one worker showed signs of extensive acne and four still complained of bronchitis. Urinary pentachlorophenol analysis may prove helpful in diagnosis, but knowledge and history of work exposure to the substance is required.

In a plant manufacturing pentachlorophenol, Glauser[35] described "a complete plant study" of 305 workers, emphasizing use of the blood chemistry profile ("SMA 24"), and noted 45 workers with "two or more abnormalities" with low-level exposures to pentachlorophenol. Glauser reported exposures to be within the TLV, although no measurements were presented. There were no clinical illnesses, no chloracne, and BUN and creatinine levels and renal clearances were normal. Eight of 145 nonexposed workers had similar abnormal findings. The workplace was improved by engineering controls.

A strongly acidic phenol, pentachlorophenol is mainly excreted unchanged in human urine. Urinary concentrations of pentachlorophenol above 10 mg/L may be considered an indicator of excess absorption. Tetrachlorohydroquinone is also excreted in the urine of workers exposed to pentachlorophenol.[1] (Additional discussion on related substances is presented in Chapter 47.)

Copper Compounds

Copper (cupric) sulfate is used as an algicide and fungicide. This substance is a relatively nontoxic chemical; reports of irritation or other toxic effects from occupational exposure are lacking. Copper 8-hydroxyquinoline is a greenish yellow crystalline powder used as a fungicide in the treatment of textiles, but also used in paper and wood preservation and in agriculture. There is no established TLV.

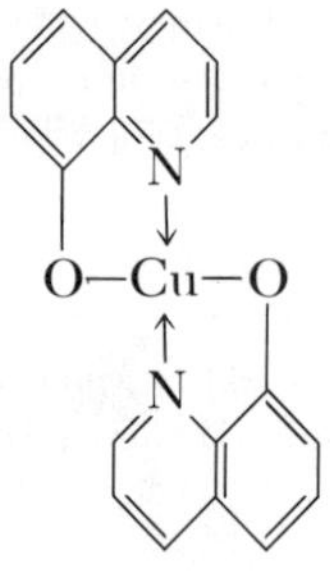

It is found in many interior paints as a protection against fungus where mercurial compounds cannot be used because of their toxicity. In the United States it is approved for use as a fungicide on wooden containers that may have contact with food products, beverage boxes, field crates, hampers, pallets, and wooden containers for fruits and vegetables. The minor uses include incorporation into plastics and paper. Generally, it is used in liquid concentrates or pastes, containing from 0.25% to 10% of the main material and 5%–30% in pastes. With liquid concentrate use, copper 8-hydroxyquinoline may be used in combination with 17% pentachlorophenol and 2.5% tetrachlorophenol. Other uses are for textile treatment of fabrics, webbing and cordage, rope and threads, and fishing nets. No occupational health problems resulting from exposure have been reported.

Ferbam

The TLV is 10 mg/cu m.

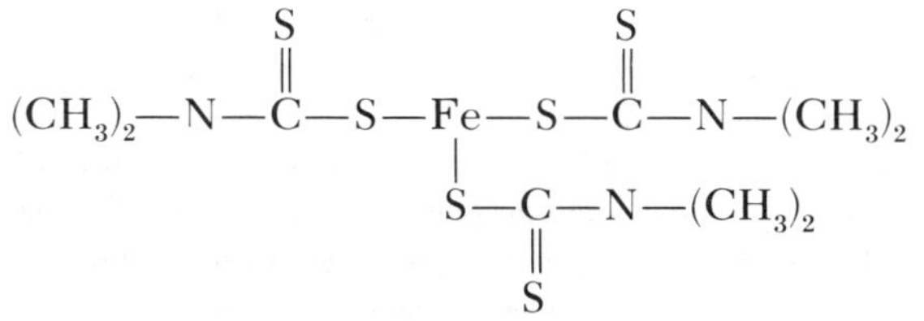

$$(CH_3)_2{-}N{-}\overset{\overset{\displaystyle S}{\|}}{C}{-}S{-}\underset{\underset{\displaystyle S{-}\underset{\underset{\displaystyle S}{\|}}{C}{-}N{-}(CH_3)_2}{|}}{Fe}{-}S{-}\overset{\overset{\displaystyle S}{\|}}{C}{-}N{-}(CH_3)_2$$

In humans, the dust is irritating to the eyes and respiratory tract; it can cause dermatitis in individuals sensitized to sulfur compounds. Large oral doses cause gastrointestinal disturbances. Ten of 20 rats died from a diet containing 0.5% ferbam for 30 days; there was a slight and ill-defined tendency toward anemia. At autopsy there was no evidence of a regularly appearing tissue injury; minor abnormalities of the lung, liver, kidney, and bone marrow were observed in a few animals.[52]

Thiram

The TLV is 5 mg/cu m.

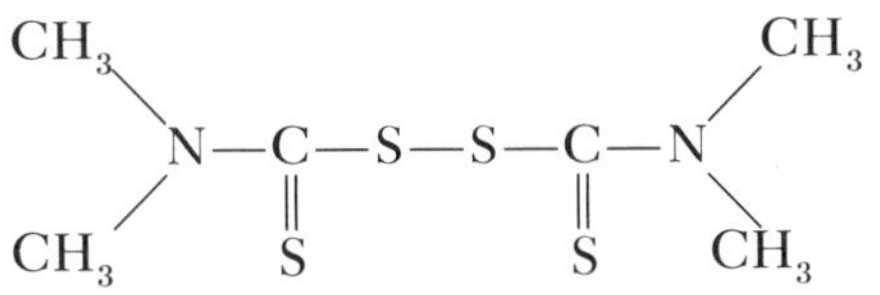

$$(CH_3)_2N{-}\underset{\underset{\displaystyle S}{\|}}{C}{-}S{-}S{-}\underset{\underset{\displaystyle S}{\|}}{C}{-}N(CH_3)_2$$

Thiram (tetramethylthiuram disulfide) dust is an irritant to the respiratory tract, eyes, and skin and causes sensitization dermatitis. Thiram was teratogenic (causing skeletal malformations) in hamsters given a single oral dose of 250 mg/kg during the period of organogenesis and in mice given oral doses of 5–30 mg daily between days 6 and 17 of pregnancy.[116, 120] In exposed humans, sensitization dermatitis in the form of eczema has occurred on the hands, forearms, and feet.[121] Ingestion of ethanol by workers exposed to thiram has caused a rapid skin response of a nonallergic nature characterized by flushing, erythema, pruritus, and urticaria (see Chapter 14).

FUMIGANTS

A fumigant is a substance or mixture of substances that produces a gas, vapor, fume, or smoke intended to destroy insects, bacteria, or rodents.

Fumigants may be solids, volatile liquids, or substances already in the gaseous state. They may be used to disinfect the interiors of buildings, objects, and materials that can be enclosed so as to retain or entrap the fumigants.

Other chemicals used as insecticides and as fumigants are acrylonitrile, calcium cyanide (cyanogas), carbon disulfide, carbon tetrachloride, dichlorobenzene, ethylene dibromide, ethylene dichloride, hydrogen cyanide, naphthalene, and sulfur dioxide. Since these substances are widely used in industry for other purposes and occupational exposures are common, a more detailed discussion for selected compounds will be found in Chapter 14.

Methyl Bromide ($BrCH_3$)

The TLV is 5 ppm.

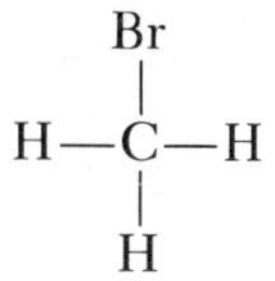

$$H{-}\underset{\underset{\displaystyle H}{|}}{\overset{\overset{\displaystyle Br}{|}}{C}}{-}H$$

Methyl bromide is also known as bromyl methane, Embafume, isobram, and monobromomethane. At room temperatures and normal pressures, it is a colorless gas, liquefying at 3° C, used chiefly as a fumigant-insecticide. It also is used as a rodenticide and in the synthesis of other chemicals and dyes. Because of its rapid action and significant toxicity, methyl bromide must be handled with special care. The vapor is more than three times as dense as air, and sometimes pockets of the gas may collect in low spots as well as poorly ventilated places. Occupational exposures may occur during fumigation of warehouses, storage areas, railroad cars, or buildings. Methyl bromide is used for preserving flour, cereals, rice, grain, seeds, dates, and nuts. Methyl bromide is commercially packed, compressed to a liquid, in various-sized metal containers for ease in handling and storage. The main routes of absorption are through inhalation and the skin. Contact with either the gas or liquid may induce eye irritation. Dry, scaling, and itching dermatitis may result from chronic but less concentrated exposures. The gas can act as a pulmonary irritant and also as a neurotoxin; high concentrations cause pulmonary edema and convulsions; chronic exposures have caused peripheral neuropathy.[51] Human intoxication arises from accidental occupational exposures and during use as a fumigant. The onset of toxic symptoms often is delayed, having a latency period of from 30 minutes to several hours. Initial symptoms may include malaise, headache, nausea, vomiting, visual disturbances, and, in some cases, eye irritation, dizziness, and tension tremors of the hands. Tremors may progress to twitchings and, in some instances, to convulsions. Greenburg[42] reported convulsions of the jacksonian type, first restricted to one extremity but gradually spreading to the entire body. Severe exposure has caused pulmonary edema, and tubular damage to the kidneys has been reported in fatal cases. Concentrations estimated to have caused human fatalities have ranged from 8,000 ppm for a few hours' exposure to 60,000 ppm for shorter exposures. Hine[51] has reported that those who have recovered from severe intoxications have had persistent central nervous system defects, including vertigo, anxiety, depression, hallucinations, and inability to concentrate.

Kantarjian and Shaheen[69] reported that eight of 14 workers repeatedly exposed to the vapor (concentration unmeasured) for three months developed peripheral neuropathy, but all recovered within six months after exposure ceased. Hine[51] observed that the determination of bromide in human blood for the purpose of estimating degree of exposure has been inconsistent. Blood bromide levels are not recommended for routine monitoring of occupational exposure.

Verberk et al.[134] studied 33 men employed in soil disinfection inside greenhouses using only methyl bromide, applied from fumigating tubes (23 workers) or from cans (ten men). Slight electroencephalographic changes were found in ten workers and a small increase in serum transaminases was found that could not be related to bromine concentration in the blood.

Workers dispensing methyl bromide, checking on concentration, or using the compound must wear approved respiratory protective equipment and must not work alone. Periodic medical examinations are advisable for employees regularly working with methyl bromide, with emphasis on the respiratory and neurologic systems.

All contaminated clothing must be promptly removed and the contaminated skin should be rapidly and thoroughly washed. (*Special admonition:* methyl bromide can penetrate ordinary rubber gloves. Therefore, adequate protective equipment [polyvinyl alcohol, neoprene, or nitrile latex composition] and instructions must be provided in advance to all workers.) Special therapy must be directed to prevent acidosis, pulmonary edema, bronchial spasm, respiratory paralysis, and/or kidney failure.

Sulfuryl Fluoride

The TLV is 5 ppm.

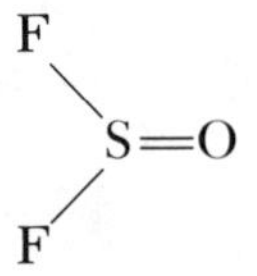

$$\begin{matrix} F \\ & \searrow \\ & & S{=}O \\ & \nearrow \\ F \end{matrix}$$

Sulfuric oxyfluoride, trade name Vikane (SO_2F_2), is a colorless, odorless gas used as an insect fumigant, with occupational exposure occurring by inadvertent inhalation. This compound is a central nervous system depressant and a pulmonary irritant. Taxay[129] described findings in a worker exposed to an unknown concentration of a mixture of sulfuryl fluoride and 1% chloropicrin for four hours who developed nausea, vomiting, abdominal pain, pleuritis with diffuse rhonchi, and paresthesia of the right leg, all rapidly subsiding after pulmonary exposure. The exact role of the sulfuryl fluoride was not known, but the cyanotic symptoms are those expected of chloropicrin overexposure. Limited other human exposure has been reported; by analogy, its toxicity has been derived from animal studies. High but unspecified concentrations of the gas to exposed animals caused signs of narcosis and, in some animals, tremors, convulsions, and pulmonary edema; with repeated exposure, lung and kidney damage was found. Animal exposures of 1,000 ppm for three hours or of 15,000 ppm for six minutes were fatal to fewer than 5% of animals tested. The oral LD_{50} for rats and guinea pigs was 100 mg/kg. There are no special tests, and strict work controls to prevent exposure are necessary.

Phosphine Fumigants

The phosphine fumigants are aluminum phosphide (Celphos, delicia, phostoxin). These compounds are highly toxic on inhalation; the main target organs are the lungs. Phosphine (PH_3), a colorless gas, is an insecticide fumigant also known as hydrogen phosphide, phosphorated hydrogen, and phosphorus trihydride. Phosphine has a fishy or garlic-like odor, detectable at about 2 ppm, but this odor threshold does not provide sufficient warning of toxic exposure. The 1979 ACGIH TLV for phosphine is 0.3 ppm for an eight-hour TWA exposure.

Jones et al.[67] described findings in workers engaged in wheat fumigation with aluminum phosphide who were exposed intermittently to concentrations up to 35 ppm but averaging below 10 ppm and who complained of nausea, vomiting, diarrhea, chest tightness, cough, headache, and dizziness, but no evidence of cumulative effects was noted.

Harger and Spolyar[45] reported that single severe exposures caused similar symptoms and signs, as well as excessive thirst, muscle pains, chills, sensation of pressure in the chest, dyspnea, syncope, and stupor, and, in some cases, dizziness and staggering gait. Since 1900, 59 cases of phosphine poisoning, with 26 deaths, have been reported, and the most frequently seen effect was marked pulmonary edema. If it is known that phosphine has been inhaled, immediate hospitalization is recommended for observation for up to 72 hours to guard against delayed onset of pulmonary edema. There are no specific tests for use in diagnosis.

ARSENICALS (INORGANIC)

The TLV for arsenic and compounds (as arsenic) is 0.2 mg/cu m for an eight-hour TWA.

$$O{=}As{-}O{-}As{=}O$$

Arsenic Trioxide

$$K{-}O{-}As{=}O$$

Potassium Arsenite

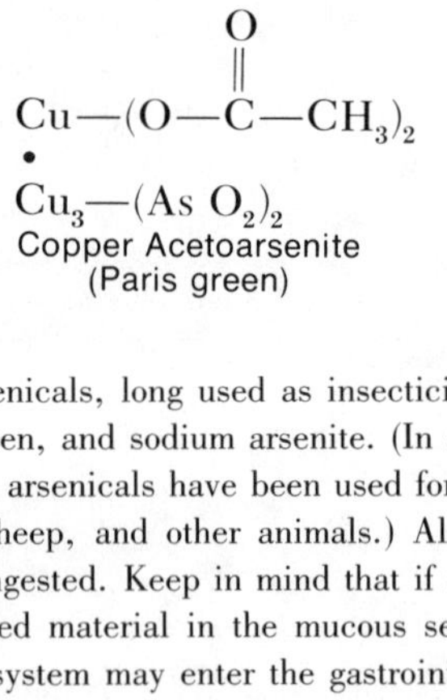

$$\begin{matrix} & & O & \\ & & \| & \\ Cu{-}(O & {-} & C & {-}CH_3)_2 \\ \bullet \\ Cu_3{-}(As\ O_2)_2 \end{matrix}$$

Copper Acetoarsenite
(Paris green)

Inorganic arsenicals, long used as insecticides, include lead arsenate, Paris green, and sodium arsenite. (In addition to use as insecticides, these arsenicals have been used for control of worms in cattle, goats, sheep, and other animals.) All are highly toxic when inhaled or ingested. Keep in mind that if inhalation occurs, accumulated inhaled material in the mucous secretions from the upper respiratory system may enter the gastrointestinal system by normal swallowing of the mucus. Prolonged overexposure to lead arsenate can cause arsenic and/or lead intoxication. With acute intoxication, symptoms and signs of arsenic intoxication usually predominate. With chronic exposure to lead arsenate, symptoms of lead poisoning may occur. The effects of acute arsenic poisoning are nausea, vomiting, diarrhea, inflammation and ulceration of the mucous membranes, and kidney damage. Chronic effects of arsenic poisoning are increased pigmentation and keratinization of skin, patchy dermatitis, and epidermoid carcinoma.[94]

Ingestion rarely is encountered during occupational exposure, but symptoms may occur 30 minutes to many hours after ingestion. In addition to those symptoms mentioned earlier, there may be bloody diarrhea later; colicky pains in the abdomen, thirst, dizziness, dehydration, muscle cramps and cyanosis may occur, as well as toxic effects leading to delirium and convulsions. Eventually, marked weakness, shock, muscle paralysis, liver and kidney damage, and death due to circulatory failure occur.

Diagnosis of arsenic intoxication requires an accurate history of the substances inhaled or ingested. Analysis of urine has indicated a great variation in levels of excreted arsenic. Some studies have reported that 0.7–1.0 mg/L in the urine of exposed workers may be considered an indication of exposure. However, dietary factors may confound these urinary levels of arsenic, since certain seafoods, especially shellfish, are high in arsenic content. The analytic procedures for arsenic are difficult to perform, and not all laboratories can perform such analyses. If severe arsenic intoxication is diagnosed, BAL (British anti-Lewisite compound) is valuable in treatment (promptly administered BAL intramuscularly as a 10% solution in vegetable oil).

The recommended dosage schedule is presented in Table 46–4.

The NIOSH has designated arsenic and its compounds as human carcinogens and has recommended restricting employee arsenic exposure to the lowest level that can be reliably measured (0.002 mg/cu m for a 15-minute duration). No increase of urinary arsenic above the "background" level (100 μg/L) is to be permitted. Arsenic determination in hair is considered unreliable for monitoring worker exposure, since it is difficult to distinguish between externally deposited arsenic and that systemically incorporated.(See Chapter 31 for further details.)

RODENTICIDES

Rodenticides are preparations intended for the control of rats, mice, gophers, porcupines, and closely related animals (such as rabbits). Rodenticide chemicals include Pival, warfarin, ANTU, sodium fluoroacetate, strychnine, and thallium.

Warfarin

The TLV is 0.1 mg/cu m.

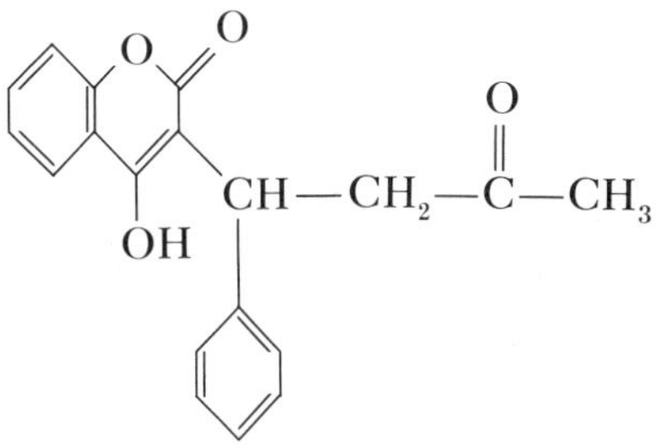

Warfarin ($C_{19}H_{16}O_4$) is a colorless, odorless, and tasteless crystalline-like substance, most commonly absorbed into the body by inhalation and skin absorption. Its usefulness as a rodenticide is its inherent ability to cause hypoprothrombinemia and vascular injury, resulting in hemorrhages. Warfarin is known to suppress the liver formation of prothrombin and other factors essential for blood clotting. A marked reduction of prothrombin activity of the blood also occurs as well as dilatation and engorgement of blood vessels, with an increase in capillary fragility. There is a latency period of several days following absorption, and acute ingestion reveals hemorrhage or depression of plasma prothrombin. Fristedt and Sterner[33] reported a farmer who had skin exposure of a 0.5% solution of warfarin over a period of 24 days and developed gross hematuria two days following the last contact with the solution. He developed spontaneous hematomas on the arms and legs. Within four days, other effects were noted, such as epistaxis, hemorrhages of the palate and mouth, and bleeding from the lower lip. After appropriate treatment, normal blood findings occurred.

Flint[32] reported a potentially dangerous drug interaction between cimetidine (trademark name Tagamet in the United States) and warfarin (Coumadin, Panwarfarin, and others). Of 17 patients stabilized on warfarin, their prothrombin time increased by 20% when 1 gm daily of cimetidine, a drug used to treat peptic ulcers, was added to the drug regimen. With increasing prescribing of cimetidine, those following workers stabilized on warfarin must be warned to watch for early signs of bleeding, such as easy bruising, bleeding gums, or dark stool.

TABLE 46–4.
Recommended Dosage Schedule for the Treatment of Arsenic Intoxication With BAL*†

	MILD POISONING	SEVERE POISONING
Days 1 and 2	2.5 mg/kg q6hr × 8 doses	3.0 mg/kg q4r × 12 doses
Day 3	2.5 mg/kg q12 hr × 2 doses	3.0 mg/kg q6hr × 4 doses
Succeeding 10 days	2.5 mg/kg q24hr × 10 doses	3.0 mg/kg q12hr × 20 doses

*From Morgan DP: *Recognition and Management of Pesticide Poisoning.* Washington, DC, US Environmental Protection Agency, Office of Pesticide Programs, 1982.

†CAUTION: *Dimercaprol* can cause troublesome side effects (hypertension, tachycardia, nausea, headache, paresthesias and pain, lacrimation, sweating, anxiety, and restlessness). Although usually not so severe as to handicap treatment, these manifestations may require antihistaminic therapy for adequate control.

Pival

The TLV is 0.1 mg/cu m.

Pival, 2-pivalyl-1,3-indandione ($C_{14}H_{14}O_3$), a yellow powder, also labeled Pindone, Pivalyl Valone, and Triban, is commonly used as a rat killer. Pival is a vitamin K antagonist, inhibiting prothrombin formation, resulting in hemorrhages. In rats, ingestion of a single large dose causes death due to multiple internal hemorrhages. There have been no reports of effects in man. If accidental ingestion occurs, the symptoms and signs are anticipated to be similar to those caused by warfarin, which may include hematuria, spontaneous hematomas on the arms and legs, epistaxis, bleeding from the lips, punctate hemorrhages from mucous membranes, abdominal and back pain, vomiting, blood in the feces, petechial rash, and abnormal blood findings, such as increased prothrombin time and blood plasma, blood in urine and feces, and hypochromic and microcytic anemia. Hypoprothrombinemia may be treated with vitamin A_1 or parenteral injections of aquamephyton or similar products—20–40 mg, repeatable every four hours until the prothrombin time returns to normal.[11]

Antu

The TLV is 0.3 mg/cu m.

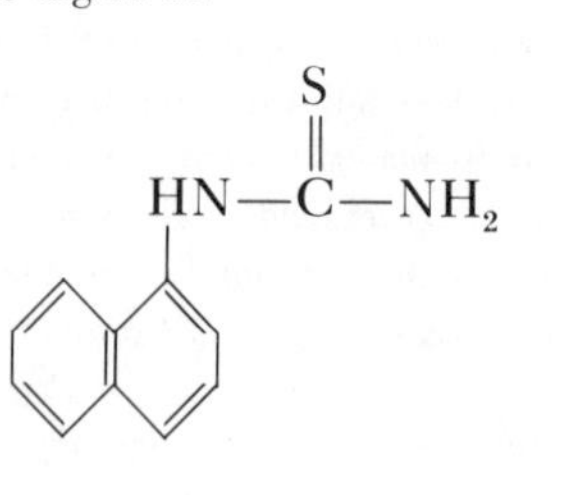

S
||
HN—C—NH_2

ANTU (α-naphthyl-thiourea) is a blue or grayish rodenticide powder, and exposure may occur by inhalation but most commonly by ingestion; occupational exposures are rare. ANTU dust may cause pulmonary edema and pleural effusion in animals. Accidental ingestion in humans has shown that the lethal dose is about 4 gm/kg. Intoxication in man has been reported in one case, by accidental ingestion involving 80 gm of a rat poison containing 30% ANTU. Signs were vomiting, dyspnea, cyanosis, and pulmonary rales, without evidence of pleural effusion, the pulmonary signs clearing on supportive therapy.[80]

Sodium Fluoroacetate

The TLV is 0.05 mg/cu m.

Sodium fluoroacetate (CH_2FCOON_a) is a fine white rodenticide powder, commonly known as Compound 1080, fluoroacetic acid, or sodium monofluoroacetate. Exposure may occur through inhalation, skin absorption, and ingestion. This is one of the most acutely toxic substances known to man, causing convulsions and ventricular fibrillation. The lethal oral dose in humans has been estimated to be 5 mg/kg. Fluoroacetate is metabolized to fluorocitrate, inhibiting the oxidation of acetate in the tricarboxylic acid cycle. On accidental poisoning, symptom onset may occur within 30 minutes or up to two hours, with central nervous system effects noted as apprehension, tingling sensation of the nose, numbness of the face, facial twitching, vomiting, auditory hallucinations, and, in severe instances, epileptiform convulsions. There are no special tests to detect this compound in man. Rigid precautions and instructions must be used in handling this compound.[46, 47]

Strychnine

The ACGIH TLV is 0.15 mg/cu m.

Strychnine ($C_{21}H_{22}N_2O_2$), a white crystalline powder, is commonly used as a poison bait for the larger animals. Human exposure may occur through inhalation but more commonly by accidental ingestion. Strychnine is a poison well known to act as a potent and long-lasting convulsant. The human lethal oral dose has been estimated to vary between 100 and 120 mg. Symptoms following ingestion may occur within 10–30 minutes and include stiffness of face and neck muscles, exaggerated reflexes, and excitability. Convulsions may ensue rapidly along with cyanosis. Without prompt treatment, convulsions may be followed by an asphyxic death. If it is known that strychnine has been swallowed and the person is conscious, vomiting may be induced unless convulsions are imminent. Treatment consists of supportive therapy, such as artificial resuscitation, oxygen, and endotracheal intubation. Convulsions may be controlled with diazepam or sodium phenobarbital given intravenously or intramuscularly. Sensory stimulation must be reduced by keeping the poisoned subject in a quiet, warm, and darkened room, with hospital observation imperative.[37]

Thallium Compounds

The TLV for soluble thallium compounds is 0.1 mg/cu m.

The thallium salts have had long-standing use as a rodenticide and may be inhaled or absorbed through the skin, with most common poisonings occurring through accidental ingestion. Toxic effects are primarily on the nervous system, but occupational exposures are rare and usually have not been fatal.

Thallium salts are used less frequently in the United States because of the known severe toxicity. Richeson[113] studied 15 workers who had handled organic thallium salt solutions over a 7½ year period, finding that six workers presented some form of thallium intoxication, the chief complaints being abdominal pain, fatigue, weight loss, pain in the legs, and nervous irritability. Three workers displayed albuminuria and one had hematuria. Thallium may be detected in the urine but is not a conclusive indicator of true systemic absorption. There is no good form of treatment; therefore, exposure prevention is mandatory. (See Chapter 45 for additional details.)

NATURALLY OCCURRING INSECTICIDES

Nicotine

The TLV is 0.5 mg/cu m.

Nicotine — 1-methyl-2-(1 pyridyl)pyrrolidine—is a liquid insecticide with high toxicity and rapid action ($C_{10}H_{14}N_2$). The route of entry is by inhalation, skin absorption, and ingestion. Nicotine causes a transient stimulation, followed by depression or paralysis of the central nervous system; it also directly stimulates smooth muscle. Many fatal human cases of nicotine intoxication have occurred, usually as a result of accidental or suicidal ingestion of nicotine insecticides. Nicotine is readily absorbed through the skin; in fatal cases of intoxication, death nearly always occurs within one hour and has occurred within one minute. The fatal adult dose is about 60 mg. Symptoms include nausea, salivation, abdominal pain, vomiting, diarrhea, cold sweat, headache, dizziness, disturbed hearing and vision, confusion, weakness, and incoordination. Initially, respiration is deep and rapid, blood pressure is elevated and the pulse is slow; intense vagal stimulation may cause transient cardiac standstill or paroxysmal atrial fibrillation; the pupils generally are constricted. Excitation of the central nervous system results in tremor and sometimes clonic-tonic convulsions. As central nervous system depression ensues, the pupils dilate, the blood pressure falls, and the pulse becomes rapid and often irregular; faintness, prostration, dyspnea, and paralysis of respiratory muscles are followed by death.[41] Recovery usually occurs if the victim survives one to four hours. Skeletal system malformations occurred in the offspring of pregnant mice injected subcutaneously with nicotine between days 9 and 11 of pregnancy.[103]

Pyrethrum

The TLV is 5 mg/cu m.

Pyrethrum is an insecticide obtained from flowers of the genus *Chrysanthemum* and is used as a dusting powder. Pyrethrum dust causes dermatitis and occasionally sensitization. In animals, effects of intoxication are excitation, convulsions, muscle fasciculations, and tetanic paralysis. The chief effect in humans from exposure to pyrethrum is dermatitis. The usual lesion is a mild erythematous dermatitis, with vesicles, papules in moist areas, and intense pruritus; a bullous dermatitis may develop.

In a study of workers engaged in processing pyrethrum powder, 30% had erythema, skin roughening, and pruritus, which subsided on cessation of exposure. One of these workers had an anaphylactic type of reaction; shortly after entering a dust-laden room, the facial skin turned red and the person felt a sensation of burning and itching; the cheeks and eyes rapidly became swollen; the pruritus became severe. The entire condition disappeared in two days after removal from exposure. Some persons exhibit sensitivity similar to pollinosis, with sneezing, nasal discharge, and nasal stuffiness. A few cases of asthma due to pyrethrum mixtures have been reported; some of the individuals involved had a previous history of asthma, with allergy to a wide spectrum of substances.[18]

Rotenone

The TLV is 5 mg/cu m.

Rotenone is the active constituent of the cube and derris plants and several other leguminous plants. It is highly toxic to insects but presents a relatively low hazard to mammals, making it a widely used insecticide. It is about one half as toxic as pyrethrum. Rotenone dust affects the nervous system and causes convulsions in animals. Animals repeatedly fed derris powder (the botanical source containing 9.6% rotenone) at levels from 312 to 4,000 ppm developed focal liver necrosis and mild kidney damage. Of 40 female rats given daily intraperitoneal injections of rotenone in sunflower oil of 1.7 mg/kg for 42 days, more than 60% developed mammary tumors 6–11 months after the end of treatment; most of the tumors were mammary adenomas and one was a differentiated adenocarcinoma; none of the control animals had tumors when examined 19 months after treatment.[39] The lethal oral dose in humans is estimated to be 0.3–0.5 gm/kg. In humans, inhalation of dust is suspected to cause pulmonary irritation. Symptoms of absorption in humans (inferred mostly from animal studies) may include numbness of oral mucous membranes, nausea, vomiting, and abdominal pain. There may be muscle tremors, incoordination, clonic convulsions, and stupor. The dust is irritating to the eyes and skin.

MISCELLANEOUS REPELLENT INSECTICIDES

Dibutyl Phthalate

The TLV is 5 mg/cu m.

Dibutyl phthalate ($C_{16}H_{22}O_4$) is used as the active ingredient in many insect repellents applied to the skin; it is also used as a plasticizer. Extensive experience with dibutyl phthalate as an insect repellent has shown that it is relatively nonirritating to the skin, eyes, and mucous membranes. Aerosols from heated dibutyl phthalate may cause irritation of the eyes and upper respiratory tract. In one report of a human case, accidental ingestion of 10 gm of this compound by a chemical operator produced nausea and dizziness, with lacrimation, photophobia, and conjunctivitis, but recovery was prompt and uneventful. Animal experiments to determine dermal and oral toxicity of dibutyl phthalate showed that extremely high doses were required to produce toxic effects. Dibutyl phthalate was found to be teratogenic by intraperitoneal injection in female rats.[123]

Dimethyl phthalate ($C_{10}H_{10}O_4$) is also used as a skin-applied insecticide, but it is slightly more irritating to the eyes and mucous membranes. (See Chapter 64 for greater clinical details.)

PRINCIPLES FOR CONTROLLING WORKPLACE HEALTH HAZARDS

The foundation for a comprehensive occupational health program is the continuing effort to ensure that workers and line and staff managers appreciate the impact of their actions on the overall health/safety performance of the organization. The successful program must integrate both industrial hygiene and medical aspects with other functions at all levels of the organization. One means of integration involves the formation of a "health and safety committee" composed of workers, line and staff facility managers, and occupational health professionals (nurse, physician, safety engineer, industrial hygienist, etc.).

The basic industrial hygiene principles involving the recognition, evaluation, and control of potential health hazards in the workplace are directly applicable to pesticide-handling situations (for specific details, refer to Fundamentals of Industrial Hygiene, National Safety Council[104]). Several specific items require additional emphasis.

Care must be taken to ensure that all potential routes of employee exposure to pesticides are evaluated and controlled.

A great majority of the pesticides can be readily absorbed through intact skin. In many cases where various routes of exposure have been quantified, skin absorption has much greater potential for exposure than inhalation. Therefore, care must be taken to minimize the frequency and duration of skin contact with these materials (Figs 46–5 and 46–6). Impervious protective clothing must be used whenever skin contact is likely. Suitable work clothing must be provided, with the employer responsible for its laundering. Contaminated work clothing can be cleaned at the facility or sent outside to a contract industrial laundry that has been informed of the potential hazards. Routine washing of hands, face and neck prior to breaks or lunch must be emphasized. Daily showers at the end of the work shift are required. Showers should be immediate for unplanned situations in which overt overexposures can occur such as spills or leaks.

Many pesticides also have significant oral toxicity and this route of exposure must be considered. Storage or consumption of food/cosmetics/smoking materials must not occur in unsanitary areas or work areas potentially contaminated with pesticides.

In most instances of pesticide manufacture, formulation, or use, several chemicals are present and therefore additive or synergistic toxic effects always must be considered. Also, the presence of many different chemicals and the use of the same equipment require care to be taken to eliminate significant cross-contamination from one product to another and to identify all containers as to contents.

Housekeeping procedures must be effective. Routine periodic decontamination procedures for both work areas and general areas (lunchroom, locker room, quality control labs, offices) should be initiated. Wet mopping or vacuum cleaning with a vacuum designed for handling toxic dusts is preferable to dry sweeping to minimize contamination. Swipe testing to evaluate the degree of surface contamination may be an important component of an overall contamination evaluation program.

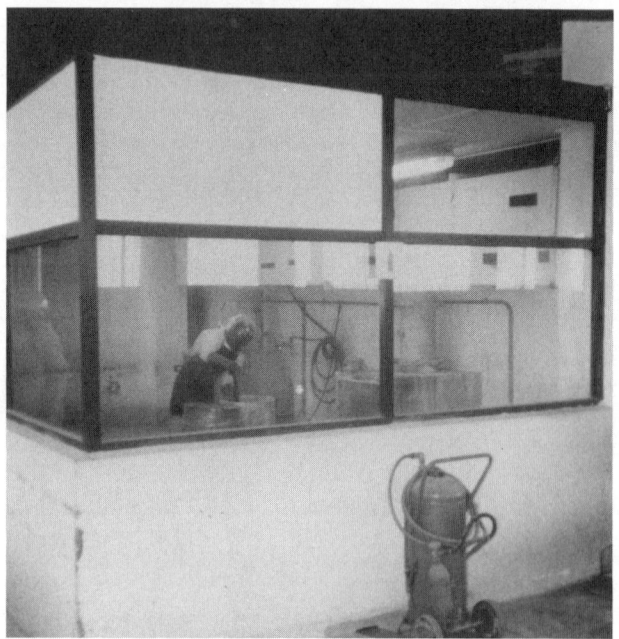

FIG 46–5.
A specially enclosed room permits the addition of a highly irritating component in a herbicide manufacturing plant (Cyanuric acid).

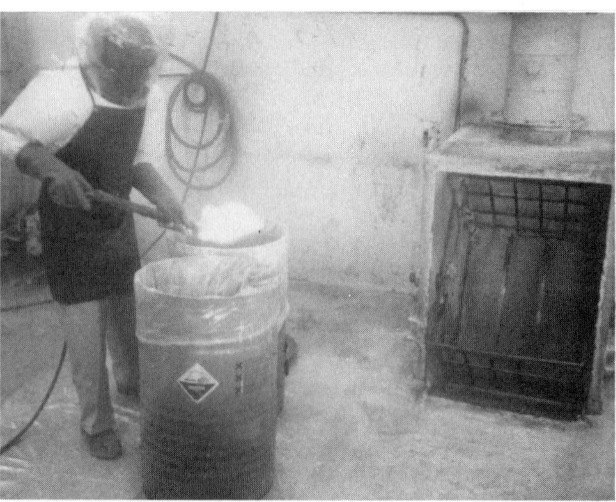

FIG 46–6.
A close-up of the hand-shoveling of cyanuric acid into the hopper. Note the air-supplied helmet provided for the worker for this delicate task. This substance has no TLV and is probably more irritating than methyl-isocyanate.

Effective control ultimately is composed of considering the health implications of a seemingly infinite number of details. This consideration can and should transcend "typical" industrial hygiene concerns and impact on related areas.

The potential health hazards associated with the performance of typical maintenance activities (welding, abrasive blasting, solvent cleaning) can be drastically increased if the equipment is potentially contaminated with a pesticide (Figs 46–7 and 46–8). The problem is further compounded if the work is being performed by an outside contractor.

Emergency planning for fires, explosions, spills, and leaks is mandatory if employees and the surrounding community are to be protected from untoward health effects (Fig 46–9). In this regard, a National Agricultural Chemicals Association brochure, *Pre-Fire Planning and Guidelines for Handling Agricultural Chemical Fires* is very informative.[90]

Effective 24-hour-a-day security prevents the entry of unauthorized personnel, such as vandals or juveniles, into areas where chemicals are stored or handled.

Environmental aspects of occupational exposures must be considered. Air-cleaning devices should be utilized on all exhaust ventilation systems. Waste materials, including empty containers, must be permanently disposed of in an environmentally secure manner.

Employee training should be designed to influence employees to comply with appropriate work practices. Such training should be conducted for all newly hired persons and periodically for all employees.

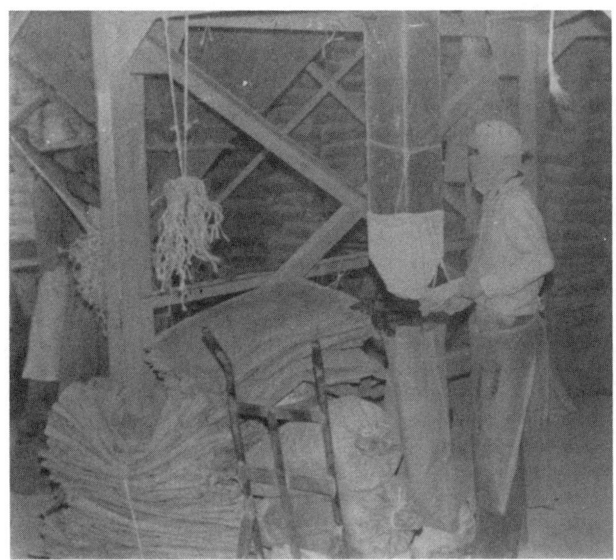

FIG 46–7.
Packaging pesticides in a small factory without worker protection of any kind (not unusual!).

Training should include the following areas:

1. Qualitative and quantitative identification of materials handled (Fig 46–10)

2. Potential risks of overexposure

3. Description of signs and symptoms that might occur

4. The importance of industrial hygiene and biologic monitoring and notification of test results

5. Description of work practice controls, including personal protective equipment (respirators, gloves, etc.)

6. First-aid and emergency training

The medical aspects of the occupational health program should parallel the ongoing industrial hygiene activities, since both are vital for a successful program. Preplacement medical examinations are important because they

1. Establish a baseline for each employee's health status

2. Identify preexisting illnesses or other conditions so that individuals can be placed in occupational settings consistent with their health and other physical capabilities

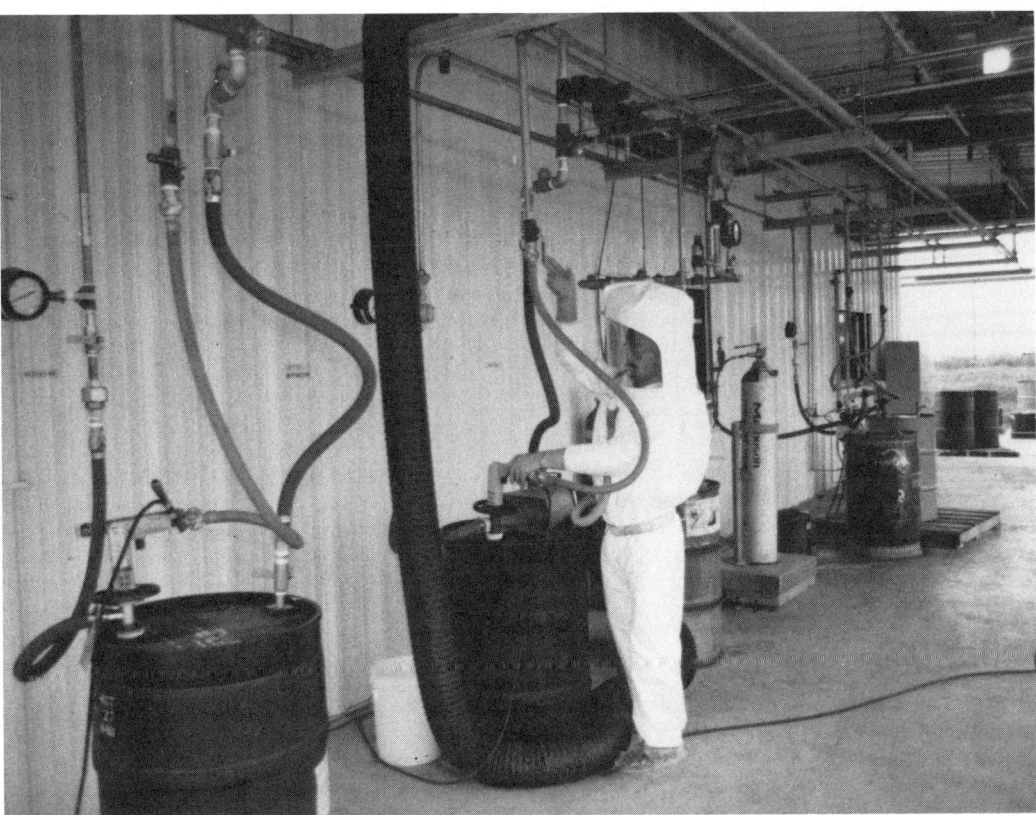

FIG 46–8.
Filling drums with concentrated insecticide showing modern controls.

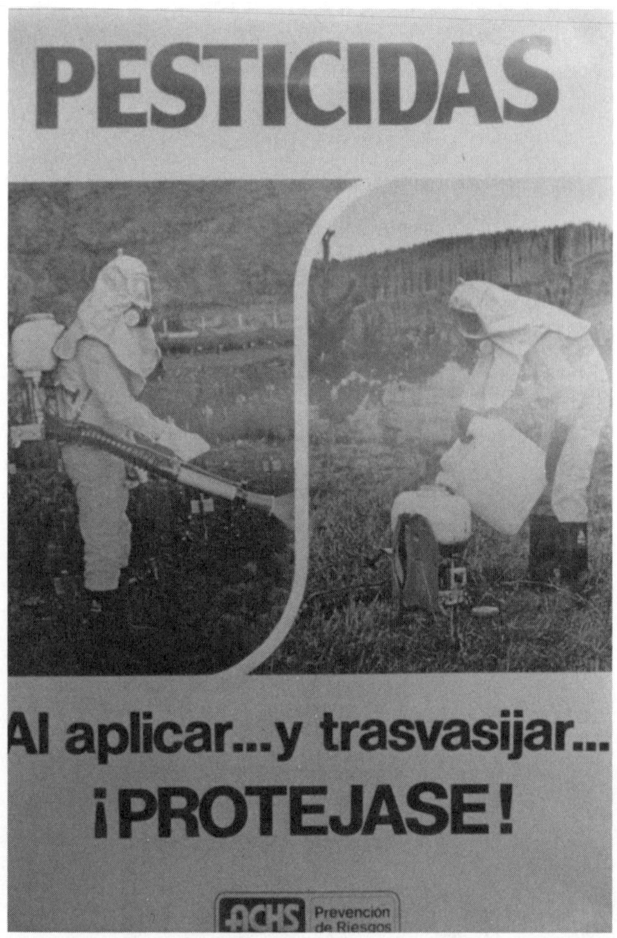

FIG 46–9.
An excellent education poster.

3. Provide a data base for determining incidence and prevalence of any adverse effects stemming from the job

The preplacement evaluation should include a comprehensive medical, family, and occupational history and a reproductive history, if indicated. The physical examination should be complete, and at the time of the examination the employer should provide the physician with a description of the employee's prospective job and identification of any hazards that might be encountered. The physician should order appropriate tests based on this information and the results of the physical examination. After a review of the type of work and any potential exposure, clinical tests such as urinalysis, pulmonary function, chest x-ray, liver enzyme determinations, complete blood count (CBC), and other tests may be carried out at the discretion of the responsible physician, but these tests need not be done routinely.[143, 146]

At the same time, a judgment of the worker's ability to use negative- and positive-pressure respirators may be made (see Chapter 14). If the person will be or has been exposed to the ChE-inhibiting pesticides as indicated in Table 46–1, red blood cell (RBC) ChE activity shall be measured for determination of a preexposure baseline.

"Preexposure baseline" for the RBC ChE is defined as the mean of two ChE activity determinations, each of which is derived from separate samples of blood taken at least one day apart after a period of at least 60 days without known exposure to any ChE-inhibiting compounds. If the determinations produce values differing by more than 15%, additional determinations on new samples must be performed until successive tests do not differ by more than 15%.

"Working baseline" for the ChE is defined as the mean of two ChE activity determinations, each of which is derived from a separate sample of blood taken at least one day apart and differing by no more than 15%, or the arithmetic mean of normal values for an appropriate control population of adults for that laboratory, whichever is higher. A "working baseline" is determined only for an individual whose work history does not permit a preexposure baseline to be determined as specified in this section.

"Mean or normal values" is defined as the arithmetic mean of ChE activities for healthy adults as determined by the laboratory's experience with repeated analyses.

Periodic examinations shall be made available on at least an annual basis and shall include at least:

1. Interim medical and work histories
2. Physical examination as described

Periodic measurement of RBC ChE activity shall be made available to workers exposed to organophosphate insecticides at more frequent intervals, depending on hygienic surveys. These intervals may be as frequently as every day or may be increased after three weekly determinations to testing as frequently as every eight weeks, based on the decision of the responsible physician after consideration of the following for each employee:

1. The degree of workplace contamination
2. The toxicity of the pesticides to which the employee may be exposed
3. The potential duration and concentration of the pesticide exposure
4. The state of health of the employee
5. The results of previous ChE determinations
6. The extent of ongoing workplace improvements

Each employee shall be given a copy of the results of his initial periodic test and of any special ChE test results as soon as possible after the test and an interpretation.

The scope of the examination is to be determined by the physician designated as the medical advisor for that plant. Community medical relationships must not be overlooked, and results of the examinations and attendant studies, whether clinically positive or negative, may be forwarded to the employee's personal physician.

During examinations, applicants or employees found to have medical conditions such as skin disease, chronic lung disease, or abnormalities of the central or peripheral nervous system that could be directly or indirectly aggravated by exposure to pesticides

VELSICOL **MATERIAL SAFETY DATA SHEET**

Revised 12/21/77 *"Essentially Similar" to U. S. Department of Labor Form, OSHA-20, Rev. May '72*

SECTION I IDENTIFICATION OF PRODUCT

MANUFACTURER'S NAME	EMERGENCY TELEPHONE NO.
Velsicol Chemical Corporation	(312) 670-4500
ADDRESS 341 E. Ohio Street, Chicago, Illinois 60611	
TRADE NAME AND SYNONYMS BANVEL Tech. Dicamba	
CHEMICAL NAME AND SYNONYMS 2-methoxy-3, 6-dichlorobenzoic acid	
CHEMICAL FAMILY Organic herbicide	MOLECULAR FORMULA $C_8H_6Cl_2O_3$

SECTION II HAZARDOUS COMPONENTS OF MIXTURES

COMPONENT	%	THRESHOLD LIMIT VALUE (UNITS)	COMPONENT	%	THRESHOLD LIMIT VALUE (UNITS)

Technical Banvel

Acute oral LD_{50} (rats) 1707 mg/kg
Acute dermal LD_{50} (rabbits) 200 mg/kg
Acute inhalation LD_{50} > 9.6 mg/l (4-hour exposure)
Not a skin irritant but extremely irritating and corrosive to the eye

SECTION III PHYSICAL DATA

BOILING POINT (°F.)			SPECIFIC GRAVITY (H_2O=1)	30°C (86°F)	1.565
VAPOR PRESSURE (mm Hg)	100°C (212°F)	3.75 x 10	PERCENT VOLATILE BY VOLUME(%)		
VAPOR DENSITY (AIR=1)		7.64	EVAPORATION RATE (______=1)		
SOLUBILITY IN WATER		0.5%	Melting Point °F (900-100°C)		194-212
APPEARANCE AND ODOR	Light tan granular solid—practically odorless.				

SECTION IV FIRE AND EXPLOSION HAZARD DATA

FLASH POINT Does not flash.	FLAMMABLE LIMITS BY VOLUME (%)	LOWER	UPPER

FIRE-EXTINGUISHING MEDIA
Fog or water spray, foam, carbon dioxide.

SPECIAL FIRE-FIGHTING PROCEDURES Wear full protective clothing, self-contained breathing apparatus. Use water spray to keep containers cool. Heat from fire can cause decomposition with the evolution of toxic and irritating fumes.

UNUSUAL FIRE AND EXPLOSION HAZARDS

(SEE OTHER SIDE)

96.30-030

FIG 46–10.
A sample material safety data sheet, which has widespread use throughout industry. *(Continued.)*

shall be counseled as to the possible increased risk of impairment of their health from working with certain substances. Employees should be further counseled about reproductive effects that have been noted in male workers and in laboratory animals involving certain pesticides, pointing out that the significance to humans of the effects in laboratory animals are not fully known but that they do indicate that exposure should be minimized, particularly in men and women of reproductive age. As has been discussed in preceding chapters, residues of some organochlorine (OC) and carbamate pesticides have been found in human breast milk.

The NIOSH recommends that a complete examination, including all findings, shall be offered to all employees within one month after employment ends. All medical and hygienic records should be kept for at least 30 years.

One of the most important responsibilities of an agricultural chemicals manufacturer is to provide correct instructions on how

SECTION V HEALTH HAZARD DATA
THRESHOLD LIMIT VALUE Has not been established.
EFFECTS OF OVEREXPOSURE Nonspecific. Severe eye injury can occur. "Skin irritation may occur when handling finely ground material."
EMERGENCY AND FIRST AID PROCEDURES EYE CONTACT: Flush with water for at least 15 minutes; get prompt medical attention. SKIN CONTACT: Wash with mild soap and water. INGESTION: Induce vomiting, saline emetic; call a physician. INHALATION: Remove to fresh air.

SECTION VI REACTIVITY DATA			
STABILITY	UNSTABLE		CONDITIONS TO AVOID
	STABLE	XX	
INCOMPATIBILITY *(Materials to avoid)*			
HAZARDOUS DECOMPOSITION PRODUCTS Thermal decomposition may yield HCl, organochloride products, carbon monoxide, carbon dioxide.			
HAZARDOUS POLYMERIZATION	MAY OCCUR		CONDITIONS TO AVOID
	WILL NOT OCCUR	XX	

SECTION VII SPILL OR LEAK PROCEDURES
STEPS TO BE TAKEN IN CASE MATERIAL IS RELEASED OR SPILLED Contain spill, sweep and collect in drums; follow by thoroughly washing down with detergent and water. Collect washings; do not allow in drainage ditches or sewers.
WASTE DISPOSAL METHOD Controlled incineration, designated landfill, or disposal in accordance with applicable local, state and federal regulations.

SECTION VIII SPECIAL PROTECTION INFORMATION		
RESPIRATORY PROTECTION *(Specify type)* Low levels—MESA/NIOSH-approved chemical cartridge respirator for pesticides.		
VENTILATION	LOCAL EXHAUST	SPECIAL
	MECHANICAL *(General)*	OTHER
PROTECTIVE GLOVES Rubber gloves or the equivalent.	EYE PROTECTION Chemical goggles.	
OTHER PROTECTION EQUIPMENT Shower, daily change of clothing.		

SECTION IX SPECIAL PRECAUTIONS
PRECAUTIONS TO BE TAKEN IN HANDLING AND STORING Store in area away from seed fertilizers, insecticides or fungicides.
OTHER PRECAUTIONS Treat as with any pesticide. Self-contained breathing apparatus and protective clothing should be available in case of severe fire.

The information presented herein, while not guaranteed, was prepared by technically knowledgeable personnel and to the best of our knowledge is true and accurate. It is not intended to be all-inclusive and the manner and conditions of use and handling may involve other or additional considerations.

FIG 46–10 (cont.).

to handle and apply the products. The information must be readily available, easy to understand (in the language of the farmer or pest control operator), and must contain the necessary educational elements. It is imperative that these products be handled properly and that the correct dosages be applied. This means that the user must know the sensitivity and compatibility of his or her crop and the proper dosage of the crop-protection product and must follow the recommendations of the manufacturer to prevent potentially harmful effects in workers.

Acknowledgment

Grateful appreciation is given to Harvey V. Davis, Ph.D., for his support and advice.

GLOSSARY

Common Pesticides

COMMON NAME	CHEMICAL NAME	MAIN USES
Abate	0,0-dimethyl phosphorothioate 0,0-diester with 4,4′-thiodiphenol	insecticide
acrylonitrile	acrylonitrile	fumigant
alachlor	2-chloro-2′-6′ diethyl-*N*-(methoxy-methyl)-acetanilide	herbicide
aldrin	1,2,3,4,10,10-hexachloro-1,4,4a,5,8,8a-hexahydro-1,4-endoexo-5,8-dimethanonaphthalene	insecticide
allidochlor	*N,N*-diallyl-2-chloroaceteamide	herbicide
aluminum phosphide	aluminum phosphide	insect fumigant
Amiben	amino-2,5-dichlorobenzoic acid	herbicide
amitrole	3-amino-1,2,4-triazole	herbicide
ammonium sulfamate	ammonium amidesulfate	herbicide
ANTU	alpha-naphthyl-thiourea	rodenticide
atrazine	2-chloro-4-ethylamino-6-isopropylamine-s-ariazine	herbicide
azinphosmethyl	0,0-dimethyl S[4-oxo-1,2,3-benzotriazin-3, 4 methyl] phosphorodithioate	fungicide
Azodrin	3-hydroxy-*N*-methyl-cis-crotonamide dimethyl phosphate	insecticide
Baygon	0-isopropoxyphenyl methyl carbamate	insecticide
benomyl	methyl-1-(butylcarbamoyl)-2-benzimidazole-carbamate	fungicide
benzene hexachloride	1,2,3,4,5,6-hexachlorocyclohexane (mixture of isomers)	insecticide
Bidrin	3-hydroxy-*N,N*-dimethyl-cis-crotonamide dimethyl phosphate	insecticide
Binapacryl	2-sec-butyl-4,6-dinitrophenyl-3-methyl-2-buteneate	insecticide
borax	sodium biborate	fungicide, herbicide
Brassicol	pentachlorophenol	fungicide
bromacil	5-bromo-3-*sec*-butyl-6-methyluracil	herbicide
bromophos	0-(4-bromo-2,5-dichlorophenyl)-0,0-dimethylphosphorothioate	insecticide, acaricide
bromoxynil	4-hydroxy-3,5-dibromobenzonitrile	herbicide
butylate	S-ethyl diisobutylthiocarbamate	herbicide
Buvinol	mixture of TCPE and atrazine	herbicide
cacodylic acid	dimethylarsinic acid	herbicide, defoliant
calcium arsenite	mono-calcium arsenite	insecticide
calcium cyanide	calcium carbimide	herbicide
carbaryl	1-naphthyl-*N*-methylcarbamate	insecticide
carbofuran	2,3-dihydro-2,2-dimethyl-7-benzofuranyl methyl carbamate	insecticide, nematocide
carbon tetrachloride	CCl_4	fumigant
carbophenothion	S-((*p*-chlorophenylthio) methyl)-0,0-diethyl phosphorodithioate	acaricide, insecticide
Carzol	*N,N*-dimethyl, N′-(2-methyl-4 chlorophenyl)-formanidine	acaricide, insecticide
CDAA	*N,N*-diallyl-2-chloroacetamide	herbicide
chlordane	1,2,4,5,6,7,8,8-octachlor-2,3,3a,4,7,7a-hexahydro-4,7-methanoindane	insecticide
chlorophyrifos	0,0-diethyl 0-(3,5,6-trichloro-2-pyridyl) phosphorothioate	insecticide
chlorprophan	isopropyl *m*-chlorocarbanilate	herbicide
Chlorthion	0,0-dimethyl 0-(3-chloro-4-nitrophenyl) phosphorothioate	insecticide
copper-8-hydroxy-quinoline	copper (II) 8-quinolinol	fungicide
copper sulfate	cupric sulfate pentahydrate	fungicide, algicide
cryolite	sodium hexafluoroaluminate	insecticide
cube (root)	rotenone	insecticide
2,4-D	2,4 dichlorophenoxyacetic acid	herbicide
dalapan	2,2-dichloropropionic acid, sodium salt	herbicide
DBCP	1,2-dibromo-3-chloropropane	soil fumigant for nematode control
DDA	bis (chlorophenyl) acetic acid (degradation product of DDT)	
DDE	1,1-bis (*P*-chlorophenyl)-2,2-dichloroethylene (degradation product of DDT)	
DDT	1,1,1-trichloro-2,2-bis (chlorophenyl) ethane	insecticide

(continued)

GLOSSARY—*Continued*

Common Pesticides

COMMON NAME	CHEMICAL NAME	MAIN USES
DEF	S,S,S,-tributylphosphorotrithioate	defoliant
demeton	mixture of 0,0-diethyl S(and 0)-[2-(ethylthio) ethyl] phosphorothioates	insecticide
Dexon	sodium [4-(dimethylamino)phenyl] diazenesulfonate	soil fungicide, seed treatment
Diazinon	0,0-diethyl 0-(2-isopropyl-4-methyl-6-pyrimidyl) phosphorothioate	insecticide
dicamba	3,6-dichloro-0-anisic acid	herbicide
dicapthon	0-(2-chloro-4-nitrophenyl)-0,0-dimethyl phosphorothioate	insecticide
dichlone	2,3-dichloro-1,4-naphthoquinone	fungicide, herbicide
dichloropropene	1,3-dichloropropylene	soil fumigant, herbicide, insecticide, fungicide, nematocide
dichlorvos (DDVP)	0,0-dimethyl-2,2-dichlorovinyl phosphate	insecticide
dicofol	4,4′-dichloro-alpha-(trichloromethyl)-benzhydrol	insecticide
dieldrin	1,2,3,4,10,10-hexachloro-6,7-epoxy-1,4,4a,5,6,7,8,8a-octahydro-1,4-endoexo-5,8-dimethanonaphthalene	insecticide
dimethoate	0,0-dimethyl S-(*N*-methylcarbamylmethyl) phosphorodithioate	systemic acaricide, insecticide
dinitrocresol	4,6-dinitro-0-cresol	insecticide, herbicide
diphacinone	2-diphenylacetyl-1,3 indandione	rodenticide
diquat	1,1′-ethylene-2,2′-dipyridinium dibromide	herbicide, desiccant
disulfiram	bis(diethylthiocarbamoyl) disulfide	fungicide
disulfoton	0,0-diethyl S-[2-(ethylthio) ethyl]phosphorodithioate	insecticide
diuron	3-(3,4-dichlorophenyl)-1,1-dimethylurea	herbicide
DMPA	0-(2,4-dichlorophenyl)0′-methyl-*N*-isopropylphosphoroamidothioate	fly larvicide
DN-111	dicyclohexylamine salt of 2-cyclohexyl-4,6-dinitrophenol	insecticide
DNBP (dinitrobutylphenol)	2,4-dinitro-6-sec-butylphenol	herbicide, insecticide
DNOC	2-methyl-4,6 dinitro phenol	herbicide
2,4-DP (dichlorprop)	2-(2,4-dichlorophenoxy) propionic acid	herbicide
DSMA	disodium methanearsonate	herbicide
endosulfan	6,7,8,9,10,10-hexachloro-1,5,5a,6,9,-9a-hexahydro-6,9-methano-2,4,3-benzodioxathiepin-3-oxide	insecticide
endothall	7-oxabicyclo (2,2,1)heptane-2,3 dicarboxylic acid, sodium salt	herbicide
endrin	1,2,3,4,10,10-hexachloro-6,7-epoxy-1,4,4a,5,6,7,8,8a-octahydro-1,4-endo-endo-5,8-dimethanonaphthalene	insecticide
EPN	0-ethyl-0-*p*-nitrophenyl phenylphosphonothioate	insecticide
EPTC	S-ethyl-*n*,*n*-dipropylthiocarbamate	herbicide
ethion	0,0,0′,0′-tetraethyl S,S′-methylenebisphosphorodithioate	insecticide
ethylene dibromide	1,2-dibromoethane	fumigant, nematocide
ethylene dichloride	1,2-dichloroethane	insecticide
ethylene oxide	ethylene oxide	herbicide
ethyl formate	ethyl formate	fumigant
fenthion	0,0-dimethyl [0-4-(methylthio)-m-tolyl] phosphorothioate	acaricide, insecticide, bird control
fenuron	3-phenyl-1,1-dimethylurea	herbicide
ferbam	ferric dimethyldithiocarbamate	fungicide
Fumarin	3(a-acetonylfurfuryl)-4-hydroxycoumarin	rodenticide
Fumazone	1,2-dibromo-3-chloropropane	soil fumigant, nematocide
Haloxon	0,0-di-(2-chloroethyl)-0-3-chloro-4-methyl-coumarin-7-yl) phosphate	anthelmintic

(continued)

GLOSSARY—*Continued*

Common Pesticides

COMMON NAME	CHEMICAL NAME	MAIN USES
heptachlor	1,4,5,6,7,8,8-heptachloro-3a,3,7,7a-tetrahydro-4,7-endo-methanoindene	insecticide
hydrogen cyanide	hydrocyanic acid	insect fumigant
Kepone	decachlorooctahydro-1,3,4-metheno-2H-cyclobuta(cd)pentalene-2-one	insecticide
lead arsenate	diplumbic hydrogen arsenate	insecticide, fungicide
leptophos	0-(4-bromo-2,5 dichlorophenyl)-0-methylphenylphosphonothioate	insecticide
lime sulfur	30% calcium polysulfide and various small amounts of calcium thiosulfate plus water and free sulfur	acaricide, fungicide, insecticide
lindane	gamma isomer of 1,2,3,4,5,6-hexachlorocyclohexane of 99%	insecticide
linuran	3-(3,4-dichlorophenyl)-1-methoxy-1 methylurea	herbicide
malathion	S-[1,2-bis(ethoxycarbonyl) ethyl] 0,0-dimethyl phosphorodithioate	insecticide
maneb	manganese ethylene bisdithiocarbamate	fungicide
MCPA	4-chloro-2-methyl-phenoxyacetic acid	herbicide
MCPB	4-chloro-2-methylphenoxy butyric acid	herbicide
MCPP	2-(4,chloro-2-methyl-phenoxy) propionic acid	herbicide
Merphos	tributyl phosphorotrithioite	defoliant
metaldehyde	metaldehyde	insecticide
metalkamate	mixture of m-(ethylpropyl) phenyl methylcarbamate and m-(1-methylbutyl) phenyl carbamate in approximate ratio of 1:3	insecticide
methomyl	S-methyl-*N*-((methyl carbamoyl) oxy) thioacetimidate	insecticide, nematocide
methoxychlor	1,1,1-trichloro-2,2-bis (*p*-methoxyphenol) ethane	insecticide
methyl bromide	bromomethane	fumigant
methyl chloride	chloromethane	aerosol propellent
methyl formate	methyl formate	insect fumigant
methyl parathion	0,0-dimethyl 0-*p*-nitrophenyl phosphorothioate	insecticide
Methyl Trithion	S-[[(*p*-chlorophenyl) thio] methyl] 0,0-dimethyl phosphorodithioate	insecticide
mevinphos	methyl 3-hydroxy-alpha-crotonate dimethyl phosphate	insecticide
mipafox	*N,N′*-diisopropylphosphorodiamidicfluoride	insecticide
mirex	dodecachlorooctahydro-1,3,4-metheno-2H-cyclobuta[Cd] pentalene	insecticide
monuron	3-(*p*-chlorophenyl)-1,1-dimethylurea	herbicide
Morestan	6-methyl-2-oxo-1,3-dithio(4,5-b)quinoxaline	acaricide, fungicide
MSMA	monosodium methanearsonate	herbicide
nabam	disodium ethylene bisdithiocarbamate	fungicide
naled	1,2-dibromo-2,2-dichloroethyl dimethyl phosphate	insecticide
naphthalene	naphthalene	insecticide
neburon	3-(3,4-dichlorophenyl)-1-methyl-1-*n*-butylurea	herbicide
Nemacide	0-(2,4-dichlorophenyl)-0,0-diethyl ester of phosphorothionic acid	insecticide
nicotine	1-methyl-2-(1 pyridyl)pyrrolidine	insecticide
ovex	*p*-chlorophenyl *p*-chlorobenzene-sulfonate	insecticide
paradichlorobenzene	*p*-dichlorobenzene	insect fumigant
paraquat	1,1′-dimethyl-4-4′dipyridylium cation	herbicide
parathion	0,0-diethyl-0-*p*-nitrophenyl phosphorothioate	acaricide, insecticide
Paris green	copper acetoarsenite	insecticide
Patoran	4-(4-bromophenyl)-1-methyl-1′-methoxyurea	herbicide
pentachlorophenol	pentachlorophenol	herbicide, wood preservative, molluscicide
Perthane	1,1-dichloro-2,2-bis (*p*-ethylphenyl) ethane	insecticide
petroleum oils		acaricide, insecticide, herbicide

(continued)

GLOSSARY—*Continued*

Common Pesticides

COMMON NAME	CHEMICAL NAME	MAIN USES
phorate	0,0-diethyl S-[(ethylthio)methyl] phosphorodithioate	insecticide
phosphamidon	2-chloro-2-diethylcarbamoyl-1-methylvinyl dimethyl phosphate	insecticide
pindone	2-pinaloyl-1,3-indandione	rodenticide, insecticide
piperonyl butoxide	butyl carbitol (6-propyl piperonyl)ether	insecticide synergist
Pival	2-pivalyl-1,3 indandione	rodenticide
PMA	phenylmercuric acetate	fungicide, herbicide
propachlor	2-chloro-*N*-isopropylacetanilide	herbicide
propanil	3′,4′-dichloropionanilide	herbicide
propylene dichloride	1,2-dichloropropane	fungicide, herbicide, insecticide, nematocide, soil fumigant
propylene oxide	propylene oxide	insecticide synergist
pyrazon	5-amino-4-chloro-2-phenyl-3 (2H) pyriadazione	herbicide
pyrethrins	the active insecticidal constituents of pyrethrum	insecticide
pyrethrum	dalmation insect flowers	insecticide
red squill	inner bulb scales of *Urquinea maritima*	rodenticide
ronnel	0,0-dimethyl 0-(2,4,5-trichlorophenyl)-phosphorothioate	insecticide
rotenone	the primary active compound of derris and cube roots	insecticide
Ruelene	4-tert-butyl-2-chlorophenyl methyl methylphosphoramidate	insecticide
ryania	powdered stemwood of *Ryania speciosa*	insecticide
sabadilla	ground seeds of sabadilla containing veratrine, a complex mixture of alkaloids	insecticide
sarin	isopropylmethyl phosphonofluoridate	nerve gas
Silvex	2-(2,4,5-trichlorophenoxy)propionic acid	herbicide
Simazine	2-chloro-4,6-bis(ethylamino)-5-triazine	herbicide
Smithion	0,0-dimethyl 0-(4-nitro-m-tolyl) phosphorothioate	insecticide, space fumigant
sodium arsenite	sodium meta-arsenite	herbicide, insecticide, poison bait ingredient
sodium chlorate	sodium chlorate	herbicide (desiccant)
sodium fluoroacetate	sodium monofluoroacetate	rodenticide
sodium *N*-methyldithiocarbamate	sodium *N*-methyldithiocarbamate	fungicide, herbicide, nematocide
Strobane	terpene polychlorinates	insecticide
strychnine	nux vomica alkaloid	rodenticide; used in poison baits for birds, moles and other rodents
sulfur (brimstone)	sulfur	acaricide, fungicide
sulfuryl fluoride	sulfuryl fluoride	insecticide, fumigant
2,4,5-T	2,4,5-trichlorophenoxyacetic acid	herbicide
tabun	dimethylamidoethoxyphosphoryl cyanide	nerve gas
tartar emetic	antimony potassium tartrate	herbicide
2,3,6-TBA	2,3,6-trichlorobenzoic acid	herbicide
TCA	sodium trichloroacetate	herbicide
TCPE	2,4,5-trichlorophenoxyethanol	herbicide
TDE (DDD)	2,2-bis (*p*-chlorophenyl)-,1-dichloroethane	insecticide
Telodrin	isobornyl thiocyanoacetate	insecticide
telone	mixed dichloropropenes	insecticide
Temik	2-methyl-2(methylthio)propionaldehyde 0-(methyl carbamoyl)oxime	insecticide, acaricide, nematocide
TEPP	tetraethyl pyrophosphate	insecticide
terbacil	3-tert-butyl-5-chloro-6-methyluracil	herbicide

(continued)

GLOSSARY—*Continued*

Common Pesticides

COMMON NAME	CHEMICAL NAME	MAIN USES
tetradifon	*p*-chlorophenyl 2,4,5-trichlorophenyl sulfone	insecticide
thallium sulfate	thallium sulfate	insecticide, rodenticide
thiram	tetramethylthiuram disulfide	fungicide, animal repellent
TME	0,0,S-trimethyl phosphorodithioate	by-product of malathion
toxaphene	chlorinated camphene	insecticide
trichlorfon	0,0-dimethyl (1-hydroxy-2,2,2-trichloro-ethyl) phosphonate	systemic insecticide
2,4,5-trichlorophenol	sodium 2,4,5-trichlorophenate	fungicide
trifluralin	a,a,a-trifluoro-2,6-dinitro-*N,N*-dipropyl-*p*-toluidine	herbicide
Valone	2-isovaleryl-1,3 indandione	rodenticide
warfarin	3-(1′-phenyl-2′-acetylethyl)-4-hydroxycoumarin	rodenticide
white arsenic	arsenic trioxide	animal dip, herbicide, ingredient in insect baits
zectran	4-dimethylamino-3,5-xylyl *N*-methylcarbamate	pesticide for control of snails and slugs
zinc white	zinc oxide	ingredient in animal remedies
zineb	zinc ethylene bisdithiocarbamate	fungicide
Zinophos	0,0-diethyl 0-2-pyrazinyl phosphorothioate	insecticide, fungicide, nematocide
Ziram	zinc dimethyldithiocarbamate	fungicide

REFERENCES

1. Ahlborg UG, Lindgren JE, Mercier M: Metabolism of pentachlorophenol. *Arch Toxicol (Berl.)* 1974; 32:271.
2. Aldridge WN, Bares JM, Johnson MK: Studies on delayed neurotoxicity produced by some organophosphorus compounds. *Ann NY Acad Sci* 1969; 160:314.
3. Aldridge WN, Johnson MK: Side effects of organophosphorus compounds: Delayed neurotoxicity. *Bull WHO* 1971; 44:259.
4. Arsenic, medical and biological effects on environmental pollutants. Washington, DC, National Academy of Sciences, 1977, pp 216–223.
5. Arterberry JD, et al: Exposure to parathion—measure by blood cholinesterase level and urinary *p*-nitrophenol excretion. *Arch Environ Health* 1961; 3:476.
6. Axelson O, Sundell L: Herbicide exposure, mortality and tumor incidence. An epidemiological investigation on Swedish railroad workers. *Scand J Work Environ Health* 1974; 11:21.
7. Baader EW, Bauer HJ: Industrial intoxication due to pentachlorophenol. *Ind Med Surg* 1951; 20:286.
8. Baker EL, et al: Epidemic malathion poisoning in Pakistan malaria workers. *Lancet* 1978; 1:31.
9. Berg GL (ed): *Farm Chemicals Handbook*. Willoughby, Oh, Meister Publishing Co. 1977.
10. Bergner H, et al: Industrial pentachlorophenol poisoning in Winnipeg. *Can Med Assoc J* 1965; 92:448.
11. Berkow R (ed): *The Merck Manual of Diagnosis and Therapy*, ed 14. Rahway, NJ, Merck & Co, Inc, 1982.
12. Best EM Jr, Murray BL: Observations on workers exposed to Sevin insecticide: A preliminary report. *J Occup Med* 1962; 10:507.
13. Bidstrup PL, Bonnel JA, Beckett AG: Paralysis following,poisoning by a new organic phosphorus insecticide (mipafox). *Br Med J*, 1953; 1:1068.
14. Bleiberg J, Wallen M, Brodkin R, et al: Industrially acquired porphyria. *Arch Dermatol* 1964; 89:793.
15. Brown VHK, Hunter CG, Richardson A: A blood test diagnostic exposure to aldrin and dieldrin. *Br J Ind Med* 1964; 21:283.
16. Brown VK: Solubility and solvent effects as rate-determining factors in the acute percutaneous toxicities of pesticides. *Soc Chem Ind Monogr*. 1968; 29:93.
17. Bullivant CM: Accidental poisoning by paraquat: Report of two cases in man. *Br Med J*, 1966; 1:1272.
18. Casida JE (ed): *Pyrethrum—the Natural Insecticide*. New York, Academic Press, 1973, pp 123–142.
19. Cavanaugh JB: Peripheral neuropathy caused by chemical agents. *Crit Rev Toxicol* 1973; 2:365.
20. Clark DG, et al: The toxicity of paraquat. *Br J Ind Med* 1966; 23:126.
21. Coble Y, et al: Acute endrin poisoning. *JAMA* 1967; 202:153.
22. Committee on Toxicology, Board on Toxicology and Environmental Health Hazards, Commission on Life Sciences. National Research Council: *An Assessment of the Health Risks of Seven Pesticides Used for Termite Control*. Washington, DC, National Academy Press, 1982.
23. Culver D, et al: Studies of human exposure during aerosol application of malathion and chlorthion. *AMA Arch Ind Hyg* 1956; 13:37.
24. Czeizel E, Király J: Chromosome examinations in workers producing Klorinol and Buvinol, in Bánki L (ed): *The Development of a Pesticide as a Complex Scientific Task*. Budapest, Medicina, 1976, pp 239–256.

25. Davies JE, et al: An epidemiologic application of the study of DDE levels in whole blood. *Am J Public Health* 1969; 59:435.
26. Derbes VJ, et al: Fatal chlordane poisoning. *JAMA* 1955; 158:1367.
27. Drenth HJ, et al: Neuromuscular function in agricultural workers using pesticides. *Arch Environ Health* 1972; 25:395.
28. Duffy FH: Long-term effects of pesticides on the brain—a new finding. Annual Meeting of the Society for Occupational & Environmental Health, Dec 10–13, 1978, Washington, DC.
29. Edmundson WF, Davies JE: Occupational dermatitis from naled—a clinical report. *Arch Environ Health* 1967; 15:89.
30. Federal Insecticide, Fungicide and Rodenticide Act ("Federal Environmental Pesticide Control Act of 1972"), amended, 1978, United States Environmental Protection Agency, Office of Pesticide Control Programs, Washington, DC.
31. Firestone D: The 2,3,7,8-tetrachlorodibenzo-para-dioxin problem: A review, in Ramel C (ed): Chlorinated phenoxy acids and their dioxins: Mode of action, health risks and environmental effects. *Ecol Bull* 27 *(Stockholm)* 1977; 27:39–52.
32. Flint A: Cimetidine and oral anticoagulants. *Br Med J* 1978; 2:1367.
33. Fristedt B, Sterner N: Warfarin intoxication from cutaneous absorption. *Arch Environ Health* 1965; 11:205.
34. Gage JC: Toxicity of paraquat and diquat aerosols generated by a size-selective cyclone: Effect of particle size distribution. *Br J Ind Med* 1968; 25:304.
35. Glauser SC: Early reversible health effects from pentachlorophenol. Annual Meeting of the Society for Occupational & Environmental Health, Dec 10–13, 1978, Washington, DC.
36. Golz HH: Controlled human exposures to malathion aerosols. *AMA Arch Ind Hyg* 1959; 19:516.
37. Goodman LS, Gilman A: *The Pharmacological Basis of Therapeutics,* ed 7. New York, Macmillan Publishing Co, 1985.
38. Gordon M, et al: Recommendation for prevention of flight crashes resulting from factors impairing performance of agricultural spray pilots. An outline statement of medical policy. Civil Aviation Authority, Ministry of Transportation, Israel, 1978.
39. Gosalvez M, Merchan J: Induction of rat mammary adenomas with the respiratory inhibitory rotenone. *Cancer Res* 1973; 33:3047.
40. Gosselin RE, Hodge HC, Smith PP, et al: *Clinical Toxicology of Commercial Products,* ed 5. Baltimore, Williams & Wilkins Co, 1982, sect II.
41. Gosselin RE, et al: *Clinical Toxicology of Commercial Products,* ed 4. Baltimore: Williams & Wilkins Co, 1976, Sect III, pp 168–171.
42. Greenburg JO: The neurological effects of methyl bromide poisoning. *Ind Med* 1971; 40:27.
43. Gribetz B, et al: Heat stress exposure of aerial spraying. *Aviat Space Environ Med* 1980; 5:68.
44. Hardell L, Sandström A: Case control study: Soft tissue sarcomas and exposure to phenoxyacetic acids or chlorophenols. Annual Meeting of the Society for Occupational & Environmental Health, Dec 10–13, 1978, Washington, DC.
45. Harger PN, Spolyar LW: Toxicity of phosphine, with a possible fatality from this poison. *AMA Arch Ind Hyg* 1958; 18:497.
46. Harrisson JWE, et al: Acute poisoning with sodium fluoroacetate (Compound 1080). *JAMA* 1952; 149:1520.
47. Harrisson JWE, et al: Fluoroacetate (1080) poisoning. *Ind Med Surg* 1952; 21:440.
48. Hayes WJ Jr: Clinical Handbook on Economic Poisons. Washington, DC, Public Health Service Publ 476, Government Printing Office, 1963, pp 47–50, 71–73.
49. Hayes WJ Jr: Studies on exposure during the use of anticholinesterase pesticides. *Bull WHO* 1971; 44:277.
50. Hayes WJ Jr: *Toxicology of Pesticides*. Baltimore, Williams & Wilkins Co, 1975.
51. Hine CH: Methyl bromide poisoning. *J Occup Med* 1969; 11:1.
52. Hodge HC, et al: Acute and short-term oral toxicity tests of ferric dimethyldithiocarbamate (ferbam) and zinc dimethyldithiocarbamate (ziram). *J Am Pharmacol Assoc* 1952; 41:662.
53. Holmes JH, et al: Short-term toxicity of mevinphos in man. *Arch Environ Health* 1974; 29:84.
54. Howard JK, East NJ, Chaney JL: Plasma cholinesterase activity in early pregnancy. *Arch Environ Health* 1978; 33:2775.
55. International Agency for Research on Cancer: Some organochlorine pesticides. *IARC Monogr Eval Carcinog Risk Chem Man* 1974; 5:90–124.
56. International Agency for Research on Cancer: Some organochlorine pesticides. *IARC*.
57. Ishikawa S.: Chronic optico-neuropathy due to environmental exposure of organophosphate pesticides (Saku disease). Clinical and experimental study, Nippon Ganka Gakkai Zasshi 77:1835, 1973.
58. Ishikawa S: Eye injury by organic phosphorus insecticides (preliminary report). *J Ophthalmol* 1971; 15:60.
59. Ishikawa S: Optico-autonomic-peripheral neuropathy due to chronic organophosphate pesticide intoxication, in *Proceedings of 22d International Congress on Ophthalmology*. Paris, Masson, 1976.
60. Jager KW: *Aldrin, Dieldrin, Endrin and Telodrin—An Epidemiological and Toxicological Study of Long-Term Occupational Exposure*. Amsterdam, Elsevier Publishing Co, 1970, pp 78–87, 217–218, 225–234.
61. Jager KW: Organophosphate exposure from industrial usage, electroneuromyography in occupational medical supervision of exposed workers. Paper presented at the EPA seminar on "Pesticide induced delayed neurotoxicity," Feb 19–20, 1976.
62. Jager KW, Roberts DV, Wilson A: Neuromuscular function in pesticide workers. *Br J Ind Med* 1970; 27:273.
63. Jirásek L, et al: Acne chlorina, porphyria cutanea tarda and other manifestations of general intoxication during the manufacture of herbicides, I. *Cesk Dermatol* 1974; 49:145.
64. Johnson MK: A phosphorylation site in brain and the delayed neurotoxic effect of some organophosphorus compounds. *Biochem J* 1969; 111:487.
65. Johnson MK: Organophosphorus esters causing delayed neurotoxic effect. Mechanism of action and structure/activity studies. *Arch Toxicol (Berl)* 1975; 34:259.
66. Johnson MK: The delayed neuropathy caused by some organophosphorus esters: Mechanism and challenge. *Crit Rev Toxicol* 1975; 3:289.
67. Jones AT, et al: Environmental and clinical aspects of bulk wheat fumigation with aluminum phosphide. *Am Ind Hyg Assoc J* 1964; 25:376.
68. Kantantzis G, et al: Poisoning in industrial workers by the insecticide aldrin. *Br J Ind Med* 1964; 21:46.
69. Kantarjian AD, Shaheen AS: Methyl bromide poisoning with nervous system manifestations resembling polyneuropathy. *Neurology* 1963; 13:1054.
70. Kolmodin-Hedman B, et al. Yskesmedicinsk kontrol av berörd personal vid lindanresp DDT- behandling av barrträdsplantor, En jämförelse, *Arbete och Hälsa:* 7, Arbetarskyddsstyrelsen, 17184 Solna, Sweden, 1977.
71. Kolmodin-Hedman B, Erne K, Håkansson M, et al: Kontrol av yrkesmässig exponering för fenoxisyror (2,4-D and 2,4,5-T). *Arbete och Hälsa:* 17, Arbetarskyddsverket, Stockholm, 1979.
72. Kolmodin-Hedman B, Ny V, Lidblom A, et al: Försöksverksamhet med lindanbehandling av tall—och granplantor, Hösten, 1974—Yrkeshygieniska Aspekter. Arbetarskyddsstyrelsen, Fack, 100 27 Stockholm. *Arbete och Hälsa:* 5, 1975.
73. Kolmodin-Hedman B, Palmer L, Götel P, et al: Plasma levels of lindane, p,ṕ-DDE and p,ṕ-DDT in occupationally exposed persons in Sweden. *Work Environ Health* 1973; 10:100.

74. Laws ER Jr, et al: Long-term occupational exposure to DDT. Effect on the human liver. *Arch Environ Health* 1973; 27:318.
75. Laws ER Jr, et al: Men with intensive occupational exposure to DDT—a clinical and chemical study. *Arch Environ Health* 1967; 15:766.
76. Lindgren S, Collste P, Norlander B, et al: Gas chromatographic assessment of the reproducibility of phenazone plasma half-lives in young healthy volunteers. *Eur J Clin Pharmacol* 1974; 7:381.
77. Lores EM, Bradway DE, Moseman RF: Organophosphorus pesticide poisoning in humans: Determination of residues and metabolites in tissues and urine. *Arch Environ Health* 1978; 33:270.
78. Maibach HI, Feldmann RJ, Milby TH, et al: Regional variation in percutaneous penetration in man. *Arch Environ Health* 1971; 23:208.
79. May G: Chloracne from the accidental production of tetrachlorodibenzodiozin. *Br J Ind Med* 1973; 30:276.
80. McClosky WT, Smith MI: Studies on the pharmacologic action and the pathology of alphanaphthylthiourea (ANTU). *J Pharmacol Public Health Reports* 1945; 60:1101.
81. McCollister DD, et al: Toxicological studies of O-O-dimethyl-O-(2,4,5-trichlorophenyl) phosphorothioate (Ronnel) in laboratory animals. *Agricultural and Food Chemistry* 1959; 7:689.
82. McGee LC: Accidental poisoning by taxaphene. *JAMA* 1952; 149:1124.
83. Menz M, et al: Long-term exposure of factory workers to dichlorvos (DDVP) insecticide. *Arch Environ Health* 1974; 28:72.
84. Mestitzova M: On reproduction studies and the occurrence of cataracts in rats after long-term feeding of the insecticide heptachlor. *Experientia* 1967; 23:42.
85. Michel HO: An electrometric method for the determination of red blood cell and plasma cholinesterase activity. *J Lab Clin Med* 1949· 34:1564.
86. Milby TH: Does chronic exposure to organophosphate insecticide cause eye complications? *JAMA* 1976; 236:1891.
87. Milby TH: Prevention and management of organophosphate poisoning. *JAMA* 1971; 216:2131.
88. Morgan DP: *Recognition and management of pesticide poisoning*. Washington, DC, US Environmental Protection Agency, Office of Pesticide Programs, August, 1982.
89. Morse DL, Baker EL, Landrigan PJ: Cut flowers: A potential pesticide hazard. *Am J Public Health* 1969; 69:1.
90. National Agricultural Chemicals Association: *Pre-Fire Planning and Guidelines for Handling Agricultural Chemicals Fires, 1979*.
91. National Cancer Institute, National Institutes of Health: *Vet Hum Toxicol* 1977; 19(4):304.
92. National Institute of Occupational Safety and Health: Aldrin/Dieldrin—*Special Occupational Hazard Review*. Cincinnati, Oh, NIOSH, Dept of Health, Education, and Welfare, PHS, Center for Disease Control, 1978.
93. National Institute of Occupational Safety and Health: *Agricultural Chemicals and Pesticides—a subfile of the Registry of Toxic Effects*, 1977.
94. National Institute of Occupational Safety and Health: *Criteria for a Recommended Standard: Occupational Exposure to Inorganic Arsenic*, US Dept of Health, Education, and Welfare. Washington, DC, 1973.
95. National Institute of Occupational Safety and Health. Washington, DC, *Criteria for a Recommended Standard: Occupational Exposure to Carbaryl*. US Dept of Health, Education, and Welfare, 1976.
96. National Institute of Occupational Safety and Health: *Criteria for a recommended standard: Occupational Exposure during the Manufacture and Formulation of Pesticides*. US Dept of Health, Education, and Welfare (NIOSH), No 78-174, 1978.
97. National Institute of Occupational Safety and Health: *Health and Safety Guide for Pesticide Formulation*. Cincinnati, Oh, US Dept of Health, Education, and Welfare, PHS, Center for Disease Control, Division of Technical Services, 1977.
98. National Institute of Occupational Safety and Health: *Criteria for a Recommended Standard: Occupational Exposure to Malathion*. Washington, DC, US Dept of Health, Education, and Welfare, 1976.
99. National Institute of Occupational Safety and Health: *Criteria for a Recommended Standard: Occupational Exposure to Methyl Parathion*. Washington, DC, US Dept of Health, Education, and Welfare, 1976.
100. National Institute of Occupational Safety and Health: *Criteria for a Recommended Standard: Occupational Exposure to Parathion*. Washington, DC, US Dept of Health, Education, and Welfare, 1976.
101. National Institute of Occupational Safety and Health: *Pesticide-Residue Hazards to Farm Workers*. Proceedings of a Workshop, 1976.
102. Negberbon WO (ed): *Handbook of Toxicology*. Philadelphia, WB Saunders Co, 1957, vol III, p 665.
103. Nishimura H, Nakai K: Developmental anomalies in off-spring of pregnant mice treated with nicotine. *Science* 1958; 127:877.
104. Olishifski JB (ed): Fundamentals of Industrial Hygiene, ed 2. Chicago, National Safety Council, 1979.
105. Ottolenghi AD, et al: Teratogenic effects of aldrin, dieldrin and endrin in hamsters and mice. *Teratology* 1974; 9:11.
106. *Paraquat Poisoning—A Physician's Guide*. San Francisco, Chevron Environmental Health Center, 1975.
107. Pasi A: *The Toxicology of Paraquat, Diquat and Morfamquat*. Bern, Stuttgart, Vienna, Hans Huber Publishers, 1978.
108. Peaslee CH: Spotlight on paraquat and marijuana. *Lab Med Pract Physicians* 1978; pp 29–31, July/Aug.
109. Plestina R, Piukovic-Plestina M: Effect of anticholinesterase pesticides on the eye and vision. *CRC Crit Rev Toxicol* 1978; pp 1–23, December.
110. Quinby GE, Doornink GM: Tetraethylpyrophosphate poisoning following airplane dusting. *JAMA* 1965; 191:95.
111. Ramel C (ed): Chlorinated phenoxy acids and their dioxins. Mode of action, health risks and environmental effects. Report from a conference arranged by the Royal Swedish Academy of Sciences, Stockholm, Sweden, Feb 7–9, 1977.
112. *Report on Carcinogenesis Bioassay of Chlordane and Heptachlor, Technical Background Information*. Bethesda, MD, US Dept of Health, Education and Welfare, National Institutes of Health, National Cancer Institute, 1977.
113. Richeson EM: Thallium poisoning, *Arch Neurol* 1972; 26:456.
114. Rider JA, Hodges JL Jr, Swader J, et al: Plasma and red blood cell cholinesterase in 800 "healthy" blood donors. *J Lab Clin Med* 1957; 50:376.
115. Roan CC, Morgan DP, Cook N, et al: Blood cholinesterases, serum parathion concentrations and urine P-nitrophenol concentrations in exposed individuals. *Bull Environ Contam Toxicol* 1969; 4:382.
116. Robens JF: Teratologic studies of carbaryl, diazinon, norea, disulfiram, and thiram in small laboratory animals. *Toxicol Appl. Pharmacol* 1969; 15:152.
117. Roberts DV: A longitudinal electromyographic study of six men occupationally exposed to organophosphorus compounds. *Int Arch Occup Environ Health* 1977; 38:221.
118. Roberts DV: EMG voltage and motor nerve conduction velocity in organophosphorus pesticide factory workers. *Int Arch Occup Environ Health* 1976; 36:267.
119. Roberts DV: Theoretical and practical consequences of the use of organophosphorus compounds in industry. *J Soc Occup Med* 1979; 29:15.
120. Roll R: Tetratologische untersuchungen mit thiram (TMTD) an zwei Mausestammen. *Arch Toxikol* 1971; 27:173.

121. Shelly WB: Golf-course dermatitis due to thiram fungicide. *JAMA* 1964; 188:415.
122. Silver A: A biology of cholinesterases, in Neuberger A, Tatum EL (eds): *Frontiers of Biology*. North-Holland Research Monographs. Amsterdam, North-Holland, 1974, vol 36.
123. Singh AR, et al: Teratogenicity of phthalate esters in rats. *J Pharm Sci* 1972; 61:51.
124. Special Pesticides Review Group (Fitzhugh OG, Fairchild HE, chairmen): Pesticidal aspects of chlordane in relation of man and the environment. US Environmental Protection Agency, Government Printing Office, Washington, DC, 1975.
125. Spiotta EJ: Aldrin poisoning in man. *AMA Arch Ind Hyg* 1951; 4:560.
126. Stålberg E, et al: Effects of occupational exposure to organophosphorus insecticides on neuromuscular function. *Scand J Work Environ Health* 1978; 4:255.
127. Surveillance Summary—Paraquat Contamination of Marijuana—United States. Center for Disease Control, *MMWR* 1979; 28:8, March 2.
128. Swan AAB: Exposure of spray operators to paraquat. *Br J Ind Med* 1969; 26:322.
129. Taxay EP: Vikane inhalation. *J Occup Med* 1966; 8:425.
130. Technical Background Information Report on Carcinogenesis Bioassay of Toxaphene. Bethesda, Md, National Institutes of Health, National Cancer Institute, 1979.
131. Thiess AM, Goldmann P: Über das Trichlorophenol-Dioxin-Ungallgeschehen in BASF AG vom 13, November, 1953, in Vortrag, auf dem IV. Medichem-Kongress, Haifa, 1977.
132. Vandekar M, Wilford K: The effect of cholinesterase activity of storage of undiluted whole blood sampled from men exposed to 7-isopropoxyphenyl methylcarbamate (OMS-33). *Bull WHO* 1969; 40:91.
133. Vaziri ND, et al: Nephrotoxicity of paraquat in man. *Arch Intern Med* 1979; 139:2.
134. Verberk MM, Rooyakkers-Beemster M, De Vlieger M, et al: Bromine in blood, EEG and transaminases in methyl bromide workers. *Br J Ind Med* 1979; 36:59.
135. Verberk MM, Salle HJA: Effects on nervous function in volunteers ingesting mevinphos for one month. *Toxicol Appl Phamacol* 1977; 42:351.
136. Wang HH, MacMahon B: Mortality of workers employed in the manufacture of chlordane and heptachlor. *J Occup Med* 1979; 21:11.
137. Warraki S: Respiratory hazards of chlorinated camphene. *Arch Environ Health* 1963; 7:137.
138. Wills JH: Percutaneous Absorption, in Montagna W, Van Scott J, Stoughton RB (eds): *Pharmacology and the Skin*. New York, Appleton-Century Crofts, 1972, Chap 12, pp 169–176.
139. Wolfe HR, Durham WF, Armstrong JF: Urinary excretion of insecticide metabolites: Excretion of paranitrophenol and DDA as indicators of exposure to parathion and DDT. *Arch Environ Health* 1970; 21:711.
140. Wolfsie JH, Winter GD: Statistical analysis of normal human red blood cell and plasma cholinesterase activity values. *Am Ind Hyg Assoc J* 1952; 6:43.
141. Xintaras C, et al: *NIOSH Survey of Velsicol Pesticide Workers—Occupational Exposure to Leptophos and Other Chemicals*. DHEW (NIOSH) Publ 78–136, 1977.
142. Yamamura Y: *n*-Hexane polyneuropathy. *Folia Psychiatr Neurol Jpn* 1969; 23:45.
143. Zenz C: The occupational physician, in Olishifski JB (ed): *Fundamentals of Industrial Hygiene*. Chicago, National Safety Council, 1979, pp 827–860.
144. Zenz C: Internal communications to and from Velsicol Chemical Corp., Chicago, Ill, 1978–1986.
145. Zenz C: Personal communication from Calo CJ, 1985.
146. World Health Organization: *Environmental Health Criteria (Chordane-no. 34; Chlordecone-no. 43; Heptachlor-no. 38; Mirex-no. 44; Paraqual and Diquat-no. 39; Carbamate Pesticides-no. 64)*. Geneva, 1984 and 1986.

47

Other Important and Widely Used Chemicals*

Alexander Blair Smith, M.D., M.S.

Carl Zenz, M.D.

With expanding uses of new materials such as are found in adhesives, coatings (paints and finishes), a multitude of plastics and other synthetic entities, more workers are potentially exposed, at various levels of risk, often unintentionally. Those concerned with occupational health practices (preventive programs) should and must be aware of the more commonly encountered substances and have some knowledge of what is going on in the factories near them. The immense quantities of certain hazardous materials used are awesome. Indeed, some chemicals being produced and used for other processes range into and beyond millions to billions of kilograms each year. For example, phosgene, used as an intermediate to make isocyanates, has an annual production in the United States in excess of 300 million kg; sodium hydroxide produced each year in the United States is more than 10 billion kg. In the smaller workshops particularly, points of concern may be found in processing and formulating, packaging, storage, shipping, reformulating, applications, maintenance work, and laboratory testing. Often overlooked is that these varied activities occur over geographically widely scattered areas and mainly involve small numbers or groups of workers. Despite technologic advances in the highly industrialized countries, some occupational exposures continue and are troublesome: exposures to carbon monoxide, hydrogen sulfide, and other irritating agents such as acids and caustics and oxides of nitrogen, which are all found in varying amounts in certain occupational settings. Methods of treatment and prevention are discussed, and the principles and practices described in this chapter are applicable to many other occupational exposures.

Terms used to describe "exposure limits" are found in Appendix A. The American Conference of Governmental Industrial Hygienists (ACGIH) publishes annually the threshold limit values for chemical substances and physical agents in the working environment and also prepares and publishes at appropriate intervals documentation of these values, which should be consulted for a better understanding of the TLVs. (See Appendix A for 1986–1987 TLVs.)

*Appreciation for assistance with this chapter is given Louis S. Beliczky, M.S., M.P.H., Vernon N. Dodson, M.D., Joseph LaDou, M.D., and Robert H. Wheater, M.S.

Significant information, such as health effect or effects, is considered in the National Institute for Safety and Health (NIOSH) reports and criteria documents. It should be noted that this chapter is not intended to provide details of these publications, and reference to the full documents is recommended for those requiring elements of a recommended standard, work practices, sampling, analytic methods, engineering control measures, and complete references. These documents have been published after critically evaluating all known and available medical, biologic, engineering, chemical, and trade data and any other information that may be relevant to recommending a standard. Included as part of the standard is a permissible exposure level, i.e., the concentration of a substance in the occupational environment that will not cause adverse effects in exposed persons. Historical reports and extent of occupational exposures always have been part of the criteria documents. Since 1976, the NIOSH has incorporated animal and human data, if available, on the effects of reproduction, carcinogenicity, mutagenicity, and teratogenicity. Attempts are made to correlate these adverse reactions with exposures and effects, where possible. For discussions on other pertinent substances, refer to specific chapters in this book, especially Chapter 29, *Occupational Exposure Limits for Chemical Agents*, by R.L. Zielhuis.

In this chapter there will be no attempt to discuss all of the known hazardous chemicals in the working environment, the coverage being limited to those substances that are most widely found and which have produced known occupationally associated illness. While reviewing the noxious characteristics of these chemicals, it is important that the reader be aware of what may constitute a toxic effect. It is this definition that dictates the level of control that must be provided for workers working in the proximity of a chemical that may cause these toxic effects.

For example, if the toxic effect to be prevented from exposure to carbon monoxide were considered to be the death of a healthy individual, the level, including whatever margin is considered necessary to protect particularly susceptible healthy people, would be between 50 and 100 ppm. On the other hand, if the toxic effect were considered to be the increased susceptibility of people with myocardial disease, it would be the time-weighted average (TWA) of 35 ppm, the level of which was recommended by the NIOSH to the U.S. Department of Labor.

Similarly, if the toxic effect from exposure to sulfur dioxide to be prevented were selected to be the irritation of the mucosa of the nose or eyes of adapted workers, the level would be a TWA of 5 ppm. However, if the toxic effect is selected to be the increased resistance to the passage of air in the respiratory tract of adapted or nonadapted workers, the level would be a TWA of 2 ppm, the level recently recommended by NIOSH. A toxic effect, therefore, can be defined as any bodily injury, reversible or irreversible; any tumor, benign or malignant; any mutagenic or teratogenic effect; irritation or allergic effect; a lessening of mental alertness or motivation; or death of a normal or disabled person who has been exposed to a substance via the respiratory tract, skin, eye, mouth or any other route. This definition thus responds to the directive offered by the Occupational Safety and Health Act of 1970, Public Law 91–596, which established a policy of ensuring every working man and woman a safe and healthful working condition in which none will suffer diminished health, functional capacity, or life expectancy as a result of his or her work experience.

Another important aspect that must be kept in mind is that a toxic material seldom is found in the work environment as a single pure chemical substance and that a worker seldom is exposed to a single hazard. Thus, a welder may be working in an occupational environment in which he or she could be exposed to several oxides of nitrogen, to fumes of cadmium, zinc, and beryllium, to ultraviolet light as well as to the stress of a hot, cold, or hyperbaric environment in the course of daily activity, simultaneously or sequentially. It is this multiplicity of exposures that has complicated the investigation and identification of noxious effects produced by chemical substances.

Another complication in identifying toxic effects from chemical exposure is the increased mobility of the working population, which prevents accurate identification of the population at risk.

And, last, as we shift our attention of the past from the dramatic effects of immediate primary irritation and disabling or lethal immediate effects, we are discovering toxic effects that have latent periods after exposure of as much as 50 years, with recorded exposures of as short duration as seven months, as is the case with asbestos exposure reported by Knox *et al.* in 1968. (See Levy, Chapter 14.)

The bases of accepted standards and occupational exposures are undergoing rigorous reevaluation to determine whether there may be different effects that have been presenting themselves and which need to be considered to ensure safe working conditions.

REFERENCES

1. Aitio A, Riihimäki V, Vainio H (eds): *Biological Monitoring and Surveillance of Workers Exposed to Chemicals*. New York, Hemisphere, 1984.
2. American Conference of Governmental Industrial Hygienists: *Documentation of the Threshold Limit Values for Substances in Workroom Air*, ed 5. Cincinnati, Oh, ACGIH, 1986.
3. Considine D, Considine G (eds.): *The Encyclopedia of Chemistry*, ed 4. New York, Van Nostrand Rheinhold Co, 1984.
4. Lauwerys RR: *Industrial Chemical Exposure: Guidelines for Biological Monitoring*. Davis, Cal, Biomedical Publishers, 1983.
5. NIOSH Recommendations for Occupational Health Standards. *MMWR* 1986; 35(1S). US Dept of Health and Human Services, Public Health Service, National Institute for Occupational Safety and Health, Centers for Disease Control, Atlanta, Ga, 30333.
6. *The Merck Index*, ed 10. Rahway, NJ, Merck & Co, Inc, 1983.
7. The microelectronics industry, in LaDou J (ed): *State of the Art Reviews. Occupational Medicine 1986*. Philadelphia, Hanley & Belfus, Inc, 1986, vol 1.
8. World Health Organization: Health effects of combined exposures in the work environment. Technical report series 662, Geneva, 1981.

ACRYLAMIDE

$$CH_2 = CHCONH_2$$

Synonyms for acrylamide include propenamide, acrylic amide, and akrylamid. The terms *acrylamide* and *acrylamide monomer* are used interchangeably. The major application for monomeric acrylamide is in the production of polymers as polyacrylamides. Polyacrylamides are used for soil stabilization, gel chromatography, electrophoresis, paper-making strengtheners, and clarification and treatment of potable water and foods. Approximately 40 million kg of acrylamide were produced in 1984 in the United States. The NIOSH estimates that approximately 20,000 workers in the United States are potentially exposed to acrylamide.

Toxic manifestations of exposure to acrylamide involve both localized and systemic effects. Localized effects include peeling and redness of the skin of the hands and, less often, of the feet, numbness of the lower limbs, and excessive sweating of the feet and hands. The systemic effects due to acrylamide intoxication involve central and peripheral nervous system damage manifested primarily as ataxia, weak or absent reflexes, a positive Romberg sign, and loss of vibration and position senses.

Since skin contact with the substance may result in localized or systemic effects, the NIOSH recommends that medical surveillance be made available to all employees working in an area where acrylamide is stored, produced, processed, or otherwise used, except as an unintentional contaminant in other materials at a concentration of less than 1% by weight. The present federal standard is 0.3 mg/cu m as a time-weighted average concentration for up to a ten-hour workday, 40-hour workweek.

REFERENCES

1. National Institute for Occupational Safety and Health: *A Recommended Standard for Occupational Exposure to Acrylamide*. Cincinnati, Oh, US Dept of Health, Education, and Welfare, PHS, Center for Disease Control, NIOSH, 1976.
2. World Health Organization: Acrylamide. Environmental Health Criteria no. 49, Geneva, 1985.

ACRYLIC AND METHACRYLIC ACIDS AND THEIR ESTERS

CH_2 $CHCO_2H$ (acrylic acid)

The esters of acrylic and methacrylic acid are acrylic acid, methyl acrylate, ethyl acrylate, butyl acrylate, methacrylic acid, methyl methacrylate, ethyl methacrylate, butyl methacrylate, and isobutyl methacrylate.

Occupational Aspects

At room temperature, acrylic and methacrylic acids and their esters are liquids with a strong and, for some, pleasant odor. Each has a different vapor pressure and boiling point. They easily polymerize, which accounts for their widespread use in the manufacture of lacquers and paints, as bonding agents for leather, paper, and textiles, and as solvents. Methacrylates have similar uses and are used widely in construction, and in the automobile and airline industries, where the combination of strength and transparency is important. Methyl methacrylate has found great use as "plexiglass" and floor coverings; in dentistry, to fill teeth and to make bridges; for contact lenses; and as a "bone cement" in certain orthopedic procedures.

Potentially exposed workers are those who lay floor covering, dental technicians and dentists, operating room personnel (during bone cementing), laboratory personnel, and some painters.

Absorption, Metabolism, and Excretion

Data on absorption, metabolism, and excretion are mainly derived from animal experiments. Uptake from the digestive tract is rapid and nearly total.[8, 6] Organ damage has been seen in experimental animals after inhalation of the acids or esters, indicating that the substances are absorbed through the lungs.[7, 9] Skin absorption is slow. In guinea pigs, total absorption to the substances are fairly slowly via the skin. In one, total absorption of methyl acrylate occurred after 16 hours.[6] Acrylates and methacrylates are lipophilic and accumulate in fatty tissues.[1]

In guinea pigs, it was shown that about 35% was excreted via the lungs in the form of carbon dioxide, with splitting of the ester bond, and oxidative breakdown seems to occur. Approximately 25% was recovered in urine as thioether during the next three days and most during the first 24 hours. Conjugation with glutathione is thus one step in the biotransformation.[6] In rats,[8] about 85% of a given dose of methyl methacrylate is recovered as carbon dioxide in expired air following exposure over the next ten days, most in the first two hours (65%). Acrylates and methacrylates are hydrolyzed in the presence of carboxyl esterase subjected to oxidative breakdown, and unhydrolyzed esters can also be conjugated to reduced glutathione and excreted in urine as thioethers.

Organ Effects

Skin.—Methacrylates are less irritating than are the acrylates. Irritation from monomethacrylates (methyl, ethyl, and butyl methacrylate) has not been reported with skin contact. Patch tests made with 100% methyl methacrylate (direct skin contact for 48 hours) resulted in no skin irritation in most subjects; a third developed slight redness. In similar tests with acrylates, there was marked irritation.[10]

Lungs.—Rats exposed to 75 ppm of acrylic acid for 14 days revealed damage to nasal mucosa. Mice showed similar damage at levels as low as 5 ppm.[4] Rabbits exposed to about 90 ppm methyl and ethyl acrylate for 50 days showed slight irritation of eye and nose mucous membranes; ethyl acrylate had a lesser effect than methyl acrylate.[9]

Kidneys.—Acrylates and methacrylates produce degenerative changes in the kidneys but only at an exposure level much higher than that which triggers other symptoms, and damage to other organs is predominant.[7, 9]

Digestive Tract.—Dogs exposed to 2,000 ppm methyl methacrylate showed a pronounced reduction of intestinal peristalsis, probably due to direct toxic effects on the smooth muscles of the intestinal wall.[8]

Heart.—With in vitro studies, slower heartbeats and weaker contractions were associated with methacrylic acid and several other methacrylates, at concentrations as little as 1:100,000.[4]

Central Nervous System.—Approximate odor thresholds: methylacrylate, 5 ppm; ethyl acrylate, 1 ppm; butyl acrylate, 0.1 ppm; methacrylic acid, 3 ppm; methylacrylate, 0.01 ppm. Studies with electrodes implanted in the brains of animals for 60 minutes to 400 ppm ethyl methacrylate in air showed reduction in electric discharges measuring points in the brain.[3]

Peripheral Nervous System.—Twenty dental technicians who worked with methyl methacrylate in direct contact with their hands were examined to measure transmission speed in the sensory nerves of the fingers.[5] Nerve transmission speed was significantly reduced in those fingers used most in their work with contact with methyl methacrylate. This appeared to be a matter of direct attack on nerve fibers via skin absorption.

Since acrylates and methacrylates are irritating to the skin-sensitizing agents and can cause allergic contact reactions, as well as causing localized peripheral nerve damage, exposures must be controlled. No skin contact should be permitted. The TWA is 10 ppm (skin) for methyl methacrylate.

REFERENCES

1. Bechtel A, Willert H-G, Frech H-A: Bestimmung des monomergehalts von Methacrylsaure-methylester in Knochenmark, Fett und Blut nach dem Ausharten verschiedener "Knochenzemente." *Chromatographia* 1973; 6:226–228 (in German).
2. Bratt H, Hathway DE: Fate of methyl methacrylate in rats. *Br J Cancer* 1977; 36:114–119.
3. Innes KL, Tansy MF: Central nervous system effects of methyl methacrylate vapor. *Neurotoxicol* 1981; 2:515–522.
4. Miller RR, Ayres JA, Jersey GC, et al: Inhalation toxicity of acrylic acid. *Fund Appl Toxicol* 1981; 1:271–277.
5. Seppäläinen AM, Rajaniemi R: Local neurotoxicity of methyl methacrylate among dental technicians. *Am J Ind Med* 1984; 5:471–477.
6. Seutter E, Rijntjes NVM: Whole-body autoradiography after systemic and topical administration of methyl acrylate in the guinea pig. *Arch Dermatol Res* 1981; 270:273–284.
7. Spealman CR, Main RJ, Haag HB, et al: Monermic methyl methacrylate—Studies on toxicity. *Ind Med* 1945; 14:292–298.
8. Tansy MF, Martin JS, Benhaim S, et al: GI motor inhibition associ-

ated with acute exposure to methyl methacrylate vapor. *J Pharm Sci* 1977; 66:613–618.

9. Treon JF, Howard S, Wright H, et al: The toxicity of methyl and ethyl acrylate. *J Ind Hyg Toxicol* 1949; 31:317–326.
10. van der Walle HB: Sensitizing potential of acrylic monomers in guinea pigs. Thesis, Krips Repro Meppel, Nijmegen, the Netherlands, 1982.

ACRYLONITRILE

$$CH_2 = CHCN$$

Acrylonitrile is an explosive, flammable liquid having a normal boiling point of 77° C and a vapor pressure of 80 mm (20° C). The chemical structure of acrylonitrile, $CH_2 = CHCN$, resembles that of vinyl chloride. Synonyms for acrylonitrile include acrylon, carbacryl, cyanoethylene, fumigrain, 2-propenenitrile, VCN, ventox, and vinyl cyanide.

Almost three quarters of a billion kg of acrylonitrile are manufactured annually in the United States by the reaction of propylene with ammonia and oxygen in the presence of a catalyst.

The major use of acrylonitrile is in the production of acrylic and modacrylic fibers by copolymerization with methy[1] acrylate, methyl methacrylate, vinyl acetate, vinyl chloride, or vinylidene chloride. Acrylic fibers, marketed under various trade names, such as Acrilan, Creslan, Orlon, and Zefran, are used in the manufacture of apparel, carpeting, blankets, draperies, and upholstery. Some applications of modacrylic fibers are synthetic furs and hair wigs.

Other major uses of acrylonitrile are manufacture of acrylonitrile-butadiene-styrene (ABS) and styrene-acrylonitrile (SAN) resins (used to produce a variety of plastic products), nitrile elastomers and latexes, and other chemicals (e.g., adiponitrile and acrylamide). Acrylonitrile is also used as a fumigant. The U.S. Food and Drug Administration recently has banned the use of an acrylonitrile resin for soft-drink bottles.

The NIOSH estimates that 125,000 persons are potentially exposed to acrylonitrile in the workplace. The acute toxic effects of acrylonitrile are similar to those from cyanide poisoning. Toxic effects of acrylonitrile inhalation that have been noted in animals include damage to the central nervous system, lungs, liver and kidneys. Embryotoxic effects in mice have also been reported. However, more recent evidence of acrylonitrile's chronic toxicity has caused a reassessment of the hazard to workers of acrylonitrile. In April, 1977, the Manufacturing Chemists Association reported interim results of two-year feeding and inhalation studies (conducted by the Dow Chemical Company) of acrylonitrile in laboratory rats. By both routes of administration, acrylonitrile caused the development of central nervous system tumors and Zymbal gland carcinomas; no such tumors were seen in control animals. Exposure to 80 ppm of acrylonitrile also revealed an increased incidence of mammary region masses.

Acrylonitrile has been tested for mutagenic effects by in vitro and in vivo test systems. The results obtained have been conflicting, and the data are not adequate for quantitative assessment of mutagenic potential, suggesting that mutagenic activity may be very weak. There is no relevant human reproductive data reported. No increase in the number of chromosome aberrations was noted in lymphocyte cultures of 18 workers exposed to levels of acrylonitrile ranging from 1.5 ppm (1957 to 1977) to 5 ppm (1963 to 1974) and unknown levels (prior to 1963).[4]

Acrylonitrile may be teratogenic in rats at levels that are maternally toxic, with a toxic response occurring at 40 ppm.[3] There is no evidence to indicate that acrylonitrile exposure presents a reproductive risk.

A preliminary epidemiologic study conducted by the E. I. Du Pont de Nemours & Company, Inc., of a cohort of 470 acrylonitrile polymerization workers from the company's Camden, South Carolina, textile fibers plant indicates an excess risk of lung and colon cancer among workers with potential acrylonitrile exposure. A total of 16 cancer cases occurred between 1969 and 1975 among the cohort first exposed between 1950 and 1955; only 5.8 cancer cases would have been expected, based on Du Pont Company rates (excluding the cohort). Although the epidemiologic findings are preliminary in nature and may not alone provide definitive evidence of the carcinogenicity of acrylonitrile in man, when considered in light of the laboratory experiments demonstrating carcinogenicity in rats, a serious suspicion is raised that acrylonitrile is a human carcinogen. Thus, the NIOSH believes that acrylonitrile must be handled in the workplace as a suspected human carcinogen.

The ACGIH TWA for occupational exposure to acrylonitrile is an eight-hour time-weighted average of 2 ppm.

REFERENCES

1. *Acrylonitrile*, NIOSH, Current Intelligence Bulletin No 18. Cincinnati, OH, Dept of Health, Education, and Welfare, PHS, Center for Disease Control, 1977.
2. *Acrylonitrile: Environmental Health Criteria 28*. Geneva, World Health Organization, 1983.

2a. Bertelli G, Berlin A, Roi R, et al, in Alessio L, Berlin A, Boni M, et al (eds): *Acrylonitrile in Biological Indicators for the Assessment of Human Exposure to Industrial Chemicals*. Varese, Italy, Joint Research Centre Ispra Establishment 1984.

3. Murray F, Schwetz B, Nitschke K, et al: Teratogenicity of acrylonitrile given to rats by gavage or inhalation. *Food Cosmet Toxicol* 1978; 16:547–551.
4. Thiess A, Fleig I: Analysis of chromosomes of workers exposed to acrylonitrile, in Barlow S, Sullivan F (eds): *Reproductive Hazards of Industrial Chemicals*. New York, Academic Press, 1982, pp 52–53.

AMINES (ALIPHATIC AND AROMATIC)

J. STEVEN MOORE, M.D., C.I.H.

Aliphatic amines are alkaline compounds that have a characteristic fish or ammonia odor and are normal constituents of biologic tissues, especially fish. Compounds of lower molecular weight are water-soluble and volatile; higher analogs decrease in water solubility, volatility, and odor. Their alkaline nature makes them severe irritants to the respiratory tract, skin, and eyes. Deep necrotic skin burns and permanent eye damage have been reported, and certain compounds are known sensitizers.

Amines are compounds that are derived from an ammonia molecule (NH_3) and may be primary ($R\text{-}NH_2$), secondary ($R_2\text{-}NH$), or tertiary ($R_3\text{-}N$), according to the number of hydrogens substituted. Their uses are varied and include dyestuff and pharmaceutical manufacture, rubber products, catalysts or curing agents in plastics, ion exchange resins, cutting fluids, corrosion inhibitors, flotation agents, finishing agents, stabilizers, soaps and emulsifiers, photographic processing, and additives for petroleum, paints, paint strippers, and leather tanning. Figure 47–1 gives an indication of the bulk quantities typically in use.

Toxicology

Below six carbons, the aliphatic amines are sympathomimetic in that they elicit elevation of the blood pressure, contraction of smooth muscle, salivation, and pupillary dilatation. With aliphatic amines of seven carbons or more, the sympathetic activity decreases and cardiac depression is noted. Repeated administration leads to an altered response in that the cardiac stimulation is replaced by cardiac depression and vasodilaitation. In humans, these pressor effects are most noticeable with the pentylamines (C-5), also called amylamines, and hexylamines (C-6). Heptylamine (C-7) has been used as a nasal vasoconstrictor.

Aliphatic amines can stimulate the release of histamine and thus elicit a classical "wheal and flare" reaction under appropriate circumstances. When administered intravenously, an octylamine (compound "48/80") causes typical histamine-like responses such as decreased blood pressure, tachycardia, headache, erythema, itching, urticaria, and facial edema. Peak histamine activity occurs with monoamines of ten carbons. For diamines, activity increases steadily from six-carbon molecules to 14-carbon molecules. Since histamine aerosol can produce bronchoconstriction and wheezing, these amines may be capable of inducing asthmatic-like responses.

Animal Studies

Pathologic studies have shown that the aliphatic amines can affect the lungs, kidneys, liver, and heart. Myocardial damage has been reported for ethylamine, ethylenediamine, and alylamines. Spermine (diaminopropyltetramethylenediamine) has a notably high degree of nephrotoxicity, manifested as proteinuria and tubular damage. Diethylenetriamine, triethylenediamine, 1,3-diaminopropane, and 1,2-diaminopropane were also nephrotoxic, but to a lesser degree. Monoamines (C-1 through C-10), diamines (C-4 through C-10), and other triamines did not produce renal lesions or proteinuria.

Human Responses

The majority of reactions are limited to local effects secondary to their irritant and sensitizing properties. Vapors may cause eye irritation, including lacrimation, conjunctivitis, and corneal edema (halos around lights). Inhalation can lead to irritation of the nose and throat as well as lung effects, manifested as dyspnea and cough; vapors may also cause a primary irritant dermatitis.

Liquid preparations can produce severe damage to the eyes and skin because of their alkalinity. Systemic symptoms are related to their pharmacologic activity and may include nausea, faintness, and anxiety, in addition to the effects described earlier.

Cutaneous sensitization has been reported in association with the use of epoxy resins and polyurethanes. Ethylenediamine, diethylenetriamine, and triethylenetriamine are used as curing agents in these processes and are known skin sensitizers as well as potent irritants. These products can be released during the curing process as well as during grinding, sanding, or polishing of the

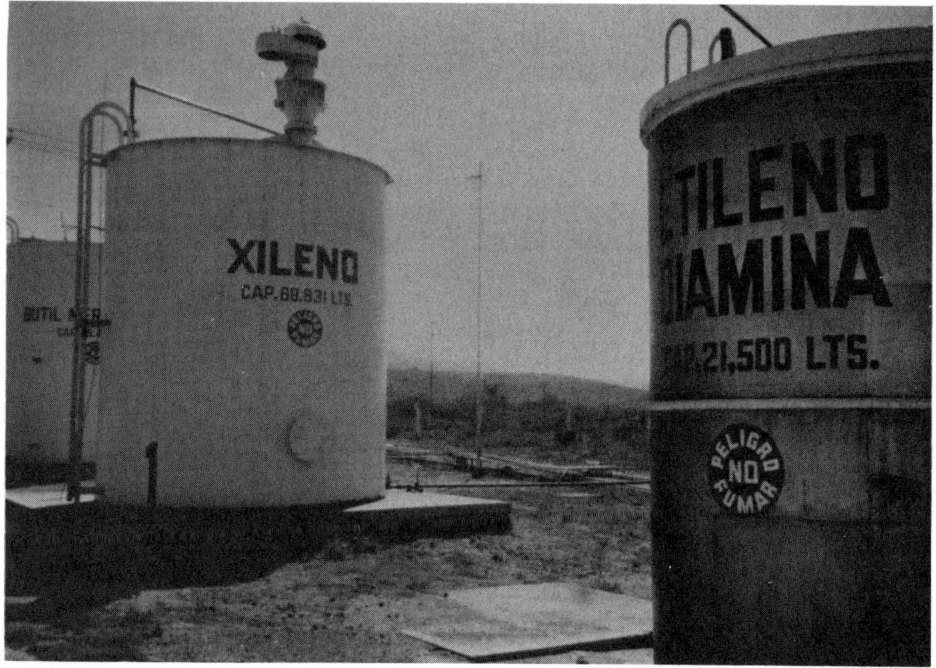

FIG 47–1.
Clear labeling of storage tanks indicates the widespread and heavy use of certain chemicals, here ethylenediamine compounds.

hardened molds. In sensitized individuals, this may lead to occupational asthma.

Aliphatic amines are metabolically altered in the body via two enzymes according to the number of amine groups present. Monoamine oxidase (MAO) acts on primary, secondary, and tertiary amines as follows:

$$2\ R\text{-}CH_2\text{-}N\text{-}R'R'' + O_2 + 2H_2O \rightarrow 2\ RCHO + 2\ NH\text{-}R'R'' + H_2O_2$$

Activity is greater for primary over secondary amines and for straight chains over branched or tertiary amines. This enzyme has no activity on methylamine, slight activity for ethylamine, and a maximum activity on amines of five to six carbons. Diamine oxidase has maximum activity on the four-carbon compound putrescine (tetramethylene diamine). It also creates piperidine, a cyclic compound, from cadaverine (pentamethylenediamine). Its reaction is as shown:

$$NH_2\text{-}R\text{-}CH_2\text{-}NH + O_2 + H_2O \rightarrow NH_2\text{-}R\text{-}HO + NH_3 + H_2O_2$$

The ammonia is transformed to urea.

Alkylamines

Of the numerous alkylamines known, only 14 have permissible exposure limits (PEL) or threshold limit values (TLV). Of these 14, seven have "skin" notations reflecting their potential toxicity via percutaneous absorption. Recommended limits are listed with the specific compounds of interest.

Methylamine

$$CH_3\text{-}NH_2$$

The PEL is 10 ppm. The TLV is 10 ppm also.

A flammable gas at normal temperature and pressure, methylamine is generally supplied as a liquid under pressure or a strong solution in water. It is a stronger base than ammonia and is used in tanning and organic synthesis. Its odor is faint at 10 ppm, strong at 20–100 ppm, and intolerable at higher levels. Olfactory fatigue occurs readily at nonirritating doses. Irritation to the eyes and respiratory tract are evident at 20–100 ppm with a no-effect level of 10 ppm.

Dimethylamine

$$(CH_3)_2\text{-}NH$$

Both the PEL and TLV are set at 10 ppm.

Supplied in the same form as methylamine, diethylamine exerts the same effects. It is used as an accelerator in the rubber industry and in the manufacture of soaps. The odor threshold is 0.6 ppm.

Ethylamine

$$CH_3\text{-}CH_2\text{-}NH_2$$

Generally supplied as a strong alkaline solution in water but readily vaporizes. It is used as a dye intermediate and as a stabilizer for rubber latex.

Triethylamine

$$(C_2H_5)_3N$$

```
   C2H5
  /
N—C2H5
  \
   C2H5
```

The TLV is 25 ppm.

Aside from irritation of the eyes and respiratory tract, triethylamine also stimulates the central nervous system, because it inhibits monoamine oxidase. In animals, myocardial degeneration was evident at 100 ppm—an effect not seen with mono- or diethylamines.

n-Butylamine

$$CH_3\text{-}CH_2\text{-}CH_2\text{-}CH_2\text{-}NH_2$$

The PEL and TLV are 5 ppm.

N-Butylamine is supplied as a liquid but will vaporize. Its odor is slight at 1 ppm, noticeable at 1–2 ppm, strong at 5–10 ppm, irritating at more than 10 ppm, and intolerable at 25 ppm with complaints of headache and irritation of the eyes, nose, and throat.

Isobutylamine

```
              CH3
               |
CH3 = CH2 = CH = NH2
```

The TLV is 5 ppm.

Isobutylamine induces nausea and unpleasant salivation in man at 40 mg/kg orally. In animals, it is sympathomimetic, a cardiac depressant, and a convulsant. It is used as a dehairing agent and as a solubilizer for 2,4-D.

Allylamine

$$CH_2 = CH = CH_2 = NH_2$$

A potent irritant, allylamine is intolerable at 14 ppm, with a recognizable odor and chest and mucous membrane discomfort at 2.5 ppm.

Cyclohexylamine

(cyclohexane ring)—NH_3

The TLV is 10 ppm (skin).

A liquid with a strong, fishy amine odor, cyclohexylamine is used as a corrosion inhibitor, insecticide, plasticizer, chemical intermediate, and dry-cleaning soap. It is severely irritating to skin, is a moderate sensitizer, and is a weak methemoglobin former. It has alleged carcinogenic, mutagenic, and embryotoxic effects in animals at levels far above those encountered in industry. For man, the no-effect level is 4–10 ppm.

Ethylenediamine

$$H_2N\text{-}CH_2\text{-}CH_2\text{-}NH_2$$

The PEL is 10 ppm.

A colorless, fuming liquid used as a solvent for albumin, casein, and shellac. It also stabilizes rubber latex and inhibits antifreeze. It is an important compound because of its ability to both irritate and sensitize the skin and lungs. At 125 ppm, an unsensitized individual reports no effects. At 200 ppm, tingling of the face and irritation of the nose are reported. At 400 ppm, the nose and respiratory tract are irritated, including some bronchospasm. It causes severe eye damage on contact.

Diethylenetriamine

$$H_2N\text{-}CH_2\text{-}CH_2\text{-}NH\text{-}CH_2\text{-}CH_2\text{-}NH_2$$

The TLV is 1 ppm.

A commonly used catalyst for epoxy resins, diethylenetriamine is an irritant of the skin and respiratory tract. It is a definite skin sensitizer and a probable pulmonary sensitizer. It is severely damaging to the eye.

Alkanololamines

This class of chemicals are alkaline solutions that are used as intermediates in the production of emulsifiers, drugs, detergents, solubilizers, cosmetics, and textile finishing agents.

Ethanolamine

$$H_2N\text{-}CH_2\text{-}CH_2\text{-}OH$$

The PEL is 3 ppm and the short-term exposure limit (STEL) is 6 ppm.

Ethanolamine is a colorless liquid with a mild ammonia odor that is detectable at 3–4 ppm. It is a normal urine constituent in man, excreted at a rate of 5–23 mg/day. In the body, it can be methylated to choline or converted to serine or glycine. Forty percent of an administered dose is deaminated and excreted as urea. Its irritant effects are more severe than those expected from its alkalinity. In animals, low doses cause hypertension, diuresis, salivation, and pupillary dilatation. At higher doses, one sees sedation, coma, and death from hypotension and cardiovascular collapse. There are no reported human injuries.

Diethanolamine

$$CHO\text{-}CH_2\text{-}CH_2)_2\text{-}NH$$

A viscous liquid used in the manufacture of rubber chemicals, herbicides, and demulsifiers, diethanolamine is also used to scrub gases and as an emulsifier and dispersing agent for herbicides, cosmetics, and pharmaceuticals. It is less potent in inducing the systemic effects noted for monoethanolamine and is an irritant of the skin and mucous membrane in man.

Triethanolamine

$$(HO\text{-}CH_2\text{-}CH_2)_3\text{-}N$$

Triethanolamine is a very viscous alkaline liquid used for the manufacture of surface active agents, waxes, polishes, herbicides, and cutting oils. No industrial injuries have been recorded. Toxic effects are predicted to be limited to mild skin irritation.

Aromatic Amines

Aromatic amines, as aliphatic amines, are categorized as being primary, secondary, or tertiary. In addition, the aromatic component may have more than one amine group (i.e., a di- or triamine). The principal route of absorption is via skin contact, which explains why the adverse health effects observed were largely unexpected. Inhalation is possible, but vapor pressures are generally low at normal temperatures. The salt forms of these compounds may be inhaled as dust during the manipulation of solid products.

Toxic effects are exerted through metabolites. Parent compounds, such as benzidine, β-naphthylamine, and aminodiphenyl, are activated to their carcinogenic forms. In contrast, aniline interacts with the red blood cells to produce methemoglobin, thus inducing a form of chemical asphyxia. Skin, respiratory, and liver effects are also notable and are discussed with the specific compounds.

Aniline

$$C_6H_5\text{—}NH_3$$

The TLV is 2 ppm, with an eight-hour time-weighted average (TWA) of 5 ppm.

Aniline is used in the manufacture of dyestuffs, rubber, and p,p′-methylenebisphenyldiisocyanate (MDI). It is readily absorbed via inhalation or skin absorption. The major acute toxic effect is the formation of methemoglobin. Mucosal cyanosis is evident at 10%–15%, with symptoms beginning at levels of 30%. Biologic monitoring is possible through hemoglobin analysis (action recommended at 5% methemoglobin), investigation for reticulocytes, or measuring urinary excretion of p-aminophenol (should not exceed 50 mg/L).

Aminophenols

$$HO\text{—}C_6H_4\text{—}NH$$

While aminophenols exist in three isomeric forms, p-aminophenol is the most important. All have low volatility and are poorly absorbed through the skin. The o- and p- isomers are skin sensitizers. Since they do not have ready access into the body, they do not pose a methemoglobin hazard.

Chloroanilines

$$Cl\text{—}C_6H_4\text{—}NH$$

This compound also exists as three isomers, with the ortho and para forms being used in the manufacture of dyes, pharmaceuticals, and pesticides. Both can be absorbed through the skin. p-Chloroaniline is capable of inducing methemoglobin. Neither are animal carcinogens.

Dimethylaniline and Diethylaniline

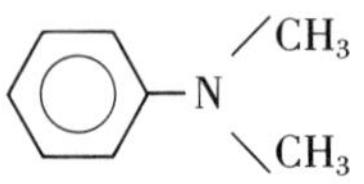

Both of these compounds are used in the manufacture of dyestuffs and other intermediates. They are readily absorbed through the skin as well as by inhalation of vapors. They are potent methemoglobin-formers.

Nitroanilines

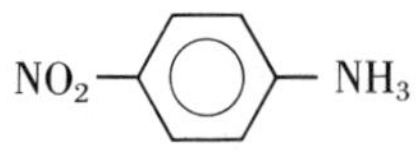

All isomers are used as dye intermediates, with para being the predominant industrial product. It is readily absorbed through the skin as well as by inhalation of dust or vapor. In addition to being powerful methemoglobin-formers, nitroanilines are capable of inducing hemolysis and liver damage. Chloronitroanilines, aside from being more potent for the above effects, are also skin sensitizers.

Phenylenediamines

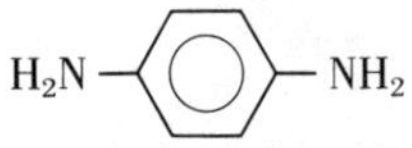

The PEL is 0.1 mg/cu m (skin).

The para isomer is used as a dyestuff intermediate as well as a dye for hair and furs. It is a potent skin and respiratory tract sensitizer. It does not induce methemoglobin in vivo. Carcinogenicity assays are negative or inconclusive.

Toluidines

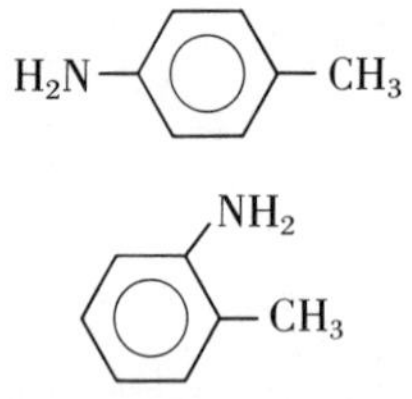

The PEL is 5 ppm (skin); the TLV is 2 ppm (skin).

The ortho and para isomers of toluidine are used in the production of dyes and other organic chemicals. They are readily absorbed through the skin and may also be inhalation hazards. They are potent methemoglobin-formers and also cause gross or microscopic hematuria in acute poisoning via bladder irritation. o-Toluidine is a suspected carcinogen, but results have not been conclusive.

5-CHLORO-o-TOLUIDINE

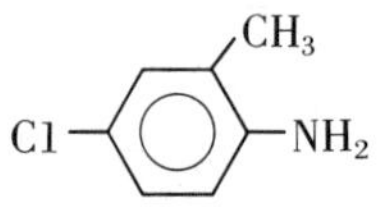

This chemical is notable for its ability to irritate the urinary tract and induce hemorrhagic cystitis. Microscopic hematuria may precede the development of symptoms. It is not a carcinogenic hazard.

Benzidine

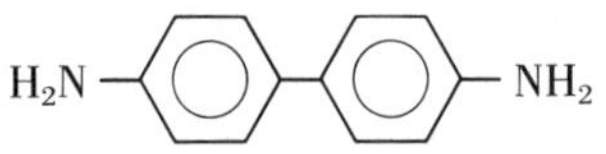

Benzidine is used in the manufacture of azo dyes and recognized as a human carcinogen. It has induced papillomas and carcinomas of the urinary bladder. Skin absorption predominates, but inhalation is possible.

Diphenylamine

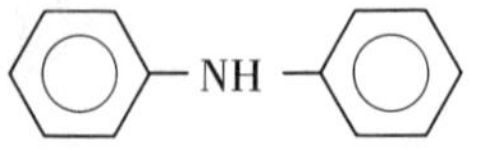

It is used in the manufacture of dyestuffs, antioxidants, pharmaceuticals, explosives, and pesticides. There are no definite cases of industrial poisoning. Impurities, especially 4-aminodiphenyl, may pose a carcinogenic risk.

Naphthylamines

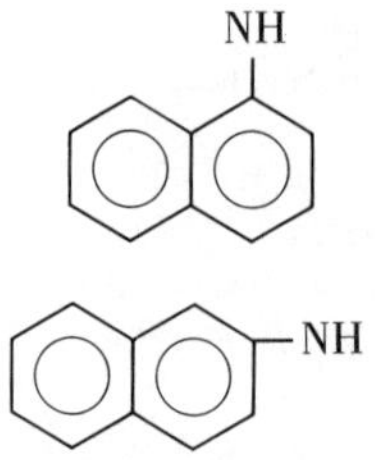

2-Naphthylamine has been almost entirely abandoned throughout the world because of its high carcinogenic potency for the bladder. 1-Naphthylamine is absorbed through the skin. Its role as a carcinogen is in doubt because of the presence of 2-naphthylamine as a contaminant.

Phenylnaphthylamines

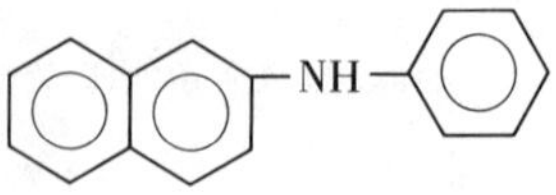

These are used as antioxidants in the rubber industry. Acne and leukoderma have been reported as well as dermatitis. The carcinogenic potential of phenylnaphthylamines is questionable because of the presence of naphthylamine as a contaminant.

Methylene Dianiline (MDA)

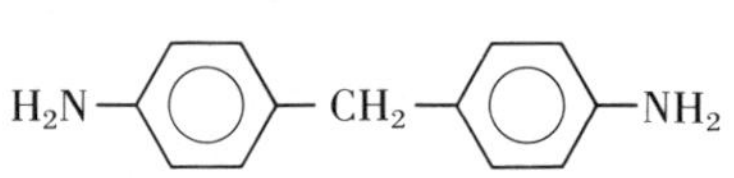

This chemical is notable for its use in the production of isocyanates, polyisocyanates, and polyurethanes. It can cause allergic contact dermatitis and has been associated with toxic hepatitis via skin absorption (occupational) and ingestion of contaminated bread (environmental). While MDA itself has not been shown to be carcinogenic, methylene-o-chloroaniline (MOCA) is carcinogenic for animals. (See further details for MDA in this chapter and chapter 63 for MOCA.

REFERENCES

1. American Conference of Governmental Industrial Hygienists: *Documentation of Threshold Limit Values for Substances in Workroom Air,* ed 5. Cincinnati, Oh, ACGIH, 1986.
2. Clayton GD, Clayton FE (eds): *Patty's Industrial Hygiene and Toxicology,* ed 3. New York, John Wiley & Sons, 1982.
3. International Labor Organization: *Encyclopedia of Occupational Health and Safety,* ed 3. Geneva, International Labour Office, 1983.

AMMONIA

Ammonia (NH_3) is a colorless gas and is one of the most widely used industrial chemicals, ranking fourth in volume of production after sulfuric acid, lime, and oxygen. Production in the United States is about 15 million metric tons. The principal uses of ammonia are direct-application fertilizer (26%), conversion to other chemical fertilizers (48%), fibers and plastics (8%), explosives and plastics (4%), and animal feeds (3%). It also is used in producing other chemicals, as a food additive, in detergents, in insecticides, and as a major commercial refrigerant. No precise figure is available as to the extent of employee exposure to ammonia; however, the NIOSH estimates that 500,000 workers have potential exposure. Occupational exposure to ammonia may occur in a number of industries, including laboratories, nitriding furnaces, fertilizer manufacturing, explosives manufacturing, coke making, diazotype reproducing operations, commercial refrigerator repair, and in various plants producing other materials mentioned earlier.

Ammonia vapor is a severe irritant to the eyes, respiratory tract, and skin. Inhalation of concentrations of 2,500–6,500 ppm causes severe corneal irritation, dyspnea, bronchospasm, chest pain, and pulmonary edema that may be fatal; production of pink, frothy sputum often occurs. Complications can include bronchitis or pneumonia; some residual reduction in pulmonary function has been reported.

In a human experimental study that exposed ten subjects to various vapor concentrations for five minutes, 134 ppm caused irritation of the eyes, nose, and throat in most subjects and one person complained of chest irritation; at 72 ppm, several reported the same symptoms; at 50 ppm, two reported nasal dryness; and at 32 ppm, only one reported nasal dryness. In a survey of eight workers in a blueprint shop, ammonia concentrations of 4–29 ppm caused "barely noticeable" to "moderate" eye irritation; no respiratory irritation was reported.

Tolerance to usually irritating concentrations of ammonia may be acquired by adaptation, a phenomenon frequently observed among workers who become inured to the effects of exposure. No data are available on concentrations that are irritating to workers who are regularly exposed to ammonia and who presumably have a higher irritation threshold.

Liquid anhydrous ammonia in contact with the eyes may cause serious eye injury or blindness; on the skin, it causes first- and second-degree burns that often are severe and, if extensive, may be fatal. Vapor concentrations of 10,000 ppm are mildly irritating to the moist skin and 30,000 ppm or greater cause a stinging sensation and may produce skin burns and vesiculation.

Wherever ammonia is used in quantity, respiratory equipment should be available for emergencies. Explosive concentrations of ammonia can be produced when the contents of a tank or a refrigeration system are released into an open flame, boiler fire, or arc.

Treatment

There should be prompt removal from exposure; if liquid splash has occurred, immediately flush eyes and skin with water. Recommendations for ammonia spills are as follows:

1. Following ammonia ingestion, a conscious person should immediately be given large quantities of water to dilute the ammonia.
2. Persons who have inhaled ammonia should be observed closely for visual disturbances, upper airway obstruction, and hypoxia.
3. The area of the ammonia spill or leak should be ventilated to disperse the gas. A flow of gaseous ammonia should be stopped; liquid ammonia should be allowed to vaporize.
4. Persons not wearing protective equipment and clothing should be restricted from areas of spills or leaks until the cleanup has been completed.

Consideration should be given to hospitalization and observation for 72 hours for delayed onset of pulmonary edema.

A TLV of 25 ppm has been selected to protect against irritation to eyes and the respiratory tract.

REFERENCES

1. American Conference of Governmental Industrial Hygienists: Ammonia, in *Documentation of the Threshold Limit Values for Substances in Workroom Air,* ed 5, Cincinnati, Oh, ACGIH, 1986.
2. Exposure to ammonia, proposed standards. *Federal Register,* 40:54684–54693, Nov 25, 1975.
3. Hygienic Guide Series: Anhydrous ammonia. *Am Ind Hyg Assoc J* 1971; 32:139.
4. National Institute for Occupational Safety and Health, US Dept of Health, Education, and Welfare: *Criteria for a Recommended Standard . . . Occupational Exposure to Ammonia, NIOSH,* US Government Printing Office, Washington, DC, 1974.
5. *Occupational Health Guidelines for Ammonia.* US Dept of Health and Human Services, US Dept of Labor, September 1978.

BENZIDINE-DERIVED DYES

The National Occupational Hazard Survey (NOHS), conducted between 1972 and 1974 by the National Institute for Occupational Safety and Health, indicates that workers are occupationally exposed to Direct Black 38, Direct Brown 95, and Direct

Blue 6 in a variety of industries, including: paper and allied products, petroleum and related industries, rubber and plastic products, leather and leather products, instrumentation and measuring devices, and banking. In addition, the textile industry accounts for a substantial occupational exposure. It is estimated that 25% of the benzidine-derived azo dyes are applied to textiles, 40% to paper, 15% to leather, and the remainder to other diverse applications.[3] The *Color Index*,[2] a reference by Great Britain's Society of Dyers and Colorists, reports the following uses for the three dyes.

Direct Black 38: Dyeing or staining of wool, silk, fibers for rope and matting, hog hair, cellulose, acetate, nylon, and biologic stains.

Direct Brown 95: Dyeing or staining silk, cotton, acetate, cellulose, wood, nylon, leather, paper, and certain plastics.

Direct Blue 6: Dyeing or staining silk, wool, cotton, nylon, leather, paper, biologic stains, and writing inks.

Benzidine has been an important intermediate in dye production since its introduction to the dyestuff industry around 1890. In 1948, production of benzidine-derived dyes was 16 million kg, which accounted for 25% of all domestic dyes manufactured and almost all of the direct-class dyes. Domestic production of direct benzidine-derived dyes dropped to 6 million kg in 1971. Domestic production in 1978 was limited to 12 benzidine dyes. The latest domestic production figures for Direct Black 38 show 3 million kg in 1971, down to 1 million kg in 1975, which rose to 2 million kg in 1976. Direct Brown 95 showed an increased production to 300,000 kg in 1976, which was up from 200,000 kg in 1975 and 150,000 kg in 1974. Domestic production figures for Direct Blue 6 indicated that 150,000 kg were produced in 1973, which is the last available figure for that dye.

In the general population, unspecified exposure levels to the three dyes are thought to occur through the use of retail packaged dyes for home dyeing and for home and school use in art and craft projects such as tie-dyeing or batik. The Art Hazards Project of the Center for Occupational Hazards, New York City, has reported that packaged dyes sold in supermarkets, variety stores, and hardware stores are combinations of direct, acid, and basic dyes, and thus may contain benzidine-derived dye components.[4] Two of these dyes, Direct Black 38 and Direct Blue 6, have been used in hair dyes.[11]

Caution is also indicated by preliminary results from the NIOSH field studies showing that humans working with these same dyes also excrete higher than expected levels of benzidine in their urine. Both laboratory and field studies indicate that these benzidine-derived dyes can be metabolized to benzidine, which is present in the urine of animals and humans. Based on the data from the short-term study, National Cancer Institute (NCI) scientists believe that a cancer-causing potential exists on exposure to the benzidine-derived dyes, most likely through the mechanism of metabolic conversion of the dyes to benzidine in the animal system.

NIOSH Field Studies

Preliminary results from NIOSH studies indicate the presence of benzidine or monacetylbenzidine (MAB), a metabolite of benzidine, in the urine of workers in four of five industrial facilities in which urine samples were collected. The facilities surveyed to date include two benzidine dye manufacturers, two textile-finishing companies, and a leather tannery.

In one dye manufacturing plant, benzidine and MAB were found in all dye workers who worked solely with the finished dyes. Bulk benzidine-based dyes were quantitatively analyzed for residual free benzidine content, which ranged from less than 1 to 19 ppm. It was conservatively estimated that about 20 times more benzidine and up to 200 times more MAB were present in the urine of these dye workers than if they had been exposed only to the residual benzidine content in the dyes. The concentrations of benzidine found in the urine of these workers were significant fractions of those concentrations associated with a high incidence of bladder cancer as reported in the scientific literature. Among tex-

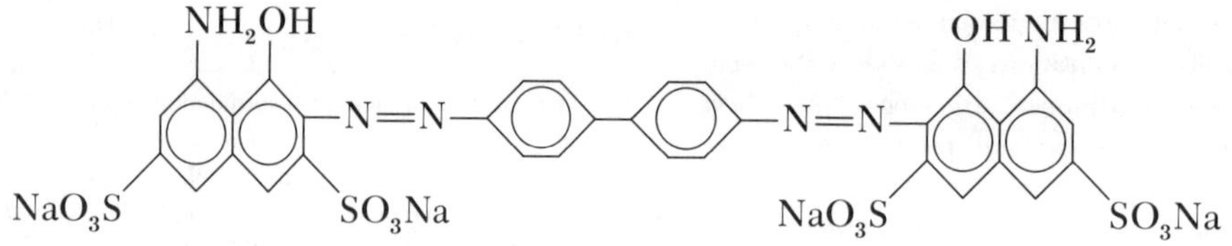

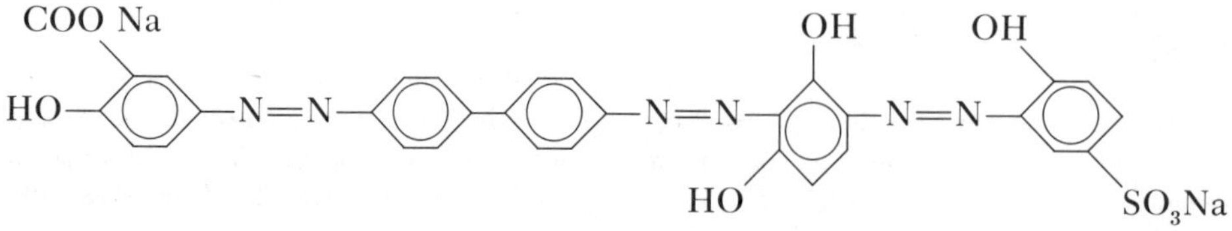

NH_2 OH — N=N — — N=N — OH NH_2

NaO_3S SO_3Na NaO_3S SO_3Na

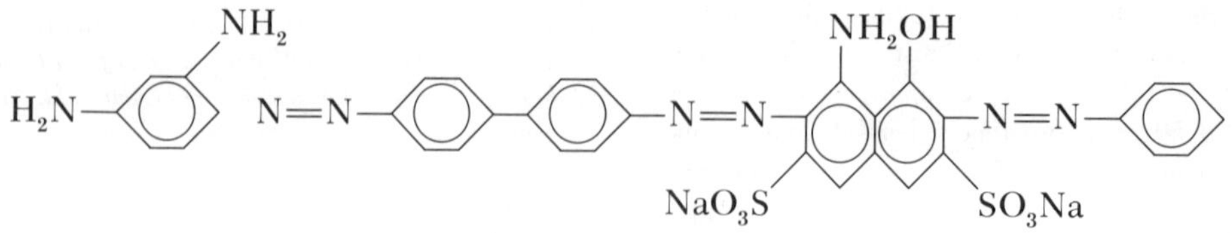

NH_2 NH_2 OH

H_2N — N=N — — N=N — — N=N —

NaO_3S SO_3Na

COO Na OH OH

HO — N=N — — N=N — — N=N —

HO SO_3Na

tile dyers included in the NIOSH study, four of ten had benzidine or MAB present in their urine and all had elevated aromatic amine levels. No benzidine or MAB was detected in urine samples collected at a leather tannery where good work practices were observed. Although there was biologic variability in body burden tolerance and differences in metabolism among those studied, it appears likely that work practices and personal hygiene played a major role in minimizing exposure. Analyses of data from these NIOSH studies are ongoing.

The relatively large particle size of the dry dye powders causes inhaled dyes to be deposited largely in the upper respiratory tract and then ingested. Prevention of worker inhalation or ingestion of these dyes would greatly reduce absorption into the body and subsequent benzidine exposure.

A strong association relating human exposure to benzidine-based dyes with the subsequent development of bladder tumors was presented after a case-control mortality study of 200 bladder cancer patients in Japan.[14] The patients were found to have been predominantly kimono painters and dyers. The kimono painters had a habit of forming a point on their brushes by drawing the brush between their lips, which allowed for ingestion of the dyes. Several other case-control mortality studies indicate an increased risk of developing bladder cancer in the textile and leather industries, both large users of direct dyes. However, only a few references have been made concerning benzidine-derived dyestuffs. In Russia, a medical study concerning the early detection of bladder tumors among textile dyers using benzidine-derived dyes revealed an unusual incidence of bladder lesions, some of which were suggested as being of a precancerous nature. The greatest number of such lesions were found in those workers with the highest potential exposure to these dyes.[5]

The NIOSH recommends that it would be prudent to handle Direct Black 38, Direct Brown 95, and Direct Blue 6 in the workplace as if they were human carcinogens. Exposure to Direct Black 38, Direct Brown 95, and Direct Blue 6 should be limited to as few employees as possible, while minimizing workplace exposure levels. The area in which they are used should be restricted to only those employees essential to the process or operation.

Exposure Monitoring

Initial and routine employee exposure surveys should be made by competent industrial hygiene and engineering personnel. These surveys are necessary to determine the extent of employee exposure and to ensure that controls are effective.

Minimizing Employee Exposure

There are four basic methods of limiting employee exposure; none of these is a simple industrial hygiene or management decision and careful planning and thought should be used prior to implementation of any of them.

Product Substitution.—The substitution of an alternative material with a lower potential health and safety risk is one method. However, extreme care must be used when selecting possible substitutes. Alternatives to Direct Black 38, Direct Brown 95, and Direct Blue 6 should be fully evaluated with regard to possible human effects. Unless the toxic effects of the alternative have been thoroughly evaluated, a seemingly safe replacement may be found to induce serious health effects, possibly only after years of use.

Contaminant Controls.—The most effective control of Direct Black 38, Direct Brown 95, and Direct Blue 6, where feasible, is at the source of contamination by enclosure of the operation and/or local exhaust ventilation. If feasible, the process or operation should be enclosed with a slight vacuum so that any leakage will result in the flow of air into the enclosure. The next most effective means of control would be a well-designed local exhaust ventilation system that physically encloses the process as much as possible, with sufficient capture velocity to keep the contaminant from entering the work atmosphere. To ensure that ventilation equipment is working properly, effectiveness (e.g., air velocity, static pressure, or air volume) should be checked at least every three months. System effectiveness should be checked soon after any change in production, process, or control that might result in significant increases in airborne exposures to Direct Black 38, Direct Brown 95, and Direct Blue 6.

Employee Isolation.—A third alternative is the isolation of employees. It frequently involves the use of automated equipment operated by personnel observing from a closed control booth or room. The control room is maintained at a greater air pressure than that surrounding the process equipment so that air flow is out of, rather than into, the room. This type of control will not protect those employees who must do process checks, adjustments, maintenance, and related operations.

Personal Protective Equipment.—The least preferred method is the use of personal protective equipment. This equipment, which may include respirators, goggles, gloves, and other devices, should not be used as the only means to prevent or minimize exposure during routine operations. Exposure to Direct Black 38, Direct Brown 95, and Direct Blue 6 should not be controlled with the use of respirators except during the time period necessary to install or implement engineering or work practice controls, or in work situations in which engineering and work practice controls are technically not feasible, or for maintenance, or for operations that require entry into tanks or closed vessels or in emergencies.

REFERENCES

1. Benzidine derived dyes. *Current Intelligence Bull* 24, Joint NIOSH/NCI. Cincinnati, Oh, US Dept of Health, Education, and Welfare, PHS, Publications Dissemination, DTS, National Institute for Occupational Safety and Health, April 17, 1978.
2. *Color Index*, ed 3. London, The Society of Dyers and Colorists, 1975.
3. Environmental Protection Agency, 40 CFR Pt 129, Benzidine: Proposed toxic pollutant effluent standards. *Federal Register* 41: No 127, June 30, 1973.
4. Jenkins C: *Dye Hazards Report*. Raleigh, NC, American Association of Textile Chemists and Colorists, 1978.
5. Korosteleva T, Kljuckareu B, Belokhuostave A, et al.: Immunological diagnosis in early stages of occupational cancer of the urinary bladder. *Probl Oncol* 1973; 19:28–32.

6. Lubs H.: *The Chemistry of Synthetic Dyes and Pigments*, Monograph 127. Washington, DC, American Chemical Society, 1952.
7. *Synthetic Organic Chemicals: United States Production and Sales*. Washington, DC, US International Trade Commission Report, 1973.
8. *Synthetic Organic Chemicals: United States Production and Sales*. Washington, DC, US International Trade Commission Report, 1974.
9. *Synthetic Organic Chemicals: United States Production and Sales*. Washington, DC, US International Trade Commission Report, 1975.
10. *Synthetic Organic Chemicals: US Tariff Commission, Report on Synthetic Organic Dyes*, Series 6-2, 1948.
11. 13-Week Subchronic Toxicity Studies of Direct Blue 6, Direct Black 38, and Direct Brown 95 Dyes. National Cancer Institute. Carcinogenesis Technical Report. DHEW Publ NIH 78-1358, 1978.
12. Synthetic Organic Chemicals: United States Production and Sales. Washington, DC, US International Trade Commission Report, 1971.
13. Venkataraman K: *The Chemistry of Synthetic Dyes*. New York, Academic Press, 1952, pp 506–514.
14. Voshida O, Miyakaqa M: Etiology of Bladder Cancer: "Metabolic" Aspects, in Nakahara W, Hirayama T, Nishioka K, et al. (eds): *Analytic and Experimental Epidemiology of Cancer*. Baltimore, University Park Press, 1974, pp 31–39.

BENZOYL PEROXIDE

—C—O—O—C—
‖ ‖
O O

Benzoyl peroxide, also called dibenzoyl peroxide, is a flammable solid that may decompose explosively if subjected to excessive heat, friction, or sudden shock. If benzoyl peroxide is exposed to temperatures of 75°–80° C for prolonged periods, it becomes unstable and may decompose spontaneously. This type of sudden decomposition, a deflagration, is the rapid spreading of fire through a mass of reactive material. Such decomposition is accompanied by a 200-fold increase in volume and yields a dense white smoke consisting of benzoic acid, phenyl benzoate, terphenyls, biphenyls, benzene, and carbon dioxide. The resulting biphenyls promote the further decomposition of benzoyl peroxide into products that can catch fire and ignite the remaining benzoyl peroxide.

Benzoyl peroxide is synthesized commercially by a reaction of benzoyl chloride, sodium hydroxide, and hydrogen peroxide. Water, plasticizers, corn starch or other diluents are added to make the numerous commercial products containing benzoyl peroxide. Benzoyl peroxide has been produced commercially in the United States since 1927, 4 million kg being produced in 1982. It is used in a number of industrial processes, particularly in the manufacture of plastics. Benzoyl peroxide is a curing agent for silicone rubber, a source of free radicals in the resin cements used in dentistry, automobile body putty, and roof bolting systems in the mining industry, and an initiator in the synthesis of polyvinyl chloride. It is also a component of flour and cheese bleaches. In the early 1900s, benzoyl peroxide was used to bleach edible oils, but this practice now is rare. In the past, textiles and paper were also treated with it. In medicine, it is used in the treatment of acne and of decubitus ulcers. Formerly, it was applied in the treatment of poison ivy.

The NIOSH estimates that 25,000 workers in the United States are potentially exposed to benzoyl peroxide or its formulations. Occupations involving possible exposure to benzoyl peroxide are automobile body repair workers, bakers, benzoyl peroxide makers, cheese makers, dentists, dental assistants, flour-mill workers, miners, nurses, pharmaceutical products makers, pharmacists, physicians, plastic product makers, polyester makers, printers, silicone rubber makers, styrene makers, and telephone repair workers.

Inhalation is the main route of exposure. Benzoyl peroxide dust causes both primary irritation and sensitization dermatitis. Application to the face as a lotion for the treatment of acne in two individuals caused facial erythema and edema; patch tests with benzoyl peroxide were positive. It may produce eye irritation and, if allowed to remain on the skin, inflammation. No systemic effects have been reported in man.[1, 2] The 1986 TLV: 5 mg/cu m. The present federal standard for exposure to benzoyl peroxide in the workplace is an eight-hour TWA concentration limit of 5 mg/cu m, based on the 1968 ACGIH TLV.

REFERENCES

1. Eaglestein WH: Allergic contact dermatitis to benzoyl peroxide—report of cases. *Arch Dermatol* 1968; 97:527.
2. Grant WM: *Toxicology of the Eye*, ed 2. Springfield, Ill, Charles C Thomas, Publisher, 1974, pp 183, 1196.
3. *NIOSH Criteria for a Recommended Standard: Occupational Exposure to Benzoyl Peroxide*. US Dept of Health, Education, and Welfare, PHS, Center for Disease Control, DHEW (NIOSH) Publ 77-166, June, 1977.

COAL TAR PITCH VOLATILES

Gordon R. Reeve, Ph.D.

Although, for regulatory purposes, the definition of the U.S. Occupational Safety and Health Administration (OSHA) of the term *coal tar pitch volatiles* (CTPVs) includes "the fused polycyclic hydrocarbons which volatilize from the distillation residues of coal, petroleum (excluding asphalt), wood, and other organic matter,"[1] the following discussion is limited to CTPVs that are evolved during the destructive distillation of coal, and the production and use of coal tar and coal tar pitch.

The chemical composition of coal tar pitch is complex and variable. The number of compounds present in most coal tar pitches is estimated in the thousands.[2] Because of variation in source materials and manufacturing processes, including different temperatures and times of carbonization, no two coal tars or pitches are chemically identical.[3] In general, however, approximately 80% of the total carbon present in coal tars exists in aromatic form.[4] Volatile fumes, designated coal tar pitch volatiles, are emitted when coal tar, coal tar pitch, or their products, are heated. They contain lower molecular-weight polycyclic hydrocarbons such as naphthalene, fluorene, anthracine, acridine, and phenanthrene, and higher molecular-weight polycyclic hydrocarbons, including known carcinogens such as benzo(a)-pyrene, benzo(a)-anthracene, benzo(j)-fluoranthrene, chrysene, and dibenz(a,b)-anthracene.[3, 5] Additional aliphatics and heterocyclic hydrocarbons are

are also present, which may enhance the carcinogenic potential of other compounds present in CTPVs.[5]

Occupational Exposures

The NIOSH estimated that approximately 78,800 workers were potentially exposed to CTPVs in 80 occupations in 1974. Approximately 250,000 workers were also estimated to be potentially exposed to coal tar and/or coal tar pitch.[18] Industrial processes which typically entail CTPV exposure include (but certainly are not limited to) metallurgical coke production, chemical and tar recovery from by-products of coke and coal gas production, primary aluminum reduction, pipe coating, and the roofing and paving industries. Reference 17 provides a more comprehensive compendium of other occupations and industrial processes which are not hereafter discussed.

Coke Production and Coke By-product Recovery.—Metallurgic coke is produced by heating bituminous coal to temperatures ranging from 1,100° to 1,400° C in the absence of oxygen for 18 hours or longer.[27] Modern coke ovens are long and narrow, measuring up to 40 ft in length and 15–24 inches in width, grouped together in batteries of up to 100 ovens to conserve space and heat. Each coke oven has up to four ports on its topside and removable doors at both ends. Coal is loaded or "charged" into each oven through the topside ports. After coking is completed, the doors at both ends of the ovens are removed, and the coke is pushed out onto a quenching car, to be subsequently sprayed with water.[28] During the coking process, much of the coal mass is volatilized. Workers with the greatest exposure to the volatiles work on the topside of the ovens. Workers at the oven sides, or at the station where coke is quenched, experience lesser exposures[12, 14] (Fig 47–2).

Coke-oven gas is condensed and piped to a by-product recovery plant, where coal tar, oils, and chemicals are recovered from the condensed coke oven volatiles. Coal tar pitch is the residual from the fractional redistillation of coal tar. Coke by-products recovery operations are similar to other chemical plants, in that the processes are enclosed, usually continuous, and not labor-intensive.[27, 28] Therefore, exposures to CTPVs in such facilities are intermittent and of lesser magnitude than those of coke oven workers.

Aluminum Production.—Aluminum is produced in large, carbon-lined steel pots by electrolysis of alumina (Al_2O_3) in cryolite at approximately 900° C to aluminum metal and oxygen. Both the anodes and the cathodes consist of carbon seamed together with coal tar and/or petroleum pitch. There are two varieties of electrolytic cells: prebaked and Soderberg. For the prebaked cells, anodes are produced in a separate facility by pressing anode paste (from coke) and coal tar pitch into the desired dimensions, and then baking them at approximately 1,200° C for five to seven days, after which they are ready to be installed in the production areas or potrooms. For the Soderberg cells, anode paste with coal tar pitch is supplied to the electrolytic cell and baked in situ. The cathode of either type of cell is the potliner and may be either carbon blocks seamed together with coal tar or petroleum pitch, or a carbonaceous monolithic lining. Exposures to coal tar pitch volatiles result from baking the anodes (prebaked cell process) and from the electrolytic process in the production area or potroom.[9, 25]

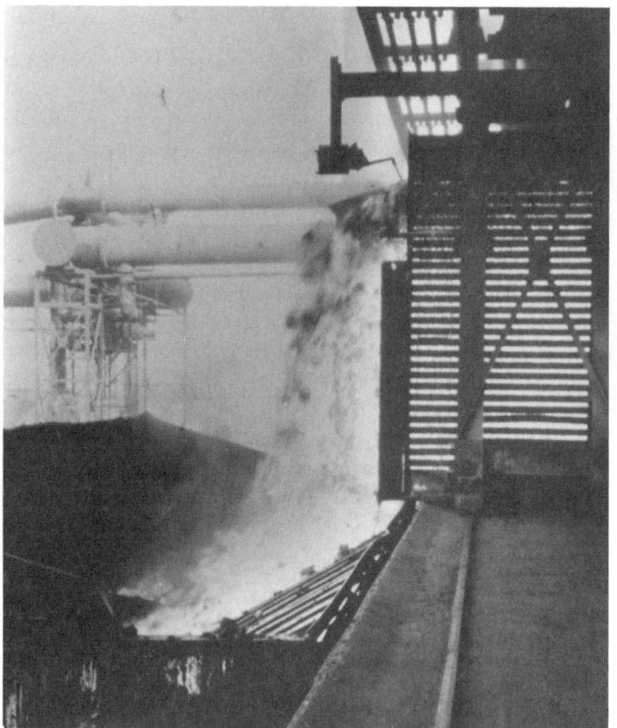

FIG 47–2.
View of coking oven being emptied, one of the major processes in steel making.

Pipe Coating.—Coal tar enamels have long been applied to steel pipe to inhibit corrosion, and such linings now are used for approximately 75% of all underground oil, gas, and municipal water pipelines currently in service.[11] Coal tar enamel is a blend of coal tar pitch and mineral fillers, usually pulverized talc.[29] In these coating operations, cleaned and primed pipe is passed and rotated under a stream of coal tar enamel heated to 260° C. The coated pipe is then wrapped with a bonded asbestos felt and a layer of paper.[15]

Workers near the coating apparatus typically have the greatest CTPV exposure. Other workers who patch imperfections in the finished coating also receive exposure to CTPVs. Anyone inside the coating building or shed similarly may be exposed if local exhaust ventilation is inadequate.

Roofing and Paving.—The use of coal tar in roofing and paving has been substantially reduced by the substitution of asphalt in many applications. Despite this, coal tar is still used in special circumstances.[16] In contrast to coal tar pitch and CTPVs, asphalt fume is generally less than 1% aromatic and greater than 99% aliphatic straight-chain unbranched hydrocarbons. Concern has been expressed that this latter fraction may account for the carcinogenic effects of asphalt fumes through a cocarcinogenic mechanism.[19]

Effects of Exposure

The major routes of coal tar pitch and CTPV exposure are dermal and inhalational. Diffuse erythema of exposed skin, with the sensation of burning and pruritus, may be temporarily disabling. Areas of folliculitis with comedones are common.[1, 26] Phototoxic keratoconjunctivitis occurs among roofers with coal tar pitch exposure.[4] Keratoacanthomas (pitch warts) occur after prolonged exposure; some of these may develop into squamous cell carcinomas.[1] Malignant skin lesions among CTP- and CTPV-exposed workers are primarily squamous cell carcinomas, with only 2.5% of malignant lesions being basal cell carcinomas in one series of 3,700 cases.[7] A survey of pitch workers identified keratotic papillomas among 10% of the group. Greater than 90% of the same group had some form of acneiform lesion.[8] In Great Britain from 1920 through 1945, nearly 5,000 persons were affected with CTP- and CTPV-associated skin cancer.[7] More recently, a fourfold excess of nonmelanotic skin cancer deaths was reported among U.S. roofers using hot pitch and asphalt compounds.[6] No skin cancer deaths were observed during a study of 3,500 coke oven workers, however; this was attributed to screening and intervention programs of the steel companies.[12, 13]

Except in coke by-product recovery workers,[3, 24] excess lung cancer mortality is consistently found in epidemiologic studies of CTPV-exposed workers. Coal tar pitch volatiles evolved from coal tars and coal tar pitches distilled at higher temperatures are associated with greater lung cancer mortality than CTPVs evolved at lower temperatures.[12] Lung cancer mortality among Japanese gas producers operating generators at 1,500° C had an 800% increased lung cancer mortality.[10] Among workers at the top of the gas retorts, a 3,200% excess in lung cancer was reported. Among U.S. coke oven workers operating ovens at temperatures from 1,200 to 1,400° C, a 250% lung cancer excess has been seen, with a 1,000% excess among workers at the top of the ovens.[12, 14, 23] British gas workers operating retorts from 400 to 900° C had lung cancer excesses of approximately twice that expected.[3] Lung cancer excesses ranging from 127% to 323% have also been reported in the aluminum industry workers for both the prebake and Soderberg processes.[5, 25] Among roofers who had used coal tar pitch, a 60% excess was seen among workers with at least 20 years of latency.[6]

Excesses of kidney cancer ranging from 450% to 750% have been reported among U.S. coke oven workers.[23] A 200% excess has been reported for British gas works and coke oven workers.[3] Excesses of bladder cancer deaths have been seen among gas producers[3] and Soderberg process aluminum workers.[25] A possible causal agent is β-naphthylamine, low levels of which (1 ppm) have been reported in the general atmosphere of gas works, with the suspicion that affected workers had received much higher exposures. Detectable amounts also have been identified in pitch derived from coal.[3] An excess of pancreatic cancer has been reported among workers in the aluminum industry[25] and in coke by-products and coal handling segments of the coking industry.[24]

Applicable Standards

Coal tar pitch volatile exposures should be limited to no greater than the permissible limits specified by regulation.[20] In the U.S., there are two standards applied by OSHA to CTPVs. The "coke oven standard," applicable only to CTPV exposures resulting from coking operations, limits allowable CTPV exposures to 150 μg/cu m (benzene soluble fraction) for an eight-hour time-weighted average (TWA). Numerous engineering and operational controls are specified, which are designed to limit CTPV exposures. Extensive medical screening is stipulated at initial employment and at specified subsequent intervals and should include medical and work history, chest x-ray, pulmonary function tests, weight, skin examination, urine analysis, sputum cytology, and urinary cytology. The CTPV standard applicable to all other exposures[20] is the 1968 American Conference of Governmental Industrial Hygienists' (ACGIH) TLV for airborne contaminants, adopted in 1971 by OSHA. Under this standard, occupational exposure to CTPVs is 200 μg/cu m as an eight-hour TWA. Unlike the coke oven standard, this standard does not specify engineering and operational controls and medical screening procedures. In 1977, the NIOSH recommended that occupational exposure to coal tar products be limited to 100 μg/cu m as a TWA for up to a ten-hour workday, 40-hour workweek.[17] The NIOSH has concluded that coal tar products, derived from carbonization of coal, are carcinogenic; and the recommended permissible exposure limit represents the lowest concentration that could reliably be detected by the then-recommended method of environmental monitoring.

REFERENCES

1. Adams RM: *Occupational Skin Disease*. New York, Grune & Stratton, 1983.
2. Bingham E, Falk HL: Environmental carcinogens. The modifying effect of cocarcinogens on the threshold response. *Arch Ind Health* 1969; 19:779–783.
3. Doll R, Vessey MP, Berarley WR, et al: Mortality of gasworkers—Final report of a prospective study. *Br J Ind Med* 1972; 29: 294–406.
4. Emmett EA, Stetzer L, Taphorn B: Phototoxic keratoconjunctivitis from coal-tar pitch volatiles. *Science* 1977; 198:841–842.
5. Gibbs GW, Horowitz I: Lung cancer mortality in aluminum reduction industry. *J Occup Med* 1983; 21:347–353.
6. Hammond EC, Selikoff JJ, Lawther PL, et al: Inhalation of benzpyrene and cancer in man. *Ann NY Acad Sci* 1983; 271: 116–124.
7. Henry SA: Occupational cutaneous cancer attributable to certain chemicals in industry. *Br Med Bull* 1947; 4:389–401.
8. Hodgson GA, Whiteley HJ: Personal susceptibility to pitch. *Br J Ind Med* 1970; 27:160–166.
9. Karsten KP: Aluminum, in Cralley LV, Cralley LJ (eds): *Industrial Hygiene Aspects of Plant Operations. Vol I. Process Flows*. New York, MacMillan Publishing Co, 1982, pp 47–59.
10. Kawai M, Amamoto H, Harada K: Epidemiologic study of occupational lung cancer. *Arch Environ Health* 1983; 14:859–864.
11. Larson B: Occupational exposure to coal tar pitch volatiles at pipeline protective coating operations. *Am Ind Hyg Assoc J* 1978; 39:250–255.
12. Lloyd JW: Long-term mortality study of steel workers. V. Respiratory cancer in coke plant workers. *J Occup Med* 1971; 13: 53–60.
13. Lloyd JW: Personal communication, 1981.

14. Mazumdar S, Redmond C, Sollecito W, et al: An epidemiology study of exposure to coal tar pitch volatiles among coke oven workers. *J Am Poll Control Assoc* 1975; 25:382–389.
15. McManus JJ, Pennie WL, Davies A: Hot applied coal tar coatings. *Ind Eng Chem* 1966; 58:43–46.
16. McNeil D: The physical properties and chemical structure of coal tar pitch, in Hoiberg AJ (ed): *Bituminous Materials: Asphalts, Tars, and Pitches*. New York, Interscience Publishers, John Wiley & Sons, 1966, pp 139–216.
17. National Institute for Occupational Safety and Health: *Criteria for a Recommended Standard: Occupational Exposure to Coal Tar Products*, NIOSH Publ 78–107. Cincinnati, Oh, US Dept of Health, Education, and Welfare, NIOSH, 1977.
18. National Institute for Occupational Safety and Health: *National Occupational Hazard Survey. Vol III. Survey Analysis and Supplementary Tables*, DHEW(NIOSH) Publ 78–114. Cincinnati, Oh, US Dept of Health, Education, and Welfare, National Institute for Occupational Safety and Health, 1978.
19. Niemeier RW, Thayer PS, Menzies KT, et al: *A Comparison of the Skin Carcinogenicity of Condensed Roofing Asphalt and Coal Tar Pitch Fumes*. Cincinnati, Oh, US Dept of Health and Human Services, National Institute for Occupational Safety and Health, 1984.
20. Occupational Safety and Health Administration. *General Industry: OSHA Safety and Health Standards* (29 CFR 1910). Washington, DC, US Government Printing Office, 1981.
21. Occupational Safety and Health Administration: Occupational exposure to coal tar pitch volatiles; Modification of interpretation. *Federal Register* 1983; 48:2764–2768.
22. Puzinauskas VP, Corbett LW: *Differences Between Petroleum Asphalt, Coal-Tar Pitch, and Road Tar*, Research Report 78–1. College Park, Md, The Asphalt Institute, 1978, p 25.
23. Redmond C, Ciocco A, Lloyd JW, et al: Long-term study of steelworkers. VI. Mortality from malignant neoplasms of coke oven workers. *J Occup Med* 1972; 14:621–629.
24. Redmond CK, Strobine BR, Cypress RH: Cancer experience among coke by-products workers. *Ann NY Acad Sci* 1976; 271:102–115.
25. Rockette HE, Arena VC: Mortality studies of aluminum reduction plant workers: Potroom and carbon departments. *J Occup Med* 1983; 25:549–557.
26. Schwartz L, Tulipan L, Peck SM: *Occupational Diseases of the Skin*. Philadelphia, Lea & Febiger, 1947.
27. Smith FA, Eckle TF, Osterholm RJ, et al: Manufacture of coal tar and pitches, in Hoiberg AJ (ed): *Bituminous Materials: Asphalts, Tars, and Pitches*. New York, Interscience Publishers, John Wiley & Sons, 1966, pp 57–116.
28. Webster DL: Steel Production, in Cralley LV, Cralley LJ (eds): *Industrial Hygiene Aspects of Plant Operations. Vol I. Process Flows*. New York, MacMillan Publishing Co, 1982, pp 457–487.
29. Whittier F: Pipeline coatings, in Hoiberg AJ (ed): *Bituminous Materials: Asphalts, Tars, and Pitches*. New York, Interscience Publishers, John Wiley & Sons, 1966, pp 291–322.

α-CHLORINATED TOLUENES

Shiro Tanaka, M.D.

α-Chlorinated toluenes are commercially important chemical intermediates. Four closely related compounds in this series are identified by the degree of α-chlorination of toluene or benzaldehyde: benzyl chloride, benzal chloride, benzotrichloride, and benzoyl chloride. They are discussed here together, since they are chemically related to one another and exist concomitantly in most industrial-exposure situations.

Benzyl chloride	$C_6H_5\text{-}CH_2Cl$	(benzene ring)—CH_2Cl
Benzal chloride	$C_6H_5\text{-}CHCl_2$	
Benzotrichloride	$C_6H_5\text{-}CCl_3$	(benzene ring with CCl_3)
Benzoyl chloride	$C_6H_5\text{-}COCl$	(benzene ring)— COCl

These compounds are colorless to slightly yellowish liquids. They are all highly reactive chemicals and thus are used extensively as chemical intermediates.

Benzyl chloride, benzal chloride, and benzotrichloride are all manufactured by direct chlorination of toluene in the presence of light; benzoyl chloride is produced by hydrolysis of benzotrichloride, or by reacting benzotrichloride with benzoic acid.

Benzyl chloride is used as an intermediate in the manufacture of benzyl phthalates, quaternary ammonium salts, benzyl alcohol, pharmaceuticals, and various other end products. Benzal chloride and benzotrichloride are used predominantly for manufacturing benzaldehyde and benzoyl chloride, respectively. Benzoyl chloride is used primarily to manufacture benzoyl peroxide, herbicides, dyes, plasticizers, and pharmaceuticals.

It is estimated that annual production volume is in the range of 50–100 million lbs for benzyl chloride and 2–20 million lbs for benzal chloride. Based on data from the National Occupational Hazard Survey (NOHS), the NIOSH estimates that approximately 30,000 workers are potentially exposed to benzyl chloride and 1,000 to benzoyl chloride.[5]

Toxicity

All of the chlorinated toluenes have strongly irritant properties. In an acute toxicity study of benzyl chloride, benzal chloride, and benzotrichloride in rats and mice, Mikhailova reported that all were highly irritating to mucous membranes and caused damage to the nervous system, liver, kidneys, and myocardium and loss of body weight. It was noted that acute toxicity increased as the number of chlorine atoms in the molecule increased.[4]

Studies of workers employed in benzoyl chloride manufacture have demonstrated increased risks of respiratory tract cancer[9, 10] and of all cancers combined.[11] Although these findings indicate clearly the hazards associated with occupational exposure to this process, they do not permit epidemiologic identification of a single causative agent, in that the workers have potential exposure to all three chlorinated toluenes and to benzoyl chloride.

Carcinogenicity bioassays by oral administration and by skin painting suggest that of the four chlorinated toluenes, benzotrichloride is probably the most highly carcinogenic.[2] Benzal chloride has also produced skin cancer by direct application, and benzyl chloride has produced sarcomas at the site of injection, with statistically nonsignificant increases in skin tumors.[1, 8] The International Agency for Research on Cancer (IARC) has concluded, on the basis of these currently available data, that evidence for animal carcinogenicity is "limited" for benzyl chloride and for benzal chloride, "sufficient" for benzotrichloride, and "inadequate" for benzoyl chloride. The IARC has concluded further that the evidence for human carcinogenicity is "limited," based entirely on exposures occurring through benzoyl chloride manufacture.[3]

Limiting Exposure

For protection of workers against both acute and chronic exposures to the chlorinated toluenes, processes using these materials must be enclosed, and local exhaust as well as general dilution ventilation must be provided. Since sporadic high exposures may occur from accidental leaks at the time of taking samples from reactors or during maintenance work, workers performing these activities should be equipped with a certified respirator that will adequately protect them against these compounds. Exposures during sampling can be minimized through the use of automatic, closed-system sampling devices. Frequencies of exposures resulting from leaks can be reduced through vigorous programs of scheduled plant maintenance.

Because of their high irritancy, even a mild exposure to the chlorinated toluenes would give a sufficient warning to prevent further exposure. However, if a severe respiratory exposure occurs inadvertently, a worker should be watched medically for at least 12 hours to guard against possible delayed onset of pneumonitis and pulmonary edema. If eye or skin contact occurs, the contaminated surface should be immediately washed thoroughly with water and brought to medical attention.

Currently in the United States, an occupational exposure limit has been established only for benzyl chloride, which is 1 ppm (5.0 mg/cu m) as a time-weighted average.[7] In the NIOSH criteria document for benzyl chloride, it is recommended that exposure to benzyl chloride should not exceed 5 mg/cu m determined as a ceiling concentration during any 15-minute sampling period. This recommended short-term limit is designed to safeguard exposed workers from irritation of the eyes, skin, or mucous membranes and to reduce the risk of long-term systemic effects.[6]

REFERENCES

1. Druckrey H, Kruse H, Preussman R, et al: Carcinogenic alkylating substances. III. Alkyl halogenides, sulfates, sulfonates, and ring-strained heterocyclic compounds. *Z Krebsforsch* 1970; 74:241 (in German).
2. Fukuda K, Matsushita H, Sakabe H, et al: Carcinogenicity of benzyl chloride, benzal chloride, benzotrichloride, and benzoyl chloride in mice by skin application. *Gann* 1981; 72:655.
3. International Agency for Research on Cancer: Some Industrial Chemicals and Dyestuffs. *IARC Monogr Eval Carcinog Risk Chem Hum* 1982; 29:49–91.
4. Mikhailova TV: Comparative toxicity of chloride derivatives of toluene: Benzyl chloride, benzal chloride, and benzotrichloride. Gigiena Truda i Professional'nye Zabolevaniya, 8:14, 1964; *Fed Proc* 1965; (translation supplement) 24:T877.
5. National Institute for Occupational Safety and Health: Computer printout from the National Occupational Hazard Survey (NOHS) data base collected during the period 1972–74. Cincinnati, Oh, NIOSH, Hazard Section, Surveillance Branch, 1975.
6. National Institute for Occupational Safety and Health: *Occupational Exposure to Benzyl Chloride, Criteria for a Recommended Standard*, DHEW (NIOSH) Publ 78–182. Washington, DC, Superintendent of Documents. US Government Printing Office, 1978.
7. Occupational Safety and Health Administration: Air contaminants. US Code of Federal Regulations, Title 29, Pt 1910.1000.
8. Preussman R: Direct alkylating agents as carcinogens. *Food Cosmet Toxicol* 1968; 6:576.
9. Sakabe H, Matsushita H, Koshi S: Cancer among benzoyl chloride manufacturing workers. *Ann NY Acad Sci* 1976; 271:67.
10. Sakabe H, Fukuda K: An updating report on cancer among benzoyl chloride manufacturing workers. *Ind Health* 1977; 15:173.
11. Sorahan T, Waterhouse JAH: A mortality study of workers in a factory manufacturing chlorinated toluenes. *Ann Occup Hyg* 1983; 27:173.

CHLORINE

At workplace temperatures and pressures, chlorine is a yellowish green gas with a distinctive, irritating odor. Because of its reactivity, it is not found in the uncombined state in nature, but commonly as salt (NaCl). Chlorine is produced commercially by electrolysis of brine, electrolysis of fused sodium chloride, or by oxidation of chlorides using chemical methods. By far the most important production method is the electrolysis of brine using diaphragm cells or mercury cells. U.S. chlorine production was estimated at 11 million short tons in 1976.

The pulp and paper industry uses chlorine primarily in the elemental form for bleaching pulp and paper; chlorine is used in the production of plastic and resins to make chlorinated solvents, to make ethylene glycol antifreeze, and ethylene chloride (used in antiknock additives). Chlorine is also used in textile and household bleaches, refrigerants, pharmaceuticals, cosmetics, in the beneficiating of ores, and in metal extraction. Exposure to chlorine can occur in any of these operations. In addition, exposure to chlorine can occur when hypochlorites are mixed with materials such as toilet bowl cleaners or vinegar and when chlorinated hydrocarbons are decomposed thermally or by actinic rays from welding[6,7] (Fig 47–3).

Some occupations with potential exposure to chlorine are aerosol propellent makers, alkali salt makers, aluminum purifiers, benzene hexachloride makers, bleachers, bleaching powder makers, bromine makers, broom makers, carpet makers, chemical synthesizers, calcium chloride makers, chlorinated solvent makers, chlorinated hydrocarbon insecticide makers, chlorine workers, color makers, disinfectant makers, dye makers, ethylene glycol makers, ethylene oxide makers, flour bleachers, fluorocarbon makers, gasoline additive workers, gold extractors, ink makers, iodine makers, iron detinners, iron dezincers, laundry workers, methyl chloride makers, paper bleachers, petroleum refinery workers, phosgene makers, photographic workers, pump bleachers, rayon makers, refrigerant makers, rubber makers, sewage treaters, silver extractors, sodium hydroxide makers, submarine workers, sugar refiners, sulfur chloride makers, swimming pool maintenance workers, tetraethyl lead makers, textile bleachers, tin recovery workers, vinyl chloride makers, vinylidene chloride makers, water

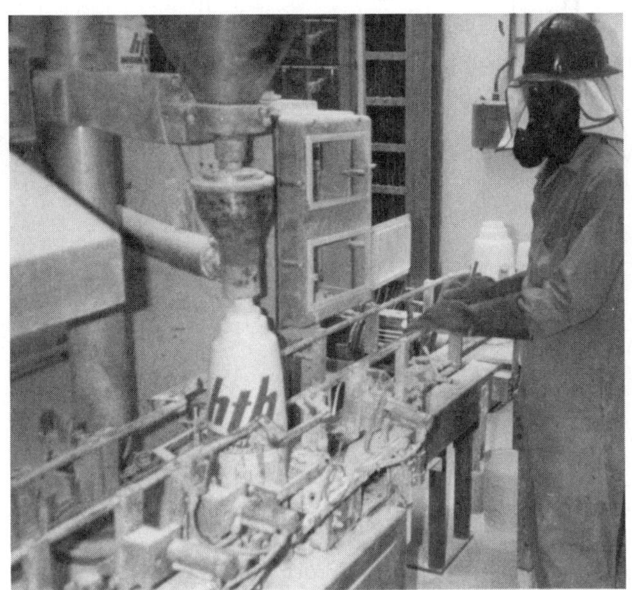

FIG 47–3.
Packaging a chloride product for home use. Note exhaust ventilation as well as respiratory protection.

treaters, and zinc chloride makers. The NIOSH has estimated that 26,000 persons are employed in the chlor-alkali manufacturing industry, and about 15,000 workers have potential occupational exposure to chlorine.[5]

The main occupational exposure is by inhalation. Chlorine gas is a severe irritant of the eyes, mucous membranes, skin, and respiratory system. Mild upper respiratory irritation may occur at 0.2–16 ppm; at 7–8 ppm, eye irritation; and cough at 30 ppm; 1,000 ppm has proved fatal after a few breaths.[4] A major accidental exposure (community) to unmeasured but high concentrations for a brief period caused burning of the eyes with lacrimation, burning of the nose and mouth with rhinorrhea, cough, choking sensation and substernal pain.[1] These symptoms frequently were accompanied by nausea, vomiting, headache, dizziness and sometimes syncope. Of the 33 persons hospitalized, all suffered tracheobronchitis; 23 progressed to pulmonary edema and, of those, 14 developed pneumonitis. Respiratory distress and substernal pain generally subsided within the first 72 hours; cough increased in frequency and severity after two to three days and became productive of thick mucopurulent sputum; cough disappeared after 14 days. In another accidental exposure of five chlorine plant workers and 13 nonworkers, pulmonary function tests showed airway obstruction and hypoxemia; these cleared within three months except in four of the chlorine plant workers who still showed effects after 12–14 months.[7] In high concentrations, chlorine irritates the skin and causes sensations of burning and pricking, inflammation, and vesicle formation. Liquid chlorine causes eye and skin burns on contact.

Treatment.—Immediate removal from exposure and hospitalization and observation for three days is advisable to guard against delayed pulmonary edema. Administer oxygen, and provide clear airway by intubation and mechanical ventilation, if needed. Positive end-expiratory pressure breathing may be indicated and helpful. If the eyes are irritated, flush with water; if there is skin contact, lightly wash with mild soap and water.

The 1986 TLV is 1 ppm.

REFERENCES

1. Chasis H, et al: Chlorine accident in Brooklyn. *Occup Med* 1947; 4:152.
2. Kaufman J, Burkons D: Clinical, roentgenologic and physiologic effects of acute chlorine exposure. *Arch Environ Health* 1971; 23:29.
3. Manufacturing Chemists Association, Inc: Chemical Safety Data Sheet SD-80, Washington, DC, 1970, pp 23–26.
4. National Research Council, Committee on Medical and Biological Effects of Environmental Pollutants: *Chlorine and Hydrogen Chloride*. Washington, DC, National Academy of Sciences, 1976, pp 116–123.
5. *NIOSH Criteria for a Recommended Standard: . . . Occupational Exposure to Chlorine*. HEW (NIOSH) Publ 76-170. Atlanta, US Dept of Health, Education, and Welfare, PHS, Center for Disease Control, 1976.
6. Rinzema LC: Behavior of chlorohydrocarbon solvents in the welding environment. *Int Arch Arbeitsmed* 1971; 28:151.
7. Rinzema LC, Silverstein LG: Hazards from chlorinated hydrocarbon decomposition during welding. *Am Ind Hyg Assoc J* 1972; 33:35.
8. World Health Organization: Environmental health criteria 21. Chlorine and hydrogen chloride. Geneva, WHO, 1982.

CHLOROETHANES

Chloroethanes are chlorinated organic compounds structurally related to ethane in which one or more of the hydrogen atoms have been replaced by a chlorine atom or atoms. Monochloroethane, for example, is shown to result from the replacement of one hydrogen atom in ethane by a chlorine atom.

At room temperature, monochloroethane is a gas, hexachloroethane is a solid, and the eight other chloroethanes are liquids. Some of the chloroethanes are manufactured on a large scale and used extensively because of their low cost and excellent solvent properties.

Pentane (C_5H_{12}), hexane (C_6H_{14}), heptane (C_7H_{16}), and octane (C_8H_{18}) are members of a homologous series of aliphatic hydrocarbons with the empirical formula C(n)H(2n + 2). At room temperature, these four classes of alkanes are colorless, neutral liquids with a light petroleum odor. Pentane, hexane, heptane, and octane are produced almost exclusively from crude petroleum by catalytic cracking, thermal cracking, hydro-cracking, and catalytic re-forming. In the processes of catalytic and thermal cracking, high molecular weight hydrocarbons are broken down at high temperatures either with or without a catalyst into lower molecular weight mixtures. During the process of hydro-cracking, high molecular weight hydrocarbons are broken down with hydrogen at high pressures and temperatures without a catalyst. In catalytic re-forming, high molecular weight hydrocarbons are passed over a platinum catalyst at elevated temperatures in the presence of high-pressure hydrogen to produce lower molecular weight mixtures, which then are separated by distillation into high-purity fractions that include pentane,

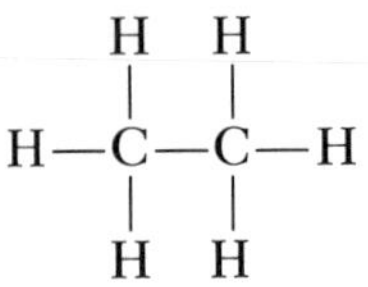

```
        H  H                      H  H
        |  |                      |  |
     H—C—C—H                 H—C—C—Cl
        |  |                      |  |
        H  H                      H  H
       Ethane                Monochloroethane

   H  H              H  Cl              H  H
   |  |              |  |               |  |
H—C—C—Cl          H—C—C—H           Cl—C—C—Cl
   |  |              |  |               |  |
   H  H              H  Cl              H  H
Chloroethane       1,1-Dichloroethane   1,2-Dichloroethane
(Ethyl Chloride)                        (Ethylene Dichloride)

   H  Cl             H  Cl              H  Cl
   |  |              |  |               |  |
H—C—C—Cl         Cl—C—C—H           Cl—C—C—Cl
   |  |              |  |               |  |
   H  Cl             H  Cl              H  Cl
1,1,1-Trichloroethane  1,1,2-Trichloroethane  1,1,1,2-Tetrachloroethane
(Methyl Chloroform)

   Cl Cl             Cl Cl              Cl Cl
   |  |              |  |               |  |
H—C—C—H           H—C—C—Cl          Cl—C—C—Cl
   |  |              |  |               |  |
   Cl Cl             Cl Cl              Cl Cl
1,1,2,2-Tetrachloroethane  Pentachloroethane  Hexachloroethane
```

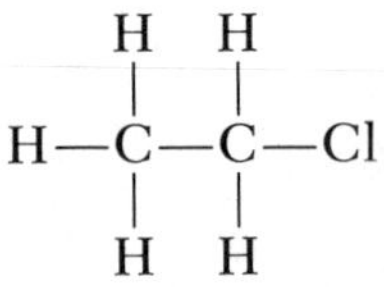

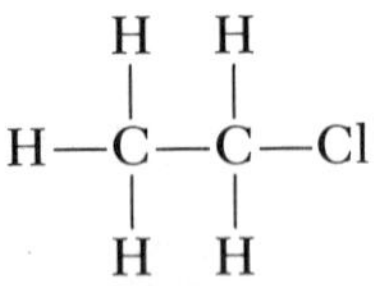

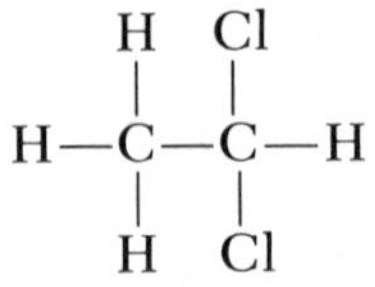

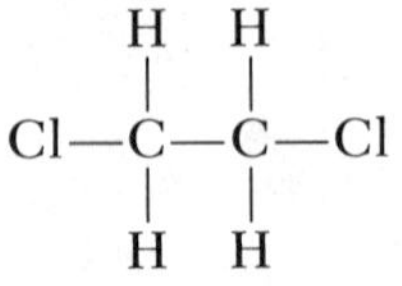

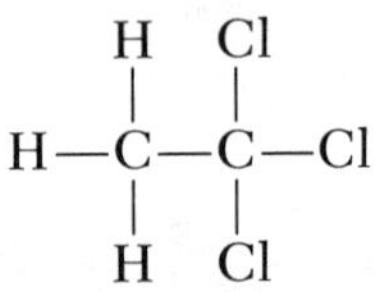

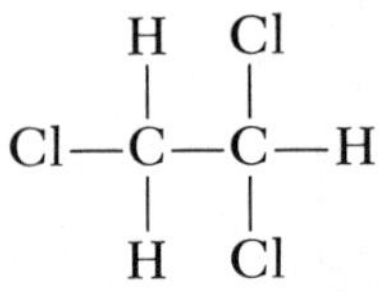

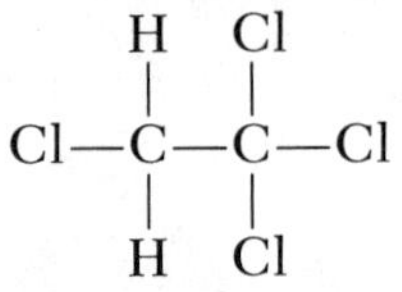

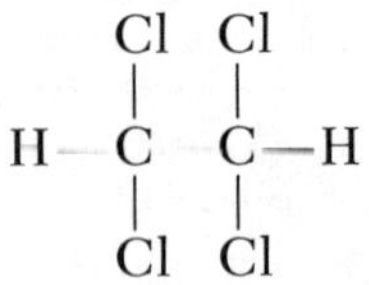

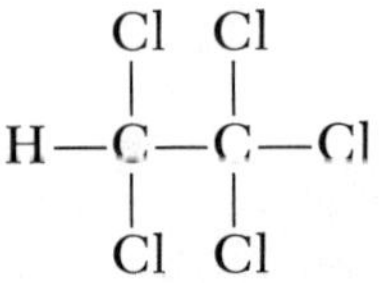

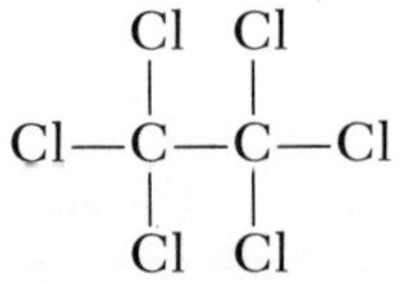

hexane, heptane, and octane. One-third of the pentane produced in the United States comes from another source, fractional condensation of natural gas. Natural gas in the United States contains an average of 0.4% pentane by volume.

The estimated U.S. production of *n*-pentane and methylbutane (isopentane) in 1967 was 310,000 and 499,000 barrels per day, respectively. This is equivalent to approximately 48 million L per day of *n*-pentane and 80 million L per day of methylbutane. In 1974, the U.S. Tariff Commission reported an annual production of 280 million liters of hexane.

Alkanes are used in a variety of industrial applications and processes. A major use of pentane is in the formulation of gasoline. Hexane is used commercially as a solvent in glues, varnishes, cements, and other products such as inks and also used in the seed oil industry to extract the natural oils from various seeds, including soybeans and cottonseed. Heptane and octane are used principally as solvents and to some extent in the formulation of gasoline.

Occupations with potential exposure to pentane, hexane, heptane, and octane are adhesive workers, automobile fuel handlers, aviation fuel handlers, cabinet finishers, degreasing workers, farm fuel handlers, furniture makers, glue fabrication workers, gluing machine operators, laboratory workers (chemical), lacquerers, lacquer makers, laminators, leather cementers, metal degreasers, petrochemical process workers, petroleum distillation workers, petroleum extraction workers, petroleum refinery workers, plastics manufacturing workers, polyethylene laminating workers, printers, printing ink production workers, resin makers, rubber cement workers, show factory workers, spray painters and stainers, stain makers, synthetic chemical production workers, synthetic rubber workers, thermometer makers (low temperature), varnish makers, vegetable oil extraction workers, and vinyl production workers. The NIOSH estimates that 10,000 workers in the United States are potentially exposed to pentane and heptane and 300,000 workers are potentially exposed to octane. It is not clear if these estimates take into account fuel handling operations. The NIOSH estimates that 2.5 million workers are potentially exposed to hexane.

Chloroethane production is estimated to be in excess of 4 billion kg in the United States. Although chloroethanes have been associated with cancer in laboratory animals, the NIOSH is unaware of any definitive evidence indicating that chloroethanes are carcinogenic in humans. The chloroethanes have long been known to be capable of producing harmful local and systemic effects. As summarized in Table 47–1, the chloroethanes may affect a variety of human organs and/or systems. The effects of chloroethane exposure vary from one compound to another, but most manifestations and laboratory findings associated with chloroethane toxicity are similar for the major routes of entry: inhalation, skin absorption, and ingestion. Liver and/or kidney injury, pulmonary irritation, and damage to the blood-forming system have been associated with inhalation of chloroethanes. Repeated or prolonged skin exposure can defat the skin and cause dermatitis.

In addition to the toxic effects of chloroethanes and their metabolites, the oxidative decomposition of products produced in the presence of open flames, hot metals, or lighted cigarettes should be taken into account. The chloroethane compounds may degrade to phosgene, hydrogen chloride, and dichloracetylene. Phosgene is considered to be dangerous to life in 30–60 minutes at 12.5 ppm.[12]

TABLE 47–1.
Adverse Effects of Chloroethane on Human Organs and Systems*†

CHEMICAL	IMMUNOLOGIC-ALLERGIC	HEMATOLOGIC	CARDIOVASCULAR	PULMONARY	RENAL-UROLOGIC	GASTROINTESTINAL	HEPATIC-BILIARY	MUSCULOSKELETAL	NEUROLOGIC	DERMATOLOGIC	OPHTHALMOLOGIC	OTHER
Monochloroethane	x		x	x		x			x	x	x	x
1,1-Dichloroethane				x					x	x		
1,2-Dichloroethane		x	x	x	x	x	x	x	x	x		x
1,1,1-Trichloroethane		x	x			x	x		x	x	x	x
1,1,2,2-Tetrachloroethane		x	x	x	x	x	x		x	x		x
Hexachloroethane									x		x	

*Data from Gosselin et al,[2] NIOSH,[8–11] and The US Trade Commission.[15]
†Adverse human health effects have not been reported to the NIOSH for 1,1,2-trichloroethane, 1,1,2-tetrachloroethane and pentachloroethane.

Laboratory Animal Studies

Carcinogenicity

As of July, 1978, four of the eight chloroethanes selected by the NCI for testing have been shown to be carcinogenic in laboratory animals. Each compound was studied separately in male and female Osborne-Mendel rats and male and female $B_6C_3F_1$ mice. Each experiment consisted of a high-dose and a low-dose group of 50 animals each. Twenty animals of each species/sex combination served as untreated controls and 20 animals of each species/sex combination served as vehicle controls. The chloroethane compounds were administered to the test animals in a corn oil vehicle by gastric intubation (stomach tube) five days a week for 78 weeks. The vehicle controls were intubated with pure corn oil at the same rate as the high-dose animals.

The National Cancer Institute has concluded that under the conditions of the bioassay, 1,2-dichloroethane, 1,1,2-trichloroethane, 1,1,2,2-tetrachloroethane, and hexachloroethane are carcinogenic in mice, inducing liver cancer in both sexes.[3–6] In addition, results of the NCI bioassay of 1,2-dichloroethane indicate that this compound also causes cancer in male and female rats. In mice, 1,1,2-trichloroethane was also associated with increased adrenal pheochromocytoma, a tumor that gives rise to high blood pressure and hyperglycemia. Toxic kidney damage was observed in all groups of both mice and rats treated with hexachloroethane.[4]

Although the occurrence of cancer in mice is highly significant, the results do not provide conclusive evidence that 1,1,2-trichloroethane, 1,1,2,2-tetrachloroethane, or hexachloroethane causes cancer in rats. A statistically significant association between increased dosage and accelerated mortality was observed in rats treated with hexachloroethane. The NCI has concluded that early mortality may have obscured a carcinogenic effect in these animals.

Other Adverse Effects in Animals

All of the chloroethane compounds are known to cause central nervous system depression in laboratory animals. This usually is expressed as abnormal weakness, intoxication, restlessness, irregular respiration, muscle incoordination, and unconsciousness. Chloroethanes generally are irritating to the eyes and skin. Damage to the liver and/or kidneys has been demonstrated in various animal species following exposure to these compounds.[13]

It has been reported that some of the chloroethanes and their metabolites are mutagenic in bacterial systems.[1, 6] Mutagenic activity, per se, should be considered a substantial liability. In addition, research suggests a correlation between mutagenicity in some bacterial strains and carcinogenicity in higher animals. Other adverse effects of the chloroethanes may vary from one compound to another.

Summaries of the current Department of Labor–Occupational Safety and Health Administration (OSHA) exposure standards[14] and the NIOSH recommended exposure standards for the chloroethane compounds are given in Table 47–2.

The OSHA exposure standards and the NIOSH recommended standards and control measures for the chloroethanes were developed before the carcinogenic potential of these compounds was recognized. Therefore, an assessment of the carcinogenicity of these compounds was not included. The levels currently recommended or adopted may not provide adequate protection from potential carcinogenic effects.

REFERENCES

1. Fishbein L: Industrial mutagens and potential mutagens I. Halogenated aliphatic derivatives. *Mutat Res* 1976; 32:267.
2. Gosselin RE, Hodge HC, Smith SP, et al (eds): *Clinical Toxicology of Commercial Products: Acute Poisoning*, ed 5. Baltimore, Williams & Wilkins Co, 1984.
3. National Cancer Institute: *Bioassay of 1,2-Dichloroethane for Possible Carcinogenicity*, DHEW Publ (NIH) 78-1305. US Dept of Health, Education, and Welfare, PHS, National Institute of Health, National Cancer Institute, Carcinogenesis Testing Program, Jan 10, 1978.
4. National Cancer Institute: *Bioassay of Hexachloroethane for Possible Carcinogenicity*, DHEW Publ NIH 78-1318. US Dept of Health, Ed-

TABLE 47–2.
Chloroethane Exposure Standards

CHEMICAL	OSHA EXPOSURE STANDARD (ppm)	NIOSH RECOMMENDED EXPOSURE STANDARD (ppm)	ACGIH TLV (ppm) 1985–86
Monochloroethane	1,000	none	none
1,1-Dichloroethane	100	none	200
1,2-Dichloroethane	50	5	10
1,1,1-Trichloroethane	350	350	350
1,1,2-Trichloroethane	10	none	10 (skin)
1,1,1,2-Tetrachloroethane	none	none	none
1,1,2,2-Tetrachloroethane	5	1	1 (skin)
Pentachloroethane	none		none
Hexachloroethane	1		10

ucation, and Welfare, PHS, National Institute of Health, National Cancer Institute, 1978.

5. National Cancer Institute: *Bioassay of 1,1,2-Trichloroethane for Possible Carcinogenicity*, DHEW Publ (NIH) 78-1324. US Dept of Health, Education, and Welfare, PHS, National Institute of Health, National Cancer Institute, 1978.
6. National Cancer Institute: *Bioassay of 1,1,2,2-Tetrachloroethane for Possible Carcinogenicity*, DHEW Publ (NIH) 78-827. US Dept of Health, Education, and Welfare, PHS, National Institute of Health, National Cancer Institute, 1978.
7. National Cancer Institute: *Chemicals Being Tested for Carcinogenicity by the Carcinogenesis Testing Program*. Division of Cancer Cause and Prevention, National Cancer Institute, June 1, 1978.
8. National Institute for Occupational Safety and Health: *Criteria for a Recommended Standard:. . . Occupational Exposure to Ethylene Dichloride (1,2-Dichloroethane)*, DHEW (NIOSH) Publ 76-139, US Dept. of Health, Education, and Welfare, PHS, Center for Disease Control, National Institute for Occupational Safety and Health, March, 1976.
9. National Institute for Occupational Safety and Health: *Criteria for a Recommended Standard:. . . Occupational Exposure to 1,1,1-Trichloroethane (Methyl Chloroform)*, DHEW (NIOSH) Publ 76-184. US Dept of Health, Education, and Welfare, PHS, Center for Disease Control, National Institute for Occupational Safety and Health, July, 1976.
10. National Institute for Occupational Safety and Health: *Criteria for a Recommended Standard: Occupational Exposure to 1,1,2,2-Tetrachloroethane*, DHEW (NIOSH) Publ 77-121. US Dept of Health, Education, and Welfare, PHS, Center for Disease Control, National Institute for Occupational Safety and Health, December, 1976.
11. National Institute for Occupational Safety and Health; NIOSH *Current Intell Bull* 25: Ethylene Dichloride, DHEW Publ (NIOSH) 74-149. US Dept of Health, Education, and Welfare, PHS, Center for Disease Control, National Institute for Occupational Safety and Health, April 19, 1978.
12. Patty FA, Fassett DW, Irish DD (eds): *Industrial Hygiene and Toxicology*, ed 2. New York, Interscience Publishers, 1963.
13. Sax NI: *Dangerous Properties of Industrial Materials*. New York, Van Nostrand Reinhold Co, 1985.
14. United States Department of Labor, Occupational Safety and Health Administration: General Industry Standards (29 Code of Federal Regulations 1910), January, 1976.
15. US International Trade Commission: *Synthetic Organic Chemicals, United States Production and Sales, 1976*. US International Trade Commission, USITC Publ 833, 1976.

CRESOLS

OH CH$_3$ OH CH$_3$ OH CH$_3$

o-Cresol *m*-Cresol *p*-Cresol

The cresol isomers ($CH_3C_6H_4OH$) are monomethyl derivatives of phenol (or hydroxy derivatives of toluene) that have the methyl group ortho, meta, or para to the hydroxyl group. The three isomers can occur alone or in various mixtures, either with one another or with other compounds. A mixture containing all three isomers often is referred to as tricresol and has a boiling range between 191° and 203° C. Commercial cresylic acids generally are defined as mixtures in which 50% of the material boils above 204° C. The cresol isomers usually are the major components of cresylic acids. Although some of these properties differ among the isomers, the oil/water partition coefficients suggest that their biologic distribution may be similar. Most nonsynthetic cresol used in industry is derived from petroleum or coal tar acids. Petroleum-based cresol is a by-product of the naphtha-cracking process and is present in the spent caustic liquor used to wash petroleum distillate. Coal tar acids are obtained from coke oven by-products, gas-retort oven tars and distilled tar by-products. The initial fractionation of petroleum or coal tar acids yields a phenolic mixture composed mainly of cresol, phenol, and xylenols. Pure *o*-cresol can be obtained by further distillation of this mixture, but because of their similar boiling points, the meta and para isomers of cresol must be separated by other methods. Generally, these two isomers are used industrially as a mixture containing 40%–65% *m*-cresol. Only small amounts of pure natural meta and para isomers are produced. There also are several methods of synthesizing the cresol isomers, particularly *p*-cresol. The catalyzed methylation of phenol is one of the methods used most often.

It is estimated that 80 million kg of cresol and cresylic acids were produced in the United States in 1982. The consumption of synthetic cresol varies to some extent from that of the natural products. Industry sources estimated that, in 1982, 28% of natural cresol was used for the production of wire enamel solvents, 20% for phosphate esters, 18% for phenolic resins, 6% for agricultural chemicals, 3% for disinfectants, 3% for ore flotation, 10% for miscellaneous purposes, and 12% for export. In 1969, 29% of synthetic cresol was consumed for phenolic resins, 26% for tricresyl phosphate, 11% for disinfectants, 17% for antioxidants and automotive products, 7% for ore flotation, and 10% for other purposes. A major use of *o*-cresol is in the manufacture of the herbicides dinitro-*o*-cresol (DNOC) and 2-methyl-4-chlorophenoxyacetic acid (MCPA). *p*-Cresol is used largely to produce the antioxidant 2,6-*ditert*-butyl-*p*-cresol (BHT), which is added to plastics and to food. Cresylic acids and *m,p*-cresol mixtures are used to make phenolic resins, tricresyl phosphate, and cresyl diphenyl phosphate, the last two used mainly as plasticizers. Some minor uses of cresols are in the production of azo dyes and as perfume additives, nylon solvents, metal degreasing agents, and synthetic tanning agents.

The NIOSH estimates that 11,000 people in the United States are occupationally exposed to cresol. This estimate is low, however, because it does not include workers who are intermittently exposed to a widely used commercial degreasing agent that contains cresol. Some representative occupations are: antioxidant producers, coal tar workers, cresol soap makers, cresol workers, cresylic acid makers, deodorant workers, disinfectant makers, disinfectors, DNOC producers, dye makers, enamel makers, flotation agent makers, flotation workers, foundry workers, glue workers, ink makers, ink remover makers, ink removers, insecticide workers, insulation enamel workers, oil additive makers, paint remover makers, paint removers, perfume makers, phenolic resin producers, phosphate ester producers, photographic developer workers, pitch workers, resin makers, roofers, rubber makers, scouring compound makers, stainers, stain makers, surfactant makers, tanning agent makers, tar distillery workers, textile sizers, varnish remover makers, varnish removers, veterinarians, and wood scourers.

The ability of cresols to be absorbed through the skin and produce local and systemic effects has been demonstrated in humans.[5, 11–13, 16, 18, 24] The skin, considered to be the primary route of occupational exposure, is the site of most of the worker injuries reported from cresols. Skin contact with cresols has resulted in skin peeling on the hands,[16] facial peripheral neuritis,[16] severe facial burns,[13] and damage to internal organs, including loss of kidney function[5] and necrosis of the liver and kidneys.[12] Cresols also have caused sensitization of the skin.[11, 24] Dermatitis developed on the fingers of workers who had been using a solution containing cresol and cresylic acid.[11] Of 30 workers in a synthetic plastics plant, six developed dermatitis on the hands and face resulting from exposure to cresol and phenol.[24] Although the information in these reports was insufficient to allow determination of dose-response relationships, industrial experience indicated that only small quantities of cresols were needed to produce chemical burns of the skin.

Animal studies also have indicated that cresols can cause local irritation and be absorbed after skin contact.[1, 4, 20] Discoloration of the skin, convulsions, and death occurred in rats given dermal applications of 1 ml/kg of various coal tar-derived cresylic acids.[4] In rabbits that had any of the three cresol isomers applied dermally in doses of 1 ml/kg for 24 hours, severe edema, erythema, or subdermal hemorrhaging developed.[1] Other effects included salivation, lacrimation, hypoactivity, tremors, convulsions, sedation, and death.[1] Shelley[20] reported that repeated dermal application of 0.5% *p*-cresol caused depigmentation of the hair and epidermis and local corrosion of the skin in mice.

Appreciable concentrations of cresol vapors rarely are generated in industry because all three cresol isomers have low vapor pressures. However, a hazardous concentration of vapor may be generated at elevated temperatures, and there have been a few reports in the literature[6, 22] describing effects from inhalation of cresol vapor. Corcos[6] reported that seven workers exposed to airborne cresol at an unspecified concentration developed headaches and nausea. Some workers also had hypertension, muscle irritability, convulsions, and decreased kidney function.[6] Interviews with workers exposed to cresol and phenol at concentrations of 0.02–10 ppm (0.08–38 mg/cu m) in air did not delineate effects on the eyes, nose, and throat.[8] The airborne concentration was reported as total phenols, so the actual exposure to cresol was not known. However, Uzhdavini et al.[22] found that eight of ten subjects experimentally exposed to *o*-cresol vapor at a concentration of 6 mg/cu m complained of dryness of the throat and the sensation of an unspecified taste. Despite the lack of specific details regarding methodology, this is the only reference of human inhalation exposure to a pure cresol and should not be ignored. Although no reports of effects in humans from long-term exposure to cresols were found, toxic effects have been observed in animals repeatedly exposed by inhalation.[4, 17, 22] Campbell[4] reported irritation of the nose and eyes and some deaths in mice that inhaled coal tar- or petroleum-derived cresylic acid vapors at "saturated" air concentrations for one hour per day on ten consecutive days. Uzhdavini et al.[22] observed some microscopic changes in mice exposed to *o*-cresol vapor aerosol at an average concentration of 50 mg/cu m for two hours per day, six days per week for one month and in rats and guinea pigs exposed to *o*-cresol vapor at a concentration of 9 mg/cu m for six hours per day, five days per week for two months and four hours per day, five days per week for another two months. These authors also reported irritation of the upper respiratory tract in humans exposed to airborne *o*-cresol at 6 mg/cu m and in cats exposed at 5–9 mg/cu m. They did not comment on whether similar effects were found in rats and guinea pigs. Kurlyandskiy et al.[17] found that 0.05 mg/cu m of tricresol vapor was the lowest concentration at which effects, including CNS excitability and protein denaturation, were noted in rats exposed for three months.

Several cases of cresol ingestion and its intravaginal applications have shown cresol to be corrosive to body tissues and to cause toxic effects on the vascular system, liver, kidneys, and pancreas. Cresol introduced into the uteri of pregnant women has produced abortion,[19, 23] extensive hemolysis,[19] erosion of blood vessels,[23] damage to the kidney tubules,[19] necrosis of the liver,[19] and death.[19] Most cases of cresol ingestion have been the result of attempted[3, 14, 15] or successful[10, 14] suicides. The smallest amount of cresol that produced death was 4 ml of a 25%–50% cresol solution in an 11-month-old child.[14] Systemic effects observed after cresol ingestion reflected those observed after its use as an abortifacient and included elevated blood pressure,[15] damage to the vascular system[15] and kidneys,[10, 14, 15] and acute pancreatitis.[10, 15]

Although no data were found that compared the effects of *o*-, *m*- and *p*-cresol in humans, several animal studies[1, 2, 9, 21] suggest that their biologic actions are similar. Mortality studies using dermal, oral, subcutaneous, or intravenous administration generally have shown that *o*- and *p*-cresol are about equal in toxicity but that *m*-cresol is less toxic. The only inhalation study[1] that compared the three isomers showed no difference in effect between *m*- and *p*-cresol at identical concentrations; *o*-cresol was given at a somewhat higher concentration. The toxic effects other than mortality observed in these studies[1, 9, 21] were qualitatively similar for the three isomers and included skin irritation, CNS disturbances, and liver and kidney damage. The urinary metabolites of the three isomers have also been found to be similar.[2] Compounds conjugated at the hydroxyl group accounted for the majority of the metabolites.

In summary, the most frequently observed effects resulting from occupational exposure to cresols are burns of the skin and eyes. In addition to being strong tissue irritants, cresols may cause impairment of kidney and liver function and CNS and cardiovascular disturbances. The NIOSH recommends that an environmental limit for cresol of 5 mg/cu m as a TWA concentration be established. It is believed that a TWA concentration of 5 mg/cu m will protect the worker from the occupational health hazards associated with cresol, considering the limited information available, and, in addition, it will reduce the probability of cresol acting as a promoter. The workplace environmental limit recommended for cresol applies to the individual cresol isomers when they occur alone or to any mixture of the isomers. (The ACGIH TLV guide has a "skin" note. See Appendix A.)

REFERENCES

1. *Bio Fax Techniques—Methods Used in Determining Biological Activity of Chemicals*. Northbrook, Ill, Industrial Bio-Test Laboratories, Inc, 1969, vols 3–5, 4–5, 5–5.
2. Bray HG, Thorpe WV, White K: Metabolism of derivatives of toluene—4. Cresols. *Biochem J* 1950; 46:275.
3. Burg K: Double central pneumonia in a case of Lysol poisoning. *Med Klin* 1929; 23:1134 (German).
4. Campbell J: Petroleum cresylic acids—A study of their toxicity and the toxicity of cresylic disinfectants. *Soap Sanit Chem* 1941; 17:103, 121.
5. Cason JS: Report on three extensive industrial chemical burns. *Br Med J* 1959; 1:827.
6. Corcos A: Contribution to the study of occupational poisoning by cresols. Dissertation. Paris, Vigot Freres Editeurs, 62 pp, 1939 (French).
7. *Criteria for a Recommended Standard: Occupational Exposure to Cresol*, DHEW (NIOSH) Publ 78-133. Cincinnati, Oh, US Dept of Health, Education, and Welfare, PHS, Center for Disease Control, National Institute for Occupational Safety and Health, 117 pp, 1978.
8. Cummins Northeastern Incorporated—Dedham, Massachusetts, Health Hazard Evaluation/Toxicity Determination Report 73-5-110. Cincinnati, Oh, US Dept of Health, Education, and Welfare, PHS, Center for Disease Control, National Institute for Occupational Safety and Health, Hazard Evaluation Services Branch, 7 pp, 1974.
9. Deichmann WB, Witherup S: Phenol studies–VI. The acute and comparative toxicity of phenol and *o*-, *m*- and *p*-cresols for experimental animals. *J Pharmacol Exp Ther* 1944; 80:233.
10. Dellal V: Acute pancreatitis following Lysol poisoning. *Lancet* 1931; 1:407.
11. Goodman H: Silk handler's disease of the skin. Dermatitis venenata due to isomers of cresol. *Med J Rec* 1933; 138:349.
12. Green MA: A household remedy misused. Fatal cresol poisoning following cutaneous absorption (a case report). *Med Sci Law* 1975; 15:65.
13. Herwick RP, Treweek DN: Burns from anesthesia mask sterilized in compound solution of cresol. *JAMA* 1933; 100:407.
14. Isaacs R: Phenol and cresol poisoning. *Ohio State Med J* 1922, 18:558.
15. Klimkiewicz E, Klinger M, Kurbiel A, et al: A case of liquid phenol poisoning complicated by acute pancreatitis and acute renal failure. *Wiad Lek* 1974; 27:1211 (Polish).
16. Klinger ME, Norton JF: Toxicity of cresylic acid-containing solvent. *US Nav Med Bull* 1945; 3:438.
17. Kurlyandskiy BA, Partsef DP, Chernomorskiy AR: Methods for determination of mean daily MPC of tricresol in the atmosphere. *Gig Sanit* 1975; 5:85 (Russian).
18. Plant observation reports and evaluation. Menlo Park, Calif., Stanford Research Institute, 146 pp. (submitted to NIOSH under Contract No. CDC-99-74-31, October, 1977).
19. Presley JA, Brown WE: Lysol-induced criminal abortion. *Obstet Gynecol* 1956; 8:368.
20. Shelley WB: *p*-Cresol. Cause of ink-induced hair depigmentation in mice. *Br J Dermatol* 1974; 90:169.
21. Uzhdavini ER, Astafyeva NK, Mamayeva AA: The acute toxicity of lower phenols. *Gig Tr Prof Zabol* 1974; 18:58 (Russian).
22. Uzhdavini ER, Astafyeva NK, Mamayeva AA, et al: Inhalation toxicity of *o*-cresol. *Tr Ufim Nauchno Issled Inst Gig Prof Zabol* 1972; 7:115 (Russian).
23. Vance BM: Intrauterine injection of Lysol as an abortifacient. Report of a fatal case complicated by oil embolism and Lysol poisoning. *Arch Pathol* 1945; 40:395.
24. Zalecki M: The results of examination of Cracow plant employees for detection of occupational skin diseases. *Med Pregl* 1965; 16:385 (Polish).

4,4′-DIAMINODIPHENYLMETHANE (DDM)

$$H_2N-C_6H_4-CH_2-C_6H_4-NH_2$$

DDM, 4,4′-diaminodiphenylmethane, also known as *p,p*′-methylenedianiline (MDA), is an important chemical intermediate. More than 100 million kg per year of DDM are manufactured in the United States. DDM is produced by the condensation of aniline with formaldehyde in the presence of an acid catalyst. Approximately 99% of the DDM produced is consumed in its crude form (occasionally containing not more than 50% DDM and polyDDM) at its production site by reaction with phosgene in the preparation of isocyanates and polyisocyanates. These isocyanates and polyisocyanates are used in the manufacture of rigid polyurethane foams that find application as thermal insulation. Polyisocyanates are also used in the preparation of the semiflexible polyurethane foams used for automotive safety cushioning. DDM is also used as an epoxy hardening agent, a raw material in the production of polyurethane elastomers, in the rubber industry as a curative for neoprene,[5] as an antifrosting agent (antioxidant), in footwear, a raw material in the production of Qiana Nylon, and a raw material in the preparation of poly (amide-imide) resins (used in magnet wire enamels).

It is estimated that 2,500 workers are exposed to DDM. Many of these exposures to DDM are in the preparation of isocyanates and polyisocyanates and on construction sites in the application of epoxy coatings. In 1965, the hepatotoxic effects of DDM in humans were first seen in the so-called Epping Jaundice outbreak in Great Britain. In this incident, 84 people who had eaten DDM-contaminated bread experienced hepatocellular damage evidenced by elevated SGOT and SGPT levels.[3, 4] DDM also has been shown to produce liver lesions in a group of intragastrically fed rats[2] and has caused liver degeneration and spleen lesions in another group of DDM-fed rats.[8]

DDM in the occupational environment has been implicated in a number of cases of toxic hepatitis. During an 18-month period beginning April, 1972, six cases of hepatitis developed among about 300 men who used epoxy resins in the construction of a nuclear power plant in Alabama. Two chemicals, DDM and 2-nitropropane, were held suspect in this study.[11, 12] In another study, 13 cases of hepatitis developed between 1966 and 1972 among workers who added DDM to a mixture to produce a hard plastic insulating material. All of these men became ill within a few days of working intensively with DDM.[6] One other case of hepatitis, possibly associated with DDM, was reported by a person who wrote to the Environmental Protection Agency describing an episode of acute hepatitis as well as CNS and pulmonary symptoms he experienced following exposure to a surfacing agent containing DDM.

The carcinogenic effects of DDM have also been studied. In one study, 16 rats were given 4 or 5 20-mg DDM doses by stomach tube over eight months. A hepatoma and a hemangioma-like tumor of the kidney were found in one rat after 18 months and an adenocarcinoma of the uterus was found in another after 24 months.[9] In another report, of 48 rats given DDM intragastrically five times weekly, all developed liver cirrhosis, four developed hepatomas (two benign), and others developed miscellaneous tumors.[7] In a third report, 50% of 50 DDM-injected rats developed tumors (four hepatomas) compared with 26% of a control group.[10] There have been no reported human cancers associated with DDM.

If, as hypothesized in the Center for Disease Control study of nuclear power plant construction workers, not all workers are susceptible to liver injury after exposure to DDM, and if the 1%–2% incidence of liver disease seen in this study were applied to all workers with possible exposure to DDM, we would expect to see 25–50 cases of DDM-associated toxic hepatitis a year.[1] The 1985–86 ACGIH TLV guide lists DDM at 0.1 ppm, with intended change to that of "suspect carcinogen" (see Appendix A).

REFERENCES

1. *DDM—Background Information on 4,4′-Diaminodiphenylmethane*. Cincinnati, Oh, Technical Evaluation and Review Branch Office of Extramural Coordination & Special Projects, National Institute for Occupational Safety and Health, Jan 30, 1976.
2. Gohlke R, Schmidt P: 4–4′-Diaminodiphenylmethane: Histological, enzyme, histochemical and autoradiographic investigations in acute and subacute experiments in rats with and without the additional stress of heat. *Int Arch Arbeitsmed* 1974; 32:217.
3. Kopelman H, Robertson MH, Sanders PG, et al: The Epping jaundice. *Br Med J* 1966; 1:514.
4. Kopelman H, Scheuer PJ, Williams R: The liver lesion of the Epping Jaundice. *QJ Med* 1966; 35:553.
5. Lloyd JW, DeCoufle P, Moore RM Jr: Current intelligence—background information on chloroprene. *J Occup Med* 1975; 17:263.
6. McGill DB, Motto JD: An industrial outbreak of toxic hepatitis due to methylenedianiline. *N Engl J Med* 1974; 291:278.
7. Munn A: Occupational bladder tumors and carcinogens: Recent developments in Britain, in Deichmann W, Lampe KF (eds): *Bladder Cancer. A Symposium*. Birmingham, Ala, Aesculapius, 1974, p 187.
8. Pludro G, Karlowski K, Mankowska M, et al: Toxicological and chemical studies of some epoxy resins and hardeners. I. Determination of acute and subacute toxicity of phthalic acid anhydride, 4-4′-diaminodiphenylmethane and of the epoxy resin Epilox EG-34. *Acta Pol Pharm* 1969; 26:352.
9. Schoental R: Carcinogenic and chronic effects of 4-4′-diaminodiphenylmethane, an epoxy resin hardener. *Nature* 1968; 219:1162.
10. Steinhoff D, Grundmann E: Zur Cancerogenen winkung von 4-4′-diaminodiphenylmethan und 2,4′-diaminodiphenylmethan. *Naturwissenschaften* 1970; 57:247.
11. Unpublished data. Center for Disease Control, 1974.
12. Williams SV, Bryan JA, Wolf FS: Toxic hepatitis and methylenedianiline. *N Engl J Med* 1974; 291:1256.

DIOXINS, CHLOROPHENOLS, AND PHENOXY HERBICIDES

MARILYN A. FINGERHUT, PH.D.
PATRICIA L. MOODY, M.D., M.P.H.
WILLIAM E. HALPERIN, M.D., M.P.H.

Dioxins are a family of 75 isomers which arise predominantly as unintended contaminants during the synthesis of the chlorophenols and the phenoxy herbicides. The isomers are chlorinated at various positions, but have a general structure (Fig 47–5).

The most toxic isomer, 2,3,7,8-tetrachlorodibenzo-p-dioxin (2,3,7,8-TCDD) is generated during production of the fungicide 2,4,5-trichlorophenol (TCP) and also during synthesis of several phenoxy herbicides, such as 2,4,5-trichlorophenoxy acetic acid (2,4,5-T), which are derived from trichlorophenol. The major route of formation of 2,3,7,8-TCDD is illustrated in Figure 47–6. A colorless crystalline solid at room temperature, 2,3,7,8-TCDD is sparingly soluble in most organic solvents and is essentially insoluble in water. It is stable in heat, acids, and alkali and will decompose when exposed to ultraviolet light.[37]

Two commercially important polychlorophenols contaminated with dioxin isomers are trichlorophenol and pentachlorophenol (Fig 47–4). Although trichlorophenol is no longer manufactured in the United States, about 50 million lb were produced in 1970.[12] From the 1940s until 1979, most trichlorophenol was used as the starting material in the manufacture of 2,4,5-T and the bactericide hexachlorophene. The process is illustrated in Figure 47–5. Accidents resulting in occupational and/or community exposure have been reported in several countries during the production of trichlorophenol.[27] A listing of these accidents appears in Table 47–3.

Pentachlorophenol has been widely used as a wood preservative and bacteriostatic agent since the 1930s. About 40 million lb were produced in the United States in 1977. Pentachlorophenol contains no 2,3,7,8-TCDD, but it is contaminated by hexa-, hepta- and octa-chlorinated dioxins.[12]

The phenoxy acid herbicides are derived by alkaline hydrolysis of the chlorinated phenols. The two best known herbicides are

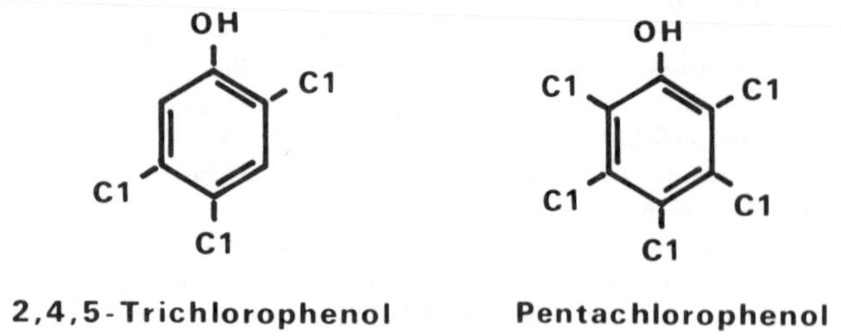

FIG 47–4.
2,4,5-Trichlorophenol and pentachlorophenol.

illustrated in Figure 47–6. During synthesis of the herbicides, the particular dioxin isomers which arise are determined by the positions to which chlorine atoms are attached in the chlorinated phenols and by the conditions of the reaction. 2,4-D has been used since the 1940s for control of broadleaf weeds in crops and along railroads and highways. Analyses of 2,4-D for its contaminating dioxins have detected some di-, tri-, and tetrachlorinated isomers, but 2,3,7,8-TCDD has not been found.[5]

The herbicide 2,4,5-T has been used for control of woody and herbaceous weeds since 1944. As shown in Figure 47–7, the 2,3,7,8-TCDD is generated as a contaminant during the synthesis of 2,4,5-T. Annual production of 2,4,5-T increased steadily from 1960 until it peaked in 1968 at 17.4 million lb,[28] when much of the herbicide was used to formulate Agent Orange. Agent Orange, a 50:50 mixture of 2,4-D and 2,4,5-T esters, and other formulations of 2,4,5-T known as Herbicides Purple, Pink, and Green, were used from 1962 until 1971 to defoliate jungle areas in South Vietnam. In the stocks of Agent Orange destroyed in 1977, the amounts of 2,3,7,8-TCDD ranged from 0.02 to 47 ppm, with an average of about 2 ppm.[56]

Occupational and Environmental Exposure

Except in research laboratories,[40] human beings never have exposure to pure dioxin. Usual exposure occurs only to the dioxin-

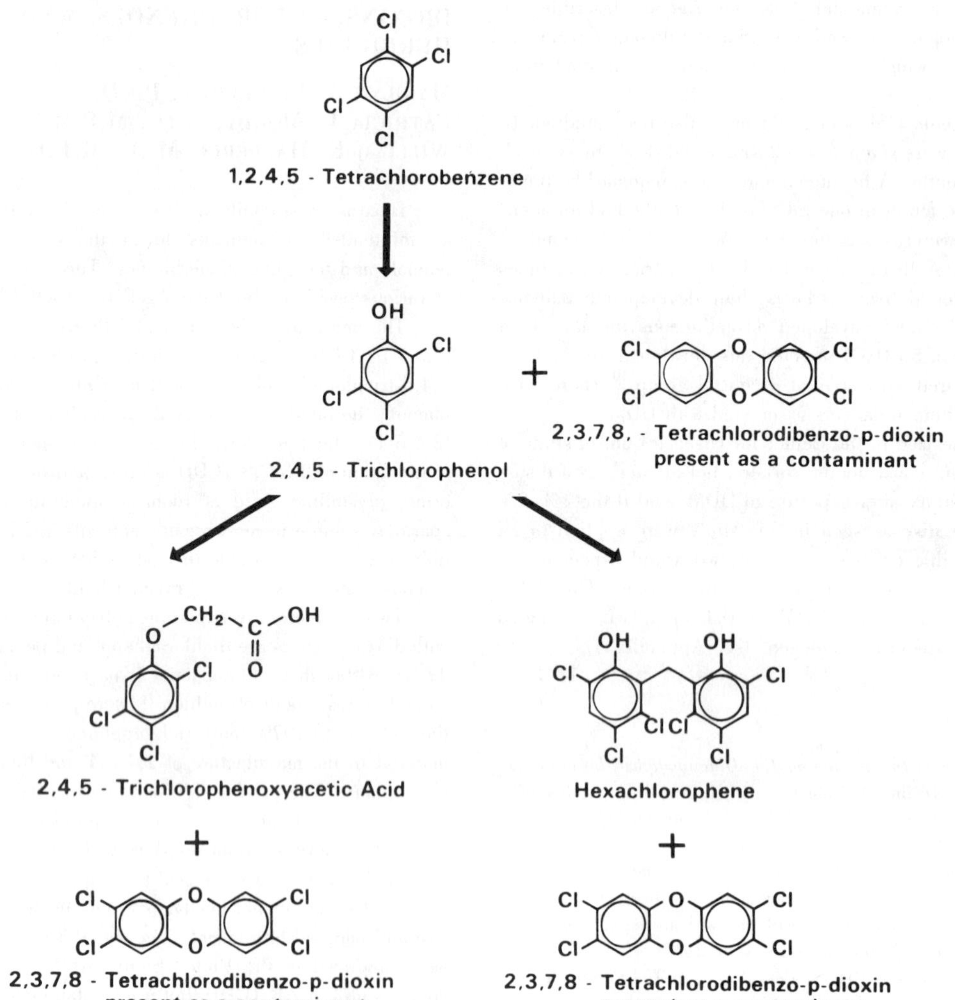

FIG 47–5.
The major route of formation of 2,3,7,8-TCDD.

TABLE 47–3.
Accidents Resulting in Occupational or Community Exposure During Production of Trichlorophenol*

LOCATION	YEAR	NUMBER OF EXPOSED PERSONS	PUBLISHED STUDIES OF EXPOSED PERSONS
Federal Republic of Germany	1953	75	Mortality
Netherlands	1963	106	None
Seveso, Italy	1976	?	Medical
United Kingdom	1968	90	Mortality, medical
West Virginia, U.S.A.	1949	228	Mortality, medical

*Table adapted from the International Agency for Research on Cancer: Long-term hazards of polychlorinated dibenzodioxins and polychlorinated dibenzofurans. *IARC Internal Technical Report* 781001, Lyon, France, June 1978, p 35.

contaminated products or to wastes. Table 47–4 lists the products contaminated with dioxin isomers and summarizes the occupational groups with potential exposure to these products.

Two major occupational groups may experience risk of exposure to 2,3,7,8-TCDD: production workers who synthesize or mix the dioxin-contaminated commercial products or dispose of the wastes, and herbicide applicators who spray 2,4,5-T.[37] These activities have now ceased in the United States. In contrast, the production and use of pentachlorophenol in the United States is widespread. Wood preservers who treat wood or wood products with pentachlorophenol have a potential for exposure to the product and its contaminant hexa-, hepta-, and octadioxin isomers.[12]

The current potential for environmental exposure to dioxin results from past production of dioxin-contaminated products and inadequate disposal of the dioxin-contaminated wastes. Residual 2,3,7,8-TCDD has been found in the production buildings as well as in the residential areas surrounding former production sites of 2,4,5-T. Sizeable tracts of residential land in the State of Missouri remain contaminated by 1 to 1,000 ppb 2,3,7,8-TCDD because oily dioxin-contaminated wastes were sprayed in rural areas for dust control.[30] Persons who consume fish from water into which dioxin-contaminated wastes escaped and settled into the soil bottom may also be exposed. Many U.S. citizens may have had exposure to dioxin-contaminated 2,4,5-T from 1946 until at least 1979, since homeowners as well as farmers used brands of herbicides containing dioxin-contaminated 2,4,5-T.[12]

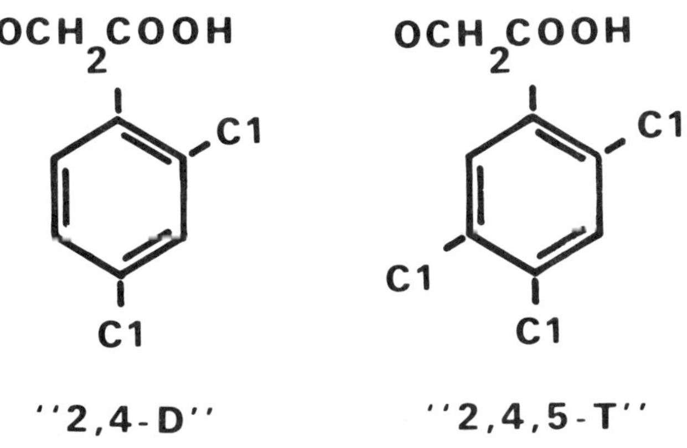

FIG 47–6.
Herbicides 2,4-D and 2,4,5-D.

Animal Toxicity

Although toxicity varies with species, dose, and length of exposure, animal studies indicate that 2,3,7,8-TCDD is one of the most potent known chemical toxins. The single acute LD_{50} for animal species ranges from 0.6 μg/kg body weight in the guinea pig to 5,000 μg/kg in the hamster.[32] Other chlorinated isomers of dioxin, by contrast, are orders of magnitude less toxic.[48]

General classes of toxicologic effect or injury caused by dioxin in animals include debilitation and wasting, skin lesions, enzyme induction, hepatoxicity, lymphoid hypoplasia, and immunologic disturbances, teratogenesis, fetotoxicity, and carcinogenesis.[27] When female rhesus monkeys were fed 2,3,7,8-TCDD, they developed alopecia, periorbital edema, thrombocytopenia, anemia, and epithelial hyperplasia and metaplasia of the salivary gland, bile duct, lung, and stomach.[1] Skin lesions in animals include hyperkeratosis and transformation of sebaceous glands to keratin cysts in mice, rats, and monkeys, and chloracne in rabbits.[26] Although liver damage after a single fatal dose is not universal, it occurs in several species.[21] Thymic atrophy has been observed in the young of all experimental species at doses which do not kill the animal,[30] and 2,3,7,8-TCDD suppresses several cell-mediated immune functions.[13]

The biochemical mechanism by which 2,3,7,8-TCDD exerts its toxic effects has not yet been established, but several lines of evidence suggest that 2,3,7,8-TCDD binds to a cytosol receptor molecule, which then translocates as a ligand-receptor complex to the nucleus, subsequently causing altered gene expression.[44]

2,3,7,8-TCDD is teratogenic in certain strains of mice when

FIG 47–7.
Dioxin nucleus, illustrating eight possible positions for chlorine atoms.

TABLE 47–4.
Occupational Exposure to Dioxin-Contaminated Products

COMMERCIAL PRODUCTS	DIOXIN ISOMERS	USES	PERIOD OF UNITED STATES PRODUCTION	MAJOR OCCUPATIONAL EXPOSURES
Trichlorophenol	2,3,7,8-TCDD	Chemical precursor fungicide	1946–1979	Production workers
2,4,5-T	2,3,7,8-TCDD	Herbicide	1947–1979	Production workers Herbicide applicators
2,4-D	di- tri- tetra-	Herbicide	1944–present	Production workers Herbicide applicators
Pentachlorophenol	hexa- hepta- octa-	Wood preservative Pesticide	1937–present	Wood preservers Pesticide applicators

pregnant females are exposed.[17] Diminished fertility, increased fetal mortality, and decreased growth rates of living offspring were the prominent findings in a three-generation mating study in rats.[36] In contrast, male mice fed 2,3,7,8-TCDD showed no adverse reproductive effects when mated with unexposed females in a simulated Agent Orange exposure study.[34]

Mutagenicity is an inconstant finding in 2,3,7,8-TCDD bioassays,[17] but carcinogenicity has been demonstrated in several species. When rats were fed diets containing 2,3,7,8-TCDD, the investigators observed a dose-dependent effect ranging from no observed change in the low-dose group to significantly increased hepatic nodules in female rats in the middle-dose group, and a significant increase in carcinomas of the liver, lung, hard palate, nasal turbinates, and tongue, as well as adenomas of the liver and adrenal cortex in the high-dose group.[33] Studies conducted by the National Toxicology Program have demonstrated the carcinogenesis of 2,3,7,8-TCDD in both dermal and gavage studies of mice and rats.[38, 39]

The toxicity of purified phenoxy herbicide and chlorophenol products has been less thoroughly studied. Existing animal studies suggest that both 2,4,5-T and 2,4-D may be neurotoxic, hepatotoxic, and produce renal lesions. 2,4,5-T apparently induces myocardial lesions and hypocellularity of the spleen and bone marrow.[60] Pentachlorophenol causes local irritation to the eyes and nose, as well as systemic effects that may result from its ability to uncouple mitochondrial oxidative phosphorylation.[59] Hepatic and chloracnegenic effects have generally been attributed to the contaminants.[19] Teratogenic and fetoxic effects have been attributed both to pentachlorophenol and to its contaminants.[4]

Human Health Effects

Human health effects have been reported chiefly in groups occupationally exposed to the manufacture of products containing 2,3,7,8-TCDD as a contaminant. Investigators from several European countries,[2, 10, 18] from England,[35] and from the U.S.[52] have described workers affected by acute exposures during industrial accidents, as well as groups of workers chronically exposed during the synthesis of herbicides and biocides.[3, 29, 42, 45, 53] Other discrete incidents involving exposure to TCDD-contaminated materials have included illness in laboratory workers following TCDD exposure,[40] and in community residents and animals in Seveso, Italy,[43, 46] and the state of Missouri.[31]

Health effects in human beings which have been associated with exposure to 2,3,7,8-TCDD-contaminated materials include chloracne, hepatotoxicity and hepatic porphyria, disordered lipid metabolism, neurotoxicity, abnormal pulmonary function, decreased libido, increased coronary heart disease, ulcer disease, and immunologic changes.[2, 3, 10, 18, 29, 35, 42, 45, 52, 53, 57, 58] Reproductive effects are also of concern, although the evidence in human populations is contradictory.[14, 17, 20, 43, 53, 55]

Chloracne is a persistent form of acne caused by exposure to a number of chlorinated organic compounds, including tetrachlorodibenzodioxins and dibenzofurans, chlorinated naphthalenes, chlorinated biphenyls, tetrachloroazobenzene, and tetrachloroazoxybenzene.[8] The first outbreak of chloracne associated with 2,3,7,8-TCDD exposure occurred in West Virginia in 1949 in the aftermath of a trichlorophenol containment vessel explosion.[52] Crow found the persistence of chloracne among some of these workers in 1979, 30 years later.[9] Hundreds of workers have developed chloracne as a result of similar exposures to TCDD-contaminated materials.[2, 3, 35, 45, 53]

Although hepatotoxicity was recognized in some of the West Virginia workers following the accident, hepatic dysfunction in 2,3,7,8-TCDD-exposed workers was not carefully documented until 1964. In employees of a New Jersey chemical plant manufacturing pesticides and herbicides, Bleiberg found abnormal hepatic function, abnormal liver biopsies, and hepatic porphyria.[3] Similar alterations of hepatic function have been described by other authors.[2, 18] Follow-up of most groups of workers, however, reveals an apparent decrease in the severity of hepatotoxic effects with time following cessation of exposure.[42, 45]

Abnormalities of serum lipids are consistently reported in studies of occupationally exposed workers. Elevated triglycerides, total cholesterol, changes in the very low density lipoprotein fraction, as well as diminished high density lipoproteins, have all been observed, although not all findings have been reported simultaneously in the same groups.[40, 42, 53, 57]

Neurotoxic effects have not been noted in animal studies, but both central and peripheral nervous system effects have been reported in humans. Twenty-seven of 36 West Virginia workers complained of persistent symptoms of pain and weakness in the lower extremities two years after the 1949 accident.[52] "Neuritis" was described in a group of German workers engaged in pentachlorophenol production, and the same author identified "psychopathic and permanent" damage among trichlorophenol workers.[2] Other signs include slowed nerve conduction velocities,[15, 49] persistent neuropathy by electromyography, and neuroses without depression ten years after exposure to trichlorophenol.[42]

Although there are extensive data on dioxin-induced immunologic changes in experimental animals, a paucity of information exists on humans. A transient decrease in peripheral lymphocytes was noted among a group of persons exposed at Seveso.[46] An unpublished study of a ten-year follow-up of British workers found diminished levels of IgM and IgD and diminished mitogen responsiveness in a subgroup of workers with a history of chloracne.[58]

Finally, several other human health effects with no consistent or recurrent pattern have been linked to exposure to 2,3,7,8-TCDD-contaminated materials, including hemorrhagic cystitis,[31] increased frequency of diabetic glucose tolerance tests,[42] gastritis or disturbances of gastric acidity,[2] and deaths from cirrhosis, bronchogenic carcinoma, fulminant atherosclerotic disease, and acute pancreatitis.[18, 42] For many of these effects, insufficient corroborating evidence from dioxin-related animal and other human illness exists to suggest a causal relationship with dioxin exposure, but such an association cannot be ruled out.

Epidemiologic Studies

Until recently, there were few mortality studies among persons exposed to dioxin-contaminated substances. Two case control studies conducted in Sweden found a five- to sixfold increased risk of soft tissue sarcoma,[11, 22] and a third Swedish study noted a sixfold increased risk of lymphoma among persons exposed to phenoxy herbicides and chlorophenols.[23]

Several small U.S. mortality studies have been conducted of chemical workers who made trichlorophenol or 2,4,5-T.[6, 7, 41, 61, 62] A reanalysis of death certificate data from these studies suggested that there may be an excess risk of soft-tissue sarcoma among these workers.[25] Expert review of their tissue specimens, however, has demonstrated that several cases are not soft-tissue sarcoma, raising questions about the adequacy of death certificate data for evaluation of this outcome.[16] Several epidemiologic studies have failed to show an association between dioxin exposure and soft-tissue sarcoma,[24, 41, 47, 50, 54] but all were limited by size of the population, incomplete exposure data, or inadequate latency. Definitive conclusions concerning the carcinogenicity of dioxin-contaminated products in human beings await the completion of large epidemiologic studies under way in the United States and elsewhere.

Conclusion

Research in animal toxicology and human clinical studies suggests that health effects of dioxin-contaminated substances include chloracne, hepatic damage, altered lipid metabolism, and immunologic and neurologic toxicity. Adverse reproductive effects have been demonstrated in exposed female animals. Epidemiologic studies suggest that persons exposed to phenoxy herbicides and chlorophenols may be at increased risk of soft-tissue sarcoma and lymphoma. Further investigations are needed to provide definitive answers.

REFERENCES

1. Allen JR, et al: Morphological changes in monkeys consuming a diet containing low levels of 2,3,7,8-TCDD. *Food Cosmet Toxicol* 1977; 15:401–410.
2. Bauer H, Schulz KH, Spiegelberg U: Industrial poisoning in the manufacture of chlorophenol compounds. *Arch fur Gewerbepathologie und Gewerbehygiene* 1961; 18:538–555.
3. Bleiberg J, et al: Industrially acquired porphyria. *Arch Dermatol* 1964; 89:793–797.
4. Cirelli D: Pentachlorophenol, Position Document 1. *Federal Register* 1978; 40:48446–48477.
5. Cochrane WP, Singh J, Miles W, et al: Determination of chlorinated dibenzo-p-dioxin contaminants in 2,4-D products by gas chromatography-mass spectrometric techniques. *J Chromatog* 1981; 271:289–299.
6. Cook RR: Dioxin, chloracne and soft tissue sarcoma. *Lancet* 1981; i:268–269.
7. Cook R, Townsend J, Ott MG, et al: Mortality experience of employees exposed to 2,3,7,8-tetrachlorodibenzodioxin (TCDD). *J Occup Med* 1980; 22:530–532.
8. Crow KD: Chloracne. *Semi Dermatol* 1982; 1:305–314.
9. Crow KD: Chloracne and its potential implications. *Clin Exp Dermatol* 1981; 6:243–257.
10. Dugois P, Colomb L: Acne chlorique au 2,4,5-trichlorophenol. *Lyon Med* 1956; 88:446–447.
11. Eriksson M, Berg N, Hardell L, et al: Soft tissue sarcomas and exposure to chemical substances, a case-referent study. *Br J Ind Med* 1981; 38:27–33.
12. Esposito MP, Tiernan TO, Dryden FE: Dioxins, EPA—600/2-80-197. Cincinnati, Oh, US Environmental Protection Agency, 1980.
13. Faith RE, Luster MI: Investigations of the effects of 2,3,7,8-TCDD on parameters of various immune functions. *Ann NY Acad Sci* 1979; 320:564–571.
14. Field B, Kerr C: Herbicide use and incidence of neural tube defects. *The Lancet* 1979; i:1341–1342.
15. Filippini G, et al: Relationship between clinical and electrophysiological findings and indicators of heavy exposure to 2,3,7,8-tetrachlorodibenzo-dioxin. *Scand J Work Environ Health* 1981; 7:257–262.
16. Fingerhut M, Halperin W, Honchar P, et al: An evaluation of reports of dioxin exposure and soft tissue sarcoma pathology in U.S. chemical workers. *Scand J Work Environ Health* 1984; in press.
17. Friedman JM: Does Agent Orange Cause Birth Defects? *Teratology* 1984; 29:193–221.
18. Goldman PJ: Critically acute chloracne caused by trichlorophenol decomposition products. *Arbeitsmedizin Sozialmedizin Arbeitshygiene* 1972; 7:12–18.
19. Goldstein J, Frieson M, Linder R, et al: Effects of pentachlorophenol on hepatic drug-metabolizing enzymes and porphyria related to contamination with chlorinated dibenzo-p-dioxins and dibenzofurans. *Biochem Pharmacol* 1977: 26:1549–2557.
20. Griffith J, Health R, Frankenburg M (eds): Report of Assessment of a Field Investigation of Six Year Spontaneous Abortion Rates in Three Oregon Areas in Relation to Forest 2,4,5-T Spray Practices. Environmental Protection Agency, 1979.
21. Gupta BN, et al: Pathologic effects of 2,3,7,8-tetrachlorodibenzo-p-dioxin in laboratory animals. *Environ Health Perspect* 1973; 5:125–140.
22. Hardell L, Sandstrom A: Case-control study: Soft tissue sarcoma and

exposure to phenoxyacetic acids or chlorophenols. *Br J Cancer* 1979; 39:711–717.

23. Hardell L, Eriksson M, Lenner P, et al: Malignant lymphoma and exposure to chemicals, especially organic solvents, chlorophenols and phenoxy acids: A case control study. *Br J Cancer* 1981; 43:169–176.
24. Hogstedt C, Westerland B: Cohort study of causes of death of forestry workers with and without exposure to phenoxy acid preparations. *Lakartidningen* 1980; 19:1829–1831.
25. Honchar P, Halperin W: 2,4,5-trichlorophenol and soft tissue sarcoma. *Lancet* 1981; 1:269–270.
26. Huff JE, et al: Long-term hazards of poly-chlorinated dibenzodioxins and polychlorinated dibenzofurans. *Environ Health Perspect* 1980; 36:221–240.
27. International Agency for Research on Cancer: Long-term hazards of polychlorinated dibenzodioxins and polychlorinated dibenzofurans. *IARC Internal Technical Report* 781001, Lyon, France, June 1978, p 275.
28. International Agency for Research on Cancer: Some fumigants, the herbicides 2,4-D and 2,4,5-T, chlorinated dibenzodioxins and miscellaneous industrial chemicals. *IARC Monogr Eval Carcinog Risk Chem Man* 1977; vol 15. Lyon, France.
29. Jirasek L, et al: Chronic poisoning by 2,3,7,8-tetrachlorodibenzo-p-dioxin. *Cesk Dermatol* 1974; 49:145–157.
30. Kimbrough RD (ed): Halogenated Biphenyls, Terphenyls, Naphthalenes, Dibenzodioxins and Related Products. New York, Elsevier North-Holland Biomedical Press, 1980.
31. Kimbrough R, et al: Epidemiology and pathology of a tetrachlorodibenzodioxin poisoning episode. *Arch Environ Health* 1977; 32:77–86.
32. Kociba RJ, Schwetz BA: Toxicity of 2,3,7,8-tetrachlorodibenzo-p-dioxin (TCDD). *Drug Metab Rev* 1982; 13:387–406.
33. Kociba RJ, et al: Results of a two-year chronic toxicity and oncogenicity study of 2,3,7,8-TCDD in rats. *Toxicol Appl Pharmacol* 1978; 46:279–303.
34. Lamb JC, Moore JA, Marks TA: Evaluation of 2,4-D, 2,4,5-T, and 2,3,7,8-TCDD toxicity in C57BBL mice: Reproduction and fertility in treated mice and congenital malformations in their offspring, National Toxicology Program, Document NTP-80-44. Research Triangle Park, NC, 1980.
35. May G: Chloracne from the accidental production of tetrachlorodibenzodioxin. *Br J Ind Med* 1973; 30:276–283.
36. Murray FJ, et al: Three generation reproduction study of rats given 2,3,7,8-TCDD in the diet. *Toxicol Appl Pharmacol* 1979; 50:241–252.
37. National Institute for Occupational Safety and Health: 2,3,7,8-Tetrachlorodibenzo-p-dioxin. *NIOSH Curr Intell Bull* 1984; 40.
38. National Toxicology Program: *Carcinogenesis Bioassay of 2,3,7,8-tetrachlorodibenzo-p-dioxin in Swiss Webster Mice* (Dermal Study), NIH Publ 82-1757. Bethesda, Md, National Institutes of Health, 1982.
39. National Toxicology Program: *Carcinogenesis Bioassay of 2,3,7,8-tetrachlorodibenzo-p-dioxin in Osborne-Mendel Rats and B6C3F Mice (Gavage Study)*, NIH Publ 82-1765. Bethesda, Md, National Institutes of Health, 1982.
40. Oliver RM: Toxic effects of 2,3,7,8-tetrachlorodibenzodioxin in laboratory workers. *Br J Ind Med* 1975; 32:49–53.
41. Ott M, Holder B, Olson R: A mortality analysis of employees engaged in the manufacture of 2,4,5-trichlorophenoxy acetic acid. *J Occup Med* 1980; 22:47–50.
42. Pazderova-Vijlupkova J, et al: The development and prognosis of chronic intoxication by tetrachlorodibenzo-p-dioxin in men. *Arch Environ Health* 1981; 36:5–11.
43. Pocchiari F, Silano V, Zampieri A: Human health effects from accidental release of tetrachlorodibenzo-p-dioxin (TCDD) at Seveso, Italy. *Ann NY Acad Sciences* 1979; 275:311–320.
44. Poland A, Glover E: 2,3,7,8-tetrachlorodibenzo-p-dioxin: Segregation of toxicity with the Ah locus. *Mol Pharmacol* 1980; 17:86–94.
45. Poland A, et al: A health survey of workers in a 2,4-D and 2,4,5-T plant. *Arch Environ Health* 1971; 22:316–327.
46. Reggiani G: Medical problems raised by the TCDD contamination in Seveso, Italy. *Arch Toxicol* 1978; 40:161–188.
47. Riihimaki V, Asp S, Hernberg S: Mortality of 2,4-dichlorophenoxyacetic acid and 2,4,5-trichloroacetic acid herbicide applicators in Finland. *Scand J Work Environ Health* 1982; 8:37–42.
48. Schwetz BA, et al: Toxicology of chlorinated dibenzo-p-dioxins. *Environ Health Perspect* Sept 1973; pp; 87–99.
49. Singer R, et al: Nerve conduction velocity studies of workers employed in the manufacture of phenoxy herbicides. *Environ Res* 1982; 29:297–311.
50. Smith AH, Fischer DO, Pearce N, et al: Do agricultural chemicals cause soft tissue sarcoma? Initial findings of a case control study in New Zealand. *Commun Health Studies* 1982; 6:114–119.
51. Smith AH, et al: Congenital defects and miscarriages among New Zealand 2,4,5-T sprayers. *Arch Environ Health* 1982; 37:197–200.
52. Suskind RR: Chloracne and associated health problems in the manufacture of 2,4,5-T. Institute of Environmental Health, University of Cincinnati Report to IARC, Lyon, France, 1978.
53. Suskind RR, Hertzberg VS: Human health effects of 2,4,5-T and its toxic contaminants. *J Am Med Assoc* 1984; 251:2372–2380.
54. Thiess AM, Frentzel-Beyme R, Link R: Mortality study of persons exposed to dioxin in a trichlorophenol process accident that occurred in the BASF AG on Nov 17, 1953. *Am J Ind Med* 1982; 3:179–189.
55. Thomas HF: 2,4,5-T use and congenital malformation rates in Hungary. *Lancet* 1980; i:214–215.
56. Tremblay JW: The Design, Implementation and Evaluation of the Industrial Hygiene Program Used During the Disposal of Herbicide Orange, in *Human and Environmental Risks of Chlorinated Dioxins and Related Compounds*. New York, Plenum Press, 1982.
57. Walker A, Martin J: Lipid profiles in dioxin-exposed workers. *Lancet* 1979; i:446–447.
58. Ward A: Investigation of the immune capability of workers previously exposed to 2,3,7,8-tetrachlorodibenzo-para-dioxin (TCDD). Hallamshire Hospital, Sheffield, U.K. (unpublished), 1983.
59. Williams PL: Pentachlorophenol, an assessment of the occupational hazard. *Am Ind Hyg Assoc J* 1982; 43:799–810.
60. Young AL, Cacagni JA, Thalken CE, et al: *The Toxicology, Environmental Fate, and Human Risk of Herbicide Orange and Its Associated Dioxin*. United States Air Force Document OEHL TR-78-92. Texas, 1978.
61. Zack JA, Gaffey WR: A mortality study of workers employed at the Monsanto Company plant in Nitro, West Virginia. *Environ Sci Res* 1983; 26:575–591.
62. Zack J, Suskind R: The mortality experience of workers exposed to tetrachlorodibenzodioxin in a trichlorophenol-process accident. *J Occup Med* 1980; 22:11–14.

DISULFIRAM

$$(CH_3CH_2)_2N-C(=S)-S-S-C(=S)-N(CH_2CH_3)_2$$

Disulfiram is a prescription drug used as an alcohol deterrent and *also is an accelerator used in the manufacture of rubber*. Disulfiram also may be used as a fungicide and insecticide. Disulfiram is widely used in alcoholism control programs under the trade names Antabuse and Ro-Sulfiram. The intake of even small quantities of ethanol (ethyl alcohol) while on disulfiram results in flushing, breathing difficulty, nausea, vomiting and low blood pressure. This violent and unpleasant reaction reinforces an individual's resolve to abstain from alcohol. The human therapeutic dose of disulfiram ranges from 125 to 500 mg per day; disulfiram therapy may continue for many months, even years.

Disulfiram was first noted for its effects on workers in a rubber plant, and its toxicity in the presence of ethyl alcohol was reported by Hald et al.[3] Disulfiram acts by inhibiting cytoplasmic and mitochondrial dehydrogenases in the liver, interfering with the ethanol-acetaldehyde-acetic acid pathway. The blocking action of disulfiram on aldehyde dehydrogenases led Plotnick[5] to investigate the effects of this on the detoxification or biotransformation of ethylene dibromide in the liver. Although the literature does not contain reports of carcinogenic effects of disulfiram in laboratory animals, the International Agency for Research in Cancer (IARC) has concluded that "the limited data available do not allow an evaluation of the carcinogenicity of disulfiram to be made."[4] The NIOSH estimates that approximately 70,000 workers have occupational exposure to disulfiram. This estimate is based on the NIOSH National Occupational Hazard Survey that was conducted between 1972 and 1974 and included more than 500,000 employees at 4,775 facilities. In addition, there may be as many as 100,000 people on disulfiram therapy for alcoholism.

Laboratory Animal Study of Toxic Interaction[2]

In the NIOSH-sponsored research, laboratory rats exposed to 20 ppm ethylene dibromide by inhalation (the current eight-hour TWA OSHA exposure standard) and also receiving a diet containing 0.05% disulfiram experienced exceedingly high mortality levels as well as a high incidence of tumors (including hemangiosarcomas of the liver, spleen and kidney). Even in those sites where tumors often occur spontaneously in rats, such as the mammary gland in females, the incidence of tumors appears to be increased and the tumors are occurring at an earlier-than-expected age. Although the clinical significance of the data has not yet been evaluated, great caution is indicated. The extent to which this toxic interaction is specific for ethylene dibromide and disulfiram is not known. Similar toxic interactions may occur between disulfiram, as well as chemicals structurally related to disulfiram, and other halogenated hydrocarbons.

NIOSH Recommendations

It is recommended, as an interim and prudent measure, that no worker be exposed to both ethylene dibromide and disulfiram. Workers should not be exposed to ethylene dibromide during the course of disulfiram therapy. Disulfiram (Antabuse, RoSulfiram) should not be administered to workers having potential occupational exposure to ethylene dibromide except in those cases where, in the best judgment of the responsible physician, the benefit of disulfiram therapy strongly outweighs the risk to the particular patient. Whenever disulfiram (bis[diethylthiocarbamoyl] disulfide, tetraethylthiuram disulfide) is used in the workplace (e.g., as an accelerator in rubber production, as a fungicide or insecticide), precautions should be taken so that no worker is exposed to both ethylene dibromide and disulfiram.

The TWA for disulfiram is 2 mg/cu m.

REFERENCES

1. *Criteria for a Recommended Standard: Occupational Exposure to Ethylene Dibromide*. Cincinnati, Oh, US Dept of Health, Education, and Welfare, PHS, Center for Disease Control, National Institute for Occupational Safety and Health, August, 1977.
2. Current Intelligence Bulletin 23: Ethylene dibromide and disulfiram toxic interaction, DHEW (NIOSH) Publ 78-145. National Institute for Occupational Safety and Health, Robert A. Taft Laboratories, 4676 Columbia Parkway, Cincinnati, Oh, April 11, 1978.
3. Hald J, Jacobson E, Larsen V: The sensitizing effect of tetraethylthiuram disulphide (Antabuse) to ethyl alcohol. *Acta Pharmacol Toxicol* 1948; 4:285.
4. *IARC Monog Eval Carcinog Risk Chem Man* 1976; 12:85.
5. Plotnick HB: Carcinogenesis in rats of combined ethylene bromide and disulfiram. *JAMA* 1978; 239:1609.
6. Yodaiken RE: Ethylene dibromide and disulfiram—a lethal combination (editorial). *JAMA* 1978; 239:2783.

ETHYL ETHER

$$C_2H_5OC_2H_5$$

Ethyl ether (ether, diethyl ether) is the well-known anesthetic agent. It is a highly volatile and flammable liquid and is the most important of the ethers (i.e., methyl ether; isopropyl ether; Bis [2-chloroethyl] ether, which is a solvent and intermediate, not a vesicant, although its sulfur analog is mustard gas; ethylene oxide; diethylene glycol; dipropylene glycol; and polyethylene glycol). Ethyl ether is produced in excess of 125 million kg per year in the United States. Important uses are as a solvent for fats, oils, gums, resins, perfumes, and nitrocellulose, in pharmaceutical making, and as a general reactant medium in the chemical industry. Nearly all of the ethers find major uses in adhesives, coatings, plastics, and expoxy resins. Occupational exposures are from inhalation.

Ethyl ether is a mild skin irritant, due to its rapid and complete defatting action. Repeated exposure will cause drying and cracking. The vapor is irritating to the eyes. Undiluted liquid in the eyes causes painful but transitory inflammation. Human subjects found 200 ppm irritating to the nose but not to the eyes or throat.[4] There is a large margin of safety between the concentration causing nasal irritation and concentrations causing anesthesia, permanent damage, coma, or death.[4] Regular exposure to the TLV concentration should cause no irritation or central nervous system depression.[1]

Concentrations of 100,000 ppm or greater may be fatal to human beings. Continued inhalation of 2,000 ppm in human subjects may produce dizziness; however, concentrations up to 7,000 ppm have been tolerated by some workers for variable periods of time without untoward effects. Initial symptoms of acute overexposure include vomiting, pallor, and irregular respiration. Temporary after-effects are vomiting, respiratory tract irritation, headache, and either depression or excitation. In some persons chronic exposure results in anorexia, headache, drowsiness, dizziness, excitation, and psychic disturbances. Albuminuria has been reported. Tolerance may be acquired through repeated exposures.

The 1986 TLV is 400 ppm.

REFERENCES

1. ACGIH: Ethyl ether. Documentation of the TLVs for Substances in Workroom Air, ed 5. Cincinnati, Oh, American Conference of Governmental Hygienists, 1986.
2. Hygienic Guide Series: Ethyl ether. *Am Ind Hyg Assoc J* 1966; 27.

ETHYLENE GLYCOL DINITRATE AND NITROGLYCERIN

CHRISTER HOGSTEDT, M.D.

History

"Dynamite or Nobel's Security Powder" was the name of Alfred Nobel's first Swedish patent in 1867 of an explosive consisting of 75% nitroglycerin and 25% silica guhr. The important contribution by Alfred Nobel was to absorb nitroglycerin on silica guhr (diatomaceous earth) to reduce the explosion hazard and still be able to bring the explosive to detonation.

Nitroglycerin was primarily synthesized by an Italian chemist in 1847 and introduced in medicine in 1879 as a remedy for angina pectoris.

Although the number of dynamite workers always has been comparatively small, the occupational hazards in the explosives industry have captured considerable interest, as reflected in the occupational medical literature. The first published report on occupational health effects from dynamite seems to be from 1882, describing a worker who got headache and flushing of the face when he carried, bare-handed, a leaking dynamite cartridge.[22]

The modern history of occupational health hazards from dynamite production might be thought of as starting in 1952, when Hans Symanski[24] published a report on three male dynamite workers who died suddenly on a Monday or Tuesday morning. In some of the "Monday death" case reports there were also speculations on chronic vascular effects from occupational exposure to nitrate esters, but as late as the mid-1970s very little was known about the long-term effects of occupational exposure to organic nitrate esters.

The Manufacturing Process and Exposure

Originally, nitroglycerin (NG) was the only component of the "blasting oil," but since the late 1920s, ethylene glycol dinitrate (EGDN) has been added. Nitroglycerin freezes at 13° C, and frozen, stiff NG is unreliable in its explosive characteristics. Frozen NG might detonate even from light pressing, e.g., during filling of a drill hole or on cleaning rests after incomplete blasting, whereas unfrozen NG is much more insensitive and, for example, can fall from considerable height without detonation. In 1905, EGDN was suggested as an additive to lower the freezing point, but it was not until the mid-1920s that a large production of ethylene glycol also made EGDN commercially attractive. Since the late 1920s, EGDN has contributed an increasing proportion to all dynamite produced.

Nitroglycerin and EGDN are produced by nitration of glycerin and ethylene glycol, respectively, with a mixture of sulfuric and nitric acids to form the so-called blasting oil. After washing and separation of surplus acid ("spent acid"), the blasting oil goes to the mix-houses (knead-houses) where it is mixed with oxidizing salts (mostly ammonium nitrate and sodium nitrate), nitrocellulose, and fillers such as sawdust and chalk (Figs 47–8 and 47–9). The well-known red color of dynamite is obtained by adding rhodamin. Until the late 1960s, trinitrotoluene (TNT) was also a component of the dynamite but was then replaced by dinitrotoluene (DNT) to reduce explosion hazards.

Manufactured dynamite consists today of about 60% ammonium and sodium nitrate, 20%–25% EGDN, 0%–5% NG, 10% DNT, 3% nitrocellulose, and a few percent sawdust, chalk, and rhodamin.

In early times, all types of work brought about direct exposure to the various compounds of dynamite. Kneading was done bare-handed, and bare-breasted in summertime, and dynamite sticks were rolled and packed by hand. No ventilation was installed until the 1950s, and at this time the use of protective gloves came into regular use. Today, much of the manufacturing process is automated in industrialized countries and supervised by TV monitors. Exposure to the workers occurs mainly in the cleaning-up operations, repairing, and sample-taking. However, bigger cartridges are still usually filled semi-automatically and such operators may be exposed to organic nitrate esters around 1 mg/cu m for EGDN (Fig 47–10).

The mean eight-hour time-weighted average (TWA) concentrations of nitrate esters for different job types during seven-year periods in 1958–1978 were calculated from a large number of semi-annually measured short-time samples in a Swedish factory.[14] The air concentrations were estimated to have been in the range of 0.2–1.1 mg/cu m, with the highest levels for cartridge fillers and mix-house workers.

The NIOSH[20] has reviewed the international literature on exposure conditions in the dynamite industry, but the comparison

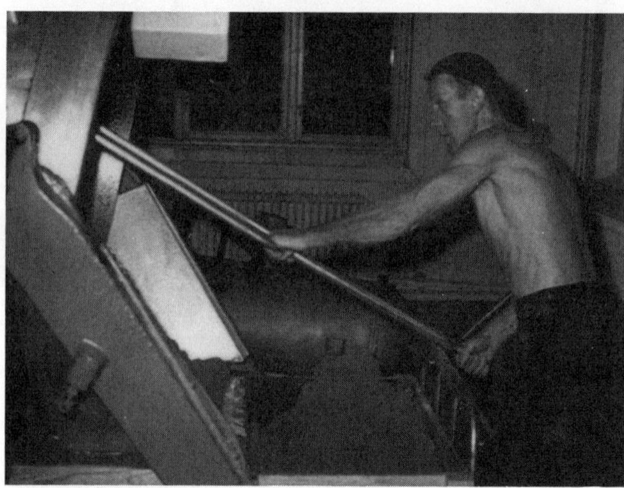

FIG 47–8.
A dynamite kneader from the 1950s. No protective equipment was used in that era.

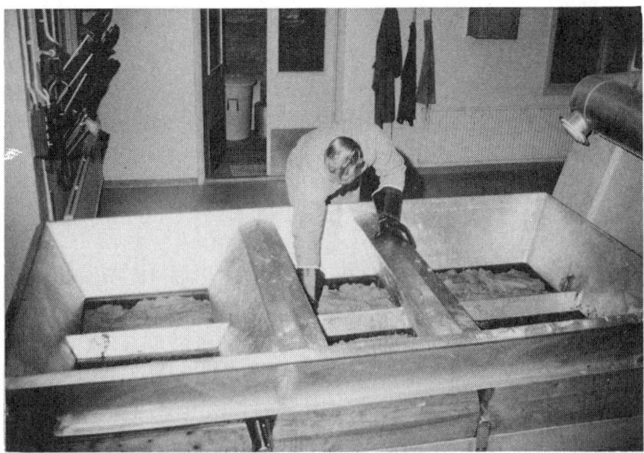

FIG 47-9.
A dynamite worker inspecting the kneaded mass.

between factories in various countries is difficult due to different sampling procedures and analytic methods.

Absorption and Metabolism

Nitroglycol and, to a lesser extent, nitroglycerin are absorbed through the skin as well as through the lungs. The air concentration will influence the uptake from both these routes of absorption, but direct skin contamination plays an important role for the total uptake.

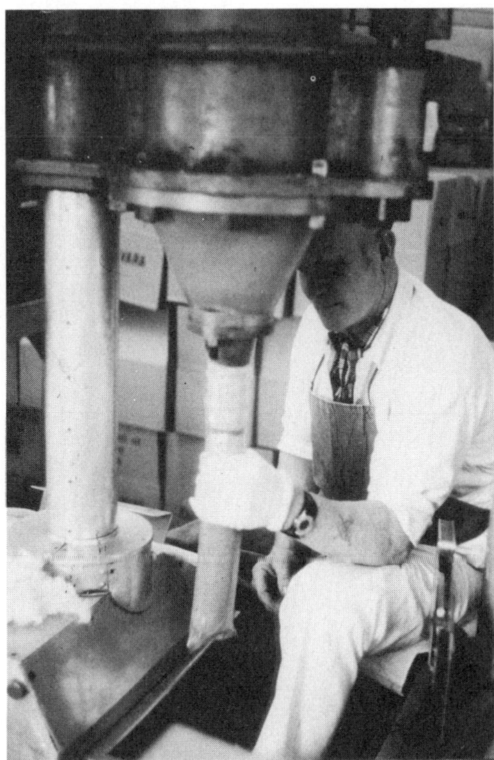

FIG 47-10.
Dynamite is packed in plastic tubes by a semi-automatic procedure.

There is only one animal study reported[4] concerning lung absorption of EGDN. High concentrations of hundreds of milligrams of EGDN per cubic meter were used, and the lung absorption seemed to be moderate.

Gross et al.[5–7] studied the absorption of EGDN and NG through the skin of cats and rabbits. The authors found that EGDN was absorbed more rapidly through the skin than NG and that EGDN caused more severe toxic effects to develop more quickly. The EGDN absorption rate in human beings was considerably less than found in rats. Later studies have indicated that skin absorption is a more important route of entry than inhalation.[15]

After administration of nitrate esters to human beings or animals, degradation of the parent molecule occurs by stepwise detachment of the organic nitrate groups from the carbon skeleton, resulting in the appearance of inorganic nitrite and nitrate.[19] The time course of metabolism for EGDN has been studied in rats by measuring blood concentrations of the compound and its metabolites after subcutaneous injection.[2] Ethylene glycol mononitrate (EGMN) was produced as the result of the initial denitration of the dinitrate, and the blood level peaked after two to three hours. Ethylene glycol dinitrate reached the maximal concentration within 30–60 minutes. Some limited human experiments suggest that the venous blood concentration is approximately halved in 30 minutes.[15]

The metabolism of NG, EGDN, and EGMN appears to involve reduced glutathione in a reaction catalyzed by an enzyme known as organic nitrate reductase, which is predominantly located in the soluble fraction of liver homogenate.[21] However, in vitro experiments with rat blood also showed that EGDN was metabolized in erythrocytes and in whole blood, but not in plasma.[1]

Health Effects From EGDN and Nitroglycerin

Acute Effects

In 1898 Laws[18] gave a very accurate description of the acute effects from vasodilation caused by nitrate ester exposure: throbbing headache, increased pulse rate, palpitations, nausea, vomiting, and alcohol intolerance. Laws mentioned also that the workers became accustomed to nitroglycerin after a week of exposure, although the symptoms recurred when they returned to work after two or more days' absence. Also, the families of the dynamite workers got similar symptoms when the workers brought their clothes home for washing and ironing.

In 1952, Hans Symanski published a report on three male dynamite workers, aged 42–50 years, who had died suddenly on a Monday or Tuesday morning. Symanski argued strongly that these sudden deaths were attributable to dynamite exposure, especially to EGDN, and stated that he had third-hand, unpublished information about six to eight similar cases from Scotland, and also 37 cases of sudden death from the dynamite industry in the U.S.A. during 1927–1936, confirmed 26 years later by Foulger.[3] The factors in common for all these cases of sudden death were that they had occurred one or two days after the last exposure to dynamite (in the "abstinence" or withdrawal phase) among fairly young and apparently healthy workers.

Symanski's report was later followed by other case reports on the "Monday death" from many other countries. The etiology of this excess has not been discovered, but based on animal studies, the hypothesis might be entertained that the increased risk of sudden deaths among dynamite workers could be caused by ventricular fibrillation due to an increased sympathetic activity during the abstinence phase in combination with a relatively ischemic myocardium because of coronary spasm in sensitive individuals. However, long-term electrocardiography in dynamite workers did not reveal more ectopic beats than in a reference group.[16]

Long-Term Effects

Two different Swedish populations of dynamite workers have been studied with attention to patterns of mortality, especially cardiocerebrovascular diseases.[11, 12] The reports on sudden deaths from the explosives industry had been somewhat conflicting with regard to the occurrence of coronary sclerosis in the victims, most of them being comparatively young men.[9] Indeed, an increased mortality from ischemic heart disease was found among long-term male dynamite workers in a case-referent study.[12] An extension of the case-referent study has recently been published[13] and the results from the original study have reinforced the evidence of excess mortality from ischemic heart disease among men with long-time exposure to explosives from nitroglycerin and nitroglycol. There was also an increased risk ratio for cerebrovascular diseases during the full study period of 1955–1980. Among 25 men who were deceased before the age of 70 and had been exposed more than 20 years, only one died from anything else but a cardiocerebrovascular disease. The results are in agreement with the results from a small cohort study of dynamite workers from another Swedish plant using national mortality for reference.[11] The excess mortality was statistically significant only with a requirement for 20 years of induction-latency time and most pronounced among those with long-term employment.

Results from a Scottish cohort study[2a] on 659 blasting workers with exposure to EGDN and NG, and 224 propellants workers with exposure to only NG were similar to Swedish findings. Further support for the observation that occupational exposure to nitrate esters increase the risk for heart disease is delivered from a U.S. Navy study of 1,2 propylene dinitrate exposed torpedo men.[2b] In the Scottish study,[2a] an increased rate of lung cancer was found among the high exposed blasting workers. In a mutagenicity study the frequency of mutations was increased in bacteria treated with EGDN compared to untreated bacteria.[17] No reports have been found concerning the carcinogenic potential of EGDN in animal experiments. A tendency to increased numbers of benign tumors has been found in animal tests for NG, however.[24, 25]

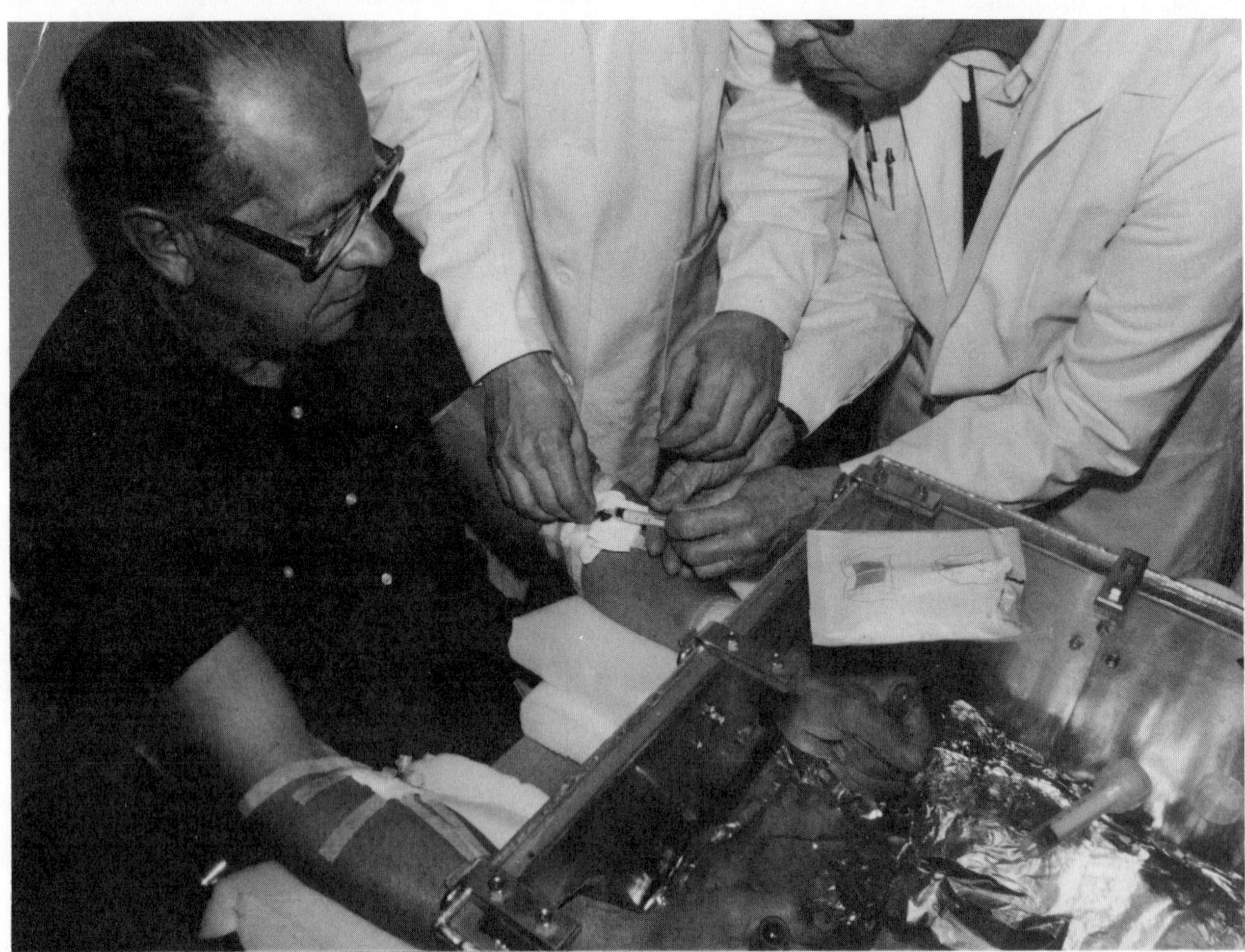

FIG 47–11.
Testing skin absorption from dynamite by blood sampling under experimental conditions.

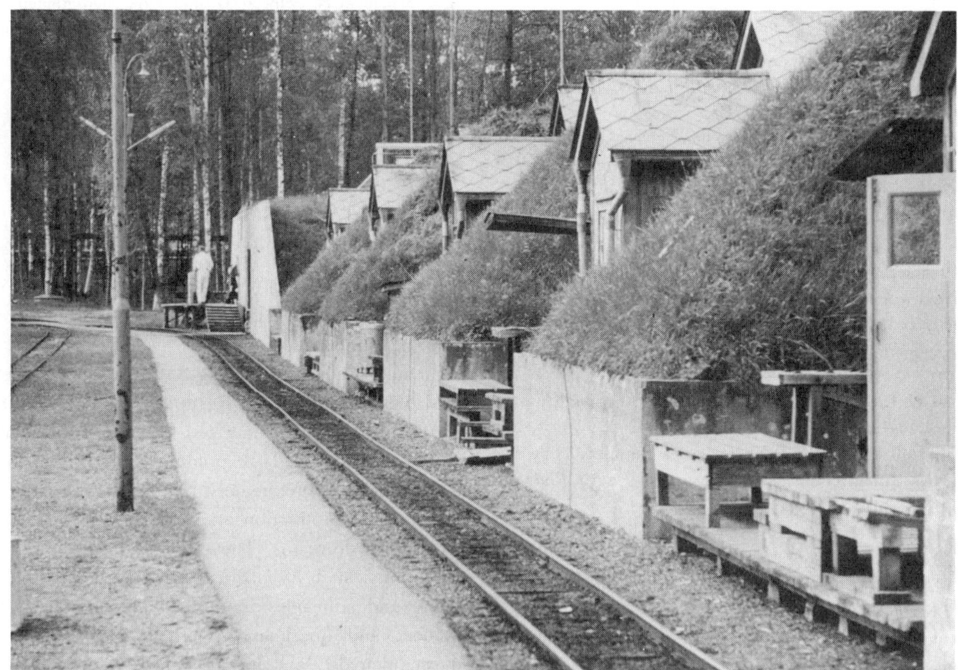

FIG 47–12.
Dynamite production units are separated by thick earthen walls in order to reduce the number of casualties in the event of an explosion.

Prevention and Industrial Hygiene

From the medical preventive point of view, a preemployment examination should exclude cardiac diseases of different types (congestive heart disease, arrhythmias, and signs of valvular dysfunction). Individuals suffering from incipient or a manifest hypertension or those complaining about migraine should not be accepted in exposed jobs. Regular surveillance might be of value to protect workers, and indications of unfitness revealed in the history, blood pressure, or in ECG findings should result in removal of the worker from exposure.

Blood samples containing EGDN indicate that uptake has occurred and could therefore be used as a qualitative measurement as applied in a study of absorption through protective gloves (Fig 47–11).[15] However, venous blood samples from cubital veins primarily seem to reflect the local concentration due to absorption distal to the sampling spot and could not be used for biologic monitoring at the workplace, since contact with solid dynamite is very hard to avoid.[10] The types of protective gloves normally used in the dynamite industry do not eliminate percutaneous absorption.[15] Considering the presented facts, it is not surprising that no correlation was found between blood samples and the air concentration of EGDN.[8]

Ethylene glycol dinitrate can be detected in urine of dynamite workers, but no study has been reported in which the feasibility of biologic monitoring by urine samples has been studied and evaluated. No EGDN was detected in exhaled air in spite of very high blood concentrations during experimental conditions with a human being.[15]

Hygienic prevention should focus on eliminating skin contact. Clean gloves that are resistant to nitrate esters are necessary, and the hygienic routines should be vigorous. Glove changes as often as hourly may be required for some work assignments. Effective measures to prevent skin absorption include easy access to washrooms for cleanup after spills or before breaks, meals, or toilet use.

Again, it must be pointed out that the internal exposure level of the workers is not reflected in measurements of the air concentrations of nitrate esters unless skin contact with the compounds is completely avoided. Headache seems to be induced in sensitive individuals at air concentrations of about 0.1 mg/cu m, whereas the TLVs proposed in different countries are about 1–2 mg/cu m for nitroglycol and 2–5 mg/cu m for nitroglycerin.

Explosion prevention requires the use of explosion-proof, nonsparking, dust-tight electric fixtures and wiring (Fig 47–12). There should be no smoking and no use of open sparks or flames, including welding in nonsecured areas. Antifriction motor bearings should be used, and conductive materials should be grounded. No maintenance work should be done without proper cleanup and entry permits. Where the use of motorized equipment is required, it must be specifically designed for use in explosive atmospheres.

These specific safety measures are aimed at explosion containment:

1. Detached buildings with explosion-venting systems, further subdivided by fire- and pressure-resistant walls
2. Limited personnel access and census in potential explosion areas
3. Limited explosives accumulation in well-ventilated storage areas
4. The use of tightly sealed storage containers
5. Planned, practiced evacuation and emergency measures.

REFERENCES

1. Clark DG, Litchfield MH: Metabolism of ethylene glycol dinitrate and its influence on the blood pressure of the rat. *Br J Ind Med* 1967; 24:320–325.
2. Clark DG, Litchfield MH: Metabolism of ethylene glycol dinitrate (ethylene dinitrate) in the rat following repeated administration. *Br J Ind Med* 1969; 26:150–155.

2a. Craig R, Gillis CR, Hole DJ, et al: Sixteen year follow up of workers in an explosives factory. *Soc Occup Med* 1985; 35:107–110.

2b. Forman SA, Helmkamp JC, Bone CM, et al: Cardiac morbidity and mortality associated with occupational exposure to 1,2 propylene glycol dinitrate. *J Occup Med* 1987; 29:445–450.

3. Foulger JH: The industrial nitroglycerine-nitroglycol question. *J Occup Med* 1978; 20:789–792.
4. Frimmer M, Gross E, Kiese M, et al: Resorption von Äthylenglykoldinitrat durch die Lunge. *Arch Toxikol* 1960; 18:200–204.
5. Gross E, Bock M, Hellrung F: Zur Toxikologie des Nitroglykols im Vergleich zu der des Nitroglycerins. *Arch f experiment Path u Pharmakol* 1942; 200:271–304.
6. Gross E, Kiese M, Resag K: Resorption von Äthylenglykoldinitrat durch die Haut. *Arch Toxikol* 1960; 18:194–199.
7. Gross E, Kiese M, Resag K: Resorption von Glycerintrinitrat durch die Haut. *Arch Toxikol* 1960; 18:331–334.
8. Gӧtell P: Environmental and clinical aspects of nitroglycol and nitroglycerin exposure. *Occup Health Saf* 1976; 45:50–51.
9. Hogstedt C: Dynamite—Occupational exposure and health effects. Linköpings University Medical Dissertations No 84, 1980.
10. Hogstedt C: Ethylene glycol dinitrate, in Aitio A, Riihimäki V, Vainio H (eds): Biological monitoring and surveillance of workers exposed to chemicals. Washington, Hemisphere Publishing Corp, 1984; 187–192.
11. Hogstedt C, Andersson K: A cohort study on mortality among dynamite workers. *J Med* 1979; 21:553–556.
12. Hogstedt C, Axelson O: Nitroglycerine-nitroglycol exposure and the mortality in cardio-cerebrovascular diseases among dynamite workers. *J Med* 1977; 10:675–678.
13. Hogstedt C, Axelson O: Mortality from cardio-cerebrovascular diseases among dynamite workers—An extended case-referent study. *Ann Acad Med (Singapore)* 1984; 13:399–403.
14. Hogstedt C, Davidsson B: Nitroglycol and nitroglycerine exposure in a dynamite industry 1958–1978. *Am Ind Hyg Assoc J* 1980; 41:373–375.
15. Hogstedt C, Ståhl R: Skin absorption and protective gloves in dynamite work. *Am Ind Hyg Assoc J* 1980; 41:362–367.
16. Hogstedt C, Söderholm B, Bodin L: 48-hour ambulatory electrocardiography in dynamite workers and controls. *Br J Ind Med* 1980; 37:299–306.
17. Kononova SD, Korolev AM, Eremenko LT, et al: Mutagenic effect of some esters of nitric acid on bacteriophage T4B. *Genetica* 1972; 8:101–108.
18. Laws CE: The effects of nitroglycerin upon those who manufacture it. *JAMA* 1898; 31:793–794.
19. Litchfield MH: Recent views on the mechanisms of nitrate ester metabolism. *Drug Metab Rev* 1973; 2(2):239–264.
20. National Institute for Safety and Health: *Criteria for a Recommended Standard: Occupational Exposure to Nitroglycerine/Nitroglycol*. Rockville, Md, US Dept of Health, Education and Welfare, NIOSH, 1978.
21. Needleman P, Hunter FE: The transformation of glycerol trinitrate and other nitrates by glutathione-organic nitrate reductase. *Mol Pharmacol* 1965; 1:77–86.
22. Nevitt, Barington (1882): from Munch JC, Friedland B, Shepard M: Glyceryl trinitrate. II. Chronic toxicity. *Ind Med Surg* 1965; 34:940–943.
23. Suzuki K, Sudo K, Yamamoto T, et al: The carcinogenicity of N-ethoxycarbonyl-3-morpholinosydnonimine (Molsidomine) in comparison with nitroglycerin in C57BL/6Jms mice. *Pharmacometrics* 1975; 9:229–242.
24. Symanski H: Schwere Gesundheitsschädigungen durch berufliche Nitroglykoleinwirkung. *Arch Hyg Bakterol* 1952; 136:139–158.
25. Takayama S: Carcinogenicity of Molsidomine and nitroglycerin in rats. *Pharmacometrics* 1975; 9:217–228.

Formaldehyde

LESLIE STAYNER, M.S.

HCHO

Formaldehyde (HCHO) is a colorless, flammable gas with a strong, pungent odor. It is usually marketed as formalin, an aqueous solution containing 35%–50% formaldehyde (by weight), and 6%–15% methanol to suppress polymerization. It is also marketed in a solid polymerized form as paraformaldehyde, or trioxane. In 1976, the U.S. produced 6.4 billion lb of aqueous formaldehyde.[40] Approximately half of the formaldehyde produced is used in the production of urea-, acetal-, melamine-, and phenol-formaldehyde resins. These resins have numerous commercial applications, such as fabric finishes to produce crease-resistant textiles, and adhesives in the manufacture of particle boards, plywoods, and fiberboards, and in foams for thermal insulation. Formaldehyde itself has numerous applications in medicine as a bactericide and tissue preservative.

Because of its widespread use, a relatively large number of workers are exposed to formaldehyde. The National Institute for Occupational Safety and Health (NIOSH) has estimated that 1.6 million workers are potentially exposed to formaldehyde: of these workers, approximately 57,000 were exposed for greater than four hours per day.[25]

Health Effects

A summary of the dose-response relationship between formaldehyde and its acute effects is presented in Table 47–5. Sensitized individuals may react to even lower concentrations of formaldehyde than those shown in the table. The odor threshold for formaldehyde has been reported to be as low as 0.05 ppm.[10] Irritation of the mucosal membranes of the eyes and upper respiratory tract leading to lacrimation, rhinitis, and pharyngitis are the most common symptoms reported with formaldehyde exposure. Adaptation to the odor and irritant effects of formaldehyde is known to occur, although this tolerance is short-lasting and may be lost after removal from formaldehyde exposure for one hour.[21] Extremely high concentrations of formaldehyde (50–100 ppm) may result in pulmonary edema and hemorrhage[4] and death.[5] Fortunately, the odor and irritant effects of formaldehyde make it difficult for individuals to remain in areas with exposures greater than 3 ppm.

Ingestion of large quantities of formaldehyde may result in severe corrosive damage to the gastrointestinal tract,[4, 15, 32, 41] irritation of the respiratory passages,[32] and death.[7a] In most instances, ingestion of formaldehyde has been reported to result in the development of corrosive gastritis, with little if any involvement of the esophagus and lower gastrointestinal tract.[4a, 15, 32, 41] Formaldehyde is rapidly metabolized to formic acid, potentially resulting in metabolic acidosis.[7a]

Formaldehyde is a sensitizing agent capable of inducing asthma and allergic contact dermatitis. Episodes of contact der-

TABLE 47–5.
Acute Effects of Airborne Formaldehyde Exposure*

EFFECT	AIRBORNE FORMALDEHYDE CONCENTRATION, PPM
Odor detection	0.05–1.0
Eye irritation	0.01–2.0
Upper respiratory tract irritation	0.10–25
Lower airway and pulmonary effects	5–30
Pulmonary edema, inflammation, pneumonia	50–100
Death	100+

*Adapted from National Research Council: *Formaldehyde and Other Aldehydes.* Washington, DC, National Academy Press, 1981, p. 186.

matitis have been observed among workers exposed to formaldehyde in the production of formaldehyde resins,[35] textiles,[30] shampoos,[4] and in hospitals.[37, 31] Contact urticaria has also been reported as a result of formaldehyde exposure.[16, 13]

Although dermal allergies to formaldehyde have been recognized for some time, respiratory allergy has only recently begun to be accepted as a clinical entity. There have been reports of occupational asthma resulting from exposure to formaldehyde in hospital laboratory workers,[33] in carpenters working with urea formaldehyde particle board,[7] and in nurses in a renal dialysis unit.[17] Diagnosis of formaldehyde-induced asthma in these reports was established using provocative inhalation testing with a formaldehyde aerosol. All of the asthma cases identified in these reports did not respond positively to this test, and it has been suggested that formaldehyde may increase the susceptibility to other provoking agents, or induce a hyperactive responsiveness of the airways.[17]

It is unclear whether long-term exposure to formaldehyde has a chronic effect on pulmonary function. Exposure of guinea pigs to formaldehyde concentrations as low as 0.3 ppm resulted in transient increases in airway resistance and decreased compliance.[3] Results from epidemiologic investigations have been contradictory. Lower than expected values for pulmonary function tests taken before work on Monday morning, suggestive of chronic obstructive lung disease, were observed in two studies of workers exposed to formaldehyde.[34, 38] In contrast, in three other epidemiologic studies of formaldehyde-exposed workers, pulmonary function measurements taken prior to exposure were judged to be within normal limits.[2, 11, 19] Decrements in pulmonary function over a work shift, indicative of an acute reversible effect on lung function, were present in three studies[2, 11, 38] and absent in one study.[34]

Carcinogenic and Teratogenic Effects

Although results from experiments in rodents indicate that formaldehyde is a carcinogen, the results from epidemiologic investigations are inconclusive. In a recent study sponsored by the Chemical Industry Institute of Toxicology (CIIT), rats exposed to 6 and 15 ppm, and mice exposed to 15 ppm, developed squamous-cell carcinomas of the nasal passages.[6] These findings were later supported by experiments in which inhalation of 14.7 ppm formaldehyde alone or in combination with 10.6 ppm hydrogen chloride induced squamous-cell carcinomas in rats.[1]

A few mortality studies of workers exposed to formaldehyde have been recently reported.[9, 14, 18, 20, 23, 39, 42, 43] None of these studies have detected an association between nasal cancer and formaldehyde exposure. However, these studies were all extremely limited in their ability to detect an excess of nasal cancer because of limited sample size, intermittent exposures, and insufficient documentation of exposures. A few of these studies have detected statistically significant excesses of other cancer sites. In particular, excesses of the following cancer sites have been observed: cancers of the skin, kidney, and brain, and lymphatic neoplasms among embalmers;[18, 42] cancers of the prostate, digestive system, and buccal cavity among chemical workers involved in the production of formaldehyde or formaldehyde resins;[9, 20, 23, 43] brain cancers and lymphatic neoplasms among pathologists;[14] and multiple myelomas, parotid gland, and gallbladder cancers among garment workers who work with cloth treated with formaldehyde resins.[39] The lack of consistency between these studies in terms of the cancer sites observed, and with the animal experiments, undermines the interpretation of their etiologic significance. Larger epidemiologic studies, which should provide more definitive results, are now in progress.

To date, formaldehyde has not been demonstrated to be teratogenic in any animal species, although the experiments conducted thus far have been inadequate and further research is needed.[29] Physiologic and biochemical effects have been observed in the concepti of animals exposed in utero, such as decreased nucleic acid and ascorbic acid content,[27] and increased fetal weight.[12, 28] The relationship of these findings to developmental abnormalities has not been established. Increased incidences of fetal resorptions, suggesting an embryotoxic effect, have been observed in mice receiving high concentrations of formaldehyde by gavage.[22]

There is also no evidence that formaldehyde has a teratogenic effect in humans, although there is limited evidence that it may have an adverse impact on reproductive function. An investigation of reproductive function in female workers exposed to formaldehyde in the garment industry revealed that, compared to nonexposed controls, workers exposed to formaldehyde had an increased incidence of menstrual disorders, inflammatory disease of the reproductive tract, sterility, anemia, and low birth weights among their offspring.[36]

Permissible Exposure Limits

The Occupational Safety and Health Administration (OSHA) standard for formaldehyde requires that exposures not exceed an eight-hour time-weighted average of 3 ppm, a ceiling concentration of 5 ppm, and an acceptable peak above the ceiling concentration of 10 ppm for no more than a total of 30 minutes during an eight-hour shift.[26] The NIOSH recommended in 1976, based upon the irritant effects of formaldehyde, that employee exposure not exceed 1 ppm for any 30-minute sampling period.[24] More recently, the NIOSH[25] recommended that formaldehyde be handled as a potential human carcinogen and that appropriate controls be used to limit worker exposure. This latter recommendation was primarily based on the evidence that formaldehyde exposure induces nasal cancers in rats.[1, 6]

REFERENCES

1. Albert RE, Sellakumar AR, Laskin S, et al: Gaseous formaldehyde and hydrogen chloride induction of nasal cancer in the rat. *J Nat Cancer Inst* 1982; 68:597–603.
2. Alexandersson R, Kolmodin-Hedman B, Hedenstierna G: Exposure to formaldehyde: Effects on pulmonary function. *Arch Environ Health* 1982; 37:279–284.
3. Amdur MO: The response of guinea pigs to inhalation of formaldehyde and formic acid along with a sodium chloride aerosol. *J Air Pollut* 1960; 3:201–220.
4. Ancona-Alayon A, Jimenez-Castilla JL, Gomez-Alvarez EM: Dermatitis from epoxy resin and formaldehyde in shampoo packers. *Contact Dermatol* 1976; 2:356–364.

4a. Bartone NF, Grieco RV, Herr BS: Corrosive gastritis due to ingestion of formaldehyde. *JAMA* 1968; 203:(1)104–105.

5. Bohmer K: Formalin poisoning. *Dtsch Z Gesamte Gerichtl Med* 1934; 23:7–18 (in German).
6. Chemical Industry Institute of Toxicology: *Summary of Final Report on a Chronic Inhalation Toxicology Study in Rats and Mice Exposed to Formaldehyde*. Research Park, NC, Chemical Industry Institute of Toxicology Activities, 1982, vol 2, pp 8–10.
7. Cockroft DW: Occupational asthma caused by urea formaldehyde. *Chest* 1982; 82:49–53.

7a. Eels JT, McMartin KE, Black K, et al: Formaldehyde poisoning. Rapid metabolism to formic acid. *JAMA* 1981; 246:1237–1238.

8. Epstein E: Formaldehyde allergy. Incidence and patch testing problems. *Arch Dermatol* 1966; 94:186–190.
9. Fayerweather WE, Bell S, Bender JR: Case control study of cancer deaths in DuPont workers with potential exposure to formaldehyde. May 17, 1982, unpublished.
10. Fel'dman YG, Bonashevskaya Y: On the effects and low concentrations of formaldehyde. *Hyg Sanit* 1971; 36:174–180.
11. Gamble JF, McMichael AJ, Williams T, et al: Respiratory function and symptoms: An environmental epidemiological study of rubber workers exposed to a phenol formaldehyde type resin. *Am Ind Hyg Assoc J* 1976; 37(9):499–513.
12. Gofmekler VA: Effect on embryonic development of benzene and formaldehyde in inhalation experiments. *Hyg Sanit* 1968; 33(3):327–332.
13. Guyot JD: Report of a case of formalin urticaria. *South Med J* 1921; 14:115.
14. Harrington JM, Shannon HS: Mortality study of pathologists and medical laboratory technicians. *Br Med J* 1975; 4:329–332.
15. Heffernon ED, Hajjar JJA: Corrosive gastritis after formaldehyde ingestion. *Lahey Clin Found Bull* 1964; 13:293–296.
16. Helander I: Contact urticaria from leather containing formaldehyde. *Arch Dermatol* 1977; 113:1443.
17. Hendrick DJ: Occupational formalin asthma. *Br J Ind Med* 1977; 34:(1)11–18.
18. Levine RJ, Adjelkovich DA, Shaw LK, et al: Mortality of Ontario undertakers: A first report, in Clary JJ, Gibson JE, Waritz RS (eds): *Formaldehyde: Toxicology and Mechanisms*. New York, Marcel Dekker Inc, 1983.
19. Levine RJ, Dalcorso RD, Blunden PB, et al: The effects of formaldehyde exposure on the respiratory health of West Virginia morticians, in Gibson JE (ed): *Formaldehyde Toxicity*. Washington, DC, Hemisphere Publishing Corp, 1983.
20. Liebling T: *Mortality in Relation to Occupation: A Study of Workers at the Monsanto-Springfield Chemical Plant*. Thesis presented for the degree of Master of Science at the University of Massachusetts, Amherst, February 1982.
21. Loomis TA: Formaldehyde toxicity. *Arch Pathol Lab Med* 1979; 103:321–324.
22. Marks TA, Worthy WC, Staples RE: Influence of formaldehyde and sonacide (potentiated acid glutaraldehyde) on embryo and fetal development in mice. *Teratology* 1980; 22(1):51–58.
23. Marsh GM: Proportionate mortality patterns among chemical plant workers exposed to formaldehyde. *Br J Ind Med* 1982; 39:313–322.
24. National Institute for Occupational Safety and Health: *Criteria for a Recommended Standard: Occupational Exposure to Formaldehyde*, DHEW(NIOSH) Publ 77–126, 1976.
25. National Institute for Occupational Safety and Health (NIOSH): Formaldehyde: Evidence of Carcinogenicity. *Curr Intell Bull* 34, April 15, 1981.
26. Occupational Safety and Health Administration: *General Industry OSHA Safety and Health Standards* (29CFR 1910). OSHA Publ 2206, Washington, DC, pp 554 (Revised Nov 7, 1978).

26a. Partanen T, Kauppinen T, Nurminen M, et al: Formaldehyde exposure and respiratory and related cancers: A case-referent study among Finnish woodworkers. Scandinavian Jour. of Work, Environ. & Health, Vol. 11, No. 6, 1985.

27. Pushkina NN, Gofmekler VA, Klevetsova GN: Changes in content of ascorbic acid and nucleic acids produced by benzene and formaldehyde. *Bull Exp Biol Med* 1968; 66:868–870.
28. Ranstroem S: Stress and pregnancy. *Acta Pathol Microbiol Scand* 1956; (Suppl) 111:113–114.
29. Report of the Federal Panel on Formaldehyde. *Environ Health Perspect* 1982; 43:139–168.
30. Romaguera C, Grimalt F, Lecha M: Occupational purpuric textile dermatitis from formaldehyde resins. *Contact Dermatol* 1981; 7:152–153.
31. Rostenberg A, Bairstow B, Luther TW: A study of eczematous sensitivity to formaldehyde. *J Invest Dermatol* 1952; 19:459–462.
32. Roy M, Conje MA, Mouton R: Corrosive gastritis after formaldehyde ingestion. Report of a case. *New Engl J Med* 1962; 266:1248–1250.
33. Sakula A: Formalin asthma in hospital laboratory staff. *Lancet* 1975; 2:816.
34. Schoenberg JB, Mitchell CA: Airway disease caused by phenolic (phenol-formaldehyde) resin exposure. *Arch Environ Health* 1975; 30:574–577.
35. Schwartz L, Peck SM, Duine JE: Dermatitis from resin glue in war industries. *Pub Health Rep* 1943; 58:599–604.
36. Shumilina AV: Menstrual and reproductive functions in workers with occupational exposures to formaldehyde. *Grig Tr Prof Zabol* 1975; 12:18–21.
37. Sneddon JB: Dermatitis in an intermittent haemodialysis unit. *Br Med J* 1968; 1:183–184.
38. Sparks MJ, Peters JM: Respiratory morbidity in workers exposed to dust containing phenolic resins. *Int Arch Occup Environ Health* 1980; 45:221–229.
39. Stayner LT, Smith AB, Reeve G, et al: Proportionate mortality study of workers in the garment industry exposed to formaldehyde. In press.
40. US International Trade Commission: *Synthetic Organic Chemicals—United States Production and Sales, 1978*, USITC Publ 1001. Washington, DC, USITC, 1979, p 311.
41. Vinson PP, Harrington SW: Involvement of the esophagus following ingestion of a solution of formaldehyde. *JAMA* 1929; 93:917–918.
42. Walrath J, Fraumeni JF: Mortality patterns among embalmers. *Int J Cancer* 1983; 31:407–411.
43. Wong O: An epidemiologic mortality study of a cohort of chemical workers potentially exposed to formaldehyde, with a discussion on SMR and PMR, in Gibson JE (ed): *Formaldehyde Toxicity*. Washington, DC, Hemisphere Publishing Corp, 1983.

HYDRAZINES

The biologic effects of hydrazines on humans and on animals described here include those of five compounds: hydrazine (H_2NNH_2), methylhydrazine (CH_3NHNH_2), 1,1-dimethylhydrazine ($(CH_3)_2NNH_2$), 1,2-dimethylhydrazine ($CH_3NHNHCH_3$), and phenylhydrazine ($C_6H_5NHNH_2$). All these hydrazines are at least slightly basic and polar, and they are strong reducing agents. The hydrazine bases are used in the production of salts and hydrazones that are used in surfactants, detergents, plasticizers, pharmaceuticals, insecticides, and herbicides. Three of the hydrazines (hydrazine, methylhydrazine, and 1,1-dimethylhydrazine) have been used as rocket propellants.

Hydrazines are very reactive and have wide use, and they are capable of causing a variety of biologic effects. There has been great interest in the toxicologic implications of the hydrazines, and there have been many animal studies conducted on the three hydrazines used as rocket fuels. Comprehensive reviews have been prepared by various groups, including the U.S. Air Force[1, 2, 9] and the International Agency for Research on Cancer (IARC).[10] The Committee on Toxicology of the National Academy of Sciences[6] also provided documentation on establishing guidelines for short-term community air exposures. The NIOSH has expressed concern about the possible tumorigenicity of a number of chemicals, including several hydrazines. In the 1976 edition of the *NIOSH's Registry of Toxic Effects of Chemical Substances*,[3] several hydrazines were listed as animal carcinogens, based primarily on the 1974 report of studies by the IARC.

Little information is available on the decomposition of the hydrazines in air and water. Hydrazine is thermodynamically unstable and may decompose into hydrogen, ammonia, and nitrogen. The reaction rate reportedly is slow at room temperatures but increases at elevated temperatures, particularly in the presence of metals such as copper.

Hydrazine, methylhydrazine, 1,1-dimethylhydrazine, and 1,2-dimethylhydrazine are characterized by a fishy, ammonia-like odor. These four compounds are clear, colorless, flammable or combustible, hygroscopic liquids that are soluble in water, ethanol, and other polar solvents. Phenylhydrazine has a faint aromatic odor and occurs as yellow monoclinic crystals or oil. It is miscible with alcohol, ether, chloroform, and benzene but only sparingly soluble in water.

Occupations with potential exposure to hydrazines are agricultural chemical workers, analytical chemists, anticorrosion additive workers, boiler operators, catalyst reclaimers, chlorine scavenger makers, drug makers, dye makers, explosives makers, foamed plastic makers, fuel cell makers, herbicide makers, hydraulic fluid workers, hydrazine and hydrazine-derivative makers, insecticide makers, jet fuel handlers, jet fuel makers, nitron makers, organic chemical synthesizers, oxygen scavenger makers, photographic developer makers, rocket fuel handlers, rocket fuel makers, rubber workers, silverplating workers, solder flux makers, solderers, textile dyers (acrylic and vinyl), vat dye makers, and water treaters.

Effects of Exposure

The potential for worker exposure to the hydrazines is primarily through two routes of exposure—inhalation and contact with skin or eyes. Hydrazine, methylhydrazine, and 1,1-dimethylhydrazine were readily absorbed through the shaved skin of dogs. Each compound was detectable in the blood in 30 seconds, and signs of acute toxicity ensued. Two drops of anhydrous hydrazine applied to the shaved skin of rats, as well as 3 ml applied to rabbits, were lethal, suggesting that even a small spill on the skin of workers could be toxic. In general, the compound with the highest vapor pressure, 1,1-dimethylhydrazine, should be the least toxic by skin absorption because of rapid evaporation. Since 1,1-dimethylhydrazine is toxic by this route, other hydrazines are likely to have a similar effect.

In regard to eye damage, as little as two drops of a 25% solution of hydrazine applied to the eyes of animals caused permanent damage.[11] Methylhydrazine, 1,1-dimethylhydrazine, and 1,2-dimethylhydrazine, however, produced only temporary mild effects. These effects probably are pH-dependent, since alkaline compounds would be expected to cause more damage to eye surfaces; thus, the eye damage expected for phenylhydrazine and the salts of hydrazines may be similarly related to pH. The salts would be at least as water-soluble, if not more so, than the free bases, and many are acidic, suggesting that they would be more readily removed by tear formation or induced flushing.

Hydrazine as the vapor or liquid is a severe skin and mucous membrane irritant, a convulsant, a hepatotoxin, and a carcinogen in animals. In animals, hydrazine is absorbed through the skin as well as by inhalation and orally; systemic effects include weight loss, weakness, vomiting, excited behavior, and convulsions; the chief histologic findings are fatty degeneration of the liver and nephritis. In dogs, hemolysis occurs after intravenous injection but not from inhalation of the vapor. Inhalation by animals results in bronchitis, pulmonary edema, and damage to the liver and kidneys. In humans, the vapor is immediately irritating to the nose and throat and causes dizziness and nausea; itching, burning, and swelling of the eyes develop over a period of several hours. Severe exposure of the eyes to the vapor causes temporary blindness lasting for about 24 hours. The liquid in the eyes or on the skin causes severe burns. Recurrent exposure to hydrazine hydrate has been reported to cause contact dermatitis of the hands without systemic intoxication. Hydrazine or hydrazine salts are carcinogenic in mice after oral administration (pulmonary adenocarcinoma, hepatocarcinoma) or intraperitoneal injection (pulmonary carcinoma) and in rats after oral administration (pulmonary adenocarcinoma). There are no special tests.

Limiting Exposure

The worker must be protected to minimize the risks of systemic toxicity, eye damage and sensitization, which can result from contact with the hydrazines and their salts, and of cancer, which is predicted to be a possible result of contact with or inhalation of these hydrazines. For these reasons, occupational exposure to hydrazines is defined as work in any area where one or more of the hydrazines is stored, produced, processed, transported, handled, or otherwise used and present in such a manner that vapors or aerosols may be released into workroom air or that the hydrazines may spill or splash onto the skin or into the eyes. Because even small spills of hydrazines on the skin can result in severe systemic toxicity, all employees assigned to such a work area, even temporarily, for any purpose, including maintenance or repair, should be regarded as occupationally exposed. Workers in areas where hydrazines are used, in either open or closed systems, should be considered to be occupationally exposed, since there is no effective way to demonstrate that a closed system remains completely free from leaks. Conversely, workers assigned only to control rooms in which no air from other hydrazine-containing areas is present should not be considered occupationally exposed.

The TLV for hydrazine is 0.1 ppm, with "skin" and "suspected carcinogen" mutations (1985–1986 ACGIH).

REFERENCES

1. Back KC, Carter VL Jr, Thomas AA: Occupational hazards of missile operations with special regard to the hydrazine propellants, in *JANNAF Working Group on Safety and Environmental Protection—Minutes of April 10-77 Meeting—John F Kennedy Space Center, Florida*. Laurel, Md. Johns Hopkins University, Chemical Propulsion Information Agency, Applied Physics Laboratory, 1977, pp 25–47.
2. Clark DA, et al: Pharmacology and toxicology of propellant hydrazines, in *Aeromedical Reviews*, review 11-68. Springfield, Va, US Dept of Commerce, National Technical Information Service (NTIS AD 688 500), 1968.
3. Christensen HE, Fairchild, EJ, Carroll BS, et al: *Registry of Toxic Effects of Chemical Substances*, 1976 ed, Publ DHEW NIOSH 76-191. Rockville, Md, US Dept of Health, Education, and Welfare, PHS, Center for Disease Control, National Institute for Occupational Safety and Health, 1976, pp 594–598,
4. *Criteria for a Recommended Standard: Occupational Exposure to Hydrazines*. US Dept of Health, Education, and Welfare, PHS, Center for Disease Control, DHEW (NIOSH) Publ 78-172. Cincinnati, Oh, National Institute for Occupational Safety and Health, June, 1978.
5. *Evaluation of Atmospheric Concentrations of Hydrazine and Unsymmetrical Dimethylhydrazine in and around the Rocky Mountain Arsenal*, Hydrazine Facility, Industrial Hygiene Special Study No. 35-0101-77. Aberdeen Proving Ground, Aberdeen, Md, US Dept of the Army, US Army Environmental Hygiene Agency, 1977.
6. *Guides for Short-Term Exposures of the Public to Air Pollutants. V. Guide for Hydrazine, Monomethylhydrazine, and 1,1-Dimethylhydrazine*. Springfield, Va, US Dept of Commerce, National Technical Information Service (NTIS PB 224 337), 1974.
7. Haun CC, Kinkead ER: Chronic inhalation toxicity of hydrazine, in *Proceedings of the 4th Annual Conference on Environmental Toxicology*. Springfield, Va, US Dept. of Commerce, National Technical Information Service (NTIS AD 781 031), 1973, pp 351–363.
8. Haun CC, MacEwen JD, Vernot EH, et al: *The Acute Inhalation Toxicity of Monomethylhydrazine Vapor*, Report No. AMRL-TR-68-169. Wright-Patterson Air Force Base, Ohio, US Air Force, Air Force Systems Command, Aerospace Medical Division, Aerospace Medical Research Laboratories, Toxic Hazards Division, Toxicology Branch, 1969.
9. Melvin WW, Johnson WS: *Survey of Information Relevant to Occupational Health Standards for Hydrazines*. Springfield, Va, US Dept of Commerce, National Technical Information Service (NTIS AD AO22 851), 1976.
10. Some aromatic amines, hydrazine and related substances *n*- nitroso compounds and miscellaneous alkylating agents. *IARC Monogr Eval Carcinog Risk Chem Man*. Lyon, France, International Agency for Research on Cancer, 1974; 4:127–172.
11. Thienes CH, et al: *Final Report on Acute and Chronic Toxicity of Hydrazine*. Dept of Pharmacology and Toxicology, University of Southern California School of Medicine, University Park, Los Angeles, 1948.
12. Toth B, Wilson RB: Blood vessel tumorigenesis by 1,2-dimethylhydrazine dihydrochloride (symmetrical). Gross, light and electron microscopic descriptions, I. *Am J Pathol* 1971; 64:585.
13. Toxic Hazards Research Unit Annual Technical Report—1975. Springfield, Va, US Dept of Commerce, National Technical Information Service (NTIS AD AO19 546 LLC), 1975, pp 101–111.
14. Wattenburg LW: Inhibition of dimethylhydrazine-induced neoplasia of the large intestine by disulfiram. *J Natl Cancer Inst* 1975; 54:1005.
15. Wilson RB: Species variation in response to dimethylhydrazine. *Toxicol Appl Pharmacol* 1976; 38:647.

HYDROGEN CYANIDE AND CYANIDE SALTS

Synonyms for hydrogen cyanide (HCN) are hydrocyanic acid, prussic acid, and formonitrile. For the purpose of this document, cyanide salts are defined as sodium cyanide (NaCN), potassium cyanide (KCN) and calcium cyanide ($Ca[CN]_2$). The word cyanide or the symbol CN is used to designate salts as well as hydrogen cyanide.

Hydrogen cyanide is used primarily in the production of chemical intermediates and in fumigation. It can be produced in electroplating, metallurgy, photographic development, and various other occupations. The estimated United States consumption of HCN for 1973 was approximately 310,000 short tons. The number of workers with potential exposure to HCN has been estimated by the NIOSH to be approximately 1,000. Sodium cyanide and potassium cyanide are used primarily in the extraction of ores, electroplating, metal treatment, and various manufacturing processes. The number of workers with potential exposure to NaCN has been estimated by the NIOSH to be 20,000. The number of workers potentially exposed to KCN and $Ca(CN)_2$ has not been estimated.

Hydrogen cyanide and its sodium, potassium, and calcium salts manifest their toxicity by way of a common mechanism, namely, inhibition of the respiratory enzyme cytochrome oxidase. This inhibition causes cellular anoxia and, if a large enough dose is received, results in death. Skin contact with a solution of cyanide salts can cause itching, discoloration, or corrosion, which most likely is due to the alkalinity of the solution. Cyanide salt aerosols can cause upper respiratory irritation. Enlargement of the thyroid glands and changes in the chemical and cellular composition of the blood of employees exposed to cyanide have also been reported. An increased occurrence of the subjective symptoms of headache, weakness, changes in taste and smell, irritation of the throat, vomiting, effort dyspnea, lacrimation, abdominal colic, precordial pain, and nervous instability has been noted among workers having long-term occupational exposure to low concentrations of HCN. The NIOSH recommends that workers occupationally exposed to cyanide have comprehensive preplacement and annual medical examinations. Engineering controls should be used wherever feasible to maintain cyanide concentrations at or below the prescribed limits and respirators should be used only in certain nonroutine or emergency situations.

Medical Surveillance and Treatment

Medical surveillance shall be made available as specified below for all workers occupationally exposed to HCN or cyanide salts.

1. Preplacement and annual medical examinations shall include:

   A. An initial or interim work and medical history with special attention to skin disorders and those nonspecific symptoms, such as headache, nausea, vomiting, dizziness, or weakness, that may be associated with chronic exposure

   B. A physical examination giving particular attention to skin, thyroid, and the cardiovascular and upper respiratory systems

   C. An evaluation of the advisability of the worker's use of negative- or positive-pressure respirators

2. Initial medical examinations shall be made available to currently employed workers within six months of the promulgation of a standard.
3. The responsible physician and the employer shall be aware of substances used in the workplace and shall ensure that employees trained in first-aid measures are on duty whenever there is potential occupational exposure to HCN or a cyanide salt.
4. Two physicians' treatment kits shall be immediately available to trained medical personnel at each plant where there is a potential for the release of or for contact with hydrogen cyanide or cyanide salts, accidental or otherwise. One kit should be portable in order that it may be carried by medical personnel while accompanying a patient to the hospital. The other kit should be kept under lock and key to ensure that it is intact and available when and if needed. The key should be readily available at all times to the work supervisor on duty, and the storage place should be of such construction as to allow accessibility in the event of loss of the key.
5. First-aid kits shall be immediately available if there is a potential for exposure to cyanide salts. This kit shall contain as a minimum two boxes of ampules (2 dozen), each containing 0.3 ml of amyl nitrite. Ampules shall be replaced biannually or sooner if needed to ensure their potency. The amyl nitrite ampules should be protected from high temperatures. In all cases, the contents of the medical and first-aid kits shall be replaced before the manufacturer's assigned expiration dates.

In case of contact, immediately flush skin or eyes with plenty of water for at least 15 minutes; get medical attention. Remove contaminated clothing and wash before reuse.

Carry patient to fresh air.

Have patient lie down.

Remove contaminated clothing but keep patient warm.

Start artificial respiration if breathing stops.

Administer antidote (amyl nitrite ampule).

Transport patient to the nearest medical treatment facility. Hyperbaric oxygen therapy has proved helpful (see Chapter 25).

If cyanide gas is inhaled: Break an amyl nitrite ampule in a cloth and hold lightly under nose for 15 seconds. Repeat at about 15-second intervals.

If cyanide is swallowed: Break an amyl nitrite ampule in a cloth and hold lightly under nose for 15 seconds. Repeat inhalation of amyl nitrite five times at about 15-second intervals. If patient is conscious or when consciousness returns, give emetic (1 tablespoonful of salt to each glass of warm water) and repeat until vomit fluid is clear. Do not give an emetic to an unconscious or barely conscious person.

More recently, physicians have used 100% oxygen together with hydroxocobalamin given intravenously. Hydroxocobalamin combines with cyanide to form cyanocobalamin (vitamin B_{12}). Graham et al.[1] have reported their results with this newer form of treatment in acute cases.

The following warning sign shall be affixed in a readily visible location at or near entrances to areas containing HCN and where there is reasonable potential for emergencies:

DANGER
CYANIDE HAZARD AREA
UNAUTHORIZED PERSONS
KEEP OUT
DO NOT WORK ALONE
IN THIS AREA

IN EMERGENCY: (Here include, as applicable:

1. Location of gas masks and other emergency equipment
2. Instructions for sounding emergency alarm
3. Location of first-aid equipment and supplies
4. Instructions for summoning medical aid)

The sign shall be printed both in English and in the predominant language of non-English-reading workers. All workers shall receive training and information on the hazards and safe work practices in handling HCN and cyanide salts and on first-aid procedures in poisoning by these compounds.

The NIOSH recommends the promulgation of new federal standards so that employee exposure to hydrogen cyanide and the cyanide salts does not exceed 5 mg/cu m of air (expressed as CN), determined as a ceiling concentration based on a ten-minute sampling period. Because of the ready hydrolysis of calcium cyanide in humid air, it is required that whenever the air is analyzed for cyanide salts, a concurrent analysis be made for HCN. Neither respective ceiling value may be exceeded nor may the combined values exceed 5 mg/cu m measured as CN during a ten-minute sampling period.

REFERENCES

1. Graham DL, Laman D, Theodore J et al: Acute cyanide poisoning complicated by lactic acidosis and pulmonary edema. *Arch Intern Med* 1977; 137:1051.
2. National Institute for Occupational Safety and Health: *A Recommended Standard for Occupational Exposure: Hydrogen Cyanide and Cyanide Salts*. US Dept of Health, Education, and Welfare, PHS, Center for Disease Control, NIOSH, 1975.

HYDROGEN FLUORIDE (HF)

Anhydrous hydrogen fluoride is a colorless liquid or gas that fumes in moist air and has a pungent, irritating odor. Its aqueous solutions also are colorless and fume above a concentration of 40%–48%. It is manufactured by allowing sulfuric acid to react with acid-grade fluorspar (97% calcium fluoride) in heated rotary or stationary kilns. Hydrogen fluoride is evolved as a gas, purified, and then condensed as liquid anhydrous hydrogen fluoride. Between 1876 and 1931, considerable quantities of aqueous hydrofluoric acid were produced and used for cleaning sand from castings and for etching glass. In 1931, anhydrous hydrogen fluoride was first produced commercially and use of anhydrous hydrogen fluoride as a catalyst in alkylation processes for making high-octane fuel blends began in 1942. Prior to 1954, the steel industry was the largest consumer of fluorspar, from which hydrogen fluoride is generated. Since then, the quantity of fluorspar used for the manufacture of hydrogen fluoride has surpassed that used in the steel industry. In 1958 and 1971, approximately 52% of all fluorspar consumed in the United States was used for making hydrogen fluoride. In 1974, production reached 375,000 tons.

Currently, the major uses of hydrogen fluoride are in the production of cryolite for the aluminum industry, in the manufacture of fluorocarbon compounds, as a catalyst in alkylation processes, in steel pickling, uranium processing, enamel stripping, glass and quartz etching and polishing, and in various electroplating operations. Hydrogen fluoride often is produced by other industrial processes using fluorides, e.g., welding and aluminum production. Some occupations with potential exposure to hydrogen fluoride include aircraft workers, alkylation plant workers, alloy steel cleaners, alloy steel makers, aluminum fluoride makers, aluminum workers, ammonium fluoride makers, bleachers, brass cleaners, brewers, brick cleaners, casting cleaners, ceramic workers, chemists, copper cleaners, cryolite makers, crystal glass polishers, dye makers, electric arc welders, electroplaters, enamel etchers, fermentation workers, fertilizer makers, filter paper makers, fluoborate makers, fluoride makers, fluorine makers, fluorocarbon makers, fluorochemical makers, fluosilicate makers, freon makers, genetron makers, glass etchers, graphite purifiers, hydrogen fluoride workers, incandescent lamp frosters, isotron makers, laundry workers, metal cleaners, metal polishers, neon sign makers, oil well acidizers, ore dissolvers, petroleum refinery workers, phosphate rock workers, phosphoric acid makers, plastic makers, polish workers, quartz crystal makers, rocket fuel handlers, rocket fuel makers, stainless steel cleaners, stainless steel makers, steel casting picklers, stone cleaners, uranium refiners, and yeast makers.

Toxic Effects

Occupational exposure main routes of entry are by inhalation and skin contact. Hydrogen fluoride as a gas is a severe respiratory irritant, and in solution causes severe and painful burns of the skin. Animals repeatedly exposed to 17 ppm showed damage to the lungs, liver and kidneys, but at 8.6 ppm there was only occasional lung injury.[1] Fatalities occurred in three of six workers exposed to spills of 70% solutions on the skin and inhalation of the vapor; despite prompt showering with water for skin burns, death from pulmonary edema occurs two hours after exposure.[6] A chemist exposed to hydrogen fluoride splashed on the face and upper extremities developed pulmonary edema three hours after exposure and died 10 hours later.[4] In human subjects, 120 ppm was the highest concentration that could be tolerated for one minute due to onset of conjunctival and respiratory irritation with stinging of the skin. Repeated experimental human exposures to concentrations of 2 ppm for six hours daily caused a slight stinging of the eyes and skin of the face, with nasal irritation.[5] Repeated exposures to low concentrations at work may produce chronic irritation of the nose, throat, and bronchi. Hydrogen fluoride solutions in contact with skin, if untreated, result in marked tissue destruction; the fluoride ion readily penetrates skin and deep tissue, causing necrosis of soft tissues and decalcification of bone.[2] When skin contact is with solutions of less than 20% hydrogen fluoride, the burns do not become manifest for several hours; burns from solutions greater than 20% generally are felt in a matter of minutes, and severe eye injuries from splashes may occur. In one case of eye burns from a fine spray of hydrofluoric acid in the face, considerable loss of corneal epithelium occurred despite immediate and copious flushing with water and irrigation for three hours with a 0.5% solution of benzethonium chloride; within 19 days there was recovery of normal vision.[3]

The determination of fluoride concentration in the urine may be utilized to gauge the degree of absorption of hydrogen fluoride following suspected overexposure.

Treatment

Persons who have had contact with hydrofluoric acid should be subjected immediately to a drenching shower of water. Contaminated clothing should be removed as rapidly as possible, even while the person is under the shower. The high risk of either immediate or delayed onset of pulmonary edema following inhalation of the gas requires that oxygen be administered under pressure immediately after a severe exposure and continued as long as necessary; close observation should be continued for 24–48 hours. It is essential that the exposed area be washed with copious quantities of water for a sufficient period of time to remove all hydrofluoric acid from the skin or eyes. Skin burns have been treated with immediate application of iced hyamine chloride or Zephiran solution and continued application for one to four hours; severe, deep or especially painful burns have been treated by local infiltration with 10% calcium gluconate following block anesthesia of the affected part.[2, 8] The 1986 TLV is 3 ppm.

REFERENCES

1. ACGIH: Hydrogen Fluoride as HF, in *Documentation of TLVs for Substances in Workroom Air*, ed 5. Cincinnati, Oh, American Conference of Governmental Hygienists, 1986.
2. Dibbell DG, et al: Hydrofluoric acid burns of the hand. *J Bone Joint Surg (Am)* 1970; 52:931.
3. Grant WM: *Toxicology of the Eye*, ed 2. Springfield, Ill, Charles C Thomas, Publisher, 1974, pp 557–559.
4. Kleinfeld M: Acute pulmonary edema of chemical origin. *Arch Environ Health* 1965; 10:942.

5. Largent EJ: The metabolism of fluorides in man. *AMA Arch Ind Hyg* 1960; 21:318.
6. Mayer L, Guelich J: Hydrogen fluoride (HF) inhalation and burns. *Arch Environ Health* 1963; 7:445.
7. NIOSH: *Criteria for a Recommended Standard: Occupational Exposure to Hydrogen Fluoride*. US Dept of Health, Education, and Welfare, PHS, Center for Disease Control, HEW (NIOSH) Publ 76-143, March, 1976.
8. Reinhardt CF, et al: Hydrofluoric acid burn treatment. *Am Ind Hyg Assoc J* 1966; 27:166.

HYDROGEN SULFIDE

H_2S

Hydrogen sulfide is a ubiquitous, acute-acting toxic substance and a leading cause of sudden death in the workplace. Brief exposures to hydrogen sulfide at high concentrations have caused conjunctivitis and keratitis, and exposures at very high concentrations have caused unconsciousness, respiratory paralysis, and death. Eye irritation, cough, sore throat, vague gastrointestinal symptoms, and photophobia may occur with low-level exposures; with overwhelming exposures, collapse and respiratory arrest can develop within minutes.

Hydrogen sulfide is used as a common reagent in chemical laboratories in the preparation of sulfide and organic sulfur compounds such as sulfuric acid and 1-dodecanethiol. The potential for release of high concentrations of hydrogen sulfide in work areas where the gas occurs as a by-product (e.g., petroleum wellheads, petroleum refineries, tanneries, and sulfur products processing) has been a major cause of concern for worker safety. Hydrogen sulfide occurs naturally in most petroleum and natural gas deposits and as a bacterial decomposition product of protein. The NIOSH estimates that 125,000 workers in the United States are exposed or potentially exposed to hydrogen sulfide.

To provide a sufficient margin of safety in protecting against the immediate acute effects (and possible chronic effects) of hydrogen sulfide, a ceiling concentration of 15 mg/cu m is recommended as an occupational exposure limit. Due to the rapid, often lethal effects of exposure to a high concentration of hydrogen sulfide, a work practice requirement for continual monitoring is recommended in situations in which there is potential exposure to a concentration of 70 mg/cu m hydrogen sulfide or greater.

Hydrogen sulfide is especially dangerous when it occurs in low-lying areas or confined work spaces or when it exists in high concentrations under pressure. As a result, work practices, such as continual monitoring and the use of specified respiratory protective equipment in certain work situations, are of great importance.

Liquid manure systems in the United States are increasing as farms modernize and become more concerned with the efficient recycling of energy-rich waste. Numerous deaths in swine, beef, and dairy animals have been associated with these systems. Furthermore, several farm workers have died after entering recently emptied liquid manure tanks or have drowned after falling into full tanks.[6]

Case Report.—A 16-year-old farm worker collapsed and died on Dec. 8, 1977, while steam cleaning gutters inside a calf barn in Eau Claire, Wisconsin. The apparent cause of his death was the inhalation of toxic gases, with hydrogen sulfide (H_2S) the probable active agent. The source of the gases was decomposing liquid manure that had been agitating for 30–60 minutes in a 50,000-L tank beneath the barn. The boy had been working inside the barn approximately 30 ft from the tank for about ten minutes when he was overcome by gases. While trying to rescue him, two other workers experienced syncopal episodes but recovered. No animals died during the incident; however, no calves were in the affected area of the barn at the time of exposure.

The farm worker had been in good health. He had no chronic illnesses, took no medication, and had no history of drug abuse. Autopsy findings were consistent with inhalation of a toxic gas resulting in emesis and aspiration. Hydrogen sulfide was implicated as the causative agent by air tests done under similar conditions two days after the incident. The tests showed that hydrogen sulfide concentrations at the site of death after eight minutes of manure agitation were 70 ppm. (By comparison, the NIOSH recommends a maximal exposure concentration of no more than 10 ppm over a ten-minute period; when concentrations reach 50 ppm, evacuation is recommended.) Other gases, such as nitric oxide, nitrogen dioxide, and sulfur dioxide, which have been associated with deaths in silos, were not detected. Carbon monoxide was ruled out at autopsy by blood tests, methane was thought not to have been present, since two open-flame heaters were in use, and ammonia was considered unlikely to have existed in high concentrations because its odor and irritation properties act as excellent warning signals.

Several factors appear to have contributed to the hazardous conditions present at the time of the incident. For example, the manure tank was full and the contents had been agitating longer than usual before pumping began. The barn was inadequately ventilated that day (outside temperature was −16° C). Only one of its five fans was in use, and then only intermittently, and a westerly wind blew through the only open door. In addition, the calves' high-protein diet made the formation of hydrogen sulfide more likely.

A number of toxic gases are released from decomposing manure, but hydrogen sulfide, carbon dioxide, methane, and ammonia are of principal concern. Several preventive measures may be taken to reduce farm workers' risk of toxic gas exposure from liquid manure systems. These steps include improving ventilation and developing contingency plans for evacuating animals and workers from enclosed farm buildings while the manure is agitating. In addition, agricultural authorities have recommended that workers who must enter a closed space containing a manure tank should wear self-contained air packs and safety harnesses, and that reserve workers should be stationed outside.[6]

Slowly decaying fish may deplete a ship's hold of oxygen and lead to the production of toxic quantities of hydrogen sulfide (H_2S), ammonia (NH_3), and carbon dioxide (CO_2). From 1966 to 1971, reports of three deaths and four cases of unconsciousness from asphyxia among Danish commercial fishermen led to a survey of the air content in the holds of 13 large industrial fishing cutters.[1] In seven of these ships, the oxygen concentration was found to be dangerously low (7 vol. %, range 3–20). There were concentrations of carbon dioxide greater than 20 vol. % (range 0–40) and ammonia (200 ppm) in nine vessels. These high concentrations are sufficient to cause immediate toxicity or asphyxia in man, and the median levels are above the threshold limit values recommended for occupational exposure in industrial workplaces. Whereas most large fishing craft have equipment to ventilate the holds of ships before crewmen enter, small vessels do not. The toxicity of air in the holds of small vessels has not previously been viewed as a potential hazard.

Sodium bisulfate and sodium metabisulfite have been used in a 1¼% solution since 1956 as a dip for the preservation of fresh shrimp. The white powder emits a pungent odor of sulfur dioxide, particularly when it is not kept cool, and this odor may be enhanced when mixed with warm salt water. The finding of measurable levels of sulfhemoglobin in the blood of the crewmen in the absence of methemoglobin suggests that their sulfur exposure may have been due in part to the inhalation of a high concentration of sulfur dioxide gas.

During July, 1978, two crewmen of a shrimp fishing vessel died and the captain was hospitalized following toxic exposure to the atmosphere of the ship's hold. The hold was refrigerated with ice and contained approximately 4,000 lb of shrimp caught in the preceding 11 days at sea. Both crewmen previously had been involved in dipping the shrimp into a sodium bisulfite solution used routinely to control "black-spot," a discoloration associated with decay. When the first crewman descended into the hold to pack the freshly caught shrimp on ice, he collapsed immediately into coma. The captain went into the hold to resuscitate the first crewman and also fell unconscious. The second crewman followed the first two men into the hold and also collapsed. The captain regained consciousness long enough to climb out of the hold and notify the Coast Guard; shortly thereafter he was evacuated by helicopter and brought to the hospital.

At autopsy of the crewmen who died, no specific gross pathologic changes were noted. The bodies and blood samples smelled distinctly of sulfur. Sulfhemoglobin determinations performed on frozen blood specimens showed levels of 6% and 12% (normal level is zero); neither carboxyhemoglobin nor methemoglobin was present. Inquiries by the Coast Guard and the Louisiana Department of Health and Human Resources have identified four similar episodes since 1970 that resulted in nine deaths and two hospitalizations. Two of these episodes involved shrimpers exposed to the sodium bisulfite dip. Four other deaths in ships' holds occurred in two separate incidents involving government inspectors.

Treatment

Immediately remove person from exposure and ensure that the airway is clear. Give 100% oxygen by tight-fitting oronasal mask or endotracheal tube. Hyperbaric oxygen at 3 atm has been successful (see the section on Carbon Monoxide for details).

Because of the acute toxicity of hydrogen sulfide, any person who might be exposed to sudden high concentrations of the gas or is controlling the handling of the gas should not be subject to episodes of fainting, epileptic seizures, or other conditions that might alter his state of consciousness and endanger himself or others. A person with chronic conjunctivitis, asthma, or other chronic respiratory diseases may be more sensitive to the effects of hydrogen sulfide exposure, and the physician should consider those potential effects in determining whether individuals with such histories should be subject to exposure, even at low levels.

REFERENCES

1. Dalgaard JB, et al: Fatal poisoning and other health hazards connected with industrial fishing. *Br J Ind Med* 1972; 29:307.
2. Donham KJ, Rubino M, Thedell TD, et al: Potential health hazards to agricultural workers in swine confinement buildings. *J Occup Med* 1977; 10:383.
3. Fletcher WJ: Safety hazards associated with livestock waste. Presented at the winter meeting of the American Society of Agricultural Engineers, Chicago, December, 1971.
4. *Hydrogen Sulfide: Environmental Health Criteria 19*. Geneva, World Health Organization, 1981.
5. Idyll PP: How to use sodium bisulfite to control "black-spot" on shrimp. Florida State Board of Conservation and the Marine Laboratory, University of Miami, Coral Gables, Florida, Special Services Bulletin No 12, August, 1956.

5a. Lundholm M, Rylander R: Work related symptoms among sewage workers. *Br J Ind Med* 1983; 40:325.

6. Midwest Plan Service: *Livestock Waste Facilities Handbook*. Ames, Iowa, Iowa State University, 1975.
7. *Morbidity and Mortality Weekly Report:* Deaths from asphyxia in fishermen. Center for Disease Control, Vol 27, No 34, pp 309–315, Aug 25, 1978.
8. Muehling AJ: Swine housing and waste management: A research review. Urbana, Ill, Cooperative Extension Service, University of Illinois, 1969, pp 65–78.
9. National Institute for Occupational Safety and Health: *Criteria for a Recommended Standard: Occupational Exposure to Hydrogen Sulfide*, DHEW (NIOSH) Publ 77-158. Cincinnati, Oh, NIOSH, 1977, pp 1–149.

METALWORKING FLUIDS

There is enormous use of "cutting oils" or "cutting fluids" in nearly all industries that cut, grind, or machine metals. Most commonly, these fluids are proprietary preparations and are formulated to cool cutting tools and parts and to flush away metal chips and particles to enhance machinability and speed production. The quantities used are beyond measurement and beyond billions of liters per year; most, to some degree, are reused in a machine (Fig 47–13).

Cutting oils are divided into two types—inactive and active. The active oils act as a lubricant under lower temperatures (400°–500° F) and the inactive are oils that perform best at higher temperatures (700°–900° F).

Inactive types are:

Straight mineral oils
Fatty oils
Fatty oil-mineral oil blends
Sulfurized fatty-mineral blends
Sulfurized-chlorinated fatty-mineral blends

The sulfurized or "leaded screw" stocks can also be machined with these oils. Such steels have the lubricant "built into" them, so they can machine easily without significant breakdown with use.

Most straight mineral oils contain some combined sulfur but this sulfur is so tightly bound that it does not act as a lubricant in use.

The fatty oils, although widely used at one time, are limited

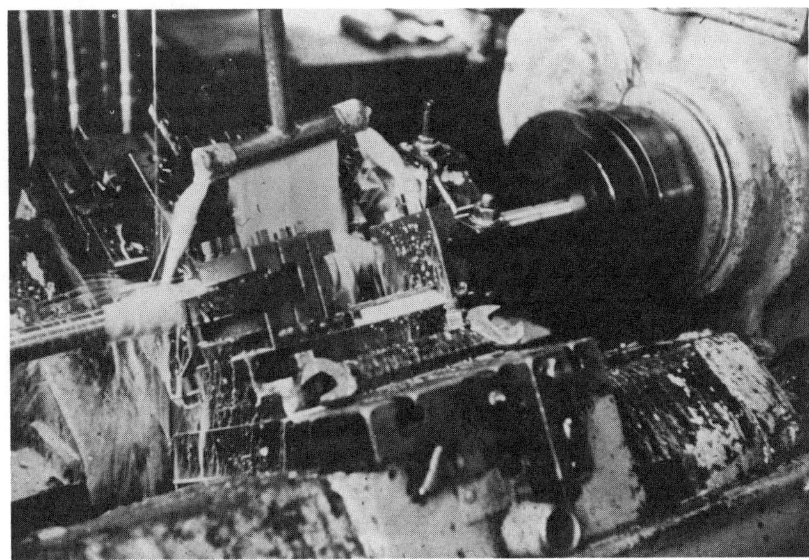

FIG 47–13.
Lathe operating with coolant pumped to area being machined.

in use today as cutting fluids, primarily because of their high price. Blends of fats and mineral oil perform almost as well as the straight, fatty oils.

Fatty oil-mineral oil blends are compounded with 10%–30% of fatty oil with varying viscosities of mineral oils. Fats and mineral oils reduce the interfacial tension of oil to metal—similar to soaps and wetting agents in water. Fats also act as mild lubricants because of their ability to form metal soaps at the tool-chip interface.

Sulfur can be combined chemically with fatty oils (usually lard oil or sperm oil) under carefully controlled conditions of temperature, pressure, and time interval. The resulting product then is "cut" with a variety of viscous mineral oils to make finished products of controlled concentrations of the fat and sulfur. Such oils will not react chemically at lower temperatures but will be active above 700° F and best under the pressure conditions at the chip-tool interface.

The sulfurized chlorinated fatty oil-mineral oil blend is interchangeable with the sulfurized fatty mineral oil in most cases but has a better antiweld property at lower pressures and temperatures.

Active types are:

Sulfurized mineral oil
Sulfochlorinated mineral oil
Sulfo or sulfochlorinated fatty oil blends

With the sulfurized mineral oil, sulfur can be dissolved hot in a mineral oil up to 1%; above this amount, it will settle out and crystallize in the cooling to room temperature. The sulfur content usually is 0.5%–0.8% and this type of oil probably is the most widely used. Because they are of high chemical activity, they are effective when steels of high ductility, low-carbon, plain steels, and materials of low machinability ratings are machined because of the lower temperature conditions existing when machining them.

Sulfochlorinated mineral oils usually contain up to 3% sulfur and 1% chlorine. The combination of sulfur and chlorine makes the product effective over a wider temperature range—the chlorine for low temperature and the sulfur for high temperature conditions. These oils are more effective than the sulfurized mineral oils for machining the tough, low-carbon steels and chrome-nickel alloy.

The sulfo or sulfochlorinated fatty oil blends, because of the fats present, combine more sulfur than the sulfomineral oil blends. They also contain more sulfur and are more active at lower temperatures than the inactive type of sulfo or sulfochlorinated fatty oil products of the inactive type. They have high oiliness properties and high extreme pressure properties. They are especially effective for slow-speed cutting of extremely tough alloys.

Commercial cutting fluids can be divided into four categories:

1. Cutting oils or straight oils, containing mineral oil, fat and additives. These oils are water insoluble.

2. Soluble cutting oils, containing mineral fat, emulsifiers (may include amines), additives (rarely nitrite*), and water.

3. Semisynthetic cutting oils containing mineral oil, water, fat, a soluble base (usually including amines), emulsifiers (may include amines), and additives (usually including nitrite).

4. Synthetic cutting fluids, containing a soluble base (usually including amines), additives (usually including nitrite), and water.

Various proprietary cutting fluids are produced by more than 1,000 companies in the United States. The NIOSH estimates that 780,000 persons are occupationally exposed in the manufacture and use of cutting fluids. Synthetic cutting fluids, semisynthetic cutting oils, and soluble cutting oils may contain nitrosamines and are found either as contaminants in amines or as products from the reaction of amines (e.g., triethanolamine) with nitrite. Straight oils do not contain nitrites or amines but may contain polynuclear aromatic compounds.

*Some consumers may incorporate additives containing nitrite into the soluble cutting oil while preparing it for use.

Although *N*-nitrosamines are thought to be an important group of human carcinogens, their role as an increased occupational risk factor has not been established. The formation of diethanolnitrosamine in cutting fluids was first postulated and reported from Sweden by Zingmark and Rappe,[4] who measured diethanolnitrosamine in a specifically formulated "grinding fluid" containing nitrite and triethanolamine.

$$\begin{matrix} R \\ & \diagdown \\ & & N{-}N{=}O \\ & \diagup \\ R \end{matrix}$$

They surmised that the potential hazard of working with these types of products should not be underestimated. Four hundred to more than 1,000 ppm diethanolnitrosamine in eight commercial cutting fluids produced by different manufacturers has been found.[1] Studies conducted during an actual machining operation showing the presence of 1,000 ppm diethanolnitrosamine in the diluted cutting fluid prior to use and 384 ppm after use strongly suggest that machine operators may be continually exposed to nitrosamines.

In 1977, Zingmark and Rappe[4] presented further evidence of formation of *N*-nitrosamines from secondary and tertiary amines with nitrite in acidic solution, noting that the acid catalyzes the reaction by forming nitrous acid, which then participates in the *N*-nitrosation. The reaction proceeds very slowly under alkaline conditions because of the low concentration of nitrous acid. Nevertheless, analyses of grinding fluid concentrates containing triethanolamine, nitrite, and water show that small amounts of *N*-nitrosodiethanolamine are formed during storage even though the pH values of the fluids are between 10.2 and 11.4. The fluids Zingmark and Rappe tested had been stored for five to seven months and showed an *N*-nitrosamine concentration ranging from 400 to 800 ppm. These analyses clearly show that the mixing of nitrite and an amine in a technical product always should be regarded with some suspicion as to *N*-nitrosamine formation, especially if the product is stored. *N*-nitrosodiethanolamine has been shown to induce cancer in rats, although high doses are required.[2, 3]

Contaminants in "Cutting Fluids"

Many materials may soil a lubricant during its use. Factory dust, waste, cigarettes, rubbish, dead insects, small rodents, and urine, as well as sputum, collect in dirty sumps.

Solvents such as paraffin and trichloroethylene might find their way into liquid oils in emulsion coolants. Chromate sensitization occurs from prefabricated cement mold oils or cutting oils soiled by priming paints, and nickel sensitization occurs from contaminated lubricants.

Microbial-Bacterial Contamination

Resident saprophytic bacteria, anaerobic staphylococci, and diphtheroids are found mostly on the exposed skin of the hands, face, and neck. They can be displaced by transient pathogens colonizing injured and eczematous skin or skin wetted by aqueous lubricants. Normally, dryness and the static bacterial action of fatty acids and low pH inhibit most nonsporing bacteria. Such oils, in sealed containers, should be clear, but contamination develops rapidly in their use, and soluble cutting oils allow some growth, but emulsified and aqueous coolants become rapidly contaminated by pathogenic colonies of *Staphylococcus aureus* and such gram-negative organisms as *Pseudomonas pyocyanea, Escherichia coli,* and *Proteus*. Hemolytic streptococci also are potential contaminants, and, rarely, cultured *Clostridium welchii* from a dirty lathe sump.

Sources of pyogenic staphylococci are nasal carriers, sneezing and spitting, infected clothing or towels, and air carriage by aerosols of streptococci from throat carriers. Infection may be conveyed from those with otitis externa and coliforms from those with poor personal habits.

Viruses and Fungi

Warts also have been conveyed by contaminated oil. Most fungal infections of the skin are personal infections from infected sites—Candida from the mouth, tinea dermatophytes from the feet. Emulsion oil-wetted skin encourages Candida infections and growth.

Prevention of Dermatitis From Cutting Oils

The most important element is cleanliness of shop personnel. Close personal attention to hygiene and cleanliness is the best means of avoiding and preventing dermatitis. Frequent and thorough cleansing of the hands and arms with soap and warm water removes accumulations of oil and dirt, and plugging of skin pores can be avoided. Quick changing from street to shop clothes and wearing oil-impervious aprons are of some help. It is important to wash with warm water and a mild soap before beginning work in the morning and after lunch as well as at the end of the work shift. If the skin has become oil-soaked, it should be mandatory that showers are taken at the close of work. Workers should put on clean clothing at least once or twice a week and more often when clothing begins to become oil-saturated. Splash guards are helpful attachments to cutting machines in protecting against flying chips and oil sprays, and these should be cleaned frequently. If the above measures do not suffice, workers with sensitive skin, after washing, may apply a suitable oil-resistant protective cream before starting work in the morning and again after lunch. Spitting into drains and oil pans is absolutely prohibited and, if necessary, cuspidors should be supplied to the machine operators, with provision for cleaning these daily. The use of kerosene and other solvents to remove oil and grease from the hands of workers should not be permitted, as this causes further defatting of the skin. New, coarse, clean, dry wipe rags should be handed out daily to the workers, and the rags should be laundered or discarded after use to remove oils as well as metal particles and slivers (Fig 47–14).

When a worker with suspicion of cutting oil dermatitis is first seen, he may be allowed to work in the same area if the dermatitis is not severe and if a protective cream is used. However, if this problem persists and is aggravated, he may be moved to another clean, dry working area; then, when the dermatitis clears, he again may be exposed to his prior work conditions. If there is a flare or exacerbation of the dermatitis, even if all the above details are

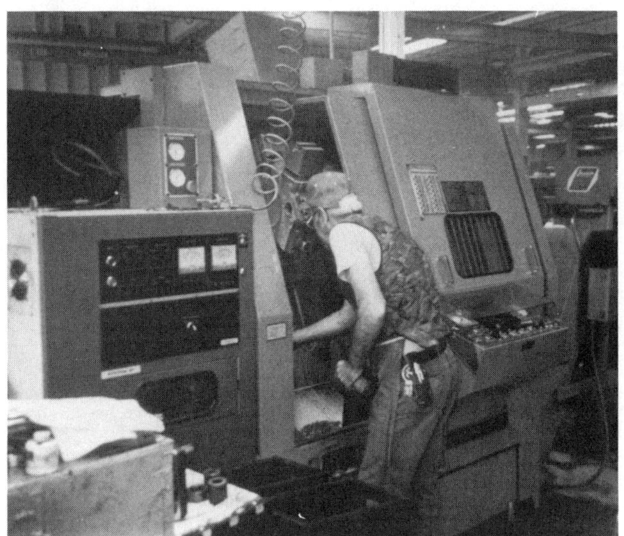

FIG 47–14.
A semi-automatic lathe with complete enclosure to protect the worker from cutting and cooling fluids.

strictly observed, the worker may have to be transferred to other work.

Practical industrial hygiene practices that can minimize dermal and respiratory exposures to cutting fluids are as follows:

Engineering controls.—The most effective control of any contaminant is control at the source of generation. Effective engineering measures include the use of local exhaust ventilation, with a suitable collector.

Substitution.—The substitution of a cutting fluid that does not contain either nitrosamine amines or the necessary ingredients (amines and nitrites) for nitrosamine formation is another possible control measure. Since many of the proprietary ingredients of cutting fluids have not undergone complete toxicologic evaluation, caution should be used when contemplating any change from one cutting fluid formulation to another, giving full consideration to the potential hazards of the substitute.

Respirators.—Personal respiratory protective devices should be used only as an interim measure while engineering controls are being installed, for nonroutine use and during emergencies. Considering the carcinogenic potential and the lack of a standard for nitrosamines as a group, the only available personal respiratory protective measure is the use of a positive-pressure-supplied air respirator or a positive-pressure self-contained breathing apparatus (see section on Respiratory Protection, Chapter 20.

Protective Clothing.—Impervious clothing should be provided and should be replaced and properly maintained. Nonimpervious clothing is not suggested, but, if used, it should be removed and laundered frequently to remove all traces of cutting fluids before being reworn. (Laundry personnel should be made aware of the potential hazard from handling contaminated clothing.)

Personal Cleanliness.—All exposed areas of the body and any area that becomes wet with cutting fluids should be washed with soap or mild detergent. Frequent showering is recommended, and these facilities should be made available in the workplace.

Isolation.—Where possible, any operations involved with cutting fluids should be placed in an isolated area to reduce exposure to employees not directly concerned with the operations.

Barrier Creams.—Barrier creams may provide limited protection against dermal irritation and skin absorption; however, the barrier cream should not contain secondary or tertiary amines (which may react to form nitrosamines in the presence of nitrites). Reliance must not be placed solely on such preparations for hygienic controls.

REFERENCES

1. Current Intelligence Bulletin: Nitrosamines in cutting fluids. Cincinnati, Oh, US Dept. of Health, Education, and Welfare, PHS, Center for Disease Control, National Institute for Occupational Safety and Health, October, 1976.
2. Fan TY, et al: *N*-nitrosodiethanolamine in synthetic cutting fluids: A part-per-hundred impurity. *Science* 1977; 196:70.

2a. Järvholm B: Mineral Oils—Studies on Health Effects in the Engineering Industry. Dissertation, University of Linköping and University of Göteborg, 1981.

3. Lijinsky W: Health problems associated with nitrites and nitrosamines. AMBIO, Royal Swedish Academy of Sciences/Universitetsforlaget (Sweden), 1976, vol 5, pp 67–72.

3a. Metalworking Fluids. *AARBETARSKYDDSFONDEN*, Tunnelgatan 31, S-111 81 Stockholm, 1983.

4. Zingmark P-A, Rappe C: On the formation of *N*-nitrosodiethanolamine from a grinding fluid under simulated gastric conditions. AMBIO, Royal Swedish Academy of Sciences/Universitetsförlaget (Sweden), vol 5, pp 237–238.

METHYL ISOCYANATE

CH_3NCO

This compound has been made in large quantities for use in organic synthesis (example follows) and as an additive to adhesives in polymer technology. "MIC" is a colorless liquid with a sharp odor causing immediate lacrimation; therefore, low-level chronic exposure information for man is unknown. It has a high vapor pressure, 348 mm Hg at 20° C (68° F) and is highly reactive. Elevated temperatures may cause methyl isocyanate to polymerize and burst container; contact with water causes formation of carbon dioxide and methylamine gases. The reaction is much more rapid in the presence of acids, alkalies, and amines. Contact with iron, tin, copper (or salts of these elements) and with certain other catalysts (such as triphenylarsenic oxide, triethylphosphine, and tributyltin oxide) may cause violent polymerization and produce hazardous decomposition products: toxic gases and vapors (such as hydrogen cyanide, oxides of nitrogen, and carbon monoxide) may be released in a fire involving methyl isocyanate. Odor threshold: *The Documentation of TLVs*[1] states that humans exposed to 0.4 ppm methyl isocyanate for periods up to 5 minutes could not detect the odor. Even at a concentration of 2 ppm, the odor was not perceived. Irritation levels: at a concentration of 0.4 ppm, eye, nose, and throat irritation was not experienced by human subjects who were exposed for periods up to 5 minutes. *The Documentation of TLVs*[1] states that "at 2 ppm no odor was detected, but the subjects experienced irritation and lacrimation. At 4 ppm the symptoms of irritation were more marked. Exposure was unbearable at 21 ppm." Since the odor and irritation thresholds of methyl isocyanate are not within 3 times the permissible exposure limit, methyl isocyanate is treated as a material with poor warning properties.

Summary of Toxicology

Methyl isocyanate vapor is an intense lacrimator and irritates eyes, mucous membranes, and skin. The liquid in contact with the eye may cause permanent damage. It can cause pulmonary irritation and sensitization. Exposure of man to high concentrations can cause cough, dyspnea, increased secretions, and chest pain. Isocyanates cause pulmonary sensitization in susceptible individuals. Should this occur, further exposure should be avoided, since extremely low levels of exposure may trigger an asthmatic episode; cross sensitization to unrelated materials probably does not occur. Experimental exposure of four human subjects for 1 to 5 minutes caused the following effects: 0.4 ppm, no effects; 2 ppm, lacrimation, irritation of the nose and throat; 4 ppm, symptoms of irritation more marked; 21 ppm, unbearable irritation of eyes, nose, and throat. A cotton plug saturated with the liquid was applied to the ear of a rabbit for 30 minutes and caused erythema, edema, necrosis, and perforation; a few drops of the liquid on the ear of a rabbit caused destruction of tissue. In rats exposed for 4 hours, the LC50 was 5 ppm; effects were injury to the lungs and subsequent pulmonary edema.

Because of the magnitude of community contamination, with over 2,000 known deaths of people of all ages, and many more thousands becoming acutely and chronically ill, the Bhopal methyl isocyanate accident in India is a striking example of the effects of massive methyl isocyanate exposure.

For about 18 years, Union Carbide Corporation's plant in Bhopal, India had been producing a widely used insecticide, carbarylb, utilizing common chemical materials and standard production procedures with methyl isocyanate (MIC) as a main ingredient.

The chemical equations for MIC production are:

(1) $COCl_2 + CH_3NH_2 \longrightarrow CH_3NHCOCl + HCl + Heat$
Phosgene — Monomethylamine (MMA) — Methylcarbamoyl Chloride (MCC) — Hydrogen Chloride

(2) $CH_3NHCOC \xrightarrow{Heat} CH_3NCO + HCl$
(MCC) — Methyl Isocyanate (MIC)

The raw materials used to make MIC are monomethylamine (MMA) and phosgene. Phosgene was produced on site by reacting chlorine and carbon monoxide, the latter being produced by an adjacent facility within the plant. The MMA and chlorine were brought by tank trucks from other plants in India, stored, and used as needed, with chloroform as the solvent throughout the process.

Early on Dec. 3, 1984, a safety valve opened as a result of a chemical reaction in the MIC storage tank, which contained approximately 41,000 kg (90,000 lb) of MIC. It was estimated that a safety valve remained open for about two hours, allowing the escape of about 24,500 kg (54,000 lb) of MIC in vapor and liquid form into the plant atmosphere. With prevailing wind velocity and direction at that time, the MIC swept from the plant confines directly into the adjacent (mainly residential) community. The few workers on night duty were not harmed.

The current U.S. standard for occupational exposure limits to MIC is 0.02 ppm averaged over an eight-hour shift (this assuming healthy adults are exposed). This level can also be expressed as 0.05 mg of MIC per cubic meter of air (mg/cu m).

Contact or inhalation of MIC causes irritation of eyes, nose, throat, and respiratory system. Liquid splashed in the eyes can cause permanent damage. MIC has a sharp odor and is extremely irritating, hence little information from low-level, chronic exposures is known.

For perspective, other highly irritating and potentially toxic substances along with currently established TLV Guides (1985–1986; See Appendix A) are listed in Table 47–6.

REFERENCES

1. American Conference of Governmental Industrial Hygienists: "Methyl Isocyanate, in *Documentation of the Threshold Limit Values for Substances in Workroom Air*, ed 5. Cincinnati, 1986.
2. Rye WA: Human responses to isocyanate exposure. *J Occup Med* 1973; 15:306–307.

TABLE 47–6.
Threshold Limit Values for Highly Irritating and Potentially Toxic Substances

SUBSTANCE	PPM	MG/CU M
Acrolein	0.1	0.25
Ammonia	25.0	18.0
Arsine	0.05	0.2
Bromine	0.1	0.7
Chlorine	1.0	3.0
Ethylene oxide	1.0	2.0
Fluorine	1.0	2.0
Formaldehyde	2.0	3.0
Hydrogen chloride	5.0	7.0
Hydrogen cyanide	10.0	10.0
Hydrogen fluoride	3.0	5.0
Hydrogen selenide	0.05	0.2
Hydrogen sulfide	10.0	14.0
MIC	**0.02**	**0.05**
Nickel Carbonyl	0.05	0.35
Nitric acid	2.0	5.0
Ozone	0.1	0.2
Phosgene	**0.1**	**0.4**
Sulfur dioxide	2.0	5.0
Sulfuric acid	—	1.0

MONOHALOMETHANES
(Methyl Chloride, Methyl Bromide, Methyl Iodide)

Production, Use, and Potential for Occupational Exposure

Commercially, methyl chloride, methyl bromide, and methyl iodide have been used as methylating agents, laboratory reagents, refrigerants, aerosol propellants, pesticides, fumigants, fire-extinguishing agents, anesthetics, degreasers, blowing agents for plastic foams, and chemical intermediates. Because of their high volatility, they are frequently contained in closed systems. Approximately 146,000 U.S. workers are potentially exposed, an estimate based on data collected by NIOSH.[13]

Methyl Chloride

Methyl chloride is produced primarily by the hydrochlorination of methanol, with primary use in the manufacture of silicones, a closed-system process. The manufacture of tetramethyl lead and triptane (2,2,3-trimethyl butane), both antiknock fuel additives, is the next largest use of methyl chloride. Other uses of methyl chloride include the production of butyl rubber; di-, tri-, and tetra-halogenated methanes; methyl cellulose; quaternary ammonium compounds; methyl mercaptan; methionine; and fungicides and pesticides (primarily methyl arsenate herbicides). The former high volume use of methyl chloride as a refrigerant and propellant has declined with the substitution of chlorofluorinated alkane derivatives. In 1981, approximately 362 million pounds of methyl chloride were produced in the United States, and domestic consumption is projected to expand by approximately 6.5% per year through the mid-1980s.

Methyl Bromide

Methyl bromide is produced by direct bromination of methane and by the hydrobromination of methanol. In the United States, methyl bromide is used primarily as a soil and spore fumigant. Methyl bromide is also used as a disinfectant, rodenticide, methylating agent, and wool degreaser and in ionization chambers (see Pesticides, Chapter 46). Most of the exposure data available on methyl bromide come as a result of the uses of methyl bromide as an agricultural fumigant. These include use as a nematocide, fungicide, herbicide, and insecticide. Methyl bromide is applied into the soil under plastic sheets or used in space fumigation under tarpaulins. It is also applied to a variety of agricultural commodities in specially designed fumigation chambers. Worker exposure may result from leaks in the plastic sheets or the tarpaulin or from failure to allow adequate time for the methyl bromide to dissipate following fumigation. In 1979, the latest year for which any production quantities are available, between 60 and 80 million pounds of methyl bromide were domestically produced for use as a pesticide; however, approximately 50% of this amount was exported to other nations. Approximately 105,000 U.S. workers are potentially exposed to methyl bromide. Methyl iodide is used primarily as a methylating agent with approximately 400 U.S. workers involved.[13]

Health Effects in Man

Most of the information related to the toxic effects on humans exposed to methyl chloride, methyl bromide, methyl iodide is derived from accidental exposures to relatively high concentrations. Symptoms of acute exposure to these compounds are similar, consisting of headache, nausea, vomiting, drowsiness, dizziness, giddiness, diarrhea, confusion, ataxia, slurred speech, paralysis, convulsions, delirium, coma, and death.[7, 8, 9, 10, 12] The lungs, liver, kidney, and brain appear to be the primary target organs in cases of severe poisoning. Liquid methyl bromide and methyl iodide have been reported to cause burning and blistering upon contact with the skin[4] and conjunctivitis when splashed into the eyes.

No human studies to evaluate the possible mutagenic, carcinogenic, or teratogenic effects from exposure to these compounds are currently available. Methyl chloride has been tested in mice and found to be a teratogen. Based on this evidence, NIOSH recommends that methyl chloride, methyl bromide, and methyl iodide be considered as potential occupational carcinogens and that methyl chloride be considered a potential occupational teratogen.[11] The excess risk of cancer to workers or the induction of a teratogenic response in the children of workers exposed to specific airborne concentrations of these compounds has not yet been determined, but the probability of developing these adverse effects would be decreased by reducing exposure. NIOSH is particularly concerned that the occupational exposure to methyl bromide may increase as a result of using this compound as a substitute fumigant for the recently restricted use of the fumigant ethylene dibromide (EDB).[6] Chronic toxicology studies of methyl bromide are currently being conducted, and NIOSH recommends that the results of these studies be thoroughly evaluated before significantly expanding the use of methyl bromide.

Exposure Standards and Guides

The current Occupational Safety and Health Administration (OSHA) permissible exposure limits (PELs) (29 CFR 1910.1000) for occupational exposure to these monohalomethanes are as follows:[5]

Methyl chloride	100 ppm, 8-hr time-weighted average (TWA) concentration
	200 ppm, acceptable ceiling concentration
	300 ppm, acceptable maximum peak for 5 minutes in any 3-hr period above the acceptable ceiling for an 8-hr shift
Methyl bromide	20 ppm (80 mg/m^3), ceiling concentration; skin
Methyl iodide	5 ppm (28 mg/m^3), 8-hr TWA; skin

The OSHA PELs for occupational exposure to methyl chloride and methyl iodide are intended to protect against the neurotoxic effects of these compounds. For methyl bromide, the OSHA PEL is intended to protect against the development of pulmonary edema as well as neurotoxic effects. The PEL for methyl chloride is based upon ANSI Z37.18-1969 as developed by the American National Standards Institute (ANSI),[3] while the PELs for methyl bromide and methyl iodide are based upon the 1968 Threshold Limit Values (TLVs) of the American Conference of Governmental Industrial Hygienists (ACGIH). At the present time, NIOSH has no recommended exposure limit for the monohalomethanes.

ACGIH, in its 1985-1986 edition of TLVs, makes the following recommendations:[2]

Methyl chloride	50 ppm (105 mg/m^3), 8-hr TWA; 100 ppm (205 mg/m^3), 15-minute TWA short term exposure limit (STEL)
Methyl bromide	5 ppm (20 mg/m^3), 8-hr TWA; 15 ppm (60 mg/m^3), 15-minute STEL; skin
Methyl iodide	2 ppm (10 mg/m^3), 8-hr TWA; 5 ppm (30 mg/m^3), 15-minute STEL; A2; skin

The ACGIH has included methyl iodide in its list of suspected carcinogens, designated as Appendix A2 in the TLV listing.[2]

The "skin" notation for methyl bromide and methyl iodide in both the OSHA PELs and the ACGIH TLVs refers to the potential contribution to the overall exposure by the cutaneous route by either airborne or direct skin contact with the substance.

REFERENCES

1. American Conference of Governmental Industrial Hygienists: *Threshold Limit Values of Air-borne Contaminants for 1968, Recommended and Intended Changes*. Cincinnati, Ohio, 1968.
2. American Conference of Governmental Industrial Hygienists: *Threshold Limit Values for Chemical Substances and Physical Agents in the Work Environment and Biological Exposure Indices with Intended Changes for 1986–87*. Cincinnati, Ohio, 1986.
3. *American National Standard-Acceptable Concentrations of Methyl Chloride*, No Z37.18-1969. New York, American National Standards Institute, Inc, 1970, p 8.
4. Butler ECB, Perry KMA, Williams JRF: Methyl bromide burns. *Br J Ind Med* 1945; 2:30–31.
5. *Code of Federal Regulations*. U.S. Department of Labor, Occupational Safety and Health Administration, No 20 CFR 1910.1000, 1982, Table Z-1.
6. *Federal Register*, Environmental Protection Agency, Part VIII, 48(197):46248, October 11, 1983.
7. Jones, AM: Methyl chloride poisoning. *Q J Med* 1942; 11:29-43.
8. Hygienic guide series—Methyl chloride: Chloromethane. *Am Ind Hyg Assoc J* 1961; 22(6):515–516.
9. MacDonald JDC: Methyl chloride intoxication—Report of 8 cases. *J Occup Med* 1964; 6:81–84.
10. Gaultier M, Fournier E, Gervais P, et al: Two hundred five cases of accidental acute poisonings by industrial compounds seen in the emergency ward of the Fernand-Widal Hospital from 1964–1973. *J Eur Toxicol* 1974; 6(6):263–265.
11. Monohalomethanes (methyl chloride CH_3Cl, methyl bromide CH_3BR, methyl iodide CH_3I). *Current Intelligence Bulletin 43*, NIOSH, Cincinnati, Ohio, 1984.
12. Scharnweber HC, Spears GN, Cowles SR: Case reports. Chronic methyl chloride intoxication in six industrial workers. *J Occup Med* 1974; 16(2):112–113.
13. Skutilova J: Acute impairment due to methyl iodide. *Prac Lek* 1975; 27(10):341–342.
14. Sundin DS: Workers potentially exposed to chloromethane, bromomethane, and iodomethane. Unpublished data available from U.S. Department of Health, Education, and Welfare, Public Health Service, Center for Disease Control, National institute for Occupational Safety and Health, Division of Surveillance, Hazard Evaluations and Field Studies, National Occupational Hazard Survey data base, Cincinnati, Ohio (data collected 1972–1974).

NAPHTHALENE

$C_{10}H_8$

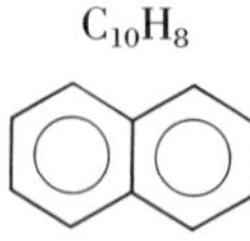

This colorless, crystalline substance has the familiar odor of "moth balls," derived chiefly from coal tar and has enjoyed long use as a household fumigant, since it readily volatilizes at room temperature. It is sold as flakes or "moth balls," and is effective against "cloth moths" and "carpet beetles" and is an excellent repellant for rats, skunks, and squirrels in confined spaces. Although several millions of kilograms are consumed in the United States, less than 2% is used to make moth balls. More than 80% is converted to phthalic anhydride, important in resin manufacturing. The remainder is used as naphthalene compounds for dye intermediates, and tanning and surface-active agents. Paradichlorobenzene has largely replaced naphthalene as an insecticide, because it possesses a more pleasant odor, but it offers less lasting protection for prolonged woolen storage. Skin contact may cause a hypersensitivity dermatitis in some persons, but chronic dermatitis is rare. As little as 15-ppm exposure to the vapor causes eye irritation, accidental contact with particles can result in conjunctivitis, and superficial corneal damage and cataracts can result from prolonged, uncontrolled exposure. Inhalation of the vapor is the main occupational risk, with severe intoxication resulting in hemolysis. Early findings include eye irritation, headache, confusion, excitement, malaise, profuse sweating, nausea, vomiting, abdominal pain, and irritation of the bladder. There may be progression to jaundice, hematuria, hemoglobinuria, renal tubular blockade, and acute renal shutdown. Hematologic features include red blood cell fragmentation, icterus, severe anemia with nucleated red cells, leucocytosis, and dramatic decreases in hemoglobin, hematocrit, and red blood cell count; sometimes there are Heinz bodies and methemoglobin. Individuals with a deficiency of glucose-6-phosphate dehydrogenase in erythrocytes may be more susceptible to hemolysis by naphthalene.[6] Cataracts and ocular irritation have been produced experimentally in animals and have been described in human beings. Of 21 workers exposed to high concentrations of fume or vapor for five years, eight had peripheral lens opacities; in other studies, no abnormalities of the eyes have been detected in workers exposed to naphthalene for several years.

The current OSHA standard for naphthalene is 10 ppm averaged over an eight-hour work shift (or 50 mg/cu m).

REFERENCES

1. American Conference of Governmental Industrial Hygienists: Naphthalene, in *Documentation of the Threshold Limit Values for Substances in Workroom Air*, ed 5. Cincinnati, Oh, ACGIH, 1986.

2. Gleason MN, et al: *Clinical Toxicology of Commercial Products*, ed 5. Baltimore, Williams & Wilkins Co, 1984.
3. Grant W: *Toxicology of the Eye*, ed 2. Springfield, Ill, Charles C Thomas, 1974.
4. Harden RA, Baetjer AM: Aplastic anemia following exposure to paradichlorobenzene and naphthalene. *J Occup Med* 1978; 20:820–822.
5. Hygienic Guide Series: Naphthalene. *Am Ind Hyg Assoc J* 1967; 28:493–496.
6. Zinkham WH, Childs B: A defect of glutathione metabolism in erythrocytes from patients with a naphthalene-induced hemolytic anemia. *Pediatrics* 1958; 22:461–471.

NITRIC ACID

HNO_3

Nitric acid is a powerful oxidizing agent, reacting with most metals, and is used in enormous quantities to produce fertilizer, dyes, and plastics. The well-known "Ostwald process" produces ammonia (NH_3) from atmospheric nitrogen, which is oxidized to nitrogen dioxide. Nitric acid is unstable, decomposing on contact with heat and exposure to light, water, nitrogen dioxide, and oxygen.

Occupational exposures may occur by inhalation and/or skin contact. Nitric acid vapor or mist is a severe irritant to the eyes, mucous membranes, and skin. When nitric acid is exposed to air or comes into contact with organic matter, it decomposes to yield a mixture of oxides of nitrogen, including nitric oxide and nitrogen dioxide, both equally or more hazardous than nitric acid. Exposure to high concentrations of nitric acid vapor or mist causes pneumonitis and pulmonary edema, which may be fatal; onset of symptoms may be delayed for 4–30 hours. In contact with the eyes, the liquid produces severe burns, which may result in permanent damage and visual impairment. On the skin, the liquid in concentrated solutions may cause deep ulcers and stain the skin a bright yellow or yellowish brown color. The vapor and mist may erode teeth. Ingestion of the liquid will cause immediate pain and burns of the gastrointestinal tract.

Treatment.—Promptly remove the worker from exposure and immediate flushing with water. Consider hospitalization for observation for the possible delayed onset of pulmonary edema.

The TLV of 2 ppm was set mainly to prevent irritation and erosion of teeth.[1]

REFERENCES

1. American Conference of Governmental Industrial Hygienists: Nitric Acid, in *Documentation of the Threshold Limit Values for Substances in Workroom Air*, ed 4. Cincinnati, Oh, ACGIH, 1980 pp 181–182.
2. Hygienic Guide Series: Nitric acid. *Am Ind Hyg Assoc J* 1964; 25:426.
3. Manufacturing Chemists Association, Inc: Chemical Safety Data Sheet, DS-5, Nitric Acid, Washington, DC, pp 15–17, 1961.
4. National Institute for Occupational Safety and Health. Cincinnati, Oh, US Dept of Health, Education, and Welfare: *Criteria for a Recommended Standard: Occupational Exposure to Nitric Acid*, NIOSH Publ 76-141 (HEW), 1976.

2-NITROPROPANE

$CH_3CHNO_2CH_3$

A recently completed inhalation study indicates that 2-nitropropane, a widely used solvent in industrial coatings and printing inks, causes liver cancer in rats. In this study, sponsored by the National Institute for Occupational Safety and Health (NIOSH), all laboratory rats exposed to 207 ppm 2-nitropropane over a six-month period developed hepatocellular carcinoma or hepatic adenoma. Although this study suggests that 2-nitropropane is carcinogenic, its carcinogenic potential in man has not yet been researched.[1] Solvent systems containing 2-nitropropane are used in coatings (e.g., vinyl, epoxy, nitrocellulose, and chlorinated rubber), printing inks, and adhesives. Occupational exposure to these products may occur in various industries, including industrial construction and maintenance, printing (rotogravure and flexographic inks), highway maintenance (traffic markings), shipbuilding and maintenance (marine coatings), furniture, food packaging, and plastic products. The NIOSH estimates that 185,000 workers are potentially exposed to 2-nitropropane in these and other industries.

Synonyms for 2-nitropropane include dimethylnitromethane, isonitropropane, nitroisopropane, and 2-NP. Trade names under which 2-nitropropane is marketed include NiPar S-20th (commercial grade 2-nitropropane) and NiPar S-30th (mixtures of 1- and 2-nitropropane). 2-Nitropropane (in concentrations ranging from approximately 5% to 25%) is used in a number of solvent systems to contribute desirable properties such as improved drying time, more complete solvent release, better flow and film integrity, retardation of blushing, greater wetting ability, improved electrostatic spraying and increased pigment dispersion. Of the estimated 30 million kg of 2-nitropropane produced annually in the United States, 6 million kg are sold domestically; the remainder is either used internally by the companies producing it, or exported.

At least five occupationally related deaths have resulted from exposure to 2-NP.[3, 4] Typically, workers coated the surface of an enclosed structure (tank, vault, or shiphold) with sealant containing 2-NP. No forced ventilation or personal protection was used. After many hours of exposure, they complained of headache, nausea, vomiting, dyspepsia, and chest pain. A few days later, acute jaundice, hematemesis, enlarged liver, edema, and oliguria/anuria developed, followed by coma and death. One nonfatal case involved a 30-minute exposure to 2-NP vapor caused by a spill.[4] No estimate concerning the frequency of 2-NP-induced hepatitis is available; however, a review of 62 cases of liver transplant recipients showed that two patients had liver failure secondary to 2-NP exposure.[2]

In short-term toxicologic experiments, high concentrations of 2-NP (700 ppm for several hours) have produced parenchymal degeneration and focal necrosis of the liver in experimental animals.[6] In chronic-exposure studies, 2-NP has produced hepatomas in rats at 207 ppm for six months, and it is considered a potential human carcinogen.[7] Although the current permissible exposure limit as determined by the Occupational Safety and Health Administration (OSHA) is 25 ppm or 90 mg/cu m (eight-hour, time-weighted average), NIOSH has recommended that, based on the evidence of animal carcinogenicity, occupational exposure to 2-NP be reduced to the lowest feasible levels.[1]

The following control measures should be considered for preventing acute toxicity and potential long-term health consequences of 2-NP exposure:

1. Paint, sealant, or other coating materials must not be applied in confined spaces without sufficient forced ventilation and respiratory and cutaneous protection.
2. Products containing 2-NP should be labeled to reflect its toxicity; workers should be warned that odor does not serve as a warning sign, since toxic levels are below the odor threshold of 83 ppm.[6]
3. 2-NP should be replaced whenever possible by other less toxic solvents in paint and coating formulations. Reportedly, 2-NP has been replaced by 1-NP in many paint formulations.[6] However, since these two chemicals have very similar characteristics, the same precautions should be taken in handling them.

Case Report.—Acute hepatic failure after occupational exposure to 2-nitropropane. On June 28, July 1, and July 2, 1985, two construction workers applied an epoxy resin coating to a water main in an underground concrete vault in San Jose, California.

During the three workdays, the men applied 10 gallons of the resin coating. The vault was unventilated, and the workers used no respiratory or skin protection.

On the evening of July 2, both men went to a local hospital because of persistent nausea, vomiting, weakness, and dizziness. Initial laboratory tests showed slightly elevated serum glutamic-oxaloacetic transaminase (SGOT) levels—60 units/L for worker 1 and 79 units/L for worker 2 (normal SGOT is less than 40 units/L). The men were admitted for observation and discharged the following day, after their symptoms had subsided.

Three days later, worker 1 returned to the hospital with persistent nausea, vomiting, anorexia, and onset of scleral icterus. Laboratory tests showed marked hepatic dysfunction (SGOT and serum glutamicpyruvic transaminase [SGPT] levels greater than 10,000 units/L, and hyperbilirubinemia), severe metabolic acidosis, and renal insufficiency. He was transferred to a university medical center, where his hospital course was marked by gastrointestinal bleeding, arrhythmia, pulmonary edema, and renal failure. He died nine days after his initial presentation. Autopsy findings were consistent with fulminant hepatic necrosis.

Worker 2 has remained clinically well, although for at least six weeks he continued to have elevated liver enzymes (SGOT and SGPT) in a range of 1.5 to two times the normal maximum. Both men had histories of moderate alcohol use (12 cans of beer per week); neither had significant past medical histories, including previous hepatic disease.

According to the manufacturer's label, the coating material contained a mixture of cyclohexanone, toluene, tri(dimethylaminomethyl)phenol, and 2-nitropropane (2-NP), combined with coal tar pitch and epoxy resin. Analysis of the leftover compound by the California Department of Health Services confirmed the presence of 2-NP.

The analysis of serum samples obtained on July 2 showed 13 μg/mL and 8.5 μg/mL of 2-NP for workers 1 and 2, respectively; 2-NP was undetectable in all subsequent samples. No other volatile compounds, including ethanol, were detected in the serum samples.

(Reported by RJ Harrison, MD, G Pasternak, MD, Division of Occupational and Environmental Medicine; P Blanc, MD, P Basuk, MD, Division of Gastroenterology, University of California, San Francisco; G Letz, MD, Hazard Evaluation System and Information SVC, California State Department of Health Services, Division of Surveillance, Hazard Evaluations, and Field Studies, Division of Safety Research, National Institute for Occupational Safety and Health, Centers for Disease Control.)[1]

REFERENCES

1. Centers for Disease Control: Acute hepatic failure after occupational exposure to 2-Nitropropane. *MMWR* 1985; 34:43–47.
2. Demetris AJ, Lasky S, Van Thel DH, et al: Pathology of hepatic transplantation: A review of 62 adult allograft recipients immunosuppressed with a cyclosporine/steroid regimen. *Am J Pathol* 1985; 118:151–161.
3. Gaultier M, Fournier PE, Gervais P, et al: Intoxication par le nitropropane. *Arch Mal Prof* 1964; 25:425–428.
4. Hine CH, Pasi A, Stephens BG: Fatalities following exposure to 2-nitropropane. *J Occup Med* 1978; 20:333–337, 1978.
5. Lewis TR, Ulrich CE, Busey WM: Subchronic inhalation toxicity of nitromethane and 2-nitropropane. *J Environ Pathol Toxicol* 1979; 2:233–249.
6. National Paint and Coatings Association (NPCA): Information released from NPCA's data bank, 1985.
7. Occupational Safety and Health Administration, National Institute for Occupational Safety and Health: *Health Hazard Alert: 2-Nitropropane*, DHHS (NIOSH) Publ 80-142, 1980.
8. Treon JF, Durta FR: Physiological response of experimental animals to the vapor of 2-nitropropane. *Arch Ind Hyg Occup Med* 1952; 5:52–61.

OXIDES OF NITROGEN (NITROGEN DIOXIDE AND NITRIC OXIDE)

Nitrogen dioxide (NO_2) is one of several oxides of nitrogen. It is a reddish brown or dark orange gas; its dimer, nitrogen tetroxide (N_2O_4), is colorless. At temperatures between −9.3° C and 135° C, nitrogen dioxide and nitrogen tetroxide coexist as a mixture of gases. Below −9.3° C, a colorless solid consisting of nitrogen tetroxide is formed, whereas above 135° C, the gas consists mostly of nitrogen dioxide. In evaluations of occupational exposures to the mixtures of these two compounds, however, the results customarily are expressed in terms of nitrogen dioxide. The conversion of molecular nitrogen into nitrogenous compounds is known as fixation of nitrogen. In the upper atmosphere, this is brought about through photochemical processes in which nitrogen and oxygen atoms from dissociated molecules combine to form nitric oxide. At ground level, the combination of nitrogen and oxygen takes place thermally in flames, explosions, and electric discharges.

Ultraviolet energy or sufficiently high temperatures to accomplish this in the occupational environment are encountered in electric or gas welding, in the combustion of fuels, for example, in furnaces or internal combustion engines, and in the detonation of explosives. Nitric oxide is also produced when nitrogen dioxide is dissolved in warm water. Both nitric oxide and nitrogen dioxide are formed when nitric acid reacts with reducing agents. For dilute nitric acid, the resultant mixture contains predominantly nitric oxide, whereas for concentrated nitric acid more nitrogen dioxide is produced. However, nitric oxide and nitrogen dioxide rarely exist independently in the occupational environment.

Elkins[7] calculated that with a nitric oxide concentration of 200 ppm, nitrogen dioxide would be formed at a rate of about 11 ppm per minute. If the nitric oxide concentration were 100 ppm, the oxidation rate could drop to 2.8 ppm per minute, whereas with 25 ppm of nitric oxide, it would take more than five minutes of 1 ppm of nitrogen dioxide to be formed. For this reason, both nitric oxide and nitrogen dioxide should be sampled simultaneously. The presence of other factors, such as moisture, metal fumes, or ultraviolet radiation, may either accelerate or slow down the actual rate of oxidation of nitric oxide in air.[17] As a result, it is not practicable to estimate the concentration of one of the nitrogen oxides solely on the basis of a measurement of the other. Mixtures of the oxides of nitrogen are also produced in other ways, such as from the combustion of nitrogen-containing materials or from reactions of nitric acid with metals or organic matter. At the time of release, these mixtures may contain substantial percentages of nitrogen dioxide. Somewhat more nitrogen dioxide is to be expected where nitrogen-containing compounds are decomposed. Where nitric acid is a reactant in acid dipping, nitrogen dioxide will be the predominant oxide released.

Sources of Exposure

Although nitric oxide is the oxide of nitrogen initially produced in the welding arc or flame, its concentration in such operations is only rarely reported. In many field studies and controlled laboratory experiments, concentrations of nitric oxide have been reported as "nitrous gases" or "nitrogen oxides," whereas other field investigations and controlled studies have expressed concentrations of nitric oxide as "nitrogen dioxide." Differences in describing environmental levels, coupled with the variety of sampling and analytic methods used to assess the environments, virtually preclude direct comparison and interpretation between these studies. In a simulation of cutting torch operations causing toxicity, Norwood et al.[16] reported separate figures for concentrations of nitric oxide and nitrogen dioxide in two of ten samples. This study showed nitrogen dioxide to be 13% of the total oxides found 15 minutes after cutting began. The nitrogen dioxide increased to 33% after an additional 25 minutes. Nitrogen dioxide is dissociated by ultraviolet radiation, producing nitric oxide plus oxygen atoms. The oxygen atoms, in turn, react with nitrogen dioxide at a very rapid rate, producing nitric oxide and oxygen molecules.[10] Thus, according to Silverman and Husain,[17] ultraviolet rays emitted in arc welding would counteract the oxidation of nitric oxide to nitrogen dioxide. On the other hand, ozone produced in the arc could oxidize nitric oxide to nitrogen dioxide or to even higher oxides, such as nitrogen pentoxide. They also pointed out that iron and moisture present could have a converse influence, reducing nitrogen dioxide to nitric oxide and possibly to ammonia or nitrogen. In addition, freshly formed iron fumes may react with nitrogen oxides to produce particulate nitrites and nitrates, with a consequent reduction in the amount of gaseous oxides present.[17] In their own welding experiments, conducted in a test chamber, Silverman and Husain[17] found that approximately equal concentrations of nitric oxide and nitrogen dioxide totaling approximately 30 ppm showed no appreciable changes in the ratio of the gases after a period of two to three hours (Table 47–7).

In general, it has been found that hot metals decompose nitric oxide, forming the metal oxide and nitrogen.[17] This may explain the higher rate of formation of oxides of nitrogen when an oxyacetylene flame does not touch metal.[16, 18] Norwood et al.[16] found that as much as 250 ppm of nitrogen oxides were formed where the flame was not in contact with metal and only 47 and 71 ppm in tests where stainless steel was being melted. Similarly, Steel and Sanderson[18] reported that the concentrations of nitrogen dioxide produced by flame alone were several times greater than the concentrations observed when metals were being flame-cut. Another example[1] of occupational hazard concerns exposure to exhaust gases from ice-resurfacing machines in ice arenas. Such exposures made the machine operators, as well as arena patrons, ill on a number of occasions. Investigations of 45 ice arenas in Minnesota showed nitrogen oxides concentrations (reported as nitrogen dioxide) as high as 40 ppm. However, concentrations of carbon monoxide were elevated, suggesting that nitrogen oxides were not the only cause of adverse effects. Since the form of nitrogen emitted from internal combustion engines exists largely as nitric oxide at the time of discharge, workers employed in automobile parking or repair garages may have occupational exposures. The production of nitric oxide by the catalytic oxidation of ammonia is the first step in the manufacture of nitric acid. Kennedy[12] reported that underground blasting operations with both nitroexplosives and gunpowder produce levels of the oxides of nitrogen up to 88 ppm after normal firing of a commonly used blasting explosive and up to 167 ppm after "misfires" (incomplete detonation). Conventional powder shots may cause momentary concentrations of up to 56 ppm and concentrations as high as 150 ppm after multiple firings. Commins et al.[3] noted that concentrations of nitric oxide and nitrogen dioxide reaching several hundred ppm were produced in a freshly filled agricultural silo during various stages of the decomposition process. The maximal concentrations of nitric oxide and nitrogen dioxide were found on the fifth day after loading the silo. At that time, a distinct layer of brown gas was observed at the center of the silo. In general, concentrations decreased with increased height above the surface of the silage. Measurements were also made before and after operation of the silo-filling blower. Use of the blower did reduce the levels of nitric oxide and nitrogen dioxide; however, high concentrations of these gases still remained near the surface of the silage.

TABLE 47–7.
Approximate Distribution of Nitrogen Oxides Generated From Various Operations*

SOURCE	NO_2 %	NO %
Carbon arc	9	91
Oxyacetylene torch	8	92
Cellulose nitrate combustion	19	81
Diesel exhaust	35	65
Dynamite blast	52	48
Acid dipping	78	22

*From NIOSH Criteria Document.[4]

It is difficult to estimate how many people are exposed to oxides of nitrogen, since hazardous occupations also involve all workers located in the vicinity of operations or processes having conditions conducive to the generation of nitrogen oxidation, i.e., furnaces, boilers, welding, internal combustion engines, and nitrogen oxides produced from numerous chemical processes. The difficulty in delineating the incidence of exposure has been shown by Storlazzi[19] in a study of welding and burning operations in U.S. naval shipyards. Although only 6,000 workers were directly engaged in such activities, approximately 60,000 workers were indirectly exposed to the by-products of these operations. The NIOSH estimates that 1.5 million workers are potentially exposed to the oxides of nitrogen. In view of the factors mentioned, this figure is low.[4] An estimated[15] 300,000 tons of nitrogen oxides are produced annually from industrial processes and 10 million tons result from fuel combustion. These are rough estimates at best and do not distinguish between the various nitrogen oxides. From the many cases found in the medical literature, it is known that serious, even lethal, concentrations of nitrogen oxides may be encountered. Similar serious consequences have been reported from chemical processes.[2, 5, 6, 11, 20]

Health Effects

Cases of marked illness from nitrogen dioxide have been from accidental exposures to arc or gas welding (in confined spaces), in unventilated farm silos, following explosions, using nitrogen-containing explosives and with the use of nitric acid. Nitrogen dioxide gas is a respiratory irritant; it causes pulmonary edema and rarely, among survivors, bronchiolitis obliterans. Brief exposure of humans to concentrations of about 250 ppm causes cough, production of mucoid or frothy sputum, and increasing dyspnea. Within one to two hours, the person may develop pulmonary edema with tachypnea, cyanosis, fine crackles and wheezes throughout the lungs, and tachycardia. Alternatively, there may be only increasing dyspnea and cough for several hours; the symptoms then gradually subside over a two- to three-week period. The condition then may enter a second stage of abruptly increasing severity; fever and chills precede a relapse, with increasing dyspnea, cyanosis, and recurring pulmonary edema. Death may occur in either the initial or second stage of the disease; a severe second stage may follow a relatively mild initial stage. The subject who survives the second stage usually recovers over two to three weeks; however, some do not return to normal but experience varying degrees of impaired pulmonary function. The radiographic features in the acute initial stage vary from normal to those of typical pulmonary edema; most reports mention a pattern of nodular shadows on the chest film at the outset. The roentgenogram then may clear, only to show miliary mottling as the second stage commences, progressing to the development of a confluent pattern. Results of pulmonary function tests in the acute stage show reduction in lung volume and diffusing capacity; similar findings are recorded in the volume and diffusing capacity. The same findings are recorded in the second stage. Pathologic examination of the acute lesion shows extensive mucosal edema and inflammatory cell exudation. The delayed lesion shows the histologic appearance of bronchiolitis obliterans; small bronchi and bronchioles contain an inflammatory exudate that tends to undergo fibrinous organization, finally obliterating the lumen.[4, 13] The effects expected in humans from exposure to nitrogen dioxide for 60 minutes are: 100 ppm, pulmonary edema and death; 50 ppm, pulmonary edema with possible subacute or chronic lesions in the lungs; 25 ppm, respiratory irritation and chest pain. A concentration of 50 ppm is moderately irritating to the eyes and nose; 25 ppm is irritating to some persons.

Exposure causes cough, mucoid or frothy sputum production, increasing dyspnea, chest pain, signs and symptoms of pulmonary edema with cyanosis, tachypnea, tachycardia, and eye irritation. Consideration should be given to hospitalization and observation for the possible delayed onset of pulmonary edema and to treatment with corticosteroids if pulmonary edema occurs.

Permissible Exposure Limits

Occupational exposure to nitrogen dioxide (NO_2) shall be controlled so that workers are not exposed to nitrogen dioxide at greater than a ceiling concentration of 1 ppm by volume (1.8 mg/cu m) as determined by a sampling time of 15 minutes. Nitric oxide (NO) causes narcosis in animals. Exposure of mice to 2,500 ppm for six or seven minutes caused narcosis, and death occurred within 12 minutes. Some early reports attributed the toxicity of nitric oxide to the formation of methemoglobin; however, more recent studies indicate that nitric oxide reacts in vitro with normal (ferrous) hemoglobin but, in exposed animals, this interaction does not occur and no methemoglobin is formed. Nitric oxide is converted spontaneously in air to nitrogen dioxide; hence, some of the latter gas invariably is present whenever nitric oxide is found in the air. At concentrations below 50 ppm, however, this reaction is slow, and frequently substantial concentrations of nitric oxide may occur with negligible quantities of nitrogen dioxide. Nitrogen dioxide causes delayed pulmonary edema.

REFERENCES

1. Anderson DE: Problems created for ice arenas by engine exhaust. *Am Ind Hyg Assoc J* 1971; 32:790.
2. Charleroy DK: Nitrous and nitric gas casualties. *US Naval Med Bull* 1945; 44:435.
3. Commins BT, Raveney FJ, Jesson MW: Toxic gases in tower silos. *Ann Occup Hyg* 1971; 14:275.
4. *Criteria for a Recommended Standard: Occupational Exposure to Oxides of Nitrogen (Nitrogen Dioxide and Nitric Oxide).* Cincinnati, Oh, US Dept of Health, Education and Welfare, PHS, Center for Disease Control, National Institute for Occupational Safety and Health, HEW (NIOSH) Publ 76-149, March, 1976.
5. Darke CS, Warrack AJN: Bronchiolitis from nitrous fumes. *Thorax* 1958; 13:327.
6. Desgranges JB: Observation and comments on a sudden death caused by nitrous gas. *J Med Chir Pharm* 1804; 8:487 (French).
7. Elkins HB: Nitrogen dioxide. Rate of oxidation of nitric oxide and its bearing on the nitrogen dioxide content of electric arc fumes. *J Ind Hyg Toxicol* 1946; 28:37.
8. Gleason, MN, et al: *Clinical Toxicology of Commercial Products*, ed 5. Baltimore, Williams & Wilkins Co, 1984.
9. Gray EL: Oxides of nitrogen: Their occurrence, toxicity hazard. *AMA Arch Ind Hyg* 1959; 19:479.

10. Harris L, Siegel BM: Reactions of nitrogen dioxide with other gases. *J Am Chem Soc* 1941; 63:2520.
11. Hortsch W: Nitric oxide poisoning with motor hemiparalysis. *Arch Gewerbepathol Gewerbehyg* 1942; 11:402 (German).
12. Kennedy MCS: Nitrous fumes and coalminers with emphysema. *Ann Occup Hyg* 1972; 15:285.
13. Levy SA: Occupational pulmonary diseases, in Zenz C (ed): *Occupational Medicine: Principles and Practical Applications.* Chicago, Year Book Medical Publishers, 1975, pp 117–155.
13a. Lindvall T: Health effects of nitrogen dioxide and oxidants. *Scand J Work Environ Health* 1985; 11(3):10–28.
14. Miles FD: *Nitric Acid Manufacture and Uses.* London, Oxford University Press, 1961, pp 1–8.
15. Nationwide Inventory of Air Pollutant Emissions 1978, NAPCA Publ AP-73. Raleigh, NC, National Air Pollution Control Administration, 1970, pp 14–16.
16. Norwood WD, et al: Nitrogen dioxide poisoning due to metal-cutting with oxyacetylene torch. *J Occup Med* 1966; 8:301.
17. Silverman L, Husain SL: A study of nitrogen oxide concentrations during arc. *Arch Ind Hyg Occup Med* 1951; 3:135.
18. Steel J, Sanderson JT: The thermal degradation of protective coating. A basic study. Part I. Zinc-rich epoxy primers. *Am Ind Hyg Assoc J* 1965; 26:449.
19. Storlazzi ID: Hygiene of welding in US naval shipyards. *Arch Ind Health* 1959; 19:307.
20. Zadek J: Mass poisoning by the inhalation of nitrous fumes (nitrite intoxications). *Berl Klin Wochenschr* 1916; 53:246 (German).

OZONE

O_3

Ozone is a highly reactive gas that can form during inert gas-shielded arc welding; it is formed in and around electrical equipment at high voltages, especially during pulse testing of motors, generators, and other devices (usually above 600 volts); it is found in air- and water-purifying devices and infrequently with certain copy and reproductive devices using powerful ultraviolet light sources.

An important industrial use for ozone is to permit the adherence of the printing inks to the surface of plastics. The surface tension of the materials must be increased for adherence of the inks. This is done by oxidizing the surface, which is achieved by ozone treatment. A high voltage of ± 12 KV (at a frequency of 40 kHz.) is used. The resulting ultraviolet spark emitted generates sufficient ozone on the surface of the cup. (This treatment is approximately 0.17 of a second, during which time, a plastic cup rotates 30 times.) The adherence of the ink achieved, the object passes through a drying tunnel where it is subjected to strong ultraviolet rays emanating from UV lamps; here, again, ozone is generated incidentally. Established concentrations of ozone reached 0.03 ppm. It was decided to install an exhaust system for ozone extraction, which consisted of a stainless steel exhaust system. (Figures 47–15 and 47–16).

Airline flight attendants on trans-Pacific flights reported an increased incidence of respiratory symptoms, attributed to high-altitude ozone exposure. An epidemiologic survey of flight attendants on three airlines with differing potential for ozone exposure was evaluated by Ostrov.[5] They were (1) an international carrier ("high exposure"), (2) a mixed domestic/foreign carrier ("intermediate exposure"), and (3) a domestic carrier ("low exposure"). Respiratory questionnaires and flight diaries were completed by 1,330 flight attendants on the three airlines. For symptoms that had been preclassified as ozone-related—chest pain, dyspnea, persistent cough, sore throat, and nosebleeds—a gradient in age-adjusted incidence with that airline was noted. A gradient was not evident for 12 nonspecific symptoms considered unrelated to ozone. Flight diaries for 5,008 flight days showed that the incidence of ozone-related symptoms increased with duration and altitude of flights, two indirect measures of ozone exposure. Although lacking environmental ozone data, these results suggest that ozone exposure is an occupational hazard for flight attendants and that more efficient in-flight air-treatment systems must be installed on high-altitude aircraft.

Typically irritated are mucous membranes, especially the eyes, nose, and throat and the lungs. The characteristic odor is readily detectable at low concentrations (0.01–0.05 ppm). Ozone produces local irritation of the eyes and mucous membranes. At low levels, a disagreeable irritation and dryness of the eyes, mouth, and throat occur at concentrations of 0.05–0.1 ppm for 10–30 minutes. At high levels, marked eye irritation, cough, a choking sensation with substernal pain, and dyspnea develop. Pulmonary edema can occur and, within several hours, signs of bronchopneumonia. Lung function can be impaired up to 24 hours following exposure to 0.6–0.8 ppm for two hours.[2, 4] If substantial exposure has occurred or is suspected, hospitalization is advisable because of delayed-onset pulmonary edema.

The 1986 TLV is 0.1 ppm, a level thought to prevent radiomimetic effects.[1]

REFERENCES

1. American Conference of Governmental Industrial Hygienists: Documentation of the TLVs for Substances in Workroom Air, ed 5. Cincinnati, Oh, ACGIH, 1986.
2. Committee on Medical and Biologic Effects of Environmental Pollutants: Ozone and other photochemical oxidants. Washington, DC, National Academy of Sciences, 1977, pp 402–415.
3. Jaffe LS: Photochemical air pollutants and their effects on men and animals. II. Adverse effects. *Arch Environ Health* 1968; 16:241.
3a. Lindvall T: Recommendations for air quality standards for nitrogen dioxide and ozone. *Scandinavian J Work Environ Health* 1985; 11(3): 3–9.
4. Nasr ANM: Ozone poisoning in man: Clinical manifestations and differential diagnosis—a review. *Clin Toxicol* 1971; 4:461.
5. Ostrov P: Ozone exposure in airline flight attendants. Epidemiology and Intelligence Service Bulletin, Atlanta, Ga, CDC, 1979.
6. Tabershaw IR, Ottoboni F, Cooper WC: Oxidants: Air quality criteria based on health effects. *J Occup Med* 1968; 10:464.

SELECTED PETROLEUM-DERIVED SOLVENTS

Almost all occupational health specialists have been confronted with workers who have had some contact or exposure to Stoddard solvent, mineral spirits, petroleum ether, kerosene, rubber solvent, varnish makers' and painters' naphtha, and benzene.

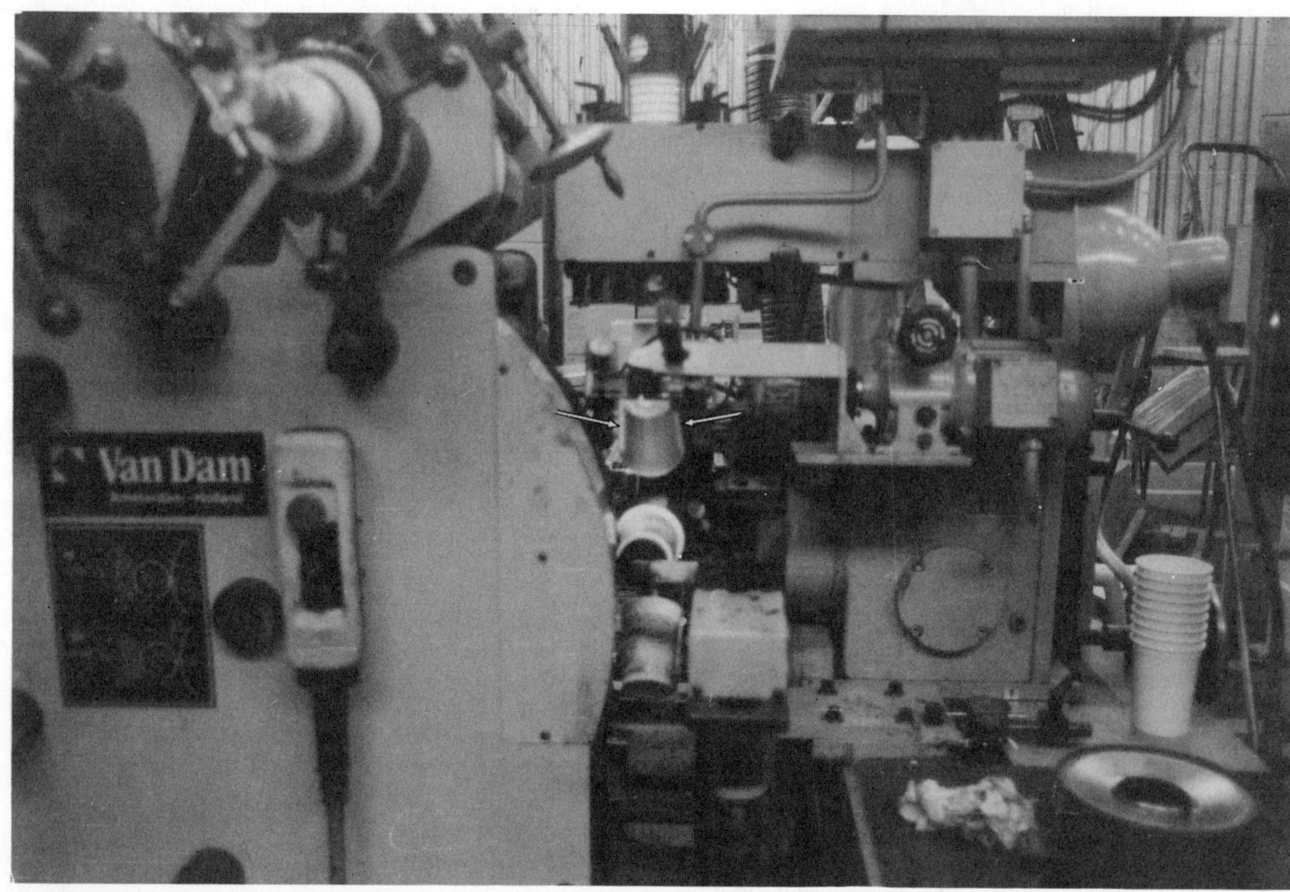

FIG 47–15.
A plastic cup labeling machine. Note the concentrated ultraviolet generated by the high voltage in close contact with the cup *(arrows)*. (Courtesy of Mr. Phil Koekemoer.)

These chemicals are used in enormous quantities in virtually all industries.

Occupations with potential exposure to these refined petroleum solvents are adhesive makers, ammonia synthesis workers, asphalt coating workers, ceramic production workers, degreasers (metal), detergent makers, dry cleaners, enamel makers (synthetic), farmers, fat and oil processors, fungicide handlers, garage workers, heating fuel handlers, herbicide handlers, hydrogen manufacturing workers, ink production workers, insecticide handlers, jet fuel handlers and makers, kerosene handlers, laboratory workers (chemical), lacquerers, leather japanners, metal cleaners, naphtha workers, oil processors, painters, paint makers, perfume extraction workers, petrochemical workers, petroleum refinery workers, photographic chemical makers, printers, resin makers, rocket fuel handlers and makers, rubber coaters and makers, stainers, stain makers, typesetters, varnish makers, wax makers, wood preservation makers, and wool process workers.

Eyes, nose, and throat irritation, dermatitis, and effects on the nervous system have been found in workers exposed to some refined petroleum solvents.

Benzene

Benzene is derived primarily through the refinement and fractionation of crude petroleum, has a boiling point of 80.1° C (176° F) at 760 mm Hg and may be a contaminant of some refined petroleum solvents, especially if the solvent has a boiling range near or encompassing the boiling point of benzene. The extent of this contamination will also vary, depending on the inherent chemical composition of the crude oil and the method of distillation in the refinery. It has been shown that the vapor pressure of benzene in mixtures deviates from Raoult's law and, therefore, the benzene vapor concentration resulting from handling such mixtures frequently will be higher than would be expected from the composition of the solvent. If the benzene content of a solvent ranged from 1% to 4% in volume, ordinary use of the solvent would not produce benzene vapor hazards, but if the concentration of benzene were greater than 5%, the possibility of "substantial" exposure to benzene vapors resulting from "free" use of the solvent must be considered.

Benzene has been recognized as causing serious deleterious effects such as blood dyscrasias in humans and experimental ani-

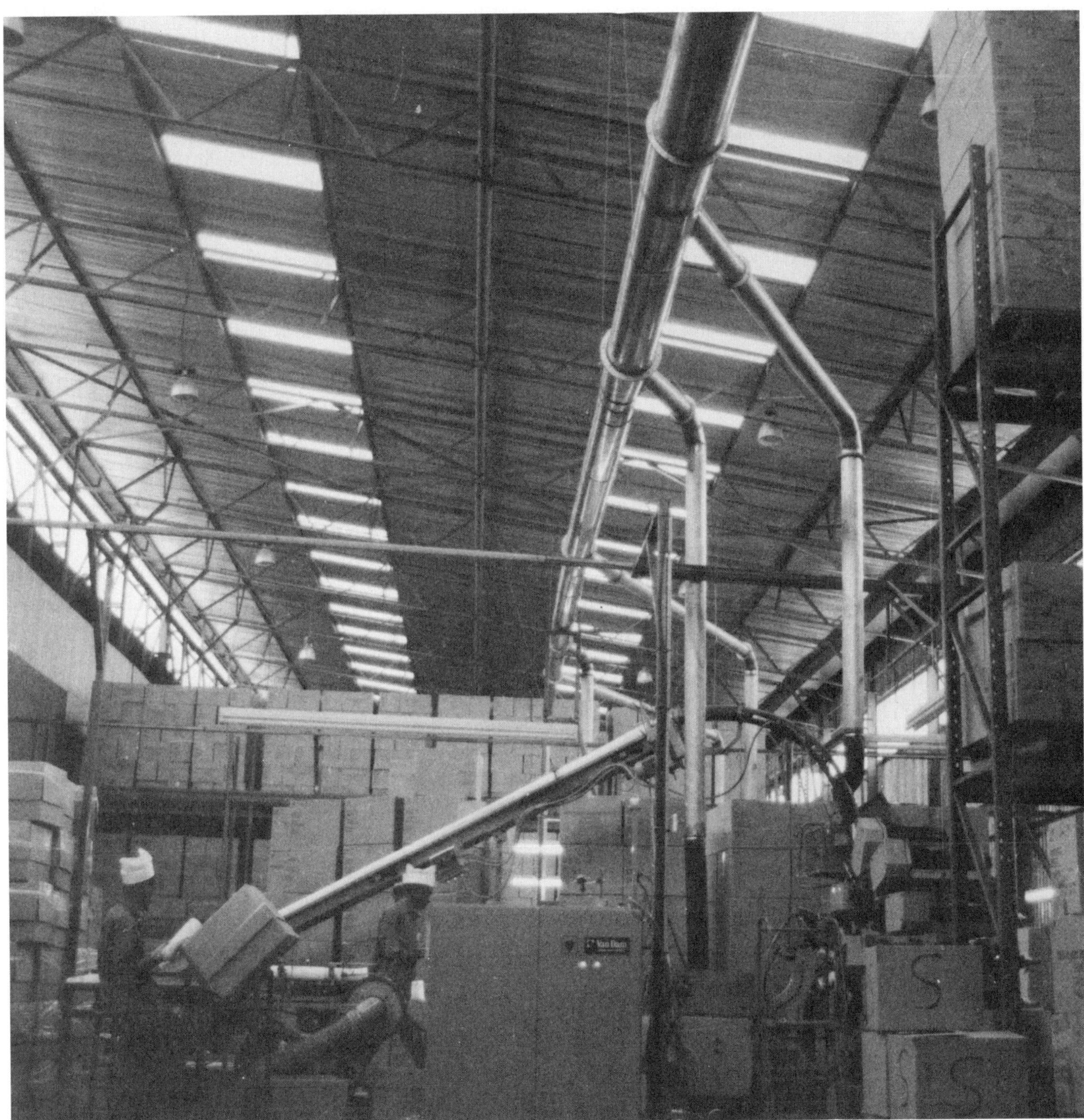

FIG 47–16.
The stainless steel exhaust system to remove any potential excess ozone produced by the ultraviolet printing operation. (Courtesy of Mr. Phil Koekemoer.)

mals, and, in 1974, the NIOSH issued criteria and recommendations for occupational exposure to this compound. Acute poisoning by benzene results primarily from its narcotic action. The inhalation of a high concentration of benzene (i.e., 3,000 ppm for 0.1–1.0 hour) may cause a state of excitation and euphoria (benzol jag), followed by drowsiness, fatigue, vertigo, nausea, and vomiting. With higher concentrations (i.e., 7,500 ppm for 0.5–1.0 hour) or longer exposure times, convulsions followed by paralysis, loss of consciousness and death from respiratory failure may result. The inhalation of small amounts of benzene over long periods has caused blood dyscrasias, including aplastic anemia, leukopenia, and thrombocytopenia. Additional signs and symptoms of chronic toxicity may include headache, dizziness, fatigue, loss of appetite, irritability, nervousness, and nosebleed, and other hemorrhagic manifestations. In 1976, the NIOSH issued an *Update Criteria and Recommendations for a Revised Benzene Standard* and recognized that there now was sufficient evidence to conclude that benzene is leukemogenic. Since benzene causes progressive, malignant diseases of the hematopoietic system, the NIOSH recommended that, for regulatory purposes, benzene should be considered carcinogenic in man and also recommended that the use of benzene as a solvent or diluent in open operations should be prohibited. The NIOSH recommended that occupational exposure be controlled so that no worker will be exposed to benzene in excess of 3.2 mg/cu m (1 ppm) in air as determined by an air sample collected at 1 L/min for two hours.

As a consequence of the toxicity and carcinogenic potential of benzene, the benzene content of a solvent should be determined, and, if it is found to be present, air monitoring should be instituted to ensure compliance with the federal standard.[52]

Stoddard Solvent

Stoddard solvent is a mixture of hydrocarbons, predominantly C9 to C11, that has a boiling range between 160° and 210° C (320°–410° F). Chemically, Stoddard solvent is a mixture of 30%–50% straight and branched chain paraffins, 30%–40% naphthenes, and 10%–20% aromatic hydrocarbons. Although Stoddard solvent and mineral spirits are not always considered the same petroleum products and are used differently for different purposes in industry, their boiling ranges (Stoddard solvent, 160°–210° C; mineral spirits, 150°–200° C) are almost identical and, therefore, their chemical compositions are similar. In fact, many investigators use the terms mineral spirits and Stoddard solvent interchangeably, and some consider Stoddard solvent to be a specific type of mineral spirits. Currently there are four classes of Stoddard solvent: regular Stoddard solvent, 140 flash solvent, odorless solvent, and low end-point solvent. Stoddard solvent, used primarily as a dry cleaning agent, can be produced from a straight-run distillate of paraffinic or mixed base crude. It was reported in 1964 that U.S. industry used 700 million liters of Stoddard solvent. Four liters of Stoddard solvent will clean about 12–16 kg of clothes. It was estimated in 1964 that 55% of the volume of dry cleaning in the United States is carried out in Stoddard solvent. The NIOSH estimates that 75,000 workers in the United States are potentially exposed to Stoddard solvent.

Braunstein[3] reported follicular dermatitis on the hands and arms of a worker after two weeks of dermal exposure to liquid Stoddard solvent. This worker also complained of nausea when initially inhaling the solvent. Eventually, he developed obstructive jaundice and subacute yellow atrophy of the liver.

Scott et al.[41] observed four cases and Prager and Peters[37] one case of aplastic anemia after dermal exposure to liquid Stoddard solvent.

In 1974, Markel and Shmunes[30] cited the results of a Stoddard solvent hazard evaluation of a greeting card company. Workers were exposed to Stoddard solvent at 99–1,906 mg/cu m (average 438 mg/cu m) in their working environment and the authors concluded that, under the conditions found at the time of the survey, Stoddard solvent was not toxic and did not constitute a hazard to health.

In 1974, Larsen and Shmunes[25] found that Stoddard solvent used to clean polishing machines probably was the cause of dermatitis in several industrial workers. These workers also complained of headache and eye and nose irritation. Although Stoddard solvent concentrations of less than 20 ppm (115 mg/cu m) were detected, the authors believed that higher concentrations could have occurred immediately after the polishing machines were cleaned with Stoddard solvent and could have been the cause of the headache and eye and throat irritation.

Carpenter et al.[5] determined both the odor and the sensory thresholds for Stoddard solvent. The odor threshold was found to be between 0.5 and 5.0 mg/cu m (0.09 and 0.9 ppm). The sensory threshold was found to be between 850 and 2,700 mg/cu m (150 and 470 ppm) for a 15-minute exposure. No irritation was noted at 140 mg/cu m (24 ppm) whereas slight, transient eye irritation occurred in one volunteer at 850 mg/cu m and in all at 2,700 mg/cu m, some with tearing. Slight dizziness also was reported at 2,700 mg/cu m by some of the subjects. The volunteers experienced olfactory fatigue at all of the concentrations tested, but recovered fully within ten minutes after exposure ended.

Nelson et al.[34] similarly observed that volunteers exposed to Stoddard solvent for three to five minutes at air concentrations in excess of 400 ppm (2,290 mg/cu m) suffered irritation of the eyes, nose, and throat.

Carpenter et al.[7] described odor threshold sensory irritation in humans exposed to 140 flash aliphatic solvent. The odor threshold was about 4 mg/cu m (0.6 ppm). Minor eye irritation was the only discomfort noted by subjects exposed to 140 flash aliphatic solvent at either 110 or 310 mg/cu m (17 or 47 ppm) for 15 minutes. This response was expressed by the same subjects during each inhalation period and did not persist after exposure. All subjects reported olfactory fatigue at both concentrations. The subjects believed that 310 mg/cu m (49 ppm) could be an acceptable concentration for an eight-hour day.

As mentioned below in the discussion of mineral spirits, dermal exposure to Stoddard solvent has been associated with several cases of aplastic anemia[37, 41] but, from present knowledge concerning benzene-free solvents, this seems unlikely to occur. But the benzene content of Stoddard solvents should be evaluated to ensure that the federal exposure limit for benzene is not exceeded.

Mineral Spirits

Mineral spirits are a mixture of hydrocarbons that have a boiling range of 150°–200° C (302°–392° F). These compounds have also been termed white spirits, petroleum spirits, and light petrol. As mentioned above, Stoddard solvent is considered by some investigators to be synonymous with mineral spirits. Mineral spirits are clear, colorless liquids with a "pleasant sweetish odor" and contain about 30%–65% paraffins, 15%–55% naphthenes and 10%–30% aromatic hydrocarbons. Mineral spirits are used as a general-purpose thinner, a solvent for paint and varnish industries and a dry cleaning agent. The NIOSH estimates that 61,000 workers in the United States are potentially exposed to mineral spirits.

In 1975, Åstrand et al.[2] reported on the effects of white spirits (mineral spirits) on human alveolar air and blood solvent concentrations during rest and exercise. The white spirits used in the study consisted of 83% aliphatic and 17% aromatic compounds. In the initial trials, men were exposed at 2,500 or 5,000 mg/cu m for an unspecified period. Nausea and vertigo were apparent at both concentrations. No differences were noted in heart rate, alveolar ventilation, or oxygen uptake either at rest or during exercise at an intensity of 50 watts during exposure at 1,250 and 2,500 mg/cu m of white spirits. In addition, their studies[2] indicated that more solvent reaches the blood during exercise than during rest. This finding, in the absence of changes in alveolar ventilation, suggests changes in the respiratory transport.

In 1975, Gamberale et al.[14] reported the effects of exposure to white spirits (mineral spirits) on humans. Performance tests were conducted in perceptual speed, reaction time, short-term memory, numerical ability, and manual dexterity. Men exposed to white spirits at 625, 1,250, 1,875 and 2,500 mg/cu m for four continuous 30-minute periods showed no impairment in the five performance tests. Exposure to 4,000 mg/cu m of white spirits for 50 minutes had no effect on perceptual speed, numerical ability, and manual dexterity. There was, however, a definite prolongation of reaction time and a possible impairment of short-term memory as a result of exposure at 4,000 mg/cu m. The authors concluded that there was a risk of subjective distress and adverse effects on psychomotor and intellectual functions in a worker exposed at 2,500 mg/cu m who is doing light industrial work, since the alveolar air concentrations of white spirits in workers at rest exposed at 4,000 mg/cu m were similar to the white spirits alveolar air concentrations of workers exposed at 2,500 mg/cu m engaged in light physical activity.[2, 14]

Since the composition of mineral spirits and Stoddard solvents is similar, it is recommended that dermal exposure to mineral spirits be avoided. The benzene content of mineral spirits should be evaluated to ensure that the federal exposure limit for benzene is not exceeded.

Petroleum Ether

Petroleum ether is a mixture of volatile aliphatic hydrocarbons with a boiling range of about 30°–60° C (86°–104° F). Petroleum ether sometimes is referred to as benzin, benzine, petroleum benzin, canadol, light ligroin, and "Skellysolve." Reference sometimes is made to high-boiling petroleum ether; this terminology is essentially synonymous with ligroin or varnish makers' and painters' naphtha.

Physically, petroleum ether is a clear, colorless, nonfluorescent, volatile liquid. It has a characteristic odor and is highly flammable. Chemically, petroleum ether consists primarily of pentane and isohexane. It typically contains no aromatics. It is a low-boiling fraction obtained from the fractional distillation of petroleum. Petroleum ether is used as a solvent for oils, fats, and waxes; a detergent; a fuel; in paints and varnishes; an insecticide; and in photography.

In 1970, Spruit et al.[42] reported that dermal exposure to petroleum ether caused disruption of the horny layer of the skin in humans. The average time of exposure before the appearance of irritation was about 20 minutes. No other reports have been found concerning the dermal toxicity of petroleum ether, but Oettel[36] conducted a study using pentane and hexane, the major constituents of petroleum ether, to evaluate the toxicity of these compounds and reported in 1936 that dermal exposure to pentane or hexane for up to one hour resulted in the development of irritation in humans characterized by erythema, hyperemia, swelling, and pigmentation. After five hours of exposure, these alkanes produced skin blisters.

Several studies have related industrial exposure to hexane with the development of polyneuropathy.[20, 45, 50, 51] In 1969, Yamamura[51] reported the effects on workers after exposure to hexane, a constituent of the glue used in the production of sandals. The concentration of hexane in the air ranged from 1,759 to 8,793 mg/cu m. The initial symptoms included sensory impairment in the distal portion of the extremities. Inoue et al.,[22] in a follow-up study on the sandal workers, indicated that polyneuropathy could have developed as a result of exposure at concentrations of *n*-hexane below 1,759 mg/cu m. In 1971, Herskowitz et al.[20] examined employees working in a furniture factory who were exposed to *n*-hexane. Air samples of hexane were found to average 2,286 mg/cu m and peaked at 4,573 mg/cu m. The patients complained of one or more of the following symptoms: abdominal cramps, burning sensations, numbness and weakness of the distal extremities, and paresthesia.

In 1972, Yamada[50] investigated 17 workers reporting symptoms of intoxication from exposure to hexane vapor. Six were employed by a pharmaceutical company and used a 95% hexane solution to remove oil from the surface of tablets. The airborne hexane concentration in the center of the workroom was 1,759 mg/cu m, but, in the immediate work area, the concentration was 3,517 mg/cu m. The initial worker complaints were fatigue and loss of appetite, followed by paresthesia in distal parts of the extremities, and difficulty in walking. In 1975, Takeuchi et al.[45] reported on four persons exposed to petroleum benzine who worked in a brocade sash cleaning shop in a poorly ventilated workroom. In general, within one to nine months, the workers experienced fatigue, loss of appetite, difficulties in walking, muscle weakness, paresthesia, irritability, insomnia, and weight loss. Although determination of the air concentrations of petroleum benzine was not made at the time the workers developed their illness, analysis of the concentrations of petroleum benzine and its major constituents in the workroom air was made subsequently. The concentration of petroleum benzine and *n*-hexane did not exceed 4,400 and 844 mg/cu m, respectively. The authors indicated that if the concentration of petroleum benzine rose higher than 4,400 mg/cu m irritation of mucous membranes would have become unbearable and a narcotic effect would have occurred. The effects of dermal exposure were not measured, but such a route could not be disregarded as a potential mode of intoxication. In all the above cases, the authors[20, 22, 40, 50, 51] concluded that the workers had signs and symptoms of polyneuropathy. Gaultier et al.[15] stated that alkanes other than *n*-hexane may also cause polyneuropathy.

In 1967, Miyagaki[32] reported the neurotoxic effects of *n*-hexane exposure in mice. The animals exposed at *n*-hexane concentrations greater than 879 mg/cu m for 24 hours per day, six days per week for one year developed signs of neurotoxicity whereas mice similarly exposed at 352 mg/cu m of hexane showed no abnormalities.

Truhaut et al.[47] exposed rats to a technical grade of hexane at a concentration of 2,000 ppm, five hours per day, five days per week for one to six months. The hexane contained 0.3% *n*-pentane, 25.1% 2-methylpentane plus cyclopentane, 18.4% 3-methylpentane, 48.8% *n*-hexane, 8% methylcyclopentane, 1.2% methylhexane and 1.2% benzene. Studies on the sciatic and saphenous nerves indicated that this solvent caused a decrease in the conduction rate, an increase in the refractory period, and a decrease in the excitability of the nerves.

The TWA concentration limit for all C5–C8 alkanes recommended by the NIOSH is 350 mg/cu m; the NIOSH also recommends that a TWA concentration for petroleum ether, a mixture of 80% *n*-pentane and 20% isohexane, be set at 350 mg/cu m. This recommended standard assumes additive toxic effects between hexane and pentane, which is a premise consistent with data and analysis presented in the NIOSH criteria document on alkanes.[11]

Kerosene

Kerosene is a mixture of petroleum hydrocarbons, with carbon chain lengths that range from C9 to C16 carbon atoms per molecule, and distills between 175° and 325° C (347°–617° F). Synonyms for kerosene include astral oil, coal oil, and No. 1 fuel oil. Physically, kerosene usually is a pale yellow or water-white, mobile, low volatile, oily liquid that has a flashpoint (closed cup) of about 38°–74° C (100°–165° F) and therefore is considered a combustible compound. The composition of kerosene varies, depending on the source of crude oil and the method of refining. Kerosene is a complex mixture of aliphatic, naphthenic, and alkylated aromatic hydrocarbons. A typical analysis of kerosene indicates that there are about 25% normal paraffins, 12% branched paraffins, 30% monocycloparaffins, 12% dicycloparaffins, 1% tricycloparaffins, 16% mononuclear aromatics, and 5% dinuclear aromatics. The aromatic content of kerosene ranges from 5% to 20%. The predominant aromatic molecular types include indenes, diphenyls, methylnaphthalenes, and tetralins. Additional chemical and physical properties of kerosene are given in the NIOSH criteria document.[12]

Kerosene can be produced in a refinery using a straight-run-treated distillate from paraffinic or mixed crude, a solvent-treated distillate from paraffinic or mixed crude or a solvent-treated distillate from aromatic crude. Deodorized kerosene (washed with fuming sulfuric acid, followed by a sodium plumbite solution and sulfur) is a highly refined product of low aromatic content, often used in insect sprays.

Kerosene is used as a fuel, as a carrier for pesticides, as a weed-killer, as a mold-release agent in the ceramic and pottery industry, as a cleaning solvent, and in asphalt coatings, enamels, paints, thinners and varnishes. In 1975, the United States produced 55,673,000 barrels of kerosene. The NIOSH estimates that 310,000 workers in the United States are potentially exposed to kerosene.

Several investigators have shown that kerosene can cause dermatitis.[13, 40, 44] In addition, several studies have examined the mechanism of action of the kerosene-induced skin irritation.[26, 28, 29]

In 1955, Johnson[23] investigated a presumable sensitivity of a person to kerosene. The patient developed hypoplastic anemia with a deficiency of all cell elements and hypoplastic marrow after recurrent exposure to kerosene for a three-year period. The author suggested, however, that aromatic hydrocarbons of the benzol series present in kerosene may have been responsible for the myelotoxicity in this individual.

Hiebel et al.[21] observed bone marrow depression after dermal exposure to kerosene in one patient and by a combination of dermal and oral routes in two patients.

In 1946, Carpenter and Smyth[9] related that the application of 0.5 ml of deodorized kerosene into the eye of rabbits produced no adverse effects. However, Volkova et al.[48] found that animals exposed to unpurified kerosene in an aerosol developed conjunctivitis.

In 1969, Volkova et al.[48] noted that aerosols of purified kerosene were less toxic than aerosols of unpurified kerosene. Exposure to unpurified kerosene at 500 mg/cu m caused respiratory irritation and leukocytosis.

In 1976, Carpenter et al.[8] determined the odor and sensory thresholds for deodorized kerosene determined in a group of volunteers. The odor threshold was approximately 0.6 mg/cu m (0.09 ppm). Fifteen-minute exposures to kerosene at a mean measured vapor concentration of 140 mg/cu m (20 ppm) were easily tolerated without sensory irritation. A slight decrease in olfactory acuity, but not total fatigue, was noted in two subjects. The 140 mg/cu m concentration of deodorized kerosene was deemed by the subjects to be acceptable for an eight-hour workday, based on the 15-minute exposure.

Light petroleum hydrocarbons, such as kerosene, have a low toxicity when ingested and retained in the stomach, but if the solvent is aspirated directly into the lungs, extensive lung damage and death can occur.[18] Several investigators[17, 18, 40, 43] have reported that 0.1–0.2 ml of kerosene administered into the trachea can cause death. In addition, there are numerous cases of kerosene poisoning in humans by aspiration or ingestion of the liquid.[31, 35, 36] There is no present reason for suggesting that these solvents, if they are free from carcinogenic aromatics such as benzene, would cause cancer, birth defects, or germinal mutations.

Kerosene has been shown to cause skin irritation[8, 13, 24, 29, 44] and possibly bone marrow depression,[10, 21, 23] probably from benzene absorption,[10, 23] after dermal exposure. Therefore, when this substance is used, care must be taken to prevent dermal exposure. Thirty minutes of dermal kerosene exposure has caused changes in skin structure.[29] The skin has developed a burning sensation during the first hour of kerosene exposure, erythema by the second hour, and blister formation by the twelfth hour.[27] A solution of 40% kerosene has been shown to be innocuous to the human skin, but 55%, 70%, and 85% kerosene solutions caused dermatitis in 24%, 85%, and 100% of volunteers, respectively.[44] Naphthenic-type kerosene has a greater skin-irritating potential than paraffinic-type kerosene.[24] Kerosene has also been shown to augment the toxicity of a skin-sensitizing agent.[38] Thus, it is possible that other sensitizing agents that may come into contact with the worker's skin may heighten the response to dermal kerosene exposure. Kerosene never should be ingested, since, in addition to its oral toxicity,[33] aspiration can occur and result in pneumonitis and possibly death.[1, 16, 17, 19, 46, 49] The benzene content of the kerosene also should be evaluated to ensure that federal exposure limits are not exceeded.

Varnish Makers' and Painters' Naphtha

Varnish makers' and painters' (VM and P) naphtha is a mixture of hydrocarbons that has a boiling range of approximately 95°–

160° C (203°–320° F). Sometimes it is known as benzine, Naphtha 76, ligroin, or high-boiling petroleum ether. Physically, VM and P naphtha is a colorless to yellow liquid that has an aromatic odor and it is composed of about 45%–60% paraffins, 30%–45% naphthenes, and 5%–13% aromatics. A sample of VM and P naphtha showed 55% paraffins, 30% monocycloparaffins, 2% dicycloparaffins, and 12% alkylbenzenes. It is used as a quick-evaporating paint thinner of moderate solvent power. The NIOSH estimates that about 600,000 workers in the United States are potentially exposed to all "specialized" naphthas.

Carpenter et al.[4] reported the effects of exposure to VM and P naphtha on human odor and sensory responses. The authors concluded that the odor threshold was about 5 mg/cu m (0.86 ppm). In assessing the sensory responses to VM and P naphtha, Carpenter et al. subjected volunteers to 15-minute exposures to the naphtha at concentrations ranging from 660 to 4,100 mg/cu m (140–880 ppm). Olfactory fatigue was noted at all concentrations. Solvent concentrations up to 2,100 mg/cu m (450 ppm) caused only slight or transitory eye and throat irritation in two of seven subjects, which the authors considered "sporadic sensory responses." At the highest concentration tested, 4,100 mg/cu m (880 ppm), definite throat and eye irritation was produced.

Since C5–C8 alkanes, Stoddard solvent, and mineral spirits are primary irritants,[3, 11, 25] VM and P naphtha, whose boiling range overlaps the ranges of these solvents, has solvent properties similar to these other solvents. VM and P naphtha is, accordingly, also considered to be a dermal irritant. Thus, contact of the skin as well as the eyes should be avoided. The benzene content of VM and P naphtha should be evaluated to ensure that federal exposure limits are not exceeded.

Rubber Solvent

Rubber solvent is a mixture of hydrocarbons that boils in the range of 45°–125° C (113–257° F). This solvent sometimes is referred to as benzene and lacquer diluent.

Physically, rubber solvent usually is a clear, colorless liquid and is less volatile than petroleum ether. Rubber solvent is primarily a mixture of paraffins (chiefly C5–C8) and aromatics. The actual composition will vary, depending on the boiling range, the refinery stocks from which the solvent is produced, and the method of preparation. In general, rubber solvent has 70%–90% paraffins, 11%–22% naphthenes, and 9%–22% aromatics. Rubber solvent can be produced from a straight-run petroleum distillate of paraffin base crude. It is used as a rubber cement diluent and as an agent in rubber dope mixing and rubber spreading. In 1965, the United States produced 28,857,000 barrels (1 barrel = 159 L or 42 gal) of what was described as special naphthas (including rubber solvent and varnish makers' and painters' naphtha), which represented 0.7% of the total production of petroleum products and, in 1975, 27,325,000 barrels of naphthas.

The NIOSH estimates that about 600,000 workers in the United States are potentially exposed to all "specialized" naphthas.

Carpenter et al.[6] exposed volunteers for about ten seconds to rubber solvent vapor to determine its odor threshold. The authors concluded that the most probable threshold concentration was about 40 mg/cu m (10 ppm) given the determined range of 6.4–64 mg/cu m (1.6–16 ppm). Volunteers were also exposed to rubber solvent vapor at one of a series of concentrations from 1,700 to 8,100 mg/cu m (430–2,000 ppm) for one 15-minute period per day. Slight transitory eye, nose and throat irritation responses were noted at concentrations of 3,100 mg/cu m (780 ppm) and above, as well as four cases of light-headedness and one of headache at the 8,100 mg/cu m concentration, both of which were reported to have subsided within ten minutes after exposure. At the 3,100 mg/cu m concentration, one volunteer reported eye irritation and two others throat irritation. One of six exposed to rubber solvent at 8,100 mg/cu m reported eye and throat irritation.

The authors[6] also reported the toxic effects of rubber solvent inhalation in animal toxicity studies. Groups of rats were exposed at 11,000, 21,000, 39,000, or 96,000 mg/cu m (2,800, 5,300, 9,800, or 24,200 ppm) for a single four-hour period. Impairment of coordination and eye irritation were observed at concentrations greater than 11,000 mg/cu m. Convulsions and death occurred at 96,000 mg/cu m. The calculated four hour LC_{50} was reported to be 61,000 mg/cu m (15,000 ppm). Female beagles were exposed to rubber solvent vapors at concentrations of 5,900, 12,000 or 25,000 mg/cu m (1,500, 3,300, or 6,300 ppm) for a single four-hour period. Loss of coordination was observed at concentrations of 13,000 and 25,000 mg/cu m. No observable effects occurred at 5,900 mg/cu m.

The acute CNS effects of a four-hour exposure to rubber solvent vapors at 49,000 mg/cu m (12,400 ppm) were examined in male cats.[6] A time-related and sequential pattern of events occurred that included ataxia, loss of proprioception, salivation, relaxation of the nictitating membrane, unconsciousness, tremors, and convulsions. Gross and microscopic examination of tissues showed no lesions related to solvent exposure.

Male rats and beagles were exposed to either 0, 1,900, 3,700, or 7,900 mg/cu m (0, 480, 930, or 2,000 ppm) of rubber solvent six hours per day, five days per week for up to 62–63 days.[6] There were no animal deaths attributed to rubber solvent. There were no changes in body weight gain, blood chemistry, or hematology that resulted from exposure to the solvent. Serum alkaline phosphatase was higher after 62 days in all rats exposed to rubber solvent, but the authors suggested that this finding was an artifact that resulted from very low control alkaline phosphatase levels. Microscopic examination of various organ sections showed no tissue damage that could be attributed to the solvent vapors. There was a significant increase in the specific gravity of the urine of dogs exposed at 7,900 mg/cu m for 62 days. The significance was not reported by the investigators.

Although no specific data on the dermal effects of rubber solvent have been found, alkanes and solvents that boil below 232° C (450° F) are known to be primary irritants[11, 21] and, therefore, rubber solvent should be considered to be a dermal irritant. Dermal exposure to this solvent, therefore, should be minimized. The benzene content of rubber solvent should be evaluated to ensure that the federal exposure limit for benzene is not exceeded.

General Control Measures

It is recommended that 350 mg/cu m be adopted as a TWA concentration limit for up to a ten-hour work shift in a 40-hour workweek for petroleum ether, rubber solvent, varnish makers' and painters' naphtha, mineral spirits, and Stoddard solvent. On a volume/volume basis, these concentrations are equal to about 114 ppm for petroleum ether, 88 ppm for rubber solvent, 75 ppm for varnish makers' and painters' naphtha, 55 ppm for mineral spirits, and 59 ppm for Stoddard solvent. The recommended TWA concentration limit for kerosenes is 100 mg/cu m (about 14 ppm). In addition, a ceiling concentration limit of 1,800 mg/cu m (about 590 ppm of petroleum ether, 454 ppm of rubber solvent, 386 ppm of varnish makers' and painters' naphtha, 282 ppm of mineral spirits, and 306 ppm of Stoddard solvent), based on a sample collection period of 15 minutes, is recommended to protect workers from short-term exposures that might cause effects, such as vertigo or other adverse reactions, that could result in accidents. No ceiling limit is believed needed for kerosene.

It is recognized that many workers handle small amounts of petroleum ether, rubber solvent, varnish makers' and painters' naphtha, Stoddard solvent, mineral spirits, and kerosene or work in situations where, regardless of the amount used, there is only negligible contact with these substances. Under these conditions, it should not be necessary to comply with many of the provisions of these recommended standards, which have been prepared primarily to protect workers' health under more hazardous circumstances. Concern for the workers' health requires that protective measures be instituted below the enforceable limit to ensure that exposures stay below that limit. For these reasons, an action level for petroleum ether, rubber solvent, and varnish makers' and painters' naphtha has been defined as 200 mg/cu m (about 66 ppm for petroleum ether, 50 ppm for rubber solvent, and 43 ppm for varnish makers' and painters' naphtha), thereby delineating those work situations that do not require the expenditure of health resources for environmental and medical monitoring and associated record keeping. The action levels for Stoddard solvent, mineral spirits, and kerosene are identical to the TWA concentration for these solvents because of the lower volatility of these solvents and the lower likelihood of developing toxicity. The action levels have been chosen on the basis of professional judgment rather than on quantitative data that delineate nonhazardous areas from areas in which a hazard may exist. Because of nonrespiratory hazards such as those resulting from skin or eye contact or from ingestion of petroleum ether, rubber solvent, varnish makers' and painters' naphtha, mineral spirits, Stoddard solvent, and kerosene, it is recommended that appropriate work practices and protective measures be required regardless of the air concentration.

REFERENCES

1. Albert WC, Inkley SR: The efficacy of steroid therapy in the treatment of experimental kerosene pneumonitis. *Am Rev Respir Dis* 1968; 98:888.
2. Åstrand I, Kilbom A, Övrum P: Exposure to white spirit. I. Concentration in alveolar air and blood during rest and exercise. *Scand J Work Environ Health* 1976; 1:15.
3. Braunstein LE: Subacute yellow atrophy of the liver due to solvent. *JAMA* 1940; 114:136.
4. Carpenter CP, et al: Petroleum hydrocarbon toxicity studies. II. Animal and human response to vapors of varnish makers' and painters' naphtha. *Toxicol Appl Pharmacol* 1975; 32:263.
5. Carpenter CP, et al: Petroleum hydrocarbon toxicity studies. III. Animal and human response to vapors of Stoddard solvent. *Toxicol Appl Pharmacol* 1975; 32:282.
6. Carpenter CP, et al: Petroleum hydrocarbon toxicity studies. IV. Animal and human response to vapors of rubber solvent. *Toxicol Appl Pharmacol* 1975; 33:526.
7. Carpenter CP, et al: Petroleum hydrocarbon toxicity studies. VIII. Animal and human response to vapors of 140 flash aliphatic solvent. *Toxicol Appl Pharmacol* 1975; 34:413.
8. Carpenter CP, et al: Petroleum hydrocarbon toxicity studies. XI. Animal and human response to vapors of deodorized kerosene. *Toxicol Appl Pharmacol* 1976; 36:443.
9. Carpenter CP, Smyth HF: Chemical burns of the rabbit cornea. *Am J Ophthalmol* 1946; 29:1363.
10. Cavanagh JR, Wilner PR: Aplastic anemia due to kerosene. *M Ann DC* 1939; 8:140.
11. *Criteria for a Recommended Standard: Occupational Exposure to Alkanes (C5-C8)*. US Dept. of Health, Education and Welfare, PHS, Center for Disease Control, National Institute for Occupational Safety and Health, 1978.
12. *Criteria for a Recommended Standard: Occupational Exposure to Refined Petroleum Solvents*. DHEW (NIOSH) Publ 77-192. Cincinnati, Oh, US Dept of Health, Education, and Welfare, PHS, Center for Disease Control, National Institute for Occupational Safety and Health, 247, 1977.
13. Deichmann WB, Kitzmiller KV, Witherup S, et al: Kerosene intoxication. *Ann Intern Med* 1944; 21:803.
14. Gamberale F, Annwall G, Hultengren M: Exposure to white spirit. II. Psychological functions. *Scand J Work Environ Health* 1976; 1:31.
15. Gaultier M, Rancurel G, Piva C, et al: Polyneuritis and aliphatic hydrocarbons. *J Eur Toxicol* 1973; 6:294 (French).
16. Gerarde HW: Kerosine. Experimental and clinical toxicology. *Occup Health Rev* 1964; 16:17.
17. Gerarde HW: Toxicological studies on hydrocarbons. IX. The aspiration hazard and toxicity of hydrocarbons and hydrocarbon mixtures. *Arch Environ Health* 1963; 6:329.
18. Gerarde HW, Eckardt RE: Aspiration hazards of petroleum products, in XIVth International Congress of Occupational Health, Madrid, Spain, Sept 16–21, 1963. International Congress Series No. 62. New York, Excerpta Medica Foundation, 1964, vol. II, pp 723–727.
19. Gross P, McNerney JM, Babyak MA: Kerosene pneumonitis. An experimental study with small doses. *Am Rev Respir Dis* 1963; 88:656.
20. Herskowitz A, Ishii N, Schaumburg H: *N*-hexane neuropathy. A syndrome occurring as a result of industrial exposure. *N Engl J Med* 1971; 285:82.
21. Hiebel J, Gant HL, Schwartz SO, et al: Bone marrow depression following exposure to kerosene. A report of 3 cases. *Am J Med Sci* 1963; 246:91.
22. Inoue T, et al: Industrial health survey of high incidence of *n*-hexane intoxication among vinyl sandal manufacturers. *Jpn J Ind Health* 1970; 12:73 (Japanese).
23. Johnson DE: Hypoplastic anemia following chronic exposure to kerosene. *J Am Med Wom Assoc* 1955; 10:421.
24. Klauder JV, Brill FA: Correlation of boiling ranges of some petroleum solvents with irritant action on skin. *Arch Dermatol Syphilol* 1947; 56:197.
25. Larsen LB, Shmunes E: Occupational health case report, No. 6—Stoddard solvent. *J Occup Med* 1974; 16:276.
26. Lupulescu AP, Birmingham DJ: Effect of lipid solvents on protein, DNA, and collagen synthesis in human skin. An electron microscopic autoradiographic study. *J Invest Dermatol* 1975; 65:419.
27. Lupulescu AP, Birmingham DJ: Effect of protective agent against lipid-solvent-induced damages. Ultrastructural and scanning electron microscopical study of human epidermis. *Arch Environ Health* 1976; 31:33.

28. Lupulescu A, Birmingham D, Habowski J et al: Electron microscopic autoradiography of 3H-kerosene in human epidermis. *J Cell Biol* 1973; 59:204A.
29. Lupulescu AP, Birmingham DJ, Pinkus H: An electron microscopic study of human epidermis after acetone and kerosene administration. *J Invest Dermatol* 1973; 60:33.
30. Markel HL, Shmunes E: *Health Hazard Evaluation,* Report 72-33-129 (Barker Greeting Card Co). Cincinnati, Oh, US Dept of Health, Education, and Welfare, National Institute for Occupational Safety and Health, Hazard Evaluation Services Branch, 15 pp, 1974.
31. McNally WD: Kerosene poisoning in children. A study of 204 cases. *J Pediatr* 1956; 48:296.
32. Miyagaki H: Electrophysiological studies of the peripheral neurotoxicity of *n*-hexane. *Jpn J Ind Health* 1967; 9:660 (Japanese).
33. Narasimhan MJ Jr, Ganla VG: Experimental studies on kerosene poisoning. *Acta Pharmacol Toxicol* 1967; 25:214.
34. Nelson KW, et al: Sensory response to certain industrial solvent vapors. *J Ind Hyg Toxicol* 1943; 25:282.
35. Nunn JA, Martin FM: Gasoline and kerosene poisoning in children. *JAMA* 1934; 103:472.
36. Oettel H: Effect of organic liquids on the skin. *Arch Exp Pathol Pharmakol* 1936; 83:641, 649, 693 (German).
37. Prager D, Peters C: Development of aplastic anemia and the exposure to Stoddard solvent. *Blood* 1970; 35:286.
38. Rebello JA, Suskind RR: The effect of common contactants of cutaneous reactivity to sensitizers. *J Invest Dermatol* 1963; 41:67.
39. Rector DE, Steadman BL, Jones RA, et al: Effects on experimental animals of long-term inhalation exposure to mineral spirits. *Toxicol Appl Pharmacol* 1966; 9:257.
40. Schwartz SI, Breslau RC, Kutner F, et al: Effects of drugs and hyperbaric oxygen environment on experimental kerosene pneumonitis. *Dis Chest* 1965; 47:353.
41. Scott JL, Cartwright GE, Wintrobe MM: Acquired aplastic anemia. An analysis of thirty-nine cases and review of the pertinent literature. *Medicine* 1959; 38:119.
41a. *Selected Petroleum Products: Environmental Health Criteria* 20. Geneva, World Health Organization, 1982.
42. Spruit D, Malten KE, Lipmann EWRM: Horny layer injury by solvents. II. Can the irritancy of petroleum ether be diminished by pretreatment?, *Berufs-Dermatosen* 1970; 18:269.
43. Steele RW, Conklin RH, Mark HM: Corticosteroids and antibiotics for the treatment of fulminant hydrocarbon aspiration. *JAMA* 1972; 219:1434.
44. Tagami H, Ogino A: Kerosene dermatitis. *Dermatologica* 1973; 146:123.
45. Takeuchi Y, Mabuchi C, Takagi S: Polyneuropathy caused by petroleum benzine. *Int Arch Arbeitsmed* 1975; 34:185.
46. Truffa O, Montalenti P: Acute pneumopathy and icterus from accidental ingestion of kerosene. *Minerva Med* 1969; 60:1403 (Italian).
47. Truhaut R, et al: Preliminary electrophysiologic results following experimental poisoning with technical hexane and heptane in white rats. *Arch Mal Prof* 1973; 34:417 (French).
48. Volkova AP, Tsetlin VM, Zhuk EB, et al: Toxicity of kerosene as a solvent used in aerosol cylinders. *Gig Sanit* 1969; 34:24 (Russian).
49. Wolfsdorf J, Kundig H: Kerosene poisoning in primates. *S Afr Med J* 1972; 46:619.
50. Yamada S: Polyneuritis in workers exposed to *n*-hexane, its cause and symptoms. *Jpn J Ind Health* 1972; 9:651 (Japanese).
51. Yamamura Y: *N*-hexane polyneuropathy. *Folia Psychiatr Neurol Jpn* 1969; 23:45.
52. Zenz C: Benzene—attempts to establish a lower exposure standard in the United States. A review. *Scand J Work Environ Health* 1978; 4:103.

PHOSGENE

$COCl_2$

This highly toxic substance can be found as gaseous or liquefied phosgene, with inhalation as the main route of exposure; it also is highly irritating to skin. Synonyms for phosgene include carbonyl chloride, carbon oxychloride, chloroformyl chloride and CG (designation used by military agencies).

Phosgene, originally known as a war gas during World War I, today is used primarily as a chemical intermediate in the manufacture of isocyanates. In the United States, more than 300 million kg are produced, with approximately 85% of this used in isocyanate manufacture, most isocyanate manufacturers producing phosgene for their own use. The NIOSH estimated that 10,000 workers have potential occupational exposure to phosgene during its manufacture and use. Also, phosgene can be formed by the decomposition of chlorinated hydrocarbons when these compounds are exposed to heat or ultraviolet radiation.

Phosgene gas is a severe respiratory irritant, and skin contact with the liquid may cause severe burns. In concentrations of 1–2 ppm, phosgene causes eye discomfort, and at higher concentrations, lacrimation and conjunctivitis can produce severe eye irritation. Three ppm is thought to be the least concentration capable of causing immediate irritation to the human throat; 4 ppm causes immediate irritation of the eyes; 4.8 ppm causes cough, and even brief exposure to 50 ppm may prove rapidly fatal. With moderate exposure, the presenting symptoms often are a dryness or a burning sensation in the throat, vomiting, pain in the chest, and dyspnea. The onset of symptoms of severe respiratory distress may be delayed for up to 72 hours, the latent interval depending on the concentration and duration of exposure. Delayed onset of pulmonary edema is characterized by cough, abundant "foamy" sputum, progressive dyspnea, and severe cyanosis. Pulmonary edema may progress to pneumonia, and cardiac failure may intervene.

Because of the often-delayed onset of symptoms following potentially lethal exposures to phosgene, education of employees and medical observation following suspected overexposures are extremely important. Medical examinations, including pulmonary function tests, are necessary to evaluate recovery from overexposure and to detect chronic lung changes.

In case of known or suspected overexposure to phosgene, first-aid measures must be taken immediately, followed by prompt medical evaluation and care. Overexposed persons should not be permitted unnecessary physical exertion and should be carried to a vehicle to receive medical assistance. Pressurized oxygen and attendants trained in its use shall be available in the event that they are needed for persons in respiratory distress. In case of skin or eye contact with liquid phosgene, contaminated clothing must be removed quickly and the exposed body areas flushed with copious amounts of water. Because of the often-delayed onset of symptoms following overexposure to phosgene, surveillance or monitoring of the patient by a physician or by trained paramedical personnel is required for the 24-hour period following overexposure. A posteroanterior chest film should be taken in each instance of known or suspected overexposure to phosgene for comparison with preplacement chest films. Pulmonary function tests may be useful during convalescence.

Occupational exposure to phosgene shall be controlled so that no worker is exposed to phosgene at a concentration greater than one-tenth part phosgene per million parts of air (0.1 ppm) determined as a TWA concentration for up to a ten-hour workday, 40-hour workweek, or to more than two-tenths part phosgene per million parts of air (0.2 ppm) as a ceiling concentration for any 15-minute period.

REFERENCE

1. NIOSH: *A Recommended Standard for Occupational Exposure to Phosgene.* Cincinnati, Oh, US Dept of Health, Education, and Welfare, PHS, Center for Disease Control, National Institute for Occupational Safety and Health, Robert A. Taft Laboratories, 1976.

PHOSPHORUS (YELLOW) AND SOME PHOSPHORUS COMPOUNDS

Yellow Phosphorus

P

Yellow phosphorus, also known as white phosphorus, WP, phosphorus, or elemental phosphorus, is a white to yellow, soft, waxy solid which gives off acrid fumes on exposure to air.

Yellow phosphorus finds use in the synthesis of high-purity phosphoric acid salts for use as fertilizers, water treatment chemicals, food products, beverages, and dentifrices. It is used in the synthesis of inorganic phosphorus compounds for use as pesticides, flame retardants for plastics and fibers, and gasoline and lube oil additives and in the synthesis of inorganic and organic compounds. Yellow phosphorus is used in the manufacture of phosphorus alloys for introduction into low-carbon steel, copper alloys, copper pipe, and bronze, and in the manufacture of explosives, munitions, and pyrotechnics for military use. It serves as a catalyst in the synthesis of acrylonitrile and organic bromine compounds. Yellow phosphorus is converted to red phosphorus for the manufacture of wood and paper safety matches and it has been used as an ingredient in rat poison and roach powders.

Toxicology.—Yellow phosphorus spontaneously burns in air, and the vapors released are irritating to the respiratory tract. Yellow phosphorus fume irritates the respiratory tract and eyes. Solid phosphorus in contact with the skin produces deep thermal burns. Prolonged absorption of phosphorus causes necrosis of facial bones. The early signs of systemic intoxication by phosphorus are abdominal pain, jaundice, and a garlic odor of the breath. Prolonged intake may cause anemia, cachexia, and necrosis of the bone, typically of the maxilla and mandible. Complaints of possible overexposure among phosphorus workers may be toothache and excessive salivation. There may be dull red appearance of the oral mucosa. One or more teeth may loosen, followed by pain and swelling of the jaw; healing may be delayed following dental procedures such as extractions. With necrosis of bone, sequestra may develop with sinus tract formation. In a series of ten cases, the shortest period of exposure to phosphorus fume leading to bone necrosis was ten months (two cases) and the longest was 18 years. Yellow phosphorus fume causes severe eye irritation, with blepharospasm, photophobia, and lacrimation; the solid in the eye produces severe injury. Phosphorus burns on the skin are deep and painful; a firm eschar is produced and is surrounded by vesiculation.

Permissible Exposure Limit.—The current OSHA standard for phosphorus (yellow) is 0.1 mg/cu m averaged over an eight-hour work shift.

REFERENCES

1. Hughes, JPW, et al: Phosphorus necrosis of the jaw: A present-day study. *Br J Ind Med* 1962; 19:83–99.
2. Hunter D: *Diseases of Occupations*, ed 4. Boston, Little, Brown & Co, 1969.
3. *Hygienic Information Guide No. 62 - Phosphorus (Yellow)*. Commonwealth of Pennsylvania, Department of Environmental Resources, Bureau of Occupational Health, 1969.
4. International Labour Office: *Encyclopedia of Occupational Health and Safety*, ed 3. Geneva, 1983.
5. Manufacturing Chemists Association, Inc: *Chemical Safety Data Sheet SD-16, Phosphorus (Elemental)*. Washington, DC, MCA, 1947.
6. Rubitsky H, Myerson RM: Acute phosphorus poisoning. *Arch Intern Med* 1949; 83:164–178.
7. Summerlin WT, et al: White phosphorus burns and massive hemolysis. *J Trauma* 1967; 7:476–484.

Phosphoric Acid

H_3PO_4

Phosphoric acid, also known as white phosphoric acid, orthophosphoric acid, 85% phosphoric acid, or meta-phosphoric acid, is a viscous, colorless, odorless liquid which can solidify at temperatures below 21° C (70° F).

Phosphoric acid is used in the manufacture of aluminum products in bright dipping operations, and in cleaning, electropolishing, and pickling in the manufacture of steel, brass, bronze, and copper. Phosphoric acid is used during surface treatment and rust-proofing operations, in the synthesis of intermediates in the manufacture of soil fertilizers, in the manufacture of livestock and poultry feed, and for synthesis of detergent and soap builders and water-treatment chemicals. It is an acidulant and flavor agent in the manufacture of carbonated beverages and jellies and preserves and in the manufacture of food products, intermediates, food additives. It is an antioxidant and preservative and is used in wood, textile, and polyurethane foam flame-retardant processing and production of flame-retardant agents. Phosphoric acid is used to make cleaning preparations and disinfectants, and it is a bonding agent in the manufacture of refactory bricks. It is used during lithography and photoengraving operations and as a catalyst in the synthesis of other chemicals. Phosphoric acid plays a role in the synthesis of textile and leather processing chemicals, clays, ceramics, cements, and clay-thinning agents for drilling mud formulations and in the synthesis of pharmaceuticals and pharmaceutical intermediates and in the extraction of penicillin. Phosphoric acid is used to make opal glass, dental cements, dentifrice adhesives, adhesive gums, synthetic rubber, and electric lights.

Toxicology.—Phosphoric acid mist is an irritant to the eyes, upper respiratory tract, and skin. The solid is especially irritating to skin in the presence of moisture. Unacclimated workers could not endure exposure to fumes of phosphorus pentoxide (the anhydride of phosphoric acid) at a concentration of 100 mg/cu m; exposure to concentrations between 3.6 and 11.3 mg/cu m produced coughing. Concentrations of 0.8 to 5.4 mg/cu m were noticeable but not uncomfortable. There is no evidence that phosphorus poisoning can result from contact with phosphoric acid. The risk of pulmonary edema resulting from the inhalation of mist or spray is remote. A dilute solution buffered to pH 2.5 caused a moderate, brief stinging sensation but no injury when dropped in the human eye. A 75% solution will cause severe skin burns.

Permissible Exposure Limit.—The current OSHA standard for phosphoric acid is 1 mg/cu m averaged over an eight-hour work shift.

REFERENCES

1. *Hygienic Guide Series*: Phosphoric acid. Akron, Oh, American Industrial Hygiene Association, 1978.
2. Grant WM: *Toxicology of the Eye*, ed 2. Springfield, Ill, Charles C Thomas, 1974.
3. Manufacturing Chemists Association, Inc: *Chemical Safety Data Sheet SD-70, Phosphoric Acid*. Washington DC, MCA, 1958.

Phosphorus Pentachloride

PCl_5

Phosphorus pentachloride is a pale yellow solid with an odor like hydrochloric acid. It is used as a chlorinating agent in organic synthesis or as a chemical reactant for aryl or alkyl acids and salts, ketones, and aldehydes. It is used in the synthesis of phosphorus compounds and as a catalyst in organic synthesis in the production of polyethylene from ethylene.

Toxicology.—Phosphorus pentachloride fume is a severe irritant of the eyes and mucous membranes. Exposure of mice to 120 ppm for ten minutes was fatal. In human beings, the fume causes irritation of the eyes and respiratory tract, and cases of bronchitis have resulted from exposure. Although it has not been reported, delayed onset of pulmonary edema may occur. The material on the skin could be expected to cause dermatitis.

Permissible Exposure Limit.—The current OSHA standard for phosphorus pentachloride is 1 mg/cu m averaged over an eight-hour work shift.

REFERENCE

1. American Conference of Governmental Industrial Hygienists: Phosphorus pentachloride. *Documentation of the Threshold Limit Values for Substances in Workroom Air*, ed 5. Cincinnati, Oh, ACGIH, 1986.

Phosphorus Pentasulfide

P_2S_5 or P_4S_{10}

Phosphorus pentasulfide is also known as phosphorus persulfide, regular phosphorus pentasulfide, reactive phosphorus pentasulfide, distilled phosphorus pentasulfide, and undistilled phosphorus pentasulfide.

It is a greenish-yellow solid with the odor of rotten eggs and is used in the preparation of lubrication oil additives for low-lead gas and the reduction of air pollution.

Toxicology.—Phosphorus pentasulfide dust irritates the eyes and skin. Since it is readily converted in the presence of moisture to hydrogen sulfide gas and phosphoric acid, its inhalation toxicology is based on hydrogen sulfide. The latter is a rapidly acting systemic poison that causes respiratory paralysis with consequent asphyxia at high concentrations. It is an irritant of the eyes and respiratory tract at low concentrations. Inhalation of high concentrations of hydrogen sulfide, 1,000–2,000 ppm, may cause coma after a single breath and may be rapidly fatal; convulsions may also occur. Exposure to concentrations of hydrogen sulfide above 50 ppm for one hour may produce acute conjunctivitis, with pain, lacrimation, and photophobia. In the severe form, this may progress to keratoconjunctivitis and vesiculation of the corneal epithelium. In low concentrations, hydrogen sulfide may cause headache, fatigue, irritability, insomnia, and gastrointestinal disturbances. In somewhat higher concentrations, it affects the central nervous system, causing excitement and dizziness. Prolonged exposure to 250 ppm may cause pulmonary edema. Prolonged exposure to concentrations as low as 50 ppm may cause rhinitis, pharyngitis, bronchitis, and pneumonitis. Repeated exposure to hydrogen sulfide results in increased susceptibility, so that eye irritation, cough, and systemic effects may result from concentrations previously tolerated without any effect. Rapid olfactory fatigue can occur at high concentrations.

Permissible Exposure Limit.—The current OSHA standard for phosphorus pentasulfide is 1 mg/cu m averaged over an eight-hour work shift.

REFERENCES

1. American Conference of Governmental Industrial Hygienists: Phosphorus pentasulfide, in *Documentation of the Threshold Limit Values for Substances in Workroom Air*, ed 5. Cincinnati, Oh, ACGIH, 1986.
2. Manufacturing Chemists Association, Inc: *Chemical Safety Data Sheet SD-71, Phosphorus Pentasulfide*. Washington DC, MCA, 1958.
3. Milby TH: Hydrogen sulfide intoxication—Review of the literature and report of unusual accident resulting in two cases of nonfatal poisoning. *J Occup Med* 1962; 4:431–437.

Phosphorus Trichloride

PCl_3

Phosphorus trichloride, also called phosphorus chloride, is a colorless to yellow fuming liquid with an odor like hydrochloric acid. It is used during the synthesis of plasticizers and intermediates and in the production of intermediates and during the chemical synthesis of dyes, pharmaceuticals, and other chlorinating agents. Phosphorus trichloride is used to make pesticide intermediates and the surfactants that are used during deposition of metallic coatings. It is used to treat polypropylene before drying in the manufacture of knitted fabrics.

Toxicology.—Phosphorus trichloride vapor is a severe irritant to the eyes, mucous membranes, and skin. These effects result primarily from the action of the strong acids, hydrochloric acid and acids of phosphorus, formed with water. In rats, the LC_{50} was 104 ppm for four hours—at autopsy, the chief finding was nephrosis and pulmonary damage was negligible. Inhalation by human beings could be expected to cause injury ranging from mild bronchial spasm to severe pulmonary edema; the onset of severe respiratory symptoms may be delayed for two to six hours, and after moderate exposure the onset may not occur until 12–24 hours later. Prolonged or repeated exposure to low concentrations may induce chronic cough and wheezing. Pulmonary changes are nonfibrotic and nonprogressive. Phosphorus trichloride causes severe burns in contact with the eyes, skin, or mucous membranes. Although ingestion is unlikely to occur in industrial use, it will cause burns of the mouth, throat, esophagus, and stomach.

Permissible Exposure Limit.—The current OSHA standard for phosphorus trichloride is 0.5 ppm averaged over an eight-hour work shift. This may also be expressed as 3 mg/cu m. The ACGIH has issued a Notice of Intended Changes of its recommended threshold limit value for phosphorus trichloride from 0.5 ppm to 0.2 ppm.

REFERENCES

1. American Conference of Governmental Industrial Hygienists: Phosphorus trichloride, in *Documentation of the Threshold Limit Values for Substances in Workroom Air*, ed 5. Cincinnati, Oh, ACGIH, 1986.
2. Grant WM: *Toxicology of the Eye*, ed 2. Springfield, Ill, Charles C Thomas, 1974.
3. Manufacturing Chemists Association, Inc: *Chemical Safety Data Sheet SD-27, Phosphorus Trichloride*. Washington DC, MCA, 1972.
4. Weeks MH, et al: Acute vapor toxicity of phosphorus oxychloride, phosphorus trichloride and methyl phosphonic dichloride. *Am Ind Hyg Assoc J* 1964; 25:470–475.

POLYBROMINATED BIPHENYLS (PBBs)

These highly brominated compounds have been used as flame retardants, mainly in plastics requiring high heat resistance, such as for electronic insulating materials, TV and other electric cabinets and housings, and in auto and truck plastics, where the PBB is added as a fine powder to the plastics. The PBBs have been used on synthetic fibers as well. (PBBs no longer are manufactured in the United States.)

The general formula is:

Br Br

Br Br

About 1 million kg were produced annually in the United States, but there are no reports of adverse human reactions in the manufacturing and subsequent use (Fig 47–17). When the PBBs are added to the mixing process to make various plastics (i.e., acrylonitrilebutadiene-styrene ["ABS"]), along with other materials such as pigments, the subsequent reactions yielding finished products result in plastic that has durable qualities, so that none of the ingredients originally used, and potentially hazardous, poses any problem to persons handling, fabricating, and assembling such PBB-containing products. Only very high heat may release decomposition products, which may be entirely different compounds.

In mid-1973, one of these PBB compounds was accidentally

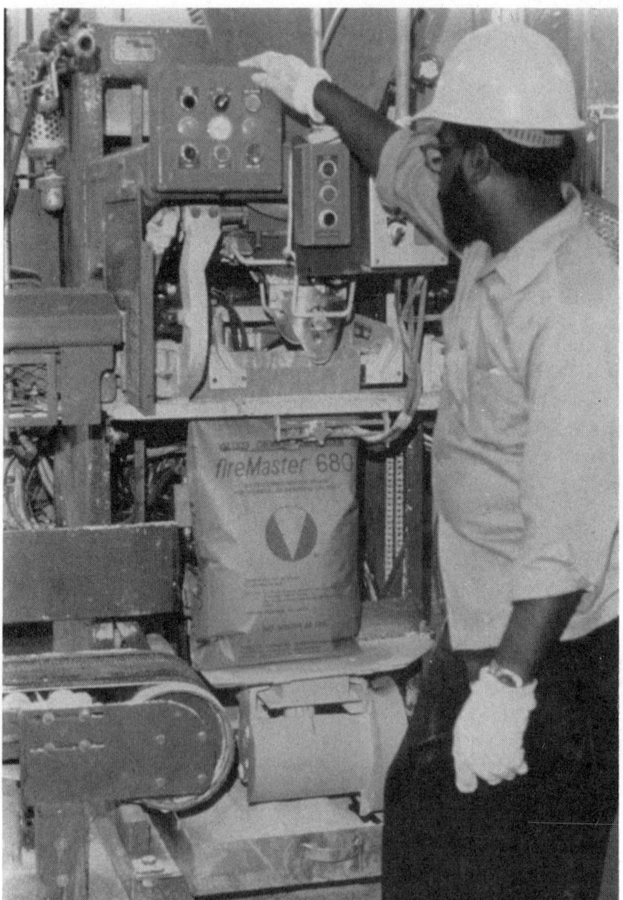

FIG 47–17.
Polybrominated biphenyl flame/fire retardent material being packaged. This compound can be safely packaged and handled with proper engineering controls, such as exhaust ventilation. If properly installed and operated, no respirators are required.

mixed into an animal feedstock, resulting in widespread distribution involving thousands of animals, including cattle, chickens, sheep, and swine. This product had an average bromine content of six bromine atoms per biphenyl molecule, also containing traces of tetra-, penta- and heptabromobiphenyls, brominated benzenes, and traces of hexa- and pentabromonaphthalene. Embryotoxicity, teratogenicity, and various degrees of neurologic dysfunctions were reported in animals and in livestock fed contaminated feed-stock. The PBBs were detected in the food chain, and a study by the Michigan Department of Public Health revealed that nearly 2,000 farm families had eaten their own contaminated meats. The range of contamination was several thousand parts per million in the meat of dairy cows to less than one part per billion in milk sold in supermarkets. Extensive studies were made of those persons involved, but no significant differences in the incidence of symptoms between the group of "heavily exposed" farmers and controls was found.

This inadvertent contamination serves to point out how potentially hazardous materials may be accidentally dissipated into the community environment, involving the population at large (see Chapter 70 for further discussion). Again, such examples illustrate the importance of physicians and others concerned with occupational health and safety having some familiarity with the materials and processes in their communities (see Chapter 13 regarding material safety data sheets—"MSDS").

No adverse occupational exposures have been reported and TLVs for the polybrominated biphenyl compounds have not been established.

REFERENCES

1. Lillis R, et al: Comparison of findings among residents on Michigan dairy farms and consumers of produce from these farms. *Environ Health Perspect* 1978; 23:105.
2. Tilson HA, et al: Some neurotoxic effects of polybrominated biphenyl (PBB) compounds in rodents. *Environ Health Perspect* 1977; 20:244.

POLYCHLORINATED NAPHTHALENE

Elizabeth Ward, M.S. Ph.D.

Polychlorinated naphthalenes (PCNs) are a class of chlorinated aromatic hydrocarbon compounds that were manufactured in the United States, primarily by the Bakelite division of the Union Carbide Corporation prior to 1960 and by the Koppers Company between 1960 and 1977, and marketed under the trade name "Halowax". U.S. manufacture of PCNs declined from over 7 million lb in 1956 to 700,000 lb in 1978, and ceased completely in 1980. In 1981, importation of PCNs totaled approximately 32,000 lb.[6] According to the National Institute for Occupational Safety and Health, in the early 1970s approximately 5,000 workers were estimated to have potential workplace PCN exposure.[6]

Polychlorinated naphthalenes are mixtures of isomers of chlorinated naphthalene homologues of varying degrees of chlorination, produced by the substitution of chlorine for hydrogen in naphthalene to the desired pour-point (determined by percent chlorination).[2] Generally, between one and three PCN homologues predominate in the finished product.[2] The physical and chemical properties of PCNs are similar to that of polychlorinated biphenyls (PCBs). It is not surprising, therefore, that PCNs and PCBs shared many of the same commercial uses, in particular as dielectric fluids in the manufacture of electrical capacitors, transformers, and cables. Some applications required melting the waxy material and using it to impregnate or coat electric parts.[2] Molten PCNs sublimate at temperatures far below their boiling point. Permissible exposure levels in the U.S. decrease with increasing chlorination, ranging from 5 mg/cu m for trichloronaphthalene to 0.1 mg/cu m for octachloronaphthalene.[10]

The most obvious toxic effect of occupational exposure to PCNs is chloracne, which is indistinguishable from chloracne associated with other halogenated hydrocarbons.[4] Chloracne outbreaks in association with PCN exposures were noted as early as World War I,[8] and as recently as 1972.[9] It appears that penta- and hexachloronaphthalene are the most potent chloracnegens. Mixtures of PCN with predominantly four and fewer, or seven and greater, chlorines per naphthalene nucleus, appear not to be acnegenic.[11] Conjunctival burning, digestive disturbances, hematuria, sexual impotence, and acute and subacute liver necrosis have also been documented in association with occupational PCN exposure.[14] During the 1930s and 1940s, a number of reports described deaths from hepatic acute yellow atrophy among PCN-exposed workers. Exposures were reportedly confounded with concomitant solvent exposures, such as carbon tetrachloride.[5, 8] Although such deaths were reportedly rare, the NIOSH has identified eight such deaths in documenting, retrospectively, an outbreak of chloracne affecting greater than 400 workers between 1942 and 1944. Consultants at the time queried if exposure to carbon tetrachloride and/or alcohol and chlorinated naphthalene might potentiate each other in causing liver damage. Experimentally, the administration of sublethal doses of carbon tetrachloride and ethanol to rats whose livers had already been injured by chlorinated naphthalene has been shown to produce massive liver necrosis and death.[1]

The hazard associated with occupational exposure to polychlorinated naphthalenes has been eliminated due to substitution of less hazardous materials in most if not all applications. In May, 1983, the U.S. Environmental Protection Agency announced[6] its intent to restrict the reintroduction of PCNs into commerce for any "significant new use" under Section 5(a)(2) of the Toxic Substances Control Act. This proposal, if finally adopted, would result in a de facto ban on significant commercial PCN use, and consequent occupational exposure.

REFERENCES

1. Bennett GA, Drinker CK, Warren MF: Morphological changes in the livers of rats resulting from exposure to certain chlorinated hydrocarbons. *J Ind Hyg Toxicol* 1938; 20:97–123.
2. Brinkman UATh, DeKok A: Production, properties, and usage, in Kimbrough R (ed): *Halogenated Biphenyls, Terphenyls, Naphthalenes, Dibenzodioxins and Related Products*. Amsterdam, Elsevier-North Holland Biomedical Press, 1980, pp 1–40.

3. Crow KD: Chloracne. A critical review including a comparison of two series of cases of acne from chloronaphthalene and pitch fumes. *Trans St Johns Hospital Dermatol Soc* 1970; 56:79–99.
4. Crow KD: Chloracne. *Semin Dermatol* 1982; 1:305–314.
5. Drinker CK, Warren MF, Bennett GA: The problem of possible systemic effects from certain chlorinated hydrocarbons. *J Ind Hyg Toxicol* 1938; 20:244–258.
6. Environmental Protection Agency: Category of chemical substances known as chlorinated naphthalenes: Proposed determination of significant new uses, 40 CFR Part 721, May 6, 1983.
7. Fulton WB, Matthews JL: A preliminary report of the dermatological and systemic effects of exposure to hexachloronaphthalene and diphenyls, Bulletin 43. Harrisburg, Penn, Commonwealth of Pennsylvania, Dept of Labor and Industry, 1936.
8. Kimbrough RD: Occupational exposures, in Kimbrough R (ed): *Halogenated Biphenyls, Terphenyls, Naphthalenes, Dibenzodioxins and Related Products*. Amsterdam, Elsevier-North Holland Biomedical Press, 1980, pp 373–397.
9. Kleinfeld M, Messite J, Swencicki R: Clinical effects of chlorinated naphthalene exposure. *J Occup Med* 1972; 14:377–379.
10. Occupational Safety and Health Administration: 29 CFR 1901.1000, 1980.
11. Shelley WB, Kligman AM: The experimental production of acne by penta- and hexachloronaphthalenes. *Arch Dermatol* 1975; 57:689–695.
12. Taylor JS: Environmental chloracne. Update and overview. *Ann NY Acad Sci* 1979; XX:295–307.
13. Taylor JS: Chloracne. A continuing problem. *Cutis* 1974; 13:585–591.
14. Von Wedel H, Holla WA, Denton J: Observations on the toxic effects resulting from exposure to chlorinated naphthalene and chlorinated phenyls with suggestions for prevention. *The Rubber Age* 1943; 53:419–426.
15. Von Oettingen WF: *The Halogenated Aliphatic, Olefinic, Cyclic, Aromatic, and Aliphatic-Aromatic Hydrocarbons, Including the Halogenated Insectacides, Their Toxicity and Potential Dangers*. Public Health Service Publ 414. Washington, DC, US Dept of Health, Education, and Welfare, 1955.

SODIUM HYDROXIDE

NaOH

Sodium hydroxide, also called caustic soda, soda lye, or white caustic, is produced commercially by electrolysis of a sodium chloride solution or from lime and soda ash. Total *United States production* of sodium hydroxide in 1974 was *10 billion kg*, attesting to the enormous use of this substance in only one industrialized country! The NIOSH estimates that 150,000 U.S. workers are potentially exposed to the alkali. It is used in the manufacture of rayon, mercerized cotton, soap, paper, aluminum, petroleum, chemicals, and dyestuffs. It is also used for metal cleaning, electrolytic extraction of zinc, tin plating, oxide coating, laundering, and bleaching.

Major hazards are by inhalation and skin contact (often concomitantly). Sodium hydroxide is a strong alkali; the mist, dust, and solutions cause severe injury to the eyes, mucous membranes, and skin (Fig 47–18). Although inhalation usually is of secondary importance in occupational exposures, the effects from the dust or mist will vary from mild irritation of the nose at 2 mg/cu m to severe pneumonitis, depending on the severity of exposure. The greatest industrial hazard is rapid tissue destruction of eyes or skin on contact with either the solid or the concentrated solutions. Contact with the eyes causes disintegration and sloughing of conjunctival and corneal epithelium, corneal opacification, marked edema, and ulceration; after 7–13 days, either gradual recovery begins or there is progression of ulceration and corneal opacification. Complications of severe eye burns are symblepharon with overgrowth of the cornea by a vascularized membrane, progressive or recurrent corneal ulceration, and permanent corneal opacification. On the skin, solutions of 25%–50% cause the sensation of irritation within about three minutes; with solutions of 4%, this does not occur until after several hours. If not removed from the skin, severe burns with deep ulceration will occur; exposure to the dust or mist may cause multiple small burns, with temporary loss of hair. Ingestion produces severe pain in the esophagus and stomach, corrosion of the lips, mouth, tongue, and pharynx and the vomiting of large pieces of mucosa; cases of squamous cell carcinoma of the esophagus have occurred with patent periods of 12–42 years after ingestion; these cancers undoubtedly were sequelae of tissue destruction and possibly scar formation rather than from a direct carcinogenic action of sodium hydroxide itself (Fig 47–19).

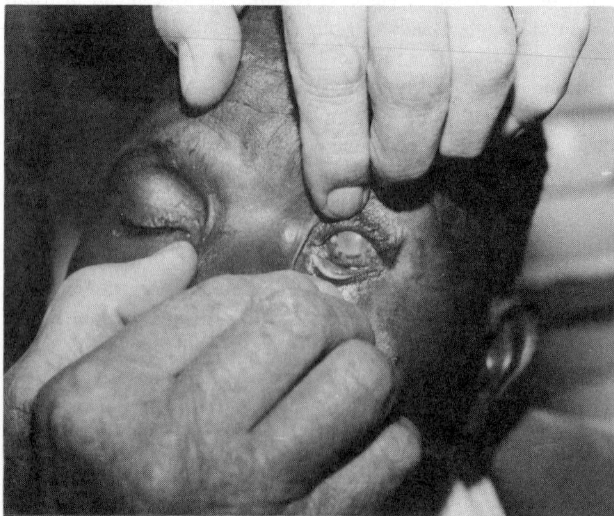

FIG 47–18.
With a broom handle, this janitor accidently bumped and shattered a small bottle containing 47% sodium hydroxide solution on a laboratory countertop. Some of the solution splashed into his eye. Despite immediate flushing and medical attention, the janitor permanently lost vision in that eye.

Treatment.—Remove from exposure. Immediately flush the eyes and skin with water. If swallowed and the person is conscious, immediately administer water orally. Consideration should be given to hospitalization and observation for the onset of pneumonitis.

The NIOSH recommends a ceiling concentration of 2.0 mg sodium hydroxide/cu m as a time-weighted average over an eight-hour workshift determined by a sampling period of 15 minutes. The present federal standard is 2.0 mg sodium hydroxide/m^3 as an 8-hour time-weighted average consideration. Samples representative of the exposure in the breathing zones of at least 25% of the

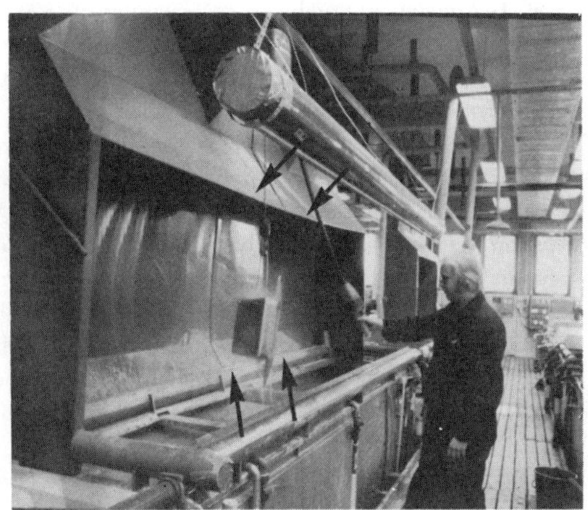

FIG 47–19.
Alkaline pickling. In order to avoid mists of sodium hydroxide in the breathing zone, yet be able to operate the lift over the bath, additional air inlets *(arrows)* were designed, constructed, and placed so that the air would blow away from the worker's face. (Courtesy of Eric Ortman, MD, LM Ericsson Co, Mölndal, Sweden.)

employees in each operation or process shall be collected. Every employee shall be included in the sampling at least once every 2 years.

The NIOSH recommends that workers subject to sodium hydroxide exposure have comprehensive preplacement medical examinations. Medical examinations shall be made available promptly to all workers with signs or symptoms of skin, eye or upper respiratory tract irritation resulting from exposure to sodium hydroxide. Containers of sodium hydroxide shall be labeled to warn of the severe burns and blindness that may result, and personal protective equipment must be made available to protect eyes, face, and skin from contact with sodium hydroxide. Engineering controls shall be used wherever feasible to maintain airborne sodium hydroxide at concentrations below the prescribed limit, and respirators may be used only in certain nonroutine or emergency situations.

REFERENCES

1. American Conference of Governmental Industrial Hygienists: "Sodium Hydroxide," Documentation of the Threshold Limit Values for Substances in Workroom Air, ed 5. Cincinnati, 1986.
2. Manufacturing Chemists Association, Inc: Chemical Safety Data Sheet DS-9, Caustic Soda, Washington, DC, pp 16–17, 1968.
3. National Institute for Occupational Safety and Health, US Dept of Health, Education, and Welfare: *Criteria for a Recommended Standard . . . Occupational Exposure to Sodium Hydroxide*. NIOSH No 76:105, Cincinnati, 1975.

SULFUR DIOXIDE

SO_2

Sulfur dioxide is a colorless gaseous by-product of processes such as smelting of sulfide ores, combustion of coal or fuel oils containing sulfur as an impurity, paper manufacturing, and petroleum refining. Industrially, sulfur dioxide is used in the manufacture of sodium sulfite and as an intermediate in the manufacture of sulfuric acid. It is also used in refrigeration, bleaching, fumigating, and preserving operations and as an antioxidant in the melting, pouring, and heat treatment of magnesium. The NIOSH estimates that 500,000 workers have potential exposure to sulfur dioxide. Occupational exposure to sulfur dioxide may occur in many industries, including petroleum refining, smelting, preserving industries, utility companies, and paper making.

Sulfur dioxide gas is a severe irritant to the eyes, mucous membranes, and skin. Its irritant properties are due to the rapidity with which it forms sulfurous acid on contact with moist membranes. Approximately 90% of all sulfur dioxide inhaled is absorbed in the upper respiratory passages, where most effects occur; however, it may produce respiratory paralysis and may also cause pulmonary edema. Exposure to concentrations of 10–50 ppm for 5–15 minutes causes irritation of the eyes, nose, and throat, rhinorrhea, choking, cough, and, in some instances, reflex bronchoconstriction with increased pulmonary resistance. Some 10–20% of the healthy young adult population are estimated to be hypersusceptible to the effects of sulfur dioxide, whereas the phenomenon of adaptation to irritating concentrations is a recognized occurrence in some workers. Workers repeatedly exposed to 10 ppm experienced upper respiratory irritation and some nosebleeds, but the symptoms did not occur at 5 ppm. In another study, initial cough and irritation did occur at 5 ppm and 13 ppm, but subsided after five minutes of exposure.[1, 4] In a human experimental study with the subjects breathing through the mouth, brief exposure to 13 ppm caused a 73% increase in pulmonary flow resistance; 5 ppm resulted in a 40% increase; 1 ppm produced no effects.[5] Exposure of the eyes to liquid sulfur dioxide from pressurized containers causes corneal burns and opacification, resulting in a loss of vision. Liquefied sulfur dioxide on the skin produces skin burns from the freezing effect of rapid evaporation.

The TLV of 2 ppm was set to prevent respiratory irritation.

Treatment.—Remove patient from exposure. Immediately flush the eyes with water and wash the skin with soap or mild detergent and water. Hospitalization is recommended for observation for possible delayed pulmonary edema.

REFERENCES

1. American Conference of Governmental Industrial Hygienists: Sulfur Dioxide. *Documentation of the Threshold Limit Values for Substances in Workroom Air*, ed. 5, Cincinnati, Oh, ACGIH, 1986.
2. Hygienic Guide Series: Sulfur dioxide. *Am Ind Hyg Assoc* 1978.
3. National Institute for Occupational Safety and Health, US Dept of Health, Education, and Welfare: *Criteria for a Recommended Standard: Occupational Exposure to Sulfur Dioxide*. Washington, DC, US Government Printing Office, 1974.
4. Occupational Exposure to Sulfur Dioxide, *Federal Register* 40:54520–54534, Nov 24, 1975.
5. Whittenberger JL, Frank RN: Human exposure to sulfur dioxide. *Arch Environ Health* 1963; 7:244.

SULFURIC ACID

James J. Beaumont, Ph.D.

Sulfuric acid is the highest volume chemical produced in the United States, with an annual production (as of 1979) of about 84 billion lb. It was estimated by the National Institute for Occupational Safety and Health (NIOSH) in its 1972–1974 survey of the United States that over 200 different occupational categories have some potential for exposure, and that these occupations include about 800,000 workers.[29]

Approximately 250 plants in the U.S. produce sulfuric acid, and approximately 30% of these plants also produce fuming sulfuric acid, also called "oleum." Most of the acid is used on site or used by industries within 200–300 miles of the supplier.[43] Major past and/or present production processes using sulfuric acid include phosphate fertilizer manufacturing, steel pickling, battery manufacturing, cellophane manufacturing, titanium dioxide manufacturing, petroleum refining, electrochemical drilling, uranium ore processing, and production of alcohol, surface active agents, ammonium sulfate, methyl methacrylate, hydrofluoric acid, and aluminum sulfate.

Exposures are relatively well-controlled in sulfuric acid manufacturing and in many processes that use sulfuric acid. Exposures that have received most attention in the scientific literature are those that have occurred to sulfuric acid mist in the manufacturing of batteries and the pickling of steel. It should be noted, however, that exposures in many industries, in particular newer industries, have not been well studied.

Types and Properties of Sulfuric Acid

Sulfuric acid is a clear to cloudy oily liquid that is soluble in water and alcohols. While it has a high boiling point and is not flammable, it reacts with metals to release hydrogen gas, which is highly flammable in the presence of oxygen. Sulfuric acid has a strong affinity for water; when it combines with water there is an exothermic reaction that can cause burning or charring of tissue.

Sulfuric acid mist is an aerosol of aqueous sulfuric acid that results from heating or bubbling of the liquid. The droplets are hygroscopic and often grow in size as they pick up moisture from the atmosphere.

Fuming sulfuric acid, or oleum, contains sulfur trioxide gas that combines with water in air and on mucous membranes to form sulfuric acid.

Most sulfuric acid is produced by the contact process, but there is still some use of the chamber and drum processes.[43] Four grades of the acid are produced: commercial, electrolyte, textile (low organic content), and reagent.

Acute Effects

Irritation.—Irritation of mucous membranes, especially those of the eyes and respiratory system, is a common symptom of sulfuric acid exposure. The mucous membranes are affected because of sulfuric acid's affinity for water and its oxidizing potential. Exposure is detectable to human beings at 0.5–0.7 mg/cu m, is irritating at 1–2 mg/cu m, and causes coughing at 5–6 mg/cu m.[7, 9, 17] Ocular irritation leads to lacrimation and conjunctivitis, most notably on hot and humid days. High humidity in particular increases the irritating properties of sulfuric acid.[38]

There is considerable variation in susceptibility to sulfuric acid: some persons become acclimatized and can tolerate three to four times as much exposure as those not regularly exposed, while others develop sensitivity and have less tolerance.[33, 38] Persons with asthma or bronchitis seem to be most sensitive.[36, 41] There is little or no allergic sensitization, in contrast to sulfur dioxide, for which about 10% of the population develops hypersensitivity.[4, 31] Smokers have been shown to be more sensitive with respect to coughing in a survey of steelworkers exposed to sulfuric acid.[42]

External Burns and Accidental Ingestion.—The effects of skin contact with sulfuric acid include burning and charring, due to the acid's exothermic reaction with and strong affinity for water.[43] Second- and third-degree burns of the face, neck, arms, and thighs have been reported after eight minutes of exposure to strong fumes from an explosion of oleum.[16]

Ingestion causes severe burns of the mucous membranes of the mouth and can affect the entire alimentary tract, with the pylorus and antrum of the stomach being particularly susceptible.[20] Alimentary tract effects include stomatitis, peritonitis, and pancreatitis; omental fat necrosis; strictures of the esophagus, gastroesophageal junction, and gastric antrum; and coagulation necrosis of the stomach, duodenum, jejunum, and ileum. Surgical intervention is sometimes indicated.[20]

Acute Respiratory Effects.—Sulfuric acid exposure can alter respiratory function, most likely as a result of a reflex bronchoconstriction mechanism.[3] Effects include increased respiration rate and decreased tidal volume,[6] decreased forced expiratory volume,[12, 15, 21, 44] increased airway resistance,[5, 15, 21] and reduced vital capacity.[12, 21] While most studies have demonstrated impaired respiratory function, there have been several reports of no effect at concentrations ranging from 0.01 to 3.0 mg/cu m.[8, 10, 35, 38] Explanations for the apparently contradictory findings include differences in particle size, humidity, and degree of ammonia neutralization in the respiratory tract which may be affected by diet, oral hygiene, time since last meal, and other factors.[21, 22, 25]

Other acute pulmonary effects include edema, hemorrhage, and loss of epithelia. Exposure to extremely high concentrations (as in the previously described explosion of oleum) has resulted in edema of the larynx, tracheobronchial tree, and lungs, followed by hemorrhagic sputum resulting from necrosis of bronchial epithelia.[16] Hyperplasia and hypertrophy of bronchiolar and bronchial epithelia, pulmonary edema, and myocardial hypertrophy have been demonstrated in monkeys exposed to concentrations ranging from 0.38 to 4.79 mg/cu m.[2] Guinea pigs exposed to 25 mg/cu m have shown collapsed, fluid-filled lungs, with edema and hemorrhage evident upon light microscopy.[11] Scanning and electron microscopy in that study showed numerous macrophages, thickening of alveolar walls, dried edema fluid, and strands of fibrin. Changes in the airways were limited to the alveolar duct region—there were no lesions of the bronchi, trachea, or larynx.

There is considerable evidence from human and animal studies that the mucociliary clearance mechanism of the respiratory system may be affected by sulfuric acid inhalation. Decreased ciliary beating frequency has been shown in hamsters,[18] decreased clearance of bacteria has been shown in mice,[13] decreased bronchial clearance half-times have been shown in donkeys,[37] and decreased clearance of radioactively labeled aerosols has been shown in two studies of human subjects.[25, 30] There is also some evidence that resistance to viral influenza may be reduced: a study of mice exposed to a sulfuric acid and carbon particle mixture showed a marked reduction in all indices of resistance to the virus.[14]

Chronic Effects

Dental Erosion.—Erosion of the teeth is a well-documented problem associated with long-term exposure to sulfuric acid. There are three grades of erosion: (1) loss or etching of the enamel, where the tooth is dull rather than shiny in appearance, (2) exposure of the dentine, and (3) exposure of the secondary dentin.[40] When pain occurs, it is usually a result of hypersusceptibility to cold.[40]

Erosion and tooth loss have been reported in workers exposed to sulfuric acid mist in storage battery manufacturing[12, 26, 40] and steel pickling.[42] In storage battery manufacturing, length of exposure has been found to be strongly associated with degree of erosion.[12, 26, 40]

Bronchitis, Emphysema, and Fibrosis.—Both short-term high exposures and long-term moderate exposures have been associated with the occurrence of respiratory disease. Pulmonary fibrosis, residual bronchiectasis, pulmonary emphysema, and chronic bronchitis have resulted from short-term high exposures caused by accidental industrial explosions.[16, 17] Increased occurrence of bronchitis has been associated with long-term moderate exposure in battery manufacturing.[12, 44] It has been hypothesized that the upper respiratory system is more affected by moderate exposure than the lower respiratory tract because of the high humidity in upper airways and the high solubility of sulfuric acid.[44]

Other Long-Term Effects.—The teratogenic potential of sulfuric acid has been studied with equivocal results. While exposure of pregnant mice and rats during the major period of organogenesis has shown little fetal toxicity and no teratogenesis,[28] exposure of chicken eggs has shown reduced embryonic weight and reduced lactic dehydrogenase (LDH) activity, which could indicate a delay in normal development.[19]

The carcinogenic or cocarcinogenic potential of sulfuric acid and sulfates has been of concern for several years.[27] Laryngeal cancer incidence in humans has been associated with sulfuric acid exposure in an ethanol manufacturing operation, in a study that controlled for the effects of cigarette and alcohol consumption,[33] and in a steel pickling operation where other acids were also used.[1] In contrast, a study of Pennsylvania steelworkers who worked in pickling operations observed no laryngeal cancer deaths, while 0.4 were expected.[34] Animal studies and one human study have shown that sulfur dioxide, a compound related to and which can convert to sulfuric acid, may have a cancer promoting effect.[23, 24, 32]

Preventive Measures

Exposure Limits.—The exposure limit used by the United States Occupational Safety and Health Administration is a time-weighted average of 1.0 mg/cu m, with no ceiling limit. This standard is based upon the irritant effects of sulfuric acid.

In 1974, NIOSH recommended that the 1.0 mg/cu m limit be kept for the reason that the limit seemed to be adequately protective.[41] In a later review of the literature, however, NIOSH stated that a decrease in the limit might be warranted on the basis of animal studies showing decreased pulmonary function, disturbances of mucociliary clearance, and microscopic pulmonary damage at levels below 1 mg/cu m.[43] It was acknowledged that extrapolation to human beings may be dangerous because most of the experimental animals were not mouth breathers.

Of the countries that have established a standard for occupational sulfuric acid exposure, all but Romania have adopted the 1.0 mg/cu m limit. Romania recommends a time-weighted average of 0.5 mg/cu m, with a ceiling of 1.5 mg/cu m.

Medical Monitoring.—The NIOSH recommends that workers be considered "exposed" for the purposes of medical monitoring and other actions at one-half the environmental standard, i.e., 0.5 mg/cu m. Medical monitoring includes preplacement and annual medical examinations directed toward, but not limited to, the teeth, eyes, skin, and the cardiopulmonary system. Particular attention should be given to dental erosion, mucous membrane irritation, and cough.[41]

Engineering Controls, Protective Equipment, and Labeling.—Engineering controls, such as ventilation, process changes, and substitution, should be used to reduce exposures wherever possible. Protective clothing and equipment should be worn to protect the skin, eyes, and respiratory system. Warning signs, for which the NIOSH has recommended specific wording, should be posted in areas where exposure to sulfuric acid, oleum, or dry sulfuric acid is likely to occur. Monitoring of exposure levels in these areas should be performed on a regular basis.

REFERENCES

1. Ahlborg G, Hogstedt C, Sundell L, et al: Laryngeal cancer and pickling house vapors. *Scand J Work Environ Health* 1981; 3:239–240.
2. Alarie Y, Busey WM, Krumm AA, et al: Long-term exposure to sulfur dioxide, sulfuric acid mist, fly ash, and their mixtures—Results of studies in monkeys and guinea pigs. *Arch Environ Health* 1975; 30:254–262.
3. Amdur MO: Aerosols formed by oxidation of sulfur dioxide: Review of their toxicology. *Arch Environ Health* 1971; 23:459–468.
4. Amdur MO: The long road from Donora—1974 Cummings Memorial Lecture. *Am Ind Hyg Assoc J* 1974; 35:589–597.
5. Amdur MO, Dubriel M, Creasia DA: Respiratory response to guinea pigs to low levels of sulfuric acid. *Environ Res* 1978; 15: 418–423.
6. Amdur MO, Schulz RZ, Drinker P: Toxicity of sulfuric acid mist to guinea pigs. *J Ind Hyg Occup Med* 1952; 5:318–329.
7. Amdur MO, Silverman L, Drinker P: Inhalation of sulfuric acid mist by human subjects. *Arch Ind Hyg Occup Med* 1952; 6:305–313.
8. Avol EL, Jones MP, Bailey RM, et al: Controlled exposures of hu-

man volunteers to sulfate aerosols. *Am Rev Respir Dis* 1979; 120:319–327.

9. Bushtueva KA: The determination of the limit of allowable concentrations of H_2SO_4 in atmospheric air, in *Limits of Allowable Concentrations of Atmospheric Pollutants*, book 3, BS Levine (tran). US Dept of Commerce, 1957, pp 20–36.
10. Chaney S, Blomquist W, Muller K, et al: Biochemical changes in humans upon exposure to sulfuric acid aerosol and exercise. *Arch Environ Health* 1980; 35(4):211–216.
11. Cockrell BY, Busey WM, Cavender FL: Respiratory tract lesions in guinea pigs exposed to sulfuric acid mist. *J Toxicol Environ Health* 1978; 4:835–844.
12. El-Sadik YM, Osman HA, El-Gazzar RM: Exposure to sulfuric acid in manufacture of storage batteries. *J Occup Med* 1972; 14:224–226.
13. Fairchild GA, Kane P, Adams B, et al: Sulfuric acid and streptococci clearance from respiratory tracts of mice. *Arch Environ Health* 1975; 30:538–545.
14. Fenters JD, Bradof JN, Aranyi C, et al: Health effects of long-term inhalation of sulfuric acid mist-carbon particle mixtures. *Environ Res* 1979; 19:244–257.
15. Gardner DE, Hazucha M, Knelson JH, et al: The effects of H_2SO_4 on men and H_2SO_4 and O_3 on laboratory animals, in *Energy/Environment III. Proceedings of the 3rd National Conference on the Interagency R&D Program Held at Washington, DC on June 1 and 2, 1978*, EPA-600/9-78-022. US Environmental Protection Agency, Office of Research and Development, 1978.
16. Goldman A, Hill WT: Chronic bronchopulmonary disease due to inhalation of sulfuric acid fumes. *Arch Ind Hyg Occup Med* 1953; 8:205–211.
17. Greenwald I: Effects of inhalation of low concentrations of sulfur dioxide upon man and other animals. *Arch Ind Hyg Occup Med* 1954; 10:455–475.
18. Grose EC, Gardner DE, Miller FJ: Response of ciliated epithelium to ozone and sulfuric acid. *Environ Res* 1980; 22:377–385.
19. Hoffman DJ, Campbell KI: Embryotoxicity of irradiated and nonirradiated catalytic converter-treated automotive exhaust. *J Toxicol Environ Health* 1977; 3:705–712.
20. Jelenko C III, Story J, Ellison RG Jr: Ingestion of mineral acid. *Am Surg* 1974; 40:97–104.
21. Kleinman MT, Bailey RM, Chang YC, et al: Exposures to human volunteers to a controlled atmospheric mixture of ozone, sulfur dioxide and sulfuric acid. *Am Ind Hyg Assoc J* 1981; 42:61–69.
22. Larson TV, Covert DS, Frank R, et al: Ammonia in the human airways: Neutralization of inspired acid sulfate aerosols. *Science* 1977; 197:161–163.
23. Laskin S, Kuschner M, Drew RT: *Studies in Pulmonary Carcinogensis*. 1970.
24. Lee AM, Fraumeni VF: Arsenic and respiratory cancer in man: An occupational study. *J Nat Cancer Inst* 1969; 42:1045–1052.
25. Leikauf G, Yeates DB, Wales KA, et al: Effects of sulfuric acid aerosol on respiratory mechanics and mucociliary particle clearance in healthy nonsmoking adults. *Am Ind Hyg Assoc J* 1981; 4:273–282.
26. Malcolm D, Paul E: Erosion of the teeth due to sulfuric acid in the battery industry. *Br J Ind Med* 1961; 18:63–69.
27. Morris SC, Morgan MG (eds): *Human Responses to Sulfur Pollutants*. Brookhaven National Laboratory, Report 20328, 1974.
28. Murray FJ, Schwetz BA, Nitschke KD, et al: Embryotoxicity of inhaled sulfuric acid aerosol in mice and rabbits, abstract. *J Environ Sci Health* 1979; 13:251–266.
29. *National Occupational Hazards Survey, vol III. Survey Analysis and Supplemental Tables,* NIOSH Publ 78–114, 1978.
30. Newhouse MT, Colobich M, Obminski G: Effect of TLV of SO_2 and H_2SO_4 on bronchial clearance in exercising man. *Arch Environ Health* 1978; 33:24–32.
31. Osebold JW, Gershwin LJ, Zee YC: Studies on the enhancement of allergic lung sensitization by inhalation of ozone and sulfuric acid aerosol. *J Environ Pathol Toxicol* 1980; 3:221–234.
32. Peacock PR, Spence JB: Incidence of lung tumors in LX mice exposed to (1) free radicals; (2) SO_2. *Br J Cancer* 1967; 21:606–618.
33. Raule A: Occupational Disease Caused by Sulfuric Acid. *Med Lav* 1954, pp 590–599 (Italian).
34. Redmond CK, Wiland HS, Rockette HE, et al: *Long-Term Mortality Experience of Steelworkers*, DHHS (NIOSH) Publ 81–120, 1981.
35. Sackner MA, Ford D, Fernandez R, et al: Effects of sulfuric acid aerosol on cardiopulmonary function of dogs, sheep, and humans. *Am Rev Respir Dis* 1978; 118:497–510.
36. Sackner MA, Reinhart M, Ford D: Effect of sulfuric acid mist on pulmonary function in animals and man, abstract. *Am Rev Respir Dis* 1977; 115[suppl]:240.
37. Schlesinger RB, Halpern M, Albert RE, et al: Effect of chronic inhalation of sulfuric acid mist upon mucociliary clearance from the lungs of donkeys. *J Environ Pathol Toxicol* 1979; 2:1351–1367.
38. Sim VM, Pattle RE: Effect of possible smog irritants on human subjects. *JAMA* 1957; 165:1908–1913.
39. Sosolne CL: *Upper Respiratory Cancer Among Refinery and Chemical Plant Workers: A Case-Control Study in Baton Rouge, Louisiana*. Ph D Dissertation, University of Pennsylvania, 1982.
40. ten Bruggen Cate HJ: *Report by the Industrial Diseases Sub-Committee of the Industrial Injuries Advisory Council*. Ministry of Social Security HMSO, London Cd. 3114, 1965.
41. US Dept of Health, Education, and Welfare, National Institute for Occupational Safety and Health: *Criteria for a Recommended Standard: Occupational Exposure to Sulfuric Acid,* 1974.
42. US Dept of Health, Education, and Welfare, National Institute for Occupational Safety and Health: *Health Hazard Evaluation Determination,* Report 77-42-452, *Cleaning House at the Wire Mill,* Johnstown, Penn, Bethlehem Steel Corp, 1977.
43. US Dept of Health and Human Services, National Institute for Occupational Safety and Health: Review and evaluation of recent literature: Occupational exposure to sulfuric acid, 1981.
44. Williams MK: Sickness, absence and ventilatory capacity of workers exposed to sulfuric acid mist. *Br J Ind Med* 1970; 27:61–66.

o-TOLIDINE

o-Tolidine (3,3′-dimethyl, 4,4′-diamino diphenyl) is a crystalline solid. *o*-Tolidine is used both as a dye and as an intermediate in the production of other dyes. It is widely used in small quantities as a laboratory analytic reagent and is a moiety of the commonly used biologic stain trypan blue. *o*-Tolidine is used in small quantities in chlorine test kits by water companies and swimming pool owners and in test tapes in clinical laboratories. Although other chemicals are preferred, *o*-tolidine has been used as a curing agent for urethane resins, in part because some of the other curing agents, e.g., 4,4′-methylene bis (2-chloraniline) (MOCA), were proposed for stringent regulation as carcinogens.

The major U.S. manufacturer of *o*-tolidine makes an average of 100,000 kg of *o*-tolidine salts, e.g., hydrochloride, each year. Smaller quantities are produced by other companies. U.S. production data on *o*-tolidine base are not available. Many chemical companies buy *o*-tolidine in bulk from other, principally foreign, manufacturers, repackage it, and sell it in smaller units; sometimes they refine it. About 150,000 kg of *o*-tolidine base and 100,000 kg of *o*-tolidine salts are imported annually.

Workers potentially exposed to *o*-tolidine are: analytical chemistry workers, artists, chemical distributors, dye makers, forest service chemists, glucose diagnostic tape makers, leather dye workers, medical laboratory workers, organic chemists, *o*-tolidine makers, sanitarians, sewage treatment plant workers, swimming pool test kit makers, swimming pool service personnel, textile dryers, toluene diisocyanate makers, urethane curers, and waterworks attendants. Workers exposed to the greatest amounts of *o*-tolidine probably are dye makers, toluene diisocyanate makers, clinical or analytical chemistry laboratory workers, and repackagers. Workers in a variety of occupations may be exposed to small quantities of *o*-tolidine for analytic purposes, among them water and sewage plant attendants, sanitarians, forest service chemists, swimming pool service representatives, and chemical test tape or kit makers. It is estimated that fewer than 100 employees are exposed to large quantities of *o*-tolidine in the United States, but as many as 200,000 may be exposed to small quantities.

Inhalation and skin absorption are main routes of entry. *o*-Tolidine absorption, whether from inhalation of the vapor or by skin absorption of the liquid, causes anoxia due to the formation of methemoglobin and hematuria. The earliest manifestations of poisoning in humans are headache and cyanosis of the lips, mucous membranes, the fingernail beds, and the tongue. As the lack of oxygen increases, there is growing weakness, dizziness, and drowsiness, leading to stupor, unconsciousness, and even death if treatment is not prompt. Transient microscopic hematuria has been observed in *o*-tolidine workers, presumably of renal origin, since no alterations in the bladder mucosa were observed by cystoscopy. In the eye of a rabbit, the liquid caused a severe burn. Excessive drying of the skin may result from repeated or prolonged contact.

Treatment.—Any *o*-tolidine on the body must be removed, including immediate removal of contaminated clothing, including shoes, washing of the entire body with plenty of soap or mild detergent and water. Shampoo the hair and scalp, clean fingernails and toenails, clean nostrils and ear canals. Give oxygen. Hospitalization is recommended. Determine methemoglobin in blood and repeat every 3–6 hours for 18–24 hours. Repeat shower and skin cleansing if methemoglobin appears to rise after 3–4 hours. Consideration may be given to the intravenous administration of methylene blue at high levels of methemoglobin in an attempt to accelerate the conversion of methemoglobin; however, the use of this agent is controversial because of its toxic effects.

REFERENCES

1. American Conference of Governmental Industrial Hygienists: *o*-Tolidine, in *Documentation of the Threshold Limit Values for Substances in Workroom Air*, ed 5. Cincinnati, Oh, ACGIH, 1986.
2. Mangelsdorff AF: Treatment of methemoglobinemia. *AMA Arch Ind Hyg* 1956; 14:148.
3. Manufacturing Chemists Association, Inc: Chemical Safety Data Sheet DS-82. *o*-Tolidine. Washington, DC, MCA, 1961, pp 13–14.
4. National Institute for Occupational Safety and Health: *Criteria for a Recommended Standard: Occupational Exposure to o-Tolidine*. US Dept of Health, Education, and Welfare, PHS, Center for Disease Control, NIOSH, 1978.

TRIMELLITIC ANHYDRIDE (TMA)

HOOC– O O O

TMA is used as a curing agent for epoxy and other resins, in vinyl plasticizers, paints and coatings, polymers, polyesters, agricultural chemicals, dyes and pigments, pharmaceuticals, surface-active agents, modifiers, intermediates, and specialty chemicals. The NIOSH estimates that approximately 20,000 American workers currently are at risk of exposure to TMA in its various applications. The sole domestic producer of TMA is Amoco Chemicals Corporation, which has a 50-million-lb-per-year plant at Joliet, Illinois.

The NIOSH recommends that TMA be handled as an extremely toxic agent in the workplace. Exposure to this compound may result in noncardiac pulmonary edema (apparently without benefit of a pulmonary irritation warning), immunologic sensitization, and irritation of the pulmonary tract, eyes, nose, and skin. There is no current OSHA exposure standard for TMA. The Amoco Chemicals Corporation, the producer, suggests a limit of "0.05 mg/cu m or less for susceptible individuals."[1]

Human Toxicity

The ability of TMA to cause pulmonary edema (lungs) has been reported by Rice et al.[4] Two workers who had been employed by the same company for only a short period (three and six weeks) received multiple inhalation exposures to an epoxy resin containing TMA when it was sprayed on heated pipes. The levels of TMA were not available to the authors. No mention was made of severe irritation of the upper respiratory tract while the workers were receiving their exposures, suggesting little or no warning of subsequent damage to the lungs. The possibility that the pulmonary edema was the result of a hypersensitivity reaction therefore must be considered. Resins can be sensitizers (e.g., toluene diisocyanate or TDI), although most of the reported effects have been those of direct irritation.

Sensitization to TMA was noted by Zeiss et al.[5] Respiratory symptoms were observed in 14 workers employed in the synthesis of TMA. The authors suggest three distinct syndromes induced by inhalation of TMA. The first, rhinitis and/or asthma, developed over an industrial exposure period of weeks to years. After this period, the sensitized worker exhibited symptoms immediately following exposure to TMA dust or fumes, which abated after the work exposure had stopped. The second syndrome, termed "TMA flu" by the workers, also required a sensitization period of exposure and was characterized by delayed onset, cough, wheezing, and labored breathing starting four to eight hours after a work shift and peaking at night. These respiratory symptoms usually were accompanied by malaise, chills, fever, and muscle and joint aches and appeared to be associated with relatively high exposures to TMA during particular work shifts. The third syndrome, which followed initial high exposure to TMA, was primarily an irritant effect. It was characterized by a "running" nose without itching or sneezing, occasional nosebleed, cough, labored breathing and occasional wheezing. Symptoms usually abated after eight hours and rarely lasted into the night.

The above studies suggest harmful respiratory effects of TMA at relatively high concentrations, but even at lower concentrations, some workers may develop an immunologic sensitization over a period of time.

Fawcett et al.[2] also observed sensitization in a worker exposed to TMA in the production of tubular steel shop fittings coated with an epoxy resin. The chemical agent responsible for asthma symptoms of six workers was identified by careful inhalation challenge testing simulating work exposure. Typical attacks that began one year after onset of TMA exposure consisted of cough and breathlessness, lasting for 30 minutes, which subsided, only to be followed the same evening by sneezing, which persisted for about 24 hours. Subsequent attacks were prevented by avoiding exposure.

Data on occupational exposures to TMA were also obtained during a NIOSH Health Hazard Evaluation of a paint and varnish company during the manufacture of an epoxy paint.[3] The Health Hazard Evaluation was conducted at the request of employees who were concerned about possible harmful effects of TMA exposure during processing and decontamination operations. The occupational airborne exposure levels averaged 1.5 mg/cu m TMA (with a range from "none detected" to 4.0 mg/cu m) during processing operations and 2.8 mg/cu m TMA (ranging from "none detected" to 7.5 mg/cu m) during decontamination operations. A total of 13 employees (five present and eight former employees) were interviewed and examined briefly. Employees' symptoms and complaints were: eye irritation, nasal irritation, shortness of breath, wheezing, cough, heartburn, nausea, headache, skin irritation, and throat irritation. Three of the former workers stated that they had left that department for health reasons. Complaints subsided when non-TMA-containing products were being formulated.

The Occupational Health and Safety Division, Department of Labor, Alberta, Canada, has reported to the NIOSH that they are aware of employee reactions in two plants using TMA-epoxy powder pipe coatings. One plant, started in 1971, had a number of employees with an immediate reaction. After instituting engineering and administrative controls, there has been no further incidence. In the second plant, begun in 1974, the first adverse reaction occurred in 1975. There have been nine cases of adverse reactions reported to date. Most of these employees were kept in intensive care while they recuperated and were advised by their physicians to seek new jobs. However, some returned to their previous jobs and became ill again. Due to the unavailability of a good analytic method for TMA, occupational levels could not be documented until November, 1977. The TMA concentrations found ranged from 0.11 mg/cu m to 0.27 mg/cu m.

The NIOSH recommends that TMA be handled in the workplace as an extremely toxic substance because it can cause noncardiac pulmonary edema, immunologic sensitization, and severe respiratory irritation. Exposure to TMA should be limited to as few employees as possible while minimizing workplace exposure levels. The area in which it is used should be restricted to those employees necessary to the process or operation. Furthermore, consideration should be given to isolating the TMA exposure area so that adjacent workers are not also exposed. The TLV is 0.005 ppm.

REFERENCES

1. Amoco-Industrial Hygiene Toxicology and Safety Data Sheet, Environmental Health Services, Medical and Health Services Dept, July 8, 1976.
2. Fawcett IW, Taylor AJ, Pepys J: Asthma due to inhaled chemical agents-epoxy resin systems containing phthalic acid anhydride, trimellitic acid anhydride and triethylene tetramine. *Clin Allergy* 1977; 7:1.
3. National Institute for Occupational Safety and Health: Health Hazard Evaluation Determination, Report 74-111-283.
4. Rice DL, Jenkins DE, Gray JM et al: Chemical pneumonitis secondary to inhalation of epoxy pipe coating. *Arch Environ Health* 1977; 32:183.
5. Zeiss CR, Patterson R, Pruzansky JJ et al: Trimellitic anhydride-induced airway syndromes: Chemical and immunologic studies. *J Allergy Clin Immunol* 1977; 60:96.

VINYL ACETATE

$$CH_3COOCH{=}CH_2$$

Vinyl acetate is a colorless, flammable liquid at room temperature with a vapor pressure of 100 mm Hg at 21.5° C. Initially, its odor is pleasant but quickly becomes sharp and irritating; the threshold of odor detection has been reported to be as low as 1 mg/cu m (0.284 ppm,), but olfactory fatigue has been reported at 19.5 ppm (68.3 mg/cu m). Vinyl acetate is produced by a vapor-phase reaction between ethylene and acetic acid in the presence of a palladium catalyst or between acetylene and acetic acid in the presence of a zinc acetate catalyst. In the United States, 800 million kg of vinyl acetate were produced in 1977. Vinyl acetate is used primarily in polymerization processes to produce polyvinyl acetate, polyvinyl alcohol, and vinyl chloride-vinyl acetate copolymer. These polymers, usually made as emulsions, suspensions, solutions, or resins, are used to prepare adhesives, paints, paper coatings, and textile finishes, and low molecular-weight polyvinyl acetate is used as a chewing gum base. Vinyl acetate is extremely flammable and forms explosive mixtures at from 2.6% to 13.4% by volume in air. Occupational exposure to vinyl acetate may occur in any work involving the production, storage, transport, or use. Occupations with potential exposure to vinyl acetate are: chemical synthesis workers, equipment cleaners, equipment repairers, maintenance workers, monomer-containing-aerosol producers, monomer loaders and unloaders, monomer production workers, monomer samplers and gagers, monomer transport workers, polymer compounders, polymer fabricators, polymer loaders and unloaders, polymer packagers, polymer processors, polymer production workers, polymer transport workers, quality-control laboratory workers, and warehouse workers. The NIOSH estimates that approximately 70,000 workers work with vinyl acetate in the United States.

Exposure to vinyl acetate occurs primarily via inhalation of the vapor and contact of the liquid or vapor with the skin and eyes. In humans, exposure to vinyl acetate vapor at lower concentrations (68.3–75.6 mg/cu m) has resulted in reversible eye and upper respiratory irritation.[7, 12] Dermal exposure to the liquid may result in irritation of the skin.[7, 13] Vinyl acetate was lethal[13] to all (presumably six) rats exposed for two hours at 28,000 mg/cu m, and four-hour LC_{50}s for exposed rats, guinea pigs, mice, and rabbits[5, 12] ranged from 5,411 to 21,753 mg/cu m. No pathologic data were reported for the animals that died from these exposures.[5, 12, 13] The one beagle exposed[12] to vinyl acetate at 13,388 mg/cu m and all of the rats exposed[13] at 3,500 mg/cu m survived. Upper respiratory difficulty, eye and nose irritation, and increased macrophages in the lungs were noted in rats exposed at 7,000 mg/cu m periodically for three weeks.[8] Deese and Joyner[7] found that each of three persons exposed to vinyl acetate at 75.6 mg/cu m experienced hoarseness or coughing and eye irritation; one person became hoarse when exposed at about 15 mg/cu m.

Ocular effects have also been reported from contact with airborne vinyl acetate. Exposure to vinyl acetate at 840 mg/cu m caused some eye blinking and reddening of the sclerae in a dog,[12] 651 mg/cu m caused eye irritation and tearing in dogs,[11] and 0.5 ml of vinyl acetate caused severe irritation or mild burns when applied to a rabbit's eye.[13] The lowest concentration that caused eye irritation in humans[7] (one of three subjects) was 20.0 mg/cu m. Two reports[7, 13] suggested that skin irritation can result in humans after dermal contact with (presumably liquid) vinyl acetate. One report[13] noted that this irritation might result in blisters. Deese and Joyner[7] reported that skin irritation or rash was noted by 3 of 31 vinyl acetate workers. Union Carbide investigators[13] reported that the dermal LC_{50} in rabbits was greater than 5 ml/kg in a 24-hour covered-skin contact test with liquid vinyl acetate, but they also stated that undiluted vinyl acetate on the skin of the shaved abdomen of a rabbit caused no reaction.

Evidence of possible adverse effects of vinyl acetate on the human nervous system is meager. Gofmekler[10] found that 0.32 mg/cu m was the minimal concentration of vinyl acetate capable of inducing EEG desynchronization as a conditioned response; 0.21 mg/cu m did not produce this effect. Goeva[9] found that rats given vinyl acetate in oral doses of 0.1 mg/kg for seven months exhibited fewer positive responses to a conditioned stimulus and took longer to develop conditioned reflexes than either controls or rats fed 0.01 mg/kg of vinyl acetate. It is questionable whether these particular studies[9, 10] demonstrated adverse changes, so it does not now seem appropriate to conclude that vinyl acetate exposure in the work environment at these concentrations will induce biologically significant effects on the nervous system.

The readily identifiable odor of vinyl acetate appears to be one means by which workers are warned of its presence in the work environment. Determinations of the threshold of odor detection have given varying results. For example, Deese and Joyner[7] reported that all of three subjects detected a marked odor of vinyl acetate at 75.6 mg/cu m; a "slight" odor was reported by three of four exposed at 14.7 and 1.4 mg/cu m. In an experimental study,[12] all of nine volunteers detected the odor of vinyl acetate at 4.6 mg/cu m but, with one questionable exception, they did not detect its odor at 2.1 mg/cu m. Minimal perceptible (threshold) and maximal imperceptible concentrations for odor detection were determined by Gofmekler[10] to be 1.0 and 0.7 mg/cu m, respectively. These findings indicate that the odor threshold of vinyl acetate probably ranges from 1.0 to 3.3 mg/cu m; their variability probably reflects differences in methods of determination and possibly in the development by the test subjects of adaptation to the odor. Although a noticeable odor of vinyl acetate may indicate a potential hazard, it is not quantitatively reliable. Olfactory fatigue has also been observed during exposure to vinyl acetate. Vinyl acetate at 68.3–250.3 mg/cu m produced olfactory fatigue in all exposed volunteers.[12] Olfactory fatigue was complete in all of three persons exposed at 68.3 mg/cu m and in one of three at 119.7 mg/cu m after 3–116 minutes; two of three subjects at the latter concentration and all of four at 250.3 mg/cu m experienced partial olfactory fatigue.

A threshold limit value (TLV) of 10 ppm or 30 mg/cu m was recommended by the Threshold Limits Committee of the ACGIH[3] in 1969 and adopted[4] in 1971. A short term exposure limit (STEL) of 20 ppm or 60 mg/cu m was recommended[2] in 1976. The *Documentation of Threshold Limit Values*[1] noted four-hour LC_{50} values in rats, mice and rabbits of 4,000, 1,550, and 2,500 ppm, respectively. No evidence of circulatory abnormalities or evidence of altered metabolism was noted in dogs exposed six hours per day to vinyl acetate for about 11 weeks at average concentrations of from 91 to 186 ppm. The documentation stated that Gage[8] had found rats unaffected by repeated exposures at 100 ppm and had recommended 50 ppm as a working standard. The documentation also noted a report of 15 years' industrial experience with 21 vinyl acetate chemical operators in whom hoarseness and coughing ("slight irritation") were observed at around 22 ppm. The medical records and multiphasic examinations were stated to have revealed no evidence of chronic effects from concentrations of 5–10 ppm. The Threshold Limits Committee recommended a TLV of 10 ppm, citing the evidence that irritation may be experienced at around 20 ppm but not at 10 ppm and in the light of evidence that neither acute nor chronic effects occur from repeated daily exposure for many years.[2] Australia, Belgium, Finland, the Netherlands, Sweden, and Switzerland have maximal allowable concentrations (MACs) for vinyl acetate of 10 ppm, or 30 mg/cu m. The ILO report noted that MACs or ceiling values are used because time-weighted averages (TWAs) should not be applied to fast-acting substances, e.g., irritants and narcotics, or to substances that are particularly toxic. There is no current U.S. federal occupational standard for vinyl acetate, but NIOSH recommends a ceiling limit of 4 ppm.[10a]

REFERENCES

1. American Conference of Governmental Industrial Hygienists, Committee on Threshold Limit Values: *Documentation of Threshold Limit Values for Substances in Workroom Air*, ed 5, 1986. Cincinnati, Oh, ACGIH.
2. American Conference of Governmental Industrial Hygienists: *TLVs—Threshold Limit Values for Chemical Substances in Workroom Air Adopted by ACGIH for 1985–86*. Cincinnati, Oh, ACGIH, 1985.
3. American Conference of Governmental Industrial Hygienists: *Threshold Limit Values of Airborne Contaminants and Intended Changes Adopted by ACGIH for 1986–1987*. Cincinnati, Oh, ACGIH, 1986.
4. American Conference of Governmental Industrial Hygienists: *Threshold Limit Values of Airborne Contaminants and Physical Agents with Intended Changes Adopted by ACGIH for 1971*. Cincinnati, Oh, ACGIH, 1971, p 27.
5. Carpenter CP, Smyth HF Jr, Pozzani, UD: The assay of acute vapor

toxicity, and the grading and interpretation of results on 96 chemical compounds. *J Ind Hyg Toxicol* 1949; 31:343.

6. *Criteria for a Recommended Standard*: Occupational Exposure to Vinyl Acetate, DHEW (NIOSH) Publ 78-205. Cincinnati, Oh, US Dept of Health, Education, and Welfare, PHS, Center for Disease Control, National Institute for Occupational Safety and Health, 78 pp., 1978.
7. Deese DE, Joyner RE: Vinyl acetate. A study of chronic human exposure. *Am Ind Hyg Assoc J* 1969; 30:449.
8. Gage JC: The subacute inhalation toxicity of 109 industrial chemicals. *Br J Ind Med* 1970; 27:1.
9. Goeva OE: Maximum permissible concentration of vinyl acetate in water basins. *Hyg Sanit (USSR)* 1966; 31:209.
10. Gofmekler VA: Maximum admissible concentration of acetates in the atmosphere. *Gig Sanit* 1960; 25:9 (Russian).

10a. NIOSH recommendations for occupational safety and health standards. *MMWR* 1986; 35(1S).

11. *Report of Toxicity of Vinyl Acetate*. Unpublished report submitted to American Conference of Governmental Industrial Hygienists by E. I. du Pont de Nemours & Co, Inc, Central Research and Development Dept, Haskell Laboratory for Toxicology and Industrial Medicine, 7 pp, January, 1967.
12. *Summary of Responses of Animals and Humans to the Vapors of Vinyl Acetate*. Unpublished report submitted to American Conference of Governmental Industrial Hygienists by Carnegie-Mellon University, Mellon Institute, Pittsburgh, 3 pp, October, 1968.
13. *Toxicology Studies—Vinyl Acetate HQ*. New York, Union Carbide Corporation, Industrial Medicine and Toxicology Dept, 2 pp, 1958.

GENERAL PRINCIPLES OF TREATMENT

A. For gases such as ammonia, chlorine, hydrofluoric acid, hydrogen sulfide, nitric acid, oxides of nitrogen and sulfur dioxide:

1. The presence of the agent when it is inhaled usually is evanescent and, therefore, cannot be washed away or otherwise removed, i.e., when only the skin is involved.

2. When the patient arrives for treatment, one is faced mainly with the problems caused by the presence of the agent.

3. Arterial blood gases are of primary importance to aid in determination of the extent of damage. Never discharge a patient significantly exposed to irritant gas without obtaining an arterial blood sample.

4. Supportive measures include suctioning (intubation may be required), volume cycle ventilator support (positive and expiratory pressure [PEEP]), steroids and antibiotics, after a culture has been taken. If the eyes are involved, an ophthalmologic consultation is recommended.

B. For gases with delayed action on the lungs:

1. Phosgene may cause severe pulmonary edema, often seen several hours after exposure. Treatment is similar to that for irritant gases described above except that PEEP may be most useful. A unique property of hydrogen sulfide is that it can kill by directly paralyzing the respiratory center within seconds of heavy exposure. Remember that hydrogen sulfide often produces olfactory fatigue, making its presence undetectable to those who have been previously exposed to lesser amounts. Delayed pulmonary edema can occur. Hyperbaric oxygen has proved to be valuable in the treatment of hydrogen sulfide poisoning (Kindwall, E. P., St. Luke's Hospital, Milwaukee, Wisconsin, unpublished).

2. Oxides of nitrogen (nitrogen dioxide and nitrogen tetroxide) have a delayed action on the lungs. A worker may be exposed for eight hours during the day with no ill effects and later, while at home, may lapse into pulmonary edema, which can be fatal. Treatment is as noted above.

48

On the Health Effects of Solvents

Olav Axelson, M.D.

Christer Hogstedt, M.D.

Solvent exposure is common in industry and constitutes a potential health hazard to millions of workers throughout the world. According to a trade union survey in the 1970s, in an industrialized country like Sweden, some 3% to 4% of the total population was reported to consider solvent exposure a problem. Estimates of specified solvent exposure in the U.S. by NIOSH (National Institute for Occupational Safety and Health) suggested about 100,000 workers to have some degree of toluene exposure and about 140,000 individuals to have potential exposure to xylene in their work. In many trades, almost every worker is exposed (e.g., painters, varnishers, and carpet layers), but there are attempts to reduce solvent exposure through the introduction of water-based paints and adhesives.

The degree of solvent exposure can vary considerably among individual workers and from time to time as in painting, varnishing, and open degreasing operations. Exposures can sometimes be extremely high, as with styrene used in the manufacturing of plastic boats under primitive conditions.[49] Furthermore, many processes require the evaporation of solvents and are therefore inherently problematic from the hygienic point of view. Good equipment and adequate work practices can decrease exposure, but even modern and well functioning equipment needs cleaning, servicing, and repair, and such work often will result in high but short-time exposures. Open handling of solvents and primitive degreasing operations are common in small shops (e.g., in automobile repairing), but also in many temporary jobs in the large and usually well-organized factories. Not to be overlooked is that hygienic concerns about solvents are applicable in the context of exposure to anesthetic gases in operating theaters as well as in the handling of gasoline and jet fuel in distribution or in the repair of equipment such as pumps and tanks.

The acute, narcotic effects of solvents have been known for a long time and some of the industrial solvents have a history of use as general anesthetics (e.g., chloroform, ether, trichloroethylene, and even gasoline).[48] Toxic effects on the blood and liver were recognized early as caused by benzene and carbon tetrachloride, respectively. Irritation of mucous membranes is another rather common, but less serious type of effect caused by, for example, styrene and isopropyl alcohol. An asthmatic condition may appear with certain solvent exposures, usually depending on a nonspecific (nonallergic) hyperreactivity, and will often require that the worker change to another job.

The long-term effects of solvent exposure have been subject to quite intensive research over the past decade, especially with regard to neurotoxicity, but also the potential carcinogenic, mutagenic, and teratogenic aspects that have attracted growing interest. There are also some more or less convincing observations on liver and kidney damage as possibly due to exposures from other solvents such as the classic, hepatotoxic halogenated aliphatics, carbon tetrachloride and chloroform. Dermatologic problems are well known to be due to skin contact with solvents and extraction of the fat from the skin, but these aspects are discussed in other chapters.

NEUROTOXIC EFFECTS

Experimental Studies

Experimental studies involving psychologic testing of volunteers after inhalation of solvent vapors have been performed to study possible effects from lower exposure levels. In one set of experiments, the specific odors were masked by menthol to obscure the absence or presence of solvents at any particular concentration.[46] Exposure times of 1.5 hours were used and the uptake of the solvent was continually measured every 20 minutes. Such tests as reaction time, short-term memory, and single arithmetic items were measured and found to be affected at surprisingly low exposures (Table 48–1). Similar studies have also been undertaken by others with fairly consistent results.[120] Prolonged reaction time appears to be a simple and reliable measurable effect of solvent exposure.

Clinical Observations and Cross-Sectional Studies

The evaluation of long-term effects of solvent exposure is associated with methodologic difficulties. Usually cross-sectional studies have been applied, i.e., the current disorders or complaints of an exposed group have been referred to existing exposure levels in comparison to an unexposed reference group. However,

TABLE 48–1.

Means of Cumulative Uptake of Solvents in Blood and Tissues for Groups of Experimentally Exposed Subjects Where Impairments in at Least One Psychologic Function Have Been Demonstrated[3]

SOLVENT	UPTAKE (MG)	NUMBER OF SUBJECTS IN THE GROUP
Toluene	170	12
Methylchloroform	330	12
Styrene	590	12
White spirit (aromatic)	240	20
(aliphatic)	1055	
Methylene chloride	1145	14
Trichloroethylene	420	15

the long-term effects might easily be overlooked in cross-sectional studies, as those individuals who become more severely affected tend to leave the job due to the symptoms or even because of disability or death, and therefore would not be present at the time of the study. Hence, nonpositive results in cross-sectional studies do not necessarily mean a safe work environment.

Another problematic aspect concerns the symptoms and signs of isolated cases in relation to solvent exposure, i.e., vague symptoms like tiredness, affect liability, irritability, memory disturbances, which are difficult to interpret in causal terms in relation to work conditions. Cases with such symptoms and histories of solvent exposure have been reported during several decades and were reviewed by Browning in 1965.[22] The symptoms characterizing these cases are usually more or less in agreement with the so-called psycho-organic syndrome or neurasthenic syndrome.[18, 86] Also, jet fuel exposure may be responsible for this syndrome, but in addition, decreased nerve conduction velocities and high vibration thresholds have been observed in this context,[77, 78] probably after quite high exposures, sometimes amounting to 500–3,000 ppm for the service personnel.

Many cross-sectional studies on the potential neurotoxic effects of solvents have been presented since the early 1970s. Those studies usually have been based on psychologic tests, sometimes neurophysiologic examinations, and also questionnaires. More or less disturbed functions with regard to visual perception, perceptual speed, hand-eye coordination, and memory have been found among individuals who have been exposed to carbon disulfide, tri- and tetrachloroethylene, toluene, xylene, and their mixtures.[54, 55, 83] Similar observations have been made among house painters[53] and workers manufacturing products of styrene-modified glassfiber-reinforced polyester plastics.[47, 51, 84] Psychologic tests also have indicated adverse effects in studies of car painters[35, 55] and jetfuel workers.[77, 78] (For further aspects with regard to these findings and the utility of psychologic tests, see Chapter 49.)

Besides psychologic tests, neurophysiologic methods have played a major role in a number of cross-sectional studies on solvent-induced disorders as reviewed by Seppäläinen.[108, 109] Electroencephalographic (EEG) recordings have been utilized in some studies and have revealed abnormalities in solvent-exposed individuals, both among patients and in active workers. Diffuse and generalized abnormalities have been seen most commonly[51, 112, 115] and even dose-response patterns have been observed as for styrene exposed workers, taking mandelic acid in the urine as the exposure parameter.[113] In other worker groups (e.g., car painters),[114] there has been less pronounced EEG changes, however. The clinical importance of EEG abnormalities in solvent-exposed individuals is somewhat unclear, but there is at least some, but not full, correlation with psychologic test results.[115] It is of interest that some 5% to 10% of solvent-exposed individuals have shown paroxysmal EEG abnormalities in the form of spikes or spike-and-wave discharges, an observation that might indicate a lowered threshold for seizures.[110] Also, some unpublished clinical observations seem to suggest the possibility of attacks of seizures as related to solvent exposure. However, the EEG is of very limited value in the examination of the individual cases of suspected solvent-induced disorders.[41]

Not only the central nervous system, but also the peripheral nerves are affected by solvents, and the experiences in this respect have been presented by Seppäläinen.[111] (See Chapter 50.)

The major effect on the peripheral nerves seems to be an axonopathy and an accumulation of neurofilaments of about 10 nm within the axons as characteristic of these damages. Microscopic changes may occur even before any major functional disturbances are seen.[23] Among the various worker groups that have been reported to show more or less pronounced signs of polyneuropathy, there are, for example, Italian shoe-workers exposed to mixtures of pentanes, hexanes and heptanes,[28, 103] U.S. workers producing plastic-coated and color printed fabrics,[3] and Swedish industrial painters and car painters;[35] similar experiences have been reported from Germany.[129] Usually a slowing of the motor and sensory conduction velocities have been registered, although the amplitudes of sensory and motor action potentials would be theoretically preferable to measure. However, such measurements are easily influenced by technical placement of electrodes, skin resistance etc., and therefore tend to be uncertain in practice.[111]

In view of the neurophysiologic findings, it is quite clear that symptoms of neuropathy should be watched among individuals exposed to solvents, especially in the context of exposure to n-hexane mixtures[63, 124] and methyl-butyl ketone,[16, 73] but also when exposure to mixtures of aliphatic and aromatic hydrocarbons has taken place as illustrated by the findings among car painters and workers with exposure to jet fuels.[35, 77, 78] Vague symptoms such as tingling and prickling sensations and even restless legs may indicate neuropathy and should be noticed carefully when examining individuals exposed to solvents. Nevertheless, such symptoms tend to be rare, whereas neurophysiologic measurements may reveal abnormalities. Not surprisingly, effects on the central nervous system tend to occur together with neuropathy, although these different manifestations are not necessarily associated.[41]

Judging from existing literature and critical reviews,[26, 32] one might conclude that polyneuropathies would be especially attributable to exposure to carbon disulfide, n-hexane, and its metabolite methyl-n-butyl ketone, also used as a solvent. To some extent, polyneuropathies may also occur as a result of exposure to mixed hydrocarbons such as the solvents used in car painting.[35, 114]

Other neurophysiologic findings of interest relate to vestibulo-oculomotor disturbances. Hence, animal experiments have shown that hydrocarbon solvents influence the vestibulo-oculomotor reflex arc, seemingly through blocking the inhibition exerted by the cerebellum. Correspondingly, solvent-exposed patients with psycho-organic syndrome have shown signs of cerebellar dysfunction, suggesting that this part of the brain might be affected early by solvent exposure.[96] Furthermore, studies of solvent-exposed individuals by a vestibulo-oculomotor test battery suggest qualitative differences between solvents with regard to the effect on the structures of the vestibulo-oculomotor reflex arc, toluene and styrene being similar, but different from trichloroethylene in their effect.[69, 81]

Epidemiology of Chronic Neuropsychiatric Disorders and Solvent Exposure

Few studies are available that elucidate the severeness of neuropsychiatric disorders due to solvent exposure, but more or less severe and even disabling symptoms might occur. A case-referent (case-control) study in a disability pension register in Sweden[12] revealed that painters, varnishers, and carpet layers (i.e., workers with considerable exposure to solvents), had a relative risk of about 1.8, to suffer from neuropsychiatric disorders in comparison to other skilled workers in various trades with some connection with construction work. To judge from this study, encompassing only one of the Swedish counties with some 250,000 inhabitants, about 3% to 4% of all neuropsychiatric disorders in men 36 to 65 years of age, and considered severe enough to potentially contribute to a sick pension, might have had a relationship to solvent exposure in the late 1960s and early 1970s.[13]

Two further epidemiologic studies from Denmark have shown quite similar results, one of them a case-referent study[99] and the other a cohort.[87] Both these studies indicated a rate ratio of about 2–3 (as dependent on the criteria applied in various subanalyses) for solvent-exposed individuals to develop a dementia-type of mental disorder. Considering isolated studies, there is always the possibility that some confounding effect has escaped control and determines the result. The remarkably good consistency between these studies makes it quite likely, however, that they reflect a true effect of solvent exposure as indicated in a quite detailed discussion of the validity of these studies.[26] In a British study, on the other hand, there was no excess of solvent-exposed individuals among those consulting general practitioners for neuropsychiatric ailments in comparison to other disorders.[27]

It might be mentioned in this context also that multiple sclerosis has been discussed on epidemiologic grounds[4] as related to solvent exposure from glues in the shoe industry, but there were only 5 exposed cases in a series of 41, which is not particularly convincing, even if the number was almost five-fold the expected. It might be mentioned also that a study on Parkinson's disease and solvent exposure has not revealed any association.[97]

Diagnostic and Health Care Aspects on Solvent Neurotoxicity

Presently, the diagnosis of solvent-induced disorders has to be based on careful history taking, particularly occupational, evaluation of the premorbid personality, and psychologic testing. Symptoms such as increased fatigue, neurasthenia, depressive complaints, and impaired memory should be specifically elicited. Personality changes and emotional dysfunctions are also characteristic for those individuals suffering from solvent-induced neuropsychiatric conditions.[41, 122] Neurophysiologic and neuroradiologic examinations tend to be insensitive and less useful in clinical examinations than in epidemiologic studies and would require rather advanced effects to provide any findings of diagnostic value. Computerized tomography of the brain seems to be of limited value as well, although it may have a place in differential diagnostics and might reveal atrophy in advanced cases.[21, 76]

It is inherent in the diagnostic situation that it can be difficult to rule out conditions with similar symptoms or other causes of a psycho-organic syndrome, such as alcoholism, endogenous depression, hereditary presenility, generalized arteriosclerosis, minor cerebrovascular disorders, post-infectious encephalopathy, brain tumors, adult hydrocephalus, late effects of electroconvulsive therapy, or "solvent sniffing," as well as exposure to lead, mercury, etc. However, anamnestic information, the gradual onset of the symptoms, the lack of specific neurologic symptoms, and the slow progress over time would be of value for the differential diagnostics.

Considering the exposure to solvents, their very nature, duration and intensity are important factors to take into account in relation to the symptoms. Sometimes it can be valuable to calculate exposure-hours per year (e.g., for a painter), thereby adjusting for outdoor painting and wallpapering, which is the task of painters in some countries. Workload during the exposure should also be considered as strongly influencing the amount of solvent absorption.[6] Sometimes records of exposure measurements are available or biologic monitoring might have been undertaken (e.g., determinations of mandelic acid in the urine of workers exposed to styrene or trichloroacetic acid in the urine after trichloroethylene exposure). Various countries have different regulations and criteria for recognizing occupational diseases, which will govern the views taken with regard to compensation. However, if the symptoms and the results from psychologic testing, as outlined in Chapter 49, are consistent with a psycho-organic syndrome, and given that there is no other reason for such a condition and the individual has had a considerable exposure to solvents during many years, it might be reasonable to support an occupational insurance claim.[41]

The prognosis for the solvent-induced psycho-organic syndrome is somewhat unclear at this time, but some improvement has been registered with regard to EEG as well as to electrophysiologic findings of neuropathies,[112] but also an unpredictable deterioration of health might occur for some individuals.[5, 21] Many feel better after cessation of exposure, however, but there might not necessarily be any improvement in psychologic tests.

Health Screening Procedures

The desirability of prevention and early detection of solvent-induced ill-health, along with the large number of solvent exposed workers, call for screening procedures that are reasonably effective and inexpensive. Attempts have been made to construct self-administered questionnaires for such primary screening of health disturbances. For such screening, a high sensitivity is desirable not to overlook relevant symptoms, but high sensitivity tends to give a considerable number of "false positives." These individuals have to be examined by ordinary clinical procedures, which is not too cumbersome in view of the benefits of not having to examine everybody in a solvent-exposed population. A screening question-

TABLE 48–2.
Results of a Validated Questionnaire of Solvent-Exposed and Nonexposed Male Workers

QUESTION	EXPOSED WORKERS (N = 229)	NONEXPOSED WORKERS (N = 173)	χ^2
1. Are you abnormally tired?	31	6	37.0
2. Do you have palpitations of the heart even when you don't exert yourself?	13	5	6.3
3. Do you often have painful tingling in some part of your body?	28	10	16.4
4. Do you often feel irritated without any particular reason?	34	13	22.8
5. Do you often feel depressed without any particular reason?	21	6	15.0
6. Do you often have problems with concentrating?	28	9	20.7
7. Do you have a short memory?	49	30	12.4
8. Do you often perspire without any particular reason?	20	10	6.5
9. Do you have any problems with buttoning and unbuttoning?	1	1	0.5
10. Do you generally find it hard to get the meaning from reading newspapers and books?	22	7	16.5
11. Have your relatives told you that you have a short memory?	42	24	13.7
12. Do you sometimes feel an oppression in your chest?	34	12	25.5
13. Do you often have to make notes about what you must remember?	28	11	16.9
14. Do you often have to go back and check things you have done such as turned off the stove, locked the door?	39	16	23.1
15. Do you have a headache at least once a week?	27	14	10.0
16. Are you less interested in sex than what you think is normal?	11	1	12.8

Notes: these questions give the percentage of symptoms among solvent-exposed male workers (a random sample from the local trade union of painters and car painters and workers exposed to solvents in the metal industry) and non-exposed male workers (a random sample of electricians and postmen). The groups were stratified for age and the chi-squares calculated according to the Mantel-Haenszel formula.
χ^2(l df) > 3.84; the p-value < 0.05 (two-tailed).

naire for neuropsychiatric symptoms is shown in Table 48–2, which—in translation from Swedish—gives 16 questions primarily based on common Scandinavian experiences and selected by a validation procedure.[64] Based on the 90th percentile for the number of symptoms among nonexposed workers, the recommendation has been made that young solvent-exposed men, i.e., less than 28 years of age, indicating more than 4 symptoms in the 16 questions, and those 28 years of age or older indicating more than 6 symptoms, should be further checked by a physician. If the physician confirms the symptoms of solvent-induced effects, further clinical examinations, with psychologic and perhaps neurophysiologic tests, are recommended to finally reach a diagnosis.[64]

CARCINOGENICITY, TERATOGENICITY, AND MUTAGENICITY

Carcinogenicity, teratogenicity, and mutagenicity are other effects besides neurotoxicity described for some solvents. Several solvents have been found to have carcinogenic properties in animal experiments, especially the chlorinated ones like carbon tetrachloride, chloroform, tetrachloroethylene, and trichloroethylene.[71] However, there are no epidemiologic studies that clearly confirm the findings from the animal experiments, although there are some studies which might indicate a human cancer risk.

With regard to the nonchlorinated hydrocarbons, there is documentation enough only for benzene to be thought of as a human carcinogen.[70, 136] The background for the possible or actual carcinogenicity of solvents might be sought in their metabolism and the formation of reactive metabolites, particularly of epoxide character. However, the benzene epoxide, as appearing early in the biotransformation, is not considered to be the ultimate carcinogen, but instead a further degradation product is held responsible, and especially a diolepoxide has been suggested in this respect.[126, 130] There is also an alternative suggestion, namely, that a depressive effect of benzene and its homologues on the T cell-dependent immunity should account for the carcinogenic activity.[89]

Another solvent, which forms reactive metabolites, is styrene as oxidized through styrene oxide. A carcinogenic effect has been suspected on the basis of results in mutagenicity tests and to some extent as based on animal experiments.[71, 132] Styrene as well as toluene and xylene seem to have some ring hydroxylation which might indicate a pathway through reactive and potentially cancer-causing intermediates.[29, 33, 98, 126]

The potential cancer risk associated with trichloroethylene exposure has been a concern since the middle of the 1970s, when the U.S. National Cancer Institute reported an increased frequency of hepato-cellular cancer in mice (males only got a significantly increased frequency of this tumor) that were fed trichloroethylene through gastric intubation.[95] Trichloroethylene like other chlorinated hydrocarbons possesses mutagenic activity in bacterial test systems after microsomal activation by added liver homogenate,[39, 50] so the mutagenic effect is probably dependent on the epoxidation that takes place in the metabolism of this compound.[19, 126] A similar indication of carcinogenicity of perchloroethylene also has been obtained[94] and methylchloroform and methylenechloride are mutagenic in bacterial test systems.[75, 116]

Except for a leukemogenic effect from benzene,[2, 70, 135] no really convincing epidemiologic reports are available on cancer hazards from solvent exposures, but indicative experience is not lacking for some of the other solvents. Hence, extensive studies based on proportional mortality[88] and case–control data,[134] respectively, have indicated an excess cancer mortality among painters with regard to malignancies of the respiratory system and the stomach, also supported by a Swedish cohort study.[36] Since the exposure pattern is complex for painters, it is not entirely clear if the indicated cancer hazard is referable to solvent exposure or to other agents such as pigments from removal of old paint or paint spraying operations. Even some asbestos exposure might have taken place through grinding on plaster. It is also noteworthy in this regard that chromosomal aberrations and sister chromatid exchanges have not been found among paint industry workers[52] who had had quite some exposure just to the solvents involved in paint, especially to xylene and toluene. The literature is not consistent and easy to evaluate, however, since chromosomal aberrations have been reported after toluene exposure by some investigators.[45] Other epidemiologic observations are of interest in this context as well, e.g., the finding of a relationship both between Hodgkin and non-Hodgkin lymphomas and occupational exposure to various organic solvents, both of the aliphatic, aromatic, and chlorinated types.[42, 56, 100] Similarly, for acute myeloid leukemia, there are also some epidemiologic indications that solvent exposure might play a role, perhaps through benzene which occurs to a greater or lesser extent in various solvents, as well as in gasoline.[20, 40] Lymphatic leukemia has been particularly associated with exposure to carbon tetrachloride and carbon disulfide in the rubber industry, but the environment is very complex in this type of industry, providing for confounding from various other rubber chemicals.[24] (See Chapter 63.)

There are also some epidemiologic observations on cancer and exposure to chlorinated solvents. Hence, in a cohort of laundry and drycleaning workers, there was a slight excess of liver cancers (4 versus 1.7 expected)[17] and in a case referent study[119] a rate ratio of 2.5 was obtained for laundering, cleaning, and other garment services. Additional case referent data have followed with an indication of a more or less clear association between exposure to a variety of solvents and liver cancer, one of them showing an association for females only,[61] whereas the other was restricted to males and found about a two-fold risk.[57]

With regard to more pure exposure to halogenated solvents there are a few studies, quite limited in size however, but these might be briefly mentioned. Hence, a proportional mortality ratio analysis and a cohort of 751 workers exposed to methylene chloride, encompassing 110 deaths in the latest followup,[59] showed no excess of cancer, nor was there any indication of an excess cancer mortality in another study of this exposure.[101] With regard to other halomethanes, a mortality study of a cohort of 539 rather young refrigerator workers with exposure to fluorocarbons might be mentioned as not showing any excess of cancer, so far.[123]

Regarding trichloroethylene, two cohort studies have been published on the potential cancer risk, one encompassing 518 men, the other 1,148 males and 969 females, none of them showing an excess of cancer,[11, 127] nor have any liver cancers been indicated in some other evaluations involving trichloroethylene.[85, 102] However, an expansion and updating of the first mentioned cohort to encompass 1,424 individuals now indicates a slight excess incidence of urinary tract cancers and malignancies in the hematolymphatic organs (11 versus 4.85 expected and 5 versus 1.20, respectively),[9] but this cohort is still rather young, so there is a need for further and more conclusive evaluations in the future.

Regarding teratogenic effects, indications of a hazard have been obtained from chicken experiments with styrene and its metabolite, styrene oxide.[131] A Czechoslovakian report[79] has suggested a relationship between various types of solvent exposure and sacral agenesis in humans and there was thought to be some support for this possibility in animal experiments, since xylene seemed to exert a teratogenic effect in chicken embryos. Observations through a case-control approach have indicated that exposure to various aromatic and aliphatic compounds might play a role in malformations in the central nervous system and also be responsible for oral clefts.[66, 67, 68] It should be recalled here as well that exposure to anesthetics, some of them halogenated aliphatics of the solvent type, has been found associated with a high frequency of spontaneous abortions.[30, 72]

The presently existing information on reproductive effects is not always consistent, however. For example, a small cohort of women with styrene exposure during pregnancy gave birth to children without any excess of malformations, nor did these women have any abnormal number of abortions.[58] On the other hand, there are also some indications toward both an abortion hazard from solvents[14, 60, 121] and a risk of malformations from styrene,[65] but definite conclusions in these respects would require further studies.

OTHER TYPES OF DISORDERS

Kidney disorders should be considered with regard to the possibility of a relationship to solvent exposure. Since the early 1970s a number of reports have appeared that suggest a possible correlation between solvent exposure and glomerulonephritis.[15, 80, 105, 138] It is not clear at present if the nephrotoxic effect from solvents is due to a long-time and low-grade exposure, or if it is merely exerted through high but short-time exposures, or to which extent only some specific solvents might be involved. However, seemingly healthy workers with exposure to styrene, toluene, and mixtures of aromatic (mainly toluene and xylene), aliphatic, and alicyclic hydrocarbons have been found to excrete more total protein or albumin, erythrocytes, and leukocytes on the average than controls,[8, 44, 92] perhaps mainly due to tubular effects rather than because of glomerular damage.

It seems as if further elucidation is needed to evaluate other factors—such as heredity or infections—that might influence the nephrotoxicity of solvents. It is interesting to note that aromatic solvents seem to decrease serum complement levels.[118]

Potential hepatotoxicity from certain solvents should also be remembered. In particular, carbon tetrachloride has long been known to cause severe hepatic damage within a few days after exposure and there also are some case reports indicating a later development of cirrhosis and hepatic tumors.[74] The use of carbon tetrachloride is now banned in many countries, severely restricted or substituted for, but there might also be toxic effects on the liver from other chlorinated solvents as well;[107] reciprocal potentiation from alcohol and solvents such as trichloroethylene and isopropyl alcohol deserves attention.[31, 126, 128] Indications of liver damage have been obtained among housepainters more or less clearly suffering from neurotoxic effects from solvent exposure.[34] Therefore, the possibility may exist that liver cirrhosis is not only caused by alcohol abuse but also by solvent exposure.[10]

Among the various effects of solvents it should also be noted that lens changes have been reported among Finnish car painters as probably dependent on solvent exposure.[104] This observation has some support from animal studies, since cataracts have been induced by exposure to alkylaromatics.[93]

Finally, it might also be recalled that solvent exposure, namely with regard to carbon disulfide, has been associated with cardiovascular disease in the rayon-viscose industry.[62, 90, 125] The cardiovascular effect is probably rather specific for carbon disulfide, but little attention has been paid to the possibility that other solvents might cause cardiovascular disorders. There are apparent problems, however, in the epidemiologic evaluation of such effects with regard to the frequent exposure to solvents and the high background morbidity from cardiovascular diseases in industrialized countries.

Health checkups concerning effects from solvents outside the nervous system are usually of little value (e.g., checking of blood or liver status), unless exposure takes place to benzene, carbon tetrachloride, and perhaps some of the aromatics, for example, styrene. Nevertheless, such tests are usually included in health checkup programs for solvent workers. Glomerulonephritis is a fairly rare disease that sometimes may result from solvent exposure, and since a simple measurement of proteinuria is convenient and inexpensive, this might be worthwhile. For painters, some other measurements should be considered (i.e., lead and chromium in blood or urine, when exposure takes place to pigments in addition to solvents, especially for many spray painters).

MONITORING SOLVENT EXPOSURE

Technical hygienic methods, as well as biologic monitoring, should be used for the control of solvent exposure (i.e., solvent concentrations in the air can be measured or, alternatively, reliance might be placed on determinations of solvent metabolites in the urine of the exposed workers). It is not the purpose of this chapter to delineate and describe methods for air measurements of solvents, but it might be briefly recalled that mixtures of various solvents can be difficult to measure. A commonly used technique is to adsorb solvents by sucking workroom air through a charcoal tube; this method is preferable for its simplicity and the possibility of sending the charcoal tubes to remote laboratories for analyses. More recently, passive samplers have appeared on the market and will probably be a good tool in the future for solvent measurements. It might be added, however, that exposure to alcohols might be underestimated through the measurements as these are difficult to dissolve from charcoal.[43] There are other problems as well, especially with regard to storing of the exposed tubes.[106] Moreover, technical hygienic monitoring is resource-demanding, since a hygienist usually cannot follow more than a few workers with measurements through the shift.

Biologic monitoring may be a convenient and preferable alternative whenever possible. A contributing factor to the usefulness of biologic monitoring is that the workload greatly influences the amount of solvent uptake, as demonstrated in experimental studies.[6] It has also been found that the solvent uptake in connection with various workloads can be fairly different for various types of solvents. For example, methylene chloride is taken up to a much lesser degree than toluene and styrene.

Biologic monitoring might be based on either a metabolite in the urine or on determination of the compound itself in alveolar air. It has been suggested that the ratio between the alveolar air concentration and the concentration in ambient air be taken as a measure of the uptake.[7] This method requires a number of samples over the workday, however, and might be somewhat uncertain if there is a great variation in the solvent concentration over the day (as would be the metabolite determinations). Nevertheless, this method of monitoring seems to be better than just using alveolar air samples at the end of the workday and during the following 12 to 16 hours. Such sampling requires the comparison of the measured concentrations in the alveolar air to so-called decay curves, which tend to be uncertain as presumably influenced by the body fat mass.[37]

The utilization of metabolites in urine, for example, trichloroacetic acid in the case of exposure to trichloroethylene and mandelic acid as a result of styrene exposure, has the advantage of permitting simple sampling methods. However, for most of the solvents, the knowledge is comparatively incomplete with regard to the relationship between exposure levels and metabolites in urine, nor is there sufficient knowledge relating the effects of solvents to metabolite concentrations in urine. For example, there could be disturbances in physiologic variables in relation to metabolite concentrations in urine and there can be some delay before excretion takes place as for trichloroacetic acid appearing in the urine as a metabolite of trichloroethylene some 24 hours after exposure.[91] Furthermore, there may be influences on the metabolism by alcohol intake as found among styrene workers.[25] The problem of dealing with low exposure levels for styrene through biologic monitoring is nowadays overcome by the available specific methods,[38, 117] which give results that are uninfluenced by various nonspecific mandelic acid derivatives in the urine.

Further information on the relationships of biologic effects and concentrations of metabolites in urine, as well as various aspects on biologic monitoring of solvents and other industrial chemicals, can be found elsewhere,[82, 126, 133, 137] and especially in a comprehensive book on this matter.[1] Presently, the authorities tend to establish standards based on air concentrations, and, therefore, the relationship between these and the levels of metabolites in urine is of the greatest interest from the compliance point of view. It would certainly be more relevant for the future, but also more demanding, to create tolerance limits with regard to metabolites or blood concentrations in direct relation to physiologic effects.

REFERENCES

1. Aitio A, Riihimäki V, Vainio H: Biological monitoring and surveillance of workers exposed to chemicals. Washington, Hemisphere Publishing Corp, 1984.
2. Aksoy M, Erdem S, Dincol G: Types of leukemia in chronic benzene poisoning. A study in thirty-four patients. *Acta Haematol* 1976; 55:65–72.
3. Allen N, Mendell JR, Billmaier DJ, et al: Toxic polyneuropathy due to methyl-n-butylketone. *Arch Neurol* 1975; 32:209–218.
4. Amaducci L, Arfaioli C, Izitari D, et al: Multiple sclerosis among shoe and leather workers: An epidemiological survey in Florence. *Acta Neurol Scand* 1982; 65:94–103.
5. Antti-Poika M: Overall prognosis of patients with diagnosed chronic organic solvent intoxication. *Int Arch Occup Environ Health* 1982; 51:127–138.
6. Åstrand I: Uptake of solvents in the blood and tissues of man: A review. *Scand J Work Environ Health* 1975; 1:199–218.
7. Åstrand I, Gamberale F: Effects on humans of solvents in the inspiratory air. A method for estimation of uptake. *Environ Res* 1978; 15:1–4.
8. Askergren A: Organic solvents and kidney function. A methodologic and epidemiologic study. *Arbete och Hälsa* 1981;5. Stockholm, Arbetarskyddsverket.
9. Axelson O, Andersson K, Selden A, et al: Cancer morbidity and exposure to trichloroethylene. *Int Conference on Organic Solvent Toxicity*. Stockholm, October 15–17, 1984, Abstracts, p 126.
10. Axelson O: Solvents and the liver (editorial). *Eur J Clin Invest* 1983; 13:109–111.
11. Axelson O, Andersson K, Hogstedt C, et al: A cohort study on trichloroethylene exposure and cancer mortality. *J Occup Med* 1978; 20:194–196.
12. Axelson O, Hane M, Hogstedt C: A case-referent study on neuropsychiatric disorders among workers exposed to solvents. *Scand J Work Environ Health* 1976; 2:14–20.
13. Axelson O, Hane M, Hogstedt C: A case-referent study on neuropsychiatric disorders among workers exposed to solvents—a review and some further aspects. *International Symposium of the Control of Air Pollution in the Working Environment*. Stockholm, International Labour Office, September 6–8, 1977.
14. Axelsson G, Lütz C, Rylander R: Exposure to solvents and outcome of pregnancy in university laboratory employees. *Br J Ind Med* 1984; 41:305–312.
15. Beirne G, Brennan J: Glomerulonephritis associated with hydrocarbon solvents. *Arch Environ Health* 1972; 25:365–369.
16. Billmaier D, Yee HT, Allen N, et al: Peripheral neuropathy in a coated fabrics plant. *J Occup Med* 1974; 16:665–671.
17. Blair A, Decoufle P, Grauman D: Causes of death among laundry and dry cleaning workers. *Am J Publ Health* 1979; 69:508–511.
18. Bleuler M: *Lehrbuch der Psychiatrie*. New York, Springer-Verlag, 1969.
19. Bonse G, Urban T, Reichert D, et al: Chemical reactivity, metabolic oxirane formation and biological reactivity of chlorinated ethylene in the isolated perfused rat liver preparation. *Biochem Pharmacol* 1975; 24:1829.
20. Brandt L, Nilsson PG, Mitelman F: Occupational exposure to petroleum products in men with acute non-lymphatocytic leukemia. *Br Med J* 1978; 4:553.
21. Bruhn P, Arlien-Soborg P, Gyldensted C, et al: Prognosis in chronic toxic encephalopathy. A two-year follow-up study in 26 house painters with occupational encephalopathy. *Acta Neurol Scand* 1981; 64:259–272.
22. Browning E: *Toxicity and Metabolism of Industrial Solvents*. New York, Elsevier North-Holland, Inc, 1965.
23. Cavanagh JB, Bennett RJ: On the pattern of changes in the rat nervous system produced by 2,5-hexanediol. *Brain* 1981; 104:297–318.
24. Checkoway H, Wilcosky T, Wolf P, et al: An evaluation of the associations of leukemia and rubber industry solvent exposures. *Am J Ind Med* 1984; 5:239–249.
25. Cherry N, Rodgers B, Venables H, et al: Acute behavioural effects of styrene exposure: A further analysis. *Br J Ind Med* 1981; 38:346–350.
26. Cherry N, Waldron HA: *The Neuropsychological effects of Solvent Exposure*. Hampshire, The Colt Foundation, 1983.
27. Cherry N, Waldron HA: The prevalence of psychiatric morbidity in solvent workers in Britain. *Int J Epidemiol* 1984; 13:197–200.
28. Chianchetti C, Abbritti G, Perticoni G, et al: Toxic polyneuropathy of shoe-industry workers. A study of 122 cases. *J Neurol Neurosurg Psychiat* 1976; 39:1151–1161.
29. Cohr K-H, Stokholm J: Toluene: A toxicologic review. *Scand J Work Environ Health* 1979; 5:71–90.
30. Corbett T: Cancer and congenital anomalies associated with anesthetics. *Ann NY Acad Sci* 1976; 271:58–66.
31. Cornish H, Adefuin J: Ethanol potentiation of halogenated aliphatic solvent toxicity. *Am Ind Hyg Assoc J* 1966; 27:57–61.
32. Couri N, Micks M: Toxicity and metabolism of the neurotoxic hexacarbons n-hexane, 2-hexanone and 2,5-hexanedione. *Annu Rev Pharmacol Toxicol* 1982; 22:145–166.
33. De Bruin A: *Biochemical Toxicology of Environmental Agents*. Amsterdam, Coronel University, 1976.
34. Dossing M, Arlien-Soborg P, Petersen LM, et al: Liver damage associated with occupational exposure to organic solvents in house painters. *Eur J Clin Invest* 1983; 13:151–157.
35. Elofsson S, Gamberale F, Hindmarsh T, et al: A cross-sectional epidemiologic investigation on occupationally exposed car and industrial spray painters with special reference to the nervous system. *Scand J Work Environ Health* 1980; 6:239–273.
36. Engholm G, Englund A: Cancer incidence and mortality among Swedish painters, in Englund A, Ringen K, Mehlman M (eds): *Occupational Health Hazards of Solvents*. Princeton, Princeton Scientific Publishing, Inc, 1982.
37. Engström J, Bjurström R: Exposure to methylene chloride. Content in subcutaneous adipose tissue. *Scand J Work Environ Health* 1977, 3:215–224.
38. Engström K, Rantanen J: A new gas chromatographic method for determination of mandelic acid in urine. *Int Arch Arbeitsmed* 1974; 3:163–167.
39. Fishbein L: Industrial mutagenes and potential mutagenes. I. Halogenated aliphatic derivatives. *Mutat Res* 1976; 32:267–308.
40. Flodin U, Andersson L, Anjou C-G, et al: A case-referent study on acute myeloid leukemia, background radiation and exposures to solvents and other agents. *Scand J Work Environ Health* 1981; 7:169–178.
41. Flodin U, Edling C, Axelson O: Clinical studies of psychoorganic

syndromes among workers with exposure to solvents. *Am J Industr Med* 1984; 5:287–295.

42. Forni A, Pacifico E, Limonata A: Chromosome studies in workers exposed to benzene or toluene or both. *Arch Environ Health* 1981; 22:373–378.
43. Fracchia M, Pierce L, Graul R, et al: Desorption of organic solvents from charcoal tubes. *Am Ind Hyg Assoc J* 1977; 38:144–146.
44. Franchini A, Cavatorta M, Falzoi M, et al: Early indicators of renal damage in workers exposed to organic solvents. *Int Arch Occup Environ Health* 1983; 52:1–9.
45. Funes-Cravioto F, Zapata-Gayon C, Kolmodin-Hedman B, et al: Chromosome aberrations and sister-chromatide exchange in workers in chemical laboratories and a rotoprinting factory and in children of women laboratory workers. *Lancet* 1977; 2:322–325.
46. Gamberale F: Behavioral effects of exposure to solvent vapors. *Arbete och Hälsa* 1975; 14. Stockholm, Arbetarskyddsverket, 1975.
47. Gamberale F, Lisper H, Anshelm-Olson B: The influence from styrene on reaction ability in plastic boat industry (English summary). Arbete och Hälsa 1975; 8. Stockholm, Arbetarskyddsverket, 1975.
48. Gerarde HW: *Toxicology and Biochemistry of Aromatic Hydrocarbons*. New York, Elsevier North-Holland, Inc, 1960.
49. Götell P, Axelson O, Lindelöf B: Field studies on human styrene exposure. *Work Environ Health* 1972; 9:76–83.
50. Greim H, Bonse G, Radwan Z, et al: Mutagenicity in vitro and potential carcinogenicity of chlorinated ethylenes as a function of metabolic oxirane formation. *Biochem Pharmacol* 1975; 24:2013–2017.
51. Guiliano G, Iannaccone A, Zappoli R: Ricerche electroencephalografiche di operai di calzaturifici esposti al rischio di intossicazione da solventi. *Lav Umano* 1974; 26:33–42.
52. Haglund U, Lundberg I, Zech L: Chromosome aberrations and sister-chromatide exchanges in Swedish paint industry workers. *Scand J Work Environ Health* 1980; 6:291–298.
53. Hane M, Axelson O, Blume J, et al: Psychological function changes among house painters. *Scand J Work Environ Health* 1977; 3:91–99.
54. Hänninen H: Psychological picture of manifest and latent carbon disulphide poisoning. *Br J Ind Med* 1971; 28:374–381.
55. Hänninen H, Eskelinen L, Husman K, et al: Behavioral effects of long-term exposure to a mixture of organic solvents. *Scand J Work Environ Health* 1976; 2:240–255.
56. Hardell L, Eriksson M, Lenner P, et al: Malignant lymphoma and exposure to chemicals, especially organic solvents, chlorophenols and phenoxy acids. A case-control study. *Br J Cancer* 1981; 43:169–176.
57. Hardell L, Bengtsson NO, Jonsson U, et al: Etiological aspects on primary liver cancer with special regard to alcohol, organic solvents and acute intermittent porphyria—an epidemiological investigation. *Br J Cancer* 1984; 50:389–397.
58. Härkönen H, Holmberg PC: Obstetric studies of women occupationally exposed to styrene. *Scand J Work Environ Health* 1982; 8:74–77.
59. Hearne T, Friedlander BR: Follow-up of methylene chloride study (letter). *J Occup Med* 1981; 23:660.
60. Hemminki K, Franssila E, Vainio H: Spontaneous abortions among female chemical workers in Finland. *Int Arch Occup Environ Health* 1980; 45:123–126.
61. Hernberg S, Korkala M-L, Asikainen U, et al: Primary liver cancer and exposure to solvents. *Int Arch Occup Environ Health* 1984; 54:147–153.
62. Hernberg S, Nurminen M, Tolonen M: Excess mortality from coronary heart disease in viscose rayon workers exposed to carbon disulphide. *Work Environ Health* 1973; 10:93–99.
63. Herskowitz A, Ishii N, Schaumburg H: n-Hexane neuropathy. *N Engl J Med* 1971; 285:82–85.
64. Hogstedt C, Andersson K, Hane M. A questionnaire approach to the monitoring of early disturbances in central nervous functions, in Aitio A, Riihimäki V, Vainio H (eds): *Biological Monitoring and Surveillance of Workers Exposed to Chemicals*. Washington, Hemisphere Publishing Co, 1984.
65. Holmberg PC: Central nervous defects in two children of mothers exposed to chemicals in the reinforced plastic industry: Chance or causal relation. *Scand J Work Environ Health* 1977; 3:212–214.
66. Holmberg PC: Central-nervous-system defects in children born to mothers exposed to organic solvents during pregnancy. *Lancet* 1979; 2:177.
67. Holmberg PC, Hernberg S, Kurppa K, et al: Oral clefts and organic solvent exposure during pregnancy. *Int Arch Occup Environ Health* 1982; 50:371–376.
68. Holmberg PC, Nurminen M: Congenital defects of the central nervous system and occupational factors during pregnancy. A case-referent study. *Am J Ind Med* 1980; 1:167–176.
69. Hyden D, Larsby B, Andersson H, et al: Impairment of visuovestibular interaction in humans exposed to toluene. *Otolaryngology* 1983; 45:262–269.
70. International Agency for Research on Cancer: *IARC Monographs on the Evaluation of the Carcinogenic Risk of Chemicals to Humans: Some Industrial Chemicals and Dye-stuffs,* Vol 29. Lyon, IARC, 1982, pp 93–148.
71. International Agency for Research on Cancer: *IARC Monographs on the Evaluation of the Carcinogenic Risk of Chemicals to Humans, Suppl 4*. Lyon, IARC, 1982.
72. International Agency for Research on Cancer: *IARC Monographs Vol II: Cadmium, Nickel, Some Epoxides, Miscellaneous Industrial Chemicals and General Considerations on Volatile Anaesthetics*. Lyon, IARC, 1976, p 285.
73. Johnson B, Setzer J, Lewis T, et al: Effects of methyl-butyl ketone on behavior and the nervous system. *Am Ind Hyg Assoc J* 1977; 38:567–579.
74. Johnstone RT: *Occupational Medicine and Industrial Hygiene*. St Louis, CV Mosby Co, 1948.
75. Jongen WMF, Alink GM, Koeman JH: Mutagenic effect of dichloromethane on salmonella typhimurium. *Mutat Res* 1978; 56: 245–248.
76. Juntunen J, Hupli V, Hernberg S, et al: Neurological picture of organic solvent poisoning in industry. A retrospective clinical study of 37 patients. *Int Arch Occup Environ Health* 1980; 46: 219–231.
77. Knave B, Anshelm-Olson B, Elofsson S, et al: Long-term exposure to jet fuel. II. A cross-sectional epidemiological investigation on occupationally-exposed industry workers with special reference to the nervous system. *Scand J Work Environ Health* 1978; 4:19–45.
78. Knave B, Persson H, Goldberg M, et al: Long-term exposure to jet fuel. An investigation on occupationally exposed workers with special reference to the nervous system. *Scand J Work Environ Health* 1976; 2:152–164, 1976.
79. Kucera J: Exposure to fat solvents: A possible cause of sacral agenesis in man. *J Pediatr* 1968; 72:857–859.
80. Lagrue G: Hydrocarbon exposure and chronic glomerulonephritis. *Lancet* 1976; i:1191.
81. Larsby B, Tham R, Ödkvist LM: Influence on the vestibular system by industrial solvents. *Acta Otolaryngol* 1982; 386:246–248.
82. Lauwerys R: Biological criteria for selected industrial toxic chemicals: A review. *Scand J Work Environ Health* 1975; 1:139–172.
83. Lindström K: Psychological performances of workers exposed to various solvents. *J Work Environ Health* 1973; 10:151–155.
84. Lindström K, Härkönen H, Hernberg S: Disturbances in psychological functions of workers occupationally exposed to styrene. *Scand J Work Environ Health* 1976; 2:129–139.

85. Malek B, Kremarova B, Rodova O: An epidemiologic study of hepatic tumor incidence in subjects working with trichloroethylene. *Pracov Lek* 1979; 31:124–126.
86. Mayer-Gross W, Slater E, Roth M: *Clinical Psychiatry*, ed 3. London, Bailliere, Tindall & Cassel, 1969.
87. Mikkelsen S: A cohort study of disability pension and death among painters with special regard to disabling presenile dementia as an occupational disease. *Scand J Soc Med* 1980; 16(suppl):34–43.
88. Milham S: Occupational mortality in Washington state, 1950–1971, Vol III. Washington, DC, US Department of Health, Education and Welfare, 1976.
89. Moszczynski P, Lisiewicz J: T and B cells and occupational exposure to benzene and its homologues (with regard to other blood cells). *Rev Esp Oncol* 1982; 29:49–55.
90. Mowe G: Coronary heart disease and occupational exposure to carbon disulfide (abstract) in Djuric D, et al (eds): *II International Symposium on Toxicology of Carbon Disulfide*. Banja Koviljaca, Yugoslavia, May 25–28, 1971. Beograd, Institute of Occupational and Radiological Health, 1971.
91. Müller G, Spassorski M, Henscher D: Trichloroethylene exposure and trichloroethylene metabolites in urine and blood. *Arch Toxicol* 1972; 29:335–340.
92. Mutti A, Lucertini S, Falzoi M, et al: Organic solvents and chronic glomerulonephritis: A cross-sectional study with negative findings for aliphatic and alicyclic C_5–C_7 hydrocarbons. *J Appl Toxicol* 1981; 1:224–226.
93. Nau CA, Neal J, Thornton M: C_9–C_{12} fractions obtained from petroleum distillates. An evaluation of their potential toxicity. *Arch Environ Health* 1966; 12:383–393.
94. National Cancer Institute: Bioassay of tetrachloroethylene for possible carcinogenicity. *Natl Cancer Inst Tech Rep* Series 13, Washington DC, Department of Health, Education and Welfare, 1977.
95. National Cancer Institute: Carcinogenesis bioassay of trichloroethylene. CAS No 79-01-6 *Natl Cancer Inst Tech Rep* Series 2, Publ No 76-802, Washington DC, Department of Health, Education and Welfare, 1976.
96. Ödkvist L, Larsby B, Tham R, et al: Vestibulo-oculomotor disturbances caused by industrial solvents. *Otolaryngol Head Neck Surg* 1983; 91:537–539.
97. Ohlson C-G, Hogstedt C: Parkinson's disease and occupational exposure to organic solvents, agricultural chemicals and mercury—A case referent study. *Scand J Work Environ Health* 1981; 7:252–256.
98. Ohtsuji H, Ikeda M: The metabolism of styrene in the rat and stimulatory effect of phenobarbital. *Toxicol Appl Pharmacol* 1971; 18:321–328.
99. Olsen J, Sabroe S: A case-reference study of neuropsychiatric disorders among workers exposed to solvents in the Danish wood and furniture industry. *Scand J Soc Med* 1980; 16(suppl):44–49.
100. Olsson H, Brandt L: Occupational exposure to organic solvents and Hodgkin's disease in men. A case-referent study. *Scand J Work Environ Health* 1980; 6:302–305.
101. Ott MG, Skori LK, Holder BB, et al: Health evaluation of employees occupationally exposed to methylene chloride. *Mortality Scand J Work Environ Health* 1983; 1(suppl):8–16
102. Paddle GM: Incidence of liver cancer and trichloroethylene manufacture: Joint study by industry and a cancer registry. *Br Med J* 1983; 286:846.
103. Passero S, Battistini N, Cioni R, et al: Toxic polyneuropathy of shoe workers in Italy. A clinical, neurophysiological and follow-up study. *Ital J Neurol Sci* 1983; 4:463–472.
104. Raitta C, Husman K, Tossavainen A: Lens changes in car painters exposed to a mixture of organic solvents. *Arch Klin Exp Ophthalmol* 1976; 200:149–156.
105. Ravnskov U, Forsberg B, Skerfving S: Glomerulonephritis and exposure to organic solvents. *Acta Med Scand* 1979; 205:575–579.
106. Saalwaechter AT, McCammon CS, Jr, Roper CP, et al: Performance testing of the NIOSH charcoal tube technique for the determination of air concentration of organic vapors. *Am Ind Hyg Assoc J* 1977; 38:476–486.
107. Schyttmann W: Zur Frage der Leberschädigung durch beruflichen Kontakt mit Triklorätylen. *Dtsch Z Verdau Stoffwechselkr* 1970; 30:43–45.
108. Seppäläinen AM: Applications of neurophysiological methods in occupational medicine: A review. *Scand J Work Environ Health* 1975; 1:1–14.
109. Seppäläinen AM: Neurophysiological findings among workers exposed to organic solvents. *Scand J Work Environ Health* 1981; 4(suppl):29–33.
110. Seppäläinen AM: Neurotoxic effects of industrial solvents. *Electroencephalogr Clin Neurophysiol* 1973; 34:702–703.
111. Seppäläinen AM: The use of clinical neurophysiological methods in studies of workers exposed to solvents, in Buser PA, Cobb WA, Okuma T (eds): *Kyoto Symposia*, EEG Suppl No 36. New York, Elsevier North Holland, Inc, 1982.
112. Seppäläinen AM, Antti-Poika M: Time course of electrophysiological findings for patients with solvent poisoning. A descriptive study. *Scand J Work Environ Health* 1983; 9:15–24.
113. Seppäläinen AM, Härkönen H: Neurophysiological findings among workers occupationally exposed to styrene. *Scand J Work Environ Health* 1976; 2:140–146.
114. Seppäläinen AM, Husman K, Mårtenson C: Neurophysiological effects of long-term exposure to a mixture of organic solvents. *Scand J Work Environ Health* 1978; 4:304–314.
115. Seppäläinen AM, Lindström K, Martelin T: Neurophysiological and psychological picture of solvent poisoning. *Am J Industr Med* 1980; 1:31–42.
116. Simmon VG, Kaukanen K, Tardiff RG: Mutagenic activity of chemicals identified in drinking water, in Scott CD, Budges BA, Sobels FH (eds): *Progress in Genetic Toxicology*. New York, Elsevier North Holland, Inc, 1977, pp 249–258.
117. Slob A: A new method for determination of mandelic acid excretion at low level styrene exposure. *Br J Ind Med* 1973; 30:390–393.
118. Smolik R, Grzybek-Hryncewicz K, Lange A, et al: Serum complement level in workers exposed to benzene, toluene and xylene. *Int Arch Arbeitsmed* 1973; 31:243–247.
119. Stemhagen A, Slade J, Altman R, et al: Occupational risk factors and liver cancer. *Am J Epidemiol* 1983; 117:443–454.
120. Stokholm J, Cohr K-H: Exposure of humans to white spirit. VI. Effect on neurophysiological functions. Copenhagen, Arbejdstilsynet, Arbejdsmiljöinstituttet. Report 4, 1979, pp 31–51.
121. Strandberg M, Sandbäck K, Axelson O, et al: Spontaneous abortions among women in hospital laboratory. *Lancet* 1978; 1:384–385.
122. Struwe G, Knave B, Mindus P: Neuropsychiatric symptoms in workers occupationally exposed to jet fuel—A combined epidemiological and causistic study. *Acta Psychiat Scand* 1983; 67 (suppl)303:55–67.
123. Szmidt M, Axelson O, Edling C: Kohortstudie av freonexponerade. *Acta Soc Med Suec Hygiea* 1981; 5:77.
124. Taheuchi Y, Mabuchi C, Tagaki S: Polyneuropathy caused by petroleum benzene. *Int Arch Arbeitsmed* 1975; 34:185–197.
125. Tiller J, Schilling R, Morris J: Occupational toxic factor in mortality from coronary heart disease. *Br Med J* 1968; 4:407–411.
126. Toftgård R, Gustafsson J-Å: Biotransformation of organic solvents. A review. *Scand J Work Environ Health* 1980; 6:1–18.
127. Tola S, Vilhunen R, Järvinen E, et al: A cohort study on workers exposed to trichloroethylene. *J Occup Med* 1980; 22:737–740.
128. Traiger G, Plaa G: Chlorinated hydrocarbon toxicity. Potentiation by

isopropyl alcohol and acetone. *Arch Environ Health* 1974; 28:276–278.
129. Triebig G, Sestler W, Baumeister P, et al: Untersuchungen zur Neurotoxizität von Arbeitsstoffen. IV. Messung der motorischen und sensorishen Nervenleitgeschwindigheit bei beruflicher Exposition gegenüber Lösenmittelgemischen. *Int Arch Occup Environ Health* 1983; 52:139–150.
130. Tunek A, Platt KL, Bentley P, et al: Microsomal metabolism of benzene to species irreversibly binding to microsomal protein and effects of modifications of this metabolism. *Mol Pharmacol* 1978; 14:920–929.
131. Vainio H, Hemminki K, Elovaara E: Styrens och styrenoxids toxicitet för utvecklande kycklingembryo (The toxicity of styrene and styrene oxide on developed chick embryos) (abstract). 26th Nordic Occupational Hygiene Meeting, Helsinki, October 24–26, 1977. Helsinki, Institute of Occupational Health, 1977, p 25.
132. Vainio H, Pääkkönen R, Rönnholm K, et al: A study on the mutagenic activity of styrene and styrene oxide. *Scand J Work Environ Health* 1976; 2:147–151.
133. Vesterberg O: General aspects on biotransformation and elimination of organic compounds in connection with occupational exposure. *Int Arch Occup Environ Health* 1975; 35:89–115.
134. Viadana E, Bross I, Houten L: Cancer experience of men exposed to inhalation of chemicals or to combustion products. *J Occup Med* 1976; 18:787–792.
135. Vigliani E: Leukemia associated with benzene exposure. *Ann NY Acad Sci* 1976; 271:143–151.
136. Zenz C: Benzene—attempts to establish a lower exposure standard in the United States, A review. *Scand J Work Environ Health* 1978; 4:103–113.
137. Zielhuis RL: Biological monitoring. (Guest lecture given at the 26th Nordic Symposium on Industrial Hygiene, Helsinki, October, 1977.) *Scand J Work Environ Health* 1978; 4:1–18.
138. Zimmerman S, Groehler K, Beirne G: Hydrocarbon exposure and chronic glomerulonephritis. *Lancet* 1975; 2:199–201.

49

Psychologic Effects of Exposure to Solvents and Other Neurotoxic Agents in the Work Environment

Kerstin Ekberg, Ph.D

Monica Hane, Ph.D.

Thomas Berggren, Ph.D.

The serious consequences of long-term work exposure to neurotoxic agents, such as solvents, lead, and mercury, are described in numerous case reports (for a review of solvent-exposed cases, see Browning[13]). Similar cases, associated with solvent exposure, still occur even in countries with advanced industrial technology.[6] Although the case reports have indicated a chronic effect of many solvents, comparably little concern was given to this aspect until the 1970s, especially regarding the chronic neurotoxic effects. The symptoms reported in connection with neurotoxic exposures, e.g., affect lability, concentration disturbances, and memory deficits, are in agreement with the so-called psycho-organic syndrome or "neurasthenic syndrome,"[12, 49] which is furthermore characterized by a decreased ability to engage in abstract thinking. The syndrome has been associated with an organic dysfunction in the central nervous system.

However, the symptoms associated with exposure to neurotoxic agents are vague and unspecific and could also be due to the stresses and strains of other conditions of social and working life. Therefore, it is necessary to supplement the frequent, but anecdotal, case reports with studies of the association between exposure and signs or symptoms. Such studies have been performed on acute effects in experimental settings and in the work environment on existing exposure levels. Epidemiologic studies have been applied for evaluation of long term, or chronic, effects.

SOLVENTS

Experimental Studies

Exposure chamber studies have been used to elucidate and quantify questions of causality between exposure and symptoms. Such studies make it possible to control and monitor exposure in terms of duration and intensity, and individual differences can be controlled for in the design.

The acute effects of isolated short-time exposures to solvents have attracted an experimental interest since the 1970s, which has resulted in better knowledge about the quantitative aspects of human solvent toxicology. Various commonly used solvents have been studied[28] by means of a uniform technique. Volunteers inhaled solvent vapors and the specific odors were masked by menthol. Exposure times of 1.5 hours were used and the uptake of the solvent was continually measured every 20 minutes. The effects were measured on various psychologic tests such as reaction time, short-term memory, and simple arithmetic items and compared to the results obtained without exposure. The overall result from these experiments seems to be that surprisingly low exposures will result in a significantly impaired performance.

Very few experiments have been reported in which the effects of simultaneous exposure to two different solvents have been studied.[2, 50, 57, 67] While Windemüller and Ettama[67] found an interactive effect between ethanol and trichloroethylene, no potentiating effect between the solvents were obtained in the other studies.

The experimental studies have shown that short-term exposure to various solvents, even at low levels, has effects on performance. However, it might be difficult to generalize from experimental situations to the complex exposure situations occurring in work settings and to effects due to long-term exposure.

Field Studies

In field studies of behavioral effects of solvent exposure, existing levels of exposure in the work environment are related to behavioral measures, e.g., before and after a work shift. The aim is to study dose-response relationships in the work environment on a pertinent population. An underlying assumption is that acute effects in the long run may lead to irreversible effects.

Prolonged reaction times or increased variability in reaction times have been related to increased levels of solvent exposure, mainly styrene or mixtures of solvents.[15, 16, 37] Exposure to methylene chloride[17] or very low levels of styrene (below 110 mg/cu m)[21] did not produce such effects. Hence, field studies may also be useful for the evaluation of solvent-specific effects and current threshold limits in the work environment.

Cross-Sectional Studies

The evaluation of long-term effects of neurotoxic exposure is associated with methodologic difficulties. Usually, cross-sectional studies have been applied, i.e., the current disorders or complaints of an exposed group are referred to existing exposure levels which may provide unreliable estimates of previous exposure. Consequently, the long-term effects might be overlooked, since those individuals who became more severely affected may have left the group of workers due to the symptoms or even because of disability or death. Thus, cross-sectional studies would underestimate the health hazard. On the other hand, in most studies the exposed group has been unexposed for only a few hours or days before investigation, causing acute and chronic effects to be confused, which possibly may overestimate the long-term health hazards.

Several studies based on psychologic testing have appeared during the 1970s, and the results from some, mainly Scandinavian, studies of workers exposed to solvents are summarized in Table 49–1. In most of these studies, comparisons are made between mean performance in exposed versus unexposed groups or between high- and low-exposure groups. The exposure indices are given in the table and will not be further mentioned in this chapter.

Hänninen[33] compared the performances on a battery of psychologic tests of 50 rayon-viscose workers who had been poisoned by carbon disulfide with 50 rayon-viscose workers exposed to carbon disulfide but without clinical symptoms of poisoning and 50 workers not exposed to carbon disulfide. There were large and statistically significant differences between the group means of the poisoned and the nonexposed group in most tests that required visuospatial ability, memory, perceptual speed and accuracy, and psychomotor coordination. Differences in some variables from the Rorschach ink blot test, for example, showed diminished rational control, and fewer emotional reactions among the poisoned workers were also found. However, it may be questionable whether a group of clinically diagnosed workers, which may be a selected group, is comparable to nonclinical materials. Since the group of exposed workers without clinical symptoms also showed impairment, although less severe, this objection may be regarded as less serious for the main conclusions.

In another study by Hänninen et al.[36] 206 male viscose-rayon workers with an average exposure time of 17 years were compared to 152 nonexposed men. The groups differed in tests measuring perceptual and psychomotor speed and in some variables from the Rorschach personality test. The differences between the groups in this study were less pronounced than in the previous study, in which the exposed group was selected for heavy exposure to carbon disulfide.

Styrene workers have been studied by Lindström et al.[45] Using a large test battery, they found impaired visuomotor speed, visual memory, vigilance and psychomotor performance among the workers. In a later study,[38] a dose-response relationship was noted between urine mandelic acid excretion and performance in perceptual and psychomotor tests.

Fifty styrene exposed and 50 unexposed subjects were studied by Mutti et al.[50] After controlling for age and for scoring on the vocabulary test, performance in visuospatial and perceptual speed tests proved to be related to the level of exposure. Perceptual speed performance was also related to duration of exposure.

In a study of printers who were solely exposed to toluene, Iregren[39] found poorer performance in a simple reaction time test as compared to an unexposed group, while the printers did not show any signs of deteriorating functions in the remaining tests. In

TABLE 49–1.
Studies of Workers Occupationally Exposed to Solvents

	EXPOSURE							
PSYCHOLOGIC FUNCTION	CS_2	STYRENE	STYRENE	TOLUENE	JET FUEL	MIXTURE	MIXTURE	MIXTURE
Verbal	–	–	+*	–		+	–	–
Cognitive: Reasoning				–			+	–
Visuospatial	+	–	+	–		+	–	–
Memory	+	–	–	–	–	+	+	+
Perceptual speed and accuracy	+	+	+	+	+	–	+	+
Eye-hand coordination/dexterity	+	+		–	–	+	+	+
Personaltiy	+	+				+		
Exposure: average number of years	9	5	8	16	17	15	14	
levels	30–132 mg/cu m	0.05–3.0 mmol/L MA	43–1,295 mg/cu m	19–573 mg/cu m	500–3,100 ppm			
Reference	33	45	50	39	41	34	31	24

*Used as matching criterion.
+ = at least one test measuring the psychologic function at issue showed differences ($P<.05$) between exposed and nonexposed.
– = the psychologic function was measured, but no significant differences were found.

a study of workers with exposure to jet fuel[41] the exposed workers had greater problems than the controls on tasks that required attention, perceptual speed, and fast reactions.

Behavioral effects of long-term exposure to a mixture of organic solvents have been studied by several authors.[34, 24] In the study of Elofsson et al., matching was performed with regard to age, education, professional status, and employment stability, while Hänninen et al. matched with regard to age only. The test batteries included tests of intelligence, memory, perception, psychomotor performance, and, in the Hänninen study, personality. Performances of the exposed groups were significantly inferior in tests measuring memory, perception, and psychomotor ability. In the Hänninen study, impairments in spatial ability and a reduced emotional reactivity were also detected, while perceptual speed was unaffected.

A study of a random sample of union-affiliated house painters was reported by Hane et al.[31] The house painters were compared on a number of medical variables and psychologic tests with a group of industrial workers having a corresponding age distribution. The groups proved to be on a par in relevant background variables, but the house painter group reported more subjective symptoms, such as fatigue, partial amnesia, and diffuse chest pain. The house painter group had significantly lower mean scores on a test measuring reasoning and on a test of psychomotor coordination than the reference group of industrial workers. The house painter group also had significantly lower performances than expected on a memory test and the reaction time test. A discriminant analysis on indicators of performance changes in the tests gave a point biserial correlation of 0.35 between the discriminant function and exposure, measured as group affinity. A stepwise multidiscriminant analysis placed the severity of the performance change among house painters between normal subjects and clinical patients.

Ekberg et al.[22] compared floor layers to unexposed referents, matched with respect to age and number of occupational years. Floor layers with more than 20 years of occupational experience performed less well than their referents in tests measuring visuospatial ability, while the performance of the two groups in vocabulary, reasoning, perceptual ability, and psychomotor speed were at the same level. Floor layers with less than ten years of occupational experience showed no visuospatial impairment.

It may be summarized that despite different methods and methodologic problems in the various studies of the effects of solvent exposure, the results are fairly consistent. The studies indicate that impaired performances on tests in which visual perception, memory, and psychomotor functions are involved may result from long-term solvent exposure.

Longitudinal Studies

In none of the cross-sectional studies of neurotoxic agents was the exposed group unexposed for more than a few days. The obtained effects may, therefore, be a combination of acute and chronic effects, which would affect the prognosis. In a Finnish study,[3] the prognosis of patients with diagnosed chronic organic solvent intoxication was studied three to nine years after having been diagnosed. Based on the clinical overall evaluation, the condition of 21 patients had deteriorated during the follow-up period, the condition of 23 had improved, and that of 43 had remained unchanged. No statistically significant correlation was found between the overall prognosis and age, sex, the duration and the level of exposure, termination of exposure after diagnosis, the presence of other diseases, or the use of alcohol.

In a Danish study,[14] 26 house painters with cerebral atrophy and/or intellectual impairment were selected for a follow-up after two years. The patients were not exposed to organic solvents during the two-year interval. The condition was unchanged for most of the subjects, and in three patients further deterioration was observed. The findings indicate that long-term exposure to organic solvents may lead to a chronic brain syndrome, since other etiologic entities were excluded in the study. To further elucidate this problem, a Swedish prospective study was recently initiated. All solvent-exposed workers who were referred to clinics of Occupational Medicine during 1982–1983 were investigated in a standardized manner. A follow-up five years after the first investigation is planned.

LEAD

Cross-Sectional Studies

The behavioral effects of exposure to inorganic lead have received increased attention during recent years (Table 49–2). Hänninen et al.[35] compared lead-exposed workers with nonexposed workers. Performance between the groups did not differ, but there was a significant negative relationship between spatial and psychomotor performance and lead uptake within the exposed group.

In an extensive study by Grandjean et al.,[30] the full Wechsler Adult Intelligence Scale (WAIS) in addition to measures of short-term memory, learning, and attention were administered to exposed and nonexposed subjects. The exposed group performed at a lower level in most tests, and there were negative correlations between level of lead absorption and test performances. However, the educational level of the groups may not have been comparable, making interpretations difficult.

In another cross-sectional study by Valciukas et al.,[63] the exposed workers performed worse on tests measuring spatial ability and perceptual speed, while no effect was detected on psychomotor performance. In a later study,[64] performance of five groups with different levels of lead absorption was studied on tests measuring spatial and perceptual ability and speed. A significant negative association between test scores and lead absorption was found.

In a study by Hogstedt et al.,[32] 49 long-term lead-exposed workers were compared to 27 low-exposed workers through a number of psychologic tests. After controlling for age, the exposed group performed worse on tests measuring memory, learning, and reaction time, while impaired performance was not detected in reasoning, perceptual speed, and psychomotor ability.

In a cross-sectional study Baker et al.[9] found impaired performances on tests of verbal concept formation, perceptual performance, and memory in a lead-exposed group with present lead concentrations between 40 and 60 μg/100 ml.

The studies are all cross-sectional, which weakens the opportunities for causal interpretations. It also appears that the results are somewhat inconsistent, making it difficult to point to characteristic features of lead-related behavioral change. However, the functions that are affected by long-term solvent exposure also ap-

TABLE 49–2.
Studies of Workers Occupationally Exposed to Lead

PSYCHOLOGICAL FUNCTION	LEAD EXPOSURE					
Verbal	−	+				+
Cognitive: Reasoning		+			−	
Visuospatial ability	+	+	+	+		
Memory	−	+			+	+
Perceptual speed and accuracy	−	+	+	+	+	+
Eye-hand coordination/ dexterity	+	+	−		−	
Exposure: average/range of number of years	2–9	0.1–25	−	−	18	
average/range of blood lead levels (μmol/L)	1.6	2.2	<2.9	1.4–2.5	2.0	1.6
Reference	35	30	63	64	32	9

+ = at least one test measuring the psychologic function at issue showed differences ($P<.05$) between exposed and nonexposed.
− = the psychologic function was measured but no significant differences were found.

pear to be vulnerable to long-term lead exposure. Several studies have provided negative associations between level of lead absorption and test performance, indicating a dose-response relationship at comparably low levels of lead exposure.

Longitudinal Study

Mantere et al.[47] made a prospective follow-up study on new lead workers. Psychologic performance was assessed before the commencement of exposure and after one, two, and four years of work. Results were compared to an unexposed reference group. Average psychologic performances were similar in the groups at the first measurement. For some of the psychologic tests there was an evident learning effect among the referents at the follow-ups, while the lead-exposed group showed no such effect. The most sensitive indicators of psychologic impairments among lead workers were the spatial block design test, the psychomotor Santa Ana test, and the Digit Span test. However, there was a large dropout of subjects at the follow-up studies: Of initially 89 lead-exposed workers, only 11 were available at the four-year follow-up. Interpretations are further complicated by the different age distributions in the exposed and reference groups.

MERCURY

Cross-Sectional Studies

A few group studies on behavioral effects of occupational exposure to mercury have been published (Table 49–3). Smith et al.[60] used two short-term memory tests on two different groups of

TABLE 49–3.
Studies of Workers Occupationally Exposed to Mercury

PSYCHOLOGIC FUNCTION	MERCURY EXPOSURE			
Verbal				−
Cognitive: Reasoning				−
Visuospatial ability				
Memory	+		+	+
Perceptual speed and accuracy	−			−
Eye-hand coordination/ dexterity	+	+		+
Exposure: average number of years	<8 years	5.3	−	16.9
U-Hg levels (nmol/L)	−	53.8 nmol/mmol crea	997	598.7
Reference	66	55	60	52

+ = at least one test measuring the psychologic function at issue showed differences ($P<.05$) between exposed and nonexposed.
− = the psychologic function was measured, but no significant differences were found.

mercury-exposed workers. They found a significant negative association between level of urine mercury and short-term memory capacity in both groups.

Williamson et al.[66] used a comprehensive test battery to compare a group of 12 long-term mercury-exposed workers with a matched control group. Matching was performed with regard to age, sex, level of education, and ethnic background. As in the previous study, short-term memory was impaired in the exposed group. In addition, the group showed poorer psychomotor coordination and premature fatigue, while motor responses, arousal, and attention remained unaffected. Impaired psychomotor performance has also been found by others.[55]

In a Finnish cross-sectional study,[52] the studied group had been exposed for at least ten years. Impairments in the memory tests were, as in the previous studies, related to exposure level. Performance of the exposed group was also inferior to that of the referents in manual dexterity, while no group differences were obtained in tests measuring verbal ability, reasoning, perceptual ability, and memory.

It appears that the most consistent behavioral effects of occupational exposure to mercury are impairment of short-term memory and psychomotor performance. However, the group studies are few, and firm conclusions should await further investigations.

OTHER AGENTS

Behavioral effects of occupational exposure to other agents have also been studied, e.g., anesthetic gases[20] and organophosphate pesticides.[54] In a review of studies on behavioral effects of organophosphate pesticides in man, Levin and Rodnitzky[42] stress the methodologic shortcomings in many of the studies. In spite of these shortcomings, the investigators generally agree on several behavioral effects of organophosphate pesticide poisoning: Such effects are impaired vigilance and reduced concentration, slowing of information processing and psychomotor speed, memory deficit, linguistic disturbance, depression, and mood defects. However, conclusive epidemiologic studies are still needed.

NEED FOR CLINICAL TECHNIQUES

Experimental and field studies have shown that short-term exposure to neurotoxic agents have acute effects on psychologic functions. Prolonged exposure to such agents may eventually produce irreversible neuropsychologic effects, as indicated by numerous cross-sectional studies and case reports. Different hypotheses have been suggested regarding the mechanisms mediating the obtained effects, e.g., neuronal degeneration or metabolic dysfunctions. No firm conclusions can, however, be drawn yet regarding the etiology of the effects or their degree of reversibility.

Organic damage to the central nervous system has to be studied by indirect methods. Psychologic tests have proved to be the most sensitive of such methods and are regularly used for clinical diagnosis of individuals with suspected brain damage due to solvent exposure.

PSYCHOLOGIC TESTS

Collaborative work between various groups of Swedish psychologists has resulted in a battery of 13 psychologic tests that have been standardized on a Swedish population.[59] The test battery consists of tests which empirically have proven to be sensitive to diffuse organic brain damage. A vocabulary test is also included. The verbal ability is generally regarded as less sensitive to diffuse organic lesions; performance in this test may therefore be used together with other information, as a rough estimate of premorbid ability. Since the battery has been used in many studies of workers exposed to various solvents in Sweden, there is a fair amount of data to be used as reference material also when the battery is used for diagnosing individuals. Presently, the battery is used in several departments of occupational medicine throughout Sweden.

The classification of tests is based on a factor analysis carried out on a sample of 99 subjects at the age of 16 and pupils in the last class of the compulsory school, thus reflecting the unrestricted variation in every variable. The first factor includes tests of vocabulary, i.e., the type of tests regarded to be less influenced in case of diffuse organic brain damage.[49] The second factor includes tests in which both visual perception and cognitive processes are supposed to be important. The third factor covers tests in which the cognitive components are supposed to be of minor importance, and the score is mainly based on perceptual speed. The fourth factor consists of tests that require eye-hand coordination, called psychomotor tests. The memory tests did not come out as a separate factor in the factor analysis due to reduced variation but was nevertheless included.

The test battery has been standardized on a group of 138 unexposed male industrial workers aged 20–66 years (mean 46 years).[27] The group was divided into five age groups, and the test results of each subgroup were transformed to a normally distributed stanine scale with nine steps (mean 5, SD 2). The scale provides a transformation matrix for the raw test scores to standardized age-corrected scores.

The test battery is briefly described below. When nothing else is marked in the description of the test, there is a time limit given for administrative reasons, but the performance is, to a very small extent, influenced by speed.

Verbal

Synonyms.—The task is to find the synonym of a given key word among five alternatives. The test includes 30 items.[19]

Cognitive

Figure Classification.—Every item consists of five geometric figures. Four figures have a common characteristic and the task in all of the 30 items is to mark the one that does not belong to the group[19] (Fig 49–1).

Block Design.—The test material consists of 16 cubes. One side of the cube is red, one side is white, and one side is divided into a white and a red triangle. The other sides of the cubes are blue and yellow. The task is to put these cubes in accordance with

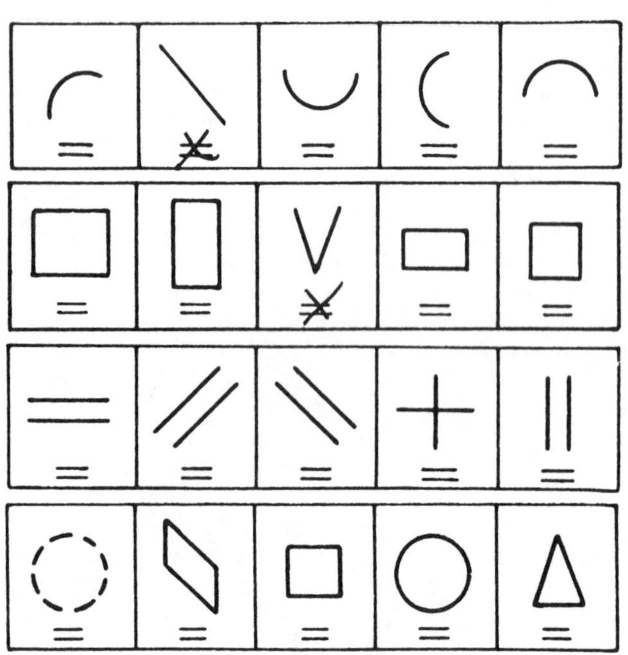

FIG 49–1.
Figure classification. Four practice items are shown.

different patterns shown on cards. Only patterns in white and red are used. The first four patterns are based on four cubes, the next two patterns on nine cubes, and the last pattern on 16 cubes. Both speed and correctness are evaluated[65] (Fig 49–2).

Unfolding.—Each of the ten items consists of a picture of a folded figure drawn in three dimensions and the same figure unfolded into two dimensions. On the folded figure, the sides and edges are numbered. The task is to transfer the numbers from the three-dimensional figure to the two-dimensional one.[27]

Perceptual Speed and Accuracy

Digit Symbols.—Each digit (1–9) is given a special symbol shown on the top of the test sheet. The task is to write the correct symbol under the digits when given in random order as quickly as possible. The score is based on performance in 90 seconds[65] (Fig 49–3).

Dots.—The test consists of six parts, and every part consists of eight lines with groups of three, four, or five dots. The task is to mark all groups that consist of four dots as quickly as possible. Speed and accuracy are evaluated and also deviation in speed and accuracy between different parts of the test, which might be an indicator of fluctuation in vigilance[27] (Fig 49–4).

Identical Numbers.—The test includes three pages with 30 columns on each page. Every column consists of eight numbers with three digits. The task is to underline all numbers that correspond to the number given at the top of each column.[27]

Eye-Hand Coordination

The Bolt Test.—The task is to take a bolt and a needle from two separate boxes, put the bolts in holes on a T bar and lock them with the needles as quickly as possible. The performance is scored every 30 seconds up to three minutes.[27] The test demands coordination of both hands and is sensitive to the size of the hands (Fig 49–5).

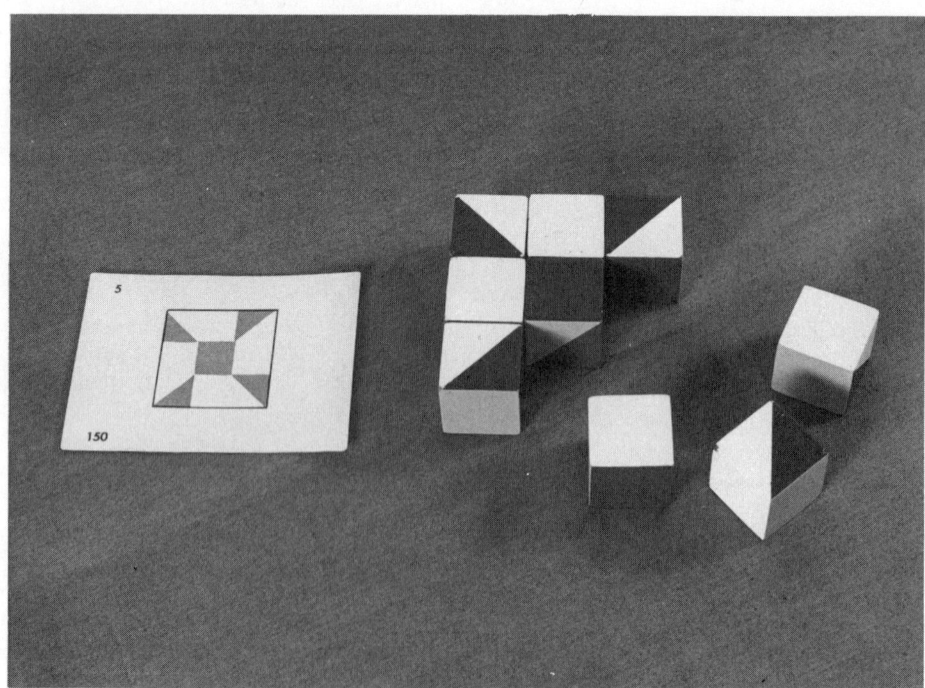

FIG 49–2.
Block design.

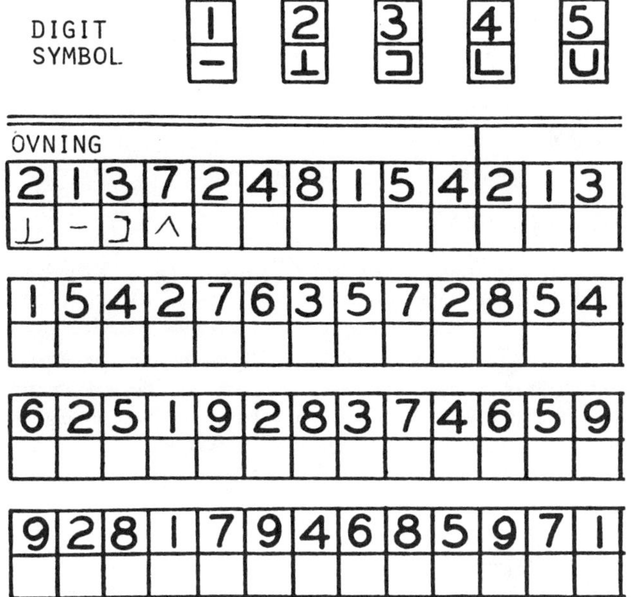

FIG 49–3.
Digit symbols.

Pins.—The task is to quickly move pins from a wooden plate to holes in a T bar by means of a pair of tweezers. The performance is scored every 30 seconds up to 90 seconds.[27] The subject works with only one hand and uses a tool, which makes the test less sensitive to the size of the hand (Fig 49–6).

Cylinders.—The test consists of two wooden plates with 60 holes in each plate. In one plate, the holes are filled with easily graspable cylinders, and the task is to move the cylinders from one plate to another as fast as possible, first with one hand and then with the other[27] (Fig 49–7).

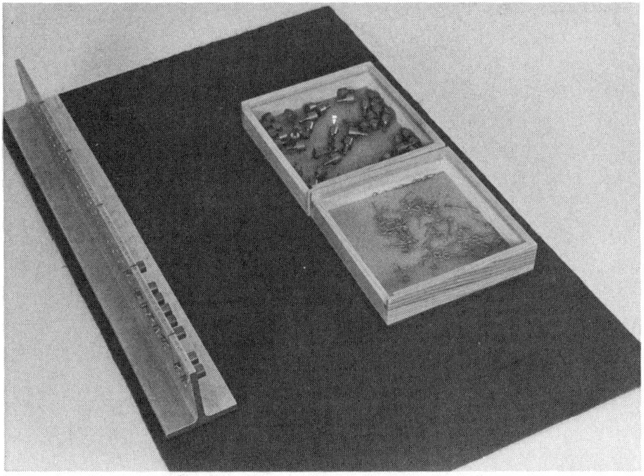

FIG 49–5.
The Bolt test.

Memory

The Benton Visual Retention test consists of ten drawings with geometric figures. Each drawing is shown for ten seconds, and the task is to reproduce the drawing immediately after its removal. Both the number of errors (more than one error can be made in each item) and the number of entirely correct reproductions are scored.[11]

"Impaired memory" is a frequent symptom among workers ex-

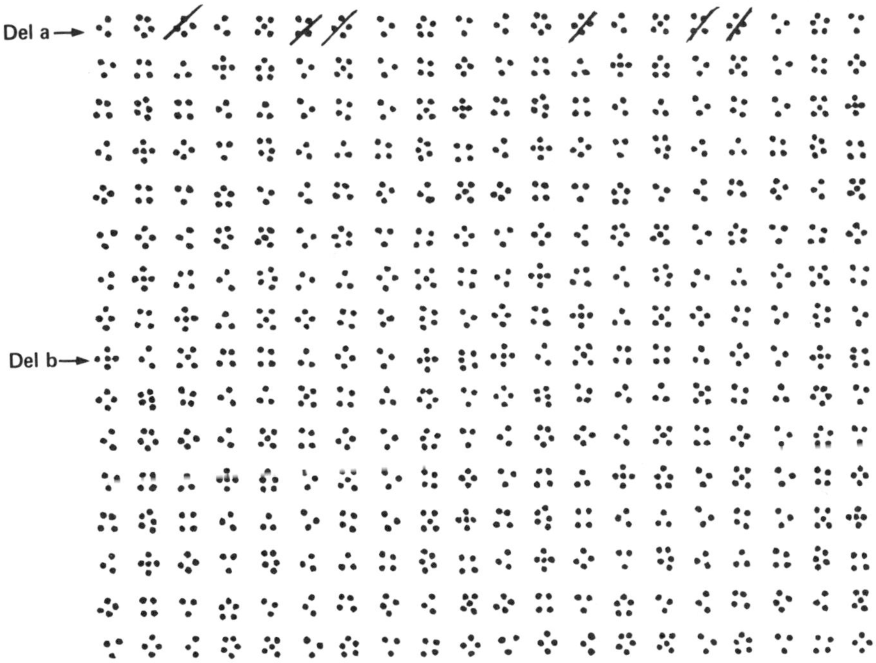

Del a →

Del b →

FIG 49–4.
Dots.

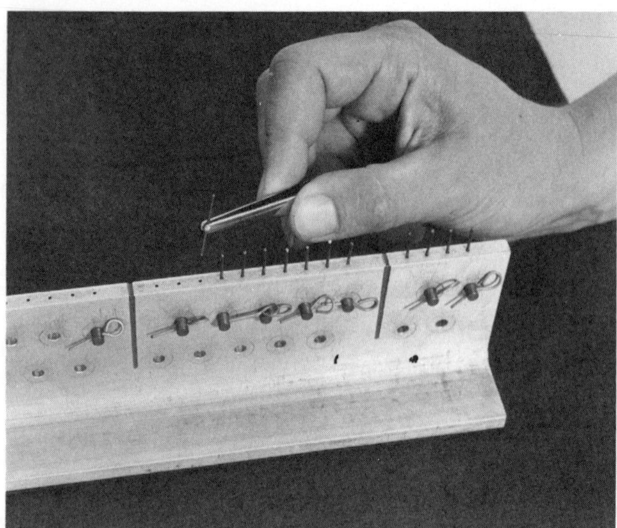

FIG 49–6.
Pins and close-up of Bolt test.

posed to solvents, but performance in the memory tests do not always correlate with the symptoms. "Memory," however, is a very broad concept including several different functions, and it is very plausible that the memory tests used cover only a limited part of the memory functions.[25]

To improve the sensitivity of the battery, a couple of new tests have been added, but they are not yet fully evaluated. One verbal learning test is presently tried.[18] It consists of up to ten presentations of a ten-word list with a recall trial after each presentation. If the subject correctly recalls all ten items on two successive trials before the tenth presentation, the learning trial is completed. In addition to the obtained learning curve, based on the number of correctly recalled items at each trial, recall may be measured after 30 or 60 minutes.

Another addition is the Trail Making test.[5] In part A of the test, the subject is presented with a sheet on which are 25 small circles, numbered 1–25, scattered over the page in an apparently random pattern. With a pencil the subject connects the circles in numerical order, working as quickly as possible. In the more complex part B, there are 13 circles numbered 1–13 and 12 circles labeled A–L. The numbers and letters are to be connected alternately, 1–A–2–B–3 and so forth. The test has proved to be sensitive to decreased efficiency in processing complex material.[43]

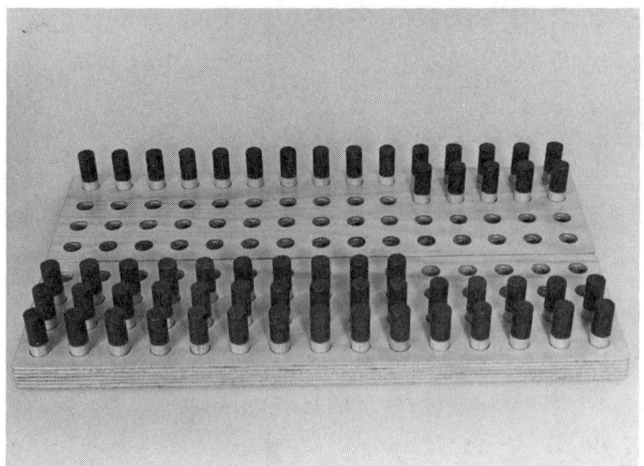

FIG 49–7.
Cylinders.

Neuropsychologic Assessment

Neuropsychologic assessment is characterized by its emphasis on identification and measurement of psychologic deficits, the rational being that brain damage carries with it behavioral changes. Psychologic tests require a combination of sensory, perceptual, and cognitive processes and motor responses, i.e., the test material has to be perceived, intellectually treated in some way or another, and the response (for example, to write down a chosen symbol) has to be given. Since neuropsychologic tests reflect such a composite behavioral or functional outcome of structural or biochemical changes, firm conclusions regarding the location and extent of the damage can not always be drawn.

Evaluation of impairments due to long-term neurotoxic exposure usually requires indirect assessment methods. Measurements of the individual's premorbid ability level are rarely available. This level must instead be estimated from a variety of sources, such as occupational career and societal and leisure time activities. Intraindividual comparisons are also common; performances in verbal and reasoning tests are assumed to be less liable to impairments of neurotoxic agents and may hence be assumed to indicate the individual's premorbid level.

New Techniques for Administration

Computers have gained popularity as a tool in neuropsychologic assessments. Numerous testing systems are under development or already in use. The advantages, such as the ease of administration and scoring of the tests, and the exactness in measurements (for example, of response times) are apparent for large scale studies of solvent exposed groups and in experimental settings. The testing procedure may also be standardized to a high degree. However, if such a system is used for clinical evaluations, the automated versions of the tests have to be validated and the reliability should be assessed.[10]

For clinical use, the technique of adaptive testing may be the most important branch of computerized testing. Adaptive testing strategies are characterized by large item pools that are only partially administered to each test taker, depending on his level of functioning.[40] A high level of flexibility is therefore built into the system.

For group studies and experimental studies, in which reference groups are used or the exposure is controlled by the experimenter, other types of computerized tests are used. Most commonly, traditional paper-and-pencil tests are automated.

At the Swedish National Board of Occupational Safety and Health (NBOSH) a test battery for administration via microcomputers has been developed. Some of the tests have been used in exposure chamber studies,[2] and others are currently implemented in the system and evaluated on clinical cases from some clinics of occupational medicine in Sweden. The validity of the tests will be evaluated against the previously described test battery. The tests that hitherto have been implemented on the computer system (LUXOR ABC 806, Motala, Sweden) are simple reaction time,[29] choice reaction time,[2] a test of Mental Arithmetic,[41] a Search and Memory test,[26] Digit Span,[60] Symbol Digit,[1] Baddeley's Logical Reasoning test,[7] and a Color Word Congruency test.[39a]

Baker and collaborators[8] have developed a computer-administered neurobehavioral evaluation system that includes a set of testing programs and questionnaires which are used to facilitate interpretation of results. The tests were selected and adapted for computer presentation following the recommendations of a WHO/NIOSH expert committee of the World Health Organization and the National Institute for Occupational Safety and Health. The system comprises tests of memory, psychomotor function, verbal ability, visuospatial ability, and mood.

Finally, new types of tests that fully utilize the computer system may be developed. Such tasks may emanate, for example, from models in experimental cognitive psychology and from artificial intelligence research. The underlying idea is that theory-guided tasks that tap basic information-processing abilities are constructed. Test performance may then be related to specific mental processes.[22]

CURRENT TRENDS IN BEHAVIORAL TOXICOLOGY

Up until now, the effects of neurotoxic substances have been looked on as impairments of normal psychologic functions and thus may be indicated by a difference in mean scores on psychologic tests between the exposed subjects and the nonexposed referents. Furthermore, the most sensitive tests to demonstrate mean differences have been chosen, although more specific changes might be found among other types of tests, i.e., those changes that are demonstrable only after more serious deterioration or heavier exposure.

As a rule, only very low correlations between exposure levels and behavioral effects have been found in nonexperimental studies. One reason may be that detailed information about exposure has not been available. More solvent-specific measurements of exposure, e.g., by using biologic measurements, may improve the correlations. Another reason may be that dysfunctions in the central nervous system must be studied by indirect methods. More direct measurements of fundamental biologic and psychologic processes may prove necessary to overcome these validity problems.[23]

Covariation between fundamental biologic mechanisms and mental activity was studied by Risberg and collaborators.[48, 53] The regional cerebral blood flow (rCBF) in 32 industrial workers who had been exposed to organic solvents was investigated. The measurements were made at rest and during the learning of associated word pairs. A comparison of groups of similar age with long and short exposure time (31 and 13 years of average exposure respectively) gave only slight differences in resting rCBF, while significant differences were seen during activation. The group with short exposure had a superior recall performance and an CBF increase during testing in task-related regions of the left hemisphere when compared to the group with long exposure. The latter group's low CBF increases during verbal learning accompanied by the low recall performance was interpreted as a likely physiologic correlate to the cerebral dysfunction that is associated with organic solvent exposure. In another study,[4] a reduced CBF in painters with slight to moderate intellectual impairment was found. The result was interpreted to indicate neuronal loss or decreased metabolism of the neurons.

Another strategy to treat the validity problems is to identify the fundamental physiologic processes that are directly related to sensoric processes with no demands on complex mental processing. In an experiment, simple attentional processes were measured by habituation of the orienting response (OR)[61] to repetitive visual stimuli indicated by electrodermal responses.[11a] A group of 18 exposed workers showing signs of intoxication (i.e., a typical test performance and symptoms) had smaller response amplitudes and faster habituation rate as compared to 18 age-matched nonexposed workers. Although the results did not reach statistical significance, the direction of differences was the same for all measures used, indicating impairment in attentional span and vigor.

Attempts are also being made to identify the basic information processes in mental activities. Performance of a cognitive task involves combinations of several interactive mental processes, such as encoding, memory matching, and response selection. Neurotoxic exposure may be more harmful to some of these processes, while others may be comparably unaffected.[66] A visual analogy test, described by Sternberg[62] is currently tried in a cross-sectional study of solvent exposed workers.[22] The different components of problem-solving in this task are identified through systematic manipulation of the number of mental processes required to solve the task. Another computerized task in the study is based on the assumption that information processing may be divided into two types; automatic and controlled.[51, 58] Case reports and clinical experience has indicated that long-term solvent exposure may obstruct conversion to automatic information processing, which would increase the processing demands and promote fatigability. This hypothesis is supported in the study.

A broadening of the types of effects to be measured, i.e., not only performance measurements, but also, for example, personality characteristics, may also improve sensitivity and specificity in the studies. The assessment of personality characteristics among workers exposed to solvents has been rare. Lindström[44] suggests that such personality factors as coping and adaptation mechanisms can influence the psychologic end state of long-term solvent exposure, and hence, act as modifiers. However, the role of personality factors as modifiers is still poorly known. In some Finnish studies[44, 46] personality measurements have been added to the measurements. The studies have indicated that changes in the personality may be an effect of long-term solvent exposure, but the results are not unambiguous. It may prove valuable to further investigate the role of personality, both as modifier of other effects of long-term solvent exposure, and as an indicator of solvent-induced effects in itself.

REFERENCES

1. Acker W: In support of microcomputer based automated testing: A description of the Maudsley Automated Psychological Screening test (MAPS). *Br J Alcohol Alcoholism* 1980; 15:144–147.
2. Anshelm Olson B, Gamberale F, Iregren A: Co-exposure to toluene

and p-xylene in man. II. Central nervous functions. *Br J Ind Med* 1985; 42:117.

3. Antti-Poika M: Overall prognosis of patients with diagnosed chronic organic solvent intoxication. *Int Arch Occup Environ Health* 1982; 51:127.
4. Arlien-Söborg P, Henriksen L, Gade A, et al: Cerebral blood flow in chronic toxic encephalopathy in house painters exposed to organic solvents. *Acta Neurol Scand* 1982; 66:34.
5. Armitage SG: An analysis of certain psychological tests used for the evaluation of brain injury. *Psychol Monogr* 1946; 60:277.
6. Axelson O, Hane M, Hogstedt C: A case-referent study on neuropsychiatric disorders among workers exposed to solvents. *Scand J Work Environ Health* 1976; 2:14.
7. Baddeley A: A 3 min reasoning test based on grammatical transformation. *Psychonomic Sci* 1968; 10:341–342.
8. Baker EL, Letz R, Fidler A: A computer-administered neurobehavioural evaluation system for occupational and environmental epidemiology: Rationale, methodology, and pilot study results. *J Occup Med* 1985; 27:206.
9. Baker EL, Feldman RG, White RA, et al: Occupational lead neurotoxicity: A behavioural and electrophysiological evaluation. *Br J Ind Med* 1984; 41:352.
10. Beaumont JG: Microcomputer-aided assessment using standard psychometric procedures. *Behavior Research Methods & Instrumentation* 1981; 13:430.
11. Benton A: *Revised Visual Retention Test. Clinical and Experimental Applications:* New York, The Psychological Corporation, 1974.

11a. Berggren T, Engman C, Nordström L, et al: Changes in primary attentional mechanisms due to long term solvent exposure. An experimental study. Department of Occupational Medicine, Örebro, 1984 (manuscript).

12. Bleuler M: *Lehrbuch der Psychiatrie*. Berlin, Springer Verlag, 1969.
13. Browning E: *Toxicity and Metabolism of Industrial Solvents*. Amsterdam, Elsevier Publishing Co, 1965.
14. Bruhn P, Arlien-Söborg P, Gyldensted C, et al: Prognosis in chronic toxic encephalopathy. A two-year follow-up study in 26 house painters with occupational encephalopathy. *Acta Neurol Scand* 1981; 64:259.
15. Cherry N, Rodgers B, Venables H, et al: Acute behavioural effects of styrene exposure: A further analysis. *Br J Ind Med* 1981; 38:346.
16. Cherry N, Waldron HA, Wells GG, et al: An investigation of the acute behavioural effects of styrene on factory workers. *Br J Ind Med* 1980; 37:234.
17. Cherry N, Venables H, Waldron HA, et al: Some observations on workers exposed to methylene chloride. *Br J Ind Med* 1981; 38:351.
18. Claeson L-E, Esbjörnsson E, Carle B-M, et al: *Claeson-Dahls Inlärningstest för Kliniskt Bruk*. Manual. Stockholm, Skandinaviska Testförlaget, 1971.
19. Dureman I, Kebbon L, Österberg E: Manual till DS-batteriet (Manual to the DS-battery). Stockholm, Skandinaviska Testförlaget, 1971.
20. Edling C: Anesthetic gases as an occupational hazard. A review. *Scand J Work Environ Health* 1980; 6:85.
21. Edling C, Ekberg K: No acute behavioural effects of styrene exposure. A safe level of exposure? *Br J Ind Med* 1985; 42:301.
22. Ekberg K, Barregård L, Hagberg S, et al: Effekter av lösningsmedelsexponering på kognitiva funktioner, neurofysiologiska funktioner och livsmönster. Slutrapport till Arbetarskyddsfonden 1984.
23. Ekberg K, Hane M (eds): Nordic conference on clinical behavioural toxicology, Örebro, Sweden, June 1–4, 1982. *Scand J Work Environ Health* 1984; 10(suppl 1).
24. Elofsson S-A, Gamberale F, Hindmarsh T, et al: Exposure to organic solvents. A cross-sectional epidemiologic investigation on occupationally exposed car and industrial spray painters with special reference to the nervous system. *Scand J Work Environ Health* 1980; 6:239.
25. Erickson RC, Scott ML: Clinical memory testing. A review. *Psychol Bull* 1977; 84:1130.
26. Folkard S, Wever RA, Wildgruber CM: Multioscillatory control of circadian rythms in human performance. *Nature* 1983; 305:223–226.
27. Frömark A, Gamberale F, Sjöborg Å: Ett psykologiskt testbatteri för beteendetoxikologiska undersökningar. En tillämpningsstudie. Stockholm, Information från Psykotekniska Institutet 1979; No. 104.
28. Gamberale F: Behavioural effects of exposure to solvent vapors. Experimental and field studies, in *Adverse Effects of Environmental Chemicals and Psychotropic Drugs, vol 2. Neurophysiological and Behavioural Tests*. Amsterdam, Elsevier Scientific Publishing Co, 1976, pp 112–133.
29. Gamberale F, Kjellberg A: Behavioral performance assessment as a biological control of occupational exposure to neurotoxic substances, in Gilioli R, Cassitto MR, Foa V (eds): *Neurobehavioral Methods in Occupational Health*.Oxford, Pergamon Press, 1983.
30. Grandjean P, Arnvig E, Beckmann J: Psychological dysfunctions in lead-exposed workers. Relation to biological parameters of exposure. *Scand J Work Environ Health* 1978; 4:295.
31. Hane M, Axelson O, Blume J, et al: Psychological function changes among house painters. *Scand J Work Environ Health* 1977; 3:91.
32. Hogstedt C, Hane M, Agrell A, et al: Neuropsychological test results and symptoms among workers with well-defined long-term exposure to lead. *Br J Ind Med* 1983; 40:99.
33. Hänninen H: Psychological picture of manifest and latent carbon disulphide poisoning. *Br J Ind Med* 1971; 28:374.
34. Hänninen H, Eskelinen L, Husman K, et al: Behavioral effects of long-term exposure to a mixture of organic solvents. *Scand J Work Environ Health* 1976; 2:240.
35. Hänninen H, Hernberg S, Mantere P, et al: Psychological performance of subjects with low exposure to lead. *J Occup Med* 1978; 20:683.
36. Hänninen H, Nurminen M, Tolonen M, et al: Psychological tests as indicators of excessive exposure to carbon disulfide. *Scand J Psychol* 1978; 19:163.
37. Härkönen H: Relationship of symptoms to occupational styrene exposure and to the findings of electroencephalographic and psychological examinations. *Int Arch Occup Environ Health* 1977; 40:231.
38. Härkönen H, Lindström K, Seppäläinen AM, et al: Exposure-response relationship between styrene exposure and central nervous system functions. *Scand J Work Environ Health* 1978; 4:53.
39. Iregren A: Effects on psychological test performance of workers exposed to a single solvent (toluene)—A comparison with effects of exposure to a mixture of organic solvents. *Neurobehavioral Toxicol Teratol* 1982; 4:695.

39a. Iregren A, Almkvist O, Kleregård M, et al: Utvärdering au sex dator-administrerade test för användning vid diagnostizering au lösnings-medelsskada (Evaluation of six computer-administered behavioral tests for use in diagnosing solvent-induced illness). *Arbete och Halsa* 1987; 13.

40. Johnson JH, Johnson KN: Psychological considerations related to the development of computerized testing stations. *Behavior Research Methods & Instrumentation* 1981; 13:421.
41. Knave B, Anshelm-Olson B, Elofsson S, et al: Long-term exposure to jet fuel. II. A cross-sectional epidemiological investigation on occupationally-exposed industrial workers with special reference to the nervous system. *Scand J Work Environ Health* 1978; 4:19.
42. Levin HS, Rodnitzky RL: Behavioral effects of organophosphate pesticides in man. *Clin Toxicol* 1976; 9:391.

43. Lezak MD: Neuropsychological assessment in behavioural toxicology—developing techniques and interpretive issues, in Ekberg K, Hane M (eds): *Nordic Conference on Clinical Behavioural Toxicology, Örebro, Sweden, June 1–4, 1984. Scand J Work Environ Health* 1984; 10(suppl 1):25.
44. Lindström K: Behavioral changes after long-term exposure to organic solvents and their mixtures. *Scand J Work Environ Health* 1981; 7(suppl 4):48.
45. Lindström K, Härkönen H, Hernberg S: Disturbances in psychological functions of workers occupationally exposed to styrene. *Scand J Work Environ Health* 1976; 3:129.
46. Lindström K, Martelin T: Personality and long term exposure to organic solvents. *Neurobehavioral Toxicol* 1980; 2:89.
47. Mantere P, Hänninen H, Hernberg S, et al: A prospective follow-up study on psychological effects in workers exposed to low levels of lead. *Scand J Work Environ Health* 1984; 10:43.
48. Maximilian VA, Risberg J, Prohovnik I, et al: Regional cerebral blood flow and verbal memory after chronic exposure to organic solvents. *Brain Cognition* 1982; 1:196.
49. Mayer-Gross W, Slater E, Roth M: *Clinical Psychiatry*, ed 3. London, Bailliere, Tindall & Cassel, 1969.
50. Mutti A, Mazzucchi A, Rustichelli P, et al: Exposure-effect and exposure-response relationships between occupational exposure to styrene and neuropsychological functions. *Am J Ind Med* 1984; 5:275.
51. Norman DA, Bobrow DG: On data-limited and resource-limited processes. *Cognitive Psychol* 1975; 7:44.
52. Piikivi L, Hänninen H, Martelin T, et al: Psychological performance and long-term exposure to mercury vapors. *Scand J Work Environ Health* 1984; 10:35.
53. Risberg J: Regional cerebral blood flow measurements by ^{133}Xe-inhalation: Methodology and applications in neuropsychology and psychiatry. *Brain Language* 1980; 9:9.
54. Rodnitsky RL, Levin HS, Mick DL: Occupational exposure to organophosphate pesticides. *Arch Environ Health* 1975; 30:98.
55. Roels H, Lauwerys R, Buchet JP, et al: Comparison of renal function and psychomotor performance in workers exposed to elemental mercury. *Int Arch Occup Environ Health* 1982; 50:77.
56. Savolainen K, Riihimäki V, Seppäläinen AM, et al: Effects of short-term xylene exposure and physical exercise on the central nervous system. *Int Arch Occup Environ Health* 1980; 45:105.
57. Savolainen K, Riihimäki V, Laine A, et al: Short-term exposure of human subjects to M-xylene and 1,1,1-trichloroethane. *Int Arch Occup Environ Health* 1981; 49:89.
58. Shiffrin RM, Schneider W: Controlled and automatic information processing: II. Perceptual learning, automatic attending, and a general theory. *Psychol Rev* 1977; 34:127.
59. Sjöborg A, Frömark A: *Standardisering av ett Psykologiskt Testbatteri för Beteendetoxikologiska Undersökningar* (Standardization of a Battery of Psychological Tests to Be Used in Behavioral Toxicological Studies). Stockholm, Information from Psykotekniska Institutet No. 93, 1977.
60. Smith PJ, Langolf GD, Goldberg J: Effects of occupational exposure to elemental mercury on short term memory. *Br J Ind Med* 1983; 40:413.
61. Sokolov EN: Perception and the conditioned reflex. Oxford, Pergamon Press, 1963.
62. Sternberg RJ: Intelligence, information processing and analogical reasoning. The componential analysis of human abilities. New York, John Wiley & Sons, 1977.
63. Valciukas JA, Lilis R, Eisinger J, et al: Behavioral indicators of lead neurotoxicity: Results of a clinical field survey. *Int Arch Occup Environ Health* 1978; 41:217.
64. Valciukas JA, Lilis R, Singer R, et al: Lead exposure and behavioral changes: Comparisons of four occupational groups with different levels of lead absorption. *Am J Ind Med* 1980; 1:421.
65. Wechsler D: *Manual for Wechsler Adult Intelligence Scale*. New York, Psychological Corporation, 1955.
66. Williamson AM, Teo RKC, Sanderson J: Occupational mercury exposure and its consequences for behavior. *Int Arch Occup Environ Health* 1982; 50:273.
67. Windemüller FJB, Ettama JH: Effects of combined exposure to trichloroethylene and alcohol on mental capacity. *Int Arch Occup Environ Health* 1978; 4:77

50

Occupational Neurotoxicology

Anna Maria Seppäläinen, M.D.

Neurotoxicology is the study of the effects of toxic substances within the nervous system. Pharmacology, especially psychopharmacology, has long used animal models for studying drug effects, especially in the brain, and in developing industrial toxicology it was soon noticed that industrial chemicals may act upon the nervous system. Toxic phenomena in other organ systems such as the liver or the hematopoietic system became fewer with improved industrial hygiene in the 1950s, but the workers still had some health problems. In 1850, an early pioneer, Delpech,[19] reported on subacute carbon disulfide poisoning with mainly psychotic symptoms and he also undertook experimental studies on this chemical. Case reports on neuropathy were published after occupational exposure to carbon disulfide[47, 76] or lead after World War II. More detailed and sensitive neurotoxicologic studies among industrial workers started slowly in the 1960s[12, 43] but began to flourish only in the 1970s. Experimental neurotoxicologic studies on industrial chemicals began in earnest in the 1970s.

The development of industrial neurotoxicology is based on a general trend of taking into consideration already minor health hazards as well as on the fact that the nervous system has poor capacity for self-repair if the damage is full-blown. The development of new methods and research instruments, especially with electronics, have furnished us with new and more accurate tools to study objectively both the central nervous system (CNS) and the peripheral nervous system (PNS). This helps us to reveal defects of structure or function, which lie behind the various and often ill-defined symptoms of nervous system dysfunction.

Neurotoxicology is not an easy field. The nervous system is complex, and wide variations, which still can be classified as normal, occur in its functions. The nervous system also shows plasticity—there are restorative mechanisms that repair incomplete damage within the PNS and CNS. Surviving neurons may also take over the duties of destroyed ones—for example, axonal sprouting for innervation of muscle fibers that have lost their neuronal connections in nerve injuries or motor neuron disease. We know less about similar phenomena in the CNS, but evidently those occur especially in younger persons. The mixture of individual variations in functions and varying degrees of damage and corrective measures is the study object in industrial neurotoxicology. Concerning especially behavioral tests and newer electrophysiologic tests of the CNS, we suffer from incomplete understanding of precisely what is being measured with certain tests.

Neurotoxicology is clearly an interdisciplinary field. Behavioral, neurophysiologic, clinical, neuropathologic, and neurochemical methods are applied. Knowledge of various occupational and nonoccupational (drugs, the effects of a multitude of food additives, chemical exposures from hobbies) exposures as well as expertise in epidemiology are employed in human studies. Chemical expertise is also needed in designing experimental exposures. With combined efforts and profound judgment of various test results, we can increase our understanding of neurotoxic phenomena and learn to prevent extraneous problems arising in the nervous system, which is the most important system for human integrity.

The research approaches in neurotoxicology may be experimental or empirical. Experimental studies can be conducted on human subjects or animals. The human studies are generally short-term studies; experimental exposure lasts for a few hours or a few days only. Animal studies can be both short- and long-term, the latter lasting several weeks to 6–12 months. For necessary reasons, the exposure levels in experimental human studies are low, usually within the threshold limit values (TLV) of the country in question. Thus, the possible effects are very slight, if any, and represent acute effects only. Toxic mechanisms can be better studied with animal models, where more intensive and longer exposures can be applied, and then also chronic effects can be detected.

Empirical studies are either clinical or epidemiologic. Clinical studies or case reports usually can give information on patients with perhaps high-level occupational exposure, but in purely clinical studies the etiologic connection to a certain chemical or even to a mixture of chemicals cannot be absolutely sure. The epidemiologic approach gives more evidence of etiologic connections, but usually in epidemiologic studies, as also in clinical studies, the past exposure can only be estimated. The varying and at times very low exposure levels within the exposed group dilute the possible toxic effects, and statistically significant differences between the exposed and reference groups are not found, although the exposed group may contain individuals with neurotoxic phenomena.

Several types of methods can be used in all the above approaches. Morphologic and neurochemical studies are mainly limited to experimental animal studies, although at times nerve biopsies may be indicated in clinical studies. Neurophysiologic methods can be applied both to the CNS and PNS, and they are used in experimental, epidemiologic, and clinical studies. Neurobehavioral studies, various psychologic tests in human studies, and observations of the spontaneous or conditioned activity as well as the learning behavior of animals, are suitable for neurotoxicology. Clinical neurologic studies completed with neuroradiologic and laboratory studies as needed are applied in case studies and epidemiologic studies. Questionnaires are applicable in all human studies.

MORPHOLOGIC METHODS

Diffuse brain atrophy as shown by pneumoencephalography[37] has been connected to long-term occupational exposure to various solvents or solvent mixtures. Prolonged toluene sniffing has caused morphologic abnormalities of the brain, as revealed by computerized tomography.[40] Gross anatomical changes are, however, infrequent as neurotoxic effects. Mainly, the lesions are on microscopic level, and electron microscopy has greatly expanded the possibilities to detect neuronal damage. The application of tissue preparation methods used in electron microscopy greatly improves the detection of neurotoxic damage in light microscopy as well. In this case, the animal should be killed with perfusion methods;[13, 71] preparations should be embedded also in plastic, and several staining methods should be used to gain most knowledge of various histologic changes. In this way, pathologic changes can be shown within the CNS after, for example, 2,5-hexanediol intoxication,[13] although it was formerly thought to cause axonal damage mainly in the peripheral nerve. Teasing of nerve fibers is laborious,[71] but offers a much greater chance to reveal focal demyelination or patchy axonal changes in peripheral nerves than do the usual transsectional slices.

Nervous system cultures can be used in toxicology testing.[58] In that application whole embryos, whole organs (a whole ganglion or hypophysis, for example), explants (a small piece, usually about 1 cu mm of nervous tissue), dispersed cell cultures, or cell lines (for example, from neuroblastomas) can be used, each method with certain advantages and disadvantages. When whole embryos are used, it is difficult to visualize toxicity at cellular and molecular levels. When using whole organs, animals may be treated with toxins in advance of organ removal and spatial relationships on a cellular level are maintained, but intercellular interactions and communications are poorly visualized, and at organ centers hypoxia may cause cellular death. Explants allow most cytoarchitecture to be maintained, myelination occurs, morphologic evaluation is usually possible with little disturbance to cell cultures, and extracellular recording of electrical activity is possible. However, the morphology is poor in the living state, and individual cells are poorly visualized. Dispersed cell cultures increase reproducibility for biochemical studies; electrophysiology, morphology, and biochemistry may be done on single identified cells, and even analysis of individual synapses is possible. However, most normal cytoarchitecture is lost and little or no myelination occurs in dispersed cell cultures. Cell lines offer large quantities of single cell types for biochemical studies and ease of electrophysiologic studies, but normal cytoarchitecture is lost and cell lines may not accurately represent their counterparts in situ.

NEUROCHEMICAL METHODS

Although the use of biochemical methods in neurotoxicology has increased greatly during recent years, little progress has been made in discovering and explaining molecular and biochemical mechanisms of toxic insults within the nervous system.

Many variables affect the brain biochemistry, starting from body temperature through dietary and nutritional factors to age, sex, and endocrine status.[16] For example, undernutrition induced by lead administration as such could explain hyperactivity and reduced dopamine levels in lead-exposed neonatal rats.[16] Even circadian and environmental factors can influence brain biochemistry and should thus be well controlled.

Neuronal and glial cell populations can be isolated from whole brain or specific brain regions, even axonal membranes can be isolated.[55] Mapping techniques with horseradish peroxidase have been widely used in recent years as a simple and reliable neuroanatomical tracing technique. Autoradiographic nerve tracing can be used, and fluorescence and immunohistochemistry can be applied to selectively visualize, for example, catecholamine- and serotonin-containing neurons.

The regional glucose utilization can be measured with labeled 2-deoxyglucose (2-DG).[70] 2-DG is taken into cells by glucose transport mechanism and subsequently phosphorylated by hexokinase to form 2-deoxyglucose-6-phosphate. This derivative cannot be further metabolized, nor can it readily leave the cell. Thus 2-DG is trapped intracellularly, and the amount in a given brain area can be determined by autoradiographic analysis or scintillation counting. The amount of labeled compound reflects the relative rate of glucose consumption and can be described as a "metabolic stain." Any impairment of glucose metabolism and energy production can have diverse effects on nervous system functioning. Specific glycolytic enzymes have been shown to be inhibited by a number of chemicals known to cause distal axonopathy—for example, acrylamide and methyl-n-butyl ketone.[52] The wider application of 2-DG method could prove useful in neurotoxicology.

Many toxic effects result from the inhibition of enzymes. Some toxic agents inhibit chemical classes of enzymes, such as those containing sulfhydryl groups, whereas other toxicants may inhibit one specific enzyme. Increases in the lysosomal enzymes β-glucuronidase and β-galactosidase are associated with Wallerian degeneration, which follows injury of a peripheral nerve. Such increases have also been noted in peripheral nerves after exposure to acrylamide and methylmercury.[16] Acid proteinase is a lysosomal enzyme responsible for protein degradation. Increase in the activity of acid proteinase has been reported in the brains of rats following exposure to solvents.[54]

NEUROPHYSIOLOGIC METHODS

In recent years, clinical neurophysiologic methods have been increasingly applied to neurotoxicologic studies among occupationally exposed workers.[59, 60] Clinical applications describe patients with various symptoms and signs, and in epidemiologic studies groups of exposed and nonexposed workers are compared, usually in one cross-sectional occasion. Follow-up studies starting at the initiation of occupational exposure are rare.[64]

The PNS can be studied with electromyography, which means the recording of electrical activity of muscles, and electroneurography, which refers to nerve conduction velocity studies of motor and sensory nerves. Both of these methods demand expertise from the examiner. Diagnostic electromyography is done with needle electrodes, and analysis is done on-line from visual and auditory displays. A well-trained electromyographer can thus gain reliable information about early neurotoxic signs in the muscles as well as the information necessary for differential diagnosis to exclude other diseases of the PNS or muscles. Automatic means to electromyographic analyses have been and are being developed, but most methods take a long time and require highly sophisticated instrumentation.[17]

Various nerve conduction velocity studies are probably the most frequently used methods in occupational neurotoxicology. Nerve conduction velocities can be measured with skin electrodes, causing only minor discomfort to the subject, especially in studies of distal sensory conduction velocities in the arm nerves. The necessary instrumentation has become portable and more reasonable in price during recent years, so methods can be applied at work sites or small clinics. The measuring technique is not very complicated, but great care and accuracy are needed in performance. The one who is evaluating the results should have a large clinical experience in electroneurography. Age, temperature close to the nerve, and, possibly, the height of the person affect the nerve conduction velocities. Various neurologic, metabolic, and autoimmunologic diseases may cause neuropathy and, consequently, slowing of nerve conduction velocities also.

The CNS can be studied with electroencephalography (EEG), which can be interpreted visually or through automatic analysis.[20] Electroencephalographic changes may occur acutely in connection with exposure;[38] thus it is also applicable to short-term experimental studies on humans as well as on animals. Spectral analysis of EEG enhances the sensitivity of the method. In measuring the effects of long-term occupational exposure, EEG has been applied to epidemiologic studies and is useful in clinical studies.[60] The EEG abnormalities are nonspecific, thus the evaluation of findings must be done together with other clinical and laboratory tests.

Evoked potentials are small electrical signals that can be detected from the scalp as responses to external stimulations, either stimulation of peripheral nerves or sensory organs.[26] The largest experience on evoked potentials concerns visual evoked potentials (VEP), either to a pattern reversal stimulus or to a bright flash stimulus. Brain stem auditory evoked potentials (BAEP) are early CNS evoked potentials to a click stimulus—the earliest response, with a latency of less than 2 milliseconds, is generated in the auditory nerve, and wave V, with a latency of 5–6 milliseconds, is generated in the brain stem structures. Auditory evoked potentials (AEP) to various sounds are recorded on the cortical areas and can be used for objective measurement of hearing. Somatosensory evoked potentials (SEP), usually in response to an electrical stimulus of a specific peripheral nerve, give information on the sensory system.

Recording of evoked potentials can be done with EEG or electromyography amplifiers. The BAEP has to be recorded with high frequency amplifiers of electromyography type. A computer system for averaging is necessary also, otherwise the small signals cannot be detected from the "noise" of brain electrical activity. Evoked potential studies are noninvasive, and visual or auditory stimuli cause no discomfort. With accurate recording and constant stimulation methods, reliable information can be derived. A large reference material for the laboratory is a prerequisite to a sensitive methodology.

Evoked potentials are suitable to experimental studies. In both human and animal studies the subject can act as his own control when the measurements are carried out in both exposed and nonexposed situations. On-going short-term exposure may cause acute small changes in evoked potentials, although the actual structural, biochemical, or functional basis of these changes cannot yet be reliably interpreted.[67] Long-term exposure to neurotoxic chemicals may cause more profound abnormalities in evoked potentials, as when occupational exposure to n-hexane caused clear attenuation of flash VEP and also prolonged latencies.[66] The availability of EEG and evoked potential studies is satisfactory, and clinical evaluation is usually done with well-established criteria. Many clinical laboratories, however, lack experience on neurotoxic syndromes, and a connection between mild abnormalities and occupational exposure to neurotoxic chemicals may thus remain undetected. With increased application of automatic analysis to epidemiologic and experimental data, we may learn more about disturbed CNS functions and various chemicals.

NEUROLOGIC EXAMINATION

Careful neurologic examination with an aim to quantitation reveals neuropathic signs and symptoms in PNS toxicity. Vibratory sensation may be diminished early, and small commercial devices are available for relatively objective testing of vibratory sense.[4] Good clinical experience is invaluable in the evaluation of higher central nervous functions. In individual cases, the neurologist plays an important role in the differential diagnosis of neurotoxicity from various neurologic diseases and in the evaluation of the remaining working capacity of the affected individual. The clinical observations of neurologists are of utmost importance when neurotoxic hazards appear and correlation to occupational or environmental exposure should be considered.[41] Neuroradiologic and clinical laboratory tests are complementary to differential diagnosis.

In epidemiologic and experimental studies, questionnaires are widely used and form one way of evaluating the subjective symptoms of workers or study subjects. Great care should be utilized in designing questionnaires so that the subjects understand what is being asked. The interpretation of questionnaire studies may be complicated; it is especially difficult to pinpoint a specific CNS or PNS area as being responsible for an admitted symptom, since many symptoms may refer to several nervous system regions.

PSYCHOLOGIC METHODS

A wide variety of psychologic test methods has been developed for testing the intellectual and behavioral functions of persons for different purposes. Some are aimed at choosing personnel for specific tasks or for selecting students most suitable for higher level education. Others measure the loss of capacities or changes of personality with disease.

The interindividual variability in test performances is very wide—it depends on the basic characteristics of the subject and his or her motivation in the test situation. Also, the standardization of the test administration and the scoring of results are often variable; thus the reproducibility of the results may be poor. Furthermore, the poor performance in specific tasks cannot yet be clearly attributed to a specific brain structural change or disease condition. The standardization of test administration is being developed by designing computerized test systems in which the tasks are given by computer display, and the computer scores the responses as well as generates a general aptitude spectrum of the individual person.

Various pencil-and-paper tests, manual dexterity tests of handling small objects in a predetermined way, oral memory tests, mood scales using questionnaires, or other personality tests and reaction time measurements have been applied to neurotoxicity studies.[7, 15, 24, 30, 75]

The original intellectual and performance level of a person cannot be unquestionably measured after a possible neurotoxic effect upon the CNS. With increasing age, diseases and other factors, such as circulatory disturbances and aging as such, may cause deterioration in brain functions that is similar to that caused by toxic factors. Some neurotoxic chemicals may enhance age-dependent changes, which consequently occur earlier than usual. Certain intelligence tests, such as those connected to verbal abilities, are little affected by diffuse brain dysfunction[42] and are accepted as indicators of original intellectual abilities. Verbal intelligence tests have revealed little deterioration in groups of workers occupationally exposed to solvents, although in solvent poisoning some deterioration may be seen even in those.[65] Deterioration caused by diffuse brain dysfunction has been evaluated by comparing scores in verbal and performance intelligence subtests and by forming neuropsychologic deficits indices based on subtest scores.[42]

Another way to overcome problems of possibly uneven original levels is to use the results of psychologic tests performed earlier in life, such as those performed in connection with military service, aptitude testing in job selection, or school reports, and thus aim to match the original intellectual levels of individuals in exposed and nonexposed groups in epidemiologic studies. This type of former information should be used when possible in the clinical work-up of individual patients suspected to suffer from neurotoxic effects.

International comparison of psychologic test results is difficult. The language and cultural differences are great and influence the scoring of test results. Subtests of Wechsler Adult Intelligence Scale (WAIS) are widely used in many countries and local standards exist. Paper-and-pencil tests for perceptual-motor speed and accuracy demand that the subject scan a test sheet row by row, searching for and marking certain target characters as fast and as accurately as possible. These tests also require the capacity for sustained concentration. They are easy and fast to score and free of language. Manual dexterity is tested by letting the subject manipulate small items, such as pegs, in special forms which must be lifted from a special plate, turned, and put back in place, or small pegs which must be picked up and placed in small holes in a specific way. Motor steadiness can be tested by having the subject aim or follow with a pencil a certain track. Many tests of the above types exist. Some probably measure very similar capacities, but differences in features may exist. International validations are often lacking, and each research group gains experience mainly of their own test batteries. (See Chapter 49.)

These variabilities may partly explain differences between epidemiologic studies, where one group reports on deficits in specific functions and another fails to show any deficits in the functions that are claimed to be the same but are tested with another, slightly different test. The vocabulary concerning neuropsychologic functions is varying. Presumably, similar functions are called by somewhat different names, causing misunderstanding among those who do not have a special psychologic education. At times, neuropsychologists have adapted terms that have a particular neurologic meaning and are used for much more minor deficits than is customary in neurology. Thus, "motor tardiness" detected in psychologic tests is not necessarily detected by a coarser test in a routine neurologic examination. "Dementia" is also a term used by some psychologists to denote a significantly smaller deficit than required for a clinical diagnosis of dementia.

Reaction time studies have been applied to experimental and epidemiologic studies. In simple reaction time studies, the subject responds as quickly as possible to a signal of one kind—light or sound stimulus, for example. In choice reaction time studies, various signals, such as red or green lights in different positions or sounds of various intensities or tones are presented to a subject, who then responds quickly in a different way (right or left hand push button, right or left foot pedal) to each signal. Reaction times depend greatly on the vigilance level of the subject, and consequently the time of day, type of work, recent exposure, and temperature and humidity affect reaction times as well as the motivation and personal interests of the subject. Possible research approaches in field situations would be to test an exposed and a nonexposed group in the morning before the work shift and right after the work shift. Lengthening of simple reaction times among styrene-exposed workers has been noted in preshift testing, and the difference in comparison to control persons was greater in postshift testing.[24]

BEHAVIORAL METHODS IN ANIMAL STUDIES

Animal studies are based on several approaches, namely, ethnologic studies,[18] motor activity measurements,[51] operant conditioning,[39] electrical self-stimulation of the brain,[1] and tests on learning and memory.[10] In ethnologic toxicologic studies, the behavior of animals is observed and reported in close to natural surroundings of the animals, assuming that a laboratory cage is a natural surrounding to a laboratory rat. The behavior should be quantitated. Thus, for example, vocalizations of the animal can be recorded on tape and the sounds can be analyzed and quantitated. Exposure to neurotoxicants may delay the maturation of the nervous system and thus induce changes in the squeals of neonatal rats.[18]

Motor activity can be measured in "open field" or in mazes of various shapes. The open field is an open area larger than the home cage and surrounded by a wall. Both horizontal locomotion (ambulation) and vertically directed locomotion (rearing) should be quantitated, either visually or using automated photoreceptors. Mazes are usually provided with automatic means of detection.

Operant conditioning and electrical self-stimulation belong actually to tests of learning. In operant conditioning, correct behavior, such as pushing a lever, is reinforced by giving a food pellet, and noncorrect behavior may be "punished" by an electric shock. In self-stimulation techniques, the reinforcement is an electric stimulus given through implanted electrodes in the posterior hypothalamus, which evidently creates a positive feeling of satisfaction in rats.[1]

Learning and memory belong together. Learning can be identified as adaptation to changes in the environment, and memory is the retention of such adaptations over some time span. If the process of learning is disturbed, memory cannot be evaluated. All learning requires memory functions, since it occurs across time. Learning functions are tested besides through operant conditioning and also through Pavlovian conditioning, in which an unconditioned stimulus, such as food, is paired with a previously neutral signal, such as sound or light, which is the conditioned stimulus. Learning is the association between the unconditioned and conditioned stimulus, such as coupling the secretion of gastric juices to the ringing of a bell, when bell ringing has been learnt to be paired with presentation of food. Also, the extinction of a conditioned reflex can be studied by replacing the earlier positive unconditioned stimulus with a new negative stimulus, such as an electric shock.

The tasks that an animal should learn in order to get a prize (food pellet) or to avoid an unpleasant sensation (electric shock) are of varying difficulty. The animal may have to respond only to a simple stimulus with one peck or touch on a lever or with a preset number of pecks, or the animal may have to learn to discriminate between different shapes of figures, different colors, or sounds. With increasing difficulty of the learning process, the sensitivity of the test may be increased, but on the other hand, a long training period is then needed, and acute, reversible dysfunctions cannot be tested. Training a rat to press a lever for food is relatively easy,[10] and this type of training can be automated. Also, more complicated operant conditioning tasks can be accomplished with a minicomputer simultaneously monitoring a dozen animals, each operating in a separate cage. Automation should lower the cost of these procedures.[39] The slow development of a toxic syndrome can be in this way monitored during a long-term dosing of a neurotoxicant such as mercury.

The correlation between behavioral dysfunctions and structural or biochemical disorders can be studied with animal models. Unfortunately, such studies are rare. Various neurophysiologic methods can be coupled to behavioral studies and/or run independently with animal models. Especially suitable are nerve conduction studies of the PNS,[55] and automated EEG analysis and evoked potentials also have been applied to animals. Studies that can be run easily on the same animal repeatedly—neurophysiologic and behavioral studies are such—are useful for following the development of neuropathy. Neurochemical and/or neuropathologic studies complete the picture after the animal is sacrificed when functional tests have shown impairment.

The extrapolation from animal data to human neurotoxicity is, of course, difficult. Toxic mechanisms can be easier studied with animal models, where longer exposure and higher exposure levels can be used, and where the exposure is better controlled and limited to one chemical or to a desired combination of chemicals than in any long-term human occupational exposure with many extraneous exposures from other sources.

NEUROTOXIC MECHANISMS

The access of toxic substances to the CNS and PNS is restricted through blood-brain and blood-nerve barriers. In the brain, this barrier is formed by capillary endothelium,[35] where the clefts between adjacent endothelial cells are blocked by tight junctions between the cells. It has been shown that the plasma membranes of adjoining cells unite to form a junctional membrane 14 nm thick. These junctions are a network of ridges on one face and corresponding grooves on the other face. There is also some evidence that endothelial cells of cerebral blood vessels do not contract, whereas vascular endothelial cells in non-neural tissues contain a contractile protein. The absence of contractile protein in endothelial cells could be a cofactor in maintaining the blood-brain barriers.

There are few descriptions of the structure of the blood-nerve barrier. Some barrier sites have been described in endoneurial blood vessels, although there seem to exist channels greater than 1 nm, which is larger than those found in the blood-brain barriers. Another barrier exists to insulate the endoneurial space from the nerve sheaths with their permeable blood vessels. This barrier is formed by tight junctions between the lamellated cells which make up the perineurial sheath.

In general, ions enter the brain slowly. The permeability of nonelectrolytes is proportional to their lipid solubility. Special transport mechanisms assist the entry of certain molecules such as glucose, the essential amino acids, lactate, pyruvate, and acetate. Some drugs may inhibit specific barriers, as, for example, mercuric ions at certain doses inhibited the passage of a glucose analog and neural amino acids through the barrier, although the blood-brain barrier remained intact according to studies with other tracers.[74]

In certain regions of the brain, capillaries with fenestrated endothelial cells allow a rapid exchange of plasma filtrate. These brain areas contain cells which produce hormones or act as hormonal or chemoreceptors, and thus direct contact with blood is required. These regions of vascular permeability border the third or fourth ventricle and include, for example, neurohypophysis and pineal body.

In the PNS the dorsal root ganglia are accessible to tracers that elsewhere are kept behind the blood-nerve barrier. Also tracer substances can pass readily across muscle capillaries and diffuse into the gap between the axon and the muscle at the myoneural junction. Thus, tracers can be taken up at axonal endings and then transported in a retrograde direction to the cell body in the spinal cord or brain.

The blood-brain barrier and blood-nerve barrier, together with other systems, also regulate the net movement of water into brain and endoneurial compartments.[49] The capacity of any blood-borne substance to reach the nervous system is related to the amount of tissue perfusion and to blood pressure. The brain is capable of regulating the cerebral blood flow. The PNS lacks the ability to automatically regulate nerve blood flow.[69]

Under normal circumstances, the tightly linked endothelial cells of the brain capillaries form the structural barrier that prevents free diffusion of proteins, electrolytes, and water-soluble nonelectrolytes. These tight junctions appear to be labile, and injection of hyperosmolar solutions can cause fluid leakage between endothelial cells and consequent extravasation.[9] When the injury is minor, extravasation of plasma proteins in hyperosmolar vasculopathy is a temporary phenomenon and no actual edema is formed. Suggested mechanisms of altered vascular permeability are mechanical distortion of endothelial cells, such as shrinkage by hyperosmolar plasma, or capillary dilatation in hypertension. Cerebral edema occurs when excess fluid accumulates within the brain sufficient to cause swelling. Edema can be general or local, and the enlargement can be confined to one or more regions, or to a particular tissue component.

Neurotoxins such as certain heavy metals (lead, mercury) and organic arsenicals cause an initial injury to cerebral capillaries and vasa nervorum by damaging the endothelial cells and disrupting their tight junctions. For example, lead poisoning causes vascular damage with plasma extravasation, which is followed by endothelial microglial and astrocytic proliferation and widespread edema.

Marked fluid accumulation can be restricted to the myelin sheath without demonstrable injury to the blood-brain barrier. This type of encephalopathy can result from experimental triethyltin administration. This organic compound penetrates blood-brain barrier readily and has an affinity for myelin. The fluid, which is protein-free but contains sodium and chloride, accumulates within the myelin sheath but not in the extracellular space. Consequently, the myelin sheath undergoes splitting, allowing fluid to accumulate between myelin lamellae without altering the chemical composition of myelin.[49]

Morphologically similar spongiform myelinopathy of the brain has been noted in premature infants who had been subjected to four or more treatments with hexachlorophene used as a topical bacteriostatic agent. Hepatic immaturity with diminished ability to conjugate hexachlorophene to glucuronide increased the vulnerability of premature infants, and often rashes or surgical wounds facilitated the entry of hexachlorophene into the patient's bloodstream. However, in these infants no generalized brain swelling developed, and death was due to other complications of prematurity.[49]

An antituberculous agent, isonicotinic acid hydrazide (INH), causes in dogs and ducklings spongy degeneration of the cerebral white matter due to intramyelinic edema, which results in vacuolization. In human beings, the most important side effect of INH is peripheral neuropathy. The latter responds to pyridoxine therapy, while encephalopathy does not respond to pyridoxine. The neuropathy is not associated with intramyelinic edema.

Edema in peripheral nerves has been much less studied than brain edema. New techniques have been developed to measure endoneurial fluid pressure.[49] Increased endoneurial fluid pressure has been found in conjunction with four morphologically different pathologic states, namely, (1) states of altered vascular permeability, such as in lead neuropathy, (2) intramyelinic edema due to myelinotoxic agents such as hexachlorophene, (3) Wallerian degeneration following crush injury, and (4) interstitial edema associated with retention in the endoneurium of osmolytically active substances such as galactitol and sorbitol.[49]

Windebank et al.[77] have shown that lead accumulated in the endoneurium of lead-treated rats during the first month of exposure, peaking at 35 days. The endoneurial water content was significantly higher in lead-treated animals 50 days after starting the lead diet. The blood-nerve barrier to lead was thus not absolute. The changes in the blood-nerve barrier to water manifested clearly later. Only at the same time as edema began to accumulate did the morphologic changes also start.

Nerve cells may have very long axons before terminating in nerve endings. Nerve endings seem to lack any major protein-synthesizing mechanisms. Therefore, neurotransmitter-related enzymes and other proteins and cellular constituents have to be synthesized in the cell body and transported down the axon to the nerve terminals. Materials replacing the components of the axonal membrane and myelin sheath or participating in the local metabolism of the axon are also transported in axons. This axoplasmic transport is "slow" or "fast" according to the rate, and it requires energy. Some materials can also migrate from the nerve endings to the cell body as retrograde axoplasmic transport; it has been suggested that, for example, lead can migrate this way to the CNS.

The distal axon is a preferential site of lesion in many toxic neuropathies. This type of degeneration often spreads in a centripetal direction. Under most circumstances, there is simultaneous involvement of the central and peripheral nervous systems, and therefore Spencer and Schaumburg[72] have used the term "central-peripheral distal axonopathy." An essential factor in the preferential vulnerability has been considered the separation of the distal axon from the site of synthetic machinery in the cell body. Precursors for both membrane-associated and soluble proteins are taken up into the cell body. The synthesis of various proteins and glycoproteins probably takes place in various cell components such as the polysomes. The synthetic processes are governed by the nucleus, where templates of deoxyribonucleic acid (DNA) direct ribonucleic acid (RNA) synthesis.

The neuronal cell processing is complex, and there are many potential sites of vulnerability. Certain drugs, such as doxorubicin (Adriamycin), interfere with DNA-dependent RNA synthesis. Doxorubicin has been identified as causing selective damage in the sensory neurons of the dorsal root ganglion.[45] Doxorubicin was quickly accepted into the cell bodies and nuclei of the dorsal root ganglion, and after six days following single dosing, there was a dispersion of the polysomes from their normal appearance in rosettes so that single scattered ribosomes were commonly found. Single ribosomes are inactive in protein synthesis. At 9–11 days, axonal degeneration could be seen clearly in the dorsal root ganglion and in the adjacent sensory nerve roots, but fewer axons underwent degeneration in the sciatic nerve and its distal branches. In this case, the spread of axonal degeneration was in a centrifugal pattern.

An increased number of neurofilaments in the axon is a characteristic finding in several toxic neuropathies. In hexacarbon neuropathies (methyl-n-butyl ketone, 2,5-hexanedione, 2,5-hexanediol, and n-hexane) 10-nm filaments accumulate in large quantities on the proximal side of the node of Ranvier,[53] and the axoplasmic transport is interfered with. It has been suggested that the impediment of axoplasmic transport is related to swelling of the proximal paranodal area of the axon which is later followed by expansion of the distal paranode as well. The proximal paranodal areas also show expansions, axonal protrusions which compress and displace the distal paranode and increase the nodal gap width.[36] This can be followed by thinning of myelin, usually on the proximal side, while on the other side of the node of Ranvier, the myelin may be split and corrugated. The axonal swelling could be analogous to multiple sites of ligation of the axon. If an axon was ligated so as only to occlude partially the axoplasmic transport, the down flow rate of radioactive leucine was only minimally slowed, while fast axoplasmic transport rate was markedly slowed.[45] In hexacarbon-induced neuropathy, there is evidence that the transport abnormality is related to axonal degeneration and that accumulation of neurofilaments precedes axonal degeneration.

In acrylamide neuropathy, Pleasure et al.[48] have suggested a defect in slow axoplasmic transport. They found injected radioactivity to accumulate in the root segments close to the cell bodies, which suggested that perikaryon protein synthesis had taken place. Histologically, changes in acrylamide intoxication consist of acute death of Purkinje cells in the cerebellum, swelling of terminals and preterminal fibers in the PNS and CNS due to the accumulation of intra-axonal organelles (neurofilaments, mixed with smooth endoplasmic reticulum and other organelles), and chromatolytic changes in primary sensory neurons and to some extent also in motor neurons.[13] The sensory symptoms and electrophysiologic signs of sensory nerve impairment are prominent in acrylamide neuropathy.

The nerve membrane plays an essential role in the propagation of nerve impulses. The resting membrane potential results from the selective permeability of the cell membrane to potassium and the potassium concentration gradient across the membrane. This potential is of the order of 80–100 mV, and the inside is negative with respect to the outside. When the membrane of an excitable cell is rapidly depolarized by an environmental change (stimulus), the membrane permeability to sodium increases and the membrane potential is changed, consequently the inside of the cell becomes positive with respect to the outside. Then the permeability ratios rechange—the sodium permeability decreases rapidly and the potassium permeability increases—and the membrane potential returns to the original resting level. Permeability changes are very fast and can be studied only with special micromethods such as voltage clamp technique.[33]

Some neurotoxicants exert their action on the cell membrane. For example, tetrodotoxin (TTX), which is the toxic principle of the puffer fish poison (a Japanese fish), selectively blocks the sodium permeability increase associated with excitation,[46] without any effect on potassium currents. The specific affinity of TTX is for the sodium channel, and it is effective only from outside of the nerve membrane. Some other natural toxins also exert unique actions on ionic channels; examples are the scorpion venom and sea anemone toxins.

DDT exerts its major toxic actions at synaptic and neuromuscular junctions. Repetitive discharges originating in the presynaptic nerve fibers cause facilitation and repetitive responses in the postsynaptic element,[46] which are due to an elevated and prolonged negative after-potential—the latter serves as a continuous stimulus. The slowing of the falling phase of sodium current is the primary cause for the increase in the negative after-potential, although there is also some decrease in outward potassium current. These phenomena could be based on interactions between the DDT molecules and the sodium channel.

Another type of damage in the peripheral nerve is segmental toxic demyelination. In this case, the myelin sheath of axons is changed, vacuoles are formed, and the myelin lamellae are split apart, while the axon itself remains intact. Secondarily, the axons suffer also and may undergo degeneration in chronic situations. This type of primary demyelination is caused by several neurotoxic compounds, for example by triethyltin, hexachlorophene, isonicotinic acid hydrazide, and salicylanilides.[11] Although the biochemical basis of primary demyelination has not been clarified, some hypothetical mechanisms have been presented, such as a direct disruptive effect on membrane structure, or an inhibition of various enzymes involved in ion or water transport (like carbonic anhydrase) or other enzymes, or an inhibition of oxidative phosphorylation, resulting in a deficit in the energy required for maintenance of myelin.[11] Some of myelinotoxic chemicals may have direct detergent-like effects on membranes (triethyltin, hexachlorophene), and these, together with disruption of the hydrophobic regions of proteins, could account for the splitting and partial dissolution of myelin.

Demyelination may also occur concomitantly with injury to myelinating cells, namely oligodendrocytes in the CNS and Schwann cells in the PNS, which synthesize and maintain the myelin sheath. Schlaepfer[57] suggested that lead neuropathy in the rat is caused by a disturbance in the supporting cells of the PNS. Dyck et al.[21] also suggested a direct toxic effect of lead on Schwann cells based on the findings that demyelinated internodes in the sural nerves of lead-poisoned rats were randomly distributed. The type of lead neuropathy varies evidently by species. In human beings, lead more likely causes axonal degeneration. Since the myelin biosynthesis, assembly, and maintenance are very complex, it is probable that even specific myelinotoxic chemicals such as triethyltin and hexachlorophene affect more than one of the biochemical systems involved in myelin structure and maintenance.

Demyelination causes marked abnormalities in the conduction of nervous impulses. At the site of demyelination the conduction velocity is considerably decreased or even blocked. In myelinated fibers the impulses are propagated in a saltatory fashion; only at the nodes of Ranvier is the membrane depolarized, and there is only a brief interval between excitation of successive nodes, so that the first node is only partially repolarized during depolarization of the next node.[50] In demyelinated fibers, continuous conduction of impulses takes place, and the node proximal to a demyelinated internode may be substantially repolarized before the ensuing node is excited. The latter results in conduction block, if the current delivered to the node distal to the demyelinated internode is insufficient to depolarize the axon to threshold for excitation. Conduction block leads to palsy of respective muscle fibers or to sensory loss in the area supplied by affected nerve fibers. Regeneration of demyelinated fibers apparently occurs by remyelination, and minor remyelination may produce dramatic improvement in clinical symptomatology, if it is sufficient to overcome conduction block.

Continuous muscle fiber activity or myokymia is occasionally seen in peripheral neuropathies. This may be caused by ectopic excitation of a demyelinated patch of a nerve fiber; this excitation then occurs in bursts.

Various combinations of lesions evidently occur in peripheral nerves after neurotoxic inference. Recently, Maxwell and Le Quesne[44] described correlations between electrophysiologic and histologic findings in experimental hexachlorophene neuropathy. Early histologic changes in animals (two weeks after starting a hexachlorophene diet) included intramyelin edema, initially located in internodal areas of several axons at several sites. Simultaneously, axonal degeneration was noted from examination of teased nerve fascicles. With time, the edema increased, and after 13 weeks segmental demyelination started to appear. Electrophysiologic studies showed slight decrease in nerve conduction velocities (7.5%) in two to three weeks, and a more substantial decrease (17%) of motor conduction velocity (MCV) was noted after one to three months of poisoning. In six to seven months, further decrease was noted in the MCV. The reduction of the MCV was noted in both the proximal and distal segments of the nerve, in animals exposed for only two weeks to hexachlorophene. The amplitude of the response dropped clearly after one to three months of exposure. The smaller reduction of MCV in the early phases of poisoning reflected axonal changes, which usually cause slight slowing only; the greater reduction later on was consistent with segmental demyelination. This type of study reflects the multiple mechanisms of vulnerability in the PNS: the more carefully we study, the more sites of lesions we detect. It also makes it clear that the types of findings we may expect depend greatly on the time point of the study—in early poisoning, the lesions may be different from those at a later stage. At a later stage, various corrective and compensatory mechanisms have also started their actions and further modify the picture of poisoning.

SOME EXAMPLES OF NEUROTOXIC PHENOMENA

A classic example of neurotoxicity in occupational settings is lead palsy, usually radial palsy with hand drop. This sign is rare if it exists at all in modern industrialized countries, but reports on the milder neurotoxic effects of lead are abundant. In human beings, neurotoxic effects probably start in axons, which is apt to cause only a slight reduction in conduction velocities. With real prospective follow-up, slight slowing was detectable at low blood lead levels (30–40 μg/100 ml),[64] and several cross-sectional human studies have shown slowing in motor conduction and, more recently in sensory conduction velocities at blood lead levels of 60–70 μg/100 ml.[2, 6, 68] Recovery of slowed conduction velocity after decrease of blood lead levels has also been reported.[3] In axonal degeneration, the slowing of conduction velocities does not become much more severe with increasing exposure levels or longer exposure time. This may partly explain the controversial findings of no demonstrable slowing in nerve conduction velocities when workers are followed up starting after two or more years of lead work and when compared to "nonexposed" workers with blood lead levels ranging up to 40 μg/100 ml.[73] In animal experiments, lead induces neuropathy in guinea pigs with axonal degeneration,[23] and in rats with demyelination.[21, 57]

Hexacarbons have been vividly studied since reports on peripheral neuropathy caused by n-hexane and methyl-n-butyl ketone appeared.[8, 32, 34] Neurotoxic effects of hexacarbons usually have occurred after repetitive and prolonged exposure to these solvents and they manifest themselves as distal symmetrical, progressive, sensorimotor polyneuropathy. Structural changes of peripheral nerves have been demonstrated in animals and human beings, and they consist of giant axonal changes secondary to aggregation of neurofilamentous masses.[5]

The neurotoxic effects of hexacarbons are not limited to the PNS, but are found also in the CNS at various sites[14, 56] where neurofilamentous masses have been detected. Human studies on the CNS toxicity of hexacarbons are rare; however, prolonged latencies and diminished amplitudes of flash-VEPs have indicated lesions in the visual pathways of n-hexane-exposed industrial workers.[66] These changes could reflect partial axonal degeneration.

Organic solvents other than hexacarbons have been claimed to induce neurotoxic changes in the CNS and in the PNS. Various symptoms, such as headache, memory loss, vertigo, pressure feelings on the thorax, and paresthesiae have been related to occupational exposure to solvents and solvent mixtures. Abnormal EEG findings have been reported among shoe workers,[25] floor layers,[27] workers exposed to various solvents,[60, 65] and boat builders exposed to styrene.[63] Psychologic tests among workers exposed to solvent mixtures have revealed impairment in verbal and visual intelligence and memory tests[29] as well as in perceptual and motor tasks.[22] When individual exposure to styrene could be measured, exposure intensity-related impairment in visuomotor accuracy and psychomotor performance was detected.[31] Qualitative differences between groups with different degrees of neurotoxic effects caused by carbon disulfide were detected by Hänninen[28] when workers with clinically manifested carbon disulfide poisoning exhibited lowered vigilance, diminished intellectual activity, retarded speech and motor disturbances, whereas exposed workers without clinical symptoms showed depressive mood, slight motor disturbances, and intellectual impairment.

Peripheral neuropathy may be found after solvent exposure. Carbon disulfide neuropathy has become less common with decreasing exposure levels in modern times.[62] The problem with polyneuropathy in various occupations with solvent exposure is, however, not yet overcome, and affected workers may suffer from neuropathic symptoms and show clear neuropathic signs in electrophysiologic tests several years after chronic solvent poisoning.[61]

While efforts to control, reduce, and minimize worker exposures continue, much can be done and should be done to study the neurotoxic effects of workplace chemicals. The mechanisms of toxic action need further clarification, as do the possible synergistic, additive, and modifying effects of complex exposures so usual in real working situations. Experimental work can help in basic considerations, but epidemiologic research and case studies are invaluable in clinical neurotoxicology.

REFERENCES

1. Annau Z: Electrical self-stimulation of the brain: A model for the behavioral evaluation of toxic agents, in *Nervous System Toxicology*. New York, Raven Press, 1982, pp 213–227.
2. Araki S, Honma T: Relationships between lead absorption and peripheral nerve conduction velocities in lead workers. *Scand J Work Environ Health* 1976; 4:225.
3. Araki S, Honma T, Yagihara S, et al: Recovery of slowed nerve con-

duction velocity in lead-exposed workers. *Int Arch Occup Environ Health* 1980; 46:151.

4. Arezzo JC, Schaumburg HH, Petersen CA: Rapid screening for peripheral neuropathy: A field study with the Optacon. *Neurology* 1983; 33:626.
5. Asbury AK, Brown MJ: The evaluation of structural changes in distal axonopathies, in *Experimental and Clinical Neurotoxicology*. Baltimore, Williams & Wilkins Co, 1980, pp 179–192.
6. Ashby JA: A neurological and biochemical study of early lead poisoning. *Br J Ind Med* 1980; 37:133.
7. Baker EL, Feldman RG, White RF, et al: Monitoring neurotoxins in industry: Development of a neurobehavioral test battery. *J Occup Med* 1983; 25:125.
8. Billmaier D, Yee HT, Allen N, et al: Peripheral neuropathy in a coated fabrics plant. *J Occup Med* 1974; 16:665.
9. Brightman MW, Hori M, Rapaport SI, et al: Osmotic opening of tight junctions in cerebral endothelium. *J Comp Neurol* 1973; 152:317.
10. Cabe PA, Eckerman DA: Assessment of learning and memory dysfunction in agent-exposed animals, in *Nervous System Toxicology*. New York, Raven Press, 1982, pp 133–198.
11. Cammer W: Toxic demyelination: Biochemical studies and hypothetical mechanisms, in *Experimental and Clinical Neurotoxicology*. Baltimore, Williams & Wilkins Co, 1980, pp 239–256.
12. Catton MJ, Harrison MJG, Fullerton PM, et al: Subclinical neuropathy in lead workers. *Br Med J* 1970; 2:80.
13. Cavanagh JB: Mechanisms of axon degeneration in three toxic 'neuropathies': Organophosphorus, acrylamide and hexacarbon compared, in *Recent Advances in Neuropathology*. Edinburgh, Churchill Livingstone, Inc, 1982, pp 213–242.
14. Cavanagh JB: The pattern of recovery of axons in the nervous system of rats following 2,5-hexanediol intoxication: A question of rheology? *Neuropathol Appl Neurobiol* 1982; 8:19.
15. Cherry N, Waldron HA, Wells GG, et al: An investigation of the acute behavioral effects of styrene on factory workers. *Br J Ind Med* 1980; 37:234.
16. Damstra T, Bondy SC: Neurochemical approaches to the detection of neurotoxicity, in *Nervous System Toxicology*. New York, Raven Press, 1982, pp 349–373.
17. Daube JR: Quantitative EMG in nerve-muscle disorders, in *Clinical Neurophysiology*. London, Butterworths, 1981, pp 33–65.
18. Davis JM: Ethological approaches to behavioral toxicology, in *Nervous System Toxicology*. New York, Raven Press, 1982, pp 29–44.
19. Delpech A: Mémoire sur les accidents que développe, chez les ouvriers en caoutchouc, l'inhalation du sulfure de carbone en vapeur. *Bull Acad Méd* 1856; 21:350.
20. Duffy FH, Burchfiel JL, Lombroso CT: Brain electrical activity mapping (BEAM): A method for extending the clinical utility of EEG and evoked potential data. *Ann Neurol* 1979; 5:309.
21. Dyck PJ, O'Brien PC, Ohnishi A: Lead neuropathy: 2. Random distribution of segmental demyelination among "old internodes" of myelinated fibers. *J Neuropathol Exp Neurol* 1977; 36:570.
22. Elofsson SA, Gamberale F, Hindmarsch T, et al: Exposure to organic solvents. A cross-sectional epidemiologic investigation on occupationally exposed car and industrial spray painters with special reference to the nervous system. *Scand J Work Environ Health* 1980; 6:239.
23. Fullerton PM: Chronic peripheral neuropathy produced by lead poisoning in guinea-pigs. *J Neuropathol Exp Neurol* 1966; 25:214.
24. Gamberale F, Lisper HO, Anshelm Olson B: The effect of styrene vapour on the reaction time of workers in the plastic boat industry, in *Adverse Effects of Environmental Chemicals and Psychotropic Drugs*. Amsterdam, Elsevier, 1976, vol 2, pp 135–148.
25. Giuliano G, Iannaccone A, Zappoli R: Ricerche elettroencefalografiche in operai di calzaturifici esposti al rischio di intossicazione da solventi. *Lav Um* 1974; 26:33.
26. Halliday AM: *Evoked Potentials in Clinical Testing*. Bath, Churchill Livingstone, Inc, 1982.
27. Hanke C, Ruppe K, Otto J: Untersuchungsergebnisse zur toxischen Wirkung von Dichlormethan bei Fussbodenlegern. *Zentralbl Gesamt Hyg Grenzgeb* 1974; 20:81.
28. Hänninen H: Psychological picture of manifest and latent carbon disulphide poisoning. *Br J Ind Med* 1971; 28:374.
29. Hänninen H, Eskelinen L, Husman K, et al: Behavioral effects of long-term exposure to a mixture of organic solvents. *Scand J Work Environ Health* 1976; 2:240.
30. Hänninen H, Lindström K: Behavioral test battery for toxicopsychological studies: Used at the Institute of Occupational Health in Helsinki. Helsinki, Institute of Occupational Health, 1979.
31. Härkönen H, Lindström K, Seppäläinen AM, et al: Exposure-response relationship between styrene exposure and central nervous functions. *Scand J Work Environ Health* 1978; 4:53.
32. Herskowitz A, Ishii N, Schaumburg, H: n-Hexane neuropathy. A syndrome occurring as a result of industrial exposure. *N Engl J Med* 1971; 285:82.
33. Hodgkin AL, Huxley AF, Katz B: Measurement of current-voltage relations in the membrane of the giant axon of Loligo. *J Physiol* 1952; 116:424.
34. Iida M, Yamamura Y, Sobue I: Electromyographic findings and conduction velocity on n-hexane polyneuropathy. *Electromyography* 1969; 9:247.
35. Jacobs JM: Vascular permeability and neural injury, in *Experimental and Clinical Neurotoxicology*. Baltimore, Williams & Wilkins Co, 1980, pp 102–117.
36. Jones HB, Cavanagh JB: Distortions of the nodes of Ranvier from axonal distension by filamentous masses in hexacarbon intoxication. *J Neurocytol* 1983; 12:439.
37. Juntunen J, Hernberg S, Eistola P, et al: Exposure to industrial solvents and brain atrophy. *Eur Neurol* 1980; 19:366.
38. Konietzko H, Elster I, Schomann P, et al: Felduntersuchungen in Lösungsmittelbetrieben. Hirnelektrische Korrelate der Trichloräthylenwirkung im telemetrisch abgeleiteten EEG. *Zbl Arbeitsmed* 1976; 26:60.
39. Laties VG: Contributions of operant conditioning to behavioral toxicology, in *Nervous System Toxicology*. New York, Raven Press, 1982, pp 67–79.
40. Lazar RB, Ho SU, Melen O, et al: Multifocal central nervous system damage caused by toluene abuse. *Neurology (Cleveland)* 1983; 33:1337.
41. Le Quesne PM: Toxic substances and the nervous system: The role of clinical observation. *J Neurol Neurosurg Psychiatry* 1981; 44:1.
42. Lezak MD: Neuropsychological assessment. New York, Oxford University Press, 1976.
43. Lukás E: Leitgeschwindigkeit peripherer Nerven bei Schwefelkohlenstoff ausgesetzten Personen. *Internat Zeitsch Klin Pharmakol Ther Toxikol* 1969; 2:354.
44. Maxwell IC, Le Quesne PM: Conduction velocity in hexachlorophene neuropathy. *J Neurol Sci* 1979; 43:95.
45. Mendell JR, Sahenk Z: Interference of neuronal processing and axoplasmic transport by toxic chemicals, in *Experimental and Clinical Neurotoxicology*. Baltimore, Williams & Wilkins Co, 1980, pp 139–160.
46. Narahashi T: Nerve membrane as a target of environmental toxicants, in *Experimental and Clinical Neurotoxicology*. Baltimore, Williams & Wilkins Co, 1980, pp 225–238.
47. Noro L: Svavelvete- och kolsvavlaförgiftningar. *Nordisk Med* 1944; 24:2015.
48. Pleasure DE, Mishler KC, Engel WK: Axonal transport of proteins in experimental neuropathies. *Science* 1969; 166:524.
49. Powell HC, Myers RR, Lampert PW: Edema in neurotoxic injury, in

Experimental and Clinical Neurotoxicology. Baltimore, Williams & Wilkins Co, 1980, pp 118–138.

50. Rasminsky M: Physiological consequences of demyelination, in *Experimental and Clinical Neurotoxicology*. Baltimore, Williams & Wilkins Co, 1980, pp 257–271.
51. Reiter LW, MacPhail RC: Factors influencing motor activity measurements in neurotoxicology, in *Nervous System Toxicology*. New York, Raven Press, 1982, pp 45–65.
52. Sabri MI, Moore CL, Spencer PS: Studies on the biochemical basis of distal axonopathies. Inhibition of glycolysis produced by neurotoxic hexacarbon compounds. *J Neurochem* 1979; 32:683.
53. Sabri MI, Spencer PS: Toxic distal axonopathy: Biochemical studies and hypothetical mechanisms, in *Experimental and Clinical Neurotoxicology*. Baltimore, Williams & Wilkins Co, 1980, pp 206–219.
54. Savolainen H, Pfäffli P, Tengen M, et al: Biochemical and behavioral effects of inhalation exposure to tetrachloroethylene and dichlormethane. *J Neuropathol Exp Neurol* 1977; 36:941.
55. Savolainen H, Seppäläinen AM: Biochemical and physiological effects of organic solvents on rat axon membranes isolated by a new technique. *Neurotoxicology* 1979; 1:467.
56. Schaumburg HH, Spencer PS: Environmental hydrocarbons produce degeneration in cat hypothalamus and optic tract. *Science* 1978; 199:199.
57. Schlaepfer WW: Experimental lead neuropathy: A disease of the supporting cells in the peripheral nervous system. *J Neuropathol Exp Neurol* 1969; 28:401.
58. Schrier BK: Nervous system cultures as toxicologic test systems, in *Nervous System Toxicology*. New York, Raven Press, 1982, pp 337–348.
59. Seppäläinen AM: Applications of neurophysiological methods in occupational medicine. A review. *Scand J Work Environ Health* 1975; 1:1.
60. Seppäläinen AM: The use of clinical neurophysiological methods in studies of workers exposed to solvents, in Kyoto Symposia, EEG Suppl No 36. Amsterdam, Elsevier Biomedical Press, 1982, pp 693–700.
61. Seppäläinen AM, Antti-Poika M: Time course of electrophysiological findings for patients with solvent poisoning. A descriptive study. *Scand J Work Environ Health* 1983; 9:15.
62. Seppäläinen AM, Haltia M: Carbon disulfide neuropathy. *G Ital Med Lav* 1981; 3:87.
63. Seppäläinen AM, Härkönen H: Neurophysiological findings among workers occupationally exposed to styrene. *Scand J Work Environ Health* 1976; 2:140.
64. Seppäläinen AM, Hernberg S, Vesanto R, et al: Early neurotoxic effects of occupational lead exposure: A prospective study. *Neurotoxicology* 1983; 4:181.
65. Seppäläinen AM, Lindström K, Martelin T: Neurophysiological and psychological picture of solvent poisoning. *Am J Ind Med* 1980; 1:31.
66. Seppäläinen AM, Raitta Ch, Huuskonen MS: n-Hexane-induced changes in visual evoked potentials and electroretinograms of industrial workers. *Electroencephalogr Clin Neurophysiol* 1979; 47:492.
67. Seppäläinen AM, Savolainen K, Kovala T: Changes induced by xylene and alcohol in human evoked potentials. *Electroencephalogr Clin Neurophysiol* 1981; 51:148.
68. Seppäläinen AM, Tola S, Hernberg S, et al: Subclinical neuropathy at "safe" levels of lead exposure. *Arch Environ Health* 1975; 30:180.
69. Smith DR, Kobrime AI, Rizzoli HV: Absence of autoregulation in peripheral nerve blood flow. *J Neurol Sci* 1977; 33:347.
70. Sokoloff L, Reivich M, Kennedy C, et al: The ^{14}C-deoxyglucose method for the measurement of local cerebral glucose utilization: Theory, procedure, and normal values in the conscious and anesthetized albino rat. *J Neurochem* 1977; 28:897.
71. Spencer PS, Bischoff MC: Contemporary neuropathological methods in toxicology, in *Nervous System Toxicology*. New York, Raven Press, 1982, pp 259–275.
72. Spencer PS, Schaumburg HH: Ultrastructural studies of the dying-back process. IV. Differential vulnerability of PNS and CNS fibers in experimental central-peripheral distal axonopathies. *J Neuropathol Exp Neurol* 1977; 36:300.
73. Spivey GH, Baloh RW, Brown CP, et al: Subclinical effects of chronic increased lead absorption. A prospective study. III. Neurologic findings at follow-up examination. *J Occup Med* 1980; 22:607.
74. Steinwall O: Transport inhibition phenomena in unilateral chemical injury of blood-brain barrier. *Prog Brain Res* 1968; 29:357.
75. Valciukas JA, Lilis R: Psychometric techniques in environmental research. *Environ Res* 1980; 21:275.
76. Vigliani EC: Carbon disulphide poisoning in viscose rayon factories. *Br J Ind Med* 1954; 11:235.
77. Windebank AJ, McCall JT, Hunder HG, et al: The endoneurial content of lead related to the onset and severity of segmental demyelination. *J Neuropath Exp Neurol* 1980; 40:692.

51

Occupational Genotoxicology

Marja Sorsa, Ph.D.

BEGINNING OF THE SCIENCE

The realization that chemicals may cause mutations was made more than 20 years after the mutagenic properties of ionizing radiation were discovered in the late 1920s by H. J. Muller in the United States. The similarity in the biologic action of certain nitrogen mustards and x-rays was confirmed in the 1940s by the work of Charlotte Auerbach in Edinburgh.

The field of chemical mutagenesis research, or genotoxicology, has developed rapidly during the last decade. There are several reasons and prerequisites for this fast progress. The first is the realization that the human chemical environment has changed rather suddenly. In a short time, tens of thousands of synthetic chemicals have been introduced into our environment, and about 1,000 new compounds appear annually. Many of these chemicals or their derivatives are highly reactive and may be potentially mutagenic in living organisms, thus causing concern about damage to the genetic material and the resulting potential to cause human ill-health.

The second major reason for this rapid progress of genotoxicology is inborn with the development of the science. The findings of Ames and his co-workers in Berkeley during the mid 1970s led to the realization of the close relationship of carcinogens and mutagens. The obvious success of the various short-term test systems developed to fit the need of rapid testing has added a certain optimism to the efforts to prevent unnecessary exposure to mutagenic and potentially carcinogenic chemicals.

DETECTION OF CHEMICAL CARCINOGENS

There are three basic methodologies leading to the identification of chemical carcinogens. The use of epidemiology is one important method providing unequivocal evidence of human carcinogenicity. However, epidemiologic approaches are always unfortunately delayed—the opportunity to prevent cancer induction has already been lost at the time when the results of the exposure can be seen as increasing cancer incidence in humans. In the occupational setting, the sizes of groups exposed are usually so small that only extremely potent carcinogens or very unusual neoplasms can be detected. The recent evaluations of the International Agency for Research on Cancer (IARC 1987) acknowledge "sufficient evidence" on human carcinogenicity with exposure to 50 chemicals or industrial processes.[20]

Secondly, the carcinogenic potential of chemicals can be detected in long-term animal bioassays. Adequately designed animal carcinogenicity tests are the closest model to human cancer induction, and most animal neoplasms are analogous to those observed in humans. The problem of animal bioassays is their insensitivity in detecting weak carcinogens. Thus, sufficient confidence in a negative result requires huge numbers of animals to be used—to overcome this problem, unnaturally high exposure levels are frequently used. The inefficiency of an animal bioassay in detecting a weak carcinogenic effect (doubling of the cancer incidence over 10% tumour rate in the control animals) is shown in Table 51–1.

It is quite evident that normal carcinogenicity bioassays are able to detect only relatively strong changes in tumor incidence (20%–30%), and such high cancer rates in the size of human populations would be totally unacceptable. The number of animal carcinogens with "sufficient evidence" is about 300, according to the latest IARC evaluations.[39]

The third type of test available in identification of chemical carcinogens predicts carcinogenicity through detection of mutagenicity or transformational properties in short-term screening tests. The use of mutagenic potential as an indication of possible carcinogenicity is based on the present knowledge of the etiologic correlation of somatic genetic damage to initiation of cancer. Also, good empirical correlations, as discussed later, exist in experimental test results of mutagenicity data and carcinogenicity in experimental animals.

DISCIPLINES OF GENOTOXICOLOGY

Concern about the increase of mutation frequency in man is the main ideologic principle in genetic toxicology. Mutations are heritable changes in the cellular genetic material, and they may occur in somatic or in germinal cells (Fig 51–1). The first concern in genetic toxicology is protection of the human gene pool, i.e., inhibition of the increase of germinal mutations in man. The second concern is the close relationship between the genotoxic and carcinogenic properties of chemicals, which enables the use of various short-term tests for genotoxicity to be used in identification of potentially hazardous chemicals.

TABLE 51–1.

Number of Animals Per Group Required to Give a 90% Chance to Detect Increase of Cancer Incidence at $P \leqslant .05$ Significance Level

INCREASE (OVER 10% CONTROL INCIDENCE) TO	NUMBER OF ANIMALS NEEDED PER GROUP
80%	12
60%	21
40%	46
20%	255
15%	826

According to experimental evidence, a large portion of the germinal mutations induced in higher organisms are deleterious or lethal to the individual. Thus, an abrupt, significant increase in the mutation frequency of any species, including man, is a serious threat to the future of the species. Due to the recessive nature of most mutations, the consequences of the genetic load, i.e., hereditary diseases and disorders, would be manifested only generations later.

Mutations that cause sterility, embryonic loss, or early lethality are detrimental in their biologic fitness value but have less impact on the society. Thus, mutations that are less dramatic biologically may actually become a heavy burden on society, if the affected persons require lifetime medical or institutional care.

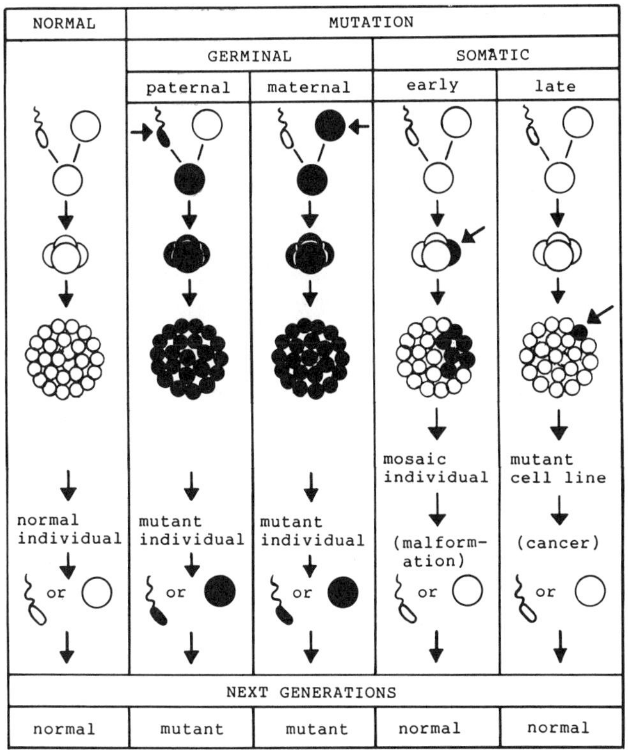

FIG 51-1.
Schematic presentation of mutations induced in germ cells (germinal) and in somatic cells during embryonic (early) or postnatal (late) development. Only germinal mutations may be passed on to the next generations, while somatic mutations can only be transmitted to the cell line derived from the mutant cell. (From Hemminki K, Sorsa M, Vainio H: Genetic risks caused by occupational chemicals. *Scand J Work Environ Health* 1979; 5:307–327. Used by permission.)

Epidemiologic studies have as yet been of little value in the effort to detect effects on human germinal mutation rates caused by exogenous exposures.

Knowledge of the biologic manifestations of somatic mutations is still partly speculative. There is firm evidence in favor of the role of chromosomal or gene mutations in the etiology of cancer.[33, 44] While tumor initiation and promotion leading to malignant transformation is a complex, multistage process, genetic mechanisms are being involved in various ways. Somatic mutations may also be involved in cellular—and finally individual—aging processes, and even in the development of some constitutional and degenerative diseases.

Induction of Mutations.—Chemicals enter the body via inhalation, ingestion, or skin absorption, and are distributed in the tissues in a manner specific to each chemical. Some chemicals may exert toxicity directly, while some are converted into active intermediates through metabolism.

Genotoxic agents are capable of causing lesions in the genetic material either directly or indirectly. Most chemical mutagens are electrophiles or are metabolized into electrophilic intermediates capable of forming covalent bonds with cellular nucleophiles.[23] Some mutagens exert their effects through other mechanisms: metals and intercalating agents form tight noncovalent associations with nucleic acids; antimetabolites may interfere with the genetic material indirectly; and spindle poisons are able to disturb the normal segregation of chromosomes during cell division. Experimental data on the mutagenicity of natural nucleosides have reemphasized the role of disturbances in nucleic acid synthesis as an additional mechanism of mutagenesis, according to Anderson et al.[3] Oxygen radicals triggered by other agents also have an important role as DNA-damaging agents.[1, 15]

Role of Repair Functions.—Cells have mechanisms that tend to remove genotoxins bound to DNA and to repair the lesions introduced. The repair mechanisms consist of several functions such as error recognition and degradative (endonuclease and exonuclease) and synthetic (polymerase and ligase) functions. Three different repair processes have been identified in mammalian cells: (1) photoreactivation repair repairing ultraviolet damage, (2) excision repair occurring throughout the cell cycle, and (3) postreplication repair confined to the period of DNA replication. The final expression of a mutation is thus always the sum of primary genetic lesions and the various repair processes. The individual efficiency in repairing mutagen-induced damage in DNA may be one of the major constitutional characteristics of inherited susceptibility to cancer.

GOALS OF GENOTOXICOLOGY IN OCCUPATIONAL MEDICINE

Possible genotoxic exposures and their detection in the occupational environment have been the object of much concern and active research during recent years. This is obviously due to the severity of the manifestations of genotoxic responses and their plausible stochastic nature. Compared to the general environment, the occupational environment often involves more easily controlled exposure conditions for research purposes, and usually also much higher chemical concentrations. The occupational genotoxicants are important for a number of reasons. Their hazards to human beings may be identified by the effects on sentinel individuals, workers who represent a risk group because of heavy exposure or because of sensitive genetic background conducive to carcinogenesis.

Furthermore, industry is the main source of many chemicals that cause environmental problems. In the overall safety evaluation of chemicals, the occupational setting thus provides indications of public health risks in general. For this reason, the surveillance of occupational health is an important component in protecting the general public from adverse health effects.

SHORT-TERM TESTS

As discussed earlier, a great majority of chemicals shown to induce malignancies in man or animals have been found positive in microbial, submammalian, or mammalian mutagenicity tests, in DNA damage assays, or in tests for cell transformation. These inexpensive tests are called short-term tests because of the relatively short time they require, compared to conventional animal carcinogenicity bioassays.

During the last years, application of short-term tests in predicting the carcinogenic hazard of chemicals has been widely accepted. Until now, at least 15,000 different chemicals have been tested in various mutagenicity assays, and the number is probably at least doubled when unpublished data on industrial chemicals in product safety development are considered.[19]

Over 100 different assay systems are more or less generally accepted for evaluation of genotoxic properties.[27] Based on the target cell type and the genotoxic end point detectable, the various tests can be divided into 13 categories, as shown in Table 51–2.

Most of the short-term test systems measure direct genetic damage in living cells. Several in vitro assays detect various injurious effects on DNA or the efficiency of its repair, thus revealing indirectly the capacities of a chemical to cause mutations. The cell transformation assays, measuring morphological transformation in specific rodent cell lines, have revealed good agreement with carcinogenicity in animal bioassays.

The predictiveness of the short-term tests has been evaluated in several studies; generally the accuracy (correct test results) is around 70% in the most frequently used tests.[38] Understanding the mechanisms of carcinogenicity as well as the end points assayed in the short-term tests is essential in evaluating the true predictive value of genotoxicity testing for human cancer risk.

TABLE 51–2.

Short-term Tests Available for Detection of Mutagens and Carcinogens

TYPE OF TEST	APPROXIMATE NUMBER OF TESTS
Bacterial point mutations	7
Bacterial growth inhibition	2
Phage tests	3
Insect mutagenesis	4
Mammalian mutagenesis	16
Mammalian cytogenetic tests	13
Other eukaryotic tests	21
Mammalian cell transformation	17
Transformation of virus-infected cells	4
DNA binding	2
DNA breakage and other damage	9
Inhibition of DNA replication	2
DNA repair	7

APPLICATION OF GENOTOXICOLOGY IN OCCUPATIONAL HYGIENE

Environmental Monitoring.—Exposures encountered in the occupational environment are usually much more extreme than those that occur in the general environment. In some occupational situations, exposures are well characterized and a hazard has been recognized as being caused by a single chemical entity: e.g., benzene production and usage. In such cases, preventive and hygienic measures can be readily selected, and actions focused on minimizing exposures. However, in most occupational environments, the spectrum of chemicals to which the population is exposed is very wide, and although there may be epidemiologic evidence of an increased frequency of disease, no firm association can be established with any single causal factor. Thus, previous experimental knowledge of the toxicology of the total array of chemicals handled would be of importance in identification of the risk factors. Mutagenic chemicals should never be handled without further studies on the nature of the hazard. If nonmutagenic substitutes are available, replacement should be recommended and implemented.

Complex Mixtures.—Complex mixtures are commonly handled in industry. Typically, complex materials, e.g., oils, tars, carbon blacks, pitches, and creosotes, contain hundreds of chemical entities with compositions that may vary, depending on the source and handling procedures. Pyrolysis, thermal degradations, and combustion of organic material in general, produces the complex emissions typically evolved in many industrial processes.

The use of mutagenicity tests has a special significance in the evaluation of complex mixtures. The complexity of, e.g., ambient air samples seldom allows the detection of specific single compounds responsible for the effect. Furthermore, the obvious synergistic, commutagenic, as well as inhibitory interactions hinder the value of testing a single compound from a mixture. The relative low cost and speed of the short-term tests permits large numbers of samples and their fractions to be tested.

A successful approach to studying complex occupational samples includes combining chemical fractionation and the bioassay techniques in order to be able to determine the responsible genotoxic component, its primary source or origin, possible spontaneous or artificial transformations, and ways to design control technology.

On-site and Off-site Methods.—Both on-site (in situ) and off-site methods have been applied in occupational situations.

On-site methods for monitoring ambient air in complex exposure situations at worksites are still in their infancy. Almost the only eukaryotic monitoring systems applied to the study of atmospheric mutagens have used plants, e.g., the *Tradescantia* staminal hair cell and the maize marker locus (waxy, yellow-green) have been applied routinely.[8] A preliminary study has been made of the use of populations of *Drosophila melanogaster*, placed at specific sites in a rubber factory, to monitor for possible exposures to mutagens in the ambient air, using sex-linked recessive lethal frequencies as the end point.[11]

Off-site methods are being used increasingly to study potential contamination of occupational environments with mutagenic agents. Bacterial mutagenicity tests have been the method used most frequently, e.g., in testing ambient air samples from vulcanizing sites in a rubber factory[16] and in testing ambient air and personal filter samples from workers in foundries.[28] Fumes collected from stainless steel welding were found to be mutagenic in the *Salmonella*/microsome test.[22] Fumes produced during the curing of different rubber polymers and mixtures of rubber in experimental vulcanizing conditions exhibited mutagenicity in various short-term bioassays.[10]

It is essential that proper sampling procedures be used when taking such complex ambient mixtures, in order to guarantee the representativity of the sample with regard to general worker exposure. Respirable particles or vapors, highly critical in human exposure, may easily escape the sampling device, causing underestimation of the real hazard.[6] Claxton reported that the extraction and fractionation methods may also be overly selective; the mutagenicity may be spread over several fractions or it may be extinguished by the toxicity of the sample.[7]

Using the approach of continuous chemical fractionation and short-term assays, the investigator can accumulate information on the actual compounds responsible for the biologic effects. Even in view of the difficulties outlined above, short-term tests provide a possibility for monitoring complex ambient exposure and are of importance in following changes in occupational conditions.

Biologic Monitoring.—Short-term tests can also be applied in evaluation of exposure to genotoxic agents from biologic specimens (usually urine or blood) of the exposed subjects.[29] The main goal of biologic monitoring in health surveillance programs is either to ensure that the current or past exposure is "safe" or to detect potential excessive exposure before the occurrence of detectable adverse health effects. Biologic monitoring is thus essentially a preventive medical activity. (See Chapter 13.)

Biologic monitoring assays are most useful when exposures are suspected but the specific genotoxic chemicals (or possible interactions between chemicals) are unknown, or when analytic techniques are not available. Such cases are not infrequent in workplaces. In situations in which the workers are exposed to complex mixtures comprising hundreds of chemical entities, the possibilities for monitoring a single chemical are limited; consequently, indicators of genotoxicity, even though unspecific as to the identity of the chemicals but specific to the nature of the health hazards, have some advantages.[40]

Covalent Modifications and DNA Adducts.—Direct information on the alkylation products of mutagens and carcinogens can be obtained with the determination of covalent modifications in proteins. This field has been pioneered by Ehrenberg and co-workers, who have measured the occurrence of alkyl groups in hemoglobin.[12] Since there is a certain relationship between the nucleophilic substitution of protein and nucleic acid residues by electrophiles (carcinogens and mutagens), the degree of protein alkylation may be used as an indirect measure of nucleic acid alkylation, according to Calleman et al.[5] The method is sensitive enough to detect, e.g., ethylene oxide residues in hemoglobin of workers exposed to 5–10 ppm of ethylene oxide. As yet, the measurement of hemoglobin alkylation has not been adapted for routine use.

In the past few years immunologic, physicochemical, and postlabeling techniques have been developed whose sensitivity approaches the levels required for the detection of DNA modifications in exposed human populations. The techniques are based on ^{32}P-labeling, fluorescence, or antibodies (usually produced in rabbits) against modified DNA, polynucleotides, nucleotides, or nucleosides.[25] Polyclonal and monoclonal antibodies can be raised and the level of DNA modifications in the human sample can be quantified by immunochemical techniques.[18] Although the DNA-adduct technique is not yet applicable for the routine monitoring of individuals exposed to genotoxic chemicals, it certainly has promising prospectives for such applications in the future.

Mutagenicity in Body Fluids.—Human body fluids, particularly urine, have been assayed for mutagenicity over ten years. The observation by Yamasaki and Ames that smokers' urine was mutagenic in the *Salmonella*/liver homogenate assay prompted a number of studies about the urinary mutagenic activity in groups of subjects exposed to various mutagens and carcinogens.[43] Studies so far have demonstrated that mutagenic activity can be detected in the urine of humans exposed to, e.g., various therapeutic drugs, industrial chemicals, and cigarette smoke (for references see review of Vainio et al.[39]). The most frequently used biologic indicators of mutagenicity have been the bacterial strains routinely applied in mutagenicity testing. In some recent attempts human lymphocyte cultures have been applied to test the urine.[36] When using this assay in monitoring occupational exposures, one has to pay special attention to possible confounding agents, such as drugs and other life-style factors. Furthermore, as most of the chemicals are excreted in conjugated "detoxified" form, the mere appearance of mutagenic activity in concentrated urine does not imply that there is a necessity for a biologic effect. Thus, the urinary mutagenicity assay should be considered as an *exposure* indicator, not an *effect* indicator.

Detection of mutagenic activity in urine can be used mainly as a nonspecific indicator of exposure to mutagenic compounds. The urinary mutagenicity assay is thus applicable to the monitoring of human exposures in specific situations. It can be used to identify hazards in the workplaces and can also be used to provide guidance in selecting appropriate hygienic measures.

POINT MUTATIONS IN LYMPHOCYTES

Recently, several attempts have been made to detect point mutational damage in human somatic cells in vivo. The most promising of these seems to be the measuring of the mutation frequency in a single marker locus, e.g., hypoxanthine-guanine-phosphoribosyltransferase (HPRT).

Strauss and Albertini have described a method which, through the determination of the frequency of 6-thioguanine-resistant peripheral blood lymphocytes, is supposed to reveal impaired activity of the X-linked HPRT locus. Even though the method is theoretically appealing, it is quite tedious in its present form, involving autoradiographic identification of 6-thioguanine-resistant cells.[37] There are, however, possibilities for automating the method with flow cytometry[2] or computer image analysis systems, which may improve the applicability of the assay system for monitoring purposes.[13]

There are still uncertainties concerning the primary molecular injury measured in the system, since azaguanine-resistant lymphocytes, and both epigenetic and mutational mechanisms may be involved.[2] Further research is needed on the basic genetic and selective mechanisms involved before judgment can be passed on the suitability of the human point mutation system for monitoring purposes.

CYTOGENETIC SURVEILLANCE

Cytogenetic damage can only be visualized in proliferating cell populations. In principle, three types of cytogenetic changes can be distinguished, i.e., structural alterations, intrachromosomal exchanges, and alterations in the chromosome number.

Chromosome Aberrations.—Somatic chromosome aberrations have been used for four decades as indicators of exposure to chromosome breaking agents. Most of the early work on induced clastogenicity dealt with radiation; in studies by Buckton et al., the dose-response relationship for ionizing radiation has been characterized well enough so that the frequency of dicentric and fragmented chromosomes can be used as a biologic dosimeter of the radiation dose received.[4]

Such quantitative measures for the monitoring of chemical exposures are far off. Mutagenic chemicals differ markedly regarding their target tissues and the type of lesions they induce. In addition, individual responses to the same chemical and the same dose may vary considerably. In the case of chromosomal aberrations caused by chemical mutagens, the lesions induced in DNA have to pass the replication phase in order to be observed. The aberrations induced are generally of the chromatid type. Despite the difficulties and the tediousness of the method, cytogenetic monitoring is at present the only practical routine possibility in screening human populations for genetic damage induced by exogenous agents.[30, 31]

Sister Chromatid Exchanges.—Sister chromatid exchanges (SCEs) reflect intrachromosomal symmetrical rearrangements of the DNA helices. Because SCE techniques are in many respects quicker, cheaper, and easier to score, many cytogenetic laboratories are turning to use them—for both in vitro and in vivo approaches—for the identification of potentially hazardous chemicals.[24] So far neither the exact nature of lesions nor the molecular mechanisms leading to SCEs are known. Even though the method is a sensitive indicator of DNA damage in vitro, the in vivo studies in humans need persistent lesions to be screened as SCEs after culturing. Also, it is clear that a high frequency of induced SCEs is not necessarily correlated with the incidence of chromosome aberrations.

Micronuclei.—Some other cytogenetic techniques not routinely used include the analysis of micronucleated cells in polychromatic erythrocytes of bone marrow, in peripheral blood lymphocytes or in exfoliated epithelial cells.[32] Micronuclei result from acentric chromosome fragments or lagging whole chromosomes. Positive responses in induction of cells with micronuclei have been obtained in studies with cells of the buccal mucosa (chewers of betel or tobacco), cultured lymphocytes of some occupationally exposed groups (styrene, ethylene oxide) or bone marrow of patients under cytostatic chemotherapy.

The knowledge on human cytogenetic surveillance is still quite limited. Currently, less than ten occupational agents have been confirmed to be chromosome damaging in human beings by several independent studies (Table 51–3). Further studies are thus urgently needed where different cytogenetic parameters would be used for the same exposure group.

Induced chromosome damage (structural aberrations, SCEs or numerical alterations) with properly documented association to specific exposure should always be considered an adverse sign of exposure to mutagenic and potentially carcinogenic environmental agents of the population studied. Even though the health consequences for the individual cannot be estimated on the basis of present knowledge, the findings, at the group level, must be interpreted as risk for potential manifestation of genotoxic end-effects.

A major reluctance in applying monitoring procedures to occupationally exposed populations is the expense and the resources

TABLE 51–3.
Human Chromosome Damaging Agents Confirmed by Several Occupational Studies

	CYTOGENETIC INFORMATION		
AGENT	CA	SCE	MN
Alkylating cytostatics	+	+	+
Benzene	+	+	+
Epichlorohydrin	+	··	··
Ethylene oxide	+	+	+
Ionizing radiation	+	−	+
Styrene	+	(+)	+
Vinyl chloride	+	+	··

CA = chromosome aberrations, SCE = sister chromatid exchanges, MN = micronucleated cells; + = confirmed positive findings, (+) = suggestive findings, − = negative findings, ·· = no data.

required. Thus, automatization of the cytogenetic analyses as well as further progress in the methods to detect induced DNA damage are urgently needed for preventive medicine in the field of occupational health.

SPERM MORPHOLOGY

Sperm counts serve as an important parameter in diagnosis of fertility in men. Recently, similar types of tests have been shown to be applicable as indicators of germinal cell damage induced in males by exposure to exogenous genotoxic agents.[42]

The most commonly used human sperm tests are sperm count, motility test, sperm morphology test, and the double-Y test. The latter measures the number of fluorescent bodies, which are expected to represent the Y-chromosome, in sperm heads, thus estimating the frequency of malsegregation of the dividing Y-chromosome during spermatogenesis.

Sperm motility and counts are unreliable and are very variable measures of quality to be used in cross-sectional studies. Recent attempts have shown that the human sperm morphology can be applied in monitoring studies.[42] Further research is needed to understand the impact of induced changes in human sperm morphology on fertility and reproductive outcome.

REPRODUCTIVE HEALTH

The concept of reproductive health, in the broad sense, includes all the aspects involved in the potential of the individual to produce offspring with full reproductive potency. Thus, worsening of reproductive health may be due to reduced fertility of either of the potential parents, but also to fetal disease in the child preventing his or her full capacity to produce offspring into the next generation.

The maldevelopment of the unborn infant may be caused either by prezygotic lesions or be due to disturbances during the embryonal and fetal periods. The latter, or postzygotic, effects may be either direct damage to the fetus, or indirect, through maternal influence to the developing fetus (Fig 51–2).

Mutational Etiology of Failures in Reproductive Health.—The prezygotic health effects to the offspring are always mutational in nature and are transmitted in conception to the zygote, giving rise to the genetic composition of the cells of the individual. The possible maldevelopment or death of the fetus due to prezygotic damage may either be caused by old mutations inherited in the germline through generations or it may be caused by newly arisen mutations during spermatogenesis or ovogenesis.

At present, it is generally estimated that some 5%–10% of newborns carry some kind of defect or illness caused by genetic etiology. Most of the deficiences are due to mono- or polygenic factors and about 0.6% are due to chromosomal aberrations, most of which are considered new mutations.[14]

Mutagenic or fetotoxic agents may also play some role postzygotically by causing somatic mutations in the cells of the developing embryo or fetus, either indirectly through the mother (transplacental mutagens) or directly (ionizing radiation). Also, simple cytotoxic effects may cause fetal damage, if the toxic chemical is able to pass through the placenta in high enough concentrations.

The frequently dividing fetal cells are known to be especially sensitive to mutational effects. Furthermore, the placental and fetal

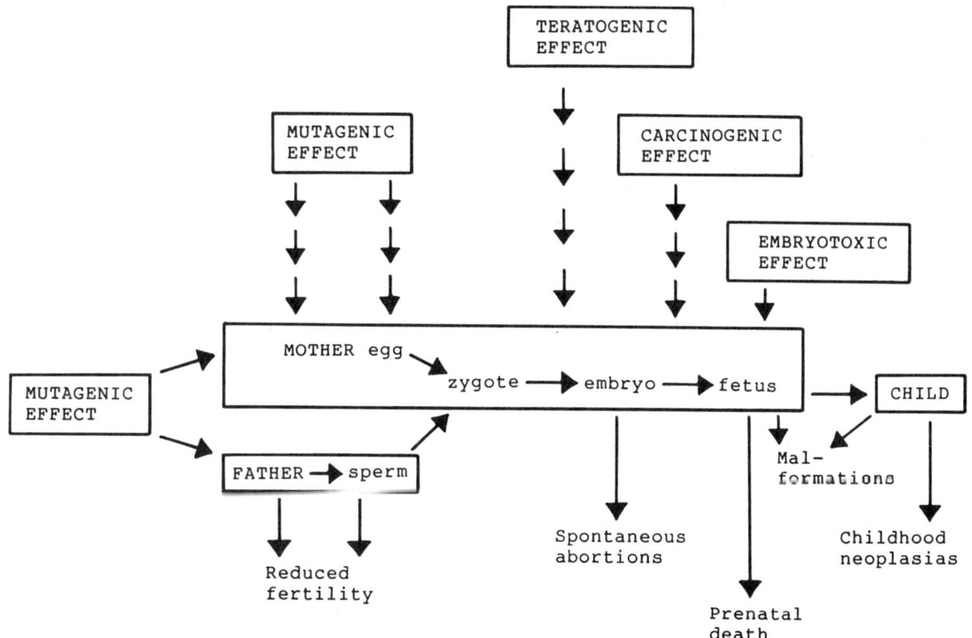

FIG 51–2.
Timing and nature of toxic effects on reproductive health and potential manifestations.

detoxification mechanisms are not comparable to the adult xenobiotic metabolism. However, the cause of transplacental mutagenicity and its possible effects as malformations, fetal death, or childhood cancer is almost entirely based on experimental data.

Teratogenicity.—Both genotoxic and fetotoxic chemicals may disturb the development of the fetus to such an extent that the pregnancy ends as miscarriage or in perinatal death. The teratogenic chemicals, which exhibit their effect as congenital malformations, are typically dependent on short, sensitive periods of the embryonal development (e.g., organogenesis). The mechanisms of teratogenicity are supposedly either genotoxic or cytotoxic.[41] Estimates of the proportion of genetic etiology in malformations vary from 20% to 80%.[9] Such a wide range of estimations points to the ignorance about the etiology of congenital birth defects. Still today the cause of about two thirds of malformations remains uncertain.

Spontaneous Abortions.—Miscarriages provide material directly relating to human reproductive damage. The abortus can be studied both cytogenetically for possible chromosomal causes and pathologically for anatomical malformations.

Chromosome karyotyping performed on spontaneous abortion material indicates that chromosomal abnormality is the etiologic cause of the miscarriage in nearly 50% of the cases.[34] The incidence of abnormal karyotypes among the abortuses is at its highest in the early abortions and gradually decreases in later stillbirths to about 0.6% among newborns (Fig 51–3). The severity of the genomic disturbance also follows this trend; trisomies of the larger human chromosomes (numbers 1–18) very rarely or never come to term. The most common of the chromosome anomalies found in spontaneous abortions is trisomy 16, which has never been found in newborns.[35]

Studies of spontaneous abortion incidences, preferably combined with cytogenetic survey programs, thus seem to be probably the most feasible way to surveillance of the effects of potential environmental and occupational genotoxins.

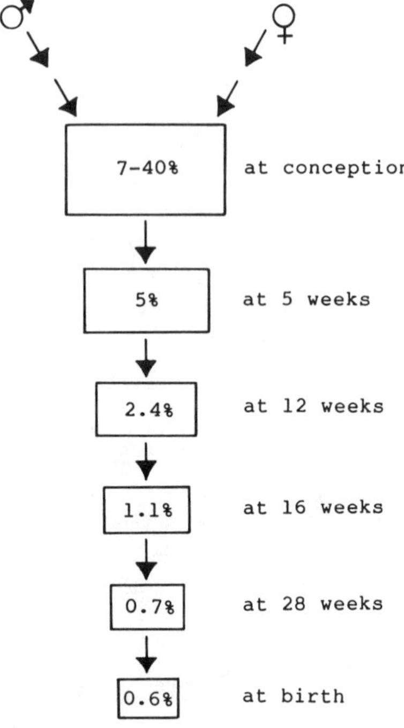

FIG 51–3.
Frequency of abnormal human karyotypes at different stages of development.

FUTURE PERSPECTIVES IN OCCUPATIONAL GENOTOXICOLOGY

Many important tasks must be performed in the field of occupational genotoxicology to make work environments healthy for the workers and their unborn offspring. Present methodologies must be made easier, cheaper, and more reliable in evaluating occupational agents and exposures. In many cases, this would mean automatizing techniques. Such progress has been seen in the automatization of the bacterial mutagenicity test, human point mutation assays, and cytogenetic scoring.

The second future perspective of occupational genotoxicology relates to the possibility of genetic screening for possible hypersusceptibility among workers. This possibility has recently become an issue, not only concerning individual health, but also involving ethical, legal, and management problems.[26] The idea that inborn genetic sensitivity might predispose workers to illness in a special exposure situation has gained support from recent findings on enzyme variants and repair deficiencies among humans.[21] However, the true value of the currently available methodologies of genetic toxicology in predicting individual differences in vulnerability to hazardous occupational exposures still needs to be established. Currently, the cytogenetic and other genotoxicologic monitoring methodologies discussed earlier in this chapter can best be applied at the group level as an early warning system of exposure to genotoxic agents, not as a tool for preemployment screening of individuals.

Knowledge of the genetic causes of human disease and its inborn predisposition has rapidly increased. Quite obviously, such monogenically inherited factors as the hemoglobinopathies (sickle-cell disease and thalassemias) predispose a fairly large risk group of the gene carriers (otherwise healthy heterozygotes) to exacerbation of lead toxicity, for example. Similarly, the X-chromosomal mutant gene for glucose 6-phosphate dehydrogenase (G6PD) predisposes the risk of acute hemolysis due to, e.g., antimalarial drugs or carbon monoxide. According to estimates, up to 3% of the general population may be genetically deficient for serum α_1-antitrypsin, a condition predisposing to emphysema due to respiratory irritants. High variations in the frequencies of such alleles may exist between ethnic and racial groups, thus making the tests vulnerable to potential discriminatory uses. The applicability of the tests, as they gradually become routine in use, thus poses serious ethical problems which each society throughout the world must solve.

REFERENCES

1. Ames BN: Carcinogens and anticarcinogens, in Sorsa M, Vainio H (eds): *Mutagens in Our Environment*. New York, Alan R Liss Inc, 1982, pp 3–19.
2. Amneus H, Matsson P, Zetterberg G: Human lymphocytes resistant to 6-thioguanine: Restrictions in the use of a test for somatic mutations arising in vivo studied by flow-cytometric enrichment of resistant cell nuclei. *Mutat Res* 1982; 106:163–178.
3. Anderson D, Richardson CR, Davies PJ: The genotoxic potential of bases and nucleosides. *Mutat Res* 1981; 91:265–272.
4. Buckton KE, Langlands AO, Smith PG, et al: Further studies on chromosome aberration production after whole body irradiation in man. *Int J Radiol Biol* 1971; 19:369–378.
5. Calleman CJ, Ehrenberg L, Jansson B, et al: Monitoring and risk assessment by means of alkyl groups in hemoglobin in persons occupationally exposed to ethylene oxide. *J Environ Pathol Toxicol* 1978; 2:427–442.
6. Chrisp CE, Fisher GL: Mutagenicity of airborne particles. *Mutat Res* 1980; 76:143–164.
7. Claxton L: Review of fractionation and bioassay characterization techniques for the evaluation of organics associated with ambient air particles, in Tice RR, Costa DL, Schaich KM (eds): *Genotoxic Effects of Airborne Agents, vol 25. Environmental and Scientific Research*. New York, Plenum Press, 1982, pp 19–34.
8. Constantin MJ: Plant genetic systems with potential for the detection of atmospheric mutagens, in Tice RR, Costa DL, Schaich KM (eds): *Genotoxic Effects of Airborne Agents, vol 25. Environmental and Scientific Research*. New York, Plenum Press, 1982, pp 159–172.
9. Dept of Health, Education, and Welfare: What are the facts about genetic disease? DHEW Publ 75–370, 1975.
10. Donner M, Husgafvel-Pursiainen K, Jenssen D, et al: Mutagenicity of rubber additives and curing fumes. *Scand J Work Environ Health* 1983a; 9[suppl 2]:27–37.
11. Donner M, Hytönen S, Sorsa M: Application of the sex-linked recessive lethal test in Drosophila melanogaster for monitoring the work environment of a rubber factory. *Hereditas* 1983b; 99:7–10.
12. Ehrenberg L, Hiesche KD, Osterman-Golkar S, et al: Evaluation of genetic risks of alkylating agents: Tissue doses in the mouse from air contaminated with ethylene oxide. *Mutat Res* 1974; 24:83–103.
13. Evans HJ, Vijayalaxmi: Induction of 8-azaguanine resistance and sister chromatid exchange in human lymphocytes exposed to mitomycin C and x-rays in vitro. *Nature* 1981; 292:601–605.
14. Evans HJ: How effects of chemicals might differ from those of radiations in giving rise to genetic ill-health in man, in Alacevic M (ed): *Progress in Environmental Mutagenesis*. Amsterdam, Elsevier North-Holland, 1980, pp 3–21.
15. Fridovich I: The biology of oxygen radicals. *Science* 1978; 201:875–880.
16. Hedenstedt A, Ramel C, Wachtmeister CA: Mutagenicity of rubber vulcanizing gases in *Salmonella typhimurium*. *J Toxicol Environ Health* 1981; 8:805–814.
17. Hemminki K, Sorsa M, Vainio H: Genetic risks caused by occupational chemicals. *Scand J Work Environ Health* 1979; 5:307–327.
18. Hemminki K: Nucleic acid adducts of chemical carcinogens and mutagens. *Arch Toxicol* 1983; 52:247–285.
19. Hoffman GR: Mutagenicity testing in environmental toxicology. *Environ Sci Technol* 1982; 16:560–574.
20. *IARC Monogr Eval Carcinog Risk Chem Hum*, suppl 7. Lyon, France, 1987.
21. Lappe M: Ethical issues in testing for differential sensitivity to occupational hazards. *J Occup Med* 1983; 25:797–808.
22. Maxild J, Andersen M, Kiel P, et al: Mutagenicity of fume particles from metal arc welding of stainless steel in the *Salmonella*/microsome test. *Mutat Res* 1978; 56:235–243.
23. Miller JA, Miller EC: Ultimate chemical carcinogens as reactive mutagenic electrophiles, in Hiatt HH, Watson JD, Winsten JA, (eds): *Origins of Human Cancer*. Cold Spring Harbor Laboratory, 1977, pp 605–627.
24. Perry P: Chemical mutagens and sister-chromatid exchange, in de Serres FJ, Hollaender A (eds): *Chemical Mutagens*. New York, Plenum Press, 1980, vol 6, pp 1–39.
25. Poirier MC: Antibodies to carcinogens—DNA adducts. *JNCI* 1981; 67:515–519.
26. Schlechter D: Genetic screening in the workplace. *Occup Health Saf* April 1983; pp 8–12.
27. de Serres FJ, Ashby J (eds): *Evaluation of Short-term Tests for Carcinogens*. Amsterdam, Elsevier North-Holland, 1981.
28. Skyttä E, Schimberg R, Vainio H: Mutagenic activity in foundry air. *Arch Toxicol* 1980; 4:68–72.
29. Sorsa M, Hemminki K, Vainio H: Biologic monitoring of exposure to chemical mutagens in the occupational environment. *Teratogen Carcinogen Mutagen* 1982; 2:137–150.
30. Sorsa M: Cytogenic methods in the detection of chemical carcinogens. *J Toxicol Environ Health* 1980; 6:1077–1080.
31. Sorsa M: Chromosomal aberrations as a monitoring method for possible genotoxic risks, in Aitio A, Riihimäki V, Vainio H (eds): Biological monitoring and surveillance of workers exposed to chemicals. Washington DC, Hemisphere Publishing Co, 1984, pp 357–370.
32. Sorsa M: Sister chromatid exchange and micronuclei as monitoring methods, in Berlin A, Draper M, Hemminki K, et al (eds): *Monitoring of Human Exposure to Carcinogenic and Mutagenic Agents*, IARC Scientific Publ 59. Lyon, France, International Agency for Research on Cancer, 1984, pp 339–349.
33. Sorsa M: Somatic mutation theory. *J Toxicol Environ Health* 1980; 6:977–982.
34. Stein Z, Susser M, Warburton D, et al: Spontaneous abortion as a screening device. The effect of fetal survival on the incidence of birth defects. *Am J Epidemiol* 1975; 102:275–290.
35. Stein Z, Warburton D, Kline J: Epidemiology of chromosomal anomalies and other malformations in spontaneous abortion, in Hemminki K, Sorsa M, Vainio H (eds): *Occupational Hazards and Reproduction*. Washington DC, Hemisphere Publishing Co, 1985, pp 163–173.
36. Stiller A, Obe G, Riedel L, et al: Mutagens in human urine: Test with human peripheral lymphocytes. *Mutat Res* 1982; 97:437–447.
37. Strauss GH, Albertini RJ: Enumeration of 6-thioguanine-resistant peripheral blood lymphocytes in man as a potential test for somatic cell mutations arising in vivo. *Mutat Res* 1979; 61:353–379.
38. Upton AC, Clayson DB, Jansen JD, et al: Report of ICPEMC Task Group 5 on the differentation between genotoxic and nongenotoxic carcinogens. *Mutat Res* 1984; 133:1–49.
39. Vainio H, Sorsa M, Falck K: Bacterial urinary assay in monitoring exposure to mutagens and carcinogens, in Berlin A, Draper M, Hemminki K, et al (eds). *Monitoring of Human Exposure to Carcinogenic and Mutagenic Agents*, IARC Scientific Publ 59. Lyon, France, International Agency for Research on Cancer, 1984, pp 247–258.
40. Vainio H, Sorsa M, Rantanen J, et al: Biological monitoring in the identification of the cancer risk of individuals exposed to chemical carcinogens. *Scand J Work Environ Health* 1981; 7:241–251.
41. Wilson JG: *Environment and Birth Defects*. New York, Academic Press, 1973.

42. Wyrobek AJ, Gordon LA, Burkhart JG, et al: An evaluation of human sperm as indicators of chemically induced alterations of spermatogenic function: A test of U.S. Environmental Protection Agency Gene-Tox Program. *Mutat Res* 1983; 115:73–148.
43. Yamasaki E, Ames BN: Concentration of mutagens from urine by absorption with the nonpolar resin XAD-2; cigarette smokers have mutagenic urine. *Proc Natl Acad Sci USA* 1977; 74:3555–3559.
44. Yunis JJ: The chromosomal basis of human neoplasia. *Science* 1983; 221:227–236.

52

Occupational Cancer Risks

Vernon N. Dodson, M.D.

Carl Zenz, M.D.

Of all the occupational health aspects of particular concern to professional workers in the disciplines involved with occupational medicine, industrial hygiene, and safety, the role of carcinogenic agents is the most vexing and perhaps the most poorly understood. A vast body of scientific evidence has been accumulated demonstrating relationships between occupational exposures and the development of cancers. Potential hazards range from the actinic or solar ultraviolet effects on outdoor workers to the effects of dust on those workers engaged in deep underground mining. Other suspected or known agents are arsenic, asbestos, beryllium, cadmium, chromium, cobalt, nickel, radioactive substances, certain aromatic amines and their derivatives, ethylene oxide,[45] vinyl chloride, phenoxy acetic acid, and chlorophenols,[56, 66] discussed in depth elsewhere in this book.

A possible occupational connection for malignant disease was first recognized when an unusually high frequency of scrotal cancer was observed among London chimney sweeps in 1775.[107, 136] Even at present, similar findings have been reported.[137] In a large-scale study of Swedish chimney sweeps (2,495 workers), Hogstedt et al.[67] found 441 deaths among the chimney sweeps studied, compared with an expected figure of 335; excess mortality was 24%. Of these, 32 had died of lung cancer against an expected figure of 12. Eight died of esophageal cancer, whereas 1.6 such deaths could normally be expected. Seven died of liver cancer, compared with an expected of 1.4. Cardiovascular diseases caused 182 deaths against an expected 152. (The expected figures were calculated on the basis of a normal Swedish male population living during the same time period and with an identical age distribution.)

Relationships between concomitant exposures from multiple exposures have yet to be systematically explored. Detailed discussions of some of the metals and their compounds and certain other substances believed to be carcinogenic are found in corresponding chapters.[43, 125]

A remarkably detailed contribution on environmental cancer hazards presenting the many variable factors regarding the elucidation of the problems of occupational carcinogenesis was published by Hueper[71] in 1972 and is a noteworthy introduction to the most complex of all occupational health problems. The prominent British investigator Doll[44] reported his concepts on established risks relating to occupational lung cancer. He began with those cancer risks that were with radiation exposure, mentioning mines that had been worked successfully for silver, nickel, cobalt, bismuth, arsenic, radium, and uranium, and referred to the well-known suggestion that lung cancer might be due to the radioactivity. This suggestion appeared in the medical literature for the first time in 1921 (the Schneeberg mines). He continued with a discussion of chromates, asbestos, combustion, and distillation products of coal for gas production, and suspected risks in the absence of radiation, such as arsenic, iron, "isopropyl oil," and beryllium. He also included views on site specificity, emphasizing in his conclusion that

> "in recent years the mortality from lung cancer due to nonindustrial causes has increased enormously; now in Britain lung cancer accounts for more than 10% of all deaths among men aged from 45 to 64 years, the ages at which a risk of industrial cancer may most readily be detected. In these circumstances, the discovery of a new risk by simple clinical observation is difficult and if any additional risks remain to be discovered, it is probable that they will be revealed by planned prospective studies, undertaken with the special object of finding out whether any risks exist. That all the existing risks have been discovered seems most unlikely. Moreover, new materials and new processes are being introduced into industry almost daily and there is no reason to suppose that they will necessarily all be free from risk. It may be expected that industrial studies will continue, as in the past, to make important advances in our knowledge of all aspects of carcinogenesis. In this respect, detailed studies of the relationship between exposure, incidence, and duration of latent period may be of particular value."

Animal studies have demonstrated clues of great importance for estimating future risk to exposed workers. Especially noteworthy in this regard is the toxicologic study of animals exposed to vinyl chloride by Torkelson et al.[127] In 1954[61] and in 1956[62] Heath reported his studies of the production of malignant tumors by cobalt in the rat. The results obtained showed that cobalt metal is capable of producing malignant tumors in the muscles of a high proportion of the rats treated, owing to neoplastic changes both in connective tissue and striated muscle. When it became evident that cobalt was a strong carcinogen, a search of the literature revealed that as early as 1942 there was a German report of malignant tumors in two out of a number of rabbits injected intrafemorally with cobalt metal (although at the time this was unknown to Heath). One of these tumors was a spindle cell sarcoma at the injection site arising six years after injection, and the other at a site remote from the injection site was a multiple adenocarcinoma of the lung with peritoneal metastases.

The results described by Heath must inevitably raise the question of what is the causative agent of the high incidence of pulmonary cancer in the Schneeberg miners. The radioactive as well as the arsenic content of the Schneeberg ores have both been incriminated as carcinogenic factors. Because a typical analysis of the Schneeberg mine dust shows 0.19% of cobalt arsenide and 0.08% of nickel cobalt, it seems likely that the cobalt might also be held suspect as believed long ago by Osler and others.[30] It also seems desirable to reinvestigate the possible carcinogenic hazards of inhalation of cobalt-bearing dusts by workers in industry. Some work on these lines with negative results in relation to the cemented tungsten carbide industry where cobalt is used as a cement has already been reported.[100]

A study of cancer mortality among uranium mill workers by Archer, et al.[9] was concerned with mortality (from all causes) for a small group of uranium mill workers. The only specific cause of death that was significantly excessive was malignant disease of the lymphatic and hematopoietic tissue, referring to data from animal experiments that suggested that this excess may have resulted from irradiation of lymph nodes by thorium 230. Earlier studies by Archer and associates[7] describing health hazards of uranium mining and milling documented an increased incidence of lung cancer in uranium miners in the United States. Subsequently, they and others reported the correlation between radon exposure and the incidence of lung cancer.[10, 47–49, 91, 142]

In Sweden, measurements of radon were carried out by the Radiological Protection Service in all mines during 1969 and 1970. These showed that 22 of 82 mines had a radon daughter level of more than 30 picocuries (pCi)/L. Following these major reports, Jörgensen[78] reported his investigation of the mortality from lung cancer among miners of the LKAB Company (Luossavaara-Kirunavaara), in Kiruna, Sweden, between 1950 and 1970. The iron ore mine in Kiruna (about 150 km north of the Arctic Circle) began as an open pit mine (the ore being mainly hematite), but in the late 1950s underground mining was started. This mine, said to be the largest of its type in the world, employs about 4,400 miners. These miners generally do not migrate from their birthplace, so available reports of deaths of miners represent nearly all deceased miners from the Kiruna mine.

From the medical and hygienic points of view, important environmental factors are brought out by Jörgensen. Diesel-powered vehicles were introduced in 1958 for subterranean transportation and were increased in numbers until today there are 75 trucks and 35 front loaders that are continually in use underground. Exhaust fumes are controlled by scrubbers and/or catalytic afterburners and by an extensive ventilation system forcing air throughout the mine. Dust measurements in the mine revealed concentrations of between 3 and 9 mg/cu m, with about 40% of the particles being less than 5 μm in diameter. Dust concentration around the loading operation at times has been between 10 and 15 mg/cu m but has decreased recently because water spraying has been introduced. "Wet drilling" has been used since the early 1930s and has practically eliminated the risk of pneumoconiosis.

Jörgensen reported, "No one realized that there could be radioactivity in the mine in Kiruna until 1970 when radon concentrations were measured." In most places, there were found concentrations of radon daughters of between 10 and 30 pCi/L. However, in some unventilated galleries, very high concentrations were found. This was attributed to the fact that the radon had not had time to evaporate in the running water. The levels of radon measured in the mine today probably are representative of the earlier conditions. On some occasions, however, and at some places near water inlets in the LKAB mine, the radon concentration previously had been considerably higher for short periods of time.

In this retrospective study, mortality among the workers revealed 13 cases of lung cancer, whereas only 4.5 were expected among the rest of the male population in this community. The lung cancer mortality rate among non-mine workers was equal to that of Sweden in general. Because the study was done at a time when concurrent exposure investigations of workers to radon daughters and diesel exhaust fumes were not possible and because there is a possibility of noxious interaction, this study should be followed up in five to ten years.

St Clair Renard[114] reported extremely high rates of mortality from carcinoma of the lung among underground miners at the Malmberget (also LKAB) iron ore mine in northern Sweden. Among the potentially causative factors were the relatively high radon levels found at various plateaus of the mine until recently, when the ventilation system was improved. The report by Boyd et al.[24] that radon 222 in a hematite mine in England had caused carcinoma of the lung (1968–1970) moved the Swedish Mine Association to collaborate with the National Institute of Radiation Protection in the examination of the content of radon 222 in the air in all Swedish mines.

The results of both these studies showed a definite tendency toward a high mortality from lung cancer among Swedish miners (underground miners: 6 expected, 26 observed). There also appeared to be a correlation between respiratory cancer in the mines and a high radon concentration in the air.

In 1968, St Clair Renard began a study of lung cancer in the Malmberget mine, reviewing all cases of respiratory cancer in all men 20–74 years of age in his community dying between 1950 and 1972. Of the 41 cases found, many once had worked in the mine. The Gällivare-Malmberget communities are north of the Arctic Circle near the LKAB Kiruna mine (the same company reported by Jörgensen), yielding essentially magnetite ore with some hematite. The mine was opened in 1809 and has conducted operations completely underground since 1930. The quartz content of the rock is 10%–20%.

Among the many potential causative factors of lung cancer listed by the author are smoking habits, quartz dust, exhaust from diesel motors, radon and its decay products, and poor ventilation. The interrelationships were too complicated to have been analyzed as part of his timely reporting.[115]

Another vital consequence from the ever-deeper mining activities was the increased need for greater volumes of artificial ventilation. To warm the air going into the mines, air was forced through great masses of crushed rocks. Thus, air exposed to rocks with low uranium content but large surface areas could be enriched with radon as it was pumped down to the depths of the mines. When the problems were identified and a possible explanation given, the ventilation system was changed and augmented. At present, the Malmberget mine is aerated with 50 million tons of air yearly (for comparison, 10 million tons of ore and rock are brought up every year).

St Clair Renard indicated that the results from the ventilation have been encouraging: remodeling measurements during recent months having showed decreasing radon levels, lower than 0.1 WL* (10 pCi/L decay products of radon), in all parts of the mine. He concluded, "The results of this study should be of interest in mining areas all over the world where uranium occurs as a trace element, either occurring directly in the mines or as fission products exposed through cracks in the surrounding rock or brought into the mines with water from outside sources."[116]

There are several classifications for identifying a substance as a carcinogen. Such classifications have been developed by the International Agency for Research on Cancer (IARC), and OSHA in its "Identification, Classification, and Regulation of Potential Occupational Carcinogens" 29 CFR 1990, also known as "The OSHA Cancer Policy." NIOSH considers the OSHA classification the most appropriate for use in identifying potential occupational carcinogens. "Potential occupational carcinogen means any substance, or combination or mixture of substances, which causes an increased incidence of benign and/or malignant neoplasms, or a substantial decrease in the latency period between exposure and onset of neoplasms in humans or in one or more experimental mammalian species as the result of any oral, respiratory, or dermal exposure, or any other exposure which results in the induction of tumors at a site other than the site of administration. This definition also includes any substance which is metabolized into one or more potential occupational carcinogens by mammals" (29 CRF 1990.103).

In the International Agency for Research on Cancer (IARC) monograph series, the term 'carcinogenic risk' is taken to mean the probability that exposure to a chemical or complex mixture or employment in a particular occupation will lead to cancer in humans. The fact that a monograph has been prepared on a chemical, complex mixture or occupation does not imply that a carcinogenic hazard is associated with the exposure, only that the published data have been examined. Equally, the fact that a chemical, complex mixture or occupation has not yet been evaluated in a monograph does not mean that it does not represent a carcinogenic hazard. Criteria used for preparing draft monographs, judging the adequacy of available data, and evaluating carcinogenic risk to humans were first established in 1971, and these criteria were adopted by the IARC Working Groups with publications of IARC Monographs (see Appendix at the end of this chapter, IARC Monograph, vol 41, 1986, Preamble, pp 13–27; and IARC Publication no. 51, 1983, pp 16–22). "The terms 'sufficient evidence' and 'limited evidence' of carcinogenicity used in those criteria refer only to the amount of evidence available and not to the potency of the carcinogenic effect nor to the mechanism involved. However, in the case of chemicals for which there is sufficient evidence of carcinogenicity in experimental animals, it was considered reasonable to recommend that, for practical purposes, such chemicals be regarded as if they presented a carcinogenic risk to humans. In the case of chemicals for which there is only limited evidence of carcinogenicity, further experimental and epidemiological research was deemed to be desirable." "The use of the expressions 'for practical purposes' and 'as if they presented a carcinogenic risk' indicates that at the present time a correlation between carcinogenicity in animals and possible human risk cannot be made on a purely scientific basis, but only pragmatically. Such a pragmatic correlation may be useful to regulatory agencies in making decisions related to the primary prevention of cancer."

Dinman[42] proposed a classification of biologic evidence for occupational carcinogenesis, identifying three major groups: group 1, *definitely* carcinogenic; group 2, *probably* carcinogenic; and group 3, *presumably* carcinogenic. Group 1 requires epidemiologic and experimental evidence of carcinogenesis. Representatives of this group are β-naphthylamine, chromium, nickel, 4-aminodiphenyl, and benzidine. Others were "uncharacterized or contaminated mixtures," such as mineral-derived tars, pitches, oil, and asbestos. In addition, arsenic, mustard gas, and hematite as an "uncharacterized mixture" were included.

The second group, probably carcinogenic based on experimental findings, included 4-nitrophenyl and α-naphthylamine as epidemiologically associated with experimental findings and the "uncharacterized or contaminated" substances auramine and magenta. Group 2 "experimental cases" also included beryllium. Group 3, presumably carcinogenic based on animal experiments only, included the following compounds: nitrosoamines (*N*-nitrosodimethylamine, alkylating agents [with the exception of mustard gas], dichlorobenzidine, *o*-toluidine and dianisidine).

According to Dinman, "there are some cautions to be applied to indicate relative levels of carcinogenic ordering even within grades of this classification. For example, where experimentation presents design problems for benzidine induction of bladder tumors in animals, the strength of the epidemiologic evidence for that compound's cancer potential in man leaves no more room for doubt of its potency than in the case, for example, of β-naphthylamine (BNA). Conversely, as regards the chromates, epidemiologic plus a single report of experimental induction[83] place chromates at the same level as benzidine in this evidentiary classification, even though it appears that the various salts and oxides of this element are less carcinogenic than benzidine."

At the Symposium on Chemical Carcinogens held in Pittsburgh in June of 1973, Weisburger[139] presented his viewpoints on the environment and cancer on the mechanism of carcinogenesis. Among the several major carcinogenesis problems pointed out by him was the carcinogenic hazard due to mixtures of agents. Often there are pronounced synergistic effects. He outlined the steps of carcinogenesis in relation to man, stating:

> "there is an essential difference between carcinogens and other toxicants and, by and large, bona fide real carcinogens do combine with DNA. Once that combination is formed, it is not reversible except by so-called repair enzymes, which, in turn, may lead to miscoding. Carcinogens are toxic, of course, kill cells, and the dead cell does not cancerize. When carcinogens react with DNA to yield a viable cell, it is an abnormal, latent tumor cell and the action is not reversible—most toxic effects are reversible. Primary carcinogens do not require metabolic activation. Others are the ethylene amines, sulfur, mustard, lactones, epoxides, or bis(chloromethyl)ether. Those do not require metabolism. Thus, with such chemicals, I would predict, although extensive studies have not really been done, age may play a lesser role in the relative hazard to agents of this type.
>
> "The other major class of agents requires biochemical activation. Thus, with these, one would predict that the major effects would hinge on the ratio of activation to detoxification. If a young person

*300 pCi/L = 1 Working Level (See Chapter 26).

has a higher ratio of activation to detoxification, he would be at a higher risk than an older person. Some of these chemicals are synthetic, some are natural products like cycasin, a plant carcinogen, or like mycotoxins. The environment contains naturally occurring as well as synthetic carcinogens. I am much more concerned about naturally occurring carcinogens that we are exposed to, eat or consume unknowingly than about synthetics. It was shown very clearly that something can be done about the synthetics. You know they are hazardous; you should and can control them. The people producing such chemicals know it is dangerous and control them, but their customers do not always appreciate the potential risk. I think this is an area where education and information are very important.

"Also, we now understand that primary carcinogens, like certain alkylating agents as β-propiolactone or bis(chloromethyl)ether, or active intermediaries obtained by host-controlled reactions, are carcinogenic because they interact with DNA structure or function. Changes in DNA may mean mutation. We know that direct alkylating agents are mutagenic as was demonstrated beautifully back in the 40s. But other experts in the field of mutagenesis, who tested not alkylating agents but procarcinogens 25 years ago, found them not mutagenic. The chemicals tested, such as polycyclic aromatic hydrocarbons or aromatic amines, were not mutagenic because they tested the procarcinogens, and they had no way of activating them in their system. Today, we know that if we activate such materials biochemically, they can be mutagenic. This gives us new tools which we are currently exploring to assess potential risks in the environment. Methods are available to resolve the question whether a product is mutagenic in two weeks, whereas it takes up to two years to find out whether a chemical is carcinogenic in an animal model. Thus, it is possible to get an inkling or a feeling for such risks in two weeks rather than two years. We need to be careful about the interpretation of the results obtained in such systems. I would not necessarily ban or recommend that a product be abolished because it is mutagenic in one system. One of you showed me a reprint where a widely used chemical expressed mutagenic properties under some conditions. If a chemical is mutagenic, I would like to recommend caution. It is a blinking yellow light. Depending on additional information, such a product might warrant testing for carcinogenicity in the conventional animal systems. At the same time, one would wish to minimize human exposure. Quick mutagenicity tests provide tools to select from the hundreds of thousands of chemicals, natural and synthetic, we concern ourselves about, as to whether they require assays in animal systems. Also, under extensive exploration is the problem of using transformation of cell cultures to develop a quick preview of possible hazards. An advantage is the possibility of using human cell systems. Again, I wish to emphasize the problem of converting into vitro the chemicals to be tested which need biochemical activation in order to detect a possibly carcinogenic material without false negatives by such abbreviated procedures."

Table 52–1 summarizes some of the main occupational cancers by industry and occupation and known substance or agents. Among occupational groups, those workers engaged in the preparation of coke and its by-products have long been recognized as being at risk for the development of skin and lung cancers.[23] These occupational and environmental observations have been comprehensively reported in the *NIOSH Criteria Document for a Recommended Standard: Occupational Exposure to Coke Oven Emissions*.[129] That there is much controversy is an understatement. Highlighted in an editorial by Nelson[102] in May, 1973 in the *New England Journal of Medicine* were several new and practical applications of chemical carcinogens. He stated, "Evidence has been accumulating in occupational settings for many years that external factors, both chemical and physical, are identifiable causes of occupational cancer. It has been estimated that possibly as much as 80% of all cancer is of environmental origin."[57] A variety of clues provide the basis for such speculation; perhaps the most persuasive stem from studies of migrant populations that clearly show that geographic differences in certain cancer rates tend to disappear in migrant populations in which the cancer rates move toward those of the native populations, clearly implying an important role in external factors in determining cancer rates.[58]

"Where occupational causes of cancer have been identified, it has been possible to intervene and prevent the disease. The implications of this simple and indeed obvious message concerning the wide role of external factors in cancer causation have been surprisingly neglected. Fortunately, however, the promise of cancer prevention is now receiving more attention. It is of interest that of the seven stated objectives of the new National Cancer Plan, the first four are aimed primarily at prevention. Of these objectives, number one is to 'Develop the means to reduce the effectiveness of external agents in increasing the probabilities of development of cancers in existing individuals or in individuals of subsequent generations.' "[108]

The American Conference of Governmental Industrial Hygienists' list of human carcinogens and suspect human carcinogens denotes "human carcinogens" as substances associated with industrial processes, recognized to have carcinogenic or cocarcinogenic potential, with an assigned threshold limit value (TLV):

SUBSTANCE(S)	TLV
Asbestos	
amosite	0.5 fiber/cm^3
chrysotile	2 fibers/cm^3
crocidolite	0.2 fiber/cm^3
other forms	2 fibers/cm^3
bis-(chloromethyl)ether	0.001 ppm
Chromite ore processing (chromate)	0.05 mg/m^3, as Cr
Chromium (VI), certain water insoluble compounds	0.005 mg/m^3, as Cr
Coal tar pitch volatiles	0.2 mg/m^3, as benzene solubles
Nickel sulfide roasting, fume and dust	1 mg/m^3, as Ni
Vinyl chloride	5 ppm
Zinc chromates	0.01 mg/m^3, as Cr

"Human carcinogens": substances associated with industrial processes, recognized to have carcinogenic potential *without* an assigned TLV:
4-aminodiphenyl-Skin
Benzidine-Skin
Beta-naphthylamine
4-nitrodiphenyl-Skin

Although there is scant animal or human data available describing quantitative skin penetration, routing, and absorption into tissues and/or systemic uptake of materials such as dusts, vapors and gases, the ACGIH substance listing refers to the potential contribution to overall exposure by the cutaneous route, including mucous membranes and eye, either by airborne, or direct contact with substance(s) with a "*skin*" notation. The rate of absorption is a

TABLE 52–1.
Selected Occupational Cancers

CONDITION	INDUSTRY/OCCUPATION	AGENT(S)
Hemangiosarcoma of the liver	Vinyl chloride polymerization	Vinyl chloride monomer
	Industry vintners	Arsenical pesticides
Malignant neoplasm of nasal cavities	Woodworkers, cabinet/furniture makers	Hardwood dusts
	Boot and shoe producers	Unknown
	Radium chemists, processors, dial painters	Radium
	Nickel smelting and refining	Nickel
Malignant neoplasm of larynx	Asbestos industries and utilizers	Asbestos
Mesothelioma (peritoneum) (pleura)	Asbestos industries and utilizers	Asbestos
Malignant neoplasm of bone	Radium chemists, processors, dial painters	Radium
Malignant neoplasm of scrotum	Automatic lathe operators, metal-workers	Mineral/cutting oils
	Coke oven workers, petroleum refiners, tar distillers	Scots and tars, tar distillates
Malignant neoplasm of bladder	Rubber and dye workers	Benzidine, alpha and beta naphthylamine, auramine, magenta, 4-aminobiphenyl, 4-nitrophenyl
Malignant neoplasm of kidney; other, and unspecified urinary organs	Coke oven workers	Coke oven emissions
Lymphoid leukemia, acute	Rubber industry	Unknown
	Radiologists	Ionizing radiation
Myeloid leukemia, acute	Occupations with exposure to benzene	Benzene
	Sterilizing of materials	Ethylene oxide
	Radiologists	Ionizing radiation
Erythroleukemia	Occupations with exposure to benzene	Benzene

function of concentration and time to which the skin is exposed and certain "vehicles" can alter this potential absorption. Substances having a "*skin*" notation and a low TLV may present a problem at high airborne concentrations, particularly if significant areas of skin are exposed for long periods of time. Respiratory tract protection, while the rest of the body surface is exposed to a high concentration, may produce such a situation. Biologic monitoring should be considered to determine the relative contribution of dermal exposure to the total dose (see Chapter 13). This is an attention-calling designation intended to suggest appropriate measures for prevention of cutaneous absorption so the respiratory threshold limit is not under-estimated, misinterpreted, or otherwise failing to provide an accurate assessment of the degree of potential worker exposure and consequent uptake, influencing substance body burden and certain physiologic functions.[2] The contributors for specific chapters in this book consider and discuss the consequences of exposure to and any absorption via the skin.

Industrial substances suspected of carcinogenic potential for man. The 1986-87 ACGIH TLV Publication indicates the following substances in this category (see Appendix A):

Acrylamine-Skin	0.3mg/m^3
Acrylonitrile-Skin	2 ppm
Antimony trioxide production	—
Arsenic trioxide production	—
Benzene	10 ppm
Benzo(a)pyrene	—
Beryllium	2 ug/m^3
1,3-butadiene	10 ppm
Carbon tetrachloride-Skin	5 ppm
Chloroform	10 ppm
Chlormethyl methyl ether	—
Chromates of lead and zinc, as Cr	0.05 mg/m^3
Chrysene	—
3,3′-dichlorobenzidine-Skin	—
Dimethyl carbamoyl chloride	—
1,1-dimenthylhydrazine-Skin	0.5 ppm
Dimethyl sulfate-Skin	0.1 ppm
Ethylene dibromide-Skin	—
Ethylene oxide	1 ppm
Formaldehyde	1 ppm
Hexachlorobutadiene	0.02 ppm
Hexamethyl phosphoramide-Skin	—
Hydrazine-Skin	0.1 ppm
4,4′-methylene bis(2-chloroaniline)-Skin	0.02 ppm
Methylene chloride	50 ppm
4,4′-methylene dianiline	0.1 ppm
Methyl hydrazine-Skin	C 0.2 ppm
Methyl iodide-Skin	2 ppm
2-nitropropane	10 ppm
N-nitrosodimethylamine-Skin	—
N-phenyl-beta-naphthylamine	—
Phenylhydrazine-Skin	5 ppm
Propane sultone	—

Beta-propiolactone	0.05 ppm
Propylene imine-Skin	2 ppm
o-Tolidine-Skin	—
o-Toluidine-Skin	2 ppm
p-Toluidine-Skin	2 ppm
Vinyl bromide	5 ppm
Vinyl cyclohexene dioxide-Skin	10 ppm

AZO DYES

The "azo" dyes form the largest class of synthetic dyes. Having been developed for coloring every fiber, both natural and synthetic, their use has been extended to the coloration of solvents and many other nontextile substances. These chemicals are derived from "aromatic hydrocarbons" typified by benzene, toluene, and xylene and have a distinctive "aromatic" odor. Originally, most were made from coal tar as by-products from coke manufacturing, but now they are obtained primarily from petroleum sources. The hydrocarbons mentioned, including naphthalene and anthracene, are basic compounds in the synthesis of most aromatic amines (see Chapter 63). Amines contain nitrogen as NH_2; of these, aniline is the best known.

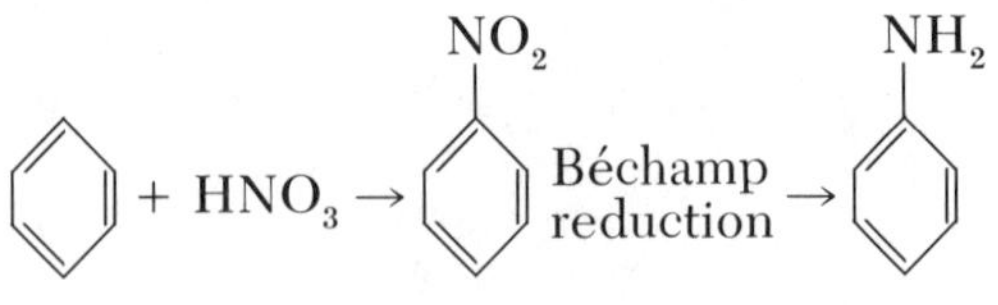

Benzene + HNO_3 → Nitrobenzene (NO_2) → Béchamp reduction → Aniline (NH_2)

Benzene   Nitrobenzene   Aniline

Unfortunately, "analine" and "aniline dyes" have become known as dangerous substances, thought capable of producing serious disturbances, such as aplastic anemia, first observed with benzene exposures (benzene was one of the first solvents isolated from the coal tar aniline compounds), and bladder tumors.

Occupational exposure to aromatic amines has long been associated with the development of bladder cancer. Historically, the population at risk has been limited to individuals employed in the "aniline" dye industry. The term "aniline cancer" was used in earlier days to denote cancer of the urinary bladder in workers engaged in the production of "aniline" dyes. Hueper[69] published a paper in 1934 in which he reviewed the history, significance, and epidemiologic evidence of "aniline cancer" in the dye industry. Hueper credited Rehn with reporting the first cases of occupational bladder tumors in 1895 in three workers in a German dye factory. In his review article, Hueper mentioned the beginning of what was to become a growing controversy concerning the etiology of occupational bladder cancer. He stated that aniline, benzidine and naphthylamine were the principal etiologic candidates, but emphasized major epidemiologic "pitfalls," including:

1. Worker exposure to more than one suspect compound, further complicated by shifting of workers between departments.

2. Different degrees of exposure hazard between processes.

3. Unsuspected impurities in trace amounts possibly more harmful than the parent compound.

4. Different composition of dyes and production methodology in different factories complicating statistical comparison.

Colors used in textile dyeing processes are considered to be generally nontoxic or of a low order of toxicity and no evidence has been shown that chronic occupational health problems have resulted from their use. The "intermediate process" or "indirect dyeing" of fibers applied by successive stages in order to attain good fixation required a number of "intermediates." Some of these intermediates are the naphthalenes and several aromatic amines that have been suspected or known to be carcinogenic. Of great concern are benzidine, some of its related compounds and α-naphthylamine. (These will be discussed further.)

In January, 1974, the U.S. Secretary of Labor of the Occupational Safety and Health Administration announced a standard for 14 carcinogens.[50] Because of this significant action, these substances are presented here in summary form. The OSHA work practices are found in this standard (Table 52–2).

2-Acetylaminofluorene (2-AAF)

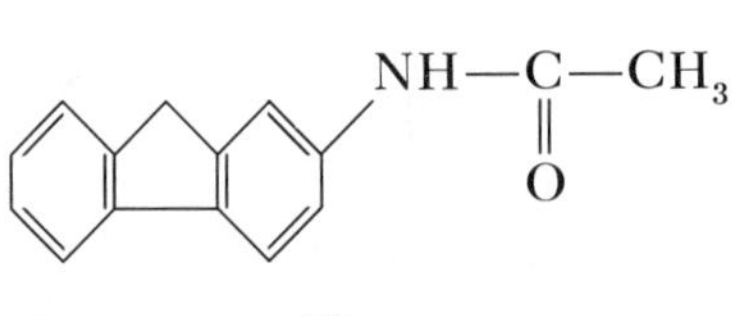

NH—C(=O)—CH_3

In 1941, Wilson et al.,[143] during a study of the toxicity in animals of a promising new pesticide, 2-acetylaminofluorene, discovered that it was a potent carcinogen. By 1961, there were more than 500 reports of studies of the carcinogenic effects of this substance or its related compounds. Although most of these studies resulted in carcinoma in rats, carcinogenic effects have been demonstrated in other laboratory animals as well. Liver and bladder tumors were produced in most animals on a dietary regimen of this substance. Weisburger et al.[140] noted from five patients treated with a single oral tracer dose of radioactive 2-AAF that man may convert 2-AAF, in part, to the potent carcinogenic metabolite, *N*-hydroxy-2-AAF. From this observation, it seems reasonable to conclude that 2-AAF, which has been shown to be carcinogenic in many animal species, probably is carcinogenic in man.

4-Aminodiphenyl

—NH_2

4-Aminodiphenyl, also known as xenylamine, has been used in rubber manufacturing as an antioxidant. Scott[118] recommended that its manufacture be terminated because its carcinogenic potency is at least equal to that of β-naphthylamine and the prospect of safe processing is remote. In 1954, Walpole et al.[138] first reported 4-aminodiphenyl to be carcinogenic in the urinary bladder of dogs. These investigators found multiple epithelial tumors in the urinary bladder of each animal. Concerning occupational exposure to 4-aminodiphenyl, they stated, "We, therefore, conclude that its manufacture and handling today would carry with it grave risks to the working population involved unless adequate precautions were taken to avoid skin contact or the inhalation of vapour or dust by

TABLE 52–2.
OSHA-Regulated Carcinogens, Completed Standards, 1986

2-acetylaminofluorene	Ethylene oxide
Acrylonitrile	3,3-dichlorbenzidine
4-aminodiphenyl	4-dimethylaminoazobenzene
Arsenic	Ethyleneimine
Asbestos	4,4-methylene(bis)2-chloroaniline†
Benzene*	Methyl chloromethyl ether
Benzidine	Beta-naphthylamine
Bis(chloromethyl)ether	Alpha-naphthylamine
Beta-propiolactone	4-nitrobiphenyl
Coal tar pitch volatiles	N-nitrosodimethylamine
Coke-oven emissions	Vinyl chloride
1,2-dibromo-3-chloropropane	

*Proposed.
†Standard vacated by legal and other technicalities.

the use of totally enclosed plant and daily changes of clothing for the operators."

In 1956[38] and in 1958,[39] Deichmann et al. published reports concerning their experiments with dogs dosed orally. Carcinomas were diagnosed in the bladders of all animals, with death occurring 4–18 months following the initial appearance of tumors.

In 1955, Melick et al.[98] presented the results of their epidemiologic investigation of the incidence of bladder cancer in workers engaged in the production of 4-ADP. Production of this aromatic amine was from 1935 to 1955 in the United States. Of 171 workers examined in several plants, 11.1% developed bladder tumors in 5–19 years following initiation of exposure. Exposure duration was 1–19 years. In a later report,[99] this range increased from 133 days to 35 years. The incidence of bladder tumors increased with time in the study group. In Plant 1, the number of workers exhibiting tumors of those examined was 12/71 in 1953 (16.9%), 23/186 in 1958 (12.4%), and 42/261 in 1970 (16.1%). In Plant 2, these statistics were 1/44 in 1953 (2.3%), 2/45 in 1958 (4.4%), and 10/54 in 1970 (18.5%). The 315 workers examined in this later report were included in a study by Koss et al.[82] of 503 workers examined who had been exposed to 4-ADP. Of the 503 workers examined, 435 had no cytologic evidence of bladder cancer, 16 had "suspicious cytology" for carcinoma, eight had conclusive cytologic diagnosis of carcinoma, nine had doubtful cytology, and 35 had histologically confirmed carcinoma of the bladder. Of the 24 workers with either suspicious or conclusive cytologic diagnosis of carcinoma, seven died of unrelated disease prior to histologic proof of bladder carcinoma, ten were lost to follow-up and the remaining seven had no histologic proof of carcinoma. Hence, it is conceivable that at the time of the report the 35 workers with histologically confirmed carcinoma of the bladder could be expanded to 52, if those workers with positive cytologic examinations were to be found histologically positive. As stated by the investigators, "as evidence from the data previously presented, many years may be required until the clinical proof of cancer is available."

From the work of Melick and Koss it is evident that more cases of bladder carcinoma will be diagnosed in this particular population. Of greater importance is the clear implication of 4-ADP in the induction of bladder tumors in workers engaged in its production. Deichmann and Radomski[37] considered 4-ADP to possess a relative carcinogenic potential for the dog six times greater than that of β-naphthylamine, 17 times greater than that of 4-nitrobiphenyl, and 27 times greater than that of benzidine. The accumulated experimental and epidemiologic evidence thus demonstrates that 4-ADP may be the most hazardous aromatic amine carcinogen.

Benzidine

$$H_2N\text{—}C_6H_4\text{—}C_6H_4\text{—}NH_2$$

Benzidine, also called 4,4′-diaminobiphenyl and *p*-diaminodiphenyl, occurs as white or slightly reddish crystals, leaflets, or as a crystalline powder and is used in the manufacture of azo dyestuffs. It is manufactured by reduction of nitrobenzene to hydrazobenzene with subsequent conversion to benzidine or its salts and coupled with other intermediates to form dyes. Benzidine base possesses a significant vapor pressure and is readily absorbed through the skin. Although its salts, such as the mono- and dihydrochloride and the sulfate, exert no significant vapor pressure, skin absorption can occur. Derivatives, such as 3,3′-dichlorobenzidine (DCB) (discussed later), are also important intermediates in the dyestuff industry.[75]

The prevalence of bladder cancer among workers in the aniline dye industry was known for many years, although the etiology of the disease was not clearly understood.[15, 18, 51, 54, 69] In 1937, Berenblum and Bonser,[19] based on their observations and review of the published literature, drew several conclusions:

> 1. Aniline cancer is associated with the handling of certain "intermediate products" used in the manufacture of dyes.
> 2. Of these intermediate products, aniline, benzidine, and alpha- and beta-naphthylamine appear to be implicated most frequently, probably the most important being benzidine and beta-naphthylamine.
> 3. Although these substances may themselves be the responsible agents, there is the alternative possibility that the disease is due to traces of unsuspected substances that are present.
> 4. The bladder tumors develop only after a long latent period (usually 10–25 years in man), and sometimes not until many years after the men have ceased work.

A confusing factor in determining whether or not benzidine, or β-naphthylamine, is a human carcinogen is that of multiple exposure, a problem that Berenblum and Bonser recognized as early as 1937. Workers in aniline dye plants usually were exposed to many aromatic amines, thereby complicating any investigation of cause-and-effect relationships. Increased incidence of bladder cancer in such plants was known but the specific causative agent was not known.

Scott[118] stated that it had been held that all stages of the manufacturing process were considered to be hazardous. Men engaged in the reduction to hydrazobenzene apparently were affected equally with those doing the conversion to benzidine and its separation. Other men engaged in other processes in the same building were affected also, and the whole operation was regarded as dangerous until Barsotti and Vigliani[15] described a factory in which hydrazobenzene was made in one building and conveyed to another factory for conversion to benzidine. No tumors had occurred among the men making hydrazobenzene, but tumors had arisen in some of the benzidine workers. So far, no tumors have been induced in experimental animals with hydrazobenzene. Scott and Williams[119] believe that the hazard exists after the conversion of hydrazobenzene to benzidine. It must be remembered that if hydrazobenzene dust or vapor is swallowed, it will be converted to benzidine by the action of the hydrochloric acid in the normal stomach.

In later years, populations of workers exposed to only benzidine were studied.[55, 94, 144] From observation of these groups, the role of benzidine as a human carcinogen became clear.

In 1954, Case et al.[26] published the results of their study of workers engaged in the manufacture and use of the dyestuff intermediates aniline, benzidine, α-naphthylamine and β-naphthylamine in the British chemical industry. They determined the incidence of tumors of the urinary bladder among such workers during a five-year field survey. Only 0.72 would have been expected from the whole male population of England and Wales ($P < .001$). The tumors appeared after an average induction period of 16 years. From the evidence of Case et al., bladder cancer is a fatal disease—only 20% of all patients having survived more than ten years from the first recognition of the disease. Processmen, pressmen, filtermen, and laborers engaged in the manufacture and use of benzidine experienced the greatest risk. The data conclusively indicated that the risk of dying of bladder cancer from benzidine exposure greatly exceeded that of the general population.

Goldwater et al.[55] studied workers in a coal tar dye plant in an effort to ascertain the association between bladder cancer induction and exposure to certain aromatic amines. The incidence of urinary bladder tumors in workers exposed to α-naphthylamine, β-naphthylamine (BNA) and benzidine, the average incubation period, the average survival time, and the incidence of malignant tumors other than those of the bladder were determined. The population studied included all male workers in the factory in question from 1912 to 1962, thus spanning a period of 50 years. The total number of workers exposed to all three compounds was 366, of whom 96 (26.2%) developed malignancies of the bladder. Of 76 workers exposed to benzidine alone, 17 (21.3%) developed bladder cancer. The incidence of bladder cancer in workers exposed to BNA plus benzidine was significantly greater than for those exposed to benzidine alone, 45.5% versus 21.3%, respectively. For the induction of bladder cancer from benzidine, the average time was 18.7 years, calculated to the first diagnosis of malignancy. Following diagnosis of bladder malignancy from benzidine, the mean survival time was approximately three years.

A cohort study of workers exposed to β-naphthylamine and benzidine was published by Mancuso and El-Attar in 1967.[94] Their primary purposes were to investigate (1) whether the previously reported[93] epidemiologic evidence of cancer of the pancreas could be substantiated over a long period, (2) the comparative carcinogenicity of β-naphthylamine and benzidine, and (3) the possibility of additive or synergistic effects. A cohort study was performed on 639 men employed during the period 1938–1939 in a company manufacturing β-naphthylamine and benzidine and who were followed in 1965 in order to determine the mortality pattern. The company cohort was characterized as containing three groups of workers: (1) exposed; (2) not exposed; and (3) exposure not known. Malignancies of the bladder and kidney constituted 35% (20/57) of all malignant neoplasms. The observed mortality rate for cancer of the bladder for white men in the company cohort, 25–64 years of age, was 78/100,000 as compared with 4.4/100,000 for white Ohio men of those ages. All cancers of the bladder for white men in the cohort occurred in the exposed group; the average annual mortality rates were 335/100,000 and 971/100,000 for the age groups 45–64 and 65 and over, respectively. Cancer of the pancreas (six cases) constituted 32% of the malignant neoplasms of the digestive system. The comparative cohort mortality rate for cancer of the pancreas was 39/100,000, whereas the rate for white men (Ohio residents) in the general population 25–64 years of age was 7.5/100,000. The incidence of cancer in workers exposed to β-naphthylamine was almost four times that in those exposed to benzidine alone. Likewise, exposure to both compounds was more hazardous than exposure to either carcinogen alone. As reported previously, benzidine was firmly implicated as a cause of human bladder cancer.

The recently published findings by Zavon et al.[144] also demonstrate that benzidine is a human carcinogen. They observed a group of 25 workers engaged in the manufacture of benzidine for an average of 10.6 years. Workers who developed tumors had an average exposure to benzidine in excess of 13 years, whereas the nontumor group averaged less than nine years of exposure. Of the 25 benzidine-exposed workers, 13 (52%) developed bladder tumors and 11 of these were malignant. The exposure time began as early as 1929, when production began, and as late as 1958, when it was discontinued. Determinations of the benzidine content of air samples from various locations in the plant were performed in 1958; the highest benzidine concentration, 17.6 mg/cu m, was obtained in the area where the final product was shoveled into steel drums. From 1929 to 1945, the final product was benzidine *sulfate;* from 1945 to 1958, the *hydrochloride* salt was prepared. The results of this study thus implicate both the hydrochloride and the sulfate salts of benzidine as human carcinogens. It should be mentioned that three of the 25 men involved in the study had approximately one year of exposure to β-naphthylamine, three had exposure to *o*-toluidine and seven had been engaged in dichlorobenzidine (DCB) production at some time. However, compared to their exposure to benzidine, their exposures to other compounds, including BNA, which also is a human carcinogen, appear insignificant. Of the workers in whom bladder cancer developed, 6/11 (55%) had no known exposure to either BNA or DCB. The authors concluded that the manufacture of benzidine was associated with a high risk of developing bladder cancer.

Epidemiologic studies[26, 55, 94, 144] of worker populations exposed to benzidine demonstrate that the compound and its salts are also human carcinogens. The incidence of bladder cancer in benzidine workers greatly exceeds the incidence of the disease in the normal population. Workers involved in the manufacture, handling, or use of this demonstrated human bladder carcinogen now are protected by current regulations promulgated by OSHA.

3,3′-Dichlorobenzidine (DCB)

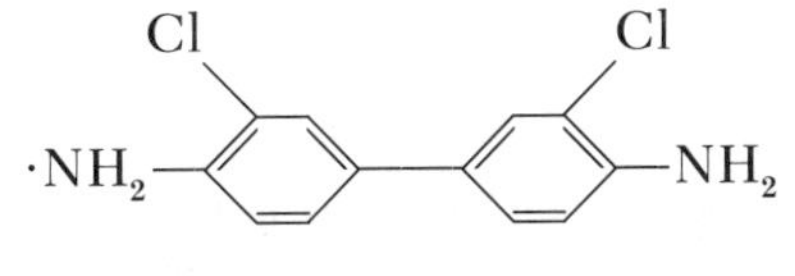

The potential of benzidine to induce cancer of the urinary bladder has precipitated inquiry into its chlorinated derivative, 3,3′-dichlorobenzidine. Today, DCB is a widely used intermediate in the organic pigment industry and is considered indispensable in the production of certain pigments. Akiyama[3] related industrial experience in Japan with finding DCB in the urine of not only the charging operators but also in the urine of dryers and crackers.

The Russian industrial experience with DCB was summarized by Lipkin[88] in a 1962 article. Lipkin stated that a 1958 hygienic study revealed ". . . very unfavorable working conditions and the presence of considerable contact of workers with dichlorobenzidine in industry." He noted that, in the following year, DCB production was halted in Russia.

The case for the carcinogenicity of DCB has rested on the validity of controlled experimental studies with several animal species because of the absence of a clearly defined worker population exposed only to DCB for any significant length of time. Where a worker population may exist, the period of actual exposure to DCB often is short and on the order of only a few years. Workers who have developed bladder tumors while working with DCB have been exposed concomitantly to such generally accepted occupational carcinogens as β-naphthylamine and benzidine. Because no significant worker population exposed exclusively to DCB has been found to exist,[100] a safe occupational exposure to DCB cannot be demonstrated. Therefore, the case for the human carcinogenicity of DCB must rely on extrapolation to human beings of the most pertinent experimental animal studies of oncogenesis.

4-Dimethylaminoazobenzene (DAB) "Butter Yellow"

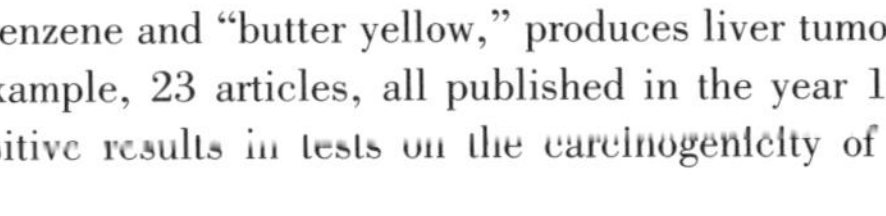

The events leading up to the demonstration by Kinosita[79] that 4-dimethylaminoazobenzene (DAB) produced cancer of the liver when added to the food of rats are well summarized by Badger and Lewis.[12] Since the initial report by Kinosita, numerous reports have confirmed the fact that DAB, also referred to as *p*-dimethylaminoazobenzene and "butter yellow," produces liver tumors in the rat. For example, 23 articles, all published in the year 1954, reported positive results in tests on the carcinogenicity of DAB in rats.[130]

In summary, DAB has been demonstrated to be carcinogenic in rats, dogs, neonatal mice, and trout. The results reported in dogs, even though quite limited, must be accorded considerable weight. In the absence of adequate epidemiologic data to the contrary, DAB must be regarded as a potential carcinogen for man.

α-Naphthylamine (1-NA)

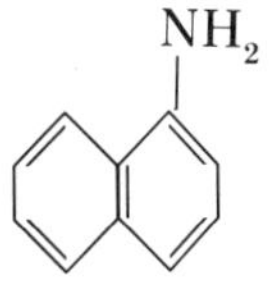

α-Naphthylamine (1-NA) is primarily used in the manufacture of azo dyes and for certain rubber processing. Scott[118] noted that under contemporary industrial practices (1962) the β-naphthylamine (2-NA) content of 1-NA was approximately 4%. It is understood that in current industrial practices this level of contamination by 2-NA can be kept below 0.5%.[80] In his evaluation of the literature and state of the art concerned with occupational exposure to 1-NA, Scott stated, "It is, therefore, difficult to escape the conclusion that alpha-naphthylamine is carcinogenic to man. . . . The standard of precautionary measures in its manufacture and use should be as high as that recommended for benzidine." It should be noted that, as concerns industrial exposure, Scott believed that 1-NA should not be considered in terms of purity but ". . . as it is found in industry, and there can be no doubt epidemiologically and theoretically of the risk attached to it."

In 1952, Barsotti and Vigliani[14] published results of an epidemiologic survey conducted among workers exposed to aromatic amines. Of the 902 workers surveyed, 30 had been exposed to 1-NA and 23 of these had been examined cystoscopically; 14 were normal, 7 had bladder congestion, and 2 had sessile papillomas. One of the papillomas appeared following four years' exposure and a 20-year latency period and the other following 25 years' exposure and one year of latency. All workers had additional exposure to toluidines, anisidines, xylidines, chloroanilines, and phenetidines.

An interesting conclusion was reached by Case et al.[26] "The average induction time is not appreciably influenced by the severity or duration of the exposure. It, therefore, appears to be a characteristic of the causal agent. This suggests that it is possible that the beta-naphthylamine content of alpha-naphthylamine is not the sole causative agent in the latter substance unless it is assumed that alpha-naphthylamine could retard the production of beta-naphthylamine tumors."

The main direction of research efforts to determine causation of bladder tumors induced by the naphthylamines has been the identification of those metabolites that possess this potentiality.

As yet, however, the ultimate carcinogenic metabolite(s) has not been clearly identified. Although the final resolution of this situation may be only academic to the occupational environment, the fact that an ultimate, active, hazardous substance has not been identified for even 2-NA precludes the dismissal of 1-NA as noncarcinogenic until it is clearly demonstrated that its metabolites are not carcinogenic for man. The demonstration that one such metabolite, *N*-OH-1-NA, was carcinogenic for rats and mice and was found to possess a greater carcinogenic potential than does its 2-NA counterpart[17] underscores this particular point. In addition, the extensive epidemiologic study in the dye industry by Case et al.[26] failed to eliminate an active role for 1-NA as a bladder carcinogen.

β-Naphthylamine (2-NA)

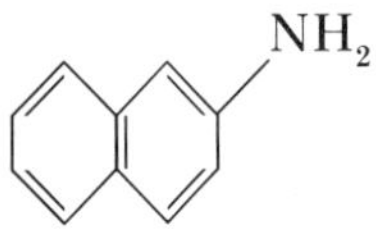

In the past, 2-NA has been used in the dye industry as an intermediate and in the rubber industry as an antioxidant. Its current commercial usage is considered minimal and its manufacture by the only known source in the United States supposedly ceased in 1972.

The induction of bladder tumors in workers exposed to 2-NA is one of the most well-established cause-and-effect relationships in occupational medicine. As mentioned earlier, Rehn is credited by Hueper as reporting the first cases of occupational bladder tumors in 1895 in three workers in a German dye factory. Many of the early epidemiologic studies were of limited usefulness as concerns specific etiologic roles, as Hueper[69] stated in 1934: "While aniline, benzidine and naphthylamine are the substances at the present time mainly accused of responsibility for the production of bladder tumors (International Labour Office), the exact chemical nature of the causative agent is not known." Thus, for some time, the term "aniline cancer" was used to describe occupational bladder cancer in dyestuff workers.

Numerous epidemiologic investigations have proceeded from these earlier reports, including limited surveys in the United States. However, the industry-wide epidemiologic survey by Case et al.[26] in 1954 is the only in-depth, comprehensive epidemiologic survey undertaken of workers exposed to 2-NA. This survey included 4,622 men who had been employed for six months or more in the dyestuffs industry. Case et al. estimated that the expected number of death certificates mentioning tumor of the bladder for this population should be three to five but actually found that of the 262 known cases of bladder tumors in this population 127 of 144 death certificates mentioned tumor of the bladder. The overall risk of death due to bladder tumor was estimated at 30 times the general population. Of 55 workers of the 262 total with bladder tumors who had received exposure to 2-NA only (excluding any exposure to benzidine or 1-NA), 26 or 27 death certificates mentioned the presence of bladder tumors. It was verified that risk of bladder tumors was present in both the manufacture and use of 2-NA. Case et al. estimated the latency period from initiation of exposure to 2-NA to development of tumors to be 16±6 years. In this regard, it was also determined that the induction period was constant with respect to age at entry and age at onset, although tumors were observed in workers exposed for fewer than five years or for more than 45 years. Based on the observation that the risk of bladder tumor development increased to a maximum and then decreased, Case et al. suggested that for a given level of risk there are both hypersusceptibles and hyposusceptibles present in the worker population and that selection might be possible by altering the level of risk. However, they considered reduction in employment time to be impractical in eliminating this risk, since tumors had been observed in workers exposed for less than one year. Case et al. considered that 2-NA was a more potent cause of bladder tumor than benzidine by a factor of 3 and 1-NA by a factor of 5.

Earlier, Barsotti and Vigliani[14] had observed in an epidemiologic study published in 1952 that 2-NA and benzidine carried the highest carcinogenic potential in the dyestuff industry.

Kleinfeld[80] published the results in 1965 and 1967 of an epidemiologic study of workers exposed to 2-NA and other aromatic amines in a dyestuffs plant. Of 376 employees examined, 109 (29%) were discovered to have bladder malignancies. Of 54 workers exposed to 2-NA only, 17 (31.5%) were discovered to have bladder malignancies. The mean latency period for workers exposed to 2-NA only was 20 years, with a range of 6–38 years. Mixed exposure to 2-NA and benzidine resulted in an incidence of bladder malignancies of 50%.

The carcinogenicity of 2-NA is well established by both animal data and human experience. Although an ultimate carcinogenic metabolite has yet to be identified, this aromatic amine is clearly implicated as a highly hazardous substance in any occupational environment.

Case et al.[26] considered the risk of bladder cancer in workers exposed to 2-NA to be 61 times greater than that in the general population. Scott[118] reported: "There is undoubtedly overwhelming evidence that beta-naphthylamine is a highly active carcinogen not only to laboratory animals but also to man in industrial conditions of manufacture and use, so much so that its manufacture has been given up in Britain and some other countries solely because of the danger associated with it." Scott considered the manufacture of 2-NA ". . . to be by far the most hazardous occupation in the dyestuffs industry." Of one group of workers distilling beta-naphthylamine who had more than five years of exposure, all reportedly developed tumors of the bladder.[105]

The American Conference of Governmental Industrial Hygienists (ACGIH) in their *Documentation of the Threshold Limit Values* (1973) noted that authorities who have studied the problem appear to be in general agreement that banning the use of this material is justifiable in view of the disastrous consequences to workers who have been engaged in its manufacture and use.

4-Nitrobiphenyl (4-NBP)

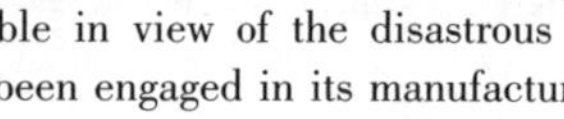

The industrial importance of 4-nitrobiphenyl (4-NBP) was intimately associated with the production of its reduced derivative, 4-aminodiphenyl (4-ADP). With the discontinuance of production of 4-ADP in 1955, due principally to the demonstration by Walpole et al.[138] in 1954 that 4-ADP produced carcinoma of the urinary bladder of dogs, the production of 4-NBP was discontinued also.

The carcinogenicity of 4-NBP is strongly supported by the induction of bladder carcinoma in dogs. The evidence that 4-NBP is metabolized in vivo to 4-ADP, which is a highly carcinogenic aromatic amine, and the possible evidence that human cases of bladder cancer attributed by Melick et al. to the exposure of 4-ADP only suggest that the carcinoma may have been induced by exposure to 4-NBP.

The carcinogenicity of 4-NBP was announced in 1958 by Deichmann at the 7th International Cancer Congress, London, July, 1958,[39] which was based on the studies by Deichmann et al.,[38] intiated in 1955.

N-Nitrosodimethylamine (DMN)

$$
\begin{array}{c} \quad\; CH_3 \\ \quad\; | \\ CH_3—N—N=O \end{array}
$$

Barnes and Magee[13] undertook the first extensive study of the toxicity of *N*-nitrosodimethylamine, also called dimethylnitrosamine (DMN), in response to the request of the medical officer of a firm that had been using it in the laboratory as a solvent. Two of three men working in that laboratory had developed cirrhosis of the liver. In their acute toxicity experiments with rats, rabbits, mice, guinea pigs, and dogs, the lethal dose was found to be in the range of 10–50 mg/kg. In chronic exposure experiments with rats, 200 ppm DMN in the diet proved lethal in approximately one month, 100 ppm required two to three months, and 50 ppm was tolerated for at least 110 days, at which time the study was terminated. The principal pathologic changes observed in the acute and in the higher-dose chronic exposure studies were hemorrhage and necrosis of the liver. In those rats surviving the longest, fibrosis and bile duct proliferation were observed also. Little change was observed in other organs.

DMN has produced cancer in a variety of sites and by several methods of administration in the rat, mouse, hamster, guinea pig, rabbit, trout, guppy, and newt. In view of this broad spectrum of carcinogenic activity in experimental animals, DMN must be regarded as potentially carcinogenic for man.

β-Propiolactone (2-oxetanone)

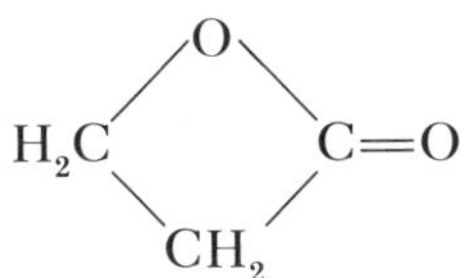

β-Propiolactone (BPL), also called 2-oxetanone, β-propionolactone, and Betaprone, is a colorless liquid with a pungent odor. It is soluble in water and miscible with ethanol, acetone, ether, and chloroform. It is formed by a reaction of ketene and formaldehyde.[60] Celanese Corporation, the only known producer, manufactures it at Pampa, Texas, primarily as an intermediate for the manufacture of acrylates.

Although its primary industrial use is in the synthesis of acrylic acid and acrylates, BPL has been shown to be an effective vapor-phase decontaminant for the treatment of enclosed spaces. Medically, BPL has also been used successfully to sterilize collagen sutures, human plasma and homotransplants, bone, and heterografts. Its value as a toxoiding agent and in preparing sterile vaccines has been reported.[96]

Celanese Corporation is constructing a new acrylate manufacturing facility not based on the BPL process, and in 1973 announced its intention to discontinue production of BPL[20]

Compounds such as BPL are highly reactive because of the strong tendency of the strained four-membered ring structure to open. BPL is an extremely corrosive chemical, the vapor being irritating to the eyes, nose, throat, and respiratory tract in general, and to other mucous membranes. In man, it is reported to be a skin vesicant, producing irritation and blister formation. Adequate protective clothing and equipment are recommended for workers likely to have dermal contact.

Results of pertinent animal experiments relating to the carcinogenicity of BPL were made available to the National Institute for Occupational Safety and Health.[41, 104, 138] Although epidemiologic evidence implicating BPL as a human carcinogen is not available, experimental animal data suggest that BPL should be a carcinogen for humans. Every precaution should be taken to prevent worker exposure.

Bis(chloromethyl)ether (BCME)

$$ClCH_2—O—CH_2Cl$$

The first accounting of a carcinogenic potential for bis(chloromethyl)ether (BCME) was made by Van Duuren et al.[131] in 1968. In this report, the authors compared the toxicity of BCME with its monofunctional analog, chloromethyl methyl ether (CMME), and discovered the former to possess much greater potential for inducing skin tumors in mice and rats than the latter. They classed BCME with such other biologically active alkylating agents as nitrogen mustards, epoxides and β-lactones.

In light of the startling incidence of lung carcinomas among rats following chronic inhalation of 0.1 ppm BCME, the National Institute for Occupational Safety and Health promptly undertook an investigation of plants producing ion exchange resins, a manufacturing process in which BCME may be found as a contaminant in the chloromethylation of polystyrene beads.[5]

Selected for study was a chemical facility that developed and had used an anion exchange production system since about 1955. An industrial hygiene survey was made of this facility in early 1972.[101] As sputum cytology was considered a sensitive method for assessing early injury to the bronchial epithelium by carcinogenic agents long before lung malignancy appears radiographically, sputum samples were obtained by standard techniques on 115 current employees at this facility. Survey results indicated that the incidence of moderate and marked atypical cytology was significantly higher. Although no malignancies were detected during this sputum survey, the results were consistent with a carcinogenic stimulus of BCME.

Further substantiation of the human carcinogenicity of BCME is provided by provisional results of a NIOSH retrospective cohort study of lung cancer incidence among all former and current employees of this plant. A significantly increased risk of lung cancer (4 observed vs. 0.54 expected, $p < .01$) was demonstrated within 15 years since onset of exposure among those individuals employed for five or more years in production-maintenance operations involving BCME. In addition to the sevenfold increase in lung cancer among this group, a preponderance of undifferentiated oat cell carcinomas was found. This pattern of risk and histology is similar to that recently reported by Figueroa et al.[52] from a study of another ion exchange facility. They reported on lung cancer found in chloromethyl methyl ether workers and suggested another occupational hazard that increases the risk of lung cancer. They surveyed and studied a chemical manufacturing plant with approximately 2,000 employees where periodic chest x-ray surveys had been carried out for many years. In 1962, the management became aware that an excessive number of workers suspected of having lung cancer were reported in one area of the plant, and promptly engaged consulting services to identify and resolve what appeared to be a serious problem. A group of 125 men were studied for the next five years. Fourteen were lost at various intervals during the investigation because of job termination, but four of the remaining 111 men developed lung cancer during the five-year period of observation. These four were from a group of 88 men in the age group from 35 to 54, giving a five-year cancer incidence of 4.54%. The best estimate of the expected number of cases must be derived from the youngest age group under investigation in the Pulmonary Neoplasm Research Project.[22] In this study, there were 2,804 men 45–54 years of age. Sixteen (0.57%) of these developed lung cancer in the first five years of observation. Smoking habits were very similar to those of the plant workers. The proportions of cigarette smokers were 78% and 74%, respectively, and the proportions of cigarette smokers using one or more packages per day were 24% and 20%, respectively. The slightly higher age of the Pulmonary Neoplasm Research Project groups makes the incidence of 0.57% an overestimate of the expected number. However, if we accept it as the best available rate, the five-year incidence was eight times higher in the plant workers. Using the binomial theorem, this difference is statistically significant at a probability of 0.0017.

While this study was in progress, plant management made a careful investigation of the work histories of several men whose lung cancers developed while they were working in the area under study. They concluded that the only common denominator was the exposure to chloromethyl methyl ether.

Further evidence that CMME could be a carcinogen was stimulated by a 44-year-old man admitted to Germantown (Pa.) Dispensary and Hospital in December of 1971 because of cough and hemoptysis. A detailed occupational history revealed that he was a chemical operator who had been exposed to CMME for 12 years. The patient stated that 13 of his fellow workers had lung cancer, and he suspected that this was his diagnosis. All had worked as chemical operators in the same building of a local chemical plant where they mixed formalin, methanol, and hydrochloric acid in two 3,800-L kettles to produce CMME. During the process, fumes often were visible. To check for losses, the lids on the kettles were raised several times during each shift. The employees considered it a good day if the entire building had to be evacuated only three or four times per eight-hour shift because of noxious fumes.

Recently, these agents have been found to be highly carcinogenic for mice and rats.[84, 86, 131, 132] Indeed, the inhalation of as little as 0.1 ppm of BCME (bis[chloromethyl]ether) has produced squamous cell carcinoma in the lungs of rats.[84] A recent report of six cases of lung cancer suspected of being due to occupational exposure to CMME in California[28] is a rare reference to a possible carcinogenic effect of this chemical for man.

The finding that all but one of the 13 histologically confirmed cases involved oat cell carcinoma of the lung, a particularly rare type of lung carcinoma in the general population, implicated an alkylating agent as the etiologic factor. Wagoner et al.[135] found in their epidemiologic study of uranium miners published in 1965 that oat cell carcinoma was the predominant type of lung cancer observed in uranium miners. In a Japanese study,[134] workers exposed to mustard gas, also an alkylating agent, were found with oat cell carcinoma. In a report, Archer, Saccomanno and Jones[8] presented evidence that the number of cases of oat cell carcinoma of the lung among uranium miners was 24 times greater than that "expected." Therefore, alkylating agents are considered to be radiometric in their biologic activity.

Figueroa et al.[52] stated in their paper that commercial-grade CMME contains 1%–8% BCME. On the basis of previous animal investigations, which demonstrated that BCME is a more potent carcinogen than CMME, it could be supposed that the BCME content of the CMME may have been responsible for the observed carcinogenic effects in humans in this study. However, the fact that substantial exposure to CMME (and, it must be presumed, to BCME also) did occur in each of the 14 cases implies that a carcinogenic role for this halo ether cannot be eliminated.

In 1973, Thiess et al.[126] reported that of 18 individuals employed in a technical research center, six died from carcinoma of the lung. In addition, 2 of 50 production facility employees died from lung cancer within the same six-year exposure period (1956–1962). The average latency period to the appearance of lung tumors was 8–16 years. Of the eight cases of lung carcinoma found, five were diagnosed as "small-cell carcinoma" ("oat cell carcinoma"). No environmental measurements were made for BCME concentration in the workplace during the period under study (1956–1962). However, the concentrations were considered minimal because of the readiness with which BCME can be detected by its strong irritant action at very low concentrations.

It is of interest that the production facility, where two of the cases of lung cancer occurred, was a "closed unit" equipped with an exhaust apparatus within which workers were required to wear air-supplied masks.

The investigators[126] concluded, "On the basis of information now available, we believe that the lung cancer cases reported by us are, with definite probability, caused by many years of breathing unknown amounts of dichlorodimethyl ether (BCME). This assertion is supported by animal tests available in the meantime and also by the known observations made in California."

Van Duuren, Laskin and Nelson[133] summarized the potential hazard associated with exposure to CMME and BCME in a letter to the Editor of *Chemical and Engineering News* on March 27, 1972:

> "Chemical carcinogens can be either direct-acting or indirect-acting. The latter type have to be metabolized in vivo to proximal carcinogens, and, hence, these indirect-acting agents are highly organ- and species-specific since the metabolic patterns vary by organ and species. The direct-acting agents, which include alkylating carcinogens such as CMME and BCME, act normally at the site of exposure and they are carcinogenic in several species and organs but usually only at the site of exposure. Since these direct-acting alkylating agents are carcinogenic in several animal species, they must be regarded as potentially carcinogenic in man. The alpha-chloro ethers should, therefore, be regarded as potentially serious occupational hazards in the chemical industry and in research laboratories where they may not always be handled with proper precautions."

An announcement[108] recently has been made that hydrogen chloride (HCl) and formaldehyde (HCHO) combine under ordinary ambient conditions, or in aqueous solutions, to form BCME. The importance of this discovery as concerns the ubiquitous availability of BCME is readily apparent. It must not be overlooked in this respect, however, that CMME rapidly decomposes both in air and in aqueous solutions to yield the above reactants.

$$ClCH_2—O—CH_3 + HOH \rightleftharpoons$$
$$CH_3OH + HCHO + HCl$$

Hence, pure CMME, even under the most rigid experimental conditions, is practically impossible to obtain or, once produced, to maintain without the subsequent formation of small amounts of BCME. Therefore, the practicability of exposure to CMME in the workplace without concomitant exposure to BCME is highly questionable.

It is very possible, based on available animal studies and epidemiologic investigations of exposed workers, that BCME may be one of the most hazardous carcinogens found in the workplace. The fact that, under ordinary conditions, BCME is formed whenever formaldehyde and hydrogen chloride are present requires continuous surveillance of workplaces where these two compounds may be present simultaneously. The hazard of lung cancer from occupational exposure to BCME requires strict measures to ensure that employees are not exposed to this substance by any route.

Chloromethyl Methyl Ether (CMME)

$$CH_3—O—CH_2Cl$$

Chloromethyl methyl ether (CMME) is used commercially in organic synthesis as a chloromethylating agent in the manufacture of ion exchange resins, in the treatment of textiles, in the manufacture of polymers and as a solvent for polymerization reactions. Because of its reactivity, CMME is highly irritating to the skin, eyes and mucous membranes.[131] With the exception of one less chloride atom, CMME is structurally identical to its highly carcinogenic bifunctional analog, bis(chloromethyl)ether (BCME). It is, therefore, of utmost importance in any consideration of the health consequences of occupational exposure to CMME that cognizance be given to concomitant exposure to BCME, which is normally present in commercial-grade CMME in quantities of 1%–7%.[52, 133] Likewise, in evaluating experimental evidence implicating CMME as a carcinogen, it is important also to know the BCME content of the CMME.

A field survey conducted by NIOSH personnel in 1972[101] revealed six cases of lung cancer in a West Coast facility that formed both BCME and CMME in the manufacture of ion exchange resins and employed approximately 75 "blue collar" workers. At least four of the six employees with lung cancer had worked in operations involving exposure to BCME and CMME. It was concluded from the field survey that an excess lung cancer risk was suspect in the worker population, and the results of a recent sputum cytologic survey among workers has demonstrated a greater than normal proportion with atypical sputum cells. Although BCME was suspected as the etiologic agent in this survey, the contributory influence of CMME was not known.

Van Duuren et al.[131] presented the first evidence for the carcinogenicity of the α-haloethers in 1968 and classified them with such other biologically active alkylating agents as nitrogen mustards, epoxides, and β-lactones. The study, which involved skin application of BCME or CMME to mice (2.0 mg/0.1 ml benzene three times weekly for 47 weeks), provided no evidence for CMME of "complete" carcinogenicity, although a slight irritating activity was elicited in mice when croton resin (0.025 mg/0.1 ml acetone) was used as a promoting agent. Of 20 rats injected subcutaneously with CMME (1–3 mg/injection three to four times monthly), 13 developed sizable palpable lesions in the treatment area. The purity of the CMME used in the study was verified by infrared spectrophotometry and gas-liquid chromatography with no BCME detected.

Although contaminating exposures to BCME have precluded conclusive evidence for the carcinogenic activity of CMME, the industrial experience with this halo ether is sufficient reason to consider CMME as a carcinogen.[97]

4,4′-Methylene-bis(2-chloroaniline) (MOCA)*

$$NH_2—C_6H_3(Cl)—CH_2—C_6H_3(Cl)—NH_2$$

A preliminary report concerning the carcinogenicity of orally introduced 4,4′-methylene-bis(2-chloroaniline) in rats was made by Grundmann and Steinhoff[56] in 1970. In 1971, these two investigators published a more extensive paper[122] of their completed findings. In the later paper, the toxicity and carcinogenicity of 4,4′-methylene-bis(2-chloroaniline) was compared with that of 4,4′-diaminodiphenylmethane (DDM). Both of these compounds are used as hardeners or curing agents for epoxy resin systems and isocyanate-containing polymers.[117, 124] Although commercial production of 4,4′-methylene-bis(2-chloroaniline) began in 1962,[87] DDM has been in production for more than 25 years.[117] The investigators quote previous work to document the strong toxic effect of DDM on both rat and human liver as well as the carcinogenic effect on rat liver. Schoental[117] has also demonstrated the carcinogenicity of DDM on the rat liver. An accidental acute poisoning episode occurred in 1965 in Great Britain in which 84 persons became ill, some seriously, with jaundice following the consumption of bread accidentally contaminated with DDM.[81]

In general, Grundmann and Steinhoff considered 4,4′-methylene-bis(2-chloroaniline) to be less toxic but more carcinogenic than the nonchlorinated compound, DDM.

Another study by Mastromatteo[95] in 1965 found two of six employees, both in their thirties, who had a mixed exposure to 4,4′-methylene-bis(2-chloroaniline), TDI and several isocyanate-containing resins, developed urinary frequency with hematuria, eye irritation, and respiratory irritation with cough and tightness in the chest. The hematuria related to the 4,4′-methylene-bis(2-chloroaniline) more than to the other substances. The author considered the conditions to be mild, but also considered that exposure to this substance, primarily by dust inhalation, was the cause of the observed cystitis.

The results of the experimental animal studies reported by several independent groups of investigators[85] clearly demonstrated

*4,4′-Methylene-bis(2-chloroaniline) or 3,3′-dichloro-4,4′-diaminodiphenylmethane has been given the registered trademark MOCA by E. I. du Pont de Nemours & Co., Inc. See Chapter 63.

an active oncogenic role for 4,4′-methylene-bis(2-chloroaniline).

Although industrial experience from reported studies is minimal,[87, 95] the positive findings in two animal studies by three independent investigators[85] firmly implicate 4,4′-methylene-bis(2-chloroaniline) as a human carcinogen.

Ethyleneimine (EI)

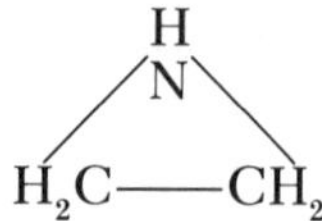

Ethyleneimine (EI), (also known as aziridine), is an extremely reactive, small-ring heterocyclic alkylating agent. The dual functionality and high degree of reactivity of EI are responsible for the synthesis of many derivatives in an increasing list of applications,[53] including textile treatment chemicals, adhesives and binders, rocket and jet fuels, chemosterilant chemicals, and chemotherapeutic agents, to name a few.

Early interest in EI centered on its possible application as an antineoplastic agent. Because of the general type of cytotoxic activity associated with EI in this role, subsequent investigators were led to question its possible role as a chemical mutagen and carcinogen.

Its high chemical activity causes it to be very irritating to the skin and mucous membranes. The renal toxicity of EI in the rat and rabbit has been described by Davies et al.,[31, 33] who also found that as little as 0.01 ml/kg body weight caused the death of rabbits from neurotoxic effects within a few hours.

A study sponsored by the National Cancer Institute in 1969 concerning the bioassay of industrial chemicals for tumorigenicity in mice was published by Innes et al.[74] The investigators' comments on their classification of liver tumors as "hepatomas" stated ". . . the term 'hepatoma' as used in this manuscript should not be considered as implying that these tumors are benign. Indeed, it seems more reasonable to conclude that the great majority had malignant potentiality." They concluded by stating, "the dose received by the mice was far above that likely to be received by humans, but there was no way to predict whether man would be more or less susceptible to tumor induction by the compound."

The case for the carcinogenicity of EI, then, rests on the possible extrapolation to human beings of the findings in two separate, controlled animal studies, one involving rats[138] and the other mice.[74]

This position is compatible with that of the NIOSH concerning the prior demonstration of carcinogenicity in at least two animal species.

OSHA WORK PRACTICES

This section applies to any activity in which a carcinogen is manufactured, processed, used, repackaged, released, handled or otherwise present in any manner.

SUMMARY

Approximately 430,000 people in the United States die annually from malignancies. The American Cancer Society estimates that some form of cancer will develop in one fourth of all Americans.[27] Cancer is the second leading cause of death and the second leading cause of lost years of potential life in the U.S. It is believed that a high proportion of all cancers are caused by "extragenetic" factors, including personal behavior patterns (e.g., cigarette smoking, alcohol and drug use, and sexual activities) and toxic environmental exposures in the workplace and the community.[46] Evidence for these relationships has been revealed principally through epidemiologic and toxicologic studies. A good example is given by Wingren and Axelson[143a] who conducted an epidemiologic study of potential cancer risks in the southeastern Swedish glassworks industry, heavily concentrated in that area. The total and specific cancer mortality in the three parishes around the glassworks were found to be approximately normal, both by comparison with national death rates and the death rates of another, similarly rural, area. More interesting results, however, were obtained in several case-referent studies also undertaken to study mortality from specific cancer sites and cardiovascular disease with regard to employment in the glassworks. A significant excess of deaths from stomach cancer, especially in glassblowers, lung cancer, and cardiovascular disease was observed among the glassworkers. Occupational exposures in the glassworks, especially to arsenic, may be of etiological importance.

The main epidemiologic observations have included differences in the incidence of cancer between groups with different exposures, changes in the incidence of cancer following migrations, changes in the incidence of cancer over time, etc. Toxicologic studies have led to the identification of specific agents that cause cancer in experimental animals.[46]

Although general agreement exists concerning the overall incidence of cancer, controversy surrounds the proportion of cancer cases attributable to occupational exposures.[40] Several characteristics of cancer contribute to the difficulty in making such estimates:

1. Latency in the development. Occupational cancer usually becomes evident long after initial exposure to the carcinogen. This interval may vary from 5 years to more than 40 years,[36] making it difficult to characterize important exposures long past.

2. Influence of exposures to multiple carcinogens. Workers may have been exposed to many carcinogens. Interaction of these agents or interactions between them and other factors may greatly increase the risk of cancer.[120]

3. Behavioral factors. Cigarette smoking, alcohol drinking, and dietary habits also influence the development of cancer.[65] Moreover, these factors—especially cigarette smoking—interact with chemical and physical agents in the working environment to increase the risk of cancer (e.g., exposure to asbestos interacts with cigarette smoking to greatly increase the risk of lung cancer) (see Chapter 14).

Further, there are many naturally occurring carcinogens and mutagens in certain fruits, vegetables, and other food stuffs. Studies of dietary practices may reveal causative connections according to Abelson[1] and Ames.[5, 6]

Also, problems with documentation of cancer and the type and extent of etiologic exposures can obscure important epidemiologic associations:

1. Errors in diagnosis and classification of cancer. Unusual neoplasms are often misdiagnosed. Even correct diagnoses may be improperly categorized according to the International Classification of Diseases (ICD); mesothelioma is an example.[120]

2. Lack of meaningful occupational histories. Information is collected on the work histories on death certificates in only a few states; hence, for many cases, crucial associations with occupational carcinogens are not apparent.

3. Difficulty in assessing exposures quantitatively. Precise measurements of levels and duration of exposures have not generally been available.[35] Consequently, the ability to delineate dose-response relationships has been very limited.

4. The frequency of specific types of cancers. The occupational etiology of a very rare cancer due to a specific agent (e.g., hemangiosarcoma of the liver due to vinyl chloride) is much more readily documented than the occupational etiology of a cancer type potentially caused by several factors (e.g., lung cancer associated with exposure to chromates).

5. The "dilution factor." Highly significant differences in the rates of cancer among small subgroups of a population may be overlooked because these rates affect the overall rate of cancer in the larger study population only slightly, if at all.[34]

Despite these shortcomings, various attempts have been made to estimate the proportion of cancers related to occupation. These estimates span a broad range, from less than 4%[4, 64] to more than 20%.[40] While these estimates are imprecise, little doubt remains that certain occupational factors are significantly related to an increased risk of cancer. Moreover, in specific groups of workers exposed to specific carcinogens, the proportion who ultimately develop occupational cancer may be large.

REFERENCES

1. Abelson PH: Dietary carcinogens (editorial). *Science* 1983; 4617:221.
2. Aitio A, Pekari K, Järvisalo J: Skin absorption as a source of error in biological monitoring. *Scand J Work Environ Health* 1984; 10:317.
3. Akiyama T: The investigation of a plant manufacturing organic pigments. *Jikeikac Med J* 1970; 17:1.
4. American Conference of Governmental Industrial Hygienists: Threshold Limit Values for Chemical Substances in Workroom Air. Cincinnati, 1986–87.
5. Ames BN: On dietary carcinogens and anticarcinogens. *Science* 1983; 4617:1256.
6. Ames BN: Peanut Butter, Parsley, Pepper and Other Carcinogens (editorial). *The Wall Street Journal* February 14, 1984.
7. Archer VE, et al: Hazards to health in uranium milling. *J Occup Med* 1962; 4:55.
8. Archer VE, Saccomanno G, Jones JH: Presented to American Association for the Advancement of Science, Salt Lake City, June 11–15, 1973.
9. Archer VE, Wagoner JK, Lundin FE, Jr: Cancer mortality in uranium mill workers. *J Occup Med* 1973; 15:11.
10. Axelson O, Sundell L: Mining, lung cancer and smoking. *Scand J Work Environ Health* 1978; 49:46.
11. Axelson O: Room for a role for radon in lung cancer causation? *Med Hypotheses* 1984; 13:51.
12. Badger GM, Lewis GE: Carcinogenic azo-compounds: Chemical constitution and carcinogenic activity. *Br J Cancer* 1952; 6:270.
13. Barnes JM, Magee PH: Some toxic properties of dimethylnitrosamine. *Br J Ind Med* 1954; 11:167.
14. Barsotti M, Vigliani EC: Bladder lesions from aromatic amines. *Arch Ind Hyg* 1952; 5:234.
15. Barsotti M, Vigliani EC: Bladder lesions from aromatic amines. *Med Lav* 1949; 40:129.
16. Battye R: Bladder carcinogens occurring during the production of "town" gas by coal carbonization. *Hyg Toxicol Occup Diseases* (XV International Congress of Occupational Medicine) 1966; 3:153.
17. Belman S, et al: Carcinogenicity and mutagenicity of arylhydroxylamines. *Proc Am Assoc Cancer Res* 1966; 7:6.
18. Berenblum I: Aniline cancer. *Cancer Rev* 1932; 7:337.
19. Berenblum I, Bonser GM: Experimental investigation of aniline cancer. *J Inc Hyg Toxicol* 1937; 19:86.
20. Beta-propiolactone. New York, Celanese Corporation of America, No N-61, 1973.
21. Blair A, Malker H, Cantor KP, et al: A review: Cancer among farmers. *Scand J Work Environ Health* 1985; 11:6.
22. Boucot KR, et al: The Philadelphia Pulmonary Neoplasm Research Project: Basic risk factors of lung cancer in older men. *Am J Epidemiol* 1972; 95:4.
23. Bowra GT, Duffield DP, Osborn AJ, et al: Premalignant and neoplastic skin lesions associated with occupational exposure to "tarry" byproducts during manufacture of 4,4-bipyridyl. *Br J Ind Med* 1982; 39:76.
24. Boyd JT, et al: Cancer of the lung in iron ore (haematite) miners. *Br J Ind Med* 1970; 27:97.
25. Boyko RW, Cartwright RA, Glashan RW: Bladder cancer in dye manufacturing workers. *J Occup Med* 1985; 27:11.
26. Case RAM, et al: Tumours of the urinary bladder in workmen engaged in manufacture and use of certain dyestuff intermediates in the British chemical industry. Part 1. The role of aniline, benzidine, alpha-naphthylamine, and beta-naphthylamine. *Br J Ind Med* 1954; 11:75.
27. Centers for Disease Control: Table V. Years of potential life lost, deaths, and death rates, by cause of death, and estimated number of physician contacts, by principal diagnosis. *MMWR* 1983; 32:411.
28. Chemical suspected in six cases of lung cancer (letter). *Occup Safety Health* 1972; 2:6.
29. Colton C: Herbicide exposure and cancer (editorial). *JAMA* 1986; 256:9.
30. Currie AN: Role of arsenic in carcinogenesis. *Br Med Bull* 1947; 4:402.
31. Davies DJ: The structural changes in the kidney and urinary tract caused by ethyleneimine ("vinylamine"). *J Pathol* 1969; 97:695.
32. Davies DJ: The early changes produced in the rabbit renal medulla by ethyleneimine: Electron-microscope and circulatory studies. *J Pathol* 1970; 101:329.
33. Davies DJ, Kennedy A, Saluja PG: Significance of the urinary ex-

cretion of the cells after experimental medullary necrosis. *Ann Rheum Dis* 1968; 27:130.

34. Davis DL, Bridbord K, Schneiderman M: Estimating cancer causes: Problems in methodology production, and trends, in Peto R, Schneiderman M (eds): *Banbury Report #9: Quantification of Occupational Cancer*. New York, Cold Spring Harbor Laboratory, 1981.
35. Davis DL, Bridbord K, Schneiderman M: Cancer prevention: Assessing causes, exposures, and recent trends in mortality for U.S. males 1968–1978. *Teratogen Carcinogen Mutagen* 1982; 2:105.
36. Decoufle P: Occupation, in Schottenfeld D, Frawmeni JF Jr (eds): *Cancer Epidemiology and Prevention*. Philadelphia, WB Saunders Co, 1982, p 318.
37. Deichmann WB, Radomski JL: Carcinogenicity and metabolism of aromatic amines in the dog. *J Natl Cancer Inst* 1969; 43:263.
38. Deichmann WB, et al: Carcinogenic action of p-aminobiphenyl in dog. Preliminary report. *Arch Ind Health* 1956; 13:8.
39. Deichmann WB, et al: Carcinogenic action of p-aminobiphenyl in dog. Final report. *Ind Med Surg* 1958; 27:25.
40. Department of Health, Education, and Welfare: Estimated fraction of cancer in the United States related to occupational factors. Bethesda, National Cancer Institute, National Institute of Environmental Health Sciences, National Institute for Occupational Safety and Health, 1978.
41. Dickens F, Jones HEH, Waynforth HB: Oral, subcutaneous and intratracheal administration of carcinogenic lactones and related substances: The intratracheal administration of cigarette tar in the rat. *Br J Cancer* 1966; 20:134.
42. Dinman DB: *The Nature of Occupational Cancer, A Critical Review of Present Problems*. Springfield, Ill, Charles C Thomas, Publisher, 1974.
43. Dodson VN: Metals intoxication as related to cancer. 18th Annual Medical-Legal-Industrial Symposium, Mount Sinai Medical Center, "Cancer and Industry," Milwaukee, 1979.
44. Doll R: Occupational lung cancer. A review. *Br J Ind Med* 1959; 16:181.
45. Doll R, Fisher REW, Gammon EJ: Mortality of gasworkers with special reference to cancers of the lung and bladder, chronic bronchitis, and pneumoconiosis. *Br J Ind Med* 1965; 22:1.
46. Doll R, Peto R: The causes of cancer: Quantitative estimates of avoidable risks of cancer in the United States today. *JNCI* 1981; 66:1191.
47. Edling C: Lung cancer and radon daughter exposure in mines and dwellings. Linköping University Medical Dissertations, No 157, Linköping University, Linköping, Sweden, 1983.
48. Edling C, Kling H, Axelson O: Radon in homes—a possible cause of lung cancer. *Scand J Work Environ Health* 1984; 10:25.
49. Edling C: Radon daughter exposure and lung cancer (editorial). *Br J Ind Med* 1985; 42:721.
50. Federal Register: Department of Labor's Occupational Safety & Health Standards, Carcinogens 1974; 39:3756.
51. Ferguson RS, et al: Symposium on aniline tumors of the bladder. *J Urol* 1934; 31:121.
52. Figueroa WG, Raszkowski R, Weiss W: Lung cancer in chloromethyl methyl ether workers. *N Engl J Med* 1973; 228:1096.
53. Fishbein L, Flamm WG, Falk HL: *Chemical Mutagens: Environmental Effects on Biological Systems*. New York, Academic Press, 1970.
54. Goldblatt MW: Occupational cancer of the bladder. *Br Med Bull* 1947; 4:405.
55. Goldwater LJ, Rosso AJ, Kleinfeld M: Bladder tumors in a coal tar dye plant. *Arch Environ Health* 1965; 11:814.
56. Grundmann E, Steinhoff D: Leber und Lungentumoren nach 3,3-Dichlor-4, 4-diaminodiphenylmethan bei Ratten. *Z Krebsforsch* 1970; 74:28.
57. Haddow A: Speech at the opening ceremony of the Ninth International Cancer Congress, Tokyo, October 23–29, 1966.
58. Haenszel W, Kurihara M: Studies of Japanese migrants. I. Mortality from cancer and other diseases among Japanese in the United States. *J Natl Cancer Inst* 1968; 40:43.
59. Hardell L, Johansson B, Axelson O: Epidemiological study of nasal and nasopharyngeal cancer and their relation to phenoxy acid or chlorophenol exposure. *Am J Ind Med* 1982; 3:247.
60. Hawley GG (ed): Beta-propiolactone, in *Condensed Chemical Dictionary*, ed 8. New York, Van Nostrand Reinhold Co, 1984.
61. Heath JC: Cobalt as a carcinogen. *Nature* 1954; 173:822.
62. Heath JC: The production of malignant tumours by cobalt in the rat. *Br J Cancer* 1956; 10:668.
63. Herndon WC: Theory of carcinogenic activity of aromatic hydrocarbons. *Trans NY Acad Sci* (Series II) 1974; 36:200.
64. Higginson J, Muir CS: The role of epidemiology in elucidating the importance of environmental factors in human cancer. *Cancer Det Prev* 1976; 1:79.
65. Higginson J: Lifestyle and cancer. *Cancer Forum* 1981; 5:4.
66. Hoar SK, et al: Agricultural herbicide use and risk of lymphoma and soft-tissue sarcoma. *JAMA* 1986; 256:9.
67. Hogstedt C, Gustavsson A, Gustavsson P: Mortality in Swedish chimney sweeps. *Arbete och Hälsa* 1986; 15.
68. Hogstedt C, Aringer L, Gustavsson A: Epidemiologic support for ethylene oxide as a cancer-causing agent. *JAMA* 1986; 255:12.
69. Hueper WC: Cancer of the urinary bladder in workers of chemical dye factories and dyeing establishments: A review. *J Ind Hyg* 1934; 16:255.
70. Hueper WC: *Occupational and Environmental Cancers of the Urinary System*. New Haven, Yale University Press, 1969.
71. Hueper WC: Environmental cancer hazards. *J Occup Med* 1972; 14:149.
72. Hueper WC, Payne WW: Experimental studies in metal carcinogenesis, chromium, nickel, iron and arsenic. *Arch Environ Health* 1962; 5:445.
73. Industrial Health Foundation, Inc: Proceedings of the Symposium on Chemical Carcinogens, Mellon Institute, Pittsburgh, June 28, 1973.
74. Innes JRM, et al: Bioassay of pesticides and industrial chemicals for tumorigenicity in mice: A preliminary note. *J Natl Cancer Inst* 1969; 42:1101.
75. International Labour Office: Benzidine ($NH_2C_6H_4C_6H_4NH_2$) in Occupational Health and Safety, Geneva, Vol 1, 1971.
76. Järvholm B, Thiringer G, Axelson O: Cancer morbidity among polishers. *Br J Ind Med* 1982; 39:196.
77. Jones DCL, Simmon VF, Mortelmans KE, et al: *In Vitro and In Vivo Mutagenicity Studies of Environmental Chemicals (Project Summary)*. United States Environmental Protection Agency, Research Triangle Park, North Carolina, EPA-600/S1-84-003, March, 1984.
78. Jörgensen HS: A study of mortality from lung cancer among miners in Kiruna, 1950–1970. *Work Environ Health* 1973; 10:126.
79. Kinosita R: Studies on cancerogenic chemical substance. *Soc Pathol Jap* 1937; 27:665.
80. Kleinfeld M, in Lumpe KF (ed): *A Symposium on Bladder Cancer*. Birmingham, Aesculapius Publishing Co, 1967.
81. Kopelman H, et al: The Epping jaundice. *Br Med J* 1966; 1:514.
82. Koss LG, Melamed MR, Kelly RE: Further cytologic and histologic studies of bladder lesions in workers exposed to para-aminodiphenyl: Progress report. *J Natl Cancer Inst* 1969; 43:233.
83. Laskin S: Inhalation Carcinogenesis. AEC Symposium Series 18, US Atomic Energy Commission, Washington, DC, 1970.

84. Laskin S, et al: Tumors of the respiratory tract induced by inhalation of bis(chloromethyl)ether. *Arch Environ Health* 1971; 23:135.
85. Lassiter DV: Hazard Review of 4,4-Methylene-Bis (2-chloroaniline). Office of Research & Standards Development, US Department of Health, Education and Welfare, National Center for Disease Control, Rockville, Md, Refs 1, 2, and 8, May, 1973.
86. Leong BKJ, MacFarland HN, Reese WH Jr: Induction of lung adenomas by chronic inhalation of bis(chloromethyl)ether. *Arch Environ Health* 1971; 22:663.
87. Linch AL, et al: Methylene-bis-ortho-chloroaniline (MOCA): Evaluation of hazards and exposure control. *Am Ind Hyg Assoc J* 1971; 32:802.
88. Lipkin IL: Carcinogenic substances in the aniline dye industry for prophylactic measures. *Labor Hyg Occup Dis* 1962; 6:19.
89. Lloyd JW: Long-term mortality study of steelworkers. V. Respiratory cancer in coke plant workers. *J Occup Med* 1971; 13:53.
90. Lloyd JW, Lundin FE Jr, Redmond CK: Long-term mortality study of steelworkers. IV. Mortality by work area. *J Occup Med* 1970; 12:151.
91. Lundin FE, Wagoner JK, Archer VE: *Radon Daughter Exposure and Respiratory Cancer, Quantitative and Temporal Aspect*. NIOSH and NIEHS joint monograph No 1, 1971.
92. Mancuso TF: Testimony to US Department of Labor Public Hearing on Possible Hazards of Vinyl Chloride Manufacture and Use, Washington, DC, February 15, 1974.
93. Mancuso TF, Coulter EJ: Methods of studying the relation of employment and long-term illness-cohort analysis. *Am J Public Health* 1959; 49:1525.
94. Mancuso TF, El-Attar AA: Cohort study of workers exposed to betanaphthylamine and benzidine. *J Occup Med* 1967; 9:277.
95. Mastromatteo E: Recent occupational health experiences in Ontario. *J Occup Med* 1965; 7:502.
96. May JR: *Hazard Review of Beta-Propiolactone (BPL)*. Office of Research and Standards Development, US Department of Health, Education and Welfare, Rockville, Md, Refs 41 to 54, July, 1973.
97. McCallum RI, Woolley V, Petrie A: Lung cancer associated with chloromethyl methyl ether manufacture: An investigation at two factories in the United Kingdom. *Br J Ind Med* 1983; 4:384.
98. Melick WF, et al: First reported cases of human bladder tumors due to new carcinogen—xenylamine. *J Urol* 1955; 74:760.
99. Melick WF, Naryka JJ, Kelly RE: Bladder cancer due to exposure to para-aminobiphenal; A 17-year follow-up. *J Urol* 1971; 106:220.
100. Miller CW, et al: Pneumoconiosis in tungsten-carbide tool industry: Report of three cases. *Arch Ind Hyg* 1953; 8:453.
101. National Institute for Occupational Safety and Health: Field Survey Report DFSCI, February 16, 1972.
102. Nelson N: Carcinogenicity of halo ethers. *N Engl J Med* 1973; 288:1123.
103. Newhouse ML, Berry G: Prediction of mortality from mesothelial tumors in asbestos factory workers. *Br J Ind Med* 1976; 33:147.
104. Palmes ED, Orris L, Nelson N: Skin irritation and skin tumor production by beta-propiolactone (BPL). *Am Ind Hyg Assoc J* 1962; 23:257.
105. Parkes HC: Identification of carcinogenic hazards from aromatic amine exposure and measures of control, in Nieburgs HE (ed): *Prevention and Detection of Cancer, Part 1: Prevention*. New York, Marcel Dekker Inc, 1978.
106. Partanen T, Kauppinen T, Nurminen M, et al: Formaldehyde exposure and respiratory and related cancers: A case-referent study among Finnish woodworkers. *Scand J Work, Environ Health* 1985; 11:6.
107. Pott P: Chirurgical observations relative to the cataract, polypus of the nose, the cancer of the scrotum, the different kinds of ruptures and the mortification of the toes and feet, in National Cancer Institute Monograph No 10, 1963, p 7.
108. Reaction of Formaldehyde and HCI Forms Bis-CME, Philadelphia, Rohm and Haas Co, December 27, 1972.
109. Redmond CK, Smith EM, Lloyd JW: Long-term mortality study of steelworkers. III. Follow-up. *J Occup Med* 1969; 11:513.
110. Reid DD, Buck C: Cancer in coking plant workers. *Br J Ind Med* 1956; 13:265.
111. Roe FJC, Salaman MH: Further studies on incomplete carcinogenesis: Triethylene melamine (TEM), 1,2-benzanthracene and b-propiolactone as initiators of skin tumour formation in the mouse. *Br J Cancer* 1955; 9:177.
112. Rutstein DD, Mullan RJ, Frazier TM, et al: Sentinel health events (occupational): A basis for physician recognition and public health surveillance. *Am J Public Health* 1983; 73:1054.
113. Salmon AG: Vinyl chloride: The evidence for human carcinogenicity in different target organs (editorial). *Br J Ind Med* 1985; 42:73.
114. St Clair Renard KG, et al: Gruvforskning B167. Svenska Gruvforeningen, 1972.
115. St Clair Renard KG: Lungcancer-dodlighet vid LKAB:s gruvor i malmberget. *Läkartidningen* 1974; 71:158.
116. St Clair Renard KG: Respiratory cancer mortality in an iron ore mine in northern Sweden. *Ambio* 1974; 3:67.
117. Schoental R: Carcinogenic and chronic effects of 4,4-diaminodiphenylmethane, an epoxy resin hardener. *Nature* 1968; 219:1162.
118. Scott TS: *Carcinogenic and Chronic Toxic Hazards of Aromatic Amines*. New York, Elsevier North-Holland, Inc, 1962.
119. Scott TS, Williams MHC: The control of industrial bladder tumours. *Br J Ind Med* 1957; 14:150.
120. Selikoff IJ: Constraints in estimating occupational contributions to current cancer mortality in the United States, in Peto R, Schneiderman M (eds): *Banbury Report #9: Quantification of Occupational Cancer*. New York, Cold Spring Harbor Laboratory, 1981, pp 3–17.
121. Silverberg E: Cancer statistics, 1982. *CA* 1982; 32:15.
122. Steinhoff D, Grundmann E: Zur Kanzerogenen Wirkung von 3,3-Dichlor-4, 4-Diaminodiphenylmethan bei Ratten. *Naturwissenschaften* 1971; 58:578.
123. Storetvedt Heldaas S, Langard SL, Andersen A: Incidence of cancer among vinyl chloride and polyvinyl chloride workers. *Br J Ind Med* 1984; 41:25.
124. Stula FF, et al: Experimental neoplasia in ChR-CD rats with the oral administration of 3,3-dichlorobenzidine, 4,4-methylenebis (2-chloroaniline), and 4,4-methylenebis (2-methylaniline). *Toxicol Appl Pharmacol* 1971; 19:380.
125. Sunderman FW Jr: Recent advances in metal carcinogenesis. *Ann Clin Lab Science* 1984; 14:2.
126. Thiess AM, Hey W, Zeller H: Zur Toxikologie von Dichlordimethylather—Verdacht auf Kanzerogene Wirkumgauch beim Menchen. Zentralbl Arbeitsmed 1973; 23:97.
127. Torkelson TR, Oyen F, Rowe VK: The toxicity of vinyl chloride as determined by repeated exposure of laboratory animals. *Am Ind Hyg Assoc J* October, 1961.
128. United States Department of Health, Education and Welfare: *Approaches and Project Area Planning Session Reports: Cancer Program Objectives*, Vol 1, Objectives 1, National Institutes of Health, National Cancer Institute, Bethesda, Md, 1972.
129. United States Department of Health, Education and Welfare: *Criteria Document for a Recommended Standard. Occupational Exposure to Coke Oven Emissions*. National Institutes of Health, Rockville, Md, 1974.
130. United States Department of Health, Education and Welfare: *Hazard Review of 4-Dimethylaminoazobenzene (DAB)*. Office of Re-

search & Standards Development, USPHS, NIOSH, Rockville, Md, Refs 3 to 25, July, 1973.
131. Van Duuren BL, et al: Alpha-halo-ethers: A new type of alkylating carcinogen. *Arch Environ Health* 1968; 16:472.
132. Van Duuren BL, et al: Carcinogenicity of Haloethers. II. Structure activity relationships of analogs of bis(chloromethyl)ether. *J Natl Cancer Inst* 1972; 48:1431.
133. Van Duuren BL, Laskin S, Nelson N: Carcinogenic alpha-chloro ethers. *Chem Eng News* March 27, 1972, p 55.
134. Wada S, et al: Mustard gas as a cause of respiratory neoplasia in man. *Lancet* 1968; 1:1161.
135. Wagoner JK, et al: Radiation as the cause of lung cancer among uranium miners. *N Engl J Med* 1965; 273:181.
136. Waldron HA: A brief history of scrotal cancer. *Br J Ind Med* 1983; 4:390.
137. Waldron HA, Waterhouse JAH, Tessema N: Scrotal cancer in the West Midlands 1936–76. *Br J Ind Med* 1984; 41:437.
138. Walpole AL, et al: Cytotoxic agents: Carcinogenic action of some monofunctional ethyleneimine derivatives. *Br J Pharmacol* 1954; 9:306.
139. Weisburger JH: Environment and cancer on the mechanism of carcinogenesis, in *Proceedings of the Symposium on Chemical Carcinogens*. Pittsburgh, Industrial Health Foundation, Inc, June 1973.
140. Weisburger JH, et al: Activation and detoxification on N-2-fluorenylacetamide in man. *Cancer Res* 1964; 24:475.
141. Weisburger JH, Williams GM: Chemical carcinogens, in Doull J, Klaassen CD, Amdur MO (eds): *Casarett and Doull's Toxicology: The Basic Science of Poisons*, ed 2. New York, Macmillan Publishing Co, 1980.
142. Whittemore AS, McMillan A: Lung cancer mortality among US uranium miners: A reappraisal. *JNCI* 1983; 71:489.
143. Wilson RH, DeEds F, Cox JA Jr: Toxicity and carcinogenic activity of 2-acetaminofluorene. *Cancer Res* 1941; 1:595.
143a. Wingren G, Axelson O: Mortality pattern in a glass producing area in southeast Sweden. *Br J Ind Med* 1985; 42:411.
144. Zavon MR, Hoegg U, Bingham E: Benzidine exposure as a cause of bladder tumors. *Arch Environ Health* 1973; 27:1.

APPENDIX

Selected Publications by the International Agency for Research on Cancer (IARC), World Health Organization, IARC Monographs on the Evaluation of the Carcinogenic Risk of Chemicals to Humans, Lyon, France:

Volume 1(1972): Some Inorganic Substances, Chlorinated Hydrocarbons, Aromatic Amines, N-Nitroso Compounds and Natural Products

Volume 1(1973): Some Inorganic and Organometallic Compounds

Volume 3(1973): Certain Polycyclic Aromatic Hydrocarbons and Heterocyclic Compounds

Volume 4(1974): Some Aromatic Amines, Hydrazine and Related Substances, N-Nitroso Compounds and Miscellaneous Alkylating Agents

Volume 5(1974): Some Organochlorine Pesticides

Volume 6(1974): Sex Hormones

Volume 7(1974): Some Anti-thyroid and Related Substances, Nitrofurans and Industrial Chemicals

Volume 8(1975): Some Aromatic Azo Compounds

Volume 9(1975): Some Aziridines, N-, S- and O-Mustards and Selenium

Volume 10(1976): Some Naturally Occurring Substances

Volume 11(1976): Cadmium, Nickel, Some Epoxides, Miscellaneous Industrial Chemicals and General Considerations on Volatile Anaesthetics

Volume 12(1976): Some Carbamates, Thiocarbamates and Carbazides

Volume 13(1977): Some Miscellaneous Pharmaceutical Substances

Volume 14(1977): Asbestos

Volume 15(1977): Some Fumigants, the Herbicides, 2,4-D and 2,4,5-T, Chlorinated Dibenzozodioxins and Miscellaneous Industrial Chemicals

Volume 16(1978): Some Aromatic Amines and Related Nitro Compounds—Hair Dyes, Colouring Agents, and Miscellaneous Industrial Chemicals

Volume 17(1978): Some N-Nitroso Compounds

Volume 18(1978): Polychlorinated Biphenyls and Polybrominated Biphenyls

Volume 19(1979): Some Monomers, Plastics and Synthetic Elastomers, and Acrolein

Volume 20(1979): Some Halogenated Hydrocarbons

Volume 21(1979): Sex Hormones (II)

Volume 22(1980): Some Non-Nutritive Sweetening Agents

Volume 23(1980): Some Metals and Metallic Compounds

Volume 24(1980): Wood, Leather and Some Associated Industries

Volume 26(1981): Some Antineoplastic and Immunosuppressive Agents

Volume 27(1981): Some Aromatic Amines, Anthraquinones and Nitroso Compounds, and Inorganic Fluorides Used in Drinking-Water and Dental Preparations

Volume 28(1982): The Rubber Manufacturing Industry

Volume 29(1982): Some Industrial Chemicals

Volume 30(1982): Miscellaneous Pesticides

Volume 32(1983): Polynuclear Aromatic Compounds, Part 1, Chemical, Environmental and Experimental Data

Volume 33(1984): Polynuclear Aromatic Compounds, Part 2, Carbon Blacks, Mineral Oils and Some Nitroarenes

Volume 34(1984): Polynuclear Aromatic Compounds, Part 3, Industrial Exposures in Aluminum Production, Coal Gasification, Coke Production, and Iron and Steel Founding

Volume 39(1986): Some Chemicals Used in Plastics and Elastomers

Volume 41(1986): Some Halogenated Hydrocarbons and Pesticide Exposures

IARC: Modulations of Experimental Carcinogenesis, publication no. 51, 1983

Supplement No. 1(1979): Chemicals and Industrial Processes Associated With Cancer in Humans (IARC Monographs, Volumes 1 to 20)

Supplement No. 2(1980): Long-term and Short-term Screening Assays for Carcinogens: A Critical Appraisal

Supplement No. 3(1982): Cross Index of Synonyms and Trade Names in Volumes 1 to 26

Supplement No. 4(1982): Chemicals, Industrial Processes and Industries Associated With Cancer in Humans (IARC Monographs, Volumes 1 to 29)

IARC Information Bulletins on the Survey of Chemicals Being Tested for Carcinogenicity, Numbers 1–10 (1973–1983), Lyon, France:
Number 1(1973)
Number 2(1973)
Number 3(1974)
Number 4(1974)
Number 5(1975)
Number 6(1976)
Number 7(1978)
Number 8(1979)
Number 9(1981)
Number 10(1983)

PART V

Selected Work Categories of Concern

53

Occupational Health Considerations for Women at Work

Jacqueline Messite, M.D.

Marcus B. Bond, M.D.

GENERAL

Three interrelated factors justify the need for separate chapters devoted to the medical interests of women at work: (1) women, *on the average*, are of smaller stature and have less physical strength than most men; (2) the woman's unique reproductive function of pregnancy means that a pregnant woman must carry her embryo and later her fetus with her into the workplace, thus possibly exposing the fetus to her occupational environment; and (3) the increased number of women at work makes them as important a component as men for consideration in occupational medicine.

In addition, major pieces of United States legislation during the past decade and a half mandate consideration of the woman at work. Among these are the Occupational Safety and Health Act of 1970 and Title VII of the Civil Rights Act of 1964 with the guidelines adopted thereunder by the Equal Employment Opportunity Commission (EEOC). The Occupational Safety and Health Act has, as its charge, the provision of a safe and healthful workplace for every worker, male or female, in this nation, and the preservation of our human resources. Title VII of the Civil Rights Act bars discriminatory practices for any reason, including sex, in the hiring of employees. Basic to the provisions of the federal regulations is the inherent assumption that tolerance to industrial stresses, susceptibilities to toxic materials, and performance capabilities are similar in all workers so that permissible levels of industrial hazards that will not endanger the health and life expectancy of any worker can be set.[22] Furthermore, "the preservation of our human resources" implies not only the protection of the health of our working men and women but also the preservation of their reproductive capacity and the products of such capacity, who will make up the human resources of the future. In order to ensure proper implementation of these pieces of landmark legislation, and to eliminate the often-stated contention that these laws have opposing goals in regard to women workers, it is meaningful to take an in-depth look at the facts concerning industrial exposures and their effects on women. Furthermore, the implementation of the guidelines of the EEOC signals a potential for substantial increases in employment of women in traditionally male jobs.

These facts are important to physicians for a proper perception of this subject. Because there may be an increasing number of women requesting placement in physically stressful and other nontraditional jobs, physicians are being asked for recommendations about placement: Is it safe? What are the differences in susceptibility to occupational stresses between men and women? What are the potential effects of the job on pregnancy and the fetus? The medical profession does not have good data on many of these questions, but the questions are currently pertinent, and the best scientific responses must be found and offered. Myths and realities about the greater susceptibility of women than men to exposures to chemical and physical agents must be separated in order to make the best judgment possible in occupational placement of female workers.

An important premise is that there is no job for which some woman, somewhere in the pool of available women workers, would not be as qualified, as competent, and of no greater susceptibility to harmful effects than any man. Fitting the individual woman to the specific job, as in the case with men, should be the primary consideration. Differences do exist between men and women in certain work capacities and physiologic responses, but these differences are, for the most part, based on averages of female and male populations and should not serve as the basis for placement recommendations for any one particular person.

TRENDS

Since about 1950, the sex composition of the civilian labor force in the United States has undergone a marked change. The proportion of the labor force made up of women 16 years of age and older rose from 29% in 1950 to 40% in 1975, a percentage point increase almost equal to that of the preceding 60 years.[46] In 1970, of all women in the United States 16 years of age and older, 43% participated in the civilian labor force. As seen in Table 53-1, by 1975 there were 37 million women workers, representing a 46.3% participation. The projected numbers and rate for 1995 are 61.4 million and 60.3% (see Table 53-1). Comparable percentages

TABLE 53–1.

Civilian Noninstitutional Population, Labor Force (% Change) and Labor Force Participation Rate by Age and Sex, Actual 1975 and Projected 1995. (Numbers in Thousands)*

SEX AND AGE	CIVILIAN POPULATION 1975 (ACTUAL)	CIVILIAN POPULATION 1995 (PROJECTED)	CIVILIAN LABOR FORCE 1975	CIVILIAN LABOR FORCE 1995	% CHANGE 1975–1995	CIVILIAN LABOR FORCE PARTICIPATION RATE 1975	CIVILIAN LABOR FORCE PARTICIPATION RATE 1995
TOTAL							
16 yrs & over:							
Women	79,865	98,003	36,998	61,417	+66.0	46.3	60.3
Men	71,403	88,031	55,615	69,970	+25.8	77.9	76.1
16–19 yrs:							
Women	8,215	6,421	4,038	3,761	−6.9	49.2	58.2
Men	8,046	6,403	4,760	4,043	−15.1	59.2	62.9
20–24 yrs:							
Women	9,471	8,139	6,069	6,796	+12.0	64.1	82.0
Men	8,747	7,580	7,398	6,530	−11.7	84.6	84.1
25–34 yrs:							
Women	15,488	19,071	8,456	16,300	+92.8	54.6	81.7
Men	14,537	18,122	13,854	18,105	+30.7	95.3	93.1
35–44 yrs:							
Women	11,632	20,384	6,493	17,427	+18.1	55.8	82.8
Men	10,756	19,236	10,288	19,446	+89.0	95.6	95.3
45–54 yrs:							
Women	12,206	15,701	6,665	11,125	+66.9	54.6	69.5
Men	11,324	14,832	10,426	13,807	+32.4	92.1	91.1
55–64 yrs:							
Women	10,347	10,637	4,244	4,671	+10.1	41.0	42.5
Men	9,215	9,738	6,982	6,311	− 9.6	75.8	64.5
65 yrs & over:							
Women	12,506	17,650	1,033	1,337	+29.4	8.3	7.0
Men	8,779	12,120	1,906	1,728	− 9.3	21.7	13.3

*From Fullerton HN Jr: *The 1995 Labor Force: A First Look.* US Dept of Labor, Bureau of Labor Statistics, Bulletin 2121, Dec 1980, and Fullerton HN Jr, Tschetter J: *The 1995 Labor Force: A Second Look.* US Dept of Labor, Bureau of Labor Statistics Bulletin 2197, Nov 1983.

for male participation in the labor force are 79.3% for 1970, 77.9% for 1975 and 76.1% projected for 1995. The percentage increase in the civilian labor force participation by sex, projected for 1995 from the 1975 data, is 66.0% for women and only 25.8% for men.

Among the factors underlying this trend is an increasing proportion of young women who are unmarried, a decline in the number of children women are bearing, and a growing participation in the labor force of women with children—even young children.[16, 26] Table 53–2 illustrates the changing percentages of women in various occupational groups from 1962 to 1983.[15, 15a] At present, women are largely employed in service industries, in white-collar clerical jobs and as semiskilled operatives in manufacturing industries. In the trade industry, women are found in the retail trades, whereas men predominate in the wholesale field. In education, women are primarily the precollege teachers, whereas men predominate in the faculties of colleges and universities, particularly at the higher levels. Manufacturing employs the largest share of the male work force.[48]

In the past 10–15 years there have been appreciable changes in attitudes and expectations of women at work. A high proportion of women currently expect salaried employment to be a major part of their lives' activities. This is consistent with, and a part of, the women's movement, which strives to increase the variety and importance of women's roles in our society. Included is a desire by many women to acquire and achieve success in jobs traditionally held by men.

Inroads are beginning to be made in some typically masculine jobs such as bartending and bus driving, although most female bus drivers work only part-time operating school buses.[15a, 48] There has been some progress in the professions. From 1962 to 1983, the proportion of physicians and surgeons who were women rose from 5.5% to 15.8% and that of lawyers and judges rose from 2.8% to 15.8%.[15, 15a] Given opportunities for training at all levels from apprenticeships in industry to education in the higher professions, it is expected that women will be moving into areas for the most part previously closed to them. With the growth of child-care facilities there will be continued increasing participation in the labor force by women in the childbearing age groups.

Table 53–3 includes examples of occupations and their exposures in which significant numbers of women presently are represented in the work force.[17] No attempt will be made in this chapter to cover the hazards associated with industries where the work force has been predominantly female but in which men can be expected to respond in similar ways, if similarly exposed. Most of the hazards associated with such industries—e.g., textile manufac-

TABLE 53–2.
Occupational Participation Rates: Women as a Percentage of the Total Number of Employed Workers, 1964–1983*

OCCUPATIONAL GROUP	1964	1983
Total Employed	33.9	43.7
Professional	35.9	48.1
Accountants	18.7	38.7
Lawyers and judges	2.8	15.8
Librarians	85.7	87.3
Chemists	8.6	23.3
Personnel and labor relations	27.4	52.3
Pharmacists	10.4	26.7
Physicians (including osteopaths)	5.5	15.8
Registered nurses	98.5	95.8
Psychologists	41.7	57.1
Social workers	60.2	64.3
Teachers, college and university	19.2	36.3
Elementary school teachers	86.5	83.3
Drafting technicians	4.1	17.5
Designers	26.3	52.7
Editors and reporters	37.8	48.4
Painters and sculptors	40.7	47.4
Public relations	20.0	50.1
Managers	15.3	21.8
Purchasing agents	10.7	23.6
Salesworkers	39.2	47.5
Huskers and peddlers	65.9	81.0
Insurance agents	10.1	25.1
News vendors	3.2	27.4
Real estate agents	28.5	48.4
Clerical workers	68.8	80.6
Bank tellers	71.5	91.0
Bookkeepers	85.4	91.0
Cashiers	82.5	84.4
Collectors, bill and account	21.2	66.4
Dispatchers, vehicle	9.1	45.7
Insurance adjusters	9.4	65.0
Mail carriers	2.9	17.1
Messengers	14.9	26.2
Payroll timekeepers	61.5	82.2
Postal clerks	14.7	36.7

OCCUPATIONAL GROUP	1964	1983
Total Employed	33.9	43.7
Secretaries	98.5	99.0
Shipping and receiving clerks	7.6	22.6
Storekeepers and stock clerks	17.4	38.7
Telephone operators	96.3	90.4
Ticket and station agents	21.1	64.7
Typists	94.8	95.6
Office machine operators	72.9	85.5
Craft workers		
Bakers	18.3	44.4
Compositors and typesetters	6.3	64.1
Painters, construction and maintenance	2.5	4.9
Operatives	25.9	26.6
Checkers, inspectors	45.4	54.9
Graders and sorters	54.8	58.6
Packers and wrappers, except meat	60.3	63.1
Photo process workers	41.2	52.4
Weavers	44.8	75.2
Welders	6.0	5.0
Bus drivers	11.9	45.5
Taxicab drivers	3.7	10.4
Farmers and farm managers	5.1	12.1
Owners and tenants	5.2	12.1
Farm laborers and supervisors	32.0	
Farm laborers (wage workers)	16.8	24.8
Farm laborers (unpaid family)	56.9	
Service workers, except private household	53.5	64.0
Bartenders	11.5	48.8
Cooks	63.6	50.8
Food counter workers	67.5	76.0
Waiters	87.4	38.8
Attendants, recreation	14.9	40.2
Hairdressers	88.1	88.7
Guards and watchers	5.0	20.6
Nursing aides	75.2	88.7

*From Garfinkle SH: Occupations of women and black workers, 1964–72, *Monthly Labor Review,* US Dept of Labor, Bureau of Labor Statistics, p 29, November 1975;[15] and Employment and Earnings, US Dept of Labor, Bureau of Labor Statistics, January 1984.[15a]

ture, laundries, food services, health services, and office workers—are covered elsewhere in this volume.

This chapter will consider sex-related differences between women and men in work capacities, responses to adverse conditions or substances in the work environment and the effects of exposure to chemical and physical agents on the pregnant woman and the fetus. The reproductive effects of chemicals on male workers also will be discussed where pertinent.

RESPONSE TO CHEMICALS

There have been a number of reports that women have a greater susceptibility than men to the effects of exposure to toxic substances in the work area. Among the specific exposures most often mentioned are lead and organic solvents. There is a dearth of information concerning studies of men and women with comparable occupational exposures to chemicals. This can be partially explained by the difficulty in obtaining adequate cohorts for study of women in jobs similar to those of men in industries where significant chemical and physical hazards exist. However, even where such working populations have existed, there has been little interest to stimulate such studies. Oliver's report[33] on women exposed to lead in the white lead industries and Hamilton's report[21] on women exposed to lead in the pottery and tile manufacturing industries are well known. One of the earliest reports of the hematologic effects of benzene exposure was made by Selling in 1916 on three young Maryland women exposed to a commercial grade of benzene used as a rubber solvent in sealing tin cans.[41] During World War II there were a considerable number of women in the work force who had significant toxic exposures, but these populations have never been investigated adequately.

In acute toxicity studies in mice and rats with oral administration of more than 200 chemical compounds, Krasovskij[27] con-

TABLE 53–3.

Examples of Possible Exposures Related to Various Occupations*

OCCUPATION	POTENTIAL EXPOSURES
1. Agriculture	
("Migrant" workers' wives work in fields while pregnant and sustain work as long as able)	Multitude of substances and conditions, including physical and biologic. Excessive work hours; intermittent and prolonged heavy work. Chemicals, especially pesticides, herbicides, insecticides, solvents, dusts, fumes, gases, heat and high humidity, infections (bacterial, viral, rickettsial) and vibration (see Chapter 59)
2. Chemical and pharmaceutical production workers	
a. Concomitant exposures and physical stressors and possible synergistic effects are factors to be considered	See text
b. Ergonomic/biomechanic deficiencies (see Chapter 28)	See text
3. Cleaning personnel	
a. Launderers	Contaminated clothing, detergents, enzymes, soaps, heat, humidity
b. Dry cleaners	Contaminated clothing, heat, perchloroethylene, Stoddard solvent, naphtha, benzene, trichloroethylene, and others
4. Clerical personnel	Carbon tetrachloride and various other cleaners, physical stresses, poor illumination, ergonomic deficiencies (see Chapter 28)
5. Domestic workers (homes, hotels, motels, office buildings)	Alkalies, bleaches, detergents, heat, cold (physiologic factors), shift work, at times hard work, and various solvents in cleaning agents
6. Electronics assemblers	Antimony, epoxy resins, lead, methyl ethyl ketone, methylene chloride, tin, trichloroethylene, and visual stresses and strain (see Chapter 28)
7. Hairdressers and cosmetologists	Acetone, aerosol propellents (freons), benzyl alcohol, ethyl alcohol, hair dyes, hair spray resins (polyvinylpyrrolidone), halogenated hydrocarbons, and other solvents of a wide variety
8. Hospital/health personnel	
a. Registered nurses, aides, orderlies, physicians, students, patients	Alcohol, anesthetic gases, ethylene oxide, infectious diseases (bacterial and viral), puncture wounds, and x-ray radiation
b. Dental hygienists	Anesthetic gases, infectious diseases (bacterial and viral), mercury, puncture wounds, ultrasonic noise, vibration, and x-ray radiation
c. Laboratory workers (clinical and research)	Infectious diseases (bacterial and viral), puncture wounds, wide variety of toxic chemicals, including carcinogens, mutagens and teratogens; and x-ray radiation. Many workers are subject to shift rotation (see Chapter 68)
9. Opticians and lens grinders	Coal tar, pitch, volatiles, hydrocarbons, iron oxide, other polishing and grinding dusts and solvents
10. Photographic processors	Bromides, caustics, iodides, iron salts, mercuric chloride, pyrogallic acid, and silver nitrate
11. Plastic fabricators	Acids, acrylonitrile, alkalies, hexamethylenetetramine, peroxide, phenol formaldehydes, styrene, urea formaldehydes, vinyl chloride, and vinylidene chloride. High heat and humidity
12. Printing operatives	Benzene, carbon tetrachloride, ink mists, lead, methanol, methylene chloride, microwave, 2-nitropropane, pigments, trace metals, toluene, and various solvents, including trichloroethylene; ultraviolet, microwave and other radiation sources. Noise and vibration
13. Sign painters and letterers	Epichlorohydrin, lead chromate pigments, lead oxide, toluene, trace metals, and xylene. A wide diversity of other chemicals as solvents and strippers
14. Textile and related operatives	
a. Textile operatives	Asbestos, dyes, flame retardants, formaldehyde, heat, noise, raw cotton dust, synthetic fiber dusts
b. Sewers and stitchers	Asbestos, cotton and synthetic fiber dusts, flame retardants, formaldehyde, noise and organic solvents
c. Upholsterers (Some specific chemicals encountered in the above occupations are benzene, carbon disulfide, chloroprene, perchloroethylene, styrene, toluene, and trichloroethylene)	Same as above
15. Transportation	
a. Bus, taxi, truck and other vehicle drivers b. Airlines	Carbon monoxide, polynuclear aromatics, lead and other combustion products of gasoline and jet fuels; circadian dysfunctions; heat; physical stresses; shift changes; and vibration (ultrasonic, noise and hypersonic) (see Chapters 19, 60, 68)

*Adapted from *Guidelines on Pregnancy and Work.* American College of Obstetrics and Gynecology, 1977.[17]

cluded that differences in susceptibility between males and females are not very great. If the susceptibility of males were taken as unity, average values of the ratios were found to be 0.92 ± 0.058 and 0.88 ± 0.036 for female mice and rats, respectively. In some cases, males were more susceptible to the poisons tested. Studies with organophosphorus pesticides indicate the female rats to be more susceptible to some organophosphorus compounds whereas male rats are more susceptible to others.[12]

Of further interest is the report that male mice of certain strains are much more susceptible to the effects of chloroform than are female mice of the same strain.[50] The female mice show virtually no effect from chloroform exposure that is lethal to the males. Castration and administration of estrogens to the males will reduce the effect whereas administration of androgens to the females increases susceptibility.[12]

Ferguson,[12] in commenting on a review by Weston Hurst of some chemicals that have been found to be more toxic in females than in males, observes that in many of the examples, the effect occurs in a single species, and often in a particular strain of that species. He proposes that where differences in susceptibility have been suggested there is some correlation with the rate of metabolism by liver microsomal enzymes of the parent compounds and the relative toxicity of the parent substance and its metabolites. He believes that the most likely explanation for any sex-related differences in toxicity, if any exists, is that the enzymatic biotransformation of the toxicant is influenced by sex hormones. When the metabolites of chemicals are more toxic than their parent compounds, the male sex, with a more rapid rate of liver metabolism, is likely to be more susceptible. On the other hand, when the parent compound is more toxic than its metabolites, the male sex is likely to be more resistant. Since estrogens have a relatively lesser stimulating effect on liver metabolism than androgens, the female of the species might be expected, in general, to be more susceptible than males to those chemicals detoxified by such metabolism. As an example of this, Ferguson[12] cites the report by Hirakawa[23] of greater sensitivity of female rabbits than males to the effect of benzene, and the reduction of the relative resistance of males after castration.

In general, the animal data are limited and often conflicting, and are difficult to relate to differences in susceptibility between men and women. Baetjer,[5] in 1946, made a critical review of the data on which conclusions were based that women were more susceptible than men to chemical exposures. She found that most of the statements were made on the basis of studies of small numbers of cases or on poorly designed studies without consideration being given to the extent and duration of exposure between men and women or, at times, by simple repeated quoting in the literature of statements made by one or two industrial health authorities. Sometimes statements were simply personal opinions. She found no significant basis for a conclusion that nonpregnant women were more susceptible than men to the effects of chemical exposure. It is noteworthy that very little new information has been added to the literature since her review.

Lead

Sir Thomas Oliver,[32] in the late nineteenth century, was a leading proponent for the abolition of female labor in the white beds, stoves, and dusty processes of white lead manufacture in England. In discussing lead poisoning in that industry, he noted that "employers cannot be too frequently reminded that the susceptibility of females to lead poisoning is greater than that of males, and that the symptoms are usually of a graver character." He indicated that women are most likely to develop poisoning between the ages of 18 and 23 years, earlier than men and after shorter exposure. He described a greater number of cases of lead poisoning in women than in men admitted to the Royal Infirmary, Newcastle upon Tyne. When Baetjer[5] compared her data to the number of men and women employed in the lead industry in the particular town during the same periods, she did not find any differences in the incidence of severe lead poisoning in the two sexes. Of note is that Oliver went on to say that "apart from the influence of sex, women's wages are smaller, and they are therefore less able, if fighting the battle alone, to obtain proper food, which is a protection to some extent against plumbism." In addition, he added that "there is not the least doubt that females had been employed in larger numbers than males in the dangerous processes."[32] From the information presented by Oliver himself, factors other than possible differences in susceptibility between the sexes, such as socioeconomic status and degree of exposure, should be considered for possible explanations for any excess in the number of cases of lead poisoning that might have existed in women in the white lead industry in England at the time of his report. After women were eliminated from the heavy exposure, the incidence of lead intoxication decreased in females and increased in males. The exclusion of women in that industry is a classic example of the emphasis for reducing occupational diseases being placed on a specific group of workers rather than on control of the environment.

Oliver[33] also reported that there was a greater incidence of lead "encephalopathy" in women with severe lead poisoning than in men. A similar finding was reported by Prendergast[36] in his review of workers with severe lead poisoning, where he found an incidence of 34.9% "encephalopathy" in women as compared to 15.0% in men. Blindness was also more common in women and "paralysis" was present in 30% of women and 59% of men. In 1975, Seppäläinen et al.[42] reported more abnormal values in the sensory conduction velocities of the ulnar and median nerves, with lower blood lead values in female than in male lead storage battery workers, although the number of female subjects was too small to be conclusive.

In Baetjer's review[5] of the U.S. Public Health Service Study of the pottery industry, she found that where there were adequate numbers of men and women workers with similar exposures, the women had a slightly lower rate of presumptive cases of lead poisoning. Hamilton's study[21] of the pottery industry showed varying results, depending on socioeconomic status. In whiteware potteries, where women had a much lower socioeconomic status than men, the rate of lead poisoning was 4.9% for men and 19.3% for women. In the tile workers, where men and women were of equal socioeconomic status, the male rate was 15.8% and the female was 11.5%. Regardless, Hamilton believed that women were more susceptible to lead than were men.

Several reports indicate that, with comparable exposure, women have lower blood and urine lead levels than do men. Table 53–4 shows the mean blood lead levels by sex of varying populations exposed to similar environmental conditions. In the reports, all blood leads of men were higher than those of women, averaging more than 30% higher. Although these studies do not generally include comprehensive assessments of exposure that could explain some of the differences, nevertheless, the consistent pattern in Table 53–4 is of interest. Similarly, Table 53–5 indicates mean urine and blood lead levels by sex with varying degrees of exposure. At any level of exposure, the mean lead levels in both blood and urine were lower in women than in men. Explanations for these differences were not offered. Roels et al.[38] studied the responses of various biologic parameters of the heme synthesis pathway in a group of male and female workers moderately exposed to inorganic lead with the identical range of blood lead levels in both groups. The women exhibited a larger increase in free erythrocyte protoporphyrin (FEP) and in δ-aminolevulinic acid than did men. Also, Stuik and Zielhuis[45] reported data on male and female volunteers who ingested 20 mg lead acetate daily for three weeks. The increase in protoporphyrin IX in the erythrocytes of women was significant as compared with men, whereas the blood lead level was consistently lower in women (30 μg/100 ml) than in men (40 μg/100 ml).

The differences in clinical response in the presence of lower blood and urine lead levels in women suggest that women may have a different distribution of lead in the body and perhaps even different target organs for lead effects than do men. However, the interpretation of these findings is not clear at this time, and it is difficult to relate them to clinically significant effects at the lower levels of exposure in the current OSHA lead standards.[9]

Organic Solvents

Reports that women are more susceptible than men to the effects of organic solvents, particularly benzene (benzol), are conflicting and often the data are inadequate to support that conclusion.

TABLE 53–4.

Blood Lead Levels in Adult Men and Women With Similar Exposures*

BLOOD LEAD LEVEL (μg/100 GM)		PERCENTAGE INCREASE IN MALE COMPARED TO FEMALE BLOOD LEAD LEVEL
Male	*Female*	
17.2	14.9	15%
19.9	12.4	60%
24.0	18.0	33%
19.0	15.0	27%
16.6	10.6	57%
16.6	12.9	29%
18.5	14.7	26%
11.8	9.1	30%
13.0	9.3	40%
14.4	10.9	24%
19.0	14.9	28%
23.7	19.2	23%
22.7	16.7	36%
16.0	9.9	62%
17.0	12.7	34%
20.6	12.7	62%
40.9	30.4	35%

*From Bridbord K: Occupational lead exposure and women. *Prev Med* 1978; 7:311.

TABLE 53–5.

Comparison of Urine and Blood Lead Content Among Men and Women Under Same Exposure*

GROUP EXPOSURES	URINE LEAD CONTENT NUMBER ANALYSES	URINE LEAD CONTENT AVERAGE μG/L ± SD	BLOOD LEAD CONTENT NUMBER ANALYSES	BLOOD LEAD CONTENT AVERAGE μG/100 ML ± SD
Low				
Men	146	35 ± 21	148	26 ± 11
Women	123	28 ± 19	124	26 ± 10
Intermediate				
Men	102	43 ± 30	108	30 ± 11
Women	25	27 ± 15	27	22 ± 10
High				
Men	386	88 ± 60	329	44 ± 16
Women	61	46 ± 25	58	34 ± 13

*From Neal PA, et al: Public Health Bulletin 267. Washington, DC, GPO, 1941.

Hunter[25] studied a group of female and male benzene-exposed workers over a period of four years and reported the findings in one factory where the male workers constituted 60.5% (26 of 43 workers) of the work force but furnished 64% of the cases of depression of the white blood cell percentages in the blood. In the total 89 cases of his study, the men comprised 85% and yet furnished less than 65% of the normal blood counts. Hunter concluded that his findings did not furnish confirmatory evidence of hypersusceptibility in women for effects of this exposure. Similarly, Savilahti[40] did not find any correlation between sex and blood effects of benzene poisoning in a study of 41 exposed women and 35 exposed men. Of these, 24 (58%) of the women and 18 (51%) of the men had positive findings.

On the other hand, in both human and animal experiments, Hirakawa[23, 24] reported a greater susceptibility of females than males to benzene effects. Among 20 men and 19 women employed in spraying wagons with a paint dissolved in a mixture of xylene and aliphatic hydrocarbons that was said to include benzene, there was a more marked diminution of red and white blood cells in the women than in the men, and recovery after removal from exposure was more prolonged in the women. Support for increased susceptibility of women was further suggested by Hirakawa's studies in rabbits injected intramuscularly with 40% benzene in peanut oil (0.2 mg/kg body weight every two days), following which he observed no significant diminution in red or white blood cells in males in contrast to a diminution in both of these cellular elements in females and castrated male animals.

Ferguson notes that "an average 20%–25% of female body weight is fat, compared with 10%–15% in men (citing Altman and Dittmer[1]). Substances such as organic solvents, which are lipophilic, may be preferentially taken up into and stored in body fat, and this might influence the rate of clearance from the body. This could explain the difference in absorption, distribution, and elimination of organic vapors observed between male and female subjects by Sato et al.[39] in Japan." On the other hand, men are larger in weight than women, and the actual amount of the fat component of their body weight may offset any greater percentage of the fat component of women.

In summary, there is no substantive evidence on which to base a conclusion that women are more susceptible than men to the effects of exposure to benzene or other organic solvents.

CANCER

The apparent difference in incidence of cancer between the sexes deserves more attention and research. In cancer incidence, other than cancer of the reproductive organs, women generally have a lower rate.[47] No single factor can explain this difference.

The higher incidence of ovarian and uterine cancer in women than prostatic and testicular cancer in men may be attributed to the greater cyclic stimulation of the reproductive organs in females.[47] The higher incidence of breast cancer in women than in men, in whom the breast is a rudimentary accessory, is not surprising. However, apart from primary and secondary sex organs, men generally have a higher incidence of cancer than do women.

Toh, in his comprehensive review of sex differences and carcinogenesis, referring to liver cancer, notes, "At first sight, the sex difference in the incidence of cancer might be thought to be due to the different environments in which the two sexes live and work. In modern Western countries, men have a greater exposure to the potentially carcinogenic substances in industry, but a higher incidence of liver cancer in men is still found in underdeveloped countries." Ferguson[12] points out that "this sex difference is not limited to areas such as Africa and Asia, where the natural incidence of this type of cancer is high, but is also seen in low-incidence areas like Europe and North America. In Singapore, the male:female sex ratio for liver cancer is about 7:1, while in Liverpool, the ratio is approximately 5:1" (citing Doll, Payne and Waterhouse[10]). In considering the possible role in cancer etiology of greater food intake (with increase in uptake of "carcinogens" in food) in males than in females, Toh[47] notes the findings in rats indicating that the sex differences in liver tumor incidence were not influenced by amount of intake of food or carcinogen, and the findings of Purchase and Steyn[37] indicating no differences between male and female rats in the absorption of carcinogens from the stomach.

Castration of adult male rats decreased liver tumor incidence, and administration of testosterone restored the susceptibility. Resistance to liver tumors was found to be of the same order among intact females, ovariectomized females, castrated males, and castrated males treated with diethylstilbestrol.[31] Administration of diethylstilbestrol to intact male rats resulted in a lower incidence of liver tumors than that of controls, whereas administration of testosterone to female rats accelerated the development of hepatic neoplasms.[13] Ferguson adds, "It is probable that the hormone does not act directly on the liver, but indirectly through effects on the thyroid and pituitary glands and perhaps on the hypothalamus. Whatever the exact mechanism, however, the general conclusion appears to be similar to that reached in the consideration of sex differences in acute toxicity, viz., that hormonally induced effects on the liver, with consequent effect on the metabolic activation of potentially carcinogenic substances, are likely to be the most important factor responsible for the higher incidence of cancer of non-sexual organs in men compared to that in women."

Skin cancer (except melanoma) is also found more frequently in males than in females and such distribution has been confirmed in animals.[47]

As for lung cancer, Toh reports that men develop lung cancer more frequently than do women, with male and female ratios ranging from 1.5:1 to 9.2:1. He suggests that a different external social environment between the sexes, particularly cigarette smoking, may be responsible for the increased incidence of lung cancer in men, but Leuchtenberger et al.[29] found that male mice still develop a greater incidence of lung tumors than do female mice after exposure to a similar amount of cigarette smoke inhalation, and Haenszel and Taeuber[19] found a greater incidence of lung cancer in men than in women among nonsmokers. These authors suggest that the sex difference in incidence of lung cancer probably is due to a steroidal factor rather than the amount of intake of carcinogen. Occupational exposure to carcinogens in jobs traditionally held by men may also contribute to the difference in lung cancer rates between men and women.

In summary, there is little evidence to suggest that the nonpregnant woman is more sensitive to the effects of toxic chemicals than is her male counterpart. While physiologic distinctions exist that could account for differences in susceptibility between men and women to certain exposures, there is no available evidence to suggest that the differences in susceptibility between the male and the nonpregnant female worker are sufficient at existing or proposed levels of exposure to be a present consideration in the occupational placement of women workers. Nonetheless, well-controlled, well-designed epidemiologic studies of cohorts of male and female populations equally exposed to low levels of toxic chemicals and physical agents should be a priority in order to provide the data to make this conclusion a certainty for the benefit of all workers.

TOLERANCE TO HEAT

Women are considered to tolerate heat less well than do men. In the 1972 NIOSH Criteria Document on working in hot environments, the proposed work standards included a lower maximal permissible environmental heat stress for unacclimatized women than for men, i.e., 79° F WBGT for men and 76° F WBGT for women (25.5° C and 24.4° C).[8]

As reported in the Criteria Document, some rest-in-heat and work-in-heat studies have indicated that women do not adjust to heat extremes as well as do men. Based on the usual methods of measuring physiologic stress from heat, women showed higher skin temperatures and pulse rates and lower sweating rates than did men exposed to the same environmental stresses. But other reports have not agreed with these findings. Weinman et al.[49] stated that their studies on men and women using treadmills in a hot environment revealed higher sweat rates in men but lower pulse rates and core temperatures in women who were physically fitter than the men. Wyndham et al.[51] tested women and men who were unacclimatized to work in a hot, moist environment. Women tolerated the heat less well than did the men and showed higher core temperatures and pulse rates but less sweating. Morimoto et al.[30] found no differences in sweat rates of men and women working in a hot, dry environment, but when relative humidity was increased to 80%, the sweat rate in women increased significantly less than in men, but core and skin temperatures remained equal.

Physiologic differences between the sexes in response to heat stress is suggested, but the evidence so far is not conclusive. Both men and women acclimatize to heat stress to a similar degree.[11] Fitness of individuals appears to play an important role. The important factor after acclimatization and fitness is the proportion of maximal capacity that a particular workload has for a particular individual, whether male or female. A person of relatively small work capacity obviously will be using more reserve capacity at a given workload than will a larger and stronger person, and will show appropriate physiologic response to such stresses—pulse, temperature, ventilation, cardiac output. If there are basic physiologic differences in heat response between the sexes, such differences probably are small and may not be sufficient to affect medical recommendations about job placement. Fortunately, there are relatively few jobs in our society that involve both strenuous physical stress and high thermal stress. Whether male or female, to be successful in such jobs, a person will have to achieve acclimatization to heat and have above-average maximal aerobic work capacity, which is based mainly on height, weight, and fitness.

AEROBIC CAPACITY AND PHYSICAL STRENGTH

Reports in the scientific literature on physical strength comparisons of men and women indicate that, on the average, women have about two thirds the physical strength of men[6, 44] (Fig 53–1).

This is of interest to those who work in job and equipment design, especially for jobs that are likely to be filled predominantly by one sex. However, the same reports indicate an appreciable overlap in individual measurements, and there are some women who have more physical strength than do some men. This is of interest to occupational health practitioners, who must evaluate *individuals* for jobs.

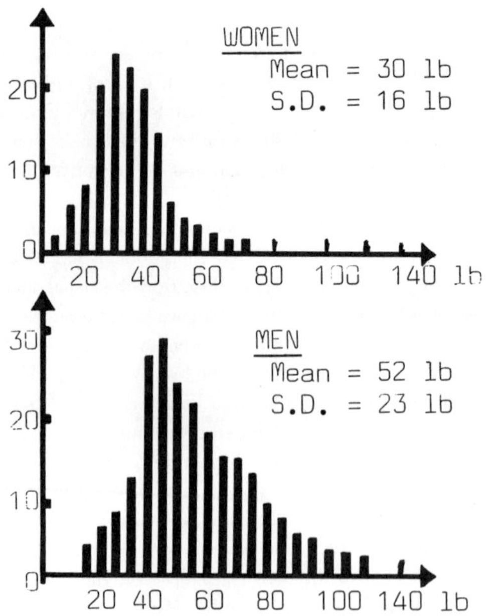

FIG 53–1.
Lifting strengths demonstrated by employees in standard position strength testing (number of people at each strength level shown on vertical lines).

Asmussen and Heeboll-Nielsen[2] reported studies that showed that isometric strength of 25 different muscle groups was maximal in women at about age 20 and in men at about age 30. There was a gradual but slow decrease in strength with increasing age, with a more rapid decrease in women than in men after age 40. Aerobic capacity also decreased with age in both sexes. Absolute values for women averaged about two thirds those of men at all ages tested. Similar results were reported by Åstrand,[4] who measured maximal aerobic capacity in L/min of oxygen using a bicycle ergometer and correlated this with heart rate. The correlations were good, and both were highest at about age 20 and declined gradually with increasing age. Mean oxygen uptake was 3.6 L/min for men and 2.7 for women. Fitness and size of the individual were responsible for most of the variation. Measurements of work production at normal jobs and usual pace of work revealed that construction workers worked at about 40% of maximal aerobic capacity and any increase above this level resulted in unacceptable fatigue.

Work capacity during various phases of the menstrual cycle in women with dysmenorrhea was tested by Gamberale et al.[14] by use of bicycle ergometers and a number of mental ability tests. Differences were minimal or none. There were no differences sufficient to affect medical recommendations about job placement. Of course, such tests are not the same as productive work at actual jobs, but rather are tests of physiologic and psychologic capacity for short periods of time in well-motivated women.

Guzman and Caplan[18] studied eight healthy pregnant women monthly to term for cardiorespiratory response to bicycle exercise. Control studies were done three months postpartum. They found oxygen consumption for a given workload to be similar at each stage of pregnancy and in the control period. But, at each workload, ventilation, heart rate, cardiac output, and stroke volume were all higher and arteriovenous (AV) oxygen differences lower during pregnancy. The rate of increase of these parameters per unit increase in work was the same in the pregnant and nonpregnant states. Also, the increases in cardiovascular dynamics were well established by the end of the first trimester and did not change appreciably during the remaining pregnancy. This latter is in contrast to the belief that blood volume increases gradually throughout pregnancy.

Pernoll et al.[34, 35] studied oxygen consumption and ventilation in 12 normal women during and after pregnancy, using a bicycle ergometer for exercise so as to minimize the differences in weight in the pregnant state. Oxygen consumption at rest and exercise was greater during pregnancy than three months postpartum, the increase being gradual throughout pregnancy. Ventilation also showed a gradual increase throughout pregnancy due to a greater tidal volume. Oxygen debt was greater from exercise during pregnancy than three months postpartum. The reports by Pernoll et al. thus are different from those by Guzman and Caplan in regard to oxygen consumption during various stages of pregnancy. Pernoll et al. concluded that there is a slightly decreased efficiency of muscular exercise during pregnancy, but were unable to offer an explanation.

All of the physiologic studies were made under laboratory

conditions that differed from actual work situations. The differences between individuals appear to be of greater importance than the differences between the sexes. But the averages of strength and aerobic capacity cannot be totally ignored. At work with moderate or greater physical strength requirements, there probably will be a greater proportion of women than men who lack the physical capacities required. The data quoted above indicate that an individual might be expected to perform satisfactorily if placed at a job in which the physical work requirements were about 40% or less of his or her maximal aerobic capacity. Measuring the physical work requirements of jobs and expressing them in kilocalories per minute, kilopondmeters (kpm), or other units is not easy, but can be done. An approximation might be satisfactory after measuring certain tasks for job components common to several jobs. Measuring the maximal aerobic capacity also is not easy but can be done. Much experience has been accumulated in estimating the maximal aerobic work capacity, and this is less difficult. Maximal aerobic capacity often is estimated by utilizing submaximal exercise and relating heart rate to amount of work done, with results expressed in ml O_2/kg body weight/min. These units are a measure of fitness but do not represent the actual physical capacity, as the latter varies directly with body weight and height. Therefore, liters per minute of oxygen uptake may be a better method to express the physical work capacity of an individual.

The work measurements and tests referred to generally have been limited to the laboratory. One of the reasons for this is that such measurements are expensive and time-consuming and require highly trained individuals to carry them out. Another practical reason is that work performance in most jobs may depend more on motivation and learning ability than on physical strength, plus many other quite subtle factors that are nearly impossible to measure. Improved mechanization of work tasks has taken away much of the sustained heavy work, but there remain many jobs requiring intermittent heavy exertion. This is discussed further in the chapter on preplacement examinations and recommendations (Chapter 56). Certain occupational ergonomic deficiencies are discussed in Chapter 28.

REFERENCES

1. Altman PL, Dittmer DS (eds): *Biology Data Book, Vol III, Section XI*, ed 2. Bethesda, Md, Federation of American Societies for Experimental Biology, 1974, p. 1528. (Cited in Ferguson[12].)
2. Asmussen E, Heeboll-Nielsen K: Isometric muscle strength in relation to age in men and women. *Ergonomics* 1962; 5:167.
3. Åstrand I: Aerobic work capacity—Its relation to age, sex, and other factors. *Circ Res*, March 1967; Suppl I, Vol XX.
4. Åstrand I: Aerobic work capacity in men and women with special reference to age. *Acta Physiol Scand* 1969; 49(Suppl 169):1.
5. Baetjer A: *Women in Industry, Their Health and Efficiency*. Philadelphia, WB Saunders Co, 1946, pp 145–156.
6. Chaffin DB: Human strength capability and low back pain. *J Occup Med* 1974; 16:248.
7. Chaffin DB, et al: Pre-employment strength testing in selecting workers for material handling jobs. University of Michigan, NIOSH (CDC-74-62) 1976.
8. *Criteria for a recommended standard: Occupational exposure to hot environments*, DHEW, PHS, NIOSH 72-10269, 1972.
9. Occupational Safety and Health Administration US Dept of Labor: Occupational exposure to lead, final standard. *Federal Register* Nov 14, 1978; 43:52952.
10. Doll R, Payne P, Waterhouse J: In *Cancer, Incidence in Five Continents*. Berlin and New York, Springer-Verlag, 1966. (Cited in Ferguson[12].)
11. Drinkwater BL: Physiological responses of women to exercise, in Wilmore JH (ed): *Exercise and Sport Sciences Reviews*. New York, Academic Press, 1973.
12. Ferguson DM: Toxicological problems related to the employment of women, in *Health of Women at Work*, Proceedings of Symposium of Society of Occupational Medicine Research Panel. London, Royal Society of Medicine, 1976, pp 41–52.
13. Firminger HI, Reuber MD: Influence of adrenocortical, androgenic, and anabolic hormones on the development of carcinoma and cirrhosis of the liver in AXC rats fed N-2-fluorenyldiacetamide. *JNCI* 1961; 27:559. (Cited in Toh[47].)
14. Gamberale F, Strindberg L, Wahlberg I: Female work capacity during the menstrual cycle: Physiologic and psychologic reactions. *Scand J Work Environ Health* 1975; 1:20.
15. Garfinkle SH: Occupations of women and black workers, 1962–74. *Monthly Labor Review*, US Dept of Labor, Bureau of Labor Statistics, 1975, p 29.

15a. Employment and Earnings, US Dept of Labor, Bureau of Labor Statistics, January 1984.

16. Grossman AS: Women in the labor force: The early years. Monthly Labor Review, US Dept of Labor, Bureau of Labor Statistics, 1975, pp 3–9.
17. *Guidelines on Pregnancy and Work*. Chicago, American College of Obstetrics and Gynecology, 1977.
18. Guzman CA, Caplan R: Cardiorespiratory response to exercise during pregnancy. *Am J Obstet Gynecol* 1970; 108:600.
19. Haenszel W, Taeuber KE: Lung cancer mortality as related to residence and smoking histories. II. White females. *J Natl Cancer Inst* 1968; 32:803. (Cited in Toh[47].)
20. Hamilton A: *Industrial Toxicology*. New York, Haifer & Bros Publishers 1934, p xv.
21. Hamilton A: Lead poisoning in potteries and tile works. US Dept of Labor, Bureau of Labor Statistics, Bull 104, 1912.
22. Henschel A: *Women in Industry—The Difference*. Transactions of the 33d Meeting of the American Conference of Governmental Industrial Hygienists, Toronto, Canada, 1971, pp 73–76.
23. Hirakawa T: Some observations on benzene poisoning. *Arch Mal Prof* 1960; 21:46. (Cited in Browning E: *Toxicity and Metabolism of Industrial Solvents*. London, Elsevier Publishing Co, 1965.)
24. Hirakawa T: Studies on poisoning by benzol and its homologues. *Jpn J Med Sci Biol* 1955; 8:275. (Cited in Browning E: *Toxicity and Metabolism of Industrial Solvents*. London, Elsevier Publishing Co, 1965.)
25. Hunter T: Chronic exposure to benzene (benzol). II. The clinical effects. *J Ind Hyg Toxicol* 1939; 21:331.
26. Klein DP: Women in the labor force: The middle years. *Monthly Labor Review*. US Dept of Labor, Bureau of Labor Statistics, 1975, pp 10–16.
27. Krasovskij GN: Species and sex differences in sensitivity to toxic substances, in *Methods Used in the USSR for Establishing Biologically Safe Levels of Toxic Substances*. Geneva, WHO, 1975, pp 109–125.
28. Lee SH, Ts'o TOT: Histological typing of lung cancers in Hong Kong. *Br J Cancer* 1963; 17:37. (Cited in Toh[47].)
29. Leuchtenberger C, et al: Cytological and cytochemical alterations in the respiratory tract of mice after exposure to cigarette smoke, influenza virus, and both. *Cancer Res* 1963; 23:555. (Cited in Toh[47].)
30. Morimoto T, Slabachova Z, Naman RK, et al: Sex differences in

physiological reactions to thermal stress. *J Appl Physiol* 1967; 22:526.

31. Morris HP, Firminger HI: Influence of sex and sex hormones on development of hepatomas and other hepatic lesions in strain AXC rats ingesting 2-diacetylaminofluoramide. *JNCI* 1956; 16:927. (Cited in Toh[47].)
32. Oliver T: *Diseases of Occupation*. New York, EP Dutton Co, 1908.
33. Oliver T: Lead poisoning and the racer. *Br Med J* 1911; 1:1096.
34. Pernoll ML, et al: Ventilation during rest and exercise during pregnancy and postpartum. *Respir Physiol* 1975; 25:295.
35. Pernoll ML, et al: Oxygen consumption at rest and during exercise in pregnancy. *Respir Physiol* 1975; 25:285.
36. Prendergast WD: The classification of the symptoms of lead poisoning. *Br Med J* 1910; 1:1164.
37. Purchase IFH, Steyn M: The metabolism of aflatoxin B in rats. *Br J Cancer* 1969; 23:800. (Cited in Toh[47].)
38. Roels HA, Lauwerys RR, Buchet JP, et al: Response of free erythrocyte porphyrin and urinary delta-aminolevulinic acid in men and women moderately exposed to lead. *Int Arch Arbeitsmed* 1975; 34:97.
39. Sato A, Nakajima T, Fujiwara T, et al: Pharmacokinetics of benzene and toluene. *Int Arch Arbeitsmed* 1974; 33:169. (Cited in Ferguson[12].)
40. Savilahti M: More than 100 cases of benzene poisoning in a shoe factory. *Arch Gerwerbepathol Gewerbehyg* 1956; 15:145 (translation).
41. Selling L: Benzol as a leucotoxin—Studies on the degeneration and regeneration of the blood and hematopoietic organs. *Johns Hopkins Hosp Rep* 1916; 17:83.
42. Seppäläinen AM, Tola S, Hernberg S, et al: Subclinical neuropathy at "safe" levels of lead exposure. *Arch Environ Health* 1975; 30:180.
43. Shinton NK: Differences in biological characteristics of various histological types of lower respiratory tract tumours. *Br J Cancer* 1963; 17:222. (Cited in Toh[47].)
44. Snook SH, Ciriello VM: Maximum weights and work loads acceptable to female workers. *J Occup Med* 1974; 16:527.
45. Stuik EJ, Zielhuis RL: Increased susceptibility of females to inorganic lead, in *Recent Advances in the Assessment of the Health Effects of Environmental Pollution*. Luxembourg, Commission of the European Communities, 1975, pp 537–541.
46. Sum AM: Female labor force participation: Why projections have been too low. *Monthly Labor Review*, US Dept of Labor, Bureau of Labor Statistics, 1977, pp 18–24.
47. Toh YC: Physiological and biochemical reviews of sex differences and carcinogenesis with particular reference to the liver. *Adv Cancer Res* 1973; 18:209.
48. Waldman E, McEaddy BJ: Where women work—An analysis by industry and occupation. *Monthly Labor Review*, US Dept of Labor, Bureau of Labor Statistics, 1974, pp 3–13.
49. Weinman KP, et al: Reactions of men and women to repeated exposure to humid heat. *J Appl Physiol* 1967; 22:533.
50. Weston Hurst E: Sexual difference in the toxicity and therapeutic amount of chemical substances, in Walpole AL, Spinks A (eds): *Symposium on the Evaluation of Drug Toxicity*. London, J & A Churchill, Ltd, 1958, pp 12–25. (Cited in Ferguson.[12])
51. Wyndham CH, Morrison JF, Williams CG: Heat reactions of male and female Caucasians. *J Appl Physiol* 1965; 20:357.

54

Reproductive Toxicology and Occupational Exposure

Jacqueline Messite, M.D.
Marcus B. Bond, M.D.

GENERAL

Research in occupational safety and health has only recently begun to focus attention on the effects of occupational exposure to chemical and physical agents on the reproductive system of either men or women.[7] This has resulted in a dearth of information to assist the occupational physician and the obstetrician in advising workers and management of the potentially deleterious effects of various agents on reproduction. Furthermore, the existing data base on the reproductive effects of occupational toxins is inadequate to serve as a guideline for the establishment of occupational health standards. With few exceptions, current standards for occupational exposures to chemical and physical agents in the work environment do not consider the reproductive effects, including mutagenesis, teratogenesis, and transplacental carcinogenesis.

The reproductive concerns, when addressed, have for the most part focused attention only on the woman's reproductive capacity and on the developmental effects in offspring solely from maternal exposures. Such a limited view fails to recognize that there are a large number of female workers of reproductive capacity who are not pregnant or currently planning pregnancy, and it does not consider the role of paternal exposure to such agents in the causation of reproductive abnormalities.

The reproductive capacity of women workers generally is in the age range of 15–45 years. During this century, most childbearing ends by the age of 35,[16] and there are many years of work outside the home for women still of childbearing capacity. According to the National Center of Health Statistics,[10] of about 3,034,000 women who had a live birth during a 12-month period in 1972–1973, an estimated 1,260,000 women (41.5%) worked during their pregnancy. This 41.5%, however, represented only about 8.8% of the estimated 14,357,000 ever-married women of reproductive age in the labor force at the time.[10] (Although the authors were not able to obtain more current data on this, it is likely that the figures would not have changed substantially.) Even if another 30% are added to include women workers whose pregnancies may not result in live births, it is clear that the number of women of childbearing age who are pregnant or who are planning pregnancies at any one time is relatively small in comparison to the total number of such women available for participation in the work force. Any sweeping policy excluding women of childbearing capacity from any particular employment is not only discriminatory but also does not allow for the participation by women workers, in cooperation with the occupational physicians, in the decision-making process concerning their employment, and also needlessly eliminates from consideration a large number of productive employees.

Many women now are employed in jobs that present no greater potential hazards than those normally encountered at home or in the community. However, a sizable number of women are currently employed in positions with significant exposures in work environments that often are not appreciated as being hazardous; e.g., laboratories and health services, the electronics industry, and dry-cleaning establishments. In addition, there is the potential that many more women may seek employment in nontraditional, hazardous jobs.

A point that needs to be emphasized is that concern for healthy offspring must include concern for paternal as well as maternal exposure. The role of paternal exposure in producing adverse effects on reproduction has been highlighted in studies of worker populations exposed to such substances as vinyl chloride and dibromochloropropane (discussed later in this chapter). Further studies may well disclose other similarly noxious agents in the work environment to which men are susceptible.

The American Medical Association's Council on Scientific Affairs' Advisory Panel on Reproductive Hazards in the Workplace prepared a report reviewing the effects of chemical exposure, in an effort to make physicians more aware of the hazards of the workplace to pregnant workers. A total of 120 chemicals were considered for reviews based on an estimate of their imminent hazard, i.e., widespread use and/or inherent toxicity. A brief introduction points out general principles, clinical applications, and aids to the recognition of a human teratogen, along with reviews and opinions for three representative chemicals (acrylonitrile, inorganic arsenic, and carbon disulfide).[4]

Table 54–1 is a graphic representation of some highlights to

TABLE 54–1.
Dynamics of Reproductive Toxicology

	STAGES OF PREGNANCY			
	PRECONCEPTION	INTRAUTERINE DEVELOPMENT		PERINATAL PERIOD
Stages of development	Gametes (sperm, ova)	1st trimester 2d trimester 3d trimester Embryo	Fetus	Infant
Vulnerable areas	Spermatogenesis Oogenesis Fertilization	Organogenesis (primarily 1st trimester)	Central nervous system late	Lactation
Major developmental effects	Mutagenesis	Teratogenesis (primarily 1st trimester)	Transplacental carcinogenesis	
Adverse manifestations	Sterility Decreased fertility Chromosomal aberrations	Implantation defects Spontaneous abortion	Premature delivery	Stillbirth Structural, behavioral or functional alterations
Parental source of exposure	Maternal and paternal		Maternal	Maternal (lactation) Paternal and maternal (home contamination)

be considered in a brief review of the dynamics of reproductive toxicology pertinent to this subject.

Preconception (Gametogenesis and Fertilization)

A chemical substance or physical agent may act directly on the germ cells so that fertilization does not take place or it may cause such severe anomalies in the zygote as to result in an early unrecognized abortion.

During the preconception period, exposure of cells to physical or chemical mutagens results in induced cytogenic damage. Damage to the germ cells of male or female workers from such exposure could result in decreased fertility, spontaneous abortion of the concepsus for which they are responsible, or to birth defects in their offspring or even in the offspring of subsequent generations. (There are only a few reports of parental exposures related to either of the latter two outcomes, although the risk is recognized.[13])

Damage to somatic cells by this exposure could possibly lead to cancer or premature aging. This damage is usually manifested as increased levels of chromosome aberrations.[4] With ionizing radiation, induction of aberrations in long-lived circulating lymphocytes has been shown to be a biologic dosimeter to estimate the absorbed dose. On the other hand, with chemicals, the situation is more complex. Mechanisms of interaction with DNA vary depending on a number of factors, including the presence of activating or deactivating enzymes, the biologic half-lives of the chemicals, and the degree of DNA repair, all of which affect the yield of aberrations. The presence of cytogenic changes cannot be used to predict specific health effects in individuals but may give an indication of the magnitude of exposure, provided the studies have been done properly and all confounding factors have been considered.[4]

It is during this preconception period that paternal exposure to mutagenic agents must be considered along with maternal exposure, for both, collectively or independently, may result in significant reproductive effects.

An unpublished NIOSH Interagency Report of a Work Group on Occupational Mutagenesis, Teratogenesis and Transplacental Carcinogenesis, in November, 1976,[13] reported that, "it is difficult to anticipate the relative sensitivity to germinal mutagenic events in men compared to nonpregnant women. Depending on the action of a particular chemical, the expected effects will differ depending on the sex of the exposed individual. Spermatogenesis involves a continuously replicating cell population with billions of cells; oogenesis is a prenatal event in mammals, and the female germ cell population is finite at birth with no further replication. Therefore, chemicals whose mechanisms of toxicity depend upon cell division would have their greatest effects in the adult on the male germ cells; chemicals affecting nonreplicating cells might have their greatest effect on the limited oocyte population. Chemical exposure which decreases the total number of germ cells would also have a more prominent effect on the female since damaged cells are not replaced as in a male." Unfortunately, our state of knowledge still is inadequate to define the mechanism of chemical mutagenesis as it relates to male and female cells. Thus, both sexes must be considered at risk from mutagenic hazards.

Most anomalous conceptions, including 95% of those with chromosomal abnormalities, rarely go to term and therefore are concentrated among spontaneous abortions. Anomalies are about 60–100 times more frequent in spontaneous abortions than in live births.[8] Errors during early intrauterine development have variously been estimated to produce a pregnancy loss in the human from 15% to 40%.[12, 15, 18] Serious defects can be detected in about 3% of newborn babies, but the number gradually rises to about 8%, including children during the first ten years of age.[12, 15] Up to 6% of these birth defects are due to known environmental agents, and at least 20%–30% have a major genetic etiology.[12] The remaining birth defects are of unknown causes and, therefore, future research into environmental components may further our awareness of these components as causes for such occurrences and in suggesting preventive measures. At least some of the causes may be found in the occupational environment.

Postconception—Maternal Organism

The maternal organism, in some ways, may be more vulnerable during pregnancy. There are alterations in detoxification mechanisms and metabolic pathways, and also there may be unusual dietary habits.[11] In addition, there are physiologic changes in blood volumes and composition, as well as alterations in lung function, the nature of which could result in increased absorption of air contaminants, particularly those that follow the inhalation route.[7]

As noted in Chapter 53, there is a progressive increase in ventilation during pregnancy, due mostly to an increase in tidal volume. There is also a decrease in arteriovenous oxygen differences, as reported by Guzman and Caplan.[5] This could mean that a pregnant woman uses a portion of respiratory and cardiovascular reserve in the pregnancy itself and, therefore, could have a reduced capacity for additional stresses. Physical factors of shift in center of gravity and resulting alterations in posture and progressively increasing weight could contribute to reduced abilities to perform physically demanding tasks. However, the *Guidelines on Pregnancy and Work*, quoted in Chapter 56, indicated that women usually have no problems continuing with work that is usual for them but may have problems adjusting to different or increased physical tasks.

In regard to increased ventilation and possible increased absorption of air contaminants, there is inadequate information on which to draw any firm conclusions.

Embryo

During the first week following fertilization, even before placental implantation, embryotoxic agents absorbed by the mother can reach the free-lying blastocyst very rapidly, and the clearance rate from the blastocyst of maternally transmitted agents is lower than their elimination rate from the maternal peripheral fluids.[19]

The first trimester, particularly the first eight-week period of embryonic organogenesis, is the time of greatest susceptibility to environmental influences, and the majority of teratologic effects are induced during this period. The drug thalidomide is a well-documented example of a substance that produces its effects only during this critical period.[9] In almost every case, the embryo is more sensitive to toxins than is the maternal organism. This is attributed to more rapid cell turnover by the embryo and fetus, their relative lack of detoxification mechanisms, and their immature biologic barriers.

Fetus

From eight weeks to term, the fetus, generally considered less vulnerable than the embryo but more susceptible than the child or adult, is subject to adverse influences that possibly could lead to physical growth retardation and postnatal behavioral and functional abnormalities. Battaglia[1] notes that the second trimester is a time of rapid fetal growth, when the placental blood flow reaches its maximum and the delivery of substances to the fetus can be very high. In general, susceptibility to teratogens decreases with gestational age, whereas susceptibility of the fetus to transplacental carcinogenesis tends to increase.[2]

Many known carcinogens can cross the placenta and result in intrauterine exposure to the embryo or fetus. Cancers that result from such exposure usually do not appear for many years (more than 15 years) after the exposure, and this latency makes the diagnosis of transplacental carcinogenesis very difficult. Cancer can be present at birth, but the environmental causes for such tumors have not been demonstrated.

Diethyl stilbestrol (DES), given as medication to pregnant women during pregnancy to avert miscarriages, has been associated with clear cell adenocarcinoma of the vagina and uterus in young adult female offspring (see section on DES). More recently, diphenylhydantoin has been suggested as a transplacental carcinogen, since four cases have been noted in 1976–1980 of neuroblastoma in newborns with fetal hydantoin syndrome. Diphenylhydantoin has occasionally caused lymphoma in adults taking the drug for epilepsy, and one would expect the children with fetal hydantoin syndrome from the same drug to also be prone to lymphoma, but this apparently is not the case.[2] To date, no known occupational exposure has been associated with transplacental carcinogenesis, but the possibility exists and should be considered in surveillance systems.

Perinatal Period—Infant

Certain developmental processes are not completed until after birth (e.g., physical growth and structural and physiologic maturation of the central nervous system and some of the endocrine glands) and may be adversely affected by environmental exposures during this period.[11] In addition, immediately following delivery, the immature metabolic system of the infant may be unable to cope with some environmental agents, thus making the infant more susceptible to their effects.

Furthermore, exposure of the infant during this period may occur from contamination of the home by the working father or mother, or from contamination of the milk in lactation. Maternal exposure to chemicals may alter the amount of lactation and the quality of the milk. Also, some chemicals may be excreted in the milk, resulting in direct exposure of the infant to potentially dangerous substances (e.g., lead, mercury, polychlorinated biphenyls) (see discussion of specific substances).

REFERENCES

1. Battaglia FC: The susceptibility of the fetus and child to chemical pollutants. Perinatal effects of chemical pollutants: Suggested studies. *Pediatrics* 1974; 53:838.
2. Bloom AD (ed): *Guidelines for Human Studies of Human Population Exposed to Mutagenic and Reproductive Hazards*. New York, March of Dimes Birth Defects Foundation, 1981, pp 84–85.
3. Bridbord K: Occupational safety and health and the reproductive process. Oral presentation at Meeting of Organization Research Counselors, Arlington, Va, May 2, 1978.

4. Council on Scientific Affairs: Effects of toxic chemicals on the reproductive system. *JAMA* 1985; 253:No. 23, June 21.
5. Guzman CA, Caplan R: Cardiorespiratory response to exercise during pregnancy. *Am J Obstet Gynecol* 1970; 108:600.
6. Hemminki K, Sorsa M, Vainio H: *Occupational Hazards and Reproduction*. New York, Hemisphere, 1985.
7. Hunt V: Pregnancy, in *Occupational Safety and Health Symposia*, 1976, NIOSH Publ 77-179, July, 1977.
8. Kline J, et al: Surveillance of spontaneous abortions. *Am J Epidemiol* 1977; 106:345.
9. Lenz W, Knapp K: Fetal malformations due to thalidomide. *Ger Med Mon* 1962; 7:253. (Cited in Strobino et al.[17])
10. National Center for Health Statistics, US Dept of HEW: Statistics needed for determining the effects of the environment on health. July 1977; *HRA* 77:1457.
11. National Center for Health Statistics, US Dept of HEW: *Advance Data, Pregnant Workers in the US*, Sept 15, 1977.
12. NIH, US Dept of HEW, PHS: *Human Health and the Environment—Some Research Needs*—2nd Task Force for Research Planning in Environmental Health Science, Publ NIH 77-1277, 1977.
13. NIOSH Interagency Report of Work Group on Occupational Mutagenesis, Teratogenesis, Transplacental Carcinogenesis, 1977 (unpublished).
14. *Principles for Evaluating Health Risks to Progeny Associated with Exposure to Chemicals During Pregnancy: Environmental Health Criteria 30*. Geneva, World Health Organization, 1984.
15. Shepard TH, Miller JR: Methods for detecting teratogenic agents in man. *Environ Health Perspect* 1976; 13:141.
16. Stellman J: *Women's Work, Women's Health, Myths and Realities*. New York, Pantheon Books, 1977.
17. Strobino BR, Kline J, Stein Z: *Chemical and Physical Exposures of Parents: Effects on Human Reproduction and Offspring. Early Human Development*. New York, Elsevier North-Holland Inc, 1978.
18. Manson JM: Human and laboratory animal test systems available for detection of reproductive failure. *Prev Med* 1978; 7:322.
19. Lutwak-Mann C: Drugs and the blastocyst, in Boréus L (ed): *Fetal Pharmacology*. New York, Raven Press, 1973.

REPRODUCTIVE EFFECTS FROM SELECTED OCCUPATIONAL EXPOSURES

Table 54–2 is a list of some of the reproductive toxins that can be found in the work environment. The substances listed have been reported to have significant reproductive effects in animals and/or human beings. It is predictable that more substances will be added as further research in this area is performed.

Substances that have been found to be mutagenic only in microbiologic systems and/or in DNA studies have not been included in this chapter. Although such findings are helpful in screening for carcinogens (which probably are related to mutagens), the findings solely in these screening tests can be regarded as suspicious, but at this time do not provide sufficient information to serve as a basis for judging the safety of occupational exposures or in predicting reproductive effects from the occupational environment.

The discussion in this chapter is essentially limited to the reproductive effects of these agents. Information on their general toxicity may be found elsewhere in this volume.

LEAD

Few substances have received as much attention in regard to reproductive effects as has lead. Lead has long been known as an abortifacient[18, 19] and, more recently, lead has been associated with premature deliveries and premature rupture of the membranes, and minor congenital abnormalities even at relatively low maternal and fetal blood lead levels.[9, 9a] The reaction to the early reports of the effects on reproduction essentially ignored effects on men. In England, women were not permitted employment in the English potteries and white lead industries. The response to more recent reports of the adverse reproductive effects on both men and women workers continues to focus on the women lead workers, and the inadequate data have resulted in conflicting opinions as to the placement of women workers in lead operations.

Lead compounds readily pass the placental barrier, and levels of lead in the fetal tissues correlate well with those of the mother. Some studies indicate fetal blood levels lower than those of the mother, but this is not a consistent finding.[3, 9–11] Regardless, embryonic and other rapidly growing tissues are more vulnerable to lead than are adult tissues and, therefore, levels of lead producing adverse effects in the embryo probably are lower than those producing adverse effects in adults.

Lead is known to be present in milk of lactating mothers who have been exposed, so further exposure to newborns is possible by this route. In addition, exposure to the infant can occur from contamination of the home by the mother or father who works with lead[2] and brings the lead-containing dust into the home on work clothing and shoes.

Several excellent reviews of the effects of lead on reproduction have been published.[1, 4, 12, 15, 20] These reviews refer to human studies that have shown lead to be associated with sterility (male and female), abnormal spermatogenesis, spontaneous abortions, stillbirths, increased infant mortality, decreased infant birth weights, slow infant development, and mental retardation. Animal studies corroborating all of the above have also been reported and emphasize the association of lead with impotency, sterility, mutagenesis, and decreased learning ability in the offspring following lead exposure of the parent.[6, 23]

It is recognized that women are more prolonged direct sources of exposure to the products of conception than are men, and lead exposure from the maternal source can continue beyond delivery through lactation; nonetheless, alterations in fertility have been reported in both men and women and genetic changes can be transmitted by either sex.[16, 18, 22]

Concern for the reproductive effects of lead exposure in male workers necessitates further research; this aspect of the problem must be clarified in order to protect the reproductive capability and the offspring of all workers. Lancranjan et al.[16] studied 150 lead storage battery workers (men) and found that at mean blood levels of 52.8 ± 21.0 μg/100 ml blood, a significant alteration from the controls was noted in spermatogenesis, namely, asthenospermia, hypospermia, and teratospermia, and they reported a decrease in libido and orgasm and an increase in "pathologic erections and ejaculations." Even in workers with slightly increased lead absorption (mean of 41 ± 12.0 μg/100 ml blood), significant differences in asthenospermia and hypospermia were found, as well as alterations in the sexual dynamics noted previously. Unfortunately, the authors were not able to obtain reliable information on reproductive performance of the subjects with respect to the number of normal pregnancies per couple or the frequency of miscarriages, spontaneous abortions, or abnormal births. Alterations in reproductive capabilities in males have been noted in animal studies. Hildebrand et al.[14] reported on the effects of lead acetate ingestion on reproduction in male rats. With blood leads of 30 μg/100 ml blood, they found a 70% reduction in testicular weight, impotency, and reduced sperm motility.

OSHA's occupational air standard is 50 μg lead/cu m of air and biologic standard of 40 μg/100 ml blood (Federal Register 10-13-78). In order to be certain that this level is protective for men, further studies in lead-exposed male workers are needed to evaluate the significance of the effects on sperm at relatively low lead exposure levels, as noted previously.

A current question is whether these proposed environmental and biologic standards provide an adequate margin of safety for occupational exposure of pregnant women. To consider this question, cognizance must be taken of the greater susceptibility of the fetus than the adult to toxic effects of lead, with particular regard to the subtle and, at times, delayed behavioral and neurologic effects and the early alterations in porphyrin metabolism associated with heme synthesis.

Lead is well recognized as a neurotoxin, with effects on both the central and peripheral nervous systems. Furthermore, it is generally agreed that the developing immature nervous system, especially in the embryo and fetus, is more sensitive to lead's neurotoxic action than is the nervous system in adults or even in older children.

Lead interferes with the biosynthesis of heme at several enzymatic steps, with the utilization of iron and with globin synthesis in erythrocytes, and an early manifestation of lead exposure in man is associated with lead's interference in heme biosynthesis. Table 54–3 summarizes the no-detected levels for various lead effects by blood leads (μg of lead/100 ml blood).[24] It is likely that a level of exposure that will prevent any significant alterations in the heme biosynthesis pathways will prevent the clinical and subclinical neurologic manifestations and probably the reproductive effects in both men and women.[24]

The earliest physiologic alteration from lead absorption is a decrease in aminolevulinic acid dehydratase (ALAD) activity, which may be found with blood lead levels as low as 10 μg/100 ml. However, hemesynthesis probably is not significantly affected even if the ALAD is markedly depressed.[25] Zielhuis reports the no-effect level for 70% ALAD inhibition to be 25–30 μg lead/100 ml blood in adults and 20–25 μg/100 ml in children.[25] After ALAD inhibition, elevations of free erythrocyte porphyrins (FEP), inhibition of erythrocyte ATPase, and elevations of aminolevulinic acid in urine (ALAU) and coproporphyrin in urine (CPU) follow in order.[24]

In 1978, the Centers for Disease Control (CDC) reported, "the statistical likelihood of childhood symptoms and permanent damage increases at least arithmetically with confirmed blood lead values above 30 μg/100 ml and EP values above 60 μg/ml."[26] Since the embryo and fetus may be more susceptible than the child, it would be prudent to maintain the exposure to lead of the products of conception in utero so that the fetal blood lead is at least below 30 μg/100 ml. However, CDC, in its latest proposal, indicated that a fetal blood level of 30 μg/100 ml affords little or no margin for safety and should be lowered to 25 μg/100 ml.[27] Blood lead levels in the working woman would have to be at or below that concentration.

How can this be translated into an acceptable exposure level for airborne lead for pregnant women? As a result of a review of epidemiologic studies on lead exposures wherein environmental and biologic data were included, Bridbord[4] estimated for adult men that occupational exposures to 50 μg lead/cu m of air would be associated with blood leads ranging from 35 to 45 μg lead/100 ml blood. Even though women at low levels of exposure have been noted to have lower blood lead levels than do men, it is not certain that the existing OSHA standard is truly protective of the fetus.

REFERENCES

1. Baetjer A: *Women in Industry, Their Health and Efficiency*. Philadelphia, WB Saunders Co, 1946, pp 145–156.
2. Baker EL, et al: Lead poisoning in children of lead workers: Home contamination with industrial dust. *N Engl J Med* 1977; 296:260.
3. Barltrop D: Transfer of lead to the human fetus, in Barltrop D, Burland WL (eds): *Mineral Metabolism in Pediatrics*. Philadelphia, FA Davis Co, 1969, pp 135–151.
4. Bridbord K: Review of lead toxicity. Conference on Women and the Workplace. Society of Occupational and Environmental Hygiene, June 17–19, 1976, pp 227–231.
5. Bridbord K: Lead exposure and women: Medical aspects, prevention. *Prev Med* 1978; 7:311.
6. Carson TL, et al: Slowed learning in lambs prenatally exposed to lead. *Arch Environ Health* 1974; 29:154.
7. Centers for Disease Control, US Dept of Health and Human Services: Increased lead absorption in children of lead workers—Vermont. *MMWR* 1977; Feb 25.
8. Centers for Disease Control, US Dept of Health and Human Services: Lead poisoning in children of battery plant employees—North Carolina. *Epidemiologic Notes and Reports* 1977; Sept 30, vol 26, no 29.
9. Fahim MS, Fahim Z, Hall DG: Effects of subtoxic lead levels on pregnant women in the state of Missouri. Presented at International Conference on Heavy Metals in the Environment, Toronto, Canada, October, 1975.
10. Gershanik JJ, Brooks GG, Little JA: Blood lead values in pregnant women and their offspring. *Am J Obstet Gynecol* 1975; 119:408.
11. Haas T, et al: Untersuchunge über die okologische bleibelastung im kindesalter (in German—English summary), in Int. Symp. Environ. Health Aspects of Lead, USEPA, October, 1972.
12. Hardy HL: What is the status of knowledge of the toxic effect of lead on identifiable groups in the population? editorial. *Clin Pharmacol Ther* 1966; 7:713.
13. Hernberg S: Lead, in Zenz C (ed): *Occupational Medicine: Principles and Practical Applications*. Chicago, Year Book Medical Publishers, 1975, pp 715–769.
14. Hildebrand D, et al: Effect of lead acetate on reproduction. *Am J Obstet Gynecol* 1973; 115:1058.
15. Infante PF, Wagoner JR: The effects of lead on reproduction, in *Proceedings of Conference on Women and the Workplace*. Society of

TABLE 54–2.
Reproductive Effects—A Summary

AGENT	SYSTEMIC EFFECTS*: NEUROLOGIC	HEPATIC	RENAL	HEMATOLOGIC	CARDIOVASCULAR	PULMONARY	OTHER SPECIAL EFFECTS	SUGGESTED BIOLOGIC TESTING	CARCINOGENESIS	PARENTAL EXPOSURE	DECREASED FERTILITY (INCLUDES DECREASED SPERMATOGENESIS)†	MUTAGENESIS (CHROMOSOMAL ABERRATION)	SPONTANEOUS ABORTION	LOW BIRTH WEIGHT (PREMATURITY)
Heavy Metals														
Lead (inorganic)	+		+					Blood lead Blood zinc protoporphyrins Urine ALA Urine coproporphyrins		Maternal	+1 +4	+7	+1 +2 +8	+3
										Paternal	+1 +5 +10	+7	+1 +8	+1 +7 +8
Cadmium		+	+	+	+	+		Urine cadmium Low molecular weight proteins in urine	? Prostate	Maternal	+1 +3 −8	+9 −10 −11	−8	+4 +8 +13
										Paternal	+1 (testicular damage) −2	−12		
Mercury	+		+					Blood mercury Urine mercury		Maternal	?2	Microbiologic +5, +6		+9
										Paternal	−7 −8 ?11 ?12			
Organic Solvents														
Benzene	+			+				CBC Urine phenols	+ Leukemia	Maternal	−1 +5	−1 +2 +3 +4		
Halogenated Hydrocarbons														
2-Chlorobutadiene (chloroprene)	+	+	+	+		+		Liver function tests	? Skin Liver	Maternal	+1	Microbiologic +4, −5, +6	?3	?3
										Paternal	+1 −2 +3		?3	
Dibromochloropropane		+	+				Azoospermia, oligospermia	Sperm count Serum testosterone	? Gastric, mammary in female rats	Maternal	+4	Microbiologic ?5		
Epichlorohydrin		+	+			+		Liver function tests	? Skin			Microbiologic +1		
										Paternal	+2 +3 +4 Single dose			

?Variable or questionable data.
*Plus signs indicate positive data; minus signs, negative data.
†Numbers throughout refer to authors listed in table.

STILLBIRTH AND NEONATAL DEATHS	CONGENITAL ANOMALIES	BEHAVIORAL OR DEVELOPMENTAL DISABILITIES	OTHER RELATED REPRODUCTIVE EFFECTS	REFERENCES FOR REPRODUCTIVE EFFECTS (SEE TEXT)	WORKPLACE AIR STANDARDS: OSHA: EXISTING	WORKPLACE AIR STANDARDS: NIOSH: RECOMMENDED	WORKPLACE AIR STANDARDS: NIOSH: REPRODUCTIVE CONSIDERATION
+1 +4 +8 +1	+11(minor)	+4 +6 +8 +9		1. Oliver 2. Pindborg 3. Fahim 4. Rom (review) 5. Lancranjan 6. Carson 7. Infante (review) 8. Bridbord (review) 9. Palmisano 10. Hildebrand 11. Needleman	50 μg/m³ air 40 μg/100 ml blood (Nov. 14, 1978)	40 μg/m³ air blood lead 60 μg/100 ml (May, 1978)	Women of reproductive age Blood Pb < 30 μg/100 ml
+4	+4 ?5 +7 +6 ?8	+13	Zinc protective action +3 +7	1. Parisek 2. Nordberg 3. Kar 4. Chernoff 5. Barr 6. Ishizu 7. Ferm 8. Tsvetkova 9. Shiraishe 10. Bui 11. Epstein 12. Galiavod 13. Webster	*Fume* 0.1 mg/m³ (ceiling—0.3 mg/m³) *Dust* 0.2 mg/m³ (ceiling—0.6 mg/m³)	40 μg/m³	?
+5 +10	+3 +9 +10	+1 +3 +4 +10		1. Harada (1968) 2. Bakir 3. Amin-Zaki 4. Pierce, Snyder 5. Ramel 6. Fahmy 7. WHO (Firman) 8. Harada (1971) 9. Oharazawa 10. Spyker 11. Suter 12. Lee	Inorganic 0.1 mg/m³ Organic 0.01 mg/m³	Inorganic 0.05 mg/m³	*WHO recom* Org. mercury none Koos and Longo review recommends elem. Hg 10 μg/m³ Inorg. and phenyl 20 μg/m³ Org. none
	+6			1. Forni 2. Vigliani 3. Tough 4. Wurster-Hill 5. Gofmekler 6. Watanabe	1 ppm	1 ppm	?
	?3 −2			1. von Oettingen 2. Culik 3. Sanotskii 4. Bartsch 5. Litton Biometics 6. Vogel	25 ppm	1 ppm	Probably
				1. Torkelson 2. Rakhmatulayeve 3. Faydysh 4. Reznick 5. Rosencrauz	10 ppb (emerg. std.)	10 ppb	Yes
−4 (single dose)				1. NIOSH Review 2. Hahn 3. Cooper 4. Epstein	1 ppm	1 ppm	?

(continued)

TABLE 54–2. *Continued*

AGENT	SYSTEMIC EFFECTS*: NEUROLOGIC	HEPATIC	RENAL	HEMATOLOGIC	CARDIOVASCULAR	PULMONARY	OTHER SPECIAL EFFECTS	SUGGESTED BIOLOGIC TESTING	CARCINOGENESIS	PARENTAL EXPOSURE	DECREASED FERTILITY (INCLUDES DECREASED SPERMATOGENESIS)†	MUTAGENESIS (CHROMOSOMAL ABERRATION)	SPONTANEOUS ABORTION	LOW BIRTH WEIGHT (PREMATURITY)
Ethylene dibromide		+	+			+			+	Maternal	+3 (avian)	microbiologic +3		
										Paternal	+1 +2			
Tetrachloroethylene (Perchloroethylene	+		+			+			?	Maternal	−2 ?1			?1
Polychlorinated biphenyls (PCBs)		+		+			Chloracne, swollen eyelids, hyperpigmentation of skin	Blood analysis Adipose tissue analysis Serum triglycerides	? + liver in animals	Maternal	+1 +6 +7	microbiologic (weak) ?9 −8	+7	+1 +2
										Paternal	+4			
Vinyl Chloride	+	+			+		Acroosteolysis	Liver function tests	+ Angiosarcoma liver	Maternal		microbiologic +1, +2, +3	+4	
										Paternal	+4	+6		
Hypoxia Carbon monoxide	+			+	+			Carboxyhemoglobin		Maternal	+8		Absorption of fetal rats	+1 +3
										Paternal			+6	+5
Anesthetic Gases Halogenated gases, e.g., halothane methoxyfluorane	+	+							? Leukemia, lymphatic system	Maternal			?2 +3 +4 +5 +7 +9 +12	?2 ?3 +9
										Paternal	−5		+3 −5 +7 +8 −9 −12	−9
Pesticides Carbaryl	+									Maternal ?	(only high doses) +10	microbiologic −1, −2, −3, ?4, ?6	−8	
										Paternal	?6 (high doses) (lower doses) −6 +10 +11			

?Variable or questionable data.
*Plus signs indicate positive data; minus signs, negative data.
†Numbers throughout refer to authors listed in table.

STILLBIRTH AND NEONATAL DEATHS	CONGENITAL ANOMALIES	BEHAVIORAL OR DEVELOPMENTAL DISABILITIES	OTHER RELATED REPRODUCTIVE EFFECTS	REFERENCES FOR REPRODUCTIVE EFFECTS (SEE TEXT)	WORKPLACE AIR STANDARDS		
					OSHA	NIOSH	
					EXISTING	RECOMMENDED	REPRODUCTIVE CONSIDERATION
	+4			1. Amir 2. Edwards 3. NIOSH Review 4. Short	20 ppm	1 mg/m³	?
?1	?1			1. Schwetz 2. Carpenter	100 ppm	50 ppm	No
+7 +1	+1 −5	−2 −5	Menstrual alteration +3, +7	1. NIOSH Review 2. Funatsu 3. Kusuda 4. Schwartz 5. Inoue 6. Allen 7. Barsotti 8. Green 9. Wyndham	42% chlorine 1 mg/m³ 54% chlorine— 0.5 mg/m³	1 µg/m³	Yes
+4	+4, −5			1. Bartsch 2. Magnussen 3. Huberman 4. Infante 5. Edmonds 6. Ducatman	1 ppm	1 ppm	?
Reported in humans, animals	Neurologic sequelae; brain damage	+5 +2, +4, +5, +6	Decreased litter size Decreased survival Decreased libido (hypoxic)	1. Astrup 2. Ginsberg 3. Grahn 4. Leway 5. Longo 6. Wells 7. Williams 8. Kamet	50 ppm	35 ppm	No
	?2 −3 ?5 +6 +7 +9 +10 +11 +12 −5 (major) +5 (minor) +7 +8 +12			1. Vaisman 2. Askrog 3. Cohen 4. Knill Jones 5. Corbett 6,7. ASA 8. Garska 9. Chang 10. Schwetz 11. Spence	Not specified	Halogenated anesthetics 2 ppm based on weight of special gas sampled not >1 hr	?
−8	−5 −6 ?7 −8 +9			1. Epstein 2. Achiyama 3. Elespuru 4. Brazeskij 5. Benson 6. Weil, 1972, 1073 7. Robens 8. Dougherty 9. Smalley 10. Shtenberg 11. Whorton	5 mg/m³	5 mg/m³	Probably

(continued)

TABLE 54–2. *Continued*

AGENT	SYSTEMIC EFFECTS*: NEUROLOGIC	HEPATIC	RENAL	HEMATOLOGIC	CARDIOVASCULAR	PULMONARY	OTHER SPECIAL EFFECTS	SUGGESTED BIOLOGIC TESTING	CARCINOGENESIS	PARENTAL EXPOSURE	DECREASED FERTILITY (INCLUDES DECREASED SPERMATOGENESIS)†	MUTAGENESIS (CHROMOSOMAL ABERRATION)	SPONTANEOUS ABORTION	LOW BIRTH WEIGHT (PREMATURITY)
Chlorinated Hydrocarbons, e.g., Chlordane				+				Fat biopsy		Maternal and childhood				
Chlordecone (Kepone)	+	+					Pleuritic and joint pains; visual disturbance	Blood analysis	? Liver	Maternal Paternal	+3 +1 +2 +3			
Estrogenic Compounds Diethylstilbestrol (DES)					+		Women—intermenstrual Men—gynecomastia	Blood analysis	+ Vaginal adenocarcinoma; ? breast	Maternal Paternal	+5 +2 +5 highest dose only +7			
Ionizing Radiation X-ray and gamma rays				+			Gastrointestinal disorder	Personal film badge or pocket dosimetry; thermoluminescent dosimetry	Blood +	Maternal	+2	+1 +2		+1
Microwaves	+						Cataract eyes			Maternal Paternal	 +1 −2	 ?5	+4 (Miscarriages)	
Miscellaneous Substances Carbon disulfide	+			+	+		Retinopathy	Urine iodine—azide test		Maternal Paternal	?1 −2 −3 +5 −7 limited exposure +3 +4	−9	?1 −2 +6	+6
Ethylene oxide				+		+	Headache; eye irritation; respiratory irritation	CBC		Maternal Paternal	+1 ?3 ?3	+ microbiologic +4 +2 +6	±5	
Ethylene thiourea							Thyroid depressant		+ Liver, thyroid	Maternal				
Glycidyl ethers	+						Skin—strong irritant and sensitizer			Paternal	Mice +4	?2		

?Variable or questionable data.
*Plus signs indicate positive data; minus signs, negative data.
†Numbers throughout refer to authors listed in table.

STILLBIRTH AND NEONATAL DEATHS	CONGENITAL ANOMALIES	BEHAVIORAL OR DEVELOPMENTAL DISABILITIES	OTHER RELATED REPRODUCTIVE EFFECTS	REFERENCES FOR REPRODUCTIVE EFFECTS (SEE TEXT)	WORKPLACE AIR STANDARDS: OSHA EXISTING	NIOSH RECOMMENDED	NIOSH REPRODUCTIVE CONSIDERATION
			? Neuro-blastoma ? Blood dys-crasias	1. Infante review	0.5 mg/m^3		Insufficient data
				1. NIOSH review 2. Good 3. Huber			
		?3 −2 +1 +5 ?3 −2	Adenosis +1, +5 Adeno-carcinoma Urinary tract (males) +4	1. Herbst 1971, 1975, 1984 2. Gill 1976, 1981 3. Lanier 4. Welch 5. McLachlan 6. Coron. Drug Project 7. Harrington 8. Greenwald	Not specified	Not specified	Insufficient data
+1	+1	+1		1. NCRP (Report No. 53) 1977 2. Voelz *(Occupational Medicine)*			NCRP Recommendation Pregnancy 0.5 rem/full pregnancy
	+3 +4		Menstrual alterations +4	1. Lancranjan 2. Siekierzynski 3. Menicke 4. Marha 5. Sigler	10 mw/cm^2		FDA/Bur. of Rad. Health recommends 1 mw/cm^2 max for pregnant women
	−2 ?8 ?8		Increased menstrual bleeding +1 +5	1. Erhardt 2. Finkova 3. Jindrichova 4. Lancranjan 5. Vasilyeva 6. Petrov 7. Wakasuki 8. Barilyak 9. NIOSH	20 ppm	1 ppm (3 mg/m^3)	?
				1. Loveless 2. Emhee 3. NIOSH Review 4. Ehrenberg 5. Hemminki 6. Yager	50 ppm	50 ppm ceiling not >75 ppm (15 min)	Inadequate data
	+1 +2			1. Stula 2. Khera	No standard (minimize exposure)	No standard (minimize exposure)	
			Testicular degeneration + 2,3,4	1. Pullin 2. NIOSH Criteria Document 3. Hine 4. Shimkin	45 mg/m^3 AGE 270 mg/m^3 BGE 2.8 mg/m^3 DGE 240 mg/m^3 IGE 60 mg/m^3 PGE	(mg/m^3) 45 AGE 30 BGE 1 DGE 240 IGE 5 PGE (all ceiling—15 min)	?

TABLE 54–3.
No-Detected Effect Levels in Terms of Pb-B (μg of Lead per 100 ml of Blood)*

NO-DETECTED EFFECT LEVEL	EFFECT	POPULATION
<10	Erythrocyte ALAD inhibition	Adults, children
20–25	FEP	Children
20–30	FEP	Adult, female
25–35	FEP	Adult, male
30–40	Erythrocyte ATPase inhibition	General
40	ALA excretion in urine	Adults, children
40	CP excretion in urine	Adults
40	Anemia	Children
40–50	Peripheral neuropathy	Adults
50	Anemia	Adults
50–60	Minimal brain dysfunction	Children
60–70	Minimal brain dysfunction	Adults
60–70	Encephalopathy	Children
>80	Encephalopathy	Adults

*From World Health Organization: *Environmental Criteria 3: Lead.* Geneva, WHO, 1977.

Occupational and Environmental Hygiene, June 17–19, Washington, DC, 1976.

16. Lancranjan I, et al: Reproductive ability of workmen occupationally exposed to lead. *Arch Environ Health* 1975; 30:396.
16a. Needleman HL, Rabinowitz M, Leviton A: The relationship between prenatal exposure to lead and congenital abnormalities. *JAMA* 1984; 251:2956.
17. Oliver T: *Diseases of Occupation*. New York, EP Dutton, 1908.
18. Oliver T: Lead poisoning and the racer. *Br Med J* 1911; 1:1096.
19. Pindborg S: Om solveroglodforgiftning i Danmark. *Ugeskr Laeger* 1945; 107:1. (Cited in Rom[20].)
20. Rom WN: Effects of lead on the female and reproduction: A review. *Mt Sinai J Med NY* 1976; 43:542.
21. *Suspected Carcinogens, A Subfile of the Registry of Toxic Effects of Chemical Substances,* ed 2. Atlanta, Ga, US Dept of Health, Education and Welfare, Public Health Service, Centers for Disease Control, NIOSH, 1977.
22. Torelli G: L'influenza cell avvelena mento cronico caprombo sulla discendexza. *Med Lav* 1930; 21:110. (Cited in Hamilton A, Hardy H: *Industrial Toxicology*, ed 2. New York, Paul B Hoeber, Inc 1949, pp 119–121.)
23. Varma MM, Joshi SR, Adeyimi, AO: Mutagenicity and infertility following administration of lead sub-acetate to Swiss male mice. *Experientia* 1974; 30:486.
24. WHO: *Environmental Health Criteria 3: Lead*. Geneva, 1977.
25. Zielhuis RL: Dose response relationships for inorganic lead. I. Biochemical and hematological responses. II. Subjective and functional responses. Chr. sequelae. No response levels. *Int Arch Occup Environ Health* 1975; 35:1–18, 19–35.
26. Centers for Disease Control, US Dept of Health, Education and Welfare: Increased lead absorption and lead poisoning in young children. Atlanta, Ga, CDC, March, 1975.
27. Centers for Disease Control: Preventing lead poisoning in young children. Atlanta, Ga, CDC, US Dept of Health and Human Services, Public Health Service, September 1984.

BENZENE (BENZOL)

Benzene is an organic solvent. It is present in such industries as gas and coke manufacturing and has enormous usage in others: chemical, printing and lithography, paint, rubber, dry cleaning, adhesives, petroleum and coatings. It is used chiefly as an intermediate in producing other organic chemicals such as phenol, cyclohexane, and styrene toluene and in the manufacture of certain detergents and pesticides, and small amounts are present in paint removers.[7] Large quantities are used in chemical laboratories and in pharmaceutical-making as a solvent, extractant, or reactant. It is present in gasoline (in the United States, 0.3%–2%; in Europe, 5%–16%) and in numerous hydrocarbon mixtures. In the United States, in 1976, benzene production was estimated to be 5 billion kg, and this vast production suggests potential widespread worker contact. NIOSH[7] estimates that about 2 million persons in the U.S. work force are potentially exposed to benzene.

Benzene is well known for its deleterious effects on the hematopoietic system, the most prominent effect, in earlier reports, being depression of single or multiple elements of the blood, including anemia, thrombocytopenia, and/or leukopenia to aplastic anemia.[1, 4] More recently, emphasis has been placed on the role of exposure to benzene in the etiology of leukemia, particularly acute myelogenous leukemia, and lymphatic and erythroleukemia. According to Vigliani and Saita,[12] the risk of death from leukemia in subjects exposed to benzene is 20-fold that of the general population. Vigliani and Forni[11] have noted from their studies in Italy that there are more cases of leukemia than of pancytopenia, which has led to the belief that the latter cases may, in fact, be examples of aleukemia or hemocytoblastic leukopenic leukemia.[10]

Studies evaluating the reproductive toxicity of male or female workers exposed to benzene have not been reported. One interesting case involving pregnancy was noted by Forni et al.,[2] in which a patient, while severely pancytopenic following exposure to benzene during the prior year and with severe hemorrhagic problems, delivered an apparently normal boy. Chromosome studies in the patient showed an increased rate of chromosome aberrations; however, a cytogenetic study of the peripheral blood performed on the newborn boy did not show chromosomal abnormalities. Subsequently, the patient had another pregnancy and delivered a normal daughter.

Chromosomal aberrations in peripheral blood lymphocytes and in bone marrow cells have been found in benzene workers with or without signs of benzene toxicity.[8, 11, 14] Vigliani and Forni,[11] in commenting on the results of cytogenic studies in subjects, including some who have, or have recovered from, benzene hemopathy as well as a number who had exposure but no toxic manifestations, noted that the rate of chromosome changes in the peripheral blood lymphocytes of workers exposed to benzene was higher than in the controls. For those with benzene hemopathy, the chromosomal aberrations were noted in the peripheral blood lymphocytes and in bone marrow cells, and the changes persisted several years after exposure ceased. No such changes were found in toluene and xylene workers as compared with controls, and no further cases of aplastic anemia were noted in the workers when these solvents replaced benzene as solvents of the inks and glues. Several investigators[11, 14] have suggested from their observations in cases of leukemia associated with benzene exposure that these workers may have a genetic predisposition for such effect.

There have been very few studies in animals on the reproductive effects of benzene. In a critical evaluation of benzene toxicity edited by Laskin and Goldstein,[5] one study is described involving groups of female rats exposed continually (24 hours) to 670, 63.3, 56.6, 20.4, 5.6 and 1 mg/cu m of benzene vapor (209.7, 19.8, 17.7, 6.4, 1.8 and 0.3 ppm) for 10–15 days before impregnation. At the highest concentration (209.7 ppm), there was complete absence of pregnancy and at 19.8 ppm, resorption of embryos was observed in 1 of the 10 treated dams. The number of offspring per female was inversely related to the benzene concentration.[3] The authors note further that there has been only one reported animal study of teratogenicity and benzene exposure. In this experiment, groups of pregnant mice were given a single subcutaneous injection of 3 ml of benzene per kilogram body weight on the 11th–15th day of gestation, respectively, and the fetuses were delivered by cesarean section of the mother on the 19th gestation day. Malformed fetuses occurred more frequently in the group treated on the 13th day of pregnancy than in other groups, and the anomalies included cleft palate, agnathia, and micrognathia. The decrease in the maternal white cell count and the increase in body weight in the mother after benzene administration during pregnancy were similar in mice with or without malformed fetuses.[13]

A Litton Bionetics Company report prepared for the EPA in 1977 revealed a study that demonstrated fetotoxic effects in rats exposed to 10 ppm of benzene during the middle trimester of gestation, the lowest dose reported for this effect. At about the same time, the Exxon Corporation submitted a notice under the Toxic Substances Control Act to the EPA that stated that benzene showed weak toxic effects in pregnant females and fetuses of experimental animals at 50 ppm, weak teratogenic effects at 500 ppm, gonadal effects in 50 male animals at a concentration of 80 ppm, and fetotoxic effects in rats at a concentration of 10 ppm. The submission reviewed two studies by Exxon and several new references. The Exxon studies concentrated on the reproductive effects of benzene inhalation in female experimental animals, apparently because Exxon's literature search failed to identify sufficient information on the reproductive effects of benzene in females. The EPA stated that the Exxon summary indicated that benzene exposure in females could lead to acquired blood dyscrasias, abnormal uterine bleeding and possibly sterility (due to ovarian disturbances), mutagenesis, and/or teratogenesis (due to benzene-induced malformed embryos that subsequently are aborted spontaneously).[9]

The NIOSH, in its revised recommendation for a benzene standard,[6] has concluded that benzene is leukemogenic and, because it causes progressive malignant disease of the blood-forming organs, should be regulated as a carcinogen. As a result, the NIOSH recommendation is that exposure to benzene be kept to a minimum and not to exceed 1 ppm (3.5 mg/cu m) for a two hour period.

The present OSHA standard is an eight-hour time-weighted average (TWA) of 10 ppm with a ceiling limit of 25 ppm and a maximum peak concentration of 50 ppm for a ten-minute period. However, in 1977, OSHA issued an emergency temporary standard reducing the permissible exposure level to 1 ppm (42 CFR 22516, May 3, 1977), but a temporary stay of this standard was granted by the Fifth Circuit Court of Appeals. (American Petroleum Institute vs. OSHA 77-1516, May 20, 1977). In 1978, OSHA promulgated a new permanent standard limiting employee exposure to 1 ppm as an eight-hour TWA. Also proposed were a ceiling limit of 5 ppm for any 15-minute period and limits on eye and skin contact as well as various industrial hygiene and medical surveillance provisions (43 CFR 5918, Feb. 10, 1978). This standard also was vacated by the Fifth Circuit Court of Appeals in 1978 (API vs. OSHA 581 F2d 493) and the decision was upheld in 1980 by the U.S. Supreme Court (Industrial Union Department, AFL-CIO vs. API, 488 U.S. 607, 1978).

In 1983, OSHA announced its intention to expedite rule-making on benzene and requested information developed since 1977 concerning the health effects of benzene and its toxicologic properties (48 CFR 31412, July 8, 1983). At this time an internal proposal to reduce the permissible eight-hour TWA level from 10 ppm to 1 is under review, but the official standard

REFERENCES

1. Erf LA, Rhoads CP: The hematologic effects of benzene (benzol) poisoning. *J Ind Hyg Toxicol* 1939; 21:421.
2. Forni A, Cappelini A, Pacifico E, et al: Chromosome changes and evolution in subjects with past exposure to benzene. *Arch Environ Health* 1971; 23:385.
3. Gofmekler VA: Effect on embryonic development of benzene and formaldehyde in inhalation treatments. *Hyg Sanit* 1968; 33:327.
4. Greenburg L, Mayers MR, Goldwater L, et al: Benzene (benzol) poisoning in the rotogravure printing industry in New York City. *J Ind Hyg Toxicol* 1939; 21:395.
5. Laskin S, Goldstein DB (eds): Benzene toxicity—a critical evaluation. *J Toxicol Environ Health* 1977; Suppl 11, pp 1–148.
6. National Institute for Occupational Safety and Health: *Revised Recommendation for an Occupational Exposure Standard for Benzene*. NIOSH, DHEW, 1976.
7. National Institute for Occupational Safety and Health: *Criteria for a Recommended Standard: Occupational Exposure to Benzene*, DHEW, PHS, NIOSH, 74–137, 1974.
8. Tough IM, Court Brown WM: Chromosome aberrations and exposure to ambient benzene. *Lancet* 1965; 1:684.
9. US Occupational Safety and Health Reporter (BNA). Washington, DC, Dec 28, 1978.
10. Vigliani EC: Leukemia associated with benzene exposure. *Ann NY Acad Sci* 1976; 271:143.
11. Vigliani EC, Forni A: Benzene, chromosome changes and leukemia. *J Occup Med* 1969; 11:148.
12. Vigliani EC, Saita G: Benzene and leukemia. *N Engl J Med* 1964; 271:872.
13. Watanabe GI, Yoshida S: The teratogenic effect of benzene in pregnant mice. *Acta Med Biol* 1970; 17:285.
14. Wurster-Hill DH, Cornwell GG, McIntyre OR: Chromosomal aberrations and neoplasm—a family study. *Cancer* 1974; 33:72.
15. Zenz C: Benzene—Attempts to establish a lower exposure standard in the United States. A review. *Scand J Work Environ Health* 1978; 4:103.

CADMIUM

A detailed discussion of cadmium and its compounds is given by Preuss in Chapter 33. There are no conclusive reports arising from occupational exposures; discussion in this section is based on animal studies.

Growth retardation and anemia have been found in young animals following chronic cadmium poisoning whereas in adult animals hypochromic microcytic anemia is characteristic. Webster[25] exposed mice to 10, 20, or 40 ppm cadmium in their drinking water throughout pregnancy. The offspring were obviously much smaller than normal and very anemic. This study confirms the extreme sensitivity of fetal growth to cadmium concentrations as low as 10 ppm. The fact that the fetuses were not only smaller than normal but were also severely anemic suggests that the two are related, the anemia perhaps being the cause of the growth retardation. Observations made during this study indicate that exposure of the nursing mother to cadmium severely limits the growth of her litter. In this respect, it is interesting that in the cadmium-treated mice, the anemia seen in the fetuses is very severe as compared with the relatively mild anemia of the mother. This suggests that cadmium might well be interfering with growth and blood formation of the fetus.

Studies in experimental animals indicate that cadmium can have destructive effects on the gonads. Necrotic effects of cadmium on testicular tissue in male rats injected subcutaneously with 1 ml of 0.03 M solution of cadmium chloride have been reported.[16, 18] Zinc acetate in large doses prevented testicular damage. Protective effects of zinc and selenium against testicular injury to rats from cadmium have also been reported.[12, 13, 24] After administering cadmium chloride subcutaneously 2.2–4.5 mg Cd/kg body weight into the interscapular region of rats and mice, Parizek[16] reported hyperemia and interstitial edema in the testes within a few hours after injection, and after 48 hours there was destruction of tubular epithelium and the interstitial tissue was hemorrhagic. A dose-response relationship was noted by Mason et al.[13] for injuries to the seminiferous tubules. Subcutaneous injection in rats of a dose of 0.57 mg/kg produced no effect, whereas a dose of 0.85 mg/kg resulted in ischemic necrosis of seminiferous tubules in 32% of the rats. At 1.1 mg/kg there was a 90% incidence and at 1.4 mg/kg 100% of rats showed these injuries. In mice and rabbits, Nordberg[15] found no testicular damage with repeated administration of cadmium at dose levels that caused slight or no kidney malfunction, suggesting that the effect of cadmium on the kidney is an earlier finding in these species.

The effect of cadmium on male gonads stimulated the study of possible effects on ovaries. Kar et al.[11] found a marked change in the rate of follicular atresia in prepubertal rats following administration of cadmium chloride subcutaneously at 10 mg/kg. After 48 hours, all follicles were destroyed and the response of the ovaries to exogenous gonadotropin was inhibited. Parizek et al.[17] injected 5-day-old female rats with either testosterone or 19-nortestosterone and after three to six months, the rats had a persistent estrus. They then were injected subcutaneously with cadmium chloride or acetate at 0.02–0.04 mmol/kg. All ovaries showed massive hemorrhages accompanied by necrosis. Kar et al.[12] found that simultaneous injection of zinc acetate or selenium oxide with cadmium chloride protected the ovaries from damage produced by cadmium chloride alone.

The animal studies indicating gonadal changes were all acute studies involving high levels of cadmium. Comparable doses in man would represent unusually high exposure, which might even be lethal.[14]

There have been several studies of the teratogenicity of cadmium in animals. Chernoff[3] administered 4–12 mg/kg cadmium chloride to CD-strain rats subcutaneously on four consecutive days, beginning on day 13, 14, 15, or 16 of gestation. There was a dose-related increase in fetal deaths, decrease in fetal weight, and an increase in the rate of anomalies, which included micrognathia, cleft palate, clubfoot, and small lungs. Barr[1] found that cadmium chloride 16 μmol Cd/kg was not teratogenic when administered subcutaneously to two different stocks of Wistar rats on days 9, 10, and 11 of gestation but was when administered intraperitoneally. Among the anomalies found were anophthalmia or microphthalmia, dysplastic or absent ears, hydrocephaly, encephalocele, exencephaly, thin abdominal wall, undescended testes, renal agenesis, diaphragmatic hernia, and atresia, dysplastic or absent tails, hydronephrosis, and a small rate of dysplastic forelimbs. The authors suggested that some of the changes might be due to cadmium interference with zinc metabolism. Teratogenic effects have also been reported in mice[10] and hamsters.[7] The protective effect of zinc for the teratogenic effects of cadmium have also been studied. Ferm and Carpenter[7, 8] found that simultaneous intravenous administration of zinc sulfate at 0.45 mg Zn/kg and cadmium sulfate at 0.88 mg Cd/kg reduced embryonic resorption and anomalies to control levels. Gradual delay of zinc injection after cadmium injection reduced the protective effect, and where the delay was 12 hours or greater there was no protective effect.

There have been very few studies on reproductive effects in human beings exposed to cadmium. Favino and co-workers[6] found one worker with impotence associated with low testosterone blood levels among ten cadmium workers studied. Tsvetkova[22] investigated effects on reproduction among 106 women workers exposed to cadmium, aged 18–48 with 2–16 years' exposure, some to cadmium oxide at concentrations of 0.1–25 mg/cu m, some to soluble cadmium salts at 0.16–25 mg/cu m. She found no significant changes in the menstrual cycle. Courses and times of pregnancies were normal. Children born weighed less than children of control workers. Four of the children born to cadmium-exposed women had signs of rickets, one had retarded eruption of teeth, and two had dental disease. These conditions were not present in children of control workers, but there were only 20 controls. No mention was made of conditions such as prenatal nutrition, maternal illnesses, maternal weight, smoking habits, and other factors that might have had a bearing on the weight of the offspring and on the other findings.[14]

Studies of the possible mutagenic effects of cadmium have been inadequate and conflicting. Shiraishi and Yosida[20] found an excess of chromosomal aberrations in cultured leukocytes among Itai-Itai patients, but these findings were not confirmed in another study of Itai-Itai patients conducted by Bui et al.[2] Itai-Itai (ouch-ouch) disease is the name given to a painful form of osteomalacia in Japan attributed to the pollution of water and crops by industrial cadmium wastes.[14] Bui et al.[2] also reported that Swedish workers exposed to cadmium were found to have a lower incidence of chromosomal changes in cultured lymphocytes than did controls. DeKnudt and Leonard[4] found chromosomal anomalies in leukocytes in workers exposed to cadmium who were also exposed to lead and some to zinc in addition. Studies of dominant lethal mutations in mice by Epstein et al.[5] and by Gilliavod and Leonard[9] revealed that cadmium was not mutagenic, and they found no aberrations in spermocytic chromosomes in male mice and their male first-generation offspring.

Further studies on the effects of cadmium on reproduction are indicated. Damaging effects on human gonads have not been investigated adequately. Although animal studies undertaken at high doses of cadmium have produced harmful effects on ovaries and testes and resulted in fetal abnormalities, there is need for further studies at lower dose levels of cadmium. Furthermore, the role of zinc and selenium in affording protection against injury by cadmium deserves attention.

The present OSHA standard for cadmium is 0.1 mg Cd/cu m TWA with a 0.3 ceiling for cadmium fume and 0.2 mg Cd/cu m TWA (0.6 ceiling) for dust. The NIOSH has proposed for all cadmium compounds an occupational environmental limit of 40 μg Cd/cu m of air as a time-weighted average exposure up to a ten-hour workday, 40-hour week and a ceiling concentration of 200 μg Cd/cu m for any 15-minute sampling period.

There is need for epidemiologic investigation and medical surveillance of cadmium worker populations, male and female, in order to obtain meaningful data relative to the effects of cadmium on reproduction, particularly at the levels of occupational exposure currently recommended as standards.

REFERENCES

1. Barr M Jr: The teratogenicity of cadmium chloride in two stocks of Wistar rats. *Teratology* 1973; 7:237.
2. Bui T-H, Lindsten J, Nordberg GF: Chromosome analysis of lymphocytes from cadmium workers and Itai-Itai patients. *Environ Res* 1975; 9:187.
3. Chernoff N: Teratogenic effects of cadmium in rats. *Teratology* 1973; 8:29.
4. DeKnudt G, Leonard A: Cytogenetic investigations on leucocytes of workers from a cadmium plant. *Environ Physiol Biochem* 1975; 5:319.
5. Epstein SS, Arnold E, Andrea J, et al: Detection of chemical mutagens by the dominant lethal assay in the mouse. *Toxicol Appl Pharmacol* 1972; 23:288.
6. Favino A, Candura F, Chiappino G, et al: Study on the androgen function of men exposed to cadmium. *Med Lav* 1968; 59:105.
7. Ferm VH, Carpenter SJ: The relationship of cadmium and zinc in experimental mammalian teratogenesis. *Lab Invest* 1968; 18:429.
8. Ferm VH, Carpenter SJ: Teratogenic effect of cadmium and its inhibition by zinc. *Nature* 1967; 216:1123.
9. Gilliavod N, Leonard A: Mutagenicity tests with cadmium in the mouse. *Toxicology* 1975; 5:43.
10. Ishizu S, et al: An experimental study of teratogenic effect of cadmium. *Ind Health* 1973; 11:127.
11. Kar AB, Das RP, Karkun JN: Ovarian changes in prepubertal rats after treatment with cadmium chloride. *Acta Biol Med Ger* 1959; 3:372.
12. Kar AB, Das RP, Mukerji FNI: Prevention of cadmium induced changes in the gonads of rats by zinc and selenium—a study in antagonism between metals in the biological system. *Proc Natl Inst Sci India* 1960; 26B(suppl):40.
13. Mason KE, Brown JA, Young JO, et al: Cadmium-induced injury of the rat testis. *Anat Rec* 1964; 149:135.
14. National Institute for Occupational Safety and Health: *Criteria for a Recommended Standard: Occupational Exposure to Cadmium,* DHEW, PHS, NIOSH, 76-192, August, 1976.
15. Nordberg GF: Effects of acute and chronic cadmium exposure on the testicles of mice—with special reference to protective effects of metallothionein. *Environ Physiol* 1971; 1:171.
16. Parizek J: The destructive effect of cadmium ion on testicular tissue and its prevention by zinc. *J Endocrinol* 1957; 15:56.
17. Parizek J, Ostadalova I, Benes L, et al: The effect of a subcutaneous injection of cadmium salts on the ovaries of adult rats in persistent oestrus. *J Reprod Fertil* 1968; 17:559.
18. Parizek J, Zahor Z: Effect of cadmium salts on testicular tissue. *Nature* 1956; 177:1036.
19. Prigge E: Inhalative cadmium effects in pregnant and fetal rats. *Toxicology* 1978; 10:297–309.
20. Shiraishi Y, Yosida TH: Chromosomal abnormalities in cultured leucocyte cells from Itai-Itai disease patients. *Proc Jpn Acad* 1972; 48:248.
21. Sutou S, Yamamoto K, Sendota H, et al: Toxicity, fertility, teratogenicity, and dominant lethal tests in rats administered cadmium subchronically. *Ecotoxicol Environ Safety* 1980; 4:51–56.
22. Tsvetkova RB: Materials concerning an investigation of the effect of cadmium compounds on the generative function. *Gig Tr Prof Zabol* 1970; 12:31. (Russian) (Cited in NIOSH Criteria Document[14].)
23. US Dept of Health and Human Services, Public Health Service, Centers for Disease Control, National Institute for Occupational Health and Safety: Cadmium (Cd). *Curr Intell Bull* 42. Cincinnati, Oh, NIOSH, 1984.
24. Webb M: Protection by zinc against cadmium toxicity. *Biochem Pharmacol* 1972; 21:2767.
25. Webster WS: Cadmium-induced fetal growth retardation in the mouse. *Arch Environ Health* 1978; 33:36.

CARBARYL

O

H_3C—NH—C—O

Carbaryl is one of the carbamate insecticides that produce most of their biologic effects by inhibiting cholinesterase enzymes. This inhibition leads to the accumulation of endogenous acetylcholine, the principal choline ester that has demonstrated physiologic significance in humans. Production in the United States was about 26 million kg (57 million lb) in 1980. Of the total produced, approximately 50% was exported. In the United States, 9.8 million kg were used for agricultural purposes, 1.8 million kg in homes and gardens, 800,000 kg by government and 600,000 kg for industrial and commercial purposes. Slightly more than half the carbaryl used nationwide was used in the Southeast and the North Central states (about 3.6 million and 2.3 million kg, respectively). An estimated 40% of the carbaryl used throughout the world is applied to the production of cotton.[9] Occupational exposure to carbaryl may occur in the development, manufacture, distribution, and mixing of insecticides, as well as in agricultural use (crops), in plant nursery operations, in spraying and dusting operations, particularly aerial spraying, soil fumigation, and extermination. Carbaryl products are widely marketed under the trade name Sevin. The NIOSH estimates that 100,000 workers are potentially exposed to carbaryl in the United States.[9]

There is limited information available concerning the effects of carbaryl on human reproduction, and reports of adverse reproductive effects in animals from this substance are limited and, at times, conflicting. Whorton et al.[16] reported on a study of 101 male carbaryl production workers, 47 of whom provided satisfactory semen samples for analysis while 36 of the 47 provided blood for hormone assay (testosterone, follicle-stimulating hormone [FSH], and luteinizing hormone [LH]).

The authors summarized their feelings as follows:

> No apparent relationships were found between sperm count and exposure category or years worked in classifications based on carbaryl exposure. Also, no relationship was found between fathering children and exposure to carbaryl. When the sperm count distribution of the carbaryl-exposed workers was compared with a distribution of sperm counts representing a nonexposed (control) population, no overall differences were observed that could be related to carbaryl exposure. There was a small excess in the number of sperm counts less than 20 million/cu ml among carbaryl-exposed men, but the excess was not significant ($P < 0.05$).

All values of the hormone immunoassays were within established laboratory normal ranges except for four elevated FSH values, and the latter did not correlate with the sperm counts.

Mutagenesis testing of carbaryl in mice[8] and bacteria[7, 13] has shown negative results. In Drosophila,[3] carbaryl has been found to be only a weak mutagen. It has been noted, however, that the nitroso compounds of the carbamates are much more strongly mutagenic in bacterial studies, and the possibility exists that nitrosation could occur from the nitrites in human saliva mixing with carbaryl in the acid medium of the stomach.[9] Since occupational exposure is more likely to be from inhalation and skin absorption rather than by ingestion, this factor is not of major occupational health concern.

Studies on the teratogenicity of carbaryl have been made in a number of animal species. Carbaryl has not been found to be teratogenic in the mouse,[2] rat,[15] rabbit,[10] hamster,[10] and monkey.[5, 6] In beagles, terata were produced.[12] In a study of 55 beagles fed carbaryl in their diets in five dosage groups ranging from 3.1 mg/kg to 50 mg/kg, the percentage of pups born alive at all dosages was fewer than the controls, with no live births at the highest dose (50 mg/kg). Of the total number of pregnant beagles from all carbaryl doses, 21% had pups showing embryotoxicity, but there were no abnormal pups in the lowest dose group (3.1 mg/kg) or in the controls. It is to be noted, however, that the dog metabolizes carbaryl differently than does man; i.e., the dog does not excrete 1-naphthol or hydroxylate carbaryl and, therefore, the effects found in this animal may not be relatable to man.[9]

In the guinea pig, Robens[10] reported skeletal defects (mostly of the cervical vertebra) with oral intubation of carbaryl at 300 mg/kg (a near-lethal dose) on days 11–20 of gestation. Fetal mortality was 17.5% in the litter of surviving treated dams as compared with 9.5% in the control litters. On the other hand, in another study of guinea pigs comparing carbaryl dosing by gastric intubation and dietary feeding. Weil et al.[14] concluded that a carbaryl dose of 300 mg/kg by diet or 200 mg/kg by intubation did not produce teratogenic effects.

In view of the apparent differences in carbaryl metabolism between man and dogs and the lack of substantial evidence of teratogenicity in rats and guinea pigs, which have carbaryl metabolism similar to man, no significant data associating carbaryl with teratogenicity has been established at this time.

In the consideration of general reproductive effects of carbaryl, of particular interest is a study by Dougherty and Coulston[6] on the rhesus monkey. In their study, including 79 female monkeys divided into three groups of 16 each given carbaryl in gelatin capsules at 0.2, 2.0, or 20 mg/kg from days 20 through 38 of gestation, one group of 16 given empty gelatin capsules, and an untreated control group of 15 animals, the authors reported that carbaryl was not associated with the production of terata, abortion, stillbirths, or any other adverse effects on reproduction.

In a multigenerational study in rats ultilizing doses as low as 2 and 5 mg/kg by gastric intubation, Shtenberg and Ozhovan[11] noted abnormal reproductive effects, including decreased spermatogenesis, decreased sperm motility, an increase in duration of estrus, a decrease in fertility of females and a decrease in the survival of pups during the first month of life. These findings should be contrasted with those of a three-generational study by Weil et al.[14] with rats utilizing varying dosages up to 100 mg/kg by oral intubation and 200 mg/kg by dietary feeding. Weil et al. concluded, "The severe effects on reproduction reported by Shtenberg and Ozhovan,[11] following repeated oral intubation (OI) at 2 mg/kg to rats were not encountered in this concurrent study even at the maximum OI level of 100 mg/kg." They suggest that the differences in the findings may be related to the identity and purity of the carbaryl used. The signs of cholinesterase inhibition, the mortality, and the reproductive effects these authors found occurred only at the maximal oral intubation dose of 100 mg/kg. The effects included a decrease in the percentage of females that littered (FO → F1b only), an increase in the number of days after first mating to birth of litter (FO → F1b only), a decrease in the number of pups born alive (F1a → F2a; F2a → F3a), a decrease in the number of fetuses and live fetuses (F2a → F3a), and an increase in the percentage of litters with resorption sites (F2a → F3b). These effects did not occur at 25 mg/kg by oral intubation or at the maximal dietary feeding level of 200 mg/kg. For the latter, the authors reported only a decrease in body weight before mating and an increase in the number of days between mating and birth of litter (F1a → F2a only).

In a comparison of mean sperm counts of 47 carbaryl workers and 90 nonexposed control workers, Avashia[1] found no evidence that carbaryl exposure impaired sperm production. Median sperm count in the workers was 92 million/ml and the median for the nonexposed 81 million/ml. Forty of 47 carbaryl workers had counts greater than 20 million/ml and 85 of 90 of the nonexposed had counts above 20 million/ml. Six workers had sperm counts below 20 million/ml and three nonexposed were below 20 million/ml, and both groups had 2% azoospermics. Carbaryl exposure levels were not reported.

The present OSHA standard for occupational exposure to carbaryl is an eight-hour time-weighted average of 5 mg/cu m of air. The NIOSH recommends this same TWA concentration for up to a ten-hour day, 40-hour workweek. The NIOSH suggests, "if humans and lower animals do not differ significantly in their susceptibility to inhaled carbaryl, the results of inhalation studies in several animal species[4, 17] would indicate that 16 mg/cu m can be considered the no-adverse-effect level with respect to toxic manifestations of cholinesterase inhibition in humans." For such effect, therefore, the proposed standard should provide an adequate margin of safety, and, with the available data, it would appear that the proposed standard should have some margin of safety for the reproductive effects as well, provided that additional exposure through the skin and by ingestion through contaminated hands, is prevented.

REFERENCES

1. Avashia BH: Testicular function among carbaryl exposed employees. Conference on Pesticides and Human Health, Society for Occupational and Environmental Health, Washington, DC, Dec 10–13, 1978.
2. Benson BW, Scott WJ, Beliles RP: Sevin—Safety Evaluation by Teratological Study in the Mouse. Unpublished report submitted to Union Carbide Corp, 1967, 19 pp. (Cited in NIOSH Criteria Document[9].)
3. Breskij VV, Vaskov VI: Studies on mutation and calculation of fertility in Drosophila melanogaster under the effect of carbaryl. *Angew Parasitol* 1971; 13:23. (German) (Cited in NIOSH Criteria Document[9].)
4. Carpenter CP, Weil SC, Palm PE, et al: Mammalian toxicity of 1-naphthyl-N-methylcarbamate (Sevin insecticide). *J Agric Food Chem* 1961; 9:30. (Cited in NIOSH Criteria Document[9].)
5. Coulston F: *The Effect of Carbaryl on Reproduction in the Rhesus Monkey*. Albany, NY: Albany Medical College, Institute of Experimental Pathology & Toxicology, 1971, 18 pp.
6. Dougherty WJ, Coulston F: Teratogenic evaluation of carbaryl in the rhesus monkey (Macaca mulatta). Unpublished report submitted to Union Carbide Corp, June 6, 1975.
7. Elespuru R, Lijinsky W, Setlow JK: Nitrosocarbaryl as a potent mutagen of environmental significance. *Nature* 1974; 247:386. (Cited in NIOSH Criteria Document[9].)
8. Epstein SS, Arnold E, Andrea J, et al: Detection of chemical mutagens by the dominant lethal assay in the mouse. *Toxicol Appl Pharmacol* 1972; 23:288. (Cited in NIOSH Criteria Document[9].)
9. National Institute of Occupational Safety and Health: *Criteria for a Recommended Standard: Occupational Exposure to Carbaryl*, DHEW, PHS, NIOSH 77–107, 1976.
10. Robens JF: Teratologic studies of carbaryl, diazinon, norea, disulfram, and thiram in small laboratory animals. *Toxicol Appl Pharmacol* 1969; 15:152.
11. Shtenberg AI, Ozhovan MV: The effect of low Sevin doses on the reproductive function of animals in a number of generations. *Vopr Pitan* 1971; 30:42. (Russian) (Cited in NIOSH Criteria Document[9].)
12. Smalley, HE, Curtis JM, Earl FL: Teratogenic action of carbaryl in beagle dogs. *Toxicol Appl Pharmacol* 1968; 13:392.
13. Uchiyama M, Tadeda M, Suzuki T, et al: Mutagenicity of nitroso derivatives in N-methylcarbamate insecticides in microbiological method. *Bull Environ Contam Toxicol* 1975; 14:389. (Cited in NIOSH Criteria Document[9].)
14. Weil CS, Woodside MD, Bernard JB, et al: Comparative effect of carbaryl on rat reproduction and guinea pig teratology when fed either in the diet or by stomach intubation. *Toxicol Appl Pharmacol* 1973; 26:621.
15. Weil CS, Woodside MD, Carpenter CP, et al: Current status of tests of carbaryl for reproductive and teratogenic effect. *Toxicol Appl Pharmacol* 1972; 21:390. (Cited in NIOSH Criteria Document[9].)
16. Whorton DM, Milby TH, Stubbs HA: Testicular function among carbaryl-exposed employees. *J Toxicol Environ Health* 1979; 5:929.
17. Yakim VS: The maximum permissible concentration of Sevin in the air of the work zone. *Gig Sanit* 1968; 32:29. (Russian) (Cited in NIOSH Criteria Document[9].)

CARBON DISULFIDE

Carbon disulfide (CS_2) is a colorless, volatile and extremely flammable liquid at room temperature. Annually, more than 350 million kg (782 million lb) of carbon disulfide are produced in the United States. Approximately half the carbon disulfide produced in the early 1970s was used in the production of regenerated cellulose (viscose rayon and cellophane) and approximately a quarter was used in the manufacture of carbon tetrachloride. Carbon disulfide is also used in vulcanizing rubber, fumigating grain, chemical analysis, degreasing, dry cleaning, and oil extraction. The NIOSH estimates that 20,000 employees are potentially exposed to carbon disulfide in the United States.[2]

Most of the studies of occupational exposure to carbon disulfide involve workers in the viscose industry, where there is concomitant exposure to hydrogen sulfide. The ratio of the concentration of evolved carbon disulfide to hydrogen sulfide is estimated at from 2:1 to 10:1. Several studies have revealed reproductive effects, including threatened abortion, spontaneous abortion, and infertility in women and spermatic disorders in men. These studies have appeared primarily in the foreign literature and are reviewed in the NIOSH Criteria Document. The following is a summary of some of the material in the Criteria Document pertinent to reproduction. For further details, the reader is referred to the Document itself.[2]

Vigliani[10] reported on occupational carbon disulfide poisoning in Italy during 1940 and 1941. Factories operated at wartime peaks and employees were exposed 10–12 hours per day at concentrations that were as high as 800 ppm (2.50 mg/L) with a mean concentration of 144–321 ppm (0.45–1.0 mg/L). Of the 100 workers examined, 16% complained of "sexual weakness."

Erhardt[3] reported on a viscose rayon factory in the German Democratic Republic that first employed women in 1950 but barred their employment six months later because of increased menstrual bleeding. The author reported that by 1966, when the maximal allowable concentration (MAC) of 17 ppm (53 mg/cu m) was not exceeded, there were no identified instances of spontaneous abortions, amenorrhea, sterility, or genital organ dysfunction. He suggests that it is not necessary to prohibit all women from exposure but that he would not expose pregnant women to carbon disulfide.

Finkova et al.[4] reported the data on 35 women exposed to carbon disulfide in a viscose rayon factory who were studied for possible gynecologic abnormalities during 1967–1969. Gynecologic examinations included inspection, palpation, and cytologic smear tests. There were no abnormalities found, nor was there any evidence of irregular menstrual function, malformed fetuses, spontaneous abortions, hormonal disorders, or altered sexual habits. The NIOSH notes that the report lacks information on methodology, quantitative data, and extent of exposure, and there is no statistical analysis of results.

Jindrichova[5] studied workers in a cord-fiber factory who were exposed to carbon disulfide at a mean concentration of 64 ppm (200 mg/cu m). There were 160 men and 23 women included in the study, and it was reported that 99 men and 11 women had symptoms of carbon disulfide "poisoning." Among the symptoms most frequently reported among the men was loss of potency. There were no specific gynecologic conditions or disturbances encountered among the women.

Lancranjan et al.[7] studied young male workers in an artificial-fiber factory who had been exposed to carbon disulfide at an average concentration of 13–26 ppm (40–80 mg/cu m), with peaks of up to 250 ppm (780 mg/cu m). There were 33 workers with a mean age of 22 years and a mean length of exposure of 21 months who were diagnosed as chronically poisoned by carbon disulfide. The controls consisted of 31 men with a mean age of 25.9 years. Seventy-eight percent of the exposed workers showed disturbances of "sexual dynamics," decreased libido in 66% and erection difficulty in 51% being the most common problems. Semen analysis revealed that the poisoned workers had higher frequencies of asthenospermia, hypospermia, and teratospermia than did the controls, and the excretion of total neutral 17-ketosteroids was lower in the exposed workers. The authors suggest that carbon disulfide may act on both the hypothalamus and directly on the gonads. In 1972, Lancranjan[6] used the same methods and examined 133 chronically poisoned male viscose workers and 50 controls, both with an average age of 30 years, for spermatic disorders. Again, significantly greater frequencies of hypospermia, teratospermia, and asthenospermia were found in exposed workers than in the controls. Vasilyeva[9] studied three different groups of female viscose rayon workers that included 500 workers in the spinning department, where the concentrations of carbon disulfide sometimes exceeded 6 ppm (20 mg/cu m) and hydrogen sulfide concentrations never were more than 7 ppm (10 mg/cu m), 209 workers in the trimming department, where the concentration of neither carbon disulfide nor hydrogen sulfide exceeded 3 ppm (10 mg/cu m), and 429 workers in the rewinding-sorting department not exposed to either substance (controls). Among the workers of both the spinning and trimming departments there were increased numbers of women with menstrual flow of more than five days, abundant and painful menstruation, and abnormal cellular composition of vaginal smears. The data suggest that exposure to carbon disulfide, even at concentrations below 3 ppm (10 mg/cu m), may affect ovarian hormone production in women and that the effect is increased in a dose-response relationship.

Petrov[8] compared a group of 189 women employed in the viscose industry who were exposed to carbon disulfide at levels of 9 ppm (28 mg/cu m) before and during pregnancy with a control group of 191 women who worked in the industry and had had no exposure to carbon disulfide. Adjustments were made for differences in age and job longevity. It was found that the exposed workers had significantly more difficulty than did controls from increased threatened abortions, spontaneous abortions, and premature births.

Wakasuki and Higashikawa[11] exposed mature male and female rabbits to carbon disulfide at 300 ppm (930 mg/cu m) 30 minutes per day for 120 consecutive days or to hydrogen sulfide at 100 ppm (140 mg/cu m) or to both substances on the same exposure schedule. The animals were killed and examined 140 days after exposure. There were no significant testicular changes in the carbon disulfide group; seminiferous tubular atrophy leading to diminished spermatogenesis was found in the hydrogen sulfide group and there was complete absence of spermatogenesis in rabbits exposed to both gases. No impairment of ovaries was found among the female rabbits. The authors believed that where there were no observable abnormalities, it was due to the fact that exposure time had been limited to 30 minutes per day or to the period of 140 days that followed exposure, which could have permitted recovery. Damage caused by the combination of vapors was not reversible during this period and suggests toxic synergism when both carbon disulfide and hydrogen sulfide are present.

Barilyak et al.[1] studied the effects of a combination of carbon disulfide and hydrogen sulfide on reproduction in rats. Groups were studied where both parents were exposed, where either the male or female was exposed prior to conception, where females were exposed for up to 20 days of gestation and where females were not exposed during gestation. The authors found that exposure to carbon disulfide and hydrogen sulfide showed definite embryotoxicity and a weak teratogenic effect compared to controls.

Reports on mutagenesis resulting from exposure to carbon disulfide or to the combination of carbon disulfide and hydrogen sulfide have not been found.

Carbon disulfide is toxic when the vapor is inhaled or when there is repeated skin contact with the liquid. Toxic effects other than on the reproductive system are discussed in Chapter 47. Exposure in combination with hydrogen sulfide may cause toxic effects that are additive or possibly synergistic.

There is a need for additional epidemiologic studies with accurate measurements of exposure to carbon disulfide and to hydrogen sulfide in the viscose industry as well as in other industries where exposure to carbon disulfide may affect the health of the worker. Well-controlled animal experiments at exposures similar to those in the workplace of carbon disulfide and hydrogen sulfide alone and in combination should be conducted. Since some studies have shown reproductive system disorders and a possible teratogenic effect on exposure, it is important that careful records be kept on reproductive problems and offspring abnormalities in both male and female industrially exposed populations.

The current federal standard for carbon disulfide specifies an eight-hour TWA value of 20 ppm (62 mg/cu m), with an acceptable ceiling concentration of 30 ppm (93 mg/cu m) for an eight-hour day, five-day workweek and an acceptable maximal peak of 100 ppm (311 mg/cu m) for 30 minutes during an eight-hour work shift.

On the basis of reported studies, the NIOSH[2] recommends that the carbon disulfide in the work environment should be controlled so that the concentration does not exceed 1 ppm (3 mg/cu m) as a TWA concentration for up to a ten-hour work shift in a 40-hour workweek and also does not exceed 10 ppm (30 mg/cu m) as a ceiling concentration for any 15-minute period. Compliance with the recommended carbon disulfide standard should also reduce exposure to hydrogen sulfide.

REFERENCES

1. Barilyak ID, Vasilyeva IA, Kalinovskaya LI: Effects of small concentrations of carbon disulfide and hydrogen sulfide on intrauterine development in rats. *Arkh Anat Gistol Embriol* 1975; 68:77. (Russian) (Cited in NIOSH Criteria Document[2].)
2. National Institute for Occupational Safety and Health: *Criteria for a Recommended Standard: Occupational Exposure to Carbon Disulfide*, DHEW, PHS, NIOSH 77-156, 1977.
3. Erhardt W: Experiences with the employment of women exposed to carbon disulfide, in Brieger H, Teisinger J (eds): *Toxicology of Car-*

bon Disulphide. Amsterdam, Excerpta Medica Foundation, 1967, p 240. (Cited in NIOSH Criteria Document[2].)

4. Finkova A, Simko A, Jindrichova J, et al: Gynecologic problems of women working in an environment contaminated with carbon disulfide. *Cesk Gynekol* 1973; 38:535. (Czech) (Cited in NIOSH Criteria Document[2].)
5. Jindrichova J: Health status of workers in the cord fiber industry. *Prac Lek* 1957; 9:10. Czech translation.
6. Lancranjan I: Alterations of spermatic liquid in patients chronically poisoned by carbon disulphide. *Med Lav* 1972; 63:29. (Cited in NIOSH Criteria Document.[2])
7. Lancranjan I, Popescu HI, Klepsch I: Changes of the gonadic function in chronic carbon disulphide poisoning. *Med Lav* 1969; 60:566. (Cited in NIOSH Criteria Document[2].)
8. Petrov MV: Some data on the course and termination of pregnancy in female workers of the viscose industry. *Pediatr Akush Ginekol* 1969; 3:50. (Russian) (Cited in NIOSH Criteria Document[2].)
9. Vasilyeva IA: Effect of low concentrations of carbon disulfide and hydrogen sulfide on the menstrual function of women and the estrual cycle in an experiment. *Gig Sanit* 1973; 7:24. (Russian) (Cited in NIOSH Criteria Document[2].)
10. Vigliani EC: Carbon disulphide poisoning in viscose rayon factories. *Br J Ind Med* 1954; 11:235. (Cited in NIOSH Criteria Document[2].)
11. Wakasuki T, Higashikawa H: Experimental studies on CS_2 and H_2S poisoning—the histological changes in hematopoietic organs and other main internal organs. *Shikoku, Igaku, Zasshi*. 1959; 14:549. (Japanese) (Cited in NIOSH Criteria Document[2].)

CARBON MONOXIDE (CO)

Eric P. Kindwall, M.D.
Carl Zenz, M.D.

This section will not consider details of acute or chronic occupational exposures to carbon monoxide or its pathophysiology and treatment. (For these specific aspects, see Kindwall, Chapter 30.) Certain aspects pertinent to both men and women working with potential exposure to carbon monoxide will be emphasized.

Insufficient knowledge exists about the biologic effects of carbon monoxide during intrauterine development and on the newborn; several studies have revealed decreased birth weights and increased mortality in the progeny of animals exposed to relatively high carbon monoxide concentrations, but few studies have reported on subtle effects of low concentrations. There is no information implicating carbon monoxide effects on the fetus from occupational exposures, but there is much information on such effects from maternal smoking. This section is intended to offer a brief overview of the potential problems involving the developing embryo, fetus, and newborn infant to carbon monoxide exposure not associated with tobacco smoking.

The carboxyhemoglobin concentration in the blood of normal nonsmoking pregnant women varies from 0.5% to 1%.[1] In addition to those factors affecting carboxyhemoglobin in the nonpregnant person,[5] maternal carboxyhemoglobin concentration (HbCOm) reflects the endogenous carbon monoxide production by the fetus and its rate of exchange across the placenta.[25] Fetal endogenous carbon monoxide production accounts for about 3% of the total carboxyhemoglobin present in the blood of a normal pregnant woman.

In 1949, Sjöstrand,[39] utilizing improved methods of measurements, demonstrated that the human body was a net producer of carbon monoxide, identifying the source as the alpha-methene bridge between the four porphyrin units in the heme molecule. During the "recycling" of the heme molecule reclaiming iron, four molecules of carbon monoxide are released for every molecule of heme catabolized.

Not only must endogenous carbon monoxide formation in the human body be considered, but other external contaminants may further compound the carbon monoxide problem. Most commonly encountered, both within industry as well as outside industry, especially the smaller working establishments and in homes, is exposure to paint removers containing a variety of hydrocarbon ingredients, a major one being methylene chloride (dichloromethane, CH_2Cl_2), which has been shown to be rapidly metabolized to carbon monoxide.[35] Under conditions of poor ventilation, such as insufficient air movement in a home garage, basement, or small workplace, concentrations of methylene chloride vapors can quickly accumulate and be readily inspired. Stewart and Hake[40] have shown that the use of such paint remover for a period of three hours can easily produce carboxyhemoglobin saturation of 5%–10% in man. It is not possible to determine the extent of use of paint removers in the private sector of the United States, and perhaps equally difficult to determine is occupational exposure to methylene chloride in the thousands of workplaces where solvents are in daily use. From the viewpoint of potential worker exposure, it is noteworthy that methylene chloride, although not the most hazardous chlorinated hydrocarbon compound, is unique in the context of a carbon monoxide source. In addition to its common use as a paint or varnish "stripper" (remover), it is widely used in degreasing, as an aerosol propellant, as a solvent for paint, plastics, and textile making, in producing photo films and in preparing certain oils and waxes. (Not to be forgotten, it has been used as a general anesthetic.) The NIOSH estimate of exposure in the United States is about 70,000 workers, excluding home use.[12]

Studies have shown that even relatively low levels of carbon monoxide as blood carboxyhemoglobin concentrations of 4%–5% result in subtle alterations in mental ability and the performance of certain functions in normal adults. Additional evidence from several extensive studies with long-term follow-up of the infants of smoking mothers demonstrates retardation of mental abilities. The pregnant woman, her fetus, and the newborn infant have been identified as subjects particularly vulnerable to the effects of low concentrations of carbon monoxide.

The relationship of carboxyhemoglobin concentrations to inspired carbon monoxide concentrations in adult humans has been experimentally determined in several studies. Recently, Longo and Hill[28] studied these relationships in pregnant sheep with catheters chronically implanted in maternal and fetal blood vessels. They exposed ewes to inspired carbon monoxide concentrations of up to 300 ppm. At 30 ppm, maternal carboxyhemoglobin concentrations increased over a period of eight to ten hours, equilibrating at about 4.6% ± 0.3% (SEM). The fetal carboxyhemoglobin concentration increased more slowly, equilibrating in 36–48 hours at about 7.4% ± 0.5%. At 50 ppm, the time courses were similar, with maternal and fetal steady-state values of 7.2% ± 0.5% and 11.3% ± 1.1%, respectively. At 100 ppm, maternal and fetal steady-state values were 12.2% ± 1.2% and 19.8% ± 1.4%, respectively. For all concentrations, the half-times for carbon monoxide uptake by maternal and fetal blood were about two and six hours, respectively.

For ethical and technical reasons, such experiments cannot be carried out with humans. The same investigators[28] examined the experimental data and theorized a mathematical model of the interrelationships of human fetal and maternal carboxyhemoglobin concentrations. The predicted changes in the carboxyhemoglobin concentrations as a function of the time of exposure to inspired carbon monoxide ranged from 30 to 300 ppm. Several points of interest are: The equilibration for fetal carboxyhemoglobin was not achieved for about 30–36 hours, the half-time of the increase in fetal carboxyhemoglobin concentration was about 7.5 hours for all concentrations, the time for fetal carboxyhemoglobin to equal the maternal value varied from 12 to 15 hours and, finally, under steady-state conditions, fetal carboxyhemoglobin concentration was about 15% greater than the maternal. The theoretic relationships in humans and the experimental data in sheep are in reasonably good agreement.

Studies have revealed the effects of carbon monoxide on fetal growth. Wells[42] exposed pregnant rats to 1.5% (15,000 ppm) carbon monoxide for from five to eight minutes ten times on alternate days during their 21-day pregnancy. This resulted in maternal unconsciousness and abortion or absorption of most fetuses. The surviving newborns did not grow normally. Similar exposure to 5,900 ppm affected only a small percentage of animals. Williams and Smith[43] exposed rats to 0.34% (3,400 ppm) carbon monoxide for one hour daily for three months, demonstrating peak carboxyhemoglobin concentrations in these animals of from 60% to 70%, and the number of pregnancies known to occur among those seven exposed animals was half the number in the controls. The number of rats born per litter decreased, and only 2 of 13 newborns survived to weaning age. There were no pregnancies in the five females exposed for 150 days to this concentration.

Astrup et al.[1] reported quantitative data on fetal weights of two groups of pregnant rabbits exposed to carbon monoxide continually for 30 days. Exposure to 90 ppm yielded maternal carboxyhemoglobin concentrations of 9%–10% from a control value of 4.5%. Mortality of the young rabbits during the following 21 days increased to 25% from a control value of 13%. Doubling the concentration of carbon monoxide to 180 ppm resulted in maternal carboxyhemoglobin concentrations of 16%–18%, birth weights decreased 20% from 53.7 to 44.7 gm, and neonatal mortality was 35% compared with 1% for the controls. Mortality during the following 21 days was the same value as for the controls, 27%.

Williams and Smith[43] studied the effects of carbon monoxide on newborn survival in animals. They exposed rats to mixtures of illuminating gas in air, with inspired carbon monoxide concentrations of 0.43%. In 22 newborn rats 12–48 hours old exposed to carbon monoxide, the average survival time was about 196 minutes, in contrast to an average survival of about 36 minutes in mature animals. McGrath and Jaeger[31] also noted that 50% of newly hatched chicks could withstand exposure to 1% (10,000 ppm) carbon monoxide concentrations for about 32 minutes. This survival time decreased to about ten minutes; by day 4 it was six minutes and by day 8 it was four minutes, where it remained for all subsequent days tested up to 21 days. Subsequently, Jaeger and McGrath[20] showed that decreasing the body temperature increased the time to last gasp from a mean value of 9.8 ± 0.5 minutes at 40° C to 20.7 ± 0.1 minute at 30° C. They noted that hypothermia caused markedly reduced heart and respiratory rates and suggested that its major benefit was a reduction in energy-requiring functions.

In 1977, Fechter and Annau[13] demonstrated reduced birth weight and decreased weight gain in rat offspring, using rats prenatally exposed to concentrations of 150 ppm of carbon monoxide. Neurobehavioral and biochemical testing of these offspring revealed lower behavioral activity levels through the preweaning period, altered central catecholamine activity, and reduction in total brain protein at birth. They suggested that the potentially more serious consequences of altered central nervous system function and biochemistry early in life or, perhaps, permanently, are only now beginning to be discovered by the use of animal models.

Several mechanisms probably account for the effects of carbon monoxide on developing tissue. As described earlier (Kindwall[22]), undoubtedly the most important of these is the interference with tissue oxygenation. Carbon monoxide also interferes with oxygen transport by displacing oxygen from the hemoglobin in arterial blood, thus decreasing the blood oxygen capacity. For the pregnant woman, these effects on blood oxygenation pose a special threat. Not only is her oxygen consumption increased 15%–25% during pregnancy,[27] but her blood oxygen capacity is decreased 20%–30% or more due to the decreased concentration of hemoglobin.[15] The woman with a significant anemia faces even more severe compromise of her oxygen delivery.

The oxygen affinity of fetal blood is greater than that of maternal blood; hence, its oxyhemoglobin saturation curve is shifted to the left. In addition, human fetal blood contains more hemoglobin than does maternal blood (16.3 vs 12 gm/100 ml); therefore, it has a greater oxygen capacity.[15] Under normal circumstances, maternal arterial oxygen tension is about 100 mm Hg and its oxygen content equals 16.1 ml/100 ml of blood. The placental exchange of oxygen extracts about 5 ml O_2/100 ml of blood, producing a uterine mixed venous oxygen tension of about 34 mm Hg. When the maternal blood contains carboxyhemoglobin, the oxygen capacity is decreased and the oxyhemoglobin curve shifts to the left. Whereas arterial oxygen tension remains essentially the same as under normal conditions, the oxygen content is reduced to 14.5 ml/100 ml. With the same placental oxygen transfer of 5 ml/100 ml blood, the venous oxygen tension would be about 27 mm Hg, a decrease from normal of about 7 mm Hg.

Ginsberg and Myers[14] studied the effects of carbon monoxide exposure on near-term pregnant monkeys and their fetuses. The anesthetized animals were acutely exposed to 0.1%–0.3% carbon monoxide, resulting in maternal carboxyhemoglobin levels of about 60%. These one- to three-hour studies showed the following: fetal blood oxygen content (pH less than 7.05), hypercapnia (P_{CO_2} = 70 mm Hg or greater), hypotension and electrocardiographic changes such as T-wave flattening and inversion.[14]

Longo and Hill[28] studied changes in oxygen tension in response to various carboxyhemoglobin concentrations in sheep in which catheters were implanted in maternal and fetal vessels. About one week following recovery from anesthesia and surgery, the ewes were exposed to various concentrations of carbon monoxide. Fifty-seven percent of the sheep fetuses in this study died when fetal carboxyhemoglobin values were greater than 15% for 30 minutes or longer (5 of 11 died at 100 ppm and three of three died at 300 ppm). These deaths were attributed to hypoxia of vital tissues. Hypoxia from carbon monoxide may interfere with tissue oxygenation by increasing the concentration of carboxymyoglobin (MbCO), in relation to carboxyhemoglobin, which is additive to the cytochrome A_3 derangement.

Coburn et al.[7] showed that when arterial oxygen tension decreases to 40 mm Hg or lower, the ratio of carboxymyoglobin to carboxyhemoglobin increases from a normal value of 1.0 to about 2.5 in the resting dog skeletal muscle and myocardium of dogs.[8] Assuming that a similar relationship exists in the fetus, where arterial blood P_{O_2} is normally 30 mm Hg or less, carboxymyoglobin concentrations would be 12.5% when the carboxyhemoglobin is 5%. This degree of carboxymyoglobin saturation may be of importance to fetal myocardial cells.

In a hog-raising building, gas-heated carbon monoxide was emitted because of improper heater function in concentrations ranging from 2.4 to 3 times the allowable 50 ppm. Although the hogs raised in these affected areas displayed no signs of carbon monoxide poisoning, those sows that were placed there a few days before farrowing gave birth to an unusually high proportion of dead piglets; in some cases, 100% were born dead. After the heating system was repaired, the loss of newborn piglets ceased immediately, according to Keller.[21]

The relationship between altitude and birth weight has been noted by Grahn and Kratchman,[16] who showed that the proportion of low birth weights increased with increasing elevation. The number of infants weighing less than 2,500 gm increased to 10.1% at 1,500–1,580 m (4,900–5,190 ft) from a control value of 6.6% at sea level. At 2,760 m (9,055 ft), the number of such newborns further increased to 16.6%. A given carboxyhemoglobin concentration may cause a more profound effect on tissue oxygenation at high altitudes than at sea level. Persons at higher altitudes would be expected to be more sensitive to the effects of carbon monoxide, and this would be especially true of a pregnant mother, whose oxygen demand is greater than when not pregnant, as well as for the newborn infant.

In the United States, approximately 2.2 million people live at altitudes at or above 1,525 m (5,000 ft), the majority of high-altitude residents living at elevations between 1,500 and 2,000 m. There are no available data concerning numbers of workers who may be exposed to carbon monoxide at work or away from work living at higher altitudes nor are there figures available for the changes of population due to tourist fluctuations with seasonal factors. A point to consider is that more and more families are using trailers and mobile homes for both living and vacationing purposes, and not all units are safely heated, which means that considerable potential for carbon monoxide exposures exists in the nonoccupational setting for these groups of people.

Longo[27] prepared an intensive review of the biologic effects of carbon monoxide on the pregnant woman, fetus, and newborn infant, describing physiologic and biochemical bases and their clinical implications, pointing out significant alterations of certain physiologic functions resulting from relatively low blood carboxyhemoglobin concentrations in pregnant women, fetuses, and newborn infants, who are particularly susceptible to carbon monoxide effects. In cases reviewed in his report, mothers exposed to high concentrations of carbon monoxide showed classic signs and symptoms of carbon monoxide poisoning and, in many of these, surviving infants subsequently developed neurologic sequelae. Infants who died at a later date showed brain damage at autopsy.[26, 29, 30] The lesions described resulted from fetal cerebral anoxia during pregnancy, labor, and delivery and also during the immediate newborn period.[4]

Longo reiterated that the pregnant woman probably is more susceptible to the effects of carbon monoxide than is the nonpregnant woman. Clearly, then, pregnant working mothers, their embryos, and newborn infants certainly constitute a population group at risk from the effects of carbon monoxide. With the increasing numbers of women entering various workplaces, occupational health physicians as well as obstetricians, pediatricians, and family practitioners and allied health personnel must recognize these new potential hazards of inadvertent exposure of the fetus and the neonate to carbon monoxide as well as other potential environmental hazards. There are no established guidelines or standards to allow for safe placement of the potentially pregnant woman worker who may be exposed to carbon monoxide concentrations to make any valid predictions to ensure the future well-being of her unborn child.[27] Rational recommendations for "safe upper limits" to exposure in the workplace to carbon monoxide will be developed to protect the unborn child. For the present, appropriate hygienic measures must not be overlooked, and adherence to the TLV for carbon monoxide of 35 ppm is recommended. Of note is that different workloads and energy expenditure were not considered in establishing the present standard (50 ppm) or the recommended one (35 ppm).

The final and most critical point is that we have no solid data regarding transport of unbound carbon monoxide across the placenta and the importance of its effect on the fetal cytochrome system.

REFERENCES

1. Astrup P, Olsen HM, Trolle D, et al: Effects of moderate carbon monoxide exposure on fetal development. *Lancet* 1972; 2:1220.
2. Ayres SM, et al: Systemic and myocardial hemodynamic responses to relatively small concentrations of carboxyhemoglobin (COHB). *Arch Environ Health* 1969; 18:699.
3. Ball EG, Strittmalter CF, Cooper O: The reaction to carbon monoxide. *J Biol Chem* 1951; 193:635.
4. Bernard C: *Lecons sur les Effets des Substances Toxiques et Meticamenteuses*. Paris, JB Baillière et Fils, 1957.
5. Caton WL, et al: The circulating red cell volume and body hematocrit in normal pregnancy and the puerperium; by direct measurement, using radioactive red cells. *Am J Obstet Gynecol* 1951; 61:1207.
6. Chance B, Erecinska M, Wagner M; Mitochondrial responses to CO toxicity. *Ann NY Acad Sci* 1970; 174:193.
7. Coburn RF, Forster RE, Kane PB: Considerations of the physiological variables that determine the blood carboxyhemoglobin concentration in man. *J Clin Invest* 1965; 44:1899.
8. Coburn RF, Mayers LB: Myoglobin O_2 tension determined from measurements of carboxyhemoglobin in skeletal muscle. *Am J Physiol* 1971; 222:66.
9. Coburn RF, Ploegmakers F, Gondrie P, et al: Myocardial myoglobin oxygen tension. *Am J Physiol* 1973; 224:870.

10. Courville CB: *Contributions to the Study of Cerebral Anoxia. Some Observations on Its History, Its Pathogenesis and Structural Characteristics, the Importance of Its Circulatory Component and Its Significance in the Evaluation of Certain Chronic Diseases of the Brain of Infancy and Early Childhood*. Los Angeles, San Lucas Press, 1953, pp 155–216.
11. National Institute for Occupational Safety and Health: *Criteria Document for a Recommended Standard: Occupational Exposure to Carbon Monoxide*, USDHEW, PHS, NIOSH (HSM 73-11000), 1972.
12. National Institute for Occupational Safety and Health: *Criteria Document for a Recommended Standard: Occupational Exposure to Methylene Chloride*, USDHEW, PHS, NIOSH 76-138, 1976.
13. Fechter LD, Annau Z: Toxicity of mild prenatal carbon monoxide exposure. *Science* 1977; 197:680.
14. Ginsberg MD, Myers RE: Fetal brain injury after maternal carbon monoxide intoxication: Clinical and neuropathologic aspects. *Neurology* 1976; 26:15.
15. Goldbaum LR, Ramierez RG, Absalon KB: What is the mechanism of carbon monoxide toxicity? *Aviat Space Environ Med* 1975; 46:1289.
16. Grahn D, Kratchman J: Variations in neonatal death rate and birth weight in the United States and possible relations to environmental radiation, geology and altitude. *Am J Hum Genet* 1963; 15:329.
17. Hellman LM, Pritchard JA: *Williams Obstetrics*, ed 14. New York, Appleton-Century-Crofts, 1971.
18. Hill EP, Hill JR, Power GG, et al: Carbon monoxide exchanged between the human fetus and mother: A mathematical model. *Am J Physiol* 1977; 232:H311.
19. Ingenito AJ, Fiedler PC, Procita L: Negative inotropic action of carbon monoxide on the isolated isovolumic heart with a hemoglobin-free perfusate. *Fed Proc* 1974; 33:502.
20. Jaeger JJ, McGrath JJ: Effects of hypothermia on heart and respiratory responses of chick to carbon monoxide. *J Appl Physiol* 1973; 34:564.
21. Keller H: Hoher kohlemonoxydgehalt der stalluft als ursache von totgeburten beim schwein. *Schweiz Arch Tierheilkd* 1976; 118:424.
22. Kindwall EP: Carbon monoxide, in Zenz, C (ed): *Occupational Medicine: Principles and Practical Applications*, ed 2. Chicago, Year Book Medical Publishers, 1988, in press.
23. Lewey FH, Drabkin DL: Experimental chronic carbon monoxide poisoning in dogs. *Am J Med Sci* 1944; 208:502.
24. Linderholm H, Lundstrom P: Endogenous carbon monoxide production and blood loss at delivery. *Acta Obstet Gynecol Scand* 1969; 48:362.
25. Longo LD: Carbon monoxide: Effects on oxygenation of the fetus in utero. *Science* 1976; 194:523.
26. Longo LD: Carbon monoxide in the pregnant mother and fetus and its exchange across the placenta. *Ann NY Acad Sci* 1970; 174:313.
27. Longo LD: The biologic effects of carbon monoxide on the pregnant woman, the fetus and newborn infant. *Am J Obstet Gynecol* 1977; 129:69.
28. Longo LD, Hill EP: Carbon monoxide uptake and elimination in fetal and maternal sheep. *Am J Physiol* 1977; 232:H324.
29. Longo LD, Power GG, Forster RE: II: Respiratory function of the placenta as determined with carbon monoxide in sheep and dogs. *J Clin Invest* 1967; 46:812.
30. Maresch R: Über einen Fall von Kohlenoxydgasschadigung des Kindes in der Gebarmutter. *Wien Med Wochenschr* 1929; 79:454.
31. McGrath JJ, Jaeger J: Effect of iodoacetate on the carbon monoxide tolerance of the chick. *Respir Physiol* 1971; 12:71.
32. National Academy of Sciences: *Carbon Monoxide, Medical & Biological Effects of Environmental Pollutants*. Washington, DC, 1977.
33. Neuburger F: Fall einer intrauterinen Hirnschadigung nach einer Leuchtgasvergiftung der Mutter. *Beitr Gerichtl Med* 1935; 13:85.
34. Pernoll ML, et al: Oxygen consumption at rest and during exercise in pregnancy. *Respir Physiol* 1975; 25:285.
35. Ratney RS, Wegman DH, Elkins HB: In vivo conversion of methylene chloride to carbon monoxide. *Arch Environ Health* 1974; 28:223.
36. Ringold A, et al: Estimating recent carbon monoxide exposures: A rapid method. *Arch Environ Health* 1962; 5:308.
37. Rylander R, Vesterlund J: Carbon monoxide criteria effects on the fetus. *Scand J Work Environ Health* 1981; 7(1):25–31.
38. Schwedenberg TH: Leukoencephalopathy following carbon monoxide asphyxia. *J Neuropathol Exp Neurol* 1959; 18:597.
39. Sjöstrand T: Endogenous formation of carbon monoxide in man under normal and pathologic conditions. *Scand J Clin Lab Invest* 1949; 1:201.
40. Stewart RD, Hake CL: Paint-remover hazard. *JAMA* 1976; 235:398.
41. US Environmental Protection Agency: *Guidelines for Air Quality Maintenance Planning and Analysis, Vol. 9. Evaluating Indirect Sources*, EPA 450/4-75-001. Research Triangle Park, NC, US EPA, Office of Air Quality, Planning and Standards, 1975.
42. Wells LL: The prenatal effect of carbon monoxide on albino rats and the resulting neuropathy. *Biologist* 1933; 15:80.
43. Williams IR, Smith E: Blood picture, reproduction and general condition during daily exposure to illuminating gas. *Am J Physiol* 1935; 110:611.

CHLORDANE AND HEPTACHLOR

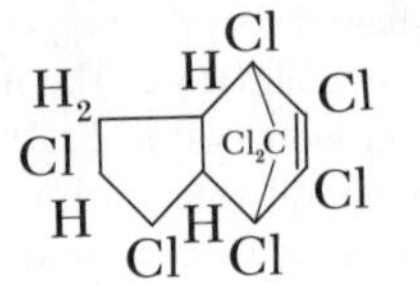

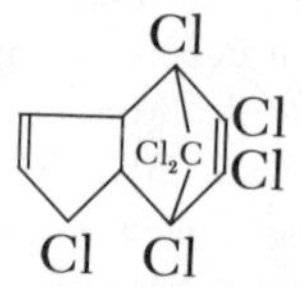

These two insecticides are members of the cyclodiene group of chlorinated insecticides, which includes aldrin, dieldrin, endrin and DDT. (See Chapter 46, showing chemical structures and their similarities.) Chlordane, first introduced in 1945, is one of the most widely used pesticides for household and garden applications. In the United States, more than 9.5 million kg are used per year, about 70% applied for termite control and the remainder in agricultural applications. Both chlordane and heptachlor are relatively persistent in the environment, with half-lives of one year (chlordane) and 0.8 year for heptachlor when used in agricultural applications. Chlordane and heptachlor have been tested under the carcinogenesis program of the National Cancer Institute, selected by the NCI for bioassay because of known biologic effects of low doses of either compound over extended periods, because of the persistence of both compounds in the environment, and the known probability of continued human exposure. In December, 1975, the Environmental Protection Agency ordered a suspension of the use of chlordane and heptachlor, which became effective in August, 1976. There were a number of specific exemptions and use still is permitted for pest control on pineapples, use against root-destroying insects on strawberries and Florida citrus crops, and other pest-control programs within specified state areas. The major current use is against termites, which is exempted from the EPA order.[9] Although there was a reduction of use of these conpounds from approximately 7.0 million kg, current usage for permitted purposes still amounts to about 3.0 million kg per year in the United States.

Exposure to chlordane and absorption into the body can occur through the intact skin, by inhalation of dust or sprays and by ingestion. Human intoxication, along with fatalities, has been reported from both dermal and oral exposures to chlordane.[1, 4, 5, 8] There are only a few reports concerning occupational exposure to chlordane, these being mainly reports in the manufacturing and handling of these substances. These reports present little data, chiefly because of the small number of workers involved or studied and the apparent high turnover in the working groups reported.[1]

Chlordane is less toxic than other cyclodiene pesticides, but acute exposure has the effect of stimulating the central nervous system. The compound metabolizes to its epoxide, oxychlordane, in which form it may be stored in body fat. It is said to be absorbable through the gastrointestinal tract and respiratory tract and directly through the skin. Both chlordane and heptachlor have been found to be mutagenic when tested in experimental organisms.

Trace amounts of heptachlor epoxide have been found in human fat tissues in most countries. The compound has been found in the blood, fat tissues, heart, adrenal gland and liver of stillborn infants, indicating that it can cross the placenta.[3] It has been found in human milk.[11] In other tests, concentrations of heptachlor epoxide in fat, liver, and brain were not found to be significantly different between cancer patients and cancer-free persons.

Under test conditions, chlordane and heptachlor both were found to be carcinogenic for the liver in mice and possibly were causes of thyroid tumors in rats.[10]

Infante et al.[6] reviewed certain blood dyscrasias and childhood tumors suspected from the histories to be related to chlordane and heptachlor. Reports of five cases of neuroblastoma related to a history of possible exposure to chlordane during prenatal and postnatal development were identified, as were three cases of aplastic anemia and three cases of acute leukemia. These authors indicated that the children with neuroblastoma were diagnosed at a single pediatric hospital between December, 1974, and February, 1976. During this period, a total of 14 patients with neuroblastoma were admitted. History of exposure to toxic agents indicated that five patients had prior exposure to chlordane formulations. Noteworthy in one case is that the mother took two Valium tablets in early pregnancy and also had received a general anesthetic for a tonsillectomy during the first month of pregnancy and that the general anesthesia was induced with sodium thiopental and was maintained with halothane and nitrous oxide. Infante et al. noted that in the nine additional cases of neuroblastoma, a history of exposure to chlordane was not known. Their report included, in addition to the cases mentioned, a review of other cases in the literature suspected to have had exposure to chlordane or heptachlor, either alone or in combination with other drugs. Infante et al. clearly indicated that in the absence of epidemiologic studies, the statistical demonstration that any chemical or drug has an etiologic relationship to blood dyscrasias is difficult to make. Reports of "associated with exposure to" from history only and lacking credible quantifying exposure data must be considered speculative.

Chlordane and heptachlor and their metabolites are persistent in the environment and their affinity for lipids makes them subject to possible bioaccumulation and transfer in the food chain, and components of technical-grade chlordane and its metabolites have been found commonly in dairy, meat, fish and poultry components of the diet. As has been the case with other chlorinated hydrocarbon pesticides, metabolites of chlordane and heptachlor may accumulate in man, and the oxychlordane and heptachlor epoxide residues have been detected in the adipose tissue in more than 90% of large samples of hospital patients studied in 1970–1972.[7]

Heptachlor epoxide residues have been detected in the organs of stillborn infants and also in samples of human milk. Because of environmental accumulation, humans may be exposed from time of conception on throughout adult life. There is a need for epidemiologic studies to further evaluate short-term and long-term health risks associated with chlordane in home use and in the agricultural setting.

The World Health Organization in 1967 established a maximal daily intake for heptachlor and its epoxide of 0.005 mg/kg of body weight. Measurement of average U.S. intake in 1970 indicated levels well below the "acceptable" level.[9]

REFERENCES

1. Alvarez, WC, Hyman S: Lack of toxic manifestations in workers exposed to chlordane. *Arch Ind Hyg Occup Med* 1953; 8:480.
2. Ambrose AM, Christensen HE, Robbins DJ, et al: Toxicological and pharmacological studies on chlordane. *Arch Ind Hyg Occup Med* 1953; 7:197.
3. Curley A, Copeland F, Kimbrough RD: Chlorinated hydrocarbon insecticides in organs of stillborn and blood of newborn babies. *Arch Environ Health* 1969; 19:628.
4. Dadey JL, Kammer AG: Chlordane intoxication, report of a case. *JAMA* 1953; 153:723.
5. Derbes VJ, Dent JH, Forrest WW, et al: Fatal chlordane poisoning. *JAMA* 1955; 158:1367.
6. Infante PF, Epstein SS, Newton WA: Blood dyscrasias and childhood tumors and exposure to chlordane and heptachlor. *Scand J Work Environ Health* 1978; 4:137.
7. International Agency for Research on Cancer: IARC monographs on the evaluation of the carcinogenic risk of chemicals to man: Some organochlorine pesticides (vol 5). Lyon, France, pp. 173–184, 1973.
8. Lensky P, Evans HL: Human poisoning by chlordane. *JAMA* 1952; 149:1394.
9. Report on carcinogenesis bioassay of chlordane and heptachlor. Technical Background Information. Bethesda, Md, USDHEW, NIH, NCI, September, 1977.
10. Special Pesticides Review Group (Fitzhugh OG, Fairchild HE, chairmen): Pesticidal aspects of chlordane in relation to man and the environment, Washington, DC, US Environmental Protection Agency, Government Printing Office, 6 pp, 1975.

CHLORDECONE (KEPONE)

Chlordecone (known under the trade name Kepone) is a chlorinated insecticide used against leaf-eating insects, ants, cockroaches, and the larvae of flies. More than 90% of the production has been for export and only 0.8% for domestic use, mainly as bait in ant traps.[8]

In 1975, an epidemiologic investigation of a Kepone manufacturing plant was initiated by NIOSH as a result of a finding by the Centers for Disease Control of a high blood level of Kepone in a worker exhibiting symptoms of marked weight loss, nystagmus, and tremors. Of 113 active and former employees studied, more than half had clinical symptoms of Kepone poisoning, including tremors ("Kepone shakes"), visual disturbances, nervousness, vertigo, insomnia, chest and abdominal pain, and weight loss. In a few cases, infertility and loss of libido were reported.[8] Manufacturing was discontinued in July, 1975.

Subsequent studies at the Medical College of Virginia of 32 former Kepone exposed employees indicated that half were unable to work at the beginning of the study because of neurologic disorders, including tremors, stuttered speech and memory lapses, and 11 patients had severely depressed sperm counts.[1]

Cholestyramine, an ion exchange resin that has been used clinically to bind bile salts and cholesterol, has been found to increase significantly the excretion of Kepone. In the Virginia study, all patients were greatly improved after six months of cholestyramine therapy and only three continue to have abnormally low sperm counts, indicating some reversibility of this effect.

Technical-grade chlordecone has been found to cause a significant increase in the incidence of hepatocellular cancer as compared to controls in high dose level rats and at both dose levels mice after oral feeding for 80 weeks at average dose levels of 8 and 24 ppm for male rats, 18 and 26 ppm for female rats, 20 and 23 ppm for male mice, and 20 and 40 ppm for female mice. Clinical signs of toxicity were observed in both species, including generalized tremors and dermatologic changes.[7]

Adverse effects of chlordecone on reproduction in mice have been reported by Good et al.[3] and Huber.[4] Huber found the reproductive capacity of treated mice inhibited or severely reduced, particularly in the female mice. Data collected by means of vaginal smears, hormone bioassays, histologic examinations, and results of matings indicated disturbances in the female hormonal system.

The author noted "the occurrence of constant estrus, the development of large follicles, the absence of corpora lutea in their ovaries, and the failure to reproduce are indications that the treated females were under a prolonged stimulation of FSH and estrogen, but insufficient LH stimulation."[4]

In August, 1975, the U.S. Environmental Protection Agency ordered the manufacturers to stop the sale and use of the compound and prohibited further manufacture.

In January, 1976, the NIOSH recommended that Kepone be considered a potential human carcinogen and that the workplace environmental level be limited to 1 μ/cu m as a time-weighted average for up to a ten-hour workday and a 40-hour workweek.

REFERENCES

1. Cohn WJ, et al: Treatment of chlordecone (Kepone) toxicity with cholestyramine. *N Engl J Med* 1978; 298:243.
2. Cueto C, Page N, Saffiotti U: *Report of Carcinogenesis Bioassay of Technical Grade Chlordecone (Kepone)*. Bethesda, Md, National Cancer Institute, 1976.
3. Good EE, Ware GW, Miller DF: Effects of insecticides on reproduction in laboratory mouse: I. Kepone. *J Econ Entomol* 1965; 53:754.
4. Huber JJ: Some physiological effects of the insecticide Kepone in the laboratory mouse. *Toxicol Appl Pharmacol* 1965; 7:516.
5. Reuber M: Carcinogenicity of kepone. *J Toxicol Environ Health* 1978; 4(5–6):895–911.
6. Reuber M: The carcinogenicity of kepone. *J Environ Pathol Toxicol* 1979; 2(3):671–686.
7. NIH-HEW Report on Carcinogenesis Bioassay of Kepone. Bethesda, Md, National Cancer Institute, April, 1976.
8. National Institute for Occupational Safety and Health. *Recommended Standard for Occupational Exposure to Kepone*. DHEW, PHS, NIOSH, 1976.

CHLOROPRENE

$$H_2C{=}\underset{\displaystyle Cl}{\underset{|}{C}}{-}CH{=}CH_2$$

Chloroprene, 2-chlorobutadiene, is used to manufacture polychloroprene latex and neoprene rubber. The NIOSH estimates that about 2,500 workers in the United States could be potentially exposed to chloroprene during its production and polymerization. In 1974, about 190 million kg (410 million lb) were produced in the United States.[3]

In 1936, von Oettingen et al.[7] reported findings of altered reproductive function in rats and mice after exposure to chloroprene by skin absorption (skin painting) and by inhalation. Exposure levels for inhalation studies over eight hours ranged from 12 ppm to 152 ppm in mice and from 121 to 6,227 ppm in rats. The animals had delays in reproduction and reduced numbers of young; some were sterile. In the rats, the testes showed pathologic changes, including epithelial degeneration with giant cell formation; the spermatic canals contained cellular debris derived from degenerated spermatozoa, and degenerative changes were described in the spermatogonia. In these initial studies of minimal lethal doses, there were no differences in susceptibility between males and females, but males were found to show altered reproductive function and histologic changes at exposure levels that produced no such changes in females. Culik et al.[4] reported that there were no effects on male reproductive function in rats at exposures of 25 ppm (90 mg/cu m) and also no histologic changes in the testes of rats.

Evidence of reproductive toxicity of chloroprene in male workers exposed to it has been reported by Sanotskii,[6] who described functional disturbances in spermatogenesis after exposure to chloroprene for six to ten years and morphologic disturbances after exposure of 11 or more years. In addition, the author found, through a questionnaire survey, a threefold incidence of spontaneous abortion in the wives of 143 chloroprene workers as compared with a control group of 100 male factory and office workers in an electrical engineering plant. Environmental data, particularly in regard to air concentrations of chloroprene, work, and health and safety practices (skin absorption), and presence of other air contaminants, were lacking. However, the author includes the findings of an inspection of a factory in the U.S.S.R., where a chloroprene-based latex was used, and indicated levels of 1–7 mg/cu m in air and low levels of ammonia (2–4 mg/cu m) as the most frequent other volatile substance in the latex.

Mutagenicity studies of chloroprene in microorganisms have shown variable results. Bartsch et al.[2] have reported positive mutagenicity findings from chloroprene (origin acetylene) in *Salmonella typhimurium* TA 1530 and TA 100; in the latter there was a linear increasing mutagenic response from 0.5% up to 8% of 2-chlorobutadiene in air. Litton Bionetics[2] reported negative mutagenicity findings of chloroprene (origin butadiene) with *Saccharomyces cerevisiae* and some Salmonella tester strains but positive findings in TA 1535. No clear data on mutagenic effects of chloroprene on mammalian cells are available.

There is no conclusion to date that chloroprene is carcinogenic, although there is evidence associating chloroprene with skin and liver cancers.[3]

Reports indicating chloroprene as a teratogenic substance are limited and somewhat conflicting. Sanotskii[6] reported that chloroprene exposure in a concentration of 4 mg/cu m (1.1 ppm) during the entire pregnancy of rats resulted in an increase in overall embryonic mortality, a decrease in fetal weight and a disturbance in vascular permeability noted in histologic sections. However, the same dose given days 5–6, 9–10, 11–12, or 13–14 of pregnancy produced teratogenic effects of cerebral hernia (mostly days 5–6) and hydrocephalus (mostly days 11–12, none days 13–14). On the other hand, Culik et al.[4] reported that inhalation during the full pregnancy of chloroprene of 1.0, 1.1, 10, or 25 ppm led to no clearly teratogenic effects, although the highest concentration used may have increased the incidence of abnormal vertebral centra in pups of the exposed pregnant rats.

The present OSHA standard for chloroprene is an eight-hour time-weighted average of 25 ppm (90 mg/cu m). The NIOSH recommended standard is a ceiling limit of 1 ppm (3.6 mg/cu m). "The adverse risk of genetic abnormalities being transmitted to subsequent generations by an agent with the mutagenic properties of chloroprene is the main reason for the NIOSH's recommendation for its current value."[3] The level of 1 ppm has been selected because it can be measured readily under field conditions by the analytic methods currently available. Studies of reproductive performance and effects on both male and female workers exposed to chloroprene are needed to elucidate the safety of 1 ppm as a standard for chloroprene.

REFERENCES

1. Appelman L, Dreef-van der Meulen H: Reproduction study with betachloroprene vapour in rats. Central Institute for Nutrition and Food Research, Report R 6225 1979. Cited in Barlow S, Sullivan F: *Reproductive Hazards of Industrial Chemicals, An Evaluation of Animal and Human Data*. New York, Academic Press, 1982, p 243.
2. Bartsch H, Malaveille C, Montesano R, et al: Tissue-mediated mutagenicity of vinylidene chloride and 2-chlorobutadiene in *Salmonella typhimurium*. *Nature* 1975; 255:641.
3. National Institute for Occupational Safety and Health: *Criteria for a Recommended Standard: Occupational Exposure to Chloroprene*. DHEW, PHS, NIOSH 77-210. 1977.
4. Culik R, Kelly DP, Clary JJ: Beta-chloroprene (2-Chlorobutadiene-1,3)—Embryotoxic and Teratogenic Studies in Rats. Wilmington, Del, EI du Pont de Nemours and Co., Haskell Laboratory for Toxicology and Industrial Medicine, 1976, 18 pp. (Cited in NIOSH Criteria Document[2].)
5. Rannug A: *Genotoxic Hazards In the Rubber Industry, Applications of Short-Term Tests in Work Environment Analyses*, doctoral thesis. Stockholm, University of Stockholm, 1984.
6. Sanotskii IV: Aspects of toxicology of chloroprene—immediate and long-term effects. *Environ Health Perspect* 1976; 17:85.
7. von Oettingen WF, Hueper WC, Deichman-Gruebler W, et al: 2-Chloro-butadiene (chloroprene)—its toxicity and pathology and the mechanism of its action. *J Ind Toxicol* 1936; 18:240.

DIBROMOCHLOROPROPANE

Dibromochloropropane (1,2-dibromo-3-chloropropane, CH_2Br-CH_2Cl) (DBCP) has been used as a fumigant and nematocide in agriculture since 1955, with about 12 million kg (25 million lb) manufactured and used in the United States each year. A complete discussion, including clinical details, is presented by Whorton in Chapter 55.

DIETHYLSTILBESTROL

$$HO{-}C_6H_4{-}C(C_2H_5){=}C(C_2H_5){-}C_6H_4{-}OH$$

Diethylstilbestrol (DES), a potent estrogenic compound, was synthesized initially by Dodds in 1938 in England. Because of a potency similar to natural estrogens and because it was inexpensive to prepare and could be administered orally, it was used extensively in women with threatened pregnancies in the late 1940s and 1950s, up to the beginning of the 1970s. Welch[11] estimated that approximately 500,000–2,000,000 women probably received DES during pregnancy in that interval. As a result of that experience, a sufficient number of cases of carcinoma of the genital tract in offspring of women treated with DES have been reported to suggest that DES is the first apparent transplacental carcinogen in humans.

Between 1966 and 1969, Herbst et al.[6] encountered seven young women and girls with clear cell adenocarcinoma of the vagina (a relatively rare tumor) and noted that all of these patients were products of pregnancies during which the mothers received DES. Subsequently, a registry for such cases was established at Massachusetts General Hospital, and Welch[11] reported the findings of 150 cases in the registry as of June, 1976. In every instance where adequate maternal histories were obtained, DES had been administered prior to the 18th week of gestation. The ages at time of diagnosis ranged from 7 to 28 years, with an average in the late teens and the majority past puberty. Vaginal bleeding and discharge were the manifestations for which medical attention was sought; however, one sixth of the patients were asymptomatic and the tumor was detected on routine gynecologic examination, including Papanicolaou smears. (Cytologic examination alone may not detect the tumor and such examination needs to be combined with adequate pelvic examination and appropriate biopsies.) Subsequently, Greenwald et al.[4] reported five additional cases of clear cell vaginal adenocarcinoma in young women, all of whose mothers received synthetic estrogens (four DES, one dienestrol) early in pregnancy. These findings can be compared with those of Lanier et al.[8] in a follow-up study of 1,719 persons (818 females, 901 males) exposed to estrogens in utero and born between 1943 and 1959. The follow-up interval ranged between 11 and 30 years and the median age was 22 years. No cases of adenocarcinoma of the vagina or cervix were found in any of the young women. On the basis of their study, the authors estimate an incidence of vaginal or cervical adenocarcinoma associated with in utero exposure to estrogens to be no greater than 4 per 1,000 cases, and for those exposed in the 1st trimester, no greater than 9 per 1,000. The authors indicated that the estrogenic dosage in their series may have been a little less than 100 mg/day, the prevailing recommended dose level at the time. Herbst, in a review of more recent studies, suggests that the risk is smaller, approximately 1 per 1,000 cases.[7] The cancers are most frequent after age 14 years, reaching a peak by age 19 years, with the oldest reported case 33 years of age.[7]

In addition to the malignancies; nonmalignant anomalies have been found in the in utero exposed populations, including vaginal adenosis and vaginal and cervical ridges.[11] In one study, Herbst et al.[6] noted that adenosis was present in 73% of offspring where the drug was administered prior to the eighth week of gestation, but in no one exposed after the 18th week. Although it has been suggested that adenosis ia a premalignant condition, malignant transformation of adenosis has not as yet been observed. Welch[11] noted that some investigators have predicted that glycogen-poor (metaplastic) squamous epithelium that is associated with adenosis will result in increased rates of squamous cell malignancy. However, for some reason, such healing has not been seen in some DES daughters.[7]

Studies by McLachlan and his associates using radioactive tagged DES in pregnant mice have indicated that DES crosses the placenta, initially very slowly, but after an appropriate time reaches the fetus in a considerable amount and accumulates in the fetal reproductive tract. In one study, analysis of selected fetal tissues for ^{3}H-DES content, a half hour after treatment, showed an approximately fourfold accumulation of parent compound relative to the fetal plasma in the genital tract.[9]

Prenatal toxicity of DES was studied in pregnant mice, using subcutaneous treatment with DES in corn oil on the ninth through 16th day of gestation, and the offspring evaluated for altered genital tract function. Altered function was reported in both female and male offspring.[9] In the females there were found dose-related decreases in reproductive capacity, ranging from minimal subfertility at the lowest dose to essential sterility at the two highest doses. Notably, the highest dose used was 100 μg/kg, which is 1/20 the maximal average daily dose based on body weight given to pregnant women therapeutically (100 mg/day). Lesions of the genital tract found in female mice included cystic hyperplasia of the endometrium, uterine adenocarcinoma, and histologic changes in epithelium resembling adenosis and/or adenocarcinoma.

Male mice exposed to DES in utero also showed impaired genital tract function,[9] but the effect occurred only at the highest dose of 100 μg/kg and not at the lower doses studied. The findings included sterility in 60%, undescended testes in 25%, epididymal cysts in 33%, and in 25% nodular enlargement of the seminal vesicles and/or coagulating glands, which were associated with squamous metaplasia.

Abnormal findings in human male offspring of DES-treated mothers have been reported by Gill et al.[2] from a follow-up study of male offspring of DES-exposed mothers, compared to placebo-exposed mothers, all of whom were participants in a prospective study at the Chicago Lying-In Hospital during the early 1950s. The more common genital lesions found were epididymal cysts, hypotrophic testes, capsular induration of the testes, and microphallus (flaccid penis less than 4 cm in length) in more than 25% of the 163 DES-exposed males, as compared to a 6.5% incidence in the 168 control males. Severe pathologic changes in spermatogenesis and abnormal spermatozoa were found in 28% and 46%, respectively, of 39 DES-exposed male children compared with 0% and 12% in 25 controls. No cases of genitourinary malignancies were found in the follow-up study of 901 males by Lanier et al.,[8] mentioned previously. In 1984, Gill et al. summarized the findings of several studies by other investigators on structural and functional genital abnormalities in DES sons and updated the findings from a further follow-up with semen analysis of the DES sons included in their original study mentioned above. Although an increased incidence of abnormal sperm continued to be noted in DES-exposed sons, a risk of infertility had not been demonstrated, and studies of larger cohorts have shown a lower incidence of the abnormalities.[3] It is noteworthy also that despite the facts that DES has been associated with uterine and vaginal cancer in DES daughters and that there is an increased risk of testicular cancer from maldescent of the testes, an increased finding in DES sons, there has not been any clear evidence of an increased risk of testicular cancer in DES-exposed sons.[3, 7]

In the late 1960s, estrogens had been used in the prevention of ischemic heart disease in men, but the practice was discontinued because of adverse side effects. Among the less severe side effects noted within a few months of treatment with doses of 5–10 mg/day of equine estrogens of 5–25 mg/day DES were breast enlargement (100%), reduced testicular size (82%), increased areolar pigmentation (77%), and decreased or absent libido (74%).

Occupational exposure to DES is largely in the pharmaceutical industry, where DES is produced and packaged and used in the production of hormonal products.[10] Hyperestrogenism has been reported in female pharmaceutical workers, manifested mostly as intermenstrual bleeding and breast enlargement and tenderness and in male workers as clinical gynecomastia with or without increased areolar pigmentation and decreased libido and impotence.[5] To date there have been no studies in the United States on the reproductive capacity and/or function in such workers or on the effects of such exposure in their offspring.

No threshold for occupational DES exposure has been established. It is recognized that DES can be absorbed through the skin as well as by inhalation. The correlative findings in both animal and human studies of the effects of DES on the genital system in both males and females and the transplacental effects reported in the offspring of exposed animals and humans indicated some dose relationship. Occupational exposure to DES should be kept to a minimum.

REFERENCES

1. Coronary Drug Project: *JAMA* 1970; 214:1303.
2. Gill WB, Schumacher GFB, Bibbo M: Structural and functional abnormalities in the sex organs of male offspring of mothers treated with diethylstilbestrol (DES). *J Reprod Med* 1976; 16:147.
3. Gill WB, Schumacher GFB, Hubby MM, et al: Male genital tract changes in humans following intrauterine exposure to diethylstilbestrol, in Herbst AL, Bern HA, (eds): *Developmental Effects of Diethylstilbestrol (DES) in Pregnancy*. New York, Thieme-Stratton, 1981, pp 103–119.
4. Greenwald P, Barlon JJ, Nasca PC, et al: Vaginal cancer after mater-

nal treatment with synthetic estrogens. *N Engl J Med* 1971; 285:390.
5. Harrington JM, Rivera RO, Lowry LK: Occupational exposure to synthetic estrogens—The need to establish safety standards. *Am Ind Hyg Assoc J* 1978; 39:139.
6. Herbst AL, Ulfeder H, Poskanzer DC: Adenocarcinoma of the vagina: Association of maternal stilbestrol therapy with tumor appearance in young women. *N Engl J Med* 1971; 284:878.
7. Herbst AL: Diethylstilbestrol exposure-1984. *N Engl J Med* 1984; 311:1433–1434, Nov 29.
8. Lanier AP, Noller KL, Decher D, et al: Cancer and stilbestrol: a follow-up of 1719 persons exposed to estrogens in utero and born 1943–1959. *Mayo Clinic Proc* 1973; 48:793.
9. McLachlan JA: Male as well as female in utero exposure to diethylstilbestrol; in *Proceedings of the Conference on Women and the Workplace*, Society of Occupational and Environmental Health, Washington, DC, June 17–19, 1976.
10. *Morbidity and Mortality Weekly Report*. Epidemiologic notes and reports: occupational exposure to synthetic estrogens, Puerto Rico, April 1, 1977, vol 26, No 13.
11. Welch WR: Transplacental carcinogenesis; Prenatal diethylstilbestrol (DES) exposure; Clear cell carcinoma and related anomalies of the genital tract in young females, in *Proceedings of the Conference on Women and the Workplace*, Society of Occupational and Environmental Health, Washington, DC, June 17–19, 1976.

EPICHLOROHYDRIN

```
              O
             / \
H2C—CH—CH2
  |
  Cl
```

Production of epichlorohydrin in the United States in 1978 was estimated at more than 320 million kg (715 million lb); 58% is used in the manufacture of synthetic glycerin and the remainder, in its refined form, to manufacture epoxy resins, surface-active agents, pharmaceuticals, insecticides, agricultural chemicals, textile chemicals, coatings, adhesives, ion exchange resins, solvents and plasticizers. The NIOSH estimates that 50,000 employees may be exposed to epichlorohydrin in the United States.[2]

Epichlorohydrin has been reported to cause sterility in animals.[1,4] Hahn[4] gave male rats of demonstrated fertility a dose of 15 mg/kg body weight orally for 12 days (total dose 180 mg/kg body weight) and evaluated the fertility of the animals after seven days by the number of uterine implantations in pre-estrus females placed in the cages of the treated males. Within one week, the males became infertile, but the effect was reversible within the succeeding week. Histologic examination of the testes, epididymis, prostate, and seminal vesicles on the 12th day of treatment showed no differences between test and control animals, and sexual libido and ability to ejaculate were unaffected.

Epstein and co-workers[3] gave a single intraperitoneal dose of 150 mg/kg of epichlorohydrin to male Swiss mice and recorded the number of total live implants and early and late fetal deaths. Late fetal deaths were very rare, and the authors reported no effects of epichlorohydrin on early fetal deaths or other reproductive characteristics, including male fertility.

Cooper et al.[1] administered epichlorohydrin orally to three groups of five adult male rats; one group received doses of 20 mg/kg for five days (total 100 mg/kg), another group was given 50 mg/kg for five days (total 250 mg/kg) and a third group 100 mg/kg as a single dose. The five doses of 20 mg/kg resulted in lost fertility during the first two weeks, but this was reversed in the third week. Five doses of 50 mg/kg resulted in sterility throughout the two-week period observed. A single dose of 100 mg/kg resulted in reduced litter size during the ten weeks and, by 12 weeks, large retention cysts were present in the ductuli efferentes and proximal caputs in four of the five test animals that were sterile.

In rats, but not mice, therefore, it appears that epichlorohydrin causes sterility that is both dose- and time-dependent.

Epichlorohydrin has been reported to produce tumors in mice at subcutaneous injection sites but not by skin painting.[8] The NIOSH Criteria Document[2] references several reports indicating that epichlorohydrin has induced a high frequency of positive results in point mutation tests in fungi, other microbial organisms, and the fruit fly. Also noted is the report that the urine of workers exposed to 25 ppm of epichlorohydrin influenced the genetic mechanisms of *Salmonella typhimurium*. The Criteria Document further states that there have been experimental attempts to cause teratogenesis by exposing pregnant animals to epichlorohydrin, but these efforts have been negative.

The present OSHA standard for epichlorohydrin is 20 mg/cu m (5 ppm). The NIOSH recommends that this be reduced to 2 mg/cu m (0.5 ppm), with a ceiling of 19 mg/cu m. This recommendation follows consideration of the limited available data on reproductive and carcinogenic effects, plus effects on the kidneys, liver, respiratory tract, and skin. Additional studies are needed on the reproductive effects, including effects on the male.

REFERENCES

1. Cooper ERA, Jones AR, Jackson H: Effect of alpha-chlorohydrin and related compounds on the reproductive organs and fertility of the male rat. *J Reprod Fertil* 1974; 38:379.
2. National Institute for Occupational Safety and Health: *Criteria for a Recommended Standard: Occupational Exposure to Epichlorohydrin*, DHEW, PHS, NIOSH 76-206, 1976.
3. Epstein SS, Arnold E, Andrea J, et al: Detection of chemical mutagens by the dominant lethal assay in the mouse. *Toxicol Appl Pharmacol* 1972; 23:288. (Cited in NIOSH Criteria Document.[2])
4. Hahn JD: Post-testicular antifertility effects of epichlorohydrin and 2,3-epoxypropanol. *Nature* 1970; 226:87.
5. Knaap A, Voogd C, Dramers P: Comparison of the mutagenic potency of 2-chloroethanol, 2-bromoethanol, 1,2-epoxybutane, epichlorohydrin and glycidaldehyde in *Klebsiella pneumoniae, Dosophila meglanogaster* and L5178Y mouse lymphoma cells. *Mutat Res* 1982; 101(3):199–208.
6. Marks T, Gerling F, Staples R: Teratogenic evaluation of epichlorohydrin in the mouse and rat and glycidol in the mouse. *J Toxicol Environ Health* 1982; 9(1):87–96.
7. Milby T, Whorton M, Stubbs H, et al: Testicular function among epichlorohydrin workers. *Br J Ind Med* 1981; 38:372–377.
8. Van Duuren BL, Goldschmidt BM, Katz C, et al: Carcinogenic activity of alkylating agents. *JNCI* 1974; 53:695.
9. Picciano D: Cytogenic investigation of occupational exposure to epichlorohydrin. *Mutat Res* 1979; 66(2):169–173.

ETHYLENE DIBROMIDE

$BrCH_2–CH_2Br$

Jennifer M. Ratcliffe, Ph.D., M.Sc.

Kyle Steenland, Ph.D.

Theodore Meinhardt, Ph.D.

Properties, Uses, and Occupational Exposures

Ethylene dibromide (EDB), correctly called 1,2-dibromoethane, is a colorless or light brown nonflammable liquid at room temperature. It boils at 135.5° C, freezes at 9.3° C, and has a vapor pressure of 11.7 mm Hg at 25° C. It is miscible with most solvents and is slightly soluble in water. EDB is readily absorbed through the skin and the lungs.[14] Because it contains two replacable bromine atoms, EDB is considered to be a bifunctional alkylating agent that reacts readily with nucleophilic biochemical constituents and may covalently bind to DNA molecules.[25] This alkylating activity is thought to be the basis of the mutagenic and carcinogenic properties of EDB.[25]

Ethylene dibromide has been in use in the United States since the 1920s. The annual U.S. production of EDB in 1981 was estimated by the National Institute for Occupational Safety and Health (NIOSH) to be approximately 300 million lb.[25] Approximately 90% of this EDB is used as a scavenger in leaded fuels, although this use has decreased since 1970 with the decline in the use of leaded gasoline. A much smaller volume of EDB is used as an agricultural pesticide. The major agricultural use of EDB is as a nematocide which is applied to the soil before planting. In granaries EDB is used as a fumigant to control insects. In fruit control, EDB is used to prevent the growth of fruit fly larvae in the crop after harvest and is also used as a soil fumigant. A small volume of EDB is also used as an intermediate in the synthesis of dyes and pharmaceuticals and as a solvent for resins, gums, and waxes.

NIOSH has estimated that approximately 108,000 workers were potentially exposed to EDB in 1981 in the U.S. during EDB production and use. Most of this exposure occurred in the agricultural uses of EDB. In addition, approximately 875,000 U.S. workers are potentially exposed to EDB in gasoline, but at very low levels.[24, 25]

The current exposure standard set by the Occupational Safety and Health Administration (OSHA) for EDB consists of a 20 ppm eight-hour TWA with a 30-ppm 15-minute ceiling and a 50-ppm 5-minute peak. However, in late 1983, OSHA proposed lowering the standard to 0.1 ppm TWA, with a 15-minute ceiling limit of 0.5 ppm.[11] The NIOSH, on the basis of the available toxicologic and epidemiologic data on EDB,[24, 25] has recommended that the occupational standard for EDB be limited to a ceiling concentration of 0.13 ppm (1.0 mg/cu m) over any 15-minute period with an eight-hour TWA of 0.045 ppm. In 1981, the state of California adopted the NIOSH ceiling limit recommendations.[35]

The U.S. Environmental Protection Agency (EPA) has jurisdiction over occupational uses of EDB when the chemical is used as a pesticide. In 1983, the EPA declared an immediate ban on the use of EDB as a soil fumigant and a gradual phase-out of its other agricultural uses.[14] In 1984, the EPA set 30 ppb by weight as the maximum safe level of EDB which could be present in grains and in the edible portions of fruits.[15]

Analytical Methods

The NIOSH recommended method for measuring EDB[20] is to collect an air sample on a charcoal tube. In low concentrations, an air flow of approximately 50 cu cm/min may be used to collect the sample. Water may displace EDB on the charcoal, and back-up tubes are recommended in humid conditions. The samples must be kept cold and analysed quickly since EDB is volatile and reactive and will off-gas from the charcoal. Analysis is conducted using gas chromatography with electron capture detection.

Toxicology and Pathology

Acute Toxicity in Animals.—The available animal data show that acute systemic effects, consisting primarily of damage to the liver, kidney, spleen, and lungs, and including central nervous system depression, occur after administration of EDB by skin application, gavage, inhalation, and injection.[24] Irritation of the mucous membranes and respiratory tract results from acute exposure to EDB vapor, and skin irritation and blistering following dermal application. In rodents, the lowest concentration of EDB reported to result in mortality is 400 ppm (by inhalation) and 250 mg/kg (by gavage).[24]

Acute Toxicity in Human Beings.—The acute toxicity of EDB in humans has been defined following cases of accidental or deliberate (suicidal) overexposures or poor work practices. On the basis of such data, OSHA estimates that doses of between 15 and 150 mg/kg can produce acute toxicity and death in humans.[11] The most prominent symptoms identified in reviewed cases are mucous membrane irritation resulting in conjunctivitis and upper respiratory tract irritation following airborne exposure and skin erythema and blistering following dermal exposure.[17, 19, 26, 29] Other reported acute symptoms include nausea, vomiting, abdominal pain, headaches, central nervous system depression, tremors, anorexia, cardiac arrhythmia, chest pain, and shortness of breath.

Limited information about the pathology of EDB poisoning in human beings can be derived from two published case reports of fatalities which included autopsy information.[19, 26] Deaths occurred 44 and 54 hours after accidental ingestion of approximately 70 and 5 ml of pure EDB, respectively. Symptoms prior to death included cardiac and pulmonary insufficiency, vomiting, diarrhea, anuria, and uterine bleeding. Autopsies revealed bronchial inflammation, extensive hepatic and renal necrosis, and mediastinal hemorrhage. At the hearings on the proposed OSHA standard for occupational exposure to EDB,[38] the case of two workers who died approximately 24 and 72 hours following acute exposure to EDB during a tank cleaning operation was cited. The level of EDB to which the men had been exposed was estimated to be approximately 30 ppm; dermal exposure was also likely.

Mutagenicity and Carcinogenicity in Plants and Animals.—EDB is mutagenic to a variety of plant and animal test systems. It has been shown to be mutagenic to the fruit fly *Drosophila melanogaster*,[40] the fungus *Neurospora crassa*,[18] *Tradescantia*,[34] *Salmonella typhimurium* bacteria,[8, 9] and mouse lymphoma cells.[10] The ability of EDB to produce chromosomal damage has been demonstrated in the Chinese hamster cell assay, in which significant dose-dependent increases in the frequency of sister chromatid exchanges and chromosomal abnormalities have been produced following exposure to EDB.[37]

Ethylene dibromide has been shown to produce significant increases in the frequency of malignancies in rats and mice as follows: (1) squamous cell carcinomas of the stomach following administration of EDB by gavage;[27, 30] (2) skin and lung tumors following skin application;[39] and (3) respiratory tract, nasal cavity, spleen, subcutaneous, pituitary gland, and mammary gland tumors following inhalation exposure.[21] In rats, a synergistic effect of concurrent administration of disulfiram (a compound widely used in alcoholism control programs and structurally related to the fungicide Thiram) and EDB exposure on the frequency of hepatocellular carcinomas has been demonstrated.[23] On the basis of these studies, the NIOSH has reaffirmed its position that EDB is a proven carcinogen in animal species and should be considered a potential carcinogen in human beings.[25]

Mutagenicity and Carcinogenicity in Human Beings.—There has been one published epidemiologic study to date of the mortality experience of workers exposed to EDB in two manufacturing plants.[25] Although a statistically nonsignificant increase in total deaths and deaths from malignancies was observed for the 161 long-term workers from both plants, the sample size is too small to draw any firm conclusions about the carcinogenic risk of EDB in human beings.

Reproductive Effects in Animals.—Oral administration of EDB has been shown to produce reversible abnormalities in sperm morphology and decreased sperm motility and concentration in bulls.[3, 4, 5] Abnormal sperm morphology and decreased sperm motility have been reported in rams given EDB subcutaneously,[13] but not after oral administration.[6] Ethylene dibromide also produces testicular atrophy and reversible changes in sperm morphology and transient infertility in rats.[12, 33] Reduced fertility in hens after oral dosing has been reported,[1, 2, 7] but cockerels given EDB orally for one year have shown no adverse effects on sperm or fertility.[2]

The teratogenicity of EDB has been investigated in a series of experiments by Short and co-workers, using rats and mice.[31–33] Significant increases in fetal malformations and resorptions were observed following exposure by inhalation during gestation. While the effect of maternal toxicity and malnutrition cannot be excluded in these studies, a comparison of the fetal abnormality rates in EDB-exposed and feed-restricted animals strongly suggest that EDB may induce malformations and heritable damage in these species.

Reproductive Effects in Human Beings.—There have been three previous reports of sperm characteristics and one fertility study of male workers exposed to EDB. Twelve workers potentially exposed to EDB at an anti-knock manufacturing plant showed a decrease in median but not in mean sperm counts and significantly elevated levels of luteinizing hormone in comparison with seven controls.[22]

No statistically significant differences in sperm concentration or motility were found among 44 citrus and soil fumigators with varied estimated potential exposure to EDB.[14, 16] Finally, Ter Haar[36] reported the distribution of sperm concentration among manufacturing workers divided according to estimated exposure, 19 receiving more than 0.5 ppm exposure and 40 receiving less than 0.5 ppm. A higher percentage of the former group had sperm concentrations of less than 40 million (42% compared to 20%), but no statistical analyses were performed on the data and no controls were used. In each of these reports, small sample sizes, lack of specification of the methods of semen sample collection and analysis, and inadequate control groups and/or poor exposure data mean that the results of these studies are unsatisfactory as a basis for conclusions.

In a study of EDB-exposed manufacturing workers,[41] the number of live births among wives of white male workers over a 19-year period were compared with U.S. national birth rates. A statistically significant decrease in the observed/expected birth ratio was found for one of the four plants. However, a number of methodologic limitations in the use of national data and the higher rate of vasectomies in this plant preclude any firm conclusions with respect to the effect of EDB on human male fertility.

No other aspects of reproductive outcome in partners of exposed men have thus far been addressed. No adequate reproductive studies of exposed female workers have been carried out to date.

Summary

Ethylene dibromide is readily absorbed through the skin, lungs, and gut and is acutely toxic at relatively low doses. The available toxicologic data indicate that EDB is strongly mutagenic and carcinogenic in a number of animal species and is toxic to the sperm of rats, bulls, and rams. Animal data also suggest that EDB has teratogenic effects and impairs fertility in male and female rats and mice. There are currently insufficient data on male or female reproductive effects and carcinogenicity of EDB in human beings.

REFERENCES

1. Alumot E, Mandel E: Gonadotropic hormones in hens treated with ethylene dibromide. *Poult Sci* 1969; 48:957–960.
2. Alumot E, Nachtomi E, Kempenich-Pinto O, et al: The effect of ethylene dibromide in feed on the growth, sexual development and fertility of chickens. *Poultry Sci* 1968; 47:1979–1985.
3. Amir D: Individual and age differences in the spermicidal effect of ethylene dibromide in bulls. *J Reprod Fertil* 1975; 44:561–565.
4. Amir D: The sites of the spermicidal action of ethylene dibromide in bulls. *J Reprod Fertil* 1973; 35:519–525.
5. Amir D, Volcani R: Effect of dietary ethylene dibromide in bull semen. *Nature* 1965; 206:99–100.
6. Bondi A, Alumot E: Effect of ethylene dibromide fumigated feed on animals, Final Technical Report PL-480. US Dept of Agriculture, 1966.
7. Bondi A, Olomucki E, Calderon M: Problems connected with ethyl-

ene dibromide fumigation of cereals. II. *J Sci Food Agric* 6:600–602.
8. Brem H, Stein AB, Rosenkranz HS: The mutagenicity and DNA-modifying effect of haloalkanes. *Cancer Res* 34:2576–2579.
9. Buselmaier W, Rohrborn G, Popping P: Pesticide mutagenicity investigated by the host-mediated assay and dominant lethal test in mice. *Biol Zentralblat* 1972; 91:311–325.
10. Clive D: Recent developments with the L5178Y TK heterozygote mutagen assay system. *Environ Health Perspect* 1973; 6:119–125.
11. Dept of Labor, OSHA: Notice of proposed rulemaking: Occupational exposure to ethylene dibromide. *Federal Register* 1983; 48:45956–46003.
12. Edwards K, Jackson H, Jones AR: Studies with alkylating esters II. *Biochem Pharmacol* 1970; 19:1783–1789.
13. Eljack A, Hrudka F: Pattern and dynamics of teratospermia induced in rams by parenteral treatment with ethylene dibromide. *J Ultrastruct Res* 1979; 67:124–134.
14. Environmental Protection Agency: EDB Position Document 4, Office of Pesticide Programs, Washington DC, Sept 27, 1983.
15. Environmental Protection Agency: Notice of decision and emergency order suspending registrations of pesticide products containing EDB, OPP-68012A, Feb 3, 1984.
16. Griffith J, Heath R, Davido R: Spermatogenesis in agricultural workers potentially exposed to ethylene dibromide. Interim report, Human Effects Monitoring Branch, Environmental Protection Agency, June 8, 1978.
17. Kochmann M: Possible industrial poisonings with ethylene dibromide. *Muench Med Wochenschr* (Ger) 1928; 75:1334–1336.
18. Malling HU: Ethylene dibromide: A potent pesticide with high mutagenic activity. *Genetics* 1969; 61:39.
19. Marmetschke G: On lethal ethyl bromide and ethylene dibromide intoxification. *Vierteljahresschr Gerichtl Med Oeff Sanitaetswes* (Ger) 1910; 40:61–76.
20. Method P and CAM 250: Ethylene dibromide, in *NIOSH Manual of Analytical Methods*, vol 4. Washington, DC, US Govt Printing Office, 1977.
21. National Cancer Institute: Carcinogenesis bioassay of 1,2-dibromoethane (Inhalation study), DHSS Publ (NIH) 81-1766.
22. National Institute for Occupational Safety and Health: Health Hazard Evaluation Report HE 77-119-481. Cincinnati, Oh, NIOSH, April 1978.
23. National Institute for Occupational Safety and Health: Ethylene dibromide and disulfiram toxic interaction. *Curr Intell Bull* 23, NIOSH Publ 78-145.
24. National Institute for Occupational Safety and Health: *Criteria for a Recommended Standard for Occupational Exposure to Ethylene Dibromide*, NIOSH Publ 77-221, August 1977.
25. National Institute for Occupational Safety and Health: Current Intelligence Bulletin 37, NIOSH Publ 82-105, Oct 26, 1981.
26. Olmstead EV: Pathological changes in ethylene dibromide poisoning. *AMA Arch Ind Hyg Occup Med* 1960; 21:45–49.
27. Olson WA, Habermann RT, Weisburger EK, et al: Induction of stomach cancer in rats and mice by halogenated aliphatic fumigants. *JNCI* 1973; 51:1993–1995.
28. Ott MG, Scharnweber HC, Langner RR: Mortality experience of 161 employees exposed to EDB. *Br J Ind Med* 1980; 37:163–168.
29. Pflesser G: Skin-damaging effect of ethylene dibromide—A constituent of the liquid from remote water gauges. *Arch Gewerbepathol Gewerbehyg* (Ger) 1938; 8:591–600.
30. Powers MB, Voelker RW, Page NP, et al: Carcinogenicity of ethylene dibromide and 1,2 dibromo-3-chloropropane after oral administration in rats and mice. *Toxicol Appl Pharmacol* 1975; 33:171.
31. Short JD, Minor JL, Ferguson B, et al: Toxicity studies of selected chemicals II. The developmental toxicity of ethylene dibromide, US EPA Report. EPA 560/6-76-018, 1976.
32. Short JD, Minor JL, Winston JM, et al: Inhalation of EDB during gestation by rats and mice. *Toxicol Appl Pharmacol* 1978; 46:174–182.
33. Short R, Winston J, Hong C, et al: Effects of ethylene dibromide on reproduction in male and female rats. *Toxicol Appl Pharmacol* 1979; 49:97–105.
34. Sparrow AH, Schairer LA, Villalobos-Pietrini R: Comparison of somatic mutation rates induced in Tradescantia by chemical and physical mutagens. *Mutat Res* 1974; 26:265–276.
35. State of California, Division of Occupational Safety and Health: Proposed emergency standard for EDB. July 28 1981 (adopted Sept. 1981).
36. Ter Haar G: An investigation of possible sterility and health effects from exposure to ethylene dibromide, in Banbury Report No 5. Cold Spring Harbor Laboratory, 1980.
37. Tezuka H, Ando N, Suzuki M, et al: Sister-chromatid exchanges and chromosomal aberrations in cultured Chinese hamster cells treated with pesticides positive in microbial reversion assays. *Mutat Res* 1980; 78:177–191.
38. Transcript of hearings on the OSHA proposed rulemaking on occupational exposure to EDB. Washington, D.C. Feb 8 1984.
39. Van Duuren BL, Goldschmidt BM, Lowewengart A, et al: Carcinogenicity of halogenated olefinic and aliphatic hydrocarbons in mice. *JNCI* 1979; 63:1433–1439.
40. Vogel E, Chandler JLR: Mutagenicity testing of cyclamates and some pesticides in Drosophila melanogaster. *Experientia* 1974; 30:113–126.
41. Wong O, Utidjian MD, Korten VS: Retrospective evaluation of reproductive performance of workers exposed to ethylene dibromide. *J Occup Med* 1980; 21:98–102.

ETHYLENE OXIDE

$$\overset{\displaystyle O}{CH_2 \;-\; CH_2}$$

Ethylene oxide (ETO) is a colorless gas used as an intermediate in the production of ethylene glycol (antifreeze), polyester fiber, and film, as an agricultural fungicide, a fumigant for foodstuffs and textiles, and for sterilization of surgical instruments, equipment, and heat-sensitive materials in medical facilities. It is one of the top 25 chemicals (by volume) produced in the United States,[16] annually about 6.1 billion lb. United States production represents about 43% of world capacity. Between 5,500 and 6,000 hospitals in the United States have ETO sterilizers, and an unknown number of industries, which are scattered throughout the country, have such sterilizers; consequently, the NIOSH estimates that up to 100,000 employees may be directly or casually exposed.[16]

Acute effects include conjunctival irritation, headaches, respiratory tract irritation, and primary irritation and sensitization of the skin.[9] Gross et al.[8] noted neurologic effects varying from incoordination to recent memory loss and delayed nerve conduction.

Hollingsworth et al.[12] and Jacobson et al.[13] studied the effects of repeated doses of ETO vapors on various animal species. There was no evidence of damage to the gonads of rats, mice, guinea pigs, rabbits, dogs, and monkeys when ETO was inhaled at dose levels of 49 ppm, 100 ppm, and 113 ppm in air for six or seven hours per day, usually on a five-day-per-week basis, with the total number of exposures per animal ranging from 122 to 157. At 204 ppm, ETO in air administered seven hours per day with 122–157 exposures over 176–226 days produced slight testicular tubal degeneration in the rat. At this dose level, 22 of 40 exposed rats died. The primary cause of death was secondary respiratory infection. At 357 ppm for seven hours per day with 123 exposures over 176 days there was degeneration of testicular tubules in male guinea pigs. All 16 exposed guinea pigs survived. Dose levels of 841 ppm given for seven hours per day with one to eight exposures over ten days were lethal to all rats, guinea pigs, rabbits, mice, and monkeys exposed.

The mutagenic potential of ETO has been studied in at least 14 different species, and in 13 of these there was an increased frequency of mutation. The exception was a bacteriophage of *Escherichia coli*.[14] Evidence of chromosomal damage has been reported in rats. Strekalova[17] found statistically significant increases in aberrations in femur bone marrow cells after the administration of a single oral dose of 9 mg ETO/kg. Embree and Hene[5] exposed rats to 250 ppm ETO in air for seven hours per day for three days. Twenty-four hours after the last exposure, they observed isochromatid and chromatid gaps and breaks in bone marrow cells. They also investigated the mutagenic potential of ETO, using the dominant-lethal assay in rats. They exposed male rats to 1,000 ppm ETO for a four-hour inhalation period. There was a significant increase in implantations that died in female rats mated to treated males at one, two, three, and five weeks after exposure.

Ethylene oxide is a highly strained three-membered ring epoxide that is broadly reactive to cellular nucleophils. Reactions with protein[6] and nucleic acid[4, 7] have been measured. Covalent chemical bonding between ETO and DNA probably can occur spontaneously to form altered biomolecules, which may account for the mutagenic properties of ETO. Furthermore, ETO exposure may saturate the detoxicating mechanisms in vivo.[1, 4] This action could be a factor contributing to the mutagenesis.

The studies on mutagenesis suggest the possibility that continual occupational exposure at significant levels of ETO may induce an increased frequency of mutations in humans. Ehrenberg and Hallstrom[3] studied a group of workers in a factory manufacturing and using ETO. Seven workers who had been exposed to high levels of gaseous ETO for two hours during an industrial accident showed a significantly higher number of chromosomal abnormalities than did a comparable control group. In 1983, Yager and co-workers reported a dose-related increase in the rate of sister chromatid exchange in human peripheral lymphocytes among a group of hospital workers exposed to ethylene oxide during sterilization procedures. The authors suggest that sister chromatid exchange may be a sensitive indicator of exposure, particularly since they appear to be related to cumulative dose in this study.[18]

In regard to teratogenic effects, Hemminki and co-workers have reported significantly increased spontaneous abortion rates among female "sterilizing" staff in 80 hospitals in Finland compared to nursing auxiliaries with no exposure. This study can only be considered suggestive at the present time because of methodologic weaknesses, particularly in regard to the definition of exposure and the retrospective design of the study for reproductive outcomes reported among the respondents.[9]

In 1979 Hogstedt and co-workers from the Department of Occupational Medicine at the Regional Hospital in Örebro, Sweden, reported their investigation and findings on a group of ethylene oxide-exposed workers from a small factory with a warehouse (storage hall) (68 women and 2 men were employed). They described one case of chronic myeloid leukemia, one case of acute myelogenetic leukemia, and one case of primary macroglobulinemia (Waldenström), which occurred between 1972 and 1977. Levels of ETO in the warehouse were 2–70 ppm with an eight-hour, time-weighted average concentration (in the breathing zone) calculated as 20 ± 10 ppm.*

The expected cumulative incidence of leukemia during that period was calculated by multiplying the person-years of observation and the sex- and age-specific national leukemia incidence for 1972.[2] Without considering any latency time or minimal exposure, a 0.2 case incidence of leukemia would have been expected. A follow-up study by Hogstedt et al.,[11] reported in 1985, showed that eight cases of leukemia have occurred among the 733 ethylene oxide-exposed workers compared with an expected 0.8 cases. Six cases of stomach cancer were reported compared to 0.65 cases expected. (Additional details are given in Chapter 52.)

Based on the conclusions of the Hogstedt report, the Swedish threshold limit value for ethylene oxide has been lowered to 10 ppm as an eight-hour, time-weighted average concentration limit. Reduction of worker exposure through improved industrial hygiene practices is vital. Continued epidemiologic studies of workers potentially exposed to ETO, including reproductive data, are urgently needed in order to assure the adequacy of the current standards.

REFERENCES

1. Arias IM, Jakoby WB (eds): *Glutathione: Metabolism and Function*. New York, Raven Press, 1976.
2. Cancer Incidence in Sweden 1972. Stockholm, National Board of Health and Welfare, 1977, p 44.
3. Ehrenberg L, Hallstrom T: Haematologic studies on persons occupationally exposed to ethylene oxide, in *International Energy Agency Report*, SM 92/26, 1967, pp 327–334. (Cited in NIOSH Criteria Document.[16])
4. Ehrenberg L, et al: Evaluation of genetic risks of alkylating agents: Tissue doses in the mouse from air contaminated with ethylene oxide. *Mutat Res* 1974; 24:83.
5. Embree JW, Hene CH: Mutagenicity of ethylene oxide. *Toxicol Appl Pharmacol* 1975; 33:172.
6. Frankel-Conrat H: The action of 1,2 epoxides of proteins. *J Biol Chem* 1944; 154:227.
7. Frankel-Conrat H: Chemical modification of viral ribonucleic acid. Part I. Alkylating agents. *Biochem Biophys Acta* 1961; 49:165.
8. Gross JA, Haas ML, Swift TR: Ethylene oxide neuropathy. *Neurology* 1978; 28:355.
9. Hemminki K, Mutanen P, Salvonemi I, et al: Spontaneous abortion in hospital staff engaged in sterilizing instruments with chemical agents. *Br Med J* 1983; 285;1461
10. Hogstedt C, Malmqvist N, Wadman B: Leukemia in workers exposed to ethylene oxide. *JAMA* 1979; 241:1132.
11. Hogstedt C, Aringer L, Gustavsson A: Epidemiologic support for ethylene oxide as a cancer-causing agent. *JAMA* 1986; 255(12) March 28.

*The authors noted that in sterilizing hospital equipment, 50% ethylene oxide and 50% methyl formate had been used since 1968 (methyl formate has much less volatility than ETO and is permitted as a food additive).

12. Hollingsworth RL, et al: Toxicity of ethylene oxide determined on experimental animals. *AMA Arch Ind Health* 1956; 13:217.
13. Jacobson KH, Hackley EB, Feinsilver L: The toxicity of inhaled ethylene oxide and propylene oxide vapors. *AMA Arch Ind Health* 1956; 13:237.
14. Loveless A: Influence of radiomimetic substances on desoxyribonucleic acid synthesis and function studied in *Escherichia coli* phage systems. Part 3: Mutation of T2 bacteriophage as a consequence of alkylation in vitro. *Proc R Soc Lond (Biol)* 1959; 150:497.
15. National Institute for Occupational Safety and Health: Ethylene oxide, in *Curr Intell Bull* 35, DHHS, PHS, NIOSH 81-130, 1981.
16. National Institute for Occupational Safety and Health: Special occupational hazard review with control recommendations: Use of ethylene oxide as a sterilant in medical facilities, DHEW, PHS, NIOSH 77-200, 1977.
17. Strekalova EE: Mutagenic action of ethylene oxide on mammals. [CA75-1077251]. Toksikil. *Nov Prom Khim Veshchesto* 1971; 12:72. (Russian) (Cited in NIOSH Criteria Document.[16])
18. Yager J, Hines C, Spear R: Exposure to ethylene oxide at work increases sister chromatid exchange in human peripheral lymphocytes. *Science* 1983; 219:1221.
19. World Health Organization: *Environmental Health Criteria*. Vol 55, *Ethylene Oxide*. Geneva, 1985.

ETHYLENE THIOUREA

```
      H
      N
    /   \
 CH2     C=S
  |      |
 CH2 ——— NH
```

Ethylene thiourea (ETU) is a white cyrstalline solid that is used extensively as an accelerator in the curing of polychloroprene (the synthetic rubber trademarked Neoprene) and other elastomers. The NIOSH estimates that approximately 3,500 workers in the rubber industry have potential occupational exposure to ethylene thiourea.[7] Not to be overlooked is that exposure to ETU can result from the very widely used ethylene bisdithiocarbamate fungicides, as ETU may be present as a contaminant in these fungicides and can also be formed when food containing the fungicides is cooked.

Ethylene thiourea is a thyroid depressant in laboratory animals, producing myxedema, goiter and other manifestations related to decreased thyroid hormone.[7] In rats, ETU has also been found to produce thyroid carcinoma.[2, 3, 9]

In addition, ETU has been found to be a significant teratogen in laboratory animals.[5, 8] Stula and Krauss[8] reported fetal malformations in all of 73 fetuses taken on the 20th day of gestation from pregnant rats in which ETU (50 mg/kg body weight) had been applied to the skin on the 12th and the 13th day of gestation, whereas no abnormalities were found in the fetuses of the controls. Their studies further demonstrated that the teratogenic effects were related to the dose and exposure time in the pregnancy. Utilizing the same dose of 50 mg ETU/kg body weight on gestation days 10 and 11 did not result in any fetal abnormalities.

At present, there is no OSHA standard for ETU exposure or a proposed limit by the NIOSH. It would be prudent, however, to minimize any exposure to this substance, including skin exposure.

REFERENCES

1. Chernoff N, Kavlock R, Rogers E, et al: Perinatal toxicity of maneb, ethylene thiourea, and ethylene bis isothiocyanate sulfide in rodents. *J Toxicol Environ Health* 1979; 5(5):821–834.
2. *IARC Monogr Eval Carcinog Risk Chem Man* 1974; 7:45.
3. Innes JRM, et al: Bioassay of pesticides and industrial chemicals for tumorigenicity in mice: A preliminary note. *JNCI* 1969; 42:1101.
4. Iverson F, Khera K, Hierlihy S: In vivo and in vitro metabolism of ethylene thiourea in the rat and the cat. *Toxicol Appl Pharmacol* 1980; 52(1):16–21.
5. Khera KS, Tryphonas L: Ethylene thiourea-induced hydrocephalus: Pre- and postnatal pathogenesis in offspring from rats given a single oral dose during pregnancy. *Toxicol Appl Pharmacol* 1977; 42:85.
6. Korhonen A, Hemminki K, Vainio H: Embryotoxicity of industrial chemicals on the chicken embryo: thiourea derivatives. *Acta Pharmacol Toxicol (Copenh)* 1982; 51:38–44.
7. National Institute for Occupational Safety and Health: Ethylene thiourea. *Curr Intell Bull* 22, DHEW, PHS, NIOSH 79-109, 1978.
8. Stula EF, Krauss WC; Embryotoxicity in rats and rabbits from cutaneous application of amide-type solvents and substituted ureas. *Toxicol Appl Pharmacol* 1977; 41:35.
9. Ulland BM, et al: Thyroid cancer in rats from ethylene thiourea intake. *JNCI* 1972; 49:583.

GLYCIDYL ETHERS

Carl Zenz, M.D.

The major use of the glycidyl ethers is as reactive diluents in epoxy resins applications. Most of the glycidyl ethers are liquids, but a few are solid and are characterized by the presence of the 2,3-epoxypropyl group and an ether linkage to another organic group. They have a generalized formula:

```
      H   H   H
      |   |   |
  H — C — C — C — O — R
       \ /    |
        O     H
```

These compounds have relatively low vapor pressures, and dermocontact is the major route of exposure, with inhalation a possible secondary route. Exposure to the epoxide moiety in certain glycidyl ethers and epoxy resins may occur until the resin is completely cured. Therefore, workers must be considered to be at some risk of exposure from the time the glycidyl ethers are synthesized until the curing process of the epoxy resin is complete.

Occupations with potential exposure to glycidyl ethers: adhesive makers and users, automobile workers, cable makers, casting and molding workers, custom-blended epoxy resin system production workers, dental laboratory technicians, dentists, electrical appliance production workers, electronic equipment production workers, flooring makers, glycidyl ether production workers, laminators, nurses, paint makers, physicians, soft drink canners, telephone production workers and telephone installers. The NIOSH estimates that 118,000 workers in the United States are exposed to glycidyl ethers and that an additional 1 million workers are exposed to epoxy resins. There are no specific diagnostic tests to determine the extent of absorption into the worker's body, and environmental controls by sampling the worker's breathing zone are necessary.

The most commonly used glycidyls, along with their acronyms and the presently allowable concentrations (1986), are presented in Table 54–4.

Because epoxy resins have such a wide range of applications, workers often must handle glycidyl ethers and the uncured resins containing them in processes such as tooling and molding, manufacturing and using adhesives, roof and floor construction, and applying protective coatings. Uncured resins used in protective coatings often are applied by spraying, so the applicators could be exposed to large quantities of vapors and mists containing glycidyl ethers. Work practices appropriate for handling glycidyl ethers should be adhered to in processes involving an uncured epoxy resin system.

Glycidyl ethers such as PGE and BGE are synthesized by adding the appropriate alcohol to epichlorohydrin in the presence of a catalyst. The intermediate chlorohydrin is not isolated and undergoes dehydrochlorination to yield a glycidyl ether. Commercial manufacture of glycidyl ethers takes place within an enclosed system, but workers may be exposed to glycidyl ethers during drumming operations at the end of the process. Very small quantities of glycidyl ethers are used for other purposes, most of which are proprietary in nature; in these instances, identification of exposed workers and estimation of their extent of exposure become difficult.

Human toxicologic data concerning these compounds are scarce, but information available reveals that glycidyl ethers are primary skin and eye irritants and that they are potential skin-sensitizing agents. There are data suggesting that di(2,3-epoxypropyl) ether should be regarded as a potential occupational carcinogen and that *n*-butyl glycidyl ether is a mammalian mutagen. Some glycidyl ethers have also produced cytotoxic effects in animals. Although there are no reports of carcinogenic, mutagenic, teratogenic, or reproductive effects of the glycidyl ethers in humans, there have been reports of animal studies demonstrating testicular degeneration in several animal species after exposure to AGE, DGE, PGE, and triethylene glycol diglycidyl ether.[3, 5, 7, 11] Necrosis of the testes was reported in rats that received six dermal applications of DGE at 250 or 500 mg/kg[5] or four injections of AGE at 400 mg/kg.[7] Testicular atrophy with decreased spermatogenic activity was seen in mice receiving high intraperitoneal doses of triethylene glycol diglycidyl ether.[11] Atrophied testes were found in two rabbits that died after a single 24-hour exposure to DGE at 24 ppm (128 mg/cu m) and possibly in a dog that received six 12.5 mg/kg intravenous doses of this compound.[5] In chronic inhalation experiments, 1 of 15 rats exposed to DGE at 3 ppm (16 mg/cu m) had necrosis of testicular tubules after 19 exposures; five of ten rats exposed at 0.3 (1.6 mg/cu m) had "poorly defined" focal degeneration in the testes after 60 exposures.[5] In rats exposed to PGE at 1.75–11.2 ppm (10–71 mg/cu m) for 19 days, focal degeneration of the seminiferous tubules was observed in 5 of 24, but the investigator considered that this damage was of questionable

TABLE 54–4.
Commonly Used Glycidyls

NAME/ACRONYM	ALLOWABLE CONCENTRATIONS (1986)
Allyl glycidyl ether (AGE)	22 mg/cu m (5 ppm)
Isopropyl glycidyl ether (IGE)	240 mg/cu m (50 ppm)
Phenyl glycidyl ether (PGE)	5 mg/cu m (1 ppm)
n-Butyl glycidyl ether (BGE)	135 mg/cu m (25 ppm)
Di(2,3-epoxypropyl)ether (DGE)	1 mg/cu m (0.2 ppm)

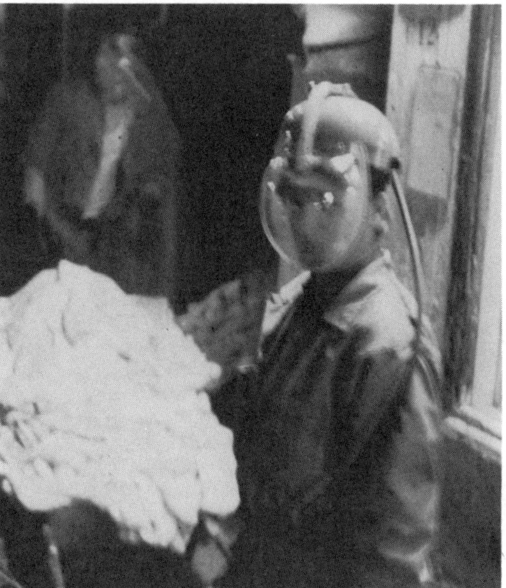

FIG 54–1.
A worker in a synthetic-fiber plant where carbon disulfide is used. Note the special air-supply helmets and facepieces provided.

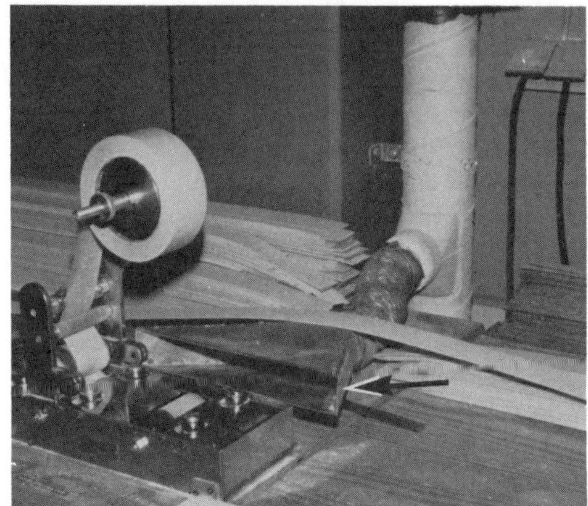

FIG 54–2.
Epoxy-fiberglass material used for manufacturing laminated skis. *Arrow* indicates the exhaust system located at this cutting stage.

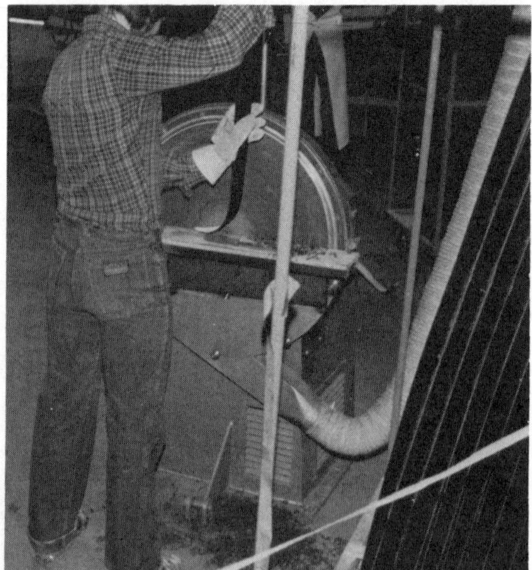

FIG 54–3.
Exhaust system at the grinding stations for manufacturing skis of epoxy fiberglass.

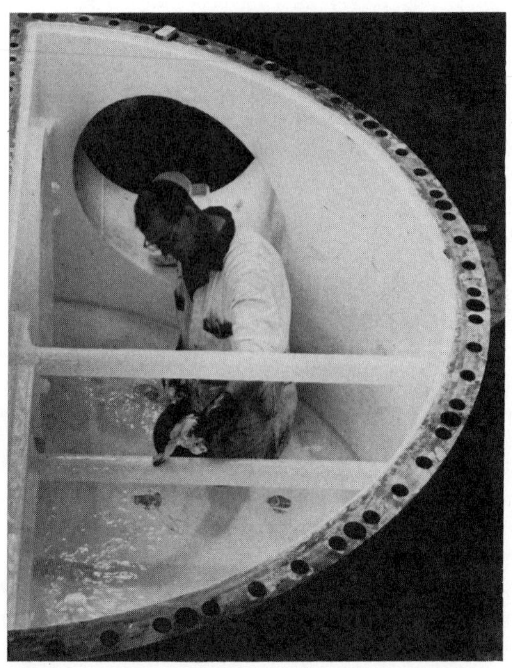

FIG 54–4.
A worker hand brushing epoxy resin on a large steel object for corrosion resistance. Note protective clothing. With down-draft exhaust ventilation, no respiratory protective equipment is needed.

significance and probably was not treatment related.[3] Only in the PGE study was any attempt made to correlate testicular damage with effects on reproduction, and this study showed no significant mutagenic or reproductive effects.[3]

Lack of data on most of the glycidyl ethers makes it difficult to correlate variations in the results of tests of their mutagenicity and carcinogenicity with differences in the structure of particular compounds within the class. Thus, only tentative conclusions can be drawn about the potential of glycidyl ethers to cause cancer or mutations.[1]

Following occupational exposures to certain substances such as styrene, for example, metabolic breakdown epoxides are formed that are very reactive and are considered to be potentially of significance in possible tumorigenesis. Since glycidyl ethers contain the epoxide group, they would be expected to undergo the types of reactions that have been demonstrated for this moiety, with potential reactions that have significance for biologic systems.[2, 9]

Experimental evidence also indicates that glycidyl ethers are very reactive biologically. They have been used for tumor inhibition because of their alkylating properties.[11] They have produced chromosomal aberrations in plants,[6, 8, 9] and Hine[5] and Kodama et al.[7] have demonstrated their radiomimetic effects on blood cells. BGE has been shown to be mutagenic in mammals,[10] and all glycidyl ethers tested have shown some mutagenic activity in bacterial systems.[3, 10, 12] However, very high doses generally were required to produce these effects, and attempts to find consistent structure-activity relationships among various glycidyl ethers have met with little success.[4, 7]

The National Institute for Occupational Safety and Health[1] states that gross skin contact with glycidyl ethers may represent an important hazard to worker health, and, because of demonstrated mutagenicity, the glycidyl ethers should, in the absence of adequate carcinogenicity test data on individual compounds, be regarded as potentially serious hazards.

Several glycidyl ethers are combustible or flammable liquids presenting fire hazards. Since many of them may polymerize violently after heating, stringent precautions must be taken to prevent fire. In addition, inhalation of the chemicals can be minimized by enclosing processes and providing suitable and adequate ventilation systems with specifically placed exhaust hoods (Figs 54–1 through 54–4) and all epoxy-based adhesives containing these substances should be used only with adequate ventilation. As with most potentially toxic substances, eating and drinking must not be permitted in the work areas nor must food or beverages be allowed to be stored in workplaces, and employees must be advised to wash their hands before eating or using toilet facilities. Workers should also be cautioned not to touch or rub their eyes with fingers or hands, which may be contaminated.

REFERENCES

1. National Institute for Occupational Safety and Health: *Criteria for a Recommended Standard: Occupational Exposure to Glycidyl Ethers,* DHEW, PHS, NIOSH 78-166, 1978.
2. Fournier PE, Gervais P: Toxicological study of epoxy resins. *Occup Health Rev* 1964; 17:19.
3. *Haskell Laboratory Reports on Glycidyl Ethers,* No. 164-75, 225-74, 133-76, 163-75. Unpublished report submitted to NIOSH by EI du Pont de Nemours & Co, Employee Relations Dept, Medical Division, February 1978, 14 pp.
4. Hendry JA, Homer RF, Rose FL, et al: Cytotoxic agents. II. Bis-epoxides and related compounds. *Br J Pharmacol* 1951; 6:235.
5. Hine CH, et al: Effects of diglycidyl ether on blood of animals. *Arch Environ Health* 1961; 2:37.

6. Kihlman BA: Factors affecting the production of chromosome aberrations by chemicals. *J Biophys Biochem Cytol* 1956; 2:543.
7. Kodama JK, et al: Some effects of epoxy compounds on the blood. *Arch Environ Health* 1961; 2:56.
8. Lane GR: Chromosome breakage by diepoxide and by x-rays, in Bacq ZM, Alexander P (eds): *Proceedings of the Radiobiology Symposium*. New York, Academic Press, 1955, pp 265–274, 277–281.
9. Loveless A: Qualitative aspects of the chemistry and biology of radiomimetic mutagenic substances. *Nature* 1951; 167:338.
10. Pullin T, Legator MS: *Integrated Mutagenicity Testing Program*. Unpublished report submitted to NIOSH by Dow Chemical Co. Midland, Mi, Dow Chemical USA, Health and Environmental Research, December 1977, 71 pp.
11. Shimkin MB, et al: Bioassay of 29 alkylating chemicals by the pulmonary-tumor response in strain A mice. *JNCI* 1966; 36:915.
12. Wade MJ, Moyer JW, Hine CH: Mutagenic Action of a Series of Epoxides, publication 78-2. San Francisco, University of California, School of Medicine, Dept of Pharmacology (Toxicology Activity), 1978, 12 pp.

GLYCOL ETHERS

Vernon N. Dodson, M.D.

Carl Zenz, M.D.

Annually, nearly 800 million lb (360 thousand metric tons) of glycol ethers are produced in the United States; about 78% of this is ethylene glycol monoethers. Ethoxyethanol has the greatest production volume, followed by butoxyethanol and methoxyethanol. These substances have a vast use as solvents in the manufacture of protective coatings for alkyd resins, baking enamels, epoxy resins, laquers, and metal coatings. Glycol ethers are found in phenolic varnishes and are used as solvents for nitrocellulose (hence, the commonly used name, "cellusolves"), leather finishes, printing inks, and textile dyes and pigments. 2-Methoxyethanol (2ME) and 2-ethoxyethanol (2EE) are used as anti-stall agents in gasoline, in aviation fuels, as anti-icing additives in brake fluids and both are used in various organic syntheses. 2EE is used to make 2-ethoxyethyl acetate (2EEA). 2EE finds use in formulating adhesives, cleaning products, cosmetics, detergents, pesticides, pharmaceuticals, thinners, varnishes, and varnish removers. In the United States, the NIOSH has estimated that about 100,000 workers may be potentially exposed to 2ME and nearly 400,000 are potentially exposed to 2EE.[14] Some structurally related glycol ethers are listed in Table 54–5.

General Effects From Occupational Exposure to 2ME and 2EE

Acute toxic effects of 2ME are irritation of the eyes, nose, and throat, drowsiness, weakness, and shaking.[13] Swallowing of 2ME may be fatal. Prolonged or repeated exposure may cause headache, drowsiness, weakness, fatigue, staggering, personality change, and decreased mental ability. In a 1978 case study report of two workers exposed to 2ME, Ohi and Wegman described clinical evidence of encephalopathy in both, bone marrow depression in one, and pancytopenia in the other. Although airborne concentrations (8 ppm) were well below the PEL, both workers had significant skin contact with 2ME. The health status of both workers returned to normal after removal from exposure and treat-

TABLE 54–5.
Structurally Related Glycol Ethers

ABBREVIATION	NAME	FORMULA
2MEA	2-Methoxyethyl acetate	$(CH_3{-}O{-}CH_2{-}CH_2{-}O{-}C({=}O){-}CH_3)$
2EEA	2-Ethoxyethyl acetate	$(CH_3{-}CH_2{-}O{-}CH_2{-}CH_2{-}O{-}C({=}O){-}CH_3)$
2BE	2-Butoxyethanol	$(CH_3{-}CH_2{-}CH_2{-}CH_2{-}O{-}CH_2{-}CH_2{-}OH)$
2PE	2-Phenoxyethanol	$(C_6H_5{-}O{-}CH_2{-}CH_2{-}OH)$
EGdiME	Ethylene glycol dimethyl ether	$(CH_3{-}O{-}CH_2{-}CH_2{-}O{-}CH_3)$
bis2ME	Bis(2-methoxyethyl)ether	$(CH_3{-}O{-}CH_2{-}CH_2{-}O{-}CH_2{-}CH_2{-}O{-}CH_3)$
2EEE	2-(2-Ethoxyethoxy)ethanol	$(CH_3{-}CH_2{-}O{-}CH_2{-}CH_2{-}O{-}CH_2{-}CH_2{-}OH)$

ment.[18] In animals, 2EE has caused liver, kidney, and lung damage, and anemia as well as eye irritation.

Effects of 2-Methoxyethanol (2ME)

Human Reproductive Effects.—In one study of a small population involved in manufacturing and packaging of 2ME, no clinically signficant differences were found between the exposed and comparison groups that could be attributed to the work environment for the fertility parameters studied. Exposures to 2ME were reported to be well below 25 ppm. 2EE and other glycol ethers were also manufactured in these facilities.

Animal Studies.—Exposure to 2ME caused dose-related adverse reproductive effects in female and male experimental animals. Pregnant mice exposed by gavage and pregnant rats and rabbits exposed by inhalation had increased incidences of embryonic deaths and abnormalities that were statistically significant. Increased incidences of testicular atrophy (decreased testicular weight) and microscopic testicular changes were observed among male mice given oral doses and male mice, rats, and rabbits exposed by inhalation. Infertility in male rats and abnormal spermhead morphology in mice have also been reported after inhalation of 2ME.

Female Animal Studies.—Adverse effects in pregnant animals and their offspring after 2ME exposure that have been reported include: significant increases in embryonic deaths, major and minor fetal abnormalities, and maternal deaths and blood effects. Dose-dependent embryomortality and gross fetal defects were observed in fetuses of mice exposed by gavage to 2ME at 250 mg/kg on days 7–14 of gestation.[10] Embryonic deaths were significantly increased among pregnant rabbits that inhaled 10 or 50 ppm of 2ME on days 6–18 of gestation. Similar results were reported after exposure at 3 ppm of 2ME, but they were not statistically significant.[5] The authors of that study noted that the embryonic death rate in the rabbit control group was less than the rate observed in their historical rabbit control groups. The authors also noted that the rate of embryonic death among rabbits exposed at 10 ppm was comparable to the rate in historical controls. Nevertheless, embryonic mortality observed in this study did increase with the exposure concentration. No evidence of teratogenicity and only minimal fetotoxicity was observed in fetuses of rats exposed to 2ME at 50 ppm;[5] another study did report fetal defects in rats after exposure at 50 ppm on days 7–15 of gestation.[15] Fetal skeletal variations, which are among the most sensitive indicators of teratogenicity, were obtained at 2ME doses as low as 31 mg/kg/day given to pregnant mice.[10] Male fetuses of pregnant mice exposed on days 6–15 of gestation at 50 ppm of 2ME had a significant increase in the incidence of unilateral testicular hypoplasia (underdevelopment of the testes).[26]

Unilateral testicular hypoplasia is considered a slight fetotoxic effect. Female rats and rabbits exposed to 2ME at 30, 100, or 300 ppm for three months had no evidence of gross reproductive or microscopic changes in the ovaries. No reduction of fertility was observed in the rats exposed at 300 ppm.[19] In mice, embryonic deaths and fetal abnormalities occurred at lower 2ME doses than required to significantly lower maternal white blood cell (WBC) counts.[10] A reduced white blood cell count was one factor for the current OSHA PEL for 2ME.

Male Animal Studies.—Significant increases in testicular atrophy, microscopic testicular changes, and blood effects were reported in mature male animals exposed to 2ME. The testicular effects found in mice[9] and rabbits occurred at lower doses of 2ME than those that caused significantly lower WBC counts.[9, 11, 12, 19] 2ME was not found to be mutagenic.

Effects of 2-Ethoxyethanol (2EE)

Human Reproductive Effects.—The only known published investigation of "reproductive performance" in a human population exposed to 2EE is difficult to interpret and is of questionable value because of mixed solvent exposures. Syrovadko and Malsheva evaluated the incidence of "gynecological disorders" and birth defects in female enameling workers.[22] The two solvent mixtures reported were chlorobenzene and 2EE (1:1) and tricresol and "solvent naphtha" (1:4). The concentrations of 2EE were reported to have been "low." There was no difference in the incidence of gynecologic disorders between the enamelers and administrative workers (a comparison group including some former enamelers), but both groups were said to have 2.6–9.4 times more gynecologic disorders than three other comparison groups. Among the disorders detected were inflammations, benign neoplasms, cervical erosions, and menstrual disorders. The rate of birth defects was significantly increased among the offspring of enamelers (10.0% vs. 3.9% in plant controls), with heart and foot defects predominant (without workroom sampling for solvent concentrations, no definite conclusions can be drawn).

Animal Studies.—Exposure of female and male animals to 2EE has caused significant dose-related adverse reproductive effects similar to the effects caused by 2ME. Oral, inhalation, subcutaneous, and dermal treatment of pregnant rats with 2EE caused increased incidences of embryonic death and abnormalities. 2EE inhalation exposure of pregnant rabbits and oral exposure of pregnant rats caused the same effects. The offspring of pregnant rats exposed by inhalation had altered behavior and neurochemical concentrations in the brain. In male mice, rats, and dogs treated orally and in rats treated subcutaneously, testicular atrophy and microscopic testicular changes have been reported.[2, 6, 9, 21, 24]

Female Animal Studies.—Significant increases in embryonic deaths, fetal abnormalities, altered behavioral test results, and changes in brain neurochemical concentrations have been reported after exposure of pregnant animals to 2EE. Embryonic deaths occurred in: rats after 2EE was given orally at 47 mg/kg/day;[21] rabbits that inhaled 2EE at 160 ppm; rats that inhaled 2EE at 765 ppm;[2] and rats that received 1.0 ml/day of 2EE dermally.[6] The resorption rate was 100% in rats receiving 2.0 ml/day.[6] Fetal cardiovascular and skeletal effects were found after inhalation exposure of pregnant rabbits at 160 ppm and pregnant rats at 200 ppm.[2] Rabbit fetuses also had kidney and ventral body wall defects. Skeletal defects were detected in fetuses of rats that received

2EE at 93 mg/kg/day orally or subcutaneously,[21] and 1.0 ml/day dermally.[6] Fetal growth retardation indicated by lower weights and shorter lengths was observed in rats exposed by inhalation.[2] Subtle teratogenic effects were reported in the offspring of pregnant rats exposed during gestation to 2EE at 100 ppm.[16] The changes included altered behavioral test results at different stages of development after birth and differences in brain neurochemical concentrations in newborn and 21-day-old rats; these differences were more pronounced in the offspring exposed earlier in gestation. Exposure of female rats to 2EE at 650 ppm for three weeks prior to mating had no effect on fertility.[2]

Male Animal Studies.—Significant increases in testicular atrophy, microscopic testicular changes, and deaths were reported in animals exposed to 2EE. Severe testicular atrophy occurred in mice given 1,000 mg/kg/day orally.[9] Testicular changes were found in rats and dogs given 2EE at 186 mg/kg/day orally and in rats given 372 mg/kg/day subcutaneously.[21] Testicular atrophy and blood effects in 2EE-treated mice were less severe than those in mice given 2ME at the same dosage levels; testicular effects in 2EE-treated mice occurred at a lower dose than the dose causing WBC effects.[9] Studies found 2EE nonmutagenic. Carcinogen studies were underway by the National Toxicology Program (NTP).

Nelson et al.[17] conducted an inhalation study with five structurally related compounds and used 15 pregnant rats in one to three concentrations for seven hours a day on gestation days 7–15; dams sacrificed on day 20. At concentrations which were apparently not maternally toxic, 2-methoxyethanol was highly embryotoxic, producing complete resorptions at 200 ppm; increased resorptions, reduced fetal weights, and skeletal and cardiovascular defects occurred at both 100 and 50 ppm. 2-Ethoxyethyl acetate at 600 ppm induced complete resorption of litters; 390 ppm reduced fetal weights and induced skeletal and cardiovascular defects, but only a single defect was observed at 130 ppm. 2-Butoxyethanol evidenced slight maternal toxicity at 200 ppm but produced no increase in congenital defects at that concentration. Neither 2-(2-ethoxyethoxy)ethanol (100 ppm) nor 2-methylaminoethanol (150 ppm) was maternally toxic or embryotoxic. They stated that shorter alkyl-chained glycol ethers produced greater embryotoxicity than those having longer chains, and the ester produced effects equivalent to the ether. Fifteen glycol ethers were tested for in vivo reproductive toxicity by Schuler et al.[20] using pregnant mice and ranked the substances for priority for further studies; they recommended (1) very high priority: triethylene glycol dimethyl ether (triEGdiME); (2) high priority: ethylene glycol (EG), ethylene glycol monomethyl ether (EGME), ethylene glycol monoethyl ether (EGEE), ethylene glycol diethyl ether (EGdiEE), and diethylene glycol monomethyl ether (deEGME); (3) middle to high priority: ethylene glycol dimethyl ether (EGdiME) and diethylene glycol dimethyl ether (deEGdiME); (4) middle priority: ethylene glycol monobutyl ether (EGBE), diethylene glycol (diEG), diethylene glycol diethyl ether (diEGdiEE), and triethylene glycol (triEG); and (5) low priority: diethylene glycol monoethyl ether (deEGEE) and diethylene glycol dibutyl ether (deEGdiBE).

Utilizing the "hydra assay"[7] as a rapid screening method, Johnson et al.[8] studied the developmental toxicity hazard of several typical glycols and glycol ethers (ethylene glycol, propylene glycol, hexylene glycol, ethylene glycol monomethyl ether, ethylene glycol monoethyl ether, ethylene glycol monobutyl ether, ethylene glycol monophenyl ether, ethylene glycol monomethyl ether monoacetate, ethylene glycol monoethyl ether monoacetate, ethylene glycol diacetate, diethylene glycol, diethylene glycol monomethyl ether, diethylene glycol monoethyl ether, and diethylene glycol dibutyl ether). Johnson and co-workers emphasized that the hydra test quickly identifies the majority of substances while ranking the minority according to their degree of hazard to developmental phenomena. The test is excellent for quantitative hazard detection because it predicts the A/D ratio. (By their protocol, this step determines to within 1/10 log those minimal effective concentrations [MEC] of the test substance capable of producing adult and developmental toxicity. The adult MEC [A] and the developmental MEC [D] are calculated as a ratio. This A/D ratio is considered as a developmental toxicity hazard index whose increasing size is directly proportional to a chemical's ability to injure embryos in the absence of adult toxicity.)

Some investigators, unfamiliar with certain occupational exposure factors, have incorporated into their reports: "Due to the low vapor pressure of 2-EEE, higher concentrations could not be tested due to probable formation of an aerosol" or "Low vapor pressure also prevented our generating high concentrations of 2-MAE." Low vapor pressures imply a lower potential risk to the worker inhalation for that substance at a given workroom temperature; aerosols are often formed and found in many processes, i.e., in mixing and spraying. Again, the reader is referred to Chapter 2, Industrial Hygiene, and pertinent sections, especially that describing typical processes and, specifically, to *vapor pressure*.

Based on these recent findings, as well as continued concern for adverse effects after percutaneous absorption, the NIOSH recommends that 2ME and 2EE be regarded in the workplace as having the potential to cause adverse reproductive effects in male and female workers and embryotoxic effects, including teratogenesis, in the offspring of the exposed, pregnant female. Although there have been animal studies conducted at concentrations at which these effects did not occur, the NIOSH does not assume that these are safe concentrations for human beings. By decreasing exposure, the potential for adverse reproductive and embryotoxic effects will decrease. Concern also extends to the structurally related glycol ethers that have not been tested adequately to assess fully their potential for causing reproductive effects. As described, test results of some structurally related glycol ethers indicate that they also have the potential for adverse reproductive effects similar to 2ME and 2EE. In light of these findings, the NIOSH recommends similar cautions be exercised to reduce worker exposure to these structurally related glycol ethers until adequate testing demonstrates their safety.[4]

Exposure Standards and Guides

The Occupational Safety and Health Administration's permissible exposure limit (PEL) for occupational exposure to 2ME is 25 ppm (80 mg/cu m), and its PEL for 2EE is 200 ppm (740 mg/cu m), both as a time-weighted average (TWA) for an eight-hour work shift (29 CFR 1910.1000).[5] The OSHA standards bear a "skin" notation, indicating the potential for skin absorption of toxic amounts of 2ME and 2EE. These standards are based primarily on reports of blood, kidney, liver, and central nervous system toxicity caused by 2ME and 2EE in animals and on case reports of human exposure to 2ME. No studies on reproductive effects of 2ME and 2EE were considered when these standards were adopted.

The American Conference of Governmental Industrial Hygienists (ACGIH) has recommended threshold limit values (TLVs) for 2ME and 2EE.[1] The TLV for 2ME as a TWA for an eight-hour work shift is 5 ppm. For 2EE, the ACGIH lowered its TLV to 5 ppm. The TLV for 2EE was lowered to prevent workers from being exposed to concentrations that had produced significant blood changes in laboratory animals. The ACGIH TLV's also bear a "skin" notation. In 1985, most manufacturers of 2ME and 2EE adopted company industrial hygiene exposure guides below current OSHA PELs. For 2ME, the eight-hour TWA exposure limits range from 2 to 10 ppm. For 2EE, manufacturers have adopted an eight-hour TWA of 5 ppm.

REFERENCES

1. American Conference of Governmental Industrial Hygienists: *Documentation of the Threshold Limit Values,* ed 5. Cincinnati, Oh, ACGIH, 1986.
2. Andrew FD, Buschbom RL, Cannon WC, et al: *Teratologic Assessment of Ethylbenzene and 2-Ethoxyethanol*. Submitted to NIOSH under Contract No 210-79-0037. Richland, Va, Battelle Pacific Northwest Laboratory, 1981.
3. Cook RR, Bodner KM, Kolesar RC, et al: A cross-sectional study of ethylene glycol monomethyl ether process employees. *Arch Environ Health* 1982; 37(6):346–351.
4. Glycol Ethers: 2-Methoxyethanol and 2-Ethoxyethanol, Current Intelligence Bulletin 39. Cincinnati, Oh, National Institute For Occupational Safety and Health, 1983.
5. Hanley TR, Yano BL, Nitschke KD, et al: *Ethylene Glycol Monomethyl Ether: Inhalation Teratology Study in Rats and Rabbits*. Midland, Mich, Toxicology Research Laboratory, Dow Chemical USA, Sept 20, 1982.
6. Hardin BD, Niemeier RW, Kuczuk MH, et al: Teratogenicity of 2-ethoxyethanol by dermal application. *Drug Chem Toxicol* 1982; 5(3):277–294.
7. Johnson EM, Gorman RM, Gabel BEG, et al: The Hydra attennata system for detection of teratogenic hazards. *Teratogen Carcinogen Mutagen* 1982; 2:263–276.
8. Johnson E, Gabel BEG, Larson J: Developmental toxicity and structure/activity correlates to glycols and glycol ethers. *Environ Health Perspect* 1984; 57:135–139.
9. Nagano K, Nakayama E, Koyano M, et al: Mouse testicular atrophy induced by ethylene glycol monoalkyl ethers. *Jap J Ind Health* 1979; 21:29–35.
10. Nagano K, Nakayama E, Oobayashi H, et al: Embryotoxic effects of ethylene glycol monomethyl ether in mice. *Toxicology* 1981; 20:335–343.
11. McGregor DB: *Tier II Mutagenic Screening of 13 NIOSH Priority Compounds, Individual Compound Report on 2-Methoxyethanol,* Report 22, submitted to NIOSH under Contract No. 210-78-0026. Musselburgh EH21 7UB, Scotland, Inveresk Research International Limited, 1980, pp 226.
12. Miller RR, Ayres JA, Calhoun LL, et al: Comparative short-term inhalation toxicity of ethylene glycol monomethyl ether and propylene glycol monomethyl ether in rats and mice. *Toxicol Appl Pharmacol* 1981; 61:368–377.
13. Miller RR, Calhoun LL, Yano BL: *Ethylene Glycol Monomethyl Ether: 13-Week Vapor Inhalation Study with Male Rabbits*. Midland, Mich, Toxicology Research Laboratory, Dow Chemical USA, March 25, 1982.
14. National Institute for Occupational Safety and Health: National Occupational Hazard Survey. 2-Ethoxyethanol, 2-Methoxyethanol, Projected Numbers by Industry, Oct 9, 1982 (printout).
15. Nelson BK, Setzer JV, Brightwell WS, et al: Comparative inhalation teratogenicity of four industrial glycol ether solvents in rats, abstract. *Teratology* 1982; 25:64A. Corrected 2-ethoxyethylacetate concentrations and new data in teratology study. BK Nelson, March 25, 1982.
16. Nelson BK, Brightwell WS, Setzer JV, et al: Ethoxyethanol behavioral teratology in rats. *Neurotoxicology* 1981; 2:231–249.
17. Nelson BK, Setzer JV, Brightwell W, et al: Comparative inhalation teratogenicity of four glycol ether solvents and an amino derivative in rats. *Environ Health Perspect* 1984; 57:261–271.
18. Ohi G, Wegman DH: Transcutaneous ethylene glycol monomethyl ether poisoning in the work setting. *J Occup Med* 1978; 20:675–676.
19. Rao KS, Cobel-Geard SR, Young JT, et al: *Ethylene Glycol Monomethyl Ether: Inhalation Reproduction and Dominant Lethal Study in Rats*. Midland, Mich, Toxicology Research Laboratory, Dow Chemical USA, Feb 10, 1982.
20. Schuler RL, Hardin BD, Niemeier RW, et al: Results of testing fifteen glycol ethers in a short-term in vivo reproductive toxicity assay. *Environ Health Perspect* 1984; 57:141–146.
21. Stenger EG, Aeppli L, Muller D, et al: The toxicology of ethylene glycol monoethylether. *Arzneim Forsch* 1971; 21:880–885.
22. Syrovadko ON, Malsheva ZV: Work conditions and their effect on certain specific functions among women who are engaged in the production of enamel-insulated wire. *Gig Tr Prof Zabol* 1977; (4):25–28.
23. TLV Airborne Contaminants Committee: *Threshold Limit Values for Chemical Substances and Physical Agents in the Workroom Environment, 1985–86*. Cincinnati, Oh, American Conference of Governmental Industrial Hygienists, 1985.
24. Uemura K: The teratogenic effects of ethylene glycol dimethyl ether on the mouse. *Acta Obstet Gynaecol Jpn* 1980; 32(1):113–121.
25. US Dept of Labor, Occupational Safety and Health Administration: *General Industry Standards,* Publ 2206, 29 CFR 1910.1000, Washington, DC, 1981.
26. Written communication. Interim report on ethylene glycol monomethyl ether submitted by EH Blair of the Dow Chemical Company to the Environmental Protection Agency under Section 8(e) of the Toxic Substances Control Act, Jan 29, 1982.

HYPOXIA

Eric P. Kindwall, M.D.

Carl Zenz, M.D.

Cabin attendants and stewardesses in commercial aircraft constitute a large body of the work force in the air transport industry, and there is the potential danger of hypoxia to the fetus of a stewardess at a normal cabin pressure. Commercial jet aircraft are pressurized to maintain a cabin altitude of about 1,500–2,100 m (5,000–7,000 ft). Hypoxic symptoms in passengers and/or crew begin above this level and are most noted above the altitude of 3,000 m (10,000 ft).[3] Fetal anomalies have been demonstrated in experimental animals exposed to very high degrees of hypoxia.[5, 12, 13, 17] Pregnant mice, when exposed to reduced pressure equivalent to 7,600 m (25,000 ft) for eight hours have delivered anomalous infants. Although the effects of high altitude on reproduction in the Bolivian Andes have been studied, there is little evidence in the literature of occupational exposure under hypoxic conditions. In addition, such conditions are encountered seldom except under unusual circumstances. There are isolated reports of defects in children born of mothers who were subjected to an acute episode of hypoxia early in pregnancy arising from exposure to an anesthesia or to carbon monoxide in suicide attempts.

Kamat[14] reported that for the first time in the 1960s, defense forces of any country were located at an altitude of 4,000 m for a prolonged period (India). In 1964, defense force personnel carried 40 male and female ducks from the plains to this altitude. The ducks were supervised with the aid of expert advice and protected from cold weather. The animals gained weight but were noticed to mate infrequently, and no eggs were laid during the first eight months. Only one egg was laid during the succeeding ten months. At the plains during this period, a comparable group laid several hundred eggs. After sacrifice, all ducks were inspected for any unlaid eggs or ova, of which none were found (unpublished observation). A two-year attempt to breed a colony of pigs at 4,000 m was also unsuccessful. The piglets were weak, small, and lethargic.

Raina[20] has reported that cows in the Himalayas experienced a vague, weak, and short period of heat. Rat species are plentiful, but diminutive, in the Ladakh area. Fertility has been shown to be impaired at altitudes above 3,200 m.[6] Weihe[23] has reported poor lactogenesis in various animals living at altitudes above 3,000 m. Several army personnel stationed at high altitudes have complained of impaired fertility, and, on investigation, scanty specimens of semen were collected, exhibiting low-count spermatozoa.

Scholten[21] summarized the oxygen requirements of the developing embryo and fetus, reviewing the work of Cameron[4] and others. The fetus normally grows at oxygen tensions that would be considered severely hypoxic for the normal child or adult.[1] The important figures to consider are the percent arterial oxygen saturation and the partial pressure of oxygen in the blood measured in millimeters of mercury. Of equal importance is the phenomenon called "oxygen cascade," a term used to describe the progressively falling partial pressure of oxygen (P_{O_2}) from the inspired air, through the circulation to the capillaries of the tissue being oxygenated at the end of the cascade.[2, 11]

At sea level, the P_{O_2} in the inspired air is about 150 mm Hg, which drops to a little over 100 mm Hg in the alveoli in the arterial blood. By the time the capillary bed is reached, the P_{O_2} is a mean of 60 mm Hg and, on return through the circulation, is 37 mm Hg in the mixed venous blood. These are the normal values at sea level.

At 2,438 m (8,000 ft), the upper limits of normal cabin pressurization, the inspired air has a P_{O_2} of about 110 mm Hg, down from the sea level of 150. The alveolar air and the arterial blood have a P_{O_2} of about 64, a considerable drop from the normal 100. Capillary levels decline from the 60 at sea level to a mean of 46 at 2,438 m (8,000 ft); on the venous side, the drop is only from 37 to 32. Thus, there is a relatively large drop in the inspired oxygen partial pressure, which results in a very much smaller decrease in the mean capillary P_{O_2}. At the same time, the oxygen saturation curve shows considerably less decline as altitude increases, because of the protective buffering features of the oxygen dissociation mechanisms in human blood.[8, 11] As the atmospheric pressure goes down, oxygen dissociates from the hemoglobin cycle at an increased rate and maintains the oxygen saturation of the blood. Oxygen saturation falls as low as 90% at an alveolar partial pressure of 50–72 mm Hg, a pressure that corresponds to about 3,048 m (10,000 ft). Most authorities would agree that hypoxia begins to be noticed only at or above this altitude.[18, 19]

The fetus normally lives in a hypoxic atmosphere.[1] At sea level it exists with a P_{O_2} of 32 in its cord arterial blood and 10.6 in the venous blood returning through the umbilical cord.[22, 24] This is in contrast to the maternal figures of 100 and 37, respectively; thus, partial pressures of oxygen in the fetal circulation are about one third those of the mother.[7]

When the mother is breathing 15% oxygen, equivalent to 2,438 m (8,000 ft), her arterial partial pressure drops to 64, but the effect on fetal oxygenation is much less. While the mother's P_{O_2} drops from 100 to 64, the fetal P_{O_2} drops from 32 to 25.6, and the oxygen saturation drops even less. This is due to several factors. First, the fetal hemoglobin dissociation curve operates at a much lower partial pressure of oxygen than the maternal and, under the same conditions, the oxygen saturation of fetal blood is greater than that of maternal blood. Second, in relatively hypoxic states there is a protective shift in pH of fetal blood to the alkaline side, which enhances the fetal dissociation curve so that more oxygen is taken up at a given partial pressure.[19]

Thus, it would appear that the fetus is able to withstand hypoxia much better than does an adult. The level of hypoxia reached by passengers and crew under normal circumstances on modern commercial jet transport aircraft has no adverse effect on the fetus. However, these studies were carried out on pregnant women who were the equivalent of sedentary passengers. There are no similar data on pregnant women doing moderate to heavy work at equivalent altitudes, as stewardesses would be. In Denver, at 1,615 m (5,300 ft), there are no greater numbers of spontaneous abortions or rates of anomalies than in seacoast cities, although the average birth weights in Denver are slightly less than in areas of lower altitudes.[9, 15, 16]

Billings[3] stated, "The question of whether hypoxia at normal cabin altitudes has a detrimental effect on the young fetus is unanswered; it is thought that it does not. I believe that pregnant women, especially early in pregnancy, should receive supplemental oxygen during flights above 3,000 m in unpressurized aircraft."

REFERENCES

1. Barcroft J: *Researches on Pre-Natal Life*. Springfield, Ill, Charles C Thomas, Publisher, 1947, p 259.
2. Bartels H, Moll W, Metcalfe J: Physiology of gas exchange in the human placenta. *Am J Obstet Gynecol* 1962; 84:1714.
3. Billings CE: Aerospace medicine—Occupational health aspects, in Zenz C (ed): *Occupational Medicine: Principles and Practical Applications*. Chicago, Year Book Medical Publishers, 1975, pp 157–190.

4. Cameron RG: Should air hostesses continue flight duty during the first trimester of pregnancy? *Aerospace Med* 1973; 44:552.
5. Carter CO: Incidence and aetiology, in Blackwell APN (ed): *Congenital Abnormalities in Infancy*. Oxford, Oxford University Press, 1963.
6. Cook SF, Krum AA: Determination of mouse strains exposed for long periods to low atmospheric pressure. *J Exp Zool* 1955; 128:561.
7. Dawes GS: Oxygen supply and consumption in late fetal life and the onset of breathing at birth, in *Handbook of Physiology*, Section 3, Vol II, *Respiration*. Washington, DC, American Physiological Society, 1965.
8. Dawes GS: The umbilical circulation. *Am J Obstet Gynecol* 1962; 84:1634.
9. Grahn D, Kratchman J: Variation in neonatal death rate and birth weight in the United States and possible relations to environmental radiation, geology and altitude. *Am J Hum Genet* 1963; 15:329.
10. Hellman LM, Pritchard JA: *Williams Obstetrics,* ed 14. New York, Appleton-Century-Crofts, 1971.
11. Hurtado A: Animals in high altitudes, resident man, in Dill DB (ed): *Handbook of Physiology,* Sect 4, *Adaptation to the Environment*. Washington, DC, American Physiological Society, 1964.
12. Ingalls TH: Environmental factors in causation of congenital anomalies, in Wolstenholme GEW (ed): *Ciba Foundation Symposium on Congenital Malformations*. London, Churchill Livingstone Inc, 1960.
13. Ingals TH: Experimental production of congenital anomalies. *N Engl J Med* 1952; 247:758.
14. Kamat SR: Fetal growth retardation and increased infant mortality at high altitude. *Arch Environ Health* 1978; 33:150.
15. Lichty JA: Studies of babies born at high altitude. *AMA J Dis Child* 1957; 93:666.
16. Lubchenco LO: Sequelae of premature birth. *Am J Dis Child* 1963; 106:101.
17. Mazess RB: Neonatal mortality and altitude in Peru. *Am J Phys Anthropol* 1965; 23:209.
18. Metcalfe J, Bartels JH, Moll W: Gas exchange in the pregnant uterus. *Physiol Rev* 1967; 47:782.
19. Metcalfe J, Novy MJ, Peterson EN: Reproduction at high altitudes, in Benirschke K (ed): *Comparative Aspects of Reproductive Failure*. New York, Springer-Verlag, 1966.
20. Raina SS: Diagnosis of early pregnancy in cows. *Indian Vet J* 1962; 39:507.
21. Scholten P: Pregnant stewardess—Should she fly? *Aviat Space Environ Med* 1976; 47:77.
22. Tominaga T, Page EW: Accommodation of the human placenta to hypoxia. *Am J Obstet Gynecol* 1966; 94:679.
23. Weihe WH: Influence of altitude and cold on pregnancy and lactation of rats on two different diets. *Int J Biometeorol* 1965; 9:43.
24. Wulf H: Gas exchange in the mature placenta in man. I. *Z Geburtsh Gynaek* 1962; 158:117.

MERCURY*

Placental transfer of mercury has been found to vary with the chemical nature of mercury compounds.[5, 6, 17, 25] Suzuki et al.[25] noted that the placenta acts as a barrier to inorganic and phenyl mercury to a similar extent but not to methylmercury. Clarkson et al.[7] studied the transplacental passage of elemental mercury in rats and found that after injection of elemental mercury, the fetal content was more than ten times greater than maternal blood and, after inhaling mercury, approximately 40 times greater than after an equivalent dose of inorganic mercury. Utilizing data from both of these studies, Koos and Longo[15] summarized the relative placental permeability for the various forms of mercury as phenyl: 1, inorganic: 2, elemental: 10–20, and methyl: 20.

After acute exposure to inorganic mercurials, the greatest concentrations are in the kidneys, liver, spleen, muscle, and blood.[5] Metallic mercury, which is more lipid soluble, can penetrate into the brain and achieve much higher levels (10×) there than ionic mercury compounds. Phenyl mercury is rapidly degraded to inorganic mercury and follows the distribution of mercuric ions.[15, 26] Methylmercury is much more stable, is lipid soluble, readily diffuses through cell membranes and can attain appreciable quantities in the brain.[10] Yang et al.[28] found by oral feeding of methylmercuric chloride in rats that the precentage of the mercury dose in all parts of the brain of the mother remained essentially the same over the five-day postfeeding period studied. On the other hand, in the fetus there was a threefold increase in uptake of mercury in brain parts from day 1 to day 5, and the fetal brain accumulated a higher concentration of mercury than did the maternal brain.

Mercury has been found in breast milk of women exposed to methylmercury through the ingestion of contaminated food. In an Iraqi experience,[4] milk levels of the total mercury correlated closely with whole blood levels and averaged 5% of simultaneous concentrations in maternal blood, consisting of 40% in the inorganic form and 60% as methylmercury. Similar findings have been reported by Skerfving[21] in 15 lactating women exposed to methylmercury found in fish, except that the methylmercury component was only 20%. Even with the relatively low concentrations of mercury in milk, suckling infants have been noted to accumulate significant amounts of mercury in the blood if their mothers had been heavily exposed.[1]

The reprodutive effects of exposure to mercury (methylmercury in particular) were brought into focus largely by the epidemic of mercury poisonings in Minamata, Japan, beginning in 1953. This epidemic resulted from the ingestion of fish and shellfish from Minamata Bay that had been contaminated with effluent containing methylmercury from a nearby factory. During the epidemic, 23 cases (more since) of prenatally exposed infants with severe psychomotor signs of brain damage (including cerebral palsy and mental retardation) were recorded. It is possible that these infants may also have had postnatal intake of mercury from breast milk. In contrast to the infants, the mothers were found to be asymptomatic or to have mild paresthesias.[12] Most of these patients were examined some time after the onset of poisoning, and no documentation on dose or maternal and fetal blood or brain levels of methylmercury was possible.

Since the 1953 epidemic, additional epidemics involving pregnancy and methylmercury poisoning from ingestion of contaminated food have been reported in Iraq[2, 4] and in the U.S.S.R.,[3] and isolated cases have also been noted elsewhere.[19, 22]

In Iraq, the source of the poisoning was traced to ingestion of homemade bread prepared from wheat treated with a methylmercury fungicide. From February, 1972 to August, 1972, there were 6,530 patients with poisoning admitted to hospitals and 459 hospital deaths in Iraq. Bakir et al.[4] observed that the admission of

*The reader is referred to Chapter 38 for a general discussion of mercury, its industrial uses, occupational exposures, biologic and toxicologic effects, diagnosis, treatment, and hygienic control measures.

pregnant women with diagnosable poisoning was low (31 observed compared to 150 expected) and that the frequency of pregnant females was also low when computed on the basis of the rural population, possibly indicative of an effect on fertility by the mercury. From this exposed population, Amin-Zaki et al.[2] reported the clinical and laboratory findings of 15 infant-mother pairs exposed to methylmercury during pregnancy. They found that in all but one case, the infants' blood mercury levels were higher than their mothers' during the first four months after birth, indicating the transplacental passage of methylmercury from the mother to the fetus and the maintenance of neonatal blood mercury levels from ingestion of mercury in mothers' milk.

Clinically, six of the 15 mothers and at least six of the infants had positive manifestations of mercury poisoning. In five severely affected infants there was gross impairment of motor and mental development. In contrast to the reported findings in Minamata, there was only one infant-mother pair in which the infant was affected and the mother free from clinical manifestations. All of the pregnancies were full term, but in five cases there was a history of unduly prolonged labor as opposed to easy deliveries in prior pregnancies. No congenital anomalies were described. Among the clinical manifestations noted in the infants were reduced head circumference, fretfulness, irritability, excessive crying, blindness, hearing impairment, altered reflexes, and mental retardation. (The investigators estimated a level of 400 ppb of mercury in blood as the level above which all mothers exhibited signs and symptoms of poisoning. The lowest infant blood mercury level associated with signs of poisoning was 564 ppb.) An attempt was made to relate the degree of effect to the period of pregnancy in which the major exposure took place. Three severely affected infants were exposed only in the third trimester and the others throughout pregnancy, particularly in the first trimester. The number of cases, however, in each trimester, namely, four, four, and eight, was too small on which to base any conclusions.[1, 2]

Of particular interest in the isolated instances of reported mercury poisonings is the experience of a family in New Mexico affected by the ingestion of meat from hogs fed seed grain treated with a methylmercury fungicide. The mother of the family was pregnant and ingested the contaminated meat from the third to the sixth month of pregnancy. Other than having elevated urinary mercury levels during the seventh and eighth months of gestation, her examination did not reveal any abnormalities, and she was without symptoms except for slight slurring of speech during a two-week period during the pregnancy. The male infant delivered at term weighed 3,062 gm, displayed intermittent, gross tremulous movements of the extremities, and had elevated urinary mercury levels. The infant had progressive neurologic abnormalities and after three months his originally normal electroencephalogram became progressively abnormal, with an epileptiform pattern. At 1 year of age, the child had normal physical growth, but he could not sit up or see. It is noteworthy that no detectable mercury was found in the urine of this infant at 6 weeks and that he was not breast fed, so the mercury exposure was solely intrauterine.[19, 22]

Genetic mutations and chromosomal aberrations have been produced by organic compounds of mercury experimentally in certain plants and Drosophila.[20] Although all of the organic mercury compounds tested produced c-mitosis, methyl and phenyl mercury are among the most active agents found to produce this effect.[9, 20] Fahmy[9] indicated that inorganic mercury is about 200 times less effective than are organic mercury compounds in producing c-mitosis. Studies on inbred CBA mice have failed to demonstrate dominant lethal mutations from organic mercury compounds,[20] but single doses given parenterally on day 10 of gestation resulted in a high frequency of resorbed litters and an increased percentage of dead fetuses.

Skerfving[21] reported a statistical increase in chromosomal breaks in blood cells of 23 human consumers of large amounts of fish containing methyl mercury (0.5–7 mg/kg) as compared with 16 people with low to moderate intake of oceanic fish. The mercury levels in blood were 1.4–11.6 μg/100 ml in the exposed group and 0.3–1.8 μg/100 ml in the nonexposed. There was a statistical relationship between blood mercury and frequency of chromosomal breaks. On the other hand, Firman, in an unpublished report to the WHO task force,[27] reported that a study in progress did not disclose a statistical difference in chromosomal breaks between mercury-exposed persons and a control population. Similarly, Harada et al.[11] reported normal chromosome patterns in seven adult victims of Minamata disease and one infant victim with severe noncongenital Minamata disease. In summary, genetic effects of mercury compounds are meager and somewhat contradictory.

There are no existing data on human exposure in utero to implicate mercury as a teratogen. However, teratogenic effects have been reported in animals. Administration of single high-level doses of methylmercury phosphate to pregnant rats on day 10 of gestation resulted in reduced birth weight of offspring and an incidence of 31.6% of cleft palates.[18] Spyker and Smithberg[23] found that single doses of methylmercury that did not affect the pregnant females of two strains of mice produced retarded growth and development, death, and congenital malformations in fetuses. Differential effects of methylmercury were dependent on strain of mice, dose, and stage of embryonic development. For both strains, only treatment on day 9 and later had significant embryocidal or teratogenic effects (cleft palates and micrognathia).

There is no information on the effects of mercury on germ cells or fertility in humans, although Bakir et al.[4] suggest that the number of pregnancies in the Iraq epidemic seemed to be low. Suter[24] has reported small but significant decreases in fertility in mice reproduction capacity studies. Male mice injected intraperitoneally with 10 mg/kg methylmercury hydroxide showed significant small reductions in numbers of implants after about 7.5 days posttreatment. Similarly treated females showed a significant small decrease in number of offspring and living embryos when mated within 4.5 days after treatment. Lee and Dixon[16] also noted reduced male fertility in mice with 1 mg/kg methylmercury hydroxide intraperitoneal doses and their studies suggested a spermatogenic effect. Studies on the reproductive capacity of men as well as women workers exposed to mercury are needed.

The present OSHA inorganic mercury standard for occupational exposure is a ceiling of 0.1 mg/cu m. In a 1973 criteria document, the NIOSH recommended 0.05 mg/cu m for a TWA over a ten-hour day.[8] The WHO task force recommends this same level for elemental and inorganic mercury compounds, but notes that this level does not consider the sensitive groups in the general population. In view of the apparent greater susceptibility of the fetus and newborn to these exposures as compared with adults, one must question whether this limit is sufficiently safe for occupational exposure of pregnant women and indirectly for the fetus in utero. For organic mercurials, the WHO task force recommends continued adherence to the advice of the 1969 MAC Committee of WHO that women of childbearing capacity not be exposed to methylmercury compounds.[27] As a result of a comprehensive review of the subject of mercury toxicity, the pregnant woman, fetus, and newborn infant, Koos and Longo[15] recommend the following as exposure limits for women of childbearing capacity: mercury vapor, < 0.01 mg/cu m; inorganic mercury salts (aerosols) and phenyl mercury compounds, < 0.02 mg/cu m and methylmercury, none.

REFERENCES

1. Amin-Zaki L, Elhassani S, Majeed MA, et al: Studies of infants postnatally exposed to methyl mercury. *J Pediatr* 1974; 85:81.
2. Amin-Zaki L, Elhassani S, Majeed MA, et al: Intra-uterine methyl mercury poisoning in Iraq. *Pediatrics* 1974; 54:587.
3. Bahulina AV: The effect of a subacute ethyl mercury coated grain poisoning on the progeny. *Sov Med* 1975; 31:60. (Cited in Koos BJ, Longo LD.[15])
4. Bakir F, Damaluji SF, Amin-Zaki L, et al: Methyl mercury poisoning in Iraq. *Science* 1973; 181:230.
5. Berlin M, Ullberg S: Accumulation and retention of mercury in the mouse, Parts I, II and III. *Arch Environ Health* 1963; 6:589.
6. Clarkson TW: The pharmacology of mercury compounds. *Annu Rev Pharmacol* 1972; 12:375.
7. Clarkson T, Magos L, Greenwood MR: The transport of elemental mercury into fetal tissues. *Biol Neonate* 1972; 21:239.
8. National Institute for Occupational Safety and Health: *Criteria Document for a Recommended Standard: Occupational Exposure to Inorganic Mercury*, DHEW, PHS, NIOSH (HSM 73-11024), 1973.
9. Fahmy FY: *Cytogenetic Analysis of the Action of Some Fungicide Mercurials*, PhD Thesis, 1951, Institute of Genetics, University of Lund, Sweden. (Cited in *Environ Res* 1971; 4:64.)
10. Friberg LT (Chairman): Expert Committee: *Maximum Allowable Concentrations of Mercury Compounds*. Report of an International Committee. *Arch Environ Health* 1969; 19:891.
11. Harada Y, et al: Clinical study (Rinshoto Kenkyu) 1971; 48:1431. (Cited in WHO *Environmental Health Criteria* I: Mercury.[27])
12. Harada Y: Congenital (fetal) Minamata disease, in Katsuna M (ed): *Minamata Disease*. Kuonamoto University, 1968, p 93.
13. Hazards of Mercury. Special Report to HEW Sec s. Pesticide Advisory Committee. *Environ Res* 1971; 4:1.
14. Knight AL: Mercury and its compounds, in Zenz C (ed): *Occupational Medicine: Principles and Practical Applications*. Chicago, Year Book Medical Publishers, 1975, pp 668–677.
15. Koos BJ, Longo LD: Mercury toxicity in the pregnant woman, fetus and newborn infant. *Am J Obstet Gynecol* 1976; 126:390.
16. Lee IP, Dixon RL: Effects of mercury on spermatogenesis studied by velocity sedimentation cell separation and serial mating. *J Pharmacol Exp Ther* 1975; 194:171.
17. Mansour MM, Dyer NC, Hossman LH, et al: Maternal-fetal transfer of organic and inorganic mercury via placenta and milk. *Environ Res* 1973; 6:479.
18. Oharazawa H: Effects of ethyl mercuric phosphate in the pregnant mouse on chromosome abnormalities and fetal malformation. *J Jpn Obstet Gynecol Soc* 1968; 29:14. (Cited in *Environ Res* 1971; 4:67.)
19. Pierce PE, Thompson JF, Likosky WH, et al: Alkyl mercury poisoning in humans. *JAMA* 1972; 220:1439.
20. Ramel C: Genetic effects of organic mercury compound. *Hereditas* 1967; 57:445.
21. Skerfving S: Conference of Environmental Effects of Mercury, Brussels, November, 1973, in *Publicaties om bet Institut voor Wiltenschappen om bet haefmilieu*, p 103. Brussels, Vrije University. (Cited in *Environ Health Criteria* I: Mercury.[27])
22. Snyder RD: Congenital mercury poisoning. *N Engl J Med* 1971; 284:1014.
23. Spyker JM, Smithberg M: Effects of methyl mercury on prenatal development in mice. *Teratology* 1971; 5:181.
24. Suter KE: Studies on the dominant-lethal and fertility effects of the heavy metal compounds methyl mercuric hydroxide, mercuric chloride and cadmium chloride in male and female mice. *Mutat Res* 1975; 30:365.
25. Suzuki T, Matsumoto N, Miyania T, et al: Placental transfer of mercuric chloride, phenyl mercury acetate and methyl mercury acetate in mice. *Ind Health* 1967; 5:149.
26. Takeda Y, Kunugi T, Hoshino O, Uketa T: Distribution of inorganic aryl and alkyl mercury compounds in rats. *Toxicol Appl Pharmacol* 1968; 13:156.
27. World Health Organization: *Environmental Health Criteria* I: Mercury. Geneva, 1976.
28. Yang MG, et al: Deposition of mercury in fetal and maternal brain. *Proc Soc Exp Biol Med* 1972; 141:1004.

POLYCHLORINATED BIPHENYLS (PCBs)

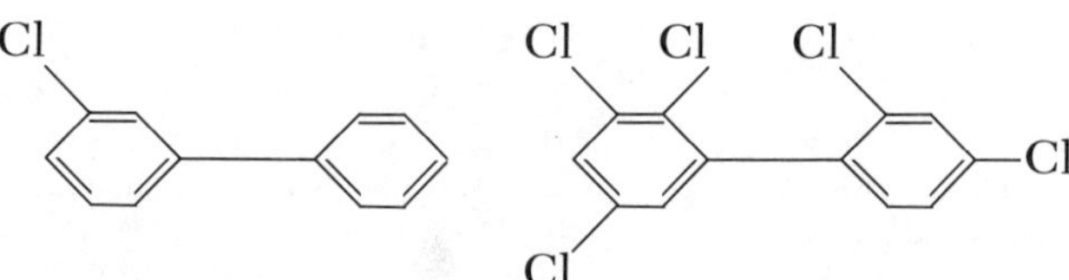

3-chlorobiphenyl 2,2′,3,4′,5-pentachlorobiphenyl

Polychlorinated biphenyls (PCBs) are groups of compounds manufactured commercially by the progressive chlorination of biphenyls in the presence of a suitable catalyst. Among the major uses are for the insulation of electric capacitors and transformers, as plasticizers, investment casting waxes and molds, and heat exchange units. PCBs have been used in "carbonless carbon paper." The NIOSH estimates that 12,000 U.S. workers currently have potential occupational exposure to these compounds, the majority in capacitor production and in investment casting processes.[5]

PCBs are very resistant to degradation and persist in the environment. Workers, in addition to their occupational exposure, may be further exposed to PCBs carried into their homes from the workplace and from general contamination of the air, water, and food supply. Within workplaces, PCBs have been shown to remain in the air and on surfaces long after their use is discontinued. The role of the impurities known to be present in commercial PCBs, namely, chlorinated dibenzofurans and chlorinated naphthalenes, in the etiology of the adverse effect of PCBs requires further clarification.

PCBs are well absorbed via the gastrointestinal tract, skin, and lungs but are poorly metabolized and can accumulate in human and animal tissues.[7] The accumulation, particularly in high-lipid tissues, seems to be greater for the penta and more highly chlorinated compounds. Surveys of human adipose tissue of nonexposed subjects in several countries have shown most samples to contain PCBs around 1 mg/kg or less in contrast to occupationally exposed men, who have shown levels up to 700 mg/kg.[20] National surveys indicate levels in blood around 0.3 μg/100 ml for nonoccupationally exposed populations and levels approaching 200 mg/100 ml in men occupationally exposed, with or without skin lesions.[20]

Placental transfer of PCBs has been found in "Yusho" patients in Japan[16] as well as in various species of animals.[5, 20] PCBs have been quantitatively measured in animal and human milk, in the latter in concentrations averaging 0.02 mg/L but reaching levels as high as 0.1 mg/L.[22]

In 1968 in Japan, numerous cases of poisoning from PCBs occurred from the ingestion of rice bran oil contaminated with Kanechlor 400, a 48% chlorinated biphenyl, which leaked through small holes in heat transfer pipes immersed in the oil during an oil purification process. The rice oil was also contaminated with chlorinated dibenzofurans, and the role of these impurities needs to be clarified.

By 1975, almost 1,300 cases of the disease called "Yusho" were registered. The major manifestations included acneiform eruptions (chloracne), enlargement and hypersecretion of the meibomian glands of the eyes, with swelling of the eyelids and hyperpigmentation of the nails and mucous membranes.[5] In addition, there were alterations in liver enzymes, an increase in serum triglycerides (up to four times normal level)[18] and changes in the microanatomy of liver cells, indicative of microsomal enzyme stimulation.[11] Offspring of "Yusho" mothers were smaller than normal and exhibited dark brown skin pigmentation, which persisted for several months after their birth. In four babies studied at birth, retarded intrauterine growth was noted in three, edematous face and exophthalmic eyes in three, retarded dentition in two, calcification of the skull and wide-open sagittal surface of the skull in 3.[9] These findings were not persistent, and postnatal mental and physical development appeared normal in these and other "Yusho" children. Only one case of "Yusho" from PCB exposure during nursing was observed.[22] In 80 female patients with "Yusho" disease, 60% had changes in their menstrual cycles after the exposure.[13] PCB levels were found for many years in the blood adipose tissue and milk of mothers and in the blood of offspring.[5, 20] This occurrence in Japan clearly indicated that PCBs can be transmitted transplacentally to the fetus and also from mothers' milk during lactation.

Data pertinent to reproductive effects from PCBs in humans other than the "Yusho" cases are very limited. In 1936, Schwartz[15] reported that impotence in men was one of the health problems associated with occupational exposure to chlorobiphenyls. Inoue et al.[12] reported on exposure to PCBs among workers in family-owned silk thread glossing factories in Japan. Among those exposed was a woman in her tenth month of pregnancy with a PCB level of 24 ppb in her blood serum. Subsequent to the birth of the child, it was found that the mother's breast milk contained 0.25 ppm PCB, and breast feeding was discontinued. At the time of the report, mother and child exhibited no abnormalities.

Animal studies have indicated such reproductive effects as increased fetal resorptions, lower fertility, decreased survival and teratogenesis, the effects occurring primarily at higher doses. Studies of rhesus monkeys are of particular interest because this animal has been found to respond to PCBs in a fashion similar to humans with "Yusho" disease.[5]

Allen et al.[2] fed female rhesus monkeys a diet containing 25 ppm Arochlor 1248 for two months. There was lower fertility in females, which persisted for at least eight months after the dose was discontinued. Barsotti et al.[3] and Allen and Barsotti[1] fed male and female rhesus monkeys 2.5 ppm and 5.0 ppm Arochlor 1248 in a commercial diet for six months. Menstrual cycles became irregular and there was prolonged and excessive menstrual bleeding. There was lower fertility and increased resorptions and abortions compared with the controls, and the offspring had lower body weights. The infants developed signs of PCB poisoning after nursing for less than two months and there was a 50% rate of infant mortality during the nursing period. (Milk levels were 0.154–0.397 ppm PCB.)

A report of the findings of a study conducted at the Karolinska Institute by Westöö and Norén[19] reiterates the persistence of PCBs in the environment. They measured levels of organochlorine pesticides and polychlorinated biphenyls (PCBs) in pooled samples of human milk from Stockholm for different periods from April, 1967 to March, 1977. These pooled milk samples were obtained from the Mothers Milk Center in Stockholm and analyzed for the pesticide levels. Reported average PCB level was 10–20 mg/kg of milk during a period from April to July, 1967, and an average level of 24–30 mg/kg of milk was found from the samples taken between April, 1976 and March, 1977. Despite the fact that PCBs have been severely restricted since June, 1972, special licenses having been required for the importation, production, sale, and use of PCBs in Sweden, the authors speculate that PCB discharges from other Baltic countries and global fallout may make a major contribution to the PCB levels in Swedish fish, which are thought to be the main source of PCBs for the mothers.

Studies in animals and microorganisms have shown PCBs to have very weak mutagenic potential. Green et al.[10] found no statistically significant chromosomal aberrations in spermatogonal or bone marrow cells or evidence of dominant lethal mutations in rats fed varying doses of Arochlor 1242 or 1254. In the Ames test, higher chlorinated PCBs showed very little activity, although 4-chlorobiphenyl showed some activity.

The carcinogenic potential of PCBs has been suggested in view of the formation of arene oxides as an intermediate in the metabolism of PCBs and the demonstration of binding of PCB metabolites to nuclear components of liver cells in monkeys, rats, and in vitro studies. Dose-related increased incidences of liver tumors, including neoplastic nodules, hepatomas, and hepatocellular carcinomas, in rats and mice were noted.[5, 20] Confirmation of carcinogenicity of the PCBs has not been obtained in humans. Follow-up of deceased "Yusho" patients indicated a possible increase in cancer incidence, but no consistency as to types of cancer found has been reported.[5]

There is no existing OSHA standard for occupational exposure to PCBs. The NIOSH proposes as the standard, a time-weighted average for up to a ten-hour workday, 40-hour workweek, 1 μg/cu m, which is the minimal detectable level with present methodology. NIOSH has considered the effects on reproduction in establishing this standard and considers that this recommended level will protect unborn babies. The WHO task force has noted that the most sensitive species to PCBs is man and that at intake rates of 0.1 mg/kg body weight per day it seems unlikely that effects on reproduction would be apparent. Based on conversion data suggested by Ferguson[6] for air concentrations and potential dose of a 1 μg/cu m for an eight-hour day, if totally absorbed, would be equivalent to 0.14 μg/kg for adult males, and 0.12 μg/kg for adult females.

Gustavsson et al.[10a] conducted an epidemiologic and medical study on the possible health impact of work in a capacitor manufacturing plant using polychlorinated biphenyls. A cohort of 142 male Swedish capacitor-making workers was studied, with 23 deaths and seven cancers noted, in agreement with anticipated numbers as calculated from national statistics. They reported results as inconclusive because the follow-up period had been relatively brief, and stated that exposure to PCBs did not present a high carcinogenic risk in this factory. One person had developed two rare tumors, a semimalignant mesenchymal tumor (desmoid) and a malignant lymphoma (the case is discussed). Some of the exposed persons had been receiving annual medical checkups, covering standard blood parameters, liver enzymes, and liver function tests. No abnormal results attributable to PCB exposure were detected.

REFERENCES

1. Allen JR, Barsotti DA: The effects of transplacental and mammary movement of PCBs on infant rhesus monkeys. *Toxicology* 1976; 6:331.
2. Allen JR, Carstens LA, Barsotti DA: Residual effects of short-term low-level exposure of non-human primates to polychlorinated biphenyls. *Toxicol Appl Pharmacol* 1974; 30:440.
3. Barsotti DA, et al: Reproductive dysfunction in rhesus monkeys exposed to low levels of polychlorinated biphenyls (Arochlor 1248). *Food Cosmet Toxicol* 1976; 14:99.
4. Bercovici B, Wassermann M, Cucos S, et al: Serum levels of polychlorinated biphenyls and some organochlorine insecticides in women with recent and former missed abortions. *Environ Res* 1983; 30:169–174.
5. National Institute for Occupational Safety and Health: *Criteria for a Recommended Standard: Occupational Exposure to Polychlorinated Biphenyls* (PCBs), DHEW, PHS, NIOSH 77-225, 1977.
6. Ferguson DM: Toxicological problems related to the employment of women, in *Health of Women at Work*. London, Society of Occupational Medicine, April, 1976.
7. Finklea J, et al: Polychlorinated biphenyl residues in human plasma expose a major urban pollution problem. *Am J Public Health* 1972; 62:645.
8. Fujiwara K, et al: Discovery of PCB pollution at a textile factory. II. Follow-up study on causes of environmental pollution. *Jpn J Public Health* 1975; 22:461. (Japanese) (Cited in NIOSH Criteria Document.[4])
9. Funatsu I, et al: Polychlorinated biphenyls (PCBs) induced fetopathy. I. Clinical observation. *Kurume Med J* 1972; 19:43. (Cited in NIOSH Criteria Document.[4])
10. Green SG, et al: Lack of cytogenetic effects in bone marrow and spermatogonal cells in rats treated with polychlorinated biphenyls (Arochlor 1242 and 1254). *Bull Environ Contam Toxicol* 1975; 13:14. (Cited in NIOSH Criteria Document.[4])

10a. Gustavsson P, Hogstedt C, Jonsson U: Hälsoeffekter Av Yrkesmässig Exponering För Polyklorerade Bifenyler (PCB) Bland Kondensatorarbetare—Epidemiologisk Och Medicinsk Undersökning. *Arbete Och Hälsa* 22, Stockholm, 1985.

11. Hirayama C, et al: Fine structural changes of the liver in a patient with chlorobiphenyls intoxication. *Fukuoka Acta Med* 1969; 60:455. (Japanese) (Cited in NIOSH Criteria Document.[4])
12. Inoue Y, et al: Discovery of PCB pollution in a textile factory. I. PCB level in blood serum of laborers and results of physical examination. *Jpn J Public Health* 1975; 22:461. (Cited in NIOSH Criteria Document.[4])
13. Kusuda M: Study on the female sexual function suffering from the chlorobiphenyls poisoning. *Sankato Fujinka* 1971; 4:1063. (Japanese) (Reviewed in WHO *Environmental Health Criteria* 2.[17])
14. Sager D: Effect of postnatal exposure to polychlorinated biphenyls on adult male reproductive function. *Environ Res* 1983; 31:76–94.
15. Schwartz L: Dermatitis from synthetic resins and waxes. *Am J Public Health* 1936; 26:586.

15a. Smith AB, Schloemer J, Lowry LK, et al: Metabolic and health consequences of occupational exposure to polychlorinated biphenyls. *Br J Ind Med* 1982; 39:361.

16. Tsukamoto H, et al: The chemical studies on detection of toxic compounds in the rice bran oils used by the patients of Yusho. *Fukuoka Acta Med* 1975; 60:496. (Japanese) (Cited in WHO Environmental Health Criteria 2.[17])
17. Urabe H, Koda H, Asahi M: Present state of Yusho patients, in Nicholson W, Moore J (eds): *Health Effects of Halogenated Aromatic Hydrocarbons*. *Ann NY Acad Sci* 1979; 320:273–276.
18. Uzawa H, et al: Clinical and experimental studies on the hyperglyceridemia induced by oral ingestion of chlorinated biphenyls. *Acta Med* 1971; 62:66. (Japanese) (Cited in NIOSH Criteria Document.[4])
19. Westöö G, Norén K: Organochlorine contaminants in human milk. Stockholm 1967–1977. *Ambio* 1978; 7(2):62.
20. WHO: *Environmental Health Criteria* 2: Polychlorinated Biphenyls and Terphenyls. Geneva, 1976.
21. Wyndham C, et al: The in vitro metabolism macromolecular binding and bacterial mutagenicity of 4-chlorobiphenyl, a model PCB substrate. *Res Commun Chem Pathol Pharmacol* 1976; 15:563. (Cited in NIOSH Criteria Document.[4])
22. Yoshimura T: Epidemiological study on Yusho babies born to mothers who had consumed oil contaminated by PCB. *Acta Med* 1974; 65:74. (Japanese) (Cited in NIOSH Criteria Document.[4])

TETRACHLOROETHYLENE (PERCHLOROETHYLENE)

$$Cl_2C{=}CCl_2$$

Tetrachloroethylene is a chlorinated organic solvent widely used as a dry cleaning agent, a degreaser, and a fumigant and as a chemical intermediate in the manufacture of other chemicals. The NIOSH estimates that approximately 500,000 workers currently are at risk of exposure to tetrachloroethylene in the United States.[4]

There have been two animal studies concerning exposure to tetrachloroethylene with reproductive effects. Schwetz et al.[5] exposed 17 rats and 17 mice for seven hours daily to 300 ppm tetrachloroethylene on days 6–15 of gestation. The controls consisted of 30 unexposed rats and 30 unexposed mice. The exposure was associated with a decrease in maternal weight gain in the rats and an increase in the maternal relative weight gain in the mice. There was a higher percentage of fetal resorptions in exposed rats but no difference in the skeletal anomalies among the exposed litters relative to the controls. Fetal mice, on the other hand, showed decreased body weights and an increased incidence of subcutaneous edema, delayed ossification of skull bones and split sternebrae, as compared with the controls.

In another study, Carpenter[3] evaluated the effects of exposures to 70 ppm, 230 ppm, and 470 ppm of tetrachloroethylene on the fertility of female rats between the ages of 70 and 250 days. There were 10 control and 12 test rats in each of the exposure groups. He found a slight drop in fertility at 70 ppm and a slight increase at the higher levels and concluded that it was unlikely that these findings were due to the tetrachloroethylene exposure.

The usefulness of the information furnished by these two animal studies in the consideration of occupational exposure of pregnant women is indeterminate at this time. The teratogenic effect of tetrachloroethylene suggested by the study of Schwetz et al. needs further evaluation, particularly in regard to the difference reported between the effects on the mice and rats. The exposure level used in the study, namely, 300 ppm, is higher than the present OSHA air standard of a time-weighted average exposure of 100 ppm and ceiling of 200 ppm and the proposed NIOSH recommendation in 1976 of 50 ppm time-weighted average and ceiling of 100 ppm (15 minutes).

Of further note is information published by the NIOSH in its 1978 *Current Intelligence Bulletin* 20, Tetrachloroethylene,[4] from a study by the National Cancer Institute (NCI) with findings of excess hepatocellular carcinomas in male and female mice exposed by forced feeding to tetrachloroethylene as compared with controls. The exposure dosages over 78 weeks were 536 or 1,072 mg/kg per day for male mice and 386 or 772 mg/kg per day for female mice. The NIOSH notes that a 70-kg man breathing a typical 10 cu m per day (over an eight-hour shift) would have an inhalation exposure equivalent to 100 mg/kg per day. Although the dosages used in the NCI studies and those in the previously mentioned animal studies referable to reproductive effects were considerably in excess of the exposure a worker might receive in work areas controlled at recommended levels, further studies are needed to determine what margin of safety, if any, exists at these levels for both the possible neoplastic and reproductive effects of tetrachloroethylene.

REFERENCES

1. Bagnell P, Ellenberger H: "Dry-cleaned" breast milk poisons baby. *Med World News* 1978; 16: Feb 20.
2. Elovaara E, Hemminki K, Vainio H: Effects of methylene chloride, trichloroethane, trichloroethylene, tetrachloroethylene and toluene on the development of chick embryos. *Toxicology* 1979; 12:111–119.
3. Carpenter CP: The chronic toxicity of tetrachloroethylene. *J Ind Hyg Toxicol* 1937; 19:323.
4. National Institute for Occupational Safety and Health: *Criteria for a Recommended Standard: Occupational Exposure to Tetrachloroethylene (Perchloroethylene)*. DHEW, PHS, NIOSH 76-185, 1976. *Current Intelligence Bulletin 20*. Tetrachloroethylene, (Perchloroethylene). NIOSH-DHEW, Jan 20, 1978.
5. Schwetz BA, Leong BKJ, Gehring PJ: The effect of maternally inhaled trichloroethylene, perchloroethylene, methyl chloroform and methylene chloride on embryonal and fetal development in mice and rats. *Toxicol Appl Pharmacol* 1975; 32:84.
6. *Tetrachloroethylene: Environmental Health Criteria 31*. Geneva, World Health Organization, 1984.

VINYL CHLORIDE

$$H_2C{=}CHCl$$

Vinyl chloride, also known as vinyl chloride monomer (VCM), chloroethylene, and chloroethene, is a gas at normal temperature and atmospheric pressure. It is the parent compound of a series of thermoplastic resin polymers and copolymers that are widely used for containers, wrapping tissues, electrical insulation, pipe, conduits, and a variety of other products. Annual world production of vinyl chloride exceeds 10 billion kg, 25% of this in the United States, where it has been produced commercially since 1939. For a detailed discussion of vinyl plastics and occupational exposures, control measures and related hygienic aspects, the reader is referred to Chapter 63.

Observations over the years have indicated toxic effects of vinyl chloride on the lung, liver, selected bones of the fingers (acro-osteolysis), and central nervous system. However, VCM has been recognized as a human carcinogen since a report made to the NIOSH in 1974 of angiosarcoma of the liver in a small number of employees at the B. F. Goodrich Chemical Company and subsequent epidemiologic studies in the United States, as well as abroad, of workers exposed to VCM, the findings of which confirmed similar data from animal studies since 1971. Both animal and human studies indicate that VCM produces excess tumors not only in the liver but also in the lung and lymphatic and central nervous systems.

Effects of VCM relative to its reproductive toxicity have also been reported. Vinyl chloride has been found to be mutagenic in microbial test systems,[1] in Drosophila[9] and in hamster cells.[6]

Excess chromosomal aberrations in lymphocyte cultures have been reported in male vinyl chloride workers.[3, 5] In a study of vinyl chloride monomer workers that compared them with an age-matched control of rubber workers with no known toxic chemical exposure, Infante et al.[7] reported a significant excess of fetal mortality in the wives of the VCM workers as compared with wives of the controls (15.8% and 6.1%, respectively). Fetal mortality (any product of conception not born alive) was not significantly different between the two groups prior to the VCM exposure (8.8% and 6.9%, respectively).

A report by Infante[8] of excess birth defects (particularly anencephaly and spina bifida) in residents of an Ohio community where a polyvinyl chloride manufacturing plant was located was followed by a subsequent case-controlled study of these birth defect cases. Comparison of subject and control data failed to indicate any relationship between occupational and geographic exposure to VCM with the birth defects noted.[4]

In view of the mutagenic responses to VCM in microbial test systems, increased chromosome aberrations in VCM male workers and increased fetal mortality in the wives of such workers, vinyl chloride can be considered a possible reproductive toxin in men. The effect in women has not as yet been evaluated.

The OSHA and NIOSH have recognized VCM as a carcinogen, and requirements of environmental and medical surveillance pertinent to known carcinogens are mandated. The present OSHA environmental limit is 1 ppm averaged over eight hours with a maximum of 5 ppm for any 15-minute period.[10]

REFERENCES

VINYL CHLORIDE

1. Bartsch H, Malaveille C, Montesano R: Human rat and mouse liver-mediated mutagenicity of vinyl chloride in *S typhimurium* strains. *Int J Cancer* 1975; 15:429.
2. Beliczky LS, Zenz C: Occupational health aspects of plastics and rubber manufacturing, in Zenz C (ed): *Occupational Medicine: Principles and Practical Applications*. Chicago, Year Book Medical Publishers, 1975, pp 786–815.
3. Ducatman A, Herschborn K, Selekoff I: Vinyl chloride exposure and human chromosome aberrations. *Mutat Res* 1975; 31:163.
4. Edmonds L: Birth defects and vinyl chloride, in *Proceedings of Conference on Women and the Workplace*. Washington, DC, Society of Occupational & Environmental Health, pp 114–119, June 17–19, 1976.
5. Funes-Cravioto F, et al: Chromosome aberrations in workers exposed to vinyl chloride. *Lancet* 1975; 1:459.
6. Huberman E, Bartsch H, Sachs L: Mutation induction in Chinese hamster V79 cells by two vinyl chloride metabolites, chloroethylene oxide and 2-chloroacetaldehyde. *Int J Cancer* 1975; 16:639.
7. Infante PF, et al: Genetic risks of vinyl chloride. *Lancet* 1976; 1:734.
8. Infante PF: Oncogenic and mutagenic risks in communities with polyvinyl chloride production facilities. *Ann NY Acad Sci* 1976; 271:49.
9. Magnussen J, Ramel C: Mutagenic effects of vinyl chloride in *Drosophila melanogaster*. *Mutat Res* 1976; 38:114.
10. OSHA US Dept of Labor: Emergency Temporary Standard for Exposure to Vinyl Chloride; *Federal Register* 1974; 39:12343.
11. Picciano D, Flake R, Gay P, et al: Vinyl chloride cytogenetics. *J Occup Med* 1977; 19:527–530.
12. Theriault G, Ituvya H, Gingras S: Evaluation of the association between birth defects and exposure to ambient vinyl chloride. *Teratology* 1983; 27:359–370.

ANESTHETIC GASES AS AN OCCUPATIONAL HAZARD

Christer Edling, M.D.

Inhalation anesthesia was introduced in 1842, when an American physician administered diethyl ether to a patient. Later on, many different compounds were used as inhalation anesthetic agents, and some of these have been utilized as industrial solvents, e.g., trichloroethylene and chloroform. Although the first report indicating that people working in operating rooms could become ill as a consequence of exposure to anesthetic gases came at the end of the 19th century, it is the physical properties of anesthetic agents that have attracted the most interest. Particularly, questions concerning volatility, flammability, and dangers of explosion have come to the fore. Thus, systems for the elimination of anesthetic gases from operating rooms were described at the beginning of the 20th century, and the anesthetic compounds have become less explosive and flammable through the introduction of halogenated anesthetic agents in the mid 1950s. During the last decade, however, interest has more and more been focused on the health hazards for occupationally exposed personnel, i.e., people manufacturing anesthetic gases, operating staff, dentists, veterinary surgeons, and ambulance personnel.

Mutagenic and Cytogenic Effects

Formula for halothane, a widely used agent:

$$F_3C{-}C(Br)(Cl)(H)$$

The studies on the mutagenicity of anesthetic agents in bacterial systems are few and contradictory. Halothane, methoxyflurane, enflurane, trichloroethylene, and isoflurane have been tested, but no evidence of mutagenicity was found.[5, 6, 80] On the other hand, fluroxene was mutagenic in the same test system,[6] and another study has reported trichloroethylene as a mutagen.[46] The urine of anesthesiologists exposed to halothane induced mutations in the conventional Ames assay,[60] and halothane has been described as an "insufficiently positive mutagen."[47] Sister chromatid exchanges (SCE) and sister chromatid exchange points (SCE points) were evaluated in lymphocytes in peripheral blood from persons exposed to anesthetics and compared to nonexposed. No indication of a mutagen effect of long-term exposure to waste anesthetic agents such as halothane and nitrous oxide was found.[49] In another study, Waksvik et al.[79] found no increase of chromosome gaps or SCE among nurses exposed to anesthetic gases such as halothane, enflurane and nitrous oxide.

Reproductive Effects

Animal Tests.—Many animal studies have been publicized indicating a teratogenic effect of nitrous oxide and halogenated anesthetic agents.[62] In most of these studies, very high exposure levels were used, and it is therefore difficult to compare the results of the animal experiments with what could be expected from the far lower exposure levels for occupationally exposed personnel. However, some recent studies have shown that, following the continuous exposure of pregnant rats to nitrous oxide in air mixtures, the threshold value for reduced litter size, skeletal anomalies, and prenatal growth retardation lies between 1,000 ppm and 500 ppm of nitrous oxide;[86, 87, 88] and following intermittent exposure, the threshold for reduction in litter size has been claimed to lie between 1,000 ppm and 500 ppm of nitrous oxide in air,[89] and the effect is dose-dependent. For halothane, it is reported that, when pregnant rats were exposed to 10 ppm of halothane, this resulted in CNS damage in the fetus.[17] On the other hand, the results of other studies do not support the hypothesis that trace levels of anesthetic agents adversely affect reproductive processes.[59, 67, 82, 83, 84, 85]

Epidemiology.—In 1967, Waisman[78] reported a Russian study of 31 pregnant anesthesiologists: one pregnancy in three had ended in spontaneous abortion, two women gave birth prematurely, and in one case the child had congenital malformations. The anesthetic gas in use during the period of exposure was mostly ether, but even nitrous oxide and halothane had been used.

This report was later followed by a Danish study[2] in which the abortion frequency was significantly higher for the exposed women (20%) in comparison with the nonexposed ones (10%). In this study, the authors even reported a higher frequency of spontaneous abortions among nonexposed women whose husbands worked as anesthesiologists. Similar results were reported in an American study,[23] in which wives of exposed dentists had a higher frequency of spontaneous abortion in comparison with nonexposed referents. In two English questionnaire surveys[52, 53] the results indicated a higher rate of spontaneous abortion among exposed women, whereas the husband's exposure did not seem to influence the outcome of pregnancy. Findings of a higher frequency of spontaneous abortion among exposed women have hitherto been reported in several studies from many countries, e.g., Czechoslovakia,[62] Finland,[69] Great Britain,[77] Sweden,[43] West Germany,[41] and the USA.[24] In a recent Swedish study, a higher, although nonsignificant, miscarriage rate was reported among women who had worked in areas with high exposure to anesthetic gases during the first trimester compared to unexposed women.[4]

In some of the aforementioned studies, a higher risk of malformations among children born to women exposed to anesthetic gases during pregnancy was also shown. In his study of English anesthesiologists, Tomlin[77] reported an increased frequency of malformations, especially in the central nervous and musculoskeletal systems.

Pharaoh et al.[66] surveyed the obstetric history of female physicians in England and Wales. They reported that, when conceptions had occurred when the mother was in an anesthetic appointment, this resulted in smaller babies, higher stillbirth rates, and more congenital malformations of the cardiovascular system than those of other female physicians. There was, however, no significant difference in the spontaneous abortion rate between the two groups. A Swedish survey[7] followed the pregnancy outcome, i.e., perinatal mortality and congenital malformations, for women working in medical occupations before giving birth. The outcome of pregnancies was checked with the aid of existing central registers and compared with the outcome of pregnancies for the whole country. There was no difference in the observed and expected number of perinatal mortality and congenital malformations among women working in anesthesia and operation departments. Neither did the results of a Finnish[71] as well as a Belgian[56] study indicate any statistically significant effects on pregnancy attributable to work in the operating theatre.

Even if there might be methodologic weaknesses in many of the epidemiologic studies using questionnaires, i.e., low response rate, response bias,[4] a lack of or poor definition of reference groups, no information on the anesthetic agents used or the environmental concentrations of the gases present, many studies indicate a higher risk for spontaneous abortion among women exposed to anesthetic gases. Less agreement is found in the information on the increased risk for spontaneous abortion among women whose husbands have been exposed to anesthetic gases, or on the increased risk of exposed women having malformed children.

Carcinogenic Effects

During the last several years, the possibility of a carcinogenic effect of anesthetic gases has attracted some attention. The anxiety about this effect is not totally unjustified, since there are many structural similarities between known human carcinogens (i.e., dibromoethane, dichloroethane, bischloromethylether, and chloromethyl methyl ether) and several of the inhalation anesthetic agents now in use. Besides, anesthetic compounds can be transformed into reactive metabolites which can combine with tissue macromolecules[21] and thereby turn into chemical carcinogens.[10]

Animal Tests.—Studies on rats and mice have demonstrated that at least some of the volatile anesthetic agents are capable of inducing cancer. In an early experiment, Eschenbrenner[37] induced hepatoma by giving mice very high doses of chloroform perorally. In 1976 the National Cancer Institute (NCI) reported[61] animal tests in which rats had been given chloroform perorally in doses of one-fifth to one-tenth of those of Eschenbrenner. A significant increase in kidney tumors, as well as hepatocellular carcinomas, was observed. However, in these studies, the methods of exposure were quite unusual when compared with occupational exposure. Therefore, no conclusion can be drawn on the basis of these studies, except that the results indicate that the tested substance might have some carcinogenic potential.

As for halogenated anesthetic gases, an animal experiment was made by Corbett[26] in which pulmonary and hepatic neoplasms were induced in the offspring of mice by repeated exposure of the mother during pregnancy and of the offspring after delivery to subanesthetic concentrations of isoflurane (0.1%–0.5% isoflurane). In another study,[36] mice were exposed, both in utero during the last half of pregnancy and after delivery, to low doses of either enflurane, isoflurane, halothane, methoxyflurane, or nitrous oxide. The result did not confirm the suggestion that isoflurane is a hepatocarcinogen, nor did the data suggest that inhaled anesthetics currently in use pose a significant threat of carcinogenicity. Coate et al.[20] studied the effects of prolonged exposure to low-concentration combinations of halothane and nitrous oxide on tumor incidence. Rats were exposed to filtered air, 1 ppm of halothane and 50 ppm of nitrous oxide or 10 ppm of halothane and 500 ppm of nitrous oxide. Histologic evaluation of the reticuloendothelial system and of other major organs did not reveal any enhancement of the spontaneous tumor rate or any unusual neoplasms.

Epidemiology.—In a retrospective cohort study,[14] the mortality among anesthesiologists in 1947–1966 was studied. An increased frequency of malignant disease in the lymphoid and reticuloendothelial system was reported among the 441 diseased persons. A later follow-up of the mortality during 1967–1971 did not, however, indicate any increase in deaths from tumors.[15] In another large American study, in which morbidity was followed in a questionnaire survey of 73,496 persons, it was found that women, but not men, who were exposed to anesthetic gases had a higher frequency of cancer, especially leukemia and lymphoma.[22] In other American studies,[27, 28] the incidence of malignant diseases among anesthetic nurses was followed. Excluding skin cancer, a higher incidence of unusual tumors, such as malignant lymphoma, leiomyosarcoma, hepatocellular carcinoma, and cancer of the pancreas, was found. Furthermore, the occurrence of cancer among children born to anesthetic nurses was studied, and for them also a higher cancer incidence was found. The same findings concerning cancer among children were also observed by Tomlin.[77]

These data could indicate that anesthetic gases can act as a transplacental chemical carcinogen, as has been reported for some other substances in man, i.e., barbiturates,[44] diethylstilbestrol,[48] chlorinated pesticides,[50] and smoking.[63] Some English studies[33, 52, 66] did not disclose any increase in cancer among anesthesiologists, nor did a recent study by Cohen et al.[24] regarding occupational diseases in dentistry.

Taken together, the results of short-term tests, genotoxic studies, animal tests, and epidemiology do not indicate any stronger risk for cancer after exposure to anesthetic agents. Howver, better epidemiologic studies are needed for a definite conclusion.

Other Organ Effects

Central Nervous System.—Some of the industrial solvents now in use have earlier been used as anesthetic agents. Solvents, as well as anesthetic agents, are fat-soluble, which is also one of the conditions for the narcotic effects. Besides, anesthetic gases can form toxic metabolites[21] in the same manner as many solvents; these metabolites react on the cellular level and can induce cell damage there.[72] The chronic damage caused by solvents has been studied to a great extent during the last ten years, and many studies have shown effects on the central nervous system as a consequence of long-term exposure to solvents.[3] Today there are no studies on the chronic nervous effects on anesthetic personnel exposed for many years to anesthetic gases. However, animal as well as human experiments indicate that exposure to anesthetic gases does affect the central nervous system (CNS).

Animal experiments have shown CNS damage in rats after exposure to halothane in concentrations of 8–12 ppm for eight hours a day five days a week during eight weeks.[18]

High levels of nitrous oxide, 20,000 ppm and above, cause a deterioration on tests of reaction time.[25, 40] After exposing volunteers to a range of concentrations, Allison et al.[1] concluded that the threshold at which nitrous oxide started to affect performance lay between 8,000 ppm and 12,000 ppm.

Controversy exists over the effects of trace levels of anesthetic gases on performance. Gamberale and Svensson[39] and Snyder et al.[74] found no acute behavioral effects of trace levels of anesthetic gases on operating theater personnel. Bruce et al.[13] and Bruce and Bach,[11] on the other hand, found that 500 ppm (0.05%) affected performance on the digit span test for short-term memory. In a later study, the same authors[12] found that 50 ppm (0.005%) of nitrous oxide caused a deterioration in the performance of an audiovisual task and that 500 ppm also caused a deterioration in the performance of vigilance and tachistoscopic tasks and the digit span test. Other studies have failed to replicate the results of Bruce and Bach using a design and a test battery which included an audiovisual task very similar or similar to that used by Bruce et al.[38, 73, 81]

In Finland, Korttila et al.[54] looked into the driving skills of operating room nurses after occupational exposure to halothane (0–43.7 ppm) and nitrous oxide (100–1,200 ppm). The driving skills of 19 nurses were measured and compared to those of 11 younger nurses working in the wards of the same hospital but with no exposure to anesthetic agents. The authors stated that no impairment of driving skills could be expected after daily exposure to halothane and nitrous oxide among long-term employees working in operating rooms.

Peripheral Nervous System.—Layzer et al.[58] reported a disabling peripheral neuropathy in three health workers who habitually abused nitrous oxide. Nerve conduction studies suggested an axonal rather than demyelinative neuropathy. The neurologic disorder improved slowly when the patients abstained from further nitrous oxide abuse. In another study, Layzer[57] reported a neurologic disorder in 15 patients after prolonged exposure to nitrous oxide. Thirteen of the patients had abused nitrous oxide to some extent for periods ranging from three months to several years, but two patients were exposed to nitrous oxide only professionally, as dentists, during work in poorly ventilated offices. Neurologic examinations showed sensorimotor polyneuropathy and a picture similar to that of subacute combined degeneration of the spinal cord.

In a dental survey in America, it was suggested that long-term exposure to anesthetics among dentists and chairside assistants might result in an increased incidence of numbness, tingling, and muscle weakness.[24] Interestingly, nitrous oxide neuropathy closely resembles the neuropathy of pernicious anemia, and it has been shown that a few hours of exposure to concentrations of nitrous oxide greater than about 1,000 ppm (1%) results in oxidation of vitamin B_{12}, causing inactivation of methionine synthase, of which it is the co-factor.[65] This inactivation also affects folate metabolism, and taken together, these changes might explain not only findings of neuropathy but also the megaloblastic changes and fetotoxicity.

Liver.—In many animal experiments, liver damage has been reported after exposure to high doses of halothane and methoxyflurance,[62] and also after long-term exposure to subanesthetic concentrations of halothane, isoflurance, and diethyl ether.[76] On the other hand, there are very few reports available on the effects on operating room personnel. A temporary increase of liver transaminases is reported among operating personnel working with halothane.[42] There are also case reports on icterus and liver cirrhosis among anesthetists exposed to halothane.[8, 51] In some of the larger epidemiologic studies made in America[22, 23, 24] and Czechoslovakia,[62] an increased frequency of liver disease among anesthesiologists or dental personnel was observed.

Nunn et al.[65] reported that the hepatic function enzyme activities (measured as aspartate transaminase and γ-glutamyl transpeptidase) showed no significant difference between a group of ten members of an operating theater staff exposed to a mean concentration of nitrous oxide ranging from 150 to 400 ppm, compared to a nonexposed group. In a Danish study,[34] no change was found in the hepatic microsomal function as assessed by the antipurine test in two groups of persons with occupational exposure of less than 10 ppm of halothane and less than 100 ppm of nitrous oxide. A third study could not either reveal any hepatic dysfunction among exposed anesthetists.[70]

Kidneys.—In animal experiments, kidney damage has been reported after exposure to low levels (100–500 ppm) of halothane.[19] An affect on man has been reported on several occasions, where side effects have been noticed in patients anesthetized with methoxyflurane.[29, 30] In 1968 there was a retrospective cohort study made among anesthetic personnel; it reported an increase in chronic kidney disease.[14] In the above mentioned American and Czechoslovakian studies, there was a higher frequency of kidney disease among exposed persons.[22, 23, 24, 62] In a Swedish report,[32] a moderate and temporary effect on kidney function was shown among patients as well as personnel exposed to methoxyflurane.

Bone Marrow.—Animal studies and clinical experience on the effect of prolonged exposure to high concentrations of nitrous oxide have shown that leukopenia may be induced.[45, 55] This effect has been used in the treatment of chronic and acute myeloic leukemia.[35] However, because of the rapid recovery of marrow, it has been ineffective as a choice of treatment for leukemia.[90] As to the effect on exposed personnel, there are no reports concerning bone marrow depression.

Exposure and Scavenging

When no scavenging is used, the levels of anesthetic gases in operating rooms are highly variable and might be rather high.[43, 43, 54, 62] Usually the levels of halothane are reported to be about 1–70 ppm and those of nitrous oxide 400–3,000 ppm. The highest levels are found in older operating rooms with poor general ventilation. However, scavenging systems have been in use for a long time and last years. New and better systems for close or local scavenging have been introduced.[9, 16, 64] With these it is possible to reduce exposure to levels well below 5 ppm of halothane and 100 ppm of nitrous oxide.

Threshold Limit Values and Monitoring

Although the adverse health effects of anesthetic gases have been discussed in many countries, quite few have set any threshold limit values for them. In 1977, the NIOSH[62] concluded (based on their compilation) that a safe level of exposure to the halogenated agents could not be defined, but recommended that exposure should be controlled to levels around 2 ppm and that the permissible level of exposure to nitrous oxide alone should be 25 ppm. In 1984, however, there was still no TLV settled in the USA, but a TWA of 50 ppm (400 mg/cu m) is proposed for halothane.

In Sweden, Denmark, and Norway a TWA of 100 ppm (180 mg/cu m) has been in use since about 1981. These countries, together with Holland, Switzerland, and West Germany, also have a TWA of 5 ppm (40 mg/cu m) for halothane.

The establishment of threshold limit values results in the requirement of simple methods for monitoring. Environmental monitoring is still the matter of choice, i.e., by pump-bag sampling and analyzing by an infrared spectrophotometer or a gas chromatograph. Methods for diffuse or "passive" sampling are a rapidly developing technology, and diffuse samples are now available for nitrous oxide[31] as well as halothane.[68] These might prove to be an important and easy tool for environmental monitoring.

Recently, some attempts have been made to use biologic monitoring as an estimate of exposure. Sonander et al.[75] found a rather high correlation between nitrous oxide in air and nitrous oxide in urine and stated that monitoring of urinary nitrous oxide with headspace extraction and gas chromatographic analysis might be a simple and accurate method for monitoring of exposure to nitrous oxide.

REFERENCES

1. Allison RH, Shirley AW, Smith G: Threshold concentration of nitrous oxide affecting psychomotor performance. *Br J Anaesth* 1979; 51:177–180.
2. Askrog V, Harvald B: Teratogen effekt af inhalationanestetika. *Nord Med* 1970; 83:498–500.
3. Axelson O, Hogstedt CH: On the health effects of solvents, in Zenz C (ed): *Developments in Occupational Medicine*, ed 2. Chicago, Year Book Medical Publishers, 1988, in press.
4. Axelsson G, Rylander R: Exposure to anaesthetic gases and spontaneous abortion: Response bias in a postal questionnaire study. *Int J Epidemiol* 1982; 11:250–256.
5. Baden JM, Brinckenhoff M, Wharton RS, et al: Mutagenicity of volatile anesthetics: Halothane. *Anesthesiology* 1976; 45:311–318.
6. Baden JM, Kelley M, Wharton RF, et al: Mutagenicity of halogenated ether anesthetics. *Anesthesiology* 1977; 46:346–350.
7. Baltzar B, Ericson A, Källen B: Delivery outcome in women employed in medical occupations in Sweden. *J Occup Med* 1979; 21:543–548.
8. Belfrage S, Ahlgren J, Axelson S: Halothane hepatitis in an anesthetist. *Lancet* 1966; 2:1466–1467.
9. Bernow J, Björdal J, Wiklund KE: Pollution of delivery ward air by nitrous oxide. Effects of various modes of room ventilation, excess and close scavenging. *Acta Anesthesiol Scand* 1984; 28:229.
10. Boyland E: Biochemistry of occupational cancer. *J Soc Occup Med* 1977; 27:97–101.
11. Bruce DL, Bach MJ: Psychological studies of human performance as affected by traces of enflurane and nitrous oxide. *Anesthesiology* 1975; 42:194–205.
12. Bruce DL, Bach MJ: Effects of trace anaesthetic gases on behavioural performance of volunteers. *Br J Anaesth* 1976; 48:871–876.
13. Bruce DL, Bach MJ, Arbit J: Trace anesthetic effects on perceptual, cognitive and motor skills. *Anesthesiology* 1974; 40:453–458.
14. Bruce DL, Eide KA, Linde HW, et al: Causes of death among anesthesiologists—A 20-year survey. *Anesthesiology* 1968; 29:565–569.
15. Bruce DL, Eide KA, Smith MJ, et al: A prospective survey of anesthesiologists mortality 1967–1971. *Anesthesiology* 1974; 41:71–74.
16. Carlsson P, Ljungqvist B, Hallén B: The effect of local scavenging on occupational exposure to nitrous oxide. *Acta Anaesthesiol Scand* 1983; 27:470–475.
17. Chang L, Dudley AW Jr, Katz J, et al: Nervous system development following in utero exposure to trace amounts of halothane. *Teratology* 1974; 9:A–15.
18. Chang LW, Dudley AW Jr, Lee YK, et al: Ultrastructural changes in the nervous system after chronic exposure to halothane. *Exp Neurol* 1974; 45:209–219.
19. Chang LW, Dudley AW Jr, Lee YK, et al: Ultrastructural changes in the kidney following chronic exposure to low levels of halothane. *Am J Pathol* 1975; 78:225–232.
20. Coate WB, Ulland BM, Lewis TR: Chronic exposure to low concentrations of halothane, nitrous oxide: Lack of carcinogenic effect in the rat. *Anesthesiology* 1979; 50:306–309.
21. Cohen EN: Toxicity of inhalation anasthetic agents. *Br J Anaesth* 1978; 50:665–675.
22. Cohen EN, Brown BW, Bruce DL, et al: Occupation disease among

operating room personnel: A national study. *Anesthesiology* 1974; 41:321–340.

23. Cohen EN, Brown BW, Bruce DL, et al: A survey of anesthetic health hazards among dentists. *J Am Dent Assoc* 1975; 90:1291–1296.
24. Cohen EN, Brown BW, Wu ML, et al: Occupational disease in dentistry and chronic exposure to trace anesthetic gases. *J Am Dent Assoc* 1980; 101:21–31.
25. Cook TL, Smith M, Starkweather JA, et al: Behavioural effects of trace and subanesthetic halothane and nitrous oxide in man. *Anesthesiology* 1978; 49:419–424.
26. Corbett TH: Cancer and congenital anomalies associated with anesthetics. *Ann NY Acad Sci* 1976; 271:58–66.
27. Corbett TH, Cornell RG, Endres JL, et al: Birth defects among children of nurse-anesthetists. *Anesthesiology* 1974; 41:341–344.
28. Corbett TH, Cornell RG, Lieding K, et al: Incidence of cancer among Michigan nurse-anesthetists. *Anesthesiology* 1973; 38:260–263.
29. Cousins MJ, Greenstein LR, Hitt BA, et al: Metabolism and renal effects of enflurane in man. *Anesthesiology* 1974; 44:44–53.
30. Cousins MJ, Mazze RI: Methoxyflurane nephrotoxicity: A study of dose response in man. *JAMA* 1973; 225:1611–1616.
31. Cox PC, Brown RH: A personal sampling method for the determination of nitrous oxide exposure. *Am Ind Hyg Assoc J* 1984; 45:345–350.
32. Dahlgren B-E: Fluoride concentration in urine of delivery ward personnel following exposures to low concentrations of methoxyflurane. *J Occup Med* 1979; 21:624–626.
33. Doll R, Peto R: Mortality among doctors in different occupations. *Br Med J* 1977; 1:1433–1436.
34. Døssing M, Weihe P: Hepatic microsomal enzyme function in technicians and anesthesiologists exposed to halothane and nitrous oxide. *Int Arch Occup Environ Health* 1982; 51:91–98.
35. Eastwood DW, Green CD, Lambdin MA, et al: Effect of nitrous oxide on the white cell count in leukemia. *N Engl J Med* 1963; 268:297–299.
36. Eager EI II, White AE, Brown CL, et al: A test of the carcinogenicity of enflurane, isoflurane, halothane, methoxyflurane and nitrous oxide in mice. *Anesth Analg* 1978; 57:678–694.
37. Eschenbrenner AB: Induction of hepatomas in mice by repeated oral administration of chloroform with observations on sex differences. *J Natl Cancer Inst* 1945; 5:251–255.
38. Frankhuizen JL, Vlek CAJ, Burm AGL, et al: Failure to replicate negative effects of trace anesthetics on mental performance. *Br J Anaesth* 1978; 50:229–234.
39. Gamberale F, Svensson G: The effect of anesthetic gases on the psychomotor and perceptual functions of anesthetic nurses. *Work Environ Health* 1974; 11:108–113.
40. Garfield JM, Garfield FB, Sampson J: Effects of nitrous oxide on decision-strategy and sustained attention. *Psychopharmacologia (Berlin)* 1975; 42:5–10.
41. Garstka K, Wagner KL, Hamacher M: Pregnancy complications in anesthesiologists. Presented at the 159th Meeting Lower Rhine, Westphalia, Gynecology and Obstetric Association, Bonn, West Germany, June 23, 1974.
42. Götell P, Ståhl R: Halothanexposition hos narkossköterskor. *Läkartidningen* 1972; 69:6179–6183.
43. Göthe C-J, Dahlgren B-E, Hultén B, et al: Narkosgaser som yrkesrisk. *Läkartidningen* 1976; 73:2553–2563.
44. Gold E, Gordis L, Tonascia I, et al: Increased risk of brain tumors in children exposed to barbiturates. *J Natl Cancer Inst* 1978; 60:1031–1034.
45. Green CD, Eastwood DW: Effects of nitrous oxide inhalation on hemopoiesis in rats. *Anesthesiology* 1963; 24:341–345.
46. Greim H, Bonse G, Radwan Z: Mutagenicity in vitro and potential carcinogenicity of chlorinated ethylenes as a function of metabolic oxyrane formation. *Biochem Pharmacol* 1975; 24:2013–2017.
47. Hemminki K, Sorsa M, Vainio H: Genetic risks caused by occupational chemicals. *Scand J Work Environ Health* 1979; 5:307–327.
48. Herbst AL, Ulfelder H, Poskanzer DC: Adenocarcinoma of the vagina: Association of maternal stilbestrol therapy with appearance in young women. *N Engl J Med* 1971; 284:878–881.
49. Husman B, Wulf HC: Sister chromatid exchanges in lymphocytes in operating room personnel. *Acta Anaesth Scand* 1980; 24:22–24.
50. Infante PF, Epstein SS, Newton WA: Blood dyscrasia and childhood tumours in exposure to chlorodane and heptachlor. *Scand J Work Environ Health* 1978; 4:137–150.
51. Klatsking G, Kimberg DW: Recurrent hepatitis attributable to halothane sensitization in an anesthetist. *N Engl J Med* 1969; 280:515–522.
52. Knill-Jones RP, Newman BJ, Spence AA: Anaesthetic practice and pregnancy: Controlled survey of male anaesthetists in the United Kingdom. *Lancet* 1975; 2:807–809.
53. Knill-Jones RP, Rodrigues LV, Moir DD, et al: Anaesthetic practice and pregnancy: Controlled survey of women anaesthetists in the United Kingdom. *Lancet* 1972; 1:1326–1328.
54. Korttila K, Pfäffli P, Linnoila M, et al: Operating room nurses' psychomotor and driving skills after occupational exposure to halothane and nitrous oxide. *Acta Anaesthesiol Scand* 1978; 22:33–39.
55. Lassen HCA, Henriksen E, Neukirch R, et al: Treatment of tetanus: Severe bone marrow depression after prolonged nitrous oxide anaesthesia. *Lancet* 1956; 1:527–530.
56. Lauwerys R, Siddons M, Mison CB, et al: Anaesthetic health hazards among Belgian nurses and physicians. *Int Arch Occup Environ Health* 1981; 48:195–203.
57. Layzer RB: Myeloneuropathy after prolonged exposure to nitrous oxide. *Lancet* 1978; 2:1227–1230.
58. Layzer RB, Fishman RA, Schafer JA: Neuopathy following abuse of nitrous oxide. *Neurology* 1978; 28:504–506.
59. Mazze RI, Wilson AI, Rice SA, et al: Reproduction and fetal development in mice chronically exposed to nitrous oxide. *Teratology* 1982; 26:11–16.
60. McCay EC, Hankel R, Robbins K, et al: Presence of mutagenic substances in the urines of anesthesiologists. *Mutat Res* 1978; 53:71.
61. National Cancer Institute: *Report on Carcinogenesis Bioassay of Chloroform*. Bethesda, Md, Carcinogenesis Program, Division of Cancer Cause and Prevention, 1976.
62. National Institute for Occupational Safety and Health: *Occupational Exposure to Waste Anesthetic Gases and Vapors*. Washington, DC, US Dept of Health, Education and Welfare, 1977.
63. Neutel CJ, Buck C: Effect of smoking during pregnancy on the risk of cancer in children. *J Natl Cancer Inst* 1971; 47:59–63.
64. Nilsson K, Sonander H, Stenqvist O: Close scavenging of anaesthetic during mask anaesthesia. Further experimental and clinical studies of a method of reducing anaesthetic gas contamination. *Acta Anaesth Scand* 1981; 25:421–426.
65. Nunn JF, Sharper N, Royston D, et al: Serum methionine and hepatic enzyme activity in anaesthetists exposed to nitrous oxide. *Br J Anaesth* 1982; 54:593–597.
66. Pharaoh POD, Alberman E, Doyle P, et al: Outcome of pregnancy among women in anaesthetic practice. *Lancet* 1977; 1:34–36.
67. Pope WD, Halsey NJ, Landsdown AB, et al: Fetotoxicity in rats following chronic exposure to halothane, nitrous oxide or methoxyflurane. *Anesthesiology* 1978; 48:11–16.
68. Purnell CJ, Wright MD, Brown RH: Performance of the porton down charcoal cloth diffusive sampler. *Analyst* 1981; 106:590–598.
69. Rosenberg P, Kirves A: Miscarriages among operating theater staff. *Acta Anaesthesiol Scand* 1973; 53:37–42.

70. Rosenberg PH, Oikkonen M: Effects of working environment on the liver in 10 anaesthetists. *Acta Anaesthesiol Scand* 1983; 27:131–134.
71. Rosenberg PM, Vänttinen H: Occupational hazards to reproduction and health in anaesthetists and paediatricians. *Acta Anaesthesiol Scand* 1978; 22:202–207.
72. Savolainen H: Some aspects of the mechanism by which industrial solvents produce neurotoxic effects. *Chem Biol Interact* 1977; 18:1–10.
73. Smith G, Shirley AW: Failure to demonstrate effect of trace concentrations of nitrous oxide and halothane on psychomotor performance. *Br J Anaesth* 1977; 49:65–70.
74. Snyder BD, Thomas RS, Gyorky Z: Behavioral toxicity of anesthetic gases. *Ann Neurol* 1978; 3:67–71.
75. Sonander H, Stenqvist O, Nilsson K: Exposure to trace amounts of nitrous oxide. Evaluation of urinary gas content monitoring in anaesthetic practice. *Br J Anaesth* 1983; 55:1225.
76. Stevens WC, Eger EI II, White A, et al: Comparative toxicities of halothane, isoflurane and diethyl ether at subanesthetic concentrations in laboratory animals. *Anesthesiology* 1975; 42:408–419.
77. Tomlin PJ: Health problems of anaesthetists and their families in the West Midland. *Br Med J* 1979; 1:779–784.
78. Waisman AI: Working conditions in surgery and their effect on the health of anesthesiologists. *Eksp Khir Anesteziol* 1967; 12:44–49.
79. Waksvik H, Klepp O, Brogger A: Chromosome analyses of nurses handling cytostatic agents. *Cancer Treatment Reports* 1981; 65:607–610.
80. Waskell LA: A study of the mutagenicity of anesthetics and their metabolites. *Mutat Res* 1978; 57:141–153.
81. Venables H, Cherry N, Waldron HA, et al: Effects of trace levels of nitrous oxide on psychomotor performance. *Scand J Work Environ Health* 1983; 9:391–396.
82. Wharton RS, Mazze RI, Baden JM, et al: Fertility, reproduction and postnatal survival in mice chronically exposed to halothane. *Anesthesiology* 1978; 48:167–174.
83. Wharton RS, Wilson AI, Mazze RI, et al: Fetal morphology in mice exposed to halothane. *Anesthesiology* 1979; 51:532–537.
84. Wharton RS, Sievenpiper TS, Mazze RI: Developmental toxicity of methoxyflurane in mice. *Anesth Analg* 1980; 59:421–425.
85. Wharton RS, Mazze RI, Wilson AI: Reproduction and fetal development in mice chronically exposed to enflurane. *Anesthesiology* 1981; 54:505–510.
86. Vieira E: Effect of the chronic administration of nitrous oxide 0.5% to gravid rats. *Br J Anaesth* 1979; 51:283–287.
87. Vieira E, Cleaton-Jones P, Austin J, et al: Intermittent exposure of gravid rats to 1% nitrous oxide and the effect on the post-natal growth of their offspring. *S Afr Med J* 1978; 53:106.
88. Vieira E, Cleaton-Jones P, Austin JC, et al: Effects of low concentrations of nitrous oxide on rat fetuses. *Anesth Analg* 1980; 59:175–177.
89. Vieira E, Cleaton-Jones P, Moyes D: Effects of low intermittent concentrations of nitrous oxide on the developing rat fetus. *Br J Anaesth* 1983; 55:67.
90. Editorial: Nitrous oxide and the bone marrow. *Lancet* 1978; 2:613–614.

RADIOFREQUENCY AND MICROWAVE RADIATION

Radiofrequency and microwave radiation (rf/microwave) refers to that portion of the electromagnetic spectrum from 10 KHz to 300 GHz. There have been thousands of reports published about the biologic effects of rf/microwave radiation, nearly all of which

TABLE 54–6.

Exposure Levels Calculated to Cause a Specific Absorption Rate of 0.4 W/kg or Less From Microwave*

1	2	3	4
FREQUENCY RANGE (MHz)	E^2 (V^2/SQ M)	H^2 (A^2/SQ M)	POWER DENSITY (mW/SQ CM)
0.3– 3	400,000	2.5	100
3 – 30	4,000 ($900/f^2$)	0.025 ($900/f^2$)	$900/f^2$
30 – 300	4,000	0.025	1.0
300 – 1,500	4,000 ($f/300$)	0.025 ($f/300$)	$f/300$
1,500 – 100,000	20,000	0.125	5.0

Note: f = frequency (MHz).
*From American National Standards Institute, 1982.

are of limited value due to lack of accurate knowledge of the dose absorbed by the study subjects. The amount of rf/microwave radiation absorbed into an object (biologic or otherwise) depends on the power output at the source, the size, shape, and composition of the object, the distance of the object from the source, and the frequency of the radiation, or more simply, the intensity of the radiation at the object and the frequency. The guides for safe exposure followed by most are those set by the American National Standards Institute (ANSI) on July 30, 1982, known as ANSI C95.1-1982.[1] Table 54–6 lists the actual exposure levels calculated to produce a specific absorption rate (SAR) of 0.4 Watts/kg or less when averaged over the whole body for any 0.1-hour period. The ACGIH has adopted a TLV of essentially the same limits but includes frequencies from 10 KHz to 300 GHz.[2] Both organizations exclude devices with power output of 7 Watts or less as being unlikely to cause harm.

Rf/microwave radiation finds its primary use in radio-TV broadcasting, telecommunications, and radar. When rf/microwave is absorbed into objects, not enough energy is absorbed to produce ionization, but rather causes heating of the object. The second most important use of rf/microwave is to heat the object into which it is beamed. It is used in the molding of thermoplastic materials and in rapid drying processes, often at frequencies near 30 MHz. It is used in medical physiotherapy to cause subcutaneous heating at 2.45 GHz, and in the cooking of food at the same frequency but at a higher power output.

Nonthermal biologic effects of rf/microwave radiation have not been shown to be significantly harmful. Hyperthermia from any cause, including such radiation, is known to cause dose-related adverse effects on the mammalian testicle[3] and embryo.[4] A few reports have been published of possible reproductive harm to men in the form of decreased fertility and/or teratogenesis from rf/microwave exposures, but without adequate information on dose, so that it is not possible to conclude that such effects were actually related to the exposures or to other causes.[5] No reports were found of harm to women or to the human conceptus from such exposures in which the exposure dose was known, and it is commonly believed there have not been significant nonthermal effects shown.

If exposure levels in the workplace are kept within the TLV and ANSI C95.1-1982, rf/microwave radiation should not cause adverse effects on human reproductive functions.

REFERENCES

1. American National Standards Institute, Inc: *Safety Levels with Respect to Human Exposure to Radiofrequency Electromagnetic Fields, 300 KHz to 100 GHz*. New York, The Institute of Electrical and Electronics Engineers, Inc, 1982.
2. American Conference of Governmental Industrial Hygienists: *Threshold Limit Values for Chemical Substances and Physical Agents in the Work Environment, 1985–86*, Cincinnati, Oh, ACGIH, 1985.
3. Council on Scientific Affairs: Effects of physical forces on the reproductive cycle. *JAMA* 1984; 251:247–250.
4. Lary JM, Conover DL, Hauser PL: Thermal threshold for teratogenesis in rats exposed to 27.12 radiofrequency radiation, abstract. *Teratology* 1981; 23:49.
5. Lancranjan I, Popescu HI, Gavanesco O, et al: Gonadic function in workmen with long-term exposure to microwaves. *Health Phys* 1975; 29:381–383.

IONIZING RADIATION

Ionizing radiation is capable of causing dose-related damage to all biologic tissues. Despite this serious potential, the radiation industry has proved to be one of the safest places to work.

The National Council on Radiation Protection and Measurements (NCRP) has for many years been considered the responsible source of recommendations about occupational exposure to ionizing radiation. The NCRP has published recommendations on exposures to fertile and pregnant women over the years, most recently in their Report No. 53.[1] Report No. 53 recommends the same exposure limits as their Report No. 39, which is reviewed by Voelz in Chapter 26.[2]

In brief, the NCRP recommends that the dose equivalent to the embryo or fetus from occupational exposure of the mother be limited to 0.5 rem. In the usual occupational setting, actual exposure measurements to an embryo or fetus within the worker's uterus are not made. Rather, the worker is monitored and the relationship of the reading of a pregnant employee's exposure badge and the dose to an embryo or fetus can vary depending on the location of the monitoring device, the geometry, type, and energy of the radiation, as well as the thickness of the overlying maternal tissues.

The occupational dose limit in effect is 5 rem per year whole body, or 1.5 rem per quarter. A pregnancy may go undiagnosed for several weeks, but if radiation exposure is within the acceptable limits and relatively stable as to dose rate, considering the attenuating effects of maternal tissues, an embryo or fetus would not be likely to receive more than 0.5 rem prior to the time of the diagnosis of pregnancy. When this occurs, the recent exposure records can be reviewed and a decision made about any further exposure as long as the estimated or calculated dose to the fetus is kept below 0.5 rem through the term of the pregnancy. The NCRP recommendations in Report No. 53 are stated to be based on limits that would not unreasonably restrict the employment of fertile women in the radiation industry, yet provide safety to the products of conception.

Ionizing radiation is considered a teratogen and a carcinogen, and the effects are dose-related. For a detailed discussion of the calculated risks, in part extrapolated from animal data, see the entire Report No. 53, and especially Chapter 26 on ionizing radiation by G. L. Voelz.[1]

REFERENCE

1. National Council on Radiation Protection and Measurements: *Radiation Dose Limits for Embryo and Fetus in Occupationally Exposed Women*. NCRP Report No. 53, 1977.

55

Male Occupational Reproductive Hazards

M. Donald Whorton, M.D., M.P.H.

Male occupational reproductive effects from radiation exposure have been recognized by the health care professions for many years; however, effects from other exposures is a more recent concern. From a regulatory point of view, the issue of male occupational reproductive effects was first addressed in the OSHA Lead Standard in 1976. However, it was not until 1977, with the discovery that exposure to dibromochloropropane (DBCP) produced infertility and sterility in men, that male occupational reproductive effects became a widely recognized issue.

The potential effects on the male reproductive system include sterility, infertility, and mutagenesis. Sterility implies an irreversible inability to procreate, while infertility involves diminished or absence of fertility, but does not imply irreversibility. Both can be caused by interference with spermatogenesis and/or function of the spermatozoa, as well as impotence. Agents which can affect nuclear material of the chromosomes during spermatogenesis can produce mutagenic effects. If conception were to occur from these mutated spermatozoa, spontaneous abortions or congenital malformations (birth defects) are possible pregnancy outcomes.

Since the mid 1970s, a number of studies have been done showing or suggesting adverse outcomes on the male reproductive system from a variety of toxic exposures. One of the most pressing issues concerning male occupational reproductive effects is how to conduct surveillance of a population. To date, a validated and sensitive method of collecting such information in a readily acceptable and simple manner has not been achieved.

BACKGROUND INFORMATION

Infertility is a relatively frequent occurrence. For instance, among married couples, some 15% are childless (involuntarily), while another 10% have fewer children than desired. In determining the cause of infertility, the man plays a significant role about 30% of the time, and a contributing role in another 20%. Any evaluation of an infertile couple must include both partners. Unfortunately, all too frequently, evaluation of the man has been either omitted or has been ignored in deference to the woman. From a practical procedural point of view, the male work-up is far easier than the female.

The current types of screening procedures for evaluation of this particular function in the occupational environment are three: (1) semen analysis; (2) blood hormonal analyses; and (3) reproductive histories.

In occupational studies, the most commonly reported parameter of the semen analysis has been the sperm count or sperm density. Hormonal analyses include serum follicle-stimulating hormone (FSH), luteinizing hormone (LH), and/or testosterone. Most of the reproductive histories thus far developed have looked at the number and timing of live births.

In the evaluation of testicular function, there are two distinct areas of the testes which must be evaluated: the seminiferous tubules and the interstitium. In the seminiferous tubules, spermatogenesis occurs. Evaluation of spermatogenesis can be done by semen analysis and serum FSH. The interstitium is best evaluated by hormones LH and testosterone. The process of spermatogenesis takes some 70–72 days in the testes. The spermatozoa then move to the epididymis for another 7–21 days of maturation. After that point, they are ready for function and ejaculation. The hormonal axes involved in the testes have been mentioned. FSH, as liberated from the pituitary, stimulates spermatogenesis. Another hormone called inhibin is liberated from the testes and goes back to the hypothalamus/pituitary as the negative feedback. LH liberated by the pituitary stimulates the interstitial cells (Leydig cells), which in turn produce testosterone which functions as the negative feedback of the hormonal axis.

There are a number of factors that can alter testicular function resulting in pathologic processes affecting production and/or transportation of sperm. Infection, trauma, varicocele, cryptorchidism, exposure to toxic agents, ionizing radiation, autoimmunity, stress, and prolonged high fever have all been shown to cause male infertility. In the majority of cases, the cause is not identified. Various therapeutic agents known to interfere with normal testicular function include antimetabolitic drugs (e.g., cyclophosphamide and chlorambucil), nitrofurantoin, and estrogens. Male fertility also depends upon the function of the prostate, seminiferous tubules, libido, and the ability to achieve erection and ejaculation. Occupational exposures to estrogens have been known to decrease libido and erectile abilities. Neurotoxins may have the effect of altering sexual performance.

EVALUATIONS REQUIRING SEMEN SAMPLES

The standard semen analyses include volume, sperm count, sperm motility, and sperm morphology. The average ejaculatory volume is 2–5 ml. The sperm count can be given as a total count or a count per milliliter (sperm density). Generally, the sperm density (count per milliliter) is used. The range can be from 0 to 400+ million/ml. The mean sperm count is approximately 100 million/ml with a median count of about 80 million/ml. Important in sperm counts is the continence time (time since last ejaculation), arbitrarily 48–72 hours. Not allowing for this continence time can result in misleadingly low sperm counts. Sperm motility is a test to evaluate the forward movement of the spermatozoa. Sperm morphology is a test to evaluate the morphological characteristics of the spermatozoa. In most laboratories, 60% or more morphologically normal spermatozoa is considered the expected.

Any occupational study requiring the examination of seminal fluid has many potential problems. Unless an imminent hazard or effect is suspected, full cooperation of the group under study may be difficult to obtain. Reasons for refusal to participate in such a study can include being beyond the child-bearing age (man or partner); impotence; medical disorders (such as retrograde ejaculation after prostatectomy); fear of possible abnormal results being interpreted by some as loss of manhood; and religious or cultural objection. Obviously, vasectomized men must be excluded. This exclusion can bias the remaining population or remove many of the men with the most exposure. For instance, in some occupational studies, the vasectomy rate has averaged 20%, with 40% seen in one study. The preferred method of collection of semen is by masturbation. The most suitable place for collection is at home with the semen then promptly brought to the workplace. Any collection area at the workplace probably will have a certain stigma attached to it and, thus, will inhibit participation and cooperation.

One must be careful in interpreting results as to normal/abnormal (normospermia/oligospermia). The current consensus is that oligospermia is the condition with less than 20 million spermatozoa per milliliter of semen.

Obtaining a suitable control population may be another problem. If current controls are unavailable, one may have to use historic control data. Table 55–1 shows a recent report of sperm count data for 861 workers and compares these data to the 1951 data of McCloud and Gold. The 1984 data would be suitable to use as an external control if concurrent controls were unavailable or insufficient in numbers.

TABLE 55–1.

Frequency Distribution of Sperm Counts for 861 Workers Compared to 1951 Data from Prenatal and Infertility Clinics

SPERM COUNTS [MILLIONS/ML]	WHORTON & MEYER [1984]	MACLEOD AND GOLD [FERTILE]	[INFERTILE]
<20	9%	5%	14%
20–39	14%	12%	13%
40–99	37%	39%	33%
100+	40%	44%	38%
Number of subjects	861	1,000	1,000
Source of subjects	Occupational studies	Prenatal clinic	Infertility clinic

Two types of studies can be done: cross-sectional or longitudinal. Cross-sectional studies have been most frequently done. Limitations of cross-sectional studies include too small a number of participants and/or an inadequate number of controls. Thus, the power of the study tends to be low. Also, there is a question as to the sensitivity of the methods, in that the range of anticipated findings is wide, sperm count more so than sperm morphology. Longitudinal studies have been done almost exclusively to study the effects of pharmaceutical agents. Advantages of such studies are that the number of participants can be far fewer and the power of the study much higher. The difficulty is to obtain participation by the individual over a long period of time. Despite these and other limitations, large cross-sectional studies requiring semen samples have been done since the discovery in 1977 of the effects of DBCP in human beings. However, obtaining repeated semen samples for routine periodic surveillance is more difficult, if not nearly impossible.

EVALUATIONS USING HORMONES

With the advent of radioimmunoassay, the precision for evaluating many body substances has improved dramatically. Serum FSH, LH, and testosterone can all be analyzed by radioimmunoassay. The sensitivity of the method depends on the particular antigen. These tests tend to be moderately expensive; however, the limiting factor for using serum hormonal analyses in lieu of sperm counts is the poor predictive value of the results. Until the individual is severely oligospermic or azoospermic, the rise of FSH does not predict sperm count. Thus, this test would be useful only in those individuals with severe damage. Similar results are true if FSH, LH, or testosterone are combined in any fashion.

STUDIES USING QUESTIONNAIRES

The questionnaire is the least invasive of the three methods described. Parameters that can be ascertained include fertility, spontaneous abortion, and birth defects. The accuracy of the information from men is highest for live children and lowest for spontaneous abortions. The information on birth defects is variable, partly depending on the definition of birth defect. The analyses for fertility have utilized an indirect standardization procedure using the number of live births. Comparative fertility data generally are taken from the National Center for Health Statistics, which are much better for women than for men. For male workers, one must know the wives' ages so the female fertility data can be used to predict male outcomes. Limitations of such procedures include number of individuals at risk, age group of individuals being evaluated, stability of the workforce, and accuracy of memory.

Advantages of using questionnaires for fertility evaluations are that they are noninvasive and inexpensive, data are easily collected (five-minute questionnaire), there tends to be high employee participation rate, and the requested information the ultimate endpoint of fertility (incidence of live births). Additionally, this type of information is suitable for long-term monitoring. Disadvantages are that national fertility rates do not consider regional differences, educational differences, socioeconomic differences, and religious or ethnic differences. Contraceptive practices in the study group may be different from the national sample. The above-cited limitations can be minimized if an internal comparison group is available. Other types of statistical analyses can also enhance the meaningfulness of the data. Using questionnaires answered solely by men concerning spontaneous abortions or birth defects is more difficult. Problems with such studies are discussed elsewhere in this text.

MAJOR REPRODUCTIVE HAZARDS IN THE WORKPLACE

A 1975 Romanian study showed that male workers exposed to lead have an apparent dose-response decrement in testicular function with decrease in sperm count and motility and change in morphology. A subsequent Swedish study and one in the U.S. have not shown such an effect, although in the latter two studies, the men had lower blood lead levels and there were fewer participants.

Dibromochloropropane (DBCP) is the best example of an agent that is toxic to the male testes. The effects on the testes were seen in men in the absence of effects on other organ systems. Of the first 25 nonvasectomized men evaluated in the initial study in a California pesticide plant, nine were azoospermic, four were oligospermic (two severely), and 12 were normospermic. There was a definite relationship between duration of employment and effect on testicular function among these men. Photomicrographs (Figs 55–1 and 55–2) show a biopsy of a normal testis compared to the biopsy of the testis of a man exposed for ten years to DBCP. In the latter, the only remaining cells within the seminiferous tubules are the Sertoli cells (Figs 55–3 and 55–4).

During 1977–78, there were a total of seven studies done in which men were then currently working with DBCP. Not all of the men in each of the studies were working with DBCP at the time of the study, but the facility or the location was handling DBCP at the time. Of the 440 subjects examined, 75 (17%) were azoospermic and 103 (23%) were oligospermic. One would have anticipated 1% azoospermic and less than 8% oligospermic. Since removal from DBCP, some of the azoospermic and oligospermic men have had improvements in sperm counts into the normospermic range and subsequently fathered children. Others have remained either azoospermic or severely oligospermic.

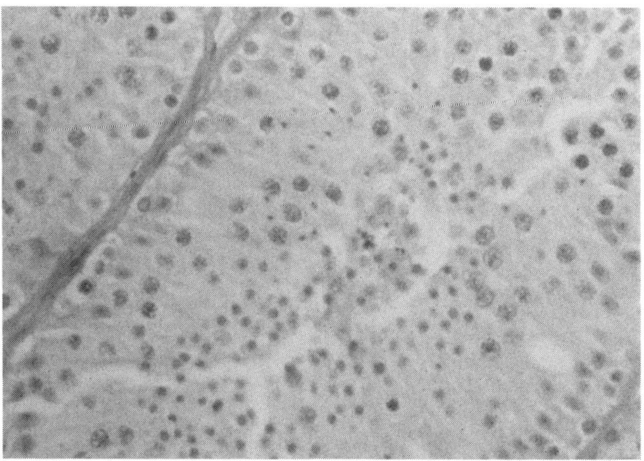

FIG 55–2.
Normal testicular tissue (×400).

On the basis of these findings, DBCP use (but not its manufacture) has been banned by the Environmental Protection Agency in the continental U.S. The temporary use allowed on pineapples in Hawaii has been discontinued. A recent longitudinal study of pineapple workers done over the course of one season has shown that there is no adverse effect on sperm count, if exposure levels are kept within current OSHA limits of 1 ppb.

Pesticides Other Than DBCP

Kepone (chlordecone) has been shown to affect semen quality among individuals who were severely poisoned and had severe neurologic disease. Improvement of the neurologic status also is accompanied by an improvement in semen quality.

Ethylene dibromide (EDB) was studied in two separate studies in 1977. Both studies had problems in definition of exposure and

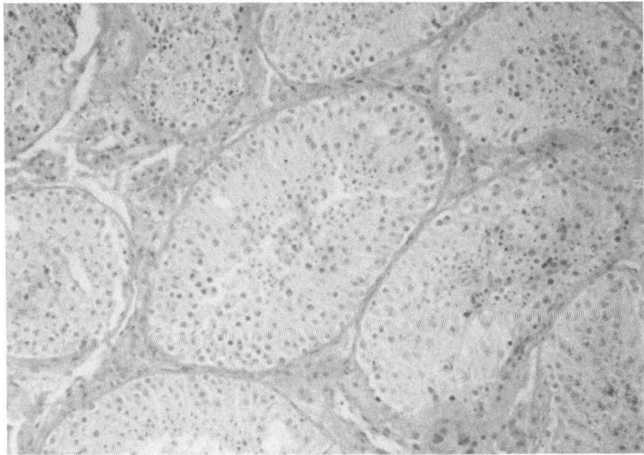

FIG 55–1.
Normal testicular tissue (×100).

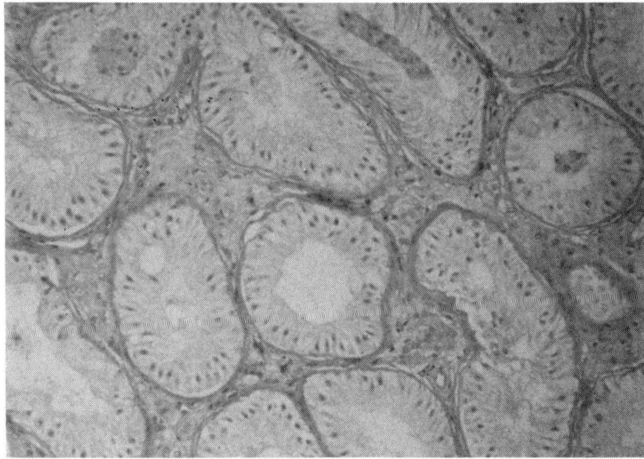

FIG 55–3.
Testicular biopsy from a man with ten years' exposures to DBCP (×100).

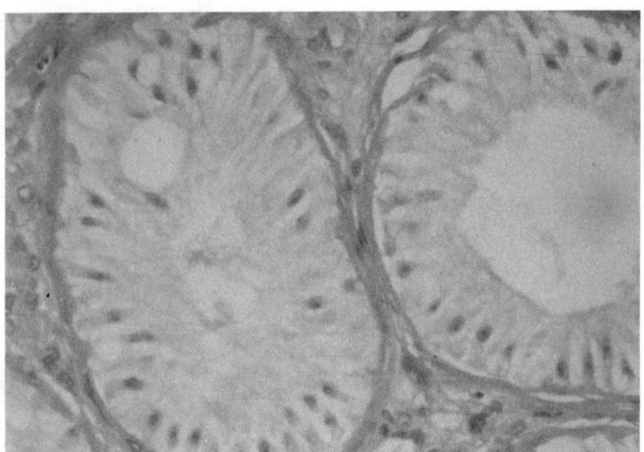

FIG 55–4.
Same patient as in Fig 55–3 (×400).

data analyses. Neither had concurrent controls; however, if compared to the worker data in Table 55–1, both show a mild, statistically significant depression in sperm count. A third positive EDB study has been recently reported on papaya workers.

Other Substances

Ionizing radiation has been well-recognized as being capable of producing severe testicular damage. A European study also implicates microwave radiation in the interference of spermatogenesis. There have been variable reports of decreased sperm count or normal sperm count with toluene diamine and carbon disulfide.

Studies of men exposed to a number of substances studied since 1977 have proven either negative or no-effect. These exposures have included: epichlorohydrin, polybrominated biphenyls, paratertiary butyl benzoic acid, glycerine products, various steroid compounds, glycol ethers, and mercuric oxide. A study of carbaryl was negative for sperm count, but positive in a non-dose-response manner for morphology.

Spontaneous Abortions

One of the difficulties in spontaneous abortion studies is the definition and the lack of medicaliy documented background rates. Estimates of spontaneous abortion rates can range from 15%–40% of all pregnancies. The lower number usually refers to pregnancies in which there was some external observer or objective evidence of pregnancy. The higher number tended to be estimates based on early pregnancies that were never seen by a medical observer. There are several studies which suggest that the male can be the cause of the spontaneous abortion. This would be similar to the dominant lethal effect seen in animals.

An Israeli study of spontaneous abortions seen in pregnancies among married banana workers living in Israel before and after exposure to DBCP showed a threefold increase in spontaneous abortions after DBCP as opposed to before exposure. A study of men exposed in a U.S. petroleum refinery waste water treatment plant showed a two- to threefold increase in relative risk of spontaneous abortions among the wives of selected craft workers. In the latter study, the husbands and wives were interviewed separately, each reporting a different number of spontaneous abortions. Husbands reported 24, while wives reported 27. The data showed agreement on 21 spontaneous abortions. Of the 21, only 3 were reported by the husband and wife as occurring in the same month. The other 18 varied by from 2 to 20 months.

A study in Finland into the incidence of spontaneous abortion in an industrialized community by the use of coded hospital discharge records and census data for occupation showed a threefold increase in risk of spontaneous abortion in women who worked in the textile industry and whose husbands worked in a metallurgical factory, as compared with any other combination of work.

Each of these studies has limitations but is described to show the difference in the types of studies currently being conducted.

Birth Defects

If a mutagenic process occurred during spermatogenesis and that mutant spermatozoan was successful in a conception that went to term, one effect could be an increase in birth defects among the offspring. The only occupational study that suggested such an occurrence was seen among the children born to male anesthesiologists. Paternal exposure to waste anesthetic gases was strongly associated with an increased rate of congenital abnormalities. On the other hand, paternal exposure had no effect on spontaneous abortion rate.

SCREENING TECHNIQUES

Screening methods for occupational reproductive surveillance is an important issue which is as yet unresolved. The criteria for such a method should be data that are simple to obtain, inexpensive, and should lend itself to relatively quick analyses. Information on all employees as to previous reproductive histories—especially number of children—could be obtained by a questionnaire. Medical payment records with coded diagnoses could be obtained and evaluated on a routine basis, as could birth certificates of all new children. Employees could be coded according to job titles or categories, as appropriate to the organization. One could use medical information to analyze for spontaneous abortions, birth weights, birth defects, and live births. If the organization was large enough, one could use internal comparisons rather than using National Center for Health Statistics data. Such a method is far easier than relying on repeated semen analyses for screening, in that such is inappropriate for long-term screening and will also not detect mutagenic effects. Reliance upon hormonal analysis is inadequate, due to the insensitivity of the method and its lack of predictability.

Much research will have to be done in this area of appropriate screening technique in order to develop meaningful and useful surveillance data. The need for other types of studies previously described would then be generated from such surveillance.

REFERENCES

1. Hemminki K, Kyyronen P, Niemi ML: Spontaneous abortions in an industrialized community in Finland. *Am J Public Health* 1983; 73:32–37.

2. Kharrazi M, Potashnik G, Goldsmith JR: Reproductive effects of dibromochloropropane. *Isr J Med Sci* 1980; 10:403–406.
3. Morgan RW, Kheifets L, Whorton MD, et al: Fetal loss and work in a waste water treatment plant. *Am J Public Health* 1984; 74:499–501.
4. Ratcliffe JM, Schrader SM, Steenland K, et al: Semen quality in papaya workers with long-term exposure to ethylene dibromide. *Br J Indust Med* 1987; 44:317–326.
5. Whorton MD: Adverse reproductive outcomes: The occupational health issues of the 1980s. *Am J Public Health* 1983; 73:15–16.
6. Whorton MD: Field studies: Lessons learned. *Teratogenesis Carcinog Mutagen* 1984; 4:25–44.
7. Whorton MD, Meyer CR: Sperm count results from 861 American chemical/agricultural workers from fourteen separate studies. *Fertil Steril* 1984; 42:82–86.
8. Whorton MD, Foliart DE: Mutagenicity, carcinogenicity, and reproductive effects of dibromochloropropane (DBCP). *Mutat Res* 1983; 123:13–30.
9. Whorton MD, Krauss RM, Marshall S, et al: Infertility in male pesticide workers. *Lancet* 1977; 2:1259–1261.
10. Wong O, Morgan RW, Whorton MD: An epidemiologic surveillance program for evaluating occupational reproductive hazards. *Am J Ind Med* 1985; 7(4): 295–306.
11. Wyrobek J, Burkhart G, Francis C, et al: Chemically induced alterations of testicular function in man as measured by semen analysis parameters. *Mutat Res* 1983; 115:73–148.

56

Preplacement Medical Evaluation and Recommendations

Marcus B. Bond, M.D.

Jacqueline Messite, M.D.

The preceding two chapters have provided considerable assurance that men and nonpregnant women do not differ sufficiently in their responses to hazardous substances or conditions in the workplace for the difference to be of major importance in recommendations about job placement. In physical strength, aerobic capacity, and tolerance to hot environments there is a wide range of capabilities in men and women, and there is much overlap. Thus, the "between individual" variations are more important than the "between sex" differences. Except for pregnancy, we believe that there are no medical reasons to make job placement recommendations solely on the basis of the sex of the worker.

NONPREGNANT WOMEN

Medical examinations prior to placement of workers in jobs that can be described as strenuous and/or potentially hazardous are required by many employers. Physicians and employers usually believe that these examinations are effective in determining those candidates whose health or safety might be adversely affected by such jobs. This is a reasonable premise insofar as it pertains to persons with gross abnormalities of structure or functions. The scope of preplacement examinations generally has been adequate to detect significant abnormalities in the special senses (especially vision and hearing), gross abnormalities in the musculoskeletal and nervous systems, such as balance and coordination, symmetry, motor power, and joint motion, the presence of significant organ or systemic disease, and gross abnormalities in mental status.

However, the absence of abnormalities in the history and physical examination in job applicants does not guarantee safe and efficient performance on the job. Other factors influence both of these important elements. In the past decade we have learned that the traditional clinical evaluation is inadequate in predicting safe job performance. Formerly there was a tendency for occupational physicians to recommend against placement of persons with deviations from usual in health status or size. Thus, there was often unfair discrimination against those persons with handicaps or those who were small or large in stature relative to the then-prevalent concepts of what was needed for the job. These facts became apparent after women began working in nontraditional jobs previously performed by men. We learned also after the passage of the Rehabilitation Act of 1973 that many persons who are handicapped can perform safely and efficiently, whereas many of them would not have been recommended for placement in the past.

In one large telecommunications company in the mid 1970s,[11] women were placed in increasing numbers in jobs designed for and previously performed only by men. Many women were successful from the start, but there was a high rate of job injuries and poor performances. An analysis of these problems revealed a need for improved selection and training, plus job modifications, and all three were attempted over a period of a few years.[11] The improved selection process will be described here and was an outgrowth of the development of a series of physical screening tests that were job-related and simple to administer. These screening procedures were validated for an important task that was common to the outside craft jobs (pole climbing). During the initial analysis of the jobs, many physical abilities were tested and found to correlate positively with job success in incumbents. However, for ease in administration, a battery of just three simple tests was adopted, consisting of static arm strength, upright balance, and skin-fold thickness. The tests were conducted by employment personnel and rated objectively. Cut-off scores were established by testing incumbents plus about 100 each of men and women prior to placement in the outside craft jobs, then following their safety and job success over a period of years. Results indicated improved job success (a higher proportion who were successfully performing at one year) and a reduction in injury as compared to those placed prior to the new screening procedures.

Lessons from this experience can be applied in other jobs and other industries. In particular where the job tasks are strenuous, thus requiring persons with above-average physical strength and agility, simple tests can be designed to measure these abilities in job candidates. Initially, the chosen tests must be validated for the particular jobs by testing successful incumbents and by testing a suitable number of persons selected for placement by the new methods. Those in the latter group should be observed over a period of weeks or months and their safety and performance correlated with test results. From these results, a pass/fail set of scores can be determined to assist in selecting those men and women with strength and agility characteristics that lead to safe and satisfactory job performance[4] (Fig 56-1).

Regulations of the U.S. Department of Labor implementing Section 503 of the Rehabilitation Act of 1973 require that any medical examinations or tests that might discriminate against persons who are handicapped, as handicapped is defined under the law, must be job-related. Thus, jobs that involve lifting of objects would be suitable for the development of lifting tests as a preplacement screening technique. Chaffin et al.,[3, 4] after research in this area for several years, working with a number of large employers, reported that the incidence and severity of low-back and other musculoskeletal on-the-job injuries vary directly with maximal weight lifted and with the frequency of lifts. Furthermore, workers with varying lifting requirements have been given static lift strength tests and the results were compared with the actual lifts required on the job. Those whose lift strength test results indicated high lifting strength as compared with lift required on the job had

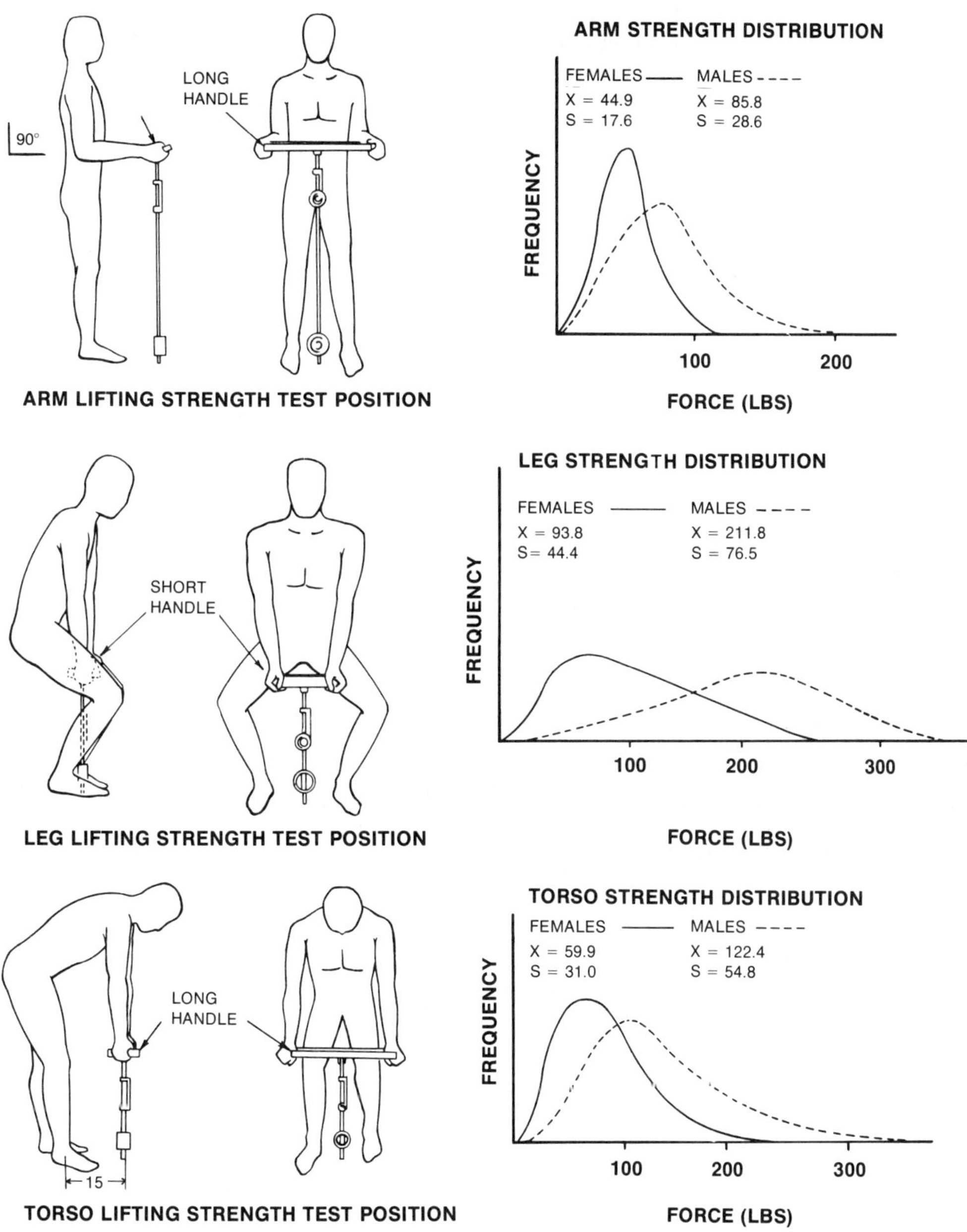

FIG 56–1.
Comparison of male and female performance on strength testing. (Adapted from Chaffin DB, et al: *Pre-employment Strength Testing in Selecting Workers for Material Handling Jobs.* University of Michigan, NIOSH Publ CDC 99–74–62, 1976.)

fewer low-back incidents than those lifting nearer their maximum. Efficiency of job performance and attrition rate were not included as study variables, but it is reasonable to think that those persons lifting at or near their maximal capacity would have less efficient production and higher attrition rates.[10]

The two techniques discussed represent a realistic approach to improving the value of preplacement screening to predict job success and safety. The testing methods apply to individuals rather than to gender and should be related to tasks required in certain jobs. A considerable degree of job analysis is required to obtain measures of lifting and carrying strength, balance, coordination, or other requirements. It is likely that simple tests and measurements will suffice and, likewise, the "person-tests" may also be simple rather than sophisticated measures such as the maximal aerobic capacity discussed earlier. Safe and efficient job performance depends heavily on factors other than strength and agility of the worker.

Job and equipment modification are additional areas that should be explored further to improve the person-machine interface. Too often, work areas and equipment have been designed for persons of average size and, in the past, primarily for men, who traditionally have predominated in the jobs. This offers barriers to persons who vary from these averages and produces artificial and adverse reasons for lack of job success.

In summary, men and nonpregnant women do not differ enough in their response to hazardous substances identified to date to justify medical recommendations for such work exposures based on gender.

PREGNANCY AND JOB PLACEMENT

Physical Stresses

As in the nonpregnant state, women who are pregnant vary greatly in ability to do physically stressful work. Therefore, it is not possible nor even legally correct to make medical recommendations about the amount of lifting, for example, that is acceptable for pregnant women as a group. The *Guidelines on Pregnancy and Work* published in 1977 by the American College of Obstetricians and Gynecologists[1] under a NIOSH contract indicate:

> The normal woman with an uncomplicated pregnancy and a normal fetus in a job that presents no greater potential hazards than those encountered in normal daily life in the community may continue to work without interruption until the onset of labor and may resume working several weeks after an uncomplicated delivery.

There was unanimous agreement among obstetric and occupational medicine representatives who prepared these guidelines on all points in the above statement except in specifying return to work after delivery, and the term "several weeks" (more than two) was chosen as a term that would recognize variations in persons. Many women may not wish to work until the onset of labor. Furthermore, some women may have minor symptoms of backache, fatigue, and/or a feeling of awkwardness, but which are not a threat to safety or health of the woman or her pregnancy and, therefore, would not require a medical recommendation to cease work. Physicians should resist requests of either employers or employees to make recommendations for nonmedical reasons.

Communication is necessary between the occupational physician and the obstetrician, particularly when the pregnancy is abnormal and/or the woman suffers from an abnormality or disease. Each case must be evaluated on the basis of the clinical status and nature of the job.

Medical recommendations about pregnant women in jobs that are strenuous require careful individualization. Strength and fitness of the individual must be considered, particularly as they relate to the proportion of maximal capacity required by the job. Pregnancy does use a portion of the reserve capacity in the cardiovascular and respiratory systems, and this must enter into clinical judgment.

Special consideration must be given to physical hazards inherent in the job. This includes working at heights (ladders, platforms, poles) and the operation of certain types of heavy equipment and machines in which an accident likely would cause serious damage to the woman and to the fetus, particularly after the uterus has enlarged out of the pelvis. Beginning about midpregnancy, posture becomes slightly distorted, and this distortion increases to term due to the increased spinal curvatures to accommodate the protruding abdomen. This may cause a potential hazard in jobs requiring frequent rapid movements of both upper and lower extremities and well-coordinated agility. The problem is compounded if the surface for footing is unsteady or slippery. Such jobs as airline flight attendants, some waitress jobs, certain factory work, and certain construction jobs have these characteristics. Many pregnant women may be uncomfortable in such jobs beyond about midterm, but each pregnant woman must be individually evaluated as to her condition and the particular job. Frequent reevaluation by the occupational physician or nurse and the obstetrician will assist women wanting to work as long as is safely possible during their pregnancy. In some jobs that are particularly strenuous or hazardous, both obstetricians and occupational physicians may agree that some women should not work beyond the first trimester in their regular jobs. Nonmedical factors also may intervene and require a change in jobs or cessation of work during pregnancy if work efficiency declines below that considered acceptable due to a combination of minor symptoms that are not truly harmful or dangerous to the woman. Transportation to and from the job, home responsibilities, and social activities are factors to be considered also.

Hazardous Substances or Conditions in the Workplace

Toxicology of the reproductive process is discussed in detail in Chapter 54. Discussion here will include only medical preplacement recommendations with respect to the embryo or fetus for women who are pregnant or who are fertile.

A dilemma exists with both medical and societal aspects in regard to undiagnosed pregnancy. Since neither the woman nor anyone else can know of the existence of pregnancy until at least several days and usually a few weeks postconception, harm to the fertilized ovum or embryo could occur from work exposures that are considered safe for the nonpregnant worker. The question that logically follows is: Are there work exposures considered acceptable for the nonpregnant woman but from which the risks of harm to the embryo are so great as to make it wise to forbid the woman of childbearing capacity to experience them? Certainly this is more than just a medical question. But it is a medical responsibility to define the risks and make recommendations based on the best scientific knowledge available. If the latter is inadequate, dependence on the informed opinion of a knowledgeable physician would be required. The "opinion" becomes increasingly important when it is realized that we do not have adequate information on the teratogenicity or fetotoxicity in humans of many substances that may be in the work environment. To a certain extent, this situation perhaps always will be with us because of new substances being introduced daily plus the difficult problem of determining whether a particular agent actually causes fetal damage. Even under existing laws and regulations (Toxic Substances Control Act, Occupational Safety and Health Act and others), we do not have assurance that required testing and surveillance will reveal information on potential harm to the embryo or fetus. Rather than conceding defeat by these discouraging words, it is suggested that the only responsible way to proceed is by more and better epidemiologic studies on humans and by cautious extrapolation from animal research. In 1974, Hernberg,[6] the scientific director of the Institute of Occupational Health in Helsinki, Finland, was one of the first investigators to address in a positive fashion the problems of women of reproductive age employed in lead industries. Gordon[5] has discussed this subject on the basis of long experience in a large chemical firm, and Lerner[8] has discussed the specific problems with lead.

For the woman who is pregnant or planning pregnancy, exposures to substances or conditions known or highly suspected to cause fetal malformations, abortions, fetal toxicity, or transplacental carcinogenesis should not be recommended unless the exposure level is known to be or can be assumed to be below the recommended standards and that such standards take into consideration the reproductive effects. Karrh, of the du Pont Company, and several representatives of other major chemical companies have presented a thorough analysis and recommendations about the risks and control of embryo-fetotoxins.[7] Dose-response data are not always known or, more frequently, the data are inconclusive, particularly as to what the threshold dose for fetal harm is. For example, the NCRP Report 53[9] recently reviewed the data on ionizing radiation and potential harm to the embryo or fetus and reaffirmed the recommended permissible total dose to the fetus of 0.5 rem, as had been provided in Report 39 in 1971. Since photon energy and dose rate are important in ionizing radiation, the Council pointed out in 1971 that if a woman were exposed to a rather steady amount of radiation within the permitted nonpregnant adult exposures of 1.25 rem per quarter, considering the intrauterine exposure to be attenuated by maternal tissues, a fetus would not receive more than 0.5 rem by the time pregnancy is diagnosed. At this time, a detailed assessment can be made of the probable dose to the fetus and exposure should be kept within 0.5 rem. Medical x-ray should be included, if known, in the calculation.

There are many data on ionizing radiation, but much less on many chemical substances known or suspected to be teratogens, abortifacients, fetotoxins, or transplacental carcinogens. Therefore, it is essential that the occupational physician keep abreast of all the pertinent toxicologic information on the exposure as it relates to pregnancy and obtain detailed information about the nature and degree of exposure associated with the particular operation(s) in question. At times, particularly where sporadic high and unanticipated exposures may occur even with good general control, it may be prudent to recommend that women who are pregnant or planning a pregnancy not be subjected to such risks to their embryos and fetuses.

For women who are not pregnant and not planning a pregnancy, but are of childbearing capacity, there is no real consensus about work exposures among those interested or even among well-informed physicians. There appear to be at least two alternatives that could be followed. One is to consider the woman capable of childbearing in the same group just discussed, viz., the pregnant or likely to be soon, and exclude them from exposure to teratogens or fetotoxins. Certainly this would be considered the safest practice to many of those concerned, including employer or legal representatives. At least a few employers have had this practice in effect with lead exposures, for example, and fertile women are forbidden in lead areas. Similar practices are in effect by many employers with substances known or suspected to be harmful to the fetus. On the other hand, in the health care and research areas, such practices are not routine, even though most laboratory and x-ray technicians and operating room personnel are women and there are potential hazards to the fetus from biologic agents, chemicals, and radiation.

Such exclusionary practices are not considered reasonable by many persons for one or more of the following reasons:

1. A large number of productive employees would be excluded from jobs.

2. This practice probably is a violation of EEOC Regulations.

3. No similar consideration is made for male workers whose reproductive function may be impaired and who may be subject to mutagenic damage to sperm from certain exposures.

4. Such exclusions are not considered in traditionally female jobs in the health industry, such as operating room personnel, nurses, and x-ray and laboratory technicians.

Therefore, an alternative is needed, and one such alternative is to make *individual* medical evaluations of the risks present, using medical judgment when precise information is not available.

Employee education is essential for all women who are or may be exposed to substances or conditions that may harm the fetus. It applies equally to women who are pregnant or who are capable of being pregnant. Information must be provided to such women in order that they may participate in decisions about when and where they work. The "right-to-know" laws in states and other jurisdictions require employers to furnish such information to employees on request. To the extent possible, information should be quantified by describing the relative toxicity of the substances or conditions concerned and to what extent they are present in the workplace, i.e., regularly, irregularly or only potentially, and at what levels relative to known effects. For example, a hazardous chemical might be present only at intervals of a week or a month and for only a few minutes or hours each time as associated with maintenance or cleanup operations. Also, a process might be completely enclosed but, with certain accidental conditions, the material could be released into the workplace, causing unavoidable exposure. Of course, the levels of potentially hazardous substances or conditions present must be known by adequate surveys and measurements and related to existing standards. With the quantitative information and a consideration of the relative toxicity of the materials, employees can be advised with reasonable confidence of the exposures and risks associated with a particular job.

The other variable of importance is the likelihood of pregnancy in a woman capable of becoming but not planning to be pregnant soon. The employee must be fully informed as described and then must be completely straightforward with the occupational physician or nurse. These conditions are necessary for frank discussion between the employee, who should be satisfied that she is not subjecting her fetus to an unusual risk, and a physician who has enough information about the employee as well as the exposures in order to make a recommendation about placement. Ultimately it is the employer who must make a decision about placement, but the physician's recommendations generally will be followed. However, in the alternative just described, the employer's legal advice may not agree with a medical recommendation to permit a fertile woman to work in an environment that is potentially hazardous to the fetus. However, provisions of EEOC Regulations and of Title VII of the Civil Rights Act may forbid such work restrictions. Reconciling such conflicting pressures is beyond the scope of this discussion. The fetus is in the workplace involuntarily and may have legal rights to sue an employer or even the mother for alleged damages during gestation.

To summarize, there may be times when women who are or expect to become pregnant soon should not be recommended for work where there are significant exposures to substances known to be or seriously considered to be abortifacients, teratogens, fetotoxins, or transplacental carcinogens. The decision to label a substance or condition as having these deleterious qualities is more difficult than deciding what to recommend once a label has been chosen.

For women not pregnant nor expecting to be soon but capable of pregnancy, the safest recommendation would be to prohibit such exposures. This is not acceptable to many in our society. A suggested alternative is to do individual medical evaluations on women subject to such exposures. An informed woman can make a judgment of the risks and decide whether or not she wishes to work at that job. But if she decides to work at that job, the physician must advise both the employee and the employer of the risks based on a medical evaluation of that individual, her pregnancy, and the particular job.

Whether a woman should be able to choose a high risk to the fetus is not really a medical question. Although it is the employer who finally must decide when a person will be placed at a particular job, it is the job of the occupational physician to adequately and properly inform both the employer and the employee of the risks involved.

REFERENCES

1. American College of Obstetricians and Gynecologists: *Guidelines on Pregnancy and Work,* NIOSH Contract 210–76–0159, 1977.
2. Bond MB: Role of corporate policy in the control of reproductive hazards in the workplace. *J Occup Med* 1986; 3:193.
3. Chaffin DB, et al: *Pre-employment Strength Testing in Selecting Workers for Material Handling Jobs*. University of Michigan, NIOSH Publ CDC 99–74–62, 1976.
4. Chaffin DB, Herrin GD, Keyserling WM: Pre-employment strength testing. *J Occup Med* 1978; 20:403.
5. Gordon HL: Placement of workers in high risk areas. *Proceedings of Conference on Women and the Workplace*. Society for Occupational and Environmental Health, 1976.
6. Hernberg S: Lead, in Zenz C (ed): *Occupational Medicine: Principles and Practical Applications*. Chicago, Year Book Medical Publishers, 1975, p 749.
7. Karrh BW, Carmody TW, Clyne RM, et al: Guidance for the evaluation, risk assessment, and control of chemical embryo-fetotoxins. *J Occup Med* 1979; 23:297–399.
8. Lerner S: Job placement of workers in the lead trades. *Proceedings of Conference on Women and the Workplace*. Society for Occupational and Environmental Health, 1976.
9. National Council on Radiation Protection and Measurements: *Radiation Dose Limits for Embryo and Fetus in Occupationally Exposed Women,* NCRP Report 53, 1977.
10. National Institute for Safety and Health: *Work Practices Guide to Manual Lifting,* NIOSH Technical Report 81-122. Cincinnati, Oh, Dept of Health and Human Services, NIOSH, 1981.
11. Reilly RR, Zedeck S, Tenopyr M: Validity and fairness of physical ability tests for predicting performance in craft jobs. *J Appl Psychol* 1979; 64:262–274.

57

Occupational Medical Considerations in the Aviation Industry*

Robert T. P. deTreville, M.D., Sc.D.

It has been estimated that the annual number of air passengers increased from 20 million in 1960 to nearly 900 million in 1984 on regularly scheduled flights (figures exclude charter flight passengers). A commercial plane lands now about every 10 seconds throughout the world. These figures do not take into account worldwide aerospace military activities, and imply that there is an enormous group of workers sustaining this complex and ceaseless working (transport) system. This chapter describes major aspects that are of consequence to the aviation and aerospace industries, discussing the relationship of occupational medicine to environmental medicine in general and providing a framework within which the occupational physician can apply occupational health principles to aerospace workers.

Aerospace medicine was recognized as a subspecialty within the field of preventive medicine in 1953. The first examinations were given by the American Board of Preventive Medicine in 1955; to date, approximately 860 physicians have been certified. The specialty of aerospace medicine was accredited and became the second subspecialty area under the American Board of Preventive Medicine (two years later, the subspecialty of occupational medicine was recognized by the Board).

Aerospace medicine deals with the medical aspects of the "normal" and "abnormal" environments, defining man's tolerance necessary for survival and ability to cope with responses to levels of stress outside the "normal microclimate." Table 57–1 lists some of the stresses and outlines some of the risks from abnormal exposures to those factors.

It has been said that flying is not inherently dangerous but that, like the sea, the air is terribly unforgiving of carelessness. The task of piloting a complex aircraft is one that, under some circumstances, demands a high level of concentration, mental integration and psychomotor skill. Pilots whose ability to perform is degraded by disease, emotional problems, drugs, fatigue or unusual physical stress are ill equipped to deal with their tasks in flight. Since World War I, physicians have recognized that illness and other problems, whether incurred on or off the job, can have disastrous consequences in flight. This recognition has led to a tradition of comprehensive care of flying personnel, which is at variance with the generally accepted tradition in occupational medicine of caring for the worker only on the job and relying on family physicians for nonoccupational health care. Because of the nature of the tasks and the environment, the practice of aerospace medicine requires knowledge in several areas of only peripheral concern to occupational physicians in other industries. Human factors in cockpit and workspace design, physiologic tolerance criteria, environmental control systems, performance psychology, selection and training, personal protective equipment and emergency escape and survival are among the areas in which the specialist flight surgeon must have knowledge if he is to fulfill his primary aim of preventing disease, injury and disability in his flying personnel.

*With admiration and great appreciation to Charles E. Billings, M.D., who set forth the principles in this chapter in 1975, a first in an occupational medical textbook. Thanks to his knowledgeable, thorough groundwork, only a few changes and additions have been made.

THE AEROSPACE ENVIRONMENT

The history of aviation is short; it was a little more than 200 years ago that man first left earth in a hot-air balloon (1783), only 80 years since the first manned flights in a heavier-than-air vehicle. During this period, progress has been measured in terms of increasing air speed, altitude, duration of flight and loads lifted.

Although speed as such has no known physiologic effect, the accelerations involved in reaching high speeds do have profound consequences. Increasing altitude involves decreases in both barometric pressure and, concomitantly, the partial pressure of oxygen in the air. Recently, the attainment of orbital velocity has brought with it periods of prolonged weightlessness. All of these pose psychologic and physiologic problems to which man must adapt, or which he must avoid, if he is to survive.

A detailed description of these and the other stresses to which man is exposed in aerial and space flight is beyond the scope of this chapter (see General References), but a brief discussion of the stresses involved in aviation is necessary for understanding of the environment in which the pilot, crew member or passenger must function while in flight.

TABLE 57–1.
The Physical Environment of Man

STRESSOR	PHYSIOPATHOLOGIC EFFECTS OF: INSUFFICIENT LEVELS	OVEREXPOSURE
The gaseous environment		
Barometric pressure	Ebullism, hypoxia	?Hypoventilation
Changes in pressure	Decompression sickness, dysbarism	Dysbarism, squeeze, blast injury
Oxygen	Hypoxia	Oxygen toxicity
Nitrogen	Atelectasis, ?developmental abnormalities	Nitrogen narcosis (toxicity)
Other inert gases	None known	Narcosis, vocal effects (He and H_2)
Electromagnetic environment	(See Chapters 26 and 27)	
Magnetism	None definite	?Growth abnormalities
Electricity	None known	Electric shock
Radio and microwave	None known	Tissue heating
Infrared	Cold stress and injury	Heat stress and injury
Light	Developmental abnormalities in CNS	Retinal and other burns
Ultraviolet	Vitamin D deficiency	Skin cancer
Ionizing radiation	None known	Mutations, cancer, radiation sickness
Kinetic environment		
Linear accelerations	Effects of weightlessness	Circulatory effects, immobility, impact injury
Angular accelerations	None known	Motion sickness, disorientation
Vibration	None definite	Physical injury to tissue
Sound	?Sensory deprivation	Hearing loss, otic trauma
Ultrasonic vibration	None known	Tissue heating, disruption
Infrasound		Nausea, increased reaction time, balance disturbance[22, 43]

Whenever an airplane leaves the earth's surface, its environment is altered. Barometric pressure declines as a geometric function of altitude, decreasing by about one half with each 5,500 m of ascent. Since the composition of the atmosphere is nearly uniform below 15,000 m, the partial pressure of oxygen in the atmosphere likewise decreases by one half with each 5,500 m of ascent. Finally, ambient air temperature drops in approximately linear fashion with increasing altitude; the lapse rate is approximately 2° C per 300 m in the troposphere, although vertical mixing at low altitudes can produce departures from this general rule.

Nearly all reciprocating engine aircraft flying today are capable of attaining altitudes well above 3,000 m. Many, equipped with superchargers, fly well at altitudes up to 7,500–9,000 m. Very few of these airplanes are pressurized; their occupants therefore must function at the pressure altitude at which the airplane is flying. Turbo-propeller-driven aircraft are most efficient in the range of altitudes between 4,000 and 9,000 m; nearly all of these are pressurized (the cabin pressure altitude is substantially lower than airplane altitude). Turbojet aircraft in current use have service ceilings between 11,000 and 15,000 m; virtually all are pressurized to maintain cabin altitudes no higher than 2,500 m when carrying passengers. Finally, spacecraft fly at altitudes above virtually all of the earth's atmosphere. Both pressure cabins and, for emergency use and extravehicular activity, pressure suits are provided to keep their occupants within tolerable pressure limits.

Oxygen

Although the upper limits of human tolerance for barometric pressure are not known, lower limits can be specified. The ultimate limit is the pressure at which water at body temperature vaporizes; this is the phenomenon of ebullism. This pressure is about 63 mb, which corresponds to an altitude of about 19,300 m. Since the alveoli can contain only water vapor at this pressure, substantially higher pressures are required if normal alveolar tensions of oxygen and carbon dioxide are to be maintained:

Water vapor	63 mb (47 mm Hg)	
Oxygen	134 mb (100 mm Hg)	
Carbon dioxide	53 mb (40 mm Hg)	
	250 mb (187 mm Hg)	= 10,400 m

if one is breathing 100% oxygen. Obviously, any nitrogen in the breathing mixture will require higher pressures if this alveolar composition is to be maintained.

The shape of the oxyhemoglobin dissociation curve allows humans a considerable degree of latitude with respect to alveolar oxygen tension and therefore arterial oxygen tension (Fig 57–1). Hemoglobin saturation drops off only slightly at oxygen tensions as low as 65–80 mb. Thus, at altitudes between sea level and 3,300–3,600 m, healthy persons can function for long periods with mini-

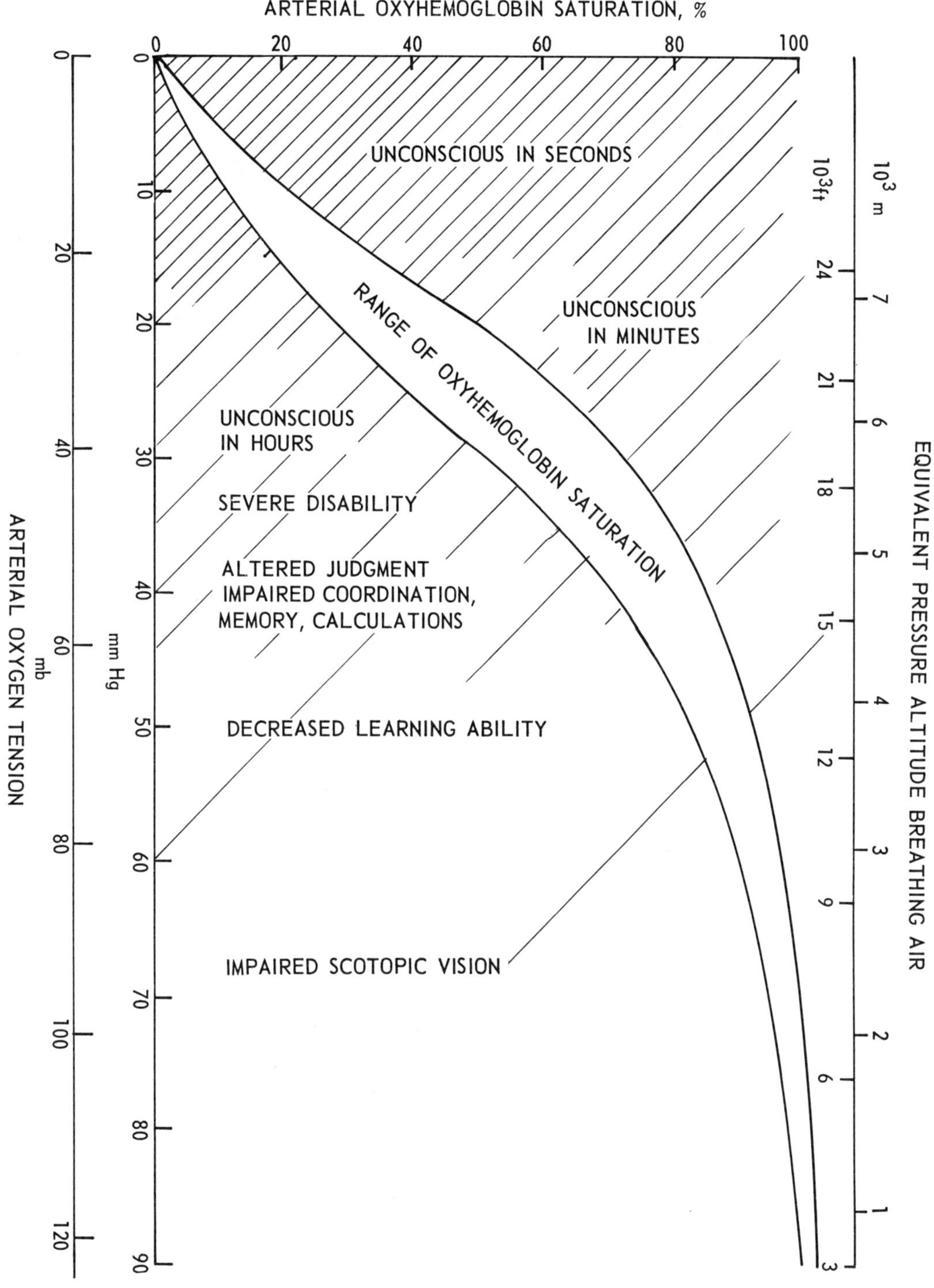

FIG 57 1.
Oxyhemoglobulin dissociation curve.

mal impairment of efficiency unless hard physical work is performed. This is true, of course, only if the entire oxygen uptake pathway from air to tissues is intact. If any part of the pathway is impaired, altitude tolerance is reduced.[9]

To provide some margin of safety for the elderly and the ill and to allow for normal human variability, virtually all transport aircraft now in service fly at altitudes such that cabin altitude does not normally exceed 2,500 m—an altitude that even moderately hypoxic patients usually can tolerate.[29] Newer wide-body jet aircraft rarely exceed 2,000 m cabin altitude.[30]

Changes in Barometric Pressure

Although man is capable of survival and productive existence at a wide range of barometric pressures, the effects of changes in barometric pressure must be considered, for such changes are responsible for the majority of clinical problems in aviation medicine. Modern jet aircraft are able to climb at rates well over 1,000 m/min; some fighters have climb rates over 7,000 m/min. Descent rates may approach 3,000 m/min.

Whenever barometric pressure on a quantity of gas decreases, its volume increases. If it is confined within a rigid container, a differential pressure is exerted across the walls of the container. The middle ear, paranasal sinuses, the lungs and the intestinal tract of man all contain air or other gases. Therefore, all will be affected by changes in pressure.

The lungs do not ordinarily represent a problem unless the rate of change of pressure is extremely rapid, because they normally are in free communication with the atmosphere. During rapid decompression of a small aircraft cabin or cockpit, however, it is possible for differential pressures to be built up across the chest wall.[9]

The intestinal tract normally contains only small amounts of gas, and presents a problem infrequently because if the gas expands enough to stimulate peristalsis, the gas usually is transported to an orifice where it can be expelled as flatus or by belching. Persons with malabsorption syndromes or hypomotile gut disorders may have substantially more trouble at moderate altitudes.

Ordinarily, the expansion of trapped gas causes trouble in two areas—the middle ear and the paranasal sinuses. The ears rarely are a problem during ascent; the architecture of the eustachian tube mucosa and orifice favors passage of gas from the ear to the nasopharynx (Fig 57–2). During descent, however, the return of gas to the middle ear does not proceed passively. As differential pressure across the eardrum increases, it may become difficult or impossible to ventilate the ear by voluntary action. Simultaneously, the relative negative pressure within the middle ear causes transudation of serous or serosanguineous fluid into the cavity. The result is the condition called *barotitis*. The condition is more common in persons whose nasal mucous membranes are swollen because of an upper respiratory infection or allergic rhinitis, although some people have considerable difficulty "clearing" or ventilating their ears even in the absence of these conditions (Table 57–2).

Sinus pain and trauma may also result from relative overpressures during ascent (if the sinus ostia are blocked by polyps or mucosal hypertrophy) or underpressures during descent if the nasal ends of the ostia are blocked. The pain produced under these circumstances may be incapacitating. Prevention and treatment of these conditions are discussed later.

Temperature Changes

As aircraft have become more sophisticated, problems due to decreased barometric pressure by environmental modification have been solved by the provision of pressure cabins. Similarly, attempts to bypass problems due to declining temperatures at altitude by providing aircraft with efficient air heaters and by insulating cabin walls have been made. Prior to pressurization, low temperatures were an almost overwhelming problem in some military aircraft. The discomfort of a waist gunner in a B-17 buffeted by windblast, chilled by temperatures of −40° C and threatened by hypoxia due to freezing of his oxygen mask valves was excruciating.

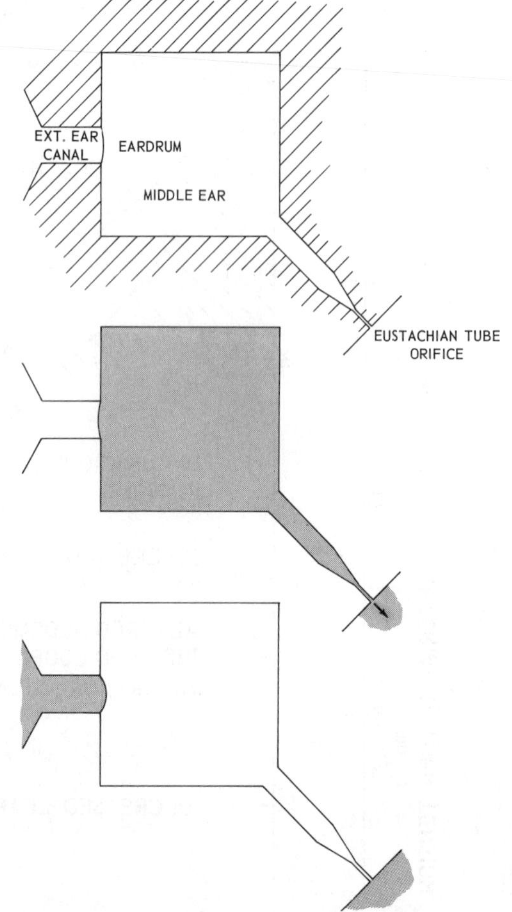

FIG 57–2.
Schematic of middle ear showing rigid structure except at semiflexible eardrum. *Center,* during ascent. *Bottom,* during descent. (See text for details.)

Cold rarely is a serious problem in flight at this time except in utility aircraft, which may have little or no insulation; in such an airplane, even though cabin air is heated, conductive and radiative heat loss to the cabin walls, floor and windows may impede human performance severely. This problem is especially severe in helicopters during winter and in all types of utility aircraft operating in arctic regions whose economy depends on air transportation.

An equally serious environmental problem in some settings may be heat, especially in military aircraft and helicopters in the tropics or desert. Visible radiation from the sun enters these aircraft through their large canopies; metal objects absorb, then reradiate this energy at longer wavelengths in the infrared portion of the spectrum to which plexiglass is opaque. This "greenhouse effect" can result in quite intolerable cockpit temperatures, causing

TABLE 57–2.
Ear Complaints Encountered During Changes in Pressure*

ASCENT (MB)	ASCENT (MM HG)	COMPLAINT	DESCENT (MB)	DESCENT (MM HG)
0	0	No sensation; hearing is normal (level flight)	0	0
4–7	3–5	Feeling of fullness in ears	4–7	3–5
13–20	10–15	More fullness, decreased sound intensity	13–20	10–15
20–40	15–30	Fullness, discomfort, tinnitus; ears usually "pop" as air leaves middle ear; desire to clear ears; if this is done, symptoms stop immediately	20–40	15–30
40+	30+	Increasing pain, tinnitus, dizziness	40–80	30–60
		Severe, radiating pain, dizziness, nausea	80–110	60–80
		Voluntary clearing difficult or impossible	130	100
		Eardrum may rupture	270	200

*Modified from Adler HF: Dysbarism. USAF SAM Review 1–64, USAF School of Aerospace Medicine, Brooks Air Force Base, Texas, 1964.
Note: During ascent, the pressure in the middle ear is greater than ambient; during descent, middle ear pressure is less than ambient.

intense crew discomfort, particularly during preflight procedures and during takeoff. These problems can be alleviated by air conditioning, but the expense and complexity of aircraft and ground systems sometimes result in less than adequate cooling for both crew and passengers.

Accelerations

Aircraft in flight enjoy freedom of motion in all three spatial axes. Accelerations, both linear and angular, are imposed on crews and passengers alike. Airline aircraft ordinarily are flown in a manner that minimizes such accelerations except during takeoff and landing. In turbulence, however, substantial linear accelerations may be imposed on the aircraft. In military aircraft, significant angular accelerations may occur also. These accelerations have a number of physiologic and psychologic effects.

When a vehicle is suddenly accelerated in rough air, an unrestrained object may become a projectile. Unrestrained passengers may also become, for short periods, free-floating objects. Serious injuries, including fractures, may be caused by the inevitable impacts.[41]

A series of such accelerations, frequently encountered in cumulus clouds or in clear-air turbulence, presents a variety of conflicting sensory stimuli to the occupants of an aircraft. The constellation of symptoms produced is called motion or air sickness; it may be a difficult and even intractable problem for some who must travel by air. There are both visual and psychologic contributions to this condition in addition to the vestibular stimuli.[47]

More important, combinations of linear and angular accelerations give rise to spurious sensations that can lead to spatial disorientation. These false sensations are not particularly troublesome if there are clear and unambiguous visual cues to spatial attitude, but in the absence of such cues, they can be catastrophic, for false cues may lead the pilot to take inappropriate corrective actions, which in turn may worsen his situation.[47]

Modern aircraft are both fast and heavy, and thus possess considerable momentum, which must be dissipated during landing. Although accident prevention is of primary concern in aviation medicine, another factor of great importance is crash survivability—the "packaging" of crew and passengers to maximize protection in the event of an aircraft accident.[41]

Noise

Although the advent of the large jet aircraft in the 1950s led to substantially lower cockpit sound levels, sound levels in earlier reciprocating engine transports had been substantially above presently accepted damage risk criteria. The sound levels in today's general aviation aircraft, helicopters and some turboprop aircraft remain above acceptable levels for occupational exposure.[42, 44, 48] Ambient noise levels around aircraft during ground operations pose a serious hazard for ground support personnel. Chapter 20 deals with noise and hearing conservation.

Other Environmental Stresses

Although nearly all civil (and military) flying still is done at altitudes below 15,000 m, some reconnaissance and special-purpose aircraft, a number of research aircraft and, more recently, supersonic transport aircraft are designed to operate in the 15,000–30,000 m altitude range. At these extreme altitudes, three additional environmental factors must be considered. Each poses a potential problem of some magnitude.

At very high altitudes, the radiation screening effect of the atmosphere is much less than at sea level. Levels of solar and cosmic ionizing radiation are substantially higher; at times of high solar flare activity, appreciable doses of ionizing radiation may be received. It is not expected that even the highest doses would present a somatic hazard; nonetheless, doses above maximal permissible levels could be received by crew members.[12, 30]

Above 15,000 m, increasing concentrations of ozone are found in the atmosphere due to the interaction of ultraviolet radiation with molecular oxygen. The concentrations at 20,000–25,000 m are well above threshold limit values for this substance.[8] Fortunately, heat and certain catalysts rapidly destroy ozone; catalytic filters in supersonic aircraft, together with heating of air during compression for use in pressurized cabins, will eliminate ozone toxicity as a hazard. (See Chapter 47.)

Nearly all aircraft that operate at very high altitudes also fly at high speeds—speeds at which frictional heating of the aircraft's metal skin is considerable. At mach 3 (three times the speed of sound), skin temperatures can reach 300° C. Cabin inner walls must be effectively isolated from fuselage outer walls and cooled by forced draft or transpiration ventilation. In spacecraft, radiant heat inputs are considerable during orbital flight; frictional heating during reentry requires the use of ablative coatings.[24]

WORK POPULATIONS SERVED BY AEROSPACE MEDICINE

Aerospace medical practitioners must meet the needs of several populations over which they exert varying degrees of control. Perhaps the most tightly controlled group is the astronaut corps, a small, highly selected group. Although even this select group is not free from known disease, it has been subjected to a searching selection process, a wide variety of psychophysiologic stress tests and to careful continuing medical surveillance.

Military pilots and other aircrewmen, numbering several thousand, are screened less extensively, but they usually are cared for on a continuing basis by flight surgeons who may tend to their medical needs (and often those of their families) and thus come to know them intimately as patients and as people.

The medical selection and surveillance of the roughly 30,000 air carrier pilots varies widely among airlines in the United States. Some of the largest carriers have extensive medical departments, see all flying personnel regularly and are available for consultation at any time. A few other carriers have smaller full- or part-time medical departments, but most of the smaller carriers have little or no direct aeromedical support. In these cases, medical selection and periodic surveillance of aircrew is limited to that required by law and is accomplished by aviation medical examiners designated by the Federal Aviation Administration's Office of Aviation Medicine.

Cabin crewmembers (pursers, stewards and stewardesses) are not required by law to undergo periodic medical evaluations. Most carriers require preemployment examinations; some either require or make available periodic examinations. The turnover in this population is high during the first years of employment, although this pattern has changed somewhat as a result of federal legislation barring discrimination on the basis of age, marital status and sex. The last prohibition has led to an influx of males to this formerly female population, and there are likely to be larger numbers of older cabin staff in the future.

Air traffic controllers are employees of the Federal Aviation Administration (FAA), with the exception of a handful of personnel employed in municipal or privately owned control towers. Nearly all of our 25,000 controllers are required to undergo medical examination and recertification annually by designated aviation medical examiners. Most are covered by a somewhat more complete medical surveillance program instituted in 1969 by the FAA. A substantial fraction of the group, employed in air route traffic control centers, is now attended by FAA flight surgeons; the agency's aim is to have a medical facility in or adjacent to each of its 27 centers in the continental United States in the immediate future.

As was noted above, airline medical coverage is far from complete. Thus, the coverage of airline ground support personnel is, at best, spotty. The majority of airport operators and corporate aviation departments in this country have no medical coverage whatsoever.

More than 450,000,000 passengers travel by air in the United States each year. Although large airlines frequently receive calls from physicians regarding transportation of seriously ill patients, the majority of the passenger population represents a physiopathologic unknown. It is probable that comparatively few airline passengers have any substantial difficulty during flight. There are specific conditions, however, in which flight, even in pressurized aircraft, poses a distinct hazard. These are discussed by Ellingson[16] and in committee reports.[29, 40]

THE NATURE AND DEMANDS OF THE JOBS

In any complex man-machine system, the nature of the interaction between man and machine must be known before the effects of the machine and environment on man can be evaluated. In aviation, a man, or a crew of several men, is required to perform a number of tasks of variable complexity in a physical environment that can affect both the machine and the man, and in an operational environment that likewise can have profound effects on the task.

The job of the astronaut perhaps is the most demanding in the aviation system. A third-generation space vehicle is an enormously complex closed ecologic system. Particularly during recent long-duration space missions, it has been necessary for astronauts to control their vehicles, monitor their guidance, navigation and orientation and manage numerous other systems. They have also had to have the knowledge to repair them, to conduct experiments and to observe and describe intelligently vehicle performance and the new environments they have encountered, as well as their own physiologic responses. This is asking a good deal; selection and training requirements for astronauts have been extremely rigid, and every man has had to fulfill many functions. It is likely that in future space flights astronauts will be either pilots, responsible for the safe conduct of the flight, or "payload specialists," responsible for the engineering and scientific experiments and tasks for which the flight is conducted. In our early space missions, we have not been able to afford that luxury.

Large military aircraft have been designed around the "pilot and payload or mission specialist" concept for many years. Although we still build single-man fighter aircraft in which the pilot is both, the increasing sophistication of modern weapons systems has increased the requirement for specialization in the cockpit. It must be realized, however, that most military airplanes are devices for inflight delivery of weapons or some other payload, often in the face of hostile action, as well as transportation of these payloads. They are utility airplanes rather than vehicles simply for the transportation of passengers or cargo. The trend toward cockpit specialization has not been reflected in civil aviation.

After World War II, when large four-engine transport aircraft began to replace the prewar airplanes in the civil fleet, a new specialty, that of flight engineer, was created. These aircraft—the Douglas DC-6 and DC-7, the Lockheed Constellation series and the Boeing Stratocruisers—had large, complicated and temperamental engines that required careful handling and close monitoring for reliable performance. By regulation, all aircraft with gross weights over 30,000 kg were required to carry engineers. For overwater flights, a navigator and, in some cases, a radio operator were added.

When jet aircraft entered civil service in the United States in 1958, it became obvious that the new engines were far simpler to operate. The jets continued to have complex environmental control and other systems, but the engineer's job became more that of a systems monitor—a task more like that of the pilots, who were themselves becoming systems managers and monitors in these highly sophisticated, highly automated aircraft. There ensued a long, acrimonious jurisdictional struggle that ended in the pilots' favor. Where three-man crews still are required, all are pilots; the second officer performs flight engineer and certain other duties. Radio operators and navigators have been eliminated, for the most part, by sophisticated electronic systems.

The task of flying is a complex one. Its metabolic demands are low, rarely requiring an oxygen consumption more than twice resting levels. Its intellectual requirements are considerably higher and include excellent short- and long-term memory, the capacity to integrate many sensory inputs into a coordinated concept of spatial orientation and position, the ability to "think ahead of the airplane" and the ability to make decisions based on a great many contingencies. A moderate level of psychomotor skill is required, as is the ability to react appropriately—although not usually with lightning speed—in emergencies.[3]

Transport flying has been described as "hours of utter boredom, punctuated by moments of utter panic." The first part of this certainly is true; a high level of tolerance for monotony and the ability to maintain one's vigilance during long, boring flights is an absolute requirement.

The air traffic control system—the operational environment within which all aircraft operate—has also undergone profound changes in the past 30 years, although its subsystems are less highly automated than those of the aircraft it controls. The ATC system has become complex, often unwieldy and moderately inflexible. Yet it controls virtually all transport aircraft from departure gate to engine shutdown. It has made the pilot's task easier in some respects and much more complex in others; except in emergencies, it has also taken from him much of the authority he once had.

The job demands on the air traffic controller are rather different from those on the pilot. Although the controller uses vision and hearing almost exclusively to acquire his targets (distant vision for tower controllers, near vision for approach and center personnel manning radarscopes), his job is almost entirely that of a monitor and decision maker. An excellent remote memory is required to master the immensely complex network of regulations, directives and decision rules within which he must operate. Good recent memory is necessary for recently acquired targets, potential conflicts, etc. He must have the capacity to integrate two-dimensional displays into a three-dimensional spatial construct rapidly and continuously and the ability to make and communicate his decisions clearly and unambiguously. He must be able to tolerate frustration, distractions and annoyance without "losing his cool"; an even temperament is an absolute necessity in the busiest facilities.

There has been much argument *pro* and *con* in recent years concerning the stressfulness of air traffic control work. (See Chapter 68.)

The job demands placed on cabin crew will have been evident to anyone who has flown as a passenger. The cabin workload varies from very low on a flight too short to permit even beverage service to extremely high on a flight just long enough to permit the serving of a meal to a full passenger load. Cabin crew must be able to work for long periods at moderately high levels of metabolic expenditure. Sustained psychomotor performance is required, along with considerable agility, especially when flying in turbulence. Psychologic requirements include a good deal of patience, tact and curiosity about and interest in people, along with a genuine desire to serve them. The public relations aspect of the job is not difficult when everything is going well but it may assume heroic proportions in the face of delays or malfunctions. Secondary tasks include assisting in the care of infants, children and the elderly, ill or handicapped as well as handling passengers during emergencies and supervising passenger egress in the event of a mishap.

Ground support personnel have different requirements, depending on their job. They include mechanics, fuelers, ramp handlers, sanitary service personnel, cabin cleaning staff, food service staff, baggage handlers, station agents, dispatchers and others. Each is concerned with some aspect of aircraft turnaround; each works under time constraints. Nearly all can affect flight or passenger safety adversely by errors of omission or commission on the job. All, without exception, can affect on-time performance and therefore operational efficiency.

Nearly all of these jobs require close adherence to standard operating procedures and stringent safety precautions. Some of the jobs require considerable strength (e.g., baggage handling), some a high level of mechanical skill, some motor dexterity. Mechanics and ramp handlers are involved in positioning and taxiing aircraft in confined spaces; visual requirements for these jobs must be considered. Noise is a constant hazard; some personnel are exposed to certain toxicologic hazards. Perhaps the most ubiquitous hazards are related to the use of large numbers of motor vehicles in the servicing of large aircraft; they present problems for drivers, riders and "pedestrians" alike. During the winter over a large part of the globe, cold, snow and ice pose additional problems for ground handling personnel.

NONOCCUPATIONAL FACTORS IN JOB PERFORMANCE

If there is any single factor that characterizes most of the tasks described, it is the requirement for concentration on the job at hand. Yet, the men and women in this field bring to their jobs all of the social, economic, physical and emotional problems that confront any working group. Illness and emotional distress are potent distracting factors. The drugs prescribed by physicians also can impair performance to a significant degree, as can many over-the-counter medications over whose use there is no control.

Health workers giving services must be wary of any factor in an employee's life that poses a threat to on-the-job performance by virtue of its distracting influence.

OCCUPATIONAL DISORDERS

Problems Due to Trapped Gas

Foremost among the disorders caused by the aerospace environment is the constellation of otolaryngologic problems caused by trapped gas. Barotitis is the most frequent complication of aerial flight, both in aircrew and in passengers. Although cabin (as opposed to aircraft) descent rates rarely exceed 100–200 m/min in commercial aircraft, some passengers have difficulty clearing their ears even at this rate. In the presence of an upper respiratory infection or allergic rhinitis, the problem is compounded.

Prevention of barotitis is easier than its later treatment. The use of chewing gum or a drink of water to induce frequent swallowing often is of help in opening the eustachian tube orifices at frequent intervals during descent. The Valsalva maneuver, in which one attempts a forced expiration while holding the nares and mouth closed, usually can elevate intrapharyngeal pressure sufficiently to force air past the closed orifice into the middle ear. This maneuver may work even after landing.

The use of nasal decongestants often is of help. It should be noted that the frequency of swallowing is sharply decreased during sleep; passengers with a history of ear trouble should ask to be awakened prior to descent. Giving infants a bottle during the descent phase of flight usually will prevent symptoms.

Although some cases of barotrauma come to the attention of airline medical personnel, the majority do not; family physicians are consulted after the patient reaches home. The history and the appearance of the eardrum by that time are diagnostic. Complaints (see Table 57–2) include deafness, fullness in the ears, dull pain, a "sloshing" sensation when the head is moved and sometimes tinnitus or vertigo. The drum is retracted, injected or inflamed and often appears to have bullae behind it; these are gas bubbles in the serous transudate and move when the head is repositioned. Very rarely, the drum may have perforated.

Treatment consists of normalizing the pressure across the drum, either by myringotomy, eustachian tube catheterization or by forcing air into the ear using a Politzer bag. Both local and systemic decongestants may be helpful; antibiotics rarely are required and the condition usually is self-limiting. A few patients with chronic serous otitis media are helped by emplacement of button fistulae in the eardrums.

Much less commonly, barosinusitis is a problem. Again, prevention is a matter of ventilating the sinuses during flight, although this may not be easy to do. After flight, treatment consists of decongestants, sinus insufflation, if necessary, and measures directed at the cause of any preexisting sinus disease.

Trapped gas poses a potential hazard for patients who must travel immediately after surgery. If at all possible, movement of such patients by air should be delayed for several days, until any air trapped at wound sites has been reabsorbed.

There have been a few cases of spontaneous pneumothorax in flight. Most of these have occurred in military operations, but they have given rise to questions concerning the role of gas expansion in closed blebs during ascent to altitude.[13] Presently it is believed that pleural blebs are not truly "closed" cavities and that they do communicate with the airway system. Nonetheless, a very rapid ascent or decompression could give rise to significant overpressures in such air spaces.

The immediate treatment of a pneumothorax in flight consists of increasing the barometric pressure by descending to decrease the volume of free gas in the thoracic cavity. Obviously, patients with a pneumothorax should not fly unless a thoracic tube is in place and connected to underwater drainage; the tube must be clamped prior to descent to avoid aspiration of fluid into the pleural space.

The recurrence rate in spontaneous pneumothorax probably is 20%–30%. Flying personnel who have had one or more episodes should be evaluated for possible surgical treatment; wedge resection of blebs and tacking of the lung to the thoracic cage has been used in a number of military aviators who later have returned to flying status.[27]

Problems Due to Hypoxia

Hypoxia unquestionably has caused a number of deaths in both military and civil aviation. It is and will remain a serious problem in flights at high altitudes in unpressurized and inadequately pressurized aircraft. Its insidious onset at moderate altitudes can lead to seriously defective judgment; at high altitudes, useful consciousness may be lost without warning in as little as 10–15 sec.

As was noted earlier, nearly all normal people can tolerate altitudes up to 3,300–3,600 m without difficulty and often without symptoms other than slight breathlessness and fatigue after some hours of exposure. In air transport, then, hypoxia usually is a problem only for passengers whose ability to obtain oxygen from the environment is impaired. This includes patients with severe obstructive lung disease, diffusion defects, impaired pulmonary or cerebral circulation, deficient hemoglobin levels or impaired tissue uptake of oxygen. Among the specific conditions in which hypoxia is tolerated poorly are congestive heart failure, pulmonary edema, berylliosis and sickle cell anemia (or, indeed, severe anemia from any cause).

The handling of problems due to hypoxia in flight is simple and specific—the provision of supplemental oxygen. Virtually all airline aircraft, and many general aviation aircraft as well, have oxygen supplies that can be used for this purpose. If a person who may need supplemental oxygen is to be transported, however, the air carrier should be notified in advance so that adequate preparations can be made.

The question of whether hypoxia at normal cabin altitudes has a detrimental effect on the young fetus is unanswered; it is thought that it does not. Pregnant women, especially early in pregnancy, should receive supplemental oxygen during flights above 3,000 m in unpressurized aircraft.

Problems Due to Accelerations

For pilots, the most serious threat posed by linear and angular accelerations is the possibility of disorientation (often incorrectly called "aviator's vertigo"). The problem is caused by inadequate or conflicting sensory cues as to the airplane's spatial orientation. It was proved long ago that flight "by the seat of the pants" is not possible, but pilots continue to attempt flight without adequate visual inputs. Most aircraft today are equipped with gyroscopic flight instruments that are not subject to the illusions that affect man. The pilot who is confronted by disorientation needs only to be able to understand the information presented by these attitude instruments and to believe them, regardless of what his proprioceptive and vestibular sensors are telling him. This takes both instruction and regular practice, however. Disorientation rarely is a problem in airline flying except during extremely severe turbulence, but it is a too-frequent cause of fatal accidents in general aviation.

As our forays into space have increased in duration, we have become aware of a constellation of problems related to weightlessness. Losses of body weight, decreases in bone density, decreases in plasma volume and red cell mass, decreases in exercise tolerance and moderate degrees of orthostatic intolerance have all been observed in returning astronauts. Most of these changes are remarkably similar to those observed in patients during prolonged bed rest. The red cell mass decreases are unexplained at this time.

For passengers, the major problem posed by accelerations is motion sickness. The problem is less frequent in jet aircraft than formerly, because jets fly at higher altitudes and usually are above most weather-induced turbulence. However, motion sickness remains a distressing syndrome, especially for those whom it affects with some regularity. The disorder has both physiologic and psychologic components. It is due to both vestibular and visual inputs and sometimes can be controlled by avoiding unnecessary head or eye movements. Its psychologic component is less predictable; mild sedation sometimes is of benefit.

It should be mentioned that a substantial fraction of military flight students is affected by motion sickness early in training. Most of these students, however, seem to adapt as training progresses (vestibular adaptation or habituation can be shown to occur). Some use has been made of the antihistamines mentioned to alleviate the problem early in dual training before it becomes a fixed response to unusual attitudes, aerobatic maneuvers, etc.

Motion sickness, or something very akin to it, has been a finding in a significant number of space flights and in those conducted by the USSR. The problem appeared early in the Russian space program and only later for the U.S. It has not occurred in all astronauts, nor has its appearance been predictable. At its worst, it has been partially incapacitating for periods of several days, and it perhaps is the most serious biomedical problem yet encountered in the weightless environment.

It is thought that this problem may be due in part to movement of crew members within their spacecraft in a weightless field. Our early vehicles were too small to permit such movement; the Russian spacecraft were substantially larger. It may also be due in part to a low level of vestibular habituation to acceleratory cues; some members of the early Russian crews were not pilots and had only very limited aerobatic flying experience. Our astronauts, in contrast, have nearly all been highly experienced pilots who remained current in high-performance military aircraft during their training. Despite this, several have had moderate or severe symptoms during space flight.

The problem does not appear to be serious in long-duration missions, since adaptation seems to occur during the first week of flight. In missions lasting only a few days, however, it poses a considerable threat to mission effectiveness.

Problems Due to Noise

Little needs to be said about noise here; the topic and methods of handling it are covered in Chapter 20. Given the importance of this stress in the aerospace environment, an effective hearing conservation program is absolutely mandatory; the use of the best available ear protection must be encouraged and enforced.

Many pilots, especially those whose careers began during World War II, have substantial noise-induced permanent threshold shifts. In some, the hearing loss is sufficient to cause a real social problem. It must not be inferred, however, that these men are necessarily handicapped in their work. Nearly all the significant auditory inputs to pilots are radio communications whose volume the pilot can control by turning up his speaker or headset volume; most of the other necessary auditory inputs are loud warning horns or bells in the cockpit. Pilots with moderate or severe hearing losses should not be grounded before being evaluated on the job to determine whether their operational effectiveness is impaired; such deafness has not posed any difficulty in flight.

Other Occupational Problems

One problem that does not neatly fit any environmental category but is real nonetheless is fatigue. There are many factors that may contribute to fatigue in aircrew; their importance and the role of fatigue in transport flying have been questioned by a number of authors.[34] Others believe that fatigue is a serious potential problem that needs careful consideration in flight scheduling.[31, 33]

Several of the factors that may produce fatigue in aircrew are related to flight schedules. Airline pilots rarely fly more than 8 hours in any 24-hour period. Preflight duties, time between legs of a flight, delays and postflight duties, however, may push duty hours to 14 or more, to which must be added travel time to and from the airport. Corporate pilots usually fly somewhat fewer hours, but their duty times may be as long, for they often must wait for passengers whose business has taken them beyond normal working hours.

Accommodations away from home may be far from ideal; food service at airports often is inadequate or may be unavailable. Compounding the problem may be time zone shifts of 5–8 hours. Although most people adapt to such changes in circadian rhythm over a few days, the pilot often is not in a zone long enough to adapt prior to going on. This is particularly true of pilots who fly around the world in the course of a tour of duty.[26, 33]

Many flight schedules do not accord with their pilots' normal diurnal schedules; in airline flying, day-night differentials in pay encourage pilots to bid for night schedules. This also may be a factor in fatigue.

The monotony of long-distance flying has been mentioned. It must be realized that a long period of time at very low work load is followed by a period of much higher work load during approach and landing, especially if the flight terminates in a busy terminal area. The effects of such considerable changes in work load and task demand on performance have not been evaluated systematically; they may be associated with problems in an already tired pilot.

"Fear of flying" is an administrative term used by the armed forces to characterize deficient motivation for flight duties in an aircrewman whose motivation formerly was adequate.[19] Regardless of the term that is used, it is a fact that a variety of specific phobias, which later may become generalized, may appear in a pilot after many years of professional flying. This phenomenon may appear during the involutional period or somewhat earlier; often it is manifested by psychosomatic symptoms or signs of emotional difficulty. It may be accompanied by increased dependence on alcohol. The flight surgeon with such a patient is in a difficult dilemma. He can hardly allow the pilot to continue flying; a frightened pilot is hardly in a position to make effective decisions under difficult circumstances. Yet, he often has no clear reason to ground the pilot, and he may properly be concerned about the cost to his employer of an indefinite period of disability. A few such cases have been denied medical certification by the FAA on the grounds that the airman's condition rendered him at least potentially unable to perform his duties safely. Other patients have simply resigned their flying positions when offered an opportunity to do so without loss of face. Some, unfortunately, remain on flying status.

Occupational Problems in Ground Support Personnel

Most of the problems observed in occupational health surveillance of ground support personnel are physical in nature, as with flying personnel. They range from severe injury or death due to rotating propellers or falling from ground vehicles through fractures incurred in falls from icy platforms or wings to eye injuries caused by safety wire, a fairly common problem in mechanics. Toxicologic problems are less common, with the exception of eye irritation and inflammation caused by certain of the synthetic hydraulic fluids. Pinch points abound in aviation, as in other industries; hand injuries are common. The problems in maintenance shops are those seen in any small manufacturing plant. It should be noted that polyurethane paints are among the best for aircraft use; exposure to toluene diisocyanate is not rare in aviation.

There is a good deal of evidence that ground support personnel are very conscious of their role in maintaining flight safety. The problem for the occupational physician is to convince his workers that ground safety is just as important to the effectiveness of the industry. It appears that the Occupational Safety and Health Act may have increased management awareness of safety problems in the industry; whether it has had a similar effect on workers, especially the semiskilled, is less certain at this time.

NONOCCUPATIONAL DISORDERS

In flying personnel, the presence of any disease or defect requires that three questions be asked. First, is the disease or defect one that may produce sudden or insidious incapacitation in flight? Second, does the disease, or its symptoms, interfere significantly with the pilot's ability to perform his duties in flight? Finally, does the treatment regimen being applied interfere with the pilot's performance?

It has been noted that physical or emotional disorders may be potent distracting influences. There are many disorders that do not pose a threat to flying safety. Evaluation of these often requires that the physician be familiar with the pilot's job, as he or she must be familiar with any industrial job in which placement is recommended.

The threat of sudden or insidious incapacitation in flight is another matter. Once an airplane has taken off, it is committed to flight until a safe landing spot can be found. One cannot simply "pull over to the side of the road" as one can in automobiles. There are few conditions that are absolutely disqualifying under current Federal Air Regulations but most of them are those that can cause sudden incapacitation. They include coronary heart disease, diabetes requiring hypoglycemic agents for control, epilepsy of all types, other convulsive disorders and psychotic disorders. Cerebrovascular disorders that have produced symptoms of cerebral ischemia are not named but fall in the same category, as do most cardiac arrhythmias. Malignant hypertension presents a similar problem because of its known complications.

The significance of these disorders in aircrew has important implications for the physician charged with medical selection of flying personnel for career positions. Is a strongly positive family history of premature death from coronary heart disease enough to rule a man out of a career slot? How about the young man whose post-exercise electrocardiogram shows "nonspecific T-wave changes"? Is it fair to exclude an obviously healthy, well-qualified young pilot based purely on statistical criteria?

One large American air carrier has estimated that each premature retirement for medical reasons requires, on the average, 13½ training and upgrading assignments for the men behind the retiree in seniority. The costs of such a premature retirement are staggering. Given a large excess of supply over demand, which is the case with airline pilots, is one not justified in seeking the best-qualified among the available applicants? It is clear that when we discuss "best-qualified," we must talk as well about "most likely to remain qualified" throughout a full working career (until age 60, in the case of airline pilots).

Air carriers are free to impose whatever medical standards they wish at the time of initial employment. Thus, the new hire may, and should, be selected using optimal standards. It is worth emphasizing that the pre-employment examination for a pilot is exactly that. He is applying for a specific job for which he must be found either qualified or unqualified.

The role of psychologic testing and psychiatric screening deserves mention. Psychiatric disorders rank second after cardiovascular diseases as a cause of premature disability retirement in airline pilots. A few corporations and some airlines include psychologic testing in their selection process for executives and for pilots. The effectiveness of such testing is hard to evaluate, if only because those not selected are lost to follow-up, but useful as a screening device, and that it probably is cost-effective as well if training costs will be high for those selected (as in airline operations).

The examination of personnel for ground support positions is similar to the preplacement medical examination in other industries. The specific demands of each job should determine the medical standards for that job. Fortunately, the range of jobs and job demands is fairly considerable; the physician and the personnel section should be able to place nearly all highly motivated applicants in some position within their physical and mental capacities.

Once flying or ground support personnel have been approved from a medical viewpoint, what factors should cause them to be suspended from their duties, either temporarily or permanently? The same factors prevail; the same questions must be asked. Is this employee affected by a disease that may incapacitate him or can cause him enough distress to interfere with the performance of his duties? Or, if his disorder is under treatment, may the drugs he is receiving interfere with his performance or with his ability to respond to stress, in the case of flying personnel?

The enormous number of medications available over the counter and by prescription makes it quite impossible to consider the latter question adequately here. A few general rules can be suggested. First, aircrew should be advised never to fly after taking medication of any kind without first checking with their flight surgeon or occupational physician. Second, flying personnel always should know the name of any drug they are taking. Third, the physician should check on the ingredients in any medication to be sure that none is a sedative, narcotic, tranquilizer, antihistamine or other central nervous system depressant or an anticholinergic agent. Finally, if doubts remain about the safety of the drug, he would be well advised to seek help from a qualified consultant.

In 1986, Engelberg et al.[17] summarized a report of a comprehensive review by the American Medical Association (AMA) of the medical standards for civilian airmen, as present standards were promulgated by the Federal Aviation Administration in 1959 (the "alcoholism" and "cardiovascular standards" were revised in 1982). The AMA report recommends new or revised standards for cardiovascular, mental and behavioral, visual, endocrine, respiratory, hematologic, hearing and equilibrium, musculoskeletal, and nervous system disorders. Special attention was given to risk factors for the development of sudden incapacitating disease, such as coronary heart disease and stroke. Their report also provides guidance for the medical certification of airmen with conditions not covered specifically by the standards and recommends a new medical history and examination form for use by aviation medical examiners. Final standards will be completed by the Federal Aviation Administration.

LEGAL CONTROLS IN CIVIL AVIATION

Since 1926, the federal government has promulgated and enforced regulations governing the skill, knowledge and medical fitness of all civil airmen in the United States. Its medical standards, Part 67 of the Federal Air Regulations, comprise a set of minimal standards for the three classes of medical certificates that it issues.

A tripartite medical standard has been with us for many years. The desirability of such an approach has been questioned; it is in part a response to the mandate to ensure the highest standard of safety and reliability in air transport while at the same time allowing any citizen the right to fly if he can do so without jeopardizing the public safety.

Part 67 contains relatively few references to specific conditions or disorders. Its general clauses allow the Federal Air Surgeon rather wide latitude in his interpretation of the regulation. Consequently, there has grown up over the years a set of policies with regard to medical certification of airmen with various conditions, in part based on the opinion of the Air Surgeon and his staff, in part the result of deliberations of the medical review boards utilized as consultants. There also has been established a set of policies regarding those drugs that may be taken safely by airmen on flying status.

From time to time, the Office of Aviation Medicine has conducted studies of the accident experience of airmen with specific classes of conditions to ascertain whether their experience has differed significantly from that of the airman population as a whole. These studies have led to modifications of certification policies in certain instances.

The Office of Aviation Medicine determines the medical policies of the FAA; these policies are implemented by the agency's Airman Certification Branch located at the FAA Aeronautical Center in Oklahoma City. It is here that periodic physical examination forms are received, reviewed, processed and coded and central record files maintained on almost 900,000 civil airmen. The Office of Aviation Medicine also provides policy guidance to Regional Flight Surgeons and their staffs. The Regional Flight Surgeons are responsible for the designation of Aviation Medical Examiners and for the occupational medical surveillance of all FAA personnel in their geographic areas.

In addition to the federal regulations governing airmen, all air carriers and many corporate aviation operations have operating manuals that contain company regulations governing operation of their aircraft. Many operating manuals contain sections pertaining to aviation medicine, as well as regulations regarding flying and duty time, crew rest requirements, etc. All air carrier pilot union contracts also contain binding provisions regarding these matters; many contain clauses pertaining to medical certification as well. The physician caring for flying personnel needs to be aware of these provisions; some may speak to the question of obtaining medical clearance after periods of illness, as an instance.

MEDICAL ROLES IN THE AEROSPACE INDUSTRY

This discussion is limited in the main to the structure of civil aerospace medicine in the United States, although certain other nations have similar structures. We noted earlier that there have been slightly more than 860 diplomas in aerospace medicine awarded by the American Board of Preventive Medicine. It should be noted, however, that aerospace medicine has been a second specialty for many, particularly those who entered the field during the 1950s. Conversely, not all of those who have received their certificates more recently are presently working in this field. Many are employed in occupational medicine and public health, and a substantial number are practicing clinical medicine.

There probably are 7,000 physicians in the United States who receive some part of their livelihood, however small, from the practice of aviation medicine. Nearly all of these are designated aviation medical examiners who perform FAA flight physical examinations. They are considered FAA employees when acting in that capacity, although they are paid by the airmen who receive the service. Approximately 2,400 of these physicians are permitted to perform class I (airline transport pilot) medical examinations. Aviation medical examiners are designated by FAA regional flight surgeons on the basis of geographic location, demonstrated interest in aviation and aviation medicine and willingness to attend periodic short training courses offered by the Aeromedical Education Branch of the Office of Aviation Medicine.

Career positions outside the armed forces exist in several areas. The Federal Aviation Administration presently employs about 50 physicians in its Office of Aviation Medicine—in Washington, at the Civil Aeromedical Institute in Oklahoma City and at regional medical offices.

The National Aeronautics and Space Administration employs physicians who function in three areas: in occupational medical surveillance of agency personnel (although much of the work at the various field centers is contracted to local groups of occupational physicians); caring for the astronaut corps in medical support of manned space missions; and several are in aviation and space medical research posts.

A few of the larger airlines have large full-time medical departments. These airlines employ physicians who are located at each of their large crew domiciles. In 1985, two U.S. airlines employed 16 full-time physicians.

During recent years, in an attempt to provide better occupational medical service for ground support personnel, more accessible aviation medical examinations for pilots and emergency medical services for passengers, a number of physicians have established airport medical clinics at large commercial air terminals. Where they have been successful, they have appreciably enhanced both the availability and the quality of medical care.[25] Such clinics presently are in operation at Boston, Chicago, Kennedy Airport in New York, Cleveland, Houston, Minneapolis, San Francisco, Los Angeles and a few other locations. Many are operated by clinically oriented aerospace or occupational physicians.

Most of the large aerospace manufacturers have medical departments headed by full-time physicians.[18] These departments generally are typical of occupational medical services in other diversified manufacturing industries. Some of them were rather large at one time; most have contracted considerably as a result of the recession in the industry during the 1980–1984 (see Chapter 7) period. Some of these corporations also employed substantial numbers of physicians and scientists in life sciences and human factors research groups during the early and middle 1960s; these groups have been sharply curtailed in recent years.

In occupational medical support to the aviation industry (in DeHart's text on aerospace medicine), deTreville reiterates the basic principles, applicable here: "The contributions of occupational medicine to the aviation industry involve the application of industrial hygiene surveys, analytic measurements, and scientific logic to the recognition, evaluation, and control of environmental hazards. Such hazards, if undetected and uncontrolled, can be expected to produce such adverse effects as illness and impaired efficiency of the aviation industry's employees, neighbors, and customers. Ideally, responsible aerospace medicine specialists will be trained and become fully qualified to direct the occupational medicine function personally. Otherwise, they must recognize the need to provide adequately for its availability and quality, to ensure its effectiveness within the total environmental and occupational health program to their respective organizations and communities."[14]

WORK AT HIGH ALTITUDES

Robert T. P. deTreville, M.D., Sc.D.

Dana Mirkin, M.D.

Not all problems of morbidity and mortality associated with exposures to the margins of physical tolerance occur in working populations served by aerospace medical specialists, although these represent an important aspect of preventive medicine. Increasingly, travel for purposes of work or pleasure (e.g., mountain climbing) will involve planned, rapid ascent to an altitude of 2,600 m (8,000 feet) or more above sea level. At these high altitudes, a variety of medical problems may be expected among normal healthy adult workers and their families. Thus, every physician preparing for certification in public health, preventive and occupational medicine (as well as those primarily interested in aerospace medicine) should become knowledgeable to offer sound advice and guidance to such individuals.

Physiologically, as the barometric pressure falls with ascent to high altitudes, so does the partial pressure of oxygen in ambient air. Reflexly, peripheral pulmonary chemoreceptors act to stimulate rate and depth of ventilation; the resulting hyperventilation "blows off" carbon dioxide, leading to respiratory alkalosis. The consequent increase in pH of cerebrospinal fluid (CSF) suppresses centrally located chemoreceptors and limits the degree of hyperventilation. After a day or more at altitude, the pH of the CSF returns to normal and several days later renal excretion of bicarbonate returns blood pH to normal. This adaptation permits maximal hyperventilation, optimizing intake of oxygen in the presence of a reduced ambient oxygen pressure.

Time needed for such physiologic adaptation or "acclimatization" varies among individuals (and may even vary in the same individual on occasions of repeated rapid ascent). Reportedly, half of unacclimatized individuals whose ascent to 3,800 m (12,000 feet) is rapid will develop a headache; and a severe, sometimes fatal, condition, "acute mountain sickness" (AMS) will occur in 10%. Depending largely on speed of ascent, onset of AMS is usually heralded by nonspecific "flu-like" malaise in 24–48 hours, or even earlier. Complaints of headache, anorexia (or nausea), weakness, imbalance and dyspnea are common. The headache is often intense and may be incapacitating. Nausea and vomiting can be severe, especially in children. During sleep, ventilation may diminish and hypoxia may be intensified, leading to more severe symptoms on awakening. Symptoms usually subside in one to five days as acclimatization occurs. Some persons seem especially susceptible to AMS, developing similar episodes on each exposure and failing to acclimatize.

Prevention of AMS involves provision for a two- to four-day stay at an intermediate altitude of 1,600 to 2,300 m (5,000 to 7,000 feet), followed by gradual ascent. Physical fitness conditioning at sea level has been shown not to be effective in preventing AMS. Symptoms of AMS can be treated by giving supplemental oxygen, especially during sleep and/or by descent to lower altitude. Pharmacologic therapy reportedly has been ineffective and remains controversial, and is summarized as follows: Acetazolamide (Diamox-Lederle) in a dose of 250 mg every 8 hours for 72 hours, beginning 24 hours before ascent to altitude, has been used and in one group of nine healthy mountaineers was thought to have caused reduced symptoms and decreased sleep hypoxia. Acting as a carbonic anhydrase inhibitor, and taken before renal compensation occurs, acetazolamide reduces renal bicarbonate reabsorption and produces a metabolic acidosis. This effect is transient, but ideally physiologic compensation should occur before its effect wears off. Mechanisms of action, however, have not been fully explored and, as it is a sulfonamide, it may cause any or all of the adverse effects associated with this class of drugs. Common side effects reported have been numbness and tingling of lips and fingers, and transient myopia can occur. In an excellent review article, Wilson[49] cautions that it is doubtful that the drug can ameliorate cerebral syndromes of AMS, once symptomatic. In this regard Wilson states that aspirin, codeine, and phenothiazines are notoriously poor at providing symptomatic relief, sometimes worsening nausea and imbalance. Wilson recommends caution with the use of furosemide (Lasix-Hoechts/Roussel), advocated by Singh et al.[37] for prevention and treatment of cerebral as well as pulmonary forms of AMS:

> "Singh and co-workers advocate the potent diuretic agent furosemide for prevention and treatment of cerebral as well as pulmonary forms of AMS. Nineteen of 24 cases with neurologic manifestations improved when given furosemide and a synthetic corticocosteroid, betamethasone. Gray and his colleagues, however, saw severe ataxia develop in five persons who were given furosemide in a study to test the efficiency of the agent for preventing AMS. It seems illogical to provoke diuresis in individuals already dehydrated from the effort of climbing, and, at times, vomiting as well, despite observations that individuals immune to altitude sickness urinate more (Hohendijrese of alpinists) on reaching altitude than those who became ill. It is more likely that the good effects observed by Singh were caused by betamethasone rather than furosemide, because betamethasone and similar corticosteroids, such as dexamethasone, are widely used in other clinical situations to reduce brain swelling. A climber with high altitude cerebral edema was recently treated with dexamethasone alone, with apparent benefit. Dexamethasone apparently lessened symptoms, abnormal physical signs, and CSF pressure and protein, but recovery in this mild case might have occurred as rapidly without medication (at sea level). Gray's warning that the use of furosemide to prevent or treat AMS may be dangerous should be heeded. The use of betamethasone or dexamethasone, 12 to 40 mg daily in divided doses for 5 to 10 days, is justified on a mountain if prompt removal of an individual with cerebral form of AMS is not possible. An unconscious person would, of course, require parenteral medication. This is often difficult to manage on a high mountain because vials of liquid medication freeze and break. Betamethasone and dexamethasone are not marketed in this country in a powdered form in vials."

Space does not permit further discussion here, but interested physicians should read the above-mentioned article as well as another by the same author[50] entitled "Death on Denali: Fatalities Among Climbers in Mount McKinley National Park From 1903 to 1976—Analysis of Injuries, Illnesses and Rescues in 1976."

In addition to AMS, the following conditions may occur following ascent to elevations above 2,600 m (8,000 feet): swelling of face, hands, and feet may begin shortly after arrival at high altitude and persist for days to weeks. More common in women, it is not prevented by gradual ascent or acclimatization. The mechanism is unknown, but salt restriction alone may be helpful. After descent, a spontaneous diuresis occurs. If taken to help prevent AMS, acetazolamide (see above), which causes diuresis, may prevent such edema.

High altitude pulmonary edema (HAPE) is a serious illness, causing many deaths annually worldwide. HAPE occurs in 0.5% of adults whose ascent above 3,300 m (10,000 feet) is rapid (in children, the incidence may rise as high as 4%). In addition to rapidity of ascent, heavy exertion and sleeping at high altitudes are important added etiologic factors. Exertional fatigue, dyspnea, cough, and altered mental status, progressing to coma, may appear from the second to fourth day after arrival at high altitude, but somnolence or coma may be the first sign, especially in children. Without treatment, death occurs in 6 to 12 hours following onset of coma. Treatment is the promptest possible removal to sea level, by rescue helicopter, if feasible. If available, oxygen by face mask at 6 to 12 L/min flow rate has been recommended, *but nothing should be allowed to delay removal to lower altitude*. Repeated attacks are common, suggesting individual predisposition. Sleeping below 2,600 m (8,000 feet) appears preventive. Fatal episodes are reported, annually, from ski resorts where lodges are located above that altitude. Gradual acclimatization and avoidance of heavy physical activity during the first few days at high altitude may prevent this disorder, but physical fitness conditioning before ascent does *not* help; in fact, the young and energetic appear most susceptible.

High altitude cerebral edema (HACE)—seen mainly in mountaineers—is a complication of rapid ascent to very high altitudes, manifested by mental dysfunction (hallucinations, bizarre behavior, obtundation (progressing to coma), and neurologic abnormalities (ataxia, paralysis, and cerebellar signs). Headache may be severe and can precede the onset of the more serious manifestations. Hypoxic injury to the brain (similar to aeroembolism) appears etiologic and cerebral edema is a secondary effect. Immediate recompression by rapid descent is essential to prevent permanent sequelae, or death, and oxygen en route is recommended (as with HAPE, above), if available.

High altitude retinal hemorrhages (HARH) may occur at altitudes above 4,500 m (14,000 feet), but are seldom symptomatic and, unless sought by funduscopic examination, may be overlooked. Noticeable defects in peripheral vision rarely occur. When discovered, treatment is oxygen, with early descent to a lower altitude. The diagnosis is good for healing (by resorption) in several weeks, without impairment of visual acuity. Rarely, persistent visual field defects may occur.

Summary

According to Wilson,[49] "Adventurers will continue to engage the great mountains. Injuries and death will inevitably come to some, but assiduous attention to party leadership, arctic experience, climbing skill, past brushes with sickness in the mountains, equipment hygiene, starting level of climbs, rate of ascent, fallback positions, willingness to assist others in trouble, and backup aircraft (including helicopters) can lessen loss of limb and life."

Addendum

No mention has been encountered by us so far, in literature reviewed on this general subject, concerning risks (of high altitude ascent) to the embryo or fetus in (fertile) women workers, or in travelers who may be pregnant. For reasons outlined in the section on hypoxia (Chapter 54), there should be careful consideration for protection of women who may be pregnant from ascent above 2,600 m (8,000 feet) equivalent altitudes, in order to avoid possible impairment of development, mental retardation, or death of the developing fetus, anoxia being a potent teratogenic influence as clearly demonstrated in experimental animal studies. This consideration has been given to altitude indoctrination in low pressure chambers; however, the brevity of exposure time would act to protect the fetus from hypoxia in any routine used in indoctrinating United States Air Force flight crews. The same cannot be assumed, however, for certain hypoxia research studies (such as the test of "Time of Useful Consciousness," especially at high altitudes). Any such proposal involving fertile female subjects requires careful review and approval in the United States Air Force by a Human Utilization Review Committee; similar review and approval capability exists in all organizations authorized to perform human research under U.S. governmental sponsorship.

REFERENCES*

1. De Hart RL (ed): *Fundamentals of Aerospace Medicine*. Philadelphia: Lea & Febiger, 1985.
2. Gillies JA (ed): *Textbook of Aviation Physiology*. Oxford, Pergamon Press, 1965.
3. McFarland RA: *Human Factors in Air Transportation: Occupational Health and Safety*. New York, McGraw-Hill Book Company, Inc, 1953.
4. Parker JF Jr, West VR (eds): *Bioastronautics Data Book*, ed 2. Washington, DC, National Aeronautics and Space Administration, NASA SP–3006, 1973. Available from US Government Printing Office.
5. Randel HW (ed): *Aerospace Medicine*, ed 2. Baltimore, The Williams & Wilkins Company, 1971.
6. Compendium of Aviation Medicine by Siegfried Ruff and Hubertus Strughold: Translated from the original German for The Committee on Aviation Medicine, Division of Medical Sciences National Research Council, for The Committee On Medical Research by the Office of Scientific Research and Development, Washington, DC, 1942.
7. Aeromedical and human factors aspects of airports. Subcommittee report. *Aerosp Med* 1971; 42:439.

*References 1–6 are texts and source books that will be stimulating and helpful to physicians who become involved in aerospace medicine. The remaining references are those specifically cited in this chapter.

8. Bennett G: Ozone contamination of high altitude aircraft cabins. *Aerosp Med* 1962; 33:969.
9. Billings CE: Atmosphere, in Parker and West,[3] pp 35–64.
10. Billings CE: Barometric pressure, in Parker and West,[3] pp 1–34.
11. Billings CE: Psychiatric disorders in military aviators. *J Aviat Med* 1959; 30:100.
12. Buley L: Provision of solar flare information in support of supersonic transport operations: A review of developments. *Aerosp Med* 1969; 40:1134.
13. Dermksian G, Lamb LE: Spontaneous pneumothorax in apparently healthy flying personnel. *Ann Intern Med* 1959; 51:39.
14. deTreville RTP: Occupational medical support in the aerospace industry, in Aerospace Medicine, in De Hart,[1] pp 904–940.
15. Dietlein LF, Johnston RS: US manned space flight: The first twenty years. A biomedical status report. *Acta Astronautica* 1981; 8:9–10.
16. Ellingson HV: Aerial transportation of patients, in Randel,[4] pp 602–613.
17. Engelberg A, Gibbons H, Doege T: A review of the medical standards for civilian airmen—Synopsis of a two-year study. *JAMA* 1986; 255(12).
18. Evans WE, Barron CI: Medical care of aircrewmen in an industrial environment. *J Occup Med* 1968; 10:688.
19. Gatto LE: Understanding the "fear of flying" syndrome. I. Psychic aspects. II. Psychosomatic aspects. *US Armed Forces Med J* 1954; 5:1093, 1267.
20. Gibbons HL, Fromhagen C: Aeromedical transportation and general aviation. *Aerosp Med* 1971; 42:773.
21. Hale HB, Williams EW, Smith BN, et al: Excretion patterns of air traffic controllers. *Aerosp Med* 1970; 42:127.
22. Handel S, Jansson P: Infra-sound-occurrence and effects. *Läkartidningen* 1974; 71:1635.
23. Harris DA, Pegram GV, Hartman BO: Performance and fatigue in experimental double-crew transport missions. *Aerosp Med* 1971; 42:980.
24. Kaufman WC: Human tolerance limits for some thermal environments of aerospace. *Aerosp Med* 1963; 34:889.
25. Kidera GJ: Physicians guide to airport medicine. *JAMA* 1967; 199:128.
26. Klein KE, Wegmann HM, Hunt BI: Desynchronization of body temperature and performance circadian rhythm as a result of outgoing and homegoing transmeridian flights. *Aerosp Med* 1972; 43:119.
27. Lamb LE: Pneumothorax, in Randel,[4] pp 510–511.
28. Medical aspects of business aviation: A guide for physicians in industry. Joint committee report, Aerospace Med Assoc and Industrial Med Assoc. *J Occup Med* 1964; 6:338.
29. Medical criteria for passenger flying. Committee report, Aerospace Med Assn. *Aerosp Med* 1961; 32:369.
30. Mohler SR: Civil aviation medicine, in De Hart,[1] pp 676–697.
31. Nicholson AN: Sleep patterns of an airline pilot operating world-wide east-west routes. *Aerosp Med* 1970; 41:626.
32. Nicogossian AE, Parker JF (eds): *Space Physiology and Medicine* (NASA SP–447). US Government Printing Office, Washington, DC, 1982.
33. Preston FS, Bateman SC: Effect of time zone changes on the sleep patterns of BOAC B. 707 crews on world-wide schedules. *Aerosp Med* 1970; 41:1409.
34. Schreuder OB: Medical aspects of aircraft pilot fatigue with special reference to the commercial jet pilot. *Aerosp Med* 1966;37.
35. Schulte JH: *E pluribus unum*. *Arch Environ Health* 1965; 11:261.
36. Sexton UAG, Wick RL Jr: Fifteen-year survey of pilots returned to flying status following a myocardial infarction. *Aerosp Med* 1973; 44:1287.
37. Singh I, Kharma PK, Srivasta MC, et al: Acute Mountain Sickness. *N Engl J Med* 1969; 280(4):175–184.

38. Sliff RS, Slaughter HH: Engineering approach to SST certification. *Aerosp Med* 1969; 40:1209.
39. Smith RC, Cobb BB, Collins WE: Attitudes and motivations of air traffic controllers in terminal areas. *Aerosp Med* 1972; 43:1.
40. Standardized criteria for carriage of the physically handicapped. Committee report. *Aerosp Med* 1962; 33:1250.
41. Stapp JP: Biodynamics of deceleration, impact and blast, in Randel,[4] pp 118–166.
42. Stone RB: Cockpit noise environment of airline aircraft, *Aerosp Med* 1969; 40:989.
43. Strandberg UK, Bjerle P, Danielsson A, et al: Studies of changes in circulation during exposure to infrasound. *Arbete och Hälsa* 1986; 19.
44. Tobias JV: Cockpit noise intensity: Fifteen single engine light aircraft. *Aerosp Med* 1969; 40:963.
45. Trites DK, Kurek A, Cobb BB: Personality and achievement of air traffic controllers. *Aerosp Med* 1967; 38:1145.
46. von Gierke HE: Noise effects and speech communication in aerospace environments, in Randel,[4] pp 224–253.
47. Waite RE, DeLucchi MR: Labyrinthine and Proprioceptive Aspects of Aerospace Medicine, in Randel,[4] pp 254–267.
48. Wick RL Jr, Roberts LB, Ashe WF: Light aircraft noise problems. *Aerosp Med* 1963; 34:1133.
49. Wilson R: Acute high-altitude illness in mountaineers and problems of rescue. *Ann Intern Med* 1973; 78:421–428.
50. Wilson R, Mills WJ Jr, Rogers DR, et al: Death on Denali: Fatalities Among Climbers in Mt. McKinley National Park from 1903–1976—Analysis of Injuries, Illnesses and Rescues in 1976. *West J Med* 1976; 128:471–476.

58

Occupational Health Programs in Clinics and Hospitals

Edward P. Horvath, Jr., M.D., M.P.H.

There are approximately 5 million persons working in 7,000 hospitals in the United States with another 330,000 employed by outpatient clinics. These health care workers have been among the last beneficiaries of our nation's renewed interest in occupational health. As recently as 1976, the National Institute for Occupational Safety and Health (NIOSH) survey revealed that almost one third of hospitals had no formal occupational health program and that only 8% satisfied minimal criteria for an effective program.[39] There have been several reasons for this dismal performance. As medical institutions, hospitals have been mistakenly assumed to be healthy places to work. Until recently, clinics and hospitals have been oriented toward the treatment of disease rather than its prevention. Economic pressures have restrained the development of non-income-generating services. The immediate proximity to health care professionals has fostered the notion that employee health matters could be handled out of hand without special planning.[17]

Although old misconceptions die slowly, the past few years have witnessed a growing emphasis on the development of effective hospital and clinic occupational health programs. There has been increased recognition of the special hazards faced by the health care worker. Articles on topics such as rubella, waste anesthetic gases, and ethylene oxide have appeared with regularity in medical journals, and have been comprehensively reviewed by Patterson et al.[57a] National occupational health meetings have featured entire sessions on the hazards of health care workers. Indeed, conferences devoted exclusively to this subject have been held.[38, 55] Monthly newsletters highlighting topics of present interest are growing in circulation. Clinic and hospital management personnel have come to the same realization as their industrial colleagues, that an effective occupational health program is important for employee well-being, satisfaction, and productivity.

Undoubtedly, some of this new-found enthusiasm has been due to pressure from regulatory agencies, unions, nurses, and attorneys. Many states have hospital codes mandating adoption of certain employee health program components such as preplacement and periodic examinations. On the national level, the Occupational Safety and Health Administration's (OSHA) general duty clause, requiring the provision of a safe and healthful work environment, would seem to apply to hospitals and clinics as well as more traditional "industries." Adoption of specific standards, e.g., ethylene oxide, will undoubtedly lead to more direct regulation. Although the Joint Commission on Accreditation of Hospitals (JCAH) does not explicitly require an institution to have an employee health service, it is difficult to imagine a hospital meeting JCAH infection control standards without one.[41] In specific instances, employee unions have been advocates of better occupational health programs. The nursing profession, whose members constitute the largest single group of health care workers, also has shown increased interest in employee health.[15, 56] Finally, legal concerns have led to heightened awareness, particularly in the areas of job discrimination and hospital-acquired infections.

While there are obvious differences between the health care industry and other businesses, both require similar occupational health services. Preplacement evaluations need to be conducted on new employees. Periodic medical surveillance is indicated for individuals who are judged to be at risk because of exposure hazards. Acute injuries and self-limited, nonoccupational illnesses require expeditious treatment. Employee education and counseling needs must be satisfied.[67]

Professional staff requirements for hospital employee health services also parallel those of other industries. The occupational health nurse is the key individual on whom day-to-day success of the program will depend. Ideally, the nurse should be trained in occupational health, but this is not an absolute prerequisite. The supervising physician is usually a primary care practitioner who provides part-time services. Less common are fully-trained occupational medicine specialists and only relatively few hospitals are large enough to justify a full-time physician. Because of differing circumstances, it is impossible to prescribe the amount of nurse and physician time required for the proper operation of an employee health service. The total number of employees served, type and location of the hospital, scope of services provided, availability of clerical assistance, and provision of cross-coverage by the emergency room during off hours are all important variables. Professional staff requirements also can be minimized by efficient interaction with administrative personnel and key hospital committees such as infection control, safety, and radiation health. Indeed, both the occupational health nurse and physician should be active members of these committees. Utilizing all the aforementioned strategies, St. Joseph's Hospital in Marshfield, Wis. has been able to provide an effective employee health program for 1,800 persons with one full-time secretary, a part-time occupational health physician, and a full-time nurse. However, our program operates in a highly cooperative atmosphere and, in most institutions, additional staff would probably be required for this number of employees.

INFECTIONS

In recent years, considerable attention has been focused on the chemical, physical, and psychological hazards of health care institutions including ethylene oxide exposure, ionizing radiation, back injuries, and stress. Yet infectious diseases continue to represent the most serious, immediate threat to the majority of employees. This risk is the most distinguishing feature between hospital workers and industrial employees, and control of infectious diseases is the major activity of most hospital employee health services. Hospital personnel may contract disease through exposure to infected patients or they may acquire infection outside the hospital environment. They may then transmit these conditions to susceptible patients, other hospital personnel, family members, or community contacts. Certain diseases such as chicken pox, which may be no more than a nuisance to a healthy individual, can be life-threatening to an immunosuppressed patient. With large numbers of young women working in hospitals, the threat from teratogenic viruses remains a constant concern.

Most hospital-acquired infections are completely preventable. One key element in any preventive effort is a formal hospital employee health service. Regardless of how such a service is organized in a particular institution, certain elements have been identified as useful in achieving infection control objectives. These include preplacement evaluations, personnel health and safety education, immunization programs, work restrictions and management of job-related illnesses and exposures, health counseling, and maintenance of health records.[77]

Preplacement Evaluations.—Personnel should undergo a preplacement evaluation to ensure they will not be placed in jobs that would pose undue risk of infection to them, patients, or fellow employees. The medical history should include a determination of the worker's immunizations status and history of any conditions which may predispose to the acquisition or transmission of certain diseases. A physical examination may provide useful supplementary information in this regard but there is little data to suggest that routine, complete physicals are essential for infection control. Similarly, there is no evidence to show that routine laboratory studies (complete blood count, serologic test for syphilis, urinalysis, or chest x-ray) or pre-employment cultures of the nose, throat, or stool are necessary. Nonetheless, the responsible physician should be free to order whatever tests seem indicated by the results of the medical history and physical examination. Serologic studies which may be useful in selected groups of hospital employees include those for rubella, hepatitis B, and chicken pox. Some of these tests may even be necessary to satisfy local or state requirements.

Personnel Health and Safety Education.—Since the reporting of many infections is dependent on individual employees and supervisors, the cooperation of hospital personnel is essential to the success of any infection control program. Such cooperation is more likely if employees are properly educated in the rationale, policies, and procedures of infection control. This material should be part of the initial job orientation and a feature of regular, ongoing educational efforts. To be optimally effective, infection control information should be geared to specific job descriptions and be presented through different modes of communication including articles in employee publications and in-service conferences. Copies of written policies and procedures should be readily available to all supervisory personnel.

Immunization Programs.—Since hospital employees have an increased risk of acquiring certain infections, maintenance of immunity is especially important not only in safeguarding their own health, but also in protecting patients. An aggressive immunization program also can reduce the pool of susceptible individuals and thereby minimize work restrictions resulting from disease exposure. The most expeditious time to administer vaccinations is during the preplacement health assessment. It is essential that the person giving the vaccine be knowledgeable about its indications, contraindications, storage, dosage, and preparation. Personnel to be immunized should be fully informed of the risk and benefits and a written note to this effect incorporated into their health record. This is particularly important for rubella and hepatitis B. Immunization recommendations for the general public are made by the U.S. Public Health Service Immunization Practices Advisory Committee (ACIP) and are published periodically in the *Morbidity and Mortality Weekly Report* (MMWR).[5]

Work Restrictions and Management of Job Related Illnesses and Exposures.—The routine surveillance of hospital infection is usually carried out by the institution's infection control office. The initial reporting of a suspected infection is primarily the responsibility of the employee and supervisor. However, once a potential problem is identified, it is the employee health service's responsibility to arrange for prompt diagnosis and treatment, to provide initial prophylaxis and to recommend appropriate work restrictions. If personnel develop a serious infection that is potentially transmissible or are in the incubation period of a disease during which infection may spread, circumstances may sometimes require that they be excluded from patient contact. Work restriction policies should be developed in close cooperation with the infection control committee and knowledgeable medical specialists. Input from hospital administration and department heads (particularly the nursing supervisor) should be sought early in this process. For any exclusion policy to be effective, it is essential that all personnel know which illnesses must be reported. To encourage such reporting, hospital administration must ensure that compliance will not result in economic penalties.

Health Counseling.—Each employee should have access to timely information about illnesses they may acquire from or transmit to patients. This is particularly important for women of childbearing age. Female personnel who may become pregnant should know about potential risks to the fetus from certain work assignments and preventive measures which might reduce those risks. Diseases with potential risk to the fetus include cytomegalovirus infection, hepatitis B, and rubella.

Maintenance of Health Records.—Maintenance of complete, confidential health records is essential. The hospital employee health record should contain the results of the initial preplacement examination, serologic studies, exposures, illnesses, and any work restrictions. In our litigious society, it is especially important that records of specific exposure incidents be kept in detail. Circumstances surrounding a disease exposure or transmission, including dates and names of personnel involved and the response by the infection control and employee health offices, should be documented in writing.

Detailed guidelines for infection control in hospital personnel have been published by the CDC.[77] Additional information on clinical manifestations, mode of transmission, and treatment can be found in other texts.[10, 44]

Selected Diseases

Rubella.—There have been numerous reports in the medical literature describing rubella outbreaks among physicians and other health care workers.[28] In our hospital, admission of an infant with congenital rubella syndrome (CRS) resulted in the exposure of 74 employees, 29 of whom were pregnant at the time. Fortunately, disease transmission did not occur but the episode did stimulate a center-wide immunization effort.[37] Cognizant of the potential risks to both health care workers and patients posed by the continued presence of rubella in the general population, professional societies,[61] associations,[58] and government agencies[62] have issued specific recommendations. Hospital or clinic employees, both male and female, who might transmit rubella to pregnant patients or other personnel, should be immune to rubella. Some states have proposed or adopted an analogous provision as part of their hospital administrative code.[64] As with any vaccination effort, objections have been raised. Although pregnancy is still a contraindication to immunization, concerns about inadvertently immunizing a pregnant woman have been shown to be much exaggerated. Since 1979, the CDC has followed prospectively 157 known rubella-susceptible pregnant women who received the RA 27/3 vaccine either within 3 months before or 3 months after conception. Although 25 elected to have induced abortions, not a single case of congenital malformations consistent with CRS was observed among the live births.[63] Fears about excessive absenteeism from adverse reactions, employee lawsuits from mandatory requirements and costs from program administration have similarly been shown to be unfounded.[37]

Tuberculosis.—Although the risk of tuberculosis (TB) has declined steadily since the turn of the century, the hospital environment remains an important site of transmission, particularly from patients with unrecognized disease. However, this risk can be reduced by an effective screening and preventive program. Screening for TB is accomplished at the time of the preplacement examination and periodically thereafter as determined by local conditions. The tuberculin skin test is the method of choice for screening and the Mantoux technique (intracutaneous injection of 0.1 ml of PPD tuberculin containing 5 TU) is the most accurate available test.[8] Multiple puncture (Tine) methods have been shown to be less sensitive.[31] A significant or positive skin test reaction is defined as 10 mm or more of induration. A two-step procedure can be used to minimize the likelihood of misinterpreting a boosted reaction as a true conversion.[73] Personnel with positive skin tests should have a chest film to exclude the presence of pulmonary disease and be placed on isoniazid (INH) chemoprophylaxis according to American Thoracic Society Recommendations.[7] After initial TB screening, policies for repeat testing can be determined after assessing the risk of acquiring infection. For employees regarded to be at significant risk, the skin test is repeated on an annual or semiannual basis. In personnel judged to be at small risk, routine skin tests are not necessary. Employees with a positive skin test who have completed an adequate course of INH chemoprophylaxis can be exempt from further screening of any kind unless symptomatic.

Personnel exposed to an infected patient need to be reevaluated. Unless a recent skin test (during the preceding three months) has been done, a baseline tuberculin test should be performed as soon as possible. All nonreactors should undergo repeat testing 10 weeks later. Personnel with significant reactions need chest x-rays to exclude pulmonary disease. All employees with active pulmonary disease must be restricted from patient care until deemed noninfectious by negative cultures or sputum smears. Personnel with positive skin tests but who cannot take preventive treatment should have their work situations evaluated. A change of assignment should be considered for those at high risk of developing active disease who also work with high-risk patients.[29]

Acquired Immune Deficiency Syndrome (AIDS).—Originally of mysterious etiology, AIDS is now known to be caused by a retrovirus, the human immune deficiency virus (HIV).[24] While no other infection has stirred such emotionalism and fear, several investigations have shown the risk of transmission of HIV to health care workers to be extremely low. In five separate studies, 666 health care workers had direct parenteral or mucus membrane exposure to the blood or body fluids of patients with AIDS or HIV infection. None of the employees whose initial serologic tests were negative developed subsequent evidence of infection. Twenty-six workers were seropositive when first tested; all but three of these persons belonged to high-risk groups. For the remaining individuals, neither a pre-exposure nor an early post-exposure serum sample was available to determine the onset of infection.[74a, 75a] A single case report from England has described a nurse who seroconverted following parenteral exposure to a contaminated needle.[8a] In spite of the extremely low risk of transmission of HIV infection, precautions are recommended to prevent spread of all blood-borne infections in the hospital environment. Care must be taken to avoid accidental wounds from needles or other sharp instruments. Contact of mucus membranes and open skin lesions with material from AIDS patients, particularly blood and blood products, should be avoided. This may require use of gloves, gowns, masks and/or eye protection. The need for emergency mouth-to-mouth resuscitation should be minimized by strategic placement of mouth pieces, resuscitation bags and other ventilation devices.[25, 34]

If a health care worker does experience parenteral or mucus membrane exposure to blood or other body fluids, the source patient should be assessed to determine the likelihood of HIV infection. If that assessment suggests infection may exist, the patient should be informed of the incident and requested to consent to serologic testing. If the source patient has AIDS or other evidence of HIV infection, declines testing or has a positive test, the exposed employee should be evaluated serologically for evidence of HIV infection as soon as possible. If seronegative, the employee should be retested after six weeks and on a periodic basis thereafter (e.g., 3, 6 and 12 months after exposure) to determine if transmission has occurred. If the source patient is seronegative and has no other evidence of HIV infection, no further follow-up of the exposed employee is necessary.[57, 57a] The difficult issue of dealing with hospital employees who refuse to care for AIDS patients has been addressed by the American Hospital Association.[1] Healthy personnel should not be excused from providing care to AIDS patients. However, intensive counseling and education are recommended for such employees before institution of disciplinary procedures.

Although there is no evidence that health care workers infected with HIV have transmitted infection to patients, risk of such transmission would exist in situations where there is both a high degree of trauma to the patient and access of blood or serous fluid from the infected health care worker to the open tissue of the patient. Employees known to be infected with HIV who do not perform invasive procedures need not be restricted from work unless they have evidence of other infection or illness for which any health care worker should be restricted. Similarly, routine serologic testing of health care workers is not recommended. Whether additional restrictions or serologic testing should be required for personnel who perform invasive procedures is currently being considered.[57a]

Herpes Simplex.—Concurrent with growing media attention on genital herpes has been increasing concern about nosocomial herpes. Employees may develop an infection of the fingers (herpetic whitlow) from exposure to oral secretions. Personnel at risk include dentists, respiratory therapists and anesthesiologists. Avoidance of direct contact with such lesions, wearing of gloves, and thorough handwashing are suggested precautions. Personnel with active, oral lesions or herpetic whitlow are considered potentially infectious, although the degree of risk is not known. It is recommended that such individuals not take care of high risk patients (newborns, burn victims, the immunocompromised, pregnant women, or patients with eczematous dermatitis) until the lesions are healed (dried and crusted). There is no evidence that employees with genital infections pose a risk to patients under usual circumstances. As with all work restrictions, the potential threat to high risk patients must be balanced against compromising patient care through suboptimal staffing. Alternate approaches to exclusionary policies have included the use of latex gloves for herpetic whitlow and application of topical antiviral agents such as acyclovir.[27]

Varicella-Zoster.—Both varicella (chicken pox) and zoster (shingles) are caused by the varicella-zoster virus (VZV). Although regarded as a common childhood disease, 5% to 10% of adults may be susceptible.[26] Because of this, nosocomial transmission of VZV among hospital personnel and patients has occurred.[45] It is advisable to identify susceptible employees at the time of the preplacement evaluation. Although most persons giving a definite previous history of chicken pox are probably immune, we have experienced an episode where a nurse with a positive past history developed chicken pox after exposure to a hospitalized case. It is now our policy to obtain a varicella zoster indirect fluoroscent antibody (VZIFA) titer on all employees who work in high risk areas. Serologic proof of immunity assists supervisors in assigning nonsusceptible personnel to care for patients with VZV infections. This avoids unnecessary work restrictions and reduces the opportunity for nosocomial transmission.

Personnel not known to be immune to chicken pox and who are exposed to an active case, either in the hospital or in the community, are advised to report to the employee health office. A VZIFA titer is drawn and results are available within 24 hours. If the VZIFA titer shows protective antibody, the employee is returned to regular duty. If the test indicates lack of immunity, the employee is restricted from working with high risk patients (immunosuppressed, pediatric, newborn, neonatal, and obstetrics) during the incubation period (10 to 21 days after exposure). While not all medical authorities would agree with the need to obtain serologic evidence of immunity in the face of a positive history, we regard this approach as prudent in view of the rapid availability of this sensitive screening test in our hospital and our past experience with a false positive history. Unfortunately, sensitive serologic screening techniques may not be readily available in all institutions. The complement fixation test is not recommended because of the high rate of false negative results. In instances where sensitive serologic studies are unavailable, it is advisable to reassign or send home recently exposed employees who have uncertain or negative histories for the duration of the infectious period.[75]

Hepatitis B.—Although nosocomial transmission of hepatitis A can occur in unusual circumstances, most outbreaks in health care personnel have been due to hepatitis B.[48] The intensity, frequency, and duration of exposures to blood and blood products place certain health workers in the high risk category including hemodialysis staff, cardiovascular and oral surgeons, laboratory technicians, phlebotomists, blood bank personnel, operating room staff, intravenous therapy nurses, and pathologists. The disease may be transmitted from persons with acute but unrecognized infections and from asymptomatic carriers of hepatitis B surface antigen (HBsAg). While the prevalence of this antigen is relatively infrequent in normal U.S. populations (0.1% to 0.5%), it may be as high as 30% in patients with Down's syndrome, lepromatous leprosy, leukemia, Hodgkin's disease, polyarteritis nodosa, or renal disease on chronic hemodialysis, or drug addicts, and male homosexuals.[16]

Prevention of hepatitis B transmission in health care institutions requires meticulous attention to the identification, care, and handling of infected patients and their clinical specimens, particularly blood.[23] Many parenteral exposures to hepatitis are the result of needle stick injuries. The risk of acquiring infection by this route from a HBsAg positive patient is approximately 6%.[69] The risk of such injuries can be reduced by proper needle disposal methods. Early administration of hepatitis B immune globulin (HBIG) is recommended for the susceptible health care worker exposed by needle-stick or mucosal contamination to specimens from a known carrier.[70] A highly efficacious vaccine against hepatitis B virus is available and should be considered for use in high risk personnel.[40] Because the actual risk of acquiring nosocomial hepatitis B varies from institution to institution, each hospital must develop an individualized strategy. Concerns to date have centered around administrative/legal issues, costs, and safety. The logistics and legalities of conducting a hepatitis B immunization program in the hospital setting have been reviewed in detail.[32] Consensus opinion is that while the decision to accept immunization is voluntary, employers may have a legal obligation to at least offer the vaccine. Although the cost of the three-injection series is approximately $125, it is considerably less expensive than the anticipated financial consequences of nosocomial hepatitis. The decision to prescreen potential vaccine recipients for susceptibility to hepatitis B is purely an economic one.

The cost of serologic tests and the prevalence of markers in the population are the two variables in determining whether screening would be cost-effective.[40] Because the plasma (Heptavax-B) vaccine is produced from human sources, which may include homosexual men, the question has arisen as to whether AIDS could be transmitted by immunization. To date, no AIDS cases in vaccine recipients have been reported outside of groups with high AIDS incidence. Nor does the risk of Guillain-Barré syndrome or other serious adverse effects seem to be increased in vaccine recipients.[72] Availability of a genetically engineered, recombinant yeast DNA vaccine (Recombivax) should obviate most concerns about disease transmission through immunization. Although the transmission of hepatitis B virus from health care professionals to patients has been reported, these persons need not be restricted from patient care responsibilities unless there is epidemiologic evidence that a specific individual is transmitting infection.[77] A carrier of HBsAg should be counseled in methods to reduce possible transmission including wearing gloves during high risk procedures and double gloving during complex surgery. Routine screening for HBsAg is not recommended except possibly in certain personnel from the high risk category such as hemodialysis staff.

Enteric Disease.—Various bacterial, viral, and protozoal agents can cause diarrhea in hospital personnel. The potential for nosocomial transmission exists, particularly if the precaution of handwashing before and after patient contact is not scrupulously observed. Employees with acute diarrhea and findings suggestive of bacterial infection (fever, abdominal cramps, bloody stools) should be excluded from patient care or food service duties pending appropriate stool cultures and treatment. Particular care is necessary in *Salmonella* enteritis because of the prolonged carriage state and risk to certain groups of patients.

When indicated by disease prevalence, all food service personnel should have appropriate cultures performed during employment exams and be required to promptly report significant gastrointestinal disease to the employee health service.[12]

Miscellaneous Infections.—Employees with an active staphylococcal skin infection (e.g., cutaneous boil) should be excluded from patient care until the lesion is healed. Because of the high carriage rate of *Staphylococcus aureus* in the anterior nares, routine cultures of nursery personnel and other hospital employees are not recommended.[47] The preferred approach is an effective surveillance program permitting prompt recognition of staphylococcal infections in patients and employees. If an asymptomatic carrier is linked to a disease outbreak, that individual should be excluded from patient contact until carriage is eradicated.

Viral upper respiratory infections present special problems because of the widespread nature of these diseases in both patients and staff. While infection of certain high risk patients is associated with significant morbidity, it may not be practical to restrict all infected personnel from taking care of such patients. The risk of transmission can be reduced by appropriate hygienic measures, particularly handwashing. Employees with influenza are usually too ill to work. Nosocomial transmission can be reduced by immunizing personnel in key areas and prophylactic use of amantadine, particularly during epidemiologic situations.

Transmission of meningococcal infection to health care workers is uncommon and usually occurs only after direct contact with respiratory secretions during intubation or mouth-to-mouth resuscitation. In such circumstances, immediate chemoprophylaxis with rifampin is indicated.

Several studies have shown that hospital employees do not have an excess risk of acquiring cytomegalovirus infection even when working in dialysis units,[74] oncology wards,[18] or pediatrics.[79] However, because of the known teratogenic potential of cytomegalovirus, some institutions have policies which prevent contact between nurses and patients with this disease.

Scabies is transmitted by direct contact with infested patients. Because an element of hysteria is often present in scabies outbreaks, proper diagnosis of pruritic skin lesions is advised before instituting treatment.

CHEMICAL HAZARDS

Waste Anesthetic Gases.—A variety of adverse health effects have been attributed to exposure to waste anesthetic gases including impaired work performance and other psychophysiologic phenomena, increased risk of spontaneous abortion and congenital anomalies, and an increased incidence of hepatic, renal, and malignant disease.[14, 49, 51] In many epidemiologic studies, these effects could not be attributed to any single anesthetic agent because various combinations had been used. In the United States, halothane and nitrous oxide are the two most common general anesthetics. Elevated ambient levels occur frequently and are usually due to inadequate scavenging systems, poor anesthetic technique, and equipment leaks. Dental, oral surgery, and outpatient operatories are less likely to have adequate ventilation and can experience ambient levels of nitrous oxide averaging 900 ppm.[76] Although there are no legal occupational exposure standards in the United States, NIOSH recommends a limit of 25 ppm nitrous oxide and 2 ppm for halogenated agents when used alone.[51] Reduction of employee exposure can be achieved through installation of scavenging systems, periodic inspection for equipment leaks, review of anesthetic technique, and annual monitoring of ambient levels.

Formaldehyde.—Exposure to formaldehyde can occur among laboratory, dialysis and housekeeping personnel. Formaldehyde is both a cutaneous irritant and skin sensitizer. Epidemics of allergic contact dermatitis have been reported among nurses[60] and dialysis employees.[71] Irritation of the eyes, nose and throat are common complaints even at relatively low concentrations. Although asthma directly caused by hypersensitivity to formaldehyde has been documented,[34] more commonly it acts as a nonspecific irritant in those with hyperreactive airways. Although formaldehyde is an animal carcinogen, whether it causes cancer in humans remains controversial. Formaldehyde has not been shown to be teratogenic in animals or humans.[11]

Asbestos.—Asbestos is generally not thought of as a hospital exposure problem. Yet some maintenance personnel do come in contact with it on an intermittent basis. Removal of friable asbestos insulation may also result in widespread environmental dissemination. Guidelines for the detection, monitoring, removal, encapsulation, and disposal of asbestos-containing building materials have been developed.[66]

Ethylene Oxide.—Ethylene oxide is used by the majority of hospitals for sterilizing medical equipment that is heat-sensitive. NIOSH has estimated that up to 100,000 employees may be exposed including those working in central supply, surgical suites, and respiratory therapy.[52] Acutely, ethylene oxide is a mucus membrane irritant and central nervous system depressant. Major concern has understandably focused on possible chronic effects, particularly adverse reproductive outcomes and neoplastic disease. Ethylene oxide has demonstrated mutagenic, cytogenic, reproductive, and carcinogenic effects in animal test systems.[43] Several studies have suggested the possibility of chronic effects in humans. Finnish investigators found an increased incidence of spontaneous abortions in ethylene oxide-exposed workers.[33] Two studies have shown an increased risk of leukemia following occupational exposure to ethylene oxide,[35, 36] but a third has failed to confirm this observation.[50] Health risks can be minimized by reducing employee exposure which occurs from opening the door after the cycle is completed, transferring sterilized goods to the aerator and changing tanks containing the gas.[65] An alarm system in the tank changing area and a written emergency protocol are also advised. OSHA has reduced the exposure limit from 50 ppm to a 1 ppm time-weighted average. It also requires periodic employee exposure monitoring and medical surveillance for personnel exposed above the "action level" of 0.5 ppm.[54]

Chemotherapeutic Agents.—The risks to patients receiving high doses of various chemotherapeutic agents are well known. Acute systemic effects and myelosuppression are relatively common. There also is considerable evidence that such agents are fetotoxic and carcinogenic in humans.[42] However, possible risks to health care personnel handling antineoplastic drugs have been recognized only recently. Studies have shown increased mutagenic activity in the urine of nurses[19] and pharmacists[53] handling chemotherapeutic agents. The health implications of these findings are unclear inasmuch as epidemiologic studies to detect increased incidence of neoplastic disease or adverse reproductive outcomes in exposed personnel are not available. Nonetheless, health care personnel should be afforded maximum protection during the preparation and administration of these drugs. Many facilities have found the National Cancer Institute's guidelines useful in establishing their own policies.[59] A vertical laminar airflow hood is recommended for areas where large volumes of drugs are prepared. In the absence of such a unit, an appropriate respirator and safety glasses are recommended. Avoidance of direct skin contact can be accomplished by polyvinyl gloves and gowns. Personnel who are at risk of exposure to these agents should be instructed as to the nature of the hazard and the precautions to be taken. Materials contaminated with cytotoxic drugs should be handled as a hazardous chemical waste. Pregnant personnel should be offered the option of transfer to other duties.

ACCIDENTS

Hospital workers have a higher incidence of job-related injuries than do office workers or employees in other service fields.[2] Nurses, food service workers, and maintenance personnel have been identified as being at highest risk.[46] At St. Joseph's Hospital in Marshfield, Wisconsin, nurses, food service workers, and housekeeping personnel account for 79% of accidents even though they represent only 65% of the work force. The most common types of incidents at our hospital are minor trauma (lacerations, bruises, abrasions), needle punctures, back injuries, and slips and falls.

While needle sticks and other local trauma tend to be the most common accidents in the hospital environment, back injuries are the leading cause of lost work time. While representing only 13% of all incidents at our hospital, back problems account for 62% of all lost work days. Nurses are especially vulnerable to back injuries during patient transfer activities. The wide variety of approaches advocated to control the incidence and severity of back injuries is prima facie evidence that no single method is clearly superior. Use of routine preplacement lumbar spine films has declined in view of their associated costs, radiation exposure, and lack of predictive value.[6] Low back x-rays should not be used as routine screening procedures but rather as a special diagnostic test available to the physician on appropriate indications for study.[30] Federal legislation and court decisions have also contributed to the decline of preplacement back x-rays by restricting the employer's right to refuse employment to those circumstances where the applicant may represent substantial risk of harm to himself or others. A bony defect on x-ray, particularly in an asymptomatic individual, is unlikely to be regarded as a substantial risk.

Nonetheless, a thorough preplacement evaluation can be useful in documenting preexisting disability for the purpose of future worker's compensation claims, particularly in those states with subsequent injury (second injury) funds. A preplacement evaluation also affords the physician the opportunity to counsel the employee about the risks of low back injury in the hospital setting and to discuss proper lifting techniques. More formal training programs, such as body mechanics courses, are becoming increasingly popular in hospital and industrial settings. While the effectiveness of such training programs has yet to be demonstrated in controlled studies, one could hardly question the potential value of knowing proper lifting techniques and the safe use of wheelchairs, lifts, rollers, and other transfer devices.

While decreasing the incidence of low back injuries has proven difficult, some hospitals have experienced success in reducing their severity by encouraging employees to return to work in light or restricted duty positions. One institution reported a 40%

decline in lost work days after such a program was instituted.[22] Isometric strength tests have been shown to be valid indicators of potential risk of future back injury.[13] These and other aspects of low back pain are discussed in detail elsewhere in this text and in a U.S. Government publication entitled "Work Practices Guide for Manual Lifting."[78]

RADIATION

Ionizing radiation is one of the most well-recognized hazards in the hospital environment and considerable effort has been directed at its control. If all radiation-emitting equipment were used exclusively in x-ray departments by trained personnel, there would be little cause for concern. However, portable x-ray equipment, radioisotopes, and the need for fluoroscopic guidance in surgical procedures and cardiac catheterization have greatly expanded the number of personnel exposed. The reduction of exposure to an individual from external sources may be achieved by any combination of the following: (1) increasing the distance of the individual from the source; (2) reducing the duration of exposure; and (3) using protective barriers (shielding) between the individual and the source. Personnel monitoring (film badges) is used to check the adequacy of the radiation protection program. The National Council on Radiation Protection (NCRP) has set the present maximum permissible whole body occupational exposure at 5 rems/year. The maximum accumulative dose cannot exceed a number designated by the formula 5(N-18), where N refers to the individual's age in years. The maximum permissible dose to the fetus from occupational exposure of the pregnant mother should not exceed 0.5 rem during the entire pregnancy.[9] In effect, this implies that such women should be employed only in situations where the annual dose is unlikely to exceed 2 to 3 rems and is acquired at a more or less steady rate. In such cases, the probability of the dose to the fetus exceeding 0.5 rem before delivery is unlikely. In our institution, pregnant technologists are not permitted to participate in fluoroscopic procedures and are given the option of complete removal from radiation exposure for the duration of their pregnancy. Increased use of diagnostic devices such as digital subtraction angiography and nuclear magnetic resonance (NMR) will reduce radiation exposure to health care personnel. Further reductions can be achieved by eliminating unnecessary preplacement and periodic x-rays, particularly those of the chest and low back. (See Chapter 26 for further details.)

WELLNESS, EMPLOYEE ASSISTANCE PROGRAMS

In an attempt to control rising costs from employee illness and to improve job satisfaction, hospital administrators have demonstrated increasing interest in programs of primary prevention, also known as wellness programs. Such efforts can include smoking cessation, hypertension screening and follow-up, exercise, diet modification, auto safety, and employee assistance programs (EAP).[20] Those components adopted in a given setting depend on the availability of financial and personnel resources, the institution's perception of need, the interest of the employee population, and the existence of similar programs in the community. Smoking cessation and hypertension screening are of proven efficacy and can be expected to provide the highest return per dollar invested.[21] Once such programs are established for a medical center's employees, they can be marketed to the rest of the community and to local industry.

Health care workers function in a high stress environment brought on by the need to care for the psychologic and physical needs of sick patients. Resultant stress may contribute to various physiologic and psychologic disorders including depression, anxiety, alcoholism, drug abuse, and even suicide. Various coping techniques have been delineated including relaxation exercises, recreational activities, and assertiveness skills.[68] Employee assistance programs also have become increasingly available to assist workers and their families in resolving health or other problems that may be affecting work performance or personal well-being. Our EAP covers a broad range of behavioral-medical problems including those related to emotional difficulties, family or marital discord, financial or legal concerns, and substance abuse. The program coordinator assists employees in determining the nature of the problem and in locating appropriate counseling or other assistance. This may be from within or outside the medical center but is always strictly confidential. While referral for diagnosis and treatment does not by itself jeopardize the employee's job security, continued poor job performance may eventuate in disciplinary action.

CONCLUSION

The occupational health concerns of those who care for the sick and disabled are finally receiving much needed attention. In times of increasing economic constraints, it can only be hoped that sufficient resources will be devoted to protecting health care workers so they can, in the words of Ramazzini, "continue to exercise their calling without harm."

REFERENCES

1. *A Hospital-Wide Approach to AIDS*. Recommendations of the Advisory Committee on Infection Within Hospitals. Chicago, American Hospital Association, December, 1983.
2. Accident Facts. Chicago, National Safety Council, 1983.
3. Acquired immune deficiency syndrome (AIDS): Precautions for clinical and laboratory staff. *MMWR* 1982; 31:557.
4. Acquired immune deficiency syndrome (AIDS): Precautions for healthcare workers and allied professionals. *MMWR* 1983; 32:450.
5. *Adult Immunization—Recommendations of the Immunization Practices Advisory Committee* (ACIP). MMWR 1984; 33:1S.
6. American College of Radiology, American Academy of Orthopedic Surgery and the Industrial Medical Association: Conference on Low Back X-rays in Pre-employment Physical Examinations. *Summary Report and Proceedings*. Tucson, Arizona, American College of Radiology/NIOSH, January 11–14, 1973.
7. American Thoracic Society, American Lung Association, and Center for Disease Control: Preventive therapy of tuberculous infection. *Am Rev Respir Dis* 1974; 110:371.
8. American Thoracic Society Executive Committee: The tuberculin skin test. *Am Rev Respir Dis* 1981; 124:356.

8a. Anonymous: Needlestick transmission of HTLV-III from a patient infected in Africa. *Lancet* 1984; 2:1376.

9. Basic Radiation Protection Criteria—NCRP Report No. 39. National Council on Radiation Protection and Measurements, 1971.

10. Beneson AS (ed): *Control of Communicable Diseases in Man*, ed 13. Washington, American Public Health Association, 1981.

11. Brooks SM, Reinhardt CF: Health effects of formaldehyde, in *Formaldehyde and Other Aldehydes*. Washington, National Academy Press, 1981.

12. Brown TC, Kreider SD, Lange WR: Guidelines for employee health services in hospitals, clinics and medical research institutions. *J Occup Med* 1983; 25:771.

13. Chaffin DB, Herrin GD, Keyserling WM: Pre-employment strength testing—an updated position. *J Occup Med* 1978; 20:403.

14. Cottrell JE (ed): *Occupational Hazards to Operating Room and Recovery Room Personnel*. International Anesthesiology Clinics, Vol 19, 1981.

15. DeRonde MM, Mason ME: Hospital employee health issues. *Occup Health Nurs* 1984; 32:44.

16. Dienstaz JL, Wands JR, Koff RS: Acute hepatitis, in Petersdorf RG, Adams RD, Braunwald E (eds): *Principles of Internal Medicine*. New York, McGraw-Hill Book Co, 1983.

17. Douglass BE: Occupational health programs in clinics and hospitals, in Zenz C (ed): *Occupational Medicine: Principles and Practical Applications*, ed 1. Chicago, Year Book Medical Publishers, 1975.

18. Duvall CP, Casozza AR, Grimley PM, et al: Recovery of cytomegalovirus from adults with neoplastic disease. *Ann Intern Med* 1966; 65:531.

19. Falch K, Grolin P, Sorsa M, et al: Mutagenicity in urine of nurses handling cytostatic drugs. *Lancet* 1979; 1:1250.

20. Fielding JE: Preventive medicine and the bottom line. *J Occup Med* 1979; 21:79.

21. Fielding JE: Effectiveness of employee health improvement programs. *J Occup Med* 1982; 24:907.

22. Fight back injury pain, costs with light duty, education. *Hospital Employee Health* 1983; 2:48.

23. Fravero MS, Maynard JE, Leger RT, et al: Guidelines for care of patients hospitalized with viral hepatitis. *Ann Intern Med* 1979; 91:872.

24. Gallo R, Salahuddin SZ, Popovic M, et al: Frequent detection and isolation of cytopathic retroviruses (HTLV-III) from patients with AIDS and at risk for AIDS. *Science* 1984; 224:500.

25. Garner JS, Simmons BP: Guideline for isolation precautions in hospitals. *Infect Control* 1983; 4:245.

26. Gershon AA, Raber R, Steinberg S, et al: Antibody to varicella-zoster virus in parturient women and their offspring during their first year of life. *Pediatrics* 1976; 5:692.

27. Greaves WL, Kaiser AB, Alford RH, et al: The problem of herpetic whitlow among hospital personnel. *Infect Control* 1980; 1:381.

28. Greaves WL, Orenstein WA, Stetler HC, et al: Prevention of rubella transmission in medical facilities. *JAMA* 1982; 248:861.

29. Guidelines for prevention of T.B. transmission in hospitals. Atlanta, US Department of Health and Human Services, Center for Disease Control, HHS Publication No (CDC)82-8371, 1982.

30. Guidelines for use of routine x-ray examination in occupational medicine—Committee Report. *J Occup Med* 1979; 21:500.

31. Hansen JP, Falconer JA, Gallis HA, et al. Inadequate sensitivity of tuberculin tine test for screening employee populations. *J Occup Med* 1982; 24:602.

32. Harben K (ed): *Hepatitis B Vaccine—Weighing the Choices*. Atlanta, American Health Consultants, 1982.

33. Hemminski K, Mutanen P, Saloniemi I, et al: Spontaneous abortions in hospital staffs engaged in sterilizing instruments with chemical agents. *Br Med J* 1982; 285:1461.

34. Hendrick DJ, Lande DJ: Occupational formalin asthma. *Br J Ind Med* 1977; 34:11.

35. Hogstedt C, Rohlen O, Berndtsson BS, et al: A cohort study of mortality and cancer incidence in ethylene oxide production workers. *Br J Ind Med* 1979; 36:276.

36. Hogstedt C, Malmquist N, Wadman B: Leukemia in workers exposed to ethylene oxide. *JAMA* 1979; 241:1132.

37. Horvath EP: The healthcare worker and rubella. *Wis Med J* 1984; 83:15.

38. Hospital employee health—Practical solutions to current and potential problems. *Proceedings of the First National Conference on Hospital Employee Health*. January 14–15, 1982, American Health Consultants, Inc, Atlanta, Georgia.

39. Hospital occupational health services study. US Department of Health, Education and Welfare, National Institute of Occupational Safety and Health, Division of Technical Services, Vol 1–7, Cincinnati, Ohio, 1976.

40. Immunization Practices Advisory Committee: Recommendations on inactivated hepatitis B virus vaccine. *MMWR* 1982; 31:317.

41. Infection control, in *Accreditation Manual for Hospitals*. Chicago, Joint Commission on Accreditation of Hospitals, 1984.

42. Jones RB, Frank R, Mass RN: Safe handling of chemotherapeutic agents: A report from the Mt. Sinai Medical Center. *Cancer J Clinicians* 1983; 33:258.

43. Landrigan PJ, Meinhardt TJ, Gordon J, et al: Ethylene oxide: An overview of toxicologic and epidemiologic research. *Am J Ind Med* 1984; 6:103.

44. Last JM (ed): *Public Health and Preventive Medicine*, ed 11. New York, Appleton-Century-Crofts, 1980.

45. LeClair JM, Zaia JA, Levin MJ, et al: Airborne transmission of chickenpox in a hospital. *N Engl J Med* 1980; 302:450.

46. Lewy R: Preventive strategies in hospital occupational medicine. *J Occup Med* 1981; 23:109.

47. Maki DG: *Solution to Common Infectious Disease Problems in Hospital Employee Health—Practical Solution to Current and Potential Problems*. Atlanta, American Health Consultants, Inc, 1982.

48. Maynard JE: Viral hepatitis as an occupational hazard in the health care profession, in Vyas GN, Cohen SN, Schmid R (ed): *Viral Hepatitis*. Philadelphia, Franklin Institute Press, 1978.

49. Messite J, Bond MB: Waste anesthetic gases and vapors, in Zenz C (ed): *Developments in Occupational Medicine*. Chicago, Year Book Medical Publishers, 1980.

50. Morgan RW, Claxton KW, Divine BJ, et al: Mortality among ethylene oxide workers. *J Occup Med* 1981; 23:767.

51. National Institute for Occupational Safety and Health: Criteria for a recommended standard: Occupational exposure to waste anesthetic gases and vapors. DHEW (NIOSH) Pub No 77-140, 1977.

52. National Institute for Occupational Safety and Health: Special occupational hazard review with control recommendations: Use of ethylene oxide as a sterilant in medical facilities. DHEW, PHS, NIOSH 77-200, 1977.

53. Nguyen TV, Theiss JC, Matuey TS: Exposure of pharmacy personnel to mutagenic antineoplastic drugs. *Cancer Res* 1982; 42:4792.

54. Occupational Safety and Health Administration: Occupational exposure to ethylene oxide, final standard. *Federal Register* 1984; 49:25734.

55. Omenn GS: Occupational hazards to health care workers: Report of a conference. *Am J Ind Med* 1984; 6:129.

56. Parker JE: Basic components of a hospital employee health program. *Occup Health Nurs* 1982; 30:21.

56a. Patterson WB, Craven DE, Schwartz DA, et al: Occupational hazards to hospital personnel. *Ann Intern Med* 1985; 102:658.

57. Prospective evaluation of healthcare workers exposed via parenteral or mucous membrane routes to blood and body fluids of patients

with acquired immunodeficiency syndrome. *MMWR* 1984; 33:181.

57a. Recommendations for preventing transmission of infection with HTLV-III/LAV in the workplace. *MMWR* 1985; 34:681.

58. Recommendations for the control of rubella within hospitals. Advisory Committee on Infections Within Hospitals, American Hospital Association, Chicago, 1981.

59. Recommendations for the safe handling of parenteral antineoplastic drugs. Prepared by the Division of Safety, in collaboration with the Clinical Center Pharmacy and Nursing Staff, and the National Cancer Institute. Bethesda, Maryland, US Department of Health and Human Services, Public Health Service, NIH Pub No 83-2621, 1982.

60. Rostenberg A, Bairstow B, Luther T: A study of eczematous sensitivity to formaldehyde. *J Invest Dermatol* 1952; 19:459.

61. Rubella—A clinical update. American College of Obstetricians and Gynecologists (ACOG) Technical Bulletin No 62, 1981.

62. Rubella prevention—Recommendations of the Immunization Practices Advisory Committee (ACIP). *MMWR* 1984; 33:301.

63. Rubella vaccination during pregnancy—United States, 1971–1983. *MMWR* 1984; 33:365.

64. Rules and regulations for licensing of hospitals (R23-16-HOSP), State of Rhode Island Department of Health, 1979.

65. Samuels TM: Exposure reduction through personnel training and safe practices and procedures. *Proceedings from In Hospital Ethylene Oxide Sterilization*. Arlington, Virginia, Association for the Advancement of Medical Instrumentation, 1984.

66. Sawyer RN, Spooner CM: Sprayed asbestos-containing materials in buildings—A guidance document. Research Triangle Park, NC: US Environmental Protection Agency, Pub No EPA 450/2-78-014, 1978.

67. Scope of occupational health programs and occupational medical practice—Committee Report. *J Occup Med* 1979; 21:497.

68. Scully R: Stress in the nurse. *Am J Nurs* 1980; 8:912.

69. Seeff LB, Wright EC, Zimmerman HJ, et al: Type B hepatitis after needle stick exposure: Prevention with hepatitis B immune globulin. Final Report of the Veterans Administration Cooperative Study. *Ann Intern Med* 1978; 88:285.

70. Seeff LB, Koff RS: Passive and active immunoprophylaxis of hepatitis B. *Gastroenterology* 1984; 86:958.

71. Sneddon JB: Dermatitis in an intermittent hemodialysis unit. *Br Med J* 1968; 1:183.

72. The Safety of Hepatitis B virus vaccine. *MMWR* 1983; 32:134.

73. Thompson NJ, Glassroth JL, Snider DE, et al: The booster phenomenon in serial tuberculin testing. *Am Rev Respir Dis* 1979; 119:587.

74. Tolhoff-Rubin NE, Rubin RH, Keller EE, et al: Cytomegalovirus infection in dialysis patients and personnel. *Ann Intern Med* 1978; 89:625.

74a. Update: Evaluation of human t-lymphotropic virus type III/lymphadenopathy associated virus infection in health care personnel—United States. *MMWR* 1985; 34:575.

75. Valenti WM: Prevention and control of nosocomial viral diseases in hospital employee health—Practical solutions to current and potential problems. Atlanta, Georgia, American Health Consultants, 1982.

75a. Weiss SH, Saxinger WC, Rechtman D, et al: HTLV-III infection among health care workers: Association with needle-stick injuries. *JAMA* 1985; 254:2089.

76. Whitcher CE, Zimmerman DC, Piziali RL: Control of occupational exposure to N_2O in the dental operatory. NIOSH Technical Information, DHEW (NIOSH) Pub No 77-171, 1977.

77. Williams WW: Guideline for infection control in hospital personnel. Centers for Disease Control. *Infect Control* 1983; 4:326.

78. Work practices guide for manual lifting. US Department of Health and Human Services, National Institute for Occupational Safety and Health, DHHS (NIOSH) Pub No 81-122, 1981.

79. Yaeger AS: Longitudinal, serological study of cytomegalovirus infections in nurses and in personnel without patient contact. *J Clin Microbiol* 1975; 2:448.

59

Agricultural Occupational Medicine

Kelley J. Donham, M.S., D.V.M.

Edward P. Horvath, Jr., M.D., M.P.H.

> Agricultural medicine encompasses the anticipation, recognition, diagnosis, treatment, prevention, and community health aspects of health problems peculiar to agricultural populations.[4]

Although the general public may perceive the farm population as a very healthy group, available information tends to dispel this misconception. Some surveys comparing them to other occupations have shown farmers experiencing the highest rate of hospital discharges[2] and the highest disease rates.[3] National data confirm that farmers have the highest rates of impairment for disorders of the back or spine, certain chronic heart conditions, serious respiratory disorders, and disabling mental conditions.[6] These health problems are present in one of the largest occupational groups in the U.S. The estimated 13.8 million people at risk include 2 million persons who report sole or primary self-employment income from agriculture, 3.1 million who report some self-employment income, 6.0 million additional farm family members,[1] and 2.7 million hired farm workers.[8]

In 1955, the University of Iowa's Institute of Agricultural Medicine was founded as the first organization at a medical school with the objective of research and service relative to occupational health concerns in agriculture. The founders of this institute realized that, relative to the size of the exposed population and the magnitude of the problem, there was little research in agricultural medicine. Also, there were only a few knowledgeable health professionals and no organized mechanism for delivery of occupational health services to the agricultural community. As the field of agricultural medicine evolved at the University of Iowa, it developed a comprehensive approach, encompassing the disciplines of industrial hygiene, safety, community health, and both human and veterinary medicine. It was felt this strategy would exert the greatest impact on existing problems given the limited resources available. However, the delivery of occupational health services to the agricultural community is ultimately in the hands of individual primary care physicians, medical clinics, and hospitals serving rural areas.

Agricultural medicine is properly a field of occupational medicine. However, occupational health issues in agriculture present unique problems. Inherent peculiarities of agriculture have resulted in a relative lack of attention to occupational health concerns.[4] Perhaps a fundamental reason is the absence of an organized labor force characteristic of such industries as mining and manufacturing, where traditional labor-management relationships prevail. In agriculture, hired workers comprise only a small portion of an industry which is dominated by family farm operations, where labor and management are one-and-the-same. Farmers are a relatively unorganized group, and their political activities have been almost entirely economic- and production-oriented.[5] Government agencies such as the Occupational Safety and Health Administration (OSHA), the National Institute for Safety and Health (NIOSH), and the U.S. Department of Agriculture (USDA) have generally paid little attention to occupational health issues in agriculture because of political considerations, absence of pressure from the farm groups, or lack of recognition and priority by the agency.[7, 9] Agriculture is geographically diverse, resulting in a variety of operations, exposures, and subsequent health hazards across the country. Agriculture is dynamic across time; so, as new processes and equipment are developed, new health hazards arise. Finally, the very nature of agricultural work (Table 59–1) complicates resolution of occupational health problems.

Although the extension agricultural safety programs at our land grant universities have been cut back in recent years, there has been increased awareness of agricultural health problems and a growing commitment to their solution in other sectors. At least three university programs deal with agricultural health concerns (the Institute of Agricultural Medicine and Occupational Health, University of Iowa, the Institute for Rural Environmental Health, Colorado State University, and the Agromedicine Program, Medical University of South Carolina). An agricultural medicine center has been established by the nation's largest rural clinic (the National Farm Medicine Center, Marshfield Clinic and Medical Foun-

TABLE 59–1
Characteristics of Agricultural Work

Agricultural practices and associated health problems vary with topography, climate, the economy, and social factors.
Rapid technologic advances in agricultural practices constantly are creating new health problems.
Farmers, who typically are stoic and independent, assume and accept rather than challenge occupational health hazards.
Agricultural work is performed by women, children, and the elderly, as well as by men 20–65 years old.
There is little formal training for farmers.
Farmers usually must do their own repairs.
There is no preplacement examination to determine "fitness for work."
It is difficult for the farmer to change jobs if not suited medically to farming.
There is no limit to the length of the workday, which often is erratic and determined by weather or machinery breakdowns.
Vacations are limited.
Farmers often work alone in an isolated environment.
Personal hygiene facilities may be few and remote.
Emergency medical services may not be accessible.
Medical benefits and workman's compensation do not apply to the self-employed farmer.
Rehabilitation after an illness or an accident often is left to the individual.
Farmers do not have access to occupational health specialists other than the Extension Agricultural Safety Specialist (one per state), whose activities are limited by scope, training, and resources to dissemination of safety information.

dation, Marshfield, Wisconsin). Economic considerations have provided additional impetus. The largest farm organization (Farm Bureau) has realized that improving occupational health and safety conditions is important in decreasing insurance claims.[5] We envision that there will be a growing demand for specialists knowledgeable in agricultural health and that the future may witness the development of a more organized occupational health delivery system to serve rural America.

REFERENCES

1. Banks VJ, Kalbacher JZ: *Farm Income Recipients and Their Families: A Socio-economic Profile*, Rural Development Research Report 30. US Dept of Agriculture, Economic Research Service, 1981, pp 1–10.
2. Data from health interview survey. National Center for Health Statistics, US Dept of Health, Education and Welfare, cited in *Health and Work in America: A Chart Book*. Washington, DC, American Public Health Association, 1975, pp 64–65.
3. *Doctor's First Report of Work Injury*. San Francisco, Cal, Agriculture and Services Agency, Dept of Industrial Relations, Division of Labor Statistics and Research, 1974, p 5.
4. Donham KJ, Mutel CF: Agricultural Medicine: The missing component of the rural health movement. *J Fam Pract* 1982; 14:511.
5. Donham KJ: Health and safety in rural areas—Whose responsibility? Presented at the American Farm Bureau Annual Meeting, Rural Health Conference, Jan 10, 1984.
6. Haber LD: Disabling effects of chronic disease and impairment. *J Chronic Dis* 1971; 24:482.
7. Higby A: Official unconcern about farm health, in Strange M (ed): *It's Not All Sunshine and Fresh Air—Chronic Health Effects of Modern Farming Practices*. Walthill, Neb, Center for Rural Affairs, 1984, pp 77–104.
8. Pollack SL: *The Hired Farm Working Force*. Agricultural Economic Report 473. US Dept of Agriculture, Economic Research Service, 1981, pp 1–20.
9. The American Conference of Governmental Industrial Hygienists, Agricultural Health and Safety Committee: Solomon's baby—The farmer (Guest editorial). *Am Ind Hyg Assoc J* 1980; 41:A–4.

CONDITIONS CAUSED BY PHYSICAL AGENTS

Accidents

Accidents are the primary cause of documented morbidity and mortality among farmers. Approximately 2,000 accidental deaths and 200,000 disabling injuries occur annually.[1] Based on rates of fatal work accidents, agriculture is either the first or second (depending on the year) most hazardous industry, rivaled only by mining and construction.[1] Agricultural technology increasingly has emphasized mechanization, and machines have been responsible for the majority of farm traumas.[4] However, farm animals are still an important source of injury.

Farm injuries present a unique challenge to the medical care system, because the farmer often works alone and may not be discovered until hours after the accident. Also, the accident may occur in a location (such as a barn lot or field) which is not easily reached by conventional emergency rescue vehicles. Emergency medical service personnel may not have the knowledge, experience, or equipment required to remove a person from under a tractor or for releasing a part of the victim's body from a machine.[5]

Besides the delay in treatment and deficiencies in emergency services, an additional unique feature of agricultural trauma is that the injury is often contaminated with soil or animal fecal material. Resultant wound infections may involve antibiotic-resistant bacteria because of the resistant microflora in the farm setting due to the common use of antibiotic-containing animal feeds.[5] Trauma induced by farm machinery is often severe; massive crushing or severing types of injuries are not unusual. Grain augers, power take-off shafts, balers, and cornpickers are all capable of producing such injuries. The cornpicker inflicts a particularly devastating wound most often involving the dominant hand and resulting in amputation, infection, and severe disability.[7]

Fatal accidents are particularly common in the rural environment. Wisconsin averaged 77 farm fatalities annually between 1976 and 1980. The incidence of 24.9 per 100,000 farm population was higher than the state's death rate for injuries related to motor vehicles.[3] These state figures are reflective of national statistics which show death rates for most unintentional injuries to be highest in rural areas.[2] Not surprisingly, these high rates are in large part due to accidents involving machinery. Of the approximately 1,500 machinery-related deaths reported nationally in

1980, more than half involved farm equipment. Detailed analysis of death certificate information on 4,500 farm machinery fatalities in the United States from 1975 to 1980 revealed that about three quarters involved tractors. The major problems were tractor overturns, falling from and/or being run over by tractors, and entanglement by the power take-off shaft. Cornpickers, augers, and combines also cause a substantial number of deaths.[6]

There are varied and complex reasons for the high accident rate in agriculture. Many of these are related to the basic characteristics of farming as listed in Table 59–1. The farm population includes very young workers who may be inexperienced, as well as elderly persons who may have physiologic impairments. Long working hours during certain seasons, such as planting and harvesting, contribute to fatigue and carelessness. Statistical analyses tend to confirm these observations. Age-specific farm machinery death rates differ markedly from rates for other machinery. Deaths from non-farm machinery peak at ages 20–24 and are rare among children. Farm machinery death rates, on the other hand, are lowest at ages 20–24; they are highest at ages 65–74, when deaths from other causes of occupational injury are uncommon.[2] A substantial number of deaths also involve children and adolescents. In Wisconsin, 22% of all fatal farm mishaps occur in those age 14 or under.[3] Analyses of farm accidents by month of death indicate that fatalities are most likely to occur during periods of peak activity such as planting and harvesting. In addition to operator error due to age-related physiologic impairment, inexperience or fatigue, the farm implement itself is a factor in many accidents. Unlike motor vehicles, home appliances and other consumer goods, farm machinery is not covered by federal product safety standards. Some equipment, particularly older models, may have been inadequately designed for safe operation. Outdated machines are common on farms, where equipment must last for 20 years or more. The fact that most family farms are exempt from OSHA enforcement standards also probably contributes to the high accident rate.

Because of the nature of farm work and the behavior of the farmer, treatment of injuries is complicated. Often the farmer will start working as soon as possible after the accident, because there is no one else to do the work. Treatment regimens must be developed and implemented with this in mind. Rehabilitation is also a very difficult task following severe injuries. Often rehabilitation services are not available and the farmer is left to his own devices. But rehabilitation to get the farmer back to his work is important because farming in many areas is still a way of life, not just a job. Also in many rural communities, there are very few other employment possibilities.

Prevention of farm accidents, especially those resulting from farm machinery, is difficult at best. Improvements have been made in machinery design in recent years, particularly in power take-off guards and tractor roll-over protection devices. However, a substantial number of older tractors do not have roll-over protection and existing power take-off shields can be circumvented during maintenance and not be replaced. Protective devices need to be developed to retrofit older machinery economically. Tractors need improved design to prevent backward or sideward overturns. Cornpickers should have a means to clear rollers jammed by cornstalks so that farmers need not risk their hands. Emergency response personnel must be better trained to handle farm accidents, particularly those requiring machinery extrication or rescue from enclosed spaces. Physicians and surgeons in rural areas must be prepared not only to treat farm injuries effectively, but also to assist in the rehabilitation process. Finally, innovative and effective programs to educate the farmer and his family are necessary to improve attitudes and behavior relative to farm safety.

REFERENCES

1. *Accident Facts*. Chicago, National Safety Council, 1981, pp 23, 24, 32, 85–88.
2. Baker SP, O'Neill B, Karpf RS: *The Injury Fact Book*. Lexington, Mass, DC Heath and Co, 1984.
3. *Fatal Farm Accidents in Accidental and Violent Deaths—Wisconsin, 1976–1980*. Madison, Wis, Dept of Health and Social Services, Division of Health, 1984.
4. Knapp LW: Agricultural injury preventions. *J Occup Med* 1965; 7:545.
5. Knapp LE, Mutel CF, Peircy L, et al: An introduction to agricultural traumas, Slide/tape presentation S-3784-X. National Library of Medicine, National Medical Audiovisual Center, 1977.
6. McKnight RH: *US Agricultural Equipment Fatalities 1975–1981: Implications for Injury Control and Health Education*. Johns Hopkins University, doctoral dissertation, 1984.
7. Melvin PM: Cornpicker injuries of the hand. *Arch Surg* 1984; 104:26.

Hearing Loss

A number of investigators have reported increased hearing loss in farmers as compared to other occupational groups or to the general population.[2, 3, 6–8, 10, 12–14] Although older farmers generally show higher hearing thresholds,[10, 12] impairment has been documented among younger individuals in their 20s.[1, 13] Those frequencies most sensitive to noise (4,000–6,000 Hz) are affected initially. With continued exposure, the loss increases in degree and extends to involve both lower and higher frequencies. Usually, the greater loss occurs in the left ear. This has been attributed to the common habit of tractor drivers looking over their right shoulder to observe their work. This directs the left ear toward the noise source, the open end of the exhaust located at the front of the tractor.[8, 10]

Among patients in rural Wisconsin referred to the Marshfield Clinic for audiometry, both farmers and their spouses showed greater hearing loss than did nonfarmers. At 4,000 Hz, the mean hearing thresholds were 54 dB and 32 dB for male and female farm workers, respectively. For nonfarming males and females of similar age distribution, the hearing thresholds at the same frequency were 30 and 22 dB, respectively. This decline in hearing among farmers was not solely attributable to aging. At 4,000 Hz, there was no significant difference in hearing loss between farmers from 20 to 29 years of age and those 50 to 69 years old.[11]

Hearing surveys and studies reported to date have exhibited various weaknesses, including selection bias, inadequate noise exposure data, technical problems with audiometry (elevated ambient noise levels, failure to test all frequencies), and inability to control for a temporary threshold shift. Despite these weaknesses, the consistency of findings cannot be ignored. Further, the fact that farmers are exposed to noise levels in excess of 90 dBA has been well documented. One survey found farm tractor noise levels ranging from 92 to 106 dB.[15] In another study, noise levels on tractors and other types of farm machinery were recorded at the operator's ear position. Overall sound pressure level for 58 tractors operating at 75% of full load ranged from 98 dB to 113 dB with a mean of 103.5 dB. Several other types of farm equipment were also evaluated, including a cornpicker, picker-sheller, snowblower, reciprocal blade power saw, combines, elevator operators, and dryers. The overall noise levels ranged from 92 dB for the electric burr mill to a high of 114 dB for a gasoline-operated reciprocal blade power saw.[5] Farmers also experience considerable noise exposure from recreational activities involving snowmobiles, speedboats, guns, and motorcycles.[14]

Although modern hearing aids can benefit most patients with sensorineural hearing loss by selective amplification of certain frequencies, they are no substitute for prevention. The nature and organization of most farm work in the United States precludes development and enforcement of an industrial-type hearing conservation program. Nonetheless, certain preventive principles can be applied to the farm setting. Sound-tight tractor cabs, improved mufflers, and other noise attenuating devices are available on newer farm equipment.[9] However, many farmers cannot afford to invest in new machinery, and continue to use older, noisier equipment.

There is clearly a need for expanded educational efforts, use of hearing protection devices, and periodic monitoring audiometry. Organizations, agencies, and extension services having regular contact with farmers are natural outlets for information on noise exposure and hearing. Use of the mass media, both print and electronic, greatly expands the available audience. Physicians practicing in rural areas have a responsibility to evaluate their patients for noise-induced hearing loss. Routine medical history should include questions about noise exposure, tinnitis, and subjective impairment, both temporary and permanent. In addition to the usual otolaryngologic examination, an air conduction audiogram should be obtained. Farmers should be educated as to the importance of hearing protection and samples of various types of hearing protectors should be available for demonstration purposes. It is especially important for young farmers to use hearing protection and to have their hearing examined regularly.[4] (See Chapter 20, Occupational Hearing Loss, Noise, and Hearing Conservation.)

REFERENCES

1. Bunch CC: The diagnosis of occupational or traumatic deafness—A historical and audiometric study. *Laryngoscope* 1937; 47:615.
2. Feldman M, Downing CGE: Tractor noise pollution on the farm. Problems and recommendations. *Can Agricul Eng* 1972; 14:2.
3. Glorig A, Wheeler D, Twiggle R, et al: 1954 Wisconsin State Fair Hearing Survey—Statistical treatment of clinical and audiometric data. Los Angeles, American Academy of Ophthalmology and Otolaryngology, Subcommittee on Noise in Industry, 1957.
4. Gregg JB: Noise. Injuries to farmers. *Agricul Eng* 1972; 53:12.
5. Jones HH, Oser JL: Farm equipment noise exposure levels. *Am Ind Hyg Assoc J* 1968; 29:146.
6. Karlovich RS, Wiley TL, Jensen DV: *Hearing Sensitivity in Farmers*. Poster presentation at the American Speech-Language Hearing Association Convention, Los Angeles, November 1981.
7. Klackhoff I, Drettner B, Svedberg A: Computerized classification of the results of screening audiometry in groups of persons exposed to noise. *Audiology* 1974; 13:326.
8. Lierle DM, Reger SN: The effect of tractor noise in the auditory sensitivity of tractor operators. *Ann Otol Rhinol Laryngol* 1958; 67:1.
9. Mutel CF, Donham KJ: *Medical Practice in Rural Communities*. New York, Springer-Verlag New York, 1983.
10. Pfeiffer S, Graham TE, Webb RDG, et al: Aspects of physical fitness and health in Ontario diary farmers. *Can J Public Health* 1984; 75:204.
11. Pierce EW, Ejercito VS, Hansen DA: Prevention of hearing loss among farmers, in Dosman JA (ed): *Health and Safety in Agriculture*. Proceeding International Symposium on Health and Safety in Agriculture, Saskatoon, October, 1985.
12. Thelin A: Work and health among farmers. *Scand J Soc Med* 1980; Suppl 22.
13. Thelin JW, Joseph DJ, Davis WE, et al: High-frequency hearing loss in male farmers of Missouri. *Public Health Rep* 1983; 98:268.
14. Townsend TH, Bess FH, Fishbeck WA: Hearing sensitivity in rural Michigan. *Am Ind Hyg Assoc J* 1975; 36:63.
15. Weston HR: A survey of tractor noise and the effects on hearing. *J Aust Inst Agricul Sci* 1963; p 15.

Vibration

Farmers, ranchers, and farm workers are at risk of becoming ill or injured from exposure to vibrating machines or tools. These vibrations transmit energy to either the whole body or segments of the body. Whole-body vibration results from riding or driving farm tractors or other self-propelled farm equipment such as combines. Segmental vibration usually involves transmission of energy to the hands from operating chain saws, operating vibrating hand tools, and grasping the steering wheel of a tractor.[2]

Illness or injury results following long-term exposure to vibration energy. Physiologic and psychologic effects may result from whole-body vibration, and specific effects depend on amplitude, frequency, intensity, and duration of vibration. Vibration of low-frequency (100 Hz or less) and high amplitude is commonly emitted by farm machines, and it causes differential vibratory movements and deformation of internal organs. The most critical frequency is 4–8 Hz, and maximum whole-body vibration occurs around 5 Hz. Some of the acute effects of whole-body vibration include fatigue, impaired vision, impaired balance, and chest pain. Chronic effects may include back pain, degenerative changes in the vertebral column, prostatitis, hemorrhoids, renal disease, and peptic ulcer.[1]

Injury from segmental vibration is thought to be less important than whole-body vibration among agricultural workers. However, long-standing vibratory exposure to the hands may result in Raynaud's phenomenon of occupational origin. This condition is a neurovascular disorder of the hands manifested by episodic spastic contraction of blood vessels in the hands and fingers, resulting in ischemia, blanching of the skin, and loss of sensation.[3] The episodes are initiated by gripping a vibrating or stationary object or by exposing the hands to cold temperatures. In the early stages of the condition, episodes last only a few minutes, but as the disease progresses they may last for up to two hours. Further progression of the disease may result in sensory and motor nerve damage, with resulting pain, numbness, and impaired manipulative skills. In the most advanced cases, the skin on the fingertips necroses, bone cysts and decalcification may occur in the carpus, radius, and ulna, and osteoporosis of the elbow may develop. (See Chapter 21 for full discussion on vibration.)

REFERENCES

1. Henderson TL, Dunn DE, Nozza MA, et al: Oscillatory vibrations, in Key MM, Henschel AF, Butler J, et al (eds): *Occupational Diseases: A Guide to Their Recognition*. DHEW (NIOSH) Publ 77-181. US Dept of Health, Education, and Welfare, Public Health Service, Centers for Disease Control, National Institute for Occupational Safety and Health, 1977, pp 515–520.
2. Mutel CF, Donham KJ: *Medical Practice in Rural Communities*. New York, Springer-Verlag New York, 1983, pp 82–83.
3. Williams N: Biological effects of segmental vibration. *J Occup Med* 1975; 17:37.
4. Wassermann DE: *Human Aspects of Occupational Vibration*. Amsterdam, Elsevier, 1987.

RESPIRATORY DISORDERS

Farmers and agricultural workers are exposed to a variety of airborne hazards including mold spores, irritant gases and particulates, many of which are capable of producing acute and/or chronic respiratory disease. A number of these conditions are briefly considered below.

Illness From Livestock Confinement Facilities

Starting in the late 1960s, many farmers changed their livestock production techniques from out-of-doors, low-volume efforts to more sophisticated, industrial mass-production operations. Today large numbers of farm animals are concentrated in semiautomated structures called "confinement buildings." Dusts, gases, and infectious agents associated with livestock production concentrate within these buildings, resulting in potential health hazards to the workers.[3, 4, 5]

An estimated 700,000 persons in the U.S. are at risk, including owner-operators, spouses, children, employees, and veterinarians.[4] In an intensive agricultural state such as Iowa, an estimated 53% of the people work on swine farms (over 80,000 persons) and in confinement buildings.[6]

Confinement operations can involve poultry, beef, swine, dairy cattle, or veal calves. From empirical evidence, the largest exposed population and the most frequent and severe health problems are associated with swine confinement houses. Health problems of swine confinement workers have been more thoroughly studied than those of workers in other types of confinement houses. Thus, much of the following information pertains specifically to swine operations. Although many of these exposures are generic to confinement operations, regardless of species, there are some general differences. Poultry confinement workers may be exposed to ammonia and to dusts similar to swine confinement workers, but generally not H_2S (hydrogen sulfide) and CH_4 (methane). Poultry workers complain of similar symptoms, but symptoms are less frequent and less severe. In sheep, beef, veal calf, and dairy confinement operations, dusts do not appear to be as concentrated, nor as irritating to the respiratory tract, as swine confinement dusts. However, exposure to NH_3 (ammonia) and to H_2S may be comparable to swine units.[3] (See Chapter 47, hydrogen sulfide case report.)

Exposures

Hazards to the respiratory system are presented by a variety of dusts and gases. Dust in swine confinement houses contains primarily dried fecal dust and feed grain dust.[7] In general, the particles in fecal dust are quite small, and constitute the major alveolar burden, while the grain dust particles are larger and form the major airways burden.[7] Also present in swine house dust are animal dander, broken bits of hair, insect parts, bacteria, bacterial endotoxins, pollen grains, and fungal spores.[6] Ammonia and possibly other toxic or irritating gases (e.g., H_2S) often are adsorbed to the dust surface.[2, 6]

Dust loads are heavy (from 2 to 15 mg/m^3 in swine houses), with loads increasing in winter when the houses are closed to conserve heat.[3, 6, 7] Dust loads also increase when animals are being moved or handled. Particle sizes range from less than 1 up to 50 microns in diameter, with a mass median diameter of around 10 microns.[7] Because of this variety of size and type of particles present, several or a combination of health effects of organic dusts (irritant, allergic and delayed hypersensitivity reactions) may be seen in workers.[3, 6, 8] Additionally, exposures to gases such as NH_3 and H_2S and to cigarette smoking can potentially complicate exposure to confinement house dusts.[6, 8, 10]

In addition to dusts, toxic, irritating, and asphyxiating gases can build to unhealthful concentrations in confinement houses. Of the 40-plus gases that may be present, those present in houses most commonly and in highest concentrations are H_2S, NH_3, CO_2, CH_4, and CO.[3, 4, 5] Concentrations of these gases in houses may exceed levels in the TLV. Carbon monoxide levels may increase in cold weather because of incomplete combustion of propane or other heating fuels within the closed structure.[1, 2, 11] Carbon dioxide from heating units, animal respiration, and the manure pit can rise to asphyxiating levels if ventilation systems fail.[4, 5] Ammonia is generated from animal wastes on the confinement house floors, and from bacterial action on animal wastes stored in manure pits under the building. Wastes within the manure pits decompose by anaerobic digestion releasing low concentrations of gases continuously. However, hydrogen sulfide can soar to acute toxic levels when the manure is agitated, which is often done to facilitate emptying manure pits.[12]

Health Hazards

Each confinement house contains a complex mixture of dusts and gases. Specific components of the mixture vary with the particular house in question, and also change through time. The following problems have been observed in surveys of swine confinement house workers from a variety of operations.

Respiratory problems of swine confinement workers can be divided into three types: acute or subacute, delayed, and chronic.[6]

Acute and subacute respiratory problems are listed in Table 59–2, along with the percentage of workers experiencing these problems. These symptoms comprise a nonspecific airway disease, usually of hyperreactive airways and bronchitis. The most common symptoms (cough, sputum production, chest tightness, and wheez-

TABLE 59–2.
Symptoms of Swine Confinement Workers

Symptom	%
Cough	67%
Sputum or phlegm	56%
Tightness of chest	36%
Shortness of breath	30%
Wheezing	27%
Scratchy throat	54%
Runny nose	45%
Headaches	37%
Burning or watering eyes	39%
Muscle aches and pains	25%

ing) are those characteristic of bronchitis.[5, 10] It appears that people become increasingly sensitive to the confinement environment with increasing exposure.[6] In general, the symptoms increase among smokers, and also increase as the number of swine raised increases.[6, 8] Problems also are greater among those with hay fever, bronchitis, heart trouble, and allergies.[6] Specific mechanisms of the respiratory problems have not been determined, but chronic airway irritation is thought to play a major role. Allergic and toxic reactions may play a role in some individuals.[6] Any one or more than one of these mechanisms may occur in any one individual.

Additional acute problems result from sudden exposure to high concentrations of H_2S gas.[12] This occurs when pits are emptied; the liquid manure is agitated and large amounts of H_2S are liberated rapidly, rather than at the slow ambient rate. This has resulted in the sudden death of several confinement house workers.

Delayed problems include a flu-like illness experienced 4 to 6 hours after working for several hours in a confinement house during particularly dusty operations such as handling, moving, or sorting animals.[6, 8] Symptoms include fever, muscle aches and pains, headache, cough, and tightness of chest. This episodic problem occurs among approximately 10% of workers in confinement buildings. The illness resembles atypical farmer's lung or grain handler's fever, but the pathophysiology remains unknown at this time. One likely cause of the flu-like illness is a non-specific reaction to inhaled endotoxins adsorbed to dust in the air.

Chronic problems are manifest as chronic bronchitis and as symptoms of airway obstruction, each of which is suffered by approximately three times as many swine confinement workers as compared to workers in conventional swine housing units.[10] Chronic bronchitis, experienced by 58% of all swine confinement workers, is the most common defined chronic health problem of this occupational group.[10] Smokers experience a greater prevalence and severity of chronic bronchitis than do nonsmokers.[10] Most workers removed from the confinement house environment return to normal within a few months, but symptoms of some workers persist for as long as two years.

Chronic or permanent respiratory tract diseases other than chronic bronchitis have not yet been recognized, presumably because swine confinement houses are a relatively new innovation. However, future chronic damage may be seen; this is suggested by the facts that pulmonary function values of most confinement house workers decrease significantly through the work day.[9] The severity of chronic bronchitis symptoms is greater in workers with a longer exposure history, and experimental animals raised in confinement buildings developed metaplasia and necrosis of the respiratory epithelium and pneumonia with a diffuse histocytic infiltrate.[13]

Table 59–3 summarizes the known health hazards associated with swine confinement.

Treatment and Prevention

There is very little medical treatment that can be prescribed, except for treatment of some of the acute illnesses, such as pulmonary edema from H_2S exposure, or asthma. The key to control of illness is protection of the worker from the environment. Protection involves first engineering and management factors, and secondly personal protective equipment. Control through engineering and management may require getting the patient in touch with a consulting veterinarian or agricultural engineer who has knowledge of environmental control. The local veterinarian or the extension service at land grant colleges should be able to refer your patient to an appropriate person. Personal protective equipment involves proper respirator selection, and education of proper fitting and maintenance of the respirator. Generally we have found a NIOSH-approved disposable half-face dust mask to be most acceptable, but more sensitive individuals may require NIOSH-approved half- or quarter-face rubber or plastic mask with replaceable filters, or a powered air-purifying respirator, such as an air helmet. (See Chapter 2, respiratory protection, pp 53–56.)

REFERENCES

1. Carson TL, Donham KJ: Carbon monoxide abortion in Iowa swine, in *21th Annual Proceedings of the American Association of Veterinary Laboratory Diagnosticians*, 1978, pp 179–184.
2. Carson TL, Donham KJ, Dominick A: Carbon monoxide-induced abortion in swine: An update, in *23rd Annual Proceedings of the American Association of Veterinary Laboratory Diagnosticians*, 1980, pp 59–66.
3. Donham KJ, Rubino MJ, Thedell TD, et al: Potential health hazards of workers in swine confinement buildings. *J Occup Med* 1977; 19:383.
4. Donham KJ, Popendorf WJ: Ambient levels of selected gases inside swine confinement buildings. *Am Indus Hyg Assoc J* 1985; 46:658–661.
5. Donham KJ, Yeggy J, Dague RR: Chemical and physical parameters of liquid manure from swine confinement facilities: Health implications for workers, swine, and the environment. *Agricultural Wastes* 1985; 14:97–113.
6. Donham KJ, Gustafson KE: Human health hazards in livestock confinement. *Annals American Conference of Governmental Industrial Hygienists* 1982; 2:137–142.
7. Donham KJ, Scallon LJ, Popendorf W, et al: Characterization of dusts collected from swine confinement buildings. *Am Indus Hyg Assoc J* 1986; 47:404–410.
8. Donham KJ, Hagland P, Peterson Y, et al: Environmental and health studies in swine confinement buildings. *Am J Indus Med* 1986; 10:289–293.
9. Donham KJ, Zavala D, Merchant J: Acute effects of the work environment on pulmonary functions of swine confinement workers. *Am J Indus Med* 1984; 5:367–375.
10. Donham KJ, Zavala D, Merchant J: Respiratory symptoms and lung function among workers in swine confinement buildings: A cross sectional epidemiological study. *Arch Environ Health* 1984; 39:96–100.

11. Donham KJ, Carson TL, Adrian BR: Carboxyhemoglobin values in swine relative to carbon monoxide exposure: Guidelines to monitor for animal and human health hazards in swine buildings. *Am J Vet Res* 1982; 5:813–816.
12. Donham KJ, Knapp LW, Monson R, et al: Acute toxic exposure to gasses from liquid manure. *J Occup Med* 1982; 24:142–145.
13. Donham KJ, Leininger JR: The use of laboratory animals to study potential chronic lung disease in swine confinement workers. *Am J Vet Res* 1984; 45:926–931.

Asthma

The agricultural environment brings the farmer into contact with allergic substances, including pollens, mold spores, grain dust, and animal dander.[4] Susceptible individuals can develop extrinsic asthma or allergic rhinitis from such exposures, oftentimes early in life. While the most severely affected sometimes leave the agricultural environment altogether, others attempt to continue farming. It is these individuals, and those who develop intrinsic or adult-onset asthma, who represent difficult clinical problems for the rural physician. Although an occasional adult asthmatic may need to leave the agricultural environment in mid-career, most are able to continue farming with proper medical management and vocational modifications.[5]

Farmer's Lung and Related Disorders

Although most farmers now recognize the potential hazard presented by airborne mold spores, cases of farmer's lung continue to occur in rural areas. However, earlier recognition of incipient disease by both the farmer and the physician has led to an apparent decrease in the number of chronic, disabling cases. Increased understanding of the natural history of the disorder and favorable experience with vocational modifications have allowed afflicted farmers to remain in agriculture without developing permanent respiratory impairment. (Farmer's lung and related disorders are covered in greater detail in Chapters 15 and 16.)

Organic dust toxic syndrome is the newly recommended term for an influenza-like illness (also referred to as pulmonary mycotoxicosis, silo unloader's disease, and atypical farmer's lung).[1] This syndrome can occur after intense exposure to a variety of agricultural dusts, including swine, fowl, and grain dusts, and moldy silage, wood chips, and grain. An acute febrile illness with a delayed onset, it is often mistaken for farmer's lung, even though it is much more common. However, organic dust toxic syndrome is clinically less severe than farmer's lung and does not appear to cause radiographic changes, permanent physiologic derangements, or progressive disease.[2]

Silo Filler's Disease

This disorder is a form of chemical pneumonitis/bronchiolitis due to inhalation of oxides of nitrogen in freshly filled silos. Once in storage, plant nitrates are eventually converted to nitrogen dioxide (NO_2) and its dimer, nitrogen tetroxide (N_2O_4) by microbial fermentation. Gas begins to form within a few hours after filling the silo, reaches a peak concentration one to five days later, and may persist in toxic quantities for two weeks or longer. Unlike most water-soluble, irritant gases which exert their strongest effects at the earliest point of contact with the mucous membranes, nitrogen dioxide hydrolizes more slowly and is capable of reaching the bronchioles and alveoli. At these locations, it undergoes almost complete hydrolysis to nitrous and nitric acids, resulting in a profound chemical pneumonitis and pulmonary edema. The onset of severe respiratory distress is usually delayed several hours after exposure, although extremely high concentrations may be rapidly fatal. An individual who survives pulmonary edema may develop widespread bronchiolitis obliterans 10–31 days after exposure.

Any patient with significant exposure to nitrogen dioxide should be observed in the hospital for 48 hours and followed closely for an additional six weeks after discharge. Corticosteroids should be started immediately in the presence of respiratory embarrassment or pulmonary edema. Therapy should be continued for a minimum of eight weeks to prevent the development of bronchiolitis obliterans.[3] Although the majority of patients who survive do not develop significant respiratory impairment, an occasional individual may exhibit persistent pulmonary dysfunction of variable severity.

Farmers are cautioned to stay out of and away from the silo immediately after filling and the following day. If it becomes necessary to enter the silo any time during the first ten days after filling, the blower should be run for at least 30 minutes prior to entering. If the silo is not known to be safe, use of an approved respirator, safety harness, and safety lines is recommended.

REFERENCES

1. Donhan KJ, Rylander R: Epilogue: Health effects of organic dusts in the farm environment. *Am J Ind Med* 1986; 10:339–340.
2. Do Pico GA: Report on diseases: Health effects of organic dusts in the farm environment. *Am J Ind Med* 1986; 10:261–265.
3. Horvath EP, do Pico GA, Barbee RA, et al: Nitrogen dioxide-induced pulmonary disease. *J Occup Med* 1978; 20:103–110.
4. Kammermeyer J: Some special aspects of pulmonary disease in a farm setting, in *Proceedings of Conference in Agricultural Health and Safety*. New York, Society of Occupational and Environmental Health, Environmental Sciences Laboratory, 1983.
5. Twiggs JT: Personal communication. Dec 18, 1984.

Grain Dust

It has been known for centuries that grain dust causes symptoms referable to the eyes, throat, and lungs.[16] The population currently at risk in North America includes grain and livestock farmers and more than 500,000 other individuals who are employed in the grain storage and transporting industry as elevator agents, dock workers, longshoremen, and mill workers.[7, 11] Grain dust is a heterogeneous mixture which may contain a large number of inorganic and organic substances (Table 59–4). The proportion of particles sufficiently small to gain entry to the peripheral airways and the alveoli (a respirable fraction) may be as high as 40% of the total suspended dust.[22] Furthermore, pesticides may adsorb onto respirable particulates, altering the site of deposition and enhancing potential toxicity.[2]

Several symptom complexes and illnesses have been attributed to grain dust exposure, including rhinitis, conjunctivitis,

TABLE 59–3.
Occupational Respiratory Conditions Associated With Livestock Confinement—Diagnosis, Treatment, and Control

CONDITION	SYMPTOMS/HISTORY	WORK EXPOSURE
Bronchitis	Cough, often with excess sputum production, possibly tightness of chest. Very frequently seen among swine confinement workers; somewhat less often in poultry workers. Smoking associated with increased frequency and more severe symptoms. Symptoms continuing for 3 or more years classified as chronic bronchitis.	Usually occurs in those who work in swine confinement for 2 or more hours per day. More frequent and severe for those who have worked 6 or more years in confinement. Generally occurs in buildings with poor environment: dusty (appears hazy and dust accumulates on horizontal surfaces), poor ventilation, older building (built before 1975). Nursery buildings and those with manure pits under slatted floors may be biggest offenders. Usually worse during cold weather.
Hyperactive airways	Chest tightness, mild dyspnea, some obstruction during breathing. Often accompanied by bronchitis. Very common in exposed workers. History identical to bronchitis.	Identical to bronchitis (above).
Asthma	Wheezing within minutes to hours following exposure. Only seen in small percentage of workers (i.e., less than 10%).	Usually a period of sensitization required, which may be anywhere from a few months to several years. Extent of exposure not important (environment may be relatively clean, and a person may spend very small amount of time in building).
Organic dust toxic syndrome	Fever, muscle aches, chest tightness, cough, malaise. Symptoms develop 4–6 hours following exposure. Self limited symptoms in 24–72 hours. Recurrent episodes common. Seen in 10–15% of the swine farming population.	Usually condition is associated with work in a totally enclosed building. Usually follows a particularly heavy exposure (e.g., 4–6 hours of very dusty work such as handling or sorting hogs).
H_2S poisoning	Sudden onset of nausea, dizziness, possibly sudden collapse, respiratory distress, apnea. May lead to sudden death. May recover if patient is removed from environment, with or without dyspnea, hemoptysis, froth expelling from trachea	Almost always occurs with agitating a liquid manure pit while emptying it.

DIAGNOSTIC AIDS	TREATMENT/CONTROL	PROGNOSIS
Symptoms usually sufficient for diagnosis. Bronchoscopy will help confirm and grade the condition. PFT may show decreased flow rates. Skin tests, or other immunological tests are *not* indicated.	Protection from environment is most important action. Medications usually are not indicated. Antihistamines, decongestants, steroids may provide temporary relief of symptoms but should not be used long-term Improved ventilation crucial. Employ management procedures to limit dust generation. Install dust and gas control technology. Establish a respirator program. Abstain from smoking.	Most improve if environmental exposure is controlled through engineering, management, and use of respirator. Temporary removal from the environment may help until other measures can be taken. Long-term or permanent damage has not been reported to date. Usually not necessary to quit working.
PFT following a workshift will show decreased flow rates, primarily FEV_1 and $FEF_{25\text{-}75}$ Respiratory tract challenge with methacholine or histamine will show decreased PFT flow rates.	Identical to bronchitis (above).	Identical to bronchitis (above).
Same as asthma from any other source: obstructive airflow patterns following exposure; skin test positive to one or more of feed grains, hog dander, hog hair, various molds, dusts; atopic status.	Medication and treatment same as for any asthmatic. Attempts to control exposures by environmental control and respirators may not be helpful. Desensitization may not be applicable, unless specific causative allergen is found for which desensitizing agents exist.	Same as for any asthmatic. Depending on degree of sensitivity, may be almost impossible to protect these people from their environment. This may be one condition where patient has to quit working in confinement house.
Elevated white blood cell count, usually neutrophilia but possibly lymphocytosis. PFT will show decreased FEV_1 and diminished flow rates. PO_2 may be decreased. Bronchioalveolar lavage may show mononuclear cells. May show serum precipitins to various molds or dust extract, but not specific. X-ray may show scattered patchy infiltrates. Lung biopsy may show interstitial mononuclear cell infiltrates.	Symptomatic treatment in acute stages includes oxygen, IV fluids to correct acid-base balance and dehydration. Aspirin may be used to control fever and myalgia. Burst and taper of corticosteroids may speed recovery.	Usually recovery period is 3–4 days, but patient may feel tired and have shortness of breath for several weeks to months. Subsequent attacks may occur in future following heavy exposure. Multiple exposures may induce interstitial fibrosis, but this has not been documented.
If patient survives: x-ray shows pulmonary edema; presence of sulfide ion in blood. If deceased, autopsy shows pulmonary edema, froth in trachea, possibly greenish tinge to viscera; blood contains sulfide and sulfhemoglobin.	Emergency treatment—removal from environment (without exposing others) and resuscitate. May have to ventilate. Watch for and control pulmonary edema. Avoid confined spaces associated with liquid manure when agitated.	If patient survives initial exposure, will probably recover with minimal loss of lung function. Recovery period may be from days to months, depending on severity of exposure.

TABLE 59–4.
Composition of Grain Dust

Cereal grains (wheat, barley, rye, oats, corn, and their disintegration products)
Pesticides (carbon tetrachloride, malathion, methyl bromide, aluminum phosphate, carbon disulfide)
Mammalian and avian debris (hairs and excreta from rodents, pigeons)
Fungi and their metabolites (alfatoxin)
Pollens
Bacterial endotoxins
Insect parts
Mites
Silica

grain fever, hypersensitivity pneumonitis, and chronic bronchitis.[3] Grain fever is a short-term flu-like illness which occurs during or shortly after exposure to high concentrations of grain dust. Headache and respiratory symptoms (substernal burning sensation, chest tightness, dyspnea, cough) develop during exposure and are followed several hours later by systemic manifestations (malaise, myalgia, fever, and chills). Attacks tend to occur for the first few days in persons who return to work after an absence, and then subside spontaneously.[8] The prevalence of grain fever varies with location. Only a few workers from Canadian terminal grain elevators complained of grain fever, or asthma hypersensitivity pneumonitis, whereas as many as one third of employees at an American facility had such symptoms.[1, 4, 9] Because of its clinical resemblance to hypersensitivity pneumonitis, grain fever has been thought to represent a Type III allergic reaction to fungi present in moldy grain. However, there are significant differences between these two disorders. Grain fever, unlike hypersensitivity pneumonitis, tends not to recur unless there is repeat, massive exposure to grain dust. There appears to be no correlation between the history of grain fever and the presence of precipitins to fungi, grain, or grain dust. Finally, physiologic or radiographic evidence of pneumonitis with grain fever has not been demonstrated.[7, 8, 19] Although hypersensitivity pneumonitis may occur in grain exposed workers,[6, 15] grain fever is probably a separate entity caused by a host reaction to bacterial endotoxins or nonallergic mediator release from grain dust or its constituents.[8]

Because grain dust contains a number of allergens, asthma has been regarded as a potential respiratory hazard of exposed workers. Immediate and late asthmatic reactions have been reported in subjects with skin hypersensitivity to grain dust.[20] However, specific allergens have been implicated only infrequently.[5] The true prevalence of grain dust asthma is unknown. Atopic or asthmatic individuals tend to leave the industry early because of their symptoms and are therefore not likely to be found in cross-sectional studies of grain handlers.[4]

Chronic bronchitis is the most prevalent and potentially serious respiratory condition resulting from exposure to grain dust.[3] Epidemiologic studies have shown that 37%–75% of grain workers experience chronic respiratory symptoms (cough, sputum, wheezing, and dyspnea).[7, 19, 21] In controlled studies, the risk of chronic bronchitis among grain workers is significantly greater than that of nonexposed subjects.[9, 12] Ventilatory impairment has been documented in some workers, even in nonsmokers.[4, 9, 12] The mechanism by which grain dust causes airways obstruction is not known. Present evidence suggests that the respiratory reaction is a nonallergic response to constituent(s) of grain dust with subsequent mediator release.[9] Atopy and α_1-antitrypsin deficiency are not regarded as significant host factors in the majority of cases.[4] However, the degree of acute change in lung function over a workweek may be a good predictor of longitudinal decline in pulmonary function.[17] Smoking contributes to the excess of both respiratory symptoms and airways obstruction. Its effects in combination with grain dust have been described as additive[4, 9] and synergistic.[10]

The present standard in the United States is OSHA's nuisance dust limit of 15 mg/cu m for total dust and 5 mg/cu m for the respirable fraction.[14] The Canadadian Labor Department has established a 10 mg/cu m exposure limit averaged over an eight-hour day and 40-hour workweek.[13] The American Conference of Governmental Industrial Hygienists (ACGIH) has adopted a specific grain dust threshold limit value (TLV) of 4 mg/cu m for total particulates.[18] In addition to environmental controls, respiratory medical surveillance and smoking cessation programs are also recommended to reduce the incidence and severity of chronic respiratory abnormalities among grain handlers.

REFERENCES

1. Broder I, Mintz S, Hutcheon M, et al: Comparison of respiratory variables in grain elevator workers of Thunder Bay, Canada. *Am Rev Respir Dis* 1979; 119:193.
2. Caplan KJ: The environment: Method of assessment and relationship to the evaluation of disease, in Dosman JA, Cotton DJ (eds): *Occupational Pulmonary Disease—Focus on Grain Dust and Health*. New York, Academic Press, 1980.
3. Chan-Yeung M, Ashley MJ, Grzykowski S: Grain dust and the lungs. *Can Med J* 1978; 118:1271.
4. Chan-Yeung M, Schulzer M, MacLein L, et al: Epidemiologic health study of grain elevator workers in British Columbia. *Am Rev Respir Dis* 1980; 121:329.
5. Davies RJ, Green M, Schofield MN: Recurrent nocturnal asthma after exposure to grain dust. *Am Rev Respir Dis* 1976; 114:1011.
6. Dennis CAR: Health hazards of grain storage, in Sinha RN, Muir WE (eds): *Grain Storage—Part of a System*. Wesport, Conn, Avi, 1971.
7. doPico GA, Reddan W, Flaherty D, et al: Respiratory abnormalities among grain handlers—A clinical, physiologic and immunologic study. *Am Rev Respir Dis* 1977; 115:915.
8. doPico GA, Flaherty D, Bhansali P, et al: Grain fever syndrome induced by inhalation of airborne grain dust. *J Allergy Clin Immunol* 1982; 69:435.
9. doPico GA, Reddan W, Tsiatis A, et al: Epidemiologic study of clinical and physiologic parameters in grain handlers of northern United States. *Am Rev Respir Dis* 1984; 130:759.
10. Dosman JA: Chronic obstructive pulmonary disease and smoking in grain workers. *Am Intern Med* 1977; 87:784.
11. Dosman JA: Chronic obstructive pulmonary disease and smoking in grain workers, in Dosman JA, Cotton DJ (eds): *Occupational Pulmonary Disease—Focus on Grain Dust and Health*. New York, Academic Press, 1980.
12. Dosman JA, Cotton DJ, Graham BL, et al: Chronic bronchitis and decreased forced expiratory flow rates in lifetime nonsmoking grain workers. *Am Rev Respir Dis* 1980; 121:11.
13. Todd H: Personal communication, 1985.
14. *OSHA Safety and Health Standards for General Industry* (29 CFR

1910). Occupational Safety and Health Administration, US Dept of Labor, OSHA220-6, March 11, 1983.
15. Pepys J: Hypersensitivity disease of the lungs due to fungi and organic dusts, in *Monograph in Allergy*. White Plains, NY, Phiebig, 1969, vol 4.
16. Ramazzini B: *Diseases of Workers, 1713*. New York, Hafner Publishing Co, 1964.
17. Tabona M, Chan-Yeung M, Enarson D, et al: Host factors affecting longitudinal decline in lung spirometry among grain elevator workers. *Chest* 1984; 85:782.
18. *Threshold Limit Values (TLVs) for Chemical Substances and Physical Agents in the Work Environment and Biological Exposure Indices with Intended Changes for 1986–1987*. Akron, Oh, American Conference of Governmental Industrial Hygienists, 1986.
19. Tse KS, Warren P, Janusz M, et al: Respiratory abnormalities in workers exposed to grain dust. *Arch Environ Health* 1973; 27:74.
20. Warren P, Cherniak RM, Tse KS, et al: Hypersensitivity reaction to grain dust. *J Allergy Clin Immunol* 1974; 53:139.
21. William N, Skoular A, Merriman JE: Exposure to grain dust. I. Survey of the effects. *J Occup Med* 1964; 6:319.
22. Yoshida K, Maybank J: Physical and environmental characteristics of grain dust, in Dosman JA, Cotton DJ (eds): *Occupational Pulmonary Disease—Focus on Grain Dust and Health*. New York, Academic Press, 1980.

ZOONOTIC DISEASES

Diseases caused by infectious agents common to animals and people are called zoonoses, and a number of these are hazards for agricultural workers. The material is presented here in two parts: *general concepts;* and essential features of *specific zoonotic diseases*. The general concepts presented are common to all agricultural zoonoses, regardless of geographic location. Tables 59–5 to 59–7 present the essential features of the most important occupational zoonoses in agriculture of North America. Over 150 zoonoses are distinguished worldwide. Of these, 40 have significance as occupational diseases in agriculture worldwide, and 25 present hazards to agricultural workers in the U.S. (Table 59–5).

Zoonotic infections are significant not only because there are so many of them, but also they are an economic burden due to loss of livestock, the expense of animal disease control,[4] and clinical care for human exposures and illness. An example of the latter is the 15 million dollars spent annually in the U.S. for administration of rabies post-exposure immunoprophylaxis to approximately 30,000 exposed individuals.[4]

Although zoonoses are recognized as a significant health problem, the actual incidence and prevalence of zoonotic infections is difficult to determine for several reasons.[10, 4] First, since many infections may be mild only the most severely ill persons may report to a physician. Second, many clinical infections are often misdiagnosed because symptoms are often protean, nonpathognomonic, and mimic severe influenza. Lack of physician awareness and of appropriate diagnostic support further increases the rate of misdiagnosis. Third, in some agriculture areas, medical services are scarce and ill persons may have little chance to see a physician, so no diagnosis is made.

Incorrect counts of zoonotic infections also result from lack of comprehensive reporting systems.[3, 4] Although states vary in their requirements for reporting infectious diseases, most include only those diseases specified by the national health authorities. These include only a few of the important occupational zoonoses. Although a few states have occupational disease reporting systems, the inherent problems previously described prevent acquisition of accurate figures. Thus, the number of zoonotic infections in agriculture is a gross underestimate.

TABLE 59–5.
The Risk to Agricultural Workers of Selected Diseases Common to Animal and Man

DEFINITE RISK	QUESTIONABLE RISK	DOUBTFUL RISK
Brucellosis	Pseudotuberculosis	Cowpox
Leptospirosis	Psittacosis/ornithosis	Taeniasis
Toxoplasmosis	Vibriosis	Dermatophilosis
Rabies	Salmonellosis	Trichinosis
Tetanus	Listeriosis	Pneumococcal infections
Anthrax	Tuberculosis	Babesiosis
Erysipeloid	Streptococcal infections (pharyngitis, erysipelas)	Fascioliasis
Q fever	Influenza and parainfluenza	Giardiasis
Histoplasmosis	Plague	
Blastomycosis	Cryptococcosus	
Ringworm	Nematodiasis (cutaneous larval migrans, visceral larval migrans, and strongyloidiasis)	
Arthropod-borne viral encephalitis	Colorado tick fever	
Newcastle disease	Pneumococcal infections	
Pseudocowpox	Encephalomyocarditis	
Vesicular stomatitis	Dirofilariasis	
Contagious ecthyma		
Staphylococcal infections		
Echinococcosis		
Collibacillosis		
Tularemia		
Acariasis		
Pasteurellosis		
Rocky Mountain spotted fever		
Sporotrichosis		
Balantidiasis		

TABLE 59–6.
Selected Agricultural Zoonoses: Risk Relative to Major Exposure Source[8, 4]

Beef Cattle	*Sheep*
Anthrax	Contagious ecthyma
Leptospirosis	Hydatid disease
Rabies	Tularemia
Dairy Cattle	*Swine*
Milker's nodules	Brucellosis
Q fever	*E. Coli* infections
Staphylococcus infections	Erysipeloid
Vesicular stomatitis	Swine influenza
Zoophilic ringworm	
Poultry	*Rural Environment*
Histoplasmosis	Blastomycosis
Newcastle disease	Arthropod-borne viral encephalidities
Ornithosis	Rocky Mountain spotted fever
	Tetanus
	Toxoplasmosis

TABLE 59–7.
Essential Features of Selected Occupationally Acquired Zoonotic Infections of Agricultural Workers

DISEASE (common names)	ETIOLOGIC AGENTS	HEALTH EFFECTS (Human and animal)	ANIMAL HOSTS A. 1 = zooanthroponosis 2 = anthropozoonosis 3 = amphixenosis B. Specific animals infected	MECHANISMS OF TRANSMISSION A. Reservoir B. 1 = direct-zoonosis 2 = meta-zoonosis 3 = sapro-zoonosis 4 = cyclo-zoonosis C. Specific mechanisms	EPIDEMIOLOGY A. Populations at risk B. Geographic distribution	PREVENTION OR CONTROL
Anthrax (Malignant pustule, wool sorter's disease)	*Bacillus anthracis*	*Human*—Persistent skin infection, usually on hands or arms Pulmonary form less common but much more severe with fairly high case fatality rate Gastrointestinal form is least common *Animal*—Usually overwhelming bacteremia and septicemia with rapid death in cattle, sheep, and goats Less acute in horse, pigs, and dogs	A. 1 B. Cattle, sheep, goats, horse, pig, dog	A. Soil Water (stagnant ponds near incubator areas) B. 1, 3 C. Direct contact with infected animals or their carcasses or body parts or animal fertilizers or feeds Inhalation of spores from hair or hide of infected animals Consumption of improperly cooked meat of infected animals	A. Sheep and goat producers Cattle producers Veterinarians and other animal health workers Hair and hide processors Abattoir workers B. Worldwide in endemic foci May be transported to distant locations with hair and hide from infected animals	Vaccination of animals in endemic areas Personal protection when handling potentially infected animals or tissues Deep burial and covering with lime of infected animal carcasses Vaccination of humans at high risk
Brucellosis (undulant fever, Malta fever, Bang's disease)	*Brucella abortus, B. suis, B. melitensis, B. canis*	*Human*—Generalized prolonged influenza-like illness, spiking fevers, myalgia, malaise Occasional chronic forms include lesions of heart valves, abscesses of bone, liver, or other body parts *Animal*—Abortions Possible chronic abscesses in bone and other tissues	A. 1 B. Cattle, swine Sheep, goats Less common: dogs, camels, deer, buffalo, and others	A. Cattle, swine, sheep, goats, dogs mainly Other susceptible animals less important B. 1 C. Direct contact with infected animals or their tissues, especially placenta and abortion products Ingestion of milk products from infected animals Possible airborne transmission	A. Sheep, goats, cattle, and swine producers primarily Abattoir workers B. Worldwide, especially in dairying areas	Eradication in primary livestock species (several countries have established such programs) Personal protection when handling infected animals, especially following abortion Sanitation of the animal environment Pasteurization of milk products)
Contagious ecthyma (orf)	Pox virus	*Human*—Skin lesions on hands and arms Start out as small papules, progress to large vesicles that then ulcerate Last 4–8 weeks *Animal*—Vesicular lesions in the mouth and on the lips	A. 1 B. Sheep mainly Goats also	A. Sheep Goats The animal environment: animal sheds, feed bunks, etc. B. 1, 3 C. Direct contact with infected animals or their environment, especially handling and examining infected animals	A. People raising or handling sheep or goats B. Worldwide, wherever sheep are raised	Isolation of infected animal Wearing protective gloves when handling infected animals or working in the environment Excellent sanitation of the animal environment

Dermatophytosis (ringworm, taenia, dermatomycosis)	*Trichophyton verrucosum, T. equinum, T. mentagrophytes, Microsporum canis, M. nanum, M. gallianae*	*Human*—Skin infection of variable severity Crusty inflamed lesions that tend to clear centrally Pustules may develop in the active portion of the lesion Lesions usually occur on face, arms, and head *Animal*—Similar to man except lesions usually much less inflamed and dry May be patches of hair loss May be subclinical infections	A. 1 B. Most animal species have their own fungal agents that cause skin infections. The infected animal species important in agriculture include cattle, goats, sheep, horse, rat, swine, and chicken	A. *T. verrucosum:* cattle mainly, sheep and goats also possible *T. equinum:* horse *T. mentagrophytes:* rat *M. canis:* dog, cat *M. nanum:* swine *M. gallianae:* chicken B. The environment (barns, feed bunks, corrals, etc) may also serve as a reservoir, because the organism lives for long periods off the host. C. Close direct contact of bare skin to infected animals or their environment	A. Farmers and livestock handlers Persons who milk infected animals are particularly at risk Children are at greater risk than adults B. Worldwide	Excellent animal health programs: sound nutrition, excellent environmental sanitation, prevent overcrowding Isolate infected animals Wear protective gloves and clothing when handling infected animals Good personal hygiene
Histoplasmosis	*Histoplasma capsulatum*	*Human*—Often subclinical Variable, depending on dose and immune response of the individual Usually a febrile illness with influenza-like symptoms, cough, pneumonitis, usually recovery in 2–3 weeks Chronic forms may be extremely severe and very difficult to treat, with chronic pneumonitis, liver infections, bone infections, or other tissues *Animal*—Often subclinical Similar to human illness	A. None of above. Animal relationship to humans comes from the fact that the organism grows particularly well in soil contaminated with fecal material of birds or bats. These species may also act to distribute the organism in nature B. Most animals have subclinical infections Dogs are the primary animal species that develop illness	A. Soil: particularly that contaminated by aged feces of birds or bats. B. 3 C. Inhalation of producing aerosols by the organism during disturbance of soil that contains the organism, e.g., cleaning or razing old chicken coops, working in areas where old bird roosts have been	A. Farmers and persons who live and work in endemic areas of the infection B. Worldwide in specific localities where soil and climatic conditions are favorable for growth of the organism	Wetting down soil and wearing a good particle filtering respirator when working in dusty environment conducive to growth of the organism (e.g., old bird roosts, old poultry house, etc.)
Influenza (grippe)	Myxovirus	*Human*—Variable effects depending on virulence of the specific strain The swine strain is the primary virus where there is good evidence for direct transmission to man from an animal source *Animal*—Mild to severe upper respiratory illness with generalized symptoms	A. 1, 2, or 3 (the various interrelationships are not yet completely understood) B. Swine, horses, poultry, domestic and wild avian species	A. Infected animals The specific roles of swine, horses, and birds as reservoirs of influenza for man are yet to be determined B. 1, possibly 4 C. Direct contact, primarily respiratory droplet from infected animals	A. Swine handlers primarily Possibly persons working with poultry or horses B. Worldwide	Excellent sanitation in the animal environment, including ventilation Vaccinate horses Swine vaccine has been successful in one European country

(continued)

TABLE 59–7. *Continued*

Essential Features of Selected Occupationally Acquired Zoonotic Infections of Agricultural Workers

DISEASE (common names)	ETIOLOGIC AGENTS	HEALTH EFFECTS (Human and animal)	ANIMAL HOSTS A. 1 = zooanthroponosis 2 = anthropozoonosis 3 = amphixenosis B. Specific animals infected	MECHANISMS OF TRANSMISSION A. Reservoir B. 1 = direct-zoonosis 2 = meta-zoonosis 3 = sapro-zoonosis 4 = cyclo-zoonosis C. Specific mechanisms	EPIDEMIOLOGY A. Populations at risk B. Geographic distribution	PREVENTION OR CONTROL
Leptospirosis (Weil's disease, swineherd's disease, swamp fever, mud fever)	*Leptospira interrogans:* many different serovars involved	*Human*—Generalized febrile, influenza-like illness of variable severity Mild cases: malaise, myalgia, symptoms of meningitis, vomiting Severe cases: hepatorenal involvement jaundiced, case-fatality ratio 20%–40% *Animal*—Abortion Hepatorenal involvement with jaundice, possible kidney failure	A. 1 B. Cattle and swine are the main livestock species infected Sheep and goats, less common Dogs, rats Wildlife including squirrels, raccoons, mice, shrew, bandicoot, fox, jackals, hedgehog, and others	A. Cattle, swine, rats mainly, but most other susceptible animals also Water, muddy soil B. 1, 3 C. Direct and indirect contact with urine from infected animals Contact with abortion products of infected animals Contact with water contaminated with urine from infected animals	A. Persons working with cattle or swine Persons working in rice paddies contaminated from urine of infected animals Abattoir workers Persons swimming in contaminated water Hunters and trappers B. Worldwide, specific serovars vary with locality	Control livestock infection with good sanitation, immunization and proper veterinary care Prevent infected animals from urinating in waters where humans have contact Personal protection of workers when handling infected animals or tissues Rat control
Milker's nodules (paravaccinia)	Paravaccinia subgroup of pox virus	*Human*—Wart-like nodules on the skin of hands and forearms *Animal*—Nodules on the teats and udders of cows	A. 1 B. Cattle	A. Infected cattle B. 1 C. Direct contact with teats and udders of cows with active lesions Hand milking or washing the udder and teats prior to machine milking are primary exposures	A. Dairy cow milkers and handlers B. Europe and the United States	Separation of infected animals Wearing protective gloves when milking or treating infected cattle
Newcastle disease (in poultry synonyms are pseudo fowl pest, pneumoencephalitis)	Paramyxovirus	*Human*—Conjunctivitis Occasionally mild influenza-like illness *Animal*—Disease varies depending on the specific virus strain 3 main forms: (1) mild respiratory illness; (2) respiratory form with nervous involvement in chicks; (3) severe highly fatal pneumoencephalitis	A. 1 B. Chickens primarily, turkeys also Many other avian species may be infected but are primarily asymptomatic	A. Infected avian species, domestic or wild B. 1 C. Direct or indirect contact with infected birds, their environment, or their tissues Direct contact with aerosolized vaccines for chickens	A. Poultry workers Those who administer aerosol vaccines to chicken flocks Poultry processing plant workers B. Worldwide	Most developed countries have eradicated the severe form and have programs to keep it out of the country Outbreaks do occur and a test and slaughter program is invoked Effective vaccines are available, but should be used with protective clothing and full face respirators with aerosol vaccine Good sanitation and personal hygiene in poultry processing plants

Psittacosis (ornithosis, fowl chlamydois)	*Chlamydia psittaci*	*Human*—Variable depending on strain Generalized febrile illness with headache, constipation and pneumonitis *Animal*—General latent or subclinical Under stress symptoms may be seen including depression, emaciation, respiratory distress	A. 1 B. Turkeys primarily Ducks, geese, and chicken also Psittacine birds Many species of wild birds	A. Subclinically infected poultry, psittacine birds, and many species of wild birds B. 1 C. Direct contact with infected birds, their tissues, or fecal material via penetration of skin or mucous membranes, or inhalation	A. Persons raising and handling poultry, particularly turkeys Poultry processing plant workers People handling psittacine birds B. Worldwide	Personal protection when handling infected birds, their environment, or their carcasses Eliminate carrier state by feeding birds tetracycline Screen animals before they enter processing plant Personal protection for poultry processing
Q Fever (query fever)	*Coxiella burnetti*	*Human*—Generalized febrile illness with pneumonitis Possible endocarditis Case fatality rate < 10% *Animal*—Often inapparent May cause abortion, especially in sheep	A. 1 B. Cattle, sheep, goats Many small wild animals	A. Cattle, sheep, goats Ticks Several species of small wild mammals B. 1 C. Inhalation of airborne organisms in dust Direct contact with infected animals, particularly placenta and placental fluids Consumption of raw milk	A. Farmers, farm workers in contact with animals, or cleaning up the animal environment, or assisting at birthing of calves or lambs Abattoir workers B. Worldwide	Personal protection when handling infected animals (especially during parturition) Respiratory protection when working in a dusty environment contaminated with the organism Immunization
Rabies	Rhabdovirus	*Human*—Progressive encephalitis with personality changes and hyperactivity to external stimuli, resulting in spastic contractions of skeletal muscles, usually resulting in dysphagia, respiratory failure, and death *Animal*—Variable encephalitis depending on species, but usually behavior changes, paralysis of muscles of mastication, death	A. 1 B. Many species of domestic and wild mammals	A. Reservoirs vary depending on geographic location, include species of canidae, mustelidae, viverridae B. 1 C. Direct contact via bite wound or contamination of preexisting wound with saliva Aerosol transmission is rare	A. Animal handlers working with bovine species Agricultural workers in outdoor areas where the disease is endemic in wild animal population B. Occurs in most areas of the world except Australia, most Caribbean islands and Hawaii	Vaccination or removal of reservoir host Vaccination of people at high risk Postexposure immunization Thorough washing of bite wounds with soap and water

(continued)

TABLE 59–7. *Continued*

Essential Features of Selected Occupationally Acquired Zoonotic Infections of Agricultural Workers

DISEASE (common names)	ETIOLOGIC AGENTS	HEALTH EFFECTS (Human and animal)	ANIMAL HOSTS A. 1 = zooanthroponosis 2 = anthropozoonosis 3 = amphixenosis B. Specific animals infected	MECHANISMS OF TRANSMISSION A. Reservoir B. 1 = direct-zoonosis 2 = meta-zoonosis 3 = sapro-zoonosis 4 = cyclo-zoonosis C. Specific mechanisms	EPIDEMIOLOGY A. Populations at risk B. Geographic distribution	PREVENTION OR CONTROL
Toxoplasmosis	*Toxoplasma gondii*	*Human*—Most infections subclinical Three forms: (1) acquired form is variable febrile disease with general lymphadenopathy; specific symptoms depend on primary affected organs; (2) congenital form is most common, resulting in abortion, stillbirth, or brain damage; (3) ocular form is a chorioretinitis *Animal*—Most infections are subclinical Abortion and central nervous system involvement most common Symptoms vary with specific organ involvement	A. 1 B. Extremely wide host range Carnivores and omnivores primarily Any mammalian or avian species may be infected Felines are the only animals in which the organism will sexually reproduce	A. Soil contaminated with feces of domestic or wild feline species Feces of feline species Improperly cooked meat of sheep, swine, cow, poultry, and many other species B. 1, 3 C. Ingestion of oocysts by hand-mouth contact or water and food contamination Ingestion of improperly cooked meat Congenital Airborne possible	A. Farmers who have a high degree of soil contact especially in warm moist climates B. Worldwide, more prevalent in warm, moist climates	Excellent personal and environmental hygiene Avoid contamination with cat feces of soil to be tilled for agriculture Sanitary disposal of cat feces Avoid consumption of uncooked meat
Tuberculosis	*Mycobacterium tuberculosis, M. bovis, M. avium*	*Human*—*M. tuberculosis* and *M. bovis:* granulomatous lesions of lungs, intestine, or other tissue. Long-standing debilitating lesions, unless treated *M. avium:* uncommon wound infections and lymphadenitis mainly, pulmonary infections rare *Animal*—Granulomatous lesions of lungs, intestines, bones and other tissues	A. *M. tuberculosis:* 2 *M. bovis:* 1 *M. avium:* 1 B. *M. bovis:* cattle mainly, especially dairy cattle *M. tuberculosis* humans *M. avium:* chickens	A. *M. bovis:* cattle *M. tuberculosis:* humans, cattle *M. avium:* chickens, soil B. 1, possibly 3 C. Inhalation of infected droplets Direct contact with infected animals Consumption of unpasteurized milk Direct contact with tissues of infected animals	A. *M. bovis:* dairy farmers, cattle producers, meat cutters, abattoir workers *M. avium:* general farm workers, especially if exposed to chickens B. Worldwide, but *M. bovis* nearly eradicated in several western countries	Eradication pnrograms based on testing herds and removing infected animals have reduced the disease in many areas Good sanitation in the animal environment, including ventilation Personal protection when handling infected animals or tissues Proper cleansing and treatment of wounds Pasteurization of milk BCG immunization of persons in high incidence countries

Although exact numbers of zoonotic diseases occurring annually are not known, general changes in incidence, or trends, can be traced.[3, 4] The importance of zoonoses and other infectious diseases has decreased compared to a rise in chronic disease. Future trends include a probable continued decrease in the number of human cases of certain zoonoses, such as brucellosis and bovine tuberculosis, where active control programs exist. Epidemics are not likely, but rather isolated sporadic outbreaks. However, natural or human-induced events that disturb ecological balances can have significant effects on disease patterns. For example, the Aswan Dam, built in the early 1930s, allowed year-round irrigation in several provinces of Egypt.[4, 10] The resulting changes in ecology and agriculture caused a 50% increase in the incidence of schistosomiasis in the human population. Some animal diseases such as influenza, campylobacteriosis, and leukemia may emerge as important occupational problems in agriculture as more is learned about the animal-human relationships involved.

Risk for specific diseases varies with the particular type of animal production and geographic location.[4, 3] For example, people working with *dairy cows* are primarily susceptible to milker's nodules, brucellosis, Q fever, and ringworm, while people working with *beef cattle* are more at risk for rabies and leptospirosis. Table 59–6 lists major types of livestock operations and the primary zoonoses for which workers are at risk.[3, 4]

Zoonoses are also occupational hazards for people in agriculturally related occupations such as veterinarians, packing plant workers, poultry processing plant workers, rendering plant workers, and hair and hide industry workers. These workers may contract diseases such as brucellosis, ornithosis, anthrax, and contagious ecthyma.[9, 12–14]

Summary of General Characteristics

The following list summarizes the general characteristics of zoonotic diseases, and capsulizes the importance of zoonoses as occupational health problems in agriculture.[4]

1. Zoonoses often cause severe economic burdens because of loss of diseased animals, and because of the cost of preventing and treating infections in animals and humans.

2. Many zoonotic infections in humans are never diagnosed. Reasons are numerous, such as the protean and nonpathognomonic symptoms, the lack of physician awareness and the lack of adequate diagnostic support. Thus, accurate figures on the rate of zoonotic disease are not available.

3. Many zoonoses mimic other diseases, especially influenza.

4. Human infections generally occur sporadically rather than in epidemics. This is because humans are accidental, dead-end hosts for infectious agents and do not transmit infections to other people.

5. The majority of zoonoses are maintained primarily by vertebrate species other than humans.

6. There are specific groups of people that have an increased risk of acquiring infection. These risk groups include persons with greater than average contact with animals: agricultural workers, abattoir workers, meat processing plant workers, veterinarians, pet owners, and people living in rural areas or engaging in outdoor activities.

7. Most zoonoses have only one or a few major host species. However, infectious agents do typically have a broad potential host range. For example, the bacterium *Francisella tularensis,* which causes tularemia, has been isolated in over 100 mammalian species and numerous other vertebrates. However, many of these species are infected only by accident and are not significant in perpetuation of the disease cycle.

8. Animals may be inapparent carriers of infection. They may pose a health hazard for humans and other livestock without offering demonstrable signs.

9. Human infections typically result in morbidity but rarely in mortality. For example, leptospirosis, brucellosis, histoplasmosis and Q fever all can cause moderate to severe illness. However, when properly treated, they rarely lead to death unless complications develop.

Occupational health professionals can increase their ability to deal with zoonotic diseases by (1) consulting local practicing veterinarians and veterinarians working for public health or agricultural sections of the government, (2) developing an awareness of specific environments and agricultural activities that increase infection risks within their geographic locations. Such an awareness is essential to be able to recognize, evaluate, and control zoonotic diseases in agriculture.

Specific Agricultural Zoonotic Diseases

Table 59–7 outlines the primary aspects of selected major zoonotic diseases that are of occupational significance for agricultural workers. These charts are meant to be used in combination with the general information presented here, and with supplementation from the references cited and with consultation with regional experts. Using this combined approach, occupational health professionals should be able to establish control programs in their individual localities.

REFERENCES

1. Acha PN, Szyfres B: *Zoonoses and Communicable Diseases Common to Man and Animal*. Scientific Pub No 354. Washington, DC, Pan American Health Organization, 1980.
2. Donham KJ: Comparative medicine addendum, in Knapp LW: *State-of-the-Art-Report on Occupational Health and Safety in Agriculture*. Prepared for the National Institute of Occupational Safety and Health. Contract HSM-99-054-145 (2), 1974, pp 1–353.
3. Donham KJ: Infectious diseases common to animals and man of occupational significance to agricultural workers, in *Proceedings of Conference on Agricultural Health and Safety*. New York, Society for Occupational and Environmental Health, Environmental Sciences Laboratory, 1975, pp 160–175.
4. Donham KJ, Mutel C: *Zoonoses: An Overview*. Slide-tape presentation No WC950, General Services Administration, National Audiovisual Center, 1978.
5. Donham KJ: Zoonotic diseases of occupational significance in agriculture: A review. *Int J Zoon* 1985; 12:163–191.

6. *Epidemiological Aspects of Some Zoonoses*. DHEW (CDC) Pub No 75-8182. Atlanta, US Dept of Health, Education and Welfare, Center for Disease Control, 1973, pp 1–12.
7. Hubbert WT, McCulloch WF, Schnurrenberger PR: *Diseases Transmitted from Animals to Man*. Springfield, Illinois, Charles C Thomas, 1975.
8. Mutel CF, Donham KJ: *Medical Practice in Rural Communities*. New York, Springer-Verlag, 1983, pp 88–96.
9. *Occupational Health Problems in Agriculture:* Joint ILO/WHO Committee on Occupational Health, WHO Technical Report Series 246, Geneva, 1962, pp 25–61.
10. Prescott NM: Shistosomiasis and development, in *World Development*. 1979; 7:1–14.
11. Schnurrenberger PR, Hubbert WT: *An Outline of the Zoonoses*. Ames, Iowa, Iowa State University Press, 1981.
12. Steele JH: Occupational health in agriculture. *Arch Environ Health* 1968; 17:267–285, and Thrower WR: Agriculture and the public health: The Milroy Lectures. *J Roy Coll Physicians (Lond)* 1970; 4:277–304.
13. Steele JH: Zoonoses in agricultural communities: Epidemiology. *Clinical Medicine* 1977; August: 24–36.
14. *Zoonoses:* Joint FAO/WHO Expert Committee on Zoonoses. Geneva, World Health Organization, 1967.

DERMATOSES

Although skin afflictions are common in many industries, agricultural workers have higher rates of skin disease than other occupational categories. In 1976, the agricultural industry employed only 1% of the work force but experienced 4% of all occupational dermatoses.[30] The nature of their activities brings farmers and other agricultural workers in contact with a broad spectrum of hazards, including climatic factors (sun, heat, cold), agricultural chemicals (pesticides, feed aditives, cleaning agents), and biologic hazards (allergenic plants, cutaneous infections, and arthropods).[35]

Skin conditions due to chronic exposure to heat and sunlight are especially common in farmers. Heat can cause miliaria and intertrigo, while excessive sunlight can result in sunburn, photosensitivity reactions, active keratoses, and cutaneous malignancies. Actinic keratoses are commonly found on the exposed skin of older farmers. Lesions tend to be multiple and, if untreated, slowly enlarge, becoming broader and more elevated. Approximately 20%–25% of these lesions will evolve into squamous cell carcinomas.[4] There is considerable evidence supporting the role of solar radiation in the etiology of human skin cancer.[2, 10, 27, 31] Although the distribution of basal cell carcinomas on the head and neck does not necessarily correspond to the sites of greatest exposure, they do tend to occur more frequently in fair-skinned individuals who experience greater overall sun exposure. The evidence for the role of sunlight in the etiology of squamous cell carcinoma is more convincing. They are distributed primarily over the head, neck, and exposed areas of the upper extremity, occur most commonly in men who work outdoors, and can evolve from preexisting actinic keratoses. Although melanomas are not concentrated on the face and neck (in contrast to squamous and basal cell carcinomas), solar exposure has also been implicated in the etiology of this cutaneous malignancy. The incidence increases with closer residence to the equator. Individuals with fair skin, blue eyes, and naturally red or blond hair seem to be at highest risk.[7, 13] It has been suggested that melanomas are more likely to occur as the result of intermittent exposure to intense sunlight as opposed to more chronic and continuous exposure more commonly associated with basal and squamous cell carcinomas.[4]

Frost nip and frostbite are constant threats to farmers in colder climates. Frost nip refers to superficial, reversible freezing of the skin, usually involving the nose, cheeks, or fingers. Unless quickly recognized and treated by rewarming, frost nip can progress to frostbite. Four categories of frostbite have been described, depending on the depth of injury.[16] The most severe degree involves the entire thickness of the skin and usually progresses to gangrene and mummification. The current treatment of choice for all forms of frostbite has been summarized (see Chapter 23).[34]

Modern-day agriculture involves exposure to a large number of chemicals, many of which are capable of producing skin reactions. Major groups of chemical agents include pesticides, animal feed additives, veterinary preparations, and miscellaneous substances (detergents, disinfectants, solvents, antioxidants, fertilizers). The resulting dermatitis may be of the allergic, irritant, or photo-contact variety.

A large number of pesticides are known to cause dermatitis.[9, 23] Dithiocarbamates (thiram) and the amine herbicide Randox (2-chloro-N,N-diallylacetomide) can produce allergic contact dermatitis.[21, 25] Other pesticides function as cutaneous irritants.[5] Porphyra cutanea tarda has occurred after exposure to hexachlorobenzene, benzene hexachloride, and the organophosphorous insecticide diazinon.[1a, 8] Chloracne from dioxin contamination of the chlorophenoxy herbicide 2,4,5-T is well known but generally occurs among heavily exposed industrial workers rather than farmers.[33]

The production of animal feeds has become a complex process requiring the addition of vitamins, minerals, hormones, antibiotics, antioxidants, and other chemicals.[3, 19] Some of these additives have caused contact dermatitis in workers manufacturing the feed and in farmers. A partial listing of causative agents includes cobalt (mineral supplement), ethylene diamine dihydroiodide (iodine source), furazolidine (growth promoting factor), hydroquinone (antioxidant), halquinol (antibacterial), and tylosin (antibiotic).[21] As with other forms of allergic contact dermatitis, cross-reactions with structurally similar compounds can occur. One farmer who acquired primary sensitization through previous use of Mycolog cream later reacted to ethylene diamine dihydroiodide which he fed to his cows.[11]

Veterinarians and farmers who administer veterinary medicines themselves may develop contact dermatitis to a variety of antibiotics, including penicillin, tylosin, spiramycin, nitrofurazone, and neomycin.[14, 15, 19, 24, 28]

Farmers also use a variety of other chemicals capable of producing contact dermatitis. Sensitivity to formalin (disinfectant), calcium ammonium nitrate (fertilizer), and N-phenyl N′-isopropyl paraphenylenediamine (rubber antioxidant) has been reported.[20, 26, 32] Other substances which tend to act as primary irritants include detergents, solvents, paints, lime, hypochlorite solutions, diesel fuel, and gasoline.

Allergenic plants, infectious agents, and arthropods are ubiquitous in the agricultural environment. Members of the genus *Rhus* (poison ivy, oak, and sumac) are well known potent cutaneous sensitizers. Chrysanthemums and daisies may be responsible for a less common form of contact dermatitis. Unusual occupations or new technical innovations can result in unusual or new forms of dermatitis. Tulip finger from handling tulip bulbs is due to a chemical allergen in the bulb itself.[29] Strimmer rash occurs in individuals operating hand-held, powered rotary grass or brush cutters. Fragments of psoralen-containing plants strike the uncovered skin of the operator and can produce a photodermatitis.[12]

Orf, a viral disease of sheep, can be transmitted to man. It produces one to a few raised pustular lesions on the hands or forearms. Milker's nodule is caused by a similar virus that is endemic among cows, usually producing lesions on the udders. In humans, the condition consists of nodules on the hands which usually heal in six to eight weeks without scarring.[18] Fungal diseases include both sporotrichosis and ringworm. Sporotrichosis produces a cutaneous ulcer with nodular lymphangitis extending proximately. It occurs in farmers, horticulturists, gardeners, and veterinarians. Sphagnum moss contaminated with the causative organism *Sporothrix schenckii* is often the source of infection.[22] Superficial fungal eruptions are extremely common. Cattle ringworm due to *Trichophyton verrucosum* usually involves the hands. An allergic reaction to the superficial fungus can lead to a kerion, a lesion commonly misdiagnosed as a bacterial abscess. Other farm animals capable of transmitting ringworm to man include cats, dogs, mice, and hedgehogs.[6, 21] Agricultural endeavors often involve contact with materials and animals infected with arthropods. Various mites and chiggers can all be causes of intensely pruritic, erythematous papules.[17]

While most forms of occupational dermatoses are amenable to treatment, prevention is the preferred approach. Principles of prevention developed in industrial settings are also applicable to the agricultural environment. Basically, one seeks to identify the risk factors in a given activity and avoid their effects either through direct elimination of the offending agent, alteration of work practices, or use of protective ointments. Sunscreening agents offering high sun protection factors are effective against solar radiation. Appropriate gloves with cotton liners can prevent hand eczema. A review of the general principles of prevention of occupational dermatoses has been published.[23] (See Chapter 10 for detailed discussion of occupational dermatoses.)

REFERENCES

1. Adams RM: *Occupational Dermatology*. New York, Grune & Stratton, 1983.

1a. Bleiberg J, Wallen M, Brodkin R, et al: Industrially acquired porphyria. *Arch Dermatol* 1964; 89:793.

2. Burmeister LF: Cancer mortality in Iowa farmers 1971–1978. *JNCI* 1981; 66:461.
3. Burrows D: Contact dermatitis in animal feed mill workers. *Br J Dermatol* 1975; 92:167.
4. Caro WA, Bronstein BR: Tumors of the skin, in Moschella LS, Hurley HJ (eds): *Dermatology*, ed 2. Philadelphia, WB Saunders Co, 1985.
5. Caplan RM: Cutaneous hazards posed by agricultural chemicals. *J Iowa Med Soc* 1969; 59:295.
6. Chmel L, Buchvald J, Valentova M: Ringworm infection among agricultural workers. *Int J Epidemiol* 1976; 5:291.
7. Climatic Impact Committee: *Environmental Impact of Stratospheric Flight*. Washington, DC, National Academy of Sciences, 1975.
8. Collins AG, Nichol AW, Elsbury S: Porphyria cutanea tarda and agricultural pesticides. *Aust J Dermatol* 1982; 23:70.
9. Cronin E: *Contact Dermatitis*. New York, Churchill Livingstone, Inc, 1980.
10. Emmett EA: Ultraviolet radiation as a cause of skin tumors. *CRC Crit Rev Toxicol* 1973; 2:211.
11. Fischer AA: Allergic contact dermatitis in animal feed handlers. *Cutis* 1975; 16:201.
12. Freeman K, Hubbard KC, Warin AP: Strimmer rash. *Contact Dermatitis* 1984; 10:117.
13. Gellin GA, Kopf AW, Garfinkel L: Malignant melanomas: A controlled study of possibly associated factors. *Arch Dermatol* 1969; 99:43.
14. Hjorth N: Occupational dermatitis among veterinary surgeons. *Contact Dermatitis Newsletter* 1967; 2:12.
15. Hjorth N, Weisman K: Occupational dermatitis among veterinary surgeons caused by spiramycin, tylosin and penethamate. *Acta Derm Venereol* 1973; 53:299.
16. Jarrett F: Frostbite: Current concepts of pathogenesis and treatment. *Rev Surg* 1974; 31:71.
17. Krinsky WL: Dermatoses associated with the bites of mites and ticks. *Int J Dermatol* 1983; 22:75.
18. Leavell UW, Phillips JA: Milker's nodules. *Arch Dermatol* 1975; 111:1307.
19. Nelder KH: Contact dermatitis from animal feed additives. *Arch Dermatol* 1972; 106:722.
20. Pasricha JS, Gupta R: Contact dermatitis due to calcium ammonium nitrate. *Contact Dermatitis* 1983; 9:149.
21. Peachey RDG: Skin hazards in farming. *Br J Dermatol* 1981; 105:45.
22. Powell KE, Taylor A, Phillips BJ, et al: Cutaneous sporotrichosis in forestry workers. *JAMA* 1978; 240:232.
23. Sanutz MH, Cohen SR: Occupational skin disease, in Maschella SL, Hurley HJ (eds): *Dermatology*, ed 2. Philadelphia, WB Saunders Co, 1985.
24. Simpson JR: Dermatitis due to neomycin in a calf-drench. *Contact Dermatitis Newsletter* 1974; 15:447.
25. Spencer MC: Herbicide dermatitis. *JAMA* 1966; 198:169.
26. TeLintum JCA, Nater JP: Allergic contact dermatitis caused by rubber chemicals in dairy workers. *Dermatologica* 1974; 148:42.
27. Urback F, et al: Genetic and environmental interaction in skin carcinogenesis, in *Environment and Cancer, Symposium on Fundamental Cancer Research, 24th, Anderson Hospital and Tumor Institute, 1971*. Baltimore, Williams & Wilkins Co, 1972.
28. Veinen NK, Hattel T, Justesen O, et al: Occupational contact dermatitis due to spiramycin and/or tylosin among farmers. *Contact Dermatitis* 1980; 6:410.
29. Verspychk Mijnssen GAW: Pathogenesis and causative agent of tulips finger. *Br J Dermatol* 1969; 81:737.
30. Wand CL: *The Problem of Skin Disease in Industry*. Washington, DC, Office of Occupational Safety and Health Statistics, US Dept of Labor, US Government Printing Office, 1978.
31. Whitaker CJ, Lee WR, Douner JE: Squamous cell skin cancer in the northwest of England (1967–69) and its relation to occupation. *Br J Ind Med* 1979; 36:43.
32. Wilkinson DS: Formalin sensitivity in mushroom farming. *Contact Dermatitis Newsletter* 1970; 7:162.
33. Zack JA, Suskind RR: The mortality experience of workers exposed to tetrachlorodibenzodioxin in a triphenol process accident. *J Occup Med* 1980; 22:11.
34. Zalar GL, Harber LC: Reactions to physical agents, in Moschella LS, Hurley HJ (eds): *Dermatology*, ed 2. Philadelphia, WB Saunders Co, 1985.
35. Zuehkle RL: Common cutaneous problems in agricultural work, in

Proceedings of Conference on Agricultural Health and Safety. New York, Society of Occupational and Environmental Health, Environmental Sciences Lab, 1975.

CANCER

The overall cancer rate for farmers is lower than that of the general population, because two of the most common malignancies (lung and breast) are less common.[5] The apparent reason for decreased lung cancer incidence is the fact that farmers smoke less than nonfarmers (approximately 17% of farmers smoke as opposed to 34% of the general population).[11, 26, 28] This theory is supported by the fact that farmers also have fewer smoking-relate cancers in general, particularly those of the mouth and esophagus.[67]

However, farmers have excess risk for several different neoplasms when compared to the general population. Milham[5, 24] noted increased risk in farmers for cancer of the stomach, brain, and kidney, and for leukemia. Burmeister[5–7] noted increased mortality rates in Iowa farmers for leukemia, lymphoma, lip cancer, multiple myeloma, and prostate cancer. Of these, excessive leukemia in farmers[1–8, 14, 15, 17, 21, 23, 24] has been consistently documented. Farming type, specific commodities produced, and agricultural chemicals have been investigated as possible risk factors. Exposure to dairy cattle, corn production, fertilizer usage, and poultry production has been implicated in one or more studies. Of these, dairy cattle and corn production have been most extensively studied. One controversial hypothesis to explain the link with dairy cattle is that farmers may become infected by the bovine leukemia virus, a common infection in cattle causing lymphosarcoma.[1, 13, 14, 20–22, 28–30]

The only certain causal association of cancer in farmers is that between excessive exposure to sun and the development of lip and skin cancer. The observed excess of stomach cancer has been attributed to the consumption of high-nitrate water, which may be converted in vivo to nitrosamines.[12, 31, 32] Other causal associations are still speculative,[5] but Table 59–8 helps to summarize potential risk factors in an area which is undergoing active research.

REFERENCES

1. Bartsch DC, Springer F, Fulk H: Acute non-lymphocytic leukemia, an adult cluster. *JAMA* 1975; 232:1333.
2. Blair A, Malker H, Cantor KP, et al: Cancer among farmers: A review. *Scand J Work Environ Health* 1985; 11:397–407.

TABLE 59–8.
Types of Cancer Common in Farmers and Possible Risk Factors

CANCER TYPE	POSSIBLE RISK FACTORS	REFERENCES
Leukemia	General farming	6, 8, 25, 26
	Beef cattle	5
	Dairy cattle	1, 3, 9, 17, 19, 21, 25, 29
	Corn production	6, 8, 9
	Poultry production	9, 24, 29
	Fertilizer usage	4, 9
	Grain farming	24
	Herbicide use	6, 9
	Insecticide use	6
Lymphoma	General farming	4, 9
	Poultry/egg production	8, 24, 27
	Dairy production	21
	Hog production	9
	Herbicide use	9
Multiple myeloma	General farming	7, 23, 24
	Poultry production (eggs)	7, 27
	Dairy production	7
	Hog production	7
	Herbicide use	7
Lip	General farming	5, 7, 23, 24
Stomach	Nitrate in water	30, 31, 32
	Cattle production	2, 7, 24
	Corn production	2, 7, 24
	Dairy production	9, 24
Prostate	General farming	6, 7, 8, 25
	Cattle ranching	24
Brain	Dairy farming	24
	Poultry farming	24
	Cattle ranching	24
Connective tissue	Phenoxy acetic acid	16, 18
	Herbicides (2-4D, 2-4-5T)	
	General farming	

3. Blair A, Thomas TL: Leukemia among Nebraska farmers: A death certificate study. *Am J Epidemiol* 1979; 110:264.
4. Blair A, White DW: A death certificate study of leukemia among farmers from Wisconsin. *JNCI* 1981; 66:1027.
5. Burmeister LF: Cancer mortality in Iowa farmers, 1971–1978. *JNCI* 1981; 66:461.
6. Burmeister LF, Van Lier SF, Isacson P: Leukemia and farm practices in Iowa. *Am J Epidemiol* 1982; 115:720.
7. Burmeister LF, Everett GD, Van Lier S, Isacson P: Selected cancer mortality and farm practices in Iowa. *Am J Epidemiol* 1983; 118:72.
8. Caldwell GG, Rosenlef RC, Lemon HM, et al: Epidemiology of leukemia-lymphoma in mid-Nebraska. *Neb Med J* 1973; 58:233.
9. Cantor KP: Farming and mortality from non-Hodgkin's lymphoma: A case control study. *Int J Cancer* 1982; 29:239.
10. Cantor K, Everett G, Blair A, et al: Farming and non-Hodgkin's. *Am J Epidemiol* 1985; 122:535.
11. Cassell J, Heyden S, Bartel AG, et al: Occupational and physical activity and coronary heart disease. *Arch Intern Med* 1971; 128:920.
12. Cuello C, Correa P, Haenszel W, et al: Gastric cancer in Columbia. I. Cancer risk and suspect environmental agents. *JNCI* 1976; 57:1015.
13. Donham KJ, Van Der Maaten MJ, Miller JM, et al: Seroepidemiologic studies on the possible relationships of human and bovine leukemia: Brief communication. *JNCI* 1977; 59:851.
14. Donham KJ, Bert JW, Sawin RS: Epidemiologic relationships of the bovine population and human leukemia in Iowa. *Am J Epidemiol* 1980; 112:80.
15. Fasal E, Jackson EW, Klauber M: Leukemia and lymphoma mortality among farm residents. *Am J Epidemiol* 1968; 87:267.
16. Hardell L, Sandstrom A: Case-control study: Soft-tissue sarcomas and exposure to phenoxyacetic acids or chlorophenols. *Br J Cancer* 1979; 39:711.
17. Heath CW Jr: Human leukemia, genetic and environmental clusters, in *Comp Leukemia Res* 1969. New York, Karger, 1970.
18. Hoar SK, Blair A, Holmes FF, et al: Agricultural herbicide use and risk of lymphoma and soft-tissue sarcoma. *JAMA* 1986; 256:1141–1147.
19. Khokhlova MP, Rakhmamin PP: Comparative study on geographical distribution of human and cattle leukosis. *Comp Leukemia Res* 1968; 31:331.
20. Kvarnfors E, Henricson B, Hugoson: A statistical study on farm and village level on the possible relations between human leukemia and bovine leukosis. *Acta Vet Scand* 1975; 16:163.
21. Linos A, Kyle RE, Elveback LR, et al: Leukemia in Olmsted County, MN, 1965–1974. *Mayo Clin Proc* 1978; 53:714.
22. McClure HM, Kelling MW, Custer RP, et al: Erythroleukemia in two infant chimpanzees fed milk from cows naturally infected with bovine C-type virus. *Cancer Res* 1974; 34:2745.
23. Milham S Jr: Leukemia and multiple myeloma in farmers. *Am J Epidemiol* 1971; 94:307.
24. Milham S: *Occupational Mortality in Washington State, 1950–1971*. Washington, DC, Dept of Health, Education, and Welfare, Public Health Service, US Government Printing Office, 1976, vols 1–3.
25. Piper CE, Abt DA, Ferrer JF, et al: Seroepidemiological evidence for horizontal transmission of bovine C-type virus. *Cancer Res* 1975; 35:2714.
26. Pomrehn P, Wallace RB, Burmeister LF: Ischemic heart disease in Iowa Farmers. The influence of lifestyle. *JAMA* 1982; 248:1073.
27. Priester WA, Mason TJ: Human cancer mortality in relation to poultry population, by county, in 10 SE states. *JNCI* 1974; 53:45.
28. Sterling TO, Weinkam JJ: Smoking characteristics by type of employment. *J Occup Med* 1976; 18:743.
29. VanDerMaaten MJ, Miller JM: Serological evidence of transmission of bovine leukemia virus to chimpanzees. *Vet Microbiol* 1976; 1:351.
30. Zaldivar R, Robinson H: Epidemiological investigation on stomach cancer mortality in Chileans: Association with nitrate fertilizer. *Z Krebsforschung* 1973; 80:289.
31. Zaldivar R, Wetterstrand WH: Further evidence of a positive correlation between exposure to nitrate fertilizers ($NaNo_3$) and gastric cancer death rates; nitrites and nitrosamines. *Experienta* 1975; 31:1354.
32. Zaldivar R: Nitrate fertilizers as environmental pollutants: Positive correlation between nitrates ($NaNo_3$ and KNO_3) used per unit area and stomach cancer mortality rates. *Experientia* 1977; 33:264.

PESTICIDES

Since the discovery of DDT in the 1940s, the use of agricultural pesticides has expanded tremendously. Today, U.S. manufacturers annually sell over 1.3 million lb of pesticides and export an additional 600 million lbs with insecticides making a large component of the pesticides used.[1] The relative amounts applied vary geographically and with type of agriculture. In row crop grain-producing areas, the amounts of herbicides used are nearly three times as great as the amounts of insecticides used.[2] In the western and southwestern United States, large quantities of insecticides relative to herbicides are used in fruit and vegetable crop production. Table 59–9 lists the major groups of herbicides and their health effects.

Data are limited regarding the frequency of pesticide poisoning. The National Clearinghouse for Poison Control Centers estimates that 5%–6% of all poisonings are due to pesticides. However, since most poison control centers are located in urban areas where they are unavailable to agricultural workers, the true proportion of pesticide poisonings may be considerably higher. One study showed that approximately 2,700 persons were hospitalized annually in the United States for pesticide poisoning between 1971 and 1973. Fifty-five percent of these hospitalizations were due to home accidents, 28% resulted from occupational exposure, and 17% were suicide attempts. Approximately 64 deaths occurred annually. Of these, 60% were suicides, 25% were from home accidents, mostly children, and 12% were from occupational exposure.[3] In addition to agricultural workers, occupational exposures may occur in several other groups, including chemical manufacturing plant employees, workers in packaging and formulation, transportation personnel, warehouse workers, and applicators.

Strategies to prevent occupational illness and injury caused by pesticides include five basic factors: (1) hygienic work practices, (2) avoidance, (3) personal protective equipment, (4) monitoring worker health, and (5) applying and enforcing regulations. Safe work practices include frequent hand washing, showering, shampooing, washing clothes that contact the chemicals, cleaning up of spills, and providing sanitary eating places. Avoidance involves developing methods to separate people from the chemicals, such as closed systems for mixing and loading, safer packaging, safer formulations, and safe time periods before workers can enter a field or orchard after the crop has been treated with pesticides. Personal protective clothing and equipment used in high-exposure jobs include rubber suits, aprons, gloves, boots, goggles, face shields, and respirators. Monitoring blood and urine of workers is done in some high-exposure jobs.[1, 4] (Refer to Chapter 46 for a thorough discussion of pesticides.)

TABLE 59–9.
Primary Use and Health Effects of Commonly Used Herbicides*†

CHEMICAL CLASS	TYPE OF HERBICIDES	MAJOR USE	TYPE EXAMPLE	TOXIC MECHANISM IN HUMANS	HEALTH EFFECTS, SYMPTOMS, CLINICAL SIGNS
Phenolic compounds	Contact and preemergent, some also used as germicides and fungicides	General weed and brush control Wood preservative Dinitroorthocresol	Pentachlorophenol	Uncouple metabolic phosphorylation resulting in excess body heat Also a direct cellular toxin	Damage liver, kidney, and brain in two ways: hyperthermia and direct chemical action Symptoms and signs include high body temperature and central nervous system disturbance
Chlorophenoxy compounds	Systemic	Control of broad-leafed plants in row crops Defoliants, general brush control	2,4-D 2,4,5-T Agent Orange	Skin irritants Generally low systemic toxicity May contain dioxins as contaminants, which have caused chloracne and neurologic damage to chemical plant workers	Irritate skin and mucous membranes Cause headache, dizziness
Arsenical compounds	Contact	Cotton defoliants Crabgrass killer	Newer products are moderately toxic organic arsenicals (e.g., arsenic acid and cacodylic acid)	The pentavalent form may be converted to trivalent arsenic in the gut, which is a potent general cellular toxin	Liver, kidney, nervous system damage

			More toxic forms (e.g., Paris green and arsenic trioxide) seldom used today		
Dipyridyl compounds	Contact	Broad spectrum Crop defoliant, used in no-till methods of row crop production	Paraquat Diquat	Contact irritant If ingested, will induce malignant pulmonary fibrosis	Superficial burns of skin and mucous membranes If ingested, cause death by asphyxiation from proliferation of alveolar connective tissue
Organonitrogen compounds	Preemergent Soil sterilants Contact	Weed control: row crops	Propachlor	Skin sensitizers Contact irritants Generally low systemic toxicity	If ingested, cause abdominal pain, nausea, and diarrhea If gotten on skin, induce irritant or allergic contact dermatitis
Phthalate compounds	Preemergent	Weed control: cotton, strawberries, beans, and other vegetable crops	Dacthal (DCPA)	Skin sensitizers Irritants Generally low systemic toxicity	If ingested, cause abdominal pain, nausea, and diarrhea Dermatitis: irritative and allergic

From Morgan DP, Mutel CF, Cain C, et al: *Pesticide Poisonings and Injuries: Where, When, and How.* Slide-tape presentation no. AO 1941. General Services Administration, National Audiovisual Center, 1979.

See also Chapters 10, 31, 46, 47, 50, 52.

REFERENCES

1. Morgan DP, Mutel CF, Cain C, et al: Pesticides poisonings and injuries: Where, when, and how (1979). Slide tape presentation No. AO 1941, General Services Administration, National Audiovisual Center.
2. Morgan DP: *Pesticide Toxicology,* vol 2. New York, John Wiley & Sons, 1982, pp 1–36.
3. National Study of Hospital Admitted Pesticide Poisonings (1976). US Environmental Protection Agency, Epidemiologic Studies Program, Health Effects Monitoring Branch, Technical Services Division, Office of Pesticide Program.
4. Prevention and management of occupational pesticide poisonings (1979), in *Guide to Health and Hygiene in Agricultural Work*. Geneva, International Labor Organization, 1979, pp 94–149.

ARTHRITIS

There are few data on the incidence or nature of arthritis in agricultural workers. A national household survey showed farmers had twice the prevalence of reported arthritis and rheumatism when compared to all other occupations combined.[6] In Minnesota, those with 20 or more years of experience as farmers were hospitalized more often for osteoarthritis than were nonfarmers.[2] Farmers also have a high proportion of Social Security Disability awards due to osteoarthritis.[3] Osteoarthritis of the hip has been reported to be increased among French farmers.[4] A Swedish study noted a 6% prevalence of "hip joint" disease determined by interview and physical examination. More cases were seen in farmers who had driven tractors for more than 20 years, a finding the author attributed to vibration, poor work position, and low environmental temperature.[5]

Farmers in the dairy region of central Wisconsin were found to have an increased prevalence of degenerative knee disease. This prevalence was more than two and one-half times that of all other workers and more than four times that of white collar workers. The increased risk observed among dairy farmers was thought to be due to the biomechanical stress placed on the knees from repetitive bending and squatting during machine milking. Modern milking parlors represent the ultimate ergonomic solution, but are not economically feasible for most farmers. Less expensive methods to reduce forces on the knee joints include strap-on, one-legged stools, and industrial knee pads.[1]

REFERENCES

1. Anderson CL, Treuhaft PS, Horvath EP, et al: Degenerative knee disease among dairy farmers, in Dosman JA (ed): *Health and Safety in Agriculture*. Proceedings International Symposium on Health and Safety in Agriculture, Saskatoon, October, 1985.
2. Burkhart JA, Egleston CF, Voss RJ: *The Rural Health Study: A Comparison of Hospital Experience between Farmers and Nonfarmers in a Rural Area of Minnesota*. DHEW (NIOSH) Publ 78-184. Dept of Health, Education and Welfare, Public Health Service, National Institute For Occupational Safety and Health, 1978.
3. Kennedy J, Fishbach TJ: *Occupational Characteristics of Disabled Workers—Social Security Disability Benefit Awards to Workers During* 1969–1972, DHHS (NIOSH) Publ 80-145. Cincinnati, Oh, Dept of Health and Human Services, National Institute for Occupational Safety and Health, 1980.
4. Louyot P, Savin R: La coxarthrose chez l'agriculteur. *Rev Rhum Mal Osteoartic* 1966; 33:625–632.
5. Thelin A: Work and health among farmers. *Scand J Soc Med* 1980; Suppl 22.
6. Woolsey TD: Prevalence of arthritis and rheumatism in the United States. *Public Health Rep* 1952; 67:505.

MENTAL HEALTH

The superiority of mental health in rural residents, as compared to their urban counterparts, has been a traditional belief. It has been argued that the faster pace and greater stress of urban life lead to more psychiatric disorders than are found in tranquil rural settings.[13] These views were supported by early studies showing higher rates of first admissions to mental institutions for persons residing in cities.[10] However, rates of treated psychiatric disorders vary with the availability of treatment facilities and with public attitudes toward their use.[4] Historically, mental hospital beds have been less available to rural people and typical rural attitudes have opposed committing "one of their family members."[7]

Subsequent epidemiologic studies have attempted to compare the prevalence of mental disorders in urban and rural areas. Unfortunately, the comparability of findings in psychiatric epidemiology is diminished by differences in data collection procedures and diagnostic criteria. For example, rates of mental disorders in rural study sites ranged from 1% to 64%.[4] It is difficult to attribute these enormous variations to true differences in the disease prevalence. It is much more likely that they are due to differences in definition of a case and of sampling methodology.[6]

Srole[12] was among the first to question the superiority of rural mental health. When comparing prevalence rates between two major epidemiologic surveys (mid-town Manhattan study and the Stirling County study), he found a statistically greater mental morbidity rate in the rural study site.[12] Srole also presented data from a national survey *(The National Center for Health Statistics Health Examination Survey, 1960–1962)* to show an inverse relationship between population size of an area and psychiatric disorder.[12] However, Mueller recently reviewed several North American studies that made urban-rural comparisons.[8] They employed symptom-screening scales assigning each respondent a numerical score and used a cut-off point to separate "cases from non-cases." No clear trend of urban versus rural differences emerged.

Regardless of whether there are true differences in the prevalence of mental disease between urban and rural areas, comparing total rates for all disorders may be misleading, because it could obscure differences in prevalence for specific diagnoses. Nine studies comparing rural versus urban prevalence rates for specific diagnostic categories were reviewed by the Dohrenwends.[5] These were all conducted outside North America, and case identification techniques varied considerably. The total rate for all psychiatric disorders combined was higher in the urban areas (seven out of nine studies) although the differences tended to be small. When specific diagnostic categories were considered separately, various trends emerged. Neuroses and personality disorders occurred more commonly in the urban environment, while total rates for all psychoses combined and for the manic-depressive subtype were higher in rural areas.

Although manic-depressive psychoses tend to occur more frequently in the rural environment, consideration of the broader category of depression shows an opposite trend. Urban centers have higher rates of depression than smaller communities, particularly for the non-psychotic depressions (neurotic and reactive).[8] A possible explanation for this phenomenon is lower levels of social and interpersonal support found in the city. However, persons living in isolated rural areas may suffer similar deprivation. Suicide rates in 12 Welch counties demonstrated a paradoxical finding in that the highest rates occurred in large communities and in isolated rural areas while the lowest rates were found in smaller communities.[3] An analysis of Minnesota's suicide data for the years 1967–1973 showed the greatest percentage of increase occurring in urban areas with one exception: rural women aged 45–64. The large increase in this group was attributed to geographic isolation and other social barriers.[1]

Stress has been defined as the generalized physiologic and psychologic reaction to anything which threatens a person's survival.[11] Farmers, like other businesspeople, are subjected to stressors from uncontrollable external events. A study of Iowa farmers shows them rating farm-related stressors such as machinery breakdown, disease outbreak, and death of an animal closely behind major personal losses such as death of a spouse or a close family member.[14] The most unique aspect of farming is that the farm family unit is also a business unit which lives and works together day after day. This close proximity makes for severe stress when economic factors, weather, or personal illness strike, particularly when family solidarity is weak.[9] The large amount of integration between home and occupational spheres may be particularly stressful for the rural housewife. Like their urban counterparts, farm women experience stress associated with role conflicts between home responsibilities and work. A recent study demonstrated a significant negative correlation between role conflict and husband support, suggesting that farm husbands can play an important role in mediating stress experienced by their wives.[2]

Rural physicians and counselors must be skilled at recognizing the signs of stess and instructing farmers how to deal effectively with the stressors in their environment. Patients suffering from stress-related symptoms can present with a wide variety of nonspecific complaints which often precipitate expensive, time-consuming and usually futile evaluations seeking an organic cause. It is increasingly common for farmers to attribute such symptoms to an exposure to a pesticide or other environmental chemical. In some instances, such an exposure event may have actually occurred, resulting in acute irritant phenomenon or transient systemic symptoms. However, the persistence of symptoms beyond the expected duration for a given chemical is often due to a psychophysiologic reaction. Key factors in the perpetuation of such a response include the individual's preexisting psychologic state, the presence of other stressors, and the perception as to whether an environmental threat still exists. The physician's role in such cases is to exclude the presence of organic disease or chronic toxicity and to counsel the farmer as to the true nature of his complaints. Depression is often an underlying cause and can be effectively managed with antidepressant medication and psychologic support.

A comprehensive overview of mental health in rural America, complete with an extensive bibliography, has been published by the National Institute of Mental Health.[6]

REFERENCES

1. Barton SN, Coombs DW, Mukherjee D: Urban-rural suicide differentials in Minnesota 1967–1973. *Minn Med* 1980; 63:415.
2. Berkowitz AD, Perkins HW: Stress among farm women: Work and family as interacting systems. *J Marriage Fam* 1984; February, p 161.
3. Capstick A: Urban and rural suicide. *J Ment Sci* 1960; 106:1327.
4. Dohrenwend BP, Dohrenwend BS: *Social Status and Psychological Disorder: A Causal Injury*. New York, John Wiley & Sons, 1969.
5. Dohrenwend BP, Dohrenwend BS: Psychiatric disorders in urban settings, in Caplan G (ed): *American Handbook of Psychiatry*, ed 2. New York, Basic Books, Inc, 1974, vol 2.
6. Flax JW, Wagenfeld MO, Ivens RE, et al: *Mental Health and Rural America: An Overview and Annotated Bibliography*, DHEW Publ (ADM) 78–753. Dept of Health, Education and Welfare, Public Health Service, National Institute of Mental Health, 1979.
7. Mott FD, Roemer MJ: Rural health and medical care. New York, McGraw-Hill Book Co, 1948.
8. Mueller DP: The current status of urban-rural differences in psychiatric disorder. *J Nervous Ment Dis* 1981; 169:18.
9. Robinson JW: Personal communication, May 24, 1984.
10. Rose AM, Stubb HR: Summary of studies in the incidence of mental disorders, in Rose A (ed): *Mental Health and Mental Disorder: A Sociological Approach*. New York, Norton, 1955.
11. Seyle N: *The Stress of Life*. New York, McGraw-Hill Book Co, 1955.
12. Srole L: The city versus town and country: New evidence on an ancient bias, in Srole L, Fischer AK (eds): *Mental Health in the Metropolis: The Midtown Manhattan Study Book Two*. New York, Harper & Row, 1977.
13. Toffler A: *Future Shock*. New York, Bantam, 1970.
14. Wiegel R: *Stress on the Farm, Cooperative Extension Circular*, Ames, Ia, Iowa State University, 1981.

60

The Health of Truck Drivers

Joseph LaDou, M.D.

OVERVIEW

There are more than 2 million truck drivers in the United States, including both line-haul (or intercity) and local pickup and delivery drivers. However, since ten times as many trucks are registered as there are full-time drivers, it appears that the total employment in trucking is far understated by traditional measures.[4] Furthermore, these numbers do not include drivers of buses, street cars, in-plant trucks, or farm vehicles, drivers in mines or in the military services, and drivers of related transport equipment, i.e., airport services, trains, and subways. With some exceptions, worldwide, train transport is decreasing and motor transport is gaining with enormous growth. The Trans European express system extends from north of the polar circle into the Middle East and Asia. U.S. industry revenues are greater than $50 billion per year.[5] By any measure, therefore, trucking is a major industry in America and throughout the world. It is also a major source of concern for the health and safety of truck drivers as well as the wider community of noncommercial drivers. In 1982, the last year for which statistics are available, interstate trucks killed 3,784 people, or three times as many Americans as all other forms of commercial transportation combined.[19]

The Motor Carrier Act of 1980 substantially deregulated the trucking industry, resulting in an increase in the number of motor carriers from 17,083 in 1979 to 27,517 in 1984.[7] Industry profits rose in 1984 by 20%, to $1.2 billion, on a 12% increase in revenues.[5] It appears that the initial period of adjustment to deregulation has occurred and that the industry is in a healthy position to give primary attention to the issue of health and safety of its drivers and of the public.

Motor carriers fall in two broad categories: private and for hire. Private carriers are shippers that use their own or leased vehicles to transport their own products. For-hire carriers provide transportation of freight for others and may operate interstate, intrastate, or locally.

Types of Trucks

In trucking, two types of vehicles are used primarily—straight trucks and tractor-trailer trucks.

Straight trucks typically are vehicles with three axles and ten wheels. They are equipped with van, flatbed, tank, dump, or similar bodies. These vehicles are used mainly for local pickup and delivery. Their drivers constitute about 70% of the nation's truckers. They frequently work a ten-hour day, with sporadic rest periods and mealtimes. Drivers who haul commodities and construction materials also follow a rigorous schedule and are required to load and unload their cargoes as well.

Tractor-trailer combinations consist of a front unit, or tractor, and one, two, or occasionally three rear units, or semitrailers. Vehicles with two semitrailers are known as "double rigs" and may exceed 70 ft in length and 40 tons in gross weight. These rigs are used for line-haul transport of goods. Their drivers are subject to any of the following work schedules, depending on the type of rig they drive.

Work Schedules

Turnaround or Short Relay.—With this type of haul, a driver leaves his home terminal at a specified time and drives for four to five hours. At a predetermined point, he meets another driver, they exchange vehicles, and he returns to his home base driving the second vehicle.

Long Relay.—Long-relay hauls are similar to short relays, except that the trucker drives for up to ten hours before reaching the exchange point and by law is required to take an eight-hour rest period before driving the exchange vehicle back to his home terminal. Truckers who have driven several long-relay hauls consecutively usually are given time off to compensate for the long work time.

Straight-Through Hauls ("Roll and Rest").—In this type of run, a driver may travel across several states or span the entire continent. He alternately drives for ten hours and rests in a motel for eight hours. At his destination, he is given a new load to be hauled to a point that may or may not be his home terminal. With succeeding cargo changes, several weeks may elapse before his cargo destination permits him to return to his home base.

Sleeper Hauls.—Sleeper hauls are a variation of straight-through hauls except that there are two drivers who alternate driving and sleeping in a sleeper berth built into the rear of the truck cab. Typically, each driver drives for four hours and rests for four hours, but they may change at longer intervals. Sleeper drivers stop regularly for rest breaks and to eat or shower. At their destination, they may be required to uncouple the trailer, hitch up to a loaded trailer that is waiting, and depart immediately for another destination. Drivers on this type of haul may be on the road for several weeks before returning to their home terminals. Owner-operators frequently follow this type of schedule.

Hazards and Stresses

The physical demands of trucking, together with a stressful work environment, may impose particular mental and physical stresses as well as psychosocial problems. Moreover, drivers have a higher rate of job-related injuries and illnesses than do workers in other fields. Vehicles were the third ranking source of injury in California in 1983, accounting for 9% of disabling work injuries. Over one third of all vehicle-related mishaps involved highway motor vehicle accidents (e.g., collisions, overturning) where the injured worker was the occupant of a motorized highway vehicle at the time of the accident. Truck drivers and deliverypersons together accounted for three fourths of all the disabling injuries among transport equipment operatives. The three leading types of accidents sustained by the group were overexertion (8,267 cases), loading and unloading injuries (5,019), and highway motor vehicle accidents (3,268 cases). As in past years, highway motor vehicle accidents were the most common cause of death, accounting for over one fourth of all work fatalities for the year.[17]

The job factors in this occupation that create mental stress include schedule shifting, irregular work/rest cycles, irregular mealtimes and poor nutrition, unsatisfactory sleeping accommodations, delays in departure and en route traffic problems, prolonged periods of driving, anxiety over meeting delivery schedules, and economic pressures.

Physically stressful factors are related to handling the big rigs. These trucks require constant visual and auditory monitoring and extreme mental alertness during driving. Stresses are compounded when driving at dusk or at night, in adverse weather, in heavy traffic, or on poorly surfaced or mountainous roads. The driving position creates another problem, because this position, when maintained for many hours, results in blood pooling in the lower extremities, postural fatigue, and stiffening of the joints and muscles. Research studies using chair rest to evaluate the physiologic effects of immobilization have shown that physical fitness deteriorates with prolonged seated immobility.[42]

To the above factors must be added the stresses of vibration, noise, heat, and the monotony of driving.

Many truckers must also perform a number of physically stressful tasks that are not related to driving, including putting on chains during heavy snow, changing tires, loading and unloading heavy cargo, coupling and uncoupling trailers, and cargo inspection and adjustment.

Finally, the schedules observed by most truckers are not conducive to a positive family or social life. Drivers may be on the road for weeks before seeing their families or sweethearts again. Wife-husband driving teams avoid the problem of separation, but other problems may occur because both are subjected to stresses. The importance of psychosocial factors cannot be ignored. In some cases, they may have tragic effects, because trucking accidents have been found to occur after drivers have experienced domestic conflicts, separation, divorce, or the serious illness or death of close friends or relatives.[34]

The tight schedules and the economic pressures associated with them are also responsible for much of the problem of drug and alcohol abuse among drivers, because some drivers attempt to drive for as long and as far as possible with insufficient sleep. The prevalent use of caffeine and nicotine among drivers also results from stressful schedules and lack of sleep.

The following discussion examines the various factors that dominate the trucker's work environment.

ACCIDENTS AND INJURIES

There are few accurate statistics on accident and injury rates among truckers, largely because of differences in the reporting methods of various agencies. The U.S. Bureau of Labor Statistics provides injury and illness data for employees in trucking and warehousing but makes no breakdown between the two occupations, nor do these statistics identify fatality cases. The U.S. National Center for Health Statistics provides information on deaths from motor vehicle accidents but does not indicate whether the figures pertain to trucks, buses, or automobiles. Reports from other agencies, both federal and state, are no more definitive. Consequently, figures on deaths and injuries among truckers, both on the highway and during loading, are at best imprecise.

The Federal Motor Carrier Safety Regulations requires accident reports to be filed when accidents result in (1) the death of a human being; (2) bodily injury to a person who, as a result, receives medical treatment away from the scene of the accident; or (3) total damage of all property aggregating $2,000 or more. Prior to 1980, reported accidents, fatalities, and injuries increased annually. During 1980, these statistics decreased and have remained relatively stable. However, during 1983, the number of injuries increased[10] (Table 60–1).

Collisions with automobiles, commercial trucks, and fixed objects accounted for 88.2% of collision accidents and accounted for 79.1% of all fatalities, 87.1% of injuries, and 88.7% of property damage (Table 60–2).

Noncollision accidents, in 91.0% of cases, were defined as ran-off-road, jackknife, and overturn. These three categories accounted for 98.2% of fatalities, 96.5% of injuries, and 90.9% of the property damage in noncollision accidents (Table 60–3).

In the absence of reliable health and safety information from

TABLE 60–1.*
Major Truck Accidents Reported 1979–1983

	1979	1980	1981	1982	1983
Accidents	35,541	31,389	32,306	31,759	31,628
Fatalities	3,072	2,528	2,810	2,479	2,528
Injuries	32,126	27,149	28,533	25,779	26,692

*From Bureau of Motor Carrier Safety: *Accidents of Motor Carriers of Property 1983.* US Dept of Transportation, Federal Highway Administration, October 1984.

TABLE 60–2.
Collision Accidents*

COLLISON INVOLVING	ACCIDENTS	FATALITIES	INJURIES	PROPERTY DAMAGE	FATALITIES PER 100 ACCIDENTS
Automobile	58.1	62.6	66.8	43.6	10.3
Commercial truck	17.1	12.0	14.6	28.7	6.8
Fixed object	13.0	4.5	5.7	16.4	3.3

*From Bureau of Motor Carrier Safety: *Accidents of Motor Carriers of Property 1983.* US Dept of Transportation, Federal Highway Administration, October 1984.

the variety of government agencies responsible for such data, it is not surprising that media inquiries often provide the public with an alarming overview of a serious situation. The following findings resulted from one investigation of interstate trucking accidents:[19]

1. One in four trucks stopped for roadside inspection by agents of the Federal Bureau of Motor Carrier Safety (BMCS) in 1983 was found to have defective brakes; 32% of these trucks were ordered off the road immediately.

2. Almost one driver in five had driven more nonstop hours than permitted by federal regulations.

3. The BMCS is so understaffed that if trucking companies' equipment and records were checked in sequence, an interstate trucker would probably be examined only once in 42 years. The BMCS has an annual budget of $14 million and 130 inspectors to oversee 1 million trucks belonging to 210,000 interstate operators. In comparison, the Federal Aviation Agency has a $2 billion budget and 22,000 employees to monitor 2,600 aircraft operated by fewer than 100 airlines.

The National Safety Council reports that passenger cars have an accident frequency rate significantly higher than that of trucks.[4] However, fatalities and injuries of greater severity are more likely to occur in accidents where trucks are involved. The Keystone-AAA Auto Club has cited statistics comparing the number of fatalities when each of three different kinds of trucks collides with a passenger vehicle. When a pickup truck collides with a passenger car, there are 3 fatalities per 1,000 persons involved; when a trailer truck collides with a passenger car, 71 persons are killed per 1,000 involved; when a tandem trailer combination collides with a passenger car, 133 persons are killed for every 1,000 persons involved. Thus, the fatality rate with the tandem trailer would be double that of a single trailer and 50 times that of a pickup truck.

TABLE 60–3.
Non-Collision Truck Accidents*

TYPE	ACCIDENTS	FATALITIES	INJURIES	PROPERTY DAMAGE
Ran-off-road	29.7	60.9	35.2	34.5
Jackknife	27.5	6.5	19.6	14.7
Overturn	33.8	30.8	41.7	41.7

*From Bureau of Motor Carrier Safety: *Accidents of Motor Carriers of Property 1983.* US Dept of Transportation, Federal Highway Administration, October 1984.

The California Highway Patrol reports that fatigue is a primary or contributing cause in 67% of truck accidents. The CHP study, conducted in 1982, found that truck drivers were driving at excessive speed, following too close, or making unsafe lane changes in 60% of the 7,673 accidents in which they were considered to be at fault. The CHP study found that 85% of drivers involved in commercial vehicle accidents had no formal truck-driving training and recommended a specific training program, a proposal not yet implemented.[41]

The lack of proper maintenance of equipment accounts for 12% of truck accidents. The CHP study agrees with BMCS experience that 30%–40% of trucks have defective brakes (which includes intercity tour buses). Other common deficiencies are defective tires, steering components, and towing connections. Although most truck-caused accidents are the fault of the driver, the nature of the vehicle contributes to the severity of the accident. In 58% of tank truck accidents, there is a rollover; and in 53% of all accidents, there is a leakage of cargo, often gasoline, with (devastating) potential fire. Furthermore, the on-board diesel fuel tank with no crash protection often ruptures and may explode on impact.[41] In 1985, the U.S. Secretary of Transportation reported that 41% of all commercial trucks were temporarily grounded and 15% of all truck drivers were temporarily suspended from driving for safety-related violations following a nationwide federal-state survey.[73]

VIBRATION

Many studies have been conducted on the physiologic effects of vibration, but few conclusive studies have been undertaken on the effects of vibration in over-the-road trucks. Vibration is the motion (oscillating, reciprocating, or otherwise) that forces a body or medium out of a position or state of equilibrium. It generally is measured in terms of frequency, amplitude, velocity, and acceleration. Frequency is expressed in cycles per second (Hz), amplitude in displacement units, velocity in displacement units per second, and acceleration in displacement units per second squared or in the nondimensional unit of g.[33] Vibration can occur from either direction in any one of three axes—front to back chest, which is designated as the x axis; front chest to lower back, designated y; and head to foot, z, which appears to be the most significant axis.

Most research has been concerned with laboratory effects of vibration along the z axis, including biodynamics, subjective evaluation, behavior and performance, and physiology.[3, 14, 24, 25, 33, 68] Biodynamic studies have revealed that human beings exhibit a major response to vibration in the z or vertical direction at about 5 Hz. The most critical frequency band is 4–8 Hz in the vertical direction, with whole-body vibration occurring at approximately 5 Hz. Sinusoidal vibration generally is uncomfortable at acceleration amplitudes above 2 g if maintained for longer than a few cycles.[33]

Vibration in the 3–7 Hz frequency range produces major physiologic effects. At about 5 Hz, chest pain may occur, balance and the ability to sit erect may be impaired, and physical fatigue results. Even very low-frequency vibration can be a problem; vibration at 1 Hz results in motion sickness and at 2 Hz can cause sleepiness. At frequencies above 10 Hz, visual acuity and coordination can be impaired.[25]

Truck cabs vibrate at a frequency of up to 20 Hz, with major structural resonances occurring anywhere within this range. In comparison, smooth-riding city buses have a mean acceleration level of 50 cm/sec or 0.05 g, whereas typical over-the road trucks have an acceleration level three to five times higher.

Although the physiologic effects of whole-body vibration on truck drivers have not been studied extensively, research to date indicates that the primary effects are related to the circulatory, gastrointestinal, genitourinary, and musculoskeletal systems. In a comprehensive comparison of the medical histories of truck drivers, bus drivers, and air traffic controllers—all of whom work in the seated position with and without vibration—truck drivers, who experience the highest degree of vibration, had a significantly higher incidence of the following problems: bone deformities and vertebrogenic pain syndrome, hemorrhoids, kidney disease, and peptic ulcer.[24]

The bone deformities observed in truck drivers are primarily spine deformities, which these drivers exhibit to a significantly greater degree than do bus drivers (less vibration) or air controllers (little if any vibration). There is more than twice the incidence of premature, degenerative deformities of the spinal column among line-haul truck drivers than there is among the bus drivers.[6]

Whole-body vibration and the faulty posture assumed by drivers to compensate for vibration discomfort, as well as the heavy manual work required of truck drivers, may contribute to the significantly higher incidence of vertebrogenic pain exhibited by these drivers as compared with bus drivers. This situation probably occurs because line-haul truck design is concerned with aspects other than riding comfort. The problems experienced are vertebrogenic pain syndrome with displacement of intervertebral disks, sacroiliac problems, and, to a lesser degree, joint ankylosis. Vibration is traumatic to the spine. The intervertebral disks serve as "shock absorbers" during vibration. If the individual is exposed to vibration over a prolonged period, the intervertebral disks appear to become susceptible to premature, degenerative deformities.

Truckers often compensate for discomfort from vibration by changing their positions. If the assumed posture is incorrect, the stress is applied along other axes, with similar effects.[57] The problem may stem not only from the exposure to vibration but also from the manual labor in trucking, as well as the cab-over-engine configuration of much truck construction, which permits greater vibration to be felt by the driver.

Truck drivers also have a significantly higher incidence of hemorrhoids than do bus drivers. This complaint may result from whole-body vibration, since large intraluminal pressures can build up in the 1–7 Hz vibration range and be transmitted to the hemorrhoidal veins, with the possibility of damage to those veins.[75] However, the poor dietary habits of truck drivers, with emphasis on low-residue foods, may also be a contributing factor.

Pain in the region of the kidneys and frequent urination with some burning have been complaints of many operators of vehicles that have a high range of vibration. Heavy seat vibrations may serve as a stimulus to diuresis, and the impact of the bladder against the pelvis and abdomen during vibration may stimulate urination. Research will be required, however, before genitourinary disease can be unequivocally attributed to truck vibration.

A higher incidence of peptic ulcer has been found among truck drivers than among either air traffic controllers or bus drivers.[24] Although whole-body vibration may be a factor in the development of peptic ulcer, there is little conclusive evidence to that end. Both air traffic controllers and bus drivers usually eat meals at regular intervals and have time to eat hot, well-prepared, and nutritious meals. Truck drivers, on the other hand, tend to eat meals hurriedly and irregularly—meals that often are high in "junk" foods and low in nutrition. The further factor of a high use of alcohol, caffeine, and nicotine among truck drivers would suggest that whole-body vibration, although it may be a factor, is not the entire cause.

Truck drivers have been found to have a high frequency of appendicitis. Although their poorer eating habits may contribute to this complaint, whole-body vibration cannot be entirely ruled out as a contributor. Increased intraluminal pressures resulting from vibration may impede the flow of blood to and from the colon and into the appendiceal mucosa, thereby contributing to appendicitis. In this regard, research has indicated that sustained intraluminal pressures in the area of the appendix can cause changes in the wall of this organ.[72]

Helmkamp, Talbott, and Marsh have provided a critical review of the literature on whole-body vibration. The total number of referenced articles is 18, indicating that interest in this important area is of very recent origin. They point out that 9% of the American work force is engaged in a variety of occupations that expose them to vibration, with a typical worker exposed to more than 40,000 hours of occupational vibration over a 30-year period. In light of this extensive exposure, it is surprising that so little investigation has taken place. Their review of the cardiovascular, digestive, and musculoskeletal problems associated with whole-body vibration in some occupations resulted in the conclusion that "causal relationships have not been established."[30]

Laboratory studies also have indicated that vibration can affect performance adversely.[34] In a series of experiments, investigators exposed 12 subjects to vibration of 6 Hz at 0.1 g, while requiring them to perform tracking tasks. The ability of the subject to perform these tasks deteriorated during vibration in both the vertical and horizontal tracking directions.

NOISE

Noise is defined as any essentially random oscillation of sound pressure with the audible frequency range of 20–20,000 Hz that does not impart information to the human ear. The measure most commonly used to assess noise intensity is related to the response curve of the human ear. It is the frequency-weighted sound level across the range of 20–10,000 Hz, with weighting values assigned according to the "A-Scaling" procedure. It is measured in decibels as a quantity 20 times (log)[10] the ratio of noise sound pressure to a specified reference pressure (0.002 dyne/cm).

The most effective short-term index of noise response is the temporary threshold shift (TTS), which indicates the immediate reaction of the human ear to excessive noise exposure. When the TTS occurs, the individual temporarily loses the ability to hear at the level where he normally would be able to hear. If temporary threshold shifts occur repeatedly over prolonged periods, permanent hearing losses may occur. When an individual is exposed to destructive noise levels over a prolonged period, noise-induced permanent threshold shifts (NIPTS) occur. A NIPTS indicates that a permanent, irreversible hearing loss has occurred.

The National Institute for Occupational Safety and Health (NIOSH) has established 90 decibels (dB) as the noise level at which hearing damage is likely to occur.[53] Exposure at this level, however, is damaging to hearing only after a long period. Exposure to high-pitched noise is also more damaging than exposure to low-pitched noise.

Cabs of older interstate trucks often reach noise levels that exceed 90 dB. Moreover, because of highway noises, drivers may be exposed briefly to noise at intensities greater than 110 dB. Exposure to this level of noise, even for brief periods, may cause temporary hearing loss that requires several days to alleviate. There are problems also at lesser levels of noise. Noise in excess of 70 dB can result in communication problems stemming from a loss of understanding of signals. Even low-to-moderate levels can create difficulties for noise-sensitive individuals, including profound emotional responses, distraction, and abnormal behavior.

In addition to hearing loss, a number of nonspecific responses have been observed following exposure to high-level noise. They include elevated heart rate, elevated blood pressure, and increased urinary excretion of adrenalin and noradrenalin.[1] These responses are indicative of a physiologic reaction to stress.

In the tracking studies referred to above, noise alone or in combination with vibration was found to have little consistent effect on performance. It has been noted in other research, however, that noise in truck driving virtually eliminates audition in the transmission of information, with even horns and sirens having only minimal effect.[31]

In an extensive study of the ergonomic and work conditions for truck drivers, Hansson et al. reported measurements and assessments on 17 different trucks manufactured in 1974–1975.[27] The trucks carried out distribution, sanitation, route traffic, long-distance traffic, oil transport, forestry haulage, and gravel haulage assignments. A questionnaire study comprising 122 drivers was conducted and included drivers of both old and new vehicles.

The questionnaire study disclosed that all the drivers were most irritated by the noise, dust, and climate in the cab and with the provisions for getting in and out of cabs. In view of the importance of these matters to them, measures are required to improve the climate (too warm in summer and too drafty in winter) and noise level in cabs, followed by measures to make getting in and out of cabs safer and more convenient. The drivers expressed concern about the driver's seat, seating position, visibility, and exhaust fumes in the cab, but these conditions were believed to be less of a problem than the four factors mentioned earlier. However, 43% of the drivers were dissatisfied with the standard lighting on their trucks, especially with dipped beams. In a number of cases, the problems perceived varied with the driving assignment. The ergonomic and hygienic measurements and assessments revealed major differences between different truck types and driving assignments.

HEAT

The NIOSH has specified that a hot environment is one in which temperature, humidity, radiation, and wind speed combine to create a wet-bulb globe temperature (WBGT) that exceeds 79° F.[52] For drivers exposed to heat for eight to ten hours, 80° F WBGT is considered to be the conservative upper limit if they take suitable rest breaks every two to three hours.

Heat stress is evidenced in a number of ways. Perspiration is the most immediate effect as the body attempts to maintain thermal equilibrium. Blood pressure declines as the blood flow shifts from the interior of the body to the skin, with systolic pressure exhibiting a greater decline than diastolic. Finally, heart rate increases, urinary excretion of 17-hydroxycorticosteroids decreases, and production of adrenalin and noradrenalin declines. All of these responses are accompanied by a rise in rectal body temperature. The decline in catecholamine production has also been observed when individuals are required to perform monotonous tasks for a long period[55] and is associated with failure to respond to important events during the extended performance of routine tasks.[56]

Fortunately, the body has a strong mechanism for adapting to heat. The primary response in this adaptive process is a shift of the blood from the interior of the body to the skin to create a heat loss through radiation and convection. This shift is accomplished by cutaneous vasodilation. Under normal conditions, 5% of the blood flow is directed to the skin. During heat adaptation, however, up to 20% of the flow will be directed to the skin. The immediate drop in blood pressure when this happens occurs because of the increased vascular space. When the blood flow is directed to the skin, it is pulled away from other organs. To compensate for this loss, cardiac output must be increased and, consequently, heart rate increases. This compensation is not sufficient in some individuals, however, and cerebral ischemia results because of inadequate blood flow to the brain. Heat exhaustion then occurs, the first indications being extreme fatigue, nausea, and dizziness. Syncope follows if the cerebral flow declines further. Although heat exhaustion generally is not a major medical problem, any reduction in cerebral blood flow is serious in motor vehicle operators because it can create serious performance problems.

The body not only begins to react immediately to a hot environment, but it also acclimatizes over a period of four to seven days, depending on the individual. Acclimatization is more effective in persons who work from one to four hours intermittently in a hot environment than in those who rest during heat exposure. It also occurs more rapidly in physically fit individuals and apparently is unaffected by age. When an individual has been acclimatized, heat discomfort disappears, body temperature and heart rate decrease, and perspiration becomes more profuse and dilute. Total blood volume and venomotor tone also increase, enhancing the refilling rate of the heart so that it need do less work to maintain normal blood pressure. Following acclimatization in hot, dry environments, total blood volume gradually returns to normal. The same is not true, however, in hot, wet environments.

Physical symptoms of heat stress appear in most individuals at a WBGT of around 79° F. At WBGTs higher than about 88° F, neither adaptation nor acclimatization is possible. Not only temperature but also sex has a bearing on response to heat stress. Thus, women are more susceptible to heat stress than are men because of the higher skin temperature at which women perspire.[32]

It has been well established that body temperature and performance are interrelated and that peak performance generally occurs at the time of peak body temperature in the circadian temperature rhythm.[13, 22] These findings, however, refer to normal body temperature rhythms, which rarely change by more than 1.2° over a 24-hour period. In contrast, during exposure to heat, body temperature rises more rapidly and to a greater degree. Current knowledge suggests that mental working capacity deteriorates progressively as body temperature exceeds 100.4°.[13, 62] It is not known, however, how long drivers would be able to function under such conditions.

Heat stress throughout much of the United States during the summer could be sufficient to impair the driving ability of truck drivers. Moreover, heat stress can exacerbate existing physiologic conditions, such as heart disease and emphysema, and many line-haul truck drivers are between 40 and 60 years of age—an age group that has a relatively high incidence of cardiopulmonary diseases. Consequently, prolonged exposure to heat must be considered a hazard to the safety and health of truck drivers.

ENGINE EMISSIONS

Truck drivers may be exposed to diesel exhaust fumes and carbon monoxide for long periods because of leaks in exhaust and ventilation systems. Exposure to fumes in truck cabs may cause dizziness, drowsiness, headache, nausea, degraded mental performance, and decrements in visual acuity. Any of these conditions could be hazardous to highwav safety.

Animal studies of the genotoxic effects of exposure to diesel emissions have resulted in considerable concern that the number of automobiles and trucks powered by diesel engines is steadily increasing. Components of diesel exhaust have been shown in laboratory tests with bacteria, animal cells, and tissues to be toxic, mutagenic, or carcinogenic.[51, 58]

Diesel engine exhaust has not been shown to cause lung cancer in humans.[15, 58] However, studies of a number of workers exposed to diesel emissions of different types and durations have shown an elevated risk of lung cancer.[36, 66, 77] There is also some recent evidence of risk of liver cancer.[77] Although a large study done in England fails to demonstrate any increase in neoplasms of exposed workers, there is sufficient evidence to warrant further study.[64]

There is considerable evidence that increasing numbers of diesel-powered vehicles will contribute to a dangerous increase in air pollution and long-term damage to respiratory health.[15, 2, 63] Workers exposed to diesel emissions have experienced significantly higher mortality rates from emphysema and accidental deaths.[77] Although few conclusions can be drawn from available studies of pulmonary and systemic effects, concern for the truck driver and the possibility of long-term diesel emissions and carbon monoxide exposure is warranted.

POSTURAL REQUIREMENTS

Line-haul truck drivers spend many hours each day in the seated position. They must cope with a multi-ton vehicle and, to control the large steering wheel, they are forced to assume a rigid, upright position. This position, when held for any length of time, causes stiffening in the neck, back, and extremity muscles. Discomfort soon results, followed by postural fatigue.

Prolonged seated immobility may also lead to the deterioration of physical fitness. Blood pooling occurs in the lower extremities, draining the blood from the upper body and heart. Orthostatic intolerance as well as metabolic and cardiovascular changes commonly occur. Studies on the physiologic effects of immobilization, using chair rest as the means of immobilization, showed that physical deconditioning occurred within a few days.[42] Total blood volume and red blood cell mass decreased and orthostatic and exercise tolerance diminished progressively the longer the chair rest was in effect. Other research has indicated that pulse frequency is reduced, blood pressure declines, and stroke volume is lowered.[71] The immediate implications for truck drivers are obvious. But the effects on the cardiovascular system of prolonged sitting posture over months or years are not known.

Considerably more is known about the effects of prolonged sitting on the musculoskeletal system. In one very comprehensive study, the medical histories of 440 subjects with back problems and 494 matched and unmatched controls without back problems were reviewed.[39, 40] The subjects ranged in age from 20 to 64 years. The study was conducted to determine whether a correlation existed between occupation and the occurrence of acute herniated lumbar intervertebral disks (HIVD). It demonstrated that truck drivers exhibited a higher incidence of HIVD than did nondrivers. Moreover, those who drove but did not drive commercially had a higher incidence of HIVD than did individuals who did not drive at all.

Twenty-two of the subjects had jobs in which they spent 50% or more of their work time seated in a motor vehicle, whereas their matched controls did not. There were also eight pairs in which the controls spent more than half of their work time in a motor vehicle, whereas the subjects did not. The difference between those who drove motor vehicles for a livelihood and those who did not was statistically significant ($P < .02$), leading the investigators to estimate that drivers of motor vehicles have a relative risk factor of 2.75. Thus, truck drivers apparently are three times as likely to experience herniated intervertebral disks as are individuals whose occupation does not require long hours of driving. The study also indicated that persons of either sex who drive are more likely to develop acute herniated lumbar disks than those who do not drive at all. The investigators could not attribute these associations to any of the other variables considered during the study—that is, age, sex, or body weight.

PSYCHOSOCIAL STRESSORS AND EMOTIONAL STRAIN

In addition to the physical stresses of commercial driving, line-haul drivers are faced with a number of psychosocial stresses, many of which can be conducive to job-related injuries and illnesses. These stresses include irregular work/rest cycles and sleep deprivation; disorganization of circadian rhythms; prolonged driving; job monotony and frustration; overburden; delays and schedule shifting; poor work, family, and social relationships; and economic pressures. The effects of many of these stressors are interrelated.

The initial response to psychosocial stress usually is emotional strain, which results as the individual tries to cope with or combat a negative life situation. With all types of stress it becomes more difficult for the individual to cope with the stressor if it occurs repeatedly or too frequently. When that happens with psychosocial stressors, the individual can suffer mental fatigue and exhaustion, decrements in performance, accidents, or illness. Particularly high accident risk factors and clusters of illnesses seem to be prevalent when motor vehicle drivers are having difficulty adapting to negative life situations.[23]

Sleep Deprivation, Fatigue, and Driving Performance

Many studies have been conducted on the effects of various psychosocial stressors on driving performance. Methods used have included driving simulators, driving vehicles on closed-circuit driving tracks, open-road driving, and driver performance tests administered both before and after prolonged driving. Much of the research has been concerned with the effects on driving performance of sleep deprivation, fatigue and prolonged periods of driving. Each of the methods used has inherent uncontrollable variables; consequently, research findings with each method may be open to question.

Study results on sleep deprivation are among the more consistent, regardless of the method used. Sleep deprivation is common among many line-haul drivers, particularly owner-operators who must drive long hours to meet deadlines. There appears to be little disagreement among investigators that sleep deprivation results in degraded performance.

One team of investigators measured the driving performance of ten subjects under two conditions of sleep deprivation—cumulative sleep deprivation (five subjects with four hours of sleep per night for three nights) and extreme sleep deprivation (five subjects with no sleep for 24–36 hours).[21] The subjects drove test vehicles for five hours, covering 200 miles over a four-lane highway during that period. The vehicle was equipped with dual braking and steering controls. All subjects served as their own controls, since they previously had driven the highway when they were not sleep deprived. The performance of those subjected to cumulative sleep deprivation did not differ significantly from that during their "normal" (no sleep deprivation) runs. For those exposed to extreme sleep deprivation, however, the differences between the normal and test conditions were significant in terms of lane drifting, unnecessary speed changes, eye blinking, and instrument checking. The findings of other studies agree with the premise that fatigue results in decrements in driver performance.

Prolonged driving time—even without sleep deprivation—also appears to have a significant deteriorative effect on driver performance. Various performance variables have been noted to change following prolonged driving. Studies using simulators have shown that the ability of drivers to maintain the proper lane position declines as a function of driving time.[29, 46, 69] The findings of these studies have been reinforced by the results of studies conducted on the open road.[18, 43, 70] Increased variability in vehicle velocity control has also been observed during prolonged driving.[48, 55, 70] Some investigators have also found that steering wheel reversal rates and judgment decrease over time on the open road.[22, 56, 65] on a closed-circuit tract[56] and in a simulator.[29] Judgmental errors, including risky maneuvers and discourteous actions, have been observed to increase as a function of driver time at the wheel.[9, 54, 61]

Physiologic changes have also been observed during prolonged driving. Electroencephalograph recordings have shown an increase in slow-frequency, 8–13 Hz, α waves.[9, 29, 49] Average heart rate has been found to decrease with prolonged driving over a closed-circuit track[8, 54] and on the open road.[44, 59] One investigator also reported that heart rate variability increased in correlation with decrements in driver performance.[43] Respiration rate has been observed to decrease,[45, 56] and changes have occurred in eye movement[38] and eosinophil counts in the blood.[46]

Circadian Desynchronosis

All physiologic systems within the human body function according to certain rhythms. Most of these rhythms approximate a 24-hour pattern and, as a result, have been termed "circadian rhythms" (meaning "about a day"). When these rhythms are disrupted—as occurs when a truck driver's schedule is shifted from driving in daylight to driving at night—a state of stress is produced that can result in impairment of physical health, emotional and behavioral problems, sleep difficulties, altered responses to medication, and decrements in work performance and safety awareness. It may also increase the individual's susceptibility to the effects of other stressors.[49, 50, 74] (See Chapter 69 for a more detailed discussion.)

Changes in circadian rhythms in motor vehicle drivers need to be studied to assess whether a measurable correlation exists between circadian desynchronization and the rate of injuries and illnesses among drivers. In view of the consistent findings that circadian desynchronosis creates both physiologic and emotional changes,[16, 50] it would seem reasonable for employers to consider carefully the advisability of shifting drivers repeatedly from day to night schedules and back.

Job Monotony and Frustration

Long-haul truck driving is a monotonous experience. The nation's carefully engineered system of highways is monotonously straight. Usually, all that the driver sees is mile after mile of highway stretching to infinity; most drivers call it a "long dreary ride." Individuals have difficulty remaining alert in a monotonous situation. Even in physically fit and healthy individuals, monotony results in drowsiness, which is followed by lethargic fatigue. Repetitive driver tasks that require intense eye fixation and scanning are also difficult to perform under monotonous conditions. The implications for highway safety, of course, are considerable. When one driver signals another in passing, he is not only observing a courtesy of the road but also "casting a lifeline" by breaking the monotony.

Frustration is another inherent part of truck driving. Frustration results from poor road conditions, heavy traffic, inconsiderate drivers, delays en route and at terminals, and shifts in schedules. It occurs when an individual is blocked from achieving his immediate goal or goals by physical obstacles, conflicts, or his own deficiencies. When frustrations occur, the individual either will react immediately or will not react at all. In the latter case, he will develop attitudes that will have more enduring consequences. Frustration usually is met either by aggression or by apathy. In aggression, the anger that is aroused when the individual is blocked tends to be expressed in some form of direct action—that is, the individual strikes back immediately at the source of the frustration. In the trucker's case, he might "tailgate" an inconsiderate driver or unleash a string of invectives at a terminal employee who caused a delay.

If the source of the frustration is impersonal, inaccessible, or too powerful to attack, displaced aggression occurs. In this case, the aggression is focused on an innocent person or an object rather than on the true source of the frustration. The implications of aggression for highway safety are serious, since aggressive driving behavior has been the cause of many accidents.

Apathy is the opposite response to frustration. When resistance to the source of frustration is futile, the frustrated individual may become sullen and withdrawn. This situation has been observed when extremely frustrating conditions persist over a long period and the individual has no hope of being free from them.[28] The apathetic person is incapable of remaining alert.

Economic Pressures

Drivers for large motor freight lines and other company-owned transport systems can earn as much as $30,000 per year and face few, if any, economic pressures. Owner-operators, however, who constitute a large proportion of the nation's truck drivers, often are faced with severe economic pressures. Most have loan payments to make on their vehicles, and the increasingly higher costs of fuel and maintenance, as well as rampant inflation, add to their financial problems. Consequently, they must work long hours at the greatest possible speed just to keep up financially. They may be known as independent operators, but, as one owner-operator expressed it, "The independent trucker today is about as free as a man in chains."

The financial risk of purchasing or leasing a truck, its costly upkeep, and the intense competition for loads and the better routes, all contribute to the stress of driving for a livelihood. Many owner-operators fail to make the financial grade and return to working as company-employed drivers. Most manage to continue on a marginal basis. Some enjoy relative success but face additional costs and stresses, as well as a greater risk to health and safety than do company-employed drivers.

Those who manage to acquire more than one vehicle employ drivers who share their goal of delivering goods the greatest distance in the shortest possible time. Drivers for small independents are relatively unsupervised and sometimes press dangerously for rapid delivery with the aid of drugs and the falsification of driving records required by the Department of Transportation. They generally lack the benefits of union representation, prefer a working life that replaces a time clock with a demanding haul, and demand a life-style free from supervision. Together with their employers, they make the maximization of distance and load their primary objectives. With the aid of amphetamines and other drugs, they may drive 1,000 miles without sleep. To such drivers, the CB radio becomes not only a means of checking the weather ahead but also a vital means of staying awake.

Economic pressures on the owner-operators who do not lease to major motor carriers are compounded by dependence on brokers for loads. Typically, such an owner-operator will be forced to pay 10% of his delivery fee to obtain a load; his profit may be even further diminished by even greater "skimming" on the part of the broker. Additional costs occur if he feels compelled to offer payment to the dispatcher to ensure prompt loading of his cargo. In some cities, particularly on the East Coast, the owner-operator's profits may be even further diminished if he is required to pay for a lumper's unloading fee.* Many drivers complain that they are subjects of extortion schemes. They are met at the loading dock by men who demand the right to load or unload their cargoes or demand payment if they are not permitted to do so. If the driver refuses to pay, he may wait days to be scheduled into a dock or warehouse. Law enforcement efforts against extortion, violence, and violation of Interstate Commerce Commission regulations are inconsistent and sometimes nonexistent.

The foregoing economic pressures place owner-operators and drivers for small for-hire trucking companies at a greater risk of serious occupational safety and health problems than those experienced by drivers employed by carriers. Owner-operators and their drivers will achieve financial rewards, such as they are, at the cost of seriously impairing their physical and mental well-being.

Mental and Emotional Illnesses

A possible correlation between mental illness, including alcoholism and drug dependence, and stressful conditions in the work environment has received increasing attention. Mental problems in the work environment take the form of job dissatisfaction, low self-esteem, job tension, impaired personal relationships, and psychosomatic illnesses. The problems stem from various stressors in the work environment, including role conflict and ambiguity, quantitative and qualitative overload, personal conflicts with supervisors and co-workers, and lack of worker autonomy.

Mental illnesses among vehicle operators have been the concern of a number of studies, with the primary objective being to determine the role played by mental disorders in traffic accidents.[14, 60, 74] A series of accident investigations conducted by the Southwest Research Institute for the National Highway Traffic Safety Administration revealed that, of 198 automobile drivers involved in accidents, 24% had severe impairment of their mental functions at the time of the accident and 72% suffered from some degree of mental disturbance ranging from mild to severe[14] (Table 60–4). In nearly 50% of those who were severely functionally impaired, the problem resulted from alcohol and drug abuse. In a similar study conducted in the District of Columbia, investigators found that drivers suffering from schizophrenia, anxiety neuroses, and depressive neuroses had 50% more accidents than did members of an appropriate control group.[60] They also had the highest accident rate of all of the impaired drivers studied. A California study showed that drivers with mental illness, other than alcoholism or drug dependence, had about twice as many accidents as did their mentally healthy counterparts.[74]

The use of alcohol is thought to be widespread among truck

*A lumper is defined as a person who controls access to a loading area and who purports to be an official loader and unloader. The Federal Bureau of Investigation has begun to investigate cases of physical abuse of truck drivers who refuse to be intimidated by this extortion scheme.

TABLE 60–4.
Diagnosed Mental Disorders of a Group of Drivers Involved in Traffic Accidents

CLASSIFICATION	NO. OF CASES	DIAGNOSIS	NO. OF CASES
Psychotic disorders	4	Paranoid schizophrenia	1
		Acute schizophrenia	1
		Schizophrenia	1
		Reactive depressive psychosis	1
Neurotic and personality disorders	19	Anxiety neurosis	1
		Depressive neurosis	1
		Hypochondriacal neurosis	2
		Cyclothymic personality	3
		Explosive personality	4
		Obsessive compulsive personality	2
		Antisocial personality	2
		Immature personalify	3
Emotional or adjustment disorders	20	Habitual excessive drinking	10
		Alcohol addiction	1
		Drug dependency	3
		Transient disturbances	3
		Epilepsy	1
		Senile brain disease	2
Mental retardation	4	Borderline mental retardation	3
		Unspecified mental retardation	1

drivers despite the fact that Federal Motor Carrier Safety Regulations prohibit commercial drivers from consuming alcoholic beverages (regardless of the percentage of alcohol content) either while on duty or for four hours prior to going on duty. During a comprehensive study of problems in the work environment conducted for the Department of Health, Education, and Welfare,[78] interviews were conducted to determine the extent of alcohol use among workers in heavy industry. Responses indicated that many workers drank heavily during the lunch break to face the sheer monotony of their jobs. The same study also revealed that there is substantial on-the-job use of drugs by younger workers, particularly assembly-line workers and long-haul truck drivers.[78]

Federal Motor Carrier Safety Regulations specify, "No person shall operate a commercial vehicle if under the influence of, or frequently using, any of the following substances: (1) a depressant drug; (2) a stimulant drug; or (3) any other substance to a degree adversely affecting arousal, mood, personality, or behavior."[23] Thus, habit-forming narcotic, barbiturate, tranquilizing, stimulating, or hallucinogenic drugs are unacceptable for use by commercial drivers.

Despite the above restrictions, it is recognized that the use of drugs, particularly stimulant drugs such as amphetamines, is widespread among truck drivers because of the need to stay awake for prolonged periods. Most drivers, of course, would not admit to using drugs, so the chances of learning how widespread the practice is are limited. One research group seeking answers to this question devised a different approach to the problem.[28] Instead of asking drivers whether they used drugs "occasionally" or "regularly," they asked, "Among other drivers that you know, what percent would occasionally use some sort of pill, like Benzedrine, to pep them up when they get tired on long hauls?" Later, the same question was asked, but with the word "frequently" substituted for the word "occasionally." Although the percentages obtained dc not represent the absolute incidence of use, they do give some indication of usage. About 45% of those interviewed stated that they knew drivers who use them regularly (Table 60–5). Those who drove more than 2,000 miles a week and those under 30 years of age were more likely to "know" drivers who used pep pills to combat fatigue.

When similar questions were asked regarding the use of alcohol, the resulting frequencies were very similar to the drug-use responses. The investigators said, "The similar patterns of response may . . . lend some credence to the assertion that there is significant use of both drugs and alcohol by some truck drivers engaged in long-haul operations."[28]

In a recent survey, Wyckoff disseminated 65,000 four-page questionnaires related to problems in trucking. Approximately 10,500 were returned, half from company drivers and half from owner-operators.[35, 79] The findings indicated that 34% of drivers 25 years of age used amphetamines and 27% of those aged 25–50 and 9% of those over 50 used "uppers."

The use of alcohol, stimulants, and barbituates by drivers has serious implications for highway safety. Moreover, not only are these drugs dangerous when a person is driving, but their physiologic impact also differs when they are taken at different times of the day. Alcohol, for example, has a much greater effect when taken early in the day. In studies of mice injected with a large amount of alcohol at various times during the day, the injections proved to be lethal when administered at the end of the animals' rest span.[26] Whereas 60% died when injected at their usual time of awakening, only 12% died when injected late in the day.

With other drugs also, there is a period during the day when the organism is highly resistant to the drug and another period when it is highly vulnerable.[50] Amphetamines, for example, have the greatest effect at the peak of an individual's activity period. In studies of rats injected with lethal amounts of amphetamine at two-hour intervals, only 6% died when injected at 0600 hours, whereas 77.6% died when injected at midnight (their activity peak).[67] Furthermore, when taken at certain times of the day, amphetamines can cause mania and psychosis, particularly when the drug has been used for prolonged periods.

Drugs not only are affected by human rhythms but also may change those rhythms. Investigators have found, for example, that sodium pentobarbital will suppress the adrenal hormone rhythms in animals.[67] When animals were given a fast-acting barbiturate in the evening, the drug blocked the morning rise in hormone levels.

TABLE 60–5.
Knowledge of Drivers Who Use Pep Pills (By Type of Carrier)

RESPONSES	OWNER-OPERATORS (N = 202)	COMMON CARRIERS (N = 100)	PRIVATE CARRIERS (N = 98)	ALL DRIVERS (N = 400)
Yes, know drivers who use pills occasionally	45	42	47	37
No, do not know drivers who use pills occasionally	32	38	38	46
Do not know whether they do or not	23	20	15	18
Yes, know drivers who use pills regularly	31	24	34	23
No, do not know drivers who use pills regularly	46	54	50	59
Do not know whether they do or not	23	22	16	18

NOTE: Numbers reflect percentage of all respondents.

This did not occur when the drug was given at other times during the day. In humans, this reaction may explain why the drug sometimes causes a hangover effect after total excretion or metabolism.

OUTLOOK FOR HIGHWAY SAFETY

Truck Traffic and Weight Increasing

Truck transportation has become a major factor in American business and industry. Truck traffic has doubled since 1960; the Highway Users Federation predicts that the figure will double again over the next 15–20 years.

Of the 4 million trucks operating in the United States, 1 million weigh up to 80,000 lb and some, by special permit, weigh up to 130,000 lb. The weight limit was raised to 80,000 lb in 1974 at the height of the energy crisis, when the 55-mile-per-hour speed limit was put into effect. The increased weight has been accepted by most states.

The introduction of more trucks, heavier trucks, and longer trucks will have a direct impact on highway safety and on the structural integrity of the nation's highways. With regard to highway safety, collisions between trucks and passenger cars result in a mortality rate that is significantly higher than that resulting from the collision of two or more automobiles. A combination of economic factors and energy issue pressures is creating larger and heavier trucks and smaller and lighter automobiles. This situation creates an extremely unequal contest when trucks collide with cars.

Independent Truckers at Risk

With regard to the safety aspects of truck drivers, Wyckoff's survey has indicated that regulated truckers have better safety records than exempt carriers and owner-operators.[79] Nearly half the drivers employed by exempt carriers reported that they "regularly" drive longer than the ten-hour limit, and about one third of them reported using multiple log books to circumvent the hours of service rules. In contrast, only about 3.5% of company drivers working for common carriers regularly violate hours of service regulations and less than 2% use multiple logs. Cruising speeds are also higher among drivers for nonregulated carriers, averaging 63 mph in contrast to the 58.85 average of drivers for regulated carriers. Similarly, moving violations, when reduced to incidents per 100,000 miles, showed the rate of exempt owner-operators to be high, at 1.33, and that for drivers for common carriers to be low, at 0.41.

Wyckoff's findings conflict with data published by the Bureau of Motor Carrier Safety, which show that regulated carriers have a higher accident rate than nonregulated carriers. In the Wyckoff survey, the rate for exempt owner-operators was high, with an accident rate of 0.70 per 100,000 miles, whereas that for drivers for common carriers was low, with 0.19 per 100,000 miles.

"My interpretation of the conflict between BMCS data and what the drivers told us is quite simple," said Wyckoff. "The only people playing by the rules or reporting accidents when they are supposed to are the regulated and private companies. The owner-operator, by his own admission, has a higher accident rate. The only time he reports an accident is when he has a major disaster."

The Department of Defense, recognizing the disparity in safety records of owner-operators, prohibits those on a trip-lease from transporting hazardous materials and ammunition or explosives.

Increasing Stress on Highway System

The integrity of the highway system must also be considered a critical factor in highway safety, because structural breakdown of U.S. highways would contribute to highway accidents. Highway engineers have predicted that, under the continual stress of 80,000-lb trucks, pavement life could be decreased by 25%–40% and bridges on interstate highways (which are stronger than non-interstate bridges) would be overstressed by up to 36%.

Smaller cars driving at lower speeds are producing less fuel tax revenue for the building and maintenance of highways. This decline of highway funds, coupled with increased use of highways by all vehicles, results in a less-than-optimistic outlook for highway safety.

Lack of Standards

Government agencies, particularly at the federal level, established few realistic standards for the health and safety of truck drivers. Although the Occupational Safety and Health Administration has established continually expanding health and safety standards for other industries, little has been done at either the federal or state level to protect the millions of individuals whose jobs require long hours of driving.

The situation in the trucking industry concerning safety and health is serious and is of considerable concern both to the industry itself and to the federal government. It may be expected to become more serious as the number of trucks and passenger vehicles increases and truck weights rise. Solutions will not be easy, and some undoubtedly will be costly. Cost presents a particularly difficult hurdle, because profit margins are narrow for much of the trucking industry, and for many owner-operators they are even more so.

Recommendations for Truck Driver Health and Safety

Four primary areas must be addressed if highway safety and health of motor vehicle drivers are to be improved—the vehicle, the driver, the highways, and the legislative standards that govern them.

Vehicle Design.—In any industry, well-designed, well-maintained equipment is essential to the well-being of the worker. In the trucking industry, it can be a matter of life and death. Design improvements that are needed in trucks include control of vibration, noise, heat, and engine emissions and better seating and cab conditions. All such improvements will contribute to the greater comfort of the driver and to his safety and health. It has been argued that providing a comfortable environment for the driver, combined with the monotony of the present highway system, will lull drivers into a soporific state that will result in fatal single-vehicle accidents. But that has not been the experience of one operator of a 1,500-truck fleet who installed air conditioning, insulation, improved seats, and engine emission controls while achieving an excellent safety record.

The relation of a truck's loaded weight to its power source is reflected in its ability to maintain speed on a grade. Results of one study have indicated that, in 7 of 8 collisions occurring on an upgrade that involved a truck, the truck was struck from the rear. Inadequate braking ability, which is also related to loaded weight, was found to be a primary factor in collisions on a downgrade or level when the truck was the striking vehicle. If such collisions involve a passenger vehicle, the occupants of the car are more likely to be killed than is the truck driver. Truck improvements in this area consequently would benefit all highway users.

In most industries, fail-safe mechanisms are incorporated into equipment to protect workers from human and other failures. Padded dashboard and air bag restraints should be provided on all trucks. One of the primary goals of vehicle design should be protection of the drivers and the occupants of passenger cars involved in collisions with trucks.

The design of heavy motor vehicles should also include doors that can be readily opened after collisions and alternative escape routes, because extrication of the occupants following collisions has been a serious problem with tractor-trailers. In one study, it was found that at least 8 of 41 truckers who died after collisions were trapped in the cab (no fire involved) for periods of up to 3½ hours. Rescuers were unable to free them because of jammed doors, smashed cabs, shifted loads, or turnover of the tractor-trailer.

Driver Education.—Drivers also need education, particularly those who have been on the road for many years or are very new to the occupation. In any field, additional training is desirable. During training, drivers should be taught newer operating methods, be conditioned to use seat belts and other safety devices, and be taught to eat properly and exercise sufficiently. They should also be taught basic life-saving techniques so that they will be able to help other truckers and passenger car occupants who are in need. This is particularly important, because most accidents occur far from sources of medical help, and the longer the accident victim remains without medical help, the less the opportunity for recovery.

Highway Standards.—These must also be improved. Highway signs are not always understandable or clear, and instructions that apply to passenger vehicles may not always be applicable to trucks. The design of some highways also is not conducive to highway safety. Divided highways that are not limited-access highways present a particular problem. Collisions occur when vehicles pull onto the highway from a side road or turn left into the path of an oncoming tractor-trailer. Road designs that permit vehicles to intersect the paths of fast-moving trucks are an invitation to fatal accidents. One study revealed that 40% of the fatal accidents surveyed were caused by vehicles entering a highway from a side road or turning left across oncoming traffic. A possible solution could lie in eliminating or modifying such intersections or restricting heavy truck traffic to limited-access highways.

Legislation.—Finally, legislation is needed to provide truckers with a working environment in keeping with the intent of the OSHA act. At present, large numbers of workers in the trucking industry have not been provided with this assurance.

REFERENCES

1. *A Study of Heat, Noise, and Vibration in Relation to Driver Performance and Physiological Status*, PB-238-829. Goleta, Cal, Human Factors Research, Inc. Prepared for the National Highway Traffic Safety Administration, December 1974.
2. *Air Quality Criteria for Particulate Matter and Sulfur Oxides*, EPA-600/882-029. Research Triangle Park, NC, US Environmental Protection Agency, 1982.
3. Allen G: Human reaction to vibration. *J Environ Sci* 1971; Sept/Oct, pp 10–15.
4. *American Trucking Trends, Statistical Supplement*. Washington, DC, Dept of Economics and Public Relations Dept, American Trucking Association, Inc, 1976.
5. Arnold B: Jackie Preser's push to halt the slide in unionized trucking. *Business Week*, 1985; Jan 21, pp 90–91.
6. Barboso E: Incidence of spine changes in drivers of one bus company. *Med Lav* 1958; 49:10.
7. Batty B: How they kept on trucking. *Nation's Business* 1984; October pp 6772.
8. Brown ID: Decrement in skill observed after seven hours of car driving. *Psychonom Sci* 1967; 7:131.
9. Brown ID, Simmonds DCV, Tickner AH: Measurement of control skills, vigilance, and performance on a subsidiary task during twelve hours of car driving. *Ergonomics* 1967; 10:665.
10. Bureau of Motor Carrier Safety: *Accidents of Motor Carriers of Property 1983* US Dept of Transportation, Federal Highway Administration, October 1984, pp 1–15.
11. Capps SA: Truckers seek another break. *San Francisco Examiner* 1984; Aug 5, pp B1, 3.
12. Collins AM: Decrements in tracking and visual performance during vibration. *Hum Factors* 1973; 15:379.
13. Colquhoun WP: Temperament, inspection efficiency and time of day. *Ergonomics* 1960; 3:377.
14. Cromack RJ, et al: *Multidisciplinary Accident Investigation*, Interim Report on Contract DOT-HS-024-1-115. Dept of Transportation, January 1973.
15. Cuddihy RG, Griffith WC, McClellan RO: Health risks from light-duty diesel vehicles. *Environ Sci Technol* 1984; 18: No 1.
16. Czeisler CA, Moore-Ede MC, Coleman RM: Rotating shift work schedules that disrupt sleep are improved by applying circadian principles. *Science* 1982; 217:460–463.
17. Division of Labor Statistics and Research: *California Work Injuries and Illnesses 1983*. San Francisco, California Dept of Industrial Relations, March 1985.
18. Ellingstad VS, Heimstra NW: Performance changes during the sustained operation of a complex psychomotor task. *Ergonomics* 1970; 13:693.
19. Editorials: Deadly Transport. *San Jose Mercury News* 1985; April 26, p 12B.
20. *Federal Register* 1978; 43: No. 90 (May 22).
21. Forbes TW, Katz MS, Cullen JW, et al: Sleep deprivation effects on component of driver behavior abstract. *Highway Res Rec* 1953; 28:21.
22. Greenshields BD: Changes in driver performance with time in driving. *Highway Res Rec* 1966; 122:75.
23. Gruber GJ: *Establishment of Guidelines to Aid Examining Physicians*. San Antonio, Tex, Southwest Research Institute, prepared for the Bureau of Motor Carrier Safety, Dept of Transportation, under Contract DOT-FH-11-8274, November 1976.

24. Gruber GJ: *Relationships between Wholebody Vibration and Morbidity Patterns among Interstate Truck Drivers*. San Antonio, Tex, Southwest Research Institute, Prepared for the National Institute for Occupational Safety and Health, under Contract CDC-99-74-22, November 1976.
25. Guignard JC, King PF: Aeromedical aspects of vibration and noise, AGARD-ograph 151. Neuilly sur Seine, France, NATO Advisory Group for Aerospace Research and Development, 1972.
26. Halberg F, Bittner JJ, Gully RJ: Twenty-four hour periodic susceptibility to audiogenic convulsions in several stocks of mice. *Fed Proc* 1955; 14:67.
27. Hansson J-E, Klussel L, Svensson G, et al: *Arbetsmiljon i Lastbilshytter*. Stockholm, *Arb och Hälsa*, 1976.
28. Harris W, Mackie RR: *A Study of the Relationships Among Fatigue, Hours of Service, and Safety of Operations of Truck and Bus Drivers*, Report PB-213 963. Goleta, Cal, Human Factors Research Inc, prepared for Bureau of Motor Carrier Safety, November 1972.
29. Heimstra NW: The effects of "stress fatigue" on performance in a simulated driving situation. *Ergonomics* 1966; 13:209.
30. Helmkamp JC, Talbott EO, Marsh GM: Whole-body vibration—A critical review. *Am Ind Hyg Assoc J* 45:162–167, March 1984.
31. Henderson RL, Berg A: *Vision and Audition in Driving*, Systems Development Corp Report TM(L)-5297/000/00, 1974.
32. Henschel A: The environment and performance, in *Physiology of Work Capacity and Fatigue*. Springfield, Ill, Charles C Thomas, Publisher, 1971.
33. Hornick RJ: Vibration, in *Bioastronautics Data Book*. Falls Church, Va, Bio Technology, Inc, 1972.
34. Hornick RJ, Lefritz NM: A study and review of human response to prolonged random vibration. *Hum Factors* 1966; 8:481.
35. How truck rules affect driver safety. *San Francisco Chronicle* 1978; June.
36. Howe GR, Fraser D, Lindsay J, et al: Cancer Mortality (1965–77) in Relation to Diesel Fume and Coal Exposure in a Cohort of Retired Railway Workers. *JNCI* 1983; 70: no 6, June.
37. *Infra and Ultra Sound*, Directions no 110:1. Stockholm, Arbetarskyddsstyrelsen, May 1978.
38. Kaluger NA, Smith GL Jr: Driver eye-movement patterns under conditions of prolonged driving and sleep deprivation. *Highway Res Rec* 1970; 336:92.
39. Kelsey J: An epidemiological study of the relationship between occupations and acute herniated intervertebral discs. *Int J Epidemiol* 1975; 4:197.
40. Kelsey J, Hardy RJ: Driving of motor vehicles as a risk factor for acute herniated lumbar intervertebral disc. *Am J Epidemiol* 1975; 102:63.
41. Kynaston E: Commercial Vehicle Safety. Speech delivered at the National Highway Safety Symposium, Williamsburg, Va, Feb 29, 1984.
42. Lamb LE, Stevens PM, Johnson RL: Hypokinesia secondary to chair rest from 40 hours to 10 days. *Aerosp Med* 1965; 36:775.
43. Lauer AR, Suhr VW: The effect of a rest pause on driving efficiency. *Percept Mot Skills* 1959; 9:363.
44. Lecret F, Pin MC, Cura JB, et al: Les variations de la vigilance au cours de conduite sur autoroute. Presented to the Sixth SELF Congress, 1968.
45. Lisper HO, Laurell H, Stening G: Effects of prolonged driving and the experience of the driver on heart-rate, respiration-rate, and a subsidiary auditory reaction time, Report 111. University of Uppsala, Sweden, 1971(b).
46. Mast TM, Jones HV, Heimstra NW: Effects of fatigue on performance in a driving device. *Highway Res Rec* 1966: 122:93.
47. McFarland RA, Moseley AL: *Human Factors in Highway Transport Safety*. Boston, Harvard School of Public Health, 1954.
48. Michaut G, Pottier M: Conduite en situation monotone. Organisme National de Securite Routiere, Bull. 8, 1964.
49. Morgan BB, Brown BR, Alluisi EA: Effects on sustained performance of 48 hours of continuous work and sleep loss. *Hum Factors* 1974; 16:406.
50. Moore-Ede MC, Czeisler CA, Richarson GS: Circadian timekeeping in health and disease, Part 1. Basic properties of circadian pacemakers. *New Engl J Med* 1983; 309:469–476, Pt 2. Clinical Implications of Circadian Rhythmicity, 1983; 309:530–536.
51. National Research Council: *Health Effects of Exposure to Diesel Exhaust*. The Report of the Health Effects Panel of the Diesel Impacts Study Committee. Washington, DC, National Academy Press, 1981.
52. *Occupational Exposure to Hot Environments. Criteria for a Recommended Standard*. US Dept of Health, Education, and Welfare, National Institute for Safety and Health, US Government Printing Office, 1972.
53. *Occupational Exposure to Noise: Criteria for a Recommended Standard*. US Dept of Health, Education, and Welfare, National Institute for Safety and Health, US Government Printing Office, 1972.
54. O'Hanlon JF: Adrenaline's effect on human vigilance: Continuous vs. pulsatile infusions. *Proceedings of the 79th Annual Convention*, American Psychiatric Association, 1971, pp 767–768.
55. O'Hanlon JF: *Fatigue as Estimated from Concurrent Performance and Psychophysiological Measures in Prolonged Driving*, Tech Rep 1712-1. Goleta, Cal, Human Factors Research, Inc, 1971.
56. O'Hanlon JF: *Vigilance, the Plasma Catecholamines and Related Bio-Chemical and Physiological Variables*, Technical Report 787-2. Goleta, Cal, Human Factors Research, Inc, 1970.
57. Osborne DJ, Boarer PA: Subjective response to whole-body vibration: The effects of posture. *Ergonomics* 1982; 25:673–681.
58. Pepelko WE, Peirano WB: Health effects of exposure to diesel engine emissions: A summary of animal studies conducted by the U.S. Environmental Protection Agency's Health Effects Research Laboratories at Cincinnati, Ohio. *J Am Coll Toxicol* 1983; 2:253–306.
59. Pin MC, Lecret F, Pottier M: Les niveaux d'activation lors de differentes situations de conduite. Organisme National de Securite Routiere, Bull. 19, 1969.
60. Pinckney TR, Rogers A: Handicapped Drivers Rated. *District of Columbia Traffic Safety Reporter* 1973; 16:1.
61. Platt FN: A new method of evaluating the effects of fatigue on driver performance. *Hum Factors* 1964; 6:351.
62. Poulton EC: *Environment and Human Efficiency*. Springfield, Ill, Charles C Thomas, Publisher, 1970.
63. *Review of the National Ambient Air Quality Standards for Nitrogen Oxides: Assessment of Scientific and Technical Information*, EPA-450/5-82-002. Research Triangle Park, NC, US Environmental Protection Agency, 1982.
64. Rushton L, Alderson MR, Nagarajah CR: Epidemiological survey of maintenance workers in London transport executive bus garages and chiswick works. *Br J Ind Med* 1983; 40:340–345.
65. Safford RR, Rockwell TH: Performance decrement in twenty-four hour driving. *Highway Res Rec* 1967; 16:30.
66. Schenker MG, Smith R, Munoz A, et al: Diesel exposure and mortality among railway workers: Results of a pilot study. *Br J Ind Med* 1984; 41:320–327
67. Scheving LE, Vedral DF, Pauly JE: A circadian susceptibility rhythm in rats to pentobarbital sodium. *Anat Rec* 1968; 160:741.
68. Shoenberger RW: Human response to whole-body vibration. *Percept Mot Skills* 1972; 34:127, monograph supplement 1-V34.
69. Suhr VW: *Driving Efficiency Over a Six-hour Period by Simulated Driving Performance*. Unpublished doctoral dissertation, Iowa State College, 1956, in Lauer AR, Suhr VW: The effects of a rest pause on driving efficiency. *Percept Mot Skills* 1959; 9:363.

70. Sussman ED, Morris DF: *An Investigation of Factors Affecting Driver Alertness*, Tech Rep VJ-28-49-B-1. Cornell Aeronautical Laboratory, 1970.
71. Vyazitsky PO, Kumanichkin SD: The effect of hypodynamia on external respiration under various microclimatic conditions. *Voen Med Zh* 1970; 7:38.
72. Wagensteen OH, Bower WF: The etiology of appendicitis. *Arch Surg* 1937; 34:496.
73. *Wall Street Journal:* Funding increase proposed to improve truck safety. Nov 8, 1985, p 17.
74. Waller JA: Chronic medical conditions and traffic safety—Review of the California experience. *N Engl J Med* 1965; 273:1413.
75. White GH, Lange KO, Coermann RR: The effects of simulated buffeting on the internal pressure of man. *Hum Factors* 1962; 275.
76. Winget CM, DeRosha BS, Markley CL, et al: A review of human physiological and performance changes associated with desynchronosis of biological rhythms. *Aviat Space Environ Med* 1984; 55:1085–1095.
77. Wong O, Morgan RW, Kheifets L, et al: Mortality among members of a heavy construction equipment operators union with potential exposure to diesel exhaust emissions. *Br J Ind* 1985; 42:435–448.
78. *Work in America, Report of a Special Task Force to the Secretary of Health, Education, and Welfare*. Cambridge, Mass, MIT Press, 1973.
79. Wyckoff driver survey shows linkage of regulation, safety. *Transport Topics* 1978; June 19.

61

An Ergonomic Checklist for Industrial Trucks

Jan-Erik Hansson

The present checklist was drawn up at the suggestion of the Transport Research Commission's (TFK) Truck Committee. Work on the checklist was supported by the Truck Committee and a reference group comprising the following members: Bertil Ulfward, Chairperson, National Swedish Board of Occupational Safety and Health, Stockholm; Lars Eriksson, AB Bygg- och Transportekonomi, Mjölby; Jan-Erik Hansson, Research Department, National Swedish Board of Occupational Safety and Health, Stockholm; Torleif Saeland, AB ASEA, Härnösand; and Nils-Erik Swartz, Transport Research Committee, Stockholm.

The main objective of the checklist was to provide buyers and manufacturers of trucks and similar equipment with "advice on ergonomic issues." The operator should participate in any evaluation of the machinery being considered for purchase. The checklist is also intended for educational usage. This checklist supersedes the checklist[18] previously published by the National Swedish Board of Occupational Safety and Health. Readers are referred to the checklist[19] published by the Logging Research Foundation for evaluation information on heavy transport and materials-handling machinery. Other important information useful to machinery evaluation will also be found in other checklists[12, 19] and standards.[11, 15, 21, 24, 28, 30] Experience derived from studies of machinery ergonomics, as performed by the Section for Technical Work Physiology at the National Swedish Board of Occupational Safety and Health and elsewhere, provided the basis for the present checklist. References to the literature and standards providing more detailed background information on proposed guidelines or special fields are provided under the various evaluation criteria.

WHICH OPERATORS ARE TO USE THE TRUCK?

Due regard must be paid to operator requirements when new machinery is designed. The objective in determining operator area specifications must be to provide operators of varying size and strength with an optimum working environment. To facilitate truck operation in, e.g., railway goods vans (i.e., freight cars) with low door openings, it may sometimes be necessary to utilize trucks too small to accommodate a large operator. Very large operators should be discouraged from using such trucks. Salespersons should be able to supply information on the operator categories for which machinery is designed.

Average height has increased considerably in Sweden and many other industrialized countries during the 20th century. The average height increase for Swedish conscripts amounted to 1.2 cm/10 years.[22] In 1974, the average Swedish conscript was 178 cm tall. This height is expected to increase to 181 cm by the year 2000. Seventy-five percent of this height increase is due to increasing leg length. Physiques are also apparently becoming slimmer.[22] Figure 61–1, A and B illustrates the manner in which height, lower leg length, elbow height, the head-to-buttocks distance, width at the elbows and hips, etc., vary in German women and men at various ages.[21] It should be noted that physical measurements in Figure 61–1 refer to measurements made with subjects in an erect, sitting position. Truck operators tend to assume a more relaxed and slumped position. A sitting height equal to about 96% of the anthropometric values specified in Figure 61–1 should be expected. Any rearward tilt of the seat and backrest influences values for elbow and sitting height.

The guideline values stated in the checklist for workplace measurements are intended for persons whose height ranges from 160 to 190 cm. Figure 61–2 illustrates the spatial requirements of a woman 160 cm tall and a man 190 cm tall. About 75% of the women and 90% of young Swedish men in a working population fit these spatial requirements.

Some trucks have controls stiff enough to cause musculoskeletal complaints in some cases. Excessive actuating force may present a safety risk by, e.g., prolonging a truck's braking distance.

Muscular strength is mainly governed by personal factors such as body size, age, and sex (Fig 61–3). But wide variations in muscular strength are found among people of the same sex, age, and body size.

So it is important to know which people are likely to operate any machinery before that machinery is purchased. If the machinery is to be operated by women and elderly men, a special check should be made to ensure that the actuating force of controls does not exceed the listed guideline values.

CHOICE OF WORK POSTURE—TRUCK TYPE

Work postures should make it possible to retain the joints in mainly neutral positions, i.e., neither heavily flexed nor extended. Work postures in which the trunk is bent and twisted or in which the joints are forced to operate at their extreme positions often give

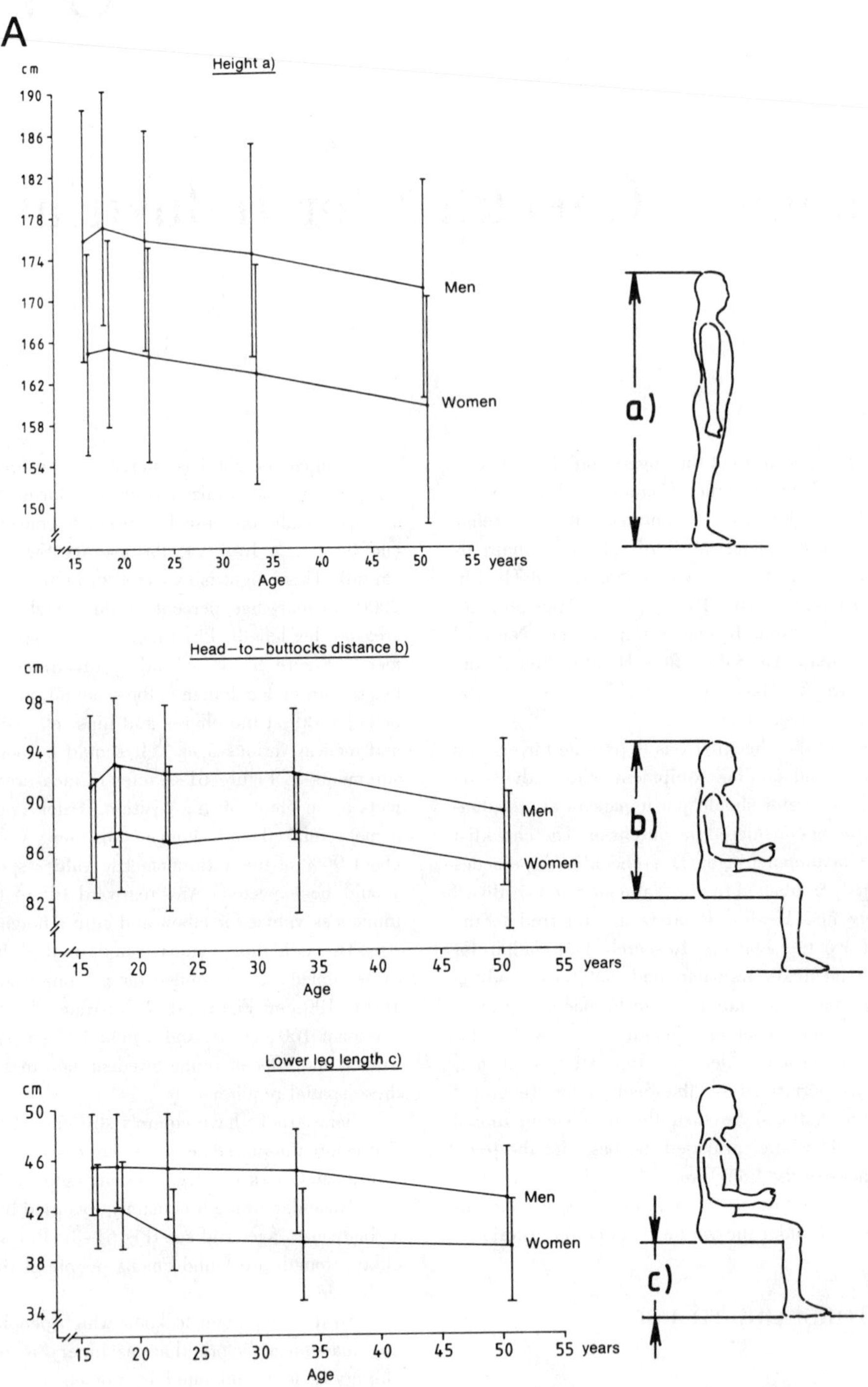

FIG 61–1.
Body measurements for German women and men. The measurements were judged to be relevant even to a Swedish population. The measurements are based on studies carried out by Jürgens et al. in the 1970s and are tabulated in the DIN 33402 standard. In figures **A,** and **B,** 5, 50 and 95 percentiles are presented.

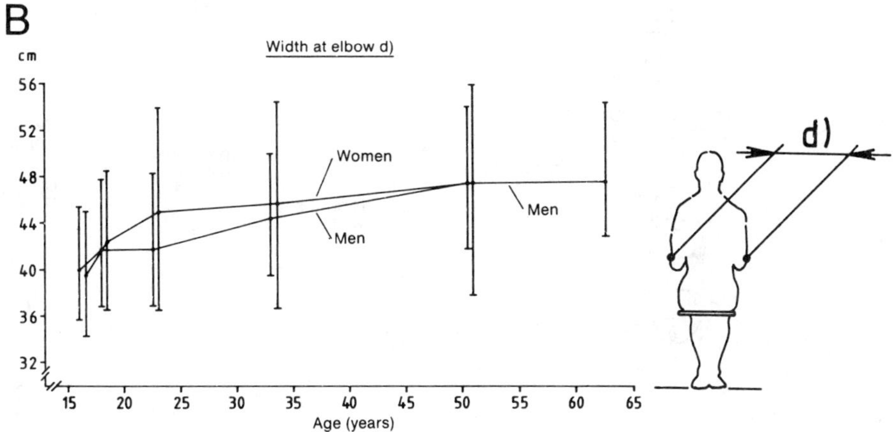

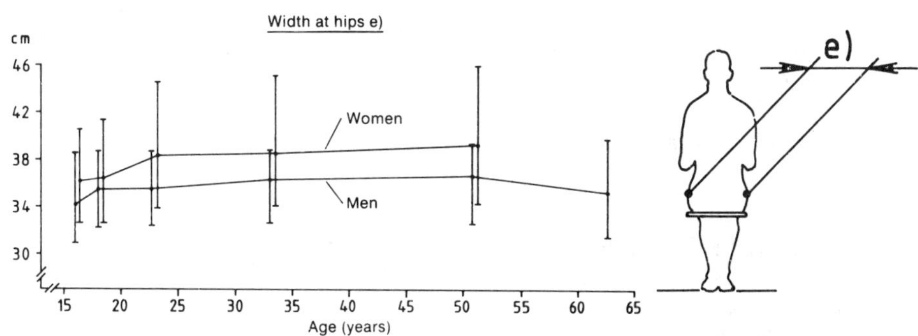

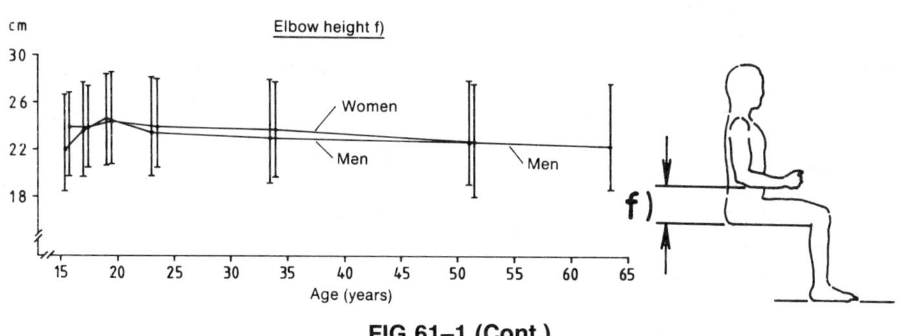

FIG 61–1 (Cont.)

rise to musculoskeletal complaints.[26] Protracted work in a sitting position, especially in fixed positions, is unsuitable. Protracted work in a standing position is unsuitable, especially for older people; efforts should be made to vary work tasks. Variations in work postures and micropauses reduce physiologic strain and the risk of overloading joints and muscles.[3] Since operators often have to remain sitting in their trucks for long periods at a time, it is especially important for them to have a work environment in which they can keep their heads, arms, shoulders and backs in acceptable work postures.

In principle, three basic types of work postures can be selected when machinery is designed or purchased: (1) a normal sitting position; (2) a high sitting position; and (3) a standing position.

A normal sitting position should be strived for. Here, the operator faces the direction in which work is performed, an especially

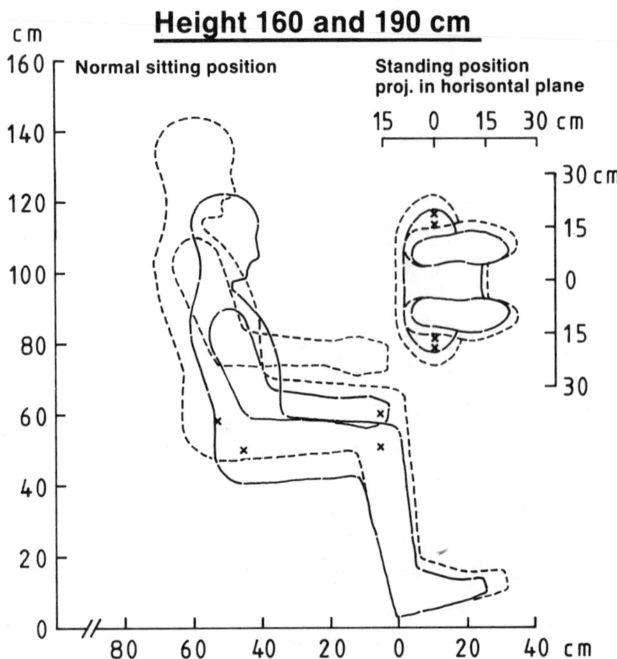

FIG 61–2.
Space requirements for large and small operator. Operator shoeless.

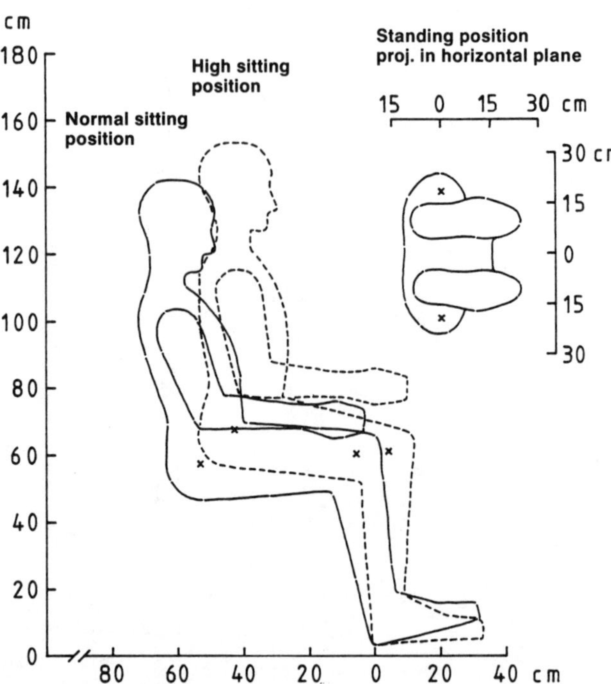

FIG 61–4.
The effect of body position on space requirements, Operator shoeless.

desirable position when the operator is forced to remain in the truck most of the day. The seat should be designed so it is easy for an operator to vary her/his work posture. It should be possible to adjust the seat to accommodate the operator's body size. A normal sitting position takes up considerable space, especially if the seat can be swiveled in different directions. When a normal sitting position cannot be attained, a high sitting position or standing position may be alternatives. These positions take up less space and make it possible to utilize smaller trucks. However, these work postures demand more vertical work space (ceiling height) and may be advantageous if an operator is frequently forced to mount and dismount. A high sitting position may be preferable when sitting space is restricted (Fig 61–4).

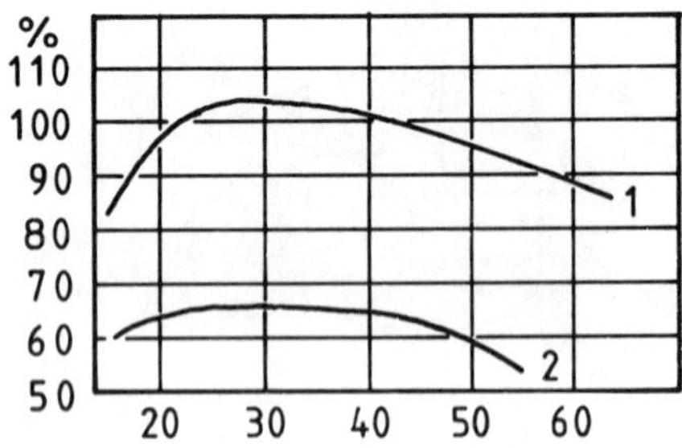

FIG 61–3.
The average strength of 25 muscle groups in relation to age. The average strength of a 22-year-old man is set at 100. *Line 1* represents male muscle strength; *line 2,* female muscle strength. The difference between men and women is even greater in the musculature of the shoulder and the arm. (Data from Asmussen E: Musklerna, in Luthman G, Aberg U, Lundgren N (eds): *Handbok i Ergonomi.* Stockholm, Almqvist & Wiksell/Gebers Förlag AB, 1966.)

From the load and stability point of view, pedal operations should be avoided in the standing and, to a certain extent, in the high sitting position. Only one foot at a time should be used for pedal operation. The two latter positions are also unsuitable, from the safety point of view, during driving operations at high speed, since they are most unstable. An operator working in a standing position should have an opportunity to leave her/his truck from time to time in order to sit down.

An operator must face the direction in which work is performed in order to assume a good work posture. The operator environment (seat and controls) or the entire cab must be capable of swiveling in more than one main work direction if required (Fig 61–5). Solutions such as these should be an objective whenever possible in 4–5-ton trucks or larger.[27]

A swiveling workplace may not be attainable when a small truck must be used because of space restrictions. A lateral sitting position can then be employed in certain instances. The lateral sitting position provides a wider field of view to the rear than a position with the operator facing the truck front, but this position demands a twisted trunk and imposes strain on the back and neck musculature. A twisted work posture in conjunction with severe whole-body vibration is particularly unsuitable.

An operator's work posture can be considerably improved if, e.g., a swiveling seat is installed and controls are laterally adjustable (see Fig 61–5). A mere 30-degree swivel can improve the work posture immensely. However, a swiveling seat does usually demand more cab space.

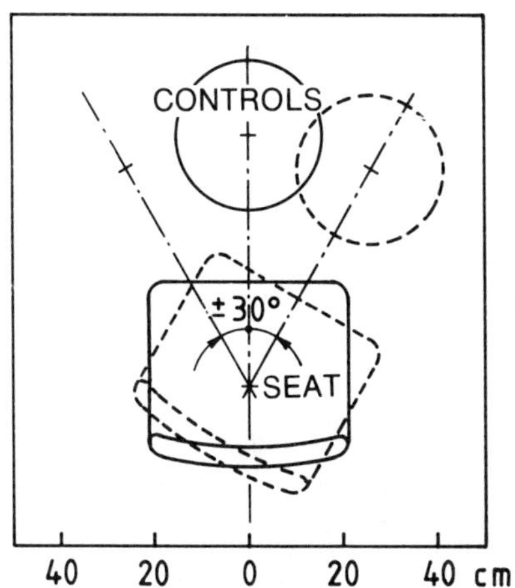

FIG 61–5.
A seat which swivels 20–30 degrees considerably improves the work position of the neck.[7] However, this may require changes in the location or design of controls.

If it is necessary to accept a truck in which certain operations require the driver to work with twisted trunk, the seat should be designed so that the torsion takes place simultaneously in the hips, back, and neck joints. A seat which is too deeply dished or has too high a backrest makes such torsion much more difficult.

Identification of the work postures capable of providing acceptable ergonomic conditions in the envisaged work is an important consideration in the evaluation of trucks.

OPERATOR WORK SPACE

The operator's work space should be large enough to enable even a large operator to find an acceptable work posture. However, the operator space must also be able to offer seat and control positions suitable for a small operator. The need for a cab and the work posture(s) desired should be included in any assessment of the factors below. If two work directions are to be possible (with a swiveling seat), the operator area must usually be considerably larger than is the case with one work direction. In many instances, even modest seat swiveling (20–30 degrees) can reduce strain on an operator.

TABLE 61–2.
Evaluating Operator Work Space

POINTS TO ASSESS	YES	NO
• Is the operator area designed and arranged so operation, loading, and unloading are not hazardous to the operator?	☐	☐
• Is there anything in the operator area which could injure the operator?	☐	☐
• Is the operator area large enough?	☐	☐

The measurements (guideline values) listed in Table 61–1 for trucks without a cab are minimum measurements for a large man. If a cramped operator area is unavoidable, the work should be reorganized so that sessions on the truck are brief. The main points to assess in evaluating operator work space are summarized in Table 61–2.

VIBRATION

Vibration is a factor important to working conditions. As a rule, test operation of a truck under normal conditions (surface, driving speed) will disclose the extent of any whole-body vibration transmitted by, e.g., the steering wheel. The manufacturer/dealer will also be able to supply details on this point. Employees and occupational health services can often supply information on vibration characteristics for similar equipment. This information is useful when machinery is designed or purchased.

Trucks generate vibration which vibrates operator's whole body, via the seat or her/his feet (whole-body vibration), and vibration that is mainly transmitted to the operator's hands and arms (hand-transmitted vibration). Both types of vibration are fatiguing and may have an adverse effect on work capacity and health. Intensity, frequency, direction, and duration must be considered in any assessment of the effect of vibration on man. The level of

TABLE 61–1.
Guideline Values for Operator Work Space

OPERATOR AREA* CM	NORMAL SITTING† POSITION			HIGH SITTING‡ POSITION		STANDING POSITION
	NONSWIVELING SEAT		SWIVELING SEAT	NONSWIVELING SEAT		
	INDOORS (NO CAB)	OUTDOORS (CAB)	OUTDOORS (CAB)	INDOORS (NO CAB)	OUTDOORS (CAB)	INDOORS (NO CAB)
Length	110	130	165	100	115	45§
Width	55	90	110	55	90	50§
Height	150	160‖	160	160‖	170‖	200

*For an operator about 160 to 190 cm tall.
†Seat height 45 cm. Adjustable ±5 cm.
‡Seat height 55 cm. Adjustable ±10 cm. The seat depth should be 5–10 cm less than the normal seat height. The normal seat height should be measured at the seat's reference point according to SMS (25).
§Spatial requirements for feet in a stand-up truck. Space allocations should be larger at hip and shoulder level. The platform width should be about 60 cm in a power pallet truck.
‖A 5–10 cm lower height may be acceptable during truck operation on a smooth surface. (See Figs 61–2 and 61–3.)

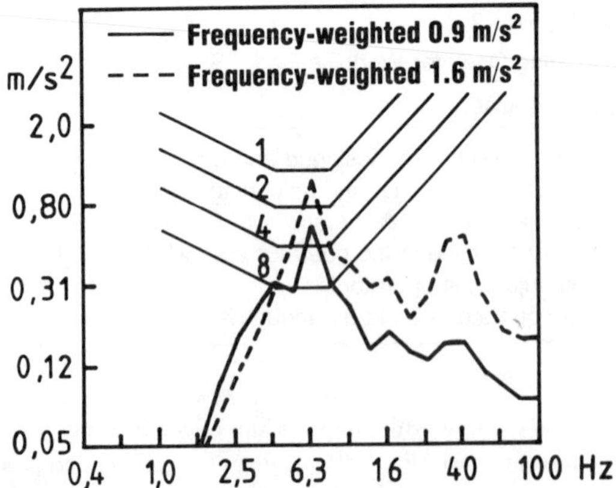

FIG 61–6.
Example of the vibration damping properties of a good driver's seat. The seat is mounted on a 2-6-ton forklift truck.[20] Driving speed: 4 m/sec. Vibration in the Z direction. *Solid line* represents the chair seat. *Dotted line* represents the vehicle floor.

vibration is governed by factors such as the surface, driving speed, engine speed, type of operator's seat, the tires and the vehicle's design. As a rule, truck suspension should be as soft as possible without impairing performance too much. So, lårge, rubber tires are favorable from the vibration point of view. However, the risk of tipping presented by certain truck designs may warrant the use of harder tires.

The operator's seat in a 2–4-ton truck should provide considerable reduction of vertical vibration (Fig 61–6). Improvements in the surface upon which the truck is operated, such as smoothing, may also considerably reduce an operator's exposure to vibration. The exposure limit values for whole-body and hand-transmitted vibration are listed in Tables 61–3 and 61–4. A vibration-reduction checklist is presented in Table 61–5.

TABLE 61–5.
Evaluating Vibration

POINTS TO ASSESS	YES	NO
• Is the truck designed so that it can be expected to expose the operator to an acceptable level of vibration during intended operations (wheel size, tire type, vibration damping of operator area, etc.)?	☐	☐
• Are suspension components (e.g., the driver's seat) sufficiently durable?	☐	☐

OPERATOR'S SEAT

The operator's seat should be designed to accommodate the sitting positions to be used. With a high sitting position, the seat depth, for example, should be shallower and the backrest more upright than in a normal sitting position (Fig 61–7). The seat should also be designed so an operator can easily change her or his sitting position and thereby relieve strain on different parts of her or his body. When items are transported long distances on

TABLE 61–3.
Guideline Values:[18] Exposure Limit Values for Whole-Body Vibration*

EXPOSURE DURATION DURING TYPICAL WORKDAY (HOURS)	ACCELERATION (M/S^2) VERTICAL Z DIRECTION	HORIZONTAL X AND Y DIRECTIONS
8	0.9	0.6
6	1.0	0.7
4	1.2	0.9
2	1.7	1.2

*The values in the table refer to acceleration of the vibrating surface in contact with the body. They are expressed as frequency-weighted RMS values (0.8–100 Hz).[29] The values are for vibration in the directions indicated in the figure.

TABLE 61–4.
Guideline Values[18]: Exposure Limit Values for Hand-Transmitted Vibration*

EXPOSURE DURATION DURING TYPICAL WORKDAY (HOURS)	ACCELERATION (M/S^2) X, Y AND Z DIRECTIONS
4	2.9
2	4.1
1	5.8
0.5	8.3

Vibration direction

*The values in the table refer to acceleration of the vibrating surface in contact with the hand. They are expressed as frequency-weighted RMS values in the 6.3–1250 Hz range.[15] The values are for vibration in the directions indicated in the figure.

Normal sitting position

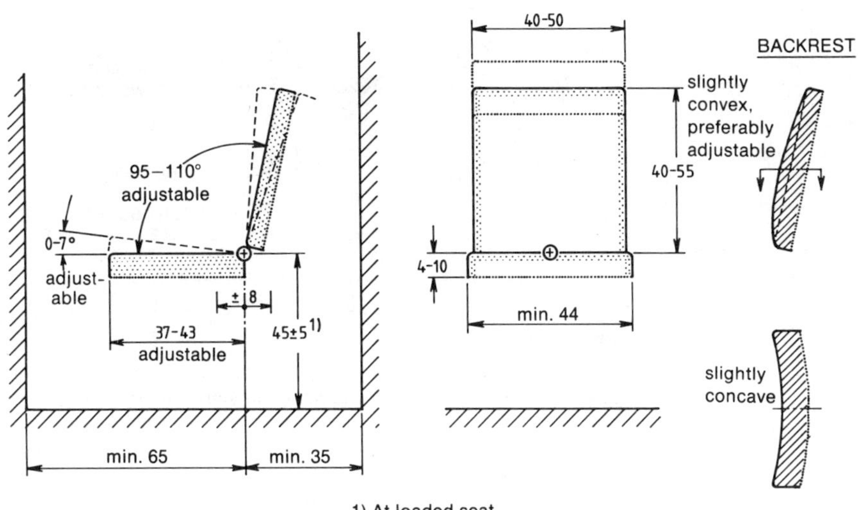

1) At loaded seat

FIG 61–7.
Optimum truck seat dimensions (in centimeters) for normal and high sitting positions.

High sitting position

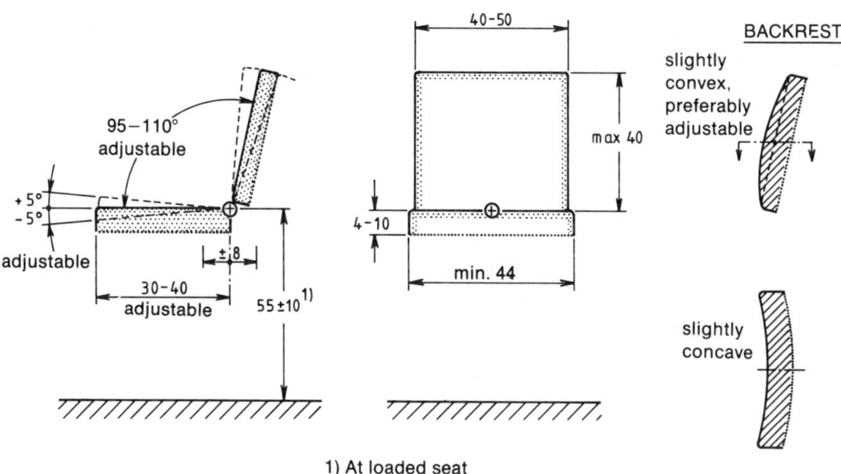

1) At loaded seat

smooth ground, a more tilted backrest than in loading work may be preferable. If the operator must have a view to the rear, the backrest should not be so high that the operator is unable to turn around and, e.g., support himself with an arm on the top of the backrest (backrest height should be less than 40 cm).

When an operator is not exposed to major vibration, e.g., as when driving at slow speeds on smooth surfaces indoors, the seat does not require any special vibration damping (shock absorbers and springs). The seat should be firmly attached to the vehicle floor.

There is considerable wear and tear on the joints of seats exposed to heavy vibration. So these joints should be sturdily made. The seat's condition (shock absorbers, stability, etc.) should be checked at least once a year.

An armrest may reduce strain on the back in certain instances. However, the armrest must not obstruct arm movements. Armrests and the seat in other respects should be readily adjustable to suit people of different physiques and weight. Simple instructions on the seat's adjustment facilities should be attached to the chair or truck. The seat cushion should contain insulating ma-

TABLE 61–6.
Evaluating the Operator's Seat

POINTS TO ASSESS	YES	NO
• Is the seat's vibration damping adequate?	☐	☐
• Is the seat sufficiently sturdy and firmly mounted?	☐	☐
• Do the seat cushion and backrest have the correct size, design, and inclination?	☐	☐
• Is adjustment of the seat cushion and any armrests adequate and sufficiently easy to modify (e.g., horizontally and vertically)?	☐	☐
• Is the seat easy to adjust?	☐	☐
• Is the thickness of the seat cushion, backrest, and upholstery suitable in terms of friction and insulation?	☐	☐

terial, permeable to air and moisture, and provide sufficient friction to prevent sliding (Table 61–6).

CONTROLS

Controls should be located at a convenient distance in all operating directions (Figs 61–8 and 61–9). This is especially true of controls bearing on safety, such as brakes and frequently used controls.

Size and shape should be such that a good grip is always provided and controls cannot be confused. The brake pedal, for example, should be to the right of the clutch.

The force required to actuate controls should be of the correct magnitude. An actuating force which is too low may be hazardous, since controls could then be affected by, e.g., vibration. On the other hand, excessive stiffness could affect the precision and speed of actuation, since greater muscular force must be mobilized. The proper actuating force is especially important for controls frequently used.[4, 10, 13, 20] Optimum actuating force is less important for controls only used sporadically.

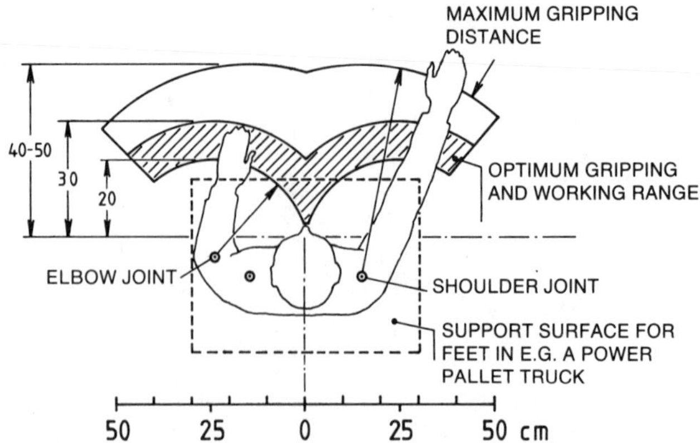

FIG 61–9.
Location of controls in a standing work posture. The optimum gripping and working range for the hands in standing work. A comfortable height for operation of hand controls is usually at elbow level when the upper arm is parallel to the trunk. It must be possible to raise and lower controls if a comfortable work height is to be attainable by both tall and short operators.

It is also important to be able to operate frequently used controls within a movement range suitable to the arms and legs.[8, 9, 14] Improper work postures can give rise to musculoskeletal complaints[26] and impair precision operation of a truck. Controls should operate in a logical pattern.

The maximum actuating forces listed in Table 61–7 are based on the circumstance that about 75% of all women in a normal sitting position should be able to actuate a control five times in rapid succession.[16]

Controls mounted in the armrest may be able to relieve strain on the shoulder during lever operation in certain instances.[23] A checklist for proper operating controls is presented in Table 61–8.

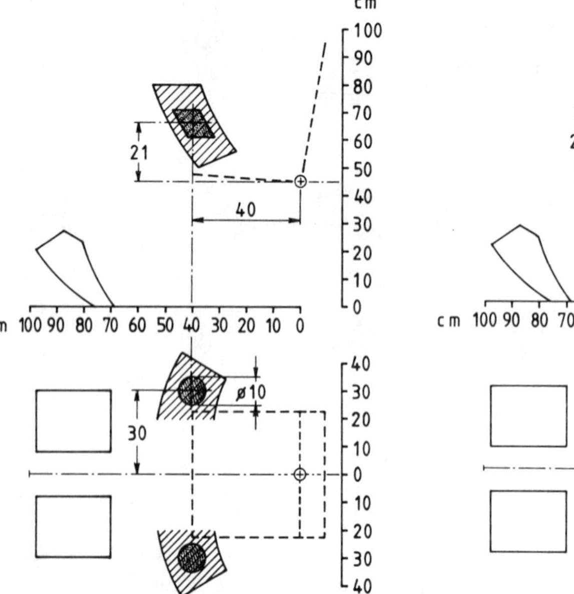

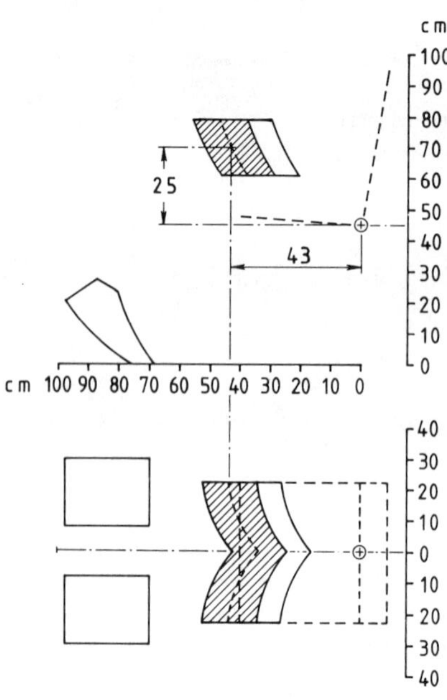

FIG 61–8.
Location of controls in normal sitting position. An optimum working range for the hands and feet in the operation with the operator in a sitting position is designated. Any change in the horizontal or vertical position of the seat should be accompanied by corresponding changes in the position of the hand controls, especially in the vertical direction, if optimum working conditions are to be preserved. **A,** *Top:* a cross-section through the center of an optimum working range *(dark area). Bottom:* Levers located at the side of the seat. The *dark area* designates the optimum area. Frequently used hand controls should be easily adjustable. **B,** levers located above the seat. Hand controls should be movable to facilitate entry and exit.

TABLE 61–7.
Guideline Values for Control Actuating Force

ACTUATING FORCES (NEWTONS)	OPTIMUM	MAXIMUM
Hand-operated lever, forward/backward	5–15	140
Hand-operated lever, lateral	5–15	60
Steering wheel, 2-hand operation	5–50	230
Steering wheel, 1-hand operation	5–15	
Finger-operated controls	3–5	
Leg-operated controls, clutch and brake	45–90	250
Toe-operated controls (e.g., accelerator)	20–30	

VISIBILITY

Visibility from the truck is governed by the design and location of the fork columns in relation to the operator. Work should be planned so that it can be carried out by the operator with a minimum of effort, e.g., with turns forward to the right (Fig 6–10). Poor visibility increases the risk of accidents and forces the operator to assume strenuous work postures.[5] Postures in which the head remains twisted or the body bent for any period of time are unsuitable.[1]

The performance of the windscreen wiper and defroster and the location of defroster nozzles are important to visibility outdoors. Favorable results have been obtained from the use of large mirrors to improve or supplement visibility upward and to the rear. Video cameras can sometimes be used to check the lift height and to ensure that there is enough space to reverse.

Visibility should be examined (forward, backward, and to the side) with and without the load the truck is intended to carry. Visibility requirements shall be assessed with a view to a truck's speed and the location in which it is to be used, considering such factors as traffic density and hidden corridors. Visibility should be checked from the operator's seat after an operator has assumed a comfortable position. It is essential for visibility through the supports to be good.

TABLE 61–8.
Evaluating Truck Controls

POINTS TO ASSESS	YES	NO
• Are frequently used controls located within a convenient working range so both tall and short operators can assume a comfortable work posture?	☐	☐
• Do controls operate in a logical pattern?	☐	☐
• Do controls have a suitable size and shape?	☐	☐
• Do controls operate with sufficient smoothness?	☐	☐
• Is the risk of involuntary actuation slight?	☐	☐

The operator should be able to see the tips of the truck forks or the equivalent while in an ordinary sitting position during loading.

An optimum work posture and movement range for the head and neck should be sought. The maximum range should be utilized only exceptionally during the workday. A checklist for evaluating visibility is presented in Table 61–9.

LIGHTING

Trucks employed in poorly lighted areas should be equipped with lighting. Satisfactory lighting must deliver sufficient light intensity within a sufficiently large area and distribute that lighting without dazzling. The lighting should be tailored to factors such as the vehicle's speed, braking distance and duties. Illuminated parts of the truck within the operator's visual field must be painted with a matte-finish paint to reduce distracting reflections. In certain instances, the truck should be equipped with running lights making it easy to detect.

Lighting should be checked during operational tests with and without loads.

Direction forward – backward

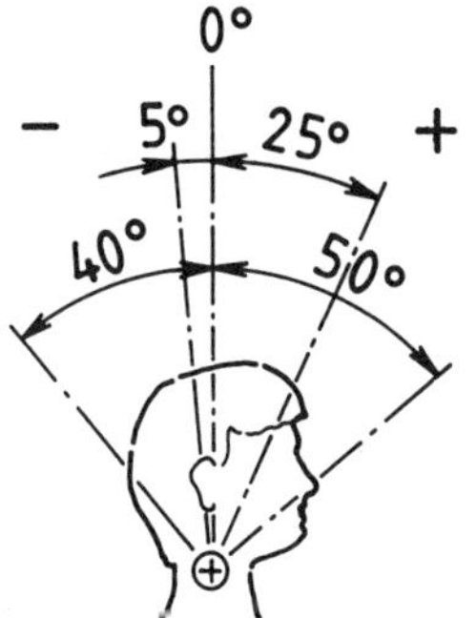

−5° – +25° = optimum range
−40° – +50° = maximum range

To the side

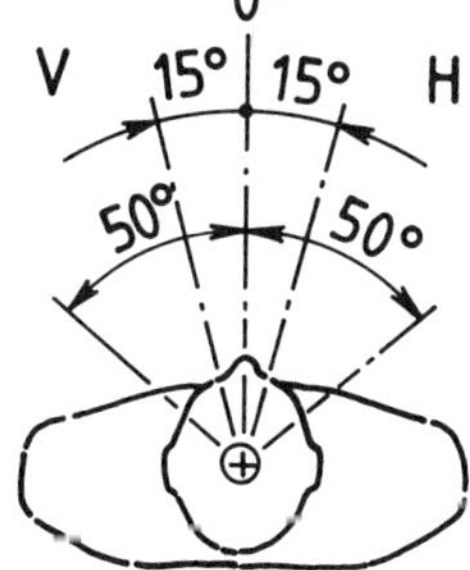

±15° = optimum range
±50° = maximum range

FIG 61–10.
Optimum and maximum ranges of operator head movement.

TABLE 61–9.
Evaluating Visibility

POINTS TO ASSESS	YES	NO
• Is visibility good when a load is being carried?	☐	☐
• Is visibility good when no load is being carried?	☐	☐
• Is visibility good during loading and unloading?	☐	☐
• Is the position of the head and neck acceptable during loading and unloading?	☐	☐
• Is the truck equipped with an efficient windscreen wiper, windscreen washer, defroster, direction indicators, rear-view mirrors, and horn?	☐	☐

Light intensity in the operator's working area should amount to at least 30 lux. The ratio between the strongest and weakest levels of illumination should be less than 1:3. A checklist for evaluating truck illumination is presented in Table 61–10.

MOUNTING AND ALIGHTING

The procedure for getting on and off trucks which frequently have to be mounted or dismounted must be convenient and without risk. This is especially important for older operators. A faulty design or improper location of a step, for example, could induce operators to jump down, thereby exposing themselves to the risk of injury. The truck must be designed so mounting and dismounting are safe and convenient with no need for uncomfortable body torsion. Consideration must be paid to:

1. The mutual location of doors, operator's seat, steering wheel and pedals

2. The location of grips and handles

3. The ground-to-floor distance and the size and location of the door opening

4. The design of the steps in relation to the risk of slipping or getting stuck

The distance to the first step should be less than 35 cm. The distance between steps should be 20–30 cm. A checklist for evaluating truck mounting and alighting is presented in Table 61–11.

TABLE 61–10.
Evaluating Illumination

POINTS TO ASSESS	YES	NO
• Is illumination acceptable during operation to the front?	☐	☐
• Is illumination acceptable during operation to the rear?	☐	☐
• Is illumination acceptable during loading and unloading?	☐	☐
• Does the truck's color contrast with the surroundings?	☐	☐
• Does the truck have a finish which does not give rise to distracting reflections from the truck's or other illumination?	☐	☐

TABLE 61–11.
Evaluating Ease of Entry and Exit

POINTS TO ASSESS	YES	NO
• Can mounting or alighting take place without the risk of an accident?	☐	☐
• Are mounting and alighting convenient?	☐	☐

NOISE

Hearing may be damaged if the sound level at an operator's ear exceeds 85 dB(A). Noise which is not damaging may still be so distracting that danger signals are not heard and may have an adverse effect on productivity. For the sake of comfort and communications, therefore, the sound level should be kept to a level much lower than the level eliciting damage.

The general criteria for action, measurement methods, and reference guideline values in the assessment of noise will be found in the noise regulations issued by the National Swedish Board of Occupational Safety and Health.

The equivalent sound level should be less than 75 dB(A). The maximum level should be 85 dB(A). A noise evaluation checklist is presented in Table 61–12.

INSTRUMENTS AND SIGNALS

The instruments should supply only necessary information. They should be of a suitable design. Signal lamps are suitable for indicating one of two conditions, such as empty–not empty, charging on–charging off, etc. Acoustic signals are suitable for brief messages, such as warnings. Instruments with dials are usually employed in other instances. A checklist for evaluating instruments and signals is presented in Table 61–13.

CAB CLIMATE

This section refers to trucks equipped with a cab and used in cold areas.

The climate inside a cab must be assessed with a view to the operator's clothing and the required level of physical activity. The cab should be designed and equipped so the operator is not exposed to drafts, dust, or severe cold, or severe heat caused by radiation/convection. Opinions vary regarding what constitutes a "good" climate (Table 61–14). The perception of climate is also

TABLE 61–12.
Evaluating Noise Level

POINTS TO ASSESS	YES	NO
• Is the noise level so low that hearing protectors are not necessary?	☐	☐
• Is noise at the driver's seat less than 75 dB(A)?	☐	☐
• Is the truck free from distracting noise?	☐	☐

TABLE 61–13.
Evaluating Instruments and Signals

POINTS TO ASSESS	YES	NO
• Does the truck have the necessary instruments/signals?	☐	☐
• Has the right type of instruments been used?	☐	☐
• Are the instruments suitably located?	☐	☐
• Are the instruments easy to read?	☐	☐

TABLE 61–14.
Guideline Values for Truck Cab Climate*

CLIMATE FACTOR	OPTIMUM VALUE	MAXIMUM VALUE
Temperature	18–22° C	32° C, 27° WBGT†
Air velocity at operator	0.1–0.3 m/s	0.4–1 m/s‡
Temperature gradient between head and feet	0–5° C	

*The guideline values may be hard to meet for equipment which has to be mounted and dismounted frequently.
†The WBGT (wet-bulb globe temperature) heat index is calculated according to the following equation:

$$WBGT = 0.7\ t_v + 0.3\ t_g$$

in which t_v = wet-bulb temperature (measured with a ventilated and radiation-shielded thermometer or psychrometer), °C, and t_g = the globe temperature (measured with a globe thermometer), °C.
‡Air velocity should not exceed 0.4–0.5 m/s at air temperatures under 25° C. Higher air velocities may be acceptable at higher temperatures.

TABLE 61–15.
Evaluating Truck Cab Climate

POINTS TO ASSESS	YES	NO
• Can the cab be ventilated?	☐	☐
• Is the operator protected from intense sunlight?	☐	☐
• Is the heating suitably designed and adequate?	☐	☐
• Is the cab insulated from the engine and gearbox?	☐	☐
• Is the cab free from the smell of oil, fuel and exhaust gases?	☐	☐

influenced by factors such as air velocity and radiation. A driver exposed to intense sunlight generally prefers a lower cab temperature.

Sensitivity to drafts and temperature gradients is reduced by the use of heavy clothing and a higher level of physical activity.

Research into the effect of heat removal systems is described in reference 25. A checklist for evaluating truck cab climate is presented in Table 61–15.

OVERALL ASSESSMENT

This checklist contains a number of different points, each of which is designed to shed light on aspects to be assessed. However, these aspects are not of equal pertinence to the final assess-

TABLE 61–16.
Overall Assessment of Truck Design

	TRUCK DESIGN*					ERGONOMIC SIGNIFICANCE OF THE ASSESSMENT POINT		
POINTS TO ASSESS	1	2	3	4	5	NOT VERY IMPORTANT	IMPORTANT	VERY IMPORTANT
Operator area								
Vibration								
Operator's seat								
Controls								
Visibility to the front								
Visibility to the rear								
Visibility—loading unloading								
Illumination								
Mounting and dismounting								
Noise								
Instruments & signals								
Cab climate, etc.								

*1 = Very bad, 2 = rather bad, 3 = neither bad nor good, 4 = rather good, 5 = very good.

ment. In this final assessment, therefore, an effort should be made to weigh the various factors in a suitable manner in which consideration is paid to when, where, how and how often the truck is to be used (Table 61–16).

ACKNOWLEDGMENT

Appreciation is given Professor Sven Carlsöö for reviewing this chapter.

REFERENCES

1. Andersson G, et al: Modell för bedömning av skada på halsrygg och axelled (skuldergördel) i enlighet med arbetsskadeförsäkringen (LAF). *Läkartidningen* 1983; 80:36.
2. Asmussen E: Musklerna, in Luthman G, Åberg U, Lundgren N (eds): *Handbok i Ergonomi*. Stockholm, Almqvist & Wiksell/Gebers Förlag AB, 1966.
3. Åstrand I: *Arbetsfysiologi*. Stockholm, Almqvist & Wiksell Förlag AB, 1986.
4. Björksten M, Jonsson B: Endurance limit of force in long-term intermittent static contractions. *Scand J Work Environ Health* 1977; 3.
5. Bjurvald M, Hansson J-E: *Ergonomiska Studier av Siktförhållanden på Industritruckar*, Investigation report AMA 111/73. Solna, National Swedish Board of Occupational Safety and Health, 1973.
6. Bottoms DJ, Barberm TS: A swivelling seat to improve tractor driver's posture. *Appl Ergonom* 1978; 9:2.
7. Caple D, Björksten M, Carlsöö S, et al: *Fordonsutformning för Bilbrevbäring. En Ergonomisk Studie*, Investigation report 29. Solna, National Swedish Board of Occupational Safety and Health, 1981.
8. Carlsöö S, Hansson J-E, Uppsäll M: Optimala arbetsområden vid manövrering av handreglage. *Arbete och Hälsa* 12. Solna, National Swedish Board of Occupational Safety and Health, 1978.
9. Carlsöö S: *Hand-Arm-Funktion vid Reglagemanövrering*, Investigation report 38. Solna, National Swedish Board of Occupational Safety and Health, 1982.
10. Corlett EN, Bishop RP: Foot pedal forces for seated operators. *Ergonomics* 1975; 18:6.
11. Determination of seat reference point, Swedish Standard SMS 2863. Swedish Standards Association, Stockholm.
12. *Ergonomic aspects. Cabins of mobile cranes*. A joint publication by Foundation Occupational Health in the Building and Construction (PO Box 8114, 1005 AC Amsterdam) and Netherlands Institute for Preventive Health Care—TNO, 1981.
13. Glass SW, Suggs CW: Optimization of vehicle accelerator-brake pedal foot travel time. *Appl Ergonom* 1977; 8:4.
14. Glencross DJ, Andersson GA: Operator response factors in the location and control of foot pedals. *Ergonomics* 1976; 19:4.
15. *Guide for the Measurement and the Assessment of Human Exposure to Vibration Transmitted to the Hand*. ISO Standard 5349-1986.
16. Gullander A, Hansson J-E: *Förmåga Till Kraftutveckling i Pedal, Ratt och Handspak*, Investigation report AMA 011/74. Stockholm, National Swedish Board of Occupational Safety and Health, 1974.
17. Hansson J-E, Kjellberg A: *Vibrationsexponering och Upplevda Besvär vid Truckkörning på Godsbangårdar*, Investigation report 1. Solna, National Swedish Board of Occupational Safety and Health, 1981.
18. Hansson J-E: *Ergonomisk Checklista för Truckar*, Investigation report 25. Solna, National Swedish Board of Occupational Safety and Health, 1983.
19. Hansson J-E, Pettersson B: *An Ergonomic Checklist for Transport and Materials-Handling Machinery*. Solna, National Swedish Board of Occupational Safety and Health, Forestry Work Research Foundation and Royal College of Forestry, 1980.
20. Hansson J-E, Suggs CW: *Lågfrekventa Vibrationers Inverkan på Reglagemanövrering*, Reports and theses 63. Stockholm, Royal College of Forestry, 1973.
21. *Körpermasse des Menschen*, DIN 33402. 1981 Deutsche Norm, Beuth Verlag GmbH, Berlin 30.
22. Levin T, Wilson O: Prognos för antropometriska mått hos svenska flygförare år 2001, FOA report C 59004-H2. Stockholm, Research Institute of the Swedish National Defence, 1982.
23. Lindbeck L: *Armstödets Betydelse för Avlastning av Skuldran* vid Spakmanövrering, Investigation report 35. Solna, National Swedish Board of Occupational Safety and Health, 1982.
24. Motorred skap och traktorer. Ordinance AFS G. Solna, National Swedish Board of Occupational Safety and Health, 1985.
25. Norén O: *Värmeavlastning och Dammreducering i förarhytter*, Summary 230. Stockholm, The Work Environment Fund, 1980.
26. Person J, Kilbom Å, Jonsson B: Unpublished data. Belastningsbesvär i skuldror och nacke—en studie över individuella riskfaktorer. Stockholm, National Swedish Board of Occupational Safety and Health, 1983.
27. *Truck Med Höj- och Vändbar Hytt*, Minireport MR 22. Stockholm, Transport Research Commission, 1982.
28. Truckar. SMS Handbook 1987. Stockholm, Swedish Standards Association.
29. *Vibration and Shock Guide for the Evaluation of Human Exposure to Whole-Body Vibration*. ISO Standard 2631-1978.
30. *Work Postures and Working Movements*, Ordinance AFS 6. Solna, National Swedish Board of Occupational Safety and Health, 1983.

62

Fire Fighters

James M. Melius, M.D., Dr. P.H.

Fire fighting is one of the most hazardous of occupations. The annual injury rate for fire fighters is among the highest of all occupational groups.[19, 51] Although accurate comparison data for occupational disease among fire fighters is not available, deaths due to myocardial infarction while on duty are quite common, and disability retirements due to cardiovascular disease, respiratory impairment, and other medical problems are also common.[19]

While some degree of hazard should be expected by the nature of the fire fighting job, the occupational health hazards of this occupation can be better understood by reviewing the potential exposures for fire fighters and the resultant medical problems described in past studies of fire fighters. These studies have focused mainly on cardiovascular, respiratory disease, and, more recently, on cancer. An understanding of these exposures and health effects and the job requirements for fire fighters provide the basis for limiting the health hazards for this occupational group.

EXPOSURES

The fire fighter is exposed to multiple toxic substances when extinguishing fires. Unfortunately, there is very little quantitative data on actual exposures during fire fighting. Carbon monoxide is the most commonly documented exposure. One study of fire fighters' exposures in Boston found carbon monoxide exposures above 400 ppm in approximately 15% of the individual exposures studied, ranging as high as 5,000 ppm.[48] Several other studies have documented elevated carboxyhemoglobin levels in fire fighters.[36, 39, 42, 43] Exposure to cyanide appears to be quite low in most fires.[23, 48] Other common exposures noted in the Boston study, included acrolein, hydrogen chloride, nitrogen dioxide, and benzene.[48] Of these, acrolein was not infrequently found at levels sufficient to produce acute conjunctivitis and respiratory irritation; 10% of the fire fighters were exposed to levels over 3 ppm. Fire fighters have also been shown to have significant noise exposure, mainly from fire fighting apparatus and sirens.[38]

The increased use of synthetic materials in building structures and furniture has raised concerns about the hazards of exposures to the combustion products of these materials.[13, 45] Laboratory studies have demonstrated that a variety of toxic substances can be emitted when plastic and other synthetic materials are burned. These include respiratory irritants, carcinogens, and acutely toxic materials such as cyanide. Also, field studies have documented acute and chronic respiratory problems in fire fighters exposed in fires involving large amounts of synthetic materials.[1, 44] However, there is relatively little documentation of the current prevalence of these exposures. Fire fighters may also be exposed to toxic substances in such situations as PCB transformer fires, chemical spills, and pesticide warehouse fires.

PHYSICAL REQUIREMENTS

In addition to toxic exposures, the physical requirements of fire fighting must be assessed in evaluating occupational hazards. Fire fighting activities are strenuous, requiring high aerobic capacity, muscular strength, and endurance.[10, 20, 22, 25] These activities require working at near maximal heart rates for prolonged periods.[5] Heart rates first increase with the fire fighter's initial reaction to an alarm.[5, 18] Tönnes et al.[47] reported a detailed study of physical loads in 15 volunteer fire fighters while carrying hose-boxes in the laboratory. Subjects walked on a treadmill at 4 km/hr, carrying one box that weighed 25 kg in each hand until completely exhausted. Exhaustion of finger and wrist flexors, shown by normalized mean frequency alterations in EMG-recordings, limited average endurance to 3.85 minutes. Compared to values obtained when subjects walked at same rate without any load, average heart rates in carrying rose from 82 beats/min (steady state) to 137 beats/min (non–steady state). Oxygen uptake rose from 22% to 49% of maximum uptake. Local muscular exhaustion was considered the limiting factor in this task rather than cardiorespiratory capacity.

In addition, Tönnes and co-workers measured muscule loading on two firefighters carrying a victim between them without using a stretcher, using a biomechanical model and a force measuring platform (Kistler). (Eleven volunteer subjects were studied.) For reference, isometric maximum strength (MVC) was measured in handgrip, elbow and shoulder flexion, and back extension. During carrying, vertical and horizontal force measurements were made with the force measuring platform under static and dynamic conditions. Appropriate limb angles and lever arms were measured. Torque at the elbow joint was calculated under static conditions for both bearers (mean and SD 45 ± 12 Nm and 40 ± 6 Nm for front and rear bearers, respectively). Shoulder torque (75 ± 33 Nm) and back torque at L5/S1 (119 ± 33 Nm) were determined for the rear bearer who carried the victim's trunk. Longitudinal tension force in forearms of rear bearer (i.e., demands on handgrip strength) was 108 ± 59 Nm. This torque at L5/S1 represents on the average 41% of MVC, limiting endurance to 1–2 min of carrying. Corresponding values for elbow and shoulder flexion of the rear bearer were 22 and 34% of MVC. (See Chapter 19 for discussion of these selected forces.) Heavy protective equipment and respirators and the heat from the fire also contribute to this physical load.[12, 25] This exertion also may increase fire fighters' accumulation of carbon monoxide and other fire contaminants.[15]

PULMONARY DISEASE

As outlined above, a fire fighter may be exposed to a variety of toxic substances which may affect the respiratory system. These include several respiratory irritants commonly found in fires such as acrolein, hydrogen chloride, and nitrogen dioxide. These irritant exposures may lead to acute and chronic respiratory problems. Disability due to pulmonary disease has long been recognized as a potential work-related hazard for fire fighters.

Intense smoke inhalation may lead to a variety of clinical respiratory problems due to injury to the bronchi and alveoli from smoke contaminants and subsequent pulmonary complications.[9] This pulmonary injury may initially be complicated by hypoxemia and cyanide or carbon monoxide intoxication. The clinical presentation varies with the type of fire and with how the fire fighter was exposed. Even asymptomatic fire fighters have been found to have significant pulmonary function changes or hypoxemia after specific fires.[14, 31] Acute episodes of smoke inhalation may also result in significant long-term pulmonary function changes and related disability.[44, 50] Acute respiratory problems have also been reported in fire fighters in incidents involving exposure to isocyanates at a polyurethane foam factory fire and to nitrogen dioxide at a chemical plant spill.[1, 49]

Chronic pulmonary changes have been demonstrated in three studies of fire fighters which have shown a significantly larger decline in pulmonary function in fire fighters than in the general population.[33, 34, 41] In a large study of Boston fire fighters, the rate of loss in pulmonary function was more than twice the expected rate (e.g., 77 ml vs. 37 ml decrease in forced vital capacity over one year).[34] This decline was significantly correlated to the frequency of fire exposures. Differences in age, smoking habits, or ethnic background did not account for these differences. Experienced fire fighters also had a higher prevalence of symptoms of chronic respiratory disease (such as cough and phlegm production) than did new fire fighters of the same age group.[40] However, follow-up studies of this large group of fire fighters three and six years after initial study found essentially normal declines in pulmonary function (mean annual decreases in FEV_1 and FVC of 36 ml and 29 ml, respectively).[29, 30] No changes in pulmonary function were found to be related to indices of fire exposure. However, increased use of respirators and job selection factors which tend to remove symptomatic fire fighters from exposure may account for the lack of significant findings in the follow-up studies. (See Chapter 14 for clinical details.)

CARDIOVASCULAR DISEASE

As outlined above, fire fighters are required to perform much of their work at near maximal heart rates. This strenuous work combined with exposures to a variety of fire contaminants (particularly carbon monoxide) places the fire fighter at increased risk from cardiovascular disease. However, the initial selection criteria for becoming a fire fighter, later selective processes which minimize exposure for symptomatic or ill individuals, and the number of other risk factors for cardiovascular disease make the study of heart disease among fire fighters quite difficult. Increased mortality from cardiovascular disease has been found in two mortality studies focusing on fire fighters, although not in a more recent mortality study of Boston fire fighters.[16, 26, 28] A study of Los Angeles fire fighters found an increased prevalence of ischemic ECG changes during exercise stress testing despite the low prevalence of other risk factors for coronary heart disease.[4] Follow-up coronary angiograms in six of the subjects with abnormal stress tests revealed only two with significant coronary artery obstruction.[3] However, the other four did show other types of cardiac abnormalities. Another recent study found no increased incidence of coronary heart disease among 171 fire fighters followed for ten years as part of a larger medical study.[11] However, the small number of fire fighters being followed, the initial selection procedure for the study, and the loss to follow-up raise questions about the generalizability of these results.

Disability due to cardiovascular disease is quite common among fire fighters. This has led to several efforts to reduce this risk by screening programs, exercise programs, and intervention efforts aimed at other risk factors such as smoking and diet. Some of these programs have been shown to improve physical conditioning and decrease post-alarm heat rate response, to help control other risk factors, and to lower the rate of back injuries.[2, 7, 8, 35, 37]

CANCER

The increased use of synthetic materials in buildings and other structures has raised concerns about the increasing exposure of fire fighters to carcinogens from the burning of these materials. Benzene is commonly found at low levels in fires.[19] Polynuclear aromatic compounds may be released by the burning of a wide variety of materials.[17, 32] Acrylonitrile and other carcinogens may be released by the burning of plastics and other materials. Fire fighters also respond to incidents such as chemical spills where exposures to carcinogenic chemicals may occur.

Unfortunately, there is relatively little information on the cancer risk for fire fighters. Two mortality studies of fire fighters have not shown an increased risk of cancer.[26, 28] However, the deaths in those studies may not reflect the effects of more recent exposures. Several more recent studies have suggested an increased risk of cancer among fire fighters—brain cancer among Washington fire fighters;[27] brain, prostate, colon, and lung cancer among Los Angeles fire fighters;[24] and digestive tract cancer.[6, 46] Further studies are needed to better define these risks.

CONCLUSION

Despite significant improvements in equipment, training, and personal protective equipment, fire fighting is still a very hazardous occupation. The medical risks of this occupation are difficult to study for a variety of reasons, including the wide variability in types and degrees of exposure, changes over time in exposures and in the use of protective equipment, and selection factors in the hiring of fire fighters and in their later job changes. While there is a need for more medical studies of fire fighters, the available exposure and medical information is sufficient to substantiate the presence of an increased risk for cardiovascular and respiratory diseases, for noise-induced hearing loss, and probably for cancer. Medical screening and prevention programs for fire fighters should focus on these diseases. Given the wide variety of exposures, particularly for fire fighters involved in hazardous materials units, documentation of significant acute exposures and appropriate medical follow-up are also needed. Medical programs for treating injuries, burns, smoke inhalation, and other acute medical problems should also be established for each fire department. Meanwhile, efforts to better understand potential exposures and to limit these exposures are needed to provide the fire fighters with as safe a working environment as possible.

REFERENCES

1. Axford A, McKerrow C, Jones A, et al: Accidental exposure to isocyanate fumes in a group of firemen. *Br J Ind Med* 1976; 33:65–71.
2. Barnard RJ, Anthony DF: Effects of health maintenance programs on Los Angeles city fire fighters. *J Occup Med* 1980; 22:667–669.
3. Barnard RJ, Gardner GW, Diaco NV: 'Ischemic' heart disease in fire fighters with normal coronary arteries. *J Occup Med* 1976; 18:818–820.
4. Barnard RJ, Gardner GW, Diaco NV, et al: Near maximal ECG stress testing and coronary artery disease risk factor analysis in Los Angeles city fire fighters. *J Occup Med* 1975; 17:693–695.
5. Barnard RJ, Duncan HW: Heart rate and ECG response of fire fighters. *J Occup Med* 1975; 17:247–250.
6. Borg J, Howell M: Occupational and bowel cancer. *J Toxicol Environ Health* 1975; 1:75–89.
7. Brown A, Cotes JE, Mortimore IL, et al: An exercise training programme for firemen. *Ergonomics* 1982; 25:793–800.
8. Cady LD, Bischoff DP, O'Connell ER, et al: Strength and fitness and subsequent back injuries in fire fighters. *J Occup Med* 1979; 21:269–272.

8a. Cahalane M, Demling RH: Early respiratory abnormalities from smoke inhalation. *JAMA* 1984; 251:771–773.

9. Cohen M, Guzzani L: Inhalation of products of combustion. *Ann Emerg Med* 1983; 12:628–632.
10. Davis PO, Dotson CO, Santa Marie DL: Relationship between simulated fire fighting tasks and physical performance measures. *Med Sci Sports Exercise* 1982; 14:65–71.
11. Dibbs E, Thomas HE, Weiss ST, et al: Fire fighting and coronary heart disease. *Circulation* 1982; 65:943–946.
12. Duncan HW, Gardner GW, Barnard RJ: Physiological responses of men working in fire fighting equipment in the heat. *Ergonomics* 1979; 22:521–527.
13. Dyer R, Esch V: Polyvinyl chloride toxicity in fires—Hydrogen chloride toxicity in fire fighters. *JAMA* 1976; 235:393–397.
14. Genovesi M, Tashkin D, Choipra S, et al: Transient hypoxemia in firemen following inhalation of smoke. *Chest* 1977; 7:441–444.
15. Griggs T: The role of exertion as a determinant of carboxyhemoglobin accumulation in fire fighters. *J Occup Med* 1977; 19:759–761.
16. Gugalnick L: Mortality by occupation and cause of death among men 20–64 years of age. United States 1950 Vital Statistics, Special Reports 53.
17. Hill T, Siedle A, Perry R: Chemical hazards of a fire fighting training environment. *Am Ind Hyg Assoc J* 1972; June, pp 423–430.
18. Hurley BH, Glasser SP, Phelps CP, et al: Cardiovascular and sympathetic reactions to in-flight emergency responses among base fire fighters. *Aviat Space Environ Med* 1980; 51:788–792.
19. International Association of Fire Fighters: *1982 Annual Death and Injury Survey*. Washington, DC, IAFF, 1983.
20. Kilbom Å: Physical work capacity of firemen with special reference to demands during fire fighting. *Scand J Work Environ Health* 1980; 6:48–57.
21. Lake J, Farmer W, Matthay R, et al: Acute and chronic effects of fire fighting on pulmonary function. *Chest* 1980; 77:369–373.
22. Lemon PW, Hermiston RT: The human energy cost of fire fighting. *J Occup Med* 1977; 19:558–562.
23. Levine M, Radford E: Occupational exposures to cyanide in Baltimore fire fighters. *J Occup Med* 1978; 20:53–56.
24. Lewis S, Bierman H, Faith M: Cancer mortality in Los Angeles fire fighters. Proceeding of American Association for Cancer Research, 1983.
25. Manning JE, Griggs TR: Heart rate in fire fighters using light and heavy breathing equipment: Simulated near-maximal exertion in response to multiple work load conditions. *J Occup Med* 1983; 25:215–218.
26. Mastromatteo E: Mortality in city firemen II: A study of mortality in firemen of a city fire department. *AMA Arch Ind Health* 1959; 20:227–233.
27. Milham S: *Occupational Mortality in Washington State 1950–1979*, DHHS (NIOSH) Publ 83-116, 1983.
28. Musk AW, Monson RR, Peters JM, et al: Mortality among Boston fire fighters, 1915–1975. *Br J Ind Med* 1978; 35:104–108.
29. Musk AW, Peters JM, Bernstein L, et al: Pulmonary function in fire fighters: A six year follow-up in the Boston fire department. *Am J Ind Med* 1982; 3:3–9.
30. Musk AW, Peters JM, Wegman DH: Lung function in fire fighters I: A three year follow-up of active subjects. *Am J Public Health* 1977; 67:626–629.
31. Musk AW, Smith TJ, Peters JM, et al: Pulmonary function in fire fighters: Acute changes in ventilatory capacity and their correlates. *Br J Ind Med* 1979; 36:29–34.
32. National Institute for Occupational Safety and Health: Health hazard evaluation report, HETA 84-044-1441. Cincinnati, Oh, NIOSH, 1984.
33. Peabody H: Pulmonary function and the fire fighters. *J Comb Toxicol* 1977; 4:8–15.
34. Peters J, Theriault G, Fine L, et al: Chronic effects of fire fighting on pulmonary function. *N Engl J Med* 1974; 291:1320–1322.
35. Puterbaugh JS, Lawyer CH: Cardiovascular effects of an exercise program: A controlled study among firemen. *J Occup Med* 1983; 25:581–586.
36. Radford E, Levine M: Occupational exposure to carbon monoxide in Baltimore fire fighters. *J Occup Med* 1976; 18:628–632.
37. Reid EL, Morgan RW: Exercise prescription: A clinical trial. *Am J Pub Health* 1979; 69:591–595.
38. Reischl U, Bair H, Reischl P: Fire fighter noise exposure. *Am Ind Hyg Assoc J* 1979; 40:482–489.

39. Sammons J, Coleman R: Fire fighter's occupational exposure to carbon monoxide. *J Occup Med* 1974; 16:543–546.
40. Sidor R, Peters J: Prevalence rates of chronic non-specific respiratory disease in fire fighters. *Am Rev Respir Dis* 1974; 109:255–261.
41. Sparrow D, Bossé R, Rosner B, et al: The effect of occupational exposure on pulmonary function—A longitudinal evaluation of fire fighters and non-fire fighters. *Am Rev Respir Dis* 1982; 125:319–322.
42. Stewart RD, Stewart RC, Stamm W, et al: Rapid estimation of carboxyhemoglobin level in fire fighters. *JAMA* 1976; 235:390–392.
43. Takano T, Maeda H: Exposure of fire fighters to carbon monoxide. *J Comb Toxicol* 1981; 8:89–95.
44. Tashkin D, Genovesi M, Chopra S, et al: Respiratory status of Los Angeles firemen—One month follow-up after inhalation of dense smoke. *Chest* 1977; 71:445–449.
45. Terrill J, Montgomery R, Reinhart C: Toxic gases from fires. *Science* 1978; 200:1343–1347.
46. Therriault G: Vital records as a data source for environmental and occupational health studies. Proceedings from Environmental Epidemiology Meeting, Association of State and Territorial Epidemiologists, October 1983.
47. Tönnes M, Behm M, Kilbom Å: Demands on the muscular strength and endurance in two heavy carrying tasks of fire fighters. *Arbete Och Hälsa* 1986; 24.
48. Treitman R, Burgess WA, Gold A: Air contaminants encountered by fire fighters. *Am Ind Hyg Assoc J* 1980; 41:796–802.
49. Tse R, Bockman A: Nitrogen dioxide toxicity report of four cases in firemen. *JAMA* 1970; 212:1341–1344.
50. Unger K, Snow R, Mestas J, et al: Smoke inhalation in firemen. *Thorax* 1980; 35:838–842.
51. Washburn A, Harlow D, Fahy R: US Fire fighter deaths—1981. *Fire Service Today*, 1982; May, pp 12–22.

63

Occupational Health Aspects of Plastics, Rubber Manufacturing, and Related Materials

Louis S. Beliczky, M.S., M.P.H.

Carl Zenz, M.D.

Chemicals and materials used and manufactured in the rubber and plastics industries constitute an incredible array: alcohols, antioxidants, ketones, isocyanates, plasticizers, and certain solvents, including carbon disulfide, chlorinated hydrocarbons, certain petroleum distillates, polyester, vinyl chloride, polyvinyl resins, and styrene are some of the most important. A few typical, widely used, and most hazardous materials are described in this chapter.

A 1980 publication by the United States Environmental Protection Agency (EPA) lists 50 chemicals produced annually in the United States in excess of 1 billion pounds (Table 63–1). Thirty-one of these are organic monomers (chiefly solvents) for plastics and rubber, or intermediates. These figures are based on production data reported in the United States. For other countries, worldwide production of these chemicals could apply to a vast work population with potential risks for exposure at various points in the production processes, and also apply to production of diversified consumer and industrial goods.

Alcohols used in the manufacture of rubber are primarily amyl, butyl, ethyl, isopropyl, and methyl. Acetates commonly in use are butyl, isoamyl, ethyl, methyl, isopropyl, and propyl. The alcohols and acetates used as solvents have similar actions and are recognized as upper respiratory irritants. To some degree, all are irritating to the eyes and, with prolonged concentrated exposures, may cause narcosis.

ORGANIC SOLVENTS

In discussing organic solvents as a class of substances used in the working environment (Fig 63–1), one toxic effect common to all solvents but seldom discussed as a toxic effect is that caused by the property of "dissolving." Although there is a nearly infinite number of substances and their combinations dissolved by solvents, the components of the skin generally are not included. With the exception of the keratolytic agents used for medicinal purposes or those industrial solvents that are overtly corrosive irritants, acids, alkalis, reducers, or oxidizers, little attention is directed to the prevention of skin injury due to defatting of the skin by solvents used in the occupations.

The defatting of the skin breaks down the barriers to the absorption of substances through the intact stratum granulosum and stratum lucidum and leads to contact dermatitis, infection, and epidermal sensitization. This is likely due to the extraction of hydrophilic material from the skin that is necessary to retain water moisture and improve the resistance to absorption.

Chronic eczematous dermatosis often follows the acute eczematous dermatitis in those patients who fail to improve. Dry, fissured, chronic dermatitis frequently is the result of reckless contact with solvents of this nature.

Further dermatologic phenomena are presented in greater detail in Chapter 10.

Because of the volatility of most solvents, coupled with the ease and rapidity of respiratory uptake, the greatest health hazards are associated with chronic exposures and the resulting central nervous system dysfunctions (see Chapters 48, 49, 50). Selected major references are listed; those especially pertinent are noted here.[78, 81, 86]

HALOGENATED HYDROCARBONS

Even though the grouping of chemical substances according to atomic components and their structural arrangement must be arbitrary, particularly when a correlation of biologic effects must

TABLE 63–1.
Production of Top 50 Chemicals*

1. Sulfuric acid (100 × 10^6)	26. Ethylene oxide
2. Lime	27. Carbon dioxide
3. Oxygen	28. Ethylene glycol
4. Ammonia	29. Ammonium sulfate
5. Nitrogen	30. Butadiene
6. Ethylene	31. P-xylene
7. Chlorine	32. Carbon black
8. Sodium hydroxide	33. Cumene
9. Phosphoric acid	34. Acetic acid
10. Nitric acid	35. Phenol
11. Sodium carbonate	36. Sodium sulfate
12. Ammonium nitrate	37. Calcium chloride
13. Propylene	38. Aluminum sulfate
14. Benzene	39. Cyclohexane
15. Urea	40. Acetone
16. Ethylene dichloride	41. Propylene oxide
17. Toluene	42. Acrylonitrile
18. Ethyl benzene	43. Isopropyl alcohol
19. Vinyl chloride	44. Adipic acid
20. Styrene	45. Vinyl acetate
21. Formaldehyde	46. Sodium silicate
22. Methanol	47. Acetic anhydride
23. Xylenes (mixed–mainly meta)	48. Sodium tripolyphos
24. Terephthalic acid	49. Titanium dioxide
25. Hydrochloric acid	50. Ethanol (1 × 10^6)

*In order by production volume, approximately 100 × 10^6 for sulfuric acid to 1 × 10^6 for ethanol.

also be considered, certain halogenated alkyl compounds have similar characteristics. One group includes the dichloro, trichloro, and tetrachloro methanes, ethanes, ethylenes, and propane. Another group, the chlorobenzenes, has importance, as has epichlorhydrin. However, for these solvents, the group is made up principally of chlorinated aliphatic compounds. Of these, the principal economically important members are closely related. The group is essentially made up of chloroform, carbon tetrachloride, ethylene dichloride, tetrachlorethane, trichloroethylene, methylene chloride, dichloropropane, tetrachloroethylene, methylchloride, isopropyl chloride, chlorobenzene, o-dichlorobenzene, and trichloroethane.

Trichloroethylene

Trichloroethylene probably is the most widely used of the halogenated hydrocarbon solvents. The National Institute for Occupational Safety and Health (NIOSH) estimates 300,000 workers in the United States are routinely exposed to trichloroethylene in their work.[2] These exposures are due, by far, to its use as a degreasing agent in metal-fabricating operations. It is used also in organic chemical processing and production and for vermin extermination.[2] It was first used commercially in the United States in 1935, which was 25 years after its introduction and use in Europe. It has been used as a general anesthetic since early in the 1930s and claims have been made about the safety and hazards of its use as an anesthetic.[7] Chemical exposures to nonindustrial workers, such as those in clinics and hospitals, often are overlooked.

Trichloroethylene is a chlorinated unsaturated hydrocarbon, $CHCl{:}CCl_2$, with a vapor pressure at 25° C of 0.1 part per 100 parts of water and a vapor density of 4.5. At ambient temperatures it is completely miscible with alcohols, ethers, and many other organic solvents. It is a clear, colorless, noncorrosive liquid with a sweet odor and is generally inert for most of the processes in which it is used.

Occupational Exposures.—Approximately 90% of trichloroethylene produced is used as a solvent in degreasing operations. It may be used in varying quantities such as in a "bucket" operation, in which the solvent is used to clean parts and tools, or in large quantities such as in major sophisticated operations in assembly lines that are well controlled against loss. The remaining 10% is used in dry cleaning operations for fabrics and in extractive processes. Consequently, the major—and possibly the only—occupationally important route of exposure to trichloroethylene has been through inhalation and absorption through the lung. Although no reports have been found of occupational intoxication via absorption of trichloroethylene through the skin, one report[7] has suggested that absorption of any trichloroethylene through the skin would be inconsequential as a source of toxic amounts in the body. However, first-degree chemical burns of the eyes as a result of hot vapors arising from a degreasing tank were reported.[85]

Toxicity.—The major occupational health problems from the exposure to trichloroethylene are the results of its depressant action on the central nervous system (CNS). Although the presence of the chlorine atoms in the molecule would suggest an effect on the liver similar to that produced by chloroform on carbon tetrachloride, this has not been the case. Reports of liver damage have been associated with massive doses at or near lethal quantities that were absorbed from accidental ingestion or by massive inhalation.[43] Suspected liver damage from exposure to high concentrations of inhaled trichloroethylene has been associated with alcohol abuse or with contaminants, such as 1,2-dichloropropane and 1,2-dichloroethane. However, liver damage from lethal concentrations has been reported where these contaminants were not contributing factors.[4, 38, 39, 85]

Other studies of workers with high, nonlethal exposures to trichloroethylene revealed some evidence of liver damage as demonstrated by hyperglobulinemia, hypercalcemia, abnormality of cephalin flocculation, and total lipids and unsaturated fatty acids. However, many studies have been reported in which no liver effects were found in workers regularly exposed in degreasing operations.[7] It can be concluded that trichloroethylene essentially has a low order of toxic effect against the liver. Such a conclusion can be supported by numerous studies of the effects of relatively large exposures on experimental animals. Rabbits were exposed for periods of time ranging up to 8 months in duration at a concentration of 6,900 ppm for a 4-hour exposure daily. Mice exposed to 1,600 ppm for 4 hours daily for as long as 24 hours a week for 8 weeks were found to have a slight degeneration of the liver. Guinea pigs exposed for more that 1,100 hours to levels of 1,200 ppm showed no significant changes in the lungs, spleen, heart, adrenals, or brain but showed some minor degenerative changes in the liver.

The most commonly reported effects caused by trichloroethylene have been those of CNS origin. The predominant signs and

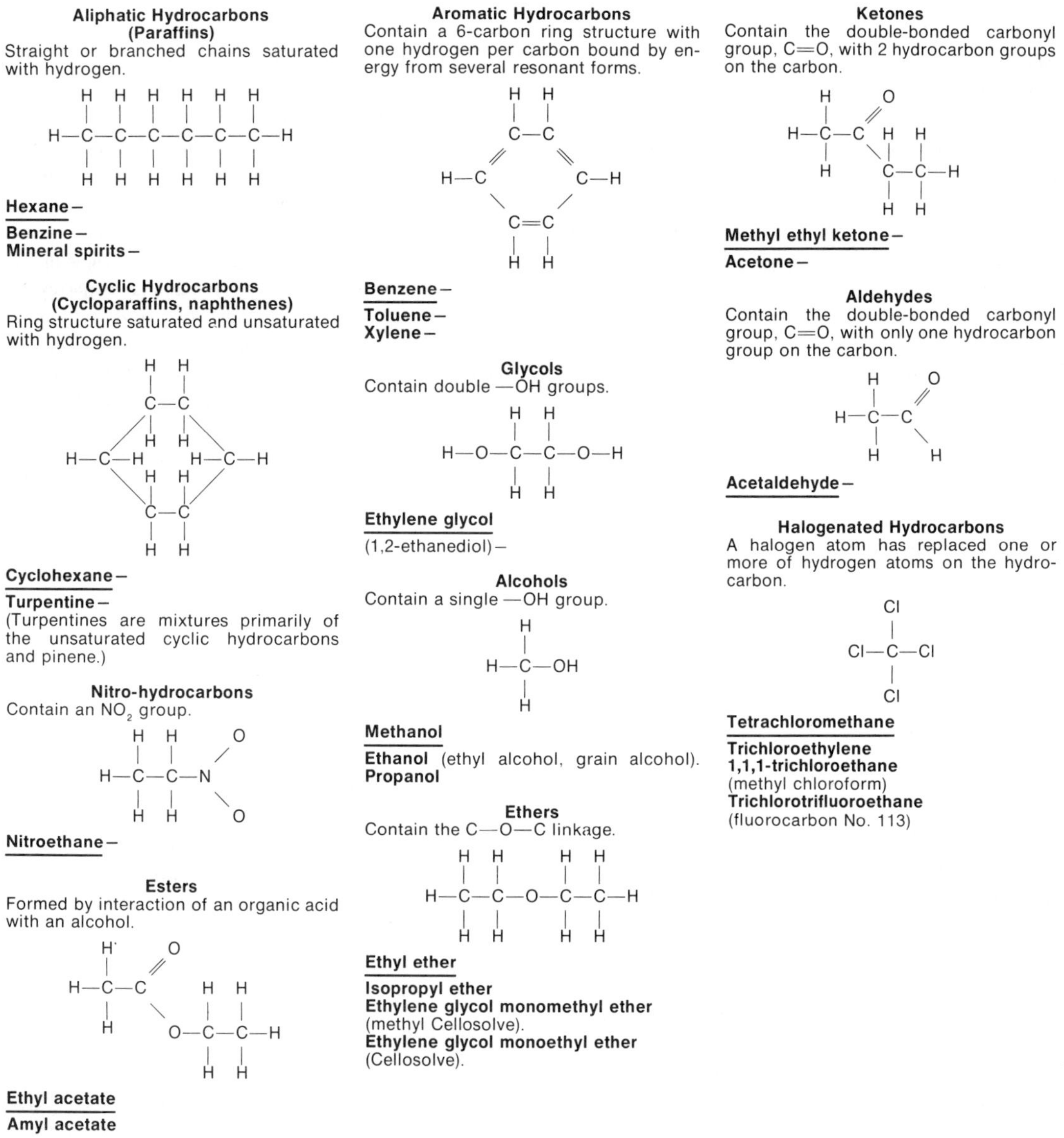

Aliphatic Hydrocarbons (Paraffins)
Straight or branched chains saturated with hydrogen.

Hexane–
Benzine–
Mineral spirits–

Cyclic Hydrocarbons (Cycloparaffins, naphthenes)
Ring structure saturated and unsaturated with hydrogen.

Cyclohexane–
Turpentine–
(Turpentines are mixtures primarily of the unsaturated cyclic hydrocarbons and pinene.)

Nitro-hydrocarbons
Contain an NO_2 group.

Nitroethane–

Esters
Formed by interaction of an organic acid with an alcohol.

Ethyl acetate
Amyl acetate

Aromatic Hydrocarbons
Contain a 6-carbon ring structure with one hydrogen per carbon bound by energy from several resonant forms.

Benzene–
Toluene–
Xylene–

Glycols
Contain double —OH groups.

Ethylene glycol
(1,2-ethanediol)–

Alcohols
Contain a single —OH group.

Methanol
Ethanol (ethyl alcohol, grain alcohol).
Propanol

Ethers
Contain the C—O—C linkage.

Ethyl ether
Isopropyl ether
Ethylene glycol monomethyl ether
(methyl Cellosolve).
Ethylene glycol monoethyl ether
(Cellosolve).

Ketones
Contain the double-bonded carbonyl group, C=O, with 2 hydrocarbon groups on the carbon.

Methyl ethyl ketone–
Acetone–

Aldehydes
Contain the double-bonded carbonyl group, C=O, with only one hydrocarbon group on the carbon.

Acetaldehyde–

Halogenated Hydrocarbons
A halogen atom has replaced one or more of hydrogen atoms on the hydrocarbon.

Tetrachloromethane
Trichloroethylene
1,1,1-trichloroethane
(methyl chloroform)
Trichlorotrifluoroethane
(fluorocarbon No. 113)

FIG 63–1.
Major classes of common organic solvents, with some typical examples. (Modified from Olishifski J (ed): *Fundamentals of Industrial Hygiene.* Chicago, National Safety Council, 1979.)

symptoms were headache, dizziness, vertigo, tremors, nausea, vomiting, fatigue, symptoms similar to alcoholic intoxication, and unconsciousness preceding death.

These CNS effects can be the result of either an immediate acute toxic exposure or a longer-term exposure of lesser concentration.

Death has resulted from progressive paralysis resulting from and following 20 hours of inhalation exposure,[4] but the usual cause of death appears to be cardiovascular failure, which can occur during exposure or shortly after.[38, 39] Of course, death can occur from massive acutely inhaled anesthetic concentrations or from ingestion causing an immediate depression of the CNS. Andersson[2] reported that 77 of 104 trichloroethylene workers showed abnormal electrocardiographic tracings, which may precede permanent heart damage.

The mechanism of this action is not understood. Lilis et al.[43] suggested that epinephrine secretion during periods of physical exertion or stress associated with hypersympathicotonia could explain such a sudden death association with trichloroethylene exposure. Trichloroethylene is converted to trichloroethanol, free and conjugated with glucuronic acid, and concluded that the initial conversion of trichloroethylene was to chloral hydrate. Trichloroacetic acid and monochloroacetic acid and trichloroethanol are found in the urine as well.

Two effects associated with exposure to trichloroethylene must be considered in the occupational environment. Although not caused directly by trichloroethylene, they cannot be ignored as a hazard to the health of the worker. The first is that common to most chlorinated alkyls—the formation of phosgene and hydrogen chloride by decomposition in the presence of hot metals, open flames, ultraviolet radiation—all of which may occur in welding operations.[69] The second is the formation of dichloroacetylene by the reaction of trichloroethylene with alkalis, such as those that may be found in rebreathing canisters of respiratory equipment.[5] In addition to the explosive potential of the dichloroacetylene formed, there is a toxic effect—that of trigeminal palsy, long associated with the use of trichloroethylene as an anesthetic. (See Chapters 48, 49, and 50 for discussion of chronic effects.)

Medical and Hygienic Controls.—NIOSH recommended that the occupational exposure to trichloroethylene shall be controlled so that workers will not be exposed to trichloroethylene at a concentration in excess of 50 ppm determined as a time-weighted average exposure for an 8-hour workday, as measured by a minimal sampling time of 10 minutes. Further, no worker shall be exposed to a peak concentration of trichloroethylene in excess of 150 ppm, as measured by a maximal sampling time of 10 minutes.

Methylene Chloride (Dichloromethane, CH_2Cl_2)

Methylene chloride, although perhaps not the most hazardous chlorinated hydrocarbon, is unique in this series of solvents. NIOSH estimates that nearly 100,000 workers are exposed to methylene dichloride and that number does not include hobbyists. Methylene chloride is used industrially as a paint stripper, a degreasing solvent, an aerosol propellant, a solvent in the textile, plastic, and paint industries, in the manufacture of photographic film, and in the preparation of heat-sensitive oils and waxes. At least 500 million pounds are used annually in the United States. It has been used as a general anesthetic.

Methylene chloride is a clear, colorless liquid with a sweet, pleasant odor and is inert under the conditions in which it is commonly used.

Occupational Exposures.—Because methylene chloride volatilizes very rapidly, its use capitalizes on this property. Thus, its use as a solvent for degreasing, paints, and paint stripping most likely causes exposure by inhalation. Of lesser occupational health importance is the absorption of the substance through the skin. Absorption through the skin, however, can occur only when methylene chloride is in direct contact with the skin. Therefore, protective equipment should be used to prevent this contact. No report of intoxication from methylene chloride absorption through the skin was found, however.

Toxicity.—As with other halogenated solvents, the principal hazardous effect is the depressant action on the CNS. The range of effects can extend from a decreased performance in psychomotor testing to narcosis and death of the individuals exposed. Although there is experimental evidence that methylene chloride produces the characteristic effects on the liver and kidney reported for other chlorinated alkyl compounds, no reports were found of liver and kidney injury to humans from occupational exposure. Irritation to the respiratory passages and eyes has been reported in humans and experimental animals from exposure to the vapor. Equivocal findings suggesting that effects similar to those caused by phosgene were reported for methylene chloride, which may have been changed by a nearby kerosene flame.[21, 31]

Within the past few years, an additional unique effect was reported in which it was ascertained that methylene chloride is rapidly metabolized to carbon monoxide.[68, 71] The amount of conversion to carbon monoxide is significant when measured by the concentration of carboxyhemoglobin, which was up to 12% measured in the blood following occupational exposure of up to 610 ppm methylene chloride. Under conditions of poor ventilation, such as insufficient air movement in a home garage, basement, or small workplace, concentrations of methylene chloride vapors can quickly accumulate and be readily inspired. Stewart and Hake[75] have shown that the use of such paint remover for a period of 3 hours can easily produce carboxyhemoglobin saturation of 5% to 10% in man.

Exposure Limits.—The ACGIH (1986) threshold limit value (TLV) is 100 ppm, the STEL (500 ppm). As the National Toxicology Program (NTP) has reported (1985), it is a suspect carcinogen, based on animal studies. NIOSH recommends the exposure limit of 75 ppm.

AROMATIC HYDROCARBONS

The aromatic hydrocarbons, such as benzene, xylene, and toluene are excellent solvents and are used extensively in the production of plastic and rubber products. These products are described later in this chapter.

KETONES

Typically, ketones include acetone (dimethyl ketone), methyl ethyl ketone (butanone) (MEK), methyl amyl ketone, and methyl isobutyl ketone. They are not especially toxic, but they do have a known narcotic action during high concentrations with prolonged exposure. Environmental concentrations must not exceed the TLVs shown in Table 63–2. As emphasized elsewhere, skin contact must be avoided because of rapid defatting action, often leading to dermatitis. Proper control of workplace exposures depends on adequate ventilation to prevent unnecessary inhalation and to minimize skin contact. Control relies on workplace atmospheric sampling to determine concentrations encountered. Blood cell counts, including differentials, cannot be relied on as an indicator of worker exposure control. Abnormal blood findings, when demonstrated, may be too late to be of value in the consideration of health protection for the worker.

The TLV for MEK is 200 ppm. Local exhaust ventilation should be used to maintain concentrations in the air below the TLV. Contact with the skin and eyes should be avoided by the use of appropriate protective clothing and eye protection. In case of

TABLE 63–2.
Typical Substances Used in Plastics and Rubber Industries*

SUBSTANCE	PPM OF AIR	MG/M^3
Acetone	1,000	2,400
Acrylonitrile	2	4.5
Amyl acetate	100	525
Amyl (iso) alcohol	100	360
Benzene	10	30
Butadiene 1, 3	10	22
Butyl acetate	200	950
Butyl alcohol	50	150
Carbon tetrachloride	5	30
Ethyl acetate	400	1,400
Ethyl alcohol	1,000	1,900
Ethylene dichloride	10	40
Gasoline	300	900
Heptane	400	1,600
Hexane	50	180
Propyl (iso) alcohol	200	500
Methyl alcohol	200	260
Methyl ethyl ketone	200	590
Methyl isocyanate	0.02	0.05
Perchlorethylene (tetrachlorethylene)	50	335
Propyl acetate	200	840
Stoddard solvent	100	575
Styrene	50	215
Toluene	100	375
Toluene diisocyanate	0.005	0.04
Trichloroethylene	50	270
Xylene	100	435
Vinyl chloride	5	10

*Based on ACGIH threshold limit values for substances in workroom air, 1986–1987 (see appendix A). Also modified from Axelson O: Solvents and the liver. *Eur J Clin Invest* 1983; 13:109; Tobia AJ, Miller CH Jr, Couri D: Aspects of solvent toxicity in mixtures, in Proceedings of the Fourteenth Conference on Environmental Toxicology, Dayton, Ohio, November 1983; and *Toxicity and Safe Handling of Rubber Chemicals 1985: Code of Practice*, ed 2. Birmingham, UK, British Rubber Manufacturers' Association, 1985

spills, persons exposed to MEK should have respiratory protection. The skin should be thoroughly washed with water after contact with MEK.

OTHER MAJOR SUBSTANCES

Reviews on the potential health hazards of filling materials compounded with plastics and rubber have been published. Fiberglass, calcium sulfate, calcium carbonate, titanium oxide, and asbestos are commonly used as fillers. Dusts of varying particulate size are generated from finishing operations, such as sawing, drilling, and grinding. Also, localized heat from these mechanical actions can form break-down products, some of which are potentially irritating and toxic in action.[82] (Further discussion is found in Chapter 67 on fibrous glass and Chapter 64 on pyrolysis products.)

Polyester resins are polymeric substances, having ester groups in chains

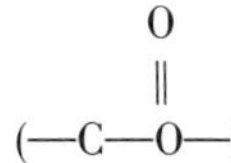

with catalyzers, and harden or cure at room temperature. Commercial products are alkyds used in paints and enamels, and unsaturated polyesters or unsaturated alkyds are used with fiberglass for some boat hulls, wall panels, and films.

POLYVINYL RESINS

Polyvinyl resins generally include polymers derived from monomers having a structure

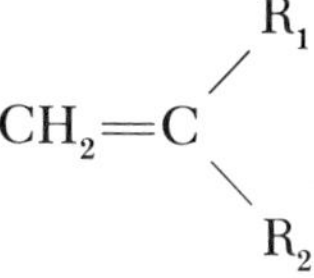

R_1 and R_2 represent hydrogen, alkyl, halogen, or other groups. Some of the polymers, such as polyvinyl chloride, polyvinyl acetate, polyvinyl acetals, polyvinyl alcohol, polyvinyl ethers, and polyvinylidene chloride, have been used for many years. Others are polyvinyl fluoride, polyvinyl pyrrolidone, and polyvinyl carbazole. These monomers are prepared by the addition of an appropriate compound combined with acetylene. Reactions of acetylene with HCl, HF and CH_3OOH are used to form vinyl chloride, vinyl fluoride, vinyl acetate, and vinyl methyl ether. Polyvinyl acetates are used in adhesives, coatings for paper, and in the leather and textile industries.

World production of vinyl chloride in 1984 was more than 15 billion kg, with U.S. production about 25% of that amount. In 1973, the EPA estimated that as much as 90 million kg escaped into the atmosphere in the U.S. per year. Polyvinyl chloride (PVC) is an exceedingly widely used material.

Polyvinyl chloride may be blended with fillers and pigments, stabilizers, and other materials, such as plasticizers, which then may be made into sheets or extruded into various shapes. These include insulation for cables and wires, packaging, tubing, pipefittings, as well as phonograph record blanks, tape cassettes, house siding, gutters and drainspouts, garden hose, furniture, upholstery, mats and tops for automobiles, footwear, raincoats, films, sheets, bottles, tools, medical equipment, etc., including acrylic resins, butadiene, styrene copolymer, polypropylene, and others. Vinyl chloride polymerized with other vinyl monomers generally carried out in closed systems is used to produce blends or alloys of PVC to form rubbery materials intended for applications in panels, other covers, including floors, and pipes with high-impact resistance. Films of polyvinylidene chloride and the copolymer containing about 15% vinyl chloride are considered resistant to moisture and many gases and have the property of being heat sealable and shrinking on heating. Many floor products are coated with this tough and resistant cover. Vinyl chloride is present in many aerosol consumer products as a propellant, especially in certain pesticides and hair sprays.

Polyvinyl ethers, soluble in organic solvents, are used in some adhesives. Vinyl stearate, a waxy material, is used for treating leather and in wax formulations (Figs 63–2 through 63–4).

Manufacturing Processes and Toxicologic Factors of Polyvinyl Chloride

Polyvinyl chloride resin is formed from the vinyl chloride (VC), a colorless gas, monomer by addition polymerization (simple addition of monomer molecules without loss of atoms from the original molecule):

$$\begin{array}{ccc} \begin{array}{cc} H & H \\ | & | \\ C & = C \\ | & | \\ H & Cl \end{array} & \xrightarrow{\text{initiators}} & \begin{array}{ccccccccc} & H & & H & & H & & H & \\ & | & & | & & | & & | & \\ - & C & - & C & - & C & - & C & - \\ & | & & | & & | & & | & \\ & H & & Cl & & H & & Cl & \end{array} \\ \text{Vinyl chloride} & & \text{Polyvinyl chloride} \end{array}$$

Vinyl chloride:
m.p. = 160°C
b.p. = 13.9°C
v.p. = 760 mm Hg (13.8°C)
vapor density = 2.15
flash point = 78°C
TLV = 5 ppm (1986)

Manufacture of VC Monomer

$HgCl_2$–catalyst; metallic mercury (reduced from $HgCl_2$ in acetylene process).

Acetylene (colorless gas, sp.gr. = 0.91, highly flammable; relatively nontoxic).

Phosphine ([impurity in acetylene]; CNS depressant and lung irritant; no evidence of cumulative effects); TLV 0.3 ppm.

Ethylene–density = 0.97; colorless gas. (Asphyxiant displacing content of air; low order of systemic toxicity.)

1,2 Dichloroethane–intermediate; clear colorless liquid; TLV 100 ppm. Skin and eye irritant; acute poisoning by inhalation has resulted in liver and kidney damage. Liver damage is more permanent and assessed by increased liver weights, changes in liver function tests and fatty liver changes in animals.

Cl_2–an intermediate; density (gas) 32; TLV 1 ppm. Mucous membrane and respiratory tract irritant; chronic effects primarily on respiratory system (bronchitis, possibly decreased pulmonary function).

HCl–an intermediate; TLV 5 ppm (corrosive; vapors are irritants to entire respiratory tract).

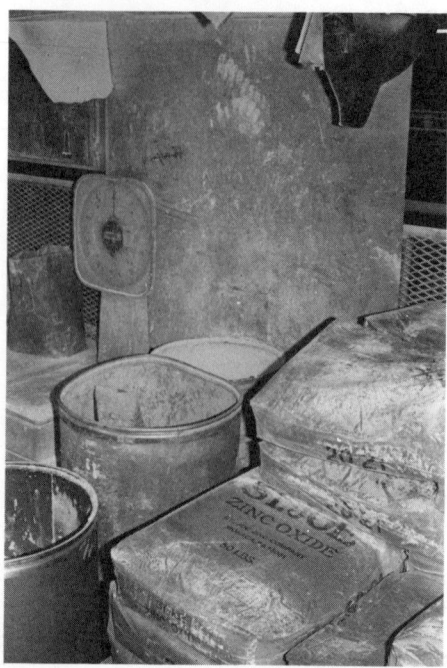

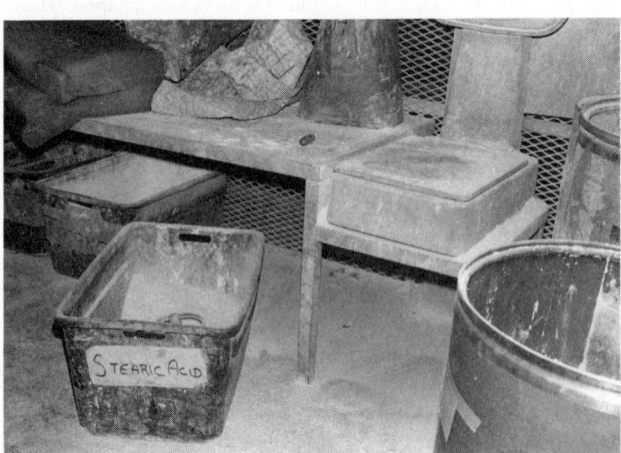

FIG 63–2.
Note the heavy use of stearic acid as a lubricant in rubber manufacturing.

FIG 63–3.
Use of zinc oxide in rubber formulations.

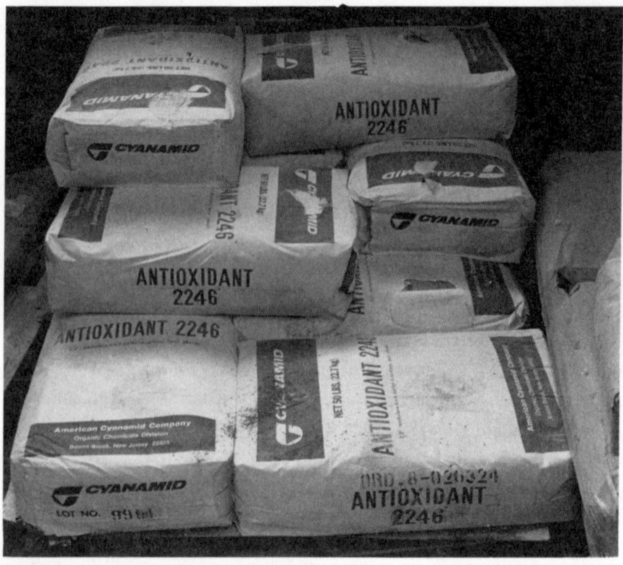

FIG 63–4.
Various antioxidants used in plastic and rubber production.

Vinyl Chloride Polymerization

The starting point of PVC resin may be either VC monomer or production of the VC monomer from either acetylene and/or ethylene (Fig 63–5).

1. Acetylene process: $CH = CH + HCl \xrightarrow{HgCl_2} CH_2 = CClH$
   (acetylene)

2. Ethylene process: $CH_2 = CH_2 + Cl_2 \rightarrow CH_2Cl - CH_2Cl$ pyrolysis $\rightarrow CH_2 = CHCl + HCl$ (1,2 dichloroethane)
   (ethylene)

3. Combination methods to utilize HCl for:
   (a) $CH_2 = CH_2 + CH = CH + Cl_2 \rightarrow 2CH_2 = CHCl$
   (ethylene) (acetylene) (VC)
   (b) $CH_2 = CH_2 + 2HCl + 1/2O_2 \rightarrow CH_2Cl - CH_2Cl + H_2 \rightarrow CH_2 = CHCl$
   (1,2 dichloroethane)

There are four major types of polymerization of VC to PVC.

1. Suspension (pearl, bead, granular) polymerization is used in the majority of general-purpose PVC manufacturing processes for the production of general-purpose resins. The VC monomer plus water is agitated to form tiny droplets, which are stabilized by "suspending agents" mixed in the water phase before agitation and introduction of monomer. VC-soluble initiating agents are added to the monomer to polymerize PVC. The compounds involved include the following: Vinyl chloride and initiating agents (lauryl peroxide, isopropyl peroxydicarbonate [IPP] [dissolved in hexane], azobisisobutyronitrile, diethylperoxydicarbonate–produced by adding ethyl chloroformate [VC phase], H_2O_2 + NaHCO [H_2O phase] and benzoyl peroxide). Suspending agents (protective colloid): gelatin, polyvinyl alcohol, and methyl cellulose. Other chemical additives: inorganic salts, buffers, and surface-active agents (Fig 63–6).

2. Bulk polymerization is carried out in the fluid monomer; no water or suspending agent is used. The monomer and initiating agent are liquefied under high pressure. After about 70% polymerization has taken place, additional monomer and initiator are added and the reaction allowed to go to 70%–85% polymerization. Thereupon, the remaining monomer is recycled and the polymer resin is pneumatically conveyed to the finishing operation for screening and storage. PVC resin produced by this process is free from polymerization residue, with excellent clarity and fusion characteristics. This resin is especially suited for blown bottles, clear films, rigid pipe, and fluidized bed coatings. The initiating compounds are the same as in suspension polymers.

3. Emulsion polymerization is used to produce fine particle size dispersion resin of about 1 μ. The monomer is emulsified in water by a surfactant (soap) and polymerized with a water-soluble initiator to form a polymer latex. The latex is degassed and then dried. The chemical compounds are monomer–VC, surfactant–0.2%–0.5%. Initiator (water soluble): potassium persulfate.

4. Solution polymerization is bulk polymerization with the

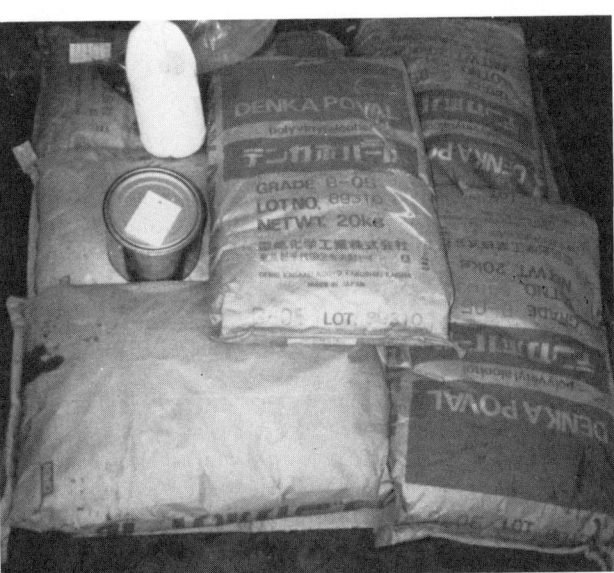

FIG 63–5.
Another lot of additives, including polyvinyl alcohol (of Japanese origin) and finely divided cobalt metal powder for special coatings.

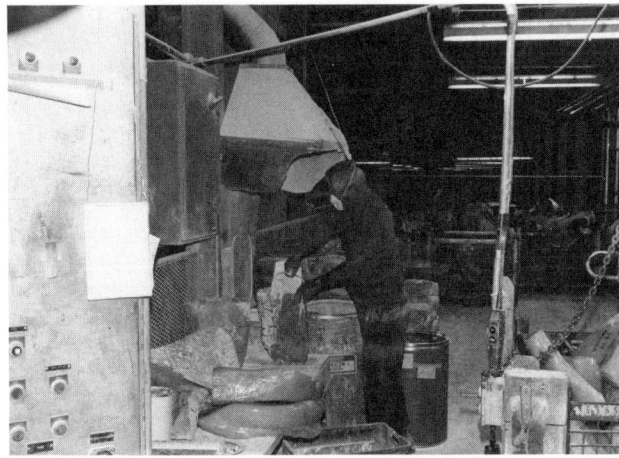

FIG 63–6.
A worker using the materials previously shown in Figures 63–2 and 63–3 for mixing to produce a special grade of adhesive or rubber.

monomer dissolved in a solvent. This process produces resins of good clarity and purity useful in the manufacture of fibers and is used to produce high-quality copolymers (e.g., vinyl chloride-vinyl acetate). The chemicals used include the following: monomer, initiators (monomer soluble)—same as for suspension polymerization—and solvents (benzene, cyclohexane, *n*-butane, chlorinated aliphatics).

Copolymers of VC with vinyl acetate, vinylidene chloride, maleic esters, vinyl ethers, and propylene are most commonly made with suspension and solution polymerization.

A summary of some properties of chemicals used in PVC production is as follows.

Initiating agents. Monomer-soluble lauryl peroxide (C_{11}, $H_{23}CO)_2O_2$, a white, coarse powder, is highly toxic by ingestion and inhalation and is a strong skin irritant and an oxidizing material.

Benzoyl peroxide $(C_6H_5CO)_2O_2$, a white granular crystalline solid, is moderately toxic and relatively safe when mixed with 25%–33% water.

Aminoethanols. 2-*N*-alkyl-substituted aminoethanols are widely used as curing agents, flotation agents, dispersants, and emulsifiers.

Organic Peroxides

Some typical and widely used examples are: benzoyl peroxide, cyclohexanone peroxide, dicumyl peroxide, and methyl ethyl ketone peroxide.

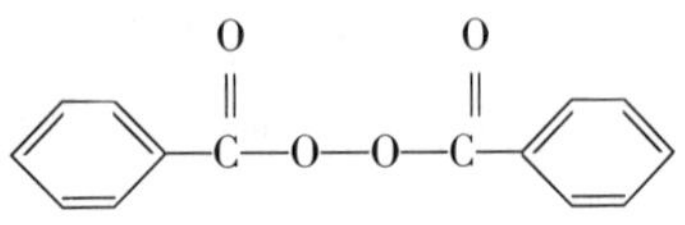

Benzoyl peroxide (dibenzoyl peroxide)

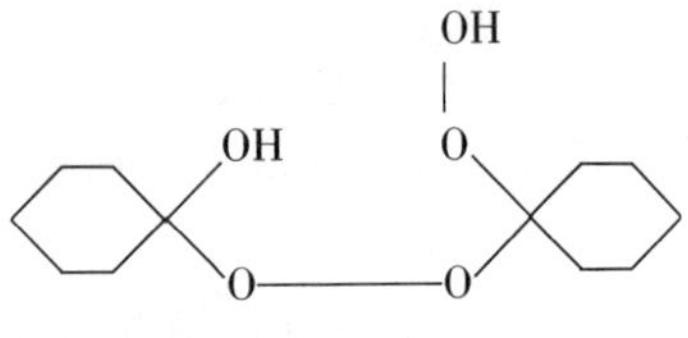

Cyclohexanone peroxide

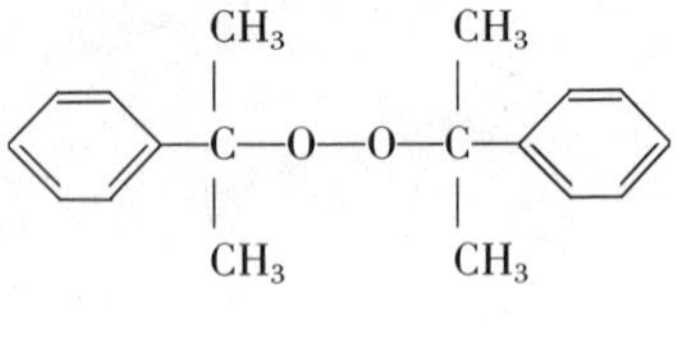

Dicumyl peroxide

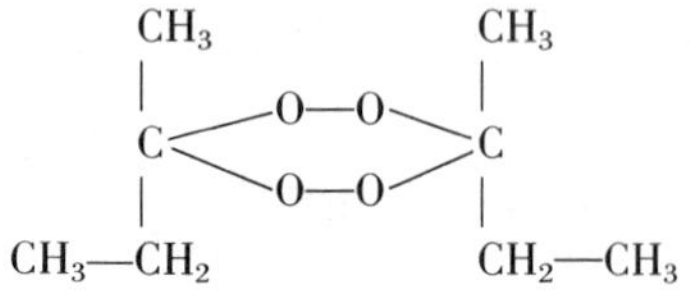

Methyl ethyl ketone peroxide

Most organic peroxides are highly reactive and powerful oxidants, characteristics that make them especially useful as catalysts in plastics and rubber polymerization. Occupational exposures are uncommon because of stringent work practices necessary, since these compounds are highly flammable and explosive. All are irritating to the skin and mucous membranes and benzoyl peroxide is allergenic (see Chapters 10, 16, and 47).

Sodium peroxide (Na_2O_2) is a yellowish white powder (highly toxic by ingestion; strong oxidizing agent).

Ethylchloroformate ($ClCOOC_2H_5$) is a colorless liquid (highly toxic; strong eye and skin irritant; chronic and acute systemic effects not known).

Azobisisobutyronitrile $(CH_3)C(CN)NNC(CN)(CH_3)_2$ is a white powder; may be toxic by ingestion; nitrile group suggests toxicity similar to other nitriles (e.g., acrylonitrile) and cyanides.

Water-soluble initiating agent. Potassium persulfate ($K_2S_2O_8$), consists of white crystals; decomposes at <100° C (liberates sulfur oxides), moderately toxic, strong irritant and oxidizing agent.

Suspending agents. Polyvinyl alcohol $(-CH_2CHOH-)_x$ is a white to creamcolored powder; low toxicity; possible carcinogen (fibrosarcomas when embedded in abdominal wall of animals).

Methyl cellulose is a grayish white, fibrous powder (nontoxic).

Solvents. Benzene (C_6H_6); TLV 10 ppm; strong irritant; anesthetic; toxic to blood-forming tissues (anemia, leukopenia, macrocytosis, reticulocytosis, thrombocytopenia, increased bleeding time; leukemia). (See section on aromatic hydrocarbons.)

Cyclohexane (C_6H_{12}); TLV 300 ppm (skin irritant, anesthetic).

n-Butane ($CH_3CH_2CH_2CH_3$) is a colorless gas (slight to moderate systemic effects from inhalation).

This is a partial list, since there are more than 227 monomers, polymers, catalysts, dispersants, inorganic compounds for coalescence regulation, emulsifying agents, surfactants, and organic solvents as well as copolymers and polymers used or produced.

POLYVINYL CHLORIDE FABRICATION (PVC RESIN TO FINAL PRODUCT)

Polyvinyl chloride plastics have hundreds of uses (Figs 63–7 and 63–8). They may be rolled into sheets and used as imitation leather or as floor covering or they may be molded into such products as electric insulators, water pipes, drug bottles, syringes, medical tubing, etc. They may be used as copolymers for such things as films or synthetic fibers or, after immersion in acetone and carbon disulfide, spun and used as "textile yarn."

Whatever the use, fabrication processes involve "compounding" the resin with other chemicals (plasticizers, stabilizers, fillers, pigments, lubricants, and modifiers) to produce the desired properties. The compounding often is done in a Banbury mixer. After mixing, the compound continues to follow a production flow similar to rubber. It may be milled, then calendered or extruded or, if a molded product, go into a mold. Compression, injection, and extrusion molding are the common processes used.

Polyvinyl chloride powder or solution is also used for coatings, such as for kitchen appliances, fabrics, metal articles, and

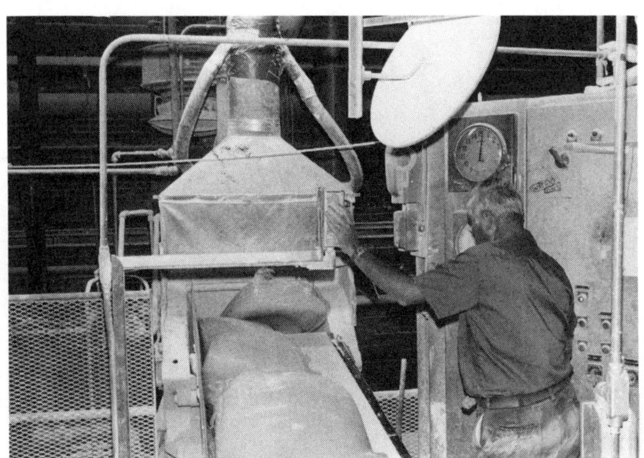

FIG 63–7.
A closeup view showing the worker adding pure latex into the hopper. The latex is packaged in vinyl plastic.

food-wrapping films, or the liquid "plastisol" may be poured directly into molds.

Polyvinyl chloride is tough and brittle with poor heat stability, so that stabilizers, antioxidants, plasticizers, etc., must be added to make the desired product. These additives may constitute up to 60% in some plastics and may produce adverse health effects in the fabrication processes and even finished articles. Potential adverse health effects in the finished product may be a result of leaching out, as has been shown, for example, in transfusion tubing. Considerable investigation has been concerned with the migration of these additives out of biologic systems (implants, cell culture studies) as well as solvent extracts evaluated by intraperitoneal and intradermal injections, cell culture, and hemolysis of red blood cells (Fig 63–9).

Plasticizers.—These are high boiling point, chemically stable liquids that reduce the intermolecular forces and lower the transition temperature of the PVC polymer (Fig 63–10). The resulting compound has decreased tensile strength but increased flexibility, softness, and elongation and is more easily processed at a lower temperature. Better than half of the plasticizers used are phthalates (diethylhexylphthalate [DOP], butyl benzyl, and diisoctyl phthalates), with phthalic acid esters comprising 20%–40% by weight in most flexible PVC plastics. The phosphoric esters also act as flame retarders.

Phthalates.—Diethylhexylphthalate, $C_6H_4(COOCH_2CH[C_2H_5]\ C_2H_{52})$; TLV 5 mg/m^3. The phthalates used are moderately volatile, liquid soluble and stable, and have been found in human tissue (lung, liver, spleen). Practically nontoxic (based on short-term oral toxicity) and poorly absorbed via skin (Fig 63–11).

Dibutyl and dioctyl phthalates.—Phthalate esters are of low level toxicity. Many of the phthalate esters have high oral lethal doses in animals and can be tolerated in relatively high levels in the diet (Figs 63–12 and 63–13).

The degree of toxicity of phthalate esters is said to be related inversely to the molecular weight and water solubility. (See Chapter 64 for clinical discussion.)

The ester of adipic acid ($COOH[CH_2]_4\ COOH$) has low toxicity, but may cause eye and skin irritation.

Phosphoric acid esters.—Tricresyl phosphate; TLV 0.1 mg/m^3; GI upset (nausea, vomiting, diarrhea, abdominal pain); soreness of lower leg muscles, numbness of toes and fingers, weakness of toes; polyneuritis, CNS degeneration; allergen. Tri (2-ethyl hexyl) phosphate; toxicity not known (low?), possibly slightly irritant.

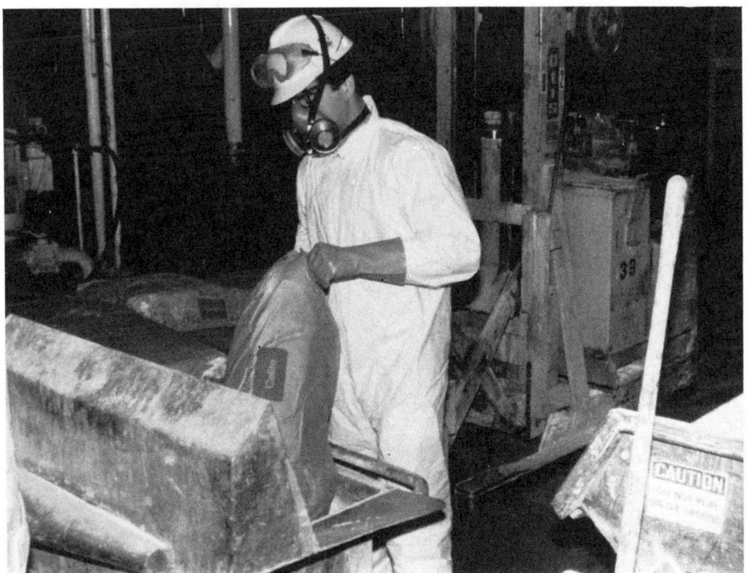

FIG 63–8.
Addition of titanium dioxide as whitening agent in paint.

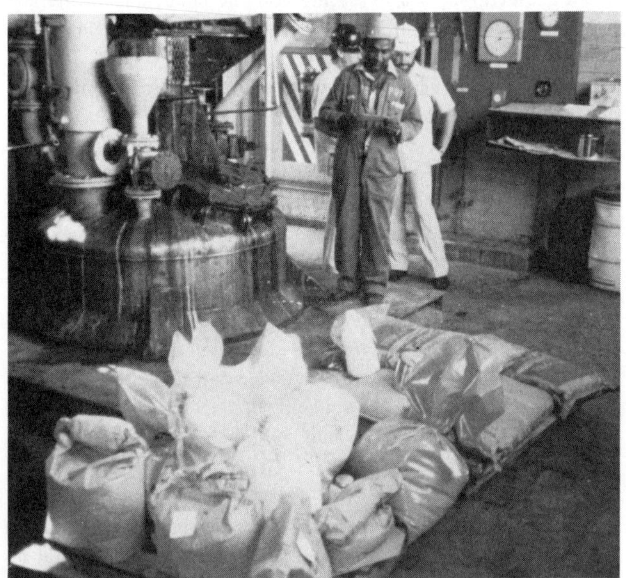

FIG 63–9.
An assortment of preweighed and packaged materials to go into the reactor vessel: pigments, plasticizers, drying agents, etc. This is the preferred method of eliminating worker contact.

Citrate esters.—Triethyl citrate, acetyl tributyl citrate; relatively toxic (soluble compounds) to nontoxic (nonsoluble).

Stabilizers.—These are metal salts or soaps that react with HCl degradation product of the heat-sensitive PVC,

$$
\text{degradation reaction} = \begin{array}{cccccccccc}
 & \text{H} & \text{H} & \text{Cl} & \text{H} & \text{Cl} & \text{H} & \text{Cl} & \text{H} & \\
 & | & | & | & | & | & | & | & | & \\
\text{Cl}- & \text{C}- & \text{C}- & \text{C}- & \text{C}- & \text{C}- & \text{C}- & \text{C}- & \text{C}- & + \text{heat} \rightarrow \\
 & | & | & | & | & | & | & | & | & \\
 & \text{H} & \text{H} & \text{H} & \text{H} & \text{H} & \text{H} & \text{H} & \text{H} &
\end{array}
$$

$$
\begin{array}{ccccccccc}
\text{H} & \text{H} & \text{Cl} & \text{H} & \text{Cl} & \text{H} & \text{Cl} & \text{H} & \\
| & | & | & | & | & | & | & | & \\
\text{HC} = & \text{C}- & \text{C}- & \text{C}- & \text{C}- & \text{C} & \text{C}- & \text{C}- & + \text{HCl} \\
 & | & | & | & | & | & | & | & \\
 & \text{H} & \text{H} & \text{H} & \text{H} & \text{H} & \text{H} & \text{H} &
\end{array}
$$

thereby providing good long-term heat stability. Organo-tin compounds are used for higher heat processing or for high-clarity objects such as clear, rigid products. Organo-phosphite chelators sequester the metal chloride formed from the metal salt. Finally, epoxidized resins or oils react with acid, thereby adding to overall compound stability.

In polymers for medical use, the toxic organo-tin compounds often are replaced with epoxidized soya oil as the primary stabilizer. The soya oil is a complex mixture containing different contaminants (e.g., peroxides, decomposition products of soya oil). In translucent compounds, light stabilizers provide protection from ultraviolet light.

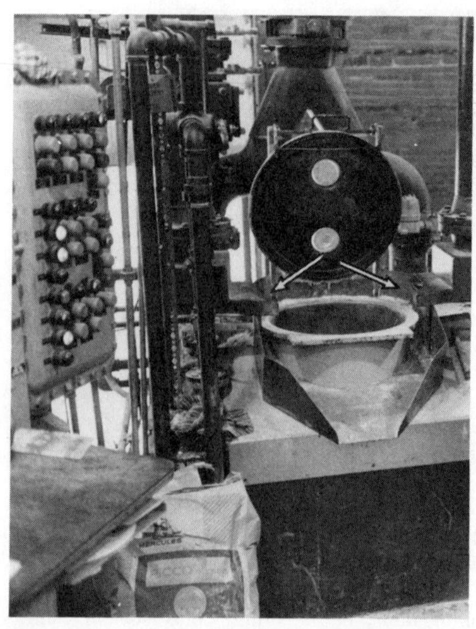

FIG 63–10.
A mixing tank for rubber formulating. Note exhaust system *(arrows).*

Stabilizers as a group may contain other agents as contaminants.

Metal salts or soaps.—(1) Lead compounds (see Chapter 36); (2) cadmium compounds or organic acids (see Chapter 33); (3) barium salts or organic acids; (4) calcium and zinc salts—used especially when nontoxic compounds are required, Cd, Ba, and Zn compounds are preferred in general processing; (5) organo-tin compounds (up to 1% of the formulation) (see Chapter 45).

Epoxidized resins or oils.—Soya oil (variable composition with many contaminants), linseed oil, epoxy stearates (toxic to cells in culture and on intracutaneous and intraperitoneal injection).

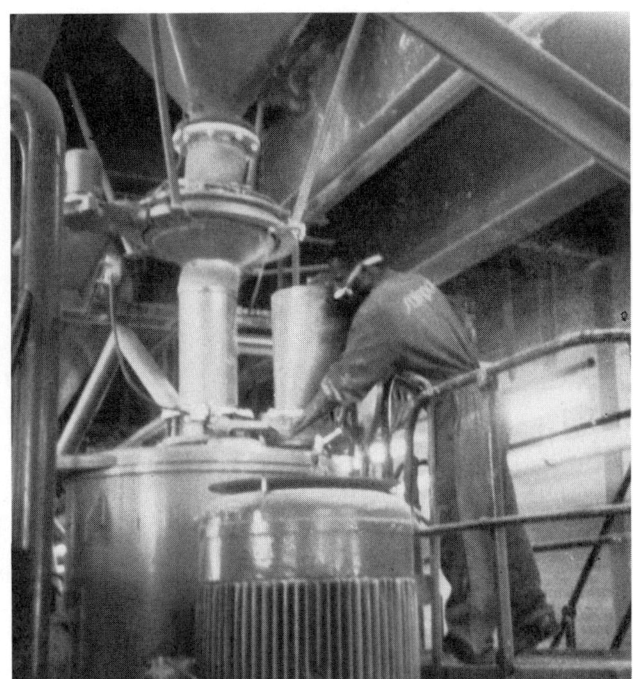

FIG 63–11.
Another view of a reactor vessel.

Light stabilizers.—Benzophenones ($C_6H_5COC_6H_5$), benzotriazoles (C_6H_4NHNN); toxicity not known; animal experiments suggest moderate toxicity by ingestion.

Fillers.—These materials are added to produce opacity and hardness and to reduce costs. They also improve electrical properties, ultraviolet light resistance and impact resistance as well as improving processing characteristics and dimensional stability by reducing elasticity. Because of their higher specific gravity (2–3 times greater than unfilled compound), they increase the density of the finished product. Unlike fillers used in rubber, which have a reinforcing effect, fillers normally lower tensile strength, elongation and tear strength in PVC.

Organic fillers.—Carbon black is used commonly. When mice were fed massive quantities of carbon black over 12 to 18 months, there was no detectable change.[14] A case of carbon black pneumoconiosis was reported in an individual who worked 32 years in carbon black storage and in the calender department of the same factory.

Hamsters, mice, guinea pigs, rabbits, and monkeys were exposed by inhalation for prolonged periods to high concentrations of channel or furnace black without significant effect other than the accumulation of the dust in the pulmonary system. No malignancies were observed.[14] A TLV for carbon black of 3.5 mg/m^3 has been recommended in the United States.

Wood fibers.—Allergenic and inhalation hazard. See Chapters 14 and 16.

Inorganic fillers (<1% silicon dioxide).—Clay, along with carbonates, the most widely used; average particle size >3μ. Calcium carbonate, mica—TLV 20 mppcf (>1% SiO_2), antimony oxide (see Antimony, Chapter 31).

Asbestos.—Talc; diatomaceous earth; titanium dioxide. (For talcosis, see Chapter 14.)

Colorants.—A wide range of colorants is used, selected on the basis of cost, processing temperature, service requirements, and color effect. Inorganic pigments do not produce a bright color but give excellent heat stability and good hiding power and are inexpensive. Organic pigments provide brightness and transparency, have a low specific gravity, and high tinting strength. They are, however, more expensive and have a poorer heat stability. Normally, only small quantities are used and, therefore, probably do not pose a hazard.

Inorganic colorants.—Titanium oxide (most commonly used) (similar to TiO_2), chromium oxide (toxic by inhalation or ingestion, see Sawyer, Chapter 34), molybdate orange (lead chromate, molybdate and sulfate), and ultramarine blue.

Organic colorants.—Phthalocyanines, with a structural unit of $4(C_6H_4)C_2N$ groups; blue-green is metal free, blue contains Cu, green contains chlorinated Cu, water-soluble green contains H_2SO_3. Benzidines (a family of pigments) (see Chapter 52). Quinacridones. Oxynaphthoic reds; moderately toxic, irritant.

Lubricants.—Usually less than 1% is incorporated into a compound to reduce internal friction and the tendency of the stock to adhere to the surfaces of the processing equipment; these are the stearic, palmitic, and oleic acids.

Metallic stearates, waxes, oils, and low molecular weight polyethylene (a polymer of ethylene [C_2H_4]; molecular weight 2,000–5,000).

Modifiers.—These are other polymers added to the PVC polymer to either reduce the melt viscosity or increase the impact strength.

Processing aids (5%–10%).—Acrylic polymers (the monomer methyl methacrylate has a TLV of 100 ppm; acrylic acid monomer is highly toxic, an irritant, and corrosive). Styrene—acrylonitrite resins, chlorinated polyethylene (nontoxic).

Impact modifiers (10%–20%).—Acrylic polymers; acrylonitrite-butadiene-styrene resins (ABS) (see separate sections); chlorinated polyethylene.

Polyvinyl chloride, as a product (resin plus additives), is more or less inert as measured by oral LD_{50}s. Inhalation of PVC dust has resulted in at least one reported case of pneumoconiosis; PVC film (as well as a number of other plastics, metals, glass, polyvinyl alcohol sponges, polyurethane, acrylic) has been shown to produce malignant tumors in rats and/or mice.

Main problem areas are mixing or milling of rubber stocks with the additives, curing or vulcanizing, and dusting of finished

Chemical Name	Structure	Functions	In Selected Applications
Benzoic Acid Technical	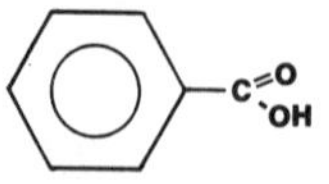 ($C_7H_6O_2$)	Intermediate in ester production	• Adhesives, plastics, rubber (Benzoate Plasticizers) • Textiles (Butyl Benzoate, Benzyl Benzoate) • Flavors & Fragrances (Benzyl Benzoate)
		Intermediate	• Pharmaceuticals (Propiophenone) • Food Preservative (Sodium Benzoate) • Benzoyl Chloride
		Diverting Agent	• Secondary Oil Well Recovery
		Chain Stopper	• Alkyd Resin Production
Benzoic Acid, USP, FCC (Regular)		Preservative	• Food, Cosmetics, Pharmaceuticals, Toiletries
Benzoic Acid, USP, FCC (Low Odor)		Preservative	• Special Applications
Benzotrichloride	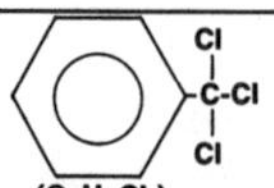 ($C_7H_5Cl_3$)	Intermediate	• Benzoyl Chloride • Other Acid Chlorides • Dyes • UV Absorbers
Benzoyl Chloride	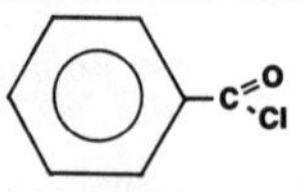 (C_7H_5ClO)	Intermediate	• Polymerization Catalyst • Food Processing, Pharmaceuticals (Benzoyl Peroxide) • Agricultural Chemicals
Benzyl Chloride	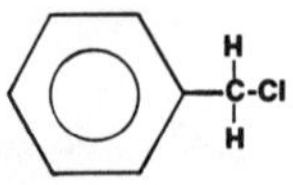 (C_7H_7Cl)	Intermediate	• Benzyl Alcohol • Benzyl Amine • Dyes • Potassium Phenylacetate • Quaternary Ammonium Compounds
PCL® Hexachloro-cyclopentadiene	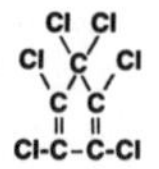 (C_5Cl_6)	Intermediate	• Pesticides • Flame Retardants
Chlorendic Anhydride, Technical & Refined Grades	($C_9H_2Cl_6O_3$)	Reactive Flame Retardant	• Polymer Systems
		Hardener	• Epoxies

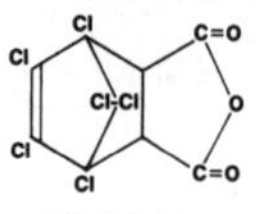

FIG 63–12.
Product summaries of the Benzoflex plasticizer product line. (Courtesy of Velsicol Chemical Corporation, Chicago.)

and semifinished products. Substances most frequently used as ingredients are shown in Table 63–3.

Rubber processing may be divided into two phases: (1) masterbatching and (2) addition of a curing agent and preparation for operations to follow. Masterbatching involves breakdown of the raw elastomer in an open-roll mill or closed mixer (Banbury) to soften the elastomer and increase plasticity. To speed the softening operation and to aid in the addition of pigments, plasticizers may be added during breakdown. When softening is complete, resins and pigments are added and mixed together until homogeneous. The batch then is extruded or formed into sheets to cool and an antitack agent is applied to the surface to prevent sticking in storage. Many of the plants included in this study purchased their rubber already masterbatched, ready for the second stage of processing in their own plants.

In the second phase, the masterbatch is added to an open-roll mill or Banbury mixer to warm up. Then the curing agent, antioxidant, plasticizer, and other ingredients called for in the formula are added and mechanically worked. This process must be carefully regulated, since both the mixing time and the heat generated govern the chemical reactions that take place within the batch (Table 63–4).

Various pigments are added to rubbers; for example, chromium compounds are used to impart the bright green colors, with generation of much dust during the milling operation.

When ready, the batch is removed and formed into shapes for

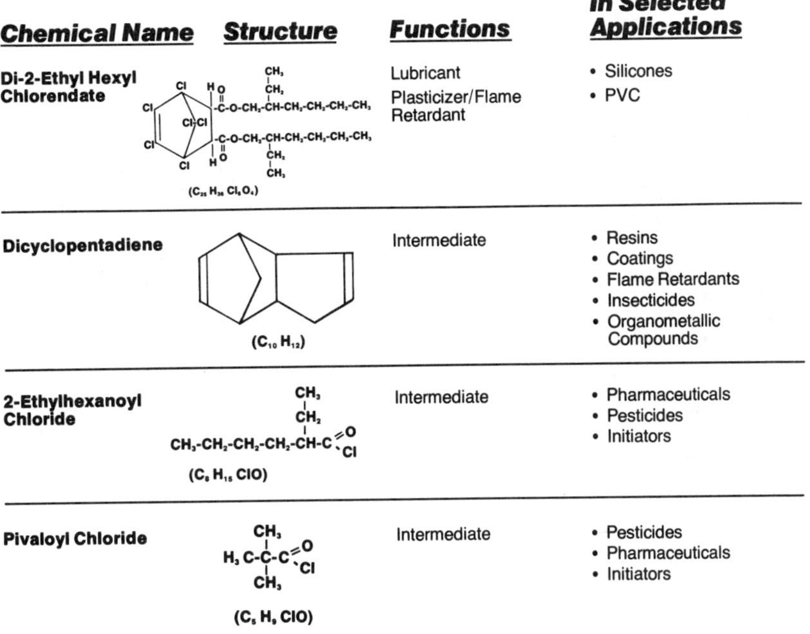

Chemical Name	Structure	Functions	In Selected Applications
Di-2-Ethyl Hexyl Chlorendate	$(C_{25}H_{36}Cl_6O_4)$	Lubricant Plasticizer/Flame Retardant	• Silicones • PVC
Dicyclopentadiene	$(C_{10}H_{12})$	Intermediate	• Resins • Coatings • Flame Retardants • Insecticides • Organometallic Compounds
2-Ethylhexanoyl Chloride	$(C_8H_{15}ClO)$	Intermediate	• Pharmaceuticals • Pesticides • Initiators
Pivaloyl Chloride	(C_5H_9ClO)	Intermediate	• Pesticides • Pharmaceuticals • Initiators

FIG 63–12 cont'd.

TABLE 63–3.
Common Rubber Additives

Accelerators	Dusting or dipping agents
Tetramethylthiuram disulfide	Zinc stearate*
Diphenylguanidine	Talc
Benzothiazyl disulfide	Soap solution
Zinc dimethyldithiocarbamate	
	"Inert" fillers
Activators	Kaolin
Zinc oxide	Whiting
Stearic acid	Silica
Magnesium oxide	Pigments
Lead monoxide	Plasticizers
	Dibutyl phthalate
Antioxidants	Dioctyl phthalate
N-isopropyl-*N'*phenyl-*P*-phenyldiamine	Reinforcing agents
	Carbon black
N-phenyl-beta-naphthylamine	
1,2-dihydro-2,2,4-trimethyl quinoline	Retarders
2,2-methylene-bis (4-methyl-6-tertiary butyl phenol)	Salicylic acid
	N-nitroso diphenylamine
Blowing agents	Vulcanizers
Sodium bicarbonate	Sulfur
Stearic acid (used in combination with sodium bicarbonate)	
Dinitrosopentamethylene tetramine	
Azodicarbonamide	

*See Chapter 45.

vulcanizing, i.e., strips, tubes, sheets, or slabs. Many articles, such as hose, belts, rolls, and footwear, are built to approximately finished form before vulcanization.

The well-known vulcanization stage is the conversion of the plastic material to impart strength and also elasticity. This reaction is completed by the addition of sulfur or sulfur compounds at temperatures above 140°C with open steam autoclaves, heated dry air ovens, or heated platen press molds, and a lubricant is necessary to ensure easy removal of the cured article from the mold. Finally, a dusting or dipping agent is supplied to eliminate surface tackiness. To add other special characteristics to rubber products, a number of aromatic amines are used, these being chiefly the "accelerators" in the vulcanization process to speed vulcanization and to make this a more efficient process. To combat the effects of aging (by sunlight and oxygen), the antioxidants used in rubbe processing are of three groups: the acetone-amino condensation products, aromatic amines or hydroquinolines, and phenolic substances.

There are several major types of synthetic rubber. Some are called butyl, ethylene-propylene, Neoprene, nitrile, polyurethane, stereoregular, and styrene-butadiene rubbers. The materials used and the occupational and hygienic aspects of importance are described below separately, some in considerable depth, such as acrylonitrile, butadiene, styrene, and the polyurethanes.

Butyl Rubber.—Butyl rubber is made by copolymerization of isobutylene and isoprene (primarily exerting a physiologic effect as an anesthetic on inhalation) in the presence of boron trifluoride and methyl chloride. Usually, these processes are closed systems, containing the hazardous materials. Boron trifluoride, highly toxic, with a TLV of only 1 ppm, has shown marked respiratory irritation in animals. Methyl chloride is described elsewhere in this book.

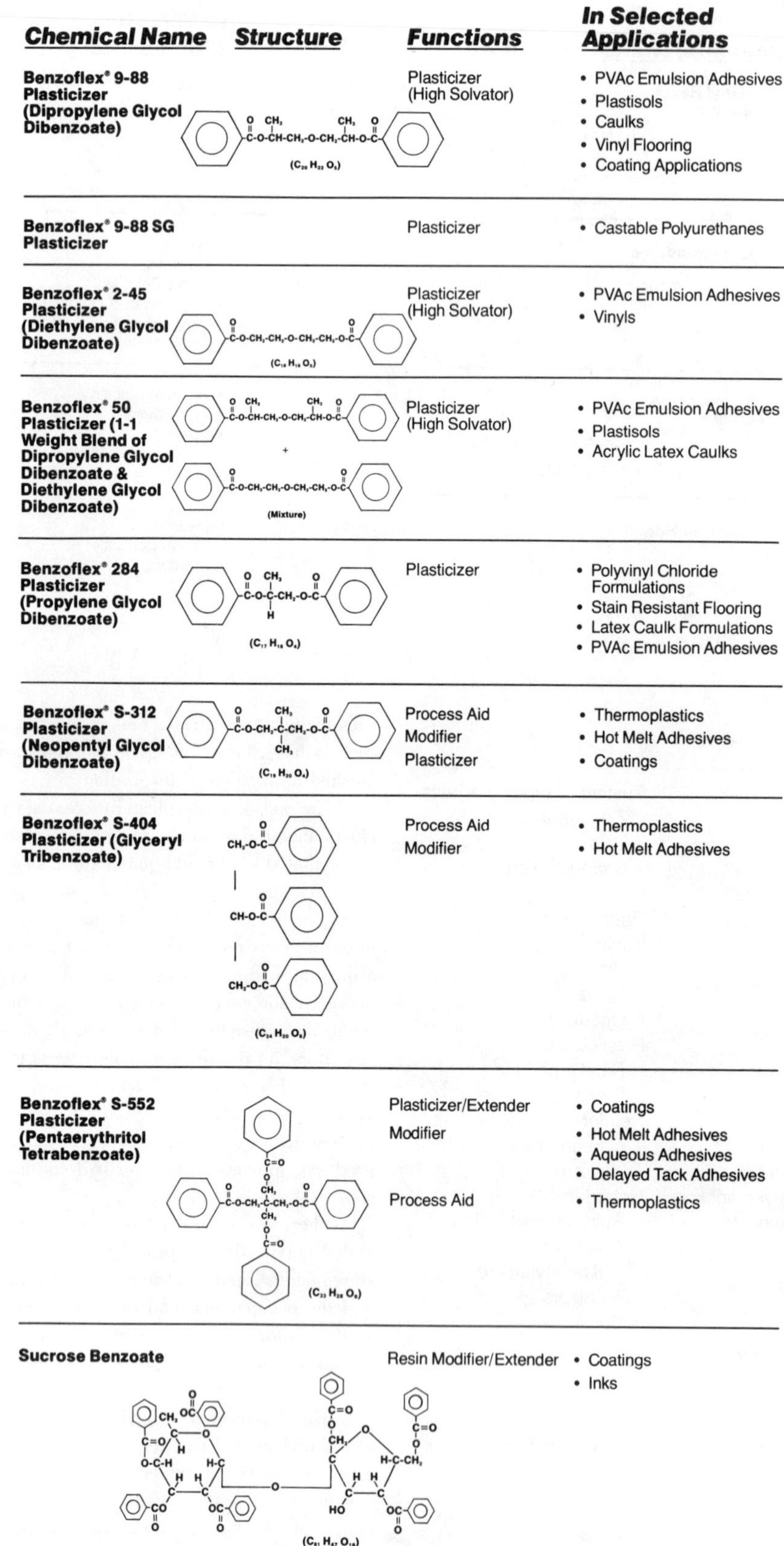

Chemical Name	Structure	Functions	In Selected Applications
Benzoflex® 9-88 Plasticizer (Dipropylene Glycol Dibenzoate)	($C_{20}H_{22}O_5$)	Plasticizer (High Solvator)	• PVAc Emulsion Adhesives • Plastisols • Caulks • Vinyl Flooring • Coating Applications
Benzoflex® 9-88 SG Plasticizer		Plasticizer	• Castable Polyurethanes
Benzoflex® 2-45 Plasticizer (Diethylene Glycol Dibenzoate)	($C_{18}H_{18}O_5$)	Plasticizer (High Solvator)	• PVAc Emulsion Adhesives • Vinyls
Benzoflex® 50 Plasticizer (1-1 Weight Blend of Dipropylene Glycol Dibenzoate & Diethylene Glycol Dibenzoate)	(Mixture)	Plasticizer (High Solvator)	• PVAc Emulsion Adhesives • Plastisols • Acrylic Latex Caulks
Benzoflex® 284 Plasticizer (Propylene Glycol Dibenzoate)	($C_{17}H_{16}O_4$)	Plasticizer	• Polyvinyl Chloride Formulations • Stain Resistant Flooring • Latex Caulk Formulations • PVAc Emulsion Adhesives
Benzoflex® S-312 Plasticizer (Neopentyl Glycol Dibenzoate)	($C_{19}H_{20}O_4$)	Process Aid Modifier Plasticizer	• Thermoplastics • Hot Melt Adhesives • Coatings
Benzoflex® S-404 Plasticizer (Glyceryl Tribenzoate)	($C_{24}H_{20}O_6$)	Process Aid Modifier	• Thermoplastics • Hot Melt Adhesives
Benzoflex® S-552 Plasticizer (Pentaerythritol Tetrabenzoate)	($C_{33}H_{28}O_8$)	Plasticizer/Extender Modifier Process Aid	• Coatings • Hot Melt Adhesives • Aqueous Adhesives • Delayed Tack Adhesives • Thermoplastics
Sucrose Benzoate	($C_{61}H_{47}O_{18}$)	Resin Modifier/Extender	• Coatings • Inks

FIG 63–13.
Product summaries. (Courtesy of Velsicol Chemical Corporation, Chicago.)

TABLE 63–4.
Rubber Formulations

TYPE OF INGREDIENT	BLACK MOLDING RUBBER		BLACK CHLOROPRENE SPONGE	
	SPECIFIC AGENT	WT (%)	SPECIFIC AGENT	WT (%)
Elastomer	Styrene-butadiene rubber	59.00	Chloroprene	68.0
			Zinc oxide	2.0
Vulcanizer	Sulfur	1.00	Calcined magnesia (MgO)	3.0
Accelerator				
Primary	Benzothiazyl disulfide	0.09	—	—
Secondary	Copper dimethyl-dithiocarbamate	0.06	—	—
Antioxidant	Octylated diphenylamines	0.06	P-(p-toluene-sulfonylamido)-diphenylamine	0.3
Activator	Stearic acid	0.60	—	—
	Zinc oxide	3.00	—	—
Processing aid	—	—	Petrolatum	2.0
Plasticizer	Mix of paraffin oil & sol. sulfonic acid	6.00	Aromatic light oil	10.0
Reinforcing agent	Thermal carbon black	18.00	Thermal carbon black	13.0
	Furnace carbon black	12.00		
Blowing agent	—	—	P,p′-oxybis-(benzene-sulfonyl hydrazide)	2.0

Ethylene-Propylene Rubbers.—Ethylene-propylene rubbers result from copolymerization of ethylene and propylene, using a hydrocarbon solvent method, along with titanium, vanadium, and alkyl aluminum compounds as catalysts. The aluminum alkyls are especially dangerous because they can ignite spontaneously in air, and extreme precautions are needed; spillage on skin results in severe or fatal burns. Ethylene and propylene display some health risks, both having anesthetic properties, and are highly flammable.

Neoprene.—Polymerization of chloroprene (2-chloro-1,3-butadiene) produces the polymer polychloroprene, best known by its trade name, Neoprene. The monomer is easily absorbed percutaneously or by inhalation, is capable of inducing CNS depression, and may be toxic to the liver. Alopecia has been noted among workers with the polymerization process, accompanied by atrophy and disappearance of the follicles and fatty glands.

Acrylamide.—The vinyl monomer acrylamide (acrylic amide, $CH_2 = CHCONH_2$) has been found to be neurotoxic. Neurotoxicity was produced in cats, rats, mice, monkeys, and dogs. Initial production experience revealed neurologic findings in workers exposed to monomeric acrylamide (see Chapter 47 for detailed discussion).

Acrylonitrile.—Acrylonitrile, or vinyl cyanide, is used in large quantities in the manufacture of synthetic rubber (based on copolymerization with butadiene, resulting in a product known for its resistance to oils and greases). It is a colorless, volatile liquid with an ethereal odor, is partly soluble in water, with a boiling point of 77.3° C. This compound, long known for its toxicity, may enter the body by ingestion, inhalation, or through the skin.

Acrylonitrile is one of the chemicals belonging to the common group called the cyanides and cyanogen compounds; the best known is hydrogen cyanide (HCN). (Refer to Chapter 47 for clinical and other discussion.)

Occupational Exposures.—Increased incidence of respiratory disease and cancer has been reported among tire workers.[42, 76] Lednar et al.[42] found that workers in curing preparation, curing and finishing, or inspection had an increased incidence of pulmonary disability retirement. Fine and Peters[23–26] reported increased respiratory morbidity among rubber workers in curing rooms and processing areas, and among workers exposed to talc. Among curing room workers, they reported increased prevalence of chronic and acute bronchitis and chronic obstructive lung disease (COLD). Workers exposed to curing fumes for more than a 10-year period were found to have statistically significant and "excessive" losses of their forced expired volume (FEV_1). In 1 year, these workers lost 173 ml of FEV_1 as opposed to 40 ml for controls. Because people typically have an FEV_1 between 2.0 and 2.5 L and because a FEV_1 of 1.5 L is indicative of COLD, Fine and Peters characterized such decreases as excessive. However, because of the small sample sizes involved, they were unwilling to estimate the future incidence of COLD among curing room workers. Among processing workers with 10 years on the job, Fine and Peters[25] found increased respiratory morbidity. Limited sampling showed that these workers were exposed to respirable general dust concentrations of 1 to 5 mg/m^3. Based on pulmonary function tests, they concluded that 40 years of exposure to processing dusts would result in clinically apparent and disabling dyspnea, and they found an average exposure concentration of 2 mg/m^3 related to definite decreases in pulmonary function. Therefore, they recommended an 8-hour TLV of 0.5 mg/m^3 of respirable dust.

Among rubber workers exposed to talc for 10 years, Fine and Peters[26] found a significantly greater prevalence of productive cough and positive criteria for COLD. On analysis of pulmonary function tests, they predicted current talc exposures would cause some workers to have significant dyspnea and pulmonary disability. Consequently, a TLV between 0.5 and 0.25 mg/m^3 for respirable talc was recommended.

Gamble[29] and Peters[64] observed the association of excess cancers (stomach, lung, and bladder) with occupational titles. Monson and Nakano[51] studied the mortality of rubber workers and found excess cancer deaths in specific sites and job classifications. They found "processing workers" had excess cancers of stomach and large intestines; "tire builders" had excess cancers of brain and lymphatic system; excess lung cancers were observed in the curing room workers; and excess leukemia occurred among all tire workers. However, in a case control study of lung cancer among rubber workers, Delzell et al.[18] observed that curing room workers did not have an excess risk of developing lung cancer relative to other workers. In a case-control study of leukemia in the U.S. rubber industry, Wolf[84] reports a significant excess of lymphatic leukemia among compounding and mixing workers at one out of four companies studied. In the British tire industry, excess stomach and lung cancer have also been reported.[3] Fox and Collier[27] analyzed records of 40,867 men employed for at least 1 year in the British rubber and cablemaking industries. They compared the mortality pattern for 1972–1974 with that previously reported for 1968–1971, noting a significant excess of deaths due to cancer of the bladder throughout the industry, including men who had not been exposed to acknowledged bladder carcinogens. The excess in deaths occurred in 1973 and 1974 in the 45–64 and 65+ year age groups. The two sectors of the industry where this excess was significant are footwear and footwear supplies, except adhesives, and the tire sector. The combined excess of all cancers noted in the study population for 1968–1971 is confirmed for 1972–1974. The same is true of the excess of lung cancer deaths. There was a greater excess in the tire sector, particularly in those men in the 55–64 year age group and those who entered the industry between 1950 and 1960. Molding, press, autoclave, pan curing, finished goods, stores, packaging, and shipping workers continue to show more lung cancer deaths than expected for 1972–1974. Fox and Collier reported this excess is no longer statistically significant. An excess of cancer of the stomach, overlooked in 1968–1971, was not confirmed in 1972–1974, but appeared high when the total period of study (1968–1974) was considered.[27] They discussed the limitations of the study with particular reference to extrapolating the results to the entire industry, but concluded that there is a higher rate of lung cancer in the tire sector, and they recommended that the hypothesis concerning the excess of bladder cancers be investigated immediately. Fox and Collier emphasized that attention must be given to control of exposures to all potential hazards in the industry.

Parkes et al.[63] reported that in the 30 years since an excess of bladder cancer was first identified in British rubber workers, fears persisted that this hazard could still be affecting men working in the industry today. Furthermore, suspicions have also arisen that other, hitherto unsuspected excesses of cancer might be occurring. For these reasons, 33,815 men who first started work in the industry between January 1, 1946, and December 31, 1960, were followed up to December 31, 1975, to ascertain the number of deaths attributable to malignant disease and to compare these deaths with the expected number calculated from the published mortality rates applicable to the male population of England, Wales, and Scotland. Their findings confirmed the absence of any excess mortality from bladder cancer among men entering the industry after January 1, 1951 (the presumed bladder carcinogens were withdrawn from British production processes in July 1949), but they found a statistically significant excess of both lung and stomach cancer mortality. A small excess of esophageal cancer was also observed in both the tire and general rubber goods manufacturing sectors. Parkes et al. commented that American reports of an excess of leukemia among rubber workers could receive only limited support based on their study.[63] A small numerical excess of deaths from leukemia resulted from the adoption of an analytical method that took into account the long latent period of induction of occupational cancer. Norell et al.[60] found a tenfold increased risk for esophageal cancer, more often localized in the upper than in the lower third of the esophagus, in a 13-year follow-up of Swedish vulcanization workers. The risk for laryngeal cancer was also significantly raised. Their study was based on a record linkage between the 1960 census and the cancer registry in Sweden. They noted the apparent increased rise in esophageal cancer could not be explained by alcohol consumption or other factors previously known to be associated with this disease.

In reviewing the world literature on cancer in the rubber industry, the World Health Organization[40] concluded that there are definite excesses of bladder, stomach, and lung cancer and leukemia in the rubber industry. Furthermore, this report stated bladder cancer was casually associated with aromatic amine exposure and leukemia was associated with solvent exposure. Limited evidence was available to casually associate stomach cancer with compounding, mixing, and milling.

OTHER POSSIBLE HEALTH HAZARDS

In addition to the occupational exposures found in the literature, potential exposures to other hazardous chemical substances have been suggested. Polyaromatic hydrocarbons (PAH) are reportedly present in carbon blacks, extender oils, and softeners used in the manufacture of tires.[14, 50] Nau[59] reported PAHs are so tightly bound to the carbon black that no hazard exists. Nutt[61] found benzopyrene in a tire manufacturing plant at concentrations not different from the outside ambient levels. In the carbon black criteria document,[14] NIOSH summarized the work of another researcher who found polynuclear aromatics on carbon black. The criteria document noted that all of the listed compounds have not been identified as carcinogens or suspected carcinogens.

Exposure to known or suspected carcinogens as tire ingredients or contaminants of tire ingredients has been reported. Monson and Fine[50] reported that several of the antioxidants and accelerators used in tire manufacturing are suspected carcinogens. Over a million pounds of phenylnaphthylamine, a metabolic precursor of alpha- or beta-naphthylamine, was used in 1975 as a rubber antioxidant.[17]

Munn[52] found certain known carcinogens as contaminants in rubber additives, but not as air contaminants in the work place. These were: diphenylamine, beta-naphthol, di-beta-naphthyl-p-phenylene-diamine and alpha-naphthol; impurities were: 4-aminodiphenyl, beta-naphthylamine, beta-naphthylamine and alpha-naphthylamine. The carcinogen beta-naphthylamine had been used in the rubber industry but its use was discontinued.[48] However, it still may be a contaminant in chemicals used by the industry.

Because tire curing "fumes" have been shown to cause respiratory disease, these fumes or "off-gas" products have been studied by several investigators. By mass, these fumes are a relatively minor emission from the tire plants. About 1% of the organic emissions are thought to be from rubber decomposition products and volatiles;[37, 83] the rest were solvents (see Chapter 64). Attempts to identify the chemical components of curing fumes have been made. By heating uncured rubber stock in the laboratory, Grote[32] identified C_5-C_8 alkanes, alkyl substituted benzenes, toluene, and tetrachloroethylene. Rappaport and Fraser[67] conducted field sampling in a tire vulcanization area, detecting styrene, toluene, ethyl benzene, and oligomers of 1,3-butadiene; concentrations of individual chemical species was found to be below 1.1 ppm.

Some n-nitroso compounds that have been identified as air contaminants near processes involving hot rubber have been reported to be potent animal carcinogens. Although the carcinogenic risk to man has not been determined, Rounbehler and Fine[70] speculate that man may not be resistant to the carcinogenic properties of these compounds. Some n-nitrosamine concentrations found in four tire plants were: n-nitroso-morpholine, n-nitroso-dimethylamine, and n-nitroso-diethylamine. Workroom air sampling locations were: mill, warm-up mill, calendar, tread tuber, extruder, curing room, and warehouse. Concentrations ranged from 0.03 to 22.0 mg/m^3. Chapter 64 includes discussions on plasticizers, vinyl chloride and polyvinyls, and pyrolysis products.

REFERENCES

1. American Conference of Governmental Industrial Hygienists: *Documentation of Threshold Limit Values for Substances in Workroom Air*, ed 5. Cincinnati, 1986.
2. Andersson A: Health dangers in industry from exposure to trichloroethylene (German). *Acta Med Scand* 1957; 157(suppl 323):7.
3. Baxter D, Werner J: *Mortality in the British Rubber Industry*. London, Health and Safety Executive Baynards House, 1980.
4. Bell A: Death from trichloroethylene in a dry-cleaning establishment. *NZ Med J* 1951; 50:119.
5. Boulton TB, Sweet RB: The place of trichloroethylene in modern anesthesia. *J Mich State Med Soc* 1960; 59:270.
6. *Cancer in the Rubber Industry: The Risks and What You Can Do About Them*. Washington, DC, US Department of Labor, Occupational Safety and Health Administration, 1980.
7. *Criteria for a Recommended Standard . . . . Occupational Exposure to Trichloroethylene*. Cincinnati, National Institute for Occupational Safety and Health, Publication no. HSM 73-11025, 1973.
8. *Criteria for a Recommended Standard . . . . Occupational Exposure to Vinyl Chloride*. Cincinnati, National Institute for Occupational Safety and Health, 1974.
9. *Criteria for a Recommended Standard . . . . Occupational Exposure to Methylene Chloride*. Cincinnati, National Institute for Occupational Safety and Health, DHEW Publication no. 76-138, 1976.
10. *Criteria for a Recommended Standard . . . . Occupational Exposure to Tetrachloroethylene (Perchloroethylene)*. Cincinnati, National Institute for Occupational Safety and Health, DHEW Publication no. 76-185, 1976.
11. *Criteria for a Recommended Standard . . . . Occupational Exposure to 1,1,1-Trichloroethane (Methyl Chloroform)*. Cincinnati, National Institute for Occupational Safety and Health, Publication no. 76-184, 1978.
12. *Criteria for a Recommended Standard . . . . Occupational Exposure to Alkanes (C_5-C_8)*. Cincinnati, National Institute for Occupational Safety and Health, 1977.
13. *Criteria for a Recommended Standard . . . . Occupational Exposure to Refined Petroleum Solvents*. Cincinnati, National Institute for Occupational Safety and Health, 1977.
14. *Criteria for a Recommended Standard . . . . Occupational Exposure to Carbon Black*. Cincinnati, National Institute for Occupational Safety and Health, Publication no. 78-204, 1978.
15. *Criteria for a Recommended Standard . . . . Occupational Exposure to Styrene*. Cincinnati, National Institute for Occupational Safety and Health, Publication no. 83-119, 1983.
16. *Current Intelligence Bulletin No. 2: Trichloroethylene*. Cincinnati, National Institute for Occupational Safety and Health, 1975.
17. *Current Intelligence Bulletin No. 16: Metabolic Precursors of a Known Human Carcinogen—Beta-naphthylamine*. Cincinnati, National Institute for Occupational Safety and Health, 1976.
18. Delzell E, Andjeklovitch D, Tyroler H: A case control study of employment experience among rubber workers. *Am J Ind Med 1982; 3:393–404*.
19. *Extent of Exposure to Styrene in the Reinforced Plastic Boat Making Industry: Technical Report*. Cincinnati, National Institute for Occupational Safety and Health, 1982.
20. Egan H, Fishbein L, Castegnaro M, et al (eds): *Environmental Carcinogens. Selected Methods of Analysis, vol 4: Some Aromatic Amines and Azo Dyes in the General and Industrial Environment*. Lyon, International Agency for Research on Cancer, Scientific Publication no. 40, 1981.
21. English JM: A case of probable phosgene poisoning. *Br Med J* 1964; 1:38.
22. Fajen JM, Carson GA, Rounbehler DP, et al: *N*-Nitrosamines in the rubber and tire industry. *Science* 1979; 205:1262–1264.
23. Fine L, Peters J: Respiratory morbidity in rubber workers: I. Prevalence of respiratory morbidity symptoms and disease in curing workers. *Arch Environ Health* 1976; 31:5–9.
24. Fine L, Peters J: Respiratory morbidity in rubber workers: II. Pulmonary function in curing workers. *Arch Environ Health* 1976; 31:10–14.
25. Fine L, Peters J: Respiratory morbidity in rubber workers: III. Respiratory morbidity in processing workers. *Arch Environ Health* 1976; 31:136–140.
26. Fine L, Peters J: Respiratory morbidity in rubber workers: IV. Respiratory morbidity in talc workers. *Arch Environ Health* 1976; 31:195–200.
27. Fox AJ, Collier PF: A survey of occupational cancer in the rubber and cablemaking industries: Analysis of deaths occurring in 1972–74. *Br J Ind Med* 1976; 33:249–264.
28. Fristedt B, Mattsson SB, Schutz A: Talcosis by exposure to granular talc in a rubber industry. *Nord Hyg Tidskr* 1968; 49:66–71.
29. Gamble J, et al: Applications of a job classification system in occupational epidemiology. *Am J Public Health* 1976; 66:768–772.
30. Gamble JF, McMichael AJ, Williams T, et al: Respiratory function and symptoms; and environmental-epidemiological study of rubber workers exposed to a phenol-formaldehyde type resin. *Am Ind Hyg Assoc J* 1976; 37:499–513.
31. Gerritsen WB, Buschmann CH: Phosgene poisoning caused by the use of chemical paint removers containing methylene chloride in ill-ventilated rooms heated by kerosene stoves. *Br J Ind Med* 1960; 17:187.
32. Grote A: Establishing a protocol from laboratory studies to be used in field sampling operations. *Am Ind Hyg Assoc J* 1978; 39:880–884.
33. Harris RL, et al: Worker exposure to chemical agents during manufacture of rubber tires and tubes. Occupational Health Studies Group, School of Public Health, Univ. of North Carolina, Chapel Hill, NC, 1977.
34. Hedenstedt A, Rannug U, Ramel C, et al: Mutagenicity and metabolism studies on 12 thiuram and dithiocarbamate compounds used as

accelerators in the Swedish rubber industry. *Mutat Res* 1979; 68:313–325.

35. Hedenstedt A: Genetic health risks in the rubber industry: Mutagenicity studies on rubber chemicals and process vapours, in *International Symposium on Prevention of Occupational Cancer*. Helsinki, Finnish Institute of Occupational Health, 1984.
36. Holmberg B, Sjöström B: A toxicological survey of chemicals used in Swedish rubber industry (investigation report 1977:19). Stockholm, National Board of Occupational Safety and Health, 1977.
37. Hoogheem TT, Chi CI, Rinoldi GM: *Draft Report: Identification and Control of Hydrocarbon Emissions From Rubber Processing Operations*. Report of Monsanto Research Corporation, Dayton, Ohio, to Environmental Protection Agency, Research Triangle Park, NC, 1977.
38. James WRL: Fatal addiction to trichloroethylene. *Br J Ind Med* 1963; 20:47.
39. Kleinfield M, Tabershaw IR: Trichloroethylene toxicity. Report of five fatal cases. *Arch Ind Hyg* 1954; 10:134.
40. International Agency for Research on Cancer: *IARC Monographs on the Evaluation of Carcinogenic Risk of Chemicals to Humans: The Rubber Industry*. Switzerland, World Health Organization, vol 28. 1982.
41. Lauwerys R: Styrene in biological indicators for the assessment of human exposure to industrial chemicals, in Alessio L, Berlin A, Boni M, et al (eds): Joint Research Centre Inspra Establishment (Varese), Italy, 1984.
42. Lednar W, et al: The occupational determinants of chronic disabling pulmonary disease in rubber workers. *J Occup Med* 1977; 19:4:263–268.
43. Lilis R, et al: Chronic effects of trichloroethylene exposure. *Med Lav* 1969; 60:595.
44. Locati G, Fantuzzi A, Consonni G, et al: Identification of polycyclic aromatic hydrocarbons in carbon black with reference to cancerogenic risk in tire production. *Am Ind Hyg Assoc J* 1979; 40:644–652.
45. *Manufacture of Paint and Allied Coating Products: Recommendations for Control of Occupational Safety and Health Hazards*. National Institute of Safety and Health, Cincinnati, 1984.
46. McCormick W: Environmental health control for rubber industry. *Rubber Chem Tech* 1971; 44:513–530.
47. McGlothlin JD, Wilcox TC, Fajen JM, et al: A health hazard evaluation of nitrosamines in a tire manufacturing plant, in Choudhary G (ed): *Chemical Hazards in the Workplace: Measurement and Control*. Washington DC, American Chemical Society, 1981, pp 283–299.
48. McMichael AJ, et al: Cancer among rubber workers: An epidemiological study. *Ann NY Acad Sci* 1976; 271:125–136.
49. *Monohalomethanes (Methyl Chloride Ch Cl; Methyl Bromide Ch Br; Methyl Iodide Ch I)*. Current Intelligence Bulletin no. 43. National Institute of Safety and Health, Cincinnati, 1984.
50. Monson R, Fine L: Cancer in rubber workers. *J Cancer Inst* 1978; 61:1047–1053.
51. Monson R, Nakano K: Mortality among rubber workers. *Am J Epidemiol* 1976; 103:284–296.
52. Munn T: Bladder cancer and carcinogenic impurities in rubber additives. *Rubber Industry* 1974; 3:19–20.
53. Mutti A, Falzoi M, Lucertini S, et al: n-Hexane metabolism in occupationally exposed workers. *Br J Ind Med* 1984; 41:533–538.
54. Nau CA, Neal J, Stembridge V: A study of the physiological effects of carbon black. I. Ingestion. *Arch Ind Health* 1958, 17: 21–28.
55. Nau CA, Neal J, Stembridge V: A study of physiological effects of carbon black. II. Skin contact. *Arch Ind Health* 1958; 18:511–520.
56. Nau CA, Neal J, Stembridge V: A study of the physiological effects of carbon black. III. Absorption and elution potentials; subcutaneous injections. *Arch Environ Health* 1960; 1:512–533.
57. Nau CA, Stembridge VA, et al: Physiological effects of carbon black. IV. Inhalation. *Arch Environ Health* 1962; 4:415–431.
58. Nau CA, Taylor GT, Lawrence CH: Properties and physiological effects of thermal carbon black. *J Occup Med* 1976; 18:732–734.
59. Nau CA: A study of the physiological effects of carbon black. Presented at the American Chemical Society, Rubber Division Symposium, Ohio, 1977.
60. Norell S, Lipping H, Ahlbom A, et al: Oesophageal cancer and vulcanization work. *Lancet* 1983; 1:462–463.
61. Nutt AR: Measurement of hazardous substances in the atmosphere of rubber factories. *Environ Health Perspect* 1976; 17:117–123.
62. Nutt AR: Toxicity of rubber chemicals. *Prog Rubber Technol* 1979; 42:141–154.
63. Parkes HG, Veys CA, Waterhouse JAH, et al: Cancer mortality in the British rubber industry. *Br J Ind Med* 1982, 39:209–220.
64. Peters J: Occupational diseases in the rubber industry. *Environ Health Perspect* 1976; 17:31–34.
65. Rannug A: Genotoxic hazards in the rubber industry: Application of short-term tests in work environment analyses. Doctoral Thesis at University of Stockholm, Sweden, 1984.
66. Rappe C, Rydsström T: Occupational exposure to N-nitroso compounds, in Walker EA, Griciute L, Castegnaro M et al (eds): N-Nitroso compounds: Analysis formation and occurrence. Lyon, International Agency for Research on Cancer, Scientific Publication no. 31, pp 565–574, 1980.
67. Rappaport S, Fraser D: Air sampling and analysis in a rubber vulcanization area. *American Industrial Hygiene Association* 1977; 38:205–209.
68. Ratney RS, Wegman DH, Elkins HG: In vivo conversion of methylene chloride to carbon monoxide. *Arch Environ Health* 1974; 28:223.
69. Rinzema LC, Silverstein LG: Hazards from chlorinated hydrocarbon decomposition during welding. *Am Ind Hyg Assoc J* 1972; 33:35.
70. Rounbehler RD, Fine D: N-nitroso compounds in the factory environment. National Institute of Safety and Health, Contract 210-77-0100, Cincinnati, 1979.
71. Sjöstrand T: Endogenous formation of carbon monoxide in man under normal and pathological conditions. *Scand J Clin Lab Invest* 1949; 1:201.
72. *Toxicity and Safe Handling of Rubber Chemicals 1985: Code of Practice*, ed 2. Birmingham, UK, British Rubber Manufacturers' Association, 1985.
73. *Special Occupational Hazard Review With Control Recommendations—Trichloroethylene*. U.S. Department of Health, Education, and Welfare, Public Health Service, Center for Disease Control, National Institute for Occupational Safety and Health, Publication no. 78-130, Bethesda, Md, 1978.
74. Spiegelhalder B, Preussmann R: Nitrosamines and rubber, in Bartsch H, O'Neill IK, Castegnaro M, et al (eds): N-Nitroso Compounds: Occurrence and Biological Effects. Lyon, International Agency for Research on Cancer, Scientific Publ. no. 41, 1984.
75. Stewart RD, Hake CL: Paint-remover hazard. *JAMA* 1976; 235:398.
76. Tyroler H: Chronic diseases in the rubber industry. *Environ Health Perspect* 1976; 17:13–20.
77. US Department of Health and Human Services: *4,4'-Methylenedianiline (MDA)*. Cincinnati, NIOSH, Current Intelligence Bulletin 47, 1986.
78. US Department of Health and Human Services: *Organic Solvent Toxicity*. Cincinnati, NIOSH, Current Intelligence Bulletin 48, 1987.
79. Van Duuren BL: Tumor-promoting and co-carcinogenic agents in chemical carcinogenesis, in Searle CE (ed): *Chemical Carcinogens*. Washington DC, American Chemical Society, ACS Monograph no. 172, pp 24–51, 1976.

80. Van Ert MP, Arp EW, Harris RL, et al: Worker exposure to chemical agents in the manufacture of rubber tires: solvent vapor studies. *AIHAJ* 1980; 41:212–219.
81. Vetenskaplig Skriftserie: Health effects from solvent exposure in the paint industry. *Arbete och Hälsa* 1985; 38.
82. Vetenskaplig Skriftserie: Criteria document for Swedish occupational standards; plastics dust. *Arbete och Hälsa* 1987; 3.
83. Williams TM, Harris RL, Arp ER, et al: Worker exposure to chemical agents in the manufacture of rubber tires and tubes: Particulates. *AIHAJ* 1980; 41:204–211.
84. Wolf PH, Andjelkovitch D, Smith A, et al: A case control study of leukemia in the U.S. rubber industry. *J Occup Med* 1981; 23:103–108.
85. World Health Organization: *Trichloroethylene*. Environmental Health Criteria 50, Geneva, 1985.
86. Åstrand I: Uptake of solvents from the lungs (editorial). *Br J Ind Med* 1985; 42: 217-218.

Benzene

D. Jack Kilian, M.D.

Early in the 19th century, coal tar naphtha was produced in the coal gas manufacturing industry, and later this naphtha was found to contain aromatic organic chemicals from which a number of valuable compounds were identified. The most important one was benzene, which is a clear, pleasant-smelling liquid that is highly flammable. Today it is one of the most essential chemicals in the chemical, pharmaceutical, and petrochemical industries. Almost 90% of benzene produced is used to create other chemicals, such as styrene, cyclohexane, and phenol. Benzene is used in the manufacturing of pesticides, adhesives, detergents, drugs, paints, explosives, and dyestuffs. Many chemical laboratories use large quantities for solvent, extraction and reaction functions.

The NIOSH[11] has estimated that approximately 2 million workers in the United States are potentially exposed to benzene. Due to the expanding appeal of self-service gasoline stations, the general public has some exposure of unknown dimensions because gasoline in the United States usually contains 0.3% to 2% benzene. In Europe the concentrations range from 5% to 16%.[46]

EXPOSURE LIMITS

Over the past four decades, there has been a growing recognition of the serious chronic health effects of benzene which has resulted in a lowering of the allowable concentrations in the workplace. In 1941 the maximum allowable concentration (MAC) was 100 ppm. This was lowered in 1947 to a 50-ppm eight-hour time-weighted average (TWA), which was further lowered in 1948 to 35 ppm TWA and 10 ppm TWA in 1969 by the ACGIH. In 1971, the Occupational Safety and Health Administration (OSHA) instituted a benzene standard of 10 ppm TWA, which allowed a ceiling of 25 ppm and an excursion to a maximum peak concentration of 50 ppm for a ten-minute period in any eight-hour shift. An emergency temporary standard was released by OSHA in May of 1977, reducing the permissible limits of exposure to 1 ppm with a ceiling of 5 ppm. Industry (through the American Petroleum Industry) challenged this rule by obtaining a temporary stay from the United States Federal Court of Appeals for the Fifth Circuit in New Orleans, Louisiana. This stay was upheld by the United States Supreme Court on July 2, 1980. Many experts in the field of occupational health believe that the present 10-ppm standard does not adequately protect the work force, since benzene is a recognized leukemogen, and no threshold of inducibility exists for a leukemogen.[45]

TOXICITY

Acute overexposure to benzene may result in toxicity which depresses the central nervous system and may produce dizziness, headache, loss of consciousness, convulsions, and death. In a workplace where uncontrolled exposure exists, this hazard can easily be present, since benzene has a pleasant odor and minimal respiratory irritative warning signs. Maibach et al. in 1981[27] and Franz[16] in 1982 demonstrated that absorption of this material through the skin was dependent on concentration and time of contact with the skin. Repeated exposure to the skin may also produce a dry, desquamating type of defatting dermatitis typical of other aromatic and chlorinated hydrocarbons.

By far the greatest health hazard from exposure to benzene is produced by chronic exposure. The main effects are : (1) suppression of one or more elements of the hematopoietic system and (2) malignant transformation of some of these elements into leukemia or possibly lymphoma. The suppression of hematopoiesis can be documented fairly well as to the level of safety from concentration and time, but many arguments exist as to a safe level that would prevent leukemia.

Benzene is characterized by considerable individual differences in toxic response which are probably due to variations in metabolic pathways in different people. Vigliani and Forni[42] have one of the larger groups of human subjects studied for the relationship between leukemia and benzene, and they postulate that the effect may be due to one or a combination of the following factors: "Benzene is a clastogen and the induced chromosomal aberrations may lead to the development of abnormal cell clones with selective growth advantages. The compound may activate a latent leukemogenic virus, or suppress the immunological surveillance system so that abnormal cell clones are allowed to exist." The complexity and interrelationship of the possible responses make the determination of the exact mechanism of action almost an unobtainable goal. Many believe that the toxic effects are mediated by the benzene metabolites such as phenol, catechols, hydroquinone, muconic acid, or others.[12] Thus far it has been impossible to establish convincing human evidence regarding which one or ones are responsible for the effect, but it offers an exciting avenue of research, since identification might well lead to the important goal of identifying individuals whose metabolism puts them at increased risk from benzene exposure.

Hematologic Effects.—Before the turn of the century, benzene was recognized as producing a toxic effect on the bone marrow. Since that time, many studies[2, 4, 5, 20] have established the fact that red blood cells, white blood cells, and platelets are the main elements affected by benzene. Careful evaluation of these elements is essential to detect those individuals who have a more sensitive response to benzene exposure. Their records should be compared to previous studies each time a blood study is run. Group analysis of the data from exposed workers should be done to detect shifts within the normal ranges so that corrective environmental changes may be instituted at the earliest possible moment to reduce the risk of an adverse hematologic health effect.

Important hematologic surveillance tests include complete blood counts, packed red blood cell volume, platelet count, blood indices, and reticulocyte count if any suppression of the red blood cell elements is seen. With benzene toxicity there may be an inappropriate lowering of reticulocyte response due to the depression of erythropoiesis.[44] Normochromic or normocytic patterns are usually seen with the developing anemia, but an increase in the mean corpuscular volume (MCV) may be a valuable early sign. There may be any combination of anemia, leukopenia or thrombocytopenia.[43] Aplasic anemia is one of the most serious manifestations of the process and carries a high mortality rate with only 30% survival after five years. Half of the deaths are likely to occur within the first six months.[44] In addition to the blood monitoring, appropriate liver and kidney function tests should be run, since benzene is metabolized in the liver and most of the metabolites are excreted through the kidney.

Mutagenicity and Carcinogenicity.—The mutagenic activity of benzene is chiefly from its colchicine-like effect[44] on marrow cells and its ability to break chromosomes in exposed humans. A colchicine effect interferes with the spindle mechanism in dividing cells and can cause an unequal segmenting of chromosomes in daughter cells or cell death. The latter effect probably plays a significant role in the development of the hypoproliferative state of the hematopoietic system in exposed humans. Benzene has shown little or no activity in the *Salmonella* bacterial tester strains presently used, or the dominant lethal test in experimental animals. Cytogenetic studies in exposed workers have been extensive and also caused considerable disagreement as to their role in establishing a safe level of exposure. A review of these studies[6, 9, 13-15, 21, 35, 40, 41] leaves little doubt that benzene has the ability to increase chromosomal aberrations in exposed workers.

However, it is still not clear why some individuals have evidence of increased chromosome breakage and others do not. It could be due to individual sensitivity, faulty information regarding exposure, or the biostatistical problem of evaluating a hundred or so lymphocytes out of several billion circulating cells. It needs to be pointed out that this biostatistical problem is no different from doing a differential count, which has been a cornerstone of medical diagnosis for decades. Group analysis of cytogenetic data with comparable controls is essential to provide statistical validity to any such study. Evaluation of cytogenetic data on one benzene-exposed individual does not yield significant information unless repeated many times over a given period of measured exposure.

Although there have been many cytogenetic studies on individuals who have developed leukemia from benzene, few studies exist which attempt to establish the levels of exposure necessary to produce increased cytogenetic aberration rates in a work force large enough to produce statistical significance. In 1965, Tough, et al.[40] reported increased aberration rates in two groups of factory workers exposed to 25–150 ppm. However, no increases were seen in a third group exposed to approximately 12 ppm. Girard, et al.[19] in 1970 reported a cytogenetic study on 50 workers exposed to benzene and solvents in a French paint factory where the concentrations of benzene were from a trace to 14 ppm. Twenty-one had evidence of increased chromosomal breaks and four had a large number of chromosomal abnormalities. Picciano[34] in 1979 reported on a group of 52 benzene-exposed workers and compared the data on 44 preemployment controls. He concluded that the study demonstrated a cytogenetic effect to exposures less than 10 ppm, and that there was a dose-related effect at exposure levels below 2.5 ppm.

The fact that benzene can produce increased chromosomal aberrations and also increased risk of malignancy in exposed human beings illustrates an important new tool in preventive medicine. Diagnosing a compound as a human carcinogen from epidemiology studies leaves much to be desired, since such studies cannot be accomplished until a latency period of many years has passed. Properly conducted cytogenetic studies[26] can serve as an early warning instrument so that corrective environmental steps can be accomplished to lower the risk of future malignancies. Many of the human carcinogens known at this time have had group cytogenetic studies accomplished, and the correlation between abnormal cytogenetic studies and increased malignancy has been strong. Many investigators have called attention to this correlation in environmentally induced situations[8, 17, 18, 24, 25] and in certain diseases.[33]

Benzene began to become suspect as the etiologic agent of leukemia in the early 1930s. More cases were reported throughout the years, and in 1977 testimony was presented to OSHA which identified benzene as a leukemogen. However, some members of the chemical and petrochemical industries, along with Tabershaw,[38] challenged the lowering of the benzene standard from 10 ppm to 1 ppm. Infante et al.[22] published an epidemiology study which strongly identified benzene as the etiologic agent for seven cases of leukemia out of a cohort of 746 workers in two pliofilm plants. Tabershaw[39] was critical of the methodology of Infante and stated: " . . . only the acute leukaemias of the cells that derive from the primitive haematoblast of the bone-marrow (acute non-lymphocytic leukaemia) may be attributable to benzene." His reanalysis of the Infante data has been criticized[23, 36, 37] by a number of health scientists, and evidence has been accumulating that benzene may play a role in other types of leukemia.

Lymphocytic leukemias, both the acute and chronic forms, have been reported[1, 7, 28-32] in benzene-exposed individuals, and the etiologic association is possible but not yet conclusive. Likewise, the relationship between benzene and lymphoproliferative disorders[1, 3, 32, 42] appears to be growing stronger but still lacks a conclusive decision. Acute myelocytic and monocytic leukemia appear to have a firm relationship with benzene exposure. Evidence is close to being established that diGugliemo's erythroleukemia may also be associated with benzene exposure.[10]

Benzene like asbestos was firmly entrenched in the chemical production world before the impact of potentially serious health effects was realized. In both instances, animal toxicology warning signals were not adequate, and the experience with these compounds should provide industry with the wisdom to reallocate some of its chemical safety resources to more human clinical evaluations.

REFERENCES

1. Andjelkovic D: Mortality experience of a cohort of rubber workers, 1964–1973. *J Occup Med* 1976; 18(6):387–394.
2. Aksoy M: Benzene (benzol) toxicity and its effect on the hematopoietic system, *Istanbul Faculty of Medicine Monograph Series*, No 51:7–68. Istanbul, Sermet Press, 1970.
3. Aksoy M: Different types of malignancies due to occupational exposure to benzene: A review of recent observations in Turkey. *Environ Res* 1981; 23:181.
4. Aksoy M, Dincol K, Erdem S, et al: Details of blood changes in 32 patients with pancytopenia associated with long-term exposure to benzene. *Br J Ind Med* 1972; 29:56.
5. Aksoy M, Dincol K, Akgun T, et al: Haematological effects of chronic benzene poisoning in 217 workers. *Br J Ind Med* 1971; 28:296.
6. Aksoy M, Erdem S, Dincol G: Leukemia in shoe-workers exposed chronically to benzene. *Blood* 1974; 44(6):837–841.
7. Aksoy M, Erdem S, Dincol G: Types of leukemia in chronic benzene poisoning. A study in thirty four patients. *Acta Haematol* 1976; 55:65–72.
8. Awa AA: Cytogenetic and oncogenic effects of the ionizing radiation of the atomic bomb, in German J (ed): *Chromosomes and Cancer*. New York, John Wiley & Sons, 1974.
9. Capurro PU: Hydrocarbon exposure and cancer. *Lancet* 1976; 2:253–254.
10. Craft BF: Solvents and related compounds, in Rom WN (ed): *Environmental and Occupational Medicine*. Boston, Little, Brown & Co, 1983.
11. *Criteria for a Recommended Standard: Occupational Exposure to Benzene*, DHEW Publ (NIOSH) 74-137. Washington, DC, US Government Printing Office, 1974.
12. Dean BJ: Genetic toxicology of benzene, toluene, xylenes and phenols. *Mutat Res* 1978; 47(#2):75–97.
13. Dobrokhotov VB: The mutagenic effect of benzol and toluol under experimental conditions. *Gig Sanitariia* 1972; 37:36–39.
14. Erdogan G, Aksoy M: Cytogenetic studies in thirteen patients with pancytopenia and leukaemia associated with long term exposure to benzene. *New Istanbul Contrib Clin Sci* 1973; 10(4):230–247.
15. Forni A, Moreo L: Cytogenetic studies in a case of benzene leukaemia. *Eur J Cancer Clin Oncol* 1967; 3:251–255.
16. Franz TJ: Percutaneous absorption of benzene in MacFarland H, et al (eds): *The Toxicology of Petroleum Hydrocarbons*. Washington, DC, American Petroleum Institute, May 1982.
17. German J: Clinical implications of chromosome breakage, in Berg K (ed): *Genetic Damage in Man Caused by Environmental Agents*. New York, Academic Press, 1979.
18. German J: Oncogenic implications of chromosomal instability, in McKusick V (ed): *Medical Genetics*. New York, HP Publishers, 1974, p 39.
19. Girard R, Tolot F, Bourret J: Hydrocarbures benzeniques et hemopathies graves. *Arch Mal Prof* 1970; 311(12):625–636.
20. Greenburg L, Mayers MR, Goldwater L, et al: Benzene (benzol) poisoning in the rotogravure printing industry in New York City. *J Ind Hyg Toxicol* 1939; 21:395.
21. Hartwich G, Schwanitz G, Becker J: Chromosomenaberrationen bei einer benzol-leukamie. *Deutsche Med Woch* 1969; 94:1228–1229.
22. Infante JW, Wagoner JK, et al: Leukemia in benzene workers. *Lancet* 1977; 2:76–78.
23. Infante PF, Rinsky RA, et al: (Letter) *Lancet*. 1977; 2(2):868–869.
24. Key MM, Kilian DJ: Counseling and cancer prevention programs in industry, in Newell G (ed): *Cancer Prevention in Clinical Medicine*. New York, Raven Press, 1983.
25. Kilian DJ: Medical surveillance, in Shaw C (ed): *Prevention of Occupational Cancer*. Boca Raton, Fla, CRC Press, 1980.
26. Kilian DJ, Picciano D: Cytogenetic surveillance of industrial populations, in Hollaender A (ed): *Chemical Mutagens*. New York, Plenum Publishing Corp, 1976, vol 4.
27. Maibach HI, Mark D: Percutaneous penetration of benzene and benzene contained in solvents used in the rubber industries. *Arch Environ Health* 1981; 36(5):256–260.
28. McMichael AJ, Anjelkovic DA, et al: Cancer mortality among rubber workers: An epidemiologic study. *Ann NY Acad Sci* 1976; 271:125–137.
29. McMichael AJ, Spirtas R, et al: Mortality among rubber workers: Relationship to specific jobs. *J Occup Med* 1976; 18(3):178–185.
30. Meinhardt T, Lemen RA, et al: Environmental epidemiologic investigation of the styrene-butadiene rubber industry. *Scand J Work Environ Health* 1982; 8:250–259.
31. Meinhardt TJ, Young RJ, et al: Epidemiologic investigation of styrene-butadiene rubber production and reinforced plastics production. *Scand J Work Environ Health* 1978; 2:240–248.
32. Monson RR, Fine LJ: Cancer mortality and morbidity among rubber workers. *J Nat Cancer Inst* 1978; 61(4):1047–1053.
33. Mulvihill J: Congenital and genetic diseases, in Fraumeni JF (ed): *Persons at High Risk of Cancer*. New York, Academic Press, 1975.
34. Picciano D: Cytogenetic study of workers exposed to benzene. *Environ Res* 1979; 19:33–38.
35. Pollini G, Colomi R: Lymphocyte chromosome damage in benzene blood dyscrasia. *Med Lav* 1964; 55:641–654.
36. Rinsky RA, Young RJ, Smith AB: Leukemia in benzene workers. *Am J Ind Med* 1981; 2:217–245.
37. Rosenstock L: Leukemia and benzene. *Ann Intern Med* 1982; 97(2):275–276.
38. Tabershaw IR: Protection from adverse effects of benzene. *Tex Rep Biol Med* 1978; 37:162–169.
39. Tabershaw IR, Lamm SH: Benzene and Leukemia. *Lancet* 1977; 2:867–869.
40. Tough IM, Brown WMC: Chromosome aberrations and exposure to ambient benzene. *Lancet* 1965; 1:684.
41. Vigiani EC, Forni A: Benzene, chromosome changes, and leukemia. *J Occup Med* 1969; 11(3):148–149.
42. Vigliani EC, Forni A: Benzene and leukemia. *Environ Res* 1976; 11:122–127.
43. Vigiani EC, Saita G: Benzene and leukemia. *N Engl J Med* 1964; 271:872.
44. Ward JH, Rothstein G: The hemic system and occupational hazards, in Rom WN (ed): *Environmental and Occupational Medicine*. Boston, Little, Brown & Co, 1983.
45. White MC, Infante PF, Walker B: Occupational exposure to benzene: A review of carcinogenic and related health effects following the U.S. Supreme Court Decision. *Am J Ind Health* 1980; 1: 233–243.
46. Zenz C: Benzene, in Zenz C (ed): *Developments in Occupational Medicine*. Chicago, Year Book Medical Publishers, 1980, p 73.

Toluene

Joe A. DeLeon, M.D., P.A.

Frank B. Stern, M.S.

Leela I. Murthy, Ph.D.

Toluene (toluol, methyl benzene), is a clear, colorless liquid with a benzene-like odor. The boiling point is 110.6° C, which is higher than benzene but lower than xylene; its vapor pressure is 28 mm Hg at 25° C. The volatility of toluene is lower than benzene but higher than xylene.

During the latter part of the 19th century, toluene was produced as a by-product of the carbonization of coal. Today, however, toluene is derived primarily from petroleum and petrochemical processes.[7] The production of toluene has increased steadily in the United States from 31 million gallons in 1940 to 694 million gallons in 1970.[8, 40] In 1981, approximately 4,700 metric tons of toluene were produced in the United States.[1] Approximately 70% of toluene produced today is converted into benzene.[8] Another 15% is consumed in the production of chemicals such as toluene diisocyanate, phenol, benzyl alcohol and benzyl derivatives, benzoic acid, toluene sulfonates, nitrotoluenes (particularly trinitrotoluene), vinyl toluene, and saccharin. The remainder is used as a solvent for paints or as a component of gasoline.

Highly purified toluene contains less than 0.01% benzene as a contaminant and is used in many commercial applications. Industrial grade toluene, however, may contain up to 25% benzene.

The NIOSH conducted a walk-through survey of approximately 5,000 United States occupational establishments during 1972–1974. This survey, The National Occupational Hazard Survey (NOHS) showed that an estimated 4 million workers were potentially exposed to toluene in 271 occupations.[25] The NIOSH recently completed a second national survey, the National Occupational Exposure Survey (NOES), in 1983.[26] Ingredients of trade name products are not yet available; however, approximately 287,700 workers were potentially exposed to toluene (actual exposure), of whom approximately 68,400 were women. The total number of potentially exposed workers will undoubtedly be much higher, when the ingredients in trade name products are resolved.

ABSORPTION, METABOLISM, EXCRETION

As is the case of most industrial exposures, the main route of entry of toluene into the body is through the respiratory system. Ingestion of toluene is rare, occurring primarily as the result of accidental swallowing. The absorption of toluene through the skin is believed to be minimal.[15] Studies with human volunteers indicate that the total amount of toluene absorbed is proportional to the concentration of toluene in inspired air, the length of exposure, and the volume of pulmonary ventilation, which in turn depends on the level of physical activity. Approximately 50% of inspired toluene is retained in the body. Zenz and Berg[39] found that it was not sufficient to state the concentration of a substance in inspiratory air and the duration of exposure without also looking at the biologic reaction to physical activity, i.e., increased pulmonary ventilation and blood circulation. This was also shown in a study by Åstrand et al.,[4] who found that toluene concentrations in alveolar air and arterial and venous blood were the same after exposure at 200 ppm at rest as to 100 ppm during light exercise.

The initial step in the metabolism of toluene is a side-chain hydroxylation by the hepatic mixed-function oxidase system, followed by oxidation to benzoic acid. Benzoic acid is then conjugated with glycine to form hippuric acid which is excreted in the urine.[30] About 80% of the absorbed toluene can be accounted for as hippuric acid in the urine, with the remainder exhaled as unchanged toluene. The excretion of toluene is rapid, with the major portion being excreted within 12 hours of inhalation.

Toxicity.—Toluene splashed into the eyes may cause conjunctivitis and a keratitis. These damages are reversible. Toluene may cause irritation of the eyes, respiratory tract, and skin. Repeated or prolonged contact with liquid toluene may remove the natural lipids from the skin, resulting in a dry, fissured dermatitis.

The predominant toxic affect of toluene is on the central nervous system. The acute exposure results in central nervous system depression, headaches, dizziness, inebriation, exhilaration, verbosity, lassitude, drowsiness, incoordination, staggering gait, and nausea. With exposures greater than 200 ppm, the effects are more pronounced, and confusion, paresthesias of the skin, dilatation of pupils, impaired light accommodation, and insomnia may occur. At very high concentrations of toluene exposure collapse, coma, and death may result.[5, 28, 29] Psychophysiologic functions in humans have been impaired by occupational and experimental exposures.

Toluene has become a "social or recreational poison" because of the euphoria induced by inhalation or "sniffing." In prolonged abuse, diffuse encephalopathy with abnormal electroencephalograms and cerebral and cerebellar atrophy have been documented.[18, 24, 25] Individuals who inhale or sniff toluene-containing substances have experienced weakness and unconsciousness and hepatotoxic and nephrotoxic effects. Some of these individuals have demonstrated hyperchloremic acidosis, renal tubular acidosis, high anion gap metabolic acidosis, hypokalemia, and hypobicarbonatemia.[10, 11, 28, 38] Toluene abusers are at risk of "sudden sniffing death." These deaths are most likely precipitated by cardiac arrhythmias secondary to sensitization of the myocardium to endogenous catecholamines.[15, 17, 19, 24, 28, 33, 38]

Human Exposure Studies.—Based on a few studies involving controlled exposures of humans to toluene vapor, as well as reports of occupational exposures and voluntary abuse ("glue sniffing"), the dose-response relationships for the acute effects in human beings of single short-term exposures to toluene can be estimated as shown in Table 63–5. However, because of the deficiences in the studies on which these estimates are based, as well as variations in sensitivity to toluene that may be expected in

TABLE 63–5.
Acute Effects in Humans Following Short-Term Exposures to Toluene*

EXPOSURE	EFFECT
37 ppm	Probably perceptible to most humans
50–100 ppm	Subjective complaints (fatigue or headache), but probably no observable impairment of reaction time or coordination
200 ppm	Mild throat and eye irritation
100–300 ppm	Detectable signs of incoordination may be expected during exposure periods up to eight hours
400 ppm	Lacrimation and irritation to the eyes and throat
300–800 ppm	Gross signs of incoordination may be expected during exposure periods up to eight hours
1,500 ppm	Probably not lethal for exposure periods of up to eight hours
4,000 ppm	Would probably cause rapid impairment of reaction time and coordination; exposures of one hour or longer might lead to narcosis and possibly death
10,000–30,000 ppm	Onset of narcosis within a few minutes; longer exposures may be lethal

*Adapted from *Health Assessment Document for Toluene,* EPA-600/8-82-008. US Environmental Protection Agency, Office of Health and Environmental Assessment, 1982.

the human population, these estimates of effects should be taken as approximations only.

The effect of chronic exposure to toluene has been reported in various occupational studies and consists primarily of central nervous system depression,[38] manifested by such symptoms as fatigue, drowsiness, confusion, and incoordination. Other reported central nervous system effects included headache, lassitude, and loss of appetite. Von Oettingen's reports[28, 29] describe the only documented exposures of human subjects to essentially pure toluene. His studies on three human subjects found that an eight-hour exposure to purified toluene at 200 parts per million (ppm) produced mild fatigue, muscular weakness, impaired coordination, moderate dilation of the pupils, and paresthesias of the skin (Table 63–6). Concentrations less than 200 ppm produced no substantiated effects, while levels above 200 ppm produced increasingly severe adverse health effects. These conclusions were supported by Wilson,[37] who stated that vapor concentrations of toluene should never exceed 200 ppm. Greenburg et al.[18] reported studying 61 workers exposed to toluene concentrations ranging from 100 ppm to 1,100 ppm for periods extending from two weeks to five years. Effects of mild intoxication included enlarged livers, macrocytosis, mild depression of the erythrocyte level, and elevation of the hemoglobin level and of the mean corpuscular hemoglobin concentration. The investigators concluded that early chronic toluene intoxication in man is evidenced by hepatomegaly and macrocytosis.

Another study investigated changes in the chromosomes of peripheral blood lymphocytes of rotogravure plant workers exposed to toluene at 200 ppm for 3–15 years.[13] Although the results showed a somewhat higher rate of unstable chromosome changes in peripheral blood lymphocytes for exposed workers than for controls, the differences were not statistically significant. The authors concluded that chronic inhalation of toluene vapor at concentrations of approximately 200 ppm did not significantly increase the rate of chromosome changes in peripheral lymphocytes. The opposite result was, however, obtained in a study by Bauchinger et al.,[6] wherein toluene exposures averaging 200–300 ppm over a period of 16 years for 20 rotogravure plant workers produced significantly higher chromatid breaks, chromatid exchanges, and gaps than in unexposed controls. The discrepancy of the findings between these two studies may have been due to the difference in (1) the number of subjects, (2) the amount of toluene concentration, and/or (3) the number of cells scored.

Girard et al.[17] conducted a case-control analysis of 401 hospital patients with serious blood disorders and a similar number of patients without blood disorders. Those who had a previous exposure to benzene and toluene had a significantly higher occurrence of acute leukemia (13.6%) and aplastic (20%) and chronic lymphatic leukemia (14.7%) than did the control group (4%). Due to the unknown amount of benzene contamination, the results that pertain to toluene toxicity should be viewed with caution.

Animal Studies.—Animals exposed to various airborne concentrations of toluene showed toxic effects on the central nervous system at levels exceeding 1,000 ppm. Purified toluene, however, produced no ill effects on the blood and blood-forming organs even at very high concentrations[10, 31] except in earlier studies when the benzene content was unknown. A recent report by the Chemical Industry Institute of Toxicology (CIIT)[16] showed no evidence that toluene caused chronic marrow toxicity or oncogenicity in Fischer-344 rats at concentrations of 300 ppm after two years exposure.

Mutagenicity testing of toluene to induce DNA damage similarly produced negative results.[12, 23] Likewise, frequencies of sister chromatid exchange were not increased in Chinese hamster ovary cells.[9]

The teratogenic effect of toluene exposure has been studied in various animal species with differing results. Toluene induced cleft palates in offspring of pregnant mice exposed on days 6–15 of gestation in addition to loss of fetal weight,[27] while other studies have concluded that toluene was not teratogenic in mice or rats.[21, 32]

Industrial Hygiene and Biologic Monitoring.—In 1973, the NIOSH recommended for toluene exposure a TWA of 100 ppm (375 mg/m^3) for an eight-hour work day, 40-hour week with a ceiling of 200 ppm (750 mg/m^3) for a ten-minute sampling period. The current OSHA standard is 200 ppm as an eight-hour TWA with an acceptable ceiling concentration of 300 ppm and with an acceptable peak above the standard of 500 ppm for a duration of ten minutes. In human beings, the odor threshold has been determined at 2.5 ppm (10 mg/m^3) and the sensory threshold at 480 ppm (1.9 mg/l). Biologic monitoring for exposure to toluene can be achieved by measuring the toluene level of the exhaled air and blood, and by measuring urinary hippuric acid excretion.[2, 34, 35, 39]

Medical Surveillance.—Comprehensive pre-employment and annual physical examination should be provided for all work-

TABLE 63–6.

Effects of Controlled Eight-Hour Exposures to Pure Toluene on Three Human Subjects*

CONCENTRATION	NUMBER OF EXPOSURES	EFFECTS†
0 ppm (control)	7	No complaints or objective symptoms
50 ppm	2	Mild headache (1)
100 ppm	4	Moderate fatigue (3)
200 ppm	3	Fatigue (3), muscular weakness (2), confusion (2), headache (2)
300 ppm	2	Severe fatigue (3), headache (2), muscular weakness (1)
400 ppm	2	Fatigue and mental confusion (3), headache (2)
600 ppm	1	Extreme fatigue, mental confusion, nausea, headache, and dizziness (3)
800 ppm	1	Severe fatigue and after 3 hours, pronounced nausea, confusion, lack of self-control, and staggering gait (3)

*Adapted from Oettingen WF von, Neal PA, Donahue DD: The toxicity and potential dangers of toluene—Preliminary report. *JAMA* 1942; 118:579. Also from Oettingen WF von, et al: The toxicity and special dangers of toluene with special reference to its maximal permissible concentration. *Public Health Serv Bull* 279, 1942.

†The number of subjects affected is noted in parenthesis.

ers exposed to toluene. Special attention should be focused on possible effects of toluene exposure on the skin, blood, liver, kidneys, and central nervous system. A complete blood count, routine urinalysis, and appropriate liver and renal function studies should be obtained. Each employee should be informed of the hazard of exposure to toluene and provided with proper clothing, eye protection, and an appropriate respirator when engineering controls are inadequate to prevent exposure above the TWA. Toluene-wet clothes should be changed promptly to prevent prolonged skin contact and fire hazard.

REFERENCES

1. Abshire AD, Hughes CS: *Chemical Economics Handbook, Marketing Research Report*. Menlo Park, Cal, Stanford Research Institute, 1982.
2. American Conference of Governmental Industrial Hygienists: *Threshold Limit Values for Chemical Substances and Physical Agents in the Workroom Environment*, with intended changes for 1986–1987. Cincinnati, Oh, ACGIH, 1986.
3. American National Standards Institute: *Acceptable Concentration of Toluene*, z37. 12-1967, New York, ANSI, 1968.
4. Åstrand I, et al: Toluene exposure. I. Concentration in alveolar air and blood at rest and during exercise. *Work Environ Health* 1972; 9:119.
5. Batchelor JJ: The relative toxicity of benzol and its higher homologues. *Am J Hyg* 1927; 7:276.
6. Bauchinger M, Schmid E, Dresp J, et al: Chromosome changes in lymphocytes after occupational exposure to toluene. *Mutat Res* 1982; 102:439.
7. Cier HE: Toluene, in Standen A (ed): *Kirk-Othmer Encyclopedia of Chemical Technology*, ed 2. New York, John Wiley & Sons, 1969, vol 20, p 528.
8. Erskine MG: *Chemical Economics Handbook, Organic Chemicals P-Z*, 696.503D. Menlo Park, Cal, Stanford Research Institute, 1967.
9. Evans EL, Mitchell AD: An evaluation of the effects of toluene on sister chromatid exchange frequencies in cultured Chinese hamster ovary cells. Prepared by SRI International, Menlo Park, Cal, under contract 88-02-2947 for the US Environmental Protection Agency, Research Triangle Park, NC, 1980.
10. Fabre R, Truhaut R, Laham S, et al: Toxicological research on substitute solvents for benzene—II. Study of toluene. *Arch Mal Prof* 1955; 16:197.
11. Ferguson T, Harvey WF, Hamilton TD: An inquiry into the relative toxicity of benzene and toluene. *J Hyg* 1933; 33:547.
12. Flunk ER, et al: Evaluation of DNS polymerase-deficient mutant of *E. coli* for the rapid detection of carcinogens. *JAMA* 1976; 241(16):1713.
13. Forni A, Pacifico E, Limonta A: Chromosome studies in workers exposed to benzene or toluene or both. *Arch Environ Health* 1971; 22:373.
14. Gafafer WM (ed): Acceptable concentrations of contaminants in workroom atmospheres, in *Manual of Industrial Hygiene*, US PHS. Philadelphia, WB Saunders Co, 1943.
15. Gerarde HW: *Toxicology and Biochemistry of Aromatic Hydrocarbons*. New York, Elsevier North-Holland, Inc, 1960.
16. Gibson JE, Hardisty JF: Chronic Toxicity and Oncogenicity bioassay of inhaled toluene in Fisher-344 rats. *Fundam Appl Toxicol* 1983; 3:315.
17. Girard R, Tolot F, Bourret J: Benzene hydrocarbons and serious blood diseases. *Arch Mal Prof* 1970; 31:625.
18. Greenburg L, Mayers MR, Heimann H, et al: The effects of exposure to toluene in industry. *JAMA* 1942; 118:573.
19. *Health Assessment Document for Toluene*, EPA-600/8-82-008. US Environmental Protection Agency, Office of Health and Environmental Assessment, 1982.
20. *Hygienic Guide Series, Toluene*. Akron, Oh. American Industrial Hygiene Association, Hygiene Guide Committee, 1957.
21. Litton Bionetics, Inc: *Teratology Study in Rats. Toluene*, LBI Project 20698-4. Final Report Submitted to American Petroleum Institute, Washington, DC. Kensington, Md, Litton Bionetics, Inc, 1978.
22. Manufacturing Chemists Association: *Chemical Safety Data Sheet SD-63, Toluene*. Washington, DC, Manufacturing Chemists Association, 1956.
23. Mortelmans KE, Riccio ES: In vitro. *Microbiological Genotoxicity As-*

says of Toluene. Prepared by SRI International, Menlo Park, Cal, under Contract 68-02202947 for the US Environmental Protection Agency, Research Triangle Park, NC, 1980.
24. National Institute for Occupational Safety and Health (NIOSH): *Criteria for a Recommended Standard: Occupational Exposure to Toluene*, USDHEW Publ (NIOSH) 73-11023. Washington, DC, US Government Printing Office, 1973.
25. *National Occupational Hazard Survey*. Cincinnati, USDHEW Publ (NIOSH) 74-127, 77-213, 78-114. National Institute for Occupational Safety and Health, 1978.
26. *National Occupational Exposure Survey*. Cincinnati, National Institute for Occupational Safety and Health, US Dept of Health and Human Services, 1983.
27. Nawrot PS, Staples RE: Embryo-fetal toxicity and teratogenicity of benzene and toluene in the mouse. *Teratology* 1979; 19:41A.
28. von Oettingen WF, Neal PA, Donahue DD: The toxicity and potential dangers of toluene—Preliminary report. *JAMA* 1942; 118:579.
29. von Oettingen WF, Neal PA, Donahue DD: The toxicity and special dangers of toluene with special reference to its maximal permissible concentration. *Public Health Serv Bull* 279, 1942.
30. Ogata M, Tomokuni K, Tokatsuka T: Urinary excretion of hippuric acid and m- or p-methylhippuric acid in the urine of persons exposed to vapors of toluene and m- or p-xylene as a test of exposure. *Br J Ind Med* 1970; 27(1):43.
31. Svirbely JL, Dunn RC, von Oettingen WF : The acute toxicity of vapors of certain solvents containing appreciable amounts of benzene and toluene. *J Ind Hyg Toxicol* 1943; 25:366.
32. Tatrai E, Hudak A, Ungvary C: Simultaneous effect on the rat-liver of benzene, toluene, xylene and CCL4. *Acta Physiol Acad Sci Hung* 1979; 53(2):261.
33. *Transactions of the Ninth Annual Meeting of the American Conference of Governmental Industrial Hygienists*. Cincinnati, Oh, ACGIH, 1947, p 44.
34. Wallén M, Holm S, Byfält Nordquist M: Coexposure to toluene and p-xylene in man: Uptake and elimination. *Br J Ind Med* 1985; 42:111–116.
35. Wallén H, Näslund P, Byfält Nordquist M: The effects of ethanol on the kinetics of toluene in man. ACGIH International Symposium on Occupational Exposure Limits, Copenhagen April 16–19, 1985. Cincinnati, ACGIH, 1986.
36. Weast RC (ed): *Handbook of Chemistry and Physics*, ed 52. Boca Raton, Fla, The Chemical Rubber Co, 1971.
37. Wilson RH: Toluene poisoning. *JAMA* 1943; 123:1106.
38. World Health Organization: *Toluene*. Environmental Health Criteria 52, Geneva, 1985.
39. Zenz C, Berg BA: The influence of submaximal work on solvent uptake. *J Occup Med* 1970; 12:367.
40. 1970 Chemical production data. *Chem Eng News* 1971; 49:12A.

Xylene

Joe A. DeLeon, M.D., P.A.

Xylene (xylol, dimethylbenzene, $C_6H_4(CH_3)_2$) is a highly flammable, clear, colorless liquid with a sweet, pungent odor. Commercial xylene is produced from the distillation of petroleum crude oil or coal tar. Three isomeric forms exist, ortho-, meta-, and para-xylene, but meta-xylene is the predominant isomer of commercial xylene. The isomers have distinct but similar physiochemical properties. Xylene is very soluble in alcohol and ether and insoluble in water. The volatility of xylene is much less than that of toluene and benzene. In addition to the three isomers, commercial xylene contains 6%–15% ethylbenzene and small quantities of benzene, toluene, and other contaminants.[28, 37]

Xylene is typically used as a chemical solvent in paint, lacquer, varnish, adhesives, ink, dye, cleaning fluids, as a fuel component, and as a chemical feedstock for the synthesis of chemicals, plastics, and synthetic textile fabrics. Xylene is also used as a solvent and emulsifier for agricultural products and in the manufacture of quartz crystal oscillators, hydrogen peroxide, perfumes, insect repellents, epoxy resins and pharmaceuticals, and in the leather industry.[37, 38] The NIOSH estimates that in the United States approximately 140,000 workers are potentially exposed to xylene.[37]

Possible toxic exposures may occur in pathology laboratories during routine histologic work;[4] however, there is disagreement as to the hazard.[6] One liter of xylene was improperly discarded in a sink in a pathology laboratory, causing an outbreak of xylene intoxication in a small community hospital.[16] Four laboratory technicians chronically exposed to xylene experienced chronic severe headaches, fever, malaise, leukopenia, chest pain, electrocardiographic abnormalities, dyspnea with impaired lung functions, cyanosis of the hands, decreased work performance, mental aberrations, and disability.[15]

HUMAN ABSORPTION, DISTRIBUTION, METABOLISM, ELIMINATION

The most important route of absorption of xylene is by inhalation, although absorption may occur by accidental eye or skin contact or by ingestion. Pulmonary retention of inhaled xylene ranges from 59% to 64% depending on the level of exposure and physical activity.[1, 2, 25, 26, 31] In 1970, Zenz and Berg[41] studied the uptake of trichloroethylene during submaximal treadmill exercise and noted an increased concentration in the expired air in relation to the intensity of the exercise. This important study demonstrates that augmentation of pulmonary ventilation and circulation by exercise increases absorption of a solvent. They emphasize that it is inadequate to consider only the ambient air concentration and the duration of exposure.

Åstrand et al.[2] also supports the view that physical activity is an important and necessary complement to the measurement of ambient air concentration of a solvent. They found that pulmonary retention was about 60% of the inhaled concentration and the ratio between the concentration in arterial blood and the alveolar air varies with physical activity. At rest the ratio was 15:1 and increased to 30–40:1 with different workloads. The blood xylene concentration increased about 1.5 times above the control level during exercise at a constant workload and exposure concentration. A simultaneous increase in concentration and workload increased the blood xylene concentration about three to four times more.

Percutaneous absorption of xylene is generally considered to be minimal and probably insufficient to produce systemic poisoning.[13] However, Dutkiewics and Tyras[8] demonstrated considerable absorption of liquid m-xylene applied to the forearm of man. The rate of absorption of m-xylene was calculated at 2.0 to 2.45 μg/sq cm/min.[15] Interestingly, one subject with a previous history of atopic dermatitis developed a toxic eczema postimmersion and revealed a threefold increase in absorption over the average for the group.[15] Two barrier creams applied as recommended by the manufacturers failed to prevent the percutaneous absorption of pure m-xylene.[18] Percutaneous absorption of solvent vapors from the ambient air through the undamaged skin appears to be insignificant.[23]

Absorbed xylene is transported in the blood mainly with the serum proteins and only a small portion in the red blood cells.[25] Xylene is very soluble in blood[29] and in lipids,[33] and adipose tissue has a high capacity to retain and accumulate xylene. The amount of xylene uptake was highly correlated to body fat, but a negative correlation between the concentration in adipose tissue and the degree of obesity was noted.[9] The estimated cumulated uptake of m-xylene in adipose tissue has been shown to vary from 3.7% to 8.0%.[10, 39]

The biotransformation of xylene is via a major and a minor pathway.[3, 17, 40] In the major pathway, one of the two methyl groups of xylene is oxidized to methylbenzoic acid (toluic) and conjugated with glycine to methylhippuric acid (toluric) before urinary excretion. This occurs mainly for m- and p-xylene. The o-xylene isomer is almost completely oxidized to o-tolyglucuronic acid before urinary excretion. In the minor pathway, the aromatic nucleus is hydroxylated to the corresponding o-, m-, p-xylenols (dimethylxylenols). The xylenols are excreted unchanged in the urine or undergo sulfate or glucuronic acid conjugation before urinary excretion.

Approximately 95% of the pulmonary retention of xylene undergoes biotransformation to methylhippuric acid.[31] Only about 5% of the xylene is exhaled unchanged and only a negligible amount is excreted in the urine unchanged.[31] The excretion of xylenols is approximately 1%–2% but may increase with physical activity. Percutaneous absorbed xylene was 80%–90% biotransformed and eliminated as methylhippuric acid.[11, 18]

Toxicity.—Xylene is a dermal irritant, and repeated or prolonged contact with the skin causes erythema, dryness, defatting, burning, blistering, cracking, and eventually a dermatitis.[3, 13] Xylene vapors may cause irritation of the eyes, nose, and throat, and conjunctivitis and corneal burns have been reported following direct contact with xylene.[13, 38]

Inhalation and ingestion of xylene may cause reversible hepatic and renal toxicity, severe abdominal distress with anorexia, nausea, abdominal pain, and vomiting if aspirated, chemical pneumonitis, pulmonary edema, and hemorrhage.[13, 19, 37, 38]

Xylene has a varied effect on the central nervous system and may elicit headaches, slight inebriation, dizziness, vertigo, drowsiness, irritability, insomnia, staggering, unconsciousness, coma, and a narcotic and anesthetic effect.[1, 27, 30, 37] One painter experienced an epileptic convulsion following an exposure to a solvent containing 80% xylene but was found to have normal reflexes and a normal electroencephalogram.[14] One fatality occurred among three shipyard painters exposed to xylene concentration at about 10,000 ppm in a poorly ventilated confined space. Two painters demonstrated mental confusion and retrograde amnesia after regaining consciousness.[19] A brief exposure to 300 ppm of xylene impaired the short-term memory and prolonged the reaction time whenever the subjects exercised, but did not, under similar conditions, when the subjects were sedentary.[12] Impairment to psychophysiologic performance corresponds to the rapid rise of blood xylene.[27] Slight exercise augments the adverse effects of xylene and tolerance develops at a constant concentration within a few days.[30] Forty-five employees manufacturing xylene from gasoline demonstrated that 20% suffered from "neuroasthenic syndrome," and 13% suffered from "autonomic vascular dysfunction."[35]

Hematopoietic and bone marrow toxicity previously attributed to xylene was probably related to benzene contamination of the xylene.[37] Minor hematologic disturbances have been reported in various animal species and in humans, but severe myelotoxicity has not been a feature of excessive xylene absorption.[36] To date, xylene has not been proven conclusively to be carcinogenic, mutagenic, teratogenic, or embryotoxic, except when maternal toxicity occurs.[7]

Industrial Hygiene and Biologic Monitoring.—In 1975, the NIOSH recommended for xylene exposure, a TWA of 100 ppm (435 mg/cu m) for a ten-hour work day, 40-hour workweek, with a ceiling concentration of 200 ppm (868 mg/cu m) as determined by a ten-minute sampling period.[37] The current OSHA standard for xylene was enacted in 1976 at 100 ppm.[20] The odor-threshold detection for xylene in air is 0.47 ppm, and in water, 2.12 ppm.[34] The odor-threshold has been determined at 1 ppm (4.5 mg/cu m).[5] Biologic monitoring has not been widely utilized, although the metabolites of xylene are well documented. Xylene can be determined in the expired air and blood by gas chromatography.[21, 22, 24, 32]

Medical Surveillance.—Comprehensive preplacement and biennial examinations should be provided for all workers exposed to xylene. Particular attention should be focused on possible effects on the skin, blood, central nervous system, gastrointestinal tract, liver, and kidneys. A complete blood count, routine urinalysis, and appropriate liver function studies should be obtained at the biennial examination. Air and biologic monitoring programs should be established at the worksites, and evaluated regularly. The worker should be informed of the hazard of exposure and provided with proper face and eye protection, proper clothing, and an appropriate respirator when industrial hygiene methods are inadequate to maintain the ambient air concentrations within the OSHA standard. Xylene-wet clothes should be changed promptly to avoid a fire hazard and prolonged skin contact.[37]

REFERENCES

1. *API Toxicological Review of Xylene*. New York, American Petroleum Institute, 1960.
2. Åstrand I, Engström J, Övrum P: Exposure to xylene and ethylbenzene. I. Uptake, distribution, and elimination in man. *Scand J Work Environ Health* 1978; 4:185–194.
3. Browning E: *Toxicity and Metabolism of Industrial Solvents*. New York, Elsevier North-Holland, Inc, 1965.
4. Bush CL, Nelson GE: Xylene—Dangers of its use in the histology and cytology laboratory. *Lab Med* 1977; 8:16.
5. Carpenter CP, Kinkead ER, Geary DL Jr, Sullivan LJ, King JM: Pe-

troleum hydrocarbon toxicity studies. V. Animal and human response to vapors of mixed xylene. *Toxicol Appl Pharmacol* 1975; 33:543–558.

6. Clark WE: Xylene hazards in perspective. *Am J Clin Pathol* 1978; 68:425–426.
7. Dean BJ: Genetic toxicology of benzene, toluene, and xylenes and phenols. *Mutat Res* 1978; 47:75–97.
8. Dutkiewics T, Tyras H: Skin absorption of toluene, styrene, and xylene by man. *Br J Ind Med* 1968; 25:243.
9. Engström J, Bjurström R: Exposure of xylene and ethylbenzene. II. Concentration in subcutaneous tissue. *Scand J Work Environ Health* 1978; 4:195–203.
10. Engström J, Riihimäki V: Distribution of m-xylene to subcutaneous adipose tissue in short-term, experimental human exposure. *Scand J Work Environ Health* 1979; 5:126–134.
11. Engström K, Husman K, Riihimäki V: Percutaneous absorption of m-xylene in man. *Int Arch Occup Environ Health* 1977; 39:181–189.
12. Gamberale S, Annwall G, Hultengren M: Exposure to xylene and ethylbenzene. III. Effects on central nervous system function. *Scand J Work Environ Health* 1978; 4:204–211.
13. Gerarde HW: *Toxicology and Biochemistry of Aromatic Hydrocarbons*. New York, Elsevier North-Holland, Inc, 1960.
14. Goldie I: Can xylene (xylol) provoke convulsive seizures? *Indian J Med-Surg* 1960; 29:33–35.
15. Hipolito RM: Xylene poisoning in laboratory workers: Case reports and discussion. *Lab Med* 1980; 1:593–595.
16. Klaucke DN, Johansen M, Vogt RL: An outbreak of xylene intoxication in the hospital. *Am J Ind Med* 1982; 3:173–178.
17. Latham S: Metabolism of industrial solvents. I. The biotransformation of benzene and benzene-substitutes. *Occup Health Rev* 1970; 21:24–28.
18. Lauwerys RR, Dath T, LaChapelle JM: The influence of two barrier creams on the percutaneous absorption of m-xylene in man. *J Occup Med* 1978; 20(1):17–20.

18a. Lauwerys R, Xylene, in Alessio L, Berlin A, Boni M, et al (eds): *Biological Indicators for the Assessment of Human Exposure to Industrial Chemicals*. Joint Research Centre Ispra Establishment (Varese), Italy, 1984.

19. Morley R, Eccleston GW, Douglas CP: Xylene poisoning: A report on one fatal case and two cases of recovery after prolonged unconsciousness. *Br Med J* 1970; 3:442–443.
20. *Occupational Safety and Health Standards*, Subpart Z—Toxic and Hazardous Substances, CFR, Title 29, Section 1910 93. Washington, DC, Occupational Safety and Health Administration, 1976.
21. Ogata M, Tomokuni K, Takatsuka Y: Urinary excretion of hippuric acid and m- or p-methylhippuric acid in the urine of persons exposed to vapours of toluene and m- or p-xylene as a test of exposure. *Br J Ind Med* 1970; 27:43–50.
22. Ogata M, Takatsuka Y, Tomokuni K: Excretion of hippuric and m- or p-methylhippuric acid in the urine of persons exposed to vapours of toluene and m- or p-xylene in an exposure chamber and in workshops, with specific reference to repeated exposures. *Br J Ind Med* 1971; 28:382–385.
23. Riihimäki V, Pfäffli P: Percutaneous absorption of solvent vapors in man. *Scand J Work Environ Health* 1978; 4:73–85.
24. Riihimäki V: Conjugation and urinary excretion of toluene and m-xylene metabolites in a man. *Scand J Work Environ Health* 1979; 5:135–142.
25. Riihimäki V, Pfäffli, Savolainen K: Pekari K: Kinetics of m-xylene and man: General features of absorption, distribution, biotransformation and excretion in repetitive inhalation exposure. *Scand J Work Environ Health* 1979; 5:217–231.
26. Riihimäki V, Pfäffli P, Savolainen K: Kinetics of m-xylene and man. Influence of intermittent physical exercise and change in environmental concentrations of kinetics. *Scand J Work Environ Health* 1979; 5:232–248.
27. Riihimäki V, Savolainen L: Human exposure to m-xylene. Kinetics and acute effects on the central nervous system. *Ann Occup Hyg* 1980; 23:411–422.
28. Sandmeyer EE: Aromatic hydrocarbons, Chapter 47 in Clayton GD, Clayton FE (eds): *Patty's Industrial Hygiene and Toxicology*, ed 3. New York, John Wiley & Sons, 1981, pp 3253–3431.
29. Sato A, Fujiwara Y, Nakajima T: Solubility of benzene, toluene, and m-xylene in various body fluids and tissues of rabbits. *Jpn J Ind Health* 1974; 16:30–31.
30. Savolainen K, Riihimäki V, Seppäläinen AM, et al: Effects of short-term m-xylene exposure and physical exercise on the central nervous system. *Int Arch Occup Environ Health* 1980; 45:105–121.
31. Sedivek V, Flek J: The absorption, metabolism, and excretion of xylenes in man. *Int Arch Occup Environ Health* 1976; 37:205–217.
32. Sedivek V, Flek J: Exposure tests for xylenes. *Int Arch Occup Environ Health* 1976; 37:219–232.
33. Sherwood RJ: Ostwald solubility coefficients of some industrially important substances. *Br J Ind Med* 1976; 33:106–107.
34. Stahl WH: *Compilation Odor and Taste Threshold Values, Data*. Philadelphia, American Society for Testing and Materials, 1973.
35. Suhanova VA, Makarivea LM, Boiko WI: Investigation of functional properties of leukocytes of workers engaged in manufacture of xylene. *Hyg Sanit* 1969; 34:448–452.
36. Swanson M, Cook R: *Drugs, Chemicals and Blood Dyscrasias*. Hamilton Ill, Drug Intelligence Publications, 1977.
37. US Dept of Health, Education, and Welfare: *Criteria for Recommended Standards for Occupational Exposure to Xylene*. Washington, DC, US PHS, National Institute for Occupational Safety and Health, Government Printing Office, 1975.
38. US Dept of Health, Education, and Welfare: *Occupational Diseases: A Guide to Their Recognition*, Publ 1097. Washington, DC, US PHS, US Government Printing Office, 1964.
39. Wallén M, Holm S, Byfält Nordquist M: Coexposure to toluene and p-xylene in man: Uptake and elimination. *Br J Ind Med* 1985; 42:111–116.
40. Williams RF: *Detoxication Mechanisms*. London, Chapman and Hall, 1959.
41. Zenz C, Berg BA: The influence of submaximal work on solvent uptake. *J Occup Med* 1970; 12:367–369.

Carbon Disulfide

Sanford Leffingwell, M.D., M.P.H.,

Carbon disulfide (CS_2) is used extensively to manufacture a variety of products. U.S. production increased from 200 million kg in 1948 to well over 450 million kg in 1970 but dropped to an estimated 323 million kg in 1977. Its greatest use is in the preparation of rayon viscose fibers. In the rubber industry, it is used as a solvent for sulfur, as a solvent for rubber cement, and also in the vulcanizing process. It has been used as an insecticide and in the chemical industries as a general solvent for such substances as phosphorus, fats and oils, resins, and waxes. Other uses include manufacture of lacquers and paints.

ABSORPTION, METABOLISM, EXCRETION

Carbon disulfide is absorbed chiefly through the lungs, entering the bloodstream and being distributed through the body. It can also be absorbed through the skin and is rapidly absorbed from the gastrointestinal tract if swallowed. People not previously exposed absorb about 80% of inhaled vapor during the first 15 minutes, but the proportion falls to about 40% after 45 minutes and remains at that level for some time. In workers previously exposed, about 55% of inhaled vapor is absorbed during the first 15 minutes. Excretion through the lungs and urine is small, with about 92% retained in the tissues and metabolized.[2]

Toxicity.—Among acute responses, the chief effect at very high concentrations (ranging from 200 to 500 ppm) is narcosis, which may result in respiratory failure and death. Exposures to lower concentrations (under 100 ppm) may have little or no evident immediate effect, but some workers may experience headache, dizziness, and some respiratory irritation, and gastrointestinal disturbances such as nausea, vomiting, and abdominal discomfort. Conjuctivitis and keratitis have been reported. Carbon disulfide has a distinct irritating or vesicant action on the skin.

The chronic effects of long-term exposure are of concern in carbon disulfide processes; since it is regarded as a very toxic substance.

Classic effects, such as those in the 1938 study by the Pennsylvania Department of Labor and Industry[24] are not often seen now, probably because exposure levels are usually much lower than 50 years ago. Chronic carbon disulfide intoxication can involve all parts of the central and peripheral nervous systems. There may be damage to cranial nerves, with a decrease in corneal and pupillary reflexes; a Parkinson-like syndrome can occur, characterized by speech disturbance, muscle spasticity, tremors, loss of memory, and even severe mental depression. Involvement of the peripheral nerves may be similar to a polyneuritic syndrome. Severe ocular disturbances have been observed. Gastrointestinal changes, including chronic gastritis, achlorhydria, and liver damage have been reported. There have been reports of individuals exhibiting symptoms of a presenile type of cerebral arteriosclerosis at an early age—from 40 to 55 years—after many years of exposure. Cerebral, renal, and myocardial sclerosis have been observed. Brieger[3] reported that actual knowledge of the developmental mechanism of the carbon disulfide atherosclerosis is fragmentary. The blood concentration of lipids, the inhibition of the lipolytic activity of the arterial wall, and the cholesterol content of the arterial wall resembled the findings in experimental atherosclerosis.

The medical literature has stressed the occupational risk of exposure to carbon disulfide and the development of mental illness among viscose rayon workers. In Mancuso and Locke's study,[15] a higher rate of suicides was found among 4,899 white men and women aged 25–64 years in certain departments and occupations. They postulated that delayed biologic effects of abnormal mental and social behavior may occur in subsequent years in response to further environmental and social stresses.

Savitz, working with the same cohort studied by Mancuso and Locke, found:

> In comparison to national rates, mental hospitalization was rarer than expected and criminal charges, accidents, suicide, and coronary heart disease were approximately equal to the expected level. . . . Comparisons within the cohort of rayon workers identified excess risk of behavioral abnormalities in departments and occupations having higher carbon disulfide exposures. . . . There was consistency across all of the outcomes (mental hospitalization, criminal charges, felonies, accident mortality, and suicide).[20]

The subtle effects of chronic exposure have been partially determined in the last decade. Coronary heart disease (CHD) associated with long-term exposure to carbon disulfide has recently been the main concern of occupational physicians in both Europe and the United States. Hernberg et al.[9, 10] and Tolonen[26] described excess mortality from coronary heart disease in viscose rayon workers exposed to carbon disulfide.

Hernberg et al. stated, "On the basis of these data, it was suggested that the Finnish TLV for CS_2 be reduced from 20 to 10 ppm. Naturally, the argument might be raised that our exposure data were too vague for such a decision, as we ourselves pointed out in 1970; however, in view of the potentially serious outcome of overexposure, it is prudent to be overcautious rather than the reverse. To find better documentation for the TLV, extreme importance is now attached to establishment of the threshold for the effects of CS_2 on CHD."

Goto et al.[5] showed frequent occurrence of microscopic aneurysms in the retina of exposed humans as revealed by flourescent angiography, finding such changes in 29% of Japanese workers exposed to carbon disulfide. Hotta and Savic[11] presented evidence that the pathogenesis of these changes may be the same as in cases of diabetes mellitus and that carbon disulfide has a slight diabetogenic effect. They also found that carbon disulfide has a toxic effect on the optic nerve, so that a considerable portion of the workers examined had a decreased adaptability to darkness and greater difficulty in discerning colors. By contrast, Raitta et al.[18, 19] found differences in peripapillary filling rate in the eyes of exposed workers and found that ocular arterioles and veins were larger in exposed workers, but overall rates of aneurysms were much lower in both exposed and comparison groups, and no effect of carbon disulfide on aneurysms could be detected. In 1976, Sugimoto et al. reported progression of retinopathy in the exposed group and regression of disease in workers removed from exposure.[22] A collaborative study between the Japanese and Finnish groups ruled out differences in protocol as an explanation for the differences in response of the two populations.[23] American workers have frequencies of aneurysms and hemorrhages intermediate between Japanese and Finnish workers. The prevalence of hemorrhages does correlate significantly with exposure.[16]

A number of studies have shown psychomotor effects[6, 7, 8, 14, 25, 27] and alterations in nerve conduction[4, 13, 21, 28, 29, 30] from carbon disulfide exposure. A recent NIOSH study found differences in the frequency with which workers generally exposed to less than 20 ppm carbon disulfide reported blurred vision, trembling of hands, memory difficulty, dizziness, insomnia, and fatigue and found differences in performance of a visual search task. But the study detected no differences in a number of other standardized tests of neurologic function. Small, but statistically significant, differences were found in some conduction velocities.[12, 17] (Refer to Chapters 54 and 55 for reproductive toxicity and Chapters 48, 49, and 50 for chronic neurologic effects.)

Medical and Hygienic Controls.—Prevention of exposure is essential. Workroom concentrations must not exceed 20 ppm (eight-hour TWA), the U.S. permissible exposure limit. The ACGIH has established a TLV of 10 ppm (eight-hour TWA). The NIOSH has recommended a standard of 1 ppm (eight-hour TWA).[16] Other nations have adopted standards lower than 20 ppm. Proper enclosures with adequate exhaust ventilation must be provided, since carbon disulfide is highly volatile. Regular hygienic surveys should be made in workplaces to ascertain concentrations and deviations from allowable limits. Periodic physical examinations of workers have been recommended and continued.

Analytic tests to determine carbon disulfide levels in blood, urine, and expired air are not recommended as a basis for monitoring a workplace. The urinary iodine-azide test, used in the past to augment environmental monitoring, does not correlate well with exposure levels below 20 ppm.[1] Temporary preventive measures are the use of air-supplied respirators and suitable protective equipment for the eyes and skin, e.g., solvent-resistant rubber gloves or aprons. If proper engineering controls are instituted and maintained, most persons can work safety with carbon disulfide.

REFERENCES

1. Boillat M-A: La reaction iode-azide en cas faible exposition au sulfure de carbone. *Soz Praventivmed* 1980; 25:203–204.
2. Boillat M-A: *The Use of the Iodine-Azide Test on Urine of Workers Exposed to Levels of Carbon Disulfide at or Below the Current [US] Federal Standard*. Masters thesis submitted to the University of Cincinnati, November, 1979.
3. Brieger H: Chronic carbon disulfide poisoning. *J Occup Med* 1961; 3:302–8.
4. Gilioli R, Bulgheroni C, Bertazzi PA, et al: Study of neurological and neurophysiological impairment in carbon disulfide workers. *Med Lav* 1977; 69:130–143.
5. Goto S, Hotta R, Sugimoto K: Studies on chronic carbon disulfide poisoning—Pathogenesis of retinal microaneurysm due to carbon disulfide, with special reference to a subclinical defect of carbonhydrate metabolism. *Int Arch Arbeitsmed* 1971; 28:115–26.
6. Hänninen H, Nurminen M, Tolonen M, et al: Psychological tests as indicators of excessive exposure to carbon disulfide. *Scand J Psychol* 1978; 19:163–174.
7. Hänninen H: Behavioral study of the effects of carbon disulfide, in Xintaras C, Johnson BL, deGroot I (eds): *Behavioral Toxicology*, Cincinnati, Oh, NIOSH, 1974, pp 73–80.
8. Hänninen H: Psychological picture of manifest and latent carbon disulfide poisoning. *Br J Ind Med* 1971; 28:374–381.
9. Hernberg S, Nurminen M, Tolonen M: Excess mortality from coronary heart disease in viscose rayon workers exposed to carbon disulfide. *Work Environ Health* 1973; 10:93–99.
10. Hernberg ST, Partanen CH, Nordman P, et al: Coronary heart disease among workers exposed to carbon disulfide. *Br J Ind Med* 1970; 27:313–325.
11. Hotta R, Savic S: Fluorescein angiography in ophthalmodynamometric study on carbon disulfide exposure. Presented at the Second International Symposium on Toxicology of Carbon Disulfide, Yugoslavia, Banja Koviljaca, May 1971, p 23.
12. Johnson BL, Boyd J, Burg JAR, et al: Effects on the peripheral nervous system of workers' exposure to carbon disulfide. *Neurotoxicology* 1983; 4(1):53–66.
13. Knave B, Kolmodin-Hedman B, Persson HE, et al: Chronic exposure to carbon disulfide: Effects on occupationally exposed workers with special reference to the nervous system. *Scand J Work Environ Health* 1974; 11:49–58.
14. Lilis R: Behavioral effects of occupational carbon disulfide exposure, in Xintaras C, Johnson BL, deGroot I (eds): *Behavioral Toxicology: Early Detection of Occupational Hazards*, HEW Publ (NIOSH) 74-126. Washington, DC, US Government Printing Office, 1974.
15. Mancuso TF, Locke BZ: Carbon disulfide as a cause of suicide. Epidemiological study of viscose rayon workers. *J Occup Med* 1972; 14:595–606.
16. NIOSH: *Health Effects of Exposure to Carbon Disulfide*. Cincinnati, Oh, National Institute for Occupational Safety and Health, 1984.

16a. Nurminen M, Hernberg S: Effects of intervention on the cardiovascular mortality of workers exposed to carbon disulphide: A 15-year follow up. *Br J Ind Med* 1985; 42:32–35.

17. Putz-Anderson VR, Albright BE, Lee ST, et al: A behavioral examination of workers exposed to carbon disulfide. *Neurotoxicology* 1983; 4(1):67–78.
18. Raitta C, Tolonen M, Nurminen M: Microcirculation of ocular fundus in viscose rayon workers exposed to carbon disulfide. *Albrecht V Graefes Arch Klin Exp Ophthalmol* 1974; 191:151–164.
19. Raitta C, Tolonen M: Ocular pulse wave in workers exposed to carbon disulfide. *Albrecht V Graefes Arch Klin Exp Ophthalmol* 1975; 195:149–154.
20. Savitz DA: *Behavioral Effects of Carbon Disulfide Exposure in Viscose Rayon Workers*. PhD Dissertation submitted to the University of Pittsburgh, 1982.
21. Seppäläinen AM, Tolonen M: Neurotoxicity of long-term exposure to carbon disulfide in the viscose rayon industry: A neurophysiological study. *Scand J Work Environ Health* 1974; 11:145–154.
22. Sugimoto K, Goto S, Hotta R: Studies on chronic carbon disulfide poisoning. A 5-year follow-up study on retinopathy due to carbon disulfide. *Int Arch Occup Environ Health* 1976; 37:233–248.
23. Sugimoto K, Goto S, Taniguchi H, et al: Ocular fundus photography of workers exposed to carbon disulfide. A comparative epidemiological study between Japan and Finland. *Int Arch Occup Environ Health* 1977; 39:97–101.
24. *Survey of Carbon Disulfide and Hydrogen Sulphide Hazards in the Viscose Rayon Industry*, Bull 46. Harrisburg, Pa, Dept of Labor and Industry, Occupational Disease Prevention Division, 1938.
25. Szymankova G: Observations on the effects of carbon disulfide on vision in workers engaged in the manufacture of synthetic fibers. *Klin Oczna* 38:41–44. Quoted in *Criteria for a Recommended Standard: Occupational Exposure to Carbon Disulfide*. NIOSH Report 77-156, 1968, p 70.
26. Tolonen M, Hernberg S, Nordman C, et al: Angina pectoris, electrocardiographic findings and blood pressure in Finnish and Japanese workers exposed to carbon disulfide. *Int Arch Occup Environ Health* 1976; 37:249–264.
27. Tuttle TC, Wood GD, Grether CB: *Behavioral and Neurological Evaluation of Workers Exposed to Carbon Disulfide*, Publ 77-128. Cincinnati, Oh, DHHS, National Institute for Occupational Safety and Health, 1977.
28. Tuttle TC, Wood GD, Grether CB: *Behavioral and Neurological Evaluation of Workers Exposed to Carbon Disulfide*, Report 77-128, Cincinnati, Oh, National Institute for Occupational Safety and Health, 1977.
29. Vanhoorne M: Preliminary study on toxicity of carbon disulfide and hydrogen sulfide in the Belgian viscose industry. *G Ital Med Lav* 1981; 3:57–68.
30. Vasilescu C: Sensory and motor conduction in chronic carbon disulphide poisoning. *Eur Neurol* 1976; 14:447–457.

Toluene Diisocyanate and Other Isocyanates

Teresa Schnorr, Ph.D.

David Egilman, M.D., M.P.H.

The diisocyanates and polyisocyanates may be considered together, since they have similar commercial applications and present similar toxicologic problems.

Isocyanates react with a wide variety of compounds containing active hydrogen atoms to produce such products as rigid or flexible foams, surface coatings, adhesives, rubbers, and fibers. Wide application of the products ranges from packaging, insulation materials, upholstery in automobiles, furniture and shoe soles. Most of the flexible foams are produced in large-scale operations in the form of slabs, blocks, or sheets, which, after curing, should contain no free isocyanates. Such operations generally are quite amenable to engineering controls. A significant proportion of the rigid polyurethane foams, however, is generated with portable equipment, or virtually no equipment at all, by mixing the polymerizing ingredients, resins, polyols, polyethers, emulsifiers, catalysts, water, and sometimes "frothing" or "blowing" agents on site and pouring them into the mold or structural cavity that is to be filled with the rigid foam.

Another method of application of rigid foam is by spraying the polymerizing ingredients immediately after mixing onto a surface that is to be coated with a layer of foam. In such situations, the problems of limiting concentration in the breathing zone are difficult.

Occupations with potential exposures are: abrasion-resistant rubber makers, adhesive workers, aircraft builders, insulation workers, lacquer workers, mine tunnel coaters, organic chemical synthesizers, plastic foam makers, plasticizer workers, polyurethane sprayers, polyurethane foam makers, ship burners, ship welders, spray painters, textile processors, upholstery makers and wire coating workers. The NIOSH has estimated the number of workers with potential exposure to be approximately 40,000. Vapor pressures have a particular importance in the assessment of the relative toxicity of different isocyanates, since the principal industrial hazard is a respiratory hazard arising from the inhalation of atmospheric isocyanate.

In addition, it should be borne in mind that isocyanates may enter the respiratory tract not only in the vapor phase but also as airborne dusts and aerosols.

TDI (TOLUENE DIISOCYANATE)

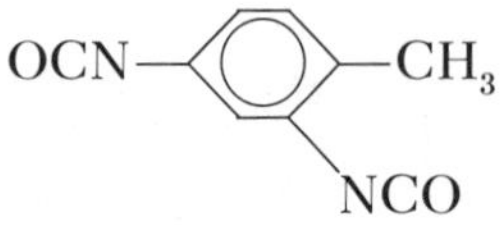

OCN—⟨benzene ring⟩—CH_3

NCO

TDI is manufactured from toluene diamine by reaction with carbonyl chloride (phosgene). Isocyanates are chemical compounds containing the N=C=O group. The two isomers most commonly used are 2,4-toluene diisocyanate and 2,6-toluene diisocyanate; commercially available are three isomer ratios: (1) 100% 2,4; (2) 80% 2,4:20% 2,6; and (3) 65% 2,4:35% 2,6.

TDI is the most widely used isocyanate, being utilized in almost all the applications in which isocyanates are used, as precursors in the production of polyurethanes, polyureas, polyamides, allophanates, and simple polymers of the isocyanates themselves. All these compounds are collectively referred to as "polyurethanes" or "polyurethane plastics." In 1979, an estimated 653 million lb of TDI was produced in the United States. Of the 475 million lb used domestically, nearly 90% was used in the production of polyurethane foams in the automobile and furniture industries.[24] Other uses include surface coatings, such as floor varnishes, sealants, and elastomers. Estimates from the National Occupational Hazards Survey indicate that between 50,000 and 100,000 workers are potentially exposed to diisocyanates.[18] TDI is highly volatile and has poor olfactory warning properties since its odor threshold of 0.4 ppm[30] is well above the OSHA ceiling limit standard of 0.02 ppm. With a vapor pressure of 0.05 atmospheres at 25° C, TDI can reach levels as high as 30 ppm in unventilated rooms; such concentrations are 1,500 times the OSHA standard. TDI is highly reactive. In the presence of reactive hydrogen, it reacts exothermally to form toluenediamine and to evolve carbon dioxide. The amine may react further with excess isocyanate to form a urea.[15] Polyurethane foams are produced by combining liquid polyhydroxy compounds and TDI, which polymerize to a cellular mass. The carbon dioxide evolved during the polymerization reaction can carry unreacted TDI, toluenediamine, and other byproducts into the atmosphere above the foam.[25]

Exposure Limits

The current OSHA standard for exposure to TDI of 0.02 ppm as a ceiling limit is based on the threshold limit value established by the American Conference of Governmental Industrial Hygienists in 1963. This exposure is based on a 1962 study by Elkins et al., which reported respiratory irritation and asthma-like symptoms in several plants where TDI concentrations were below 0.1 ppm, but none in plants where levels were below 0.07 ppm.[8] In a 1973 criteria document, the NIOSH recommended that an appropriate standard would be 0.005 ppm as a time-weighted average (TWA) with a ceiling limit of 0.02 ppm. These values are based on a careful review of the Elkins study[8] which revealed cases of respiratory illness below 0.01 ppm and upon another study[11] which found respiratory symptoms in workers after one week of exposure to TWA concentrations ranging from 0.03 to 0.07 ppm. More recent studies not included in the NIOSH criteria document present additional data which show that acute and chronic respiratory effects may occur at levels as low as 0.003 ppm, which is below the NIOSH recommended standard.[6, 17, 27, 29]

Acute Effects

At high concentrations, TDI causes irritation of the eyes, upper respiratory tract, and skin. The irritation, if severe, can lead to bronchitis and pulmonary edema, which may be fatal. Prolonged contact of liquid TDI with the skin can produce redness, swelling, and blistering.[19]

Exposure to TDI has produced acute effects ranging from a asthmalike response in nonsensitized individuals,[3, 8, 9] an asthmatic reaction in sensitized individuals,[1, 9, 31] and decreases in pulmonary function during a workshift.[10, 12, 26]

Among nonsensitized persons, the most well recognized acute response to TDI is an asthmalike reaction.[3, 9] The number of persons affected increases in a dose-dependent manner.[11, 25] Symptoms resemble those of an upper respiratory infection and may include chest tightness, chills, cough, fever, headache, wheezing, and shortness of breath. The onset of these symptoms can be delayed up to eight hours.[1, 3] The symptoms usually resolve within 24–48 hours.

Sensitization to TDI is defined as a tendency to be susceptible to the respiratory effects of TDI at concentrations much below those which affect most persons. The symptoms which develop in sensitized individuals are much the same as classical asthma, including dry cough, chest tightness, wheezing, and shortness of breath. Once sensitized, persons can exhibit symptoms at doses as low as 0.001 ppm.[5] Following development of this state, the worker usually cannot return to the workplace. Studies of occupationally exposed groups have found sensitization rates of 4% to 15%.[1, 5] Some people exhibit the sensitized allergic reaction upon first exposure to TDI, others may become sensitized to TDI years after initial exposure.[1, 28] Studies have found that neither atopy nor smoking served to identify persons at high risk of TDI sensitivity.[1, 28] It has generally been thought that sensitization occurs after brief exposure to high doses. However, sensitivity to TDI has been observed in workers with no known high exposures.[20, 29] One study found that sensitization occurred at a dose of 0.003 ppm among workers whose only exposure was in trimming and sewing polyurethane cushions.[29] Since the urethane foam was manufactured elsewhere, a possibility of accidental high exposures was unlikely.

The mechanism of asthma induced by TDI is not yet understood, and in fact, multiple mechanisms may be responsible for production of the syndrome. An immunologic basis for asthmatic reactions has received support because of the small number of workers sensitized, the variation in latent period between exposure and sensitization, and the markedly reduced threshold level which induces response in sensitized individuals. Possible immune mechanisms include IgE-mediated pathogenesis. Some investigators have found TDI-specific IgE antibody in sensitized workers.[13] However, other studies suggest that a pharmacologic mechanism is also involved, demonstrating that TDI interfered with pharmacologic-mediator control mechanisms in vitro.[4, 28] Weill[28] and Butcher[4] found no correlation between TDI-specific IgE antibody and TDI sensitivity, identifying IgE antibodies in only 15%–18% of sensitized workers.

TDI can produce loss of ventilatory capacity over a work shift in asymptomatic workers both at high concentrations (over 0.9 ppm)[10] and also at low levels (below 0.02 ppm[26] and 0.001 ppm[12]). Acute loss of forced expiratory volume (FEV_1) of 0.18 L over eight hours occurred in workers exposed to an estimated 0.9 ppm.[10] Among the same workers, no change in FEV_1 occurred on days when isocyanate processes were not in operation. Workers exposed to relatively low levels (0.013 ppm[26] and 0.001 ppm[12]) also showed significant loss of FEV_1 over a work shift. The implications of acute decline in pulmonary function on long-term ventilatory function have been the subject of several studies.[1, 6, 17, 21–23, 27, 28]

Chronic Effects

TDI may cause chronic respiratory impairment both in sensitized and nonsensitized persons. Sensitization to TDI may lead to long-term impairment in respiratory function. Men who had been removed from TDI exposure because of sensitization were found to have significantly lower than predicted FEV_1 values when tested 2–11 years after cessation of exposure.[1, 28] Because these were not longitudinal studies, these data are insufficient to determine if this decline in lung function is a continuing process or a fixed deficit.

TDI may cause development of chronic obstructive lung disease at low exposure levels in workers who are not sensitized. Several studies found that chronic exposure to TDI levels was associated with excess annual decline in ventilatory function.[6, 27, 21–23] Exposure levels in these studies ranged from TWAs of 0.0035 to 0.014 ppm with some excursions above the OSHA standard of 0.02 ppm ceiling limit. One of these studies noted a significantly greater decline in FEV_1 for those in the high exposure category compared to those in the lower category.[6] One study found a no-effect level for chronic decline in lung function at levels below 0.003 ppm.[17] Another study found no effect at levels near the OSHA standard. This study differed from the other studies in that symptomatic individuals were excluded.[1]

Mutagenicity and Carcinogenicity.—TDI causes frameshift and base-pair mutations when assayed using the Ames test.[2] Because metabolic activation is required, this effect is ascribed to the TDI amine analogue, 2,4 toluenediamine, formed during the hydrolysis of isocyanates. The formation of toluenediamine may occur when isocyanate vapors come in contact with moist surfaces, skin, or respiratory mucosa. Toluenediamine is a frameshift and base-pair mutagen[16] and has been shown to produce liver cancers in rats.[13a]

Two animal studies to evaluate the carcinogenicity of TDI have been conducted.[7, 14] A gavage study of rats found that TDI caused dose-related subcutaneous fibromas or fibrosarcomas in males and females, pancreatic acinar-cell adenomas in males, and pancreatic islet-cell adenomas, neoplastic nodules of the liver, and mammary gland fibroadenomas in females.[7] TDI caused hemangiomas or hemangiosarcomas and hepatocellular adenomas in female mice. It was not carcinogenic for the male mice.[7]

An inhalation study of rats and mice found no statistically

significant increase in tumor incidence.[14] However, exposure levels were quite low for an animal bioassay. The low and high exposure groups (0.05 ppm and 0.15 ppm) received doses similar to human occupational exposures in the 1960s (0.01–0.10 ppm).[3]

No epidemiologic studies of TDI workers have been published that examine the question of possible heightened cancer risk in exposed worker groups.

NDI (NAPHTHALENE DIISOCYANATE)

—NCO

OCN—

NDI is a solid isocyanate at room temperature that is used in the manufacture of urethane elastomers. It is relatively nonirritating to the skin in crystalline form. Having a low volatility, it is unlikely to present a vapor hazard unless heated, but at the elevated temperatures required for processing, the vapor pressure is such that a number of cases of respiratory sensitization due to contact with the heated material have been recorded.

MDI (DIPHENYLMETHANE DIISOCYANATE)

OCN— —CH_2— —NCO

MDI is an isocyanate that may vary in physical form, being produced either as a viscous liquid or as a solid material. It is extensively and increasingly used in the manufacture of polyurethane foams, adhesives, and solid urethane elastomers. It is also suitable for use in certain spray applications. Having a low volatility, it constitutes much less of a practical hazard than TDI and at room temperature can be handled without fear of a vapor hazard. When airborne spray droplets are inhaled, respiratory irritation and sensitization may result. The main toxic effect of MDI is the development of respiratory sensitization, leading to asthma and allergic bronchitis. The asthmatic response may be delayed several hours after the last exposure and a reduction in the FVC and FEV_1 may occur. At high levels, irritation to the nose and throat, chest tightness, and pain may occur. Sensitive individuals may also develop dermatitis. There are no specific diagnostic tests, although some physicians find hematocrit and white blood cell count, with differential cell count to determine eosinophils, to be useful to rule out infection or other allergies. The demonstration of isocyanate-specific antibodies in sera has been investigated as a possible biologic test of sensitization, but this test has not become standardized for routine use. There is no specific treatment.

TRIPHENYLMETHANE TRIISOCYANATE

This isocyanate, which usually is in liquid form as a 20% solution in methylene chloride, is used chiefly in bonding applications.

In general, its toxicity is comparable to that of MDI, but it is a more potent skin irritant because of the solvent. It usually contains a trace of free phenyl monoisocyanate, which may contribute to its irritant properties and frequently it is used in combination with other diisocyanates. It may constitute a respiratory hazard (as in the case of MDI) when used in spray applications.

POLYMETHYLENE POLYPHENYLISOCYANATE

This high molecular weight, low volatile polyisocyanate is a viscous liquid used chiefly in the manufacture of surface coatings, adhesives, and polyurethane foams. Polymethylene polyphenylisocyanate has a low order of hazard, since, in normal conditions of industrial use, vapor concentrations are unlikely to approach the TLV of 0.02 ppm. During spray operations, however, great care will be required to ensure protection against inhalation of airborne droplets (Figs 63–14 and 63–15). It does not appear to have any significant irritant properties in contact with the skin.

Polyurethane paints are those in which an organic isocyanate is used as a constituent. The most likely source of free isocyanate is the two-pack paint system, which separates the active isocyanate-containing catalyst from the inert base material. Respiratory problems have been reported from the use of single-pack moisture-cured surface coatings. Toluene diisocyanate, hexamethylene diisocyanate, diphenyl methane diisocyanate, and isophorone diisocyanate may be incorporated in polyurethane paint systems. The volatile isocyanates usually are modified to reduce their vapor pressure but always will contain a small percentage of residual free

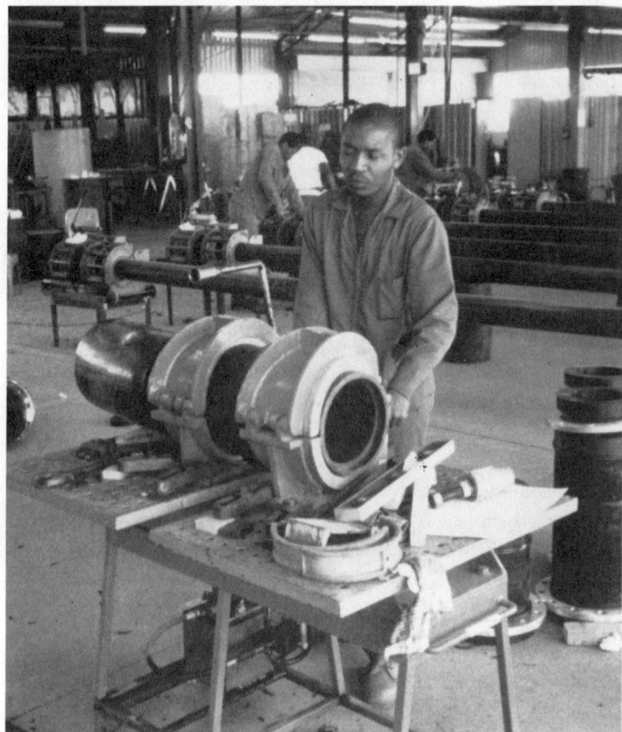

FIG 63–14.
Making special pipes and fittings of polyethylene. This involves hand cementing (see pages 749–750 for details of worker exposures).

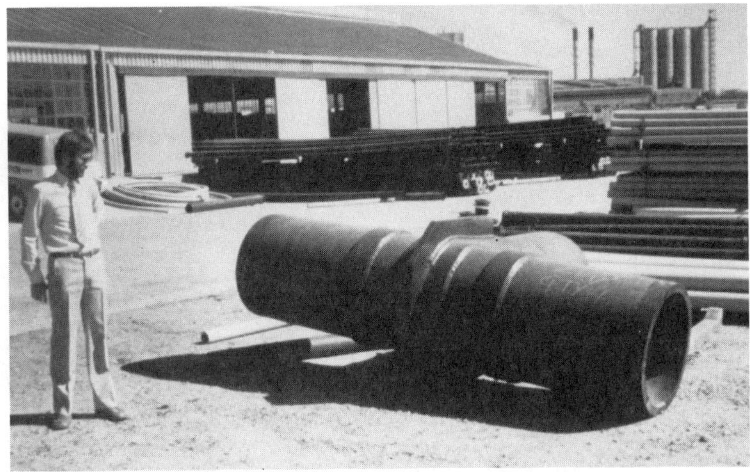

FIG 63–15.
Another example of the use of plastics for large pipes and valves.

volatile parent isocyanate (this usually is less than 0.7% residual isocyanate related to 100% of the polyisocyanate used as a catalyst in the paint system). A health hazard may arise from the inhalation of free volatile parent isocyanate when the paint is applied by brush at room temperature. A greater hazard, however, arises when the paint is spray-applied, for, in addition to the free parent isocyanate, the paint also contains a high proportion of nonvolatile isocyanate groups, which, although chemically combined in the paint, will cause respiratory problems if the paint spray is inhaled. An oronasal mask fitted with cartridges effective against dust and 1% organic vapors is satisfactory if the paint is applied by brush. A compressed-air-fed respirator should be worn if the polyurethane paint is spray-applied (Figs 63–16 and 63–17).

POLYURETHANE PREPOLYMERS

Prepolymers are manufactured by reacting a polyol with a molar excess of diisocyanate in the absence of water. The prepolymer itself, therefore, is a large molecule of very low volatility with reactive isocyanate groups at its ends. The commercial prepolymer, however, will contain traces of the diisocyanate used to make it, and this will be far more volatile. Prepolymers are used in the manufacture of semirigid and rigid foams, surface coatings, and elastomers. They are also used as binding agents in the manufacture of reconstituted polyether foam. Surface coatings with nonyellowing characteristics can be produced only from prepolymers based on aliphatic or alicyclic diisocyanates (methylene bis-4 cyclohexylene isocyanate, isophorone diisocyanate, or hexamethylene diisocyanate, etc.). It is possible to mask the isocyanate groups of diisocyanates or prepolymers by reacting them reversibly with other chemicals, e.g., phenolic compounds or tertiary alcohols. In this way, the free isocyanate is safely held in chemical combination until the masking is unblocked by heating or chemical displacement of the blocking agent with compounds containing more highly reactive hydrogen atoms. *Isocyanate prepolymers and marked isocyanates always should be handled with the same precautions as the isocyanate itself.*

Medical Surveillance

To prevent the development of serious pulmonary impairment, a medical surveillance program should be provided to TDI-exposed employees.

Comprehensive preplacement medical examinations should be given to each employee.[18] The examination should include a pul-

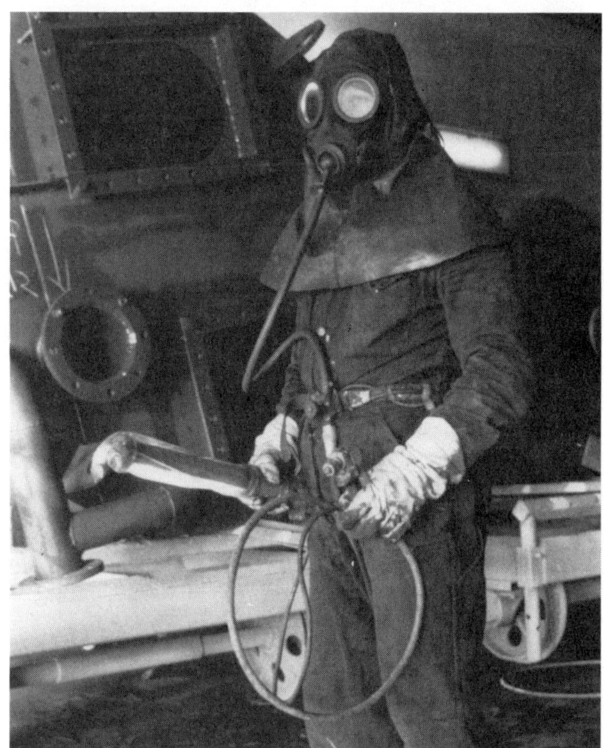

FIG 63–16.
A suitably equipped paint sprayer in a shipyard that uses acrylic, epoxy, and vinyl resins. (Courtesy of Thelma Aro, Institute of Occupational Health, Helsinki, Finland.)

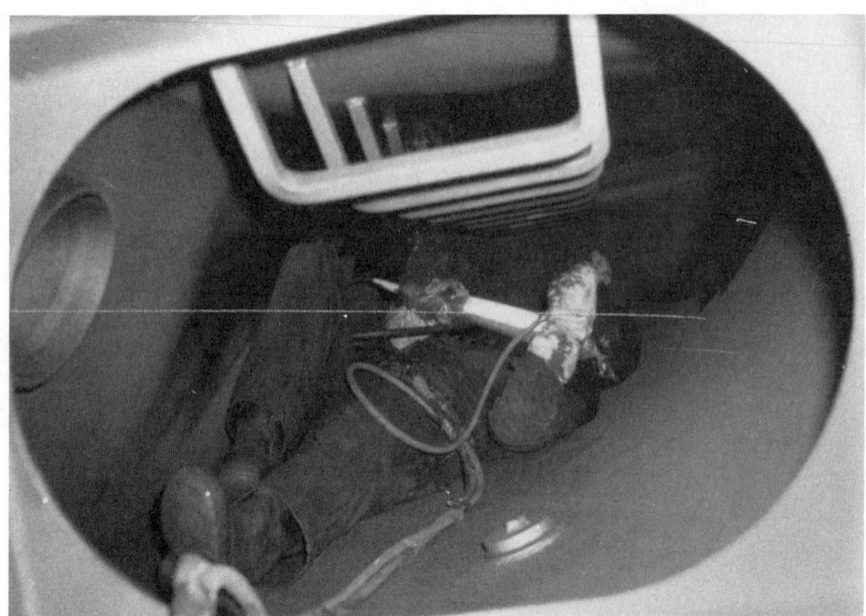

FIG 63–17.
Work in confined spaces of ships requires special and stringent health and safety controls. (Courtesy of Thelma Aro, Institute of Occupational Health, Helsinki, Finland.)

monary function test including FEV_1, FVC, and FEV_1/FVC, a history of diisocyanate exposure, smoking history, and history of respiratory conditions. The medical data obtained in the preplacement examination can be used as a base line for periodic examination. Periodic examinations may be useful in detecting a reduction in lung function. Lung function tests, pulmonary history, and pulmonary physical exam should be repeated at least annually. All medical records, including pulmonary function and related medical tests, should be maintained for 30 years.[18]

Any employee who begins to experience shortness of breath during a shift should be removed from work immediately and should not return to work until pulmonary function tests have returned to base line. As is the case with asthma of any type, pulmonary function recovery may lag behind symptom recovery and take up to eight weeks to return to normal. If sensitized, the individual should not return to work in a TDI area or work with any other isocyanate.

Industrial Hygiene Controls

Engineering controls should be used when needed to keep airborne levels of TDI below the NIOSH recommended standard of 0.005 ppm TWA.[18] As noted earlier in the chapter, respiratory effects have been observed at levels of exposure below both the OSHA standard and the NIOSH recommended standard (Fig 63–18).[21–23, 6, 17, 27, 29] These studies indicate that chronic respiratory effects occur at levels as low as 0.003 ppm.

Chemical cartridge respirators should not be used because isocyanates have poor olfactory warning properties.[18] Supplied air respirators should be used only during emergencies, during installation and testing of engineering controls, during spray painting with isocyanate-based paints, nonroutine maintenance or repair, or in confined spaces.[18] If a major spill occurs, the area should be evacuated immediately. Clean-up crews must wear air-supplied respirators, eye protection, and protective clothing.

Environmental monitoring should be routinely (at least every six months) conducted to determine whether there is occupational exposure to airborne TDI. These monitoring records should be kept for at least 30 years after the last exposure.[18]

Details for the protection of TDI-exposed workers are provided in the NIOSH Criteria Document on isocyanates.[18]

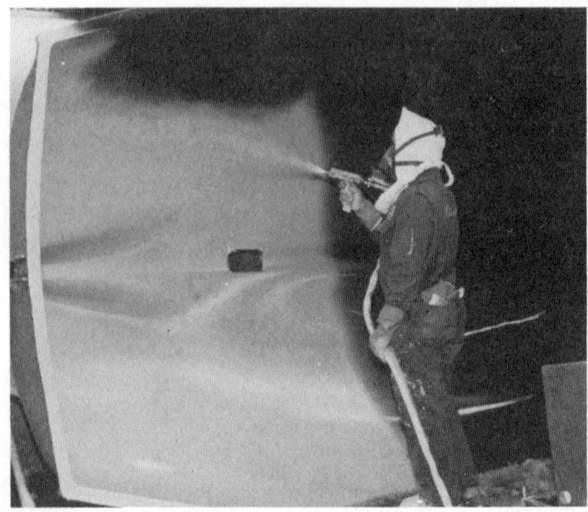

FIG 63–18.
Spray application of special coating. Worker has proper clothing and suitable respiratory protective equipment.

REFERENCES

1. Adams WG: Long-term effects on the health of men engaged in the manufacture of toluene diisocyanate. *Br J Ind Med* 1975; 32:72–78.
2. Anderson M, Binderup M, Kiel P, et al: Mutagenic action of isocyanates used in the production of polyurethanes. *Scand J Work Environ Health* September 1980; 6(3):221–226.
3. Brugsch HG, Elkins HB: Toluene diisocyanate (TDI) toxicity. *N Engl J Med* 1963; 268:353–357.
4. Butcher BT, Karr RM, O'Neill CE, et al: Inhalation challenge and pharmacologic studies of toluene diisocyanate (TDI)-sensitive workers. *J Allergy Clin Immunol* 1979; 64:146–152.
5. Carroll KB, Secombe CJP, Pepys J: Asthma due to non-occupational exposure to toluene (toluene) di-isocyanate. *Clin Allergy* 1976; 6:99–104.
6. Diem JE, Jones RN, Hendrick DJ, et al: Five-year longitudinal study of workers employed in a new toluene diisocyanate manufacturing plant. *Am Rev Respir Dis* 1982; 126:420–428.
7. Dieter MP: *NTP Technical Report on the Carcinogenesis Bioassay of Toluene Diisocyanate,* NIH Publ 82-2507. Research Triangle Park, NC, National Toxicology Program, August 1982.
8. Elkins HB, McCarl GW, Brugsch HG, et al: Massachusetts experience with toluene diisocyanate. *Am Ind Hyg Assoc J* 1962; 23:265–272.
9. Fuchs S, Valade P: Clinical and experimental study of several cases of intoxication by Desmodur T (toluene diisocyanate 1-2-4 and 1-2-6). *Arch Mal Prof* 1951; 12:191–196 (French).
10. Gandeiva B: Studies of ventilatory capacity and histamine response during exposure to isocyanate vapour in polyurethane foam manufacture. *Br J Ind Med* 1963; 20:204–209.
11. Hama GM: Symptoms in workers exposed to isocyanates—Suggested exposure concentrations. *AMA Arch Ind Health* 1957; 16:232–233.
12. Holness DL, Broder I, Corey PN, et al: Respiratory variables and exposure-effect relationships in isocyanate-exposed workers. *J Occup Med* 1984; 26:449–455.
13. Karol MH, Alarie Y: Antigens which detect IgE antibodies in workers sensitive to toluene diisocyanate. *Clin Allergy* 1980; 10:101–109.

13a. Ito N, Hiasa Y, Konishi Y, et al: The development of carcinoma in liver of rats treated with m-toluylenediamine and the synergistic and antagonistic effects with other chemicals. *Cancer Res* 1969; 29:1137–1145.

14. Loeser E: Long-term toxicity and carcinogenicity studies with 2,4/2,6 toluene-diisocyanate (80/20) in rats and mice. *Toxicol Lett* 1983; 15:71–81.
15. Lowe A: The chemistry of isocyanates. *Proc R Soc Med* 1970; 63:367–368.
16. McCann J, Choi E, Yamasaki E, et al: Detection of carcinogens as mutagens in the Salmonella/microsome test: Assay of 300 chemicals: Discussion. *Proc Nat Acad Sci* 1976; 73:950–954.
17. Musk AW, Peters JM, DiBerardinis L, et al: Absence of respiratory effects in subjects exposed to low concentrations of TDI and MDI. *J Occup Med* 1982; 24:746–750.
18. National Institute for Occupational Safety and Health: *Criteria for a Recommended Standard of Occupational Exposure to Diisocyanates,* Publ 78-215. US Dept of Health, Education and Welfare, NIOSH, September 1978.
19. *Occupational Diseases: A Guide to Their Recognition*. DHEW (NIOSH) Publ 77-181. Cincinnati, Oh, US Dept of Health, Education, and Welfare, National Institute for Occupational Safety and Health, 1977.
20. Pepys J, Pickering CAC, Breslin ABX, et al: Asthma due to inhaled chemical agents. *Clin Allergy* 1972; 2:225–236.
21. Peters J: Cumulative pulmonary effects in workers exposed to toluene diisocyanate. *Proc R Soc Med* April 1970; 63:372.
22. Peters J, Murphy R, et al: Respiratory impairment in workers exposed to "safe" levels of toluene diisocyanate. *Arch Environ Health* 1970; 20:364–367.
23. Peters J, Murphy R, et al: Ventilatory function in workers exposed to low levels of toluene diisocyanate. A six month follow-up. *Br J Ind Med* 1969; 26:115–120.
24. Stanford Research Institute: *Chemical Economics Handbook*. December 1980.
25. Walworth HT, Virchow WE: Industrial hygiene experiences with toluene diisocyanate. *Am Ind Hyg Assoc J* 1959; 20:205–210.
26. Wegman DH, Pagnotto LD, Fine LJ, et al: A dose-response relationship in TDI workers. *J Occup Med* 1974; 16:258–260.
27. Wegman DH, Peter J, et al: Chronic pulmonary function loss from exposure to toluene diisocyanate. *Br J Ind Med* 1977; 34:196–197.
28. Weill H, Butcher B, et al: Respiratory and immunologic evaluation of isocyanate exposure in the new manufacturing plant, NIOSH Contract 210-75-0006, Final Report, 1981.
29. White WB, Morris MJ, Sugden E, et al: Isocyanate-induced asthma in a car factory. *Lancet* 1980; 1(8171):756–760.
30. Wolf CR: *Isocyanates: Their Occupational Health Aspects*. Berkeley, Cal, Occupational Health Technical Information Service, Bureau of Occupational Health and Environmental Epidemiology, Dept of Health, 1970.
31. Woolrich PF: Toxicology, industrial hygiene, and medical control of TDI, MDI, and PMPPI. *Am Ind Hyg Assoc J* 1982; 43:89–97.

Butadiene

Vernon N. Dodson, M.D.

(1, Butadiene—$CH_2=CH-CH=CH_2$)

1-3 Butadiene (biethylene, bivinyl, butadiene, buta-1, 3-diene, alpha-gamma-butadiene, divinyl, erythrene, pyrrolylene, vinylethylene) is a liquid below 23.5° F and a colorless, irritating, flammable gas at higher temperatures. Approximately 4,000 million pounds of butadiene are manufactured in the United States; 78% is produced as a coproduct in the manufacture of ethylene, and 22% is produced by dehydrogenation of n-butene and n-butane. Styrene-butadiene rubber (SBR) and polybutadiene rubber (BR) account for the two largest uses in the U.S., primarily in the tire industry; polychloroprene (neoprene) rubber production ranks third. Other uses are in styrene-butadiene copolymer latexes used as carpet backing and paper coating materials; in acrylonitrile-butadiene-styrene (ABS) resins used to make high impact resistant pipes and parts for automobiles and appliances; in the production of nitrile rubber, adiponitrile/hexamethylenediamine for nylon, polybutadiene polymers, thermoplastic elastomers, and methyl methacrylate-butadiene-styrene and nitrile resins. As an intermediate, 1,3-butadiene is used in the production of various chemicals such as 1,4-hexadiene, 1,5-cyclooctadiene, and fungicides such as tetrahydrophthalic anhydride.[8] About 65,000 U.S. workers are exposed to butadiene, mostly at levels below 40 ppm, which is well below the TLV of 1,000 ppm, according to a recent NIOSH survey.[16] Despite the number of those employed, only a few intoxications have been reported from butadiene workers, organic chemical synthesizers, fuel handlers and makers, and synthetic rubber makers.[10] Since such workers are usually exposed to other agents simultaneously, their clinical features are multiple, mixed, and often confusing. The accrued medical experience in humans and animals suggests a relatively benign toxicity primarily irritation and narcosis even at 8,000 ppm.[10] Excessively high vapor concentrations can produce unconsciousness and death. Liquid skin contacts have produced frostbite.

ABSORPTION, METABOLISM, AND EXCRETION

Human experience and animal data readily attest to absorption of butadiene gas by inhalation. Few data are available for other portals of entry. Distribution is ubiquitous but by no means uniform. Fat tissues are favored. Shugaev and Yaroslavl[15] determined the LD_{50} to be 270 and 285 mg/L in mice and rats respectively. As an example of comparative tissue concentrations to controlled exposure of rats, they presented the figures shown in Table 63–7.

Narcosis effects paralleled brain concentrations. Animals in deep narcosis returned to normal coordination 1 hour after removal from butadiene exposure. No cumulative effects were demonstrated.

TOXICITY

Carpenter et al.[1] reported that the toxicity is not very great for man. Two humans exposed to 8,000 ppm displayed no greater narcosis than when exposed to 200 ppm of toluene. At high concentrations, humans note burning of the eyes and coughing. As the exposure continues, narcosis begins and is accompanied by headache, drowsiness, fatigue, and vertigo. Ultimately, loss of consciousness, respiratory paralysis, and death can occur, paralleling the effects observed in rats and mice. Physical examination reveals a lethargic, somewhat ataxic person with normal vital signs. There are no specific laboratory tests.

Checkoway and Williams[2] surveyed workers in a styrene-butadiene synthetic rubber manufacturing plant and found no pronounced evidence of hematological abnormality. Duverser et al.[6] studied the mutagenicity and metabolic activation of butadiene with other vinylic monomers using multiple micro-organism in vitro tests and found no certain or convincing evidence related to butadiene. A very significant study by Crouch et al.[3] exposed rats for 6 hours per day, 5 days per week, for 13 weeks at up to 8,000 ppm of 1,3-butadiene with no ill effects.

TABLE 63–7.
Controlled Tissue Concentrations of Butadiene (mg/100 ml)

BRAIN	LIVER	KIDNEY	SPLEEN	PERINEPHRIC FAT	HYPODERMIC FAT
50.8	51.4	36.3	45.0	152.1	—

Owen[12] exposed rats to butadiene by inhalation to concentrations from 1,000 ppm to 8,000 ppm 6 hours per day, 5 days per week, for 2 years and found benign and malignant tumors at various sites, including testicular Leydig adenomas in the males, and thyroid mammary and uterine adenomas, carcinomas, and sarcomas in the females. A corroboration and extension of these observations was made by Powers[14] in mice exposed by inhalation over 61 weeks. Early evidence by Owen[13] in pregnant rats exposed to 200 ppm to 8,000 ppm of butadiene by inhalation resulted in retarded fetal growth and significant major skeletal defects.

It is recommended that 1,3-butadiene be regarded as a potential occupational carcinogen, teratogen, and as a possible reproductive hazard. Consequently, appropriate engineering and work practice controls should be used to reduce worker exposure. These recommendations are based on long-term animal studies that demonstrated carcinogenicity, teratogenicity, and adverse effects on the testes and ovaries.[4]

The ACGIH included 1,3-butadiene in their *Notice of Intended Changes* for the 1985–1986 threshold limit values, based upon reported animal carcinogenicity data. The *Notice* identified 1,3-butadiene as an industrial substance suspect of carcinogenic potential for man with a TLV of 10 ppm.

The present NIOSH-OSHA standards of 1,000 ppm TLV stands, but will be reexamined in the near future.

REFERENCES

1. Carpenter CP, et al: Studies on the inhalation of 1,3-butadiene with a comparison of its narcotic effect with benzol, toluol, styrene, and a note on the elimination of styrene by the human. *J Ind Hyg* 1944; 26:69.
2. Checkoway H, Williams TM: A hematology survey of workers at a styrene-butadiene synthetic rubber manufacturing plant. *Am Ind Hyg Assoc J* 1982; 43:164–169.
3. Crouch CN, Bullinger DH, Gaunt IF: Innovation toxicity studies with 1,3 butadiene: II. 3 month toxicity study in rats. *Am Ind Hyg Assoc J* 1979; 40:796–802.
4. *Current Intelligence Bulletin 41: 1,3-Butadiene*. Publication no. 84-105, Cincinnati, National Institute for Occupational Safety and Health, 1984.
5. Dieter MP: *NTP Technical Report on the Carcinogenesis Bioassay of Toluene Diisocyanate*. NIH Publication no. 82-2507, National Toxicology Program, Research Triangle Park, NC, 1982.
6. Duverser M, Lambotte M, Malvoisin E, et al: Metabolic activation and mutagenicity of four vinylic monomers. *Toxicol Eur Res* 1981; 3:131–140.
7. Ito N, Hiasa Y, Konishi Y, et al: The development of carcinoma in liver of rats treated with m-toluylenediamine and the synergistic and antagonistic effects with other chemicals. *Cancer Res* 1969; 29:1137–1145.
8. Killilea TF: *CEH Marketing Research Report on Butadiene*. SRI Chemical Economics Handbook. SRI International, Menlo Park, Calif, pp 300, 5800A-300.5803U, 1979.
9. Loeser E: Long-term toxicity and carcinogenicity studies with 2,4/2.6 toluene-diisocyanate (80/20) in rats and mice. *Toxicol Lett* 1983; 15:71–81.
10. Mackison FW, Stricott RS, Partridge LJ, Jr: *Occupational Health Guidelines for Chemical Hazards*. US DHHS, USPHS, CDC, NIOSH and USDL, OSHA January 1981; DHHS (NIOSH) Publication no. 81, 123.

11. McCann J, Choi E, Yamasaki E, et al: Detection of carcinogens as mutagens in the *Salmonella*/microsome test: Assay of 300 chemicals: Discussion. *Proc Nat Acad Sci* 1976; 73:950–954.
12. Owen PE: The toxicity and carcinogenicity of butadiene gas administered to rats by inhalation for approximately 24 months. Final Report. Volumes 1–4, Addendum. Unpublished report submitted to The International Institute of Synthetic Rubber Producers, Inc. by Hazleton Laboratories Ltd., Harrogate, England, November 1981.
13. Owen PE, Irvine LFH: 1,3-Butadiene: Inhalation teratogenicity study in the rat. Final Report. Unpublished report submitted to The International Institute of Synthetic Rubber Producers, Inc. by Hazleton Laboratories, Harrogate, England, November, 1981.
14. Powers M: Board Draft on NTP technical report on the toxicology and carcinogenesis studies of 1,3 butadiene (CAS No. 106-99-0) in B6C3F mice (inhalation studies). NTP-83-071/NIH Publication no. 84-2544. U.S. Department of Health and Human Services, Public Health Service, National Institutes of Health, National Toxicology Program, October 28, 1983.
15. Shugaev BB, Yaroslavl BS: Concentration of hydrocarbons in tissues as a measure of toxicity. *Arch Environ Health* 1969; 18:878.
16. Sundin DS: Workers potentially exposed to 1,3 butadiene. Unpublished data available from U.S. Department of Health, Education and Welfare, Public Health Service, National Institute for Occupational Safety and Health, Division of Surveillance, Hazard Evaluations and Field Studies, National Occupational Hazard Survey data base, Cincinnati, data collected 1972–1974.

4,4°-Methylene-bis-(2-chloroaniline)

Elizabeth Ward, M.S., Ph.D.

Cl Cl

NH_2—⟨ring⟩—CH_2—⟨ring⟩—NH_2

4,4°-Methylene-bis-(2-chloroaniline) (MBOCA) is an aromatic amine used commercially as a curing or hardening agent for certain castable polyurethane elastomers (such as tires, gaskets, belts, and rollers) and polyurethane surface coatings. MBOCA manufacture in the United States peaked between 5.5 and 7.7 million lb in the early 1970s. U.S. production ceased in 1979. However, 0.5 to 3.5 million lb are estimated to be imported each year.[3] Estimates of the number of U.S. workers potentially exposed to MBOCA range from 1,400[1] to 33,000,[12] in an estimated 500[1] to 2,868[12] worksites. In general, fewer than ten workers are estimated to be exposed directly to MBOCA at any particular facility.[7] MBOCA is purchased either as solid pellets or as a prepolymer solution. MBOCA has a low vapor pressure (less than 0.000036 mm Hg at 100° C). Workplace exposures are therefore primarily related to dust generated in the manual handling of solid MBOCA prior to mixing it with polyurethane prepolymers.[3] The primary route of absorption is thought to be percutaneous, since there is little or no correlation between MBOCA levels measured in workroom air and MBOCA levels in the urine of exposed workers.[9]

TOXICITY

Case reports have documented urinary frequency, hematuria,[11] and transient inability to reabsorb low molecular weight proteins and concentrate urine[6] among exposed workers. While MBOCA produces methemoglobinemia in rats and dogs,[13] cyanosis has not been observed among MBOCA-exposed workers. MBOCA is weakly carcinogenic in mice and strongly carcinogenic in rats[8, 18] and dogs.[19] The target organs for tumor induction differ by species, being the liver in mice,[16] the lung, liver, and mammary gland in rats,[8, 18] and the urinary bladder in dogs.[19] There have been no adequate epidemiologic studies from which to assess MBOCA's carcinogenicity in human beings. However, based on its carcinogenicity in several animal species, and the concordance between bladder tumor induction by structurally similar aromatic amines in dogs and humans,[19] MBOCA is considered to be a potential human carcinogen whose most likely target organ is the urinary bladder.

Exposure Limits.—A standard promulgated in 1974[2] by OSHA, regulating MBOCA as a carcinogen, was remanded for procedural errors.[20] The Court did not dispute the scientific basis for the standard or its provisions. After the MBOCA standard was remanded, OSHA continued to issue citations for MBOCA exposure under the general duty clause of the Occupational Safety and Health Act, holding that the prior existence of a comprehensive standard had raised MBOCA to the level of a "recognized hazard." However, three such citations for employee MBOCA exposure were overturned in Occupational Safety and Health Review Commission judgments,[17] based on the argument that use of the general duty clause for MBOCA was an attempt to impose the vacated MBOCA standard without following the procedural requirements of the Occupational Safety and Health Act regarding promulgation of health standards. Except for the state of California, workplace MBOCA exposure is unregulated at this time.

In 1978, NIOSH recommended that occupational exposure to MBOCA be limited to 3 μg/cu m of workroom air, as a ten-hour time-weighted average. This was the lowest level considered to be reliably measurable. In practice, however, workplace monitoring by air-sampling of MBOCA has not proved to be useful, since surface contamination and appreciable dermal exposures may occur in the absence of detectable air levels.[9] Wipe sampling has also been used for compliance purposes by the state of Michigan OSHA. Wipe samples have limited value for compliance purposes, however, because of the difficulty in designing standard sampling protocols. The NIOSH has also recommended that urinary monitoring be used to assess percutaneous MBOCA absorption.[13] Urinary monitoring for MBOCA has been incorporated in the state California standard and is widely accepted by the U.S. polyurethane manufacturing industry. Commercial laboratories offer a semiquantitative assay for MBOCA using thin-layer chromatography.[5] The NIOSH has developed a gas chromatographic assay which detects MBOCA in urine at levels as low as 1 μg/L.[15] There is considerable uncertainty, however, about what urinary MBOCA concentration should be considered a "safe" level. The relationship between MBOCA exposure, absorption, and urinary excretion in human beings is unknown, since the assays measure parent

MBOCA, not its metabolites. Parent MBOCA is known to be less than 1% of total MBOCA excreted in the urine of rats and dogs.[4, 10]

Industrial Hygiene and Medical Surveillance.—MBOCA-exposed workers should be informed of its known animal and suspected human carcinogenicity. Control guidelines recommended by the NIOSH for handling MBOCA in the workplace include engineering controls to keep air levels below the NIOSH-recommended exposure limit; wearing of protective clothing (gloves, aprons, boots, and overshoes) made of butyl rubber, neoprene, or spun-bonded olefin; and use of air-supplied or self-contained respiratory protection for nonroutine operations. The NIOSH has developed a method for MBOCA air measurement.[14] Periodic medical screening of MBOCA-exposed workers should include annual urine analysis for hematuria and cytology, with referral to a urologist if there is the suspicion of bladder malignancy.

REFERENCES

1. Centaur Associates, Inc: *Economic and Market Analysis of MOCA and the Polyurethane Industry*. Contract 68-01-6412, task order 8, Office of Toxic Substances, US Environmental Protection Agency, Washington, DC, August 1982.
2. Dept of Labor, Occupational Safety and Health Administration: Carcinogens. Occupational Health and Safety Standards. *Federal Register* 39:(20) pt III (Jan 29) 1974.
3. Environmental Protection Agency: *Risk Assessment on MBOCA (4,4′-Methylene-bis-(2-chlorobenzamine)*. Washington, DC, Office of Toxic Substances, US Environmental Protection Agency, 1983.
4. Groth DW, Wiegel WW, Tolos WP, et al: 4,4′-Methylene-bis-(ortho-chloroaniline) (MBOCA): Absorption and excretion after skin application and gavage. *Environ Res* 1984 (in press).
5. Health Evaluation Programs, Inc. 808 Busse Hwy, Park Ridge, Ill.
6. Hosein HR, Van Roosmalen PB: Acute exposure to methylene-bis-orthochloroaniline (MOCA). *Am Ind Hyg Assoc J* 1978; 39:496–497.
7. JRB Associates, Inc: Final draft report: *Phase II Study of 4,4′-Methylene-bis-(2-chloroaniline)*, prepared for the US Dept of Labor.
8. Kommineni C, Groth DH, Frockt IJ, et al: Determination of the tumorigenic potential of methylene-bis-orthochloroaniline. *J Environ Pathol Toxicol* 1979; 2(5):149–171.
9. Linch AL, O'Conner BG, Barnes JR, et al: Methylene-bis-ortho-chloroaniline (MOCA): Evaluation of hazards and exposure control. *Am Ind Hyg Assoc J* 1971; 32:802–810.
10. Mannis M, Braselton E: Pharmacokinetics of MBOCA in dogs, in *MBOCA—Research Results and Recommendations for Environmental and Occupational Levels*. Lansing, Mich, Michigan Toxic Substance Control Commission, 1982.
11. Mastromatteo E: Recent occupational health experiences in Ontario. *J Occup Med* 1965; 1:502–511.
12. National Institute for Occupational Safety and Health: *National Occupational Hazards Survey*, Publ DHEW (NIOSH) 77-114. Cincinnati, Oh, US Dept of Health, Education, and Welfare, Public Health Service, 1977.
13. National Institute for Occupational Safety and Health: *Special Hazard Review with Control Recommendations for 4,4′-Methylene-bis-(2-chloroaniline)*, Publ DHEW (NIOSH) 78-118. Cincinnati, Oh, US Dept of Health, Education, and Welfare, Public Health Service, 1978.
14. National Institute for Occupational Safety and Health: *Manual of Analytical Methods*, ed 2, vol 1, P & CAM 236, Publ DHHS (NIOSH) 77-157A. Cincinnati, Oh, US Dept of Health, Education, and Welfare, Public Health Service, 1977.
15. National Institute for Occupational Safety and Health: *Manual of Analytical Methods*, ed 2, vol 1, P & CAM 342, Publ DHHS (NIOSH) 77-157A. Cincinnati, Oh, US Dept of Health, Education, and Welfare, Public Health Service, 1977.
16. Russfield AB, Homburger F, Boger E, et al: The carcinogenic effect of 4,4′-methylene-bis-(2-chloroaniline) in mice and rats. *Toxicol Appl Pharmacol* 1975; 31:47–54.
17. Secretary of Labor, V Kastalon, Inc, and Conap, Inc, Consolidated OSHRC Docket Nos 79-3561 and 79-5543. Aug 26, 1982. Brief of the Secretary of Labor.
18. Stula EF, Sherman H, Zapp JA Jr, et al: Experimental neoplasia in rats from oral administration of 3,3′-dichlorobenzidine, 4,4′-methylene-bis-(2-chloroaniline), and 4,4′-methylene-bis-(2-methylaniline). *Toxicol Appl Pharmacol* 1975; 31:159–176.
19. Stula EF, Barnes JR, Sherman H, et al: Urinary bladder tumors in dogs from 4,4′-methylene-bis-(2-chloroaniline) (MOCA). *J Environ Pathol Toxicol* 1977; 1:31–50.
20. *Synthetic Organic Chemical Manufacturers Association vs. Brennan*. Third Circuit Court of Appeals. 506 F 2d 385, 1974.

Styrene

Carl Zenz, M.D.

Louis S. Beliczky, M.S., M.P.H.

$$H_2C{=}CH{-}C_6H_5$$

Styrene, or vinylbenzene, is one of the most widely used chemicals, with the highest production nearing 7,500 million pounds in the United States in 1979 and 6,600 million pounds in 1981. Styrene is a liquid with a low vapor pressure (2.34 mm Hg at 10° C [50° F] to 14.30 mm Hg at 40° C [104° F] and has a low odor threshold (<1 ppm). First successful production was begun by I. G. Farbenindustrie in 1925 and by the Dow Chemical Company in 1930 (Fig 63–19).

Most styrene is produced by the catalytic dehydrogenation of ethyl benzene, but styrene has also been produced as a coproduct with propylene oxide. In this latter process, ethyl benzene is first oxidized to its peroxide, then reacted with propylene, yielding propylene oxide and alpha-methylphenyl carbinol; the carbinol is dehydrated to styrene. Nearly all of the ethyl benzene used in styrene production in the U.S. is obtained by on-site alkylation of benzene with ethylene. A small amount (10–15 ppm) of p-tert-butyl catechol is added to the styrene monomer to prevent spontaneous polymerization. (See specific chapters on different metals and their compounds utilized as catalysts for these reactions.) This vast production is the greatest single use of benzene (50% of world capac-

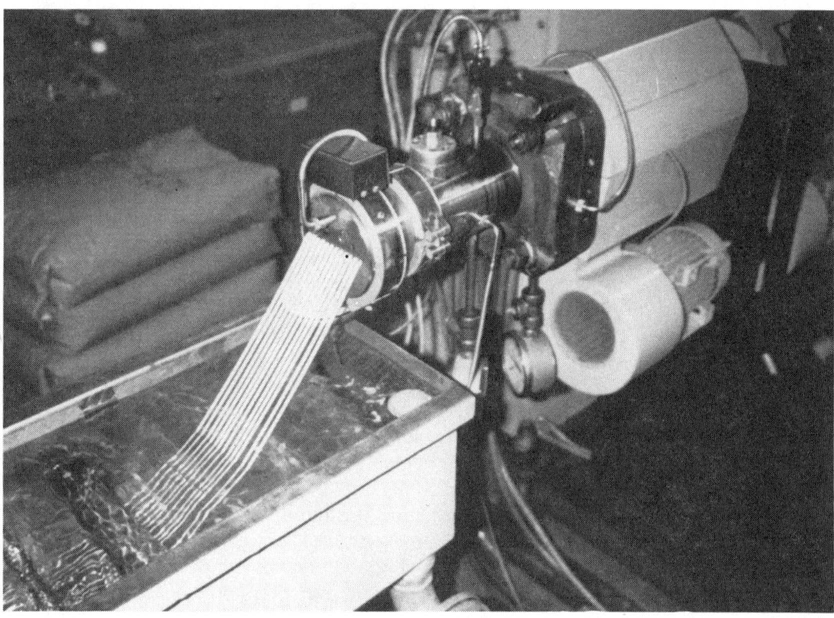

FIG 63–19.
Continuous polystyrene extruding (into water bath).

ity) and the third greatest use of ethylene next to polyethylene and polyvinyl chloride production. About 62% is consumed in polystyrene production, 22% in copolymers such as styrene-acrylonitrile (SAN) and acrylonitrile butadiene styrene (ABS), 7% in styrene-butadiene rubber (SBR), 7% in unsaturated polyester resins, and 2% miscellaneous uses (see Table 63-8 for the different uses of styrene).

Considerable quantities of styrene are used in spraying and hand rolling of styrene-modified polyester plastics with fiberglass reinforcement in manufacturing boats of all sizes, swimming pools, and various large and small containers. Much manufacturing goes on in small factories, especially in the numerous shops for boat-building that often employ women in these semiskilled activities (Figs 63–20 and 63–21). It is estimated that more than 1 million workers, worldwide, are exposed to detectable styrene concentrations.

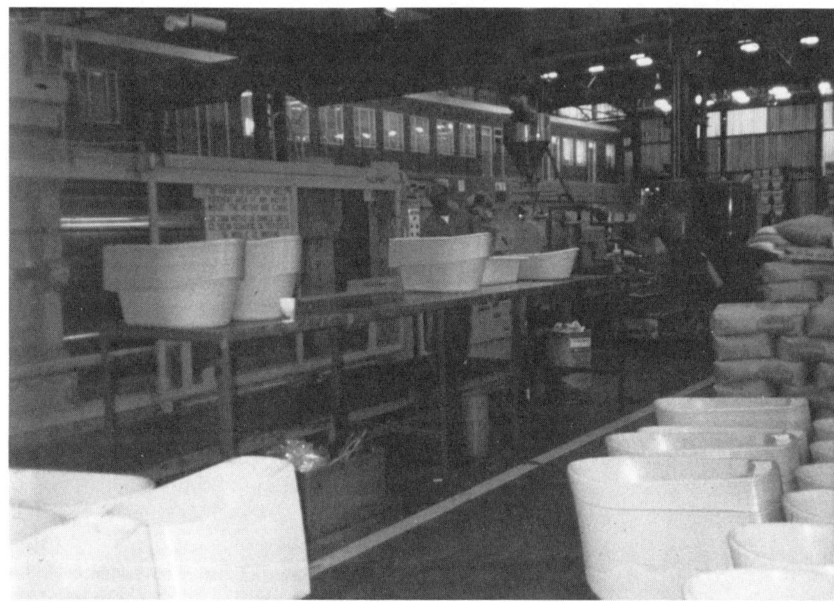

FIG 63–20.
Polystyrene tub production. The tubs are produced in various colors.

TABLE 63–8.
Typical Uses of Styrene*

Polystyrene	Audio and video cassettes, brushes, combs, disposable dinnerware, drain pipes, eyeglasses, food containers, furniture parts, games, hobby kits, housings for room air conditioners, insulation board, light diffusers, loose-fill packaging, molded shutters, picnic coolers, room dividers, shower doors, small hand-held appliances, television cabinets, toys, tubing, soap dishes, watering cans
Acrylonitrile butadiene styrene (ABS)	Automotive components (instrument panels, consoles, front radiator grilles, headlight housings, etc.), conduit, hobby kits, luggage and cases, margarine tubs, pipefittings, piping (drain, waste, and vent), radio chassis, refrigerator doorliners and food compartments, shower stalls and bathroom fixtures for mobile homes, telephones, toys
Styrene-acrylonitrile (SAN)	Battery cases, blender jars and covers, dishes, drinking tumblers, instrument panel lenses
Styrene-butadiene latexes	Binder for felt base or vinyl floor tile, binder for paper coatings, cement additive, component of latex paints, tufted carpet and upholstery backcoatings
Other copolymers	Ion-exchange resins (divinylbenzene-modified polystyrene), paints, paper coatings, and floor polishes (styrene-acrylic copolymer emulsions), footwear and adhesives (styrene block copolymers)
Styrene-butadiene rubber (SBR)	Passenger car tires, industrial tubing and hoses, conveyer belts, appliance parts, wire and cable insulation, footwear, coated fabrics, car bumpers, weatherstrips, additive in cements and adhesives
Unsaturated polyester resins (reinforced plastics/composites)	Boats, open storage tanks, recreational vehicles, truck camper tops, tub and shower units, wall panels

*Adapted from Criteria for a Recommended Standard: Occupational Exposure to Styrene. DHHS (NIOSH) Publication No. 83-119. Cincinnati, National Institute for Occupational Safety and Health.

MAIN POTENTIAL OCCUPATIONAL EXPOSURES

As noted in Figures 63–22 through 63–31, styrene has enjoyed early and heavy use in boat building for diluting polyester resins during construction, especially for the laminating stages of the fiberglass-reinforced-polyester resin (FRP). The resin system used in the FRP boat industry is a mixture of styrene monomer, glycols (propylene glycol or diethylene glycol), phthalic anhydride or isophthalic anhydride, maleic anhydride, and inhibitors. Handling of resins after manufacture does not produce other than trace level-exposure to these chemicals, since they are substantially converted to polyester. The styrene content in the resin is approximately 40% (by weight), and it is both a reactant and a diluting solvent. During spraying and hand lay-up, 10% to 15% of the styrene can evaporate into the workplace air. The remainder is consumed in the reaction. The hardening system used may contain a cobalt salt (cobalt haphthenate) as an initiator and a hydroperoxide (methyl ethyl ketone peroxide [MEKO] or benzoyl peroxide) as a catalyst. Acetone is the only other compound likely to be present in high concentrations in the vapor phase, as it is heavily used as a solvent for cleaning tools, spraying equipment, and workers' hands. Because of the small size of many shops, control measures such as adequate ventilation may be insufficient for economic and technical reasons.

In a reinforced plastics fabrication plant, Götell et al.[31] found 8-hour time-weighted average (TWA) concentrations of 235–292 ppm. Based on the extensive Swedish factory studies, Götell et al. judged skin absorption to be low. In a later study of a reinforced plastic factory, Brooks et al.[11] reinforced this finding, noting that workers wearing gloves and protective clothing with a respiratory device did not have more protection than the use of respiratory protection alone. Their study did not show any major contribution of percutaneous absorption to the body burden in these workers.

The National Institute for Occupational Health and Safety (NIOSH) undertook an extensive industrial hygiene study of seven FRP boat manufacturing plants scattered throughout the United States.[25] This study was designed to quantitate worker exposure patterns and work categories involving styrene monomer (exposure to acetone was also measured). Four hundred sixty-four personal air samples were collected, and 96 of these were found to be above the Occupational Safety and Health Administration (OSHA) eight-hour TWA (100 ppm). The exposures across all plants were substantially variable, ranging from 2 to 183 ppm. Most exposures predominated in a few plants. It was shown that the mean expo-

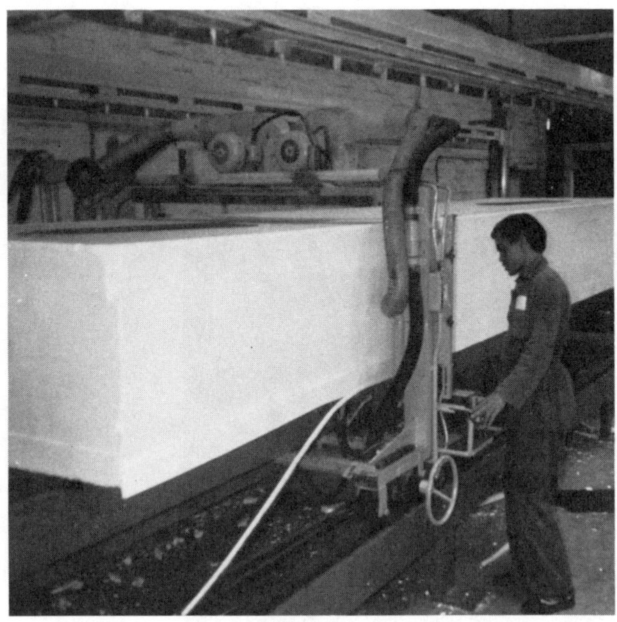

FIG 63–21.
Trimming a large polystyrene block that will be used in building, packaging, or insulation.

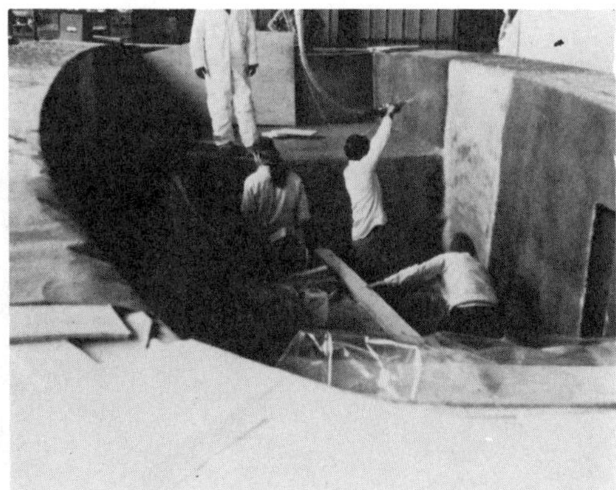

FIG 63–23.
Young men and women building the large boat hull shown in Figure 63–22, using fiberglass polyester resins. Boat builders use from 41% to 44% styrene in these laminating stages that is mostly hand applied. Exhaust ventilation and respiratory protective equipment are absent.

sures for the major job categories of hull, deck, small parts, and gelcoat were different from each other and that the magnitude of these averages followed resin consumption patterns (styrene exposure is proportional to the amount of catalyzed resin used in the job). When chopper and hand lay-up counterparts in the hull, deck, and small parts categories were compared, the results were mixed. Exposures were not consistently higher for either task, and seemed to be related to the divison of labor between them in the particular plant.

It was demonstrated by the survey results that for some plants dilution ventilation techniques could adequately control exposure to styrene and application of local exhaust ventilation in two plants could be practical.

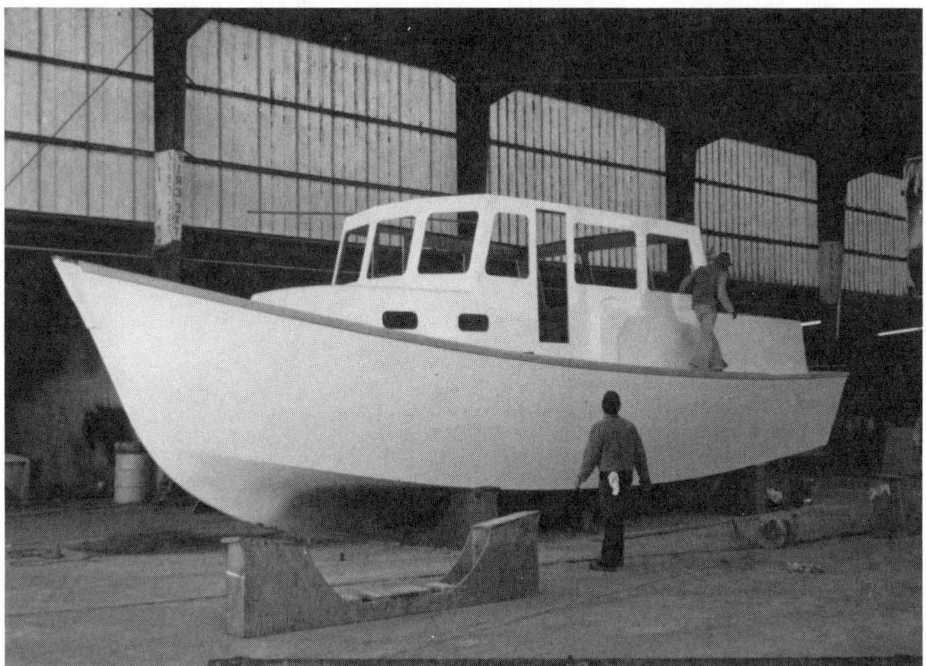

FIG 63–22.
A boat of the trawler type made almost entirely of fiberglass and polyester resins using styrene as a major component.

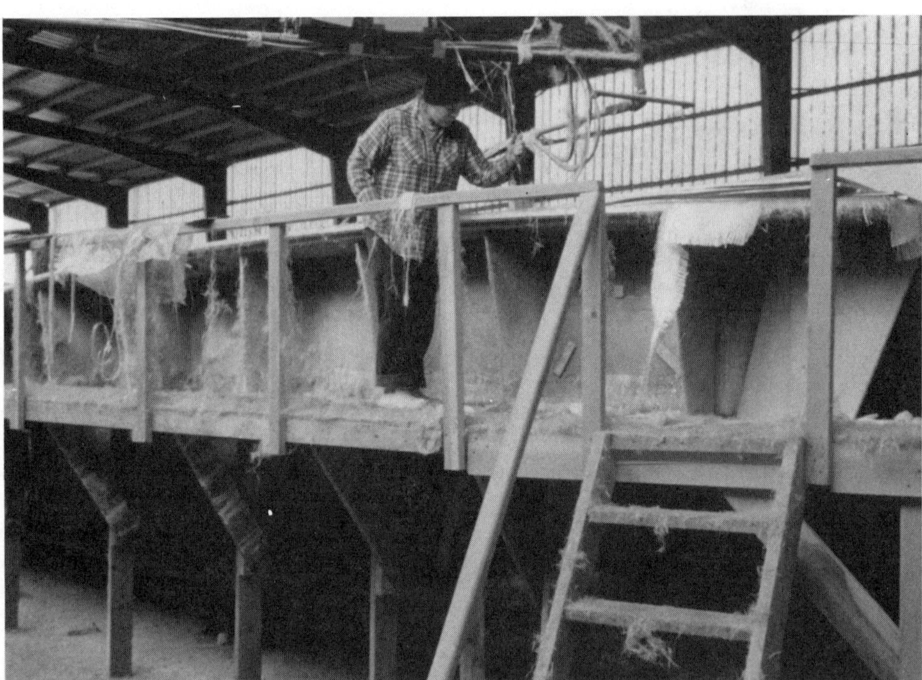

FIG 63–24.
Young woman building the hull of the trawler shown in Figure 63–22.

UPTAKE, METABOLISM, STORAGE, AND ELIMINATION

Styrene is readily absorbed by inhalation, and skin absorption has been shown to occur, more with the liquid than vapor. After inhalation, retention in the body is reported to be from 60% to 75%. In humans, styrene is excreted mainly in urine as metabolites, but some lung excretion occurs. Styrene is metabolized with formation of hippuric acid as a main metabolite in the rabbit but styrene glycol and mandelic acid are also found in the urine. Experiments with subcutaneous injections of radioactive styrene in rats showed styrene to be rapidly metabolized and, to the greater

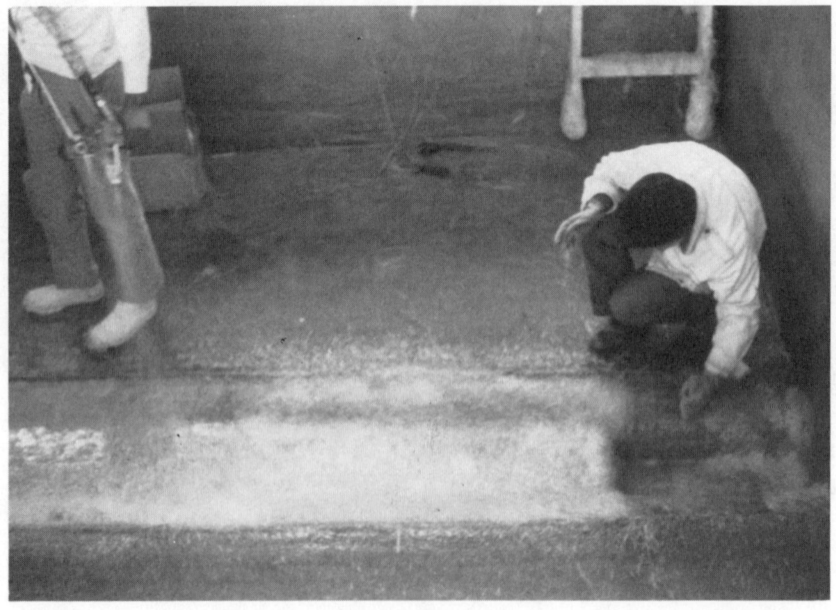

FIG 63–25.
Applying layers of fiberglass polyester diluted with styrene. No respiratory protection used.

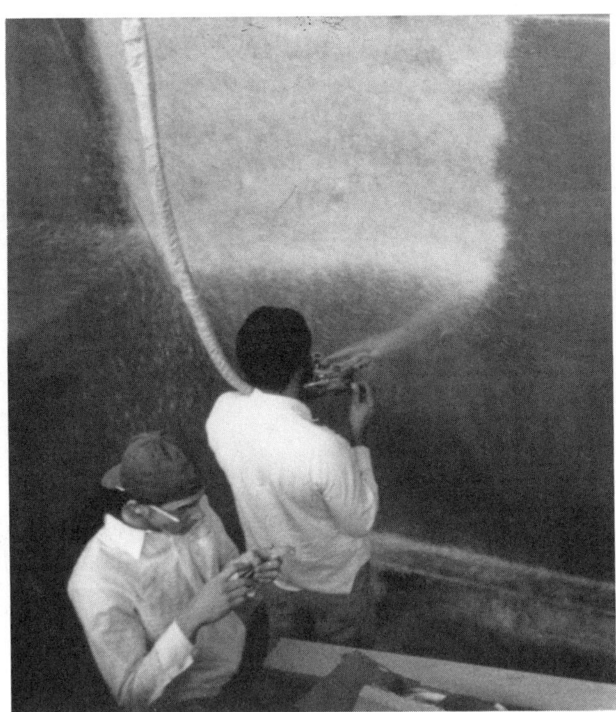

FIG 63–26.
Applying layers of fiberglass polyester diluted with styrene. No respiratory protection used.

extent, recovered as follows: 71% of the radioactivity appeared in the urine, 12% as respiratory CO_2 and 3% was exhaled unchanged through the lungs.[17] Based on animal studies, mice, human volunteers, and factory workers, the principal biotransformation as shown in Figure 63–32 has been proposed.[77]

O
CH—CH$_2$

Styrene oxide

Styrene is converted by liver microsomes to its epoxide, styrene oxide, which is further metabolized by epoxide hydratase to styrene glycol.[77] In humans, however, styrene metabolism seems to be somewhat different, at least from a quantitative point of view. Thus, human studies have revealed mandelic acid and phenylglyoxylic acid to be the major metabolites, whereas hippuric acid has not been found to increase,[6] and similar results have been obtained in several investigations.[7, 70] At high exposure levels, however, some formation of hippuric acid also seems to occur in humans,[43] as was proposed previously,[12] although the "hippuric acid branch" seems to be of minor importance in humans. This is also indicated in inhalation studies,[6] as 60% of inspired styrene (at 22 ppm) was found to be retained in the respiratory tract. Of this amount, 85% was metabolized to mandelic acid and some 10% to phenylglyoxylic acid. These metabolites may be used for

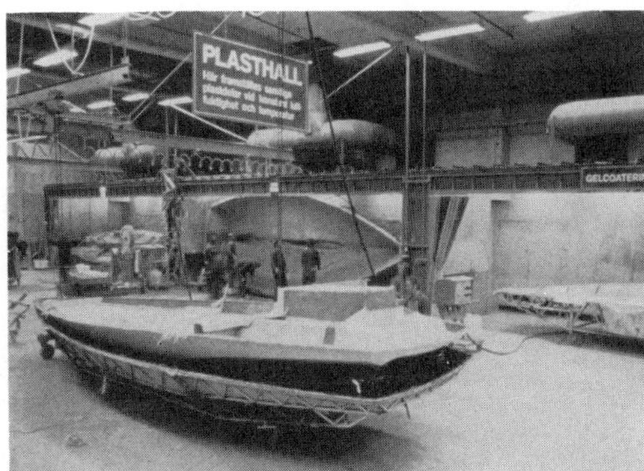

FIG 63–27.
A modern plastic boat-building factory. Note extensive exhaust system. (Courtesy of Mr. Håkan Widman, Mölnycke Marin, Mariestad, Sweden.)

surveillance of styrene exposure, as proposed by several authors.[6] Although Bardodej and Bardodejova[7] proposed 1,500 ppm of mandelic acid to correspond to exposures of workplace levels of 50 ppm of styrene and 3,000 ppm to correspond to 100 ppm, studies on workers by others[31] have suggested 1,000 ppm of mandelic acid in urine in the afternoon to correspond to an 8-hour TWA exposure of 50 ppm styrene and 2,000 ppm to correspond to 100 ppm of styrene in the air. (These values for mandelic acid refer to urine adjusted to a specific gravity of 1.024.) At exposures above 150 ppm TWA for 8 hours there seem to be uncertain relationships between concentration of styrene in the air and mandelic acid as well as phenylglyoxylic acid in the urine; i.e., the metabolites perhaps should be considered in the light of the possible range of exposure.[31] Similar experiences have been encountered in animal studies (rats), as mandelic acid shows a good correlation with styrene exposure up to about 100 ppm in the air during 8 hours.[43] Above this styrene concentration, however, the excretion of mandelic acid forms a plateau, whereas hippuric acid continues to increase with increasing styrene exposure. As workload increases, the absorption of styrene and (possibly the excretion of mandelic acid) will vary with performance of the worker.[5] The relationship between styrene exposure and mandelic acid excretion given above refers to moderate or light work.

Engström et al.[23] determined the uptake, distribution, and elimination of styrene in male subjects, with special reference to storage in cutaneous adipose tissue, exposing seven men to styrene vapor concentrations of 210 mg/m^3 (50 ppm) in inspired air, using a bicycle ergometer to simulate work intensities of 50, 100, and 150 watts. (Exposures were 30 minutes at rest and three 30-minute periods at work.) Styrene was found to be highly soluble in blood and tissues, and the equilibrium between concentrations in arterial blood and alveolar air was not achieved during short-term exposure. The mean uptake was 490 mg, corresponding to 63% of the amount inspired. Respiratory elimination of styrene 19 hours after exposure revealed that about 3% of the styrene was retained in the body during exposure. Needle biopsies of subcutaneous adipose tissue were made before exposure and ½, 2, 4, and 20–24 hours after exposure in all subjects. In four of the subjects, biopsies were obtained 1 to 2 weeks after exposure to styrene. The concentrations of styrene in adipose tissue were determined by gas chromatogra-

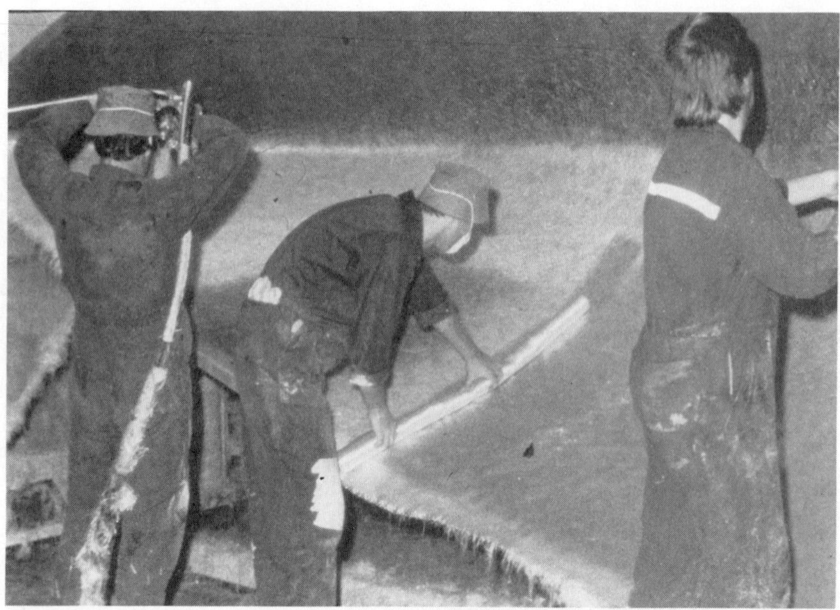

FIG 63–28.
Extensive hand work in applying the many layers of fiberglass in boat building; see Fig 63–29.

phy after evaporation into nitrogen at a high temperature. Twenty-four hours after exposure ceased, the mean concentration of styrene in adipose tissue was at about the same level as 2 to 4 hours after exposure, i.e., about 3.5 mg/kg. Of considerable interest was that the retention of styrene in adipose tissue was found as late as 13 days after this short experimental exposure at a concentration in inspired air that closely corresponds to the Swedish TLV (40 ppm). Engström and coworkers estimated the half-life of the concentration of styrene in adipose tissue to be about 2 to 4 days, despite the rapid metabolism of styrene, and they considered oc-

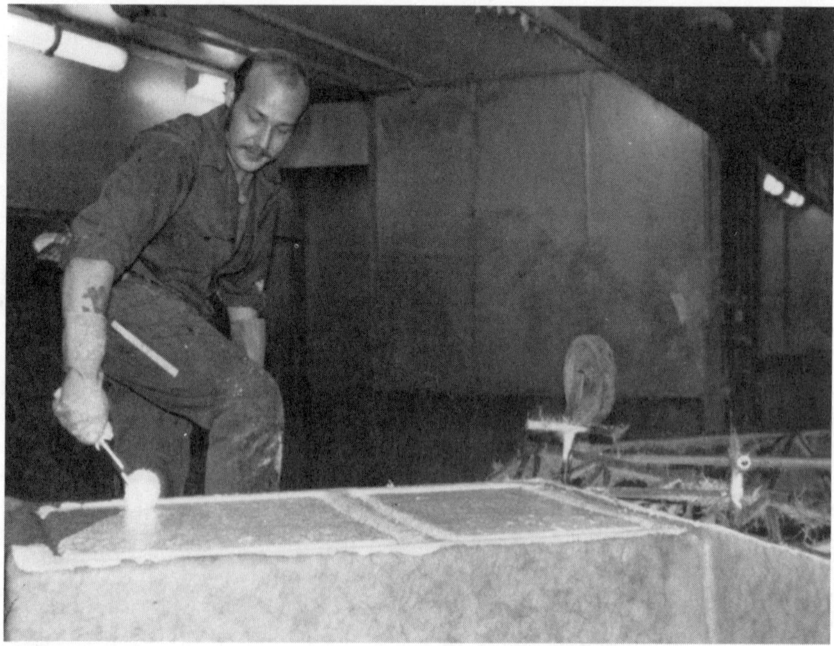

FIG 63–29.
Application of the many layers of fiberglass in boat building involves extensive hand work.

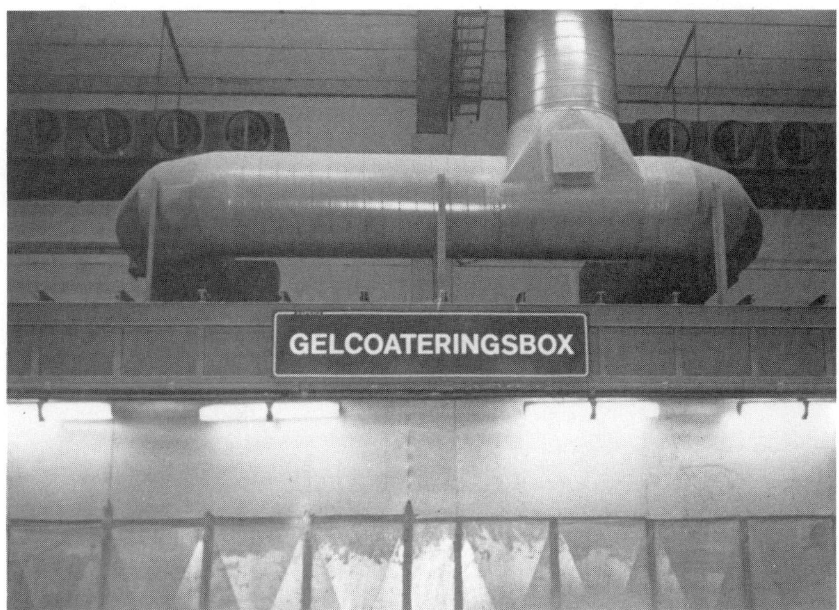

FIG 63–30.
Close-up of massive ventilating system in factory shown in Figure 63–27.

cupational exposure to be accompanied by a risk of accumulation of styrene in adipose tissue because of the slow elimination. Clearly, the results of these investigations focus on a reorientation of the concepts of the absorption, metabolism, and excretion of styrene and other similar substances with lipid affinity.

Parallels can be drawn between styrene and other commonly used solvents, previously thought to be relatively "safe" in terms of acute and chronic exposures. This means that the traditional concepts of "metabolism" of many substances must be reconsidered, since immediate metabolism may not occur, but instead a "storage" or "retention" may occur, an added factor for concern because of lipid affinity for many substances and potential effects on the nervous system. Metabolism and elimination following the ordinary work shift of 8 hours, along with weekends, may prove to be insufficient time for long-term work under existing limit values for many substances, especially when work effort is at an energy

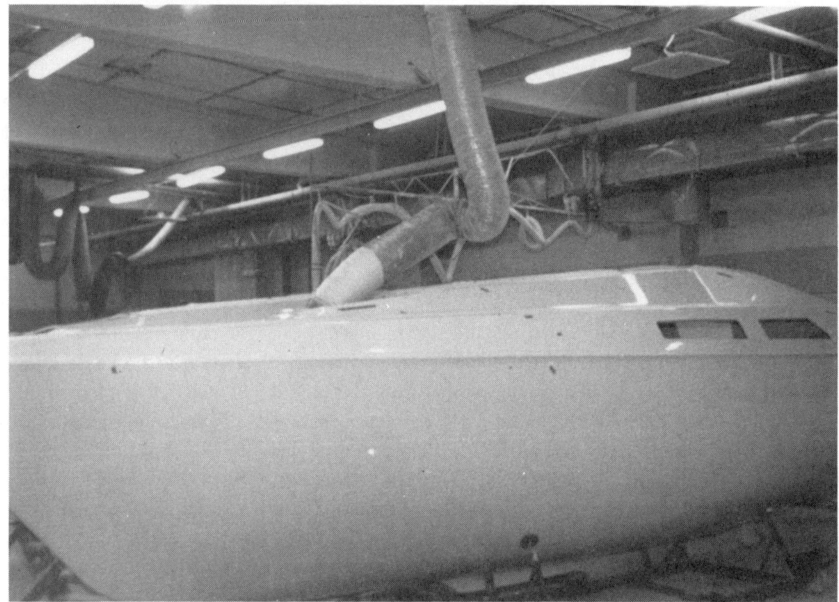

FIG 63–31.
Each hull has a clean air supply; same factory as in Figure 63–27.

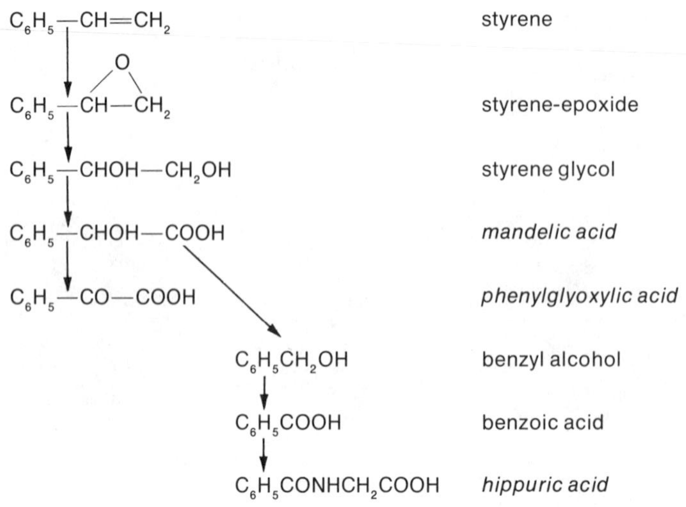

$C_6H_5-CH=CH_2$	styrene
$C_6H_5-CH(O)CH_2$	styrene-epoxide
$C_6H_5-CHOH-CH_2OH$	styrene glycol
$C_6H_5-CHOH-COOH$	*mandelic acid*
$C_6H_5-CO-COOH$	*phenylglyoxylic acid*
$C_6H_5CH_2OH$	benzyl alcohol
C_6H_5COOH	benzoic acid
$C_6H_5CONHCH_2COOH$	*hippuric acid*

FIG 63–32.
Metabolism of styrene.

level far above a "sedentary," "sitting," or "resting" level. This storage or retention of styrene was further demonstrated in workers fabricating polyester storage tanks. Engström et al.[24] studied three male employees during a workweek, monitoring from Tuesday to Friday the concentration of styrene in the ambient air continually in the breathing zone. The uptake was estimated as the product of the TWA concentration in inspiratory air, the mean 8-hour pulmonary ventilation and the percentage uptake in the lungs measuring pulmonary ventilation with a respirometer. The percentage styrene uptake was estimated on the basis of the concentrations in inspiratory and alveolar air. The amount of body fat was estimated by an anthropometric method. Concentrations of styrene in subcutaneous adipose tissue were determined by gas chromatography after needle biopsy before and after the work shift of Monday, Wednesday, and Friday. They found that the TWA concentration of styrene in inspiratory air during the workweek was 32 to 85 mg/m^3, i.e., below half of the Swedish TLV (210 mg/m^3), and the mean daily uptake was 193 to 558 mg. On Monday morning, the concentration of styrene in adipose tissue was 2.8 to 8.1 mg/kg and on Friday afternoon 4.7 to 11.6 mg/kg. The concentrations were higher in the two subjects with a higher exposure of longer duration, as compared to the concentrations in a recently employed worker, who was exposed to lower concentrations in inspiratory air.

Both of the two former workers had a large estimated amount of body fat (27 and 41 kg). The calculated half-life of the concentration of styrene in adipose tissue after the end of exposure was 5.2 and 2.8 days in these two men and an elimination time of about 5 weeks in the subject with the slowest elimination, before the limit of detection (0.1 mg/kg) was reached. Increased cardiorespiratory and vascular demands during pregnancy, described in other sections in this chapter, imply that the transport and potential storage in fetal tissues to a variety of chemicals must be viewed in the light of the investigations by Engström et al., who distinctly revealed a "half-life" of styrene in male workers after exposure ceased to be in excess of 5 days.

HEALTH EFFECTS AND TOXICITY

Prolonged skin contact with the liquid can cause chapped skin, rash, and dermatitis due to styrene's fat-solvent properties.

At 100 ppm, workers developed eye, nose, and throat irritation within 20 minutes of exposure. Workers in plastics applications exposed to styrene for several years complained of eye and respiratory tract irritation but were able to tolerate exposure in excess of 500 ppm for several hours at a time. Bodner et al.[10] reported that workers exposed for almost 4 years at 45 to 550 ppm complained of eye, nose, and throat irritation, and about half of them complained of shortness of breath. In a factory where reinforced plastics were made, Rosensteel and Meyer[65] found that workers exposed at concentrations greater than 100 ppm had eye irritation, and 30% to 50% of them had upper respiratory tract irritation. Complaints of wheezing and chest tightness have been noted in workers during an investigation of a styrene and polystyrene production plant[51]; however, spirometric studies of airway effects did not suggest significant changes, nor was there any radiologic evidence of changes in the lungs. In a factory where reinforced plastics were made, workers exposed to TWA styrene concentrations of 9 to 111 ppm (average 69 ppm) complained of chest tightness (23% of the workers), wheezing (18%), and shortness of breath (54%), but ventilatory function was significantly changed during the shift only in those workers who smoked.[65]

Among 21 workers exposed to styrene at about 75 ppm for about 10 years at another reinforced plastics/composites (RP/C) plant, there were four cases of reduced FEV_1, but whether the cause was age, styrene exposure, or other factors was not clear.[15] As compared to controls, a significantly greater number of RP/C workers in another clinical study had abnormal pulmonary function.[11] From these reports it is clear that irritation of the eyes and upper respiratory tract has occurred in some workers and experimental subjects at styrene concentrations well below 200 ppm, indicating the need for follow-up of potential long-term respiratory effects from styrene.

EFFECTS ON THE NERVOUS SYSTEM

The neurotoxic effects of styrene have been known for some time, both in animals and in humans. Klimkova-Deutschova[44] reported that styrene in occupational exposure induces electroencephalogram (EEG) abnormalities more often than several other chemicals. Seppäläinen and Härkönen[68] described neurophysiologic findings among 96 men occupationally exposed to styrene and concluded that the EEG examination is useful in the study of the neurotoxic effects of styrene. Experimental exposures in humans to styrene have demonstrated that styrene causes CNS depression.[12, 30, 59, 70] Within minutes of exposure at 800 ppm, two men experienced listlessness, drowsiness, and impaired balance.[12] During a 1-hour exposure to 376 ppm, decrements in balance, coordination, and manual dexterity tests were measured, and subjective complaints of headache, nausea, and a feeling of slight inebriation were reported.[70] A significant difference in reaction time was noted in 12 subjects after a 2-hour exposure that included consecutive 30-minute styrene exposures of 50, 150, 250, and 350 ppm.[29] Slower reaction times were found in two or three subjects during 90-minute exposures of 50, 100, and 200 ppm; loss of balance was found for three subjects during the 90-minute exposure at 200 ppm.[59] Subjective complaints reported by six subjects during 90-minute styrene exposures at 50, 100, or 200 ppm included headache, fatigue, sleepiness, malaise, difficulty in concentrating, and a feeling of intoxication.[59] During a study lasting a couple of weeks that included a series of styrene exposures at 20, 100, and 125 ppm for 7.5 hours, there were some changes in three of six subjects in both visual evoked response and EEG amplitude, which the investigation deemed to be consistent with central nervous system depression. Loss of balance was not found during 90-minute exposures to 50 or 100 ppm and no significant optokinetic changes were noted in five subjects exposed to 300 ppm of styrene for 1 hour.[58, 59]

Workers exposed to styrene have experienced weakness, increased reaction times,[30] abnormal EEGs,[36, 44, 45, 68] and headache, fatigue, malaise, tension, or dizziness.[9, 51, 52] Styrene exposures in many of these studies were either not determined, or were at times greater than 100 ppm for some of the workers.[8, 9, 14, 30, 44, 64, 65] However, at one RP/C facility where the average styrene exposure was estimated from urinary mandelic acid measurements to be about 30 ppm, 24% of the workers had EEGs judged to be abnormal.[68]

There is some evidence of styrene-induced peripheral neuropathy. In an investigation of workers at a U.S. styrene and polystyrene production plant (with potential exposures to styrene, benzene, ethyl benzene, and toluene), radial and peroneal nerve conduction velocities were said to be reduced, but comparative data on normal velocities were not given.[46] It was also reported in the same study[46] that radial and peroneal nerve conduction velocities decreased with increasing duration of exposure, but because appropriate corrections for age were not made, it is not evident whether the decrement with longer exposure was due to the longer exposure, increasing age, or a combination of both. In a Swedish study,[64] 10 of 33 workers exposed to about 5 to 125 ppm of styrene had evidence of a mild sensory neuropathy with polyphasic sensory responses; these 10 workers were older than those not having signs of neuropathy, and they were more heavily exposed. The investigators speculated that age alone did not cause these effects, but that the effects of age and styrene exposure might have been synergistic.[64]

MUTAGENICITY

Chromosomal changes were found to be more frequent in the lymphocytes of styrene-exposed workers in several European RP/C factories than among controls.[2, 27, 39, 54, 55] An increased frequency of sister chromatid exchanges (SCE) in the lymphocytes of styrene-exposed workers has been reported.[2] However, other studies of workers exposed to styrene have shown no significant increases in either chromosomal aberrations or SCE. In a study of unscheduled DNA synthesis in lymphocytes of styrene-exposed workers, styrene did not alter the efficiency of DNA repair,[74, 81] but rather predisposed the lymphocytes to an increased risk for DNA damage from subsequent exposures to genotoxic agents (see Chapter 51). A variety of in vitro and in vivo animal experiments have yielded conflicting results, and no conclusions have been set forth implicating styrene as a definite mutagen.

REPRODUCTIVE EFFECTS

Congenital defects in children whose mothers had been occupationally exposed to styrene were reported by Holmberg[40]; further investigations are underway to verify the implications of these findings. The finding of styrene, at unstated concentrations, in umbilical cord blood[18] suggests that styrene can cross the placenta; in these cases, the source of the styrene exposure of the mothers was not found. Placental transfer of styrene in rats has also been noted. An increased rate of spontaneous abortions observed among Finnish styrene workers[38] might be compatible with findings of cytogenetic effects or of terata; thus, despite lack of confirmation of this study, the finding warrants concern. A later study, however, found no difference in the number of spontaneous abortions between styrene workers and a group of age-matched and social class–matched controls with no solvent exposures.[37] At present, styrene does not appear to be teratogenic, embryotoxic, or fetotoxic in humans, and further investigations of the reproductive outcomes of workers are needed for greater proof.

CARCINOGENICITY

The possible carcinogenicity of styrene has been investigated by long-term administration to rodents, which yielded weak evidence for carcinogenic action. Mortality studies of workers exposed to styrene have not shown an excess cancer mortality.[28, 52, 56, 60] There have, however, been suggestions of an excess of leukemia. Nicholson et al.[56] studied the mortality experience in one U.S. styrene and polystyrene production plant, and found no excess of deaths from cancer or from any of the nonneoplastic diseases examined such as cardiovascular or respiratory disease. The investigators concluded that the information found regarding leukemia was not definitive.

In a U.S. styrene production plant, Ott et al.[60] found fewer total deaths (303 vs. 425) and fewer cancer deaths (58 vs. 76.5) among 2,904 workers at four plants than would be expected from the U.S. white male population. Most of these workers had been exposed to low levels of styrene during their employment (TWA concentrations were 10 ppm or less). The mortality data on the styrene workers (i.e., production and nonprofessional research) were also compared with previous mortality experiences from that company, and the styrene workers had a lower total mortality and a lower cancer mortality. However, there was a significant excess ($P < 0.05$) of leukemia deaths compared with other company workers (6 observed vs. 1.6 expected), although the excess was not significant when compared with the U.S. population (6 vs. 2.9). Most of the excess was due to lymphatic leukemia. Some workers had been exposed many years earlier to high levels of benzene, but whether those men with leukemia had been exposed to benzene was not evident.

Excess cancer was not seen in a German styrene and polystyrene plant.[28] In that study, 74 death certificates were examined, and there were 12 deaths from cancer and 3 from lung cancer. Neither statistic is significantly different from the comparison groups.

In a study of 1,205 reinforced plastics workers in Sweden[1] where exposure levels were thought to be 150 to 300 ppm styrene in recent years and higher in the past, a slight but nonsignificant decrement in cancer incidence from that expected in the Swedish population was found. The latency period was not high for many of the workers; further follow-up might reveal more cases of cancer.

While it does not seem appropriate from presently available evidence to conclude that styrene can cause cancer among exposed workers, there is enough reason to suggest it might be at least a weak carcinogen, and priority should be given to further studies of this problem, according to NIOSH.[16]

STANDARDS

The MAK value (maximum concentration value in the workplace) for styrene in the Federal Republic of Germany is 100 ppm.[53] In 1981, Sweden adopted a TWA styrene standard of 25 ppm with a 15-minute short-term value of 75 ppm; styrene was designated as being easily absorbed into the body.[42]

The OSHA standard for styrene is 100 ppm (420 mg/m^3) for an 8-hour TWA, 200 ppm (840 mg/m^3) for a ceiling concentration, and 600 ppm (2,520 mg/m^3) for 5 minutes in any 3-hour time period. The American Conference of Governmental Industrial Hygienists (ACGIH) threshold limit values (TLVs) for styrene are 50 ppm (215 mg/m^3) for an 8-hour TWA, and 100 ppm (425 mg/m^3) for a short term exposure limit (STEL) (the maximum exposure concentration for a continuous 15-minute period).

MEDICAL AND HYGIENIC CONTROLS

The difficulties in evaluating the risks of chronic styrene exposure may to some extent be reflected in the different TLVs proposed throughout the world, most often ranging from 25 to 100 ppm but also as low as 1 ppm (USSR, 1979). Although the validity of the reports referred to above may be doubted, in certain respects they imply careful precautions to be undertaken to avoid undue exposures. Central and peripheral nervous system disturbances should be kept in mind in monitoring workers exposed to styrene.

Control of work exposures demands adequate ventilation at all times. Because of the large sizes and shapes of objects fabricated in styrene-modified polyester plastic, difficulties in providing and construction of adequate exhaust systems are encountered. Some type of air-supplied helmet or face mask should be used where there is insufficient general ventilation, and medical monitoring of the workers as a backup measure to detect individual worker sensitivity and as a control of the efficacy of the plant hygienic engineering methods should be installed. The determination of mandelic acid in the urine offers a fair correlation between styrene in the workplace air, but note that alcohol ingestion inhibits styrene metabolism, making urine mandelic acid determination useless. For details of these biologic monitoring aspects, refer to Chapter 13 on Biologic Monitoring.

REFERENCES

1. Ahlmark A: *Styrene Research: Epidemiological Report*. Stockholm, Swedish Plastics Federation, 1978.
2. Andersson HC, Tranberg EA, Uggla AH, et al: Chromosomal aberrations and sister-chromatid exchanges in lymphocytes of men occupationally exposed to styrene in a plastic-boat factory. *Mutat Res* 1980; 73:387.
3. Astrand I, Kilbom A, Wahlberg I, et al: Exposure to styrene. I. Concentration in alveolar air and blood at rest and during exercise and metabolism. *Arbete och Hälsa:* 3, Stockholm; Arbetarskyddsverket (Swedish with English summary).
4. Axelson O, Fröbärj G, Wedefelt U: Kan styrenexposition orsaka cer ebrolesionella tillstand? *Läkartidningen* 1974; 71:137.
5. Axelson O, Gustavson J: Some hygienic and clinical observations on styrene exposure. *Scand J Work Environ Health* 1978; 4(suppl 2):215.
6. Bardodej Z, Bardodejova E: The metabolism of ethylbenzene, styrene and alpha-methylstyrene. *Proceedings of the 15th International Congress of Occupational Health*, vol. II-1. Vienna, 1966, pp 457–460.
7. Bardodej Z, Bardodejova E: Biotransformation of ethylbenzene, styrene and alpha-methylstyrene in man. *Am Ind Hyg Assoc J* 1970; 31:206.
8. Bergman K, Lindberg E: Styrene exposure in the plastic boat industry. *Arbete Och Hälsa* 1977; 3.
9. Bernard PL: Contribution to the study of polystyrene toxicity. *Arch Mal Prof Med Trav Secur Soc* 1966; 27(12):891 (French).
10. Bodner AH, Butler GJ, Okawa MT: Health Hazard Evaluation/Toxicity Determination Report No. 73-103-128—American Standard Fiberglass Inc., Stockton, Calif, Cincinnati, Oh, US Department of Health, Education and Welfare, National Institute for Occupational Safety and Health, 1974.
11. Brooks SM, Anderson L, Emmett E, et al: The effects of protective equipment on styrene exposure in workers in the reinforced plastics industry. *Arch Environ Health* 1980; 35(5):287.
12. Carpenter CP, Schaffer CB, Weil CS, et al: Studies on the inhalation of 1,3-butadiene with a comparison of its narcotic effect with benzol, toluol and styrene, and a note on the elimination of styrene by the human. *J Ind Hyg* 1944; 26:69.
13. Carrard D: Study on styrene—toxicity, urinary metabolites based on a survey of four factories. Thesis, University of Lausanne, School of Medicine 1975.

14. Cherry N, Waldron HA, Wells GG, et al: An investigation of the acute behavioural effects of styrene on factory workers. *Brit J Ind Med* 1980; 37:234.
15. Chmielewski J, Renke W: Clinical and experimental studies on the pathogenesis of toxic effects of styrene—Part II. The effect of styrene on the respiratory system. *Bull Inst Marit Trop Med Gdynia* (Engl) 1975; 26:299.
16. Criteria for a Recommended Standard: Occupational Exposure to Styrene. DHHS (NIOSH) Publication No. 83-119. Cincinnati, National Institute for Occupational Safety and Health, 1983.
17. Danishefsky I, and Willhite M: The metabolism of styrene in the rat. *J Biol Chem* 1954; 211:549.
18. Dowty BJ, Laseter JL, Storer J: The transplacental migration and accumulation in blood of volatile organic constituents. *Pediatr Res* 1976; 10:696.
19. Droz PO, Guillemin MP: Human styrene exposure. *J Int Arch Occup Environ Health* 1983; 53:19.
20. Dutkiewicz T, Tyras H: Skin absorption of toluene, styrene and xylene by man. *Br J Ind Med* 1967; 24:243.
21. Engström K, Rantanen J: A new gas chromatographic method for determination of mandelic acid in urine. *Int Arch Arbeitsmed* 1974; 33:163.
22. Engström K, Härkönen H, Kalliokoski P, et al: Urinary mandelic acid concentration after occupational exposure to styrene and its use as a biological exposure test. *Scand J Work Environ Health* 1976; 2:21.
23. Engström J, Bjurström R, Åstrand I, et al: Uptake, distribution and elimination of styrene in man. *Scand J Work Environ Health* 1978; 4:315.
24. Engström J, Astrand I, Wigaeus E: Exposure to styrene in a polymerization plant. *Scand J Work Environ Health* 1978; 4:324.
25. Extent of Exposure to Styrene in the Reinforced Plastic Boat Making Industry: DHHS (NIOSH) Publication No 82–110. Cincinnati, Oh, National Institute for Occupational Safety and Health, 1983.
26. Fiserova-Bergerova V, Teisinger J: Pulmonary styrene vapor retention. *Ind Med Surg* 1965; 34:620.
27. Fleig I, Thiess A: Mutagenicity study of workers employed in the styrene and polystyrene processing and manufacturing industry. *Scand J Work Environ Health* 1978; 4(Suppl 2):254.
28. Frentzel-Beyme R, Thiess AM, Wieland R: Survey of mortality among employees engaged in the manufacture of styrene and polystyrene at the BASF Ludwigshafen works. *Scand J Work Environ Health* 1978; 4(Suppl 2):231.
29. Gamberale F, Hultengren M: Exposure to styrene. II. Psychological functions. *Arbete Och Hälsa* 1973; 3. Stockholm: Arbetarskyddsverket (Swedish with English summary).
30. Gamberale F, Lisper HO, Anshelm-Olson B: Styrene exposure effects on plastic boat industry workers. *Arbete Och Hälsa* 1975; 8.
31. Götell P, Axelson O, Lindelöf B: Field studies on human styrene exposure. *Scand J Work Environ Health* 1972; 9(2):76.
32. Guillemin MP, Bauer D: Biological monitoring of exposure to styrene by analysis of combined urinary mandelic and phenylglyoxylic acids. *Am Ind Hyg Assoc J* 1978; 39(11):873.
33. Härkönen H, Kalliokoski P, Hietala S, et al: Concentrations of mandelic and phenylglyoxylic acid in urine as indicators of styrene exposure. *Scand J Work Environ Health* 1974; 11:162.
34. Härkönen H: Symptoms and findings among workers exposed to styrene with special reference to the central nervous system, in Kahn H, Hernberg S (eds): *Detection of Early Effects of Toxic Substances—Collection of Scientific Papers*. Tallinn, Estonia, Institute of Experimental and Clinical Medicine of the Ministry of Health of the Estonian SSR and Institute of Occupational Health, Helsinki, 1977.
35. Härkönen H: Styrene, its experimental and clinical toxicology: A review. *Scand J Work Environ Health* 1978; 4(Suppl. 2):104.
36. Härkönen H, Lindström K, Seppäläinen AM, et al: Exposure-response relationship between styrene exposure and central nervous functions. *Scand J Work Environ Health* 1978; 4:53.
37. Härkönen H, Holmberg PC: Obstetric histories of women occupationally exposed to styrene. *Scand J Work Environ Health* 1982; 8:74.
38. Hemminki K, Franssila E, Vainio H: Spontaneous abortions among female chemical workers in Finland. *Int Arch Occup Environ Health* 1980; 45:123.
39. Hogstedt B, Hedner K, Mark-Vendel E, et al: Increased frequency of chromosome aberrations in workers exposed to styrene. *Scand J Work Environ Health* 1979; 5:333.
40. Holmberg PC: Central nervous defects in two children of mothers exposed to chemicals in the reinforced plastics industry—chance or a causal relation? *Scand J Work Environ Health* 1977; 3:212.
41. Horiguchi S, Teramoto K: The upper limits of mandelic and phenylglyoxylic acids normally excreted in the urine as an index of styrene exposure. Studies on industrial styrene poisoning—Part III. *Sangyo Igaku* 1972; 14(4):288.
42. Hygieniska Gränsvärden: Directives concerning limit values for air contaminants at places of work. National Board of Occupational Safety and Health, Stockholm, Sweden, May, 1981.
43. Ikeda M, Imamura T: Evaluation of hippuric, phenylglyoxylic and mandelic acids in urine as indices of styrene exposure. *Int Arch Arbeitsmed* 1974; 32:93.
44. Klimkova-Deutschova E: Neurologische Befunde in der Plasticindustrie bei Styrol-Arbeitern. *Int Arch Gewerebepath Gewerebehyg* 1962; 19:35.
45. Klimkova-Deutschova E, Dandova D, Salomanova Z, et al: Recent advances on the neurological picture of occupational exposure to styrene. *Cesk Neurol Neurochir* 1973; 36(1):20.
46. Lilis R, Lorimer WV, Diamond S, et al: Neurotoxicity of styrene in production and polymerization workers. *Environ Res* 1978; 15:133.
47. Lindström K, Härkönen H, Hernberg S: Disturbances in psychological functions of workers occupationally exposed to styrene. *Scand J Work Environ Health* 1976; 3:129.
48. Lindström K, Härkönen H, Mantere P: Alcohol consumption and tolerance of workers exposed to styrene in relation to level of exposure and psychological symptoms and signs. *Scand J Work Environ Health* 1978; 4(Suppl 2): 196.
49. Loprieno N, Prescuittini S, Sbrana I, et al: Mutagenicity of Industrial Compounds—VII; Styrene and Styrene Oxide—II; Point Mutations, Chromosome Aberrations and DNA Repair Induction Analyses. *Scand J Work Environ Health* 1978; 4(Suppl 2):169.
50. Loprieno N, et al: A. Mutagenicity of industrial compounds: Styrene and its possible metabolite styrene oxide. *Mutat Res* 1976; 40:317.
51. Lorimer WV, Lilis R, Nicholson WJ, et al: Clinical studies of styrene workers—initial findings. *Environ Health Perspect* 1976; 17:171.
52. Maier A, Ruhe R, Rosensteel R, et al: Health Hazard Evaluation/Toxicity Determination Report No. 72-90-107–Arco Polymer Incorporated (Sinclair-Koppers Company, Inc.), Monaca, Pa, Cincinnati, Oh, US Department of Health, Education, and Welfare, National Institute for Occupational Safety and Health, 1974.
53. Maximum Concentrations at the Workplace and Biological Tolerance Values for Working Materials, Commission for Investigation of Health Hazards of Chemical Compounds in the Work Area, Report No. XVIII. Bonn, Federal Republic of Germany, German Science Foundation, 1982.
54. Meretoja T, Vainio H, Sorsa M, et al: Occupational styrene exposure and chromosomal aberrations. *Mutat Res* 1977; 56:193.
55. Meretoja T, Jarventaus H, Sorsa M, et al: Chromosome aberrations in lymphocytes of workers exposed to styrene. *Scand J Work Environ Health* 1978; 4(Suppl 2):259.
56. Nicholson WJ, Selikoff IJ, Seidman H: Mortality experience of sty-

rene-polystyrene polymerization workers—initial findings. *Scand J Work Environ Health* 1978; 4(Suppl 2):247.

57. Norppa H, Vainio H, Sorsa M: Chromosome aberrations in lymphocytes of workers exposed to styrene. *Am J Ind Med* 1981; 2:299.
58. Odkvist LM, Astrand I, Larsby B, et al: Does styrene disturb the balance apparatus in man? *Arbete Och Hälsa* 1979; 1980:2.
59. Oltramare M, Desbaumes E, Imhoff C, et al: Toxicology of Monomeric Styrene—Experimental and Clinical Studies on Man, Geneva, Editions Medecine et Hygiene, 1974.
60. Ott MG, Kolesar RC, Scharnweber HC, et al: A mortality survey of employees engaged in the development or manufacture of styrene-based products. *J Occup Med* 1980; 22(7):445.
61. Pero RW, Bryngelsson T, Hogstedt B, et al: Occupational and in vitro exposure to styrene assessed by unscheduled DNA synthesis in resting human lymphocytes. *Carcinogenesis* 1982; 3(6):681.
62. Pfäffli P, Vainio H, Hesso A: Styrene and styrene oxide concentrations in the air during the lamination process in the reinforced plastics industry. *Scand J Work Environ Health* 1979; 5:158.
63. Riihimaki V, Pfäffli P: Percutaneous absorption of solvent vapors in man. *Scand J Work Environ Health* 1978; 4:73.
64. Rosén I, Haeger-Aronsen B, Rehnström S, et al: Neurophysiological observations after chronic styrene exposure. *Scand J Work Environ Health* 1978; 4(Suppl 2):184.
65. Rosensteel RE, Meyer CR: Health Hazard Evaluation Determination Report No. 75-150-378—Reinell Boats, Inc, Poplar Bluff, Mo, Cincinnati, Oh, US Department of Health, Education, and Welfare, Center for Disease Control, National Institute for Occupational Safety and Health, 1977.
66. Rossavainen A: Styrene use and occupational exposure in the plastics industry. *Scand J Work Environ Health* 1978; 4(Suppl 2):7.
67. Scandinavian Expert Group on Limit Value Documentation—4: Styrene, *Arbete Och Hälsa* 1979; 14.
68. Seppäläinen AM, Härkönen H: Neurophysiological findings among workers occupationally exposed to stryene. *Scand J Work Environ Health* 1976; 3:140.
69. Seppäläinen AM: Neurotoxicity of styrene in occupational and experimental exposure. *Scand J Work Environ Health* 1978; 4(Suppl 2):181.
70. Stewart RD, Dodd HC, Baretta ED, et al: Human exposure to styrene vapors. *Arch Environ Health* 1968; 16:656.
71. Thiess AM, Fleig I: Chromosome investigations on workers exposed to styrene/polystyrene. *J Occup Med* 1978; 20(11):747.
72. Thiess AM, Friedheim M: Morbidity among persons employed in styrene production, polymerization and processing plants. *Scand J Work Environ Health* 1978; 4(Suppl 2):203.
73. Thiess AM, Friedheim M: Morbidity study in co-workers of the polyester laboratory and of the technical service, exposed to styrene. *Zentralbl Arbeitsmed Arbeitsschutz* 1979; 9:238.
74. Thiess AM, Schwegler H, Fleig I: Chromosome investigations in lymphocytes of workers employed in areas which styrene-containing unsaturated polyester resins are manufactured. *Am J Ind Med* 1980; 1:205.
75. Tossavainen A: Styrene use and occupational exposure in the plastics industry. *Scand J Work Environ Health* 1978; 4(Suppl 2):7.
76. Vainio H, Paakkonen R, Ronnholm K, et al: A study on the mutagenic activity of styrene and styrene oxide. *Scand J Work Environ Health* 1976; 3:147.
77. Vetenskaplig skriftserie: Toxicokinetics of styrene-biotransformation and covalent binding by Löf, A. *Arbete Och Hälsa* 1986; 6.
78. Vivoli G, Vecchi G: Study of the urinary excretion of mandelic acid as a test of styrene exposure. *Lav Um* 1974; 26(1):1.
79. Waldron HA, Cherry N, Johnston JD: The effects of ethanol on blood toluene concentrations. *Int Arch Occup Environ Health* 1983; 51:365.
80. Watabe T, Hiratsuka A, Aizawa T, et al: Studies on metabolism and toxicity of styrene. IV. 1-vinyl-benzene-3, 4-oxide, a potent mutagen formed as a possible intermediate in the metabolism in vivo of styrene to 4-vinylphenol. *Mutat Res*. 1982; 93(1):45.
81. Watanabe T, Endo A, Sato K, et al: Mutagenic potential of styrene in man. *Ind Health* 1981; 19(1):37.
82. Zielhuis RL, Hartogensis F, Jongh J, et al: The health of workers processing reinforced polyesters. XIVth International Congressional Occupational Health, vol 111:1092. Madrid, Spain, September 16–21. 1963.

Leather Manufacturing

Bruce Hills, M.S.

John Fajen, M.S.

In the United States, approximately 19,800 workers are employed in leather manufacturing, one of the oldest industries in the world.[2, 4] This section will summarize information on occupational exposures to chemical and physical agents in leather manufacturing and also will discuss briefly the health problems associated with employment in this industry.

Tanning is the chemical process that transforms hides and skins into nonputrescible leather. The epidermis and subcutaneous layer of the animal hide is removed, and the collagen fibers of the dermis are stabilized. Tanning can be grouped into four major stages: (1) preparing the hide in the beamhouse; (2) tanning in the tanyard; (3) modifying the hide by retanning, coloring, and fat liquoring; and (4) finishing. Figure 63–33 shows these steps for the two major types of processes, vegetable and chrome tanning. This general diagram does not take into account all the possible variations required to give various leather products their different desired properties.

In the beamhouse, hides are prepared for tanning by washing, soaking, defleshing, unhairing, deliming, and bating. Washing and soaking removes blood, manure, dirt, and the salt used to preserve the hide. Unhairing is usually accomplished by soaking the hide in a lime solution of calcium oxide and sodium sulfide, to destroy the hair. Dimethylamine sulfate is used as a catalyst in the dehairing operation. Hides are then delimed and bated with buffering salts, such as ammonium sulphate or ammonium chloride, and proteolytic enzymes, such as trypsin. The bate and the buffering salts also reduce swelling and soften the hide texture by removing residual chemicals used in the unhairing process. Hides that are to be chrome tanned are then pickled, usually in a mixture of sodium chloride and sulfuric acid.

Stabilization of the dermis is accomplished either by vegetable or chrome tanning. Vegetable tanning is used for heavier leather, such as belts and shoe soles. The hides are immersed in progressively concentrated tanning baths in a series of large pits

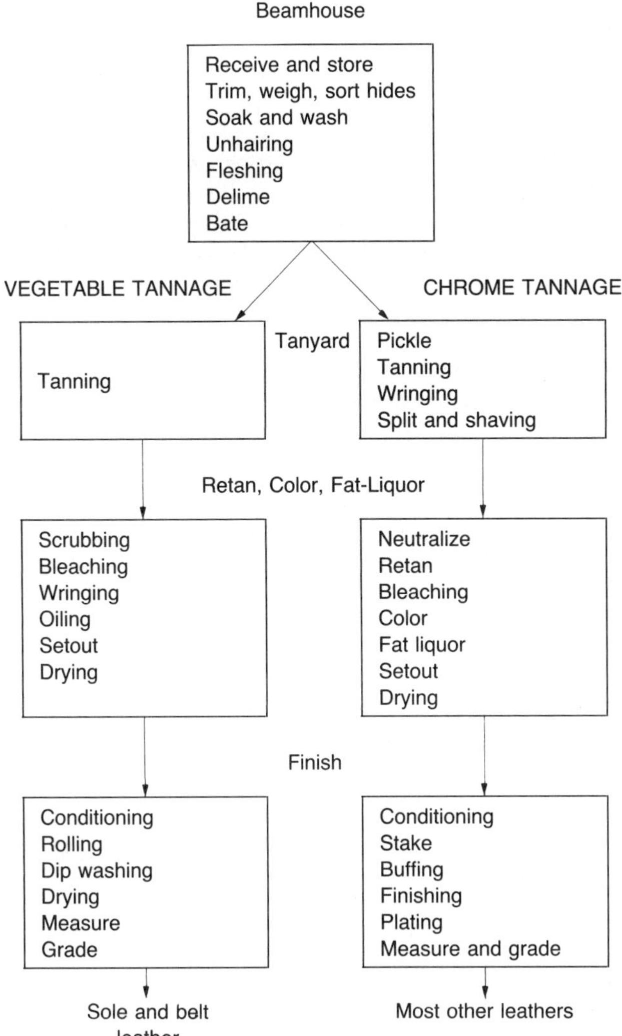

FIG 63-33.
General process flowsheet of leather tanning and finishing.

over a period of approximately three weeks. Aqueous extracts of various woods and barks are utilized to penetrate the hide and to cross-link collagen. Synthetic tanning agents (syntans) may also be used, alone or in combination with vegetable tannings. Most syntans are condensation products of formaldehyde, sulfonated phenols, diaryl sulfones, urea, melamine, and dicyandiamide.

Chrome tanning is accomplished by either a one-bath or two-bath method. The "one bath" method is the most commonly used procedure, in which the hide is tanned with trivalent chromium sulfate. Sodium dichromate, sulfuric acid, and glucose are the most commonly used reducing agents. The hides are then milled in a colloidal solution of basic sulfate of chromium until tanning is complete. In the "two-bath" method, which is now obsolete, the hide is immersed in a bath of hexavalent chromium salts. Following impregnation, it is placed in a second bath of sodium thiosulfite and acid, which reduces the hexavalent chromium to its trivalent state. The "one-bath" method is more rapid and eliminates the handling of hides saturated with chromic acid.

Other tanning methods use zirconium, oxidizable oil, sulfonyl chloride, formaldehyde, gluteraldehyde, iron, or aluminum, depending on the desired final product.

After tanning, excess water is removed from the hide by wringing. The chrome tanned hides are then split and shaved to adjust their thickness. During this mechanical process, workers may be exposed to airborne dust which contains many of the chemicals used in tanning.

The retanning, coloring, and fat liquoring stages modify the hides after tanning to impart desirable properties. Most leathers are colored with one of three major types of dyes: acid, basic, and direct. Acid dyes are usually azo-, triarylmethane, or anthraquinone dyes with acid substituents such as nitro-, carboxy-, or sulphonic acid. Benzidine, o-toluidine, and o-diansidine-based dyes are in this family. Basic dyes contain free amino groups. Direct dyes are principally water-soluble salts of sulphonic acids of azo-dyes.

Fat liquoring lubricates the leather to impart strength and flexibility. Oils and natural fats and their transformation products, mineral oils, and several synthetic fats are incorporated into the leather in an aqueous suspension. Drying operations are used to eliminate excess water from the hide.

Finishing, the last step in the process, involves smoothing the grain surface and applying film-forming materials to protect the leather and enhance the color. Chrome leather is subjected to a sequence of mechanical and chemical operations to produce a specific look and feel. Buffing the leather to improve appearance results in leather dust being generated in the work area.

The application of the film coat on the leather may use an aqueous or solvent-based finish. The most common film coats are aqueous dispensed synthetic resins, such as acrylic resins, methylacrylic resins, and synthetic rubbers based on butadiene. Other finishing materials include dyes, pigments, waxes, proteins, lacquers, plasticizers, solvents, nitrocellulose, polyurethane, and formaldehyde.[6–8, 12]

In summary, the manufacturing of leather requires the use of numerous toxic chemicals and results in multiple exposures to workers. The following is a list of the toxic chemicals commonly encountered in tanneries. Detailed discussion of their effects on workers are presented elsewhere in this volume.

TOXIC EXPOSURES

Calcium Oxide.—This is used to burn the hairs from hides. Because of its caustic properties, lime can burn the skin and eyes on contact.

Sodium Sulfide.—This is also used in the dehairing operation and has similar caustic effects as lime. An additional hazard develops when sodium sulfide comes in contact with an acid, in which the resulting reaction forms hydrogen sulfide.

Ammonia.—Ammonia gases and vapors are generated in the beamhouse from the reaction of ammonium salts with acids and from the putrefaction of decaying flesh and other waste products.

N-Nitroso Compounds.—These include the human carcinogen, N-nitrosodimethylamine (NDMA), and have been found in airborne samples from the beamhouse. There is evidence that dimethylamine sulfate, which is used in some hide unhairing processes, is nitrosated by airborne nitrogen oxides to produce NDMA.[9]

Chromium (Chromic Acid, Sodium Dichromate, and Chromium Compounds).—Chromium is the most commonly used tanning agent for leather. In the obsolete "two-bath" tanning system, the hide was soaked in a solution of hexavalent chromium salts (potassium or sodium dichromate) and then reduced to trivalent chromium salt by immersing the hide in a second "bath" containing sodium thosulfate and mineral acid. Workers would be exposed to hexavalent chromium during the transfer of the hides from one vat to another. The current "one-bath" method eliminates this handling by using trivalent chromium. Since the introduction of the "one-bath" method and greater mechanization of the tanning process, there has been a decrease in the incidence of burns, skin irritation, and dermatitis caused by dermal contact with the chromium.

Biocides.—These are added at nearly every step of the tanning process to prevent loss due to microbial infestation. The most common biocides are: 1,2- and 1,4-dichlorobenzenes, phenols such as tri- and pentachlorophenols, and paranitrophenol in military leather.[5]

Benzidine Analogue-Based Dyes.—These are used in the coloring of the leather. Benzidine is a regulated human carcinogen,

TABLE 63–9.
Current U.S. Department of Labor Exposure Limits for Chemical Substances in the Tanning Industry*

SUBSTANCES	8-HOUR TIME-WEIGHTED AVERAGE EXPOSURE LIMIT		ACCEPTABLE CEILING CONCENTRATION	ACCEPTABLE MAXIMUM PEAK ABOVE THE ACCEPTABLE CEILING CONCENTRATION FOR AN 8-HOUR SHIFT	
	PPM	MG/M^3		CONCENTRATION	MAXIMUM DURATION
Acetone	1,000	2,400			
Ammonia	50	35			
Benzidine-dyes	Exposure should be reduced to lowest feasible level.				
Carbon Monoxide	50	55			
Chromium sol. chromic, chromous salts as Cr	--	0.5			
Metal as insol salts	--	1			
Chromic acid and chromates	--	--	1 mg/10 cu m		
o-Dichlorobenzene	50	300	Ceiling level		
p-Dichlorobenzene	75	450			
Formaldehyde	3	--	5 ppm	10 ppm	30 minutes
Formic acid	5	9			
Hydrogen peroxide (90%)	1	1.4			
Hydrogen sulfide	--	--	20 ppm	50 ppm	10 minutes once only if no other measurable exposures occur
Isobutyl alcohol	100	300			
Methyl ethyl ketone	200	590			
Methyl isobutyl ketone	100	410			
Pentachloroethylene				300 ppm	5 minutes in any 3 hours
Sulfur hexafluoride	1,000	6,000			
Sulfuric acid	--	1			
Toluene	200	--	300 ppm	500 ppm	10 minutes
1,1,1-Trichloroethane	350	1,900			
Trichloroethane	100	--	200 ppm	300 ppm	5 minutes in any 2 hours
Leather dust (inert or nuisance dust)					
Respirable fraction			15 mppcf		5 mg/cu m
Total dust			50 mppcf		15 mg/cu m

*From General Industry OSHA Safety and Health standards (29 CFR 1910.1000) US Dept of Labor, OSHA 2206, revised June, 1981.

and the analogues of benzidine, such as o-tolidine and o-dianisidine, which have similar chemical structure, exhibit carcinogenic properties in animals.[3] Exposure to these dyes occurs mainly in the finishing department.

Organic Solvents.—These are widely used throughout the finishing process. These solvents include: acetone, benzene, xylene, toluene, methanol, formaldehyde, trichloroethane, and dichloromethane.

Leather Dust.—This dust can comprise both fibers and grains, and may be in the respirable range. Buffing is the main source of dust, requiring local ventilation equipment to control exposure levels. The hazards associated with breathing leather dust is linked with the chemicals used to treat the leather. Trivalent and hexavalent chromium are present in dust from chrome-tanned leathers.[12]

Infectious Biologic Agents.—Infection is a constant hazard for tannery workers. In the wet operations, the hides and excess tissue serve as the media for numerous microorganisms. The disinfectants and biocides used to disinfect the hides inhibit the development of bacteria, fungi, and yeast colonies. The vaccination of livestock against anthrax as well as the use of biocides has prevented cases of anthrax in tannery workers which was common before the turn of the century.[10]

Table 63–9 contains a list of the chemical substances which are commonly encountered in the tanning industry, for which the Occupational Safety and Health Administration has issued legally enforceable exposure limits.

Other Health Hazards

Accidents are a leading cause of disability in leather tanning workers. Slips and falls on wet, soiled floors are common, as are knife cuts from the trimming of hides. The machinery used to process the hides also presents a hazard to workers with the capability of inflicting bruises, scrapes, crushing, abrasions, or amputations of the upper extremities.

According to the Bureau of Labor Statistics, leather tanning and finishing had the highest incidence of dermatoses of any working group in the United States.[11] Wet hides are still handled manually throughout the tanning process in many plants. Even though workers wear cotton gloves to get a firm grip on the slippery hides, these gloves offer no protection from the continuous exposure to the tanning chemicals.

Although one study dealing specifically with leather tanners demonstrated a nonsignificant increase in bladder cancer,[1] it has been suggested that leather tanners may have an increased risk for nasal, lung, and bladder cancer, since they have potential or actual exposure to many known or suspected mutagens and carcinogens.[12] These include hexavalent chromium, formaldehyde, benzidine-analogue dyes, and N-nitroso compounds.

The International Agency for Research on Cancer (IARC) of the World Health Organization has evaluated the limited epidemiologic evidence. The IARC noted that the association between lymphomas as well as cancer of the lung, larynx, buccal cavity, pharynx, kidneys, and bladder came from hypothesis-generating studies, and referred to employment in the leather industry but not specifically tanneries.[12]

REFERENCES

1. Cole P, Hoover R, Friedell GH: Occupation and cancer of the lower urinary tract. *Cancer* 1972; 29:1250–1260.
2. *Employment and Earnings*. US Bureau of Labor Statistics, October 1979, vol 26.
3. Health Hazard Alert, OSHA, NIOSH, Benzidine-, o-Tolidine-, and o-Dianisidine-Based Dyes, DHHS (NIOSH) Publ 81-106. US Dept of Labor, US Dept of Health and Human Services, December 1980.
4. *Industry Wage Survey: Leather Tanning and Finishing, March 1973*. US Bureau of Labor Statistics, Bull 1835, 1975.
5. Lallor RM: Report on a study and the development of a mold resistant treatment for leather. *J Am Leather Chemists Assoc* 1944; 39:(1)12–24.
6. Leather, in *Kirk-Othmer Encyclopedia of Chemical Technology*, ed 3. New York, Wiley-Interscience Publisher, vol 14, 1981.
7. *Leather Facts*. Peabody, Mass, New England Tanners Club, 1965.
8. O'Flaherty F, Roddy WT, Lollar RM (eds): *The Chemistry and Technology of Leather*. Malabar, Fla, Tanners' Council Laboratory, Robert E Krieger Publishing Co, 1978, vol 1–4.
9. Rounbehler DP, Krull IS, Goff EU, et al: Exposure to N-nitrosodimethylamine in a leather tannery. *Fd Cosmet Toxicol*, 1979; 17:487–491.
10. Sommer D, et al: Occupational pathology in tanneries. *Arch Mal Prof Med Travial Securite Sociale (Paris)* 1971; 32(12):723–732.
11. Stevens CS: Assessing skin problems of occupational origin. Occupational Health and Safety Nov/Dec 1979; 79 48(8):18, 39–43.
12. World Health Organization, International Agency for Research on Cancer: Wood, leather and some associated industries. *Eval Carcinog Risk Chem Hum, IARC Monogr* 25:201–247. Lyon, France, IARC Publishers, 1981.

64

Plasticizers, Vinyl Chloride, Polyvinyls, and Pyrolysis Products: Biochemical and Clinical Aspects

Edward M. Cordasco, M.D.

Julius Kerkay, Ph.D.

Stephen L. Demeter, M.D.

Karl Pearson, Ph.D.

Vernon N. Dodson, M.D.

Today, about 300 different plasticizers are manufactured, and about 100 of these, including phthalates, phosphates, and epoxides, have great industrial use. A plasticizer is defined in terms of the desired properties of a given polymer system. For coating of films, it is defined as a compound that gives flexibility, shock resistance, a feeling of hardness, etc. For an elastomeric material, a plasticizer changes the properties by reducing stiffness and permitting easier milling and mixing. Depending on how plasticizers are compounded into the polymers, there are two kinds of plasticizers: internal and external. External plasticizers are compounds of low vapor pressure that, without chemical reaction, interact with the polymer by means of their solvent or swelling power at elevated temperatures. Internal plasticizers are actually part of the polymer molecule. Because external plasticizers are more efficient, have more solvent power and have higher compatibility, they are more commonly used in the polymer industry. Phthalate esters are external plasticizers.

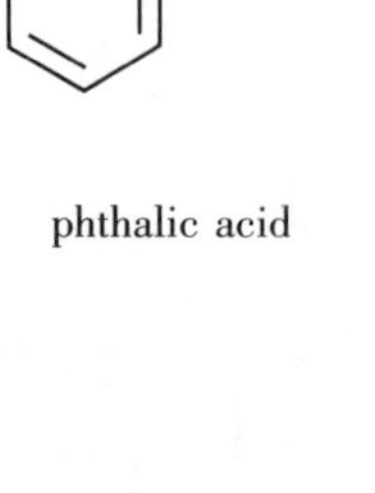

COOH, COOH

phthalic acid

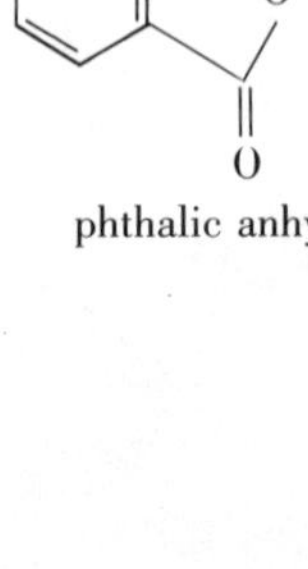

O, O, O

phthalic anhydride

PHTHALATE ESTERS

Phthalate esters are prepared by reacting phthalic anhydride with a specific alcohol to produce the desired ester. Phthalic acid is made by catalytic oxidation of *o*-toluic acid and oxidation of xylene. Phthalic anhydride is prepared from naphthalene by oxidation with a mixture of $HgSO_4$ and $CuSO_4$ in the presence of H_2SO_4 and V_2O_5 as a catalyst. Exposures may occur by inhalation or skin contact. The diesters of methanol, ethanol, butanol, isobutanol, isooctanol, isononanol, 2-ethylhexanol, etc., are irritants and sensitizers of the skin and respiratory tract (see Chapters 10 and 16).

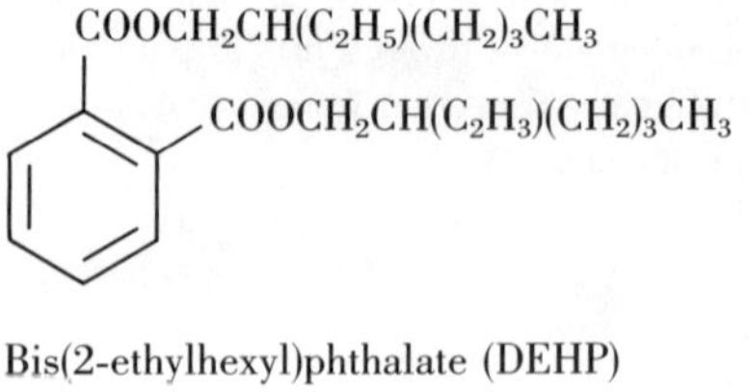

$COOCH_2CH(C_2H_5)(CH_2)_3CH_3$

$COOCH_2CH(C_2H_3)(CH_2)_3CH_3$

Bis(2-ethylhexyl)phthalate (DEHP)

Bis(2-ethylhexyl)phthalate (DEHP) is one of the most commonly used industrial phthalate esters. In a finished product, the composition of a phthalate ester may be up to 40% by weight of plastic. DEHP is probably the most widely used plasticizer. It is used extensively in polyvinyl chloride (PVC) products. In 1970, an estimated 160 million kilograms of DEHP were produced in the

United States; by 1980, two and a half million metric tons of PVC were produced in the United States. About 87% of these substances are consumed by the plastics industry for production of "soft polyvinyl chlorides." Other uses are for producing or as additive for cellulose, in many colors, lacquers, lubricants, insect repellants, in perfumes, and in some explosives as binders.

Industrial and consumer products of the PVC type will generally contain one of the phthalate esters as a plasticizer. Common household goods, food packagings, medical tubings, catheters, blood and blood product containers, and even coatings of drugs contain phthalate esters. Incineration of these waste products may be a factor for concern for potential health risks to humans.[1a]

Draviam et al.[21] studied the human metabolism of DEHP, and found that the urine of dialyzed nonuremic patients contained phthalic acid, mono(2-ethylhexyl)phthalate (MEHP), and DEHP. Other compounds identified were p-hydroxybenzoic acid, m-hydroxybenzoic acid, o-hydroxyhippuric acid, o-hydroxybenzoic acid, and benzoic acid. The levels of phthalic acid and DEHP found in the urine of patients who were on total body oxygenators were comparable to levels of phthalic acid in the urine of uremic patients, while MEHP and DEHP were present only in small amounts or were not detected.

To examine the toxic effects in animals, Chen et al.[9] injected DEHP into dogs. Among adipose tissue, brain, heart, kidney, liver, lung, and spleen, lung tissue was found to have the highest concentration of DEHP. Lung tissues had extensive presence of intra-alveolar fluid compared to lung tissues from non-DEHP-treated controls. Toxicity of phthalate esters appeared to be of low order, described as "subtle" by Lawrence and Tuell.[34] However, toxicity is the major concern for those chronically exposed to DEHP and who develop pulmonary dysfunction, because low levels of DEHP have been demonstrated to produce "shock lung" syndrome in animals.[48]

Airborne DEHP exists in trace amounts in metropolitan areas. Bove et al.[6] found that the average yearly concentrations of DEHP were 10.20, 16.79, and 14.10 ng/m^3, respectively, at three sampling stations located in the metropolitan area of New York City. They found that there were higher levels of DEHP in urban than in suburban air. These authors suggest that DEHP as an air pollutant is probably associated with the activities characteristic of city living. The subtle toxicity of phthalate esters suggests that it is necessary to continue to study the relationship between environmental pollution by phthalate esters and their toxicity.

Milkov et al.[45] studied the effect of chronic exposure to phthalate plasticizers on the health of workers. One hundred and forty-seven people (87 women and 60 men) were studied. The duration of occupational contact with plasticizers was 1 to 5 years for 54 people, 6 to 10 years for 28 people, and 10 to 29 years for 65 people. The levels of vinyl chloride, carbon monoxide, and hydrogen chloride in the working zones were found to be either less than maximum allowable levels or not detectable. Various subjective and other findings were reported in those subjects: pain and weakness in the extremities, polyneuritis, and other central nervous system disorders.

Dioctyl adipate (DOA) is another additive used with DEHP in PVC products intended for low-temperature use, as in films, sheeting, and extrusions. This agent has induced dominant lethal mutations and reduced fertility in mice, but no adverse effects in rats or other animal species.

Clinical Aspects of DEHP Leachability

The most widely used polymer in medical applications is plasticized PVC, even though large quantities of the plasticizer, mainly DEHP, leach out into blood. Although DEHP seems to have low acute toxicity as described earlier, its long-term effects, including carcinogenicity, are still debated.[64] In any event, the large amount of DEHP leaching out into patients represents added burden on the liver and kidney. Also, the more toxic MEHP, one of the DEHP metabolites, increases the concern of this aspect. Lewis et al.[37] found that serum levels of DEHP were being absorbed by a patient undergoing cardiac bypass surgery. Draviam et al.[21] found that the average DEHP excretion into the urine of cardiac bypass surgery patients was 52 μgrams per 24 hours and 161 μgrams 48 hours post surgery.

Concern over risk of exposure to DEHP needs to be kept in proper perspective, especially since many biomedical devices incorporating DEHP-plasticized PVC provide often lifesaving therapeutic benefit.

Vinyl Chloride
$H_2C{=}CHCl$

The earliest studies on vinyl chloride (vinyl chloride monomer = VCM) were limited to acute exposures. These observations led to its consideration as a surgical anesthetic. About 30 to 35 years ago, during the earlier work exposures, the chief concern was to keep workroom atmospheric concentrations below the explosive limit (3.5% or about 30,000 ppm). Men commonly worked at exposure levels of 3,000 to 4,000 ppm (near the narcosis level), and it was not at all unusual to have men leave the work place for relief and fresh air outside. Generally, these studies showed vinyl chloride to be low in acute toxicity, to be anesthetic in action, and to have little capacity to cause liver injury from exposures of a few hours. Mastromateo[44] and Lester et al.[36] studied acute exposures of animals and humans. They reported very little effect until exposure concentrations approached 10,000 ppm, when humans experienced dizziness after 5 minutes of exposure.

Torkelson et al.[59] conducted animal studies to determine chronic toxicity to assess the hazards to humans. Vinyl chloride was found to have a slight capacity to cause liver and kidney injury on repeated exposures. Male and female rats showed micropathologic changes after repeated 7-hour exposures at 500 ppm for 4.5 months. Repeated 7-hour exposures at 200 ppm for 6 months resulted in micropathologic changes in the livers of rabbits and statistically significant increases in the average weight of the livers of male and female rats but no detectable changes in dogs and guinea pigs. Repeated 7-hour exposures at 100 ppm resulted in slight increases in the average weight of rat livers; the other species were not affected. All species studied tolerated repeated daily 7-hour exposures to 50 ppm for 6 months with no detectable injury.

Repeated daily 1-hour exposures at 200 and 100 ppm of vinyl

chloride were without effect; longer exposures caused a slight increase in liver weight.

The standard for evaluating regular daily 7- to 8-hour exposures may be defined as the concentration below which practically all analytic results must fall. The value of 100 ppm was suggested as the standard for vinyl chloride, with a time-weighted average for all exposures not to exceed 50 ppm (Fig 64–1).

Acro-osteolysis

Acro-osteolysis consists of localized areas of bone necrosis and absorption. These lesions are nontender and are not associated with a periosteal reaction. The hands and fingers are most commonly involved. In a majority of cases, acro-osteolysis is associated with Raynaud's phenomenon and sclerodermatous skin changes.

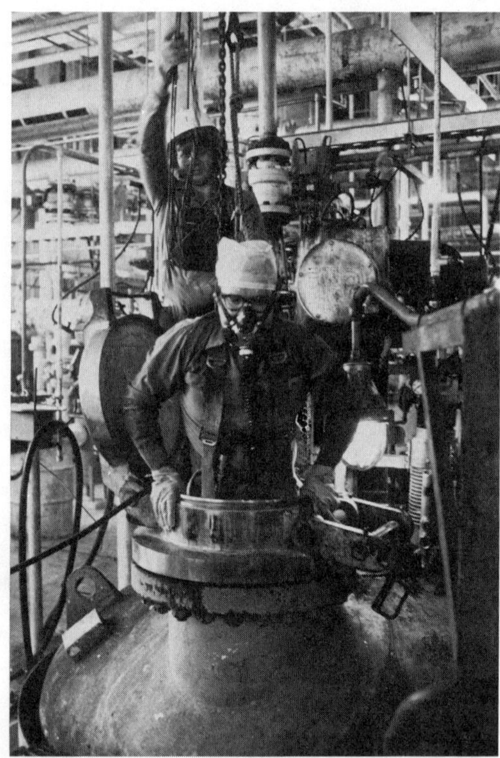

FIG 64–1.
A worker entering a PVC reactor vessel to clean out caked polymer adhering to the inner surfaces. During the polymerization reaction, sludge from the slurry has a tendency to form a crust on the impeller mechanism as well as the tank inner surfaces. The caked polymer is periodically hand-chipped by workers inside the tank, and this is the operation that subjected workers to the highest concentrations of vinyl chloride. Current practice requires that flexible ducts be used for purging with clean air before the worker enters. In addition, workers in this operation must be provided with positive-pressure air-supplied respirators, preferably the hood type. Demand-type respirators have been used, but may not offer the same protection as the continuous-flow type of hood respirator. (Courtesy of Maurice N. Johnson, M.D., B.F. Goodrich Company, Akron, Ohio. Photographer–H. Groskinski.)

Harris and Adam[28] studied workers engaged in the polymerization of vinyl chloride and reported two cases in which autoclave cleaners in the vinyl chloride polymerization process were scraping the walls of the autoclave to remove the PVC with considerable hand/skin contact. Acro-osteolysis was reported to have occurred in two workers.

Of the 588 PVC workers in this plant, including 150 autoclave cleaners, two cases were identified based on x-rays of the hands of these workers. The terminal phalanges of the hands, the patella, and the phalanges of the feet were involved. Two other workers, also autoclave cleaners, demonstrated early changes accompanied by Raynaud's phenomenon.

Wilson[68] studied 31 cases of occupational acro-osteolysis of the hands of workers engaged in vinyl chloride polymerization processes. Most of these workers had worked as cleaners of vessel walls and other equipment in the polymer process. The acro-osteolysis was localized to the distal phalanges of hands and frequently was associated with Raynaud symptoms. They reported that the disorder resulted from a combination of physical insult, chemical insult, and personal idiosyncrasy, and were unable to name specific causes. Prevalence was reported to be less than 3% among employees performing similar work, and no cases were found in workmen processing the polymer or manufacturing commercial resins. More than 100 workers handled the finished resin; those who processed it into plastic products did not demonstrate findings of acro-osteolysis.

In 1970 and 1971, Dinman[19] of the Institute of Environmental and Industrial Health at The University of Michigan, conducted a comprehensive study of acro-osteolysis in workers producing and compounding vinyl and PVC. The epidemiologic population represented more than 5,000 workers in 32 plants. Thirty-one cases were discovered, of which 25 had a definite diagnosis; there were 16 suspicious diagnoses of acro-osteolysis clearly associated with hand cleaning of the polymerizers.

Dodson[20] determined that work practices, rather than any specific agent or combination of agents, appeared to relate to the occurrence of the disease. He thought the disease to be of systemic rather than localized in nature, but was unable to define the etiologic agent or portal of entry, suggesting some idiosyncratic "sensitization of susceptibility." An industrial hygiene survey of this epidemiologic investigation[9] revealed vinyl chloride concentrations in the reactor before ventilating to be about 3,000 ppm. After aeration of the containers, the vinyl chloride concentration inside the reactors during scraping was found to be under 100 ppm and usually around 50 ppm. It was found that scraping released some unpolymerized vinyl chloride so that levels of 600 to 1,000 ppm were found close to the hands during these operations, implying the potentially high worker respiratory inhalation. Other possible constituents of the scrapings of the reactor vessels were thought to be polymerized resins, unreacted catalysts, additives and, of course, the polymerized vinyl chloride. No serious disability had been reported in any of the above-mentioned cases but a few men had been partially disabled because of hand soreness, with some restriction in manual activity. With proper protective equipment and careful hygienic measures, all these cases are preventable (Fig 64–2).

Veltman et al.[62] reported findings in 70 workers cleaning autoclaves and centrifuges, during drying and sifting processes, and

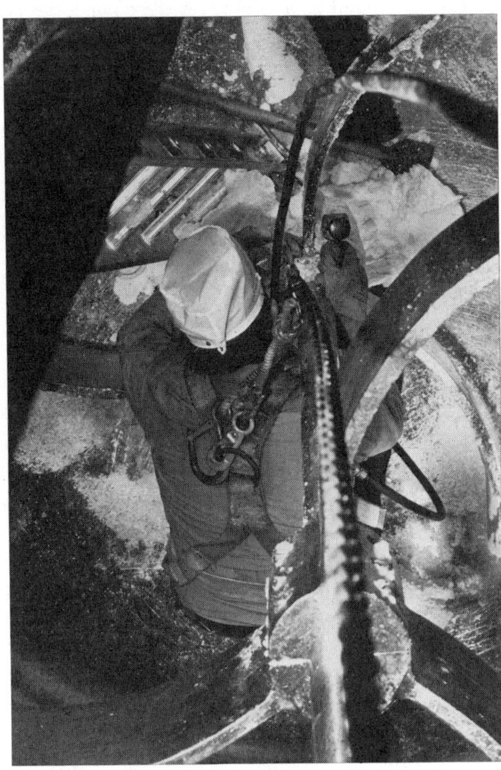

FIG 64–2.
The solid, caked polymer must be removed by chisels, hammers, and handpicks. Neither workers nor management may be aware of the hazard involved when a spark is generated by steel on steel. It is not uncommon to open a pocket of the cake lining the vessel. The pocket may contain liquid vinyl chloride monomer. It is very possible that the lower explosive limit for vinyl chloride monomer (33,000 ppm) can be reached during the chipping with steel on steel. Reactor vessels have exploded, leaving nothing but a crater in the ground where the plant once stood. Reactor chipping or cleaning tools should be of the nonsparking type. To minimize worker entry, some companies use high-pressure water guns to remove the caked polymer. These water guns may operate from 9,000 to 13,000 pounds of pressure per square inch. This in itself may produce a serious safety hazard. Some attempts in the United States to remove the caked slurry have utilized closed solvent cleaning systems in which solvents such as tetrahydrofuran are used. To date, such solvent cleaning systems have been relatively unsuccessful. Recently completed production systems using 30,000-gallon reactor vessels have been utilizing automatic high-pressure water cleaning guns and solvent systems to minimize or eliminate the need for worker entry into reactor vessels. Older reactor vessels, which contain cooling vanes of heat exchangers, complicate the cleaning process and high-pressure water guns and solvent systems cannot be used in these tanks. (Courtesy of Maurice N. Johnson, M.D., B. F. Goodrich Company, Akron, Ohio. Photographer–H. Groskinski.)

wrapping dry PVC as an end product for a 7.7-year average. Sclerodermatous-like skin changes were seen in 8 patients, acro-osteolysis in 6, and Raynaud's phenomenon in 6.

Lilis et al.[38] believed that a vascular abnormality was the primary lesion leading to secondary skin and bone changes. In many people in a group of 267 workers and 87 former workers of a vinylchloride polymerization plant, they found clinical symptoms and signs of abnormal peripheral circulation. These effects were seen much more frequently in those with greater than 10 years exposure. Findings included numbness, tingling, excessive sensitivity to cold, pain, cyanosis, involvement of the toes, and Raynaud's syndrome. An abnormal Allen test was seen in 26.6% of all workers, pseudoclubbing in 8.75%, and sclerodermatous-like skin changes in 6.4%.

The specific effect of VCM on the peripheral circulation that culminates in neural, dermal, and skeletal manifestations has long been in doubt. The superficial resemblance to progressive systemic sclerosis (scleroderma) has prompted immunologic investigation. In a report of 22 PVC workers by Langauer-Leowowick et al.[32] in 1976, 6 workers had prodromal symptoms of Raynaud's phenomenon, 10 had typical Raynaud's syndrome, and an additional 6 had scleroderma-like changes in the upper extremities with acro-osteolysis of the distal phalanges and Raynaud's syndrome. Raynaud's syndrome was described as symptoms of cold intolerance and paresthesia in the fingers with increased vasospastic tendencies in the digital arteries. Cryoglobulinemia (83.8%) and increased levels of immunoglobulins (22.7%) were found as well as changes in other plasma proteins. Those with more pronounced symptoms were more likely to have immunologic abnormalities. IgG was elevated in 5 of 22 and IgM in 1 of 22. In another study, IgG was found to be elevated in 67%.[54]

Cryoglobulins were also seen in a study of 88 workers by Ward et al.[27] These workers were divided into three groups: 9 patients with vinyl chloride disease (VCD) with a spectrum of clinical findings encompassing abnormalities of the liver, spleen, blood, nervous system, lungs, as well as acro-osteolysis; 44 with possible VCD; and 35 vinyl chloride "exposed only" workers. Cryoglobulins were seen in 66%, 44%, 0%. Immune complexes were found in 55%, 27%, and 0%. The cryoglobulin was composed of IgG, C3, and fibrinogen. Rheumatoid factor was negative in all patients when measured by the latex agglutination method but was positive in low titer by hemagglutination in 90% of workers with definite VCD and 22.7% of those with possible VCD. Immunofluorescent examination of skin and muscle biopsies in those patients with definite VCD showed the presence of IgG, C3, and fibrinogen within the lumen of small blood vessels and adherent to the vascular endothelium. These authors proposed that a metabolite of VCM binds to IgG-producing aggregates that can precipitate as immune complexes during cold exposure. These complexes then stimulate complement activation and cause platelet aggregation and the conversion of fibrinogen to fibrin, thus occluding capillaries and small blood vessels.

Liver

A hepatitis-like effect has been long associated with PVC exposure. In a study of 70 workers,[62] 14% had elevated liver enzymes including SGOT, alkaline phosphatase, and LDH. Hepatomegaly was found in 15% of patients in Lilis' series,[38] although no direct associations could be found with elevated liver enzymes. In a study of vinyl chloride and liver disease, Thomas et al.[58] identified hemangiosarcomas in 15 of 26 patients studied. This was a nonconsecutive series, but all patients had at least 2 years' exposure. In addition to the tumors, histologic changes included hypertrophy and hyperplasia of both hepatocytes and hepatic splenic mesenchymal cells. Portal tract fibrosis was seen. Varices in the esophagus or fundus of the stomach were seen in 11.4% of 70 workers[62] although no mention was made of alcohol ingestion history. In a review of liver biopsies in 51 PVC production workers,[26] degenerative lesions in the hepatocytes were seen in 46 of 50, septal or perisinusoidal fibrosis in 16 and 37 patients, and activation and proliferation of sinusoidal cells in nearly all the patients. Hemangioendothelioma or sarcoma was seen in 2 patients. Thus, vinyl chloride-PVC exposure appears to encompass the spectrum of hepatic injury from hepatitis with a simple enzyme deviation to hepatic fibrosis and tumor.

In January 1974, a manufacturer of PVC and copolymers notified its employees, the National Institute for Occupational Safety and Health, the Kentucky State Department of Labor, and the public that three workers had died of angiosarcoma of the liver. These cases had a common denominator: employment in the manufacture of PVC resins. The report by Creech and Johnson[17] has resulted in an enlarged scope of knowledge and eventually uncovered more than 75 known angiosarcomas connected with vinyl chloride exposures from other workplaces in later years.

Thomas[57] proposed a pathogenetic scheme involving the "stimulation" of hepatic cells in vinyl chloride workers that leads to the various inflammatory, fibrotic, or neoplastic states. It has been shown that PVC can be directly cytotoxic.[18, 49] In a study of the fate of inhaled VCM in rats, Hefner[29] reported that small but significant amounts were retained in tissue, particularly the liver. Inhaled VCM has been shown to produce hepatic inflammation and fibrosis in guinea pigs.[48, 69] These effects can be seen with relatively low exposures (50 ppm) but are dependent on the duration of exposure. Other animal studies have shown the induction of various tumors including lung adenoma and adenocarcinomas, lymphomas, mammary gland tumors, skin tumors (including papillomas and mucoepidermoid carcinomas), osteochondromas, tumors of the zymbal glands, nephroblastomas, and neuroblastomas, in addition to the hepatic tumors.[35, 63]

With the exception of hemangioma of the liver, no firm conclusions can be found in epidemiologic studies. Increased numbers of tumors in PVC workers were found in the respiratory, central nervous, and the lymphatic/hematopoietic systems,[8, 30, 56, 65,] but had not reached a significant level. However, Falk and co-workers[24] found a change in the expected cell types of lung tumors with more large cell undifferentiated and adenocarcinomas. The total number of deaths due to malignancy was increased in Waxweiler's report,[65] but this association could not be found in other series.[22, 24, 50] Duck et al. reported a significant excess deaths in the category of malignant brain neoplasms[22] and Cooper[13] reported excess deaths from brain tumors.

OSHA and the NIOSH have recognized VCM as a carcinogen, and requirements of environmental and medical surveillance pertinent to known carcinogens are mandated. The present OSHA environmental limit is 1 ppm averaged over 8 hours with a maximum of 5 ppm for any 15-minute period.[61]

Pulmonary Effects

Exclusive exposure to vinyl chloride or PVC can result in acute or chronic effects; symptoms of acute bronchitis have been found by some and not by others.[25, 46] Airflow limitation has been found to be associated with either the production or degradation (decomposition) of vinyl chloride or PVC. In 1973, Sokol[52] coined the term "meal wrapper's asthma" to describe a syndrome of acute airflow obstruction associated with tightness in the chest, wheezing, dyspnea, and cough, suggesting that these findings were associated with the liberation of PVC fumes during the pyrolysis of PVC film. Falk and Portnoy[23] found that meat wrappers had increased respiratory tract problems: wheezing, shortness of breath, chest pain or tightness, and a large number of meat wrappers probably had mild symptoms with some progressing to severe respiratory impairment or clinical asthma. They found a group of 145 meat wrappers who were working with mechanical blade machines did not develop respiratory tract symptoms related to work. While the existence of this syndrome[7] or the specificity of PVC as the offending agent[5] has been disputed, it has been shown that workers exposed to vinyl chloride-PVC fumes do have both acute and chronic airflow obstruction. These effects have been shown to be both dependent[25, 46] and independent[3, 53] of smoking status. Greater abnormalities in pulmonary function testing were found usually in workers with the longest exposures. Impaired flow rates were seen in 84% of workers with greater than 20 years of exposure,[46] and in 50% of workers in another series.[3] These findings were not independent of cigarette smoking and could not be corroborated by another study.[25] Restrictive abnormalities were found in 8% of 37 patients[33] and abnormal chest x-rays compatible with early interstitial lung disease were seen in 6% of 818 patients,[53] 8% of 37 workers,[33] 31.9% of 1,216 workers,[42] up to 30% of workers after 20 years of exposure,[39] and 50% of 985 patients.[3] These changes were not usually extensive and were not independent of smoking status. Pneumoconiosis was diagnosed in 2.7% of 852 exposed PVC workers.[43]

Some histologic lesions due to PVC dust were described in humans.[55] In 1981, Lilis[40] reviewed pulmonary effects of PVC and vinyl chloride exposure. She suggested that interstitial pulmonary fibrosis is a possible effect of vinyl chloride exposure. However, in a large epidemiologic study of 818 men working in a PVC manufacturing company, Soutar showed that exposure to respirable PVC dust with particle diameter less than 7 μm was associated with some deterioration of lung function, slight abnormalities of the chest radiograph, and complaints of slight dyspnea.[53] These authors ruled out that the symptoms were the effects of vinyl chloride, and the results agreed with the findings of Waxweiler et al.[66] Chivers and co-workers[10] conducted a study involving 509 male workers exposed to PVC dust. They concluded that work with PVC dust did not produce deleterious effects on ventilatory function.

Recently, Antti-Poika et al. have demonstrated interstitial changes from PVC dust characterized by profuse accumulation of macrophages, some intra-alveolar hemmorhage, and increased elastic and collagen fibers.[1]

In an experiment simulating meat wrapping in a supermarket, Boettner and Ball[5] found that during hot wire cutting of film, plasticizer values ranged from 1 to 100 mg per cut with up to 300 mg per cut when there were smoky cuts in the series. They found that DEHP was one of the major plasticizers. Airborne DEHP particulates are generally breathable. In an experiment, Pegg and Soderholm[47] demonstrated that the size of airborne DEHP particulates ranged from 0.1 to 10.0 μm with mass median aerodynamic diameter (MMAD) less than 2.0 μm. Smith and co-workers[51] reported that poor cutting techniques could produce substantially higher emissions than those produced by a good technique. They suggested that plasticizer particulate aerosol may act as a carrier of hydrogen chloride deep into the lungs of the exposed workers. Although DEHP has a low vapor pressure and low water solubility tends to be stabilized within a polymer matrix, when it is heated, volatilization of DEHP can occur at an increased rate, resulting in elevated atmospheric concentration different from the processing of PVC. Wheeler[67] suggested that in a study of PVC-linked occupational hazards, the type of process of PVC plant must be identified, something not done in the past.

Twenty-four pulmonary patients who reported having work-related exposure to PVC, either as volatile chemicals or solid particulates, were subjects to determine DEHP levels in their body fluids and tissues. These patients were diagnosed as having acute or chronic interstitial lung disease (ILD) or bronchial asthma.

In most patients, blood and 24-hour urine specimens were collected, and in 5 patients, lung biopsy specimens were available. DEHP was present in the serum of 13 of the 22 patients, and the concentration of DEHP ranged from 12.5 to 400.0 ng/ml. The detection limit was 5.0 ng/ml. DEHP levels in 24-hour urine specimens of 14 patients ranged from 9.0 to 292 ng/ml with 5.0 ng/ml as the detection limit. Two of the five lung biopsy specimens had DEHP concentrations of 59.7 and 1090.0 ng/gm, respectively, with a detection limit of 30.0 ng/gm. Serum DEHP levels were below the detection limit for 10 healthy individuals whose age ranged from 28 to 39 years old and who were not exposed to DEHP in job-related environments. DEHP concentrations in 24-hour urine specimens were at or below detectable levels for 2 healthy individuals aged 30 and 32 years old, respectively, who also participated as controls in the serum DEHP levels study. Table 64–1 shows the DEHP levels of these patients and the type of exposure that probably caused their pulmonary dysfunction. Five of these patients with negative results had been away from exposure for several years, which perhaps accounts for those negative results. Additionally, 3 patients were not involved with PVC fumes or dust for several months.

Patients 10, 11, and 19 (see Table 64–1) had asbestos exposure confirmed from biopsy specimens examined by an electron microscopy specialist. DEHP levels in patient 10 were very high (400.0 ng/ml serum). During 29 years of work, this patient was exposed to talc and other chemicals of plastic monomer types, including styrene, vinyl toluene and methylacrylate, besides asbestos. However, his stated history did not reveal any PVC related exposure. Begin et al.[4] found that lung biopsy specimens demonstrated peribronchiolar alveolitis and fibrosis with obliteration and narrowing of the small airways in 3 out of 17 asbestos workers. Patient 5 was exposed to MDI (diphenylmethane diisocyanate), TDI (toluene diisocyanate), methylene chloride, and other fumes and aerosols. Blood sample of this patient was not available, but there was 18.0 ng DEHP/ml in his urine sample. The diagnosis of the patient was chemical bronchitis and occupational asthma; nevertheless, it is uncertain that DEHP or PVC exposure contributed

TABLE 64–1.
DEHP Levels*

PATIENT CODE	NAME	OCCUPATION	AGE	SEX	SERUM (NG/ML)	URINE	TISSUE (NG/GM)
1	BS	Meat wrapper	35	F	63.9	124.7	
2	JS	Butcher	42	M	170.0	37.0	
3	BB	Meat wrapper	54	F	54.0	25.0	
4	NK	Retired RN	63	F	NA	35.0	
5	AL	Carpenter	46	M	NA	18.0	
6	JT	PVC (cables and sewer ducts)	31	M	95.0	28.0	1090.0
7	OO	Meat cutter	50	M	81.0	30.0	
10	RP	Foreman	51	M	400.0	9.0	
11	DS	Estimater	52	M	25.0	9.6	
12	LL	Press operator	43	F	ND	ND	
13	RB	Paint mixer	46	M	170.0	292.0	
14	JN	Const. worker	34	M	ND	ND	
15	TF	Const. worker	56	F	110.0	ND	
16	ML	Meat wrapper	57	F	82.8	40.9	ND†
17	GB	PVC worker	55	F	12.5	58.0	
18	BL	Mechanic	35	M	84.0	32.0	59.7
19	HH	Packer	59	F	25.0	30.0	QNS
20	AW	Chem. worker	37	M	NA	ND	
21	BM	Rubber worker	47	F	ND	ND	
22	FB	Retired film processor	67	F	ND	ND	
23	TT	Press operator	52	M	ND	ND	
24	WT	PVC worker	57	M	ND	ND	ND†

*ND = none detected (less than 5.0 ng/ml); NA = specimen not available;
†ND = none detected (less than 30.0 ng/gm); QNS = quantity not sufficient (less than 0.3 gm).

to the cause of the symptoms (further study of the aerosols to which he was exposed were indicated). Patient 18 was working for a vinyl plant as a maintenance mechanic for 2 years when pulmonary symptoms developed. He had 84.0 ng DEHP/ml serum and 32.0 ng DEHP/ml urine. The lung biopsy specimen of this patient contained 59.7 ng/gm. Although no plasticizer exposure was identified in the history of this patient, the results of DEHP analyses suggest that he was possibly exposed to DEHP in his working environment.

Patient 21 was exposed to 1,1,1-trichloroethane (which when heated may evolve hydrogen chloride, phosgene, and carbon monoxide). Both serum and urine DEHP levels were nondetectable, which correlated well with the type of patient exposure. DEHP was absent (below 5 ng/ml) in both serum and urine specimens from patient 12, who inhaled xylene fumes as a drill press operator. Occupational chronic bronchitis was the diagnosis for this patient.

Table 64–2 tabulates the type of exposure and corresponding DEHP levels of serum and urine of the patients. There were 11 subjects exposed to PVC in manufacturing factories (patients 6, 13, 14, 17, 19, 20, 22, 23, 24) and in living environment (patient 15). No serum DEHP was found in the urine of this uremic patient who was undergoing chronic dialysis using PVC tubings. Draviam et al.[21] found that there were very low levels (less than 28 ng/ml) of DEHP in the urine of uremic patients undergoing routine hemodialysis. Our patient's result agreed with their findings.

In the group consisting of patients with PVC exposure only, patient 22 and patient 24 had nondetectable levels of serum and urine DEHP. Patient 22, who had interstitial lung disease and rheumatoid arthritis, had been a moderate (¼ pack per day) smoker for 28 years, and was a light (7 packs per year) smoker recently. She was exposed to PVC when working with plastic photomaterial in a copying process that required hot wire cutting of the material. Patient 24 was a PVC plant worker; he had chronic inflammation and organizing alveolitis with some slight alveolar lining cell desquamation and arteriosclerosis. The clinical findings strongly suggested a PVC and/or vinyl chloride exposure. DEHP might be not the plasticizer used in the PVC materials with which patients 22 and 24 worked and may be the reason for the nondetectable amount of DEHP in these patients' specimens.

In this study, DEHP levels of patients who worked in supermarket meat cutting and wrapping processes show the most significant correlation between patient DEHP levels and the type of exposure. In the group, including a butcher and a meat cutter, DEHP levels ranged from 54.0 to 170.0 ng/ml serum and 25.0 to 124.7 ng/ml urine.

Patient 16 was a typical example of this group. The woman had been employed as a meat wrapper for 20 years. Besides cutting and sealing the plastic wrap by melting it on a hot wire, she worked with adhesive stamping. She experienced cough and shortness of breath in relation to her work, and reported more pronounced fatigue as the week went by. It was found that she had interstitial pulmonary fibrosis that accounted for her symptoms. DEHP levels of her serum and urine were 82.8 and 40.9 ng/ml, respectively. DEHP concentration of her lung biopsy specimen, however, was below 30.0 ng/gm, which is the minimum detectable level.

As discussed earlier, DEHP tends to accumulate in lung tissues, and in high concentration is shown to cause lung infiltrates in animals.[9, 48] The effect observed in animals is similar to that observed in ILD in humans caused by chemicals, for which PVC and/or DEHP may be etiologically responsible. In the environment where inhalation exposure of heated PVC is the major concern, DEHP, which is lipophilic and breathable, should be considered as a pathogenic agent.

Recently, Cook[12] reported that PVC film now used in meat wrapping operations contains bis(2-ethylhexyl)adipate (DOA) as its major plasticizer. Smith et al.[51] found that 100% of particulates emitted from the wire cutter in the meat wrapping process was DOA. Boettner and Ball[5] found that DOA was one of three plasticizers commonly used in food-wrapping films, while DEHP and acetyl tributylcitrate (ATBC) are the other two. Experiments done in our laboratory to determine the DEHP content of meat wrap film confirmed the presence of this agent in seven different sample rolls. The mean concentration was 37.5 μg/gm of film, .038% by weight (Table 64–3). Since 1956, DOA has been classified as a "slightly toxic" substance;[41,60] however, more toxicological studies need to be performed, especially for its chronic toxicity from inhalation and ingestion. Analyses of DOA in pulmonary patients who are chronically exposed to fumes generated from PVC products may be clinically significant.[47a]

Exposure-type injuries to lung tissue with long latency periods and causation chains have presented new pathologic challenges.

TABLE 64–2.
DEHP Levels According to Type of Exposure

TYPE OF EXPOSURE	NUMBER OF PATIENTS	RANGE OF DEHP LEVEL IN NG/ML* SERUM	URINE
Supermarket meat wrapping	5	54.0–170.0	25.0–124.7
PVC	7	ND–170.0	ND–292.0
Chemicals including PVC	4	ND– 25.0	ND– 35.0
Chemicals excluding PVC	6	ND–400.0	ND– 32.0

*ND = nondetectable (less than 5.0 ng/ml).

TABLE 64–3.
DEHP Analyses of Plastic Film*

SAMPLE NO.	LOCATION FROM OPEN END	WEIGHT OF SAMPLE (GM)	DEHP FOUND (μG/GM)
1	9.14 m†	0.3096	30.7
2	18.29 m†	0.2760	34.5
3	27.43 m†	0.4265	27.2
4	332.23 m†	0.2057	60.3
5	362.71 m (side)	0.4625	33.5
6	362.71 m (edge)	0.3064	53.8
7	362.71 m (middle)	0.2900	22.8
Mean			37.5
Standard Deviation			14.0
% RSD			37.3

*Make: Goodyear (The Goodyear Tire and Rubber Co., Akron, OH 44361)
Product: Prime-Wrap II 12" Stretch Meat Film 5000 ft.
Catalog #: 423-85-4012
Lot #: 1118827
†Side to side.

Results of DEHP analyses in our pulmonary patients revealed significant correlation between DEHP exposure and both acute and chronic interstitial pulmonary abnormalities.

It is suggested that DEHP analysis in PVC exposed patients is useful as a screening test, provided the information of occupational exposure has been studied in detail.

Acknowledgments

The administrative assistance of Patricia Senor in preparation of this chapter and the assistance of Sue Simms are greatly appreciated by the authors.

REFERENCES

1. Antti-Poika M, Nordman N, Nichels J, et al: Lung disease after exposure to PVC dust. *Thorax* 1986; 41:566–567.
1a. Arnaud A, Pommier De Santi P, Garbe L, et al: Polyvinyl chloride pneumoconiosis. *Thorax* 1978; 33:19.
2. Austian J: Toxicity and health threats of phthalate esters: Review of the literature. *J Environ Health Perspect* 1973; 4:3.
3. Barnes AW: Vinyl chloride and the production of PVC. *Proc R Soc Med* 1976; 69:277.
4. Begin R, Cantin A, Berthiaume Y, et al: Airway function in lifetime-nonsmoking older asbestos workers. *Am J Med* 1983; 75:631.
5. Boettner EA, Ball G: Thermal degradation products from PVC film in food-wrapping operations. *Am Ind Hyg Assoc J* 1980; 41:513.
6. Bove JL, Dalven P, Kukreja VP, et al: Airborne di-butyl and di-(2-ethylhexyl)-phthalate at three New York City air sampling stations. *Int J Environ Health Anal Chem* 1978; 5:189.
7. Brooks SM, Vandervort R: Polyvinyl chloride film thermal decomposition products as an occupational illness. *J Occup Med* 1977; 192.
8. Byren D, Engholm G, England A, et al: Mortality and cancer morbidity in a group of Swedish VCM and PVC production workers. *Environ Health Perspect* 1976; 17:167.
9. Chen WS, Kerkay J, Pearson KH, et al: Tissue bis(2-ethylhexyl)phthalate levels in uremic subjects. *Anal Lett* 1979; 12:1517.
10. Chivers CP, Lawrence-Jones C, Paddle GM: Lung function in workers exposed to polyvinyl chloride dust. *Br J Ind Med* 1980; 37:147.
11. Cook WA: Occupational acroosteolysis. II. An industrial hygiene study. *Arch Environ Health* 1971; 22:74.
12. Cook WA: Industrial hygiene evaluation of thermal degradation products from PVC film in meat-wrapping operations. *Am Ind Hyg Assoc J* 1980; 41:508.
13. Cooper C: Personal communication, May 1983.
14. Cordasco EM, Lira R, Demeter SL, et al: Industrial technology includes hazardous inhalants. *J Occup Health Safety* 1980; 49:42.
15. Cordasco EM, Demeter SL, Kerkay J, et al: Pulmonary manifestations of vinyl and polyvinyl chloride (interstitial lung disease). *Chest* 1980; 78:828.
16. Demeter SL, Cordasco EM, Kerkay J, et al: Interstitial lung disease associated with plastic fume exposure. Presented at The American Occupational Medical Conference, Washington, DC, 1987; *Am J Ind Med* in press.
17. Creech JL Jr, Johnson MN: Angiosarcoma liver in the manufacture of polyvinyl chloride. *J Occup Med* 1974; 16:150.
18. Dehaan RL: Toxicity of tissue culture media exposed to polyvinyl chloride plastic. *Nature* 1971; 231:85.
19. Dinman BD: Occupational acroosteolysis. I. An epidemiological study. *Arch Environ Health* 1971; 22:61.
20. Dodson VN: Occupational acroosteolysis. III. A clinical study. *Arch Environ Health* 1971; 22:83.
21. Draviam EJ, Pearson KH, Kerkay J: Human metabolism of bis(2-ethylhexyl)phthalate. *Anal Lett* 1982; 15:1729.
22. Duck BW, Carter JT, Coombes EJ: Mortality study of workers in a polyvinyl-chloride production plant. *Lancet* 1975; 4:1197.
23. Falk H, Portnoy B: Respiratory tract illness in meat wrappers. *JAMA* 1976; 235:915.
24. Falk H, Waxweiler RJ: Epidemiological studies of vinyl chloride health effects in the United States. *Proc R Soc Med* 1976; 69:303.
24a. Fishbein L: *Industrial Hazards in Plastics and Synthetic Elastomers*. New York, Alan R Liss, 1984.
25. Gamble J, Kiu S, McMicheal AJ, et al: Effect of occupational and non-occupational factors on the respiratory system of vinyl chloride and other workers. *J Occup Med* 1976; 18:650.
26. Gedigk P, Muller R, Bechtelsheimer H: Morphology of liver damage among polyvinyl chloride production workers. *Ann NY Acad Sci* 1975; 246:278.
27. Grainger RG, Walker AE, Ward AM: Vinyl chloride monomer-induced disease, in Preger L (ed): *Clinical, Radiological and Immunological Aspects in Induced Disease*. New York, Grune & Stratton, 1980, p 191.
28. Harris DK, Adam WGF: Acroosteolysis occurring among men engaged in the polymerization of vinyl chloride. *Br Med J* 1967; 3:712.
29. Hefner RE, Watanabe PG, Gehring PJ: Preliminary studies of the fate of inhaled vinyl chloride monomer in rats. *Ann NY Acad Sci* 1975; 246:135–149.
30. Infante PF, Wagoner JK, Waxweiler RJ: Carcinogenic, mutagenic and teratogenic risks associated with vinyl chloride. *Mutat Res* 1976; 41:131.
31. Jaeger RJ, Rubin RJ: Migration of a phthalate ester plasticizer from polyvinyl chloride blood bags into stored human blood and its localization in human tissues. *N Engl J Med* 1972; 287:1114.
32. Langauer-Lewowika H, Dudziak Z, Byczkowska Z, et al: Cryoglobulinemia in Raynaud's phenomenon due to vinyl chloride. *Int Arch Occup Env Health* 1976; 36:197.
33. Lange CE, Juhe S, Stein G, et al: Further results in polyvinyl chloride production workers. *Ann NY Acad Sci* 1975; 246:18.
34. Lawrence WH, Tuell SF: Phthalate esters: The question of safety—an update. *Clin Toxicol* 1979; 15:447.
35. Lee CC, Bhandari C, Winston JM, et al: Carcinogenicity of vinyl chloride and vinylidene chloride. *J Toxicol Environ Health* 1978; 4:15.
36. Lester D, Greenberg LA, Adams WR: Effects of single and repeated exposures of humans and rats to vinyl chloride. *Am Ind Hyg Assoc J* 1963; 24:265.
37. Lewis LM, Flechtner TW, Kerkay J, et al: Determination of plasticizer levels in serum of hemodialysis patients. *Trans Am Soc Artif Intern Organs* 1977; 13:566.
38. Lilis R, Anderson H, Nicolson WJ: Prevalence of disease among vinyl chloride and polyvinyl chloride workers. *Ann NY Acad Sci* 1975; 246:22.
39. Lilis R, Anderson H, Miller A, et al: Pulmonary changes among vinyl chloride polymerization workers. *Chest* 1976; 69(S):229.
40. Lilis R: Review of pulmonary effects of polyvinyl chloride and vinyl chloride exposure. *Environ Health Perspect* 1981; 41:167.
41. Limiting doses according to route of administration to experimental animals causing death. In *Registry of Toxic Effects of Chemical Substances*. Rockville, Md, National Institute for Occupational Safety and Health, 1977, vol 1.
42. Mastrangelo G, Manno M, Marcer G, et al: Polyvinyl chloride pneumoconiosis: Epidemiological study of exposed workers. *J Occup Med* 1975; 21:540.
43. Mastrangelo G, Saia B, Marcer G, et al: Epidemiological study of pneumoconiosis in the Italian polyvinyl chloride industry. *Environ Health Perspect* 1981; 41:153.

44. Mastromateo E: Acute inhalation toxicity of vinyl chloride to laboratory animals. *Am Ind Hyg Assoc J* 1960; 21:394.
45. Milkov LE: Health status of workers exposed to phthalate plasticizers in the manufacture of artificial leather and films based on PVC resins. *Environ Health Perspect* 1973; 3:175.
46. Miller A, Teirstein AS, Chuang M, et al: Changes in pulmonary function in workers exposed to vinyl chloride and polyvinyl chloride. *Ann NY Acad Sci* 1975; 246:42.
47. Pegg DG, Soderholm SC: An apparatus for production of submicron radio-labeled di-2-ethylhexyl phthalate aerosol. *Am Ind Hyg Assoc J* 1982; 43:333.
47a. Pfaffli P: *Int Arch Environ Health* 1986; 58:209–216.
48. Prodan L, Suciu I, Pislaru V, et al: Experimental chronic poisoning with vinyl chloride (monchloroethene). *Ann NY Acad Sci* 1975; 246:159.
49. Salthouse TN, Matlaga BF, O'Keary RK: Microspectrophotometry of macrophage lysosomal enzyme activity: A measure of polymer implant tissue toxicity. *Toxicol Appl Pharmacol* 1973; 25:201.
50. Smith TJ, Cafarella JJ, Chelton C, et al: Evaluation of emissions from simulated commercial meat wrapping operations using PVC wrap. *Am Ind Hyg Assoc J* 1983; 44:176.
51. Sokol WN, Aelony Y, Beall GN: Meat-wrapper's asthma. *JAMA* 1973; 226:639.
52. Soutar CA, Copland LH, Thornley PE, et al: Epidemiological study of respiratory disease in workers exposed to polyvinyl chloride dust. *Thorax* 1980; 35:644.
53. Suciu I, Prodan L, Ilea E, et al: Clinical manifestations of vinyl chloride poisoning. *Ann NY Acad Sci* 1975; 246:53.
54. Szende B, Lapis K, Nemes A, et al: Pneumoconiosis caused by the inhalation of polyvinyl chloride dust. *Med Lav* 1970; 61:433.
55. Tabershaw IR, Gaffey WR: Mortality study of workers in the manufacture of vinyl chloride and its polymers. *J Occup Med* 1974; 16:509.
56. Thomas LB: Pathology of angiosarcoma of the liver among vinyl chloride/polyvinyl chloride workers. *Ann NY Acad Sci* 1975; 246:268.
57. Thomas LB, Popper H, Berk PD: Vinyl chloride induced liver disease. *N Engl J Med* 1975; 292:17.
58. Saric M, Kulcar Z, Zorica M, et al: Malignant tumors of the liver and lungs in an area with a PVC industry. *Environ Health Perspect* 1976; 17:189.
59. Torkelson TB, Oven F, Rowe VK: The toxicity of vinyl chloride as determined by repeated exposure of laboratory animals. *Am Ind Hyg Assoc J* 1961; 22:354.
60. Toxicity information. St Louis, Monsanto Company, 1976.
61. U.S. Department of Labor Recommended Standard for Occupational Exposure to Vinyl Chloride. Rockville, Md, National Institute for Occupational Safety and Health, 1974.
62. Veltman G, Lange CE, Juhe S, et al: Clinical manifestations and course of vinyl chloride disease. *Ann NY Acad Sci* 1975; 246:6–18.
63. Viola PL, Bigotti A, Caputo A: Oncogenic response of rat skin, lungs and bones to vinyl chloride. *Cancer Res* 1971; 31:516.
64. Villeneuve DC: Conference on Phthalates, National Toxicology Program Interagency Regulatory Liason Group, Washington, DC, US Department of Health and Human Services, 1981.
64a. Vinyl chloride: Nordic expert group for documentation of occupational exposure limits (Storetvedt Heldaas S, ed). *Arbete och Hälsa* 1986:17.
65. Waxweiler RJ, Stringer W, Wagoner JK, et al: Neoplastic risk among workers exposed to vinyl chloride. *Ann NY Acad Sci* 1975; 291:40.
66. Waxweiler RJ, Falk H, McMichael A, et al: A cross-sectional epidemiological survey of vinyl chloride workers. Cincinnati, National Institute for Occupational Safety and Health, Center for Disease Control, 1977.
67. Wheeler RN: Polyvinyl chloride processes and products. *Environ Health Perspect* 1981; 41:123.
68. Wilson RH: Occupational acroosteolysis. *JAMA* 1967; 201:577.
69. Winell M, Holmberg D, Kronev IT: Biological effects of vinyl chloride: An experimental study. *Environ Health Perspect* 1976; 17:211–216.

Combustion Products From Plastics and Natural Polymers

Vernon N. Dodson, M.D.

Since the first edition of this book, concerns for and information about the composition of combustion and pyrolysis products, not only from plastics, but from natural polymers, has increased. These latter concerns include the thermal degradation of wood, tobacco, and fossil fuels. Discussion of the petroleum fuels and coal are dealt with elsewhere in this volume. Personal air pollution (smoking various materials) and community air pollution, often of domestic origin, continue to compound workers' respiratory exposures will be discussed in this section.

PYROLYSIS OF PLASTICS

Toxicity resulting from the massive use of plastics in our modern society is not restricted to exposures sustained by workers during synthesis, formulation, or manufacture. Rapid and nearly complete oxidation of plastic products occurs with the application of extreme heat during a conflagration, resulting in carbon dioxide, water, and oxides of nitrogen. Even so, partially degraded molecules result and these may recombine to form new molecular species. The application of lower heat results in a host of compounds, as depicted in Tables 64–4 through 64–7.[2, 8] Thermal degradation often begins at relatively low temperatures (200–400°C), producing hydrogen chloride, carbon dioxide, carbon monoxide, and some hydrocarbons. Neoprenes release sulfur dioxide and hydrogen sulfide.[8] Rigid urethanes and isocyanates also produce CO_2, CO, and small amounts of $CFCl_3$, HCN, HCl, and hydrocarbons.[8]

Although the expected toxicity results from those compounds released in greater amounts, those emitted in smaller quantities

TABLE 64–4.
Combustion Products of Polyurethane Foam at Several Combustion Conditions

Air flow, cc/min	100	100	100
Oxygen flow, cc/min	0	40	0
Heating rate, c/min	5	5	50
Carbon dioxide	591.0	836.0	480.0
Carbon monoxide	165.0	235.0	241.0
Cyanide ion (as HCN)	34.7	32.5	11.6
Ammonia	0.23	0.09	0.01
Methane	2.40	2.41	27.3
Ethylene	1.57	3.08	15.5
Ethane	0.23	0.32	3.5
Propylene	3.58	10.60	61.1
Propane	0.37	0.68	8.3
Methanol	26.4	19.7	26.0
Acetaldehyde	27.1	32.5	53.9
Propionaldehyde	2.4	3.1	16.2
Acetone	12.4	11.1	39.8
% Nitrogen accounted for	32.3	30.3	10.8
% Plastic accounted for	34.3	44.5	49.8

cannot be disregarded for three major reasons: (1) they are very toxic, e.g., benzene and hydrogen cyanide; (2) certain workers are hypersusceptible for some reason, e.g., allergy to isocyanates and pharmacobiochemical sensitivity as encountered occasionally with amines and certain halogenated hydrocarbons; and (3) the toxicity of some substances is not yet recognized and therefore not studied.

TABLE 64–5.
Combustion Products Identified by Gas Chromatrography

POLYPHENYLENE OXIDE	POLYPROPYLENE	POLYCARBONATE
Benzene	Carbon dioxide	Carbon dioxide
Toluene	Carbon monoxide	Carbon monoxide
Ethylbenzene or xylene	Methane	Methane
	Ethylene	Ethylene
Styrene	Ethane	Ethane
Trimethylbenzene*	Propylene	Propylene
Indan	Propane	Propane
Indene	z-Butene	Methanol
Unidentified	Butane	Acetaldehyde
Unidentified	trans-2-Butene	1-Butene
Phenyl propynyl ether*	cis-2-Butene	Butane
	1-Pentene	Benzene
o-Cymene*	Pentane	Toluene
Naphthalene	1,3-Pentadiene?	Ethylbenzene
o-Cresyl ethyl ether*	1-Hexene	Styrene
Dimethylindan		
Unidentified		
Unidentified		
Methylnaphthalene		
2,6-Dimethylphenol		
o-Cresol		
Trimethylphenol		
2,4-Dimethylphenol		
2-(x-Xylyloxy) ethanol?		
Trimethylphenol		
Unidentified		

*Or isomer.

TABLE 64–6.
Identification of Polysulfone Residue Chromatogram Peaks

PEAK NUMBER	MOLECULAR WEIGHT	SUBSTANCE DETECTED
1	92	Toluene
2	106	Ethylbenzene (or xylene)
3	104	Styrene
4	120	Methyl ethylbenzene*
	126	Chlorotoluene?
5	106	Benzaldehyde
	118	Benzofuran
	116	Indene
6	132	Methylbenzofuran
	130	Methylindene
	120	Trimethylbenzene*
7	128	Naphthalene
	142	Methylnaphthalene
8	94	Phenol†
	154	Biphenyl
9	170	Diphenyl ether (or phenyl phenol)
10	108	Cresol
11	168	Dibenzofuran
	184	Phenyl-p-tolyl ether†
	156	Dimethylnaphthalene
	122	Ethylphenol
12	198	aryl-Ethylphenyl phenyl ether*
13	212	2-Hydroxyphenol1-2-phenyl propane
14	226	Unidentified
15	224	Unidentified

*Or isomer.
†Major component.

Not only should the major parent compounds be considered but also additives, such as accelerators, catalysts, copolymers, dyes, fillers, mold lubricants, pigments, plasticizers, solvents, stabilizers, and ultraviolet absorbers.

There are a number of syndromes being reported that appear to result from thermal degradation products of plastics. *Teflon fume fever* has been reported, especially in smokers exposed to Teflon fume generated by temperatures far in excess of those achieved during the cooking with Teflon coated utensils.[4, 6, 9, 13] *Meat wrapper's asthma* is another alleged syndrome that appears to be associated with exposure to heated plastics, in this instance, hot wire cutting of polyvinyl chloride film.[11] There are instances of adverse reactions when urethane foams, polystyrene, and other plastics are thermally degraded.

COMBUSTION PRODUCTS OF WOOD

The products released by wood are more difficult to measure because of (1) the tendency for some to incinerate more rapidly at high temperatures; and (2) the composition and density vary from heavy, hard tropical ebonies to resinous pines and light weight balsas. In real exposures the air effluents may contain wood preservatives such as arsenic copper, chromium or pentochlorophenol. Table 64–8 portrays chromatogram peaks identified by Boettner et al. under controlled conditions.[2]

TABLE 64–7.
Identification of Polyvinyl Chloride Chromatogram Peaks

PEAK NO.	SUBSTANCE DETECTED
1	Methane
2	Ethylene
3	Ethane
4	Propylene
5	Propane, methyl chloride
6	Vinyl chloride
7	1-Butene, isobutane, butadiene
8	Butane
9,10	trans-2-Butene, cis-2-Butene
11	3-Methyl-1-butene
12	Isopentane, 1,4-Pentadiene
13	1-Pentene
14	Pentane
15,16	trans-2-Pentene, cis-2-Pentene
17	2-Methyl-2-butene
18	cis or trans-1,3-Pentadiene
19	cis or trans-2-Pentadiene
20	Cyclopentene
21	Cyclopentane
22	2-Methylpentane
23	1-Hexene, 3-methylpentane
24	Hexane
25	2-Hexane
26	Methylcyclopentane
27	1-Methylcyclopentene
28	Benzene
29	Cyclohexane
30	1-Heptene
31	1,4-Dimethylcyclopentene
32	Heptane
33	Unidentified
34	3-Ethylcyclopentene
35	Methylcyclohexane
36	Ethylcyclopentane
37	1,2-Dimethylcyclopentene
38	1-or 4-Ethylcyclopentene
39	1-Methylcyclohexene
40	Toluene
41,42	Unidentified
43	Octane
44–47	Unidentified
48	Ethylbenzene
49–51	o-, m-, p-Xylene

PYROLYSIS PRODUCTS RELEASED DURING THE MANUFACTURE OF RUBBER PRODUCTS

Volatile air pollutants liberated during the pyrolysis of rubber vulcanization and extrusion are legion and have been extensively identified by Rappaport and Frazer in 1976–1977. More recently over 100 organic substances ranging from 25-27,000 μg/cu m were identified by gas chromatography and mass spectroscopy (GC/MS). Table 64–9 portrays these compounds by chemical families.[3] The toxicity resulting from the rubber industry is dealt with elsewhere in this volume.

TABLE 64–8.
Identification of Wood Chromatogram Peaks

SCAN NUMBER	MOLECULAR WEIGHT	IDENTIFICATION
1	44	Carbon dioxide
2	28	Ethylene
3	30	Ethane
4	18	Water
5	—	Unidentified
6	42	Propylene
7	32	Methanol
	44	Propane
8	32	Methanol
	50	1,3-Butadiyne?
	52	1-Buten-3-yne?
9	44	Acetaldehyde
10	60	n-Propanol
11	54	Butadiene
	56	Butene or Isobutene
12,13	56	Butene (Isomer?)
14	56	Butene (Isomer?)
15	58	Butane
	68	Pentadiene

COMBUSTION PRODUCTS OF TOBACCO

Tobacco smoke is also the combustion product of natural polymers and is mentioned because workers and nonworkers alike are often exposed to it and because analyses of the smoke provides clues to its complex mixture of toxicants. The contaminants vary as a function of the manner in which the tobacco is burned (cigarettes, cigars, and various types of pipes) and the presence of numerous additives. Table 64–10 provides data on the composition of mainstream smoke.[10] Table 64–11 portrays the ratio of side stream smoke (SS) to mainstream smoke (MS) indicating greater concentrations from side stream smoke.[10] It is worth noting that other air pollutants in the work area may be simultaneously burned by the smoking process.

The combustion of natural polymers such as wood, tobacco, and fossil fuels have been studied in relationship to combustion products and community pollution. Murphy et al. analyzed air pollution in Telluride, Colorado, from primarily wood combustion heating that gave averages of 61 μg/cu m and 7.4 ng/cu m of total suspended particulate matter and benzo(a)pyrene respectively, which was several times higher than most metropolitan areas in the United States.[7] Beck and Brain studied the pathological changes resulting from the intratracheal installation of respirable products of wood burning stoves in hamsters and they appear dose-related producing macrophage impairment, pulmonary edema, and patterns resembling pneumoconiosis.[1]

That the pyrolysis or combustion products of natural or manmade synthetic polymers are toxic has been confirmed by numerous controlled studies even though the precise toxicants have not been clearly identified. These products have produced effects ranging from adverse to lethal *in vitro* tests, *in vivo* animal studies, and in human study series. Such studies tend to affirm some anecdotal reports in humans.

Newer analytical techniques offer more precise and rapid

TABLE 64–9.

Chemical Families of Identified Compounds: Number of Observed Compounds, Mean and Range of Environmental Concentrations (μg/cu m)

SAMPLING SITE:	A*			B1†			B2‡			C§		
NUMBER OF SAMPLES:	13			6			6			10		
		CONCENTRATION			CONCENTRATION			CONCENTRATION			CONCENTRATION	
FAMILY (NO. OF COMP.)	NO. OF COMP.	MEAN	RANGE	NO. OF COMP.	MEAN	RANGE	NO. OF COMP.	MEAN	RANGE	NO. OF COMP.	MEAN	RANGE
Alkanes (16)	9	3,560	20–14,200	13	190	7–920	11	33	2–80	13	26	4–70
Cycloalkanes (11)	10	2,120	350–8,100	7	304	1–1,220	7	24	4–58	2	1	0–5
Cycloalkanes (10)	6	138	0–830	6	485	0–2,600	6	17	0–30	2	5	0–25
Aromatic hydrocarbons (32)	20	605	0–3,130	23	813	16–3,730	16	187	58–420	13	50	0–300
Chlorinated (4)	0	—	—	0	—	—	0	—	—	4	4	0–11
Phenols (6)	6	73	0–230	2	178	4–860	2	21	0–86	0	—	—
Esters (6)	3	70	0–200	4	545	10–3,000	2	10	5–15	4	32	1–85
Miscellaneous (14)‖	6	165	0–800	3	95	1–475	1	0.2	0–1	7	37	0–145
TOTAL (99)	60	6,700	960–27,000	58	2,700	60–13,000	45	300	100–490	45	140	25–550

*Shoe-sole factory, vulcanization area.
†Tire retreading factory, vulcanization area.
‡Tire retreading factory, extrusion area.
§Electrical cables insulation plant, extrusion area.
‖Ethers, sulfur- and nitrogen-compounds, aldehydes, alcohols, ketones, peroxides, and quinones.

TABLE 64–10.

Some Constituents of the Mainstream of Cigarette Smoke (μg/Cigarette)

GAS PHASE	
CO	13,400
CO_2	50,600
NH^3	80
HCN	240
C_5H_8	582
$CH_2{=}CH{-}CHO$	84
CH_3-CHO	770
C_6H_5-CH_3	108
CH_3-CN	210
$(CH_3)_2N{-}N{=}O$	0.08
$(CH_3)(C_2H_5)N{-}N{=}0$	0.03
$NH_2{-}NH_2$	0.03
$CH_3 - NO_2$	0.5
$C_2H_5{-}NO_2$	1.1
$(CH_3)_2CO$	578
$C_6H_5{-}NO_2$	25
C_6H_6	67
PARTICULATE PHASE	
TPM, wet	31,500
TPM, dry	27,900
TPM, FTC	26,100
Nicotine	1,800
Phenol	86.4
o-Cresol	20.4
m- and p-Cresol	49.5
2,4-Dimethylphenol	9.0
p-Ethylphenol	18.2
β-Naphthylamine	0.028
N-Nitrosonornicotine	0.14
Cholesterol	14.2
Campesterol	24.5
Stigmasterol	53
β-Sitosterol	37
Carbazole	1.0
N-Methylcarbazole	0.23
Indole	14
N-Methylindole	0.42
Benz[a]anthracene	0.044
Benzo[a]pyrene	0.025
Fluorene	0.42
Fluoranthene	0.26
Chrysene	0.04
DDD	1.75
DDT	0.77
4,4'-DCS	1.73
HCN	74

methods of identifying, quantifying these complex products and their unique physical and chemical characteristics even infinitesimal quantities. These new techniques are reviewed in several articles in a recent issue of *Science* (226[4672]:249–318, October 18, 1984).

Knowledge in this field is expanding rapidly and one can expect increasing awareness of the influence on the health of humans, animals, and plants resulting from combustion products in the future.

TABLE 64–11.

Constituents of Cigarette Smoke Ratios of Sidestream (SS) to Mainstream (MS) Concentration Levels (SS/MS)

	SS/MS
Nicotine	2.7
Phenol	2.6
Benzo[a]pyrene (mg)	3.4
Benzo[a]pyrene (ppm)	2.1
Dry Condensate	1.7
3-Vinylpyridine	43.0
Water	24
Ammonia	106
Methane	3.1
Acetylene	0.81
Propane-propene	4.1
Methylchloride	2.1
Hydrazine	3
Methylfuran	3.4
Propionaldehyde	2.4
2-Butanone	2.9
Butanedione	1.0
Pyridine	20.3
Carbon monoxide	2.5
Carbon dioxide	8.1
Toluene	5.6
Hydrogen cyanide	0.66
Acetonitrile	3.9
Acetone	2.5
Cholesterol	0.8
Campesterol	0.9
Stigmasterol	0.8
β-Sitosterol	0.8

REFERENCES

1. Beck BD, Brain JD: Prediction of the pulmonary toxicity of respirable combustion from residential wood and coal stoves, in Frederick ER (ed): *Resid. Wood Coal Combust. 5th Conf. Proc.* APCA, Pittsburgh, 1982, pp 264–80.
2. Boettner EA, Ball GL, Weiss B: *Combustion Products from the Incineration of Plastics*. Final Report to U S Environmental Protection Agency, Research Grant No. E.C.-00386, Ann Arbor, The University of Michigan, February, 1973.
3. Cochea V, Bellamo ML, Bumbl G: Rubber manufacture: Sampling identification of volatile pollutants. *Am J Ind Assoc* 1983; 44(7):521.
4. Coleman WE, et al: The identification of toxic compounds in the pyrolysis products of polytetrafluorethylene (PTFE). *Am Ind Hyg Assoc J* 1968; 29:33.
5. Cornish HH, Abar EL: Toxicity of pyrolysis products of vinyl plastics. *Arch Environ Health* 1969; 19:15.
6. Lewis CE, Kerby GR: An epidemic of polymer fume fever. *JAMA* 1965; 191:375.
7. Murphy DJ, Buchan RM, Fox DG: Ambient total suspended particulate matter and benzo[a]pyrene concentrations from residential wood combustion in a mountain resort community. *Am Ind Hyg Assoc J* 1984; 45(7):431–5.
8. Pacioreck KL, Kratzer RH, Kaufman J: *Coal Mine Combustion Products, Identification and Analysis*. U S Department of Commerce, Bureau of Mines, PB-214-124, July 1972.
9. Robbins JJ, Ware RL: Pulmonary edema from Teflon fumes: A report of a case. *N Engl J Med* 1964; 271:360.
10. Schmeltz I, Hoffmann D, Wynder EL: Influence of tobacco smoke on indoor atmospheres. *Prevent Med* 1975; 3:66–82.
11. Sokol WN, Aelony Y, Beall GN: Meat wrapper's asthma. *JAMA* 1973; 226:639.
12. Sterling TD: Indoor by-product levels of tobacco smoke. *J Air Pullution Cont Assoc* 1982; 32:250–7.
13. Tepper LB: Hazards to health. *N Engl J Med* 1962; 276:349.

65

Effects of Gases and Particles in Welding and Soldering

Bengt Sjögren, M.D.

The American Welding Society defines welding as "a metal-joining process wherein coalescence is produced by heating to suitable temperatures with or without the use of filler metal." Welding and cutting are often grouped together because these processes are related to each other and because cutting precedes welding and involves the same personnel in many manufacturing operations. The number of welders was estimated to be about 500,000 in the U.S. in 1976[71] and in England and Wales together there were 117,000 welders in 1971.[28] Thus, welders are an important occupational group in industrialized countries.

Soldering and brazing are allied activities. These processes consist of metal joining by using a lower-melting-point metal to alloy with the surfaces to be joined.

METHODS

Welding and cutting can be performed with a great variety of methods in many different materials. In this text only the more common methods and exposure situations will be mentioned.

Gas Welding

In gas welding, a burning gas is used as the source of heat to produce metal melting. Gas welding is used for welding thin material and for applications requiring low gradients of temperature to avoid cracking as in welding cast iron. The oxyacetylene flame, consisting of a mixture of equal volumes of oxygen and acetylene, has a higher temperature than any other commercially available fuel gas combination. When adding oxygen, the flame can be used for cutting low-alloy steel.

An oxyacetylene flame burning in air produces nitrogen dioxide from nitrogen and oxygen in the atmosphere. The concentrations of nitrogen dioxide can reach high levels (200–400 ppm) when the flame is used in confined spaces and this exposure might cause pulmonary edema.[43, 53]

Shielded Metal-Arc Welding

Shielded metal-arc welding is defined as a process in which fusion is produced by heating with an electric arc established between the coated electrode and the base metal (Fig 65–1). The shielding required for the arc and molten weld metal is obtained from the decomposition of the electrode coating. Electrodes are often classified according to their coatings. Among the most commonly used electrodes are acid, basic, and rutile electrodes. Acid electrodes produce acid slag while basic electrodes, which contain fluorides, give a basic slag. Rutile electrodes contain rutile (TiO_2).

The shielded metal-arc welding process is the most widely used method of welding since its introduction in the late 1920s.[2] About half of all the welders in Sweden used this method in carbon steel in 1974,[81] and the proportion has probably been about the same in many industrialized countries.

In general, the welding fume concentrations are higher when welding is performed in confined spaces compared to welding in open air. In open-air welding of railway tracks in Sweden, 25%–50% of the measured total particulate concentrations inside the welding helmet exceeded 5 mg/cu m,[81] and in confined spaces in Danish shipyards, 50% of the measurements were above 7 mg/cu m.[71] In electric-arc welding, the majority of the generated particles are smaller than 1 μ and thus respirable.[2, 81]

The main components of welding fumes are iron oxide, of which the major part is magnetite (Fe_3O_4).[36, 70] Since magnetite has magnetic properties, the inhaled iron oxide can be assessed by a method measuring induced magnetic fields of the lung-retained contaminants.[35] Due to clearance mechanisms, the amount of retained lung contaminants among welders reflects the exposure during the last five to ten years. The clearance rate has been estimated to be about 20% per year.[37] This method has been suggested for biologic monitoring of long-term welding fume exposure.

Basic electrodes coated with calcium fluoride emit fluorides in the fume. The emitted compounds are mainly in particulate form[34, 76, 79] and can amount to 25% of the total particle content.[79] Welders working with outdoor welding using basic electrodes emitting 18%–20% fluorides did not have postshift urine concentra-

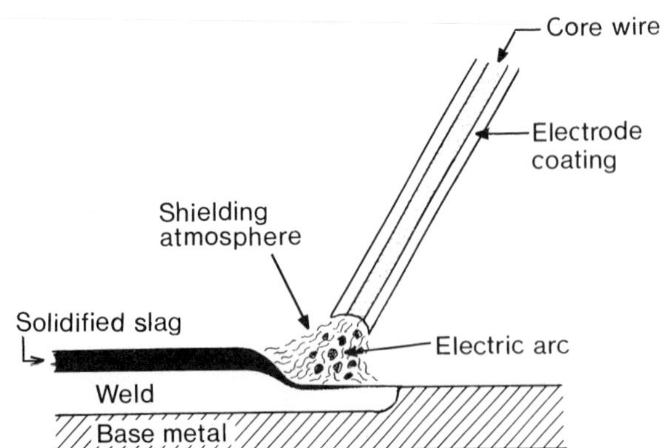

FIG 65–1.
Shielded metal-arc welding.

tions of fluorides exceeding 370 mole/L,[65] the threshold recommended by the National Institute for Occupational Safety and Health (NIOSH).[52] Welders working in confined spaces with basic electrodes might have higher postshift urine concentrations, but such a group has not been thoroughly studied.

Metal-arc welding with coated electrodes on stainless steel generates particles of easily soluble hexavalent chromium,[42, 78] and this chromium is known to be irritative to the respiratory airways.[33, 67] Urinary chromium can only be used as a weak indicator of current chromium exposure in stainless steel welding.[63, 82] (See Chapters 34 and 13.)

Gas-Shielded Metal-Arc Welding

The gas-shielded welding processes are used extensively in many areas of the industry, because one or more of these processes can be used to join any of the weldable metals and alloys.

Gas Tungsten-Arc Welding.—Gas tungsten-arc welding or tungsten inert gas (TIG) welding is a process in which fusion is produced by heating with an arc established between a nonconsumable tungsten electrode and the base metal (Fig 65–2). Shielding of the arc and the molten weld metal is obtained by an inert gas (helium or argon) or a mixture of these gases.

Gas Metal-Arc Welding.—Gas metal-arc welding is a process in which fusion is produced by heating with an arc established between a consumable electrode and the workpiece (see Fig 65–2). In metal inert gas (MIG) welding an inert gas is used for shielding. In metal active gas (MAG) welding, small amounts of gas reacting with the base metal (most often carbon dioxide) are added to helium or argon.

Gas-shielded welding of aluminum generates a characteristic ultraviolet light which produces ozone from oxygen. When MIG welding was performed in aluminum, almost 50% of the measured ozone concentrations exceeded 0.1 ppm.[81] Welders working with gas-shielded welding in aluminum have more respiratory symptoms at higher ozone concentrations than at lower concentrations[66] (Fig 65–3). Gas-shielded welding of stainless steel generates much less ozone.[81] Metal inert gas welding of aluminum raises the aluminum blood levels among the welders, but the concentrations are much lower than the levels at which neurotoxic symptoms have been seen in patients with kidney dysfunction who experience aluminum blood level elevations when treated with dialysis.[64]

Carbon monoxide can be formed when carbon dioxide is used as a shielding gas. Blood carboxyhemoglobin concentrations reaching 20% have been seen in welders working with insufficient ventilation.[19]

Plasma-Arc Welding.—Plasma-arc welding is a process which utilizes a plasma produced by the heat of constricted electric-arc-gas mixture. The shielding gas may be an inert gas or a mixture of gases. Plasma-arc welding resembles TIG-welding in its use of an inert gas but differs from it in the use of a constricting orifice.

Submerged Arc Welding

Submerged arc welding is a process in which fusion is produced by heating with an arc established between a bar electrode and the workpiece. The arc and the molten weld metal are shielded by a blanket of granular, fusible flux. In contrast to the previously mentioned processes, there is no visible evidence of the arc. The total amount of fumes generated during submerged arc welding are in general lower than those produced with coated electrodes. The generated air contaminants are dependent on the fluxes in use. Gaseous fluorides, mostly silicon tetrafluoride (SiF_4), are evolved when using some high silica-type fluxes. Carbon monoxide is formed from the carbon in the welding wire and the steel being welded. These gases might reach high levels in badly ventilated areas.[2]

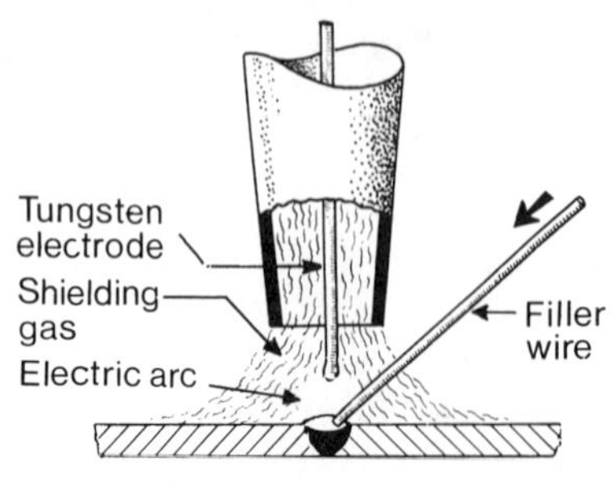

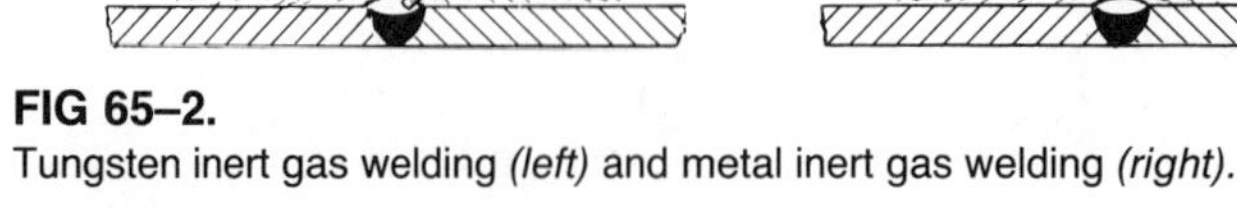

FIG 65–2.
Tungsten inert gas welding *(left)* and metal inert gas welding *(right).*

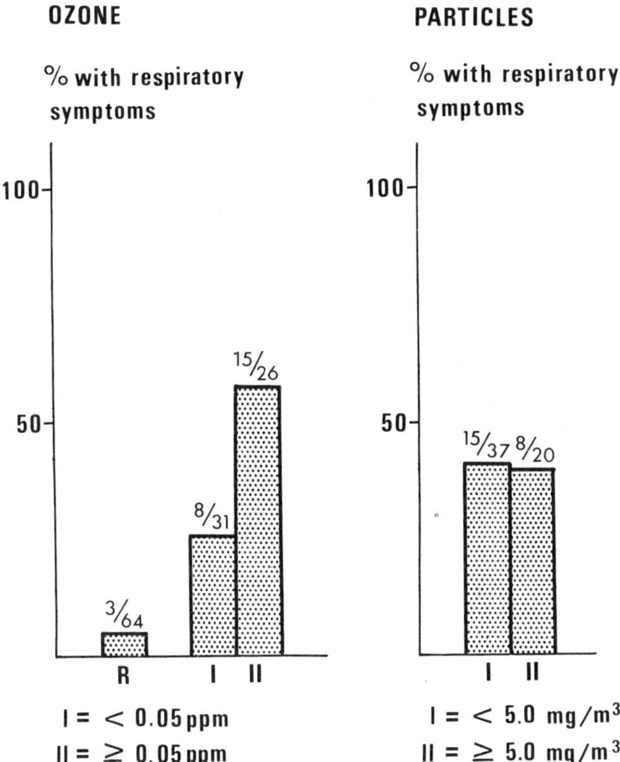

FIG 65–3.
Respiratory symptoms in nonwelding referents *(R)* and groups of welders with varying exposure to ozone and particles.

Arc-Air Gouging

The arc-air gouging process is a method to remove excessive metal. It consists of the melting of a metal by means of an electric arc and the removal of the molten material by using a fairly powerful blast of compressed air. The electrode in most common use consists of a mixture of carbon and graphite, and it is normally coated with copper (Fig 65–4). This process produces high amounts of particles, particularly when used in confined or semiconfined spaces. The concentrations of carbon monoxide may also reach high levels (100 ppm). The method generates much noise and the sound pressure levels are often above 110 dBA.[59]

Applying this process to a manganese alloy (10%–14%) has caused manganese poisoning in some workers.[75, 83] (See Chapter 37.)

Considering this dusty and noisy process, operators must use adequate protective devices.

Soldering and Brazing

Soldering and brazing are processes of metal joining by using a lower-melting-point metal to alloy with the surfaces to be joined. Soldering or soft-soldering uses a solder which melts below 450° C. Brazing uses an alloy or hard-solder which melts above that temperature.

Soft-solders often contain lead and tin. The lead exposure is most often low or moderate when these solders are used. (See Chapter 36 on Lead.) Fluxes are used to protect the metal surfaces and to dissolve oxides. Corrosive fluxes contain zinc chloride and ammonium chloride, while noncorrosive fluxes often contain colophony, a pine resin. Colophony-containing fluxes have caused asthma in English electronics factories.[13] Other fluxes have also been responsible for the development of asthma. (See Chapter 16.)

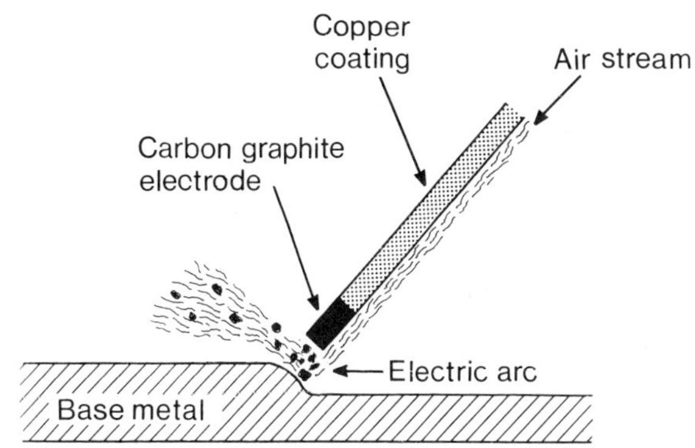

FIG 65–4.
Arc-air gouging.

Hard-solders usually contain copper and zinc. Silver and cadmium are added to decrease the melting temperature. When cadmium-containing solders are used, the cadmium exposure can be quite high when large splices are brazed, since local exhaust ventilation often is difficult to apply.[46]

Welding or Cutting in Painted or Plated Materials

Welding or cutting of cadmium-plated materials can cause life-threatening effects due to cadmium exposure.[10] (See also Chapter 33.)

Lead-painted steel emits high concentrations of lead when subjected to welding or cutting. Shipbreaking is a well-documented, although often poorly controlled, hazard. (See Chapter 36.)

Cutting or welding of zinc-coated or galvanized steel has often been accompanied by zinc fume fever some hours later.[58]

Arc welding with a rutile electrode of mild steel coated with a zinc epoxy primer did not significantly affect pulmonary function when measured before and after a working shift. However, in that study, a positive correlation was found between the increase of residual volume and the fume concentrations in the breathing zone of the welders.[22, 49]

Arc welding with basic electrodes of steel coated with a shop primer that contains iron oxide, zinc chromate, polyvinylbutyral and phenol resins emits several organic as well as inorganic compounds. In one study of nonsmoking welders, no significant relationship between fume exposure and pulmonary function was revealed during a working shift.[54]

Welding in Atmospheres Contaminated With Halogenated Hydrocarbons

Halogenated hydrocarbons such as trichloroethylene, perchloroethylene, and methyl chloroform are often used as degreasing agents in the metal industry. The ultraviolet radiation emitted from welding arcs might decompose these hydrocarbons to phosgene when welding is performed in such atmospheres.[3, 17, 18] Welding methods emitting more ultraviolet light, such as MIG-welding of aluminum, generate more phosgene compared with methods emitting less ultraviolet light, such as coated electrodes on mild steel.[16] Dichloroacetyl chloride is formed when trichloroethylene decomposes, and this substance has a very irritating odor which acts as a warning.[17] Welding in atmospheres containing these chlorinated hydrocarbons should be avoided. Air contaminated with perchloroethylene is regarded as the most hazardous.[3, 17, 18]

Dichlorodifluoromethane is a common cooling agent in refrigerators. This gas can decompose to phosgene during repair work when an open flame is used. A phosgene concentration of 0.04 ppm was measured when the concentrations of dichlorodifluoromethane varied between 13 and 223 ppm.[74]

DISORDERS

Several disorders are associated with different welding exposures. Shoulder pain has been associated with the static working situation which is a common feature of welding.[29]

The electromagnetic radiation from welding arcs are strong enough to cause damage to the skin and the eye. In a Swedish shipyard with approximately 3,000 workers, more than 7,000 eye hazards were reported in one year. About 30% of these were caused by exposure to ultraviolet radiation.[77] Particles that stick to the cornea must often be removed surgically. Welders working in a lying position have occasionally been exposed to hot particles which have penetrated the eardrum and injured the labyrinth, causing a severe acute vertigo. The following disorders are however associated with exposure to gases or respirable particulates[2, 81] generated by welding, soldering, or cutting.

Pulmonary Edema

Welders exposed to nitrogen dioxide when using an oxyacetylene flame in confined spaces have developed pulmonary edema (see Gas Welding).

Inhalation of ozone generated from gas-shielded welding has also caused pulmonary edema.[40] Metal inert gas welding of aluminum is the most powerful combination of process and method for the generation of ozone (see Gas Metal-Arc Welding).

Concerning the formation of phosgene, see Welding in Atmospheres Contaminated with Halogenated Hydrocarbons.

High concentrations of cadmium oxide are known to produce pulmonary edema. Cadmium oxide generated from the cutting of cadmium-plated material and from brazing with cadmium-containing solders has caused several fatal cases of pulmonary edema.[10, 11] Such exposures have also produced pneumonitis.[45, 80] (See Chapter 33.)

Chronic Bronchitis and Emphysema

For epidemiologic purposes, chronic bronchitis may be defined as a condition with productive cough at some time of the day for at least three months in two consecutive years. According to the degree of airway obstruction, one may distinguish between two forms of this disease: Nonobstructive chronic bronchitis and chronic bronchitis with airways obstruction. Emphysema is a pathologic condition of the lungs characterized by an increase beyond the normal size of the air spaces, distal to the terminal bronchioles with destruction of the walls.[84]

TABLE 65–1.
Relative Risk of Chronic Bronchitis Among Different Groups of Welders

EXPOSURE	RELATIVE RISK	STUDY
Mainly low-alloy steel		
Shipyard (More than 50% of the welders)	1.2	Fogh et al. (1969)
Shipyard	1.5	Barhad et al. (1975)
Shipyard	2.0	Oxhöj et al. (1979)
Engineering shops	1.0	Keimig et al. (1983)
Engineering shops	1.7	Antti-Poika et al. (1977)
Engineering shops	3.1	Axelson (1974)
Railway track	3.3	Sjögren & Ulfvarson (1985)
Stainless steel	2.1	Sjögren & Ulfvarson (1985)
Gas-shielded welding of aluminum	2.2	Sjögren & Ulfvarson (1985)

Practically all studied groups of welders report an increased frequency of chronic bronchitis (Table 65–1). In general, smoking welders report more frequent symptoms than smoking referents and nonsmoking welders have more frequent symptoms compared with nonsmoking referents.

Chronic bronchitis may be associated with airway obstruction. Airway obstruction can be measured in different ways, FEV% being one of them.* The FEV% is not related to height, and the mean decrease is at most 0.4% per year.[9] Table 65–2 summarizes the largest published studies including 100 or more welders working mainly in low-alloy steel. The differences between FEV% in nonsmoking shipyard welders and the referent groups were 0%–5%, while smoking welders had average values 1%–10% less than their referents. These differences can only to a minor extent be explained by differences in age. Obstructive changes have not been seen in non-shipyard welders. The explanation might be that shipyard welders inhale more air contaminants in semiconfined or confined spaces than other welders. In railway track welding, for instance, 25%–50% of the measured total particle concentrations in the welding helmet exceeded 5 mg/cu m,[81] and in Danish shipyards, 50% of the measurements in confined spaces were above 7 mg/cu m.[71]

A study of closing volume and closing capacity in nonsmoking and ex-smoking shipyard welders revealed higher values compared with referents, and these changes are regarded as an expression of obstruction in the small airways.[54]

Nonobstructive chronic bronchitis has been observed in weld-

*See Chapter 18 for explanations.

TABLE 65–2.
FEV% Based on Mean Spirometric Results From Welders and Referents in Different Studies

WELDERS FEV%	REFERENTS FEV%	REMARK	STUDY
		Shipyard Welders	
72	77	Nonsmokers	Hunnicutt et al (1964)
67	77	Smokers	
78	78	Nonsmokers	Oxhöj et al. (1979)
75	77	Smokers	
77	79	Nonsmokers	Akbarkhanzadeh (1980)
74	75	Smokers	
		Non-Shipyard Welders	
80	81	Equal proportion of smokers and nonsmokers Engineering shops	Antti-Poika et al. (1977)
80	80	Nonsmokers	Sjögren & Ulfvarson (1985)
77	77	Smokers Railway track (Original figures not presented in the reference)	

ers working in different materials and airway obstruction has been demonstrated in shipyard welders.

An increased frequency of deaths due to chronic bronchitis and emphysema has also been observed in welders and flame cutters.[8, 51]

Pneumonia

Some studies of welders have demonstrated an increased risk of deaths due to pneumonia,[8, 50] but this risk has been decreasing in England and Wales during the latest decades.[50] This decrease might be an expression of gradually improved working conditions since World War II.

Asthma

Bronchial asthma is a condition characterized by acute attacks of bronchial obstruction which is totally or partially reversible between the attacks.[84]

Hexavalent chromium is generated in manual metal arc stainless steel welding, and this exposure has been associated with immediate and nonimmediate types of asthmatic reactions.[39]

Soldering in the electronics industry is often performed with a colophony-containing flux. Colophony is a pine resin, which has been used as a soldering flux since ancient times. In an English electronics factory, 20% of the workers exposed to solder flux fumes had work-related breathlessness and wheeze, and an equal proportion of workers had rhinitis.[13] On provocation, there was a low correlation between the reaction to colophony fumes and the nonspecific reactivity to histamine, suggesting that colophony fumes were causing specific sensitization.[14]

In aluminum soldering, a flux containing amino-ethyl ethanolamine has been used. Fumes from this flux have produced bronchoconstriction in several workers.[48, 55, 69]

One electronic assembler experienced bronchoconstriction shortly after a new soldering flux containing 95% alkyl aryl polyether alcohol and 5% polypropylene glycol had been introduced in the workshop.[73]

Toluene di-isocyanate is a well-known asthmatic agent, and such fumes have been formed from soldering polyurethane coated wires.[56]

"Welder's Lung"

Welders inhale freshly formed iron oxide during their work. Doig and McLaughlin in 1936[20] drew attention to the abnormal appearances found in the x-ray films of six such workers, which they suggested might be due to the presence of aggregates of iron oxide particles in the lungs. A decade later, the same authors described one welder in whom the abnormal x-ray appearance had disappeared after cessation of exposure and one case in whom the abnormality of the x-ray picture had diminished after being less exposed.[21] Such lung changes are supported by a Polish study of dockyard welders. A marked improvement of previous x-ray pictures was demonstrated in four out of 13 welders with siderosis after three years of diminished exposure. A slight improvement was seen in four, no change was observed in four, and in one welder a progression was demonstrated.[25]

In 661 British welders working in heavy industry in West Scotland, small rounded opacities were noted on chest x-ray examination (category 0/1 or greater). The prevalence of these changes was 5% after 20 years of welding and 20% after 35–40 years of exposure.[5]

Large cross-sectional studies including more than 100 welders working in low-alloy steel have not revealed restrictive pulmonary changes (Table 65–3). Restrictive changes have, however, been demonstrated in other studies, e.g., Peters et al.[57] observed restrictive as well as obstructive changes in shipyard welders despite normal x-ray films. Fibrosis and restrictive impairment have been described in several case reports.[12, 15, 24, 68]

TABLE 65–3.

Mean Values and Ratios of Vital Capacities in Welders of Low-Alloy Steel and Referents

WELDERS	REFERENTS	RATIO	STUDY
4.16	4.12	1.01	Hunnicutt et al. (1964)
4.95	4.83	1.02	Antti-Poika et al. (1977)
5.20	5.32	0.98	Oxhöj et al (1979) (Corrected to age and height according to Berglund et al. (1963)
5.00	5.22	0.96	Akbarkhanzadeh (1980)
5.12	5.17	0.99	Sjögren & Ulfvarson (1985)

Prolonged inhalation of high concentrations of iron oxides may cause siderosis which is a benign condition not associated with fibrosis of the lung. (See Chapters 14 and 45.) However, welding has been associated with exposure to many different substances, such as nonchrystalline silicon dioxide,[68] asbestos,[20] and fluorides from the electrode coatings, metals such as aluminum, cadmium, chromium, manganese, and nickel from the electrode cores, or the base metals and gases such as nitrogen dioxide, ozone, and phosgene generated in the welding process. Welders may also be exposed to chrystalline silicon dioxide when working close to sand-blasting operations and to asbestos when working in shipyards[61] and in other heavy industries.[5] Combinations of these agents might be responsible for the occasional occurrence of mixed dust fibrosis seen in welders.

"Metal Fume Fever"

Exposure to metal welding fumes can cause "metal fume fever." Almost 40% of welders above the age of 30 have been estimated to experience metal fume fever. Welding galvanized steel was the most common cause for this disorder.[58]

Genotoxic Effects

Mutagenic activity has been demonstrated in *Salmonella* and *Escherichia coli* test systems after exposure to fumes from metal-arc welding of stainless steel.[27, 47] Particles from MIG-welding of stainless steel were much less mutagenic in the same bacterial test systems, and this welding method is known to produce much less hexavalent chromium. Welding fumes generated from metal-arc welding with coated electrodes and MIG-welding of mild steel have not been mutagenic in bacterial test systems.[27, 47]

Cultured Chinese hamster cells were exposed to stainless steel welding fumes. Cells exposed to metal-arc welding with coated electrodes demonstrated higher frequencies of chromosome aberrations and sister chromatid exchanges compared with cells exposed to MIG-welding fumes. The increase of sister chromatid exchanges was dependent on concentrations of hexavalent chromium but not on concentrations of trivalent chromium or nickel, suggesting that hexavalent chromium is responsible for the increase of sister chromatid exchanges.[41]

Welders working with metal-arc welding with coated electrodes of stainless steel had equal amounts of sister chromatid exchanges and chromosome aberrations in their peripheral blood lymphocytes compared with nonexposed referents.[32, 44] In contrast, electroplaters had an increased amount of these genetic indicators when exposed to chromium acid mist.[60]

The fact that stainless steel fumes from metal-arc welding with coated electrodes are mutagenic to bacteria and to Chinese hamster cells in vitro but not to human peripheral blood lymphocytes in vivo might be explained by a slow clearance of chromium from the lungs and a relatively rapid clearance from the blood, which has been demonstrated in rats.[36] The slow passage from the lungs to the blood might also be accompanied by a reduction of hexavalent chromium into trivalent, but this has not yet been demonstrated.

Tumors

Several studies have reported a 30%–40% increased incidence of pulmonary tumors among welders.[72] The reason for this increase is not quite clear, but asbestos exposure is probably of some importance. About 40% of the welders in heavy industry in Scotland had been exposed to asbestos from mats and cloths made of asbestos in order to retain heat. To a lesser extent, they were exposed to asbestos from other workers using this material.[5] Pleural plaque and parenchymal fibrosis as expressions of asbestos exposure were very common among American welders and burners in the ship repair industry.[61] Welders have also an increased incidence of mesothelioma,[50, 62] which adds further to the assumption that the excess of pulmonary tumors may be at least partly caused by asbestos exposure.

Hexavalent chromium is a well-known occupational carcinogen causing lung cancer. This compound is formed during stainless steel welding with coated electrodes. In a small cohort of 234 Swedish stainless steel welders, five pulmonary tumors were seen versus two expected.[67] About 1% of all welders in Sweden have been working with coated electrodes in stainless steel for more than half of their daily working time. However, many more were exposed to a lesser degree.[26, 81]

Exposures other than asbestos and hexavalent chromium might also cause an increased risk of pulmonary tumors among welders, but epidemiologic evidence is lacking at present.

A well-conducted case-referent study showed an increased risk for nasal and sinonasal tumors in welders. These welders had been exposed to chromium as well as nickel.[30]

REFERENCES

1. Akbarkhanzadeh F: Long-term effects of welding fumes upon respiratory symptoms and pulmonary function. *J Occup Med* 1980; 22:337–341.
2. American Welding Society: *The Welding Environment*. Miami, Fla, American Welding Society, 1973.
3. Andersson HF, Dahlberg JA, Wetterström R: Phosgene formation during welding in air contaminated with perchloroethylene. *Ann Occup Hyg* 1975; 18:129–132.
4. Antti-Poika M, Hassi J, Pyy L: Respiratory diseases in arc welders. *Int Arch Occup Environ Health* 1977; 40:225–230.
5. Attfield MD, Ross RS: Radiological abnormalities in electric-arc welders. *Br J Ind Med* 1978; 35:117–122.
6. Axelson O: Bronchitis in welders. *Läkartidningen* 1974; 71:479–482. (In Swedish with English abstract.)

7. Barhad B, Teculescu D, Craciun O: Respiratory symptoms, chronic bronchitis and ventilatory function in shipyard welders. *Int Arch Occup Environ Health* 1975; 36:137–150.
8. Beaumont JJ, Weiss NS: Mortality of welders, shipfitters, and other metal trades workers in boilermakers local no. 104, AFL-CIO. *Am J Epidemiol* 1980; 112:775–786.
9. Berglund E, Birath G, Bjure J, et al: Spirometric studies in normal subjects. Forced expirograms in subjects between 7 and 70 years of age. *Acta Med Scand* 1963; 173(fasc 2):185–192.
10. Beton DC, Andrews GS, Davies HJ, et al: Acute cadmium fume poisoning. Five cases with one death from renal necrosis. *Br J Ind Med* 1966; 23:292–301.
11. Blejer HP, Caplan PE, Alcocer AE: Acute cadmium fume poisoning in welders—A fatal and a nonfatal case in California. *Calif Med* 1966; 105:290–296.
12. Brun J, Cassan G, Kofman J, et al: La sidero-sclerose des soudeurs a l'arc a forme de fibrose interstitielle diffuse et forme conglomerative pseudo-tumorale. *L Poumon Coeur* 1972; 28:3–10.
13. Burge PS, Perks W, O'Brien IM, et al: Occupational asthma in an electronics factory. *Thorax* 1979; 34:13–18.
14. Burge PS, Harries MG, O'Brien I, et al: Bronchial provocation studies in workers exposed to the fumes of electronic soldering fluxes. *Clin Allergy* 1980; 10:137–149.
15. Charr R: Pulmonary changes in welders: A report of three cases. *Ann Intern Med* 1956; 44:806–812.
16. Dahlberg JA: The intensity and spectral distribution of ultraviolet emission from welding arcs in relation to the photodecomposition of gases. *Ann Occup Hyg* 1971; 14:259–267.
17. Dahlberg JA, Myrin LM: The formation of dichloroacetyl chloride and phosgene from trichloroethylene in the atmosphere of welding shops. *Ann Occup Hyg* 1971; 14:269–274.
18. Dahlberg JA, Christiansen VO, Eriksson EA: On the formation of phosgene by photo-oxidation of methyl chloroform in welding. *Ann Occup Hyg* 1973; 16:41–46.
19. De Kretser AJ, Evans WD, Waldron HA: Carbon monoxide hazard in the CO_2 arc-welding process. *Ann Occup Hyg* 1964; 7:253–259.
20. Doig AT, McLaughlin AIG: X-ray appearances of the lungs of electric arc welders. *Lancet* 1936; i:771–775.
21. Doig AT, McLaughlin AIG: Clearing of x-ray shadows in welders' siderosis. *Lancet* 1948; i:789–791.
22. Evans MJ, Ingle J, Molyneux MK, et al: An occupational hygiene study of a controlled welding task using a general purpose rutile electrode. *Ann Occup Hyg* 1979; 22:1–17.
23. Fogh A, Frost J, Georg J: Respiratory symptoms and pulmonary function in welders. *Ann Occup Hyg* 1969; 12:213–218.
24. Friede E, Rachow DO: Symptomatic pulmonary disease in arc welders. *Ann Intern Med* 1961; 54:121–127.
25. Garnuszewski Z, Dobrzynski W: Regression of pulmonary radiological changes in dockyard welders after cessation or decrease of exposure to welding fumes. *Pol Med J* 1967; 6:610–613.
26. Hallne U, Erlandsson A: *The Occurrence of Welding in Aluminum and Stainless Steel and Brazing with Silver-Containing Solders in Swedish Manufacturing Industry*. Investigation report 6. Stockholm, Swedish National Board of Occupational Safety and Health, 1977 (in Swedish).
27. Hedenstedt A, Jenssen D, Lidesten B-M, et al: Mutagenicity of fume particles from stainless steel welding. *Scand J Work Environ Health* 1977; 3:203–211.
28. Her Majesty's Stationary Office: *Occupational Mortality*, The Registrar General's decennial supplement for England and Wales, 1970–1972. London, 1979.
29. Herberts P, Kadefors R, Högfors C, et al: Shoulder pain and heavy manual labor. *Clin Orthop* 1984; 191:166–178.
30. Hernberg S, Westerholm P, Schultz-Larsen K, et al: Nasal and sinonasal cancer. Connection with occupational exposures in Denmark, Finland and Sweden. *Scand J Work Environ Health* 1983; 9:315–326.
31. Hunnicutt TN Jr, Cracovaner DJ, Myles JT: Spirometric measurements in welders. *Arch Environ Health* 1964; 8:661–669.
32. Husgafvel-Pursiainen K, Kalliomäki P-L, Sorsa M: A chromosome study among stainless steel welders. *J Occup Med* 1982; 24:762–766.
33. Jindrichova J: Chromschäden bei Elektroschweissern. *Z Gesamte Hyg ihre Grenzgebiete* 1978; 24:86–88.
34. Jones RC: Selective tests for contaminants in welding fumes from electric arc welding—An environmental assessment. *Ann Occup Hyg* 1967; 10:369–373.
35. Kalliomäki K, Aittoniemi K, Kalliomäki P-L, et al: Measurement of lung-retained contaminants in vivo among workers exposed to metal aerosols. *Am Ind Hyg Assoc J* 1981; 42:234–238.
36. Kalliomäki P-L, Junttila M-L, Kalliomäki K, et al: Comparison of the behavior of stainless and mild steel manual metal arc welding fumes in rat lung. *Scand J Work Environ Health* 1983; 9:176–180.
37. Kalliomäki P-L, Kalliomäki K, Rahkonen E, et al: Follow-up study on the lung retention of welding fumes among shipyard welders. *Ann Occup Hyg* 1983; 27:449–452.
38. Keimig DG, Pomrehn PR, Burmeister LF: Respiratory symptoms and pulmonary function in welders of mild steel: A cross-sectional study. *Am J Ind Med* 1983; 4:489–499.
39. Keskinen H, Kalliomäki P-L, Alanko K: Occupational asthma due to stainless steel welding fumes. *Clin Allergy* 1980; 10:151–159.
40. Kleinfeld M, Giel C, Tabershaw IR: Health hazards associated with inert-gas-shielded metal arc welding. *AMA Arch Ind Health* 1957; 15:27–31.
41. Koshi K: Effects of fume particles from stainless steel welding on sister chromatid exchanges and chromosome aberrations in cultured Chinese hamster cells. *Ind Health* 1979; 17:39–49.
42. Lautner GM, Carver JC, Konzen RB: Measurement of chromium VI and chromium III in stainless steel welding fumes with electron spectroscopy for chemical analysis and neutron activation analysis. *Am Ind Hyg Assoc J* 1978; 39:651–660.
43. Lindqvist T: Nitrous gas poisoning among welders using acetylene flame. *Acta Med Scand* 1944; 118(fasc I–III):210–243.
44. Littorin M, Högstedt B, Strömbäck B, et al: No cytogenetic effects in lymphocytes of stainless steel welders. *Scand J Work Environ Health* 1983; 9:259–264.
45. Lucas PA, Jariwalla AG, Jones JH, et al: Fatal cadmium fume inhalation. *Lancet* 1980; II:205.
46. Lundberg I, Sjögren B, Hallne U, et al: Environmental factors and uptake of cadmium among brazers using cadmium-containing hard-solders. *Am Ind Hyg Assoc J* 1984; 45:353–359.
47. Maxild J, Andersen M, Kiel P, et al: Mutagenicity of fume particles from metal arc welding on stainless steel in the Salmonella/microsome test. *Mutat Res* 1978; 56:235–243.
48. McCann JK: Health hazard from flux used in joining aluminium electricity cables. *Ann Occup Hyg* 1964; 7:261–268.
49. McMillan GHG, Heath J: The health of welders in naval dockyards: Acute changes in respiratory function during standardized welding. *Ann Occup Hyg* 1979; 22:19–32.
50. McMillan GHG, Pethybridge RJ: The health of welders in naval dockyards: Proportional mortality study of welders and two control groups. *J Soc Occup Med* 1983; 33:75–84.
51. Milham S Jr: Cancer mortality patterns associated with exposure to metals. *Ann NY Acad Sci* 1976; 271:243–249.
52. National Institute for Occupational Safety and Health: *Criteria for a Recommended Standard: Occupational Exposure to Inorganic Fluorides*. Washington DC, US Dept of Health, Education and Welfare, 1975.

53. Norwood WD, Wisehart DE, Earl CA, et al: Nitrogen dioxide poisoning due to metal-cutting with oxyacetylene torch. *J Occup Med* 1966; 8:301–306.
54. Oxhöj H, Bake B, Wedel H, et al: Effect of electric arc welding on ventilatory lung function. *Arch Environ Health* 1979; 34:211–217.
55. Pepys J, Pickering CAC: Asthma due to inhaled chemical fumes—Amino-ethyl ethanolamine in aluminium soldering flux. *Clin Allergy* 1972; 2:197–204.
56. Pepys J, Pickering CAC, Breslin ABX, et al: Asthma due to inhaled chemical agents—Toluene di-isocyanate. *Clin Allergy* 1972; 2:225–236.
57. Peters JM, Murphy RLH, Ferris BG, et al: Pulmonary function in shipyard welders. *Arch Environ Health* 1973; 26:28–31.
58. Ross DS: Welders' metal fume fever. *J Soc Occup Med* 1974; 24:125–129.
59. Sanderson JT: Hazards of the arc-air gouging process. *Ann Occup Hyg* 1968; 11:123–133.
60. Sarto F, Cominato I, Bianchi V, et al: Increased incidence of chromosomal aberrations and sister chromatid exchanges in workers exposed to chromic acid in electroplating factories. *Carcinogenesis* 1982; 3:1011–1016.
61. Selikoff IJ, Nicholson WJ, Lilis R: Radiological evidence of asbestos disease among ship repair workers. *Am J Ind Med* 1980; 1:9–22.
62. Sjögren B, Hogstedt C, Malker H: Chromium and asbestos as two probable risk factors in lung cancer among welders, letter to the editor. *J Occup Med* 1982; 24:874–875.
63. Sjögren B, Hedström L, Ulfvarson U: Urine chromium as an estimator of air exposure to stainless steel welding fumes. *Int Arch Occup Environ Health* 1983; 51:347–354.
64. Sjögren B, Lundberg I, Lidums V: Aluminium in the blood and urine of industrially exposed workers. *Br J Ind Med* 1983; 40:301–304.
65. Sjögren B, Hedström L, Lindstedt G: Urinary fluoride concentration as an estimator of welding fume exposure from basic electrodes. *Br J Ind Med* 1984; 41:192–196.
66. Sjögren B, Ulfvarson U: Respiratory symptoms and pulmonary function among welders working with aluminum, stainless steel and railway tracks. *Scand J Work Environ Health* 1985; 11:27–32.
67. Sjögren B, Gustavsson A, Hedström L: Mortality in two cohorts of welders exposed to high- and low-levels of hexavalent chromium. *Scand J Work Environ Health* 1987; 13:247–251.
68. Slepicka J, Kadlec K, Tesar Z, et al: Beitrag zur Problematik der Elektroschweisserpneumokoniose. *Int Arch Arbeitsmed* 1970; 27:257–280.
69. Sterling GM: Asthma due to aluminium soldering flux. *Thorax* 1967; 22:533–537.
70. Stern RM: Production and characterization of a reference standard welding fume. Copenhagen, The Danish Welding Institute, 1979.
71. Stern RM: Process-dependent risk of delayed health effects for welders. *Environ Health Perspect* 1981; 41:235–253.
72. Stern RM, Berlin A, Fletcher AC, et al: *Health Hazards and Biological Effects of Welding Fumes and Gases*. Amsterdam, Excerpta Medica International Congress Series 676. Proceedings of the International Conference, Copenhagen, 1985. Elsevier Science Publishers BV, 1986.
73. Stevens JJ: Asthma due to soldering flux: A polyether alcohol-polypropylene glycol mixture. *Ann Allergy* 1976; 36:419–422.
74. Svensson E, Alexandersson R, Bergman K, et al: No chronic changes after exposure to Freon 12. *Läkartidningen* 1982; 79:198–199. (In Swedish.)
75. Tanaka S, Lieben J: Manganese poisoning and exposure in Pennsylvania. *Arch Environ Health* 1969; 19:674–684.
76. Tebbens BD, Drinker P: Ventilation in arc welding with coated electrodes. *J Ind Hyg Toxicol* 1941; 23:322–342.
77. Tengroth B, Vulcan J: Welding light. *Strahlentherapie* 1977; 153:267–272.
78. Thomsen E, Stern RM: A simple analytical technique for the determination of hexavalent chromium in welding fumes and other complex matrices. *Scand J Work Environ Health* 1979; 5:386–403.
79. Thrysin E, Gerhardsson G, Forssman S: Fumes and gases in arc welding. *Arch Ind Hyg Occup Med* 1952; 6:381–403.
80. Townshend RH: A case of acute cadmium pneumonitis: Lung function tests during a four-year follow-up. *Br J Ind Med* 1968; 25:68–71.
81. Ulfvarson U: Survey of air contaminants from welding. *Scand J Work Environ Health* 1981; 7 (Suppl 2).
82. Welinder H, Littorin M, Gullberg B, et al: Elimination of chromium in urine after stainless steel welding. *Scand J Work Environ Health* 1983; 9:397–403.
83. Whitlock CM, Amuso SJ, Bittenbender JB: Chronic neurological disease in two manganese steel workers. *Am Ind Hyg Assoc J* 1966; 27:454–459.
84. World Health Organization: Early detection of chronic lung disease. Report on a WHO meeting. *EURO Reports and Studies* 24. Copenhagen, WHO, 1980.

66

Hazardous Waste Sites

James M. Melius, M.D., Dr. P.H.

Richard J. Costello, P.F., C.I.H.

David L. Dahlstrom, B.S., M.S.

Throughout the world, industrialized societies are producing effluents and wastes in gigantic quantities, now recognized as potential environmental hazards, but also of great concern about the health and safety of workers who clean up hazardous waste sites or who respond to chemical spills and other hazardous waste emergencies. At present, we have very little quantitative data on the occupational exposures and resultant health effects for these workers. Fortunately, the available information provides the basis for designing effective programs to protect these workers. Such efforts should provide an integrated program of employee training, industrial hygiene, and medical testing, appropriate engineering controls and protective equipment, and occupational safety measures in order to ensure appropriate health protection for these workers.

EXPOSURE

Exposure monitoring at these sites must assess potential exposures to multiple toxic substances and to physical hazards, such as noise and heat stress. Low-level chronic exposures to multiple substances are common and short-term acute exposures, as in accidental releases, may also occur. Contaminants may be in the form of particulates, particulate-bound toxic substances, bulk liquids, mists, gases, or vapors. Inhalation, ingestion, and skin contact are all important routes of exposure.

Due to the complexity of these work environments, the application of typical workplace industrial hygiene monitoring techniques may not be totally effective in identifying the hazards present. In most cases, the precise chemical composition of the wastes (especially barrelled wastes) is known for only a small percentage of the wastes prior to ultimate site closure, and waste analysis during cleanup is frequently limited to compatibility tests and a broad classification of the wastes (i.e., ignitability, corrosiveness, reactivity, and toxicity) prior to transport from the site. Generally, prior to the initiation of cleanup procedures, compounds present on the site can only partially be identified by conducting a thorough background review of facility records, waste manifests, site history, and prior site investigation records. To identify and quantify these often diverse contaminants for industrial hygiene evaluation, a variety of sampling techniques and multiple sampling media must be chosen and adapted to the environment in which these materials are found. Typically, these sampling techniques are combined with the use of direct reading instrumentation (e.g., flame ionization, photoionization and infrared detection, and respirable particulate monitors) to assist in the characterization of the site environment, the location of "hot spots" or high hazard areas, and the subsequent identification of contaminants in the work environment. The application of these techniques, however, requires the recognition of instrument and sampling limitations and interferences before any definitive conclusions can be derived regarding contaminant composition.

During the last three years, the National Institute for Occupational Safety and Health (NIOSH) has characterized exposures at four hazardous waste sites, including two remedial actions,[1, 2] a municipal landfill,[3] and a waste treatment facility.[4] Of the 500 samples analyzed, no contaminant concentration has exceeded 10% of the appropriate Occupational Safety and Health Administration's time-weighted average standard. The only acute medical problem found by the NIOSH investigators during these investigations have been heat stress,[2] acute dermal exposure to solvents due to improper selection of protective clothing,[5] and eye and respiratory irritation due to particulate-bound polynuclear aromatic compounds.[4] However, this is not to say that more severe conditions do not exist on waste sites as a whole, for every waste site cleanup is different in character and degree of hazard (Fig 66–1).

MEDICAL CONSIDERATIONS

A medical surveillance program for hazardous waste workers should prescribe specific fitness criteria in conjunction with periodic medical evaluations to ensure that only medically sound individuals participate in field operations and that the health status of these individuals is maintained. Therefore, the purpose of this

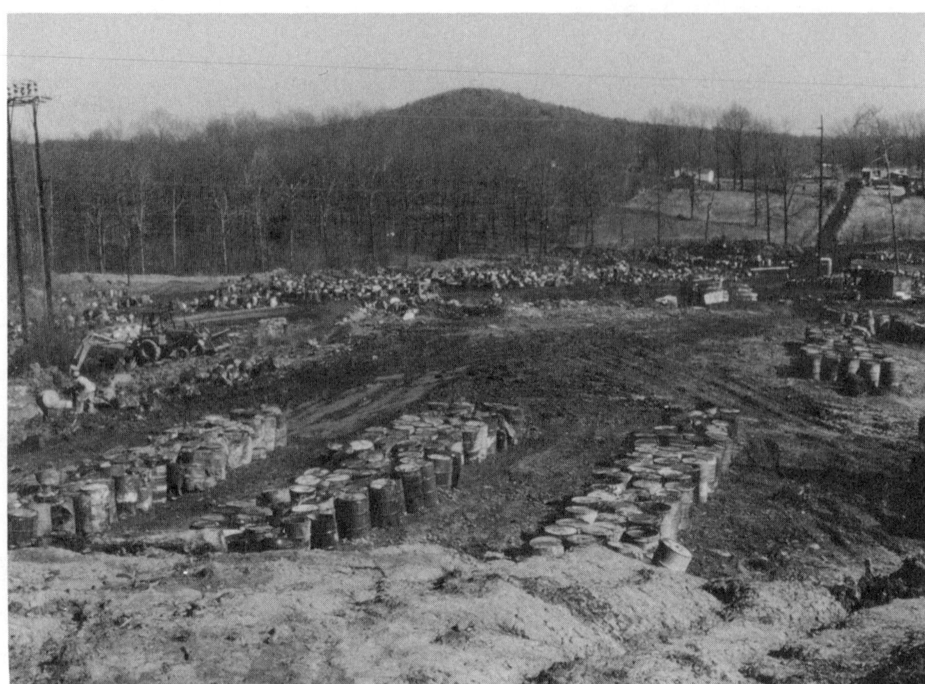

FIG 66–1.
General view of the task facing hazardous waste cleanup workers.

system is to detect any changes in health status of individuals or employee groups which might be related to the nature of the job performed and/or the substances to which the employee comes into contact. In consideration of the nature and variety of chemicals and mixtures related to hazardous waste sites and the frequency for potential exposure to these chemicals, it is extremely important to provide a means by which the health of personnel who work at hazardous waste sites can be periodically assessed.

A medical surveillance program for hazardous waste workers should include several components: comprehensive preplacement examinations, periodic testing and evaluation, episodic and emergency medical care, exit examinations, record keeping, and periodic program review. Given the nature of possible exposures and injuries at these sites, the medical program must be integrated with the industrial hygiene, safety, and employee training programs in order to provide a basis for appropriate medical monitoring and to assure that lapses or defects in the protection of workers are identified (Fig 66–2).

Preplacement and Periodic Screening

The major focus of the preplacement examination should be to determine whether the worker is mentally and physically fit to perform the assigned work at hazardous waste sites. Such work often requires strenuous activity while wearing a wide array of respiratory and protective equipment and clothing (Figs 66–3 and 66–4). Ambient temperatures of 70° F and above pose an additional stress for the worker. Currently there is little sound information available to provide for a good quantification of these added physiologic burdens, particularly for the purpose of preplacement screening. Preplacement screening should include a comprehensive medical and employment history and physical examination, focusing on health problems which may impair the worker's ability to handle this burden safely (Table 66–1). Information regarding past illnesses and chronic diseases such as asthma, allergies, diabetes, epilepsy, pulmonary disease, cardiovascular disease, and related risk factors should be obtained and assessed. Characteristics which may make an individual more susceptible to injury or severe physiologic stress, such as obesity or poor exercise tolerance, should also be ascertained. Further medical testing such as chest x-rays, pulmonary function testing, electrocardiograms, stress testing, and the routine analysis of body fluids or excreta for direct or indirect evidence of exposure to toxic chemicals will be useful in assessing a worker's overall health status over time.

Criteria for the exclusion of workers are not always clear-cut and will depend upon specific job requirements. Workers with symptomatic lower back problems or heart or lung disease should usually be excluded from heavy physical work at hazardous waste sites, particularly when that work requires the use of respirators with other protective equipment. Medical judgment based on knowledge of the required working conditions must play a large role in these decisions.

Another purpose for implementing a program of pre-employment medical screening is to establish an individual base line of useful medical data. This information will be important in evaluating the possible adverse health effects resulting from chronic exposure to low concentrations of chemicals and mixtures characteristic of waste site operations. Given the potential number of toxic substances which the typical waste site worker may be exposed to, the selection of the appropriate medical parameters to be tested

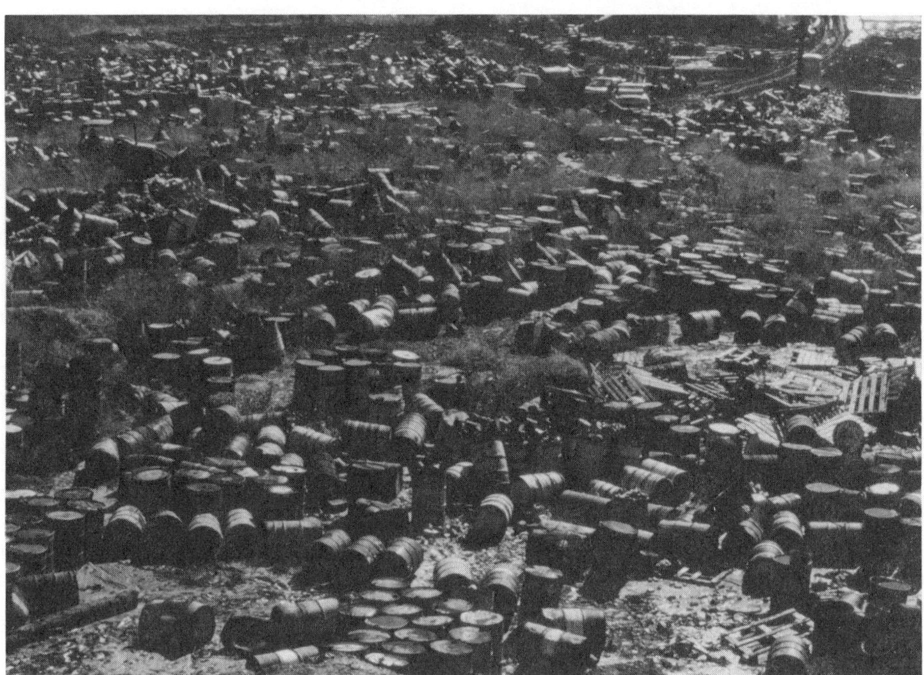

FIG 66–2.
Close-up view of enormous task of cleaning up hazardous wastes shown in Figure 66–2.

may be difficult but must be comprehensive. Further, these tests must be sensitive enough to detect even small changes in individual physiologies respective of these types of exposures. It is important to recognize that, physiologically, the chemicals and mixtures typically confronted at waste sites (solvents, pesticides, sludges, radionuclides, heavy metals, corrosives, and biologic agents) can be absorbed, transformed into metabolites, distributed throughout the body, concentrated in particular organs, or excreted. In each way, exposure to even low concentrations of these materials over time can significantly affect the worker's health and overall well-being. Consequently, the selection of specific tests to be performed should not be based upon individual exposures to a particular substance or even a chemical category, as would be the case in traditional occupational medicine, but upon the multiple chemicals and their variety of forms which may be confronted.

Consideration of the specific job(s) of the employee may also be useful when defining the specific parameters to be tested during the pre-employment examination (Figs 66–5 and 66–6). For ex-

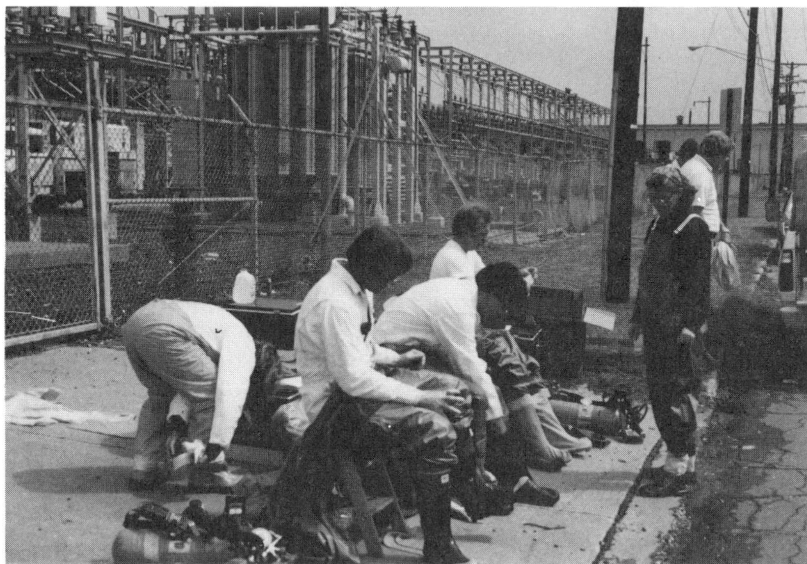

FIG 66–3.
"Suiting up" with proper protective equipment.

TABLE 66–1.
Suggested Occupational Medical Examination Parameters

Medical & Occupational History
(Self-administered and physician reviewed, taken during initial examination and updated by the physician during all subsequent examinations)

To determine each employee's
- Previous work involvement with chemicals and possible exposures;
- Pre-existing physical condition including allergies, sensitivities, physical abnormalities, current medications, and immunization history.

Vital Signs and Physical Examination Screen
(initial and all subsequent examinations)

A record of height, weight, body frame type, blood pressure (supine and standing), pulse rate (supine and standing), respiratory rate, and oral temperature.

A complete assessment of skin, eyes, ears, nose, throat; and respiratory, cardiovascular, genitourinary, musculoskeletal, abdominal, and neurologic systems.

Maximal Stress—Treadmill Exercise Test
With 12-lead ECG
(initial exam only)

Provides baseline information regarding each individual's physical status and ability to withstand physical stress related to field work while wearing a variety of protective equipment.

Pulmonary Function (Initial Exam Only) and Spirometry Testing (All Subsequent Exams)

To determine overall health of the pulmonary system and assess one's ability to use respiratory equipment. It is used to detect restrictive or obstructive lung diseases and chronic disorders such as bronchitis and emphysema.

Chest X-Ray (PA and Lateral)
(initial examination and periodically thereafter, depending upon age and exposure history)

To assist in determining the presence of lung disease.

Audiometry
(initial and all subsequent examinations)

To determine hearing acuity in the range of 500–8,000 Hz.

Vision Screening—Titmus
(initial and all subsequent examinations)

To screen individual's visual acuity. Tests should include an assessment of muscle balance, eye coordination, depth perception, peripheral vision, color discrimination, and tonometry.

Hematology Survey
(initial and all subsequent examinations)

This survey is used to screen for disorders of the blood and hematopoietic system.

Urinalysis
(initial and all subsequent examinations)

This test should include a chemical analysis for albumins, glucose, bilirubin, ketones, and occult blood as well as a measurement of pH, specific gravity, color, and character; and a microscopic review. The purpose of this analysis is to assess the overall function of the complete urinary system.

Heavy Metal Screens
(initial and subsequent examinations dependent upon exposure potential)

This screen is used to assess the quantity of lead in the blood and cadmium, mercury, and arsenic in the urine. (These heavy metals are most frequently encountered during work activities on waste sites.)

Blood Chemistry Screen
("SMA–20", 12-hour fasting required)
(initial and all subsequent examinations)

The value of this screen is to assess the overall functioning of the hepatic, renal, endocrine, and other metabolic systems.

Stool Sample for Occult Blood

ample, heavy machinery operators and drillers may experience significant exposures to noise and vibration and should consequently have appropriate baseline and periodic audiometric, visual acuity, and nerve conduction tests.[4] Traditionally, however, employees do not perform only one job function on-site, thereby requiring the examination protocols to be comprehensive rather than job-specific.

The purpose of the periodic screening examinations to be performed on hazardous waste site workers is to detect any deleterious effects due to exposure and to assure the employee remains physically fit to perform the tasks for which he has been hired. The content of these examinations, therefore, will be dependent upon the type of work performed, the worker's health status, and the materials to which he has been exposed since the previous examination. Accurate ambient or personal monitoring data reflective of actual site conditions where the employee has worked may be helpful in selecting the appropriate tests. In any case, the data derived from these examinations should be correlated to the employee's baseline data for indications of exposure or degradation of health status.

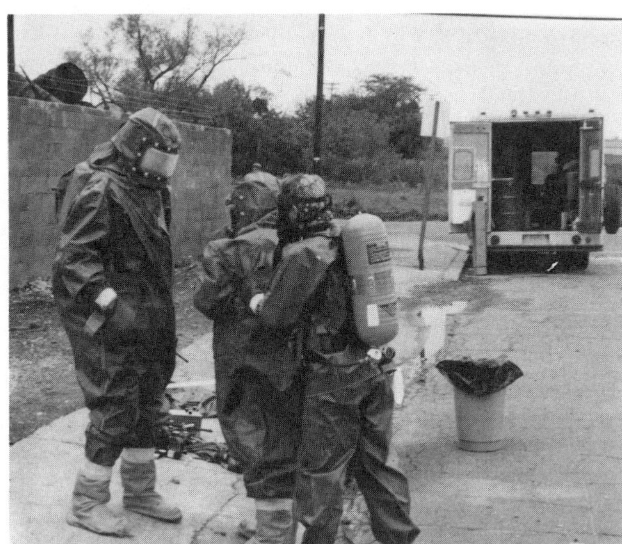

FIG 66–4.
Workers properly garbed, usually in teams of two or more.

The medical surveillance program developed for hazardous waste site workers should also provide for exit/termination examinations. Similar in content to the pre-employment and periodic examinations, the purpose of this examination is twofold. First, the data derived, when compared to previous examination data, defines the employee's health status at the time of termination, thus completing the employee's medical history during the time of employment. Secondly, it allows for the timely identifications of any medical abnormalities which may have resulted from chemical exposure or injuries during the period of employment and the implementation of specific treatment regimes to return the individual to pre-employment status prior to final discharge, thus alloying, to a large extent, any future liabilities on the part of the employer.

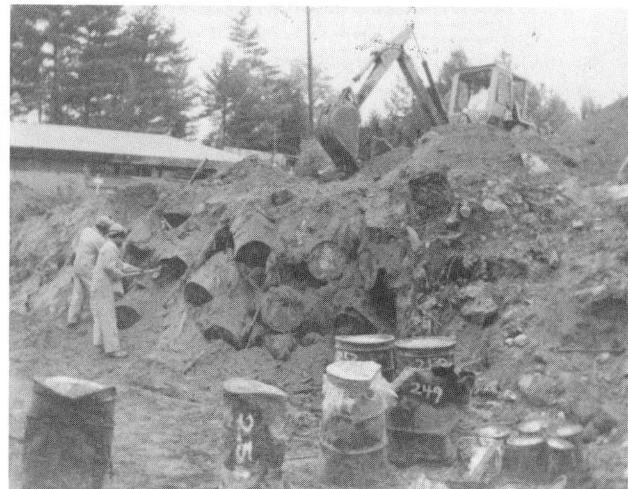

FIG 66–5.
Another view showing the difficulties encountered in disposing of hazardous waste fills.

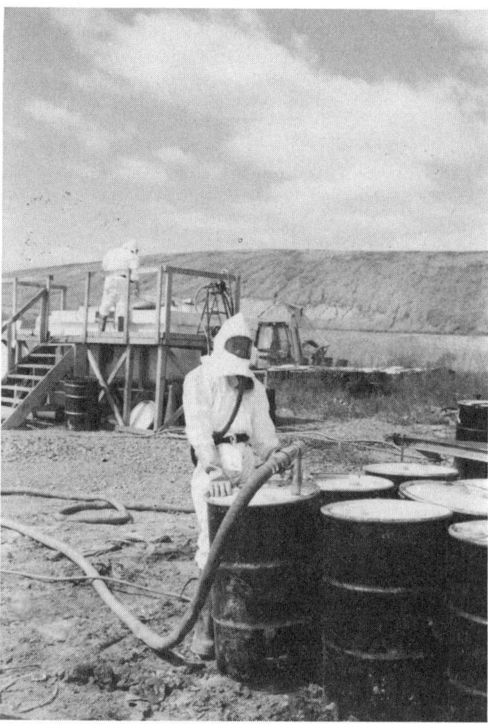

FIG 66–6.
Close-up view operation involving the complete removal of the materials found in discarded tanks.

Medical Contingencies

Medical contingencies for acute exposure, injuries, and periodic medical exclusion of workers should also be provided for in the design of a complete medical surveillance program for hazardous waste site workers. In preparation for an acute exposure to chemicals on-site, it is imperative that appropriate treatment facilities and medical resources be designated prior to the initiation of on-site activities. Hospital and emergency medical support services should be informed of the potential exposures at each specific site and appropriate preparations made for receiving these patients. Specific protocols for providing emergency first aid, decontamination, and emergency extrication of injured or exposed individuals should be known by all on-site personnel. Equally important is the designation of local analytical services to provide for the rapid identification of the chemical constituents to which the individual has been exposed. This information will prove invaluable to the attending physician and toxicologists in developing and implementing the most effective diagnostic and treatment schemes.

Provisions for the periodic medical exclusion of employees from hazardous waste site work should also be implemented. These provisions should not necessarily provide a basis for termination, but only for disability leave implemented in the best interest of the employee. Examples for the need of such provisions include physical injuries that limit mobility, medical abnormalities resulting from chemical exposure, and pregnancy. Implementation of these medical exclusions must be justifiable, well-documented, and periodically assessed.

Arrangements for episodic medical care for these workers may be difficult, due to the remote location of many of these sites. It is important to ensure that all possible occupationally-related symptoms or illnesses are appropriately evaluated in the context of the worker's exposures at the site and that other nonoccupationally related illnesses, such as colds or flu, do not place the worker at risk due to the physical requirements of hazardous waste site work.

Heat stress is a major acute medical problem at most sites.[2] Monitoring of heat stress is particularly difficult, due to the use of protective clothing. A heat stress prevention program will need to be established at most cleanup sites. This program should include appropriate screening for individuals at increased risk from heat stress; monitoring of heat stress by parameters such as surface body temperature, pulse rate, and body weight loss; provisions for periodic rest breaks and rehydration; and, if necessary, alteration of work schedules.

Police, fire fighters, and other emergency support personnel may also be exposed in responding to incidents at hazardous waste sites.[2] Prior to the initiation of work operations at these sites, these groups should be informed of the potential hazards and procedures defined to limit unnecessary exposures and to insure the availability of appropriate protective equipment. These arrangements should also include considerations for access to the site and decontamination of personnel and equipment involved in mitigating the incident.

Record Keeping and Program Review

The evaluation of employee medical records and occupational exposure and bodily injury records is an important aspect of any medical surveillance program. Periodic (e.g., by site or monthly) reviews of these records is also important, especially for hazardous waste site workers whose exposures are difficult to define. This review should critically evaluate the efficiency and effectiveness of the present medical surveillance program in the context of the available information on exposures at these sites. Medical protocols may require modification based upon the types of chemicals or conditions to be confronted at specific waste sites for ease in detecting exposures to particular compounds (e.g., dioxins versus heavy metals versus organophosphates). In any event, the medical surveillance program implemented to protect hazardous waste site workers must not be considered a static program but must be continually evaluated and revised, based upon the rapid changes in the medical sciences and current technologies, in order to assure that the worker's health is continually protected.

CONCLUSION

Protecting the health of hazardous waste workers is a difficult task. These workers are potentially exposed to a multitude of toxic substances. Often these exposures are not known at the time of exposure and may never be completely identified or quantitated. Protecting workers at these sites is dependent on careful planning, use of appropriate engineering controls and personal protective equipment, careful work practices, and appropriate environmental monitoring in order to identify and quantify exposures. Medical programs must assure that workers are fit for this type of work and are appropriately monitored for any adverse health effects during the course of the work. Finally, this health and safety program must be coordinated to assure a safe and healthful workplace in what may seem to be the opposite—a hazardous waste site.

REFERENCES

1. Costello R: *Triangle Chemical Site,* Health Hazard Evaluation Report 83-417-1357. NIOSH, 1983.
2. Costello R, Melius J: *Chemical Control,* Health Hazard Evaluation Report 80-077-853. NIOSH, 1981.
3. Costello R, Singal M, Liss G: A health hazard evaluation of waste disposal operators at a municipal landfill. Paper presented at the American Industrial Hygiene Conference, May 1983.
4. Costello R, Froneberg B, Melius J: *Rollins Environmental Services,* Health Hazard Evaluation Report 81-037-1055. NIOSH, 1981.
5. Reed L: *Taylor Borough Drum Site,* Health Hazard Evaluation Report 84-010-1445. NIOSH, 1984.
6. Tanaka M, Brisson G, Volle M: Body temperature in relation to heart rate for workers wearing impermeable clothing in a hot environment. *Am Ind Hyg Assoc J* 1978; 39:885–890.
7. US Department of Health and Human Services, National Institute for Occupational Safety and Health: *Occupational Safety and Health Guidance Manual for Hazardous Waste Site Activities*. Washington, DC, Superintendent of Documents, US Government Printing Office, 1985.

67

Observations on Fiberglass in Relation to Health

Jon L. Konzen, M.D.

The term *fiberglass* conjures different images to different people. To the sportsman it may be a boat, to a homeowner it may be window screening or draperies, to an engineer it may be an air transmission system, and to a builder it may be batts of insulation. Each of these products may contain a high percentage of fiberglass.

Modern fiberglass materials are manufactured into a wide variety of products suitable for specific applications. Fiberglass products frequently are classified into two broad categories: wools and textiles. Wool products are made into commercial, industrial, and residential insulation; acoustical ceiling panels; air conditioning ducts; and mats, by varying the product's compression, density, and amount of binder. Textile fibers are used in glass fiber yarns and rovings and chopped strand mats for applications such as decorative and industrial fabrics; reinforcements for plastic, rubber, and paper; electrical insulation; and filtration and roofing materials.

TYPES OF MORPHOLOGY OF FIBERGLASS

Most fiberglass is produced in a glass furnace, using a borosilicate batch. The diameters of fibers in each product vary, so the diameter of the majority of fibers in the products determines the *nominal diameter*. If the actual diameters of fiberglass produced by a particular process are plotted on a graph, the overwhelming majority of them will be "near" the nominal diameter. Although the majority of all fiber glass wool products have a nominal diameter of 3.5 μ or greater, all products contain some fibers with diameters equal or less than 3.5 μ (respirable fibers) and a small percentage are in the less than 1 μ diameter range. These respirable-size fibers have been present since fiberglass production began over 40 years ago.[22]

Wool fibers are generally manufactured by the centrifugal process in a range of nominal diameters from approximately 3 to 8 μ.

Fine-diameter fiberglass wool may include fibers that have a nominal diameter as small as 1 μ. These fibers have been produced on a commercial basis since the early 1940s in limited quantity.[49]

Very fine-diameter fiberglass with a nominal diameter of less than 1 μ is manufactured for certain highly specialized applications such as aerospace insulation and sophisticated filtration and represents less than 1% of all production.

Textile fiberglass products generally have larger nominal diameters than wool-type products. These fibers are drawn or extruded from holes in the base of the fiberizing equipment in a process that produces continuous fibers of infinite length. The nominal diameters range from approximately 6 to 25 μ, with a very narrow range of diameter distribution. The majority of textile fiberglass is used in reinforcement applications, where a larger fiber diameter is desired for superior reinforcing properties. For this reason, most of the textile fiberglass produced is the larger diameter fibers. The finest diameter textile fiber has a nominal diameter of 3.5 μ, is produced in relatively small quantities, and is used for specialized fabric applications. Because of the nature of the manufacturing process, even this textile fiberglass contains only a small amount of fiber with diameters of less than 3.5 μ.

Practically all fiberglass products are coated with bindings, sizings, and lubricants. During the past 40 years, there has been little change in the basic chemical composition of the principal ingredients of insulation bonding resins (wool). The most significant change has been the progressive replacement of a bonding material that consisted largely of phenol formaldehyde resin and insoluble wood resin by-products by a bonding material made up mainly of phenol formaldehyde resin with urea-containing components. Although originally a water-soluble resin, it remains after "cure" as an insoluble and infusable resin film on the fiber surfaces. The wool binder coating is cured in high temperature ovens immediately after application. Formaldehyde off-gassing from the cured binder is insignificant.[29] Since the 1930s, high flash-point paraffinic mineral oils have been used in the production of all wool products, with little change in composition or percentage of total product weight (0.5%–1.0%). The oil reduces lint generation in the cured insulation.

Sizes or binding agents for textiles are of the starch, cationic, lubricant vegetable oil type for yarns that are woven into decorative fabrics such as curtains and drapes. This starch-base binding agent is removed from the woven fabric by heat treatment. Textile fibers destined for reinforcement applications are coated with a polyvinyl acetate-chrome chloride, polyvinyl acetate-silane, polyester-silane, or epoxy-silane size appropriate to the reinforcement application.

INDUSTRIAL HYGIENE CONSIDERATIONS

Several industrial hygiene studies have been reported.[8, 9, 16, 35, 39, 43] The results of these studies are remarkably consistent. In general, the respirable airborne fiber concentration in manufacturing operations, especially in wool-type operations, has the greatest potential to contribute respirable fiber, usually less than 0.1 f/ml. The airborne concentration in many fabrication operations is essentially the same. In areas where fiberglass is being installed in buildings, the airborne concentration in most applications parallels manufacturing operations. The exception to this is when the material is blown or applied in a closed space such as an attic. In such installations, the airborne concentration has been noted to be in an average range of 0.4 f/ml to 3 f/ml. The effect of fiberglass-lined air transmission systems in buildings demonstrates that properly installed systems do not contribute any significant amount of fiber to the indoor air.[1] Rather, the indoor airborne concentration in these situations reflects the outdoor air fiberglass concentration.

Fiberglass with intentionally produced finer average diameters deserves comment. Fine-diameter glass may include fibers that have a nominal diameter as low as 1 μ. These fibers, which represent less than 1% of all fiberglass production, have been produced since the early 1940s for use in filtration and aviation insulation.[49] In even more limited production is very fine-diameter fiberglass, having a nominal fiber diameter of less than 1 μ which is manufactured for highly specialized applications such as aerospace insulation and sophisticated filtration. It has been produced since the 1950s. The airborne exposure to respirable-size fibers in manufacturing operations making or using fine-diameter fiber generally is less than 1 f/ml and 2 to 10 f/ml for very fine fibers.[8, 9]

Fiberglass and the Skin

Fiberglass is capable of producing a mechanical transitory skin irritation. The most common symptom of fiberglass irritation is an itching or prickling of the skin, especially in the skin folds where clothing comes into tight contact with the skin or where an exposed skin surface such as the forearm comes in contact with a surface contaminated with fiberglass. The hallmark of fiberglass irritation is a varying degree of pruritus without objective findings that occurs upon contact with the material.[21] The macular or maculopapular rash frequently described in relation to fiberglass irritation is less frequently seen. A visible sign of irritation (other than scratch marks) is usually a macular eruption over pressure points, especially the forearms and between the fingers. Problem cases may involve secondary infection from scratching. However, this is an infrequent complication in most cases of fiberglass irritation.

Good personal hygiene practices are essential for reducing the irritation from fiberglass, since there are no specific methods of fully preventing skin contact in workers exposed to the material. Individuals usually become acclimatized to the material after working with it for several consecutive days. This acclimatization is marked by a reduction of irritation. Good personal hygiene includes rinsing the exposed surface of the skin occasionally during the workday and showering at the end of the day. A washcloth is helpful in removing any adherent fiberglass lint. Initially, work clothes should be long sleeved and loose fitting. As acclimatization occurs, it is reasonable to wear short-sleeved, open-necked attire. In most situations where fiberglass is handled, it is appropriate to wear gloves. Work clothes should be changed frequently and washed separately from other clothing. The washer should be wiped out with a damp cloth. Since irritation from fiberglass is a mechanical irritation, barrier creams are of little use. The reason that barrier creams seem to aid in lessening irritation is related to the increased skin care occasioned by applying the material and washing it off at the end of the work period. Barrier creams do have a place in operations where various plastic resins are used in hand lay-up operations during fabrication of reinforced plastic products. They will help prevent chemical dermatitis. If treatment is required for the mechanical irritation, simple emollient lotions are effective. Steroids, either local or systemic, are usually not indicated.

With the exception of a few specialty applications, the resin binder in insulation products has been cured before the products leave the factory and will not cause dermatitis. However, uncured resin binders on insulation products have the potential to cause chemical dermatitis and skin sensitization. Most physicians will not encounter workers who come in contact with insulation products containing the uncured resin binder, since this market is limited.

Fiberglass and the Eye

Fiberglass may be deposited in the eye by contaminated fingers or deposition of such fibers from the air. In contrast to skin irritation, involvement of the eye is uncommon.[27] Plant experience suggests that there have been few serious consequences. Most foreign bodies are nonadherent and are readily removed with a moistened cotton swab. The foreign body can be located more easily after staining with fluorescein.

Although most foreign bodies will lie in the inferior conjunctival sac or on the globe, it is not unusual to locate the offending material on the inner surface of the upper lid just posterior to the lid's margin.

Safety glasses, goggles, or a face shield should be worn as appropriate when handling or applying the materials.

Fiberglass and the Pulmonary System

Fiberglass can, if the airborne concentration is high enough, cause an upper respiratory irritation. Such irritation occurs much less frequently than skin irritation. It is manifested by a tickling or prickling sensation in the pharynx. Nasal irritation is an uncommon symptom. Asthma-like symptoms, while possible in theory, in fact occur very rarely. A NIOSH or MSHA approved air purifying respirator such as the 3M Model 8710 or Model 9900 (in high humidity environments) or equivalent should be used when working with fiberglass wool products under the following conditions: installing loosefill, in any confined or poorly ventilated space, fabrication involving power tools, and any installation operation or fabrication operation that creates a dusty working environment.

Exposed Workers Studies.—The mortality studies reported prior to the International Conference on Man-Made Mineral Fibers in October 1986 demonstrated no consistent evidence of malignant or nonmalignant disease in man.[2, 4, 6, 7, 33, 41, 45] At the conference, three studies, all follow-ups of previously reported mortality studies (one U.S., one Canadian, and one European), reported a statistically significant excess of lung cancer in fiberglass wool manufacturing workers (reported as respiratory cancer in the U.S. study).[6, 44, 46] There was no excess of mesotheliomas reported. The excess in the wool manufacturing workers was based on national death rates in the U.S. and European studies and provincial rates in the small Canadian study. Local rates were reported for the European study. The use of local rates reduced the excess death rate in the European study to a nonsignficant level for glass wool (93 overserved vs. 90.5 expected). Subsequently, the local rates for respiratory cancer in the U.S. study were reported (267 observed vs. 244.3 expected) and as in the European study were not statistically significant.[6, 46] It should be noted that both the American and European studies showed an elevated standarized mortality ratio with time since first exposure for glass wool manufacturing workers that became statistically significant 30 or more years and time of first exposure when national rates were used. However, when local mortality rates were used, neither the excess nor the slope of the increase was statistically significant.

Manufacturing workers exposed to textile fibers were also evaluated in the U.S. and European studies but not in the Canadian study.[44] The numbers of workers studied were much smaller than in glass wool. There were no excess deaths from lung cancer (79 observed vs. 84.6 expected). Also, lung cancer mortality did not increase with time since first exposure.

The most pertinent mortality studies evaluating nonmalignant respiratory disease were those reported at the International Conference on Man-Made Mineral Fibers in October 1986 that incorporated the cohorts of previously reported studies. The European and Canadian studies reported no excess of nonmalignant respiratory disease.[44, 46] The American study did demonstrate a statistically significant excess of nonmalignant respiratory disease other than pneumonia and influenza in fiberglass wool manufacturing workers with no relation to duration of employment, time from first exposure, or intensity of exposure. When local rates were calculated for nonmalignant respiratory disease other than pneumonia and influenza (available only since 1962) from data obtained from Enterline, the excess became nonsignificant for glass wool.[50] Continuous filament demonstrated no statistically significant excess of nonmalignant respiratory disease.

There have been seven pertinent cross-sectional morbidity studies of populations exposed to fiberglass.[10, 17, 18, 28, 34, 52, 53] In four of these studies, there was no adverse effect attributable to exposure to fiberglass. One study noted upper respiratory irritation but no fibrosis or pulmonary function changes.[28] In one of the other two studies, no effect related to exposure was observed with respect to symptoms or pulmonary function measurements.[18] The slight excess of small densities observed radiologically was related to previous occupational dust exposure (coal and silica) and to never having lived in a smoke-free zone. None of the radiologic or other findings were directly attributable to cumulative exposure to fiberglass. The other fiberglass study included five fiberglass manufacturing plants.[52] The study employed roentgenography, a questionnaire for symptoms, and pulmonary function measurements. No adverse effects were observed with repect to symptoms or pulmonary function measurements. There was a low prevalence of the lowest profusion categories for small irregular densities observed radiologically. These were described as requiring further evaluation, but not as indicative of disease.

Lung tissue obtained at autopsy from 20 individuals occupationally exposed from 16 to 32 years was analyzed and no effects attributable to fiberglass were observed based on a direct comparison with tissue from 26 urban dwellers not exposed to fiberglass.[13] Although this is a very small study, one would expect if dust disease was going to be caused by fiberglass, the earliest manifestation would have been seen.

Animal Studies.—Prior to 1982, four studies of rodents exposed by inhalation to fiberglass for periods of 12 to 24 months were reported.[14, 24, 25, 42] No diffuse interstitial fibrosis was observed to develop. The reaction was primarily that of dust storage in foci of macrophages and also in regional lymph nodes. No excess of pulmonary or pleural tumors was observed. Recently, two studies (one in Europe and the other in the United States) were reported that used the same samples of fiberglass and the same strain of animals.[30, 40, 51] Both studies exposed rats by inhalation. The airborne concentration was approximately 10 mg/cu m. Exposure was for 12 months, and the animals were permitted to live out their lives. A few malignant tumors of the lung developed in both the experimental and control groups, but there was no significant differences noted in their frequency. A cellular dust response consisting of macrophage aggregates was noted at the end of 2 years but no true fibrosis. The lung reaction was not progressive and tended to regress. The minimal to mild reaction appears to be a nonspecific response common to any dust. Another study has been reported that exposed rats and monkeys for 18 to 20 months to various lengths and diameters of fiberglass. No evidence of pulmonary fibrosis, lung cancer, or mesothelioma was noted. Again, a nonspecific dust response was noted.[31]

Smith reported in 1986 on a study that exposed rats and hamsters by inhalation to very fine glass fibers (.45 μ) as well as glass fibers of average diameters (3.1 μ, 5.4 μ, and 6.1 μ, respectively).[47] The airborne concentration of fibers with an average diameter of 0.45 μ was approximately 3,000 f/ml. The thicker average diameter material (3.1 μ and 5.4 μ) produced airborne concentrations of 100 f/ml and the largest diameter fiber (6.1 μ) could only be lofted at a maximum of 25 f/ml. Survival of the exposed and sham and unmanipulated controls varied from 2 to 3 years. No primary lung tumors or mesotheliomas were found in any of the animals exposed to fiberglass. A few tumors did occur in chrysotile asbestos-exposed animals, but not at a rate that was statistically significantly greater than the controls. There was no unusual disease pattern or evidence of pulmonary fibrosis in the animals exposed to fiberglass as compared to the control animals.

Studies to determine the deposition pattern and ultimate fate of fiberglass introduced by inhalation and by multiple intratracheal injection have been reported.[3, 11, 15, 20, 23, 26, 32] These and an additional study demonstrate that short fiberglass is rapidly picked up by macrophages and stored in regional lymph nodes and in those at the hilum of the lung.[54] Many fibers also are completely removed from the respiratory system. These studies indicate that fewer than 10% of the fibers originally deposited remain in the lung for a substantial period of time. Longer fibers undergo marked changes. Many are fractured transversely and thus are more easily removed or stored. Others undergo great reduction in diameter, losing approximately 50% of their volume in 18 months. In other words, these fibers appear to be dissolved by the lung fluids. This phenomenon may explain partially the observation of minimal cellular and fibrotic reaction in the lung tissue of heavily exposed experimental animals.

One inhalation study not yet completed has reported some lung changes after exposure of primates to very fine fiber at extremely high concentrations (1,000 f/ml).[12] There were no controls reported, and the findings were reported on biopsy samples. Further evaluation of this ongoing study is necessary before any final conclusions can be drawn.

Intratracheal injection studies from one center have produced pulmonary fibrosis, lung cancer, and mesotheliomas.[36, 37] Other investigators using the intratracheal injection method of administering fine diameter fiberglass have been unable to produce malignant tumors, but have reported mild pulmonary fibrosis.[3, 38, 48, 54] This fibrosis is believed to be an artifact created by the technique of administration.

Recent animal implantation studies reaffirm previously published findings that the use of highly artificial methods of exposure can cause mesotheliomas in animals.[51] It must be remembered that the epidemiologic and animal inhalation studies have not reported that fiberglass causes mesothelioma.

IARC EVALUATION

In June 1987, the International Agency for Research on Cancer (IARC) classified fiberglass wool as a possible cancer causing agent to humans.[19] This classification was based on a combined evaluation of published human studies and animal studies. The human studies included large scale mortality studies of U.S. and European fiberglass wool factory workers. The IARC concluded that the human studies did not provide sufficient evidence that fiberglass wool caused cancer in humans. The classification of fiberglass wool as a "possible" carcinogen to humans was based substantially on experimental studies in which animals were exposed to wool glass fibers through nonnatural routes, such as injection or implantation. The IARC regards it as prudent to treat a material for which there is sufficient evidence of carcinogenicity to animals as if it is a possible carcinogen in humans.

The IARC categorized fiberglass continuous filament (textile) as not classifiable with respect to human carcinogenicity.[19] The evidence from human as well as animal studies was evaluated by IARC as insufficient to classify fiberglass continuous filament as a possible, probable, or confirmed cancer causing material.

SUMMARY

Fiberglass is manufactured in two forms: textile and wool. Textile fibers are used primarily in fabric or in reinforcing applications, while wool-type fiberglass is used in acoustical and thermal applications. Fiberglass can cause a temporary mechanical irritation that usually lessens over a period of days with continued exposure. Good personal hygiene, the appropriate use of gloves, long-sleeved, loose-fitting garments, and eye protection, and, in some cases, the use of a respirator will protect the worker handling the material. The airborne concentration of fiberglass consistently has been demonstrated to be low in most manufacturing applications. Animal studies demonstrate with remarkable consistency a notable lack of malignant or nonmalignant disease development in animals exposed by inhalation to fiberglass. Human morbidity and mortality studies of workers exposed to fiberglass demonstrate no consistent evidence of disease either malignant or nonmalignant in this material, which has been in use for well over 40 years.

REFERENCES

1. Balzer JL, Cooper WC, Fowler DP: Fibrous glass-lined air transmission systems: An assessment of their environmental effects. *Am Ind Hyg Assoc J* 1971; 32:512–518.
2. Bayliss DL, Dement JM, Wagoner JK, et al: Mortality patterns among fibrous glass production workers. *Ann NY Acad Sci* 1976; 271:324–334.
3. Drew RT, Bernstein DM, Kuschner M: The deposition, translocation, and fate of sized man-made mineral fibers in rats. Final report to TIMA of the Brookhaven National Laboratory, Upton, Long Island, New York, September 30, 1985.
4. Enterline PE, Henderson V: The health of retired fibrous glass workers. *Arch Environ Health* 1975; 30:113–116.
5. Enterline PE, Marsh GM: The health of workers in the MMMF industry; in *Biological Effects of Man-Made Mineral Fibres*. Proceedings of a WHO/IARC Conference, 1984; 1:311–339.
6. Enterline PE, Marsh GM, Henderson V: Mortality update of a cohort of U.S. man-made mineral fiber workers. *Ann Occup Hyg* (accepted for publication).
7. Enterline PE, Marsh, GM, Esmen NA: Respiratory disease among workers exposed to man-made mineral fibres. *Am Rev Respir Dis* 1983; 128(1):1–7.
8. Esmen N, Corn M, Hammad Y, et al: Summary of measurements of employee exposure to airborne dust and fiber in sixteen facilities producing man-made mineral fibres. *Am Ind Hyg Assoc J* 1979; 40:108–117.
9. Esmen N, Sheehan M, Corn M, et al: Exposure of employees to man-made vitreous fibers: Installation of insulation materials. *Environ Res* 1982; 28:386–398.
10. Fibrous glass manufacturing and health: Report of an epidemiological study: Parts I and II, in Proceedings of the 35th Annual Meeting of the Industrial Health Foundation, Pittsburgh, 1970.
11. Forster H: The behavior of mineral fibres in physiological solutions, in *Biological Effects of Man-Made Mineral Fibres*. Proceedings of a WHO/IARC Conference, 1984; 2:27–59.
12. Goldstein B, Rendall REG, Webster I: A comparison of the effects of exposure of baboons to crocidolite and fibrous-glass dusts. *Environ Res* 1983; 32:344–359.
13. Gross P, et al: Lungs of workers exposed to fiber glass: A study of their pathologic changes and their dust content. *Arch Environ Health* 1971; 23:67–76.
14. Gross P, deTreville RTP, Cralley LJ, et al: The pulmonary response to fibrous dusts of diverse compositions. *J Am Ind Hyg Assoc* 1970; 30:125–132.
15. Hammad YY: Deposition and elimination of MMMF, in *Biological Effects of Man-Made Mineral Fibres*. Proceedings of a WHO/IARC Conference, 1984; 1:126–142.
16. Hammad YY, Esmen NA: Long-term survey of airborne fibres in the United States, in *Biological Effects of Man-Made Mineral Fibres*, Proceedings of a WHO/IARC Conference, 1984; 1:118–132.

17. Hill JW, et al: Absence of pulmonary hazard in production workers. *Br J Ind Med* 1973; 30:174–179.
18. Hill JW, Rossiter CE, Foden DW: A pilot respiratory study of workers in a MMMF plant in the United Kingdom, in *Biological Effects of Man-Made Mineral Fibres*. Proceedings of a WHO/IARC Conference, 1984; 1:413–426.
19. IARC (International Agency for Research on Cancer): IARC working group on the evaluation of carcinogenic risk to humans: Man-made mineral fibres and radon, Lyon, France, June 1987.
20. Johnson NF, Griffiths DM, Hill RJ: Size distribution following long-term inhalation of MMMF, in *Biological Effects of Man-Made Mineral Fibres*. Proceedings of a WHO/IARC Conference, 1984; 2:102–125.
21. Konzen JL: Fiberglas and the skin, in Maibach HI (ed): *Occupational and Industrial Dermatology*. Chicago, Year Book Medical Publishers, Inc, 1987, pp 282–285.
22. Konzen JL: Production trends in fibre sizes of MMMF insulation, in *Biological Effects of Man-Made Mineral Fibres*. Proceedings of a WHO/IARC Conference, 1984; 1:44–64.
23. LeBouffant L, et al: Distribution of inhaled MMMF in the rat lung: Long-term effects, in *Biological Effects of Man-Made Mineral Fibres*. Proceedings of a WHO/IARC Conference, 1984; 2:143–168.
24. Lee KP, Barras CE, Griffith FD, et al: Comparative pulmonary responses to inhaled organic fibers with asbestos and fiberglass. *Environ Res* 1981; 24:167–191.
25. Lee KP, Barras CE, Griffith FD, et al: Pulmonary response to glass fiber by inhalation exposure. *Lab Invest* 1979; 40:123.
26. Leineweber JP: Solubility of fibres *in vitro* and *in vivo*, in *Biological Effects of Man-Made Mineral Fibres*. Proceedings of a WHO/IARC Conference, 1984; 2:87–101.
27. Lucas J: The cutaneous and ocular effects resulting from worker exposure to fibrous glass. A symposium, in *Occupational Exposure to Fibrous Glass: Proceedings of a Symposium*. NIOSH, April 1976, pp 211–219.
28. Maggioni A, Meregalli G, Sala C, et al: Respiratory and cutaneous pathology in workers engaged in the production of glass fibers (spun glass). *Med Lav* 1980; 3:216–227.
29. Matthews TG, Westley RR: *Determination of Formaldehyde Emission Levels for Ceiling Panels and Fibrous Glass Insulation Products*. Washington, DC, Consumer Product Safety Commission, 1983.
30. McConnell EE, Wagner JC, Skidmore JW, et al: A comparative study of the fibrogenic and carcinogenic effects of UICC Canadian chrysotile B asbestos and glass microfibre (JM 100), in *Biological Effects of Man-Made Mineral Fibres*. Proceedings of a WHO/IARC Conference, 1984; 2:234–250.
31. Mitchell RI, Donofrio DJ, Moorman WJ: Chronic inhalation toxicity of fibrous glass in rats and monkeys. *J Am Coll Toxicol* 1986; 5(6):545–575.
32. Morgan A, Holmes A: The deposition of MMMF in the respiratory tract of the rat, their subsequent clearance, solubility *in vivo* and protein coating, in *Biological Effects of Man-Made Mineral Fibres*. Proceedings of a WHO/IARC Conference, 1984; 2:1–7.
33. Morgan RW, Kaplan SD, Bratsberg JA: Mortality in fibrous glass production workers, in *Biological Effects of Man-Made Mineral Fibres*. Proceedings of a WHO/IARC Conference, 1984; 1:340–346.
34. Nasr ANM, Ditchek T, Scholtens PA: The prevalence of radiographic abnormalities in the chests of fiberglass workers. *J Occup Med* 1971; 13:317–376.
35. Ottery J, Cherrie JW, Dodgson J, et al: A summary report on environmental conditions at 13 European MMMF plants, in *Biological Effects of Man-Made Mineral Fibres*. Proceedings of a WHO/IARC Conference, 1984; 1:83–117.
36. Pott F, Ziem U, Reiffer FJ, et al: Carcinogenicity studies on fibres, metal compounds, and some other dusts in rats. *Exp Pathol* (to be published).
37. Pott F, Ziem U, Mohr U: Lung carcinomas and mesotheliomas following intratracheal instillation of glass fibres and asbestos. Proceedings of the VIth International Pneumoconiosis Conference, 1983; 2:746–756, Bochum, Bergbau Berufsgenossenschaft.
38. Renne RA, Eldridge SR, Lewis TR, et al: Fibrogenic potential of intratracheally instilled quartz, ferric oxide, fibrous glass, and hydrated Alumina in hamsters. *Toxicol Pathol* 1985; 13(4):306–314.
39. Riediger G: Measurements of mineral fibres in the industries which produce and use MMMF, in *Biological Effects of Man-Made Mineral Fibres*. Proceedings of a WHO/IARC Conference, 1984; 1:133–177.
40. Rossiter CE: The MRC and NIEH studies: A further analysis (appendix), in *Biological Effects of Man-Made Mineral Fibres*. Proceedings of a WHO/IARC Conference, 1984; 2:251–252.
41. Saracci R, et al: The IARC mortality and cancer incidence study of MMMF production workers, in *Biological Effects of Man-Made Mineral Fibres*. Proceedings of a WHO/IARC Conference, 1984; 1:279–310.
42. Schepers GWH, Delehant AB: An experimental study of the effects of glass wool on animal lungs. *Arch Ind Health* 1955; 12:276–279.
43. Schneider T: Review of surveys in industries that use MMMF, in *Biological Effects of Man-Made Mineral Fibres*. Proceedings of a WHO/IARC Conference, 1984; 1:178–190.
44. Shannon H, Jamieson E, Julian J, et al: Mortality experience of glass fibre workers: Extended follow-up. *Ann Occup Hyg* (accepted for publication).
45. Shannon H, Hayes M, Julian J, et al: Mortality experience of glass fibre workers, in *Biological Effects of Man-Made Mineral Fibres*. Proceedings of a WHO/IARC Conference, 1984; 1:347–349.
46. Simonato L, Fletcher A, Saracci R, et al: The man-made mineral fibers (MMMF) European historical cohort study: Extension of the follow-up. *Ann Occup Hyg* (accepted for publication).
47. Smith DM, Ortiz LW, Archuleta RF: Long-term exposure of Syrian hamsters and Osborne-Mendel rats to aerosolized 0.45 μm mean diameter fibrous glass, in *Biological Effects of Man-Made Mineral Fibres*. Proceedings of a WHO/IARC Conference, 1984; 2:253–272.
48. Smith DM, Ortiz LW, Archuleta RF, et al: Long-term health effects in hamsters and rats exposed chronically to man-made vitreous fibers. *Ann Occup Hyg* (to be published).
49. Smith HV: Manufacturing and uses of fibrous glass: One company's experience, in *Symposium on Occupational Exposure to Fibrous Glass: Proceedings of a Symposium*. NIOSH, April 1976.
50. Unpublished Enterline data analyzed by TIMA (Thermal Insulation Manufacturers Association), 1987 (7 Kirby Plaza, Mt Kisco, NY).
51. Wagner JC, Berry GB, Hill RJ, et al: Animal experiments with MMM(V)F fibres: Effect of inhalation and intrapleural inoculation in rats, in *Biological Effects of Man-Made Mineral Fibres*. Proceedings of a WHO/IARC Conference, 1984; 2:209–233.
52. Weill H, Hughes JM, Hammad YY, et al: Respiratory health in workers exposed to man-made vitreous fibers. *Am Rev Respir Dis* 1983; 28:104–112.
53. Wright GW: Airborne fibrous glass particles: Chest roentgenograms of persons with prolonged exposure. *Arch Environ Health* 1968; 21:175–181.
54. Wright GW, Kuschner M: The influence of varying lengths of glass and asbestos fibers on tissue response in guinea pigs, in Walton WH (ed): *Inhaled Particles*. New York, Pergamon Press, vol 4, 1977.

PART VI

Psychosocial Considerations

68

Stress at Work: An Interactive Model for Work Environment Analysis

Tomas Berggren, Ph.D.

Monica Hane, Ph.D.

Kerstin Ekberg, Ph.D.

Recent reviews have indicated the serious effects of factors in the work environment associated with stress on both psychologic and somatic well-being.[16, 25, 40, 45, 63] Certain elements inherent in the work content or related to work organization that either tax the capacities of the individual or are of relevance for fulfillment of psychologic needs and resources have been associated with stress at work. There has been a tendency to consider almost every aspect of work content and work organization as a potential stressor. This tendency has, however, blurred the original meaning and made the stress concept less useful as a guide for research and understanding of how work content and organization can affect psychologic and physiologic functioning. To ascertain a special meaning for the concept, it is therefore important to limit its use to those factors in the environment that trigger physiologic, psychologic, or behavioral arousal from those that do not. This is in accordance with the definition of stress as an unspecific physiologic, psychologic, and behavioral arousal response to any kind of demand.[91, 92] For example, to have too little to do, to be underutilized, or to be lacking in control, may be boring or frustrating, and has detrimental psychologic effects, but does not cause increased arousal levels, and thus should not be regarded as an example of a stress-relevant factor. However, as will be shown, factors in the environment that are relevant to the fulfillment of needs and aspirations, though not primarily associated to arousal level, can modify the effects of stress involving environmental factors.

Occupational stress research varies in the choice of effect variables studied. The variation ranges from mortality in psychosomatic illness to physiologic reactions to self-reported well-being or discomfort. There is also a large variability in definitions and choice of environmental variables studied; many studies are based only on comparisons between different occupations. Various occupations differ in many respects and, as a rule, the different "exposures" are not well analyzed. In some studies, the "exposure" is defined by the worker's appraisal of different aspects of the work environment. These studies are in line with the conception of stress as a response system not directly activated by characteristics in the environment but by the threats or expectations to which they give rise. In this chapter, the latest research and concepts in the area will be discussed, and as a conclusion, a model of occupational stress is presented. The chapter will focus on studies of the effects of various demands taxing the capacities of the individual at work. Investigations of modifying effects of factors in the environment and within the individual are considered and organized according to the type of effect studied. First, it is necessary to define the "stress concept," since it has been used in different ways by various investigators.

STRESS AS A RESPONSE SYSTEM

Several studies of occupational stress have used the stress concept to denote an external demand or the psychologic appraisal of that demand.[23, 35, 60, 69] The immediate reaction to the demanding situation in these studies have been called psychologic or physiologic "strain." Here, we will adhere to Seleye's original definition, in which stress is considered an unspecific reaction or response process to any kind of environmental demand.[91, 92] In this sense, "stress" as a response belongs to normal life. Only when triggered too often and at too high a degree do serious problems for well-being and health arise. The stress response has different phases, consisting of at least three different dimensions: psychologic, physiologic and behavioral responses. These different response dimensions sometimes vary together and sometimes do not, and have been shown to be triggered by physical and chemical agents, as well as by psychologic threats and demands.[76, 77] The common factor binding these diverse agents together has been shown to be aversion or threat, rather than the physical impact.[78] The fact that the demand has to be perceived in some way before triggering the stress response is important for measuring environmental factors and leaves room for individual differences in appraising a given situation.

Modern experimental stress research has shown that the character of acute physiologic reactions depends on the kind of environmental agent used. Difficult, but not impossible, tasks seem predominantly to trigger arousal from the sympathetic branch of the autonomic nervous system which affects cardiovascular regulation, fat metabolism, and blood clotting, either directly or via stimulation of the adrenal medulla to excrete adrenalin and noradrenalin. Impossible tasks with aversive consequences for failure, novelty, and a high degree of uncertainty, have been shown to affect the sympathetic nervous system and adrenal medulla and also to activate the pituitary-adrenal-cortical axis with excretion of corticosteroid hormones, which affects protein metabolism, cardiovascular mechanisms, and the immune system.[73, 78, 95, 96] Differences in the character of the psychologic reaction system in parallel with these endocrinologic differences have also been shown. Impossible or uncontrollable tasks, in some circumstances, have been shown to give rise to negative emotional arousal accompanied by feelings of helplessness and rather long-lasting intellectual impairment.[13, 73, 93] Heavy, but manageable demands, give rise to positive experiences of arousal.[73] Cognitive and behavioral aspects of acute stress have not been extensively studied. However, high, as well as low, stress levels have been associated with impaired cognitive and perceptual performance.[27, 82] The interplay between the different dimensions and phases in the stress response system, together with some modifying factors can be illustrated by the scheme in Figure 68–1.[56,69]

From this scheme it is clear that the effects can be measured at different phases and the environmental agents may be defined either in the actual objective environment or at the psychologic appraisal level. In much of the earlier stress research, the complex interrelations between the different response dimensions have been neglected. In some investigations, characteristics in the work environment, such as overload, role ambiguity, and role conflict, have been associated with emotional states such as anxiety and tension.[63,75] Others have related these factors to behavioral variables, such as smoking, alcohol consumption, absenteeism, and turnover, and still others to indices of somatic ill health, but the interplay between these different dimensions has seldom been studied. Overload, role ambiguity, or lack of control may, for example, initiate a sense of psychologic tenseness leading to lowered job satisfaction and/or increases in smoking and alcohol consumption, which, in combination with increased physiologic reactivity, would add to the "wear and tear" of the organism, over and above their effects on the psychologic functioning. The structural scheme also suggests a temporal character of the stress process, differentiating between acute reactions, intermediate responses, or states of adaption and the end state of exhaustion consisting of long-lasting pathologic changes. However, response characteristics in the later stages in this process are not fully known and relations between them are far from perfect, depending on specificities in the biologic program or differences in the psychologic coping processes. In some experimental animal studies, the acute stress responses have, however, been linked to pathologic changes in the heart muscle and blood vessels.[38, 44, 58, 67]

ACUTE PHYSIOLOGIC REACTIONS

The rationale behind investigations of acute effects is that these can be precursors of later ill health (see Fig 68–1). This

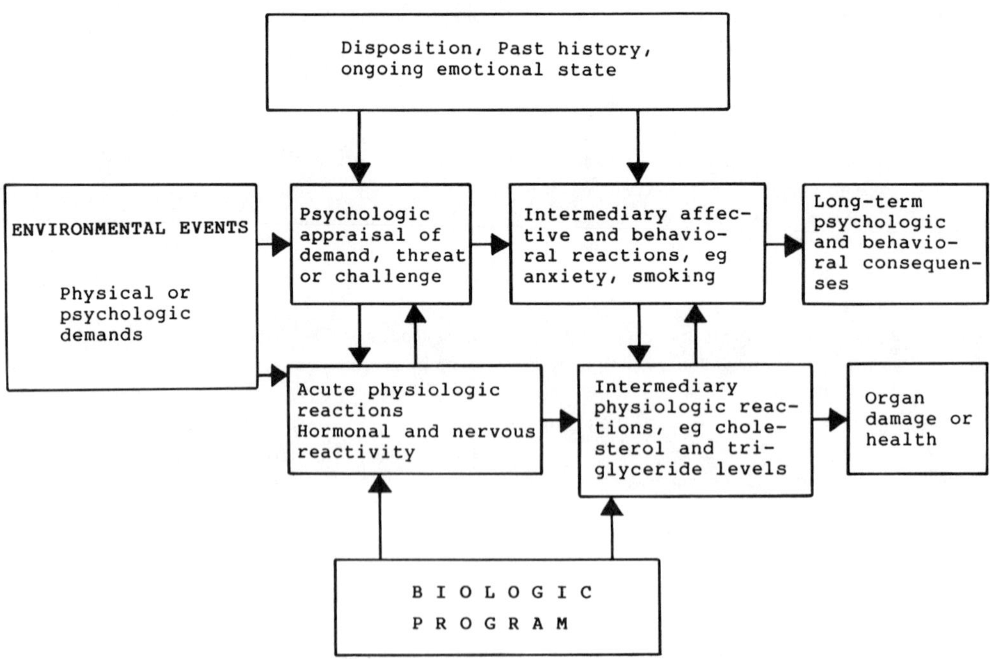

FIG 68–1.
Structural scheme of phases and dimensions in the stress response and some biologic and psychologic factors modifying the response.

hypothesis is supported by indirect evidence from animal studies and can also get support, although indirect, from research linking different diseases to demands in the work environment.[44, 58, 67]

Experimental Studies

The experimental research that seems most relevant for the occupational stress area is research using human subjects in situations varying in psychological rather than physical demands.

Underload–Overload.—In an experiment by Frankenheuser et al.,[31, 32] it was shown that a monotonous task requiring attention to infrequently occurring signals or a highly demanding task (color-conflict) gave rise to increased catecholamine excretion as compared to rest periods. Simulating an assembly line in the laboratory, Cox et al.[20] reported increased adrenalin excretion in two repetitive tasks as compared to a nonrepetitive task. One of the repetitive tasks consisted of inspections for faults and demanded similar attention strategies as that of the monotonous vigilance task used by Frankenheuser et al. The tasks used by both Frankenheuser and Cox are in some ways analogous to the tasks of a worker on the assembly line requiring unfailing attention while in a monotonous situation.[22, 23] A necessary condition for the observed increases in endocrine reactions in these tasks may be the conflict between attentional requirements and the lack of stimulus variation. Monotonous surroundings without attentional requirements may not provide such conflicting demands but would rather lead to a decreased physiologic arousal level and a sense of experienced boredom.[11, 21, 97]

Controllable vs. Uncontrollable Demands.—The different, acute physiologic effects of a self-paced task as compared to a forced reaction time task has been demonstrated by Lundberg and Frankenheuser.[73]

In the self-paced task, as compared to a resting state, elevations of catecholamine excretion were observed, while the forced task was accompanied by elevation of both catecholamines and corticosteroid hormones. The two tasks were further accompanied by differences in mood, the self-paced task with sensations of positive arousal, such as alertness, and vigor, and the forced task by negative stress sensations, such as tenseness and irritation. These differences in physical arousal and emotional quality could not be explained by differences in the physical activities required. Laboratory as well as field studies of controllability of aversive events have demonstrated acute as well as long-term emotional and intellectual impairments resulting from uncontrollable as compared to manageable demands.[13, 93, 105, 106]

Field Studies

The sensitivity of both the pituitary-adrenal-cortical reaction system and the sympathetic-adrenal-medullary reaction system to demanding situations or even the anticipation of various demands has been shown in several investigations (for reviews, see references 76 and 77). For example, increasing levels of both cortisol and catecholamine have been observed in students the day before a final exam and in army trainees and in aircraft personnel while being in, or preparing for, difficult operations.

Parachute Trainees: Threat and Uncertainty.—Following the training program of parachute trainees, Ursin, Baade et al.[99] showed how both the corticosteroids and the catecholamines react in different phases of a tower training program. The corticoid responses were more pronounced early in training, perhaps reflecting the greater uncertainty of possible danger, but adapted rather quickly as the training proceeded, while the catecholamine responses did not adapt as a function of training.

Bus Drivers: Time Pressure, Responsibility, and Attentional Demands.—Rissler and Aronsson[84] studied psychophysiologic and psychologic responses in a group of urban bus drivers. In comparison with other groups studied, e.g., office staff, saw mill workers, maintenance, and process minding personnel,[30] the bus driver group had catecholamine levels that were almost twice as high. The demands of urban bus driving consist of high time pressure, especially in heavy traffic hours, the responsibility of the passengers' welfare, and emotional demands relating to passenger complaints. A significant positive relation was found between experienced demands and reports of psychologic stress reactions. For the shift-work group, there was a significant positive relation between experienced demands, indices of psychologic stress, and levels of adrenalin, noradrenalin and serum triglyceride levels. Thus, the extra load of working during inconvenient hours strengthened the relation between experiences of external demands and physiologic reactivity.

Office Clerks: Extra Workload.—In a study of young women working as invoicing clerks in an insurance company, elevated levels of adrenalin and noradrenalin were found when working on piece-work as compared to a salaried schedule.[70] Simulating an assembly line in the laboratory, Cox et al. found similar differences between working under a flat payment rate compared to a bonus pay system.[20] Raised levels of cholesterol and blood clotting have been shown for U.S. tax accountants as workloads go up before the April 15 deadline approaches.

Rissler et al.[83] found elevated levels of adrenalin and noradrenalin in weeks with overtime as compared to a normal work period for a group of secretaries. They also observed a displacement of maximum levels in adrenalin excretion toward the end of the day and thus a slower decrease during the free hours in the evening. Experienced tension was positively associated to catecholamine levels.

Assembly-Line Work: Monotonous Working Conditions, Predetermined Work Pace.—Assembly line workers in a saw-mill had elevated catecholamine levels as compared to other workers with comparable physical conditions in the same plant.[53] The tasks of the assembly-line worker group required high and unfailing attention in connection with extremely short work-cycle periods (five to ten seconds), repetition of the same movements, and working at a high predetermined speed. Increases in catecholamine excretion was associated with shorter work-cycle periods and increased repetitiveness of the work. A displacement in maximum levels of catecholamine excretion to the late part of the working day was shown for the assembly-line group. Positive relations between subjective reports of tenseness and a measure of general well-being and catecholamine excretion were also reported.[53] However, in a recent field experiment, Salvendi and Knight[90] could not detect any differences in blood pressure and heart rate between a machine-paced and a self-paced group of industrial operators. The machine-paced group had shorter cycle times (56–145 seconds as compared to 8–23 minutes for the self-paced task) and fewer tasks to be done in each cycle period. The lack of differences between the groups could be explained by the short time period studied (two weeks) and the novelty of the less structured self-paced task. In a study of workers in a highly automated process industry, a relation between time urgency and levels of adrenalin, heart rate, and blood pressure was found. Experience of monotony was accompanied by lower levels of adrenalin and tendencies to a relative increase of levels of cortisol.[54] The environmental variables studied have been rather complex, containing elements of time pressure, responsibility, in some instances, threats, and, for some of the groups, lack of personal control, monotony, and shift work. The extra burden of shift work seems to strengthen the link between experienced demands and physiologic reactivity. In studies where different physiologic reaction systems have been compared, there is a tendency supporting Lundberg and Frankenheuser's[73] experimental results of different physiologic reactivity for time pressure and rush as compared to repetitious work with low opportunities for personal control over the work situation.[54]

LONG-TERM SOMATIC EFFECTS

Differences Between Occupations

Long-term somatic effects have been associated with different occupations. It is often a matter of interpretation to pinpoint the factors that are critical for observed differences in health in these types of studies, although the effects of some confounders are controlled in the investigations to be discussed.

Bus Drivers: Time Pressure, Responsibility, and Attentional Demands.—In a classical cross-sectional study of bus-drivers in London, it was shown that the drivers had a higher risk for cardiovascular mortality than the conductors. This difference would not be related to differences in physical demands.[79] In a five-year follow-up study of bus drivers in Copenhagen, it was found that the drivers had a significantly higher mortality due to ischemic heart disease and an earlier incidence of first clinical episode of myocardial infarction as compared to Copenhagen men.[80] In a cross-sectional analysis, it was found that the prevalence of self-reported positive angina pectoris was twice as high for bus drivers as compared to locomotive drivers.[80] Although no explicit measures of job stressors were used in the study, indirect information can be obtained from a similar study of bus drivers.[42] In this study, it was shown that the bus and truck drivers had higher blood pressure and higher levels of serum cholesterol and serum triglyceride in comparison with a control group matched for age, dietary habits, socioeconomic status, smoking habits, and alcohol consumption. On an index of tempo-time-limit/urgency in the work, the driver groups scored significantly higher than the controls.

Air-Traffic Controllers: Time Pressure, Responsibility, and Attention Demands.—In a cross-section study,[12] it was shown that air-traffic controllers had about four times as high a prevalence of diagnosed hypertension and a greater annual incidence of hypertension as compared to a group of second-class airmen. Self-selection, differences in other confounding life-style variables, and differences in licensing standards between the groups could explain some of the differences. The most obvious of these confounding factors, different licensing practices, probably cannot explain the whole difference between the groups, since it was found that controllers working in towers with higher traffic loads had a significantly increased incidence of hypertension compared to controllers in towers with relatively less traffic density. Rose[86] found higher plasma cortisol levels in a group of air-traffic controllers as compared to values reported in the literature. This relatively higher cortisol level may, according to stress theory, be a precursor to the high prevalence of hypertension previously found in air-traffic controllers (see above). However, a three-day cortisol average was not significantly related to other biologic and psychologic risk factors. In a study by Caplan et al.,[7] the prevalence of hypertension for air-traffic controllers was not higher than for other occupational groups, e.g., machine-paced assemblers, supervisors, technicians, and controllers at large airports did not have higher blood pressure than controllers at small airports. Workload variables in the compared groups are not explicitly defined, which makes it difficult to draw any firm conclusions about relations between specific workload variables and long-term blood pressure measures from these studies.

Bank Clerks: Various Organizational and Work Demand Factors.—In a ten-year prospective study of two cohorts of middle-aged bank clerks,[65] it was shown that clerks working in semipublic savings banks had a significantly smaller incidence and lower mortality in cardiovascular diseases as compared to the clerks working in private banks. These differences could not be explained by differences in age, smoking habits, or cholesterol levels at the start of the follow-up period. The clerks in the private banks, in contrast to the clerks in the semipublic savings banks, had been exposed to large changes in management policy that among other things, encouraged competition. In a retrospective questionnaire study after the final follow-up, significant differences in self-reported job demands were found between the two cohorts.[65] However, the index of work demands on which the groups were compared was complex, including, among other things, physical work conditions, workload, responsibility, tension at work, salary, promotion, drug use, and physical exercise. From published data, it is not possible to see how these factors taken separately differ between the groups. The differences between the private as compared to semipublic savings banks are probably very complex, with differences in workload, time urgency, possibilities for personal control and responsibility, as well as differences in physical activities required and differences in recruitment policies. From studies of different occupational groups, it is evident that factors in the work content and work organization are associated with increased risk for ischemic heart disease. Since these factors are not defined in detail and are possibly confounded by different physical requirements and life-style factors, it is difficult to draw any firm conclusions as to the exact nature of the observed associations. Indirect evidence from the bus driver studies indicate that workload factors contribute to the differences in cardiovascular disease for that group. This conclusion is also supported by acute reactions reported by Rissler and Aronsson.[84]

Self-Reported Work Demands

A more direct way to relate environmental demands to health outcomes is to use self-reporting data as the independent variable. This is also more compatible with modern conceptions of stress in which the appraisal of the environment is decisive for triggering the stress reaction system. Theorell and Floderus-Myrhed,[98] in a prospective study of middle-aged building construction workers, found that an index of self-reported workload was significantly related to nonfatal myocardial infarction.

Responsibility, Role Conflict, and Work Load.—House et al.,[47] using self-reporting data on job demands and work content in a rubber manufacturing plant, found significant positive relations between high responsibility and self-reported symptoms of angina pectoris. Role conflict and work load was positively related to blood pressure as measured in a medical examination on a sample of the studied group, though not related to self-reported angina symptoms. Quality concern and responsibility pressure as defined in the study can be seen as primarily qualitative work demands, while the work load variable mirrors the quantitative demands. Positive relations with self-reported work demands and symptoms of dermatologic irritations and cough and phlegm were also reported. This effect was strengthened when high levels of self-reported exposure to gas and dust were added, indicating a synergism between job demands and the effects of physical and chemical agents. However, these relations could not be confirmed when data from the medical examination were used. This negative finding could either be caused by insensitive methods used in the medical examination or to response biases. However, the synergistic association between work demands and exposure to gas and dust could not be demonstrated for symptoms other than respiratory tract problems, thus speaking against the latter explanation.

Multivariate Combinations of Job Characteristics.—Karasek et al.[61] in a prospective study of a random sample of the male Swedish working force, used two variables, job demands and job content, to predict cardiovascular-cerebrovascular mortality and self-reported cardiovascular symptoms. In a cross-sectional prevalence analysis of reported cardiovascular symptoms, both workload and work content were related to symptoms. The workload variable consisted of both a time limit aspect ("Is your job hectic?") and a psychologic demand aspect ("Is your job psychologically demanding?"). The job content variable consisted of both an aspect of variation and utilization of skills and possibilities for personal control. The former aspect was called "intellectual discretion," and the latter, "low personal schedule of freedom." The combination of low intellectual discretion and high job demands had the highest relation to reported symptoms. Old age, heavy job demands, and low intellectual discretion were significant predictors in the six-year follow-up incidence of cardiovascular symptoms. In a case control analysis, significant increased risk of cardiovascular-cerebrovascular death was found in groups with either high demands or low intellectual discretion and in a group with low intellectual discretion and low personal schedule of freedom. The variable of low personal schedule of freedom was related to a higher rate of cardiovascular-cerebrovascular death in the subgroup with low education. The self-reported measures of job characteristics were, in general, in accordance with expert ratings of the same jobs. In addition, self-reported job characteristics were related to objective mortality data. Several indicators of the psychosocial environment, job demand, and job content were used, and tendencies for synergistic effects between job demands and aspects of job content were demonstrated. The combined effects were most pronounced for psychologic and sociologic health indices.[59, 60] Recent studies defining job demands and content in ways similar to the Karasek et al. studies[1, 2] have classified occupational groups according to earlier self-reports on work conditions, making it possible, independently of subjectively derived opinions, to investigate health risks for combinations of various aspects of work demands and content. Occupations classified (by means of earlier self-reports) as hectic and with low personal schedules of freedom and occupations classified as hectic and with low intellectual discretion were both found to have a significantly increased risk for nonfatal as well as fatal myocardial infarctions. These relations could not be explained by confounding by other risk factors, such as smoking, age, physical requirements at work, and education. The work demand and content variables taken separately were not significantly related to myocardial infarction incidence. Furthermore, psychologic work demands in combination with physical workload variables (heavy lifting) yielded increased risks for ischemic heart disease as compared to the variables taken separately.

In concluding this review of studies using objective signs of decreased somatic well-being, it can be stated that the recent and reasonably well-designed studies support earlier concepts of causal links between various occupational demands and decreased somatic well-being. However, it is difficult from most of these studies to disentangle exactly which components in the tctality of work demands have been decisive for the effects. Often, occupational groups with a similar demand structure but differing in intensity are compared. Comparisons between groups of very dissimilar occupational status may be even more complex and difficult. For example, Rose and Marmot,[85] in a large prospective investigation of British civil servants, found that the 7½-year coronary mortality was 3.6 times higher in the lowest than in the top grade. The differences could partly be explained by known risk factors, but most of the differences between the groups could not be explained. Since no detailed information about job demands or job content in the various groups were gathered, it is not possible to know exactly which job characteristics may have been decisive for the differences. But it is, for example, unlikely that qualitative demands decrease as one climbs the occupational ladder. However, the character of work demands and combinations between demands and organizational factors, as for example, possibilities for personal control, can be the decisive difference between the occupational grades studied.[61]

Personal control is a complex variable, ranging from the

power to determine when to take a break[61] to the power to participate in organizational decisions. Possibilities for control at the organizational decision level may have its effects primarily on job satisfaction, while direct personal control over factors of relevance for the actual task, such as the power to decide how the job should be done, when to take a break, or the power to adapt the pace of work to actual conditions in combination with work demands, probably have acute as well as long-lasting effects on physiologic and psychologic reactions. Siegrist et al.[94] demonstrated in a retrospective case control study that myocardial infarction patients had a higher workload level than the healthy controls. However, the nature of the workload was different for blue collar as compared to white collar patients. Inconsistent demands and high responsibility were more frequent in the white collar group, while a combination of physical environmental factors and time pressure, interruptions, and qualitative underload was more common in the blue collar group. The difference between myocardial infarction groups and the healthy control group was strengthened when a variable of previous job insecurity was added. The latter result shows the importance not only of considering current occupational stressors, but, since cardiovascular diseases probably develop over a long time, also the previous occupational history. In none of the studies cited has it been possible to study the physiologic mechanisms underlying the observed differences in health. Some suggestions regarding this issue come from the studies of acute physiologic effects reviewed above, showing increased sympaticus mediated endocrine activity to increasing demands. Of special interest are the studies in which sympaticus-mediated endocrine activity has been dissociated from pituitary-adrenal-cortical reactivity. From this research, it could be hypothesized that the observed simultaneous activity of both systems in demanding but aversive situations, without possibilities for personal control, is a mechanism underlying the increased health risks observed in occupations characterized by heavy demands and low schedules of freedom, or with little possibilities for development and variation.[62] An interesting suggestion for future research comes from the House et al. study,[47] in which tendencies were shown that psychologic workload variables may modify the effects of physical agents in the environment. This suggestion is strengthened by results from a study by Alfredsson and Theorell,[2] showing that aspects of workload and work content potentiate the effects of physical requirements on cardiovascular health.

Psychologic Reactions

Heavy quantitative demands may give rise to increased levels of tension. This has been shown for different occupational groups and different characteristics of the environmental demands.[3, 21, 52, 53, 54, 55] Repetitive, monotonous working conditions seem to strengthen the relation between work demands and experienced tension and contribute to negative emotional aspects of high arousal, e.g., distress.[39, 53, 73]

Overload-Underload: Job Satisfaction, Alienation, and Boredom.—Job satisfaction, occupational self-esteem, alienation, or boredom have often been used as signs of the intermediate or long-term psychologic effects of heavy environmental demands.[39, 63, 66] Job satisfaction may, however, not always be an effect of environmental demands taxing the capacities of the individual, but rather of other aspects of job content relevant to the fulfillment of needs and aspirations. This hypothesis may explain the sometimes conflicting results in the area. For example, Margolis et al.,[75] in a sample of different occupational groups, found no relation between a measure of workload and job satisfaction. In a recent cross-sectional study of the Finnish work force, only a slight positive association was found between workload and job dissatisfaction.[64] However, other investigations have shown a negative association between high demands and job satisfaction.[35, 59, 60]

Overload: General Affective Symptoms.—Heavy demands, as perceived by the worker, have, in many different investigations, been associated with nervous symptoms, anxiety, and depression.[35, 39, 47, 59, 75] In the study by House et al.,[47] nervous symptoms were positively associated with self-reported responsibility, pressure, role conflict, workload, and quality concern. In a study of Swedish bus drivers, Aronsson and Barklöf[3] found positive associations between experienced workload and mild nervous symptoms. French et al.[35] reported positive associations between self-reported workload and anxiety reactions. Numerous investigations of the specific workload characteristics in different occupations have associated workload factors to psychologic stress reactions.[17–19, 55, 108, 109]

Multivariate Combinations of Work Demands and Organizatoral Factors.—Aronsson and Barlköf[3] found that lack of support from fellow workers and supervisors strengthened the association between work demand factors and negative psychologic effects. In the Finnish study cited above,[64] it was found that the combined effects of high time-pressure and low levels of self-determination at work explained more of the variance in work-related exhaustion than the variables analyzed separately. Karasek[60] showed that lack of possibilities for control modified the association between workload factors and symptoms of depression and insomnia. In the French et al. study,[35] the effects of workload on affective variables were modified by the fit between preferred and experienced complexity of the work. For groups experiencing a misfit in either direction on work complexity, increasing workload was associated with nervous symptoms, when the fit between preferred and perceived work complexity was good, the relation between workload and symptoms was less clear. As was the case for the association between work demands and cardiovascular diseases, the association between work demands and nervous symptoms seems to be conditioned by aspects of job content and possibilities for control. High quantitative demands in combination with low qualitative demands and limited possibilities for control seems to be an especially disadvantageous combination for psychologic as well as somatic well-being.

FACTORS MODIFYING THE STRESS REACTIONS

In the review of the associations between various work demands and acute as well as long-term stress-related effects, the necessity of considering the combined effects of the level and characteristics of work demands, as well as factors of job content and work organization, was pointed out. Variation in the job, utilization of skills, and possibilities for participation and control are aspects of the work environment that modify the effects of heavy demands on stress-related illness.

Social Support

Social support is an aspect of the work environment that has been shown to mediate the effects of work demands on health. Epidemiologic research has repeatedly found that social support attenuates the risk for physical and mental ill health.[4, 6, 11, 46] French et al.,[35] in a cross-sectional study of men from 23 different occupations, found a significant negative association between amount of social support from co-workers and symptoms of irritation and depression. The effects of social support were independent of workload levels. La Rocco et al.,[68] in a study of men working in a rubber manufacturing plant, found selective evidence for beneficial main effects of social support on health and perceived occupational stress. The effects were dependent on the source of the social support. The main effects were only significant for supervisor support, while the buffering effects of support on health were shown especially when it came from their supervisor or wife. In a reanalysis of data from the Caplan et al. study[7] of men from 23 occupational groups, La Rocco et al.[68] showed that, while social support did not buffer effects on job dissatisfaction, it had strong effects on such general affective variables as depression and irritation and also had an effect on the amount of somatic complaints. In this study, the most effective source of social support came from co-workers, as compared to supervisors or the workers' families. Some conflicting evidence exists regarding the exact mechanisms of social support, whether it has main or predominantly buffering effects or whether it influences the individual's perception of the environment or has effects on later psychologic and physiologic coping mechanisms; in general, however, there is agreement about its beneficial health effects. Social support can have both an instrumental aspect, e.g., getting help for solving problems, and an emotional aspect. It is not fully understood which one of these is most important; it might depend on the situation. However, many studies demonstrate the importance of the emotional aspect.[6, 46]

Psychologic Coping Processes.—Differences between individuals in appraising a given situation, in preferences for different workload levels, and in coping strategies will also modify the effects of objective work demands on health. One suspicion sometimes heard is that the relation between self-reported environmental characteristics and psychologic or somatic symptoms or indices of health are artefactual, merely mirroring idiosyncratic response biases. A recent prospective study by Cherry[8] supports such a suspicion in showing that the association between job-related psychologic strain and a variety of somatic symptoms could be explained by indicators of anxiety rather than by job-related factors. However, the factors in the work environment studied consisted of different occupational groups, supervision, and shift work. The possibilities of characterizing the different aspects of the work environment that have been shown to be important for psychologic and physiologic well-being were thus severely limited. Individual factors may influence the way a given environment is appraised and valued, but many investigations have shown a good agreement between independently defined environmental factors and the perceptions of these by groups of workers.[39, 54, 61]

Person-Environment Fit.—A model considering individual differences in preferences for levels of environmental demands and complexity has been developed by French et al.[34] According to the model, the decisive factor for work stress and work satisfaction is the fit between experienced and preferred levels of characteristics in the work environment. In a cross-sectional study of a sample of 23 occupations, French et al.[35] demonstrated that the fit between perceived and preferred levels of various environmental variables was a better predictor of job satisfaction and general effective symptoms than perceived environmental characteristics alone.

Personality Differences in Coping with Stress and Vulnerability for Stress-Related Disease.—The stress scheme presented in Figure 68–1 presents an outline of different aspects of the stress response system both for the psychologic and physiologic dimensions. Psychologic coping processes are thought to mediate environmental demands to psychologic as well as somatic long-term effects. The type A behavior style is the most studied of these coping behaviors. The type A person is characterized by impatience, aggressive competition, and a hard driving nature.[9, 41]

In experimental studies, individuals characterized as high in type A behavior have been shown to react with increased cardiovascular responses to demanding situations, such as situations invoking social competition or varying in difficulty and/or controllability, and during forced periods of inactivity.[5, 14, 15, 72, 81, 100–103] In several prospective as well as retrospective studies, the type A behavior pattern has been shown to be an independent predictor of cardiovascular disease.[26, 36, 43, 50, 51, 87, 88] The psychologic mechanisms mediating this increased reactivity seem to be a continuous struggle to gain control.[41] Certain environmental conditions probably interact with the type A behavior style, thereby modifying the acute reactions and probably the long-term cardiovascular health risks. In a study by Chesney et al.,[10] type A persons who described their work as encouraging autonomy had lower blood pressure than those who did not. The reverse was found for type Bs. Ivancevich and Matteson[49] proposes an interactional model of fit between environmental demands and type A/B behavior style. It is hypothesized that an environment that is controllable, encourages autonomy, and is moderately challenging, is congruent with the type A behavior style, thus attenuating the association between the type A behavior and cardiovascular disease. That sort of situation will be incongruent for the type B behavior style, thereby elevating the health risks for type Bs.

Conclusions

In conclusion, it has been shown that environmental, social, and personality factors can modify stress responses and health risks. Though models considering the interplay between individual and environmental factors are better predictors of stress effects than environmental or personality factors alone, the problems accounted for are different. In studies showing that objective environmental or perceived environmental factors can contribute to various signs of decreased well-being, the problem is to remove or change the critical environmental factors for groups of workers regardless of the variance within the group. Most work in preventive occupational medicine is of this character.

Many recent investigations of occupational stress have shown, first, that environmental demands in certain circumstances can be detrimental for groups of workers exposed and, second, that combinations of environmental factors modify this relation. Future research in the area thus has to take the interplay between various environmental factors into account, e.g., the character and level of work demands, job complexity, possibilities for control and participation, and the social support provided at work. Results from research using interactive models, such as the person-environment fit model, and research on the effects of individual characteristics on perception of aspects in the work environment and reactions at work can guide the design of individual programs to relieve stress in a particular work environment.

A MODEL ON OCCUPATIONAL STRESS

It has been shown that various demands as they are perceived by the individual lead to psychologic and physiologic reactions, with possible deleterious effects on general health. These reactions can be modified by various coping strategies by the individual, by organizational variables in the work environment, and by aspects of job content. The type A behavior pattern does strengthen the reactions, while social support, possibilities for control, variation and utilization of skills, and possibilities for development in the job attenuates the relations. It seems as if various demands on the individual at work give rise to acute psychologic and physiologic stress reactions, while aspects of job content and organizational variables of importance for satisfying needs and aspirations give the emotional quality to this response, facilitating or obstructing successful coping behavior.

The model in Figure 68–2 pictures the individual at work influenced by different forces. Various demands and factors in the environment that can be used to control or clarify these demands contain both a threat and a promise. On the one side, the individual is under the threat of failure to meet these demands. The enormity of this threat depends both on the fit between the demands and the abilities of the individual and of the consequences for failure. On the other hand, successful fulfillment of the tasks give, according to organizational and job content factors, possibilities for satisfying needs of variation, development, autonomy and pride, variables that are seen as preconditions for a high motivation to work.[71] The balance between the negative value of failure in combination with the probability for failure on the one side and the positive value of success combined with the probability for success on the other, will, according to the model, be decisive for the emotional quality of the stress reaction. If, for example, the demands lay very near the maximum ability of the individual, he will fail meeting them if he cannot control or redistribute the environmental demands in accordance with fluctuations in his ability. This, then, is assumed to cause a continuous threat. The consequences of the threat will be modified by opportunities for social contact and the social climate at work. The variables are also influenced by the organizational structure. The emotional quality of the acute stress reactions, according to studies reviewed, will probably have different long-term outcomes. Tasks that demand working at high speed and with expenditure of great effort without at the same time fulfilling needs for variation, autonomy, or pride, may have deleterious effects on cardiovascular and mental health. On the other hand, demands at the same level accompanied by possibilities for fulfillment of these needs and aspirations probably have more benign effects on somatic and especially on psychologic well-being.

In the model, the case of not being able to cope with the demands is also outlined. The inability to cope probably gives rise to feelings of resignation and helplessness, with, according to some experimental and field studies from other areas, serious consequences for intellectual and emotional functioning.[13, 93] The demands must be of a certain magnitude to challenge the ability of the individual for the above described reactions to take place. The motivation for fulfilling the tasks must be reasonably high, either stemming from an interest in solving the tasks themselves or forced by the aversiveness of failure. The model presents a set of identifiable variables in the environment which are perceived by the individual and related to the different symptoms and outcomes in an interactive rather than additive way. For example, the effects of high demands are attenuated by possibilities for control, role clarity, resources for fulfillment of needs and aspirations and the social climate, but aggravated by the lack of these factors. This, then, represents an extension of the Karasek[60] approach in studying occupational stress and represents in greater detail the possible causative environmental factors. A program for measuring the critical factors in the work environment according to the model has been started at the Clinic of Occupational Medicine at Örebro in Sweden. Questionnaires for measuring the relevant aspects of the environment as well as psychologic and psychosomatic symptoms have been developed, and a large-scale program of validation of these methods has been started. Many local occupational health care organizations have been stimulated to use the same methods in their health control programs and work environment surveys. The data are then stored at the "data bank," to provide opportunities for developing reference data for a wide range of occupational groups and work conditions. The questionnaires have been translated into different languages and will also be used in other countries. The aim of this enterprise is, apart from developing compatible systems of measurement, to be able to predict the risk of various aspects of decreased health if the given conditions remain unaltered. The detailed information of aspects in the environment can be translated to local circumstances and thus be of help in designing necessary interventions. The model represents a program for developing a strategy for prevention in the psychosocial area similar to those developed for physical and chemical hazards. The model also contains a program for future research in considering the joint and interactive effects of many hitherto undifferentiated aspects of the psychosocial work environment. The psychologic effects of different characteristics of the work environment and their relation to mental health as well as to productivity, turnover, and absenteeism ought to be studied in more detail in the future. Furthermore, the suggestions from House et al.[47] and Alfredsson et al.[1] of the possible modifying effects of psychosocial stressors on the effects of physical and chemical hazards should be followed up.

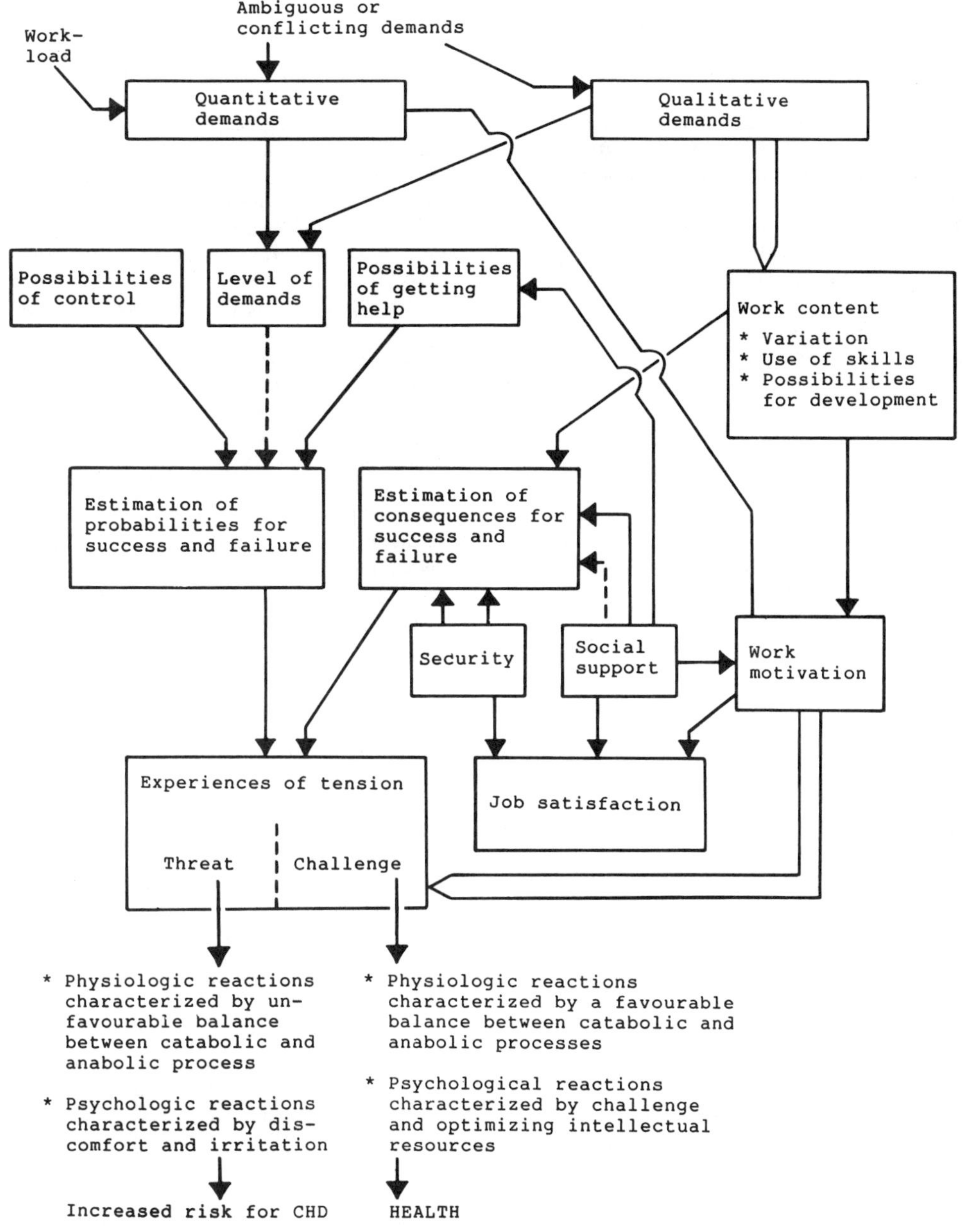

FIG 68–2.
Model picturing the interactions between factors in the work organization and work content with consequences for psychologic and physiologic functioning. (*Solid arrows* = positive associations; *dotted arrows* = negative associations; *double arrows* = conceptual relations.)

REFERENCES

1. Alfredsson L, Karasek R, Theorell T: Myocardial infarction risk and psychological work environment: An analysis of the male Swedish working force. *Soc Sci Med* 1982; 16:463–467.
2. Alfredsson L, Theorell T: Job characteristics of occupations and myocardial infarction risk effects of possible confounding factors. *Soc Sci Med* 1983; 17:1497–1503.
3. Aronsson G. Barlöf K: Att arbeta inom lokaltrafiken. Arbetsförhållanden-hälsa-fritid (The working environment for local transit personnel. Workload-health-leisure). *Rep Dept Psychol Univ Stockholm* 1980; No 26.
4. Billings AG, Moos RH: Work stress and the stress-buffering roles of work and family resources. *J Occup Behav* 1982; 3:215–232.
5. Blumenthal JA, Lane JD, Williams RB, et al: Effects of task incentive on cardiovascular response in type A and type B individuals. *Psychophysiology* 1983; 20:63–70.
6. Broadhead EW, Kaplan BH, James SA, et al: The epidemiologic

evidence for a relationship between social support and health. *Am J Epidemiol* 1983; 117:521–537.

7. Caplan RD, Cobb S, French JRP, et al: *Job Demands and Worker Health*, HEW (NIOSH) Publ 75-160. Washington DC, National Institute for Occupational Safety and Health, 1975.
8. Cherry N: Nervous strain, anxiety and symptoms amongst 32-year-old men at work in Britain. *J Occup Psychol* 1984; 57:95–105.
9. Chesney MA, Rosenman RH: The type A behaviour in the work setting, in Cooper CL, Payne R, (eds): *Current Concerns in Occupational Stress*. New York, John Wiley & Sons, 1980.
10. Chesney MA, Sevelies G, Black GW, et al: Work environment, type A behaviour and coronary heart disease risk factors. *J Occup Med* 1981; 23:551–55.
11. Cobb S: Social support as a moderation of life stress. *Psychosom Med* 1976; 38:300–314.
12. Cobb S, Rose RM: Hypertension, peptic ulcer and diabetes in air traffic controllers. *JAMA* 1973; 224:489–492.
13. Cohen S: After effects of stress on human performance and social behavior: A review of research and theory. *Psych Bull* 1980; 88:82–108.
14. Contrada JR, Glass DL, Karkoff LR, et al: Effects of control over aversive stimulation and type A behavior on cardiovascular and plasma catecholamine responses. *Psychophysiology* 1982; 19:408–419.
15. Contrada RJ, Wright RA, Glass DC: Task difficulty, type A behavior pattern, and cardiovascular response. *Psychophysiology* 1984; 21:638–646.
16. Cooper CL, Marshall J: Occupational sources of stress: A review of the literature relating to coronary heart disease and mental ill health. *J Occup Psychol* 1976; 49:11–28.
17. Cooper CL, Cooper RD: Occupational stress among international interpreters. *J Occup Med* 1983; 25:889–895.
18. Cooper CL, Grimby PJ: Stress among police detectives. *J Occup Med* 1983; 25:534–540.
19. Cooper CL, Melhuish MB: Executive stress and health. Differences between men and women. *J Occup Med* 1984; 26:99–104.
20. Cox S, Cox T, Thirlaway M, et al: Effects of simulated repetitive work on urinary catecholamine excretion. *Ergonomics* 1982; 25:1129–1141.
21. Cox, T, MacKay C, Page H: Simulated repetitive work and self-reported mood. *J Occup Behav* 1982; 3:247–252.
22. Cox T, Thirlaway M, Cox S: Repetitive work, well-being and arousal, in Ursin H, Murison R (eds): *Biological and Psychological Basis of Psychosomatic Disease*. *Advances in the Biosciences*, vol 42. New York, Pergamon Press, 1982.
23. Cummings TG, Cooper CL: A cybernetic framework for studying occupational stress. *Hum Rel* 1979; 32:395–418.
24. Davidson MJ, Cooper CL: Type A coronary-prone behaviour in the work environment. *J Occup Med* 1980; 22:375–383.
25. Davidson MJ, Cooper CL: A model of occupational stress. *J Occup Med* 1981; 23:564–574.
26. Dorian B, Taylor CB: Stress factors in the development of coronary artery disease. *J Occup Med* 1984; 26:747–756.
27. Easterbrooke JA: The effect of emotion on cue utilisation and the organisation of behavior. *Psychol Rev* 1959; 66:183–201.
28. Frankenheuser M: Psychoneuroendocrine approaches to the study of emotions, in Howe HE, Dienstbier RA (eds): *Nebraska Symposium on Motivation, 1978*. Lincoln, Neb, University of Nebraska Press, 1979.
29. Frankenheuser M: Coping with job stress, in Gardell B, Johansson G (eds): *Working Life: A Social Science Contribution to Work Reform*. London, John Wiley & Sons, 1981, pp 213–233.
30. Frankenheuser M, Gardell B: Underload and overload in working life. Outline of a multidisciplinary approach. *J Hum Stress* 1976; 2:35–46.
31. Frankenheuser M, Johansson G: On the psycho-physiological consequences of understimulation and overstimulation. *Rep Psychol Lab Univ Stockholm* 1974; Suppl 25.
32. Frankenheuser M, Johansson G: Task demand as reflected in catecholamine excertion and heart rate. *J Hum Stress* 1976; 2:15–23.
33. Frankenheuser M, Johansson G: On the psychophysiological consequences of understimulation and overstimulation, in Levi L (ed): *Society, Stress and Disease*. New York, Toronto, Oxford University Press, 1981, pp 82–89.
34. French JRP, Rogers W, Cobb S: A model of person-environment fit, in Coelho GW, Hamburgh DA, Adams JE (eds): *Coping and Adaptation*. New York, Basic Books, 1974.
35. French JR, Caplan RD, Van Harrison R: *The Mechanisms of Job Stress and Strain*. Wiley series on studies in occupational stress. New York, John Wiley & Sons, 1982.
36. Rosenman RH, Straus R, et al: Coronary heart disease in the Western Collaborative Group Study. A follow-up experience of 4½ years. *J Chronic Dis* 1970; 23:173–190.
37. Friedman MD, Rosenman RD, Carroll V: Changes in serum cholesterol and blood clotting time in men subject to cyclic variation of occupational stress. *Circulation* 1958; 17:852–861.
38. Folkow B: Central neurohormonal mechanisms in spontaneously hypertensive rats compared with human essential hypertension. *Clin Sci Mol Med* 1975; 48:205–214.
39. Gardell B: Alienation and mental health in the modern industrial environment, in Levi L (ed): *Society, Stress and Disease*, vol 1. London. Oxford University Press, 1971.
40. Gardell B: Scandinavian research on stress in working life. *Int J Health Serv* 1982; 12:31–40.
41. Glass DC: Stress, behavior patterns and coronary disease. *Am Sci* 1977; 65:177–187.
42. Hartwig P, Midtun O: Coronary heart disease risk factors in bus and truck drivers. *Int Arch Occup Environ Health* 1983; 52:353–360.
43. Haynes SG, Feinleib M, Kamrel WB: The relationship of psychosocial factors to coronary heart disease in the Framingham study III. Eight-year incidence of coronary heart disease. *Am J Epidemiol* 1980; 3:37–58.
44. Henry JP, Stephens PM: Stress, health and social environment. A sociobiological approach to medicine. New York, Springer-Verlag New York, 1977.
45. House J: Occupational stress and coronary heart disease. A review and theoretical integration. *J Health Soc Behav* 1974; 15:12–27.
46. House JS: *Work Stress and Social Support*. Reading, Mass, Addison-Wesley Publishing Co, 1981.
47. House JS, Wells JA, Landerman LR, et al: Occupational stress and health among factory workers. *J Health Soc Behav* 1979; 20:139–160.
48. Hugdahl K: The three-systems model of fear and emotion. A critical examination. *Behav Res Ther* 1981; 19:75–85.
49. Ivancevich JM, Matteson MT: A type A-B person-work environment interaction model for examining occupational stress and consequences. *Hum Rel* 1984; 37:491–513.
50. Jenkins DC: Recent evidence supporting psychologic and social risk factors for coronary disease. *N Engl J Med* 1976; 294:1033–1038.
51. Jenkins DC: Psychosocial risk factors for coronary heart disease. *Acta Med Scand* (Suppl) 1982; 660:123–136.
52. Johansson G: Subjective well-being and temporal pattern of sympathic-adrenal medullary activity. *Biol Psychol* 1976; 4:157–172.
53. Johansson G, Aronsson G, Lindstrom BO: Social psychological and

neuroendocrine stress reactions in highly mechanized work. *Ergonomics* 1978; 21:583–599.

54. Johansson G, Sandén PO: Mental belastning och arbetstillfredsställelse i kontrollrumsarbete (Mental load and job satisfaction of control room operators). *Rep Dept Psychol Univ Stockholm* 1982; No 40.
55. Johansson G, Aronsson G: Stress reactions in computerized administrative work. *J Occup Behav* 1984; 5:159–181.
56. Kagan A, Levi L: Health and environment—Psychosocial stimuli. A review. *Soc Sci Med* 1974; 8:225–241.
57. Kahn RL: Conflict, ambiguity, and overload: Three elements in job stress. *Occup Ment Health* 1973; 3:2–9.
58. Kaplan JR, Manuck SB, Clarksson TB, et al: Social stress and atherosclerosis in normocholesterolemic monkeys. *Science* 1983; 220:733–735.
59. Karasek R: Job demands, job decision latitude, and mental strain: Implications for job redesign. *Admin Sci Qtrly* 1979; 24:285–307.
60. Karasek R: Job socialisation and job strain. The implications for two related psychosocial mechanisms for job design, in Gardell B, Johansson G (eds): *Working Life. A Social Science Contribution to Work Reform*. New York, John Wiley & Sons, 1981.
61. Karasek R, Baker D, Marxer F, et al: Job decision latitude, job demands and cardiovascular disease. A prospective study of Swedish men. *Am J Public Health* 1981; 71:694–705.
62. Karasek RA, Russel SR, Theorell T: Physiology of stress and regeneration in job related cardiovascular illness. *J Hum Stress* 1982; 8:29–42.
63. Kasl S: Epidemiological contributions to the study of work stress, in Cooper CL, Payne R (eds): *Stress at Work*. New York, John Wiley & Sons, 1978.
64. Kauppinen-Toropainen K, Kandolin J, Mutanen P: Job dissatisfaction and work-related exhaustion in male and female work. *J Occup Behav* 1983; 4:193–207.
65. Kittel F, Kornitzer M, Dramaix M: Coronary heart disease and job stress in two cohorts of bank clerks. *Psychother Psychosom* 1980; 34:110–123.
66. Kornhauser A: Mental health of the industrial worker. New York, John Wiley & Sons, 1965.
67. Kranz DS, Manuck SB: Acute psychophysiologic reactivity and risk of cardiovascular disease: A review and methodologic critique. *Psychol Bull* 1984; 96:435–464.
68. La Rocco JM, House JS, French JRP: Social support, occupational stress and health. *J Health Soc Behav* 1980; 21:202–218.
69. Lazarus RS: Psychological stress and the coping process. New York, McGraw-Hill Book Co, 1966.
70. Levi L: Stress and distress in response to psychosocial stimuli. *Acta Med Scand* 1972; 191 (Suppl 528).
71. Locke EA: The nature and causes of job satisfaction, in Dunnette MD (ed): *Handbook of Industrial and Organisational Psychology*. Chicago, Rand McNally. 1976.
72. Lundberg U: Type A behavior and psychophysiological arousal. *Scand J Psychol* 1982; 23(Suppl 1): 145–150.
73. Lundberg U, Frankenheuser M: Pituitary—adrenal and sympathetic—adrenal correlation of distress and effort. *J Psychosom Res* 1980; 24:125–130.
74. McCay C: The measurement of mood and psychophysiological activity using self report techniques, in Martin J, Venables PM (eds): *Techniques in Psychophysiology*. New York, John Wiley & Sons, 1980.
75. Margolis BL, Kroes WH, Quinn RP: Job stress. An unlisted occupational hazard. *J Occup Med* 1974; 16:659–661.
76. Mason JW: A review of psychoendocrine research on the pituitary—adrenal cortical system. *Psychosom Med* 1968; 30:576–597.
77. Mason JW: A review of psychoendocrine research on the sympathetic-adrenal medullary system. *Psychosom Med* 1968; 30:631–653.
78. Mason JW, Maher JT, Hartley LH, et al: Selectivity of corticosteroid and catecholamine reactions to various natural stimuli, in Serban G (ed): *Psychopathology of Human Adaption*. New York, Plenum Publishing Corp, 1976.
79. Morris JN, Crawford MD: Coronary heart disease and physical activity at work. *Br Med J* 1958; 2:1485–1492.
80. Netterstrom B, Laursen P: Incidence and prevalence of ischaemic heart disease among urban bus drivers in Copenhagen. *Scand J Soc Med* 1981; 9:75–79.
81. Newlin DB, Levenson RW: Cardiovascular responses of individuals with type A behavior pattern and parental coronary heart disease. *J Psychosom Res* 1982; 26:393–402.
82. Persson LO. Sjöberg L: The influence of emotions on information processing. *Univ Göteborg Psychol Rep* 1978; 8 (7).
83. Rissler A: Stress reactions at work and after work during a period of quantitative overload. *Ergonomics* 1977; 20:13–16.
84. Rissler A, Aronsson G: Stressors, psychophysiological reactions and health. Unpublished manuscript. Stockholm University, Dept of Psychology, 1984.
85. Rose G, Marmot MG: Social class and coronary heart disease. *Br Heart J* 1981; 45:13–19.
86. Rose RM: Predictors of hypertension in air traffic controllers. A prospective study. *Psychosom Med* 1978; 40:86.
87. Rosenman RH, Friedman M, Straus R, et al: A predictive study of coronary heart disease: The Western Collaborative Group Study. *JAMA* 1964; 189:15–26.
88. Rosenman RH, Brand RJ, Jenkins DC, et al: Coronary heart disease in the Western Collaborative Group Study. Final follow-up experience of 8½ years. *JAMA* 1975; 233:872–877.
89. Sales SM, House J: Job dissatisfaction as a possible riskfactor in coronary heart disease. *J Chron Dis* 1971; 23:861–873.
90. Salvendi G, Knight JL: Circulatory responses to machine-paced and self-paced work: An industrial study. *Ergonomics* 1983; 26:713–717.
91. Seleye H: *The Stress of Life*. New York, McGraw-Hill Book Co, 1956.
92. Seleye H: The stress concept today, in Kutash JL, Schlesinger LB, et al (eds): *Handbook of Stress and Anxiety*. New York, Jossey-Bass, 1980.
93. Seligman MEP: *Helplessness*. San Francisco, Freeman, 1975.
94. Siegrist J, Dittman K, Rittner K, et al: The social context of active distress in patients with early myocardial infarction. *Soc Sci Med* 1982; 16:443–453.
95. Steptoe A: Psychological factors in cardiovascular disease. New York, Academic Press, 1981.
96. Steptoe A: Stress, helplessness and control: The implications of laboratory studies. *J Psychosom Res* 1983; 27:361–367.
97. Thackray RJ: The stress of boredom and monotony: A consideration of the evidence. *Psychosom Med* 1981; 43:165–176.
98. Theorell T, Floderus-Myrhed B: 'Workload' and risk of myocardial infarction—A prospective psychosocial analysis. *Int J Epidemiol* 1977; 6:17–21.
99. Ursin H, Baade E, Levine S (eds): *Psychobiology of Stress. A Study of Coping Men*. New York, Academic Press, 1978.
100. van Doornen LJP: The coronary risk personality: Psychological and psychophysiological aspects. *Psychother Psychosom* 1980; 34:204–213.
101. van Doornen LJP, Orlebeke KF: Stress, personality and serum cholesterol level. *J Hum Stress* 1982; 24–29.

102. van Egeren LF, Abelson JL, Sniderman LD: Interpersonal and electrocardiographic responses of type A's and type B's on competitive socioeconomic games. *J Psychosom Res* 1983; 27:53–59.
103. van Egeren LF, Fabrega H, Thornton DW: Electrocardiographic effects of social stress on coronary prone (Type A) individuals. *Psychosom Med* 1983; 45:195–203.
104. van Harrison R: Person-environment fit and job stress, in Cooper CL, Payne R (eds): *Stress at Work*. Wiley series on occupational stress. New York, John Wiley & Sons, 1981.
105. Weiss J: Influence of psychological variables on stress-induced pathology, in *Physiology, Emotion & Psychosomatic Illness*. *Ciba Found Symp* 8, 1972.
106. Weiss JM, Glazer HJ, Pokorecky LA, et al: Effects of chronic exposure to stressors on avoidance escape behavior and on brain norepinephrine. *Psychosom Med* 1975; 37:522–554.
107. Wells JA: Objective job conditions, social support and perceived stress among blue collar workers. *J Occup Behav* 1982; 3:79.
108. Wilkes B, Stammerjohn L, Lalich N: Job demands and worker health in machine-paced poultry inspection. *Scand J Work Environ Health* 1981; 7(Suppl 4):12–19.
109. Vredenburgh DJ, Trinkaus RJ: An analysis of role stress among hospital nurses. *J Vocation Behav* 1983; 23:82–95.

69

Shift Work

Joseph Rutenfranz, M.D., Ph.D.

Prof. Dr. Peter Knauth

According to the 1977 Bureau of Labor Statistics, approximately 18% of the U.S. labor force had to work in shift systems,[35] i.e., at "unsocial" or "unphysiologic" working times. The main reasons for the introduction of shift work are:

1. Technologic reasons.—Some technologic processes, e.g., in steel and chemical industries, need more time than a normal day worker has to work or may even require continuous production.

2. Economic reasons.—High costs of capital equipment and high demands of the market tend to increase shift work.

3. Social reasons.—Medical health care workers, safety personnel (e.g., police, fire protection), suppliers of energy and water, those in the travel, communication, and information industries (e.g., telephone, TV, newspapers), as well as the purveyors of cultural events and entertainment maintain our "quality of life."

Although many shift workers have problems (as will be discussed later), some shift workers seem to have no essential problems caused by shift work. Only a few, around 10%, like shift work, 20%–30% do not like it, and the majority tolerates it.[31]

The fact that different shift workers vary widely in their tolerance of their unnatural way of life is taken into consideration in the model of stress and strain of shift workers. Colquhoun and Rutenfranz[19] describe this model as follows: The objective stress resulting from the disruption of physiologic rhythms by shift work, and from the slow rate of re-entrainment of these rhythms to the changed wake/sleep cycle, induces a state of subjective strain in the shift worker that can potentially affect his working efficiency, his physical and psychologic health and well-being, and his family and social life. The magnitude of the effects observed in any individual will be influenced by a number of "intervening variables" acting separately, or in combination. Important intervening variables are particular characteristics of the shift worker, such as his age, his personality, his rhythmic "type," his physiologic adaptability and social circumstances such as marital status, number and age of children, or domestic situation such as housing conditions.

STRESS OF SHIFT WORKERS

One kind of stress in connection with shift work—in particular, night work—results from the discrepancy between the time structure of behavior (work, sleep) and the daily variations of physiologic functions. Biologic rhythms with a periodicity of approximate 24 hours are called "circadian rhythms" (from the Latin "circa diem," i.e., "about a day"). For more than 100 human physiologic functions and organs the existence of a circadian rhythm has been shown.

According to Aschoff,[8] the circadian rhythm is based on an endogenous component, which can be detected if all "Zeitgebers" are excluded. Zeitgebers,[7] or synchronizers[29] are periodic factors in the environment which are able to synchronize endogenous rhythms. The period of the spontaneous rhythm which occurs under free-running conditions (without Zeitgeber) may deviate from 24 hours. Wever[97] has shown that the average period of rectal temperature of 147 subjects in free-running experiments was 25 ± 0.5 hours.

In human beings, the endogenous rhythms are synchronized to a period of 24 hours, in particular by cognitive and social Zeitgebers, i.e., the knowledge of the time of day as well as the daily experience that the family and the society has another rhythm of wakefulness and sleep than the shift worker. In contrast to transmeridian flights, these Zeitgebers are not phase shifted for normal shift workers. It cannot be expected that the circadian rhythms of a shift worker adapt completely to night work, when important synchronizers are conflicting. In laboratory and field studies with data covering the 24 hours, only a partial adjustment of the circadian rhythm of body, temperature to night work was found.[17, 38, 44, 71, 80, 91]

Although the partial adjustment to night work is more advanced in connection with more consecutive night shifts than in shorter periods of night shifts, the re-entrainment always remains incomplete. Furthermore, different physiologic functions adjust with different velocity to night work which causes a dissociation between these physiologic functions. This dissociation is smallest at the day of the first night shift. In summary, when only a few consecutive night shifts are worked (i.e., only one or two), less disturbance of circadian physiologic function is observed and fewer days of recovery are needed.

From studies concerning tolerance to shift work, Reinberg et al.[73, 74] conclude that the subject tolerant to shift work for many years is likely to have a large amplitude of the circadian rhythm and is likely to adjust slowly to the "new" schedule during the night shift. These studies of rotating shift-work systems suggest that features of the circadian rhythm of temperature associated with minimal re-entrainment are also linked to a greater tolerance of shift work.

In addition to the stress caused by the phase-shift of working and sleeping times, shift workers seem to suffer more often from unfavorable environmental conditions than day workers. However, our knowledge about the combined effects of shift work and unfavorable environmental conditions is rather poor.[37, 64, 67, 79, 96]

STRAIN OF SHIFT WORKERS

Since the circadian rhythms do not adjust completely to night work, effects on performance and on well-being have to be expected, e.g., fatigue, sleep difficulties, and disturbances of appetite.

Performance

The daily variations of performances, which have been known for a long time,[11, 50] are based on physiologic functions[34] as well as on psychic processes.[27, 33]

Some field studies have shown that performance was lowest during night time (midnight to 6 a.m.) and/or during the "post lunch dip," i.e., 1 p.m. to 3 p.m.[12, 32, 68] These performances were related to simple immediate processing tasks, e.g., vigilance tasks and sensorimotor tasks.

However, different types of memory processes may show different trends over the day.[23] The precise timing of the peak depends on the level of the memory load involved as Folkard et al.[24] have shown in laboratory experiments. In a field study, process controllers with a high short-term memory-loaded task performed better at night than at day.[58]

Fatigue and Sleep Loss

Sleep difficulties are a major problem for shift workers, in particular for shift workers who have to work in night shifts. Studies concerning sleep disturbances of day and shift workers were reviewed and classified according to the type of shift by Rutenfranz et al.[76] and Knauth[37] of 18,352 persons, 10%–40% with day work, 5%–30% with rotating morning and afternoon shifts, 10%–95% with rotating shift systems including night work, and 35%–55% with permanent night shift who complained about sleep disturbances. However, the two studies mentioned above differed considerably concerning the population (age, shift experience, marital status, age of children), workers' housing conditions, and the regularity of the shift system. Complaints about sleeping difficulties refer both to the duration of sleep and to the quality of sleep. To analyze the duration of sleep dependent on the type of shift, 1,230 workers were asked to fill out diaries during one week.[40] The mean duration of day sleep between two night shifts was about six hours, i.e., significantly shorter than the night sleep. However, it was not only the night shift that created problems of sleep duration. The shortest night sleep was found before morning shifts (about seven hours). This sleep is reduced particularly when the morning shift starts early and when the time needed to travel to work is long.

Comparisons of studies with contradictory results of permanent and rotating or slowly and quickly rotating shift systems do not allow the drawing of firm conclusions.[39, 56, 71, 80, 81, 85]

There are two reasons why the day sleep after night shifts is shortened. First, many shift workers complain that the day sleep is more disturbed by noise, in particular the noise of children and traffic noise, than the normal night sleep. Secondly, the night worker has to sleep during an unphysiologic time of day.

The day sleep is not only a phase-shifted night sleep, but it also has a different sleep structure. Most electroencephalographic studies comparing night and day sleep have shown a shorter REM-latency, and a shorter amount of REM and stage-2 sleep, as well as a different distribution of REM-periods over the sleep in day sleep.[15, 26, 54, 87, 90, 95]

If a shift worker has to work several night shifts in succession, an accumulation of sleep deficits may be expected. Kiesswetter et al.[36] studied police officers with a weekly rotating shift system. They compared the quality of night sleep with the quality of the first and last day sleep in the week with night shifts. Mean sleep duration was longest in the night, shorter after the first night shift, and shortest after the last night. REM-sleep percentages were reduced in the first and last day sleep of the night shift week. Only the slow-wave sleep percentages (not the absolute amount) increased from the night sleep up to the last day sleep. Regarding the subjective ratings of sleep quality, the restorative effect of sleep was rated lowest after the last day sleep. Neglecting the increase of slow-wave sleep percentages, all other findings supported the hypothesis that there is an accumulation of sleep deficits within a week of night shifts.

In two studies of shift workers who had changed from a slowly rotating to a rapidly rotating shift system with maximal two or three night shifts, the shift workers experienced reduced fatigue in the new system.[94, 99]

Disturbances of Appetite

Besides problems with sleep, some shift workers complain about disturbances of appetite. In particular, night shifts may cause a change of the sequence and frequency of meals. Reviewing studies[37, 76] which referred to altogether 11,258 persons, the following frequencies of complaints about disturbances of appetite were found: 5%–30% with day work, 5%–20% of persons with morning and afternoon shifts, 20%–75% of persons with rotating shift systems including night shifts, and 40% of persons with permanent night shift.

Vinit et al.,[92] Debry et al.,[21] and Reinberg et al.,[72] however, showed that the disturbances of appetite did not lead to a reduction of total caloric intake. The disturbances of appetite may be influenced by the dislike of having to eat at unusual times outside the preferred social environment and by the fact that during nighttime cold food is often consumed.

Gastrointestinal Complaints

Gastrointestinal complaints may be long-term effects of irregular food intake. However, the causes for this complex of symptoms are manifold. Therefore, it is not surprising that in a review of studies referring to 22,693 persons, the groups of day workers and shift workers with and without night work did not differ clearly with respect to the frequency of gastrointestinal complaints.[37, 76]

Comparing the illness reports of 12-hour shift workers and day workers, those shift workers who changed from shift work to day work had a higher incidence rate of gastrointestinal diseases than the other shift workers and the day workers.[6]

DANGER TO HEALTH

The studies cited above show that not all types of shift work are similarly problematic, but rather that mainly shift systems that include night work are a risk factor to health. If the unavoidable disturbance of biologic rhythms caused by night work is combined with very unfavorable personal or situational factors, it might be expected that in such cases the human organism may not be able to adapt and that an increased frequency of diseases or even an excessive mortality rate should show up.

Studies of Mortality

A careful epidemiologic mortality study of shift workers and day workers has been carried out by Taylor and Pocock.[83] They analyzed the 1,578 deaths occurring in a 13-year period in 8,603 male manual workers. The results did not show a significant overall excess mortality among shift workers. The standard mortality rate of ex-shift workers was 118.9, compared with 101.5 for current shift workers.

Hannunkari et al.[30] compared 4,347 engineers, i.e., drivers of locomotives and their assistants, with two reference groups of 1,575 trainmen and 1,224 railroad clerks in a retrospective follow-up survey on invalidity and mortality over 18 years. The observed number of deaths per person years was 5.3 in the groups of engineers, 4.6 in the group of railroad clerks, and 4.1 in the group of trainmen. In an additional questionnaire study, the locomotive engineers complained about irregular working hours (including night shift), noise, vibration, draft, and poor seats. However, there is no information about the working conditions and working hours of the two reference groups.

The combination of shift work and adverse environmental effects also seems to play a role in the study of Teiger,[84] who analysed data from a professional retirement fund of four occupational groups in daily newspaper companies: 972 rotary printers (permanent night workers), 248 plate makers (permanent evening workers), 1,481 compositors (afternoon and evening workers), and 208 correctors (afternoon and evening workers).

The working conditions of the first two groups are characterized by physical load, time pressure, noise, toxic exposure, and heat. Compositors and especially correctors have better environmental conditions. Analyzing the decrease in percent of living population between ages 55 and 70, Teiger found a significant difference at age 70 between the rotary printers (63.5% survivors) compared with the other groups combined (plate makers: 66.9%, compositors: 70.5%, and correctors: 74.3%). Furthermore, there was four times as much early retirement for rotary printers (43.0%) than for correctors (10.8%); the reason for most of the early retirements was medically attested working incapacity.

Gastrointestinal Diseases

Reviewing investigations of various authors concerning ulcer incidence in a total of 34,047 persons with day or shift work, we[76] found ulcers occurring in 0.3%–7% of persons with day work, 5% of persons with morning and afternoon shifts, 2.5–15% of persons with rotating shift systems including night work, and 10%–30% of persons who had given up shift work, probably for health reasons.

The incidences of ulcer in day and shift workers are overlapping. Shift work is only one of many potential factors which may contribute to ulcers. Wolf et al.[100] reported on 17 factors that increase the probability of duodenal ulcer. Careful epidemiologic studies by Aanonsen[1] and Angersbach et al.[6] showed a much higher incidence of ulcers in former shift workers compared with other shift workers and day workers.

In the retrospective cohort study of Angersbach et al.,[6] covering a study period of 11 years, the process of self-selection in the shift workers cohort seemed to be still incomplete, because the relative risk of suffering from a gastrointestinal disease for the first time was higher in the last years of the investigation.

Cardiovascular Diseases

Only a few careful epidemiologic studies have been carried out on the possible effects of shift work on cardiovascular diseases. Aanonsen[1] observed ten times more absence attributable to cardiovascular disease in day workers compared with shift workers. No significant difference between day workers and night workers concerning cardiovascular mortality was found by Taylor and Pocock.[83] In the study by Angersbach et al.,[6] those shift workers who had changed from shift work to day work (mostly because of medical reasons) had a higher incidence rate of cardiovascular diseases compared with other shift workers and day workers. Koller et al.[49] compared day workers and "drop-outs" from a shift worker cohort, the drop-outs having a significantly higher rate of cardiovascular complaints which had occurred during the time when they had worked on shift. A Swedish cohort study of 394 subjects, the risk ratio of cardiovascular diseases was shown to increase with the years exposed to shift work.[63] After 20 years, the risk ratio dropped, probably because of self-selection.

Summing up, there is not enough evidence to conclude that cardiovascular disease is more prevalent in shift workers. More long-term studies, in particular, investigating ex-shift workers, are needed.

Other Diseases

In a review of studies concerning neurotic reactions and psychosomatic disorders, Koller et al.[48] state, "no clear conclusions about different frequencies of psychiatric disorders in shift and day workers can be drawn."

EFFECTS ON SOCIAL LIFE

The working times and leisure times of shift workers are out of sync with the "normal" social environment. This discrepancy may create problems within the family and concerning other social activities.

It is difficult for the shift worker, when working in afternoon shifts, to keep contact with the children who go to school.[60] However, rapid rotation of shift systems enables the workers to have more contact with their children than slowly rotating shift systems.[35]

In regard to the organization of household work, greater problems may occur when the spouse of the shift worker is also working outside the home, when female shift workers have to take care of small children, and when two members of the family have different shift systems.[78]

It is difficult for a shift worker to have regular contact with day working friends or to participate in regular social activities and in continuing education courses, which are often fixed to evening hours and to the weekend. Therefore, permanent evening shifts and continuous shift systems are particularly unfavorable for social contacts.[9, 10, 60]

SPECIAL HEALTH MEASURES FOR NIGHT WORKERS

Based on the recommendations by Rutenfranz,[75] special health provisions for night workers should include:

1. Pre-employment selection of workers
2. Regular health checks
3. Preventive health care
4. Additional free days
5. Provision of proper meals at night
6. Sleeping allowances during night shifts
7. Construction of shift schedules based on objective physiologic, psychologic, and social criteria
8. Reduction of unnecessary night work

Although all shift workers working in the same shift system at the same working place are exposed to the same stress, the individuals react in very different ways to shift work.

Selection of Workers

It would be desirable to have positive selection criteria at hand allowing one to predict which persons will have fewer health problems when working in particular shift systems. However, our actual knowledge only allows us to make a listing of negative criteria for the selection of night workers. According to Collier[16] and Rutenfranz,[75] the following persons should be excluded from shift work if possible:

1. People with a history of digestive tract disorders. Shift work produces special psychophysiologic problems and also involves unusual meal times, both of which may affect gastric functions.[2, 16, 22, 57, 86]

2. Diabetics and those with thyrotoxicosis. Regular food intake and correct therapeutic timing can be difficult to maintain under shift work conditions.[20, 52]

3. Epileptics. Reduction of sleep increases the incidence of fits.[20, 52]

4. People with severe mental derangements involving the whole personality. Depression is particularly important here, because this disease often starts with sleep disturbances, which indicate disruption of the sleep-wakefulness cycle and other circadian rhythms.[88]

5. All persons suffering from chronic sleep disturbances (allegedly caused by e.g., traffic noise).[52]

6. Patients with heart diseases who exhibit a significant reduction of physical performance capacity.

7. Active and extensive tuberculosis patients.

8. Alcoholics and other drug addicts.

9. Persons with marked hemeralopia, or visual impairment that is too severe for effective compensation to be possible. Illumination of many parts of factories is normally reduced at night; therefore these persons may have a particularly high risk of accidents.

Concerning positive criteria for the selection of night workers, it is not yet possible to put forward recommendations. However, there are many factors which have already been taken into consideration or which should be studied in more detail:

1. Rigidity[25, 101]
2. Extraversion/introversion[13]
3. Neuroticism[18]
4. Circadian phase position, morningness/eveningness[14, 59, 62, 65]
5. Amplitude of circadian rhythms[3, 4, 73, 74]
6. Sleep cycle properties
7. Liability to internal desynchronization[70]

Furthermore, situational factors seem to be of importance for the adaptability to shift work. In studies of chemical workers, train drivers, and air traffic controllers, 55%–80% complained about their sleep being disturbed by noise on the day after the night shift.[42, 61, 77] Shift workers reported that traffic noise and noise of children disturbed their day sleep most frequently. These kinds of noise may deteriorate the quality of sleep, as has been shown by Knauth and Rutenfranz,[41] Williams,[98] and Griefahn et al.[28] Shift workers whose day sleep was often or always disturbed by noise complained more frequently about neurovegetative and gastrointestinal symptoms than shift workers with undisturbed or rarely disturbed day sleep.[37, 51]

Another situational factor, which has not yet been studied in detail, is the attitude of the family of the shift worker toward shift work in general or toward particular negative aspects of a shift system. If, for example, the night work of a shift worker is not accepted by his or her spouse, it may be expected that this shift worker will have more problems coping with night work than a colleague who is supported by a more positive attitude from his or her spouse.

Regular Health Checks

The standard medical examinations before starting work have only limited predictive value for sickness-absence.[82] Therefore, it has been proposed that a second health examination be carried out not later than one year after starting shift work.[53] Between the two examinations the shift worker has found out what his or her most important problems concerning shift work are, and how shift work affects the worker's sleep, family, and social life.

A committee of German occupational health practitioners and scientific experts has proposed the following procedure:[75]

1. All persons working at least six hours on a regular shift system or at least five hours on an irregular shift system during the hours from 10 p.m. to 6 a.m. should have regular health checks.

2. The preplacement medical examination should exclude all persons from night work who meet the above-mentioned negative health criteria.

3. There should be a second health check 12 months, at the latest, after starting night work, and regular health checks, depending on the age of the worker, at the following intervals: aged under 25 years, 24 months; 25–50 years, 60 months; 50–60 years, 24–36 months; and over 60, 12–24 months.

Preventive Health Care

Since most problems of the shift worker are caused by the discrepancy or mismatch between the time structure of the social sphere and the work sphere, it seems to be desirable, occasionally, to give the shift workers the chance to live under normal conditions with respect to circadian rhythms. Some large German plants and communities have therefore begun to offer regular treatment for shift workers older than 50 years old in specialized hospitals for two to three weeks at two- or three-year intervals. By following a regular sleep-wake routine with proper mealtimes, these workers may normalize their circadian rhythms. Furthermore, a general health check and physiotherapeutic measures are offered. However, there are no long-term experiences with such treatments. Another way of reducing the problems of shift workers is realized by a French plant with a special organization of working time: three weeks of shift work are followed by four weeks of non-shift work, i.e., normal day work or a continuing education or holidays.

Additional Free Days

The medical reason for recommending additional free days for those who work in continuous shift systems is the same as mentioned before, namely, to give the shift workers the chance to have more "normal" days to allow the circadian system to renew. However, since there are up to now no epidemiologic longitudinal studies, nothing is known about the efficiency of these extra rest days for health.

Providing Proper Meals at Night

Complaints about disturbances of appetite are relatively frequent, particularly in connection with night work. Therefore, in France, a law obliges the industry to provide the night workers with facilities to warm up meals during nighttime. Reinberg et al.,[72] who studied the eating habits of shift workers of an oil refinery in 1974, observed five years later that the consumption of carbohydrates was reduced.[69] This change may be caused by the introduction of a cafeteria which offered warm, light meals, whereas in 1974 much bread had been consumed during night shifts. The meals should not be eaten too late in the night shift (e.g., not later than 1 a.m.). Beverages that contain caffeine should be drunk only many hours before bedtime.

Sleeping Allowances During Night Shifts

Since sleep is a major concern of night workers, any measure that will improve their sleep is important. Occupational health practitioners and scientists who have studied the problems of nightworkers know that in some work places illegal naps are taken during nighttime. Kogi[6, 47] reports that 43% of day-night (two-shift) workers and nearly half of regular (three-team or four-team) three-shift workers took naps in the form of short anchor-sleep-like sleep during midnight or early-morning hours. Many plants in Japan seem to have such more or less legalized sleeping allowances during night work and many of the nappers even had the chance to use a bed in the factory.

The main reasons for naps are prevention of fatigue and improvement of efficiency and safety.[5, 47] Problems may arise if the night worker has difficulties in falling asleep or if he has to react correctly immediately after being woken up, e.g., by an alarm bell. The nighttime nap seems to influence the following daytime sleep. Torsvall et al.[89] found that nappers had a shorter main sleep compared with non-nappers. Matsumoto et al.[55] observed that the stage-4 sleep in the subsequent day-sleep was decreased in proportion to how late the preceding nap was taken.

Constructing Shift Schedules Based on Objective Criteria

Based on the criteria concerning physiologic adjustment, performance and accidents, well-being, health, and personal and social problems, Knauth and Rutenfranz[43] have put forward nine recommendations for the construction of shift systems:

1. A shift system should have few night shifts in succession.

2. The morning shift should not begin too early.

3. The shift change times should allow individuals some flexibility.

4. The length of the shift should depend on the physical and mental load of the task, and the night shift should be shorter than the morning and afternoon shifts.

5. Short intervals of time between two shifts should be avoided.

6. Continuous shift systems should include some free weekends, with at least two successive full days off.

7. In continuous shift systems, a forward rotation should be preferred.

8. The duration of the shift cycle should not be too long.

9. Shift rotas should be regular.

In summary, the reasons for the first and most important recommendation are that re-entrainment of physiologic functions to night work seems to remain incomplete even after many night shifts in succession, and least disturbance of circadian physiologic functions is observed in connection with few consecutive night shifts.[37]

An accumulation of sleep deficits and fatigue has been observed in the course of longer periods of consecutive night shifts. Furthermore there are hints in the literature that the probability of accidents may increase after the second night shift.

In studies of groups which had changed from slowly to rapidly rotating shift systems, the majority of shift workers reported an overall preference for the new shift system[45, 66, 93] or had a higher level of job satisfaction.[99]

Reduction of Unnecessary Night Work

Since night work may be regarded as a risk factor for health and often results in negative effects on the well-being and social contacts of shift workers, ideally, the best measure would be to eliminate night work in general. However, this is an unrealistic approach. Therefore, the second-best measure would be to reduce unnecessary night work. When asking the management of a plant if some activities could be removed from the night shift and placed in morning or afternoon shifts, in general the first answer will be "that is not possible." However, if the activities are studied in more detail, in some cases it will be possible to reduce the amount of work done during the nighttime.

As an example, we gradually reduced (in cooperation with the management and the occupational health practitioner) the number of persons needed during nighttime (2–6 a.m.) for loading and unloading aircrafts from 104 to 66 in a first step, and in a second step to 38 persons.[39]

To sum up, occupational health measures for night workers and shift workers are necessary to prevent lowering of well-being and occurrence of job-related diseases. These measures should also include activities of the occupational health practitioner outside the workplace, such as advising workers on coping strategies, e.g., for organizing the social life, for sleeping and eating behavior, or supporting the amelioration of housing conditions.

REFERENCES

1. Aanonsen A: *Shift Work and Health*. Oslo, Universitetsforlaget, 1964.
2. Andersen EJ: The main results of the Danish medico-psycho-social investigation of shiftworkers, in *Proceedings of the 12th International Congress on Occupational Health, Helsinki, 1.–6.7.1957*. Helsinki, 1958, vol. 3, pp 135–136.
3. Andlauer P: Différentes modalités du travail en équipes alternantes. *Arch Mal Prof* 1971; 32:393–395.
4. Andlauer P, Reinberg A: Amplitude of the oral temperature circadian rhythm and the tolerance to shift work. *Chronobiologia* 1979; 6(Suppl 1):67–73.
5. Andlauer P, Rutenfranz J, Kogi K, et al: Organization of night shifts in industries where public safety is at stake. *Int Arch Occup Environ Health* 1982; 49:353–355.
6. Angersbach D, Knauth P, Loskant H, et al: A retrospective cohort study comparing complaints and diseases in day and shift workers. *Int Arch Occup Environ Health* 1980; 45:127–140.
7. Aschoff J: Zeitgeber der tierischen Tagesperiodik. *Die Naturwissenschaften* 1954; 41:49–56.
8. Aschoff J: Exogene und endogene Komponente der 24-Stunden-Periodik bei Tier und Mensch. *Die Naturwissenschaften* 1955; 42:569–575.
9. Baer K, Ernst G, Nachreiner F, et al: Psychologische Ansätze zur Analyse verschiedener Arbeitszeitsysteme. *Z Arbeitswiss* 1981; 35(7 NF):136–141.
10. Banks O: Continuous shift work: The attitudes of wives. *Occup Psychol* 1956; 30:69–84.
11. Bechterew W v: Über die Geschwindigkeitsveränderungen der psychischen Processe zu verschiedenen Tageszeiten. *Neurol Zbl* 1893; 12:290–292.
12. Bjerner B, Holm A, Swensson Å: Diurnal variation in mental performance. A study of three-shift workers. *Br J Ind Med* 1955; 12:103–110.
13. Blake MJF: Temperament and time of day, in Colquhoun WP (ed): *Biological Rhythms and Human Performance*. London, Academic Press, 1971, pp 109–148.
14. Breithaupt H, Hildebrandt G, Döhre D, et al: Tolerance to shift of sleep, as related to the individual's circadian phase position. *Ergonomics* 1978; 21:767–774.
15. Bryden G, Holdstock TL: Effects of night duty on sleep patterns of nurses. *Psychophysiology* 1973; 10:36–42.
16. Collier HE: *Outlines of Industrial Medical Practice*. London, Arnold, 1941; reprinted (with corrections) 1943.
17. Colquhoun WP, Edwards RS: Circadian rhythms of body temperature in shift-workers at a coalface. *Br J Ind Med* 1970; 27:266–272.
18. Colquhoun WP, Folkard S: Personality differences in body-temperature rhythm, and their relation to its adjustment to night work. *Ergonomics* 1978; 21:811–817.

19. Colquhoun WP, Rutenfranz J (eds): *Studies of Shiftwork*. London, Taylor & Francis, 1980.
20. Cook FP: *Shift Work*. London, Institute of Personnel Management, 1954.
21. Debry G, Girault P, Lefort J, et al: Enquête sur les habitudes alimentaires des travailleurs "à feux continus". *Bull Inst Natl Santé Recherche Médicale (Paris)* 1967; 22:1169–1202.
22. Dervillée P, Lazarini H-J: A propos du travail en équipe avec changement d'horaires. Incidences familiales et répercussion possible sur la santé des travailleurs. *Arch Mal Prof* 1959; 20:306–309.
23. Folkard S: Diurnal variation, in Hockey R (ed): *Stress and Fatigue in Human Performance*. Chichester, UK, Wiley, 1983, pp 245–272.
24. Folkard S, Knauth P, Monk TH, et al: The effect of memory load on the circadian variation in performance efficiency under a rapidly rotating shift system. *Ergonomics* 1976; 19:479–488.
25. Folkard S, Monk TH, Lobban MC: Towards a predictive test of adjustment to shift work. *Ergonomics* 1979; 22:79–91.
26. Foret J, Benoit O: Structure du sommeil chez des travailleurs à horaires alternants. *Electroencephalogr Clin Neurophysiol* 1974; 37:337–344.
27. Graf O: *Begriff der Leistungsbereitschaft*. *Z Arbeitswiss* 1954; 8:141–144.
28. Griefahn B, Jansen G, Klosterkötter W: *Zur Problematik lärmbedingter Schlafstörungen—eine Auswertung von Schlaf-Literatur*. Berlin, Umweltbundesamt (Hrsg), 1976. (Berichte des Umweltbundesamtes, 4/76)
29. Halberg F, Visscher MB: Some physiologic effects of lighting, in *Proceedings of the 1st International Photobiology Congress (4th International Light Congress)* Amsterdam, 1954, pp 396–398.
30. Hannunkari I, Järvinen E, Partanen T: Work conditions and health of locomotive engineers. II. Questionnaire study, mortality and disability. *Scand J Work Environ Health* 1978; 4 (Suppl 3):15–28.
31. Harrington JM: *Shift Work and Health. A Critical Review of the Literature*. London, Her Majesty's Stationery Office, 1978.
32. Hildebrandt G, Rohmert W, Rutenfranz J: 12 & 24 h rhythms in error frequency of locomotive drivers and the influence of tiredness. *Int J Chronobiol* 1974; 2:175–180.
33. Hockey GRJ, Colquhoun WP: Diurnal variation in human performance: a review, in Colquhoun WP (ed): *Aspects of Human Efficiency. Diurnal Rhythm and Loss of Sleep*. London, The English Universities Press, 1972, pp 1–23.
34. Ilmarinen J, Ilmarinen R, Korhonen O, et al: Circadian variation of physiological functions related to physical work capacity. *Scand J Work Environ Health* 1980; 6:112–122.
35. Johnson LC, Colquhoun WP, Tepas DI, et al: *Biological Rhythms, Sleep and Shift Work*. New York, Spectrum Publications, 1981, preface.
36. Kiesswetter E, Knauth P, Schwarzenau P, et al: Daytime sleep adjustment of shiftworkers, in Koella WP, Rüther E, Schulz H (eds): *Sleep '84*. New York, Stuttgart, G Fisher, 1985, pp 273–275.
37. Knauth P: *Ergonomische Beiträge zu Sicherheitsaspekten der Arbeitszeitorganisation*. Düsseldorf, VDI-Verlag, 1983. (Fortschr.-Ber. VDI-Z., Reihe 17, Nr. 18)
38. Knauth P, Emde E, Rutenfranz J, et al: Re-entrainment of body temperature in field studies of shiftwork. *Int Arch Occup Environ Health* 1981; 49:137–149.
39. Knauth P, Kiesswetter E, Ottmann W, et al: Time-budget studies of policemen in weekly or swiftly rotating shift systems. *Appl Ergonom* 1983; 14:247–252.
40. Knauth P, Landau K, Dröge C, et al: Duration of sleep depending on the type of shift work. *Int Arch Occup Environ Health* 1980; 46:167–177.
41. Knauth P, Rutenfranz J: Untersuchungen zum Problem des Schlafverhaltens bei experimenteller Schichtarbeit. *Int Arch Arbeitsmed* 1972a; 30:1–22.
42. Knauth P, Rutenfranz J: Untersuchungen über die Beziehungen zwischen Schichtform und Tagesaufteilung. *Int Arch Arbeitsmed* 1972b; 30:173–191.
43. Knauth P, Rutenfranz J: Development of criteria for the design of shiftwork systems. *J Hum Ergol* 1982; 11 (Suppl):337–367.
44. Knauth P, Rutenfranz J, Herrmann G, et al: Re-entrainment of body temperature in experimental shift-work studies. *Ergonomics* 1978; 21:775–783.
45. Knauth P, Schmidt K-H: Beschleunigung der Schichtrotation und Ausweitung der regulären Betriebszeit auf das Wochenende. *Z Arbeitowiss* 1985; 39(MNF):226–230.
46. Kogi K: Comparison of resting conditions between various shift rotation systems for industrial workers, in Reinberg A, Vieux N, Andlauer P, (eds): *Night and Shift Work. Biological and Social Aspects*. Oxford, Pergamon Press, 1981, Advances in the Biosciences, vol 30, pp 417–424.
47. Kogi K: Sleep problems in night and shift work. *J Hum Ergol* 1982; 11(suppl):217–231.
48. Koller M, Haider M, Kundi M, et al: Possible relations of irregular working hours to psychiatric psychosomatic disorders, in Reinberg A, Vieux N, Andlauer P (eds): *Night and Shift Work. Biological and Social Aspects*. Oxford, Pergamon Press, 1981, *Advances in the Biosciences*, vol 30, pp 465–472.
49. Koller M, Kundi M, Cervinka R: Field studies of shift work at an Austrian oil refinery. I: Health and psychosocial wellbeing of workers who drop out of shiftwork. *Ergonomics* 1978; 21:835–847.
50. Kraepelin E: Über psychische Disposition. *Arch Psychiatr Nervenkr* 1893; 25:466–467.
51. Küpper R, Rutenfranz J, Knauth P, et al: Wechselwirkungen zwischen lärmbedingten Störungen des Tagschlafs und der Häufigkeit verschiedener Beschwerden bei Schichtarbeitern, in Brenner W, Rutenfranz J, Baumgartner E, et al (eds): *Arbeitsbedingte Gesundheitsschäden—Fiktion oder Wirklichkeit*. Bericht über die 20. Jahrestagung der Deutschen Gesellschaft für Arbeitsmedizin e.V, Innsbruck, 27.–30.4.1980, pp 165–170. Stuttgart, Gentner, 1980.
52. LaDou J: Health effects of shift work, *West J Med* 1982; 137:525–530.
53. Loskant H, Knauth P: Kriterien zur Gestaltung der Schichtarbeit, in Brenner W, Rohmert W, Rutenfranz J (eds): *Ergonomische Aspekte der Arbeitsmedizin*. Bericht über die 15. Jahrestagung der Deutschen Gesellschaft für Arbeitsmedizin e.V., München, 24.–26.4.1975, pp 231–240. Stuttgart, Gentner, 1976.
54. Matsumoto K: Sleep patterns in hospital nurses due to shift work: An EEG study. *Waking and Sleeping* 1978; 2:169–173.
55. Matsumoto K, Matsui T, Kawamori M, et al: Effects of nighttime naps on sleep patterns of shiftworkers. *J Hum Ergol* 1982; 11 (Suppl):279–289.
56. Melton CE, Smith RC, McKenzie JM, et al: *Stress in air traffic controllers: Comparison of two air route traffic control centers on different shift rotation patterns*, Final report, FAA-AM-75-7. Washington, DC, US Dept of Transportation, Federal Aviation Administration, 1975.
57. Menzel W: *Menschliche Tag-Nacht-Rhythmik und Schichtarbeit*. Basel, Schwabe, 1962.
58. Monk TH, Embrey DE: A field study of circadian rhythms in actual and interpolated task performance, in Reinberg A, Vieux N, Andlauer P (eds): *Night and Shift Work. Biological and Social Aspects*. Oxford, Pergamon Press, 1981, *Advances in the Biosciences*, vol 30, pp 473–480.
59. Moog R, Hildebrandt G: Morning-evening-types and tolerance to shift work. *J Interdiscipl Cycle Res* 1985; 16:147–148.

60. Mott PE, Mann FC, McLoughlin O, et al: *Shift work. The Social, Psychological and Physical Consequences*. Ann Arbor, The University of Michigan Press, 1965.
61. Nachreiner F, Frielingsdorf R, Romahn R, et al: *Schichtarbeit bei kontinuierlicher Produktion*. Wilhelmshaven, Wirtschaftsverlag Nordwest, 1975 (Bundesanstalt für Arbeitsschutz und Unfallforschung, Dortmund, Forschungsbericht Nr. 141).
62. Östberg O: Circadian rhythms of food intake and oral temperature in 'morning' and 'evening' groups of individuals. *Ergonomics* 1973; 16:203–209.
63. Orth-Gomer K, Knutsson A, Jonsson B, et al: Direct and indirect evidence of ischemic heart disease in shift workers, in Bertazzi PA (ed): *4th International Symposium Epidemiology in Occupational Health, Como, Italy, 10.–12.9.1985*. Como, Italy, Ricerca scientifica ed educazione permanente, Suppl 45, 1985, p 43.
64. Ottmann W, Plett R, Knauth P, et al: Combined effects of experimental shiftwork and heat stress on cognitive performance tasks, in Haider M, Koller M, Cervinka R (eds): *Night and Shiftwork*. Frankfurt/Main, Lang, 1986, pp 361–368.
65. Pátkai P: Interindividual differences in diurnal variations in alertness, performance, and adrenaline excretion. *Acta Physiol Scand* 1971; 81:35–46.
66. Pocock SJ, Sergean R, Taylor PJ: Absence of continuous three-shift workers. A comparison of traditional and rapidly rotating systems. *Occup Psychol* 1972; 46:7–13.
67. Pokorski J, Oginski A, Knauth P: Work physiological field studies concerning effects of combined stress in morning, afternoon and nightshifts, in Haider M, Koller M, Cervinka R (eds): *Night and Shiftwork*. Frankfurt/Main, Lang, 1986, pp 369–376.
68. Prokop O, Prokop L: Ermüdung und Einschlafen am Steuer. *Dt Z Gerichtl Med* 1955; 44:343–355.
69. Quéinnec Y, Teiger C, de Terssac G: *Repères pour Négocier le Travail Posté*. Toulouse, Service des Publications UTM, 1985 (Travaux de l'Université de Toulouse-Le Mirail, Serie B, Tome 2).
70. Reinberg A, Andlauer P, De Prins J, et al: Desynchronization of the oral temperature circadian rhythm and intolerance to shift work. *Nature* 1984; 308:272–274.
71. Reinberg A, Chaumont A-J, Laporte A: Circadian temporal structure of 20 shift workers (8-hour shift—weekly rotation): An autometric field study, in Colquhoun P, Folkard S, Knauth P, et al: *Experimental Studies of Shiftwork*. Opladen, Westdeutscher Verlag, 1975, pp 142–165 (Forschungsberichte des Landes Nordrhein-Westfalen, Nr 2513).
72. Reinberg A, Migraine C, Apfelbaum M. et al: Circadian and ultradian rhythms in the feeding behaviour and nutrient intakes of oil refinery operators with shift-work every 3–4 days. *Diabete & Metabolisme (Paris)* 1979c; 5:33–41.
73. Reinberg A, Vieux N, Andlauer P, et al: Oral temperature, circadian rhythm amplitude, aging and tolerance to shift-work (study 3). *Chronobiologia* 1979a; 6 (Suppl 1):77–85.
74. Reinberg A, Vieux N, Ghata J, et al: Consideration of the circadian amplitude in relation to the ability to phase shift circadian rhythms of shift workers. *Chronobiologia* 1979b; 6 (Suppl 1):57–63.
75. Rutenfranz J: Occupational health measures for night- and shift-workers. *J Hum Ergol* 1982; 11 (Suppl):67–86.
76. Rutenfranz J, Knauth P, Angersbach D: Arbeitsmedizinische Feststellungen zu Befindlichkeitsstörungen und Erkrankungen bei Schichtarbeit. *Arbeitsmed Sozialmed Präventivmed* 1980a; 15:32–40.
77. Rutenfranz J, Knauth P, Hildebrandt G, et al: Nacht- und Schichtarbeit von Triebfahrzeugführern. 1. Mitt: Untersuchungen über die tägliche Arbeitszeit und die übrige Tagesaufteilung. *Int Arch Arbeitsmed* 1974; 32:243–259.
78. Rutenfranz J, Knauth P, Küpper R, et al: Pilot project on the physiological and psychological consequences of shiftwork in some branches of the services sector, in *Effects of Shiftwork on Health, Social Life and Family Life of the Workers*. Dublin, European Foundation for the Improvement of Living and Working Conditions, 1980b.
79. Rutenfranz J, Neidhart B, Ottmann W, et al: Circadian rhythms of physiological functions during experimental shift work with additional heat stress, in Haider M, Koller M, Cervinka R (eds): *Night and Shiftwork*. Frankfurt/Main, Lang, 1986, pp 347–359.
80. Smith P: A study of weekly and rapidly rotating shiftworkers. *Int Arch Occup Environ Health* 1979; 43:211–220.
81. Tasto DL, Colligan MJ, Skjei EW, et al: *Health Consequences of Shift Work*, DHEW (NIOSH) Publ 78–154. Cincinnati, Oh, US Dept of Health, Education, and Welfare, 1978.
82. Taylor PJ: Personal factors associated with sickness absence. A study of 194 men with contrasting sickness absence experience in a refinery population. *Br J Ind Med* 1968; 25:106–118.
83. Taylor PJ, Pocock SJ: Mortality of shift and day workers 1956–68. *Br J Ind Med* 1972; 29:201–207.
84. Teiger C: Overmortality among permanent nightworkers: Some questions about "adaptation," in Wedderburn A, Smith P (eds): *Psychological Approaches to Night and Shift Work*. International research papers, seminar paper. Edinburgh, Scotland, Heriot-Watt University, 1984, pp 15.1–15.34
85. Tepas DI, Walsh JK, Moss PD, et al: Polysomnographic correlates of shift worker performance in the laboratory, in Reinberg A, Vieux N, Andlauer P (eds): *Night and Shift Work. Biological and Social Aspects*. Oxford, Pergamon Press, 1981, Advances in the Biosciences, vol 30, pp 179–186.
86. Thiis-Evensen E: Shift work and health. *Ind Med Surg* 1958; 27:493–497.
87. Tilley AJ, Wilkinson RT, Drud M: Night and day shifts compared in terms of the quality and quantity of sleep recorded in the home and performance measured at work: A pilot study, in Reinberg A, Vieux N, Andlauer P (eds): *Night and Shift Work. Biological and Social Aspects*, Oxford, Pergamon Press, 1981, Advances in the Biosciences, vol 30, pp 187–196.
88. Tölle R: Sleep deprivation and sleep treatment, in van Praag HM (ed): *Handbook of Biological Psychiatry, Part VI*. New York, Dekker, 1981, pp 473–496.
89. Torsvall L, Åkerstedt T, Gillander K, et al: 24^h recordings of sleep/wakefulness in shift work, in Haider M, Koller M, Cervinka R (eds): *Night and Shiftwork*. Frankfurt/Main, Lang, 1986, pp 37–41.
90. Torsvall L, Åkerstedt T, Gillberg M: Age, sleep and irregular workhours. A field study with electroencephalographic recordings, catecholamine excretion and self-ratings. *Scand J Work Environ Health* 1981; 7:196–203.
91. van Loon JH: Diurnal body temperature curves in shift workers. *Ergonomics* 1963; 6:267–273.
92. Vinit F, Ract G, Audollent MC, et al: Enquete sur les travailleurs postes de l'industrie des textiles artificiels. *Bull Inst Natl Hyg (Paris)* 1962; 17:31–62.
93. Walker J: Shift changes and hours of work. *Occup Psychol* 1961; 35:1–9.
94. Walker J: Frequent alternation of shifts on continuous work. *Occup Psychol* 1966; 40:215–225.
95. Walsh JK, Tepas DI, Moss PD: The EEG sleep of night and rotating shift workers, in Johnson LC, Tepas DI, Colquhoun WP, et al (eds): *Biological Rhythms, Sleep and Shiftwork*. New York, Spectrum Publications, 1981, pp 371–381.
96. Werner E, Borchardt N, Frielingsdorf R, et al: *Schichtarbeit als Langzeiteinfluβ auf betriebliche, private und soziale Bezüge*.

Opladen, Westdeutscher Verlag, 1980 (Forschungsbericht des Landes Nordrhein-Westfalen, Nr 2974).

97. Wever RA: *The Circadian System of Man. Results of Experiments under Temporal Isolation*. New York, Springer-Verlag, 1979.
98. Williams HL: Effects of noise on sleep: A review, in Ward WD (ed): *Proceedings of the International Congress on Noise as a Public Health Problem, Dubrovnik, Yugoslavia, 13.–18.5.1973*, Washington DC, US Environmental Protection Agency, 1973, pp 501–511.
99. Williamson AM, Sanderson JW: Changing the speed of shift rotation: A field study. *Ergonomics* 1986; 29:1085–1096.
100. Wolf S, Almy TP, Bachrach WH, et al: The role of stress in peptic ulcer disease. *J Hum Stress* 1979; 5 (No 2):27–37.
101. Wynne RF, Ryan GM, Cullen JH: Adjustment to shiftwork and its prediction: Results from a longitudinal study, in Haider M, Koller M, Cervinka R (eds): *Night and Shiftwork*. Frankfurt/Main, Lang, 1986, pp 101–108.

70

Diagnosis of Absenteeism

Johann T. Mets, M.D.

> "Every industrial society generates—and must then settle—a conflict between its functions of production and of the protection of the producer, between the needs of the economy and the biological and psychological requirements of the workers and between the demands of industrial growth and the quality of individual and social life."
>
> J. Carpentier and P. Camazian
> in *Night Work*. (Geneva, International Labor Organization, 1977.)

Employees are expected to come to work when scheduled to do so, but it is generally accepted that, at times, there may be valid reasons for workers not to attend.

Absence from work, or absenteeism (without any pejorative connotation of the suffix *ism*), is defined as nonattendance when expected to work, for any reason at all, medical or other.[21] In this chapter, the three terms (absence, absenteeism, and sick-absence) will be used as synonymous in meaning and without any connotation other than that workers were scheduled and expected to attend, excluding overtime. "Sickness-absence" is a convenient term for absence from work attributed to sickness or injury and accepted as such by the employer or the social security system.

Some sickness absence and some absenteeism for other reasons may be regarded as objectively necessary and, therefore, acceptable and normal. Norms applied in respect of what extent of absence is acceptable depend on local conditions such as prevailing morbidity, labor market situation, and many other factors.

Absenteeism becomes abnormal, in medical terms "pathologic," when excessive in degree. This may refer to workdays lost or to frequency of absences, especially of unauthorized and short-term sickness incidents. The latter, if their duration is less than four days, often reflects a need for absence rather than a real necessity (incapacity to work), even though they may have been certified by a physician. Excessive nonattendance on a particular day is another abnormal manifestation of note. Excessive absenteeism may be viewed as a symptom which indicates something wrong in the person-work-enterprise-society relationship.

Absenteeism in industry is not really a medical phenomenon. To investigate it, ideally one would require a team of researchers, consisting of an occupational physician, industrial psychologist, sociologist, economist, statistician, personnel and labor relations specialist, and maybe other experts as well. Occupational medicine, in general, concerns itself with the relationship of the work environment to the health of workers in a particular socioeconomic and sociocultural setting.

The study of absenteeism, viewed as a "social" disease of workers which is symptomatic for underlying faults in their working environment, falls within the realm of occupational medicine. There might be shortcomings in the adjustment and adaptation of work and work environment to workers and vice versa. There might be adverse factors in the organizational climate or in the workers themselves. External influences are to be expected and must be taken into account.

CONCEPTUAL CONSIDERATIONS IN RESPECT TO ABSENTEEISM AND ABSENCE BEHAVIOR

Basic concepts for the study of absenteeism are the concept of meaning of work to individuals, the concept of their social role, and, for sickness absence, their concept of illness in relation to the social role and work. Illness or disease (here used as synonyms) is regarded as the objective entity, which can potentially be diagnosed by a doctor. Sickness is viewed as the perception and experience of illness by the patient, without whom illness could not exist in any case. Not all illness or sickness leads to absence. Sickness absence only occurs when the worker, who decided to assume the role of patient, also decides not to work.

Hogerzeil[9] emphasized that sickness absence will result only when a person experiences a deviation from his or her normal state of well-being that markedly impedes functioning in the work situation. The point at which this occurs depends on the person's threshold for reporting sick-absent. This threshold, markedly influenced by the personal motivation of the worker, is also determined by a host of personal, social, cultural, and economic factors. Essentially, however, sickness absence behavior is personal behavior and depends on the decision by the individual not to work. The same applies, of course, to voluntary absence that is unauthorized and not sanctioned by a sick certificate. Lack of motivation to maintain the role of worker is, among other factors, related to the meaning his work has for the individual. Under-utilization and under-stimulation are as harmful to health as excessive stress, since a modicum of stress is healthy and needed to maintain a state of well-being. Van Strien[30] views the "quality of work" as an aspect of the "quality of life." He illustrated this by discussing five facets of work, partly based on Maslow[15] and Herzberg:[7]

1. Work, as physical activity, means a regularly returning load (in the sense of taxing) on the body, which is necessary to maintain health.

2. In an economic sense, work provides the means to fulfill basic and other needs. These involve recreation and development of the worker and his or her dependents.

3. In the social and psychologic field, work provides opportunities to develop social relationships and a sense of belonging.

4. Work, or its fruits, is also a source of socioeconomic status, prestige, and power, which implies security.

5. Work forms the basis for controlling some part of the environment, mastering a skill, and acquiring a psychologic identity.

The Volvo Report[14] relates that high absenteeism, personnel turnover, and recruiting problems had been important incentives to the Volvo company to "humanize" the work there. At the Olofström factory, innovation of job design, mechanization, elimination of repetitive jobs and heavy lifting, and other measures which increased the freedom and responsibility of workers led to a 50% decrease in absenteeism. Productivity and profitability did not diminish. Job rotation and team work, allowing more social communications, were also introduced and led to similar results.

Responsibilities in the social sphere, such as having to provide for a family and feeling responsible to the work group and the employer, are particularly relevant to voluntary absence. Voluntary absence is defined as not being attributable to incapacitating illness nor to those nonmedical incidents which physically prevent a worker from coming to work. Norms prevailing in a particular society in respect to the social duty of the individual to contribute to the well-being of the community by working strongly influence absenteeism.

The views of Western Europeans in respect to work are similar to those found by Kahn[12] and others in the United States. Kahn believed his study indicated that the meaning of the job to workers shows some stability over time. He did not find evidence that the meaning of the word "work" had been transformed, for better or worse. In his critique on "Work in America," a report by a special task force to the Secretary of Health, Education, and Welfare, Kahn stated, however, that "work" failed to meet a number of criteria for many workers. Many workers, he said, did not find work intrinsically rewarding, nor did they believe that their jobs required valued skills and abilities or provided opportunities to acquire new ones; further, they did not think of their work as being socially approved and instrumentally meaningful.

O'Toole,[17] who had headed the task force, indicated the need for improvement of jobs, since "a significant number of American workers were dissatisfied with the quality of their working lives."

More recent discussions of the factors which influence individual patterns of absence of workers by Steers and Rhodes,[24] Rushmore and Youngblood,[22] as well as by Breaugh[2] throw some light on the dynamic character of these concepts. While a change in overall absence culture (the prevailing attitudes that sanction or condone absence from work) appears to occur in parts of the world, prediction of future absence behavior on the basis of an individual's historical record is often possible. This, again, emphasizes the importance of individual absence behavior, in addition to the sociologic aspects incorporated in discussions such as by Chadwick-Jones et al.[3, 4] Chadwick-Jones et al. discussed absenteeism first as a psychologic phenomenon. Their main assumption was that absence is, to some degree, voluntary withdrawal and should be distinguished from unavoidable absence. Incapacitating illness would be unavoidable absence. They indicated that part of the problem, in practice, is how to define that part of sickness absence which reflects true morbidity. They mentioned a number of theories and stated, "what attempts have been made to postulate general hypotheses to explain absence behavior are almost entirely social psychologic, at least in origin."

Withdrawal is the central explanatory concept. The hypothesis refers to the way in which the individual reacts to a stressful work situation. The quality of the person-work relationship determines whether, consciously or unconsciously, relief of stress will be sought by temporary absence from work. Absences are, therefore, seen as motivated behavior. All forms of absences, including separation (labor turnover), can be considered under this concept of withdrawal from the work situation.

Nonattendance at work depends on a necessity to absent oneself (unavoidable) or on a desire for absence (individual choice), coupled with the opportunity to absent oneself. It results essentially from an individual decision. In the case of absence behavior as defined above, it is viewed as reflecting the quality of the person-work-enterprise relationship. Unbearable perceived "stress" leads to an escape mechanism: withdrawal. Phrased in a less dramatic way, and incorporating other theoretical considerations, the concept would cover withdrawal from work resulting from a need to seek relief when the attracting forces within the work situation are not strong enough to hold the worker there. In a nutshell, one could state that employees stay away from work for one of two reasons: (1) they have to, because they are physically unable to work or to get to work, or (2) they choose to.

In a wider context, absence culture is defined as the pattern of sanctioned, condoned, and unaccepted nonattendance in a particular organization. It is influenced by the organizational climate and by such factors as the labor market and "conjuncture" of the economy. The absence culture, together with sick pay regulations, determines the opportunity to absent oneself from work and is, itself, influenced by the norms of a society with regard to the social importance attached to work.

Hogerzeil[8] pointed out that medical diagnoses listed in the International Classification of Diseases are inadequate indicators for sickness absence. They are designed to classify disease and not sickness absence, which is a social, not a medical, phenomenon. Sickness absence is viewed as a process, caused by a perceived incapacity to work as a result of a disturbance in social functioning. It is not necessarily caused by classic morbidity. Phases discernible in the process which leads to sickness absence are the incipience of a disturbance in well-being, followed by recognition, and then by either accepting the role of patient and acting upon this, or ignoring the disturbance. On return of the feeling of well-being, the reverse takes place, or else the role of patient, including absence from work, is maintained. Sickness absence results from a decision by the individual to withdraw from the work situation.

Relating these concepts to the duration of sickness absence spells, Hogerzeil argued that "being unable to work" is not a static condition but a dynamic process: "The cause and, therefore, the treatment of absences of different durations can be very different."

The influence of the physician on the decision-making of the worker is, in part, also dependent on the type of syndrome the patient displays. Absences of longer duration are characterized by the occurrence of classic diseases and, therefore, more likely to be subjected to control by physicians.

The term *absence pattern* is a concept used to indicate how the absenteeism of groups of workers is constituted in terms of level of absence (days lost in proportion to potential working days), frequency rates of incidents (certified sickness and unauthorized absence), and duration of spells. The latter aspect may be reported as average or median duration of spells of absence or, to indicate absence behavior, as the proportion of short spells (sickness absence of less than four days). Determination of the absence pattern is used as a means to arrive at a diagnosis of the type and severity of absenteeism observed in the plant or its subpopulations. Only then is it possible to attempt to indicate what actions could be taken to reduce it to acceptable levels.

Commonly used measurements for absenteeism control are:

1. *Gross absence rate (GAR):* Total days of absence expressed as percentage of potential working days (manpower strength multiplied by the number of working days).

2. *Sickness absence rate (SAR):* Total number of certified sickness absence days, again expressed as percentage of potential working days.

3. *Unauthorized absence rate (UAR):* Unauthorized absence in days, expressed in the same way as SAR and GAR.

(For the computation of these percentage rates, overtime is excluded. An average figure for the manpower strength is taken for the period under consideration. Absences for training, study, annual leave, and all other absences authorized in advance are excluded.)

4. *Absence Frequency Rate (AFR):* The average number of absence incidents (e.g., sickness spells) per person per period of time computed for individuals, groups, or the work force as a whole.

The first three absence rates can only indicate the proportion of work days lost due to unplanned nonattendance. The absence frequency rate indicates how widespread absences occur and can serve as a barometer for the working "climate."

In general, if the GAR of a particular enterprise exceeds 5%, especially if the AFR is higher than 1.0 (incidents per person per annum), absenteeism must be regarded as excessive. In such a case, full investigation and evaluation is indicated.

In different countries, or even localities, higher or lower figures may have to be determined to serve as action level. What is "normal" and "acceptable" depends on a host of factors which will have to be taken into account before a norm is decided on.

EFFECTS OF ABSENTEEISM

The study of absenteeism as a social and psychologic phenomenon is an interesting exercise. That of sickness absenteeism, which is widely, but erroneously, regarded as a "pure" medical problem, is of particular interest to the occupational physician.

The effects of absenteeism on society, mainly in economic terms, have received quite some attention, as evidenced by publications in the literature.[1, 11, 23] One might consider these effects as, in a sense, secondary to the effects of absence from work on the employing organization as the primary focus of interest.[5, 18, 25, 31]

High absence rates on a particular day may seriously disrupt the proceedings and lead to feelings of annoyance and frustration. Because of this, "morale" may be adversely affected. High absentee rates may have a very disruptive effect on production, depending on the type of industry and the processes used.

Lastly, absenteeism and, in particular, sickness absence leads to an increased workload on the staffs of personnel, administrative, and medical departments who are charged with the task of monitoring absenteeism, processing claims, and counseling returning absentees.

From the viewpoint of management, high absentee rates on particular days, high overall absence levels, and frequent or long absences of individuals are of particular interest. Absenteeism interferes with production and adds to costs.

From the viewpoint of society, the economic and social effects are most important.

From a strictly medical viewpoint, the causes of absence and contributory factors are more important than effects. The cost-benefit aspects of certain preventive actions (such as influenza vaccination), and the potential adverse effects on "morale" that excessive absenteeism may have, make it imperative for the occupational physician to pay attention to effects as well.

Personal, occupational, and organizational variables are of prime interest in considering a possible control of excessive absenteeism. The word "control" is used here to mean regulating or influencing absenteeism by specific or general measures. Not all the variables can be regarded as controllable. The effect of some personal factors could be influenced by selection of employees. That of other personal variables could indirectly be influenced by management organization policies. Occupational variables are mainly determined by the type of industry, production methods, and the size of a particular firm. Among the group of organizational factors, which one might regard as most likely to be under the control of management, some are so strongly determined by outside influences (e.g., labor market) that they also cannot all be regarded as controllable. It would appear that only a few of the internal factors are really under the direct control of management. This is particularly so when one considers an already established firm with the labor force serving it in a particular socioeconomic and sociocultural setting.

THE MICRO-CLIMATE: INTERNAL, PARTICULARLY ORGANIZATIONAL, FACTORS

Personal Variables

Absence behavior is essentially personal and motivated behavior. A well-integrated personality and older age, possibly implying greater maturity, especially if combined with social responsibilities such as having dependents, appear to be associated with a low level of absenteeism. Considerable length of service (or a high stability rate of the labor force) shows the same correlation. "Blue collar" workers with a relatively high socioeconomic status, which may well be associated with a higher degree of job satisfaction and personal motivation and a more positive attitude to the work situation, will also be absent less frequently. Personal ill-health does not necessarily imply high rates of absence frequency. Sickness absence spells attributable to "genuine" organic disease tend to be of longer duration in older workers. In general, it appears to be mainly the quality of the person-work relationship, influenced by the above-mentioned interdependent variables, which determines the extent of personal absence behavior. Frequency rates of short-term absences, unauthorized or "certified," are the most valid indicators for personal (and group) absence behavior. Excessive smoking and consumption of alcohol may be viewed as personality traits associated with high levels of absence behavior.

Occupational Variables

Occupational variables are closely interwoven with organizational as well as with personal factors. Typical occupational factors are the type of work performed, the physical working environment (for each part of the organization), the organization of production, day work or shift work, and the type of supervision. Social factors seem to be of overriding influence with regard to the influence on absence behavior of these occupational factors. In general, "good" working conditions, physical and social, appear to be associated with low levels of absence behavior. This statement is, however, too vague to be of much practical value. Autocratic, authoritarian leadership appears to be associated with higher absenteeism. The influence of shift work appears to depend on the type of rota used and on the degree of self-selection of shift workers, which would be a personal factor.[28, 29] It would appear that the stability of the social work group and the quality of its relationship with the supervisor override the influence of "pure" occupational factors.

Organizational Variables

Although a rather nebulous concept, the general "climate" prevailing in an organization appears to be a derived variable of considerable importance with regard to absenteeism in an enterprise. In the first place, that "climate" is created by the attitude of management toward its employees and the ways management attempts to achieve its goals. This is expressed in an organization's policies and procedures, including whether or not these provide for professional personnel and medical services. In the second place, the specific "absence culture" of an enterprise, although markedly influenced by external factors, is also determined by management attitudes and forms part of the "climate" concept. "Each enterprise experiences the absenteeism it deserves" puts this concept in a nutshell.

General organizational factors of note are, again, the physical working conditions, but also the "name" an organization has among the population as an employer "for whom it is good to work." This includes, of course, remuneration levels, compared with other firms in an area. In general, if organizational factors are regarded as favorable, they seem to be associated with low absenteeism levels, except that piece-rate payment tends to be associated with high absenteeism. Highly paid subpopulations of workers may also show higher-than-average absence frequency rates.

A specific organizational factor is the regulations concerning sick pay benefits. If no economic incentive to remain at work (or to return to work as soon as possible) exists, absence frequency rates and overall sickness absence tend to be higher. Smulders,[25] attempting to explain differences in absenteeism patterns in 85 Dutch enterprises by their organizational characteristics, found an average gross absence rate of 11.7% (1981–1982), with a range of 5.2%–19.2%. In general terms, he confirmed the findings of Philipsen[18] whose study he replicated, investigating 19 organizational variables, to which he added some more contemporary ones, e.g., "guest labor." In broad outline, it was found that absenteeism, measured by the sickness absence rate, was unfavorably influenced by such factors as poor financial-economic status of the enterprise (inferring a low level of security and a poor reputation of the firm), poor quality of work conditions and of human interrelationships at work, as well as a high degree of automatization, with shift work arrangements and an authoritarian type of leadership, combined with a lack of input from professional personnel management.

A higher degree of worker participation in decision-making tended to reduce absence frequency, while demonstrated attention to individuals, i.e., active involvement by personnel and medical departments, tended to reduce absence spell durations.

These findings are in agreement with the author's own studies in a large motor manufacturing plant in South Africa,[16] where variables were shown to exert a different influence on absence frequency than on spell duration and thus indirectly on sickness absence rate.

If an organization employs a heterogenous labor force, different groups of workers may be affected in a different way and to a different degree by occupational and organizational variables which, at face value, might be expected to have the same influence on all workers.

The influence of occupational and organizational variables on absenteeism of groups of workers must, therefore, be evaluated in relation to specific (in particular, socioeconomic) aspects, peculiar to each group, if one wishes to compare absence behavior of groups of workers, although standardization for personal variables is then also required.

THE MACRO-CLIMATE: EXTERNAL FACTORS, PARTICULARLY MEDICAL CERTIFICATION

Economic Factors

A literature survey would provide clear indications that unemployment is an important external variable.[16] The labor market, itself a function of the state of the economy ("conjuncture"), is regarded by some as the most potent of all the factors influencing absence behavior, but it is, of course, an uncontrollable factor.

A low level of absence behavior is to be expected in times of poor economic "conjuncture." This is especially so for those worker groups who, by virtue of low skill and earnings and the high cost of living, believe that their job security is most threatened (including opportunities to secure alternative work).

On the other hand, the expected influence of a decline in the state of the economy may be obscured in groups who enjoy a measure of preferential treatment with regard to employment opportunity.

Sociocultural and Ethnic Factors

The conclusion reached from studying the literature was that concepts of work, time, illness, and also sociocultural values must be expected to influence absence behavior. However, in industrialized, highly urbanized worker populations, even when originating from rural-tribal communities, such effects as were observed appeared to be minor.[16] The counteraction of effects which are deemed to result from adjustment to industrial life and from changes in concepts of acceptable sickness absence behavior did not allow firm conclusions about what influence on absence behavior one may expect in a particular industrial society. Smulders and others have shown that the absence behavior of "foreign guest labor" groups may differ markedly from autochthonous worker populations.

Medical Factors

Among medical factors, the prevailing and changing morbidity patterns and seasonal variation of disease incidence have received attention in the literature.[6, 20] It is self-evident that these would influence sickness absence and that socioeconomic factors, such as poor living conditions, nutritional status, and differences in exposure, would play a role.

Medical certification requirements concerning social security and sick fund regulations are a matter of interest and controversy. The role of medicine as a whole, and of the physician in particular, in preventing and curing disease would be expected to reduce sickness absenteeism. However, a study of the literature indicates that sickness absence appears to have increased so much in Western societies that any decline in absence attributable to true morbidity was overshadowed.[27, 28] Increases in sickness absence over the years have become a matter of great concern in these industrial societies. The role of the certifying doctor in this respect has received relatively little attention.

In the author's study,[16] the role of the doctor as a variable in sickness absence was examined. It was found that a doctor's awareness of the implications of issuing a sickness certificate could greatly influence sickness absence. Sickness certificates do not only sanction absence from work for incapacity to work in cases of (genuine) disease. They are also used to sanction forms of absence behavior. In other words, a sickness certificate affords a sanctioned opportunity to withdraw from work (the worker's social role) even when this escape fulfills a desire rather than a necessity. When sick pay benefits are available, a certificate implies that the absence will not only be authorized but also paid. A sickness certificate is "therapeutic" in that it is a prescription for "rest," but physicians often do not consciously use it as a prescription for "work," which should also be regarded as a form of therapy.

Certification is not an exact science but depends on how the patient-worker and doctor interact, influenced by social security regulations and norms prevailing in a particular society. Few doctors issue attendance certificates, i.e., a note that a person consulted his doctor but was not unfit to work. Doctors, as an extraneous factor, also tend to "stretch" sickness absence until Monday as a logical day to resume work. In general, patient-workers themselves decide when to stop work, and this usually is accepted as a "fait accompli" by their doctors. Only in instances of genuine illness, especially if lasting longer than four days, did doctors seem to have a determining influence on the day of resumption of work. The latter depends on clear communications and on the physician's perception that there is an optimal duration for each sickness absence—neither too short nor too long.

Physicians, in general, do not tend to treat their patients as people with a social role to fulfill. Not all doctors provide their patients with firm guidance as to when to resume their worker's role, in their own interest, as well as in the interest of the employing organization and society as a whole.

The future may well bring changes in certification requirements in advanced industrial societies. For instance, some form of self-certification already exists for certain categories of workers and in certain communities and organizations (Sweden, Holland, salaried staff). Another form of certification, advising patients that it is in their interest not to work for a period determined on medical grounds, rather than declaring them "unfit for work" is already in use in some areas (England). Such changes, however, only shift some of the responsibility and do not detract from the conclusions stated above.

Kruidenier and Bakker[13] described the apparent drop in level of absenteeism in particular worker-populations from 1978 to 1983 in Holland. Apparently, the "less healthy" workers were selected out of the work force by the recession, so the level of absenteeism was lower. However, Kruidenier and Bakker showed that there were variable positive and negative effects on absence frequency and spell duration and that the overall decrease masked a marked increase in "sickness absence" among the group of stayers, i.e., the workers who remained in employment over the five-year period they investigated.

Prins[19] discussed the difficulties in comparing sickness absence levels in different countries and questioned whether valid comparisons can, in fact, be made. He noted a decrease of a few percentage points from 1979 to 1983 for the Netherlands (to 9.5%), Italy (9.4%), but no change for Sweden (13.8%) and hardly any for the U.S.A. (3.2%). For Japan, a level of 1.5% was reported. The discrepancy in figures already indicates that no comparison with another country can be made without taking into account all known factors and methods used to calculate such figures. Since 1983, programs are in progress to find reliable methods to compare sickness absence in enterprises in the Netherlands, Belgium, and West Germany, for a start.

THE ROLE OF THE OCCUPATIONAL HEALTH WORKER IN ABSENCE CONTROL

The role of the physician in industry in "controlling" sickness absence is regarded differently in different countries. At one end of the opinion spectrum is the idea that the physician should have nothing whatever to do with this. It is argued that, as a member of the management team, industrial physicians would be seen as biased and that this, of necessity, would distort the doctor-patient (worker) relationship. They should, therefore, not be expected to "police" sickness absence. At the other end of the spectrum, there are countries in which no sickness absence can be authorized by any physician other than those at the company clinic. In between there are organizations in which the monitoring and counseling function of industrial physicians is viewed as so important that they are indirectly charged with the control of sickness absence as well, albeit in an advisory role. In whatever organization or society occupational medical officers are placed, their principal objectives remain the same. These are, in general, to investigate and understand how particular symptoms, syndromes, or disease entities arise in individuals or groups, to identify these and the factors associated with them, and to devise curative and preventive measures. Thus, occupational physicians strive to improve the physical and psychosocial working conditions of the labor force under their care, partly in an active function, partly in an advisory role.

Occupational physicians may be required to monitor sickness certificates because, under prevailing personnel policy regulations, the occupational physician must approve the certificate before sick pay is granted to the employee. Or this may be so because of regulations that deny sick pay to workers with venereal disease or an incapacity to work due to abuse of alcohol or to misconduct. A more important reason for the monitoring of sickness certificates is that they provide data about absenteeism of individuals and groups and may indicate where and when abnormal absence behavior occurs. From an epidemiologic viewpoint, data from certificates may indicate that certain groups of workers are exposed to toxic agents, unsafe working conditions, or psychologic distress. Further investigations could then lead the doctor to advise changes in occupational hygiene or, in certain instances, in labor relations. The monitoring of sickness absence, including absence behavior, is an indispensable tool for diagnosing, or at least pinpointing, "faulty" working conditions, which include unsatisfactory person- (or group) work-employer relationships.

A diagnosis of an "illness" in labor relations before the condition becomes serious is as important to management as an early diagnosis of disease is to the physician. The physician in industry, working in a close relationship with the workers in the plant, as well as with labor relations officers, is well placed to detect early symptoms when all is not well on the factory floor. Absenteeism of a part of the working population may reflect the "illness" of the whole organization.

This applies to individuals as well as to groups or to the work force as a whole. So-called "medical" (i.e., physical and mental illness) as well as psychologic and social factors (affecting the individual, family, work group) need to be taken into account. To that end, ideally, the medical department should keep records for all individuals and also be able to visualize trends of sickness absence in departments, sections of the organization, and the work force as a whole.

Individual records should be kept in such a way that, from the records of sickness absence incidents, including diagnoses and durations of absence spells, it would be possible to conclude whether:

1. The worker has had recurrent episodes of a particular, possibly progressive, chronic illness, indicating the need for assistance.

2. The worker has had frequent episodes of a few days of illness with a variety of vague, subjective diagnoses, such as headache, backache, gastroenteritis, or fibrositis, or notably on Mondays. Such frequent "grey" sickness absence spells indicate sickness absence behavior, a withdrawal pattern which could be based on alcoholism or on conflict situations at work that require counseling or intervention.

3. The worker has had a few incidents of serious medical illness requiring adaptation of the work to his or her reduced capabilities, or rehabilitation of some sort.

4. The worker needs monitoring of long-term treatment for such ailments as epilepsy (possibly needing a transfer to a safe area), hypertension, diabetes, or mental illness.

It should be accepted policy and procedure that no worker returns to work without reporting back to the occupational health department after an absence of, for example, two weeks' duration. This would ensure that all workers with serious illness will be seen and assisted on return to work, if assistance, in the form of restricted work, temporarily shorter hours, or rehabilitation, is needed. When outside physicians are aware that their patients will be assisted on return to work, they may be prepared to allow them to go back at an earlier date, in the interest of both patient and enterprise.

Grouped records, arranged in categories according to workshops, departments, or type of worker, would help to diagnose problems in an epidemiologic context. More sophisticated record systems would be needed to attain such objectives. Computerization would facilitate access to the data for analysis at any time this is required. If, for example, an accumulation of upper respiratory tract infections, dermatitis cases, or back problems would occur in a particular department, the occupational health worker could ring the alarm and, together with other involved parties, investigate the work situation. A high frequency of absences ascribed to vague subjective illnesses or complaints could point to a supervisor-foreman-workers relationship problem amenable to therapeutic intervention by the department manager and personnel department combined.

For medical staff, an important measure of sickness absence is the "spell duration," defined as the number of consecutive calendar days an employee was certified as off sick for a particular incident. Average spell durations (excluding spells of longer than 14 days which would confuse the picture), computed for groups of workers or the company as a whole, may enable one to make a group diagnosis of what is wrong:

1. If the average sickness absence spell duration is less than four days and is combined with a high absence frequency rate (incidents of absences per annum) of more than 2.0 per person, one can be sure that there is a serious flaw in the working relationship, unless, for example, an influenza epidemic accounts for these phenomena.

2. If, however, the average spell duration is in the order of seven days or more, this is an indication that there is a high degree of genuine morbidity in the worker population. If the absence frequency rate is also high (e.g., more than two incidents per person per annum), a real medical problem may exist, in the sense that the health of the worker population as a whole is below par.

In such cases, the recorded diagnoses become very important. While medical diagnoses on certificates are of great value to medical people, they should, if at all possible, be withheld from lay people and institutions so that the privacy of the worker is protected. One can preserve confidentiality and avoid circulating medical diagnoses among nonmedical administrative staff by routing all medical certificates through medical departments and separating medical data (diagnoses) from the certified sickness dates (which are the only data really needed by sick pay administrations if the medical department does the screening for them).

In conclusion, the occupational health worker's concern with regard to sickness absence would be:

1. To identify workers or groups of workers who appear to have defects in their physical, mental or social well-being at work, using sickness absence records as a diagnostic tool.

2. To assist such workers by counseling, rehabilitation measures, monitoring of their medication, and clinical or laboratory tests.

3. To assist management and the enterprise as a whole, indirectly reducing sickness absence, by preventive and curative medical programs aimed at improving conditions at work that could otherwise affect the health of the enterprise and its workers adversely.

DIAGNOSIS OF ABSENTEEISM

Absenteeism assumes abnormal, pathologic proportions if there is something wrong with the quality of the person-work-employing organization relationship (the microclimate). The norms against which absence from work is measured are, from a management viewpoint, determined by economic considerations, but they are also intricately interwoven with, and influenced by, norms and values concerning the meaning of work and the acceptability of staying away from work which pertain in a particular society (the macroclimate).

The gross absence rate is only a crude measure of absenteeism but is widely used. In general, a GAR of 5% is regarded as a sign that the situation needs to be investigated and a GAR of 10% as serious by any standard.

An AFR of over 1.0 per annum indicates absence-taking that is far too widespread and suggests a "permissive" absence policy, where absence is condoned, or even hardly noticed. Even at 0.5 there is still considerable room for improvement, and a first target should be to get AFRs below this level.

Adequate absence records are a prerequisite for attempts to diagnose absenteeism. A high gross absence rate can only serve as an indication that something is wrong. Its components, SAR and UAR, may help to point out where the main causes of the high absenteeism may be found. An excessive number of days lost due to unauthorized absence indicates that the absence culture is too lenient, while it may also indicate that the workers need frequent withdrawal from a stressful work situation. High incidence rates for such unauthorized absences are another manifestation of note (AFR (U)). If the SAR is high and a high proportion of lost days is due to sickness spells lasting longer than four days, this may indicate a high degree of morbidity in the labor force. That would point to a medical rather than a managerial problem.

Apart from the GAR, SAR, and UAR, other absence indicators, such as AFR (sickness and unauthorized), average spell duration (excluding spells longer than 14 days), and days lost per person per annum (attributable to illness or to absence behavior), are valuable. Recording of medical diagnoses is necessary to establish whether better medical care and preventive measures could help to "cure" absenteeism. For individual records, the emphasis would be on frequency and spell durations as well as on medical diagnoses. For groups and enterprises, a system of recording is needed that would indicate which broad groups of determining variables might be responsible for the observed absence patterns. For example:

1. An increase in short-term absences points to the psychosocial sphere and concerns the management of an organization because it indicates psychosocial problems, anxiety, lack of good human relations, disorganization, or social insecurity.

2. An increase in acute respiratory disease points to virologic or toxicologic problems, indicating the need for preventive measures, assistance by consultants, and, perhaps, prophylactic therapy.

3. An increase in objective syndromes points to the need for experts in somatic illnesses, such as family physicians or specialists. It can, for example, indicate toxicologic problems or bad ergonomics if a special department is concerned.

Each enterprise should organize its absence-from-work recording system, with due regard to cost-benefit consideration in relation to the absenteeism it suffers from and to the means at its disposal. Having set absence norms which are regarded as acceptable by management, the enterprise could then use its records foı the purpose of diagnosing absence patterns in its departments and of identifying controllable factors. It could then devise corrective measures. If an employing organization has computer facilities at its disposal, it could use refined methods for diagnosing its absenteeism problems. However, simple manual recording systems can be just as effective if properly designed and used, whether an enterprise is small or large. A firm's absenteeism represents an appreciable, and in part controllable, loss. The occurrence of high absentee rates on particular days is a striking and disturbing phenomenon but does not provide the means to arrive at a diagnosis of absenteeism nor can it indicate what to do about it.

CONTROL OF ABSENTEEISM

With regard to the pathogenesis of absenteeism, defined as assumed causation of nonattendance and influence of variables taken together, only a few general statements will be made. The crux of the matter is to differentiate between controllable and uncontrollable factors. It is the natural inclination of a doctor to look out for possibilities of preventing or curing a disease. Occupational physicians, serving not only their potential patient population, the labor force, but also the enterprise as a whole, will in the first place look for possibilities of preventing and curing occupational diseases and injuries. In the second place, anything in the enterprise which seems to indicate that it, itself, is "ill" will also be of concern. Abnormal absenteeism is such an indication and so falls under a broad concept of occupational health.

Personal factors, especially personality, married status, age, and socioeconomic status, are relevant, but are outside the control of the management. Education, training, and, particularly, induction of the new employee may be means to improve the quality of the person-work relationship. The length of service of an employee is influenced by both personal and organizational factors and has considerable influence on absenteeism. A high stability rate (and consequently low labor turnover) is a group characteristic associated with low levels of absenteeism. The quality of the relationship between the employees and their employing organization appears to be more important than that of the worker-supervisor-work group relationship.[18, 25] Both are partly controllable.

The organization cannot be viewed as isolated from the local area, country, and society as a whole. Norms and values prevailing in that society with regard to the value of work, social security, and acceptability of absenting oneself for particular reasons, all play a role. The state of the economy (conjuncture) and the labor market have a profound influence on absenteeism, mainly through the medium of the perceived security of earning a living. Prevailing morbidity, medical care facilities, and the attitudes of doctors are also characteristics of a particular society which influence sickness absence, adversely or favorably. Concepts of what constitutes illness warranting withdrawal from work may be influenced by ethnocultural concepts of illness and work. Most, but not all, of these factors are outside the control of the employing organizations.

The absence culture of an organization, defined as the pattern of sanctioned, condoned, and unaccepted absences, is of major importance for the absenteeism it experiences. Although partly determined by external influences, it is, or should be, the expression of its management's attitude, policies, and procedures. Whether the latter are fairly and consistently applied to all categories of workers, irrespective of job category, ethnic group, or other characteristics, influences the quality of the relationship of the workers to the organization. How management organizes its response to increased demands of production (by taking in additional labor, overtime, shift work, or other means) may also affect absenteeism appreciably. Its sick pay benefit policy is a powerful factor; if no economic incentive to work or to return to work is involved, management may have to expect a high level of sickness absence. Providing a safe place to work (complying with reasonable requirements with regard to occupational hygiene) and in-plant medical facilities, with scope for preventive health maintenance, improves the quality of the relationship of the labor force with its employing organization. Although not always directly measurable, these factors should lead to lower absenteeism. Adapting its hiring and firing policies to an objective which aims to hold its employees in its employ for years of service has the same effect. Remuneration and fringe benefits, as well as attention to the needs of the labor force outside the work situation, may have favorable effects on absenteeism.

With regard to discipline, it may prevent excess absenteeism if workers know that individual absence records are kept and that needs and necessity for absence are recognized when warranted, but that unwarranted absences invoke just and fairly applied disciplinary measures. Counseling, rather than punitive action, would fit in with a policy aimed at retaining employees when they experience personal problems, including those of physical or mental health.

Overall, if the attitude and actions of management are perceived as striving to attain a high quality in the relationship with its work force, absenteeism should be low. If workers are employed by a firm "for which it is good to work" in an environment "where it is good to work," a high degree of motivation and a high absence threshold would be expected.

Depending on the diagnosis of the prevailing manifestations of absenteeism, remedial action may have to be managerial, or medical, and should be economically justified or at least acceptable. Taylor[28] indicated the necessity of involving the employees themselves to achieve a joint acceptance of objectives. He emphasized, "All supervisors should be personally concerned with absence in their own areas and not be allowed to abdicate responsibility to personnel departments. They should play their part in making employees feel that their contribution to the working group and to the objectives of the firm is really valued."

Personnel departments (labor relations) should be charged with specific tasks in controlling absenteeism. Their expertise, for example, in the field of industrial psychology, would be invaluable.

PRIMARY AND SECONDARY PREVENTION

In general, a physician is expected to cure diseases and injuries, thereby healing the patient, to prevent illness and to promote health, a state of well-being. The field of action of occupational physicians is somewhat wider.

They advise management on issues of occupational hygiene, which includes the physical environment as well as the psychosocial climate in an enterprise. They assist in the adjustment of the work to the workers and of the workers to their work by an application of medical and behavioral sciences, ergonomics, selection of workers, and other methods. In that way, occupational physicians contribute to the quality of the person-work relationship, and to that of the worker-organization relationship, in close cooperation with other departments in a firm. The prevention of occupational diseases, monitoring potentially adverse influences in the working environment, and monitoring exposed workers, is the direct responsibility of occupational physicians. Depending on the prevailing conditions, they may be involved in promoting the safety of the work environment with regard to potential injuries resulting from unsafe conditions and unsafe acts. Through epidemiologic research, they may identify pathogenic conditions in the work environment and assist in removing these, thus preventing illness. With regard to contagious diseases, they may organize immunization campaigns and isolate or remove sources of contagion, thus reducing the incidence of such diseases. All this can be summarized as activities aimed at preventing disease, or reducing its incidence, severity, or duration.

Secondly, occupational physicians may be charged with curative actions, depending on prevailing philosophy and medical care facilities. Treatment of minor ailments at work and of potentially more serious disease or injury in an early stage indirectly reduces sickness absence from work. In-plant medical facilities reduce the necessity to seek treatment elsewhere.

Thirdly, occupational physicians have a role to play in counseling the chronically ill, especially those workers suffering from repetitive incidents of illness, or from emotional problems, particularly if they seek refuge in excessive alcohol intake. In this way, absences from work may be reduced and workers are assisted in fulfilling their social role at work.

As Howe[10] stated, "One of the functions of the physician in industry is, through his anticipatory health guidance, or preventive or constructive medical measures, to minimize cost of time lost through illness absence. . . . The significant role of the physician in contributing his aid to absence control is in working thoughtfully with those repeaters whose individual spells of absence are part of a continuum which comprises their life pattern or life style."

Fourthly, in consultation with his colleagues, private physicians, hospital doctors, and specialists, occupational physicians may promote timely return to work, e.g., by initially restricting hours of work or prescribing restricted duties to safeguard the health of a patient in a rehabilitation phase. The objective would be to guide the patient to resume his or her social role as soon as possible, after an optimal absence, in the patient's own interest and that of the work group and society.

Lastly, occupational physicians, because of their knowledge of the working situation and of the prevailing "climate" and absence culture in the organization, may assist workers in retaining their jobs when their absence behavior threatens to lead to their dismissal. By monitoring individual sickness absence records, such individuals may be identified in time to prevent further excessive absence behavior before it is too late.

All this can be summarized as activities which, although they may not be primarily aimed at reducing unnecessary sickness absence, in fact result in this effect.

REFERENCES

1. *Absence from Work, Incidence, Cost and Control*. British Institute of Management. Southampton, BIM Library 1961, Millbrook Press Ltd.
2. Breaugh JA: Predicting absenteeism from prior absenteeism and work attitudes. *J Appl Psychol* 1981; 66:555–560.
3. Chadwick-Jones JK, Brown CA, Nicholson N: Absence from work: Its meaning, measurement, and control. *Int Rev Appl Psychol* 1973; 22:137–155.
4. Chadwick-Jones JK, Nicholson N, Brown C: *Social Psychology of Absenteeism*. New York, Praeger, 1982.
5. Gadourek I: *Absences and Well-being of Workers*. Health Research, TNO Netherlands van Gorcum-Assen, 1965.
6. Gandhi HS: A study of sickness absenteeism among textile workers of Kanpur. *Indian J Med Res* 1971; 59:1467–1479.
7. Herzberg F: One more time: How do you motivate employees? *Harvard Business Rev* 1968; 36:53–62.
8. Hogerzeil HHW: Arbeidsongeschiktheid en medisch-sociaal beleid. *T Soc Geneesk* 1972; 50:538–550.
9. Hogerzeil HHW: The effects on sickness absence of personal characteristics, in *Proceedings of the Symposium on Absence from Work Attributed in Sickness, June 1968*. London, Society of Occupational Medicine, October 1977.
10. Howe HF: Organization and operation of an occupational health program. Part I. *J Occup Med* 1975; 17:360–400.
11. Jones RM: *Absenteeism*, Manpowers papers No 4. London, Her Majesty's Stationery Office, 1971.
12. Kahn R: On the meaning of work. *J Occup Med* 1974; 16,11: 716–719.
13. Kruidenier HJ, Bakker TPV: Vermindering en vervanging van personeel en de ontwikkeling van het ziekteverzuim. *T Soc Gezondheidsz* 1985; 63:302–308.
14. Lindholm R, Norstedt JP: *The Volvo Report*. Stockholm, Swedish Employers' Confederation, 1975. ISBN 91 7152 072 4.
15. Maslow AH: *Motivation and Personality*, ed 2. New York, Harper & Row, 1970.
16. Mets JT: *Absenteeism in Motor Manufacturing Plant*, PhD thesis. Pretoria, 1979.
17. O'Toole J: The great job satisfaction controversy. *J Occup Med* 1974; 16:710–715.
18. Philipsen H: *Afwezigheid wegens Ziekte*, Doct Thesis, 1968. Nederlands Instituut v Praev Geneeskunde, TNO Wolters-Noordhoff, Groningen, 1969.
19. Prins R: Ziekteverzuim in Belgie, West-Duitsland en Nederland. *T Soc Gezondheidszorg* 1985; 63:308–315.
20. Pocock SJ: Harmonic analysis applied to seasonal variations in sickness absence. *J Roy Stat Soc* 1974; Series C, 23(2):103–120.
21. Recommendations of the Sub-committee on Absenteeism. Permanent Commission on Occupational Health. *J Soc Occup Med* 1973; 23:132.
22. Rushmore CH, Youngblood SA: Medically related absenteeism. Random or motivated behaviour? *J Occup Med* 1979; 21: 245–250.
23. *Sickness Absence—A review*, OHE Briefing 16. London, Office of Health Economics 1981.
24. Steers RM, Rhodes SR: Major influences on employee attendance: A process model. *J Appl Psychol* 1978; 63:391–407.
25. Smulders PGW: *Bedrijfskenmen en Ziekteverzuim in de Jaren Zestig en Tachtig*, Publ 84014. Leiden, The Netherlands, NIPG, 1985.
26. Taylor PJ: International comparisons of sickness absence. *Proc Roy Soc Med* 1972; 65:577–580.

27. Taylor PJ: National and international trends in sickness absence. *Proc Roy Soc Med* 1970; 63:1144–1146.
28. Taylor PJ, Pocock SJ, Sergean R: Absenteeism of shift and day workers. *Br J Ind Med* 1972; 29:208–213.
29. Taylor PJ, Pocock SJ, Sergean R: Shift and day workers' absence. relationship with some terms and conditions of service. *Br J Ind Med* 1972; 29:338–340.
30. Van Strien PJ: Humanisering van de arbeid en de kwaliteit van het bestaan. *T Soc Geneesk* 1978; 56:682–689.
31. Yolles SF: Absenteeism in industry. *American Lecture Series* 969, ISBN - O - 39803302 1, 1975.

PART VII

Epidemiology: Principles and Practical Examples

71

Epidemiology in Occupational Health

Sven Hernberg, M.D., Ph.D.

Ever since 1775, when Sir Percival Pott described the extraordinarily high occurrence of scrotal cancer among chimney sweeps, who at that time were usually forced to begin work at an early age, epidemiologically oriented thinking has been infiltrating occupational medicine. Yet, with a few brilliant exceptions, most of the investigations published before the middle of this century contained severe errors. Fortunately, the past few decades have shown a favorable development in the quality of epidemiologic studies, but there is still room for improvement. Raising the quality of epidemiologic research essentially involves intensifying the education of research workers—the "producers" of data. This goal would best be achieved through formal training at public health schools or through intensive "crash" courses in combination with practical exercises under the guidance of experienced epidemiologists.

There is also another aspect to improvement, however. Not only active research workers, but all those who read epidemiologic reports—the "consumers" of data—must be familiar with at least the basic principles of epidemiology. Otherwise, they are unable to form their own critical opinions on the validity of the studies and the justifiability of the conclusions drawn by the authors. The aspect of educating the "consumers" is becoming more and more important, because a substantial part of knowledge in the field of occupational medicine is derived nowadays from epidemiologic studies, especially with respect to work-related diseases with multiple etiologies and nonspecific symptoms.

This presentation is primarily addressed to the "consumers"; for the "producers," it will be too superficial and fragmentary. For example, data analysis is not even discussed. Those who are in need of a more comprehensive treatise are referred to some of the recent textbooks on epidemiology, for example, Schlesselman,[18] Kleinbaum, Kupper, and Morgenstern,[22] Rothman,[47] and, especially, Monson.[38]

EXPERIMENTAL VERSUS NONEXPERIMENTAL RESEARCH

Epidemiologic research is nonexperimental, whereas experiments and clinical trials represent experimental research. The main distinction between experimental and nonexperimental research is that in experiments the investigators actively manipulate the conditions. They decide which individuals (usually animals) will be exposed or unexposed; furthermore, they design the exposure conditions. In a nonexperimental setting, investigators have no influence over these factors, and this is a pertinent distinction when causal relationships between two phenomena are being sought. Only experimental research can provide definite proof for a cause-effect relationship, because only under experimental conditions is there an opportunity to allocate the animals (or rarely, human beings) into exposed and unexposed categories *randomly*. This procedure tends, with increasing sample sizes, to eliminate systematic errors (biases). In addition, other factors can be strictly controlled. For example, exposure can be dosed exactly, and other concurrent exposures do not occur. Also, the effects can be measured systematically and accurately under standardized laboratory conditions.

In nonexperimental (epidemiologic) research, on the other hand, the possibilities of ensuring unbiased conditions are not so good. In particular, because randomization can rarely, if ever, be utilized, uncertainties regarding the presence or absence of systematic errors prevail. Hence, the interpretation of the results also becomes more conditional. What these uncertainties are and how they can be minimized are discussed in the section titled "Validity," in this chapter. Because perfection cannot be achieved, the cause-effect inferences drawn from epidemiologic studies must be viewed conditionally only; they are never definite. Some guidelines for judging whether an association is likely to be causal or not are given in the section titled "Guidelines for Interpreting Epidemiologic Studies."

Although experimental evidence is more definite than nonexperimental, epidemiology has its own important role in medicine. Many of the reasons are self-evident, the most central being, of course, that the study of human illness is best carried out with human beings. On the other hand, experimentation on human beings is seldom ethical, and this aspect generally rules out the experimental approach. Besides, since many environmental factors require a relatively long time to produce their effect, human experiments, even if ethically acceptable, would not be practically possible for the study of many problems.

DIFFERENT LEVELS OF EPIDEMIOLOGIC RESEARCH

Epidemiologic research can be classified into three categories, namely: (1) descriptive epidemiology; (2) etiologic or analytic epidemiology; and (3) interventive epidemiology.

Descriptive epidemiology observes the occurrence of illness in different categories of people under different circumstances. It can be used for a "community diagnosis" of workplaces, risk identification, surveillance of trends of health problems, determination of normal values, and generation of hypotheses for the study of cause-effect relationships.

Etiologic epidemiology concerns the study of causal connections between diseases and various genetic and environmental factors. Such connections are not directly observable—they must be inferred, and inferences fall in the sphere of abstractions. Etiologic epidemiology is predominantly used in the search for causal connections between occupational exposures and various adverse health effects. Hence, it can be used to determine occupational etiologic factors or preventive factors for diseases with a multiple etiology, to complete the clinical picture and, as a second-order problem, to establish exposure-effect and exposure-response relationships for known toxic agents.

Interventive epidemiology, which resembles experimental research, can be used to support cause-effect inferences and to evaluate health care processes and, in some rare cases, also the success of preventive programs.

However, it must always be remembered that epidemiology is only one of the approaches used for solving scientific problems or for implementing occupational health practices. Epidemiologic research should therefore be in close interaction with experimental research, clinical trials, and other methods for increasing knowledge and improving the quality of practice. True insight into epidemiology requires not only knowledge of its possibilities, but also a thorough understanding of its limitations and shortcomings.

SOME BASIC EPIDEMIOLOGIC MEASURES

In order for a discussion of study types and validity problems to be meaningful, some basic epidemiologic terms and concepts must be clear. Only the most essential ones are introduced here; the rest can be found in textbooks on epidemiology.

Crude Measures of Morbidity

Because epidemiology is concerned with the study of the occurrence of illness, a central event is the transition of individuals from the state of being healthy to that of being ill. When this change occurs in a population, it is referred to as the *incidence* of the particular disease. Hence, incidence is a measure of *new cases* occurring in a population during a certain period. By contrast, *prevalence* is a measure of all *existing cases* in the population at some point in time.

Incidence rate (IR) can be expressed as follows:

$$\text{IR} = \frac{\text{number of new cases occurring during a period of time}}{\text{average size of the population during the same time period}}$$

Similarly, *prevalence rate* (PR) denotes the proportion of people affected with the illness, and it can be expressed as

$$\text{PR} = \frac{\text{number of existing cases}}{\text{size of the population}}$$

The IR can be expressed in two ways. The most common expression is *incidence density* (ID), which measures the number of new cases occurring in a population during a given period of time, as already explained. However, quite often the size of the population varies over the years. Consider, for example, the occurrence of lung cancer among workers in an iron foundry. Suppose the period of follow-up began in 1950 and that the foundry employed 1,000 workers in that year. In 1957, the foundry expanded and hired, say, another 500 workers. In addition, normal turnover accounted for, e.g., 500 new employees during 1950–1970, hired at irregular intervals throughout that period. Such a situation—which is common indeed—complicates the process of defining the average population. This difficulty can be overcome, however, if every worker is given a score denoting the number of years he or she has been in the study, i.e., the number of years "at risk." If the study spans 1951 through 1976, a worker employed at the beginning of the follow-up in 1951 has a score of 25 and another who was hired in 1961 has one of 15. These scores are called *person-years*. The person-years for all workers are added, and the sum replaces the average size of the population during the time interval studied. Consequently, IR can also be expressed as follows:

$$\text{IR} = \frac{\text{number of new cases}}{\text{total number of person-years}}$$

This type of IR is conceptually similar to the ID defined before, except that the denominator is of a different type. Incidence density is an abstract measure, and sometimes its meaning may be difficult to conceptualize. Another, more easily understandable measure of incidence is the *cumulative incidence rate* (CIR). The CIR can be defined as the proportion of the population that has become ill during a certain period of time. The CIR dimension is usually expressed as a percentage. For example, if 70 persons out of 1,000 incur lung cancer in 20 years, the CIR_{20} is approximately 7%.

Often there is a silent, asymptomatic period between the onset of exposure and the manifestation of disease. This *latency period* should be taken into account, if known, in the computation of person-years at risk. If its exact length is not known, one or two periods of tentative duration may be tried. In practice, then, the person-years during the latency period are not accounted for, i.e., the person in question is not yet "at risk" because not enough time has passed for him to acquire the illness. For example, if a worker was employed as an insulator (exposed to asbestos) in 1940 and if the mean latency period is 20 years, the computation of person-years should not start earlier than, say, 1950, which represents half that time. By 1978, he will have accrued 28 person-years instead of 38. The effect of this technique is that the expected figure becomes smaller. (Fewer cases are expected to occur in 28 years than in 38.) Of course, the observed figure also becomes smaller, but, if there is indeed an occupational factor causing cancer, the effect on that figure is not so marked, since the "occupational" cases will appear after the end of the latency period. It should be stressed that allowing for a latency period does not bring about an artificial "manipulation" of the data, since this concept is based on a true biologic phenomenon.

A *rate* is a characteristic of a *population*, not of its members. In contrast, *risk* characterizes the *individual*. The risk is the probability of an individual to develop a particular illness. Being a probability measure, risk is not observable, but it can be calculated for each individual sharing the characteristics of a population for which the CIR is known.

Two rates obtained from different populations, be they PRs, IDs, or CIRs, can be compared by dividing the rate of the "exposed" group by that of the reference group. Hence, the *rate ratio* (RR) (synonyms: risk ratio, relative risk) can be defined as the rate of the exposed group over the rate of the reference category, or

$$RR = R_{exp}/R_{ref}$$

If the RR is greater than 1, the risk of contracting a particular disease is greater in the exposed group; if it is lower than 1, the risk is lower. Provided that the study is valid (see section "Validity"), exposure can be inferred to cause disease in the first case and prevent it in the second. The RR as such is a point estimate and subject to random variation (i.e., if the study were to be repeated, the RR would vary due to chance). Hence, confidence limits should also be given that indicate the probability (e.g., 95% or 99% probability) of the "true" RR being within these limits. If the lower confidence limit is greater than 1, statistically the RR is significantly greater than 1.

The difference between two rates, the *rate difference* (RD), can be computed by subtracting the rate of the reference group from that of the exposed group, i.e.,

$$RD = R_{exp} - R_{ref}$$

In a case-referent study, the *exposure* frequencies are being compared between the groups. The *odds ratio* (OR) is the ratio between the proportions of exposed to unexposed cases and exposed to unexposed referents. (The RR, the RD, and the OR are described further in this chapter, in the section "Epidemiologic Study Types and Their Applications in Occupational Health Research.")

Adjusted Measures of Morbidity

All morbidity measures are dependent on some basic characteristics of the population(s) being studied, e.g., the age and sex distributions. Crude rates are computed irrespective of the properties of the population. They are obtained simply by dividing the number of prevalent or incident cases by the size of the population. Crude RRs and RDs are computed in a similar manner. A meaningful comparison of crude rates presupposes that the populations concerned have a similar distribution of basic characteristics such as age, gender, or geographic area.

If the basic characteristics are not similar, the rates must be adjusted. An adjusted rate can be obtained if the distribution of characteristics of the population under study is changed artificially to correspond with that of some other population. For example, the age distribution of the reference category can be weighted so as to correspond to that of the exposed group, or vice versa. Standardization is a method by which the rates of two or more populations are adjusted to correspond with a common distribution—the standard. The best known standardized measure is the *standardized mortality ratio*, the SMR. This measure is often used when the mortality of an "exposed" group is compared to "expected values" derived from the general population. Hence,

$$SMR = \text{observed cases/expected cases} = O/E$$

The expected values are obtained from the actual mortality rates of the general population, but its age structure is adjusted to correspond with that of the exposed group. Consequently, the actual rates in each age category become weighted so as to describe the mortality of a hypothetical general population with the same age structure as that of the exposed group. Adjustment is usually done also for different periods of a lengthy follow-up.

Because this procedure has to be accomplished separately for each exposed group with its age distribution as the standard, two or more SMRs cannot be directly compared. They are not, in fact, mutually standardized, since the expected figures in each case depend on the age structure of the exposed group in question.[33, 49]

The SMR, obtained by dividing observed rates by the expected ones, is customarily multiplied by 100. Hence, an SMR greater than 100 denotes increased risk in the exposed group. Standardized mortality ratios of less than 100 are more difficult to interpret because of a number of factors leading to a better-than-expected mortality experience in occupationally active populations. This "healthy worker" effect is discussed in the section "Guidelines for Interpreting Epidemiologic Studies."

Computation of person-years at risk is sometimes difficult or even impossible; for example, when personnel records are deficient or lacking. When denominator data are not available, an increase in the *cause-specific* mortality can be shown by means of the *proportional mortality ratio* (PMR). The PMR compares the *proportion* (percentage) of deaths due to a particular cause occurring in an exposed population with "expected" ones, obtained from national figures. The PMR is usually adjusted for age and calendar period, if needed, in an analogous manner with the SMR. With the symbols presented in Table 71–1, the PMR can be expressed in the following way:

$$PMR = (a/a+c)/(b/b+d)$$

From this formula it is evident that any excess or defect in the other causes of death *(c)* changes the proportion (a/a + c) attributable to the cause in question *(a)*. Consequently, if one cause is in excess, there *must* be a deficit of the others, taken together. An excess of a major "other" cause, say, cardiovascular disease, may thus mask a true excess of, say, cancer. The PMR is therefore a poor substitute for the SMR. The proportion of violent deaths is greater than the average among blue-collar workers, and this results in a correspondingly lower proportion of natural causes. The bias caused by violent deaths can be avoided if the distribution of

TABLE 71–1.
Layout for the Computation of PMR

NUMBER OF DEATHS	EXPOSED	UNEXPOSED
Cause of interest	a	b
Other causes	c	d
Proportionate mortality	a/(a + c)	b/(b + d)
PMR	$\frac{a/(a + c)}{b/(b + d)}$	

natural causes of death is studied separately, but variations in the proportion of some major "other" natural cause are always a source of concern.

Proportional mortality data, despite their inherent weaknesses and a more difficult interpretation, may offer the first clue to an occupational factor leading to an elevated cause-specific mortality of some disease. For example, in 1967, our research team found that 52% of the workers in a viscose rayon factory had died of coronary artery disease during the period 1945 to 1966, the expected mortality figure being only 32%. The PMR was 163. Subsequently, a follow-up study revealed 14 coronary deaths between 1967 and 1972 among the exposed cohort (343 men) in contrast to only 3 corresponding deaths in an equal-sized matched reference cohort selected from local paper-mill workers. The RR of 4.7 was statistically significant.[52]

An alternative to the PMR has recently been suggested by Miettinen and Wang.[37] They call it the *mortality odds ratio* (MOR) and compute it by taking the *odds* for the cause of interest. Again, with the symbols given in Table 71–1,

$$\text{MOR} = (a/c)/(b/d)$$

If the rates for the "other" causes *c* and *d* are the same, the MOR gives a good estimate of the SMR. The MOR is independent of how large or small the number of "other" causes is. An alternative way of computing the MOR is to select one or a few "other" causes instead of all "other" causes. This procedure helps sharpen the criteria for the reference causes of death so that they indeed are neither caused nor prevented by the exposure of interest.

SOURCES OF INFORMATION

Many countries, among them the Nordic ones, have excellent central and local registers that make it easy to obtain data for epidemiologic research, but many other countries are not so privileged. The registers can, broadly speaking, be classified into *vital records* and *exposure registers*.

Vital Records

Vital records, the two main types of which are death and morbidity registers, are essential for epidemiologic research. Yet their shortcomings must be realized. Death registration is more or less complete in the United States, Canada, Europe, and Japan, but this is certainly not the case in many other parts of the world. As a rule, death registers are central, national ones, but there are also local registers, such as parish registers. Morbidity registers may also be national, such as the national health care registers and cancer registers of the Nordic countries, or local, such as the coronary or stroke registers in several counties and cities around the world.

Although the fact of death can be accepted as a certainty, the registered cause is less reliable. The reliability of death registers is to some extent related to the frequency of autopsies in a country—but not always, because a death certificate may be completed before the autopsy and not amended to include later findings.[28] Furthermore, different diseases are recorded in different proportions. For example, cancer usually appears on a high proportion of death certificates, whereas other diseases, such as diabetes, hypertension, and pneumonia, are not recorded to the same extent even if present at the time of death.[28] Multiple causes of death further confuse the picture. Although two or more diagnoses appear on more than half of the death certificates listed in most registers, only one is usually taken into account in mortality statistics.

The use of death statistics in the study of causal relations between disease and occupation is also hampered by the fact that the data on occupation is usually deficient. There are two main reasons. First, no satisfactory system for coding occupations for investigative purposes exists. Second, the recorded occupation seldom yields relevant information about the entire exposure history of a person. Most workers have been employed in several jobs during their lifetime, and their last employment (the end occupation) is often without any significance with respect to possible occupational risks. Therefore, crude death registers alone are of little or no value for the establishment of causal connections between occupation and disease. Morbidity statistics are even less useful for this purpose because of diagnostic uncertainties and reporting defects, and therefore they are useless as such for the study of causal connections.

Vital statistics are useful in other ways, however. First, they are the basis for the computation of expected figures. Second, they provide relevant data once the population group or disease under study has been defined from other sources. For example, it is possible to form a cohort fulfilling certain exposure criteria from, say, a paper mill and then to note the numbers and causes of death from the register during a follow-up period. From population or social security registers it is also possible in many countries to trace subjects who have "disappeared" or at least check whether they are dead or alive or have emigrated. For example, in a case-referent study, one may select from the cancer register all those who have died of a certain form of neoplasm during a given period of time, whereafter exposure data can be obtained from relatives and employers.

Exposure Registers

If an exposure is broadly defined, exposure registers include employee rolls, registers of occupational groups (e.g., physicians, dentists, divers, bricklayers), or military records. In some countries, sales and customs records are kept on toxic compounds. Moreover, International Labour Organization convention 139, concerning the prevention and control of occupational hazards caused by carcinogens, has (by the end of 1986) been ratified by more than 20 countries, among them Denmark, the Federal Republic of Germany, Finland, Hungary, Italy, Japan, Norway, Sweden,

Switzerland, and Yugoslavia, but not Canada and the United States. The ratifying countries have committed themselves to set up nationwide registers of *workers exposed to carcinogens*. However, thus far, only Finland has done so,[20] although some restricted regional compilation of exposure data is underway, at least in Ontario, Canada, and Tuscany, Italy. Because of the inexact and crude quality of the exposure data collected routinely from employers and because there should be at least a strong suspicion of carcinogenicity before a chemical is added to the list, it is doubtful if such registers can ever aid epidemiologic research on occupational cancer. New carcinogens cannot be identified, and the exposure data are too crude and inexact for the estimation of exposure-response relationships. At most, registers of this type may aid the definition of exposed groups, and they may help locate scattered and rare exposures. But their quality cannot be very good, and hence their usefulness will always be limited.

In occupational epidemiology, *population registers* are mainly used for tracing persons who have "disappeared" during a follow-up. The situation is somewhat different in public health research, which utilizes such registers for several other purposes.

An alarming trend is that the increasing public demand for privacy is progressively restricting the use of registers, especially vital records, in research work. In some countries—for example, France, the Federal Republic of Germany, and Sweden—legislation already prohibits registries from delivering individual data to "outsiders," among them research workers. Of course, personal integrity must be protected, but regulations that are too strict make the use of registers impossible for research purposes.

Linkage

The easy availability of computers has raised the problem of linking vital records with exposure registers. However, the quality control of large amounts of data is more difficult than that of more limited amounts, and no register can be more reliable than the data fed into it. Furthermore, since register data are usually compiled for some purpose other than the actual study, they do not take into account the special needs of the latter. Many of the inaccuracies may be unsystematic, i.e., misclassifications of a random type. Hence, they do not lead to false positive conclusions but they do mask true positive findings. On the other hand, systematic errors may also be involved, such as regional overreporting of some disease, different nomenclature for cause of illness, or for occupations, and overclassification or underclassification of workers exposed to, say, carcinogens. Because statistically significant P values are easily yielded from small differences in large series, such flaws may result in grossly erroneous conclusions if record linkage is (mis)used uncritically and "significances" are judged without insight. Falsely significant results can thus be due both to systematic errors and the "mass-significance" phenomenon, i.e., when enough comparisons are made without a prior hypothesis, some "significances" will result by definition (one out of 20, 100, or 1,000, depending on the criterion). Finally, in practice, setting up registers without any specified aim other than that they may be useful for linkage becomes very expensive due to the vast amount of data computerized that are irrelevant to a particular problem. All these circumstances greatly restrict the intelligent use of crude register data, and mechanical linkage of registers exposes the uncritical user to the danger of drawing too far-reaching or completely erroneous conclusions. However, the danger of overlooking true problems is even more imminent. Hence, even a small, well-planned, and controlled *ad hoc* study is preferable to the mechanical linkage of large registers. This is a well-known fact among experienced epidemiologists, but it may be hard to comprehend for those less familiar with scientific epidemiologic research.

Ad Hoc Registers

If there are no useful basic registers, which often is the case, information regarding the study population must be gathered in another way. The first task then is to define the problem in terms of the quality, minimal duration, and intensity of exposure, and the age, sex, and geographic area of the exposed population. Subsequently, employee rolls form the basis for an ad hoc register of all persons complying with the established criteria. After examining the size of the exposed population and the nature of the problem, the researcher may either select a suitable group from his or her compiled register or include all persons in the study (census). Of course, no register can be established if employee rolls are lacking or insufficient. In such a situation, the study cannot utilize retrospective data, and the only option becomes a prospective follow-up. Similarly, in case-referent studies, autopsy records, hospital records and industrial health service records can be used in the absence of basic morbidity registers. However, the use of such sources poses problems, because the diagnostic accuracy of primary health care records in particular may be rather poor. Nondifferential diagnostic misclassification always tends to mask an existing effect.

Measures of Exposure

The need to ensure good exposure data, especially when a quantitative study is being planned, cannot be stressed too much. A hierarchic order (from the point of view of usefulness in exposure-response research) of the dimension of the exposure variable can be constructed in the following way:

1. Biologic measurements (such as blood, urine, alveolar air)

2. Air samples collected from the breathing zone with the aid of portable samplers

3. Area sampling by stationary samplers

4. Classification of the exposed subjects by work area, type of work, and occupational title

5. Classification into "exposed" and "unexposed"

Exposure should not only be classified according to intensity, but also according to duration, fluctuations (peak exposures may be highly relevant), and calendar time (which is important, for example, when studying occupational cancers with a long latency). Concurrent other exposures should also be accounted for. The worst problem is usually that retrospective exposure data are lacking or inaccurate. While measuring *present* levels, at least in theory, is always possible, there is little remedy for missing data for *past* levels. This lack may, in fact, render the study completely unfeasible. Some information might, however, be obtained through a comparison of the current situation and judgments of past conditions provided by old workers, foremen, and safety personnel ("four times worse in the 1950s"). Careful history-taking of the cumulative amounts of a chemical used may also sharpen the exposure estimation. In addition, the time of major improvements, such as the installation of exhaust ventilation, is usually listed in a company's records. The result, of course, will be a coarse classification into, for example, heavy, medium, light, and no exposure, which may be sufficient for qualitative studies but quite insufficient for exposure-effect and exposure-response studies. Sometimes it has been possible to simulate past conditions by reconstructing old workplaces, but such opportunities are rare exceptions.

Inaccurate exposure data, leading to random misclassifications, always mask existing effects, that is, they produce falsely negative results. Likewise, in a study on exposure-effect or exposure-response relationships they flatten the regression slope. *Exposure* data of poor quality are therefore a very important reason for failing to find an exposure-effect or exposure-response relationship where one actually exists.

Measures of Effect

When selecting parameters for a study, the researcher should always consider the optimal "hardness." In general, the harder the parameter, the more reliable the information. As mentioned before, the event of death is subject to no ambiguity, but already the cause of death is less reliable. The softer the parameter, the greater the possibility for error. Questionnaires, for instance, may give highly misleading data in inexperienced hands, and their use requires careful standardization of the method and critical interpretation of the results. Yet it does not necessarily follow that hard parameters should always be preferred. Death is such a crude measure that a mortality study can reveal only the most severe health hazards. In addition, several ailments, such as disorders of the musculoskeletal system, mental disease, and eczema, do not appear in mortality statistics at all, and when milder health effects such as fatigue, dizziness, nausea, neurasthenia, or mucosal irritation are being studied, no better methods than interviews or questionnaires exist. Thus the ideal hardness of a parameter depends on the problem to be studied.

Some occupational disorders are characterized by *exposure-specific* symptoms and signs. For example, lead causes certain well-defined disturbances in heme synthesis, measurable, for example, as an increased excretion of Δ-aminolevulinic acid in the urine. On the other hand, quite *nonspecific* effects belong to the picture of many occupational disorders. For example, dust exposure may cause bronchitis that usually does not differ from smoking-related bronchitis. Both specific and nonspecific effects can be used for studying exposure-effect and exposure-response relationships. It is also important to study the order in which various effects appear. In general, the protection of workers should aim at the prevention of the earliest effects.

EPIDEMIOLOGIC STUDY TYPES AND THEIR APPLICATIONS IN OCCUPATIONAL HEALTH RESEARCH

Epidemiologic studies are either cross-sectional or longitudinal. In a cross-sectional study, the observation of both the cause and the effect is related to a single point in time, whereas in longitudinal studies their measurement is separated by a time interval, even though the collection of data may take place simultaneously.

Cross-sectional studies are prevalence studies, often descriptive, and their main use is in health administration (e.g., the prevalence of diabetics needing regular control, say, among plant personnel). Etiologic research, on the other hand, usually requires a longitudinal study design. A cross-sectional study is useful in etiologic research in only very few situations, namely, when the effect is immediately time-related to the exposure (as with the acute effects of irritant gases), when exposure is relatively permanent in relation to the effect (as with steady lead exposure and neurophysiologic abnormalities), or when the effect is of long duration and its selective force is negligible (as in noise-induced hearing loss in various types of work). Therefore, longitudinal studies form the basis for etiologic epidemiology.

Cross-Sectional Studies

Cross-sectional studies measure the cause (exposure) and the effect at the same point in time. They compare the rates of diseases or symptoms of an exposed and an unexposed group, e.g., the prevalence of symptoms of bronchial irritation among pulp workers exposed to chlorine and among some other group of workers not exposed to chlorine. This study type can be viewed as a cohort study where the time span is zero. Purely descriptive cross-sectional surveys, made for health administrative purposes, do not even require measurements of exposure (e.g., mere estimation of the prevalence of diabetes in a group of employees). However, as soon as other aspects become involved, some measure of the exposure—even if it is as broad as the district of habitation—must be included. Since, by definition, the exposure status is considered at the time the effects are measured, there must be a biologic rationale before a temporal relation between the two measures can be assumed. In other words, unless the current exposure intensity or, alternatively, past exposure as reflected by the current level could be responsible for the effects under scrutiny theoretically, the relationship is meaningless. For example, the prevalence of silicosis in a foundry has little to do with current dust concentrations. But current exposure to lead, measured from the lead concentration in blood or urine, can be related to the current urinary excretion of Δ-aminolevulinic acid; hence, a cross-sectional study of the interrelationship between these parameters is valid. Similarly, if no major changes in exposure have taken place over the years, the current concentration of lead in blood can then be (etiologically) related to a slowing of conduction velocities in peripheral nerves. If variations in the intensity of exposure have occurred, some other parameter, e.g., the time-weighted average concentration of lead in blood, is more representative, and a purely cross-sectional design is not suitable.

Longitudinal Studies

Longitudinal studies are conventionally divided into cohort studies, case-referent studies, and intervention studies. A dynamic population-based design, in which people move in and out of the study base, can often be applied in public health research, but it has gained little use in occupational epidemiology because of the selectiveness involved in entering a job and, especially, in leaving it.

Cohort Studies

In a cohort study (synonym: follow-up study), the groups under scrutiny—the exposed and unexposed cohorts—are defined on the basis of *exposure*. In this sense the situation is the same as in an experiment, where the investigator randomly allocates experimental animals into the exposed and unexposed groups. The basic distinctions are that, in epidemiology, unlike in experiments, no randomization is possible, the exposure intensity cannot be decided, and confounding exposures often occur.

When selected into the exposed cohort, the subject must fulfill certain criteria set up in advance (e.g., age, gender, minimum exposure). Then the cohort is followed over a period of time, or its members are traced at the end of the period, and all new cases (the incidence) of the disease(s) under study are recorded. The morbidity rate of the exposed cohort may be contrasted to "expected" figures computed from the experience of the general population and adjusted for age, sex, and calendar time, but preferably the incidence is compared to that of an unexposed cohort that is similar in as many relevant ways as possible except for the exposure (Fig 71–1). Because the cohorts are formed on the basis of exposure or its absence, only *one exposure* can usually be considered at a time. On the other hand, this design permits the study of several different diseases simultaneously.

Traditionally, a fixed cohort design is preferred in occupational health epidemiology. Alternatively, all those employed at a certain *point* in time (cross-sectional base), or those hired during a certain *period* of time (entry base), form the cohort. It is not irrelevant which approach is chosen. The effect(s) under study tend(s) to become diluted by the cross-sectional base design, while the entry base design results in high turnover and thereby short exposure times for a large proportion of subjects. All those who are accepted into the cohort must be traced irrespective of the exposure status at the end of the follow-up, and their health state must be recorded (Fig 71–2). In contrast, when the base is a *dynamic population*, new entries are accepted throughout the investigation. Those who drop out are not accounted for and, accordingly, need not be traced. Unfortunately, this effort-saving design can be utilized only rarely in occupational health research, because the turnover may be largely due to health selection. However, in public health studies, a dynamic population design is often appropriate.

A cohort study may be *retrospective* (historical) or *prospective* (concurrent). In both cases, the scientific logic is the same, the principal differences being timing and methodology. In a retrospective cohort study, the cohorts are defined at a suitable point or period in time in the past, e.g., 20–30 years earlier. The members then are *traced* over time, usually to the present (or, for practical reasons, to one or two years before the present—for example, to ensure accumulation of pertinent morbidity data in the registers). Retrospective cohort studies usually focus on mortality, since other reliable retrospective data are seldom available. Prospective cohorts are defined in the present and *followed* into the future for a number of years. This design permits the recording of a variety of morbidity data, not only deaths.

As explained previously, the various measures of disease occurrence are computed as rates, i.e., the proportion of disease in the exposed and unexposed cohorts (Table 71–2).

When two rates are compared, the *rate ratio* (risk ratio, relative risk, RR) is computed in the following way (for symbols, see Table 71–1):

$$RR = [a/(a+b)]/[c/(c+d)]$$

An RR of 1 denotes no observed difference between the cohorts. If it is greater, there is more disease, and, if lower, less disease in the exposed cohort. When no reference cohort is available (e.g., for economic reasons) the overall and cause-specific mortality (rarely morbidity) experiences of the exposed cohort can be contrasted with those of the general population and adjusted for age,

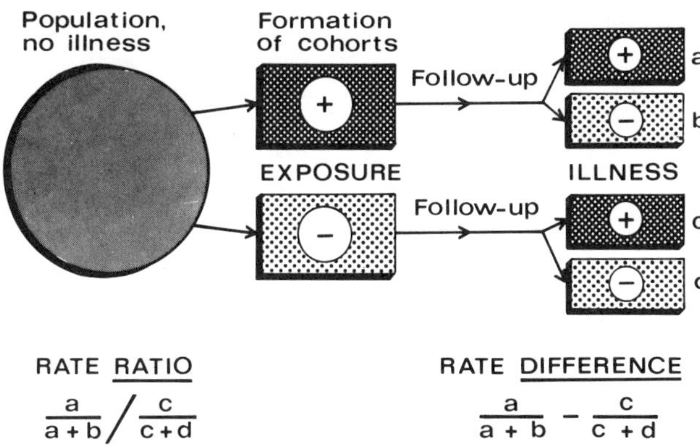

FIG 71–1.
General outline of a cohort study.

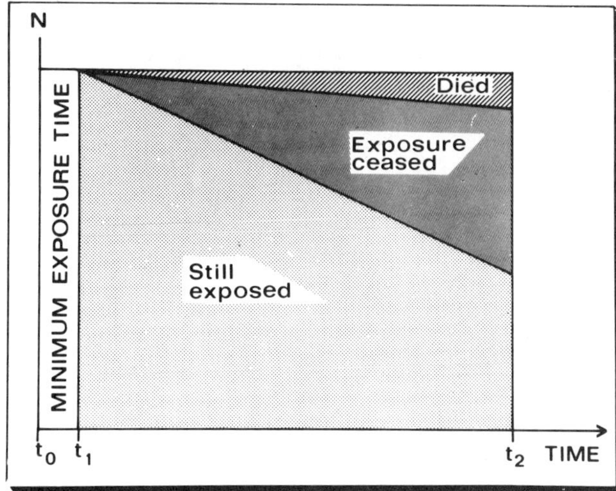

FIG 71–2.
Typical fixed cohort constellation, where the definition of the cohort is cross-sectional.

TABLE 71–2.
General Outline for Data From Cohort Studies

	DISEASE		
COHORTS	PRESENT	ABSENT	TOTAL
Exposed	a	b	a + b
Unexposed	c	d	c + d
Total	a + c	b + d	

gender, and calendar time. In this case, the rate ratio is called the standardized mortality ratio, or the SMR. An SMR in excess of 100 denotes an increased risk in the exposed cohort and one below 100 a decreased risk. (But note the "healthy worker effect" discussed later in this chapter.)

Whereas the RR gives a proportional estimate of the risk, the *rate or risk difference* (RD) yields an absolute measure of it. The RD is computed as follows:

$$RD = a/(a+b) - c/(c+d)$$

Figure 71–3 shows the difference in the information obtained with the RR and the RD. The former is a measure of the *strength* of the association, i.e., the biologic effect, the latter of the severity of the problem in terms of *number* of excess cases. Comparisons between the exposed cohort and the reference population are conventionally subjected to statistical testing but, as is discussed later, scientific inferences cannot be drawn merely from *P* values.

Case-Referent Studies

In case-referent studies (synonyms: case control study, case-history study), the groups are defined on the basis of *disease* (cases) or its *absence* (referents) (Fig 71–4). The issue is now to obtain an indirect estimate of the rate ratio by comparing the *exposure* frequencies among cases and referents.

A general outline for data from an unmatched case-referent study is shown in Table 71–3. Similar tables can be constructed for each exposure studied. From this outline the *exposure odds* can be compared for cases and referents. For the cases, the odds are a/b and for the referents c/d. Consequently, the *odds ratio* (OR) can be calculated as follows:

$$OR = (a/b)/(c/d) = ad/bc.$$

	"COMMON"		"RARE"	
	Obs.	Exp.	Obs.	Exp.
INCIDENCE DENSITY (cases / 10 000 person-years)	150	100	2	0.01
RATE RATIO	$150/100 = \underline{1.5}$		$2/0.01 = \underline{200}$	
RATE DIFFERENCE	$150-100 = \underline{50}$		$2-0.01 = \underline{1.99}$	

FIG 71–3.
Computation of rate ratio and rate difference from a cohort study. Comparison between these measures in the case of a "common" and a "rare" disease.

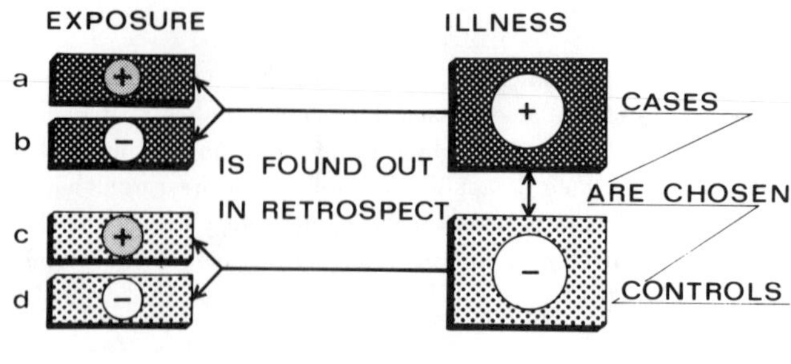

ODDS RATIO: $\frac{a}{b} / \frac{c}{d} = ad / bc$

FIG 71–4.
General outline of a case-referent study.

The OR gives a measure of how much more or less frequently the cases have been exposed to the factor under study. Under some conditions the *rate ratio* for the disease in question in the target population can be estimated from the OR. The conditions are that, first, there must be no selection bias, i.e., the cases and noncases are representative of the target population. Second, the disease must be rare in the target population. However, this second condition is not always obligatory. (See the following discussion.)

There are three types of case-referent studies.[5] In a *density type* of case-referent study, incident cases are collected during a certain period of time and compared with regard to past exposure(s) with referents drawn from an open, dynamic base population. The referents can be drawn either as a random sample of noncases or as individuals with "noncase" diagnoses. If another disease is used as the reference category, it must be a condition which is neither caused nor prevented by the exposure(s) under scrutiny; in other words, totally unrelated to it (them). In a density-type case-referent study, the OR estimates the RR without any rare-disease assumption.[35] In other words, the ratio ad/bc can be regarded as a true rate ratio.

If a sample of referents is taken from those individuals of a stable or closed population who remain healthy at the end of the study period, the study can be termed a *cumulative incidence* type of case-referent study. This type can also be thought of as a "nested" case-referent study. The ratio ad/bc is now merely an OR, and it requires the "rare-disease" assumption to be interpreted in terms of the RR.[5]

The third type can be referred to as a *prevalence type* of case-referent study. Prevalent cases and noncases are sampled. In order for the sample to be unbiased, the duration of the disease must not depend on the exposure.

In all types of studies, an alternative to using noncases as referents is to draw a random sample of the base population, including both cases and noncases. This method would yield an es-

TABLE 71–3.
General Outline for Data From Case-Referent Studies (Unmatched Series)

	EXPOSED	NONEXPOSED	TOTAL
Cases	a	b	a + b
Referents	c	d	c + d

timate of the exposure frequency in the *whole base population*, not only among the noncases. Procedurally this approach may be difficult, however.

Often the referents are *matched* to the cases with respect to some parameters, such as age, gender, and geographic area. For each case, one or more referents can be used. Their number depends on how easily available they are. However, more than four referents for each case increases the statistical efficiency of the study only slightly.[31] For unmatched series, a balanced design (i.e., equal-sized groups) is optimal.

The analysis of matched series concentrates on pairs which are discordant with respect to the exposure in question, i.e., the case is exposed but not the referent, or the referent is exposed but not the case. Concordant pairs, i.e., both the case and the referent or neither the case nor the referent (usually the largest category) are exposed, are not considered at all. Table 71–4 shows a general outline for data from a matched (one-to-one) case-referent study. In the analysis, A and D are disregarded, and the ratio B/C is the one which contains the information. Note that each cell is composed of *pairs*, not single individuals.

Since the groups of a case-referent study are defined on the basis of presence or absence of a given disease, only *one disease* can be studied at a time. In contrast, many exposures can be studied simultaneously (cf. cohort studies, where the circumstances are reversed). Exposure data in a case-referent study are usually collected by interviews and questionnaires.

A *"nested" case-referent* study is nowadays used more and more often to save costs. In this type of investigation the cohort is defined first. However, instead of all members being studied, only cases and a *sample* of noncases are compared with regard to exposure history. One requirement is that sufficient *variations* in exposure intensity and duration occur within the basic cohort. If such variations are not likely, or if the exposure data are quantitatively unreliable, unexposed categories can be included in the study base on purpose. Next, the cases (of whatever the disease under study is) and a sample of noncases are drawn, and exposure histories are collected for both groups and compared in the usual way.

The nesting is effective only when the disease is common enough (or the population large enough) to yield a sufficient number of cases. The advantage over a cohort design is that one can neglect the exposure histories of all those who are neither cases nor referents, and therefore a lot of effort is saved. In addition, compared with a conventional case-referent design, one can "enrich" exposure and thereby add efficiency. However, the more common the disease, the more the OR overestimates the true risk.

TABLE 71–4.
General Outline for Data From a Matched Case-Referent Study (One-to-One Matching)

CASES	REFERENTS EXPOSED	REFERENTS NONEXPOSED
Exposed	A	B
Nonexposed	C	D

Intervention Studies

In contrast to the study types described so far, in which the investigator passively observes what nature has accomplished (sometimes with the help of man), the intervention study utilizes active manipulation on the part of the investigator. This active approach bears some resemblance to an experiment, and therefore interventive epidemiology is often referred to as experimental epidemiology. The use of the latter term has resulted in some confusion, because some authors like to include a variety of experimentation under this heading.

In this discussion an intervention study is an investigation of what happens to an exposed cohort after a change in exposure level. In principle this change can be an increase, a decrease or a complete cessation of exposure. However, in practice, any *intended* change in exposure conditions must be downwards for ethical reasons, while unintended changes may occur in both directions. In this constellation the only thing in common with a true experiment is the change in the exposure conditions and the before-after comparison. There is no randomization (not possible in real life), and other concomitant effect modifiers can usually not be controlled.

A clinical trial is in sharp contrast to this design, being a true experiment. It is an *experimental* study, where subjects are *randomly* allocated into those receiving treatment and those who do not. The latter group usually receives a "placebo" treatment without medical effect. Neither the subjects nor the investigator should be aware of who belongs to the treated group and who receives the placebo treatment (double blinding). Alternatively, some old, established treatment can be used instead of the placebo. The confusion mentioned earlier in reference to experimental epidemiology stems from the fact that some authors include clinical trials—even certain animal experiments—in this approach (e.g., reference 26). Why not let epidemiology be epidemiology and experiments remain experiments?

According to the narrower concept, an intervention study can be thought of as a continuation of a cohort study. The baseline data of the exposed group is collected during the "cohort stage," then comes the intervention, and at the "postintervention" stage the effect of the intervention is evaluated. The data are collected in the same way during both stages, and, in addition to comparisons with a reference population, the morbidity experience within the cohort can be studied in a before-after fashion. The reference population may be one whose members have always been unexposed, or it can be another exposed group without intervention, or both. Although intervention studies, defined in this manner, can never reach the same validity as true experiments, documented changes in morbidity occurring after changes in the exposure give rather strong support for the probability of a causal relation between exposure and effect.

However, unfortunately, intervention studies are rare in occupational epidemiology, especially if public health research within an occupational setting (such as antismoking and antihypertensive campaigns) is not included. The epidemiologist rarely has the opportunity to influence exposure conditions actively to suit his or her intentions, although he or she sometimes may happen to be "on the spot" when strong enough (from the study efficiency point of view) improvements are made in work conditions for reasons other than epidemiologic research. Then an "intervention study" can be improvised. The very alert epidemiologist may even succeed in getting access to situations where the exposure levels have deteriorated unintentionally. But the literature indicates that the epidemiologist is rarely present when changes occur, and even then potential studies face difficulties, sometimes insurmountable design problems. For example, the baseline morbidity experience may be unrecorded, the intervention may cause selective turnover of the workers (e.g., if completely new technology is being introduced), the observations before and after the intervention may not be comparable, or no suitable reference groups can be found. If long latency times are involved, the effects initiated before the intervention (e.g., cancer) become manifest long after the intervention. Therefore, the possible effects of the intervention become evident after the end of the latency time, and a time span double that of a simple cohort study will be needed, possibly even up to some 60 years.

A continuation of our 1967 cohort study[52] on the connection between exposure to carbon disulfide and coronary artery disease may serve as an example of occupational interventive epidemiology. When it became clear from the results of a five-year prospective follow-up that there was a several-fold excess mortality of coronary artery disease, the exposure intensity was sharply reduced in the next two years. In addition, workers with "coronary risk factors" or early manifestations of the disease (hyperlipemia, hypertension, angina, and electrocardiographic findings) were removed to departments without exposure. These changes meant that only 17% of the original cohort was exposed in 1976. Follow-up of the coronary mortality in the period 1975–1982 revealed that no difference any longer existed between the exposed cohort and the reference group.[42]

This "intervention" illustrates some of the problems facing the occupational epidemiologist. First, it did not occur suddenly, but over a period of two years, so it is difficult to pinpoint exactly the shift from "before" to "after." Second, the intervention affected those who were totally removed from exposure (who in addition were selected according to high risk) differently than those remaining. On the other hand, our team of investigators had the opportunity to collaborate with the company at all times, and we could therefore plan the continuous follow-up rather well.

Advantages and Limitations of Different Study Designs

Longitudinal designs are in general to be preferred over cross-sectional ones in etiologic research; however, no single study type is *in principle* superior to all others. The choice of the approach depends on several factors, and quite often the same, scientifically "true" result can be obtained in different ways.

Since the limitations of cross-sectional studies have already been discussed, and longitudinal studies are by far the most important sources of epidemiologic knowledge in occupational medicine, only longitudinal designs are discussed in this section.

Prospective or Retrospective Timing?

The fact that *timing* and *design* differ conceptually may be difficult to understand, but the distinction must be kept clear. Prospective follow-up studies are always—and intervention studies usually—*timed* prospectively; i.e., they start in the present and move forward. In contrast, retrospective follow-up studies are always and case-referent studies are usually *timed* retrospectively, i.e., they deal with past events. Sometimes the collection of cases in a case-referent study can be based on incident cases, and then its timing in fact is prospective. However, the *design* of a retrospective follow-up study is prospective, because it moves *forward* to the present from some point in the past; a case-referent study is always retrospective in this regard also.

Retrospectively timed studies offer the *advantage* that the results become available rather quickly, usually within a few years. In a retrospective cohort study, whose starting point lies in the past, the end-point events (case events) have already occurred. The problem is to trace and find the cohort members, both the exposed and unexposed, rather than to wait for the development of disease. Also, in a case-referent study the cases are already at hand. Still, a *disadvantage* of retrospective timing is that past exposure data usually are scanty, unreliable, or even nonexistent. The same is usually true for data on medical risk indicators, such as blood chemistry and blood pressure. Another restraint is that a retrospective cohort study must be confined to hard indicators of disease, usually death, since data on softer indicators are rarely available or, if recorded, are often unreliable. This limitation does not concern a case-referent study, however, which can well be based on morbidity, provided the diagnostic criteria are straightforward.

The following example illustrates typical features of a retrospective follow-up study. Ott and his co-workers[44] were interested in whether or not occupational exposure to benzene causes excess mortality, especially from leukemia. To study this problem, they designed a retrospective cohort study of the mortality of employees who had been employed in three different plants and exposed to benzene.

In this investigation, the fact that only mortality data could be used probably did not distort the results because of the severe prognosis of leukemia. But had the problem been one of, for example, colonic cancer with a curability of about 40%, the observed differences in mortality figures could have been affected by systematic differences in early diagnosis and treatment, not necessarily by an occupational factor.

The investigators identified the exposed workers from annual census lists for 1938–1970. Such a procedure is usually possible only in large companies with well-kept records. They abstracted job histories from personnel records, coded them according to a standardized system, and assigned one month as the minimal exposure time for entry into the cohort. This, of course, was an arbitrary decision. Stricter criteria would have resulted in loss of material, but, on the other hand, also in an accentuation of the risk.

Because of job mobility within the units, most employees had been exposed at more than one intensity. Some workers had also been exposed to other chemicals. Both of these circumstances are typical for epidemiologic studies in occupational medicine, irrespective of study type.

Measurements of exposure levels had been performed in the past, but, since they were occasional, extrapolations had to be made for a rough classification of the average exposure intensity. Assessment of exposure is difficult, especially in retrospective studies, and Ott and his collaborators were fortunate to have accessibility to better-than-average data.

The mortality analysis covered those hired between 1940 and 1974. In this respect, a usual—and sometimes practical—deviation from the strictly fixed cohort design was made—the investigators accepted entries until the end of 1973. However, in this case, a dilution of the possible effect arose from the liberal admissibility criteria, since a latency period is involved in the development of environmental cancers. Although the exact length of the latency time is not known, some allowance should be made for it. New entries should not be accepted, person-years should not be accounted for during the latency period, and cases occurring during that period should not be included. Whenever the length of the latency time is not known for certain, two or more different tentative latencies can be tried. In this case (based on experiences from radiation-induced leukemia), five and ten years could have been tested. But the investigators did not publish such data for leukemia, although they gave results for some major disease groups, analyzed in subcategories of different intervals since the beginning of exposure.

Through the Social Security Administration, the authors traced those who had left the company; they estimated the results to be 94% successful. The difficulty in tracing resigned and retired employees varies from one country to another, but the aim should be a success rate of at least 97%–98%.

The expected number of deaths was calculated indirectly from American white male mortality statistics for seven representative years between 1940 and 1970, and the SMRs were computed from the obtained figures. The overall mortality of the exposed cohort showed no excess, but three fatal cases of leukemia were found against the 0.8 expected. Statistically, the difference was almost significant ($P = .047$), but the expected figure would have been considerably lower had a latency time been allowed for when the person-years were calculated and had the minimal exposure criteria been stricter (e.g., at least one year). Hence, a very conservative estimate was obtained.

Prospective studies offer the following advantages: (1) the study can be better designed to meet the investigator's requirements; (2) exposure data can be systematically collected; (3) several indicators of the disease can be measured; (4) the measurements can be repeated over time if needed; (5) the methodology can be standardized and its validity checked and, finally, (6) an intervention can sometimes be combined with the follow-up. The main inconvenience of prospective timing is the long period sometimes required before the results are at hand. In the study of chronic diseases, such as occupational cancer, this period may be 20–40 years.

High expenses are often said to be an obstacle to prospective follow-up studies, but this is not necessarily true in terms of *cost per amount of information*. Because a prospective follow-up, in contrast to a retrospective one, allows the collection of a variety of both exposure and morbidity data, the absolute costs will, of course, be higher. But since much more information is gained, the costs in relative terms do not necessarily differ considerably. The key to cost reduction is to confine the collection of data to the most relevant items.

Prospective follow-up studies are rare in the literature on occupational medicine, and therefore suitable teaching examples are difficult to find. The following study was chosen to illustrate the difference as markedly as possible between this type of study and a retrospective mortality study (a prospective mortality study would be rather similar); it furthermore demonstrates that prospective studies can indeed be both quick and simple.

Tola and his co-workers[51] were interested in the time sequence of the appearance of lead-induced hematologic abnormalities. They studied 33 lead workers who had no prior occupational exposure to toxic agents. Freedom from disease at entry (in this case lead-induced disease) was ascertained in a preemployment examination. The following parameters were measured: blood and urinary lead, hemoglobin, hematocrit, erythrocyte Δ-aminolevulinic acid dehydratase (ALA-D) activity, and urinary Δ-aminolevulinic acid (ALA) and coproporphyrin (CP). The methods were strictly standardized and continually controlled. The original study plan involved starting the sampling before the beginning of exposure (day 0). Subsequent samples would then be taken on the second, fourth, and sixth days of exposure, followed by weekly samplings until the end of the third month, and two additional samplings at two-week intervals during the fourth month.

In this study, some of the benefits of a prospective design became evident: repeated measurements, inclusion of several parameters of disease, precise exposure data (repeated blood and urinary lead concentrations), and method control. Yet, some practical difficulties arose. First, the planned sampling scheme could not be followed rigorously because of weekends, sick leaves, and public holidays. Second, dropouts reduced the cohort so that only 18 persons remained in the study for more than 70 days. In two cases the blood lead level rapidly increased above the recommended value, and the exposure had to be interrupted.

Having subjects drop out before the minimal exposure criteria are met is probably the most difficult complication of a prospective follow-up because it causes waste of time and money. Later dropouts are not a loss in the same sense, but tracing them is necessary and may be costly. The other problem illustrated by this example is an ethical one. The investigator must never allow his examinees to be dangerously exposed; hence, there may arise a conflict between ethical and study-efficiency aspects.

The results of this study showed that the depression of ALA occurred without a time lag, whereas the increase in ALA and CP excretion in urine was delayed by some two to three weeks. The ALA and CP values concomitant to the blood lead values corresponded well with those found in cross-sectional studies. The establishment of the time sequence for these effects was the major benefit obtained by the prospective design utilized.

The major inconvenience of a prospective follow-up study—long waiting time for the results—was no problem in this example because a rather quick phenomenon was studied. But whenever the problem involves a long latency period (e.g., occupational cancer), it is understandable that the investigator prefers a retrospective approach. However, it seems appropriate to advise research institutes and companies to initiate long-term prospective follow-up studies for future benefit by defining risk groups and by monitoring their exposure systematically. Similarly, the routine use of continuous health monitoring of the personnel of a company could be effected through the standardization of test methods and "computer-minded" record keeping. These procedures would help overcome many of the difficulties faced today in the study of diseases with long latency times.

Cohort or Case-Referent Design?

Problems related to *timing* may also affect the decision of whether to use a follow-up or case-referent study, but they will not be discussed further. Instead, questions pertinent to different types of *designs* will be dealt with.

First, the type of hypothesis is relevant. A specific hypothesis of the form "A causes B" can in principle be studied either by an exposure-based (cohort) or a disease-based (case-referent) design. Both designs are basically equally valid in solving the problem, and feasibility determines the choice. For example, the first evidence in favor of the causal connection between cigarette smoking and bronchial cancer came from case-referent studies. Later, the same conclusion was reached in numerous follow-up studies, and still later it was confirmed by intervention studies.

An important distinction is that a case-referent study is the only sensible one when the *disease* is rare, whereas follow-up studies must be preferred when *exposure* is rare. Otherwise, enormous amounts of material would be required. However, the reverse is *not* necessarily true, i.e., that case-referent studies would be unsuitable for common diseases and follow-up studies for common exposures. The major advantage of a case-referent study over a follow-up one is its relative simplicity and its low cost. In a follow-up, most cohort members do not incur the disease in question, but, despite that, they must be followed or traced, and their exposure history must be recorded. Whenever the hypothesis is semispecific, or whenever there is no clear *a priori* hypothesis, the options are reduced. If the hypothesis states "exposure A causes diseases $B_1, B_2, \ldots B_i$," or if the question is "what is caused by A?", then the only epidemiologic option is a cohort design, because this design is exposure-based. By the same token, if the *a priori* hypothesis states that "disease B is caused by exposures $A_1, A_2, \ldots A_i$," or if the question is "what are the etiologies of disease B?", then a case-referent study is the only option, because the absence or presence of a certain disease is the basis of the design. These considerations concern single studies. Of course, one can also create a whole set of different studies to test "parts" of the semispecific hypothesis, one at a time, or case-referent or cohort studies can be designed to address two or more "parts" of the hypothesis. Then one conceptually deals with multiple studies testing several specific hypotheses simultaneously.

A good example of a multiple case-referent study has been published by Axelson and his colleagues.[6] The authors investigated the connection between exposure to arsenic and lung cancer in a large Swedish copper smeltery and, using separate series of cases, also some other diseases, among them coronary artery disease and "other cancers." The cases pertinent to this example had died from malignant lung tumors, and the referents were all those subjects who had died of any of the remaining causes. Both the cases and the referents were drawn from the register of deaths and burials in the local parish. One of the problems in this study was that, since arsenic may also cause several other diseases, liberal admission criteria for the referents would dilute the results. The investigators overcame this difficulty by having *separate series of cases* for all these diseases and by using the remaining diagnoses for the reference group. As always in retrospective studies, the assessment of exposure was a problem. The authors requested an experienced safety engineer to classify the probable exposure intensity into the following three categories: (1) one considerably below the previous hygienic standard of 0.5 mg/cu m, (2) one close to it, and (3) one exceeding it. Unlike Ott and his colleagues,[44] the Swedish authors allowed for a latency period for the development of lung cancer. They applied a median latency period of 34–36 years, and in the exposure classifications only exposures occurring before half the median latency period, i.e., 17 years, were considered. In short, a 4.6-fold increase was observed in the mortality from lung cancer for workers employed in the smeltery.

The obstacle of rare exposures can be avoided if the cases and referents are drawn from a geographic area where the particular exposure is much more common than in the country, state, county, or city at large. This was exactly how Axelson and his coworkers[6] proceeded in their study.

Several other aspects help determine optimal study design, but, as validity aspects are involved, they are discussed in the next section.

VALIDITY

Validity means the lack of systematic error or bias. A systematic error is one that distorts the results of a study in such a way that hypothetical replications of it would produce the same results under the same premises, so that a false conclusion is reached. There are two dimensions of validity: *internal* and *external*.[8] The former refers to how "true" the results of a study are with respect to the study itself. The latter stands for the generalizability of the results beyond time and place, i.e., to other similar situations and, finally, to the sphere of scientific theories.

Internal Validity

The components of internal validity can be classified into validity of selection, validity of observation, and validity of comparison.

Validity of Selection

Validity of selection means that the probability of a subject being nominated for the study must not depend in a systematic way on the disease or exposure under study. The effect of selection bias in *cross-sectional studies* can be illustrated by the following example. Let the problem be: Does physically strenuous work cause low-back disease? In a cross-sectional study, the groups are chosen according to current occupation. Suppose the investigator compares the prevalence of lumbar disease (using some fixed criteria) among forest workers with that of car assembly workers. In this design, a selection bias occurs because first, workers who already have back problems, knowing that lumbering is strenuous, may prefer other types of jobs. Second, some of those who develop back trouble during lumbering may have to quit. And, third, since forest work is heavier than car assembly, the same severity of lumbar disease may cause more sickness absence in forestry than in a car assembly plant at the time of the survey. Then, because of selection, sick persons are underrepresented among lumberjacks, and the possible effect of lumbering may totally or partly escape discovery (negative bias).

By contrast, the inverse effects of selection may cause overrepresentation of lumbar disease in certain light occupations (positive bias). These examples are pertinent because the knowledge of the effects of work on lumbar disease is predominantly based on prevalence studies. (For a review, see reference 54.) Most of them, despite the inherent negative bias, show that low-back pain is associated with heavy work. Hence, the true effect must be even greater than what is revealed by cross-sectional data.

In a *case-referent study*, selection bias may arise in the following way. Suppose that there is a hospital specializing in occupational medicine where a physician wishes to study the effects of various environmental factors, among them occupational exposures, on the occurrence of gastritis. Patients with this disease (according to preset criteria) are defined as cases, and patients with, for example, lumbar disease as referents. A surprisingly high frequency of lead exposure among the cases will probably emerge. The result is an overestimate of the role of lead exposure in the etiology of gastritis *in general* (positive bias). Of course, there is no doubt that overexposure to lead causes a gastritis-like syndrome. But workers exposed to lead and having epigastric pain are more likely to be admitted to this specialized clinic because plant physicians usually suspect lead poisoning in such a situation. In this hypothetical example, the reasons for selection bias were: (1) the hospital specializes in occupational medicine, and (2) the connection between lead exposure and epigastric pain was known in advance. Had there been no specialized hospital and had the local physicians been unaware of the connection between gastric symptoms and lead exposure, a selection bias of this kind would have been unlikely.

Selection bias is seldom a problem in *cohort* studies in general. But in occupational medicine one of the most difficult factors is the assessment of self-selection into an occupation or trade. Its effects are insignificant for diseases with long, silent latency times, but they are important whenever symptoms of the disease under study are provoked or worsened by the work in question. For example, persons with chronic bronchitis are not attracted to jobs known to be dusty, and those with previous back pain avoid physically heavy work. Preemployment examinations tend to strengthen this type of selection even further. However, it should be emphasized that a true selection bias arises only when the *disease under study* is responsible for the selection. If other, concomitant diseases (e.g., bronchial asthma in a study of coronary artery disease) cause "selection," the type of bias is, in fact, a comparison bias in the sense that the exposed group may be different from the reference category.

Later health-based selection, occurring after the worker has become exposed, can be methodologically controlled by means of tracing all those who change employment or retire and by classifying them as exposed. However, from a quantitative point of view, such selection causes flattening of the exposure-response curve because those classified as being ill will have accrued short exposure times. (The disease forces them to interrupt the exposure earlier than those not affected.)

Selection bias must be avoided at the planning stage of a survey, since there exists no method to control it during data handling. If it cannot be completely avoided, its effects should be assessed and considered when conclusions are drawn. A slight selection bias does not invalidate a study, provided that its direction and magnitude are known. Effective handling of selection bias requires a thorough knowledge of the selective forces operating in every specific occupation, hospitalization process, and the scientific problem in general.

Validity of Observation

Validity of observation means that the (in)accuracy of the information gathered from both the cases and the referents, or from both the exposed and the nonexposed, is similar. Inaccuracy in itself does not necessarily affect validity, provided that it is symmetrical (i.e., only asymmetrical inaccuracy can cause bias). But the *sensitivity* of the study (the power to detect a causal association, if present) suffers from symmetrically inaccurate or crude information, and a falsely negative result may emerge. Observation bias may affect all types of epidemiologic investigations, but the problem is usually potentially the most serious in case-referent studies.

These studies derive their information from questionnaires and interviews rather than from measurements, and the greatest problem is how to ensure comparability between the histories obtained from the cases and those from the referents (or their relatives). Consider, for example, a case-referent study of congenital malformations in which the cases are mothers of malformed children and the referents are mothers of healthy babies. Data on possible harmful exposures during pregnancy would be collected by interviews. Such exposures that would provide useful data include medicines, past infections, occupational exposures, radiologic examinations, or traumas. An observation bias may arise because mothers of malformed babies may recall exposures in more detail than mothers of healthy babies, who have no reason to brood about such matters. Insofar as occupational exposures are concerned, this bias can be overcome if other sources of information are utilized—namely, employers' records. But for some other exposures—for example, alcohol, tobacco and medicines—there is no such possibility. However, as discussed further in a later section of this chapter, the effects of an observation bias should not be judged in too simplistic a way. Very few studies explicitly address this problem, and its effects may easily become exaggerated in the absence of hard facts.

Retrospective cohort studies are also subject to observation bias because of a general tendency to observe exposed populations more thoroughly than unexposed ones, by means of periodic health examinations, for example. By contrast, in a prospective cohort study one can avoid observation bias if, for example, the investigator is blinded and a similar quality of data is obtained from both the exposed and the unexposed cohorts. Special care should be taken to ensure a minimal loss of subjects from follow-up, since lost (unknown) information may be asymmetrical and hence affect validity even more than inaccurate information.

The requirement of observation validity sometimes determines the study design. For example, if it is judged that unbiased retrospective exposure data cannot be obtained by means of interviews in a case-referent design, the remaining option is a prospective follow-up study, or, sometimes, no study at all.

Validity of Comparison

The validity of comparison has two components: validity of the reference group and lack of confounding. These components are interrelated in the sense that confounding does not occur if the reference group is perfect. However, achieving this goal rarely, if ever, succeeds, and therefore some confounding must be accounted for even in well-designed studies. Sometimes it may even be economical or feasible to accept some confounding at the planning stage, as it can later be controlled when the data are analyzed.

An ideal *reference group* should share all characteristics of the study group *relevant to the problem at issue*, except for the property that defines the groups, which is the exposure in a cohort study and the disease in a case-referent study. If this goal cannot be completely achieved, emphasis should be put on those factors that most affect the actual problem in light of available knowledge. For example, in the aforementioned study on the effect of exposure to carbon disulfide on the occurrence of coronary artery disease,[19, 52] the exposed cohort was formed from workers in a viscose rayon plant and the reference cohort from paper mill workers. The assumption was that the two occupational environments had the same effect, if any, on the occurrence of coronary artery disease apart from the effect of carbon disulfide. Next, comparability had to be ensured with regard to as many known risk factors of coronary artery disease as possible. Table 71–5 summarizes the procedure followed.

The groups were intentionally not equalized with respect to blood lipids, blood pressure, and blood glucose concentration because the literature indicated that the cardiotoxic effects of carbon disulfide could be mediated through these risk factors. Matching should be avoided on the intermediate steps in the etiologic sequence from exposure to disease, since such a procedure masks a true effect.

Attention may also be drawn to the fact that the birth district had to be taken into account. This is a specifically Finnish problem. Eastern Finland has a substantially higher coronary mortality than western Finland, and we knew in advance that 40% of the viscose rayon workers were born in eastern Finland as compared with 25% of the paper mill workers. This is a good illustration of

TABLE 71–5.

Example Showing the Achievement of Comparability Between the Exposed and the Reference Group in a Study on the Effect of Carbon Disulfide Exposure on the Incidence of Coronary Artery Disease*

CHARACTERISTIC	SIMILARITY	METHOD
Age	Same	Pair-matching
Birth district	Same	Pair-matching
Type of work	Same	Pair-matching
Social structure	Same	Result of matching
District of habitation	Same	Questionnaire
Cigarette consumption	No major differences	Questionnaire
Leisure-time physical activity	No major differences	Questionnaire
Physical work capacity	No major differences	Ergometry
Relative body weight	Same	Measurement
Drug therapy	No major differences	Questionnaire
Diet	No major differences	Judgment

*Data from Hernberg S, Partanen T, Nordman C-H, et al: Coronary heart disease among workers exposed to carbon disulfide. *Br J Ind Med* 1970; 27:313.

the importance of knowing the substance of the problem under study when the reference group is defined.

Another example may illustrate the situation in a case-referent design. If patients with some other disease are used as referents, this disease should neither be caused nor prevented by the exposure(s) at issue. Consider a study on occupational factors in the etiology of nasal cancer. The cases are, of course, selected from patients with that disease. If the referents are patients with some other type of cancer, the symmetry of the data is best ensured, since healthy people probably would not give similarly accurate histories. However, the referents must have a type of cancer with an etiology completely unrelated to any occupation. Self-evidently, no respiratory cancer fulfills this requirement, and the use of several other cancer sites would also be doubtful. However, prostatic cancer is considered to be predominantly nonoccupational in origin, and therefore patients with this type of cancer could be used as referents for male cases. An empirical check of the validity of this assumption could in principle be made through a comparison of the results with another series of referents without cancer of any type. But if the results were to differ, which one would be correct? A third series would be required to solve this problem, but then economic obstacles could arise.

Lack of confounding is the other requirement for comparison validity. A confounder is an outside disturbing factor that is intermixed with a scientific problem. Because of this intermixing, the confounder disturbs the assessment of the effect under study. To have this confounding effect, the factor must be a *causal risk factor (determinant) of the illness,* and it must be *associated with the exposure* in the *particular* study. In a cohort study, confounding occurs when one or more risk factors of the disease, other than the one being studied, occur more or less frequently in the study group than in the reference group. Note that the connection to the disease is causal and "always occurring," but the connection with exposure may occur only in a particular study. In other words, if the problem is whether dust exposure causes chronic bronchitis, smoking (which is *always* a risk factor for that disease) is a confounder *only* if smokers are more (or less) frequent among the exposed workers than among the referents. In one study this may be the case, while in another the smoking habits may be uniform. In the first instance smoking is a confounder (how strong a factor depends on the magnitude of the difference in *that particular* study); in the second it is not, although it is an effect modifier. Possible asymmetries of potential confounders between the groups are not a matter for significance testing, because the degree of asymmetry has bearing only on that particular study and is no probabilistic matter. In other words, if the difference is, say, 15%, its distorting effect is exactly 15% in that study, and it is totally irrelevant if the difference is "significant" or not. In another study the difference may be something else.

Consider, once again, the aforementioned study on the connection between exposure to carbon disulfide and coronary artery disease.[19, 51] The question arises as to whether or not cigarette smoking should be considered a confounder in this specific study. It is well known that smoking is a causal risk factor for coronary artery disease; hence, it fulfills the first requirement for a confounder. To fulfill the second, it should be associated with the exposure in the particular study, i.e., viscose rayon workers should smoke more (or less) than the reference group. As the cigarette consumption is usually not known in advance, the smoking histories must be obtained, usually by a questionnaire. If smoking turns out to be more prevalent in the exposed group, it is a confounder. If not, it does not fulfill the second requirement for a confounder and, contrary to what most people think, *need not be controlled* in that particular study. In our study, the differences in smoking habits were so small that we considered it justified not to treat smoking as a confounder in the statistical analyses. However, because smoking may have been an effect modifier, it was considered necessary to compare the groups by smoking category also. The purpose of this analysis was to see if the cardiotoxic effect of carbon disulfide was *modified* (not confounded) by smoking. For example, was the excess mortality confined to smokers only, or perhaps to nonsmokers only, or was it different in different smoking categories? The analysis showed that the effect was uniform, as far as could be judged from the rather small numbers.

The effect of a confounder may be "positive," producing a false association, or "negative," masking a true association. Had smoking in the preceding example been more common among the exposed subjects, positive confounding would have arisen; had it been less common, negative confounding may have masked, partly or completely, the excess of coronary artery disease in the exposed cohort. In occupational medicine, confounding is usually a less severe problem than selection. Insofar as smoking is concerned, Axelson[4] calculated the effect of various hypothetical smoking distributions on the rate ratio of lung cancer. As can be seen from Table 71–6, the asymmetry must be rather extreme to produce serious bias. More specifically, the effects of differences in smoking habits between common categories of workers affect only slightly the rate ratio for lung cancer, as long as a population with mixed smoking habits, e.g., the general population, is used as the reference. That these considerations indeed are pertinent has recently been shown by Asp,[3] who gathered information on smoking from a sample of 1,990 men and, using Axelson's procedures, computed how much the differences in smoking habits between various occupational categories would have confounded the rate ratio under the presumption that the lung cancer incidence otherwise would have been uniform. As can be seen from Table 71–7, when compared with the average of the whole material (an approximation of "the general population"), the *confounded* rate ratio varied between 0.67 and 1.31 for the extreme groups, in spite of the fact that the strong weighing factors used exaggerated the confounding effect. These considerations clearly show that smoking as a confounder becomes an issue only when the observed rate ratio for lung cancer is between some 0.5 and 2.0—which undoubtedly is often the case in occupational epidemiology—but that one need not worry much about confounding when the observed rate ratio is higher, quite contrary to what is often claimed. For example, a study showing an exposure-related rate ratio of, say, 3 or more *cannot* be totally invalidated on the basis that smoking has been insufficiently controlled.

TABLE 71–6.

Estimated Crude Rate Ratios in Relation to Fraction of Smokers in Various Hypothetical Populations*†

POPULATION FRACTION (%)			
NONSMOKERS (1x)	MODERATE SMOKERS (10x)	HEAVY SMOKERS (20x)	RATE RATIO
100	–	–	0.15
80	20	–	0.43
70	30	–	0.57
60	35	5	0.78
50‡	40‡	10‡	1.00‡
40	45	15	1.22
30	50	20	1.43
20	22	25	1.65
10	60	30	1.86
–	65	35	2.08
–	25	75	2.69
–	–	100	3.08

*From Axelson O: Aspects on confounding in occupational health epidemiology. *Scand J Work Environ Health* 1978; 4:85. Used by permission.

†Two different risk levels are assumed for smokers, i.e., 10 times and 20 times that of nonsmokers for "moderate" and "heavy" smokers, respectively.

‡Reference population (similar to the general population in countries such as Sweden). Smoking habits in various industrial populations rarely diverge outside the broken lines.

Control of Confounding

Confounding can be controlled in a study either at the planning stage or during data analysis (in contrast to selection, which must always be controlled at the planning stage). The most effective means of controlling confounding is random allocation into the exposed and unexposed categories, which is the method used in experiments. However, epidemiologists can almost never utilize randomization; instead, they use the following procedures:

1. Restriction
2. Matching
3. Standardization
4. Stratification
5. Modeling (multivariate analysis)

Restriction.—Restriction means that the study focuses on a certain category only, such as persons over 40 years of age, men, normotensives, or smokers. Apart from improving the symmetry of the series, restriction makes a study more effective, since persons with a low risk of contracting the particular disease can be excluded. For example, a study on occupational lung cancer becomes more efficient if only persons over 50 years of age are included. Restriction can be used alone or in combination with other methods.

Matching.—Matching refers to the equalization of cases (or exposed subjects) and referents with respect to potential confounders, for example, age, gender, smoking status, or time of diagnosis. Matching is used most often in case-referent studies; it controls confounding by ensuring that the distribution of the matched property becomes practically equal among the cases and referents. There are several ways of matching, among them individual match-

TABLE 71–7.

Estimated Confounded Rate Ratios of Lung Cancer in Relation to the Fractions of Nonsmokers, Ex-smokers, and Smokers in Various Occupational Groups*

	PERCENTAGES				
OCCUPATIONAL GROUP	NONSMOKERS R† = 1	EX-SMOKERS R† = 10	SMOKERS R† = 20	TOTAL	ESTIMATED CONFOUNDED RATE RATIO
Civil servants	41	37	22	100	0.67
Business executives	30	40	30	100	0.81
Scientific and engineering personnel	27	37	36	100	0.88
All male workers	27	28	48	100	1.00
Miners and workers in the basic metal industry	20	17	63	100	1.15
Packers, loaders and depot workers	13	22	65	100	1.21
Operators of mobile machines	7	25	68	100	1.28
Construction workers	10	16	74	100	1.31

*From Asp S: Confounding by variable smoking habits in different occupational groups. *Scand J Work Environ Health* 1984; 10:325. Used by permission.

†R = assumed effect of smoking expressed as a rate ratio, i.e., ex-smokers are assumed to have a 10-fold and smokers a 20-fold lung cancer incidence as compared with that of nonsmokers, which probably is an exaggeration. Hence the true confounding effect would be even weaker.

ing, in which one or more referents matched with each case on the matching variables, or frequency matching, which involves stratifying the distribution of the confounding variable(s) among the cases and then selecting referents with the same distribution of the confounding variable(s).

A series can be matched on one or more factors. The more factors that are matched, the harder it becomes, however, to find suitable referents. Hence, unnecessary matching must be avoided. Under no circumstances is matching allowed on some intermediate step in the causal sequence of events because such "overmatching" creates a negative bias.[32] Matching may be combined with other methods of controlling confounding also; i.e., only some properties are matched, whereas others are controlled with alternative methods. In general there is a trend nowadays toward being more and more restrictive with matching. Instead, many authorities recommend control of confounding at the data analysis stage by means of stratified or multivariate analysis.

Standardization.—When an exposed cohort is compared with the general population, or when two or more different "general populations" are being compared, standardization is used. The most common standardized measure is the standardized mortality ratio.

Stratification.—Stratification represents a means of controlling confounding in connection with data analysis. Hence, it is especially suitable when restriction or matching has not been utilized. Stratification is performed by dividing the groups examined into strata according to confounders, e.g., age, sex, smoking habits, or body weight. The comparisons are then performed within the strata, and biases caused by primarily asymmetrical distributions are thereby eliminated. However, the more asymmetrical the primary populations are, the more loss of material results from stratification, since each end of the distribution will contain enough subjects from only one of the two populations (Table 71–8).

Stratification requires that both the confounding variables and the risk variables be categorical (e.g., the serum cholesterol level must be categorized into "high" and "low"). Categorizing several variables leads to many strata and hence stratification is effective only in large materials. Otherwise the strata run out of numbers. Moreover, persons with a "low high" and a "high high" value become similarly classified, and confounding can be controlled only approximately. Therefore, the investigator should, already at the planning stage, consider whether or not stratification is the optimal method and, if so, the extent to which stratification will be used. The need for stratification is one of the aspects determining the size of the study population.

TABLE 71–8.

Hypothetical Result of Stratification According to Age (Because of Asymmetrical Age Distribution, Comparisons Can Be Made for Age Categories 30–59 Years Only)

	NUMBER OF SUBJECTS	
AGE STRATUM (IN YEARS)	EXPOSED (N = 485)	REFERENTS (N = 388)
19 or younger	1	28
20–29	6	77
30–39	82	94
40–49	143	128
50–59	116	36
60–69	86	4
70 or older	51	1

Multivariate Modeling.—This is used when many confounding variables must be controlled simultaneously at the data analysis stage. Consequently, this method is often an alternative to stratification. Modeling yields an estimate of the effect of the risk factor adjusted for confounding variables. Modeling tends to be a complicated procedure that requires a skilled statistician and a computer, and interpretation of its results is often difficult.

External Validity

External validity can be defined as the generalizability of the results beyond the data. There are two distinctly different constellations, because epidemiologic research problems can be either particularistic or abstract.

Particularistic research is descriptive and deals with problems confined to time and space. For example, one may be interested in surveying the occurrence of lead exposure or of noise-induced hearing loss in some geographic area. Alternatively, one may look at how occupational health care for small industry is functioning in a particular country. Such studies should be based on representative samples from the entire populations in question (lead-exposed workers, noise-exposed workers, and units delivering occupational health services for small industry, respectively). The generalization to be made from this type of research is a sample-to-population generalization, but it is confined to the time of the survey and to the geographic area from which the sample was drawn. It tells what is currently going on and where, nothing more.

The problems of generalization in *scientific research* are profoundly different. This type of generalization goes from the study experience to the abstract-general, i.e., to "scientific truths." In this exercise it is totally irrelevant how representative the sample is of, say, workers in general. In contrast, it should describe a *particular* category of subjects submitted to a *particular* exposure, such as, for example, male viscose rayon workers exposed for five years or more to carbon disulfide. The issue is then, does carbon disulfide cause or accelerate coronary artery disease? Answering this question does not even take into consideration how representative the workers are of all Finnish men. Instead it is inferred that, given that an effect is shown, other exposed workers also run the same risk, because *carbon disulfide is cardiotoxic*. One may wish to go even further and make the scientific generalization more specific by looking at the association conditionally on other effect modifiers (coronary risk factors), such as age, smoking habits, or lipid levels. This specification of the generalization helps the understanding of the mechanisms of the effect in question. Scientific inference is, it should be pointed out, very much a question of judgment where prior knowledge is weighed against the new data obtained. It is very evident that good internal validity is an absolute requirement for any generalization.

SOME USES OF EPIDEMIOLOGY IN OCCUPATIONAL HEALTH—AN OVERVIEW

Epidemiologic methods can be, and are today, widely applied to solve occupational health problems—usually not as a single approach but together with other methods. The following presentation is intended to exemplify the main categories of problems that can best be studied with an epidemiologic approach. Roughly speaking, epidemiologic methods are best suited for detecting and quantifying medium risks—if the hazard is strong, its effects are evident without epidemiology; if it is weak, epidemiologic methods are too crude and vulnerable to bias to be of much use.

Descriptive Epidemiology

Survey of the General Health of Employees

A workplace can be considered a community with its specific health problems. Part of the problems may be induced by occupational exposures or the work conditions in general, but most health problems in working populations are actually composed of "general" morbidity. These problems of course also have bearing on occupational health, since almost any disease can interfere with the work capacity of the employee or interact with his or her capability to cope with occupational exposures and stresses. Hence, a complete picture of the "community health" of a workplace is crucial for any well-functioning occupational health service, and therefore "occupational health" must be given a broad meaning in this context.

A survey of the general health state of the employees can be designed to identify the following persons:

1. Those who are at special risk of contracting a specific disease (e.g., coronary artery disease) in order that preventive action may be taken

2. Those with minor curable or correctable disorders (e.g., iron deficiency, refraction anomalies)

3. Those in an early stage of chronic disease that requires regular health services (e.g., diabetes or hypertension)

4. Those with restrictions or contraindications for certain jobs (e.g., those with allergy, bronchitis, or low-back problems)

5. Those with unfavorable health behavior (e.g., heavy smokers, or obese and/or physically inactive persons)

Because resources are limited, the purpose of the survey should be made clear before the start. In other words, is the intention one of initiating regular health control, one of replacement, or some other? Equally important is the selection of screening methods with sufficient sensitivity and specificity. Self-evidently, insensitive methods do not detect the cases they should detect, and methods with low specificity produce a high proportion of false positive findings. Their use leads to unnecessary further examinations, which may be costly, or even pose some risk, and which may cause unnecessary anxiety. For feasibility reasons, the survey should not employ too many screening tests, either.

Furthermore, there should be guarantees that the occupational health service, or, alternatively, some other health service system, can take care of those in need of further diagnostic examinations, regular surveillance, or therapy. If transfer to less demanding tasks is impossible, there is no use in "identifying" (and worrying) handicapped individuals who themselves usually are well aware of their ailment anyway. If the scope of the survey is prevention, the disease must indeed be preventable, or its course prolongable, otherwise the survey may cause more harm in the form of unnecessary anxiety than benefit in terms of prevention. It may be noted that it is usually prudent to await the results of well-planned randomized clinical trials before initiating "prevention" at the workplace level, with the *important exception of reducing harmful exposures*.

And, finally, since the working population itself and also its health state are dynamic, any action should be planned with continuation in mind. One may repeat the survey at regular intervals, or even better, one may focus the activities on worker categories which have a high likelihood for positive findings, e.g., those 40 years and over, smokers, or obese persons. Commonly those 40, 45, or 50 years of age are selected for examination, and thereby a cyclic system covering everybody in that age range in a 5-year period is created. In addition, other risk groups may be examined more often.

Observation or Morbidity in Relation to Occupation, Work Area, or Specific Exposures

In the "community diagnosis" of workplaces, the harder indicators of morbidity, such as death and severe disease, are not usually feasible. Descriptive ad hoc studies of health problems usually employ self-administered questionnaires, interviews, the records of the occupational health services, absenteeism statistics, and a variety of clinical, functional, and biochemical tests. Since the aim of such activities is to describe morbidity in relation to work area, occupation, or some specific exposure, these variables must be well-defined. Furthermore, the tests employed must describe the type of health effects that may arise from the exposure in question. Such health effects may be rather specific (e.g., disturbances of the protoporphyrin synthesis among lead workers), semispecific (e.g., tremor among workers exposed to mercury), or quite nonspecific (e.g., chronic bronchitis in foundry workers exposed to dust).

However, as already stated several times, such cross-sectional data are invalidated by selection. This error provides an underestimate of the true prevalence, since many of those with manifest symptoms seek other employment. Study of the true effects of hazardous exposures usually requires a longitudinal design.

Risk Identification—Alarms

Sometimes descriptive epidemiologic observations may provide the first clue to hitherto unrecognized occupational health hazards. For example, a sudden increase of dermatosis in a group of workers may indicate that a new skin-toxic chemical has been taken into use. The unexpected occurrence of several cases of a rare tumor, e.g., angiosarcoma of the liver, may be the first alarm of the occurrence of a carcinogen in the work environment. Concentration of short influenza-like episodes to a certain department may suggest, e.g., contamination of the air conditioning system with an agent causing humidifier fever. Such observations require both alertness on the part of the plant physician and a good recording system.

Nationwide Occupational Morbidity and Mortality Statistics

Official statistics and national or regional morbidity and mortality registers may provide some clues to the epidemiologic study of work-related diseases. However, direct conclusions are usually difficult to draw from such registers, for reasons already discussed. In Great Britain, the Registrar General has reviewed mortality in relation to information provided by decennial censuses to deaths in a period before and after the census for more than 100 years.[12] Direct effects of some occupations are readily seen, such as various dust diseases among miners, potters, foundrymen, and cotton workers, while the influence of occupations on other, more nonspecific diseases is less clear, because factors outside work, such as social class and smoking habits, may affect the rates. Hence, national registers on occupational morbidity have their main use as starting points for etiologic epidemiologic studies, because the crude descriptive data they provide are too inexact for specific conclusions and, besides, are confounded by nonoccupational factors.

Survey of Exposure Data

Occupational epidemiology should relate indicators of illness to at least qualitative, but preferably to quantitative, measures of exposure. Furthermore, true preventive action at the workplace aims at eliminating or reducing harmful exposures or isolating the workers from them. In both instances systematic and accurate information on conditions of exposure is crucial.

Exposure surveys serve to (1) identify, locate, and quantify hazards; (2) form a base for preventive action (reduction of exposure); (3) assess the need for regular health surveillance; (4) monitor the trend of the hazard; and (5) provide data for cause-effect inferences and exposure-response relationships.

Exposure surveys may focus on samples from the ambient air (stationary or personal sampling) or on measurements of a toxic agent (or sometimes its specific effects) from biologic samples (blood, urine, exhaled breath, or hair). Assessment of the total exposure for individuals or groups and consequently their risk assessment is best achieved from biologic samples, while measurements of concentrations in the ambient air are best suited for engineering purposes, for the identification of areas with exceptionally high exposure, for the regular surveillance of workplace hygiene, and for the frequent situations when no standardized biologic tests exist.

Exposure surveys may be occasional or regular. They may cover one or a few departments, one factory, an entire type of industry or a geographic district (e.g., a city or even an entire country). The larger the source population (of workplaces or individuals) is, the more important statistical sampling procedures grow.

Generation of Hypotheses for the Study of Cause-Effect Relationships

A scientific hypothesis may arise from several different incitements, among them analogies, experiments, clinical observations, and descriptive epidemiologic data, or often they may arise from a synthesis of prior knowledge derived from many different sources. In this context only epidemiology will be considered.

Four main domains can be distinguished. First, occupational health records may initiate the first suspicion of a causal connection between disease and exposure to new—and sometimes old—hazards. Second, cross-sectional ad hoc surveys comprising differently exposed workers, as well as unexposed reference groups, may show a varying prevalence of symptoms and signs, which may relate to some specific exposure(s). Because of the well-known invalidity problems hampering cross-sectional studies, the result can usually be no more than suggestive of a cause-effect relationship, but it may generate a hypothesis for further testing. It must again be repeated that in cross-sectional studies selection bias usually tends to *mask existing relationships*, while observation bias may cause *falsely positive* results (e.g., through a tendency of exposed workers to complain more).

Third, computerized linkage of exposure and morbidity registers may occasionally provide clues for etiologic research, as already discussed. The strong diluting effects, mainly arising from nondifferential misclassification and/or crudeness of the exposure parameter, restrict their use, however, and also positive findings are difficult to interpret.

The fourth way of using descriptive epidemiology for creating hypotheses is the study of national occupational mortality or pension statistics. Such statistics may provide clues for etiologic research, but they seldom allow direct cause-effect conclusions because of many interfering factors such as misclassification and the effects of nonoccupational conditions.

In conclusion, descriptive epidemiology may generate useful hypotheses when based on good basic data, but, if these data are crude or inaccurate, it more often tends to mask existing effects. In particular, the uncritical use of data collected for other purposes is risky. The availability of computers has unfortunately increased the opportunities for malpractice. Meaningful interpretation of descriptive data requires deeper insight into epidemiology and better knowledge of the many sources of errors involved in the use of the data than what is generally realized.

Etiologic Epidemiology

Epidemiologic Hypotheses

Etiologic epidemiology is concerned with the testing of some hypothesis. Usually the problem consists of revealing a causal connection between some occupational exposure and a nonspecific disease (e.g., cancer or lumbar disorders). Quite often, the problem involves the study of multifactorial etiology, the occupational factor being only one of several causes. When the occupational exposure is the only (or clearly dominant) cause, the hypothesis is so trivial, e.g., "lead causes lead poisoning," that etiologic research is not needed. The only exception, perhaps, is in the case of newly introduced agents whose action is not completely known. Occasionally etiologic research can be initiated without any well-defined prior hypothesis. A typical example is a case-referent study with the aim of "looking at the different exposures associated with a disease," or a cohort study addressing the question of "what different diseases are caused by a certain exposure."

An *epidemiologic hypothesis* may be specific or semispecific. A specific hypothesis states that "exposure A causes disease B," e.g., asbestos exposure causes bronchial cancer. Semispecific hypotheses are of two types. The first has the form "exposure A causes diseases B_1, B_2, . . . B_i," e.g., asbestos causes bronchial cancer, mesothelioma, stomach cancer, . . . and asbestosis. The second type postulates that "disease B is caused by factors (exposures) A_1, A_2, . . . A_i," e.g., bronchial cancer is caused by smoking, asbestos, chromates, . . . and foundry dust. (Note the conceptual distinction from the "fishing expeditions" without any prior hypothesis exemplified above.)

Using Epidemiology to Test Hypotheses

The specific hypothesis "A causes B" can in principle be tested equally well by either a cohort or a case-referent design. The choice is determined by validity and feasibility aspects. If the disease is rare, a case-referent study is definitely to be preferred, and, conversely, if the exposure is rare, a cohort study is more efficient. The semispecific hypothesis of the type "exposure A causes diseases B_1, B_2, . . . B_i" can be tested (epidemiologically) only by a cohort design, or, as a subcategory of this approach, an interventive study. The main question then is whether one should choose a prospective or a retrospective cohort study. Since the basic design is the same, it is actually a matter of *timing*, not of different designs. By contrast, the semispecific hypothesis of the type "disease B is caused by exposure A_1, A_2, . . . A_i," can be tested (epidemiologically) only by means of a case-referent study, because this design is outcome-based. The alternatives for study design and their advantages and disadvantages have been discussed previously.

Completing the Clinical Picture

A common use of epidemiology is to complete the clinical picture. Many occupational diseases are insufficiently known, especially as regards early stages. Conversely, the variety of manifestations that toxic agents can cause are only partially known. This deficiency is by no means typical of occupational medicine; other fields of medicine share this defect because so much knowledge is derived from clinical studies. A thorough discussion of this problem in general can be found in J. N. Morris's book, *Uses of Epidemiology*.[39]

Multiple Causes

Classical occupational diseases are without any doubt causally related to work. However, there is now growing awareness that they represent only one end of a continuum, the other representing diseases which are only partly or occasionally caused or aggravated by work. The World Health Organization has recently included the whole of this continuum into the concept "work-related diseases."[10] The study of these conditions is a challenge for occupational epidemiology.[17] The first task is to provide qualitative evidence of a causal relationship between an exposure (in a broad sense) and a certain disease. In this context a "causal relationship" means that the exposure in question is *one* of the causes of that disease, not necessarily The Cause. The next issue is to assess quantitatively the proportion of cases among the exposed that are actually due to the exposure. This *etiologic fraction* can be calculated in the following way:[34]

$$EF = \frac{O/E - 1,}{O/E}$$

where

EF = etiologic fraction, among the exposed,
O = number of observed cases, and
E = number of expected cases.

For example, if 120 cases of bronchial cancer are observed in a cohort of chromate workers against 44 expected, the O/E ratio is about 2.8. The EF = (2.8 − 1)/2.8 = 0.64, i.e., 64% of the cases are due to chromate exposure. Quite obviously, the etiologic fraction is not generalizable, since its magnitude strongly depends on exposure intensity and duration and the specific population studied. Furthermore, it is difficult to interpret. Being a proportion, it is dependent on the effects of any other factor, e.g., smoking.[9] A reduction of that factor would lead to an increase in the etiologic fraction of interest, even if the absolute number of excess cases would remain unchanged. Furthermore, since the concept(s) of multiple etiology is (are) complex (e.g., presupposing several sufficient causes, which can be split into component causes, *contributing* to, not necessarily *causing* the disease), the sum of different etiologic fractions is often in excess of 100%. In fact, it has a lower limit of 100%, while its upper limit could be any value in excess of 100%.[9, 47]

In intervention studies, the preventive fraction (PF) for the lower category of exposure can be computed in a similar way, i.e.,

$$PF = 1 - O/E$$

For example, as described previously, our research group found a 3.2-fold coronary death rate during a seven-year follow-up of viscose rayon workers exposed to carbon disulfide.[42] A strong intervention was made by the management, who reduced exposure levels and removed workers with high coronary risk factors from exposure. During the following eight years, the rate ratio fell to unity. The hypothetical number of deaths from coronary artery disease during that period, in the absence of intervention and on the assumption of the same rate of mortality as before, would have been 59 instead of the 19 cases actually observed. Thus the preventive fraction became $1 - 19/59 = 68\%$.[42]

So far, the assumption has been that the different causes are additive. However, synergism may also occur. A well-known example is cigarette smoking and asbestos exposure. For example, Hammond et al.[14] have shown in a cohort of asbestos workers that, if the rate ratio for nonsmoking, non-asbestos-exposed workers is defined as 1, the ratio for nonsmoking asbestos workers was 5.2 and that for nonexposed smokers was 10.9. Smoking asbestos workers had a rate ratio of 53.2, which is very close to 5.2 times 10.9. These figures concerned lung cancers occurring 20 years or more after the commencement of exposure. From these figures the authors estimated that the preventive effect of eliminating (or rather avoiding ever) smoking alone would have been 92% and that of eliminating asbestos exposure alone would have been 81%.[14]

Exposure-Effect and Exposure-Response Relationships

Once the qualitative causal association between two phenomena is known, the secondary question arises of determining the quantitative relationship between different degrees of exposure and the different qualities, intensities and frequencies of its effects. Besides being scientifically relevant, this knowledge is important in the scientific-administrative procedure of standard setting.

The use of "exposure" instead of the more familiar pharmacologic concept of "dose" is motivated by the trivial fact that the dose is not measurable in occupational situations."Effect" and "response" are different concepts. The Task Group of Metal Toxicity, at its meeting in Tokyo in 1974,[40] defined effect as a biological change caused by an exposure. When data are available for both exposure and effect on a graded scale, an exposure-effect relationship can be established. One example is the relationship between blood lead levels and the concentration of Δ-aminolevulinic acid (ALA) in the urine. The term response was defined as the *proportion* of a population that demonstrates a specific effect (say, a concentration of ALA in the urine in excess of 5 mg/L), and its correlation with estimates of exposure provides the exposure-response relationship. The exposure-effect relationship exhibits an *average* effect in all individuals at the same exposure levels, and therefore may provoke the false impression that the population is homogeneous. By contrast, an exposure-response relationship takes into account the variation in susceptibility within groups of individuals since it indicates the proportion of persons affected. For preventive purposes it is extremely important to be able to define the most sensitive members of a group.

Interventive Epidemiology

For ethical reasons, an interventive investigation in occupational epidemiology can only study the *decrease* in morbidity following a *reduction* of exposure intensity. The reverse may take place involuntarily and may then offer the alert plant physician opportunities to study the adverse effects of a more intense exposure, but because of the unintendedness of such a situation, the study of accidental deterioration of work conditions cannot be regarded as interventive epidemiology.

As will be discussed later, an important aspect for judging causality in nonexperimental research is positive results of an interventive study. The provision of such arguments would be the main, scientific use of interventive epidemiology, but because of the reasons already mentioned, there are seldom possibilities for this exercise. The few "interventive" studies published are by no means pure. However, some of them may, nevertheless, add something to the credibility of the causality of an association between exposure and disease, as for example, the Finnish study on carbon disulfide and coronary mortality, already discussed several times in this chapter. This project started as a cohort study and later became an intervention study. Together with coherent data from other investigations, plausible biologic explanations, a rather high rate ratio before the intervention, and a tendency toward an exposure-response relationship, its results strengthened the possibility of causality between carbon disulfide exposure and coronary artery disease, but of course the scientific correctness of the intervention is open to criticism and this weakens the argument.

SOME GUIDELINES FOR INTERPRETING EPIDEMIOLOGIC STUDIES

The interpretation of an epidemiologic study is very much a matter of judgment, which means that it has strong subjective elements. Unfortunately, readers cannot always assume that the author's evaluation is correct. They must be able to examine the data presented critically, and their own opinions must be formed as a result of this scrutiny. In addition to sufficient knowledge of the subject matter, they must have some insight into epidemiology and scientific thinking in general. The preceding sections have illustrated questions related to the planning and execution of epidemiologic studies; this section gives some elementary guidelines for critically evaluating them. It focuses on general methodologic aspects, because all the diverse areas of occupational medicine cannot be covered in this context.

Checking the Validity

Readers can evaluate the validity of a study only if enough details of the design, material, and methods are given in the report. Articles with superficial, incomplete, or otherwise defective methods sections easily make the authors seem nonchalant or ignorant of how to ensure validity. Even worse, one may suspect that the authors avoid going into particulars on purpose because they know that the study is biased. Irrespective of the reason for the lack of detail, such papers must be regarded as scientifically uninformative, although they provide useful information of the authors' and sometimes the editor's level of sophistication.

When the ingredients for evaluating validity are present, readers will profit if they check the article systematically with respect to each of its components. They should first consider to what extent the study fulfills the criteria of valid design in general (such as "correct" study type and "sufficient" material). Next, they should turn their attention toward the components of internal validity and look for selection bias, observation bias, and comparison bias, especially confounding. The last issue may be subtle indeed and even impossible to judge without thorough knowledge of the subject matter. If systematic errors are detected, their direction and, their magnitude should be evaluated. Biases should not be regarded in black-or-white terms, but in quantitative terms. Minor biases do not necessarily invalidate a study, provided their effects are known. Enlightened authors often point out biases themselves and discuss their effects on the interpretation of the data.

Provided the validity is satisfactory, and only then, readers should consider to what extent and into what categories the results can be generalized. Do they allow the formulation of new hypotheses, or do they support or challenge existing ones? How do the conclusions of the authors influence the prevailing world view? In evaluating this point, one must be aware of the subjectivity involved. Even if the study in question provides valid, "objective" data, the world view is highly subjective. There may even exist several different world views, because experts disagree frequently. So, when the "objective" data from the study are being used to modify or strengthen some world view, the end result can only be subjective.

P-Values

The *P*-value is a statistic known to all and understood by few. It is computed from the statistical test which has been applied to the data, and it is so constructed that a low *P*-value favors the correctness of the study hypothesis and a high *P*-value that of the null hypothesis. The *P*-value depends not only on the magnitude of the difference between two groups, but also on the amount of information in the data.

If the information is scanty (very small groups, for example), the point estimate of the RR, say, is subject to great random variation and the *P*-value is rather uninformative. By contrast, if the information is very ample, even a small difference will produce a very low *P*-value. Such a small difference is usually without any biologic significance and can, besides, often be due to undetected confounding or other bias. Therefore the *P*-value is uninformative also in this situation. One can say that it is too *sensitive* to be of any use.

For example, a rate ratio of 1.5 is significant ($P = .01$) in a study of 1,000 exposed and 1,000 referents if the mortality is 10%. However, the same level of significance in a study of 50 exposed and 50 referents requires a rate ratio of 11. Assume that the issue is occupational lung cancer, caused by, say, exposure to chromates. A glance at Tables 71–6 and 71–7 shows that smoking could confound the "significance" of the larger study, whereas such confounding would be impossible in the smaller study, assuming the same level of significance in both ($P = .01$). Of course a rate ratio of 1.5 would have been far from significant in the smaller study, and a rate ratio of 11 in the large study even more convincing than in the small study.

In studies of intermediate size, the *P*-value can be interpreted in a more meaningful way. Biologically insignificant differences do not cause very small *P*-values, and the random variation (of hypothetical replications of the study) is not overly great. Intuitively, then, a very small *P*-value supports the study hypothesis, a medium small value is uninformative and a large *P*-value supports the null hypothesis. The word intuitively is used on purpose, because there are no fixed definitions of "large," "small," or "very small," neither for the amount of information nor for the magnitude of the *P*-value. The conventionally used levels of significance, i.e., $P =$ .05 or .01, are arbitrary and without any theoretical grounds.

The difficulty of interpreting the *P*-value whenever the information is very ample should of course not lead to one overlooking such data. Instead, a quantitative assessment of the group difference becomes meaningful. In other words, one should regard the rate ratio rather than the *P*-value. Hence, in large studies the magnitude of the rate ratio is more informative than the statistical significance. But the smaller the amount of information, the more the rate ratio is influenced by chance, and the more uncertain its absolute value (point estimate) is.

In almost every situation there are several alternative statistical tests that can be used. Usually tests which have the greatest *power* to detect a true difference are preferred. Therefore not only the *P*-value, but also the test yielding it should be considered.

Statistical testing presupposes that systematic errors do not exist. No significance test can separate a bias from a true effect. If biases are present, statistical testing loses its meaningfulness, and it may be highly misleading in the hands of uncritical so-called scientists. A *P*-value is therefore never a summarized package truth, but only one of the several tools we have to evaluate the data.

Supporting Evidence for Cause-Effect Inferences

It may once more be repeated that definite cause-effect conclusions cannot be derived from nonexperimental research. Causality, therefore, can be viewed in terms of *probability* only. Sir Austin Bradford Hill[7] has elaborated some rules for judging the causality of an association. Although some criticism has been raised later,[47] the general message still holds. This list, together with some amendments, follows. Its use self-evidently presupposes reasonable certainty that the study is valid.

1. The *stronger the association* (meaning that the rate ratio is high), the greater the probability of a causal association. An exception is "small" studies, because their rate ratios are subject to substantial random variation. But if a moderately large study or large study yields a high rate ratio, the probability of a causal relationship is great. It should be added that the confidence limits for rate ratios from large series are narrow; therefore, statistical significance is easily obtained even for rather low rate ratios in such instances, as has already been discussed.

2. The *consistency* of the observed association speaks in favor of causal relationship. If the observation has been made repeatedly by different persons, in different places or under different circumstances and times, the argument is strong in favor of causality.

3. The *specificity* of the association is important. If the association is limited to specific workers (say, spinners in a viscose rayon plant) and to particular sites and types of disease (say, coronary artery disease), and there is no association between the work and other diseases (say, cancer), causation is supported.

4. The *temporal relationship* of the observed association is straightforward when the effect is immediate but becomes subtle when latency times are involved. In other words, exposure must have commenced early enough to be a cause (procedurally, e.g., earlier than half of the mean latency period, if known).

5. The presence of an *exposure-response relationship* supports the causality of an association. However, confounding factors can be so intermixed with the exposure that the effects of the two cannot be separated. Therefore this argument loses much of its theoretical power, although it is hard to conceive that undetected confounding in practice would explain a strong relationship. Especially, concomitant exposure to several harmful agents in industry is difficult to separate. For example, in mixed exposure situations occurring in many smelteries, the carcinogenic effect of one metal cannot be separated from the possible effects of the others. Then the exposure-response relationship becomes severely confounded and cannot be considered to support a causal connection between cancer and a *particular* metal.

6. *Biologic plausibility* is important for the evaluation. For example, the causality of the association between exposure to carbon disulfide and coronary artery disease becomes more plausible when one considers that there are at least five biochemical mechanisms by which carbon disulfide may act.[18] On the other hand, a lack of knowledge may complicate the use of the plausibility argument. For example, there was no biologic knowledge to link Sir Percival Pott's observation in 1775 of the excess of scrotal cancer in chimney sweeps to the carcinogenic effects of soot tar. Even today, there remain many unknown biologic mechanisms.

7. *Coherence of the evidence* from, e.g., experimental work strongly supports the causality of an epidemiologic association. In contrast, it is difficult to place much confidence in associations that have no explanation. Remember, by definition, 1 in 20 associations is statistically significant at a level of 0.05, and 1 in 100 at a level of 0.01, without having any meaning at all. The availability of computers has greatly increased the production of such nonsense associations. One should use sound judgment rather than blind faith in statistical significances.

8. Perhaps the most conclusive evidence of causality is provided when a *change in the exposure brings about a change in the illness*. This type of evidence is obtained in interventive epidemiologic studies, and its strength of evidence is connected with the similarities between intervention and experiment that have already been discussed.

9. In some circumstances *reasoning by analogy* helps judge the causality of an association. For example, a compound with structural similarities to a known carcinogen, when found to be associated with excess cancer, is more easily accepted as the cause of this excess than one without structural analogy.

Looking for a Positive Bias

The most common reasons for falsely positive results are comparison bias and observation bias. Falsely positive findings may arise through confounding. Large studies are the most problematic in this respect, since even a small difference yields statistical significance. Then even a confounding factor too weak to be easily spotted may be decisive. By contrast, the difference must be so large to yield statistical significance in smaller studies that confounding is more easily revealed, as has already been discussed. Of course, there may also exist a true difference which becomes exaggerated by confounding, and then the bias is quantitative rather than qualitative.

The most important reason for falsely positive results in case-referent studies is conventionally said to be observation bias. It arises whenever cases remember better than referents, or whenever the interviewer takes a more detailed history from the cases, as discussed earlier. However, in spite of the frequent statements in favor of this view, there is astonishingly little documentation in the literature on its correctness. By contrast, Pershagen and Axelson[45] found that relatives of workers who had died of lung cancer gave a very accurate history (true positive rate 98% and true negative rate 99% regarding previous exposure in a smeltery). When exposure to arsenic was considered specifically, the true positive rate dropped to 40%, but the true negative rate remained as high as 90%. Data on smoking habits were identical to those in medical files. Of course the results of one single study cannot be generalized, but Pershagen and Axelson's findings definitely do not support the commonly held view that observation bias is a great danger in case-referent studies. One may assume that major matters, such as long employment in some industry, are in general symmetrically and correctly reported, while minor events such as use of medicines, short occupational episodes, and the like are more easily forgotten and perhaps asymmetrically recalled. The observation bias would then depend on how significant are the events which are inquired about, not on general rules. It is possible that, if present, the observation bias would be positive rather than negative, but at least in occupational epidemiology this assumption has not yet received enough documentation.

A biased study design may specifically cause positive bias, as well as much confusion in general. In a recent study,[50] liver specimens were selected from those 23 patients who had been "exposed to chemicals" *and* referred for biopsy because of liver function alterations. The basic material was 800 patients who had had a diagnostic liver biopsy. Not surprisingly, the investigators found a variety of structural nonspecific abnormalities when they applied sophisticated methods of examination. No proper control group was employed. The authors concluded that chemical exposure was the cause of the abnormalities found in the electron microscopy. It is quite clear that structural abnormalities *must* be found in a series of patients selected in this way. (Why was liver biopsy performed if not for suspicion of liver disease?) Moreover, because the source material contained *both* subjects with abnormal liver enzymes (the majority of them) *and* with exposure to chemicals, it is inevitable that there were subjects with both attributes by mere coincidence, and therefore some of the "exposed" indeed must have structural abnormalities. Any occupational activity, even office work, can be incriminated as being hepatotoxic—and toxic to whatever target organ—if such a biased study design is used.[25]

Another less well conceived possibility of positive bias concerns the literature as a whole, not single studies. It has to do with the fact that it is much easier to get positive than negative findings published. Especially first reports of a phenomenon can be heavily biased in the positive direction. Consider, for example, that a random cluster ($P < .01$) of, say, congenital malformations occurs in a group of employees working with video display terminals. Such a finding can easily become published. Similar clusters occur with a frequency of one per one hundred (by definition!), and if enough people are "exposed," several "corroborative" studies will perhaps enter the literature. A pure random occurrence can then be considered a scientific truth, and there will be a hard job to convince uncritical readers by means of true negative studies that the risk, actually, does not exist. The difficulties involved in designing and carrying out true negative studies create difficult obstacles for a balanced supply of published studies, as will be discussed later.

Finally, uncritical authors may tend to interpret their findings in an unscientific way. For example, they may fail to realize the difference between a statistical association and a causal connection. They may even deliberately suppress data on positive confounding or other errors. There are always researchers who love publicity, and although they are usually revealed sooner or later they can cause much confusion in the meantime.

Looking for a Negative Bias

The definition of safe work conditions is the main goal of research in occupational health, and therefore studies showing the absence of effect are as important as positive findings. However, in order to be meaningful, negative studies must fulfill certain requirements, and therefore a clear distinction must be made between truly negative and nonpositive studies.[16]

A *true negative study* must fulfill three criteria: (1) it must be large; (2) it must be sensitive; and (3) it must have well-documented exposure data. Obviously it must also be well-designed otherwise, and there must be a clear awareness of whether only a specific condition is to be excluded (say, cancer) or if all types of adverse health effects are to be excluded. Only negative results arising from investigations that comply with these criteria can be considered as being truly negative.

A small negative study is uninformative in the sense that it can exclude the presence of very powerful hazards only. Of course the terms large and small are diffuse concepts. If large is defined as a *"sufficient" number of exposed cases,* some specification is provided. Then large becomes a function of cohort size, length of follow-up time, and frequency of the disease under study in a cohort study, and enough cases together with common enough exposure in a case-referent study.

Insensitive studies, i.e., studies with a crude design or crude measuring methods, are also uninformative. They can be compared to an insensitive laboratory test in clinical diagnosis, e.g., the sole measurement of total urinary proteins for diagnosing cadmium poisoning.

Negative results can only be referred to the actual or lower levels of exposure; hence the availability of accurate exposure data is crucial. As is well known, this is seldom the case.

It must be realized, however, that it can be artificial to dichotomize between positive and negative studies. When the negative is a function of statistical power (size of the study), the negativity-positivity axis is a continuum. For example, even a nonpositive study can be considered to *exclude* the presence of a risk greater than the upper confidence limit of the rate ratio, of course in relation to prevailing exposure conditions and when no negative biases are present. However, as will be discussed later, there are indeed important types of negative bias which have nothing to do with statistical power, and such errors may render a negative study totally uninterpretable.

Errors Related Mainly to Sample Size and Type of Subjects

Inappropriate design results in an inefficient study that fails to reveal an existing effect. *Too small a sample size* (and/or reference group) is the most common reason. In general, such an error is easy to identify, but in spite of this the failure to obtain statistical significance is often misinterpreted as being evidence of negativity. Even seemingly large studies can, in reality, be small. For example, if the disease under study is rare in relation to the cohort size and follow-up time, *only few exposed cases* of the disease in question will occur. Such a study is actually small, although its number of person-years may seem quite impressive. Whenever the disease is rare, a case-referent study should be preferred to the cohort design.

Falsely negative results can also be produced if the study focuses on *incorrect categories* of exposed workers. For example, if retired workers are not included in occupational cancer studies, crucial information will usually be lost, and the "truth," which is actually positive, may appear negative. Likewise, if a study is restricted to retired workers only, it may fail to detect pathognomonic manifestations of the exposure in question in younger age groups. Moreover, those who have survived to the age of retirement may be selected in some way or another. For example, a mortality study of asbestos workers must consider that mesothelioma often occurs in comparatively young persons, while bronchial carcinoma is a disease of older workers.

Errors Related Mainly to Insensitivity

When the problem is *qualitative,* i.e., causation is being studied, workers with too short an exposure time and too low an exposure intensity should not be included in the exposed cohort, not even when there are difficulties in obtaining a large enough sample size, because this step leads to the dilution of any existing effect as long as the cohort is analyzed as a homogeneous population. However, such a procedure *is* appropriate when the problem is *quantitative*, i.e., for the study of exposure-response relationships. Such research is usually done when the qualitative aspects of causation are already known. But a *qualitative* negative conclusion can never be based only on the outcome of subjects with low exposure intensity and/or short exposure time.

Whenever diseases with long latency periods (e.g., occupational cancer) are studied, a falsely negative result emerges if the follow-up time is *too short* and if allowance is not made for the *latency period* in the computation of person-years. Unfortunately, however, most latency periods are unknown; therefore no fixed rules can be given. It is believed that many cancers have latency periods of several decades, especially if the exposure is low; this is a difficult practical problem, especially in prospective cohort studies. The urgency for obtaining quick results must not interfere with the requirement of allowing for a minimum latency period before the computation of person-years is begun. An arbitrary rule would be half the supposed mean latency period of the cancer in question. In this context it should be stressed that the latency period should be computed separately for each individual. The general five-year latency period proposed by Fox[11] is very likely too short in a biologic sense. For example, Koskela and her coworkers[24] have shown that the maximum lung cancer-inducing effect of foundry dust exposure becomes evident as late as 20–30 years after the commencement of exposure. Figure 71–5 illustrates that a cancer study is informative only during a certain time period.

A choice of *insensitive indicators* of illness also results in falsely negative results when the purpose of the study is to demonstrate complete safety (e.g., for the documentation of hygienic standards). For example, mortality is too crude an indicator of health risks associated with exposure to many conditions in today's industry. Failure to find increased mortality has unfortunately been misinterpreted as a total absence of health hazards. This misinterpretation becomes especially dangerous when the conclusion is based on a comparison with the general population.

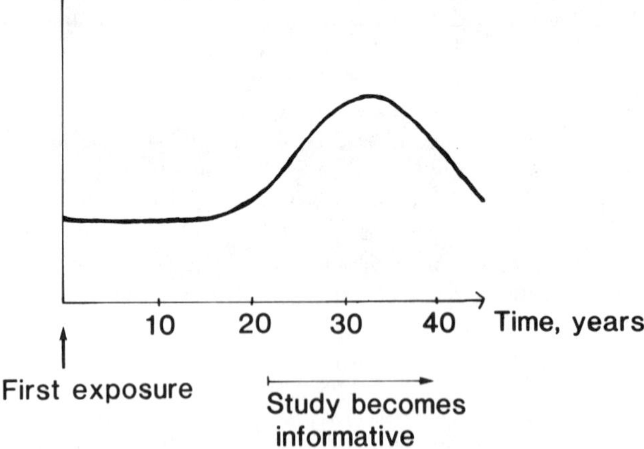

FIG 71–5.
Constructed example of how a cancer study yields information only after the latency period has been completed and how the informativeness decreases when the latency period has been passed. The numbers are arbitrary.

Errors Related Mainly to Comparison Bias

In cohort studies the reference group should reflect what would have happened in the exposed groups had there been no exposure, and in case-referent studies it should reflect the average exposure pattern in the base population. Finding such reference groups is by no means simple, and therefore occupational cohorts are very often contrasted against the general population. This procedure gives rise to a serious negative comparison bias, generally named "the healthy worker effect." How scientifically erroneous this common practice indeed is has been expressed by Wang and Miettinen[53] in the following way: "If therapeutic research were conducted in an analogous manner, treated patients would be compared with the 'general population' for any criterion of outcome. Experience would show that the treated group usually has a worse outcome than the reference population, and the difference might be referred to as the 'sick patient effect'."

The healthy worker effect has been discussed so much in a variety of books and articles (e.g., references 13, 14, 15, 29, 38, and 53) that only a short summary of its anatomy will follow.

The healthy worker effect is no interesting epidemiologic phenomenon per se, but a trivial comparison error, arising from a comparison of an exposed cohort to a completely unsuitable reference group, i.e., the general population.[15, 53] The latter is heterogeneous, is not completely free from the exposure under study, and rarely, if ever, represents the same social stratum as the exposed cohort. In other words, the general population does not fulfill even the most elementary requirements of comparison validity. The reasons for using such an invalid reference category so often, in spite of its faults, are the practicability involved and economy. An ad hoc reference cohort would double the costs of the investigation, and, besides, valid and suitable reference cohorts are hard to find.

The healthy worker effect causes the standardized mortality ratio (SMR) of the exposed cohort to fall well below 100 if no life-shortening occupational hazard exists. In fact, figures on the order of 60–90 have often been reported. These figures are obvious underestimates of the "true" mortality.[29] The main reason for the better-than-expected mortality experience of occupational groups lies in the fact that the general population also includes unemployable and unemployed persons. Among them are those in institutions, those with congenital anomalies, those handicapped during childhood, those otherwise ill at the time job-seeking commences, and those unemployed or with unstable employment. All these groups have a higher mortality rate than the active population. Kitagawa and Hauser[21] reported that those American white men unemployed in 1950 or later (4.3% of the population) had an SMR of 204. An additional 4% with no occupation showed an SMR of 125. Since occupational cohorts often contain a relatively high number of elderly workers and since the inactive part of the population increases in the older age categories, a general population adjusted to correspond to the age distribution of such cohorts may comprise up to 10% of those with exceptionally high mortality. Hence, in such a comparison, any SMR exceeding, say, 85 or 90 would indicate elevated mortality. Table 71–9 shows some published SMRs from occupationally active cohorts. Attention should be drawn to the fact that the interpretation of SMRs between, say, 90 and 110, is difficult indeed. Is it so that no life-shortening hazard exists, or does the healthy worker effect mask such a hazard? In the Finnish foundry worker study,[23] we were faced with this problem of inter-

TABLE 71–9.
Some SMRs Showing the Healthy Worker Effect (General Population = 100)

OCCUPATIONAL GROUP	SMR
Finnish foundry workers[23]	90
"Typical" foundry occupations[23]	95
American steel workers[27]	82
American rubber workers[30]	87
Finnish granite workers[2]	83
Finnish dock workers[1]	81
American chemical workers[43]	81

pretation. No certain conclusions could be drawn, but we intuitively favored the explanation that the healthy worker effect masked a slightly elevated overall mortality.

The healthy worker effect is not constant but varies depending on a number of circumstances.[29] It (1) is strongest in *younger age groups*, and declines with age until it is no longer significant (and sometimes even reversed) in the postretirement age range; (2) is *stronger for men* than for women; (3) is *stronger in higher social categories* than in lower strata; (4) is *strongest during the first years* after the beginning of employment; and even more important, (5) *is different for different causes of death*. In general, diseases with silent early stages and a rapid fatal course do not cause a healthy worker effect (except for during the first one or two years after cohort identification). Cancer is a typical example. By contrast, proneness to die from coronary artery disease can be established in advance by early diagnosis of the disease or identification of its risk factors. Furthermore, self-selection occurs because of symptoms or earlier warnings from physicians to avoid demanding jobs.

What still weakens the use of the general population as a reference group is that no details of possible confounders are known. For example, there is no information on smoking or drinking habits in national mortality statistics. Therefore the healthy worker effect poses a serious methodologic problem when occupational groups are compared with the general population. The interpretation of such studies is therefore difficult unless the effect under study is outspoken. Because systematic errors of unknown strength are involved, tests of significance are meaningless, although they are conventionally carried out. In fact, there is a danger that they mislead the unlearned reader if used uncritically.

Once all these aspects have been taken into consideration, it is evident that the healthy worker effect poses a serious methodologic problem when occupational groups are compared with the general population. Whenever possible, a more appropriate reference entity should be used. But if an ad hoc reference group cannot be utilized for practical or economic reasons, the *active* general population would form a better reference entity than the total general population. In some countries there are statistical data on this population, too. The healthy worker effect can be further decreased if the calculation of person-years does not start immediately at the time of cohort identification but, say, 5 or 10 years later. Alternatively, a separate comparison can be made at different intervals after the identification. The mortality rates should also be compared separately for different causes and within different age groups. Finally, whenever possible, comparisons should be made within the cohort itself between different categories of exposure intensity. These procedures often reduce the healthy worker effect; however, many uncertainties will still be left to the intuitive judgment of both the author and the reader of a report. But there is little help from P-values!

Errors Related Mainly to Misclassification

Random errors always tend to mask existing effects. Random misclassification is a serious diluting effect in all types of studies. For example, consider a case-referent study in which 40 out of 100 cases are exposed and 10 out of 100 referents are exposed. The "true" odds ratio is then 6.0. Suppose then that 20%, or eight cases, are misclassified, i.e., they are in fact noncases. Now the odds ratio becomes 4.8. If 50% are misclassified, it decreases to 3.9. Such misclassification may seem extreme, but it can occur when specific histologic types of tumor are being studied (e.g., mesothelioma). A misclassification of exposure causes an even stronger masking. A 10% error brings the odds ratio of the example to 3.3, a 20% error to 2.2, and a 50% error to 1. In real life it is often very difficult to obtain reliable exposure data, especially retrospectively, so this source of error may be important indeed. One can only speculate about the number of falsely negative results that have arisen from this deficiency.

Other random errors may arise from poorly standardized measuring methods. Poor analytical precision decreases existing group differences and may hence decrease or totally mask an existing effect.

Miscellaneous Errors

The effects studied may be inappropriate or irrelevant to the exposure in question. For example, an American study compared lead workers with present or five-year mean blood lead levels of 60–80 μg/100 ml (2.89–3.86 μmol/L) to those with levels below 60 μg/100 ml (2.89 μmol/L).[46] Many biochemical tests and other indicators of illness were impressively employed, among them a comprehensive list of no less than 29 laboratory tests. No statistically significant differences were found between the groups. The authors concluded that "there were no significant differences in the health of workers with blood lead concentrations between 60 and 80 μg/dl and those whose blood lead concentrations were lower than 60 μg/dl." They also stated, "It is our opinion that the current blood lead standard of 80 μg/dl can be kept, unless more data will support the OSHA proposal." A very remarkable flaw in this study was that no tests whatsoever describing direct disturbances of protoporphyrin synthesis were included and that no measurements of neurophysiologic functions or psychologic performance were performed. Making a general negative statement without studying these parameters, which are generally known to be the critical effects of lead toxicity, is a flagrant example of misinterpretation of epidemiologic data.

Conclusions

The intention of these considerations is to open the eyes of readers of epidemiologic articles to the fact that, being such a crude method, epidemiology most often is *unable to detect slight risks*. This lack stems from the fact that most of the errors of cohort and cross-sectional studies, and also some errors of case-referent studies, are toward the negative. Until now, the emphasis has been on controlling positive rather than negative bias, and conservative risk evaluations have been considered a hallmark of the author's sound judgment. In my view this is only one side of the coin. There is at least as much danger in not realizing that epidemiologic studies, when improperly conducted and wrongly interpreted, may lead to serious neglect or underestimation of the true risk. It is the worker who suffers from such errors.

ACKNOWLEDGMENTS

Although this text has not yet adapted all the new ideas in Prof. Olli S. Miettinen's present teaching, I would like to express my sincerest gratitude to him for his stimulating inspiration and pedagogical impact for more than a decade of advanced courses in epidemiology. I would also like to thank Prof. J. Malcolm Harrington, Birmingham, England, and Mr. Timo Partanen, Institute of Occupational Health, Helsinki, Finland, for their constructive criticism of my manuscript.

REFERENCES

1. Ahlman K, Backman A-L, Koskela R-S, et al: Satamatyöntekijöiden työolot ja terveydentila (The health and work conditions of dock workers). (Työterveyslaitoksen tutkimuksia no. 105). Helsinki, Institute of Occupational Health, 1975. (English summary.)
2. Ahlman K, Backman A-L, Hannunkari I, et al: Kivityöntekijöiden työolosuhteet ja terveydentila (Work conditions and health of granite workers). (Kansaneläkelaitoksen julkaisuja AL:4/1975). Helsinki, The Social Insurance Institution, 1975. (English summary.)
3. Asp S: Confounding by variable smoking habits in different occupational groups. *Scand J Work Environ Health* 1984; 10:325.
4. Axelson O: Aspects on confounding in occupational health epidemiology. *Scand J Work Environ Health* 1978; 4:85.
5. Axelson O: Elucidation of some epidemiologic principles. *Scand J Work Environ Health* 1983; 9:231.
6. Axelson O, Dahlgren E, Jansson CD, et al: Arsenic exposure and mortality: A case-referent study from a Swedish copper smelter. *Br J Ind Med* 1978; 35:8.
7. Bradford Hill A: *Principles of Medical Statistics*, ed 8. London, The Lancet Limited, 1967, chapter XXIV.
8. Campbell DT: Factors relevant to the validity of experiments in social setting. *Psychol Bull* 1957; 54:297.
9. Cole P, Merletti F: Chemical agents and occupational cancer. *J Environ Pathol Toxicol* 1980; 3:399.
10. El Batawi MA: Work-related diseases. A new program of the World Health Organization. *Scand J Work Environ Health* 1984; 10:341.
11. Fox AJ: Vinyl chloride and mortality? *Lancet* 1976; 2:416.
12. Fox AJ, Adelstein AM: Occupational mortality: Work or way of life? *J Epidemiol Community Health* 1978; 32:73.
13. Goldsmith J: What do we expect from an occupational cohort? *J Occup Med* 1975; 17:126.
14. Hammond EC, Selikoff IJ, Seidman H: Asbestos exposure, cigarette smoking and death rates. *Ann NY Acad Sci* 1979; 330:473.
15. Hernberg S: Evaluation of epidemiologic studies in assessing the long-term effects of occupational noxious agents. *Scand J Work Environ Health* 1980; 6:163.
16. Hernberg S: "Negative" results in cohort studies—How to recognize fallacies. *Scand J Work Environ Health* 1981; 7(Suppl 4):121.
17. Hernberg S: Work-related diseases—Some problems in study design. *Scand J Work Environ Health* 1984; 10:367.
18. Hernberg S, Nurminen M, Tolonen M: Excess mortality from coronary heart disease in viscose rayon workers exposed to carbon disulfide. *Work Environ Health* 1973; 10:93.
19. Hernberg S, Partanen T, Nordman C-H, et al: Coronary heart disease among workers exposed to carbon disulphide. *Br J Ind Med* 1970; 27:313.
20. Herva A: The Finnish register of employees occupationally exposed to carcinogens, in *Proceedings of the International Symposium on Prevention of Occupational Cancer, Helsinki, April 21–24, 1981* (Occupational and Safety Health Series No 46). Geneva, International Labour Office, 1982, pp 569–575.
21. Kitagawa EM, Hauser PM: *Differential Mortality in the United States*. Cambridge, Mass, Harvard University Press, 1973.
22. Kleinbaum DG, Kupper LL, Morgenstern H: *Epidemiologic Research Principles and Quantitative Methods*. Belmont, Calif, Lifetime Learning Publications, A division of Wadsworth, Inc, 1982.
23. Koskela R-S, Hernberg S, Kärävä R, et al: A mortality study of foundry workers. *Scand J Work Environ Health* 1976; 2(Suppl 1):73.
24. Koskela R-S, Järvinen E, Kolari P: Effect of cohort definition and follow-up length on occupational mortality rates. *Scand J Work Environ Health* 1984; 10:311.
25. Kurppa K, Tola S, Hernberg S, et al: Industrial solvents and the liver. *Lancet* 1983; 1:129.
26. Lilienfeld AM: *Foundations of Epidemiology*. New York, Oxford University Press, 1976.
27. Lloyd JW, Lundin FE, Redmond CK, et al: Long-term mortality study of steelworkers. IV. Mortality by work area. *J Occup Med* 1970; 12:151.
28. MacMahon B, Pugh E: *Epidemiology, Principles and Methods*. Boston, Little, Brown & Co, 1970.
29. McMichael AJ: Standardized mortality ratios and the "healthy worker effect": Scratching beneath the surface. *J Occup Med* 1976; 18:165.
30. McMichael AJ, Spirtas R, Kupper LL: An epidemiologic study of mortality within a cohort of rubber workers, 1964–72. *J Occup Med* 1974; 16:458.
31. Miettinen OS: Individual matching with multiple controls in the case of an all-or-none response. *Biometrics* 1969; 25:339.
32. Miettinen OS: Matching and design efficiency in retrospective studies. *Am J Epidemiol* 1970; 91:111.
33. Miettinen OS: Standardization of risk ratios. *Am J Epidemiol* 1973; 96:383.
34. Miettinen OS: Confounding and effect-modification. *Am J Epidemiol* 1974; 100:350.
35. Miettinen OS: Estimability and estimation in case-referent studies. *Am J Epidemiol* 1976; 103:226.
36. Miettinen OS: Design options in epidemiologic research. An update. *Scand J Work Environ Health* 1982; 8(Suppl 1):7.
37. Miettinen OS, Wang JD: An alternative to the proportionate mortality ratio. *Am J Epidemiol* 1981; 114:144.
38. Monson RR: *Occupational Epidemiology*. Boca Raton, Fla, CRC Press Inc, 1983.
39. Morris JN: *Uses of Epidemiology*. Edinburgh, Livingstone, 1970.
40. Nordberg GF (ed): Effects and dose-response relationships of toxic metals, in *Proceedings from an International Meeting on the Toxicology of Metals, Tokyo, 1974*. Amsterdam, Elsevier Scientific Publishing Co, 1976.
41. Nurminen M, Hernberg S: Cancer mortality among carbon disulfide-exposed workers. *J Occup Med* 1984; 26:341.
42. Nurminen M, Hernberg S: Effects of intervention on cardiovascular mortality among workers exposed to carbon disulfide. A 15-year follow-up. *Br J Ind Med* 1985; 42:32.
43. Ott MG: Determinants of mortality in an industrial population. *J Occup Med* 1976; 18:171.

44. Ott MG, Townsend JC, Fishbeck WA, et al: Mortality among individuals occupationally exposed to benzene. *Arch Environ Health* 1978; 33:3.
45. Pershagen G, Axelson O: A validation of questionnaire information on occupational exposure and smoking. *Scand J Work Environ Health* 1982; 8:24.
46. Ramirez-Cervantes B, Embree JW, Hine CH, et al: Health assessment of employees with different body burdens of lead. *J Occup Med* 1978; 20:610.
47. Rothman KJ: *Modern Epidemiology*. Boston, Little, Brown & Co, 1986.
48. Schlesselman JJ: *Case-Control Studies. Design, Conduct, Analysis. Monographs in Epidemiology and Biostatistics*. New York, Oxford, Oxford University Press, 1982.
49. Silcock H: The comparison of occupational mortality rates. *Popul Stud* 1959; 13:183.
50. Sotaniemi EA, Sutinen Seppo, Sutinen Sirkka, et al: Liver injury in subjects occupationally exposed to chemicals in low doses. *Acta Med Scand* 1982; 212:207.
51. Tola S, Hernberg S, Nikkanen J: Parameters indicative of absorption and biological effect in new lead exposure. A prospective study. *Br J Ind Med* 1973; 30:134.
52. Tolonen M, Hernberg S, Nurminen M, et al: A follow-up study of coronary heart disease in viscose rayon workers exposed to carbon disulphide. *Br J Ind Med* 1975; 32:1.
53. Wang J-D, Miettinen OS: Occupational mortality studies. Principles of validity. *Scand J Work Environ Health* 1982; 8:153.
54. Wickström G: Effect of work on degenerative back diseases. A review. *Scand J Work Environ Health* 1978; 4(Suppl 1):1.

Appendix A

Threshold Limit Values and Biological Exposure Indices*

CHEMICAL SUBSTANCES

Introduction

Threshold limit values refer to airborne concentrations of substances and represent conditions under which it is believed that nearly all workers may be repeatedly exposed day after day without adverse effect. Because of wide variation in individual susceptibility, however, a small percentage of workers may experience discomfort from some substances at concentrations at or below the threshold limit; a smaller percentage may be affected more seriously by aggravation of a preexisting condition or by development of an occupational illness.

Threshold limits are based on the best available information from industrial experience, from experimental human and animal studies, and, when possible, from a combination of the three. The basis on which the values are established may differ from substance to substance; protection against impairment of health may be a guiding factor for some, whereas reasonable freedom from irritation, narcosis, nuisance, or other forms of stress may form the basis for others.

The amount and nature of the information available for establishing a TLV varies from substance to substance; consequently, the precision of the estimated TLV is also subject to variation and the latest Documentation should be consulted in order to assess the extent of the data available for a given substance.

These limits are intended for use in the practice of industrial hygiene as guidelines or recommendations in the control of potential health hazards and for no other use, e.g., in the evaluation of control of community air pollution nuisances, in estimating the toxic potential of continuous, uninterrupted exposures or other extended work periods, as proof or disproof of an existing disease or physical conditions or adoption by countries whose working conditions differ from those in the United States of America and where substances and processes differ. These limits are not fine lines between safe and dangerous concentration and should not be used by anyone untrained in the discipline of industrial hygiene.

The Threshold Limit Values, as issued by the American Conference of Governmental Industrial Hygienists (ACGIH) are recommendations and should be used as guidelines for good practices. In spite of the fact that serious injury is not believed likely as a result of exposure to the threshold limit concentrations, the best practice is to maintain concentrations of all atmospheric contaminants as low as is practical.

The ACGIH disclaims liability with respect to the use of TLVs in a manner inconsistent with their intended use as stated herein.

Notice of Intent.—At the beginning of each year, proposed actions of the Committee for the forthcoming year are issued in the form of a "Notice of Intended Changes." This Notice provides not only an opportunity for comment, but solicits suggestions of substances to be added to the list. The suggestions should be accompanied by substantiating evidence. The list of Intended Changes follows the Adopted Values in the TLV booklet. Values listed in parenthesis in the "Adopted" list are to be used during the period in which a proposed change for the Value is listed in the Notice of Intended Changes.

Definitions.—Three categories of threshold limit values (TLVs) are specified herein, as follows:

1. The Threshold Limit Value–Time Weighted Average (TLV–TWA).—The time-weighted average concentration for a normal 8-hour workday and a 40-hour workweek, to which nearly all workers may be repeatedly exposed, day after day, without adverse effect.

2. Threshold Limit Value–Short Term Exposure Limit (TLV–STEL).—The concentration to which workers can be exposed continuously for a short period of time without suffering from (1) irritation, (2) chronic or irreversible tissue damage, or (3) narcosis of sufficient degree to increase the likelihood of accidental

*Reprinted with permission from American Conference of Governmental Industrial Hygienists, Inc: Threshold Limit Values and Biological Exposure Indices for 1986–1987. Cincinnati, Ohio, 1987.

injury, impair self-rescue or materially reduce work efficiency, and provided that the daily TLV–TWA is not exceeded. It is not a separate independent exposure limit, rather it supplements the time-weighted average (TWA) limit where there are recognized acute effects from a substance whose toxic effects are primarily of a chronic nature. A STEL is recommended only where toxic effects have been reported from high short-term exposures in either humans or animals.

A STEL is defined as a 15-minute time-weighted average exposure which should not be exceeded at any time during the workday even if the eight-hour time-weighted average is within the TLV. Exposures at the STEL should not be longer than 15 minutes and should not be repeated more than four times per day. There should be at least 60 minutes between successive exposures at the STEL. An averaging period other than 15 minutes may be recommended when this is warranted by observed biologic effects.

3. Threshold Limit Value–Ceiling (TLV–C).—The concentration that should not be exceeded during any part of the working exposure.

Conventional industrial hygiene practice in the assessment of a TLV–C is to sample over a 15-minute period except for those substances which may cause immediate irritation with exceedingly short exposures.

For some substances, e.g., irritant gases, only one category, the TLV–Ceiling, may be relevant. For other substances, either two or three categories may be relevant, depending upon their physiologic action. It is important to observe that if any one of these three TLVs is exceeded, a potential hazard from that substance is presumed to exist.

The Committee holds to the opinion that limits based on physical irritation should be considered no less binding than those based on physical impairment. There is increasing evidence that physical irritation may initiate, promote, or accelerate physical impairment through interaction with other chemical or biologic agents.

Time-Weighted Average vs. Ceiling Limits.—Time-weighted averages permit excursions above the limit provided they are compensated by equivalent excursions below the limit during the workday. In some instances it may be permissible to calculate the average concentration for a workweek rather than a workday. The relationship between threshold limit and permissible excursion is a rule of thumb and in certain cases may not apply. The amount by which threshold limits may be exceeded for short periods without injury to health depends upon a number of factors, such as the nature of the contaminant, whether very high concentrations—even for short periods—produce acute poisoning, whether the effects are cumulative, the frequency with which high concentrations occur, and the duration of such periods. All factors must be taken into consideration in arriving at a decision as to whether a hazardous condition exists.

Although the time-weighted average concentration provides the most satisfactory, practical way of monitoring airborne agents for compliance with the limits, there are certain substances for which it is inappropriate. In the latter group are substances which are predominantly fast-acting and whose threshold limit is more appropriately based on this particular response. Substances with this type of response are best controlled by a ceiling "C" limit that should not be exceeded. It is implicit in these definitions that the manner of sampling to determine noncompliance with the limits for each group must differ; a single brief sample, which is applicable to a "C" limit, is not appropriate to the time-weighted limit; here, a sufficient number of samples are needed to permit a time-weighted average concentration throughout a complete cycle of operations or throughout the work shift.

Whereas the ceiling limit places a definite boundary which concentrations should not be permitted to exceed, the time-weighted average limit requires an explicit limit to the excursions that are permissible above the listed values. It should be noted that the same factors are used by the Committee in determining the magnitude of the value of the STELs, or in determining whether to include or exclude a substance for a "C" listing.

Excursion Limits.—For the vast majority of substances with a TLV–TWA, there is not enough toxicologic data available to warrant a STEL. Nevertheless, excursions about the TLV–TWA should be controlled even where the eight-hour TWA is within recommended limits. Earlier editions of the TLV list included such limits chose values depended on the TLV–TWAs of the substance in question.

While no rigorous rationale was provided for these particular values, the basic concept was intuitive: in a well-controlled process exposure, excursions should be held within some reasonable limits. Unfortunately, neither toxicology nor collective industrial hygiene experience provide a solid basis for quantifying what those limits should be. The approach here is that the maximum recommended excursion should be related to variability generally observed in actual industrial processes. Leidel, Busch, and Crouse,* in reviewing large numbers of industrial hygiene surveys conducted by National Institute for Safety and Health (NIOSH), found that short-term exposure measurements were generally log normally distributed with geometric standard deviation mostly in the range of 1.5 to 2.0.

While a complete discussion of the theory and properties of the log normal distribution is beyond the scope of this section, a brief description of some important terms is presented. The measure of central tendency in a log normal description is the antilog of the mean logarithm of the sample values. The distribution is skewed and the geometric mean is always smaller than the arithmetic mean by an amount which depends on the geometric standard deviation. In the log normal distribution, the geometric standard deviation (sd_g) is the antilog of the standard deviation of the sample value logarithms and 68.26% of all values lie between m_g/sd_g and $m_g \times sd_g$.

If the short-term exposure values in a given situation have a geometric standard deviation of 2.0, 5% of all values exceed 3.13 times the geometric mean. If the process displays a variability greater than this, it is not under good control and efforts should be made to restore control. This concept is the basis for the new excursion limit recommendations, which are as follows:

> Short-term exposures should exceed three times the TLV–TWA for no more than a total of 30 minutes during a work day and under no

*Leidel NA, Busch KA, Crouse WE: *Exposure Measurement, Action Level and Occupational Environmental Variability*. NIOSH Pub 76–131, December 1975.

circumstances should they exceed five times the TLV–TWA, provided that the TLV–TWA is not exceeded.

The approach is a considerable simplification of the idea of the log normal concentration distribution but is considered more convenient to use by the practicing industrial hygienist. If exposure excursions are maintained within the recommended limits, the geometric standard deviation of the concentration measurements will be near 2.0 and the goal of the recommendations will be accomplished.

When the toxicologic data for a specific substance are available to establish a STEL, this value takes precedence over the excursion limit regardless of whether it is more or less stringent.

"Skin" Notation.—Listed substances followed by the designation "Skin" refer to the potential contribution to the overall exposure by the cutaneous route, including mucous membranes and eye, either by airborne, or more particularly, by direct contact with the substance. Vehicles can alter skin absorption.

Little quantitative data are available describing absorption of vapors and gases through the skin. The rate of absorption is a function of the concentration to which the skin is exposed.

Substances having a skin notation and a low TLV may present a problem at high airborne concentrations, particularly if a significant area of the skin is exposed for a long period of time. Protection of the respiratory tract while the rest of the body surface is exposed to a high concentration may present such a situation.

Biologic monitoring should be considered to determine the relative contribution of dermal exposure to the total dose.

This attention-calling designation is intended to suggest appropriate measures for the prevention of cutaneous absorption so that the threshold limit is not invalidated.

Mixtures.—Special consideration should be given also to the application of the TLVs in assessing the health hazards which may be associated with exposure to mixtures of two or more substances. A brief discussion of basic considerations involved in development, amplified by specific examples, are given in Appendix C.

Nuisance Particulates.—In contrast to fibrogenic dusts which cause scar tissue in lungs when inhaled in excessive amounts, so-called "nuisance" dusts have a long history of little adverse effect on lungs and do not produce significant organic disease or toxic effect when exposures are kept under reasonable control. The nuisance dusts have also been called (biologically) "inert" dusts, but the latter term is inappropriate to the extent that there is no dust which does not evoke some cellular response in the lung when inhaled in sufficient amount. However, the lung-tissue reaction caused by inhalation of nuisance dusts has the following characteristics: (1) the architecture of the air spaces remains intact; (2) collagen (scar tissue) is not formed to a significant extent; and (3) the tissue reaction is potentially reversible.

Excessive concentrations of nuisance dusts in the workroom air may seriously reduce visibility, may cause unpleasant deposits in the eyes, ears and nasal passages (Portland cement dust), or cause injury to the skin or mucous membranes by chemical or mechanical action per se or by the rigorous skin cleansing procedures necessary for their removal.

A threshold limit of 10 mg/cu m of total dust less than 1% quartz is recommended for substances in these categories and for which no specific threshold limits have been assigned. This limit, for a normal workday, does not apply to brief exposures at higher concentrations. Neither does it apply to those substances which may cause physiologic impairment at lower concentrations but for which a threshold limit has not yet been adopted. Some nuisance particulates are given in Appendix D. This list is not meant to be all inclusive; the substances serve only as examples.

Simple Asphyxiants—"Inert" Gases or Vapors.—A number of gases and vapors, when present in high concentrations in air, act primarily as simple asphyxiants without other significant physiologic effects. A TLV may not be recommended for each simple asphyxiant because the limiting factor is the available oxygen. The minimal oxygen content should be 18% by volume under normal atmospheric pressure (equivalent to a partial pressure, Po_2 of 135 mm Hg). Atmospheres deficient in O_2 do not provide adequate warning and most simple asphyxiants are odorless. Several simple asphyxiants present an explosion hazard. Account should be taken of this factor in limiting the concentration of the asphyxiant. Specific examples are listed in Appendix E. This list is not meant to be all inclusive; the substances serve only as examples.

Physical Factors.—It is recognized that such physical factors as heat, ultraviolet and ionizing radiation, humidity, abnormal pressure (altitude), and the like may place added stress on the body so that the effects from exposure at a threshold limit may be altered. Most of these stresses act adversely to increase the toxic response of a substance. *Although most threshold limits have built-in safety factors to guard against adverse effects to moderate deviations from normal environments, the safety factors of most substances are not of such a magnitude as to take care of gross deviations*. For example, continuous work at temperatures above 90° F, or overtime extending the workweek more than 25%, might be considered gross deviations. In such instances judgment must be exercised in the proper adjustments of the threshold limit values.

Hypersusceptibility.—Tests are available (*J Occup Med* 1973; 15:564, *Ann NY Acad Sci* 1968; 2:968) that may be used to detect those individuals hypersusceptible to a variety of industrial chemicals (respiratory irritants, hemolytic chemicals, organic isocyanates, carbon disulfide).

Unlisted Substances.—Many substances present or handled in industrial processes do not appear on the TLV list. In a number of instances, the material is rarely present as a particulate, vapor, or other airborne contaminant, and a TLV is not necessary. In other cases sufficient information to warrant development of a TLV, even on a tentative basis, is not available to the Committee. Other substances, of low toxicity, could be included in Appendix D pertaining to nuisance particulates. This list (as well as Appendix E) is not meant to be all inclusive: the substances serve only as examples.

In addition there are some substances of not inconsiderable toxicity, which have been omitted primarily because only a limited number of workers (e.g., employees of a single plant) are known to have potential exposure to possibly harmful concentrations.

Trade Names.—Because many chemical substances are marketed under several trade names, the trade names have been replaced with their generic equivalent in the alphabetical listing. Appendix H was created to ease this transition and the CAS number appears with the generic name to aid identification.

Operational Guidelines.—The ACGIH Board of Directors has adopted operational guidelines for Chemical Substances TLV Committee. These guidelines prescribe: charge, authority, policies, membership, organization, and operating procedures. The policies include the appeals procedures. Copies of the guidelines document are available from the Publications Office at a cost of $5 per copy.

Adopted Threshold Limit Values

	ADOPTED VALUES			
	TWA		STEL	
SUBSTANCE [CAS #]	PPM[a)]	MG/M[3b)]	PPM[a)]	MG/M[3b)]
Acetaldehyde [75-07-0]	100	180	150	270
Acetic acid [64-19-7]	10	25	15	37
Acetic anhydride [108-24-7]	C 5	C 20	—	—
Acetone [67-64-1]	750	1,780	1,000	2,375
Acetonitrile [75-05-8]—Skin	40	70	60	105
Acetylene [74-86-2]	E	—	—	—
Acetylene dichloride, *see* 1,2-Dichloroethylene				
* Acetylene tetrabromide [79-27-6]	1	15	—	—
Acetylsalicylic acid (Aspirin) [50-78-2]	—	5	—	—
Acrolein [107-02-8]	0.1	0.25	0.3	0.8
‡Acrylamide [79-06-1]—Skin	—	(0.3)	—	(0.6)
Acrylic acid [79-10-7]	10	30	—	—
Acrylonitrile [107-13-1]—Skin	2,A2	4.5,A2	—	—
* Aldrin [309-00-2]—Skin	—	0.25	—	—
Allyl alcohol [107-18-6]—Skin	2	5	4	10
Allyl chloride [107-05-1]	1	3	2	6
Allyl glycidyl ether (AGE) [106-92-3]—Skin	5	22	10	44
Allyl propyl disulfide [2179-59-1]	2	12	3	18
* α-Alumina [1344-28-1]	—	D	—	—
Aluminum [7429-90-5]				
* Metal & oxide	—	10	—	—
Pyro powders	—	5	—	—
Welding fumes	—	5	—	—
Soluble salts	—	2	—	—
Alkyls (NOC†)	—	2	—	—
4-Aminodiphenyl [92-67-1]—Skin	—	A1b	—	—
2-Aminoethanol, *see* Ethanolamine				
* 2-Aminopyridine [504-29-0]	0.5	2	—	—
3-Amino 1,2,4-triazole, *see* Amitrole				
* Amitrole [61-82-5]	—	0.2	—	—
Ammonia [7664-71-7]	25	18	35	27
Ammonium chloride fume [12125-02-9]	—	10	—	20
* Ammonium sulfamate [7773-06-0]	—	10	—	—
‡n-Amyl acetate [628-63-7]	100	530	(150)	(800)

(a) Parts of vapor or gas per million parts of contaminated air by volume at 25° C and 760 torr.
(b) Approximate milligrams of substance per cubic meter of air.
‡ See Notice of Intended Changes.
* 1986–87 addition.
Capital letters A, B, D, and E refer to Appendices; C denotes ceiling limit.

Continued.

Adopted Threshold Limit Values—*Continued*

SUBSTANCE [CAS #]	ADOPTED VALUES TWA PPM[a)]	TWA MG/M[3b)]	STEL PPM[a)]	STEL MG/M[3b)]
‡sec-Amyl acetate [626-38-0]	125	665	(150)	(800)
* Aniline [62-53-3] & homologues—Skin	2	10	—	—
Anisidine [29191-52-4] (o-, p-isomers)—Skin	0.1	0.5	—	—
Antimony [7440-36-0] & compounds, as Sb	—	0.5	—	—
Antimony trioxide [1309-64-4]				
Handling and use, as Sb	—	0.5	—	—
Production	—	A2	—	—
* ANTU [86-88-4]	—	0.3	—	—
Argon [7440-37-1]	E	—	—	—
Arsenic [7440-38-2] & soluble compounds, as As	—	0.2	—	—
Arsenic trioxide production [1327-53-3]	—	A2	—	—
Arsine [7784-42-1]	0.05	0.2	—	—
Asbestos [1332-21-4], *see* DUSTS	—	A1a	—	—
‡Asphalt (petroleum) fumes [8052-42-4]	—	5	—	(10)
Atrazine [1912-24-9]	—	5	—	—
* Azinphos-methyl [86-50-0]—Skin	—	0.2	—	—
Barium [7440-39-3], soluble compounds, as Ba	—	0.5	—	—
* Benomyl [17804-35-2]	0.8	10	—	—
‡Benzene [71-43-2]	10,A2	30,A2	(25,A2)	(75,A2)
Benzidine [92-87-5]—Skin	—	A1b	—	—
p-Benzoquinone, *see* Quinone				
Benzoyl peroxide [94-36-0]	—	5	—	—
Benzo(a)pyrene [50-32-8]	—	A2	—	—
Benzyl chloride [100-44-7]	1	5	—	—
Beryllium [7440-41-7] & compounds, as Be	—	0.002,A2	—	—
‡Biphenyl [92-52-4]	0.2	1.5	(0.6)	(4)
* Bismuth telluride [1304-82-1]	—	10	—	—
* Se-doped	—	5	—	—
Borates, tetra, sodium salts [1303-96-4]				
Anhydrous	—	1	—	—
Decahydrate	—	5	—	—
Pentahydrate	—	1	—	—
* Boron oxide [1303-86-2]	—	10	—	—
* Boron tribromide [10294-33-4]	C 1	C 10	—	—
Boron trifluoride [7637-07-2]	C 1	C 3	—	—
* Bromacil [314-40-9]	1	10	—	—
Bromine [7726-95-6]	0.1	0.7	0.3	2
* Bromine pentafluoride [7789-30-2]	0.1	0.7	—	—

(a) Parts of vapor or gas per million parts of contaminated air by volume at 25° C and 760 torr.
(b) Approximate milligrams of substance per cubic meter of air.
‡ See Notice of Intended Changes.
* 1986–87 addition.
Capital letters A, B, D, and E refer to Appendices; C denotes ceiling limit.

SUBSTANCE [CAS #]	ADOPTED VALUES TWA PPM[a]	MG/M3[b]	STEL PPM[a]	MG/M3[b]
Bromochloromethane, *see* Chlorobromomethane				
Bromoform [75-25-2]—Skin	05	5	—	—
* 1,3-Butadiene [106-99-0]	10,A2	22,A2	—	—
Butane [106-97-8]	800	1,900	—	—
Butanethiol, *see* Butyl mercaptan				
2-Butanone, *see* Methyl ethyl ketone (MEK)				
‡2-Butoxyethanol [111-76-2]—Skin	25	120	(75)	(360)
n-Butyl acetate [123-86-4]	150	710	200	950
‡sec-Butyl acetate [105-46-4]	200	950	(250)	(1,190)
‡tert-Butyl acetate [540-88-5]	200	950	(250)	(1,190)
Butyl acrylate [141-32-2]	10	55	—	—
n-Butyl alcohol [71-36-3]—Skin	C 50	C 150	—	—
sec-Butyl alcohol [78-92-2]	100	305	150	455
tert-Butyl alcohol [75-65-0]	100	300	150	450
Butylamine [109-73-9]—Skin	C 5	C 15	—	—
tert-Butyl chromate, as CrO_3 [1189-85-1]—Skin	—	C 0.1	—	—
n-Butyl glycidyl ether (BGE) [2426-08-6]	25	135	—	—
n-Butyl lactate [138-22-7]	5	25	—	—
Butyl mercaptan [109-79-5]	0.5	1.5	—	—
o-sec-Butylphenol [89-72-5]—Skin	5	30	—	—
p-tert-Butyltoluene [98-51-1]	10	60	20	120
* Cadmium [7440-43-9] Dusts & salts, as Cd	—	0.05	—	—
Cadmium oxide [1306-19-0]				
Fume, as Cd	—	C 0.05	—	—
Production	—	0.05	—	—
* Calcium carbonate/marble [1317-65-3]	—	D	—	—
* Calcium cyanamide [156-62-7]	—	0.5	—	—
Calcium hydroxide [1305-62-0]	—	5	—	—
Calcium oxide [1305-78-8]	—	2	—	—
Calcium silicate [1344-95-2]	—	D	—	—
Camphor, synthetic [76-22-2]	2	12	3	18
‡Caprolactam [105-60-2]				
Dust	—	(1)	—	(3)
Vapor	(5)	(20)	(10)	(40)
Captafol [2425-06-1]—Skin	—	0.1	—	—
* Captan [133-06-2]	—	5	—	—
* Carbaryl [63-25-2]	—	5	—	—
Carbofuran [1563-66-2]	—	0.1	—	—
* Carbon black [1333-86-4]	—	3.5	—	—
* Carbon dioxide [124-38-9]	5,000	9,000	30,000	54,000
Carbon disulfide [75-15-0]—Skin	10	30	—	—
Carbon monoxide [630-08-0]	50	55	400	440
Carbon tetrabromide [558-13-4]	0.1	1.4	0.3	4

(a) Parts of vapor or gas per million parts of contaminated air by volume at 25° C and 760 torr.
(b) Approximate milligrams of substance per cubic meter of air.
‡ See Notice of Intended Changes.
* 1986–87 addition.
Capital letters A, B, D, and E refer to Appendices; C denotes ceiling limit.

Continued.

Adopted Threshold Limit Values—*Continued*

SUBSTANCE [CAS #]	ADOPTED VALUES TWA PPM[a]	TWA MG/M3[b]	STEL PPM[a]	STEL MG/M3[b]
* Carbon tetrachloride [56-23-5]—Skin	5,A2	30,A2	—	—
Carbonyl chloride, *see* Phosgene				
Carbonyl fluoride [353-50-4]	2	5	5	15
Catechol [120-80-9]	5	20	—	—
* Cellulose (paper fiber) [9004-34-6]	—	D	—	—
Cesium hydroxide [21351-79-1]	—	2	—	—
Chlordane [57-74-9]—Skin	—	0.5	—	2
Chlorinated camphene [8001-35-2]—Skin	—	0.5	—	1
Chlorinated diphenyl oxide [55720-99-5]	—	0.5	—	2
Chlorine [7782-50-5]	1	3	3	9
Chlorine dioxide [10049-04-4]	0.1	0.3	0.3	0.9
Chlorine trifluoride [7790-91-2]	C 0.1	C 0.4	—	—
Chloroacetaldehyde [107-20-0]	C 1	C 3	—	—
α-Chloroacetophenone [532-27-4]	0.05	0.3	—	—
Chloroacetyl chloride [79-04-9]	0.05	0.2	—	—
Chlorobenzene [108-90-7]	75	350	—	—
o-Chlorobenzylidene malononitrile [2698-41-1]—Skin	C 0.05	C 0.4	—	—
Chlorobromomethane [74-97-5]	200	1,050	250	1,300
2-Chloro-1,3-butadiene, *see* β-Chloroprene				
Chlorodifluoromethane [75-45-6]	1,000	3,500	1,250	4,375
Chlorodiphenyl (42% Chlorine) [53469-21-9]—Skin	—	1	—	2
Chlorodiphenyl (54% Chlorine) [11097-69-1]—Skin	—	0.5	—	1
1-Chloro,2,3-epoxy-propane, *see* Epichlorohydrin				
2-Chloroethanol, *see* Ethylene chlorohydrin				
Chloroethylene, *see* Vinyl chloride				
* Chloroform [67-66-3]	10,A2	50,A2	—	—
bis(Chloromethyl) ether [542-88-1]	0.001,A1a	0.005,A1a	—	—
Chloromethyl methyl ether [107-30-2]	A2	A2	—	—
1-Chloro-1-nitropropane [300-25-9]	2	10	—	—
Chloropentafluoroethane [76-15-3]	1,000	6,320	—	—
Chloropicrin [76-06-2]	0.1	0.7	0.3	2
β-Chloroprene [126-99-8]—Skin	10	35	—	—

(a) Parts of vapor or gas per million parts of contaminated air by volume at 25° C and 760 torr.
(b) Approximate milligrams of substance per cubic meter of air.
‡ See Notice of Intended Changes.
* 1986–87 addition.
Capital letters A, B, D, and E refer to Appendices; C denotes ceiling limit.

SUBSTANCE [CAS #]	ADOPTED VALUES			
	TWA		STEL	
	PPM[a)]	MG/M$^{3b)}$	PPM[a)]	MG/M$^{3b)}$
o-Chlorostyrene [2039-87-4]	50	285	75	430
o-Chlorotoluene [95-49-8]	50	250	75	375
2-Chloro-6-(trichloromethyl) pyridine, *see* Nitrapyrin				
Chlorpyrifos [2921-88-2]—Skin	—	0.2	—	0.6
Chromite ore processing (Chromate), as Cr	—	0.05,A1a	—	—
Chromium [7440-47-3] Metal	—	0.5	—	—
Chromium (II) compounds, as Cr	—	0.5	—	—
Chromium (III) compounds, as Cr	—	0.5	—	—
Chromium (VI) compounds, as Cr				
Water soluble	—	0.05	—	—
Certain water insoluble	—	0.05,A1a	—	—
Chromyl chloride [14977-61-8]	0.025	0.15	—	—
Chrysene [218-01-9]	A2	A2	—	—
Clopidol [2971-90-6]	—	10	—	20
Coal tar pitch volatiles [8007-45-2], as benzene solubles	—	0.2,A1a	—	—
‡Cobalt [7440-48-4], as Co Metal, dust & fume	—	(0.1)	—	—
Cobalt carbonyl [10210-68-1], as Co	—	0.1	—	—
Cobalt hydrocarbonyl [16842-03-8], as Co	—	0.1	—	—
Copper [7440-50-8]				
Fume	—	0.2	—	—
* Dusts & mists, as Cu	—	1	—	
* Cotton dust, raw	—	0.2[(d)]	—	—
Cresol [1319-77-3], all isomers—Skin	5	22	—	—
‡Crotonaldehyde [123-73-9]	2	6	(6)	(18)
Crufomate [299-86-5]	—	5	—	20
‡Cumene [98-82-8]—Skin	50	245	(75)	(365)
Cyanamide [420-04-2]	—	2	—	—
Cyanides [151-50-8; 143-33-9], as CN—Skin	—	5	—	—
Cyanogen [460-19-5]	10	20	—	—
Cyanogen chloride [506-77-4]	C 0.3	C 0.6	—	—
‡Cyclohexane [110-82-7]	300	1,050	(375)	(1,300)
Cyclohexanol [108-93-0]—Skin	50	200	—	—
‡Cyclohexanone [108-94-1]—Skin	25	100	(100)	(400)
Cyclohexene [110-83-8]	300	1,015	—	—
Cyclohexylamine [108-91-8]	10	40	—	—
Cyclonite [121-82-4]—Skin	—	1.5	—	3
‡Cyclopentadiene [542-92-7]	75	200	(150)	(400)
‡Cyclopentane [287-92-3]	600	1,720	(900)	(2,580)
* Cyhexatin [13121-70-5]	—	5	—	—

(a) Parts of vapor or gas per million parts of contaminated air by volume at 25° C and 760 torr.
(b) Approximate milligrams of substance per cubic meter of air.
‡ See Notice of Intended Changes.
* 1986–87 addition.
Capital letters A, B, D, and E refer to Appendices; C denotes ceiling limit.
(d) Lint-free dust as measured by the vertical elutriator cotton-dust sampler described by Lynch JR: *Transactions of the National Conference on Cotton Dust.* May 2, 1970, p. 33.

Continued.

Adopted Threshold Limit Values—*Continued*

SUBSTANCE [CAS #]	TWA PPM[a]	TWA MG/M3[b]	STEL PPM[a]	STEL MG/M3[b]
* 2,4-D [94-75-7]	—	10	—	—
* DDT (Dichlorodiphenyl-trichloroethane) [50-29-3]	—	1	—	—
Decaborane [17702-41-9]—Skin	0.05	0.3	0.15	0.9
* Demeton [8065-48-3]—Skin	0.01	0.1	—	—
‡Diacetone alcohol [123-42-2]	50	240	(75)	(360)
1,2-Diaminoethane, *see* Ethylenediamine				
* Diazinon [333-41-5]—Skin	—	0.1	—	—
Diazomethane [334-88-3]	0.2	0.4	—	—
Diborane [19287-45-7]	0.1	0.1	—	—
1,2-Dibromoethane, *see* Ethylene dibromide				
* 2-N-Dibutylaminoethanol [102-81-8]—Skin	2	14	—	—
Dibutyl phosphate [107-66-4]	1	5	2	10
‡Dibutyl phthalate [84-74-2]	—	5	—	(10)
Dichloroacetylene [7572-29-4]	C 0.1	C 0.4	—	—
o-Dichlorobenzene [95-50-1]	C 50	C 300	—	—
p-Dichlorobenzene [106-46-7]	75	450	110	675
3,3′-Dichlorobenzidine [91-94-1]—Skin	—	A2	—	—
* Dichlorodifluoromethane [75-71-8]	1,000	4,950	—	—
1,3-Dichloro-5,5-dimethyl hydantoin [118-52-5]	—	0.2	—	0.4
1,1-Dichloroethane [75-34-3]	200	810	250	1,010
1,2-Dichloroethane, *see* Ethylene dichloride				
1,1-Dichloroethylene, *see* Vinylidene chloride				
‡1,2-Dichloroethylene [540-59-0]	200	790	(250)	(1,000)
Dichloroethyl ether [111-44-4]—Skin	5	30	10	60
Dichlorofluoromethane [75-43-4]	10	40	—	—
Dichloromethane, *see* Methylene chloride				
* 1,1-Dichloro-1-nitroethane [594-72-9]	2	10	—	—
1,2-Dichloropropane, *see* Propylene dichloride				
* Dichloropropene [542-75-6]—Skin	1	5	—	—
2,2-Dichloropropionic acid [75-99-0]	1	6	—	—
* Dichlorotetrafluoroethane [76-14-2]	1,000	7,000	—	—
* Dichlorvos [62-73-7]—Skin	0.1	1	—	—
Dicrotophos [141-66-2]—Skin	—	0.25	—	—
Dicyclopentadiene [77-73-6]	5	30	—	—
* Dicyclopentadienyl iron [102-54-5]	—	10	—	—
* Dieldrin [60-57-1]—Skin	—	0.25	—	—

(a) Parts of vapor or gas per million parts of contaminated air by volume at 25° C and 760 torr.
(b) Approximate milligrams of substance per cubic meter of air.
‡ See Notice of Intended Changes.
* 1986–87 addition.
Capital letters A, B, D, and E refer to Appendices; C denotes ceiling limit.

	ADOPTED VALUES			
	TWA		STEL	
SUBSTANCE [CAS #]	PPM[a)]	MG/M[3b)]	PPM[a)]	MG/M[3b)]
Diethanolamine [111-42-2]	3	15	—	—
Diethylamine [109-89-7]	10	30	25	75
2-Diethylaminoethanol [100-37-8]—Skin	10	50	—	—
Diethylene triamine [111-40-0]—Skin	1	4	—	—
Diethyl ether, *see* Ethyl ether				
Di-2-ethylhexylphthalate, *see* Di-sec, octyl phthalate				
Diethyl ketone [96-22-0]	200	705	—	—
‡Diethyl phthalate [84-66-2]	—	5	—	(10)
* Difluorodibromomethane [75-61-6]	100	860	—	—
Diglycidyl ether (DGE) [2238-07-5]	0.1	0.5	—	—
Dihydroxybenzene, *see* Hydroquinone				
Diisobutyl ketone [108-83-8]	25	250	—	—
Diisopropylamine [108-18-9]—Skin	5	20	—	—
Dimethoxymethane, *see* Methylal				
* Dimethyl acetamide [127-19-5]—Skin	10	35	—	—
Dimethylamine [124-40-3]	10	18	—	—
Dimethylaminobenzene, *see* Xylidene				
Dimethylaniline [121-69-7] (N,N-Dimethylaniline)—Skin	5	25	10	50
Dimethylbenzene, *see* Xylene				
Dimethyl carbamoyl chloride [79-44-7]	A2	A2	—	—
Dimethyl-1,2-dibromo-2-dichloroethyl phospate, *see* Naled				
* Dimethylformamide [68-12-2]—Skin	10	30	—	—
2,6-Dimethyl-4-heptanone, *see* Diisobutyl ketone				
* 1,1-Dimethylhydrazine [57-14-7]—Skin	0.5,A2	1,A2	—	—
Dimethylnitrosoamine, *see* N-Nitrosodimethylamine				
* Dimethylphthalate [131-11-3]	—	5	—	—
Dimethyl sulfate [77-78-1]—Skin	0.1,A2	0.5,A2	—	—
Dinitolmide [148-01-6]	—	5	—	—
* Dinitrobenzene [528-29-0; 99-65-0; 100-25-4] (all isomers)—Skin	0.15	1	—	—
* Dinitro-o-cresol [534-52-1]—Skin	—	0.2	—	—
3,5-Dinitro-o-toluramide, *see* Dinitolmide				
* Dinitrotoluene [121-14-2]—Skin	—	1.5	—	—
* Dioxane [123-91-1]—Skin	25	90	—	—
Dioxathion [78-34-2]—Skin	—	0.2	—	—
Diphenyl, *see* Biphenyl				

(a) Parts of vapor or gas per million parts of contaminated air by volume at 25° C and 760 torr.
(b) Approximate milligrams of substance per cubic meter of air.
* 1986–87 addition.
‡ See Notice of Intended Changes.
Capital letters A, B, D, and E refer to Appendices; C denotes ceiling limit

Continued.

Adopted Threshold Limit Values—*Continued*

SUBSTANCE [CAS #]	ADOPTED VALUES TWA PPM[a)]	TWA MG/M[3b)]	STEL PPM[a)]	STEL MG/M[3b)]
* Diphenylamine [122-39-4]	—	10	—	—
Diphenylmethane diisocyanate, *see* Methylene bisphenyl isocyanate				
Dipropylene glycol methyl ether [34590-94-8]	100	600	150	900
Dipropyl ketone [123-19-3]	50	235	—	—
* Diquat [85-00-7]	—	0.5	—	—
Di-sec, octyl phthalate [117-81-7]	—	5	—	10
* Disulfiram [97-77-8]	—	2	—	—
* Disulfoton [298-04-4]	—	0.1	—	—
‡2,6-Ditert. butyl-p-cresol [128-37-0]	—	10	—	(20)
Diuron [330-54-1]	—	10	—	—
Divinyl benzene [108-57-6]	10	50	—	—
* Emery [112-62-9]	—	D	—	—
* Endosulfan [115-29-7]—Skin	—	0.1	—	—
* Endrin [72-20-8]—Skin	—	0.1	—	—
Enzymes, *see* Subtilisins				
* Epichlorohydrin [106-89-8]—Skin	2	10	(5)	—
* EPN [2104-64-5]—Skin	—	0.5	—	—
1,2-Epoxypropane, *see* Propylene oxide				
2,3-Eposy-1-propanol, *see* Glycidol				
Ethane [74-84-0]	E	—	—	—
Ethanethiol, *see* Ethyl mercaptan				
Ethanol, *see* Ethyl alcohol				
Ethanolamine [141-43-5]	3	8	6	15
Ethion [563-12-2]—Skin	—	0.4	—	—
2-Ethoxyethanol [110-80-5]—Skin	5	19	—	—
2-Ethoxyethyl acetate [111-15-9]—Skin	5	27	—	—
Ethyl acetate [141-78-6]	400	1,400	—	—
‡Ethyl acrylate [140-88-5]—Skin	5	20	(25)	(100)
Ethyl alcohol [64-17-5]	1,000	1,900	—	—
Ethylamine [75-04-7]	10	18	—	—
Ethyl amyl ketone [541-85-5]	25	130	—	—
Ethyl benzene [100-41-4]	100	435	125	545
Ethyl bromide [74-96-4]	200	890	250	1,110
‡Ethyl butyl ketone [106-35-4]	50	230	(75)	(345)
* Ethyl chloride [75-00-3]	1,000	2,600	—	—
Ethylene [74-85-1]	E	—	—	—
Ethylene chlorohydrin [107-07-3]—Skin	C 1	C 3	—	—
Ethylenediamine [107-15-3]	10	25	—	—
Ethylene dibromide [106-93-4]—Skin	A2	A2	—	—
* Ethylene dichloride [107-06-2]	10	40	—	—
Ethylene glycol [107-21-1] Vapor	C 50	C 125	—	—

(a) Parts of vapor or gas per million parts of contaminated air by volume at 25° C and 760 torr.
(b) Approximate milligrams of substance per cubic meter of air.
‡ See Notice of Intended Changes.
* 1986–87 addition.
Capital letters A, B, D, and E refer to Appendices; C denotes ceiling limit.

SUBSTANCE [CAS #]	ADOPTED VALUES TWA PPM[a)]	MG/M[3b)]	STEL PPM[a)]	MG/M[3b)]
Ethylene glycol dinitrate [628-96-6]—Skin	0.05	0.3	—	—
Ethylene glycol methyl ether acetate, *see* 2-Methoxyethyl acetate				
Ethylene oxide [75-21-8]	1,A2	2,A2	—	—
Ethylenimine [151-56-4]—Skin	0.5	1	—	—
Ethyl ether [60-29-7]	400	1,200	500	1,500
‡Ethyl formate [109-94-4]	100	300	(150)	(450)
Ethylidene chloride, *see* 1,1-Dichloroethane				
Ethylidene norbornene [16219-75-3]	C 5	C 25	—	—
* Ethyl mercaptan [75-08-1]	0.5	1	—	—
* N-Ethylmorpholine [100-74-3]—Skin	5	23	—	—
* Ethyl silicate [78-10-4]	10	85	—	—
Fenamiphos [22224-92-6]—Skin	—	0.1	—	—
Fensulfothion [115-90-2]	—	0.1	—	—
Fenthion [55-38-9]—Skin	—	0.2	—	—
* Ferbam [14484-64-1]	—	10	—	—
Ferrovanadium dust [12604-58-9]	—	1	—	3
Fibrous glass dust	—	10	—	—
Fluorides, as F	—	2.5	—	—
Fluorine [7782-41-4]	1	2	2	4
Fluorotrichloromethane, *see* Trichlorofluoromethane				
Fonofos [944-22-9]—Skin	—	0.1	—	—
Formaldehyde [50-00-0]	1,A2	1.5,A2	2,A2	3,A2
‡Formamide [75-12-7]	(20)	(30)	(30)	(45)
Formic acid [64-18-6]	5	9	—	—
‡Furfural [98-01-1]—Skin	2	8	(10)	(40)
Furfuryl alcohol [98-00-0]—Skin	10	40	15	60
Gasoline [8006-61-9]	300	900	500	1,500
* Germanium tetrahydride [7782-65-2]	0.2	0.6	—	—
Glass, fibrous or dust, *see* Fibrous glass dust				
Glutaraldehyde [111-30-8]	C 0.2	C 0.7	—	—
Glycerin mist [56-81-5]	—	D	—	—
‡Glycidol [556-52-5]	25	75	(100)	(300)
Glycol, monoethyl ether, *see* 2-Ethoxyethanol				
‡Graphite (Natural) [7782-42-5], *see* DUSTS				
‡Graphite (Synthetic)	—	(D)	—	—
* Gypsum [10101-4-4]	—	D	—	—
* Hafnium [7440-58-6]	—	0.5	—	—
Helium [7440-59-7]	E	—	—	—
* Heptachlor [76-44-8]—Skin	—	0.5	—	—
Heptane [142-82-5] (n-Heptane)	400	1,600	500	2,000
2-Heptanone, *see* Methyl n-amyl ketone				
3-Heptanone, *see* Ethyl butyl ketone				
Hexachlorobutadiene [87-68-3]—Skin	0.02,A2	0.24,A2	—	—

(a) Parts of vapor or gas per million parts of contaminated air by volume at 25° C and 760 torr.
(b) Approximate milligrams of substance per cubic meter of air.
‡ See Notice of Intended Changes.
* 1986–87 addition.
Capital letters A, B, D, and E refer to Appendices; C denotes ceiling limit.

Continued.

Adopted Threshold Limit Values—*Continued*

	ADOPTED VALUES			
	TWA		STEL	
SUBSTANCE [CAS #]	PPM[a]	MG/M3[b]	PPM[a]	MG/M3[b]
* Hexachlorocyclopentadiene [77-47-4]	0.01	0.1	—	—
Hexachloroethane [67-72-1]	10	100	—	—
* Hexachloronaphthalene [1335-87-1]—Skin	—	0.2	—	—
* Hexafluoroacetone [684-16-2]—Skin	0.1	0.7	—	—
Hexamethyl phosphoramide [680-31-9]—Skin	A2	A2	—	—
Hexane (n-Hexane)				
[110-54-3]	50	180	—	—
Other isomers	500	1,800	1,000	3,600
2-Hexanone, *see* Methyl n-butyl ketone				
Hexone, *see* Methyl isobutyl ketone				
sec-Hexyl acetate [108-84-9]	50	300	—	—
Hexylene glycol [107-41-5]	C 25	C 125	—	—
Hydrazine [302-01-2]—Skin	0.1,A2	0.1,A2	—	—
Hydrogen [1333-74-0]	E	—	—	—
Hydrogenated terphenyls [61788-32-7]	0.5	5	—	—
* Hydrogen bromide [10035-10-6]	C 3	C 10	—	—
Hydrogen chloride [7647-01-0]	C 5	C 7	—	—
Hydrogen cyanide [74-90-8]—Skin	C 10	C 10	—	—
* Hydrogen fluoride [7664-39-3], as F	C 3	C 2.5	—	—
* Hydrogen peroxide [7722-84-1]	1	1.5	—	—
Hydrogen selenide [7783-07-5], as Se	0.05	0.2	—	—
Hydrogen sulfide [7783-06-4]	10	14	15	21
‡Hydroquinone [123-31-9]	—	2	—	(4)
4-Hydroxy-4-methyl-2-pentanone, *see* Diacetone alcohol				
2-Hydroxypropyl acrylate [999-61-1]—Skin	0.5	3	—	—
‡Indene [95-13-6]	10	45	(15)	(70)
* Indium [7440-74-6] & compounds, as in	—	0.1	—	—
Iodine [7553-56-2]	C 0.1	C 1	—	—
* Iodoform [75-47-8]	0.6	10	—	—
* Iron oxide fume (Fe_2O_3) [1309-37-1], as Fe	B2	5	—	—
Iron pentacarbonyl [13463-40-6], as Fe	0.1	0.8	0.2	1.6
* Iron salts, soluble, as Fe	—	1	—	—
‡Isoamyl acetate [123-92-2]	100	525	(125)	(655)
Isoamyl alcohol [123-51-3]	100	360	125	450
Isobutyl acetate [110-19-0]	150	700	187	875
‡Isobutyl alcohol [78-83-1]	50	150	(75)	(225)
Isooctyl alcohol [26952-21-6]—Skin	50	270	—	—

(a) Parts of vapor or gas per million parts of contaminated air by volume at 25° C and 760 torr.
(b) Approximate milligrams of substance per cubic meter of air.
‡ See Notice of Intended Changes.
* 1986–87 addition.
Capital letters A, B, D, and E refer to Appendices; C denotes ceiling limit.

	ADOPTED VALUES			
	TWA		STEL	
SUBSTANCE [CAS #]	PPM[a]	MG/M3[b]	PPM[a]	MG/M3[b]
Isophorone [78-59-1]	C 5	C 25	—	—
‡Isophorone diisocyanate [4098-71-9]—Skin	(0.01)	(0.09)	—	—
‡Isopropoxyethanol [109-59-1]	25	105	(75)	(320)
Isopropyl acetate [108-21-4]	250	950	310	1,185
Isopropyl alcohol [67-63-0]	400	980	500	1,225
Isopropylamine [75-31-0]	5	12	10	24
* N-Isopropylaniline [768-52-5]—Skin	2	10	—	—
Isopropyl ether [108-20-3]	250	1,050	310	1,320
Isopropyl glycidyl ether (IGE) [4016-14-2]	50	240	75	360
* Kaolin	—	D	—	—
Ketene [463-51-4]	0.5	0.9	1.5	3
* Lead [7439-92-1], inorg. dusts & fumes, as Pb	—	0.15	—	—
Lead arsenate [10102-48-4] as $Pb_3(AsO_4)_2$	—	0.15	—	—
Lead chromate [7758-97-6] as Cr	—	0.05,A2	—	—
* Limestone [1317-65-3]	—	D	—	—
* Lindane [58-89-9]—Skin	—	0.5	—	—
Lithium hydride [7580-67-8]	—	0.025	—	—
‡L.P.G. (Liquified petroleum gas)	1,000	1,800	(1,250)	(2,250)
* Magnesite [546-93-0]	—	D	—	—
Magnesium oxide fume [1309-48-4]	—	10	—	—
Malathion [121-75-5]—Skin	—	10	—	—
Maleic anhydride [108-31-6]	0.25	1	—	—
‡Manganese [7439-96-5], as Mn				
‡ Dust & compounds	—	(C 5)	—	—
Fume	—	1	—	3
* Manganese cyclopentadienyl tricarbonyl [12079-65-1], as Mn—Skin	—	0.1	—	—
Manganese tetroxide [1317-35-7]	—	1	—	—
* Marble/calcium carbonate [1317-65-3]	—	D	—	—
Mercury [7439-97-6], as Hg—Skin				
Alkyl compounds	—	0.01	—	0.03
All forms except alkyl				
Vapor	—	0.05	—	—
Aryl & inorganic compounds	—	0.1	—	—
Mesityl oxide [141-79-7]	15	60	25	100
Methacrylic acid [79-41-4]	20	70	—	—
Methane [74-82-8]	E	—	—	—
Methanethiol, *see* Methyl mercaptan				
Methanol, *see* Methyl alcohol				
Methomyl [16752-77-5]	—	2.5	—	—

(a) Parts of vapor or gas per million parts of contaminated air by volume at 25° C and 760 torr.
(b) Approximate milligrams of substance per cubic meter of air.
‡ See Notice of Intended Changes.
* 1986–87 addition.
Capital letters A, B, D, and E refer to Appendices; C denotes ceiling limit.

Continued.

Adopted Threshold Limit Values—*Continued*

	ADOPTED VALUES			
	TWA		STEL	
SUBSTANCE [CAS #]	PPM[a]	MG/M[3b]	PPM[a]	MG/M[3b]
Methoxychlor [72-43-5]	—	10	—	—
2-Methoxyethanol [109-86-4]—Skin	5	16	—	—
2-Methoxyethyl acetate [110-49-6]—Skin	5	24	—	—
4-Methoxyphenol [150-76-5]	—	5	—	—
Methyl acetate [79-20-9]	200	610	250	760
Methyl acetylene [74-99-7]	1,000	1,650	1,250	2,040
Methyl acetylene-propadiene mixture (MAPP)	1,000	1,800	1,250	2,250
Methyl acrylate [96-33-3]—Skin	10	35	—	—
* Methylacrylonitrile [126-98-7]—Skin	1	3	—	—
‡Methylal [109-87-5]	1,000	3,100	(1,250)	(3,875)
Methyl alcohol [67-56-1]—Skin	200	260	250	310
Methylamine [74-89-5]	10	12	—	—
Methyl amyl alcohol, *see* Methyl isobutyl carbinol				
‡Methyl n-amyl ketone [110-43-0]	50	235	(100)	(465)
* N-Methyl aniline [100-61-8]—Skin	0.5	2	—	—
* Methyl bromide [74-83-9]—Skin	5	20	—	—
Methyl n-butyl ketone [591-78-6]	5	20	—	—
Methyl chloride [74-87-3]	50	105	100	205
Methyl chloroform [71-55-6]	350	1,900	450	2,450
Methyl 2-cyanoacrylate [137-05-3]	2	8	4	16
‡Methylcyclohexane [108-87-2]	400	1,600	(500)	(2,000)
‡Methylcyclohexanol [25639-42-3]	50	235	(75)	(350)
o-Methylcyclohexanone [583-60-8]—Skin	50	230	75	345
* Methylcyclopentadienyl manganese tricarbonyl [12108-13-3]—Skin as Mn	—	0.2	—	—
* Methyl demeton [8022-00-2]—Skin	—	0.5	—	—
‡Methylene bisphenyl isocyanate (MDI) [101-68-8]	(C 0.02)	(C 0.2)	—	—
‡Methylene chloride [75-09-2]	(100)	(350)	(500)	(1,740)
4,4'-Methylene bis(2-chloroaniline) [101-14-4]—Skin	0.02,A2	0.22,A2	—	—
‡Methylene bis(4-cyclohexlisocyanate) [5124-30-1]	(C 0.01)	(C0.11)	—	—
* 4,4'-methylene dianiline [101-77-9]—Skin	0.1,A2	0.8,A2	—	—

(a) Parts of vapor or gas per million parts of contaminated air by volume at 25° C and 760 torr.
(b) Approximate milligrams of substance per cubic meter of air.
‡ See Notice of Intended Changes.
* 1986–87 addition.
Capital letters A, B, D, and E refer to Appendices; C denotes ceiling limit.

SUBSTANCE [CAS #]	TWA PPM[a]	TWA MG/M3[b]	STEL PPM[a]	STEL MG/M3[b]
	ADOPTED VALUES			
Methyl ethyl ketone (MEK) [78-93-3]	200	590	300	885
Methyl ethyl ketone peroxide [1338-23-4]	C 0.2	C 1.5	—	—
Methyl formate [107-31-3]	100	250	150	375
5-Methyl-3-heptanone, *see* Ethyl amyl ketone				
Methyl hydrazine [60-34-4]—Skin	C 0.2,A2	C 0.35,A2	—	—
* Methyl iodide [74-88-4]—Skin	2,A2	10,A2	—	—
Methyl isoamyl ketone [110-12-3]	50	240	—	—
Methyl isobutyl carbinol [108-11-2]—Skin	25	100	40	165
Methyl isobutyl ketone [108-10-1]	50	205	75	300
Methyl isocyanate [624-83-9]—Skin	0.02	0.05	—	—
Methyl isopropyl ketone [563-80-4]	200	705	—	—
Methyl mercaptan [74-93-1]	0.5	1	—	—
‡Methyl methacrylate [80-62-6]	100	410	(125)	(510)
* Methyl parathion [298-00-0]—Skin	—	0.2	—	—
Methyl propyl ketone [107-87-9]	200	700	250	875
* Methyl silicate [681-84-5]	1	6	—	—
α-Methyl styrene [98-83-9]	50	240	100	485
Metribuzin [21087-64-9]	—	5	—	—
Mevinphos [7786-34-7]—Skin	0.01	0.1	0.03	0.3
Molybdenum [7439-98-7], as Mo				
* Soluble compounds	—	5	—	—
* Insoluble compounds	—	10	—	—
Monochlorobenzene, *see* Chlorobenzene				
Monocrotophos [6923-22-4]	—	0.25	—	—
Morpholine [110-91-8]—Skin	20	70	30	105
* Naled [300-76-5]—Skin	—	3	—	—
Naphthalene [91-20-3]	10	50	15	75
β-Naphthylamine [91-59-8]	—	A1b	—	—
Neon [7440-01-9]	E	—	—	—
Nickel [7440-02-0]				
Metal	—	1	—	—
* Soluble compounds, as Ni	—	0.1	—	—
Nickel carbonyl [13463-39-3], as Ni	0.05	0.35	—	—
Nickel sulfide roasting fume & dust, as Ni	—	1,A1a	—	—
* Nicotine [54-11-5]—Skin	—	0.5	—	—
Nitrapyrin [1929-82-4]	—	10	—	20
Nitric acid [7697-37-2]	2	5	4	10
* Nitric oxide [10102-43-9]	25	30	—	—

(a) Parts of vapor or gas per million parts of contaminated air by volume at 25° C and 760 torr.
(b) Approximate milligrams of substance per cubic meter of air.
‡ See Notice of Intended Changes.
* 1986–87 addition.
Capital letters A, B, D, and E refer to Appendices; C denotes ceiling limit.

Continued.

Adopted Threshold Limit Values—*Continued*

SUBSTANCE [CAS #]	TWA PPM[a]	TWA MG/M3[b]	STEL PPM[a]	STEL MG/M3[b]
p-Nitroaniline [100-01-6]—Skin	—	3	—	—
* Nitrobenzene [98-95-3]—Skin	1	5	—	—
‡p-Nitrochlorobenzene [100-00-5]—Skin	(0.5)	(3)	—	—
4-Nitrodiphenyl [92-93-3]	—	A1b	—	—
* Nitroethane [79-24-3]	100	310	—	—
Nitrogen dioxide [10102-44-0]	3	6	5	10
* Nitrogen trifluoride [7783-54-2]	10	30	—	—
Nitroglycerin (NG) [55-63-0]—Skin	0.05	0.5	—	—
* Nitromethane [75-52-5]	100	250	—	—
* 1-Nitropropane [108-03-2]	25	90	—	—
‡2-Nitropropane [79-46-9]	(C 25, A2)	(C 90,A2)	—	—
N-Nitrosodimethylamine [62-75-9]—Skin	—	A2	—	—
Nitrotoluene [99-08-1]—Skin	2	11	—	—
Nitrotrichloromethane, *see* Chloropicrin				
‡Nonane [111-84-2]	200	1,050	(250)	(1,300)
Octachloronaphthalene [2234-13-1]—Skin	—	0.1	—	0.3
Octane [111-65-9]	300	1,450	375	1,800
Oil mist, mineral [8012-95-1]	—	5[(e)]	—	10
Osmium tetroxide [20816-12-0], as Os	0.0002	0.002	0.0006	0.006
Oxalic acid [144-62-7]	—	1	—	2
* Oxygen difluoride [7783-41-7]	C 0.05	C 0.1	—	—
Ozone [10028-15-6]	0.1	0.2	0.3	0.6
‡Paraffin wax fume [8002-74-2]	—	2	—	(6)
Paraquat [4685-14-7], respirable sizes	—	0.1	—	—
* Parathion [56-38-2]—Skin	—	0.1	—	—
Particulate polycyclic aromatic hydrocarbons (PPAH), *see* Coal tar pitch volatiles				
Pentaborane [19624-22-7]	0.005	0.01	0.015	0.03
* Pentachloronaphthalene [1321-64-8]	—	0.5	—	—
* Pentachlorophenol [87-86-5]—Skin	—	0.5	—	—
* Pentaerythritol [115-77-5]	—	D	—	—
Pentane [109-66-0]	600	1,800	750	2,250
2-Pentanone, *see* Methyl propyl ketone				
Perchloroethylene [127-18-4]	50	335	200	1,340
Perchloromethyl mercaptan [594-42-3]	0.1	0.8	—	—
Perchloryl fluoride [7616-94-6]	3	14	6	28
Phenacyl chloride, *see* α-Chloroacetophenone				
‡Phenol [108-95-2]—Skin	5	19	(10)	(38)

(a) Parts of vapor or gas per million parts of contaminated air by volume at 25° C and 760 torr.
(b) Approximate milligrams of substance per cubic meter of air.
‡ See Notice of Intended Changes.
* 1986–87 addition.
Capital letters A, B, D, and E refer to Appendices; C denotes ceiling limit.
(e) As sampled by method that does not collect vapor.

SUBSTANCE [CAS #]	ADOPTED VALUES TWA PPM[a)]	MG/M3[b)]	STEL PPM[a)]	MG/M3[b)]
* Phenothiazine [92-84-2]—Skin	—	5	—	—
N-Phenyl-beta-naphthyl—amine [135-88-6]	A2	A2	—	—
p-Phenylene diamine [106-50-3]—Skin	—	0.1	—	—
Phenyl ether [101-84-8], vapor	1	7	2	14
Phenylethylene, *see* Styrene, monomer				
Phenyl glycidyl ether (PGE) [122-60-1]	1	6	—	—
Phenylhydrazine [100-63-0]—Skin	5,A2	20,A2	10,A2	45,A2
Phenyl mercaptan [108-98-5]	0.5	2	—	—
Phenylphosphine [638-21-1]	C 0.05	C 0.25	—	—
Phorate [298-02-2]—Skin	—	0.05	—	0.2
Phosdrin, *see* Mevinphos				
Phosgene [75-44-5]	0.1	0.4	—	—
Phosphine [7803-51-2]	0.3	0.4	1	1
Phosphoric acid [7664-38-2]	—	1	—	3
* Phosphorus (yellow) [7723-14-0]	—	0.1	—	—
Phosphorus oxychloride [10025-87-3]	0.1	0.6	0.5	3
Phosphorus pentachloride [10026-13-8]	0.1	1	—	—
Phosphorus pentasulfide [1314-80-3]	—	1	—	3
Phosphorus trichloride [7719-12-2]	0.2	1.5	0.5	3
‡Phthalic anhydride [85-44-9]	1	6	(4)	(24)
m-Phthalodinitrile [626-17-5]	—	5	—	—
Picloram [1918-02-1]	—	10	—	20
Picric acid [88-89-1]—Skin	—	0.1	—	0.3
‡Pindone [83-26-1]	—	0.1	—	(0.3)
Piperazine dihydrochloride [142-64-3]	—	5	—	—
2-Pivalyl-1,3-indandione, *see* Pindone				
* Plaster of Paris	—	D	—	—
Platinum [7440-06-4]				
Metal	—	1	—	—
Soluble salts, as Pt	—	0.002	—	—
Polychlorobiphenyls, *see* Chlorodiphenyls				
Polytetrafluoroethylene decomposition products	—	B1	—	—
Portland cement	—	D	—	—
Potassium hydroxide [1310-58-3]	—	C 2	—	—
Propane [74-98-6]	E	—	—	—
Propane sultone [1120-71-4]	A2	A2	—	—
‡Propargyl alcohol [107-19-7]—Skin	1	2	(3)	(6)
‡β-Propiolactone [57-57-8]	0.5,A2	1.5,A2	(1,A2)	(3,A2)
‡Propionic acid [79-09-4]	10	30	(15)	(45)
‡Propoxur [114-26-1]	—	0.5	—	(2)

(a) Parts of vapor or gas per million parts of contaminated air by volume at 25° C and 760 torr.
(b) Approximate milligrams of substance per cubic meter of air.
‡ See Notice of Intended Changes.
* 1986–87 addition.
Capital letters A. B, D, and E refer to Appendices; C denotes ceiling limit.

Continued.

Adopted Threshold Limit Values—*Continued*

SUBSTANCE [CAS #]	ADOPTED VALUES TWA PPM[a]	TWA MG/M3[b]	STEL PPM[a]	STEL MG/M3[b]
n-Propyl acetate [109-60-4]	200	840	250	1,050
Propyl alcohol [71-23-8]—Skin	200	500	250	625
Propylene [115-07-1]	E	—	—	—
Propylene dichloride [78-87-5]	75	350	110	510
Propylene glycol dinitrate [6423-43-4]—Skin	0.05	0.3	—	—
Propylene glycol mono-methyl ether [107-98-2]	100	360	150	540
Propylene imine [75-55-8]—Skin	2,A2	5,A2	—	—
Propylene oxide [75-56-9]	20	50	—	—
n-Propyl nitrate [627-13-4]	25	105	40	170
Propyne, *see* Methyl acetylene				
‡Pyrethrum [8003-34-7]	—	5	—	(10)
‡Pyridine [110-86-1]	5	15	(10)	(30)
Pyrocatechol, *see* Catechol				
‡Quinone [106-51-4]	0.1	0.4	(0.3)	(1)
RDx, *see* Cyclonite				
Resorcinol [108-46-3]	10	45	20	90
Rhodium [7440-16-6]				
Metal	—	1	—	—
Insoluble compounds, as Rh	—	1	—	—
Soluble compounds as Rh	—	0.01	—	—
Ronnel [299-84-3]	—	10	—	—
‡Rosin core solder pyrolysis products, as formaldehyde	—	0.1	—	(0.3)
‡Rotenone (commercial) [83-79-4]	—	5	—	(10)
* Rouge	—	D	—	—
Rubber solvent (Naphtha)	400	1,600	—	—
Selenium compounds [7782-49-2], as Se	—	0.2	—	—
Selenium hexafluoride [7783-79-1], as Se	0.05	0.2	—	—
* Sesone [136-78-7]	—	10	—	—
Silane, *see* Silicon tetrahydride				
* Silicon [7440-21-3]	—	D	—	—
* Silicon carbide [409-21-2]	—	D	—	—
Silicon tetrahydride [7803-62-5]	5	7	—	—
Silver [7440-22-4]				
Metal	—	0.1	—	—
Soluble compounds, as Ag	—	0.01	—	—
Sodium azide [26628-22-8]	C 0.1	C 0.3	—	—
Sodium bisulfite [7631-90-5]	—	5	—	—
Sodium 2,4-dichloro-phenoxyethyl sulfate, *see* Sesone				
Sodium fluoroacetate [62-74-8]—Skin	—	0.05	—	0.15
Sodium hydroxide [1310-73-2]	—	C2	—	—
Sodium metabisulfite [7681-57-4]	—	5	—	—

(a) Parts of vapor or gas per million parts of contaminated air by volume at 25° C and 760 torr.
(b) Approximate milligrams of substance per cubic meter of air.
‡ See Notice of Intended Changes.
* 1986–87 addition.
Capital letters A, B, D, and E refer to Appendices; C denotes ceiling limit.

SUBSTANCE [CAS #]	TWA PPM[a)]	TWA MG/M$^{3b)}$	STEL PPM[a)]	STEL MG/M$^{3b)}$
	ADOPTED VALUES			
* Starch [9005-25-8]	—	D	—	—
* Stibine [7803-52-3]	0.1	0.5	—	—
‡Stoddard solvent [8052-41-3]	100	525	(200)	(1,050)
* Strychnine [57-24-9]	—	0.15	—	—
Styrene, monomer [100-42-5]	50	215	100	425
Subtilisins [1395-21-7] (Proteolytic enzymes as 100% pure crystalline enzyme)	—C0.00006[(f)]		—	—
* Sucrose [57-50-1]	—	D	—	—
* Sulfotep [3689-24-5]—Skin	—	0.2	—	—
* Sulfur dioxide [7446-09-5]	2	5	5	10
* Sulfur hexafluoride [2551-62-4]	1,000	6,000	—	—
Sulfuric acid [7664-93-9]	—	1	—	—
* Sulfur monochloride [10025-67-9]	C 1	C 6	—	—
* Sulfur pentafluoride [5714-22-7]	C 0.01	C 0.1	—	—
* Sulfur tetrafluoride [7783-60-0]	C 0.1	C 0.4	—	—
Sulfuryl fluoride [2699-79-8]	5	20	10	40
Sulprofos [35400-43-2]	—	1	—	—
Systox, *see* Demeton				
* 2,4,5-T [93-76-5]	—	10	—	—
‡Tantalum [7440-25-7]	—	(5)	—	(10)
TEDP, *see* Sulfotep				
Tellurium & compounds [13494-80-9], as Te	—	0.1	—	—
Tellurium hexafluoride [7783-80-4], as Te	0.02	0.2	—	—
* Temephos [3383-96-8]	—	10	—	—
* TEPP [107-49-3]—Skin	0.004	0.05	—	—
Terphenyls [26140-60-3]	C 0.5	C 5	—	—
* 1,1,1,2-Tetrachloro-2,2-difluoroethane [76-11-9]	500	4,170	—	—
* 1,1,2,2-Tetrochloro-1,2-difluoroethane [76-12-0]	500	4,170	—	—
* 1,1,2,2-Tetrachloroethane [79-34-5]—Skin	1	7	—	—
Tetrachloroethylene, *see* perchloroethylene				
Tetrachloromethane, *see* Carbon tetrachloride				
* Tetrachloronaphthalene [1335-88-2]	—	2	—	—
* Tetraethyl lead [78-00-2], as Pb—Skin	—	0.1[(g)]	—	—
Tetrahydrofuran [109-99-9]	200	590	250	735
* Tetramethyl lead [75-74-1], as Pb—Skin	—	0.15[(g)]	—	—
* Tetramethyl succinonitrile [3333-52-6]—Skin	0.5	3	—	—
Tetranitromethane [509-14-8]	1	8	—	—
Tetrasodium pyrophosphate [7722-88-5]	—	5	—	—

(a) Parts of vapor or gas per million parts of contaminated air by volume at 25° C and 760 torr.
(b) Approximate milligrams of substance per cubic meter of air.
‡ See Notice of Intended Changes.
* 1986–87 addition.
Capital letters A, B, D, and E refer to Appendices; C denotes ceiling limit.
(f) Based on "high volume" sampling.
(g) For control of general room air, biologic monitoring is essential for personal control.

Continued.

Adopted Threshold Limit Values—*Continued*

SUBSTANCE [CAS #]	ADOPTED VALUES TWA PPM[a]	TWA MG/M^{3}[b]	STEL PPM[a]	STEL MG/M^{3}[b]
* Tetryl [479-45-8]—Skin	—	5	—	—
Thallium [7440-28-0] Soluble compounds, as Tl—Skin	—	0.1	—	—
* 4,4'-Thiobis(6-tert, butyl-m-cresol) [96-69-5]	—	10	—	—
Thioglycolic acid [68-11-1]—Skin	1	4	—	—
* Thionyl chloride [7719-09-7]	C 1	C 5	—	—
* Thiram [137-26-8]	—	5	—	—
Tin [7440-31-5]				
* Metal	—	2	—	—
* Oxide & inorganic compounds, except SnH_4, as Sn	—	2	—	—
* Organic compounds, as Sn—Skin	—	0.1	—	—
* Titanium dioxide [13463-67-7]	—	D	—	—
o-Tolidine [119-93-7]—Skin	A2	A2	—	—
Toluene (toluol) [108-88-3]	100	375	150	560
Toluene-2,4-diisocyanate (TDI) [584-84-9]	0.005	0.04	0.02	0.15
o-Toluidine [95-53-4]—Skin	2,A2	9,A2	—	—
* m-Toluidine [108-44-1]—Skin	2	9	—	—
* p-Toluidine [106-49-0]—Skin	2,A2	9,A2	—	—
Toxaphene, *see* Chlorinated camphene				
* Tributyl phosphate [126-73-8]	0.2	2.5	—	—
Trichloroacetic acid [76-03-9]	1	7	—	—
1,2,4-Trichlorobenzene [120-82-1]	C 5	C 40	—	—
1,1,1-Trichloroethane, *see* Methyl chloroform				
* 1,1,2-Trichloroethane [79-00-5]—Skin	10	45	—	—
Trichloroethylene [79-01-6]	50	270	200	1,080
Trichlorofluoromethane [75-69-4]	C 1,000	C 5,600	—	—
Trichloromethane, *see* Chloroform				
* Trichloronaphthalene [1321-65-9]—Skin	—	5	—	—
Trichloronitromethane, *see* Chloropicrin				
‡1,2,3-Trichloropropane [96-18-4]—Skin	(50)	(300)	(75)	(450)
1,1,2-Trichloro-1,2,2-trifluoroethane [76-13-1]	1,000	7,600	1,250	9,500
Tricyclohexyltin, *see* Cyhexatin				
Triethylamine [121-44-8]	10	40	15	60
* Trifluorobromomethane [75-63-8]	1,000	6,100	—	—
Trimellitic anhydride [552-30-7]	0.005	0.04	—	—
Trimethylamine [75-50-3]	10	24	15	36
‡Trimethyl benzene [2551-13-7]	25	125	(35)	(170)

(a) Parts of vapor or gas per million parts of contaminated air by volume at 25° C and 760 torr.
(b) Approximate milligrams of substance per cubic meter of air.
‡ See Notice of Intended Changes.
* 1986–87 addition.
Capital letters A, B, D, and E refer to Appendices; C denotes ceiling limit.

SUBSTANCE [CAS #]	ADOPTED VALUES TWA PPM[a)]	MG/M[3b)]	STEL PPM[a)]	MG/M[3b)]
* Trimethyl phosphite [121-45-9]	2	10	—	—
2,2,6-Trinitrophenol, *see* Picric acid				
2,4,6-Trinitrophenylmethylnitramine, *see* Tetryl				
* 2,4,6-Trinitrotoluene (TNT) [118-96-7]—Skin	—	0.5	—	—
* Triorthocresyl phosphate [78-30-8]—Skin	—	0.1	—	—
Triphenyl amine [603-34-9]	—	5	—	—
* Triphenyl phosphate [115-86-6]	—	3	—	—
Tungsten [7440-33-7], as W				
Insoluble compounds	—	5	—	10
Soluble compounds	—	1	—	3
‡Turpentine [8006-64-2]	100	560	(150)	(840)
Uranium (natural) [7440-61-1]				
Soluble & insoluble compounds, as U	—	0.2	—	0.6
n-Valeraldehyde [110-62-3]	50	175	—	—
Vanadium, as V_2O_5 [1314-62-1]				
Respirable dust & fume	—	0.05	—	—
Vegetable oil mists	—	D	—	—
Vinyl acetate [108-05-4]	10	30	20	60
Vinyl benzene, *see* Styrene				
Vinyl bromide [593-60-2]	5,A2	20,A2	—	—
Vinyl chloride [75-01-4]	5,A1a	10,A1a	—	—
Vinyl cyanide, *see* Acrylonitrile				
Vinyl cyclohexene dioxide [106-87-6]—Skin	10,A2	60,A2	—	—
Vinylidene chloride [75-35-4]	5	20	20	80
Vinyl toluene [25013-15-4]	50	240	100	485
‡VM & P Naphtha [8032-32-4]	300	1,350	(400)	(1,800)
‡Warfarin [81-81-2]	—	0.1	—	(0.3)
Welding fumes (NOC†)	—	5,B2	—	—
Wood dust (certain hard woods as beech & oak)	—	1	—	—
Soft wood	—	5	—	10
Xylene [1330-20-7] (o-, m-, p-isomers)	100	435	150	655
m-Xylene α,α'-diamine [1477-55-0]—Skin	—	C 0.1	—	—
Xylidine [1300-73-8]—Skin	2	10	—	—
‡Yttrium [7440-64-5]	—	(1)	—	(3)
Zinc chloride fume [7646-85-7]	—	1	—	2
‡Zinc chromate [13530-65-9], as Cr	—	(0.05,A2)	—	—
Zinc oxide [1314-13-2]				
Fume	—	5	—	10
Dust	—	D	—	—
‡Zinc stearate [557-05-1]	—	(D)	—	(20)
Zirconium compounds [7440-67-2], as Zr	—	5	—	10

(a) Parts of vapor or gas per million parts of contaminated air by volume at 25° C and 760 torr.
(b) Approximate milligrams of substance per cubic meter of air.
‡ See Notice of Intended Changes.
* 1986–87 addition.
Capital letters A, B, D, and E refer to Appendices; C denotes ceiling limit.
† NOC = Not otherwise classified.
Radioactivity: See Physical Agents section on Ionizing Radiation.

Dusts[h]

SUBSTANCE	TLV-TWA
SILICA, SiO_2	
Crystalline	
* Quartz [14808-60-7]	0.1 mg/m^3, respirable dust
* Cristobalite [14464-46-1]	0.05 mg/m^3, respirable dust
Silica, fused [60676-86-0]	0.1 mg/m^3, respirable dust
* Tridymite [15468-32-3]	0.05 mg/m^3, respirable dust
Tripoli [1317-95-9]	0.1 mg/m^3 of contained respirable quartz dust.
Amorphous	
* Diatomaceous earth (uncalcined)[i] [68855-54-9]	10 mg/m^3, total dust
‡Precipitated silica	(5 mg/m^3, respirable dust) 10 mg/m^3, total dust
‡Silica gel	(5 mg/m^3, respirable dust) 10 mg/m^3, total dust
* *SILICATES*[i]	
Asbestos[j]	
Amosite [12172-73-5]	0.5 fiber/cc, A1a
Chrysotile [12001-29-5]	2 fibers/cc, A1a
Crocidolite [12001-28-4]	0.2 fiber/cc, A1a
Other forms	2 fibers/cc, A1a
‡Graphite (natural) [7782-42-5]	2.5 mg/m^3, respirable dust (5 mg/m^3, total dust)
* Mica [12001-25-2]	3 mg/m^3, respirable dust
Mineral wool fiber	10 mg/m^3
* Perlite	10 mg/m^3, total dust
* Portland cement	10 mg/m^3, total dust
Soapstone	3 mg/m^3, respirable dust 6 mg/m^3, total dust
Talc (containing no asbestos fibers) [14807-96-6]	2 mg/m^3, Respirable dust
Talc (containing asbestos fibers)	Use asbestos TLV-TWA. However, should not exceed 2 mg/m^3 respirable dust.
OTHER DUSTS	
* Barium sulfate [7727-43-7]	10 mg/m^3, total dust
* Grain dust (oats, wheat, barley)	4 mg/m^3, total particulate
* Graphite, synthetic	10 mg/m^3, total dust
*Nuisance particulates (see Appendix D)	10 mg/m^3, total dust
‡*COAL DUST*[j]	
‡ 2 mg/m^3 (respirable dust fraction $<$ 5% quartz). If $>$ 5% quartz, use respirable quartz value.	

‡ See Notice of Intended Changes
* 1986–1987 Addition.
(h) The concentration of respirable dust for the application of these limits is to be determined from the fraction passing a size-selector with the characters defined in Appendix F, *Other Issues,* point 1, both "c." paragraphs.
(i) For silicates, the values are for dust containing no asbestos and <1% crystalline silica in the total dust. For coal dust, the value is for coal dust containing <5% crystalline silica in the respirable fraction. For materials containing more than these percentages of crystalline silica, the environment should be evaluated against the TLV-TWA of 0.1 mg/m^3 for respirable quartz. Even where the respirable quartz concentration is less than 0.1 mg/m^3, the level of the major component should not exceed its TLV.
(j) Fibers longer than 5 μm and with an aspect ratio equal to or greater than 3:1 as determined by the membrane filter method at 400–450X magnification (4 mm objective) phase contrast illumination.

Notice of Intended Changes (for 1986–87)

These substances, with their corresponding values, comprise those for which either a limit has been proposed for the first time, or for which a change in the "Adopted" listing has been proposed. In both cases, the proposed limits should be considered trial limits that will remain in the listing for a period of at least two years. If, after two years no evidence comes to light that questions the appropriateness of the values herein, the values will be reconsidered for the "Adopted" list. Documentation is available for each of these substances.

Notice of Intended Changes—Substances

SUBSTANCE [CAS #]	TWA PPM[a)]	TWA MG/M[3b)]	STEL PPM[a)]	STEL MG/M[3b)]
Acrylamide [79-06-1]—Skin	—	0.03,A2	—	—
†Ammonium perfluoro-octanoate [3825-26-1]	—	0.1	—	—
†Caprolactam [105-60-2] Vapor & aerosol	0.25	1	—	—
Cobalt metal, dust & fume [7440-48-4], as Co	—	0.05	—	0.1
Enflurane [13838-16-9]	75	575	—	—
†Formamide [75-12-7]—Skin	10	15	—	—
Halothane [151-67-7]	50	400	—	—
†Hexamethylene diisocyanate [822-06-0]	0.005	0.035	—	—
†Isophorone diisocyanate [4098-71-9]	0.005	0.045	—	—
†Manganese dust & compounds [7439-96-5]	—	5	—	—
†Methylene bisphenyl isocyanate [101-68-8]	0.005	0.055	—	—
†Methylene chloride [75-09-2]	50,A2	175,A2	—	—
†Methylene bis-(4-cyclohexylisocyanate [5124-30-1]	0.005	0.055	—	—
†p-Nitrochlorobenzene [100-00-5]	0.1	0.6	—	—
2-Nitropropane [79-46-9]	10,A2	35,A2	(20,A2)	(70,A2)
†Stearates	—	D	—	—
†Tantalum [7440-25-7], metal and oxide, *see* DUSTS				
1,2,3-Trichloropropane [96-18-4]—Skin	10	60	—	—
†Yttrium [7440-65-5] metal and compounds, and Y	—	1	—	—
†Zinc chromates [13530-65-9; 1103-86-9; 37300-23-5], as Cr	—	0.01,A1	—	—

(a) Parts of vapor or gas per million parts of contaminated air by volume at 25° C and 760 torr.

(b) Approximate milligrams of substance per cubic meter of air.

‡ 1986–1987 revision or addition.

Capital letters A, B, D, and E refer to Appendices; C denotes ceiling limit.

Delete the Short-Term Exposure Limits (TLV-STELs) for the Following Substances

n-Amyl acetate
sec-Amyl acetate
Asphalt (petroleum) fumes
Benzene
Biphenyl
2-Butoxyethanol
sec-Butyl acetate
tert-Butyl acetate
Crotonaldehyde
Cumene
Cyclohexane
Cyclohexanone
Cyclopentadiene
Cyclopentane
Diacetone alcohol
Dibutyl phthalate
1,2-Dichloroethylene
Diethyl phthalate
2,6-Ditert. butyl-p-cresol
Ethyl acrylate
Ethylbutyl ketone
Ethyl formate
Furfural
Glycidol
Hydroquinone
Indene
Isoamyl acetate
Isobutyl alcohol
Isopropoxyethanol
L.P.G. (liquified petroleum gas)
Methylal
Methyl n-amyl ketone
Methylcyclohexane
Methylcyclohexanol
Methyl methacrylate
Nonane
Paraffin wax fume
Phenol
Phthalic anhydride
Pindone
Propargyl alcohol
β-Propiolactone
Propionic acid
Propoxur
Pyrethrum
Pyridine
Quinone
Rosin core solder pyrolysis products
Rotenone (commercial)
Stoddard solvent
Trimethyl benzene
Turpentine
VM & P naphtha
Warfarin

Notice of Intended Changes—Dusts

SUBSTANCE	TLV-TWA
SILICA, SiO_2	
Amorphous	
Precipitated silica[i]	10 mg/m^3, Total dust
Silica gel[i]	10 mg/m^3, Total dust
SILICATES[i]	
Coal dust	2 mg/m^3 respirable dust fraction[i]
Graphite (natural) [7782-42-5]	2.5 mg/m^3, Respirable dust
OTHER DUSTS	
†Stearates (Appendix D—Nuisance Particulates)	10 mg/m^3, Total dust
†Tantalum [7440-25-7], metal and oxide	10 mg/m^3, Total dust

SUBSTANCE	TLV
Asbestos	
Amosite	0.5 fiber[k]
Chrysotile	2 fibers[k]
Crocidolite	0.2 fiber[k]
Other forms	2 fibers[k]
bis-(Chloromethyl) ether	0.001 ppm
Chromite ore processing (chromate)	0.05 mg/m^3, as Cr
Chromium (VI), certain water insoluble compounds	0.05 mg/m^3, as Cr
Coal tar pitch volatiles	0.2 mg/m^3, as benzene solubles
Nickel sulfide roasting, fume and dust	1 mg/m^3, as Ni
Vinyl chloride	5 ppm
†Zinc chromates	0.01 mg/m^3, as Cr

†1986–1987 Revision or Addition.

Adopted Appendices

Appendix A: Carcinogens

The guidelines explain how the Chemical Substances Threshold Limit Values Committee classifies substances found in the occupational environment as either carcinogenic in man or experimental animals. Scientific debate over the existence of biological thresholds for carcinogens is unlikely to be resolved in the near future. For most substances determined to be carcinogenic by the Committee, a value is given to provide practical guidelines for the industrial hygienist to control exposures in the workplace.

The Chemical Substances TLV Committee considers information from the following kinds of studies to be indicators of a substance's potential to be a carcinogen in humans; epidemiology studies, toxicology studies and, to a lesser extent, case histories. Because of the long latent period for many carcinogens, and for ethical reasons, it is often impossible to base timely risk-management decisions on results from human toxicological studies. In order to recognize the qualitative differences in research results, two categories of carcinogens are designated in this booklet: A1—Confirmed Human Carcinogens; and A2—Suspected Human Carcinogens. All steps must be taken to keep exposures to all A1 carcinogens to a minimum. Workers exposed to A1 carcinogens without a TLV should be properly equipped to insure virtually no contract with the carcinogen. Please see the *Documentation of the Threshold Limit Values* for a more complete description and derivation of these designations.

The Committee lists below those substances in industrial use that have proven carcinogenic in man, or have induced cancer in animals under appropriate experimental conditions. Present listing of those substances carcinogenic for man takes two forms: Those for which a TLV has been assigned (1a) and those for which environmental conditions have not been sufficiently defined to assign a TLV (1b).

A1a. Human Carcinogens.—Substances, or substances associated with industrial processes, recognized to have carcinogenic or cocarcinogenic potential, with an assigned TLV:

A1b. Human Carcinogens.—Substances, or substances associated with industrial processes, recognized to have carcinogenic potential without an assignd TLV:

4-Aminodiphenyl—Skin
Benzidine—Skin
β-Naphthylamine
4-Nitrodiphenyl—Skin

For the substances in 1b, no exposure or contact by any route—respiratory, skin or oral, as detected by the most sensitive methods—shall be permitted. The worker should be properly equipped to insure virtually no contact with the carcinogen.

A2. Industrial Substances Suspect of Carcinogenic Potential for MAN.—Chemical substances or substances associated with industrial processes, which are suspect of inducing cancer, based on either (1) limited epidemiologic evidence, exclusive of clinical reports of single cases, or (2) demonstration of carcinogenesis in one or more animal species by appropriate methods.

Acrylamide—Skin	0.03 mg/m^3
Acrylonitrile—Skin	2 ppm
Antimony trioxide production	—
Arsenic trioxide production	—
Benzene	10 ppm
Benzo(a)pyrene	—
Beryllium	2 μg/m^3
‡1,3-Butadiene	10 ppm
Carbon tetrachloride—Skin	5 ppm
Chloroform	10 ppm
Chlormethyl methyl ether	—
**Chromates of lead and zinc, as Cr	0.05 mg/m^3
Chrysene	—
3,3'-Dichlorobenzidine—Skin	—
Dimethyl carbamoyl chloride	—
1,1-Dimethylhydrazine—Skin	0.5 ppm
Dimethyl sulfate—Skin	0.1 ppm

** See Notice of Intended Changes.
‡ 1986–1987 Adoption.

Ethylene dibromide—Skin	—
Ethylene oxide	1 ppm
Formaldehyde	1 ppm
Hexachlorobutadiene	0.02 ppm
Hexamethyl phosphoramide—Skin	—
Hydrazine—Skin	0.1 ppm
4,4'-Methylene bis(2-chloroaniline)—Skin	0.02 ppm
†Methylene chloride	50 ppm
‡4,4'-Methylene dianiline	0.1 ppm
Methyl hydrazine—Skin	C 0.2 ppm
Methyl iodide—Skin	2 ppm
2-Nitropropane	10 ppm
N-Nitrosodimethylamine—Skin	—
N-Phenyl-beta-naphthylamine	—
Phenylhydrazine—Skin	5 ppm
Propane sultone	—
β-Propiolactone	0.5 ppm
Propylene imine—Skin	2 ppm
o-Tolidine—Skin	—
o-Toluidine—Skin	—
‡o-Toluidine—Skin	2 ppm
Vinyl bromide	5 ppm
Vinyl cyclohexene dioxide—Skin	10 ppm

For the above, worker exposure by all routes should be carefully controlled to levels consistent with the animal and human experience data (*see* Documentation), including those substances with a listed TLV.

The Committee Guidelines for Classification of Experimental Animal Carcinogens

The following guidelines are offered in the present state of knowledge as an aid in classifying substances in the occupational environment found to be carcinogenic in experimental animals. A need was felt by the Threshold Limits Committee for such a classification in order to take the first step in developing an appropriate TLV for occupational exposure.

Determination of Approximate Threshold Response Requirement—In order to determine in which category to classify an experimental carcinogen for the purpose of assigning an industrial air limit (TLV), an approximate threshold of neoplastic response must be determined. Because of practical experimental difficulties, a precisely defined threshold cannot be attained. For the purpose of standard-setting, this is of little moment, as an appropriate risk, or safety, factor can be applied to the approximate threshold, the magnitude of which is dependent on the degree of potency of the carcinogenic response.

To obtain the best "practical" threshold of neoplastic response, dosage decrements should be less than logarithmic. This becomes particularly important at levels greater than 10 ppm (or corresponding mg/m^3). Accordingly, after a range-finding determination has been made by logarithmic decreases, two additional dosage levels are required within the levels of "effect" and "no effect" to approximate the true threshold of neoplastic response.

The second step should attempt to establish a metabolic relationship between animal and man for the particular substance found carcinogenic in animals. If the metabolic pathways are found comparable, the substance should be classed highly suspect as a carcinogen for man. If no such relation is found, the substance should remain listed as an experimental animal carcinogen until evidence to the contrary is found.

† 1986–1987 Addition.

‡ 1986–1987 Adoption.

Proposed Classification of Experimental Animal Carcinogens—Substances occurring in the occupational environment found carcinogenic for animals may be grouped into three classes, those of high, intermediate and low potency. In evaluating the incidence of animal cancers, significant incidence of cancer is defined as a neoplastic response which represents, in the judgment of the Committee, a significânt excess of cancers above that occurring in negative controls.

Exceptions: No substance is to be considered an occupational carcinogen of any practical significance which reacts by the respiratory route at or above 1000 mg/m^3 for the mouse, 2000 mg/m^3 for the rat; by the dermal route, at or above 1500 mg/kg for the mouse, 3000 mg/kg for the rat, by the gastrointestinal route at or above 500 mg/kg/d for a lifetime, equivalent to about 100 g T.D. for the rat, 10 g T.D. for the mouse. These dosage limitations exclude such substances as dioxane and trichlorethylene from consideration as carcinogens.

Examples: (1) Dioxane—rats, hepatocellular and nasal tumors from 1015 mg/kg/d, oral; (2) Trichloroethylene—female mice, tumors (30/98 at 900 mg/kg/d), oral.

A. *Industrial Substances of High Carcinogenic Potency in Experimental Animals.*

1. A substance to qualify as a carcinogen of high potency must fulfill *one* of the three following conditions (a, b, or c) in two animal species:

a. *Respiratory*. Elicit cancer from (1) dosages below 1 mg/m^3 (or equivalent ppm) via the respiratory tract in 6- to 7-hour daily repeated inhalation exposures throughout lifetime; or (2) from a single intratracheally administered dose not exceeding 1 mg of particulate, or liquid, per 100 ml or less of animal minute respiratory volume.

Examples: **(1)** bis(chloromethyl) ether—malignant tumors, rats, at 0.47 mg/m^3 (0.1 ppm) in 2 years; **(2)** Hexamethyl phosphoramide—nasal squamous cell carcinoma, rats at 0.05 ppm, in 13 months.

b. *Dermal*. Elicit cancer within 20 weeks by skin-painting, twice weekly at 2 mg/kg body or less per application for a total dose equal to or less than 1.5 mg, in a biologically inert vehicle.

Examples: **(1)** 7,12-Dimethylbenz(a)anthracene—skin tumors at 0.12-0.8 mg T.D. in four weeks; **(2)** Benzo(a)pyrene—mice 12 μg, 3×/wk for 18 mos. T.D. 2.6 mg, 90.9% skin tumors.

c. *Gastrointestinal*. Elicit cancer by daily intake via the gastrointestinal tract, within six months, with a six-month holding period, at a dosage below 1 mg/kg body weight per day; total dose, rat ≤ 50 mg; mouse, ≤ 3.5 mg.

Examples: **(1)** 7,12-Dimethylbenz(a)anthracene—mammary tumors from 10 mg 1X; **(2)** 3-Methylcholanthrene—tumors at 3 sites from

8 mg in 89 weeks; **(3)** Benzo(a)pyrene—mice, 3.9% leukemias, from 30 mg T.D. 198 days.

2. Elicit cancer by all three routes in at least two animal species at dose levels prescribed for high or intermediate potency.

B. *Industrial Substances of Intermediate Carcinogenic Potency in Experimental Animals.*

To qualify as a carcinogen of intermediate potency, a substance should elicit cancer in two animal species at dosages intermediate between those described in A and C by two routes of administration.

Example: Carbamic acid ethyl ester—dermal, mammary tumors, mice, 100%, 63 weeks, 500–1400 mg T.D. Gastrointestinal, various type tumors, mice 42 weeks, 320 mg T.D. Gastrointestinal, various type tumors, rats, 60 weeks, 110–930 mg T.D.

C. *Industrial Substances of Low Carcinogenic Potency in Experimental Animals.*

To qualify as a carcinogen of low potency, a substance should elicit cancer in one animal species by any *one* of the three routes of administration at the following prescribed dosages and conditions:

1. *Respiratory*. Elicit cancer from *a)* dosages greater than 10 mg/m^3 (or equivalent ppm) via the respiratory tract in 6- to 7-hour, daily repeated inhalation exposures, for 12 months' observation period; or *b)* from intratracheally administered dosages totaling more than 10 mg of particulate or liquid per 100 ml or more of animal minute respiratory volume.

Examples: **(1)** Beryl (beryllium aluminum silicate)—malignant lung tumors, rats, at 15 mg/m^3 at 17 months; **(2)** Benzidine—various tumors, rats, 10–20 mg/m^3 at $>$ 13 months.

2. *Dermal*. Elicit cancer by skin-painting of mice in twice weekly dosages of $>$ 10 mg/kg body weight in a biologically inert vehicle for at least 75 weeks, i.e., $\geqslant$ 1.5 g T.D.

Examples: **(1)** Shale tar—mouse, 0.1 ml $\times$ 50 = 5 g T.D. 59/60 skin tumors; **(2)** Arsenic trioxide—man, dose unknown, but estimated to be high.

3. *Gastrointestinal*. Elicit cancer from daily oral dosages of 50 mg/kg/day or greater during the lifetime of the animal.

Appendix B—Substances of Variable Composition

B1. Polytetrafluoroethylene* decomposition products.—Thermal decomposition of the fluorocarbon chain in air leads to the formation of oxidized products containing carbon, fluorine and oxygen. Because these products decompose in part by hydrolysis in alkaline solution, they can be quantitatively determined in air as fluoride to provide an index of exposure. No TLV is recommended pending determination of the toxicity of the products, but air concentration should be minimal.

B2. Welding Fumes—Total Particulate (NOC)† (TLV-TWA, 5 mg/m^3).—Welding fumes cannot be classified simply. The composition and quantity of both are dependent on the alloy being welded and the process and electrodes used. Reliable analysis of fumes cannot be made without considering the nature of the welding process and system being examined; reactive metals and alloys such as aluminum and titanium are arc-welded in a protective, inert atmosphere such as argon. These arcs create relatively little fume, but an intense radiation which can produce ozone. Similar processes are used to arc-weld steels, also creating a relatively low level of fumes. Ferrous alloys also are arc-welded in oxidizing environments which generate considerable fume, and can produce carbon monoxide instead of ozone. Such fumes generally are composed of discrete particles of amorphous slags containing iron, manganese, silicon and other metallic constituents depending on the alloy system involved. Chromium and nickel compounds are found in fumes when stainless steels are arc-welded. Some coated and flux-cored electrodes are formulated with fluorides and the fumes associated with them can contain significantly more fluorides than oxides. Because of the above factors, arc-welding fumes frequently must be tested for individual constituents which are likely to be present to determine whether specific TLVs are exceeded. Conclusions based on total fume concentration are generally adequate if no toxic elements are present in welding rod, metal, or metal coating and conditions are not conducive to the formation of toxic gases.

Most welding, even with primitive ventilation, does not produce exposures inside the welding helmet above 5 mg/m^3. That which does, should be controlled.

*Trade Names: Algoflon, Fluon, Teflon, Tetran.

† Not otherwise classified (NOC).

Appendix C—Threshold Limit Values for Mixtures

When two or more hazardous substances, which act upon the same organ system, are present, their combined effect, rather than that of either individually, should be given primary consideration. In the absence of information to the contrary, the effects of the different hazards should be considered as additive. That is, if the sum of the following fractions,

$$\frac{C_1}{T_1} + \frac{C_2}{T_2} + \ldots \frac{C_n}{T_n}$$

exceeds unity, then the threshold limit of the mixture should be considered as being exceeded. C_1 indicates the observed atmospheric concentration, and T_1 the corresponding threshold limit (*see* Example A.1 and B.1).

Exceptions to the above rule may be made when there is a good reason to believe that the chief effects of the different harmful substances are not in fact additive, but *independent* as when purely local effects or different organs of the body are produced by the various components of the mixture. In such cases the threshold limit ordinarily is exceeded only when at least one member of the series (C_1/T_1 + or + C_2/T_2, etc.) itself has a value exceeding unity (*see* Example B.1).

Synergistic action or potentiation may occur with some combinations of atmospheric contaminants. Such cases at present must be determined individually. Potentiating or synergistic agents are not necessarily harmful by themselves. Potentiating effects of exposure to such agents by routes other than that of inhalation is also possible, e.g., imbibed alcohol and inhaled narcotic (trichloroethylene). Potentiation is characteristically exhibited at high concentrations, less probably at low.

When a given operation or process characteristically emits a number of harmful dusts, fumes, vapors or gases, it will frequently be only feasible to attempt to evaluate the hazard by measurement of a single substance. In such cases, the threshold limit used for this substance should be reduced by a suitable factor, the magnitude of which will depend on the number, toxicity and relative quantity of the other contaminants ordinarily present.

Examples of processes which are typically associated with two or more harmful atmospheric contaminants are welding, automobile repair, blasting, painting, lacquering, certain foundry operations, diesel exhausts, etc.

Examples of TLVs for Mixtures

A *Additive effects*. The following formulae apply only when the components in a mixture have similar toxicologic effects; they should not be used for mixtures with widely differing reactivities, e.g., hydrogen cyanide and sulfur dioxide. In such cases the formula for Independent Effects (B) should be used.

1. General case, where air is analyzed for each component, the TLV of mixture =

$$\frac{C_1}{T_1} + \frac{C_2}{T_2} + \frac{C_3}{T_3} + \ldots = 1$$

Note: It is essential that the atmosphere be analyzed both qualitatively and quantitatively for each component present, in order to evaluate compliance or non-compliance with this calculated TLV.

Example A.1: Air contains 400 ppm of acetone (TLV, 750 ppm), 150 ppm of sec-butyl acetate (TLV, 200 ppm) and 100 ppm of methyl ethel ketone (TLV, 200 ppm).

Atmospheric concentration of mixture = 400 + 150 + 100 = 650 ppm of mixture.

$$\frac{400}{750} + \frac{150}{200} + \frac{100}{200} = 0.53 + 0.75 + 0.5 = 1.75$$

Threshold Limit is exceeded.

2. Special case when the source of contaminant is a liquid mixture and the atmospheric composition is *assumed* to be similar to that of the original material, e.g., on a time-weighted average exposure basis, all of the liquid (solvent) mixture eventually evaporates. When the percent composition (by weight) of the liquid mixutre is known, the TLVs of the constituents must be listed in mg/m^3. TLV of mixture =

$$\frac{1}{\frac{f_a}{TLV_a} + \frac{f_b}{TLV_b} + \frac{f_c}{TLV_c} + \ldots \frac{f_n}{TLV_n}}$$

Note: In order to evaluate compliance with this TLV, field sampling instruments should be calibrated, in the laboratory, for response to this specific quantitative and qualitative air-vapor mixture, and also to fractional concentrations of this mixture, e.g., ½ the TLV; ⅒ the TLV; 2 × the TLV; 10 × the TLV; etc.)

Example A.2: Liquid contains (by weight):

50% heptane: TLV = 400 ppm or 1600 mg/m^3
1 mg/m^3 ≡ 0.25 ppm
30% methyl chloroform: TLV = 350 ppm or 1900 mg/m^3
1 mg/m^3 ≡ 0.18 ppm
20% perchloroethylene: TLV = 50 ppm or 335 mg/m^3
1 mg/m^3 ≡ 0.15 ppm

$$\text{TLV of Mixture} = \frac{1}{\frac{0.5}{1600} + \frac{0.3}{1900} + \frac{0.2}{335}}$$

$$= \frac{1}{0.00031 + 0.00016 + 0.0006}$$

$$= \frac{1}{0.00107} = 935 \text{ mg/m}^3$$

of this mixture

50% or (935)(0.5) = 468 mg/m^3 is heptane
30% or (935)(0.3) = 281 mg/m^3 is methyl chloroform
20% or (935)(0.2) = 187 mg/m^3 is perchloroethylene

These values can be converted to ppm as follows:

heptane: 468 mg/m^3 × 0.25 = 117 ppm
methyl chloroform: 281 mg/m^3 × 0.18 = 51 ppm
perchloroethylene: 187 mg/m^3 × 0.15 = 29 ppm

TLV of mixture = 117 + 51 + 29 = 197 ppm, or 935 mg/m^3

B. Independent effects. TLV for mixture =

$$\frac{C_1}{T_1} = 1; \frac{C_2}{T_2} = 1; \frac{C_3}{T_3} = 1; \text{etc.}$$

Example B.1: Air contains 0.15 mg/m^3 of lead (TLV, 0.15) and 0.7 mg/m^3 of sulfuric acid (TLV, 1).

$$\frac{0.15}{0.15} = 1; \qquad \frac{0.7}{1} = 0.7$$

Threshold limit is not exceeded.

C. TLV for mixtures of mineral dusts. For mixtures of biologically active mineral dusts the general formula for mixtures given in A.2 may be used.

Appendix D—Some Nuisance Particulates[1]

TLV-TWA, 10 mg/m^3 of total dust[i]

α-Alumina (Al_2O_3)	Mineral wool fiber
Calcium carbonate	Pentaerythritol
Calcium silicate	Plaster of Paris
Cellulose (paper fiber)	Portland cement
Emery	Rouge
Glycerin mist	Silicon
Gypsum	Silicon carbide
Kaolin	Starch
Limestone	‡Stearates
Magnesite	Sucrose
Marble	Titanium dioxide
Vegetable oil mists (except castor oil, cashew nut or similar irritant oils)	‡Zinc stearate
	Zinc oxide dust

[i]When toxic impurities are not present, e.g., quartz <1%.
[1]As defined in the Introduction.
‡See Notice of Intended Changes.

Appendix E—Some Simple Asphyxiants[1]

Acetylene	Ethylene	Methane	Propylene
Argon	Helium	Neon	
Ethane	Hydrogen	Propane	

Appendix F—Chemical Substances and Other Issues Under Study[A]

Chemical Substances

Acetomethylchloride	Mineral wool fibers
Acetophenone	Naled
Acetylacetone	Nitrous oxide
Acrylic acid	Pentachlorophenol
Allyl chloride	Perchloroethylene
Bromodichloromethane	Persulfates
Ceramic fibers	Petroleum solvents
Dibutyl phenyl phosphate	o-Phenylenediamine
Dichlorvos	Propylene dichloride
Dinitrotoluene	Rosin core solder pyrolysis products
Epichlorohydrin	Skydrol hydraulic fluid
Ethylamines	1,1,1,2-Tetrachloro-2,2-difluoroethane
Gasoline (unleaded)	1,1,2,2-Tetrachloro-1,2-difluoroethane
Graphite fibers	1,1,2,2-Tetrachloroethane
Hexachlorocyclopentadiene	Thiram
Hydrazine	Trichloroethylene
Jet, petroleum and diesel fuels	
Malathion	
Methyl bromide	
Methyl hydrazines	

Other Issues

1. Particle Size-Selective Sampling Criteria for Airborne Particulate Matter[B]

   For chemical substances present in inhaled air as suspensions of solid particles or droplets, the potential hazard depends on particle size as well as mass concentration because of: (1) effects of particle size on deposition site within the respiratory tract, and (2) the tendency for many occupational diseases to be associated with material deposited in particular regions of the respiratory tract.

   ACGIH has recommended particle size-selective TLVs for crystalline silica for many years in recognition of the well established association between silicosis and respirable mass concentrations. It now has embarked on a re-examination of other chemical substances encountered in particulate form in occupational environments with the objective of defining: 1) the size-fraction most closely associated for each substance with the health effect of concern, and 2) the mass concentration within that size fraction which should represent the TLV.

   The Particle Size-Selective TLVs (PSS-TLVs) will be expressed in three forms, e.g.,

   a. *Inspirable Particulate Mass TLVs (IPM-TLVs)* for those materials which are hazardous when deposited anywhere in the respiratory tract.

   b. *Thoracic Particulate Mass TLVs (TPM-TLVs)* for those materials which are hazardous when deposited anywhere within the lung airways and the gas-exchange region.

   c. *Respirable Particulate Mass TLVs (RPM-TLVs)* for those materials which are hazardous when deposited in the gas-exchange region.

   The three particulate mass fractions described above are defined in quantitative terms as follows:

   a. Inspirable Particulate Mass consists of those particles that are captured according to the following collection efficiency regardless of sampler orientation with respect to wind direction:

   $$E = 50(1 + \exp[-0.06\ d_a]) \pm 10;$$
   $$\text{for } 0 < d_a \leqslant E\ 100\ \mu m$$

   Collection characteristics for $d_a > 100\ \mu m$ are presently unknown. E is collection efficiency in percent and d_a is aerodynamic diameter in μm.

   b. Thoracic Particulate Mass consists of those particles that penetrate a separator whose size collection efficiency is described by a cumulative lognormal function with a median aerodynamic diameter of 10 μm + 1.0 μm and with a geometric standard deviation of 1.5 (± 0.1).

   c. Respirable Particulate Mass consists of those particles that penetrate a separator whose size collection efficiency is described by a cumulative lognormal function with a median aerodynamic diameter of 3.5 μm ± 0.3 μm and with a geometric standard deviation of 1.5 (± 0.1). This incorporates and clarifies the previous ACGIH Respirable Dust Sampling Criteria.

   These definitions provide a range of acceptable performance for each type of size-selective sampler. Further information is available on the background and performance criteria for these particle size-selective sampling recommendations.[1–3]

REFERENCES

1. ACGIH: *Particle Size-Selective Sampling in the Workplace*, Cincinnati, Ohio, 1984, 80 pp.
2. Particle Size-Selective Sampling in the Workplace. *Ann Am Conf Govt Ind Hyg* 1984; 11:23–100.
3. Performance Considerations for Size-Selective Samplers (revised), chapter seven *Ann Am Conf Govt Ind Hyg*, submitted for publication.

2. Should the TLVs currently expressed as "total dust"[C] be changed to "inspirable particulate mass" (as defined in the above criteria) without changing the numerical value?

3. Applications of TLVs to altered work schedules.

[1] As defined in the Introduction.

[A] Information, data especially, and comments are solicited to assist the Committee in its deliberations and in the development of draft documents. Draft documentations are used by the Committee to decide what action, if any, to recommend on a given question.

[B] Includes redefinition of respirable dust and notice of additional size-selective concentrations to be used in TLVs for particulate matter under consideration for revision.

[C] As used for the mineral dusts.

Appendix G—Registered Trade Names

Trade Name	Generic Name	CAS No.
Abate	Temephos	3383-96-8
Ammate	Ammonium sulfamate	7773-06-0
Azodrin	Monocrotophos	6923-22-4
Baygon	Propoxur	114-26-1
Baytex	Fenthion	55-38-9
Bidrin	Dicrotophos	141-66-2
Bolstar	Sulprofos	35400-43-2
Butyl Cellosolve	2-Butoxyethanol	111-76-2
Cellosolve acetate	2-Ethoxyethyl acetate	111-15-9
Coyden	Clopidol	2971-90-6
Crag herbicide	Sesone	136-78-7
Dasanit	Fensulfothion	115-90-2
Delnav	Dioxathion	78-34-2
Dibrom	Naled	300-76-5
Difolatan	Captafol	2425-06-1
Disyston	Disulfoton	298-04-4
Dursban	Chlorphrifos	2921-88-2
Dyfonate	Fonofos	944-22-9
Furadan	Carbofuran	1563-66-2
Guthion	Azinphos-methyl	86-50-0
Lannate	Methomyl	16752-77-5
Methyl Cellosolve	2-Methoxyethanol	109-84-4
Methyl Cellosolve acetate	2-Methoxyethyl acetate	110-49-6
Nemacur	Fenamiphos	22224-92-6
Nialate	Ethion	563-12-2
N-Serve	Nitrapyrin	1929-82-4
Pival	Pindone	86-26-1
Plictran	Cyhexatin	1312 1-70-5
Sencor	Metribuzin	21087-64-9
Sevin	Carbaryl	63-25-2
Teflon	Polytetrafluoro-ethylene	9002-84-0
Thimet	Phorate	298-02-2
Thiodan	Endosulfan	115-29-7
Tordon	Picloram	1918-02-1
Zoalene	Dinitolmide	148-01-6

BIOLOGICAL EXPOSURE INDICES

Introduction

Biological Exposure Indices (BEIs) represent warning levels of biological response to the chemical, or warning levels of the chemical or its metabolic product(s) in tissues, fluids, or exhaled air of exposed workers, regardless of whether the chemical was inhaled, ingested, or absorbed via skin. Introduction of the BEI is a step in the evolution of the concept of TLVs. The BEI provides the health personnel with an additional tool to provide protection for the worker. Use of body fluids and appendages such as hair or nails for measuring the absorbed amount of a substance has long been a standard practice for certain substances. Lead is a classical example of a substance for which blood concentrations have long been considered the critical value in determining "safe" versus "unsafe" exposures. Two problems hindered the wider use of biological measurements as indicators of "safe" environmental exposures: 1) the relatively wide range in individual response to a substance and the wide range of "normal" that has to be considered, and 2) the lack of simple specific analytical methods of sufficient sensitivity. Both problems are capable of solution, and we believe that sufficient progress has been made to begin ultilizing selected BEIs which can be used as a guide to "safe" exposures to toxic chemicals. The BEI is considered supplementary to an airborne TLV.

TLVs are intended to provide the industrial hygienist with an additional measure to aid in the design of engineering controls or for temporary use of personnel protective equipment which will protect almost all exposed workers from untoward effects of chemical exposure. In principle, TWA-TLVs are designed to prevent exposures which may cause acute or chronic adverse effects. They are also intended to avoid attendant deterioration of normal physiological function. This approach is based on the assumption that for nearly all workers there is a tolerable exposure limt and a tolerable body burden of airborne material. If this assumption is valid, there should be a range of safe biologically insignificant changes of various measures of body function.

TLVs are a measure of the composition of the external environment surrounding the worker. BEIs are a measure of the amount of chemical *absorbed* into the body. The concept of the BEI is particularly useful in evaluating exposures to substances with significant absorption through the skin.

The biological determinant on which the BEIs are based can furnish two kinds of information useful in the control of worker exposure; (1) measure of the worker's individual response, and (2) measure of the worker's individual overall exposure. Measurements of response furnish an estimate of the physiological status of the worker and can be made by (*a*) determining changes in the amount of a critical biochemical constituent, (*b*) determining changes in activity of a critical enzyme, and (*c*) determining changes in a physiological function. Measurements of exposure can be made by (*a*) determining the chemical in exhaled air, urine, blood, hair, nails, body tissues and fluids, (*b*) determining the metabolite(s) of the chemical in tissues and fluids, and (*c*) determining the extent of specific biochemical and physiological changes induced by the chemical.

Recommended values of BEIs are based on data obtained in epidemiological and field studies or determined as bioequivalent to a TLV by means of pharmacokinetic analysis of data from controlled human studies. Most chemicals (including organic solvents) are initially absorbed and eliminated fairly rapidly—usually with initial half-life values measured in a few hours or even minutes. Rapidly changing concentrations in body fluids complicate the interpretation of data and the average body burden of a chemical attained during a work shift can easily be over-predicted or under-predicted. Furthermore, biological measurements fail in most instances to detect transient periods of over-exposure during the work shift. Because elimination of chemicals and their metabolic products, as well as biological changes induced by exposure to the chemical, are kinetic events, the listed BEIs are strictly related to 8-hour exposures and to the specified timing for the collection of biological samples.

Factors to be considered. There are other factors to be considered when the BEI is applied. Among the factors which must be considered in using BEIs are: (*a*) changes induced by strenuous physical activity; (*b*) changes induced by environmental eonditions (altitude, heat, diet, etc.); (*c*) changes induced by water intake; (*d*) changes in physiological functions induced by preexisting disease or congenital variation; (*e*) changes in metabolism induced by congenital variation of metabolic pathways; and (*f*) changes in metabolic pathway induced by simultaneous administration of another chemical (induction of inhibition of activity of a critical enzyme by medication or by preexposure or coexposure to another chemical).

For BEIs based on urine analysis, simple measurements of concentrations can provide sufficient information on exposure, but in many instances, measurements of elimination rates provide more precise information. Urinary concentrations related to creatinine represent a reasonable compromise between the accuracy of the information and the technical means of obtaining the data.

Some BEIs are not protective of an identified population, or are nonspecific. The correlation between the exposure and biological determinant is weakened by variables introduced by large interindividual variation in response to the chemical or by time factors and fluctuation of exposure concentration. In such cases the BEIs carry the following notations:

"R" Notation. Indicates that an identifiable population group might have an increased susceptibility to the effect of the chemical which leaves it unprotected by the recommended BEI. The specific documentation should be consulted for detailed information.

"" Notation*. Some determinants are nonspecific, since different chemicals may bear the same biological response. Such BEIs carry "*" notation. These nonspecific tests are preferred because they are easy to use and, in many instances, offer a better correlation between exposure and response than specific tests. In such instances, a BEI for a specific less quantitative biological determinant is recommended as a confirmatory test. The documentation shold be consulted for information on factors affecting interpretation of such a BEI.

"" Notation*. Indicates that the biological determinant is a specific indicator of exposure to the chemical but the quantitative interpretation of the measurements is very ambiguous, and that the relationship between the TLV and BEI is markedly weakened by variables or time factors, fluctuation of exposure concentrations, and by other circumstantial variables. Such biological determinants should be used as confirmatory tests; and their BEIs should be applied cautiously, mainly for confirmation of exposures indicated by nonspecific BEIs.

† Notation. The determinant is usually present in the biological specimens collected from subjects without occupational exposure. For information on background levels consult the documentation.

"G" Notation. Because of the wide interindividual variation in response to some chemicals, the BEI is in some instances recommended as a mean value of a group test for workers subjected to a similar level of occupational exposure, rather than as an index for an individual. Such BEIs carry "G" notation.

The table includes BEIs for which a sufficient data base is available and on which the committee took action. Some BEIs are more suitable for correlation with TLV-TWAs than others. Other BEIs are preferable for evaluating recent exposure or for confirmation of exposure. For specific instances the documentation should be consulted.

Workers are not expected to suffer any ill effects as long as the described measurement of the determinants are maintained within limits of the recommended BEIs. Measurements outside these limits are not necessarily indicators of a disease process. However, if these deviate measurements persist, it is an indication that the individual should be examined by a physician to determine whether there is any health effect. The workplace and work practices should be investigated further.

Note: It is strongly advisable to consult the specific documentation published in the *Documentation of Threshold Limit Values and Biological Exposure Indices*, 5th edition, before invoking the BEIs listed in the following table.

Chemical Substances Under Study to Establish BEIs

Acetone
Chromium
Fluoride
Malathion
Mercury
Nitrobenzene
Parathion
Perchloroethylene
Polychlorinated biphenyls

THRESHOLD LIMIT VALUES FOR PHYSICAL AGENTS IN THE WORK ENVIRONMENT ADOPTED BY ACGIH

Introduction

These threshold limit values refer to levels of physical agents and represent conditions under which it is believed that nearly all workers may be repeatedly exposed day after day without adverse effect. Because of wide variations in individual susceptibility, exposure of an occasional individual at, or even below, the threshold limit may not prevent annoyance, aggravation of a preexisting condition, or physiological damage.

These threshold limits are based on the best available information from industrial experience, from experimental human and animal studies, and when possible, from a combination of the three.

These limits are intended for use in the practice of industrial hygiene and should be interpreted and applied only by a person trained in this discipline. They are not intended for use, or for modification for use, (1) in the evaluation or control of the levels of physical agents in the community, (2) as proof or disproof of an existing physical disability, or (3) for adoption by countries whose working conditions differ from those in the United States of America.

These values are reviewed annually by the Committee on Threshold Limits for Physical Agents for revision or additions, as further information becomes available.

The ACGIH disclaims liability with respect to the use of TLVs in a manner inconsistent with their intended use as stated herein.

Notice of Intent–At the beginning of each year, proposed actions of the Committee for the forthcoming year are issued in the

Adopted Biological Exposure Indices

AIRBORNE CHEMICAL [CAS #] INDICES	TIMING	BEI	ADDITIONAL NOTATION
•CARBON MONOXIDE [630-08-0]			R
*Carboxyhemoglobin in blood	End of shift	less than 8%	†
*CO in end-exhaled air	End of shift	less than 40 ppm	†
•ETHYL BENZENE [100-41-4]			
*Mandelic acid in urine	End of shift and end of workweek	2 g/L	G
		1.5 g/g creat.	G
**Ethyl benzene in end-exhaled air	Prior to shift	2 ppm	
•STYRENE [100-42-5]			
*Mandelic acid in urine	End of shift	1 g/L	G
		0.8 g/g creat.	G
**Styrene in mixed-exhaled air	Prior to shift	40 ppb	
*Phenylglyoxylic acid in urine	End of shift	250 mg/L	†G
		240 mg/g creat.	G
**Styrene in mixed-exhaled air	During shift	18 ppm	
**Styrene in blood	End of shift	0.55 mg/L	
	Prior to shift	0.02 mg/L	
•TOLUENE [108-88-3]			
*Hippuric acid in urine	End of shift	2.5 g/g creat.	†G
	Last 4 hrs of shift	3 mg/min.	G
**Toluene in venous blood	End of shift	1 mg/L	
**Toluene in end-exhaled air	During shift	20 ppm	
•TRICHLOROETHYLENE [79-01-6]			
*Trichloroacetic acid in urine	End of workweek	100 mg/L	G
*Trichloroacetic acid and trichloroethanol in urine	End of workweek and end of shift	300 mg/L	G
		320 mg/g creat.	G
Free trichloroethanol in blood	End of shift and end of workweek	4 mg/L	
**Trichloroethylene in ene-exhaled air	Prior to shift and end of workweek	0.5 ppm	
•XYLENES [1330-20-7]			
Methylhippuric acids in urine	End of shift	1.5 g/g creat.	
	Last 4 hrs of shift	2 mg/min	

•1986-1987 Adoption.

form of a "Notice of Intent." This notice provides not only an opportunity for comment, but also solicits suggestions of physical agents to be added to the list. The suggestions should be accompanied by substantiating evidence.

Definitions–Two categories of Threshold Limit Values (TLVs) are specified herein, as follows:

a) *Threshold Limit Value–Time-Weighted Average (TLV-TWA)*—the time-weighted average concentration for a normal 8-hour workday and a 40-hour workweek, to which nearly all workers may be repeatedly exposed day after day, without adverse effect. Examples of their use can be found in the TLVs for Heat and Noise.

b) *Threshold Limit Value-Ceiling (TLV-C)*—the concentration that should not be exceeded even instantaneously, as in the case of 115 dBA limit for noise.

Physical Factors. It is recognized that combinations of such physical factors as heat, ultraviolet and ionizing radiation, humidity, abnormal pressure (altitude), and the like may place added stress on the body so that the effects from exposure at a threshold limit may be altered. Also, most of these stresses may act adversely to increase the toxic response of a foreign substance. Although most threshold limits have built-in safety factors to guard against adverse effects to moderate deviations from normal environments, the safety factors of most substances are not of such a magnitude as to take care of gross deviations. For example, continuous work at WBGT temperatures above 30° C (86° F), or overtime extending the workweek more than 25%, might be considered gross deviations. In such instances judgment must be exercised in the proper adjustments of the Threshold Limit Values.

Adopted Threshold Limit Values

Heat Stress

These Threshold Limit Values (TLVs) refer to heat stress conditions under which it is believed that nearly all workers may be repeatedly exposed without adverse health effects. The TLVs shown in Table 1 are based on the assumption that nearly all acclimatized, fully clothed workers with adequate water and salt intake should be able to function effectively under the given working conditions without exceeding a deep body temperature of 38° C.[1, 2]

Notice of Intent to Establish

AIRBORNE CHEMICAL [CAS #] INDICES	TIMING	BEI	ADDITIONAL NOTATION
‡ANILINE [62-53-3]			
*Total p-aminophenol in urine	End of shift	50 mg/L	G
BENZENE [71-43-2]			
*Total phenol in urine	End of shift	50 mg/L	†G
**Benzene in exhaled air	Prior to next shift		
mixed-exhaled:		0.08 ppm	
end-exhaled:		0.12 ppm	
‡CADMIUM [7440-43-9]			
Cadmium in urine	Not critical	10 μg/g creat.	†
Cadmium in blood	Not critical	10 μg/L	†
‡CARBON DISULFIDE [75-15-0]			
2-Thiothiazolidine-4-carboxylic acid (=TTCA) in urine	End of shift	5 mg/g creat.	
‡DIMETHYLFORMAMIDE [68-12-2]			
N-Methylformamide in urine	End of shift	40 mg/g creat.	
n-HEXANE [110-54-3]			
*2,5-Hexanedione in urine	End of shift	5 mg/L	G
**n-Hexane in end-exhaled air	During shift	40 ppm	
LEAD [7439-92-1]			R
Lead in blood	Not critical	50 μg/100 ml	†G
Lead in urine	Not critical	150 μg/g creat.	†G
Zinc protoporphyrin in blood	After 1 month of exposure	250 μg/100 ml erythrocytes or 100 μg/100 ml blood	
‡METHYL ETHYL KETONE (MEK) [78-93-3]			
MEK in urine	End of shift	2 mg/L	G
†PENTACHLOROPHENOL (PCP) [87-86-5]			
Total PCP in urine	Prior to the last shift of workweek	2 mg/L	†
Free PCP in plasma	End of shift	5 mg/L	†
PHENOL [108-95-2]			
*Total phenol in urine	End of shift	250 mg/g creat.	†G
	Last 2 hrs of shift	15 mg/hr	†G

‡1986-1987 Addition or Revision.

Since measurement of deep body temperature is impractical for monitoring the workers' heat load, the measurement of environmental factors is required which most nearly correlate with deep body temperature and other physiological responses to heat. At the present time Wet Bulb Globe Temperature Index (WBGT) is the simplest and most suitable technique to measure the environmental factors. WBGT values are calculated by the following equations:

1. Outdoors with solar load:

$$WBGT = 0.7\ NWB + 0.2\ GT + 0.1\ DB$$

2. Indoors or outdoors with no solar load:

$$WBGT = 0.7\ NWB + 0.3\ GT$$

where

WBGT = Wet Bulb Globe Temperature Index
NWB = Natural Wet-Bulb Temperature
DB = Dry-Bulb Temperature
GT = Globe Temperature

The determination of WBGT requires the use of a black globe thermometer, a natural (static) wet-bulb thermometer, and a dry-bulb thermometer.

Higher heat exposures than shown in Table A-1 are permissible if the workers have been undergoing medical surveillance and it has been established that they are more tolerant to work in heat than the average worker. Workers should not be permitted to continue their work when their deep body temperature exceeds 38.0° C.

TABLE A-1.
Permissible Heat Exposure Threshold Limit Values*

	WORK LOAD		
WORK—REST REGIMEN	LIGHT	MODERATE	HEAVY
Continuous work	30.0	26.7	25.0
75% Work—25% Rest, each hour	30.6	28.0	25.9
50% Work—50% Rest, each hour	31.4	29.4	27.9
25% Work—75% Rest, each hour	32.2	31.1	30.0

*Values are given in °C WBGT

Evaluation and Control

1. Measurement of the Environment

The instruments required are a dry-bulb, a natural wet-bulb, a globe thermometer, and a stand. The measurement of the environmental factors shall be performed as follows:

A. The range of the dry and the natural wet bulb thermometer shall be −5° C to 50° C with an accuracy of ± 0.5° C. The dry bulb thermometer must be shielded from the sun and the other radiant surfaces of the environment without restricting the airflow around the bulb. The wick of the natural wet-bulb thermometer shall be kept wet with distilled water for at least ½ hour before the temperature reading is made. It is not enough to immerse the other end of the wick into a reservoir of distilled water and wait until the whole wick becomes wet by capillarity. The wick shall be wetted by direct application of water from a syringe ½ hour before each reading. The wick shall extend over the bulb of the thermometer, covering the stem about one additional bulb length. The wick should always be clean and new wicks should be washed before using.

B. A globe thermometer, consisting of a 15 cm (6-inch) diameter hollow copper sphere painted on the outside with a matte black finish or equivalent, shall be used. The bulb or sensor of a thermometer (range −5° to + 100° C with an accuracy of ± 0.5° C) must be fixed in the center of the sphere. The globe thermometer shall be exposed at least 25 minutes before it is read.

C. A stand shall be used to suspend the three thermometers so that they do not restrict free air flow around the bulbs, and the wet-bulb and globe thermometer are not shaded.

D. It is permissible to use any other type of temperature sensor that gives identical reading as that of a mercury thermometer under the same conditions.

E. The thermometers must be so placed that the readings are representative of the condition where the men work or rest, respectively.

The methodology outlined above is more fully explained by Minard.[3, 4]

II. Work Load Categories

Heat produced by the body and the environmental heat together determine the total heat load. Therefore, if work is to be performed under hot environmental conditions, the workload category of each job shall be established and the heat exposure limit pertinent to the workload evaluated against the applicable standard in order to protect the worker exposure beyond the permissible limit.

A. The work load category may be established by ranking each job into light, medium, and heavy categories on the basis of type of operation. Where the work load is ranked into one of said three categories, i.e.,

(1) light work (up to 200 kcal/hr or 800 Btu/hr): e.g., sitting or standing to control machines, performing light hand or arm work,

TABLE A-2.

Assessment of Work Load[9]

Average values of metabolic rate during different activites

A. BODY POSITION AND MOVEMENT	KCAL/MIN
Sitting	0.3
Standing	0.6
Walking	2.0-3.0
Walking up hill	add 0.8 per meter (yard) rise

B. TYPE OF WORK		AVERAGE KCAL/MIN	RANGE KCAL/MIN
Hand work	*light*	0.4	0.2-1.2
	heavy	0.9	
Work with one arm	*light*	1.0	0.7-2.5
	heavy	1.7	
Work with both arms	*light*	1.5	1.0-3.5
	heavy	2.5	
Work with body	*light*	3.5	2.5-15.0
	moderate	5.0	
	heavy	7.0	
	very heavy	9.0	

(2) moderate work (200-350 kcal/hr or 800-1400 Btu/hr): e.g., walking about with moderate lifting and pushing, or

(3) heavy work (359-500 kcal/hr or 1400-2000 Btu/hr): e.g., pick and shovel work,

The permissible heat exposure limit for that workload shall be determined from Table A-1.

B. The ranking of the job may be performed either by measuring the worker's metabolic rate while performing his job or by estimating his metabolic rate with the use of Tables A-2 and A-3. Addi-

TABLE A-3.

Activity Examples[9]

- Light hand work: writing, hand knitting
- Heavy hand work: typewriting
- Heavy work with one arm: hammering in nails (shoemaker, upholsterer)
- Light work with two arms: filing metal, planing wood, raking of a garden
- Moderate work with the body: cleaning a floor, beating a carpet
- Heavy work with the body: railroad track laying, digging, barking trees

Sample Calculation

Assembly line work using a heavy hand tool.

A. Walking along	2.0 kcal/min
B. Intermediate value between heavy work with two arms and light work with the body	3.0 kcal/min
Subtotal	5.0 kcal/min
C. Add for basal metabolism	1.0 kcal/min
Total	6.0 kcal/min

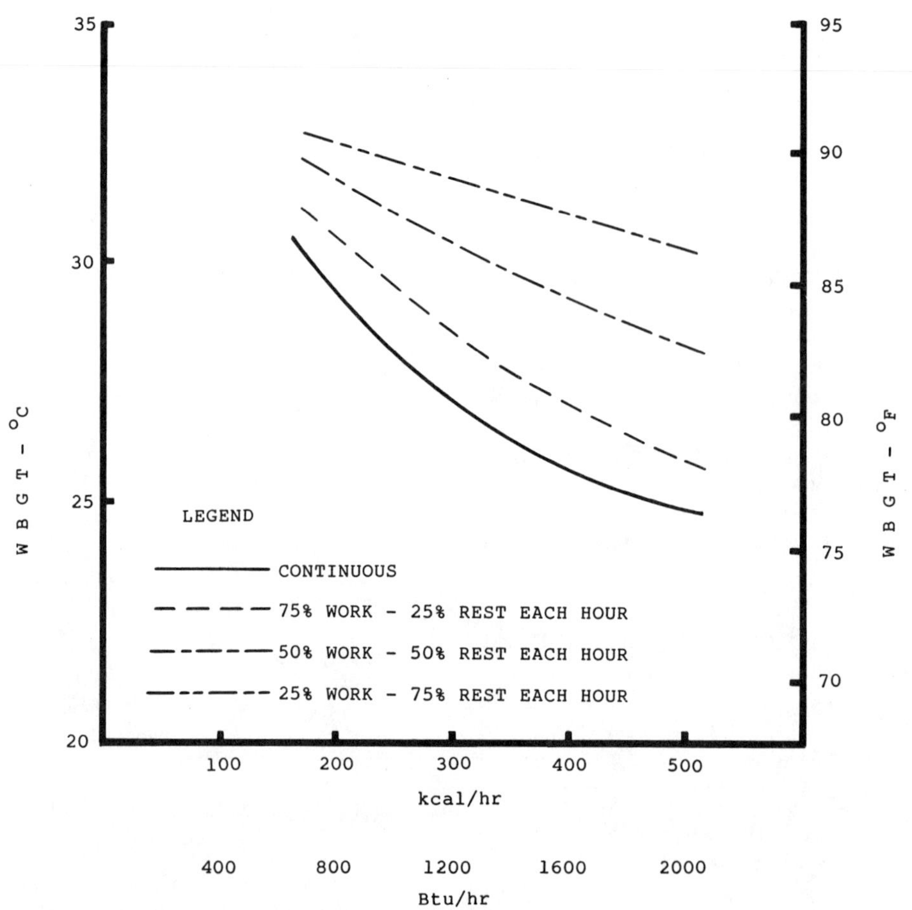

FIG A–1.
Permissible heat exposure threshold limit values.

tional tables available in the literature[5-8] may be utilized also. When this method is used the permissible heat exposure limit can be determined by Figure A-1

III. *Work-Rest Regimen*

The permissible exposure limits specified in Table A-1 and Figure A-1 are based on the assumption that the WBGT value of the resting place is the same or very close to that of the workplace. Where the WBGT of the work area is different from that of the rest area a time-weighted average value should be used for both environmental and metabolic heat. When time-weighted average values are used, the appropriate curve on Figure A-1 is the solid line labeled "continuous."

The time-weighted average metabolic rate (M) shall be determined by the equation:

$$\text{Av. M} = \frac{M_1 \times t_1 + M_2 \times t_2 + \ldots + M_n \times t_n}{t_1 + t_2 + \ldots + t_n}$$

where M_1, M_2 . . . and M_n are estimated or measured metabolic rates for the various activities and rest periods of the worker during the time periods t_1, t_2 . . . and t_n (in minutes) as determined by a time study.

The time-weighted average WBGT shall be determined by the equation:

$$\text{Av. WGBT} = \frac{\text{WBGT}_1 \times t_1 + \text{WBGT}_2 \times t_2 + \ldots + \text{WBGT}_n \times t_n}{t_1 + t_2 + \ldots + t_n}$$

where WBGT_1, WBGT_2 . . . and WBGT_n are calculated values of WBGT for the various work and rest areas occupied during total time periods t_1, t_2 . . . and t_n are the elapsed times in minutes spent in the corresponding areas which are determined by a time study. Where exposure to hot environmental conditions is continuous for several hours or the entire work day, the time-weighted averages shall be calculated as hourly time-weighted average, i.e., $t_1 + t_2 + \ldots t_n = 60$ minutes. Where the exposure is intermittent, the time-weighted averages shall be calculated as two-hour time-weighted averages, i.e., $t_1 + t_2 + \ldots + t_n = 120$ minutes.

The permissible exposure limits for continuous work are applicable where there is a work-rest regimen of a 5-day work week and an 8-hour work day with a short morning and afternoon break (approximately 15 minutes) and a longer lunch break (approximately 30 minutes). Higher exposure limits are permitted if additional resting time is allowed. All breaks, including unscheduled pauses and administrative or operational waiting periods during work, may be counted as rest time when additional rest allowance must be given because of high environmental temperatures.

IV. *Water and Salt Supplementation*

During the hot season or when the worker is exposed to artificially generated heat, drinking water shall be made available to the workers in such a way that they are stimulated to frequently drink small amounts, i.e., one cup every 15-20 minutes (about 150 ml or ¼ pint).

The water shall be kept reasonably cool (10°-15° C or 50.0°-60.0° F) and shall be placed close to the workplace so that the worker can reach it without abandoning the work area.

The workers should be encouraged to salt their food abundantly during the hot season and particularly during hot spells. If the workers are unacclimatized, salted drinking water shall be made available in a concentration of 0.1% (1 g NaCl to 1.0 liter or 1 level tablespoon of salt to 15 quarts of water). The added salt shall be completely dissolved before the water is distributed, and the water shall be kept reasonably cool.

V. *Other Considerations*

A. *Clothing:* The permissible heat exposure TLVs are valid for light summer clothing as customarily worn by workers when working under hot environmental conditions. If special clothing is required for performing a particular job and this clothing is heavier or it impedes sweat evaporation or has higher insulation value, the worker's heat tolerance is reduced, and the permissible heat exposure limits indicated in Table A-1 and Figure A-1 are not applicable. For each job category where special clothing is required, the permissible heat exposure limit shall be established by an expert.

B. *Acclimatization and Fitness:* Acclimatization to heat involves a series of physiological and psychological adjustments that occur in an individual during this week of exposure to hot environment conditions. The recommended heat stress TLVs are valid for acclimated workers who are physically fit. Extra caution must be employed when unacclimated or physically unfit workers must be exposed to heat stress conditions.

REFERENCES

1. *Health Factors Involved in Working Under Conditions of Heat Stress*. WHO Technical Report Series No 412, 1969.
2. Dukes-Dobos FN, Henschel A: Development of Permissible Heat Exposure Limits for Occupational Work. *ASHRAE Journal* 1973; 15(9):57–62
3. Minard D: *Prevention of Heat Casualities in Marine Corps Recruits, Period of 1955–60, with Comparative Incidence Rates and Climatic Heat Stresses in other Training Categories*. Research Report No 4, Contract No MR 005.01–0001.01, Naval Medical Research Institute, Bethesda, MD, Feb 21, 1961. Published in *Military Medicine* 1961; 126(44):261–272.
4. Minard D, O'Brien RL: *Heat Casualities in the Navy and the Marine Corps 1959–1962 with Appendices on the Field Use of the Wet-Bulb Globe Temperature Index*. Research Report No 7, Contract No MR 005.01–0001.01, Naval Medical Research Institute, Bethesda, MD, March 12, 1964.
5. Astrand PO, Rodahk K: *Textbook of Work Physiology*. New York, McGraw-Hill Book Co, 1970.
6. Ergonomics Guide to Assessment of Metabolic and Cardiac Costs of Physical Work. *Am Ind Hyg Assoc J* 1971; 32:560.
7. *Energy Requirements for Physical Work*. Research Progress Report No 30. Purdue Farm Cardiac Project, Agricultural Experiment Station, West Lafayette, IN, 1961.
8. Durnin JVGA, Passmore R: *Energy, Work and Leisure*. London, Heinemann Educational Books, Ltd, 1967.
9. Lehmann GE, Muller A, and Spitzer H: Der Kalorienbedarb bie Gewerblicher Arbeit. *Arbeitsphysiol* 1950; 14:166.

**Cold Stress*

These Threshold Limit Values (TLVs) are intended to protect workers from the severest effects of cold stress (hypothermia) and cold injury and to describe exposures to cold working conditions under which it is believed that nearly all workers can be repeatedly exposed without adverse health effects. The TLV objective is to prevent the deep body core temperature from falling below 36° C and to prevent cold injury to body extremities. Deep body temperature is the core temperature of the body as determined by rectal temperature measurements. For a single, occasional exposure to a cold environment a drop in core temperature to no lower than 35° C should be permitted. In addition to provisions for total body protection, the TLV objective is to protect all parts of the body with emphasis on hands, feet and head from cold injury.

Fatal exposures to cold among workers have almost always resulted from accidental exposures involving failure to escape from low environmental air temperatures or from immersion in low temperature water. The single most important aspect of life-threatening hypothermia is the fall in the deep core temperature of the body. The clinical presentations of victims of hypothermia are shown in Table A-4 (taken from Dembert in *AFP*, January 1982). Workmen should be protected from exposure to cold so that the deep core temperature does not fall below 36° C (96.8° F); lower body temperature will very likely result in reduced mental alertness, reduction in rational decision making, a loss of consciousness with the threat of fatal consequences.

Pain in the extremities may be the first early warning of danger to cold stress. During exposure to cold, maximum severe shivering develops when the body temperature has fallen to 35° C (95° F). This must be taken as a sign of danger to the workers and exposure to cold should be immediately terminated for any workers when severe shivering becomes evident. Useful physical or mental work is limited when severe shivering occurs.

Since prolonged exposure to cold air, or to immersion in cold water, at temperatures well above freezing can lead to dangerous hypothermia, whole body protection must be provided.

1. Adequate insulating clothing to maintain core temperatures above 36° C must be provided to workers if work is performed in air temperatures below 4° C (40° F). Wind

* 1986–1987 Adoption.

TABLE A-4.
Progressive Clinical Presentations of Hypothermia*

CORE TEMPERATURE		
°C	°F	CLINICAL SIGNS
37.6	99.6	"Normal" rectal temperature
37	98.6	"Normal" oral temperature
36	96.8	Metabolic rate increases in an attempt to compensate for heat loss
35	95.0	Maximum shivering
34	93.2	Victim conscious and responsive, with normal blood pressure
33	91.4	Severe hypothermia below this temperature
32	89.6	Consciousness clouded; blood pressure becomes difficult to obtain; pupils dilated but react to light; shivering ceases
31	87.8	
30	86.0	Progressive loss of consciousness; muscular rigidity increases; pulse and blood pressure difficult to obtain; respiratory rate decreases
29	84.2	
28	82.4	Ventricular fibrillation possible with myocardial irritability
27	80.6	Voluntary motion ceases; pupils nonreactive to light; deep tendon and superficial reflexes absent
26	78.8	Victim seldom conscious
25	77.0	Ventricular fibrillation may occur spontaneously
24	75.2	Pulmonary edema
22	71.6	Maximum risk of ventricular fibrillation
21	69.8	
20	68.0	Cardiac standstill
18	64.4	Lowest accidental hypothermia victim to recover
17	62.6	Isoelectric electroencephalogram
9	48.2	Lowest artificially cooled hypothermia patient to recover

*Presentations approximately related to core temperature. Reprinted from the January 1982 issue of *American Family Physician,* published by the American Academy of Family Physicians.

chill factor[A] or the cooling power of the air is a critical factor. The higher the wind speed and the lower the temperature in the work area, the greater the insulation value of the protective clothing required. The equivalent chill temperature should be used when estimating the combined cooling effect of wind and low air temperatures on exposed skin or when determining clothing insulation requirements to maintain the deep body core temperature.

2. Unless there are unusual or extenuating circumstances cold injury to other than hands, feet, and head is not likely to occur without the development of the initial signs of hypothermia. Older workers or workers with circulatory problems require special precautionary protection against cold injury. The use of extra insulating clothing and/or a reduction in the duration of the exposure period are among the special precautions which should be considered. The precautionary actions to be taken will depend upon the physical condition of the workers and should be determined with the advice of a physician with knowledge of the cold stress factors and the medical condition of the worker.

Evaluation and Control

For exposed skin, continuous éxposure should not be permitted when the air speed and temperature results in an equivalent chill temperature of −32° C (−25° F). Superficial or deep local tissue freezing will occur only at temperatures below −1° C regardless of wind speed.

At air temperatures of 2° C (35.6° F) or less it is imperative that workers who become immersed in water or whose clothing becomes wet be immediately provided a change of clothing and be treated for hypothermia.

Special protection of the hands is required to maintain manual dexterity for the prevention of accidents:

1. If fine work is to be performed with bare hands for more than 10–20 minutes in an environment below 16° C (60° F), special provisions should be established for keeping the workers' hands warm. For this purpose, warm air jets, radiant heaters (fuel burner or electric radiator), or contact warm plates may be utilized. Metal handles of tools and control bars shall be covered by thermal insulating material at temperatures below −1° C (30° F).
2. If the air temperature falls below 16° C (60° F) for sedentary, 4° C (40° F) for light, −7° C (20° F) for moderate work and fine manual dexterity is not required then gloves shall be used by the workers.

To prevent contact frostbite, the workers should wear anticontact gloves.

1. When cold surfaces below −7° C (20° F) are within reach, a warning should be given to each worker by his supervisor to prevent inadvertent contact by bare skin.
2. If the air temperature is −17.5° (0° F) or less, the hands should be protected by mittens. Machine controls and tools for use in cold conditions should be designed so that they can be handled without removing the mittens.

Provisions for additional total body protection is required if work is performed in an environment at or below 4° C (40° F). The workers shall wear cold protective clothing appropriate for the level of cold and physical activity:

1. If the air velocity at the job site is increased by wind, draft, or artificial ventilating equipment, the cooling effect of the wind shall be reduced by shielding the work area, or by wearing an easily removable outer windbreak layer garment. Wind chill cooling rates are illustrated in Figure A-2 and Table A-5.
2. If only light work is involved and if the clothing on the worker may become wet on the job site, the outer layer of the clothing in use may be of a type impermeable to water. With more severe work under such conditions the outer layer should be water repellent, and the outerwear should be changed as it becomes wetted. The outer gar-

[A]Wind chill factor is a unit of heat loss from a body defined in watts per meter squared per hour being a function of the air temperature and wind velocity upon the exposed body.

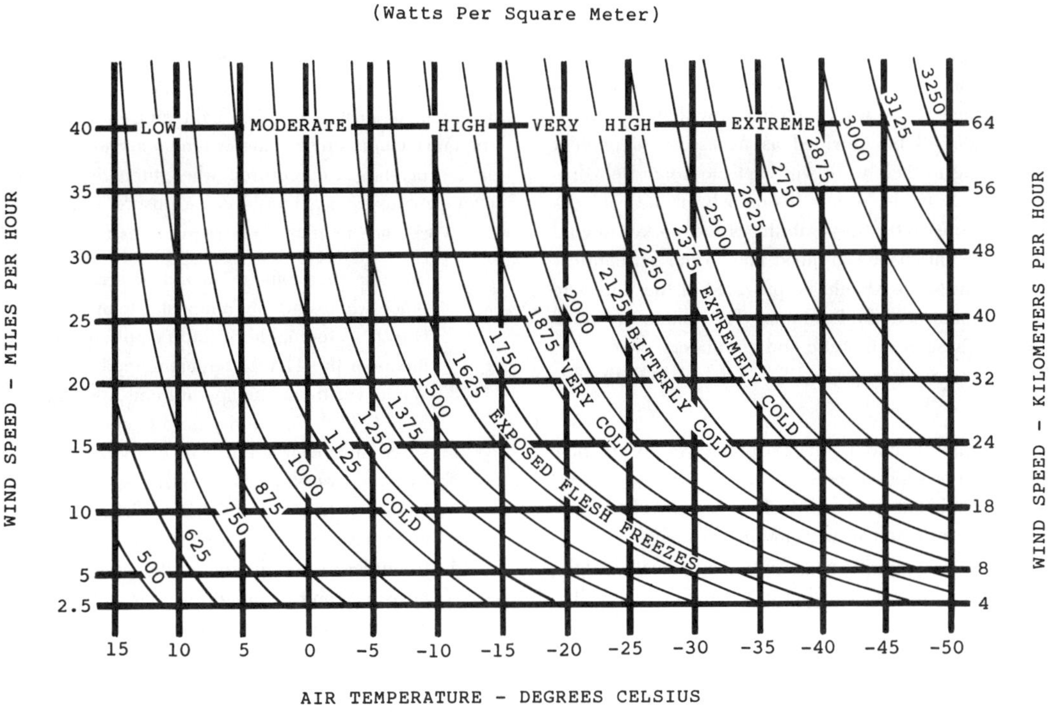

FIG A–2.
Wind chill cooling rates. Adapted from Canadian Department of the Environment, Atmospheric Environment Service.

ment must include provisions for easy ventilation in order to prevent wetting of inner layers by sweat. If work is done at normal temperatures or in a hot environment before entering the cold area, the employee shall make sure that his clothing is not wet as a consequence of sweating. If his clothing is wet, the employee shall change into dry clothes before entering the cold area. The workers shall change socks and any removable felt insoles at regular daily intervals or use vapor barrier boots. The optimal frequency of change shall be determined empirically and will vary individually and according to the type of shoe worn and how much the individual's feet sweat.

3. If extremities, ears, toes and nose, cannot be protected sufficiently to prevent sensation of excessive cold or frostbite by handwear, footwear and face masks, these protective items shall be supplied in auxiliary heated versions.
4. If the available clothing does not give adequate protection to prevent hypothermia or frostbite, work shall be modified or suspended until adequate clothing is made available or until weather conditions improve.
5. Workers handling evaporative liquid (gasoline, alcohol or cleaning fluids) at air temperatures below 4° C (40° F) shall take special precautions to avoid soaking of clothing or gloves with the liquids because of the added danger of cold injury due to evaporative cooling. Special note should be taken of the particularly acute effects of splashes of "cryogenic fluids" or those liquids with a boiling point only just above ambient temperatures.

Work-Warming Regimen

If work is performed continuously in the cold at an equivalent chill temperature (ECT) or below −7° C (20° F) heated warming shelters (tents, cabins, rest rooms, etc.) shall be made available nearby and the workers should be encouraged to use these shelters at regular intervals, the frequency depending on the severity of the environmental exposure. The onset of heavy shivering, frostnip,

TABLE A-5.
Wind Chill Cooling Rate Effects*

WIND CHILL RATES ($WATTS/M^2/HR$)	COMMENTS/EFFECTS
700	Conditions considered comfortable when dressed for skiing.
1200	Conditions no longer pleasant for outdoor activities on overcast days.
1400	Conditions no longer pleasant for outdoor activities on sunny days.
1600	Freezing of exposed skin begins for most people depending on the degree of activity and the amount of sunshine.
2300	Conditions for outdoor travel such as walking become dangerous. Exposed areas of the face freeze in less than 1 minute for the average person.
2700	Exposed flesh will freeze within half a minute for the average person.

*From Canadian Department of the Environment, Atmospheric Environment Service.

the feeling of excessive fatigue, drowsiness, irritability, or euphoria, are indications for immediate return to the shelter. When entering the heated shelter the outerlayer of clothing shall be removed and the remainder of the clothing loosened to permit sweat evaporation or a change of dry work clothing provided. A change of dry work clothing shall be provided as necessary to prevent workers from returning to their work with wet clothing. Dehydration, or the loss of body fluids, occurs insidiously in the cold environment and may increase the suscepibility of the worker to cold injury due to a significant change in blood flow to the extremities. Warm sweet drinks and soups should be provided at the work site to provide caloric intake and fluid volume. The intake of coffee should be limited because of a diuretic and circulatory effect.

For work practices at or below −12° C (10° F) ECT the following shall apply:

1. The worker shall be under constant protective observation (buddy system or supervision).
2. The work rate should not be so high as to cause heavy sweating that will result in wet clothing; if heavy work must be done, rest periods must be taken in heated shelters and opportunity for changing into dry clothing shall be provided.
3. New employees shall not be required to work full-time in cold in the first days until they become accustomed to the working conditions and required protective clothing.
4. The weight and bulkiness of clothing shall be included in estimating the required work performance and weights to be lifted by the worker.
5. The work shall be arranged in such a way that sitting still or standing still for long periods is minimized. Unprotected metal chair seats shall not be used. The worker should be protected from drafts to the greatest extent possible.
6. The workers shall be instructed in safety and health procedures. The training program shall include as a minimum instruction in:
   a. Proper rewarming procedures and appropriate first aid treatment.
   b. Proper clothing practices.
   c. Proper eating and drinking habits.
   d. Recognition of impending frostbite.
   e. Recognition signs and symptoms of impending hypothermia or excessive cooling of the body even when shivering does not occur.
   f. Safe work practices.

Special Workplace Recommendations

Special design requirements for refrigerator rooms include the following:

1. In refrigerator rooms, the air velocity should be minimized as much as possible and should not exceed 1 meter/sec (200 fpm) at the job site. This can be achieved by properly designed air distribution systems.
2. Special wind protective clothing shall be provided based upon existing air velocities to which workers are exposed.

Special caution shall be exercised when working with toxic substances and when workers are exposed to vibration. Cold exposure may require reduced limits.

Eye protection for workers employed out-of-doors in a snow and/or ice-covered terrain shall be supplied. Special safety goggles to protect against ultraviolet light and glare (which can produce temporary conjunctivitis and/or temporary loss of vision) and blowing ice crystals are required when there is an expanse of snow coverage causing a potential eye exposure hazard.

Workplace monitoring is required as follows:

1. Suitable thermometry should be arranged at any workplace where the environmental temperature is below 16° C (60° F) to enable overall compliance with the requirements of the TLV to be maintained.
2. Whenever the air temperature at a workplace falls below −1° C (30° F), the dry bulb temperature should be measured and recorded at least every 4 hours.
3. In indoor workplaces, the wind speed should also be recorded at least every 4 hours whenever the rate of air movement exceeds 2 meters per second (5 mph).
4. In outdoor work situations, the windspeed should be measured and recorded together with the air temperature whenever the air temperature is below −1° C (30° F).
5. The equivalent chill temperature shall be obtained from Table 16 in all cases where air movement measurements are required, and shall be recorded with the other data whenever the equivalent chill temperature is below −7° C (20° F).

Employees shall be excluded from work in cold at −1° C (30° F) or below if they are suffering from diseases or taking medication which interferes with normal body temperature regulation or reduces tolerance to work in cold environments. Workers who are routinely exposed to temperatures below −24° C (−10° F) with wind speeds less than five miles per hour, or air temperatures below −18° C (0° F) with wind speeds above five miles per hour should be medically certified as suitable for such exposures.

Trauma sustained in freezing or subzero conditions requires special attention because an injured worker is predisposed to secondary cold injury. Special provisions must be made to prevent hypothermia and secondary freezing of damaged tissues in addition to providing for first aid treatment.

Hand-Arm (Segmental) Vibration

These Threshold Limit Values (Table A–6) refer to component accelerations levels and durations of exposure that represent conditions under which it is believed that most workers may be exposed repeatedly without progressing beyond Stage 3 of the Taylor-Pelmear Classification System for Vibration-induced White Finger (VWF), also known as Raynaud's Phenomenon of Occupational Origin). Since there is a paucity of dose-response relationships for VWF, these recommendations have been derived from epidemiological data from forestry, mining, and metal working. These values should be used as guides in the control of hand-arm vibration exposure and because of individual susceptibility, should not be regarded as defining a boundary between safe and dangerous levels.

*1986–1987 Adoption.

TABLE A–6.

Threshold Limit Values for Exposure of the Hand to Vibration in Either X_h, Y_h, Z_h Directions

TOTAL DAILY EXPOSURE DURATION[a]	VALUES OF THE DOMINANT,[b] FREQUENCY-WEIGHTED, rms, COMPONENT ACCELERATION WHICH SHALL NOT BE EXCEEDED a_K, ($a_{K_{eq}}$)	
	M/S^2	g[c]
4 hours and less than 8	4	0.40
2 hours and less than 4	6	0.61
1 hour and less than 2	8	0.81
less than 1 hour	12	1.22

[a]The total time vibration enters the hand per day, whether continuously or intermittently.
[b]Usually one axis of vibration is dominant over the remaining two axes. If one or more vibration axis exceeds the Total Daily Exposure then the TLV has been exceeded.
[c]g = 9.81 m/s^2.

It should be recognized that the application of the TLV alone for hand-arm vibration will not protect all workers from the adverse effects of hand-arm vibration exposure. The use of (1) antivibration tools, (2) antivibration gloves, (3) proper work practices which keep the worker's hands and remaining body warm and also minimize the vibration coupling between the worker and the vibration tool are necessary to minimize vibration exposure, and (4) a conscientiously applied medical surveillance program are ALL necessary to rid VWF from the workplace.

Continuous, Intermittent, Impulsive, or Impact Hand-Arm Vibration

The measurement of vibration should be performed in accordance with the procedures and instrumentation specified by the Second Draft International Standard ISO/DIS 5349 (1984), *Guide for the Measurement and the Assessment of Human Exposure to Vibration Transmitted to the Hand,* and summarized below:

The acceleration of a vibration handle or work piece should be determined in three mutually orthogonal directions at a point close to where vibration enters the hand. The directions shall preferably be those forming the ISO biodynamic coordinte system, but may be closely related basicentric system with its origin at the interface between the hand and the vibrating surface (Fig A–3) to accommodate different handle or work piece configurations. A small and lightweight transducer shall be mounted so as to record accurately one or more orthogonal components of the source vibration in the frequency range from 5 to 1500 Hz. Each component should be frequency-weighted by a filter network with gain characteristics specified by the ISO for human-response vibration measuring instrumentation, to account for the change in vibration hazard with frequency (Fig A–4).

Assessment of vibration exposure should be made for EACH applicable direction (X_h, Y_h, Z_h) since vibration is a vector quantity (magnitude and direction). In each direction, the magnitude of the vibration during normal operation of the power tool, machine or work piece shall be expressed by the root-mean-square (rms) value of the frequency-weighted component accelerations, in units of meters per second squared (m/s^2), or gravitational units (g), the largest of which, a_k, forms the basis for exposure assessment.

For each direction being measured, linear integration shall be employed for vibrations that are of extremely short duration or vary substantially in time. If the total daily vibration exposure in a given direction is composed of several exposures at different rms accelerations, then the equivalent, frequency-weighted component acceleration in that direction shall be determined in accordance with the following equation:

$$(a_{K_{eq}}) = \left[\frac{1}{T}\sum_{i=1}^{n}(a_{K_i})^2\,T_i\right]^{1/2} = \sqrt{(a_{K_1})^2\frac{T_1}{T} + (a_{K_2})^2\frac{T_2}{T} + \ldots (a_{K_n})^2\frac{T_n}{T}}$$

where: $T = \sum_{i=1}^{n} T_i$

T = total daily exposure duration

a_{K_i} = ith frequency-weighted, rms acceleration component with duration T_i

These computations may be performed by commercially available human-response vibration measuring instruments.

Notes: Table A–6:

1. Hardly any person exposed at or below the TLVs for vibration contained in Table A–6 has progressed to *Stage 3* Vibration White Finger, in the Taylor-Pelmear classification, i.e., the point at which extension blanching of all fingers has occurred and there is definite interference at work, home, and restricted social activities.[(2–7)]
2. Acute exposures to frequency-weighted, rms, component accelerations in excess of the TLVs for infrequent periods of time (e.g., 1 day per week, or several days over a two-week period) are not necessarily more harmful.[(2–4)]
3. Acute exposures to frequency-weighted, rms, component accelerations of three times the magnitude of the TLVs are expected to result in the same health effects after between 5 and 6 years of exposure.[2–4)]
4. Preventive measures, including specialized preemployment and annual medical examinations to identify persons susceptible to vibration, should be implemented in situations in which workers are or will be exposed to hand-arm vibration.[(3–7)]

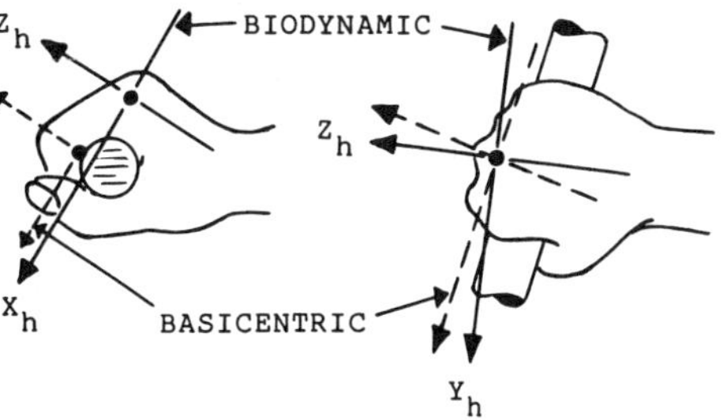

FIG A–3.
Biodynamic and basicentric coordinate systems for the hand, showing the directions of the acceleration components (ISO 5349).

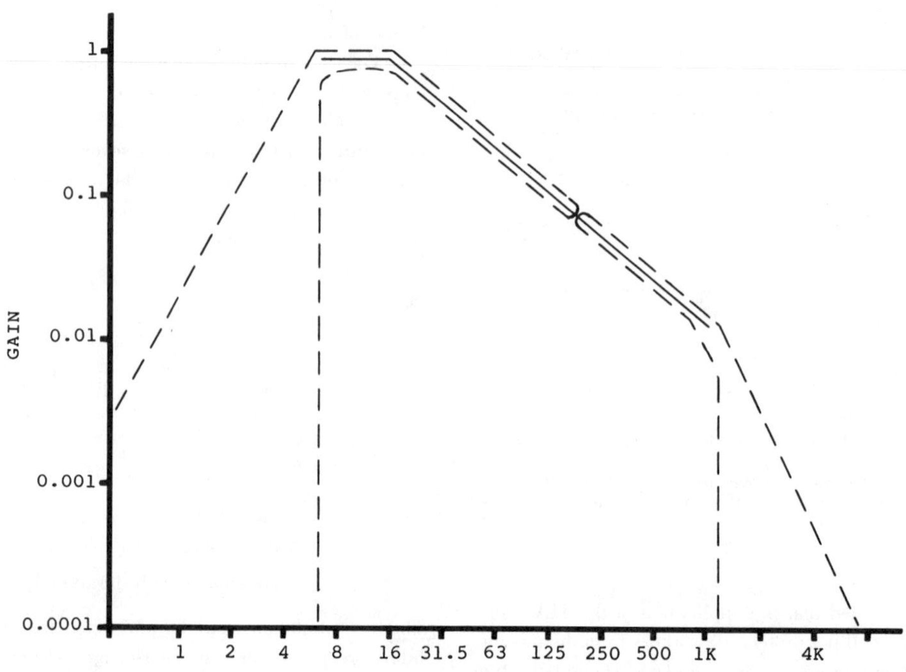

FIG A–4.
Gain characteristics of the filter network used to frequency-weight acceleration components *(continuous line).* The filter tolerances *(dashed lines)* are provisional, and are those contained in ISO 5349.

5. To moderate the adverse effects of vibration exposure, workers should be advised to avoid *continuous* vibration exposure by cessation of vibration exposure for approximately 10 minutes per continuous vibration hour.
6. Good work practices should be used, and should include instructing workers to employ a minimum hand grip force consistent with safe operation of the power tool or process, keep their body and hands warm and dry, and avoid smoking.[(2–3)]
7. A transducer and its device for attachment to the vibrating source suitable for measurement purposes together should weigh less than 15 grams, and should possess a cross-axis sensitivity of less than 10%.
8. The measurement by many (mechanically underdamped) piezoelectric accelerometers of repetitive, large displacement, impulsive vibrations, such as those produced by percussive pneumatic tools, is subject to error. The insertion of a suitable, low-pass, mechanical filter between the accelerometer and the source of vibration with a cutoff frequency of 1500 Hz or greater (and cross-axis sensitivity of less than 10%) can help eliminate incorrect readings.[(3, 4)]
9. The manufacturer and type number of all apparatus used to measure vibration should be reported, as well as the value of the dominant direction and frequency-weighted, rms, component acceleration.

REFERENCES

1. Pyykko I: Vibration Syndrome. A Review. in Dorhonen O (ed): *Vibration and Work*. Helsinki, Institute of Occupational Health, 1976.
2. Taylor W, Palmear PL (eds): *Vibration White Finger in Industry*. London, Academic Press, 1975.
3. Wasserman DE, Taylor W (eds): NIOSH: *Proceedings of International Occupational Hand-Arm Vibration Conference*, DHEW NIOSH Pub No 77–170, 1977.
4. Brammar JJ: Treshold Limit for Hand-Arm Vibration Exposure Throughout the Workday, in Brammer AJ, Taylor W (eds): *Vibration Effects on the Hand and Arm in Industry*, pp. 291–301. New York, John Wiley & Sons, 1982.
5. Wasserman DE, Taylor W: *Environmental and Occupational Medicine*, in Rom WN (ed): *Occupational Vibration*. Boston, Little, Brown & Co, 1982, pp 743–749.
6. NIOSH: *Current Intelligence Bulletin #38*: *Vibration Syndrome*, DHHS (NIOSH) pub no 83–110 (1983).
7. NIOSH: *Vibration Syndrome*. NIOSH Videotape #177 (27 minutes). Cincinnati, OH.
8. International Organization for Standardization: *Guide for the Measurement and the Assessment of Human Exposure to Vibration Transmitted to the Hand*. Second DIS 5349. International Organization for Standardization, Geneva, in press, 1983.
9. International Organization for Standardization: *Human-Response Vibration Measuring Instrumentation*. Second Draft Proposal DP 8041. ISO/TC 108/SC 3 n 99. International Organization for Standardization, Geneva, unpublished, 1982.

Ionizing Radiation

The Committee accepts the philosophy and recommendations of the National Council on Radiation Protection and Measurements (NCRP) for the ionizing radiation TLV. The NCRP is charted by Congress to, in part, collect, analyze, develop and disseminate information and recommendations about protection against radiation and about radiation measurements, quantities and units, including development of basic concepts in these areas. NCRP Report No. 39 provides basic philosophy and concepts leading to protection criteria established in the same report.[1] Other NCRP reports address specific areas of radiation protection and, collectively, provide an excellent basis for establishing a sound program for radiation control. The Committee recommends the listed references as substantive documentation of a sound basis for ionizing radiation protection. The Committee also strongly recommends that all exposure to ionizing radiation be kept as low as reasonably achievable within the stated guidance.

REFERENCES

1. *Basic Radiation Protection Criteria*. NCRP Report No 39, January 15, 1971.
2. *Maximum Permissible Body Burdens and Maximum Permissible Concentrations of Radionuclides in Air and in Water for Occupational Exposure*. National Bureau of Standards Handbook 69, June 5, 1959, with *Addendum 1*, August 1963. Available as NCRP Report No 22.

The above documents, as well as information on numerous other NCRP Reports addressing specific subjects in ionizing radiation protection, are available from: NCRP Publications, 7910 Woodmont Ave., Suite 1016, Bethesda, MD 20814.

Lasers

The Threshold Limit Values (TLVs) are for exposure to laser radiation under conditions to which nearly all workers may be exposed without adverse effects. The values should be used as guides in the control of exposures and should not be regarded as fine lines between safe and dangerous levels. They are based on the best available information from experimental studies.

Limiting Apertures

The TLVs expressed as radiant exposure or irradiance in this section may be averaged over an aperture of 1 mm except for TLVs for the eye in the spectral range of 400–1400 nm, which should be averaged over a 7 mm liniting aperture (pupil); and except for all TLVs for wavelengths between 0.1–1 mm where the limiting aperture is 10 mm. No modification of the TLVs is permitted for pupil sizes less than 7 mm.

The TLVs for "extended sources" apply to sources which subtend an angle greater than α (Table A–7) which varies with exposure time. This angle is *not* the beam divergence of the source.

TABLE A–7.
Limiting Angle to Extended Source Which May Be Used For Applying Extended Source TLVs

EXPOSURE DURATION(S)	ANGLE α (mrad)	EXPOSURE DURATION(S)	ANGLE α (mrad)
10^{-9}	8.0	10^{-2}	5.7
10^{-8}	5.4	10^{-1}	9.2
10^{-7}	3.7	1.0	15
10^{-6}	2.5	10	24
10^{-5}	1.7	10^{2}	24
10^{-4}	2.2	10^{3}	24
10^{-3}	3.6	10^{4}	24

Correction Factors A and B (C_A and C_B)

The TLVs for ocular exposure in Tables A–8 and A–9 are to be used as given for all wavelength ranges. The TLVs for wavelengths between 700 nm and 1049 nm are to be increased by a uniformly extrapolated factor (C_A) as shown in Figure A–5. Between 1049 nm and 1400 nm, the TLV has been increased by a factor (C_A) of five. For certain exposure times at wavelengths between 550 nm and 700 nm, correction factor (C_B) must be applied.

The TLVs for skin exposure are given in Table A–10. The TLVs are to be increased by a factor (C_A) as shown in Figure A–5 for wavelengths between 700 nm and 1400 nm. To aid in the determination of TLVs for exposure durations requiring calculations of fractional powers Figures A–6, A–7, and A–8 may be used.

**Repetitively Pulsed Exposures*

Scanned CW lasers or repetitively pulsed lasers can both produce repetitively pulsed exposure conditions. The TLV for intrabeam viewing which is applicable to wavelengths between 400 and 1400 nm and a single-pulse exposure (of pulse duration *t*) is modified in this instance by a correction factor determined by the number of pulses in the exposure. First calculate the number of pulses (n) in an expected exposure situation; this is the pulse repetition frequency (PRF in Hz) multiplied by the duration of exposure. Normally, realistic exposures may range from 0.25s for a bright visible source to 10s for an infrared source. The corrected TLV on a per-pulse basis is:

$$\text{TLV} = (n^{-1/4})\,(\text{TLV for single-pulse}) \qquad (1)$$

This approach applies only to thermal-injury conditions, i.e., all exposures at wavelengths greater than 700 nm, and for many exposures at shorter wavelengths. For wavelengths less than or equal to 700 nm, the corrected TLV from equation 1 above applies if the average irradiance does not exceed the TLV for continuous exposure. The average irradiance (i.e., the total accumulated exposure for *nt* seconds) shall not exceed the radiant exposure given in Table A–8 for exposure durations of 10 seconds to T_1.

Noise

These Threshold Limit Values (TLVs) refer to sound pressure levels and durations of exposure that represent conditions under which it is believed that nearly all workers may be repeatedly exposed without adverse effect on their ability to hear and understand normal speech. Prior to 1979, the medical profession had defined hearing impairment as an average hearing threshold level in excess of 25 decibels (ANSI-S3.6-1969) at 500, 1000, and 2000 Hz, and the limits which are given have been established to prevent a hear-

*1986–1987 Addition.

TABLE A–8.

Threshold Limit Value for Direct Ocular Exposures (Intrabeam Viewing) From a Laser Beam

SPECTRAL REGION	WAVE LENGTH	EXPOSURE TIME, (t) SECONDS	TLV	
UVC	200 nm to 280 nm	10^{-9} to 3×10^{4}	3 mJ · cm^{-2}	
UVB	280 nm to 302 nm	"	3 "	
	303 nm	"	4 "	
	304 nm	"	6 "	
	305 nm	"	10 "	
	306 nm	"	16 "	
	307 nm	"	25 "	
	308 nm	"	40 "	*not to exceed 0.56 $t^{1/4}$ J · cm^{-2} for t ≦ 10 s.
	309 nm	"	63 "	
	310 nm	"	100 "	
	311 nm	"	160 "	
	312 nm	"	250 "	
	313 nm	"	400 "	
	314 nm	"	630 "	
UVA	315 nm to 400 nm	10^{-9} to 10	.56 $t^{1/4}$ J · cm^{-2}	
	" "	10 to 10^{3}	1.0 J · cm^{-2}	
	" "	10^{3} to 3×10^{4}	1.0 mW · cm^{-2}	
	Light	400 nm to 700 nm	10^{-9} to 1.8×10^{-5}	$5 \times 10^{-}$J · cm^{-2}
		400 nm to 700 nm	1.8×10^{-5} to 10	1.8 $(t/\sqrt[4]{t})$mJ· cm^{-2}
		400 nm to 549 nm	10 to 10^{4}	10mJ · cm^{-2}
		550 nm to 700 nm	10 to T_1	1.8 $(t/\sqrt[4]{t})$mJ·cm^{-2}
		550 nm to 700 nm	T_1 to 10^{4}	10 C_B mJ · cm^{-2}
		400 nm to 700 nm	10^{4} to 3×10^{4}	C_BμW · cm^{-2}
	IR-A	700 nm to 1049 nm	10^{-9} to 1.8×10^{-5}	5 $C_A \times 10^{-7}$ J · cm^{-2}
		700 nm to 1049 nm	1.8×10^{-5} to 10^{3}	$1.8C_A(t/\sqrt[4]{t})$mJ· cm^{-2}
		1050 nm to 1400 nm	10^{-9} to 10^{-4}	5×10^{-6} J · cm^{-2}
		1050 nm to 1400 nm	10^{-4} to 10^{3}	$9(t/\sqrt[4]{t})$mJ · cm^{-2}
		700 nm to 1400 nm	10^{3} to 3×10^{4}	320 C_A μW · cm^{-2}
	IR-B & C	1.4 μm to 10^{3} μm	10^{-9} to 10^{-7}	10^{-2} J · cm^{2}
		" "	10^{-7} to 10	$0.56\sqrt[4]{t}$ J · cm^{-2}
		" "	10 to 3×10^{4}	0.1 W · cm^{-2}

C_A - See Fig A–5; C_B = 1 for λ = 400 to 549 nm; $C_B = 10^{[(0.015\,(\lambda - 550)]}$ for λ = 550 to 700 nm; T_1 = 10 s for λ = 400 to 549 nm; $T_1 = 10 \times 10^{[(0.02\,(l - 550)]}$ for λ = 550 to 700 n.

At wavelengths greater than 1400 nm, for beam cross-sectional areas exceeding 100 cm^2 the TLV for exposure durations exceeding 10 seconds is: TLV = (10,000/A_5) mW/cm^2 (2), where A_s is the irradiated skin area for 100 to 1000 cm^2, and the TLV for irradiated skin areas exceeding 1000 cm^2 is 10 mW/cm^2 and for irradiated skin areas less than 100 cm^2 is 100 mW/cm^2.

TABLE A-9.

Threshold Limit Values for Viewing a Diffuse Reflection of a Laser Beam or an Extended Source Laser

SPECTRAL REGION	WAVE LENGTH	EXPOSURE TIME, (t) SECONDS	TLV
UV	200 nm to 400 nm	10^{-9} to 3×10^{4}	Same as Table A-10
Light	400 nm to 700 nm	10^{-9} to 10	10 $\sqrt[3]{t}$ J · cm^{-2} · sr^{-1}
	400 nm to 549 nm	10 to 10^{4}	21 J · cm^{-2} · sr^{-1}
	550 nm to 700 nm	10 to T_1	3.83 $(t/\sqrt[4]{t})$ J · cm^{-2} · sr^{-1}
	550 nm to 700 nm	T_1 to 10^{4}	21 C_B J · cm^{-2} · sr^{-1}
	400 nm to 700 nm	10^{4} to 3×10^{4}	2.1 $C_B t \times 10^{-3}$ W · cm^{-2} · sr^{-1}
IR-A	700 nm to 1400 nm	10^{-9} to 10	10 C_A $\sqrt[3]{t}$ J · cm^{-2} · sr^{-1}
	700 to 1400 nm	10 to 10^{3}	3.83 C_A $(t/\sqrt[4]{t})$ J · cm^{-2} · sr^{-1}
	700 nm to 1400 nm	10^{3} to 3×10^{4}	0.64 C_A W · cm^{-2} · sr^{-1}
IR-B & C	1.4 μm to 10^{3} μm	10^{-9} to 3×10^{4}	Same as Table A-8

C_A, C_B, and T_1 are the same as in footnote to Table A-8.

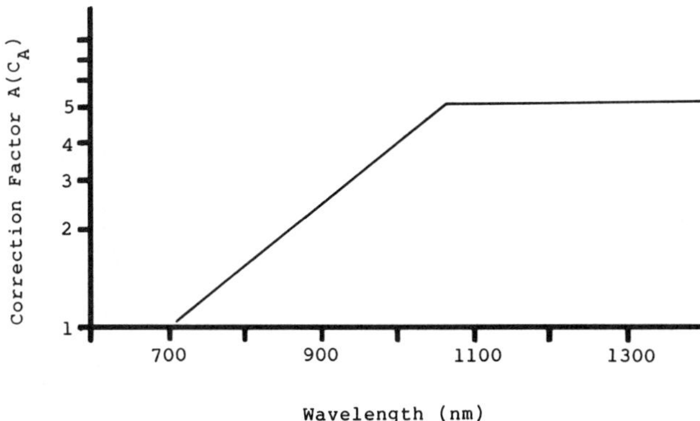

FIG A–5.
TLV correction factor for λ = 700–1400 nm.* (*For λ = 700–1049 nm, $C_A = 10^{[0.002(\lambda-700)]}$; For λ = 1050–1400 nm, C_A = 5.)

ing loss in excess of this level.[a] The values should be used as guides in the control of noise exposure and, due to individual susceptibility, should not be regarded as fine lines between safe and dangerous levels.

It should be recognized that the application of the TLV for noise will not protect all workers from the adverse effects of noise exposure. A hearing conservation program with audiometric testing is necessary when workers are exposed to noise at or above the TLV levels.

Continuous or Intermittent

The sound level shall be determined by a sound level meter, conforming as a minimum to the requirements of the American National Standard Specification for Sound Level Meters, S1.4 (1971) Type S2A, and set to use the A-weighted network with slow meter response. Duration of exposure shall not exceed that shown in Table A-11.

These values apply to total duration of exposure per working day regardless of whether this is one continuous exposure or a number of short-term exposures and does include the impact and impulsive type of noise that contributes to the sound level meter reading at slow response.

When the daily noise exposure is composed of two or more periods of noice exposure of different levels, their combined effect should be considered, rather than the individual effect of each. If the sum of the following fractions:

TABLE A-10.
Threshold Limit Value for Skin Exposure From a Laser Beam

SPECTRAL REGION	WAVE LENGTH	EXPOSURE TIME, (t) SECONDS	TLV
UV	200 nm to 400 nm	10^{-9} to 3×10^4	Same as Table 10
Light &	400 nm to 1400 nm	10^{-9} to 10^{-7}	$2\ C_A \times 10^{-2}$ J · cm^{-2}
IR-A	" "	10^{-7} to 10	$1.1\ C_A \sqrt[4]{t}$ J · cm^{-2}
IR-A	" "	10 to 3×10^4	$0.2\ C_A$ W · cm^{-2}
IR-B & C	1.4 μm to 10^3 μm	10^{-9} to 3×10^4	Same as Table A-8.

C_A = 1.0 for λ = 400–700 nm; see Figure A-5 for λ = .700 to 14 nm.

[a] In 1979 the American Academy of Ophthalmology and Otolaryngology (AAOO) included 3000 Hz in their hearing impairment formula.

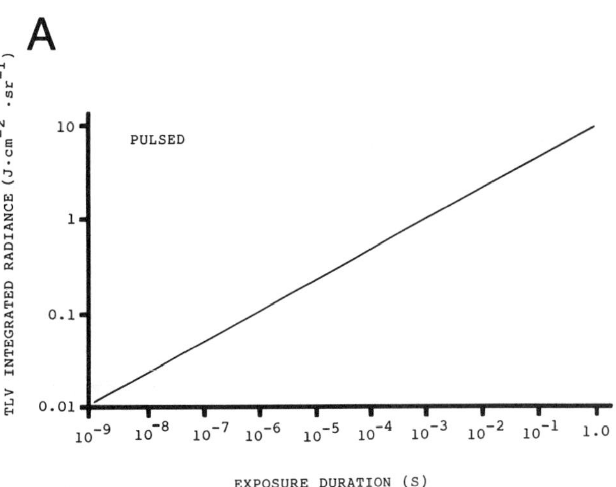

FIG A–6A.
TLV for intrabeam (direct) viewing of laser beam (400–700 nm).

$$\frac{C_1}{T_1} + \frac{C_2}{T_2} + \ldots \frac{C_n}{T_n}$$

exceeds unity, then, the mixed exposure should be considered to exceed the threshold limit value, C_1 indicates the total duration of exposure at a specific noise level, and T_1 indicates the total duration of exposure permitted at that level. All on-the-job noise exposures of 80 dBA or greater shall be used in the above calculations.

Impulsive or Impact

It is recommended that exposure to impulsive or impact noise shall not exceed the limits listed in Table A-12 or taken from Figure A-9. No exposures in excess of 140 decibels peak sound

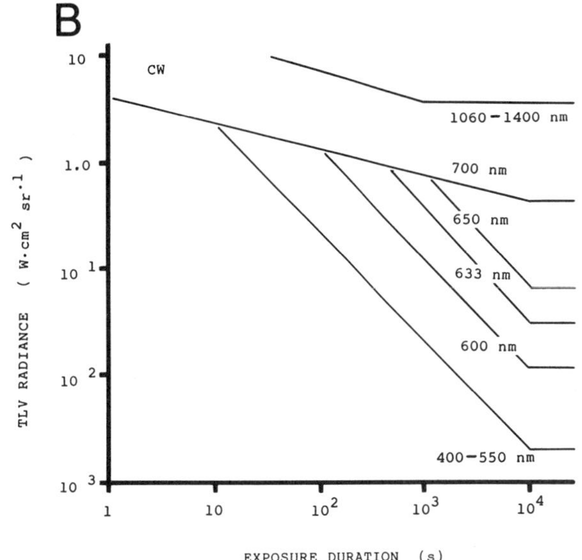

FIG A–6B.
TLV for intrabeam (direct) viewing of CW laser beam (400–1400 nm).

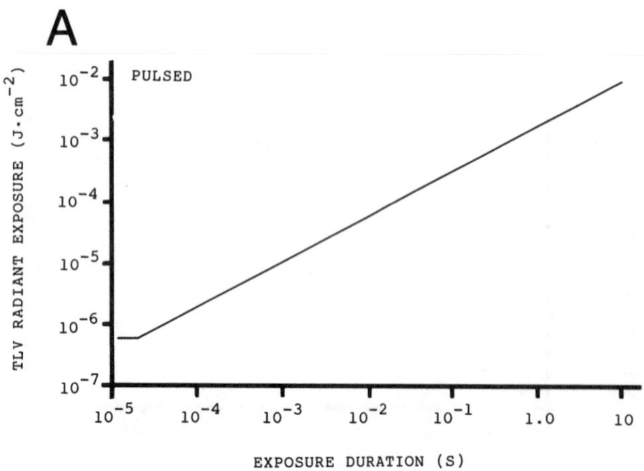

FIG A–7A.
TLV for laser exposure of skin and eyes for far-infrared radiation (wave-lengths greater than 1.4 μm).

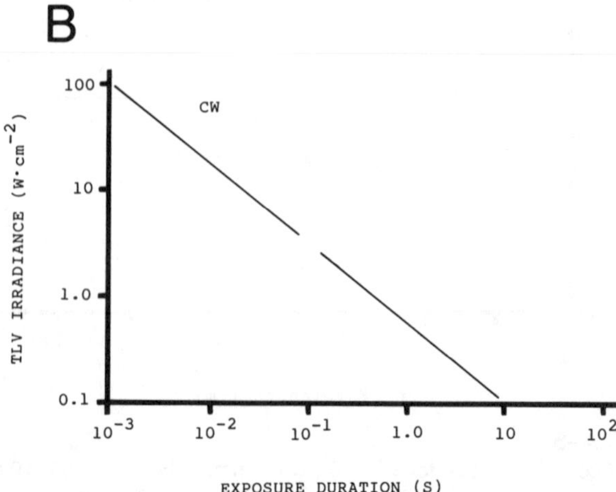

FIG A–7B.
TLV for CW laser exposure of skin and eyes for far-infrared radiation (wave-lengths greater than 1.4 μm).

pressure level are permitted. Impulsive or impact noise is considered to be those variations in noise levels that involve maxima at intervals of greater than one per second. Where the intervals are less than one second, it should be considered continuous.

Radiofrequency/Microwave Radiation

These Threshold Limit Values (TLVs) refer to radiofrequency (RF) and microwave radiation in the frequency range from 10 kHz to 300 GHz, and represent conditions under which it is believed workers may be repeatedly exposed without adverse health effects. The TLVs shown in Table A-13 are selected to limit the average whole body specific absorption rate (SAR) to 0.4 W/kg in any six-minute (0.1 hr) period for 3 MHz to 300 GHz, see Figure A-10. Between 10 kHz and 3 MHz the average whole body SAR is still limited to 0.4 W/kg, but the plateau at 100 mW/cm^2 was set to protect against shock and burn hazards (Fig A–10).

Since it is usually impractical to measure the SAR, the TLVs are expressed in units that are measurable, viz, squares of the electric and magnetic field strength, averaged over any 0.1 hour period. This can be expressed in units of equivalent plane wave power density for convenience. The electric field strength (E) squared, magnetic field strength (H) squared, and power density (PD) values are shown in Table A-13. For near field exposures PD cannot be measured directly, but equivalent plane wave power

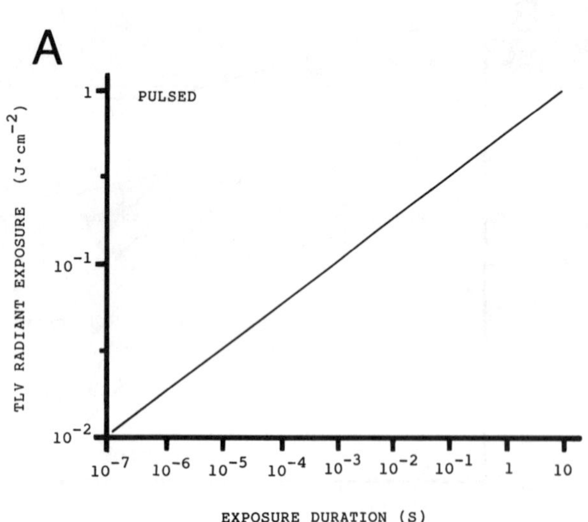

FIG A–8A.
TLV for extended sources or diffuse reflections of laser radiation (400–700 nm).

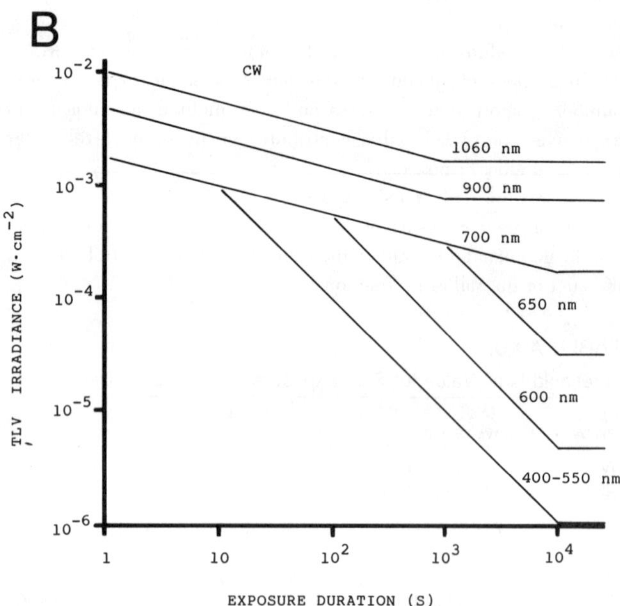

FIG A–8B.
TLV for extended sources or diffuse reflections of laser radiations (400–1400 nm).

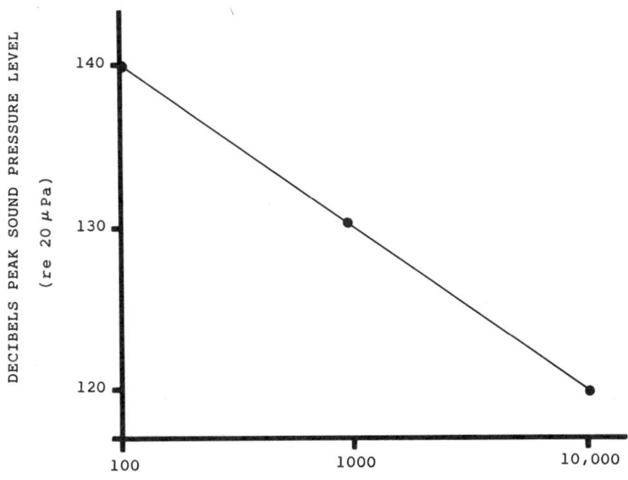

FIG A–9.
Threshold limit values for impulse/impact noise.

TABLE A-11.
Threshold Limit Values for Noise

DURATION PER DAY HOURS	SOUND LEVEL DBA†
16	80
8	85
4	90
2	95
1	100
½	105
¼	110
⅛	115*

†Sound level in decibels are measured on a sound level meter, conforming as a minimum to the requirements of the American National Standard Specification for Sound Level Meters, S1.4 (1971) Type S2A, and set to use the A-weighted network with slow meter response.
*No exposure to continuous or intermittent in excess of 115 dBA.

density can be calculated from the field strength measurement data as follows:

$$\text{PD in mW/cm}^2 = \frac{E^2}{3770}$$

where:

E^2 is in volts squared (V^2) per meter squared (m^2).

$$\text{PD in mW/cm}^2 = 37.7\ H^2$$

where:

H^2 is in amperes squared (A^2) per meter squared (m^2).

These values should be used as guides in the evaluation and control of exposure to radiofrequency/microwave radiation, and should not be regarded as a fine line between safe and dangerous levels.

Notes:

1. Needless exposure to all Radiofrequency Radiation (RFR) exposures should be avoided given the current state of knowledge on human effects, particularly non-thermal effects.
2. For fields consisting of a number of frequencies, the fraction of the protection guide incurred within each frequency level should be determined and the sum of all fractions should not exceed unity.
3. For pulsed and continuous wave fields, the power density is averaged over the six-minute period.
4. For partial body exposures at frequencies between 10 kHz and 1.0 GHz, the protection guides in Table A-13 may be exceeded if the output power of a radiating device is 7 watts or less. For example, if a hand held transmitter operating at 27 MHz has a maximum output of 5 watts, it would be excluded from any further field measurements.
5. The TLVs in Table A-13 may be exceeded if the exposure conditions can be demonstrated to produce an SAR of less than 0.4 W/kg as averaged over the whole body and spatial peak SAR values less than 8.0 W/kg as averaged over any 1.0 gram of tissue. For example, for frequencies from 3 to 30 MHz, the equivalent power density can be increased by a factor of 10 up to a limit of 100 mW/cm^2, if it can be assured that exposed individuals are not in contact with the ground plate.
6. At frequencies below 30 MHz, ungrounded objects such as vehicles, fences, etc., can strongly couple to RF fields. For field strengths near the TLV, shock and burn hazards can exist. Care should be taken to eliminate ungrounded objects, to ground such objects, or use insulated gloves when ungrounded objects must be handled.
7. No measurement should be made within 5 cm of any object.
8. All exposures should be limited to a maximum (peak) electric field intensity of 100 kV/m.

*Ultraviolet Radiation**

These Threshold Limit Values (TLVs) refer to ultraviolet radiation in the spectral region between 200 and 400 nm and represent conditions under which it is believed that nearly all workers may be repeatedly exposed without adverse effect. These values

TABLE A-12.
Threshold Limit Values Impulsive or Impact Noise

SOUND LEVEL DB*	PERMITTED NUMBER OF IMPULSES OR IMPACTS PER DAY
140	100
130	1000
120	10,000

*Decibels peak sound pressure level; re 20 μPa.

* See Laser TLVs.

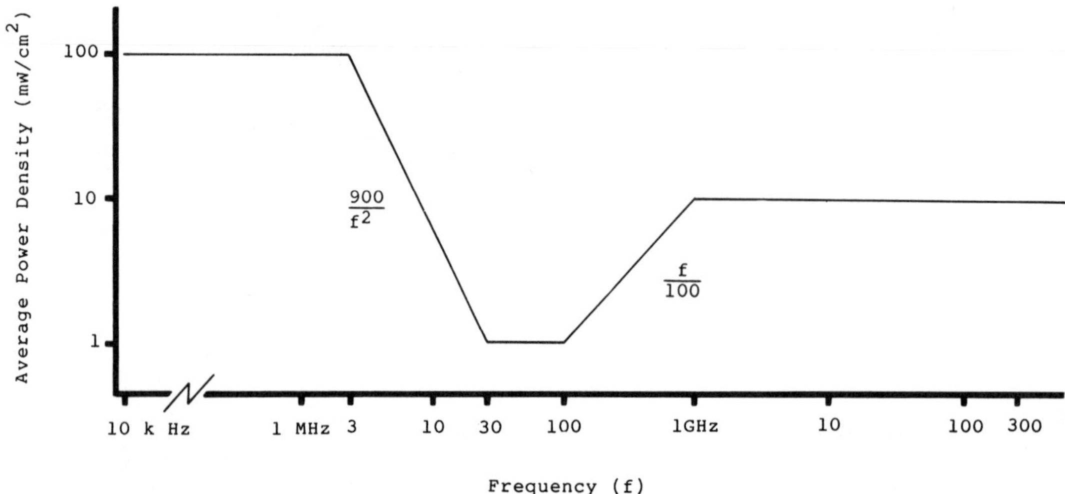

FIG A–10.
Threshold limit values (TLV) for radiofrequency/microwave radiation in the workplace (whole body SAR less than 0.4 W/kg).

for exposure of the eye or the skin apply to ultraviolet radiation from arcs, gas and vapor discharges, fluorescent and incandescent sources, and solar radiation, but do not apply to ultraviolet lasers.* These values do not apply to ultraviolet radiation exposure of photosenitive individuals or of individuals concomitantly exposed to photosensitizing agents.[(1)] These values should be used as guides in the control of exposure to continuous sources where the exposure duration shall not be less than 0.1 sec (Figure A-11).

These values should be used as guides in the control of exposure to ultraviolet sources and should not be regarded as a fine line between safe and dangerous levels.

Recommended Values

The threshold limit value for occupational exposure to ultraviolet radiation incident upon skin or eye where irradiance values are known and exposure time is controlled are as follows:

1. For the near ultraviolet spectral region (320 to 400 nm) total irradiance incident upon the unprotected skin or eye should not exceed 1 mW/cm^2 for periods greater than 10^3 seconds (approximately 16 minutes) and for exposure times less than 10^3 seconds should not exceed one J/cm^2.
2. For the actinic ultraviolet spectral region (200–315 nm), radiant exposure incident upon the unprotected skin or eye should not exceed the values given in Table A-14 within an 8-hour period.
3. To determine the effective irradiance of a broadband source weighted against the peak of the spectral effectiveness curve (270 nm), the following weighting formula should be used:

$$E_{eff} = \Sigma E_{\lambda} S_{\lambda} \Delta\lambda$$

where:

E_{eff} = effective irradiance relative to a monochromatic source at 270 nm in W/cm^2 ($J/s/cm^2$)

E_{λ} = spectral irradiance in $W/cm^2/nm$

S_{λ} = relative spectral effectiveness (unitless)

$\Delta\lambda$ = band width in nanometers

4. Permissible exposure time in seconds for exposure to actinic ultraviolet radiation incident upon the unprotected

TABLE A-13.
Radiofrequency/Microwave Threshold Limit Values

FREQUENCY	POWER DENSITY (mW/cm^2)	ELECTRIC FIELD STRENGTH SQUARED (V^2/m^2)	MAGNETIC FIELD STRENGTH SQUARED (A^2/m^2)
10 KHz to 3 MHz	100	377,000	2.65
3 MHz to 30 MHz	$900/f^{2}$*	$3770 \times 900/f^2$	$900/(37.7 \times f^2)$
30 MHz to 100 MHz	1	3770	0.027
100 MHz to 1000 MHz	f/100	$3770 \times f/100$	$f/37.7 \times 100$
1 GHz to 300 GHz	10	37,700	0.265

*f = frequency in MHz.

* See Laser TLVs.

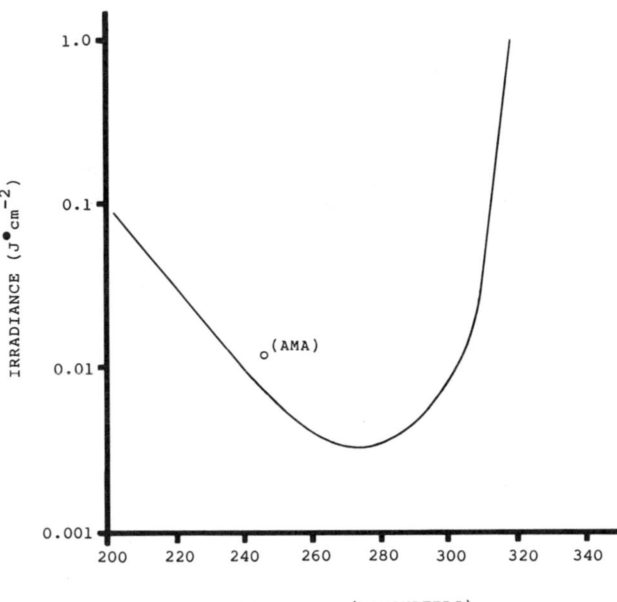

FIG A–11.
Threshold limit values for ultraviolet radiation.

skin or eye may be computed by dividing 0.003 J/cm^2 by E_{eff} in W/cm^2.
The exposure time may also be determined using Table A-15 which provides exposure times corresponding to effective irradiances in μW/cm^2.

5. All the preceding TLVs for ultraviolet energy apply to sources which subtend an angle less than 80°. Sources which subtend a greater angle need to be measured only over an angle of 80°.

Conditioned (tanned) individuals can tolerate skin exposure in excess of the TLV without erythemal effects. However, such conditioning may not protect persons against cancer.

TABLE A–14.
Relative Spectral Effectiveness by Wavelength*

WAVELENGTH (NM)	TLV (MJ/CM^2)	RELATIVE SPECTRAL EFFECTIVENESS S_λ
200	100	0.03
210	40	0.075
220	25	0.12
230	16	0.19
240	10	0.30
250	7.0	0.43
254	6.0	0.5
260	4.6	0.65
270	3.0	1.0
280	3.4	0.88
290	4.7	0.64
300	10	0.30
305	50	0.06
310	200	0.015
315	1000	0.003

*See Laser TLVs.

TABLE A–15.
Permissible Ultraviolet Exposures

DURATION OF EXPOSURE PER DAY	EFFECTIVE IRRADIANCE, E_{eff}(μW/cm^2)
8 hrs	0.1
4 hrs	0.2
2 hrs	0.4
1 hr	0.8
30 min	1.7
15 min	3.3
10 min	5
5 min	10
1 min	50
30 sec	100
10 sec	300
1 sec	3,000
0.5 sec	6,000
0.1 sec	30,000

REFERENCES

1. Fitzpatrick, et al (Eds): *Sunlight and Man*. Tokyo, Japan, University of Tokyo Press, 1974.

Notice of Intended Changes (for 1986–87)

These physical agents, with their corresponding values, comprise those for which either a limit has been proposed for the first time, or for which a change in the "Adopted" listing has been proposed. In both cases, the proposed limits should be considered trial limits that will remain in the listing for a period of at least one year. If after one year no evidence comes to light that questions the appropriateness of the values herein the values will be reconsidered for the "Adopted" list.

Notice of Intent to Establish Threshold Limit Values

Light and Near-Infrared Radiation

These Threshold Limit Values (TLVs) refer to visible and near-infrared radiation in the wavelength range of 400 nm to 1400 nm and represent conditions under which it is believed that nearly all workers may be exposed without adverse effect. These values should be used as guides in the control of exposure to light and should not be regarded as a fine line between safe and dangerous levels.

Recommended Values

The Threshold Limit Value for occupational exposure to broad-band light and near-infrared radiation for the eye apply to exposure in any eight-hour workday and require knowledge of the spectral radiance (L_λ) and total irradiance (E) of the source as measured at the position(s) of the eye of the worker. Such detailed spectral data of a white light source is generally only required if

TABLE A–16.
Spectral Weighting Functions for Assessing Retinal Hazards From Broad-Band Optical Sources

WAVELENGTH (NM)	BLUE-LIGHT HAZARD-FUNCTION B_λ	BURN HAZARD FUNCTION R_λ
400	0.10	1.0
405	0.20	2.0
410	0.40	4.0
415	0.80	8.0
420	0.90	9.0
425	0.95	9.5
430	0.98	9.8
435	1.0	10.0
440	1.0	10.0
445	0.97	9.7
450	0.94	9.4
455	0.90	9.0
460	0.80	8.0
465	0.70	7.0
470	0.62	6.2
475	0.55	5.5
480	0.45	4.5
485	0.40	4.0
490	0.22	2.2
495	0.16	1.6
500–600	$10^{[(450-\lambda)/50]}$	1.0
600–700	0.001	1.0
700–770	0.001	$10^{[(700-\lambda)/505]}$
770–1400	0.001	0.2

the luminance of the source exceeds 1 cd cm^{-2}. At luminances less than this value the TLV would not be exceeded.

The TLVs are:

1. To protect against retinal thermal injury, the spectral radiance of the lamp weighted against the function R (Table A-16) should not exceed:

$$\sum_{400}^{1400} L_\lambda \cdot R_\lambda \cdot \Delta\lambda \leq 1/\alpha t^{1/2} \qquad (1)^*$$

where L_λ is in W cm^{-2} sr^{-1} nm^{-1} and t is the viewing duration (or pulse duration if the lamp is pulsed) limited to 1 μs to 10 s, and α is the angular of the source in radians. If the lamp is oblong, α refers to the longest dimension that can be viewed. For instance, at a viewing distance r = 100 cm from a tubular lamp of length l = 50 cm, the viewing angle is:

$$\alpha = l/r = 50/100 = 0.5 \text{ rad} \qquad (2)$$

2. To protect against retinal photochemical injury from chronic blue-light exposure the integrated spectral radiance of a light source weighted against the blue-light hazard function B_λ (Table A-16) should not exceed:

$$\sum_{400}^{1400} L_\lambda \cdot t \cdot B_\lambda \cdot \Delta\lambda \leq 100 \text{ J cm}^{-2} \text{ sr}^{-1} \ (t \leq 10^4 \text{ s}) \qquad (3a)$$

$$\sum_{400}^{1400} L_\lambda \cdot B_\lambda \cdot \Delta\lambda \leq 10^{-2} \text{ sr}^{-1} \ (t > 10^4 \text{ s}) \qquad (3b)$$

The weighted product of L_λ and B_λ is termed L (blue). For a source radiance L weighted against the blue-light hazard function (L [blue]) which exceeds 10 mW cm^{-2} sr^{-1} in the blue spectral region, the permissible exposure duration t_{max} in seconds is simply:

$$t_{max} = 100 \text{ J cm}^{-2} \text{ sr}^{-1}/\text{L (blue)} \qquad (4)$$

The latter limits are greater than the maximum permissible exposure limits for 440 nm laser radiation (*see* Laser TLV) because of a 2–3 mm pupil is assumed rather than a 7 mm pupil for the Laser TLV. For a light source subtending an angle α less than 11 mrd (0.011 radian) the above limits are relaxed such that the spectral irradiance weighted against the blue-light hazard function, B_λ should not exceed E (blue).

$$\sum_{400}^{1400} E_\lambda \cdot t \cdot B_\lambda \cdot \Delta\lambda \leq 10 \text{ mJ} \cdot \text{cm}^{-2} \ (t \leq 10^4 \text{ s}) \qquad (5a)$$

$$\sum_{400}^{1400} E_\lambda \cdot B_\lambda \cdot \Delta\lambda \leq 1 \ \mu\text{W} \cdot \text{cm}^2 \ (t \geq 10^4 \text{ s}) \qquad (5b)$$

For a source where the blue light weighted irradiance E (blue) exceeds 1 μW · cm^{-2} the maximum permissible exposure duration t_{max} in seconds is:

$$t_{max} = 10 \text{ mJ} \cdot \text{cm}^{-2}/\text{E (blue)} \qquad (6)$$

3. *Infrared radiation:* To avoid possible delayed effects upon the lens of the eye (cataractogenesis), the infrared radiation (λ = 770 nm) should be limited to 10 mW cm^{-2}. For an infrared heat lamp or any near-infrared source where a strong visual stimulus is absent, the near infrared (770–1400 nm) radiance as viewed by the eye should be limited to:

$$\sum_{400}^{1400} L_\lambda \cdot \Delta\lambda \leq 0.6/\alpha \qquad (7)^*$$

for extended duration viewing conditions. This limit is based upon a 7 mm pupil diameter.

Airborne Upper Sonic and Ultrasonic Acoustic Radiation

These Threshold Limit Values (TLVs) refer to sound pressure levels that represent conditions under which it is believed that nearly all workers may be repeatedly exposed without adverse effect. The values listed in Table A-17 should be used as guides in the control of noise exposure and, due to individual susceptibility, should not be regarded as fine lines between safe and dangerous levels. The levels for the third-octave bands centered below 20

* Formulae (1) and (7) are empirical and are not, strictly speaking, dimensionally correct. To make the formulae dimensionally correct, one would have to insert a dimensional correction factor *k* in the right hand numerator in each formula. For formula (1) this would be k_1 = 1 W · rad · s½(cm^2 · sr), and for formula (7) K_2 = 1 W · rad/(cm^2 · sr).

TABLE A–17.
Permissible Ultrasound Exposure Levels

MID-FREQUENCY OF THIRD-OCTAVE BAND KHZ	ONE-THIRD OCTAVE-BAND LEVEL IN DB RE 20 μPA
10	80
12.5	80
16	80
20	105
25	110
31.5	115
40	115
50	115

kHz are below those which cause subjective effects. Those levels for ⅓ octaves 20 kHz are for prevention of possible hearing losses from subharmonics of these frequencies.

Physical Agents Under Study

The Physical Agents TLV Committee of ACGIH has examined the current literature and has not found sufficient information to propose a TLV. However, these agents will remain under study during the coming year to examine new evidence indicating the need and feasibility for establishing a proposed TLV. Comments and suggestions, accompanied by substantive documentation are solicited and should be forwarded to the Executive Secretary, ACGIH. Documentation summarizing the current status of the biological effects literature is available on those agents preceded by an asterisk (*).

1. *Extremely Low Frequency (ELF) Radiation*. Specifically, that portion of the spectrum from 0 to 300 Hz.
2. *Magnetic Fields*. Both pulsed and *continuous.
3. *Laser Radiation*. Specifically laser exposures of less than one (1) nanosecond.
4. *Vibration*. Whole-body.
5. *Pressure Variations*.

Appendix B

Selected Conversion Tables for Units of Measure in the SI System

The International System of Units (SI) has been adopted by most European countries and Canada. In the United States, occupational health data are not commonly described in SI units, exemplified by the Occupational Safety and Health Administration (OSHA), the National Institute for Occupational Safety and Health (NIOSH), the Environmental Protection Agency (EPA), most other U.S government agencies, and the majority of U.S. physicians. The American Medical Association (AMA) has brought forth action in SI usage. Since July 1986 all articles appearing in the *Journal of the American Medical Association (JAMA)* and the AMA's speciality journals express clinical laboratory data in conventional units followed in parentheses by SI units, the first phase of a 2-year conversion.[1, 2] An approved translation of the International Bureau of Weights and Measures publication entitled *Le Système International d'Unités* is available.[3] It includes relevant extracts from the International Organization for Standardization (ISO) for practical use of the system and is available in several languages.

Several conversion tables appear on the following pages.

REFERENCES

1. Editorial: Now read this: The SI units are here. *JAMA* 1986; 255:17.
2. Powsner ER: SI quantities and units for American medicine. *JAMA* 1984; 252:13.
3. *The International System of Units (SI)*. Washington, DC, National Bureau of Standards Special Publication 330, 1977, Superintendent of Documents (SD Catalog No. C13.10:330/4).
4. *Handbook of Chemistry and Physics*, ed 67. Boca Raton, Fla, CRC Press, Inc, 1987.

TABLE B–1.
SI Basic and Supplementary Units

NAME	SYMBOL	PHYSICAL QUANTITY
SI base units		
Meter	m	Length
Kilogram	kg	Mass
Second	s	Time
Ampere	A	Electric current
Kelvin	K	Thermodynamic temperature
Mole	mol	Amount of substance
Candela	cd	Luminous intensity

TABLE B–2.
Representative Derived Units

DERIVED UNIT	NAME AND SYMBOL	DERIVATION FROM BASE UNITS
Area	Square meter	m^2
Volume	Cubic meter	m^3
Force	Newton (N)	$kg \cdot m \cdot s^{-2}$
Pressure	Pascal (Pa)	$kg \cdot m^{-1} \cdot s^{-2}$ (N/m^2)
Work, energy	Joule (J)	$kg \cdot m^2 \cdot s^{-2}$ (N-m)
Density	Kilogram per cubic meter	kg/m^3
Frequency	Hertz (Hz)	s^{-1}

TABLE B–3.

Units Used Temporarily With the International System

NAME	SYMBOL	VALUE IN SI UNIT
Nautical mile*		1 nautical mile = 1,852 m
Knot		1 nautical mile per hour = (1,852/3,600) m/s
Angstrom	Å	1 Å = 0.1 nm = 10^{-10} m
Hectare	ha	1 ha = 1 hm^2 = 10^4 m^2
Standard atmosphere	atm	1 atm = 101, 325 Pa
Barn†	b	1 b = 100 fm^2 = 10^{-28} m^2
Bar†	bar	1 bar = 0.1 MPa = 10^5 Pa
Curie†	Ci	1 Ci = 3.7 × 10^{10} Bq
Röntgen†	R	1 R = 2.58 × 10^{-4} C/kg
Rad†	rad	1 rad = 1 cGy = 10^{-2} Gy

*The nautical mile is employed for marine and aerial navigation to express distances.

†For explanations and discussion in occupational health practice, refer to Chapter 26 by G. L. Voelz.

TABLE B–4.

Units Outside the International System, but Often Used With SI

NAME	SYMBOL	VALUE IN SI UNIT
Minute	min	1 min = 60 s
Hour	h	1 h = 60 min = 3,600 s
Day	d	1 d = 24 h = 86,400 s
Degree	°	1° = (π/180) rad
Minute	′	1′ = (1/60)° = (π/10,800) rad
Second	″	1″ = (1/60)′ = (π/648,000) rad
Liter*	l	1 l = 1 dm^3 = 10^{-3} m^3
Metric ton	t	1 t = 10^3 kg

*When there is a risk of confusion between the letter l and the number 1, "ltr" or "liter" may be used; in the United States, L is recommended.

TABLE B–5.

Conversion of Mass-Based Results to Molar Units (Amount in μmol That Corresponds to mg)*†

Aluminum	37.06
5-Aminolevulinic acid	7.626
Arsenic	13.35
Cadmium	8.896
Cobalt	16.97
Chromium	19.23
Fluoride	52.64
2, 5-Hexanedione	8.761
Hippuric acid	5.581
Lead	4.826‡
Mandelic acid	6.573
Manganese	18.20
Methylenebis (2-chloroaniline)	3.743
n-Methylformamide	16.93
Mercury	4.985
Methylhippuric acid	5.176
Nickel	17.04
Pentachlorophenol	3.755
Phenol	10.63
Tetrachloroethylene	6.030
Tetrachlorophenol	4.312
Thiocyanic acid	16.92
2-Thiothiazolidine (4-carboxylic acid)	6.127
Toluene	10.85
Trichloroacetic acid	6.120
1, 1, 1-Trichloroethane	7.495
Trichloroethanol	6.693
Trichlorophenol	5.064
Vanadium	19.63
Zinc-protoporphyrin	1.592

*This table was prepared by Antero Aitio, Jorma Järvisalo, Vesa Riihimäki, and Sven Hernberg for Chapter 13, "Biologic Monitoring," and is duplicated here with appreciation.

†Amounts given in mass units per excreted creatinine, i.e., mg/gm of μmol/mol creatinine, cannot be directly converted to volumetric units. The daily volume of urine is approximately 600–160 ml, and the daily excretion of creatinine approximately 1–3 gm. Thus, values expressed in mg/gm creatinine are roughly 0.5–1.0 × those expressed in mg/L. The molecular weight of creatinine is 113.12; 1 gm is thus 8.84 mmol. Values expressed in mass/gram creatinine may be converted to mass/mole creatinine by multiplying by 113.12.

‡The traditional unit for lead in blood is μgm/100 ml; to convert to μmol/L, the figure is multiplied by 0.04826.

TABLE B–6.

Other Useful Equivalents and Conversion Factors

1 kilometer = 0.6214 mile
1 meter = 3.281 feet
1 centimeter = 0.3937 inch
1 micrometer = 1/254,000 inch = 40 microinches = 100,000 Angstrom units
1 foot = 30.48 centimeters
1 inch = 25.40 millimeters
1 square kilometer = 0.3861 square mile (U.S.)
1 square foot = 0.0929 square meter
1 square inch = 6.452 square centimeters
1 square mile (U.S.) = 2,389,998 square meters = 640 acres
1 acre = 43.560 square feet = 4,047 square meters
1 cubic meter = 35.315 cubic feet
1 cubic centimeter = 0.0610 cubic inch
1 cubic foot = 28.32 liters = 0.0283 cubic meter = 7.481 gallons (U.S.)
1 cubic inch = 16.39 cubic centimeters
1 U.S. gallon = 3.7853 liters = 231 cubic inches = 0.13368 cubic foot
1 liter = 0.9081 quart (dry), 1.057 quarts (U.S. liquid)
1 cubic foot of water = 62.43 pounds (4° C)
1 U.S. gallon of water = 8.345 pounds (4° C)
1 kilogram = 2.205 pounds
1 gram = 15.43 grains
1 pound = 453.59 grams
1 ounce(avoir.) = 28.35 grams
1 gram mole of a perfect gas ≈ 24.45 liters (at 25° C and 760 mm Hg barometric pressure)
1 atmosphere = 14.7 pounds per square inch
1 foot of water pressure = 0.4335 pound per square inch
1 inch of mercury pressure = 0.4912 pound per square inch
1 dyne per square centimeter = 0.0021 pound per square foot
1 gram-caloric = 0.00397 Btu
1 Btu = 778 foot-pounds
1 Btu per minute = 12.96 foot-pounds per second
1 hp = 0.707 Btu per second = 550 foot-pounds per second
1 centimeter per second = 1.97 feet per minute = 0.0224 mile per hour
1 footcandle = 1 lumen incident per square foot = 10.764 lumens incident per square meter
1 grain per cubic foot = 2.29 grams per cubic meter
1 milligram per cubic meter = 0.000437 grain per cubic foot

To convert degrees Celsius to degrees Fahrenheit: ° C(9/5) + 32 = ° F
To convert degrees Fahrenheit to degrees Celsius: (5/9)(° F − 32) = ° C
For solutes in water: 1 mg/L ≈ 1 ppm (by weight)
For gases or vapors in air at 25° C and 760 mm Hg pressure:
To convert mg liter to ppm (by volume): mg liter (24.450/mol wt) = ppm
To convert ppm to mg liter: ppm (mol wt/24.450) = mg liter

Index

C

I

J

O

Q

R

S

T

W

X

Y

Z